Dictionary of

Medical Syndromes

Sergio I. Magalini, M.D.

Professor of Clinical Toxicology
Department of Anesthesia and Resuscitation
School of Medicine
Universita Cattolica del Sacro Cuore, Rome

Sabina C. Magalini, M.D.

Department of Surgery
School of Medicine
Universita Cattolica del Sacro Cuore, Rome

Giovanni de Francisci, M.D.

Department of Anesthesia and Resuscitation
School of Medicine
Universita Cattolica del Sacro Cuore, Rome

Dictionary of

Medical Syndromes

Third Edition

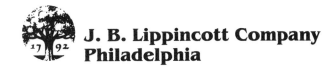

J. B. Lippincott Company
Philadelphia

Acquisitions Editor: Charles McCormick, Jr.
Developmental Editor: Mary J. Cain
Project Editor: Dina Kamilatos
Indexer: Alexandra Weir Nickerson
Design Coordinator: Ellen C. Dawson
Cover Design: Kathy Luedtke
Production Manager: Carol A. Florence
Production Coordinator: Barney Fernandes
Compositor: Bi-Comp
Printer/Binder: R. R. Donnelley & Sons Co.

Third Edition

3   5   6   4

Library of Congress Cataloging-in-Publication Data

Magalini, Sergio I.
    Dictionary of medical syndromes / Sergio I. Magalini and Sabina C. Magalini and Giovanni de Francisci.—3rd ed.
        p.   cm.
    Includes bibliographies and index.
    ISBN 0-397-50882-4
    1. Syndromes—Dictionaries.   I. Magalini, Sabina C.
II. de Francisci, Giovanni.   III. Title.
    [DNLM: 1. Dictionaries, Medical.   WB 15 M188d]
    RC69.M33   1990
    616.07'2'0321—dc19
    DNLM/DLC   89-2804
    for Library of Congress   CIP

The authors and publisher have exerted every effort to ensure that drug selection and dosage set forth in this text are in accord with current recommendations and practice at the time of publication. However, in view of ongoing research, changes in government regulations, and the constant flow of information relating to drug therapy and drug reactions, the reader is urged to check the package insert for each drug for any change in indications and dosage and for added warnings and precautions. This is particularly important when the recommended agent is a new or infrequently employed drug.

Preface

The idea that stimulated the writing of the *Dictionary of Medical Syndromes* in this format has remained valid for the almost twenty years since the first edition. Over the years the use of eponyms in medicine has not disappeared, as predicted by some authors; on the contrary, it has proliferated, thus causing some occasional confusion.

The concept of syndrome as a cluster of symptoms and signs also remains valid on the condition that we consider these clusters as entities that are alive, and like living organisms subject to be born, to live, to change in their structure by integration and fusion, and eventually to die because they no longer correspond to clinical needs.

To make a short natural history of the criteria at the basis of the structure of syndromes, we can see that initially they were represented by "clinical" data. We may call this the "Latin period" (Italian, French, Spanish). Successively they were integrated first by the morphological discoveries of histopathology (the "German period") and then by the progress of biochemistry (the "Angloamerican period"). This last stage, by contributing to understanding of the metabolic processes underlying the clinical and morphological manifestations, has allowed further revision and integration of the already established syndromes and the birth of new ones.

The branch of medicine that is most responsible for the present revision of syndromes is genetics, a discipline that with its precise codification not only contributes to the understanding of their inheritance pattern but also allows the correlation among groups of syndromes and the reclassification of many.

Genetics, in particular, seems to contribute greatly to pigeonholing of syndromes and to the attribution of numbers for syndrome classification, facts foreseen in the writing of the introduction to the first edition of this book. A final consideration is merited by the users of the eponymic system of classification, who are confronted with a mass of data based on the name of discoverer (real or alleged) or of the patient, the geographic location, as well as clinical, pathological, biochemical, and genetic data. This book has been written to come to their aid.

Sergio I. Magalini, M.D.

Preface to the Second Edition

The favorable acceptance of the first edition of *Dictionary of Medical Syndromes* and the increase in the number of syndromes in recent years have led us to prepare this greatly enlarged and completely revised second edition. This edition contains over 2,700 syndromes, 900 more than the first. The practical format and the goal of the book remain the same.

I would like to mention the great contribution of my late colleague, Professor Euclide Scrascia, M.D., who coordinated and organized the material in this edition. His untimely death not only prevented him from seeing the results of this effort but also ended a very promising medical career.

Sergio I. Magalini, M.D.

Preface to the First Edition

In presenting the information about the individual syndromes, we have followed a slightly different procedure from that currently used in most medical books. Instead of starting with the etiology and ending with the pathology, a method that attempts to force the clinical manifestations into the frame of our knowledge, we have attempted to insert this knowledge into the actual sequence of events that occurs when the patient seeks our care, and match it with the information available or obtainable.

The inputs in this system are: (1) the subjective information given by the patient, and (2) the results of our observation on the objective manifestations. With this body of information we feel that we may now attempt to postulate the number of etiologic agents that will fit into that pattern, and as we proceed in the matching, the backlog of information on the type of damage of anatomic and physiologic nature that these agents determine has to be brought forth (pathology).

Now comes the first output or the design of the objective diagnostic procedures necessary to evaluate the correlation between the information collected, and the diagnostic hypothesis. Once this information has been collected and the correlation proven, the outputs would be: (1) a therapeutic plan, that is the active implementation of a different kind of knowledge, and (2) the prognosis or hypothetical projection of the predicted outcome based on the ratio of physician knowledge : disease entity.

We believe this is a better method, since it restores the patient's complaints to the primary role. This is the way in which medicine is usually practiced.

We will see changes in the future where more and more tests will be routinely done in normal population, even before individuals present any subjective complaints (lanthanic cases), and in that instance, different input will be used in the practice of medical thinking and practice (diagnosing and treating).

Although it was far from my intention in writing this book to get involved in a polemic between "eponym defenders" and "eponym abolitionists," I feel a few words on this matter are necessary as an introduction.

Medicine is not the only science to use "eponyms." Biologists use them, although they have better systematized their use. Chemists use them to name new elements (*e.g.,* Californium or Parisium). Physicists to name their laws or phenomena. Cartographers or explorers to name countries, towns, rivers, *etc.* (*e.g.,* America, Alexandria, Amazon River). Astronomers to name planets, stars, and areas of the moon.

However, the lack of a systematic codification for the use of proper names in the field of medicine has generated a certain amount of confusion, and a part of the medical profession wants to completely reject the use of eponyms.

Two types of terminology have been created to designate a pathological entity. The cold scientific one (still complex and confusing), which follows the "Scholastic method," attempts to categorize and to give to an entity its "pigeonhole" and eventual "number." The other method, undoubtedly less scientific, designates an entity by the name of the discoverer, the name of the patient who presented the symptom complex, a geographic location, or whimsy.

The eponym has enriched medical literature down through the ages. Its function has been double: (1) to honor its discoverer and (2) to provide mnemonics for different symptoms. It is currently used in the medical literature, and if we wish to know what the author means when discussing any syndrome indicated with a particular name, we must have knowledge of his terminology. Thus, this book of quick references was designed in an attempt to bridge the gap between the two types of medical terminology and to provide a means of translation from one to the other system.

In defense of the use of eponyms, we may add that syndromes play an important role in perpetuating the "humanistic aspect" of medicine. In addition to serving the useful purpose as pointed out above, the eponym gives to the user a sense of the participation in the process of untangling the complex pattern of disease manifestation and in recognizing these "symptom complexes." And by being a sort of nickname, it provides a familiarity with the subject and establishes a sort of personal relationship between the physician using it and that particular entity. Since the human mind does not work exactly like a computer, any help or boost that may be received by the use of different types of correlation is welcomed. If we have looked at a map to see the location of Borholm Island, how can we forget the existence of pleurodynia when a patient with that set of symptoms asks for our care?

During the writing of this book we have been exposed to delightful bits of information that will never allow us to forget the associated syndromes or their stories. We covered an enormous time span that goes from the description of migraine syndrome by an Indian poet in 3000 B.C., to the story of the Dutch admiral in 1723 who ate and drank too much, and while vomiting, burst his esophagus and made his own prognosis—"I am going to die soon" (Boerhaave's syndrome)—and finally, we read of the discovery and elucidation of new syndromes by the use of the electron microscope.

Sergio I. Magalini, M.D.

Acknowledgments

The revision and updating of this new edition would not have been possible without the enthusiastic cooperation of the following people: Professor Rocco Schiavello, M.D., and Liliana Sollazzi, M.D., for reviewing the congenital heart malformations syndromes; my secretaries Stefania Croce and Nadia Bruschelli for their patience in typing, cutting, and gluing the revised pieces; and Drs. Alessandro Barelli and Angelo Chierichini for preparing the computer programs utilized in the preparation of the manuscript.

Dictionary of

Medical Syndromes

13q

Synonyms. Lele's.

Symptoms and Signs. Growth deficiency, usually of prenatal onset; mental deficiency; microcephaly with tendency toward trigonocephaly and holoprosencephaly-type of brain defects; prominent nasal bridge, hypertelorism; ptosis, epicanthal folds, microphthalmia, colobomata; retinoblastoma, usually bilateral, cardiac defects; hypospadias, cryptorchidism; small to absent thumbs, clinodactyly of fifth finger.

Etiology. Deletion of part of the long arm of a 13 chromosome.

Pathology. Several malformative findings as outlined above.

Diagnostic Procedures. *Chromosome study.*

Therapy. Symptomatic.

Prognosis. Poor.

BIBLIOGRAPHY. Lele KP, Penzose LS, Stallarf HB: Chromosome deletion in a case of retinoblastoma. Ann Human Genet 27:171–174, 1963
Smith DW: Recognizable Patterns of Human Malformations. Philadelphia, WB Saunders, 1982

18p

Synonyms. De Grouchy I.

Symptoms and Signs. Mild to moderate growth deficiency; mental deficiency; ptosis, epicanthal folds, low nasal bridge, hypertelorism, micrognathia, wide mouth, downturning corners of mouth, large, protruding ears; pectus excavatum. Five cases with holoprosencephaly arhinencephaly-type defect reported.

Etiology. Short arm 18 deletion, sometimes as part of the deficiency in a ring 18 chromosome.

Pathology. Malformative findings as outlined above.

Diagnostic Procedures. *Chromosome study.*

Therapy. Symptomatic.

Prognosis. Poor for those patients with holoprosencephaly-type defect.

BIBLIOGRAPHY. De Grouchy J, Lamy M, Thieffry S, Arthuis M, Salmon C: Dysmorphie complexe avec oligophrenie: deletion des bras courts d'un chromosome 17-18. CR Acad Sci (D) (Paris), 256:1028–1029, 1963
Smith DW: Recognizable patterns of human malformations. Philadelphia, WB Saunders, 1982

18q

Synonyms. De Grouchy II.

Symptoms and Signs. Growth deficiency, mental deficiency with hypotonia, poor coordination, nystagmus, conductive deafness; microcephaly, midfacial hypoplasia with deep-set eyes, carp-shaped mouth, narrow palate; long hands, tapering fingers, and short first metacarpal with proximal thumb; distal hypoplastic tapering of lower part of legs.

Pathology. Malformations outlined above.

Etiology. Deletion of part of the long arm of chromosome 18.

Diagnostic Procedures. *Chromosome study.*

Therapy. Symptomatic.

Prognosis. Mental deficiency, along with hearing and visual problems, makes patients severely handicapped.

BIBLIOGRAPHY. De Grouchy J, Royer P, Salmon C, Lamy M: Deletion partielle du bras long du chromosome 18. Path Biol (Paris) 12:579–582, 1964
Smith DW: Recognizable patterns of human malformations. Philadelphia, WB Saunders, 1982

AAGENAES'

Synonyms. Cholestasis-lymphedema. See Cholestatic intrahepatic, recurrent.

Symptoms and Signs. Both sexes. From and after birth. In Norwegian kindreds. Jaundice in recurrent episodes. Progressive edema of legs from school age on.

Etiology. Recessive inheritance.

Pathology. Hypoplasia of lymphatic vessels causing lymphedema; obstructive cholestasis with bouts of icterus.

BIBLIOGRAPHY. Aagenaes O, Sigstad H, Bjorn-Hausen R: Lymphedema in hereditary recurrent cholestasis from birth. Arch Dis Child 45:690–699, 1970

Aagenaes O: Hereditary recurrent cholestasis with lymphoedema—two new families. Acta Ped Scand 63:465–471, 1974

A AND V

Synonyms. A-esotropia; A-exotropia; horizontal–vertical–noncomitant strabismus; V-esotropia; V-exotropia.

Arbitrary Standards for the Syndromes to Qualify

1. A-esotropia. Esodeviation greater by 10 diopters in upward gaze than in direct forward gaze.
2. V-esotropia. Esodeviation greater by 15 diopters in downward gaze than in direct forward gaze.
3. A-exotropia. Exodeviation greater by 10 diopters in lower gaze than in direct forward gaze.
4. V-exotropia. Exodeviation greater by 15 diopters in upward gaze than in direct forward gaze.

Etiology. Unknown. Three schools: (1) Horizontal recti school; (2) vertical muscles school, (3) combined school.

Therapy. Surgical correction still not assessed.*

BIBLIOGRAPHY. Urist MJ: Horizontal squint with secondary vertical deviations. AMA Arch Ophthalmol 46:245–267, 1951

Dunlap EA: Present status of the A and V syndromes. Am J Ophthalmol 52:396–401, 1961

Roy FH: Practical Management of Eye Problems: Glaucoma, Strabismus, Visual Fields, p 132, p 144 Philadelphia, Lea & Febiger, 1975

Pesando P: Vertical retraction syndrome. Ophthalmologia 177:254–259, 1978

AARSKOG-SCOTT

Synonyms. Facial-digital-genital, FDG; facial dysplasia–short stature–penoscrotal anomalies. AAS; hypertelorism–brachydactyly–shawl scrotum.

Symptoms. Males fully affected; females exhibit partial features. Normal weight and length at birth. Good health. Developmental landmarks within normal limits. In some cases, moderately impaired intelligence or early delay in motor performance, or both. Slow maturation from 3 years on.

Signs. Short stature (100%). Craniofacial. Hypertelorism (100%); anomalous superior helices (100%); "widow's peak" (triangular point of scalp hair) (60%); ptosis (30%); hypoplastic maxilla (100%). Acral. Small, broad hands and feet (90%); short fingers with single crease (57%); simian crease (28%); mild webbing between fingers (43%); joint laxity (29%); joint restriction (35%). Abdominal. Inguinal hernia (57%); protruding umbilicus (100%); cryptorchidism (64%). Other. Abnormal cervical vertebrae (90%); pectus excavatum (21%). Shawl scrotum. A new associated anomaly recently described is cystic porencephaly with generalized seizures.

Etiology. X-linked recessive; possible X-linked semidominant mode of inheritance.

Pathology. See Signs.

Diagnostic Procedures. X-Rays. See Signs. Bone age normal. Growth hormone assay. Normal. Karyotype. Normal.

Therapy. Trials with growth hormone have failed.

Prognosis. Shortness of stature; no serious mental deficiencies.

BIBLIOGRAPHY. Aarskog D: A familial syndrome of short stature associated with facial dysplasia and genital anomalies. J Pediatr 77:856–861, 1970

Scott CJ Jr: Unusual facies, joint hypermobility, congenital anomaly and short stature: A new dysmorphic syndrome. In Bergsma D, McKusick VA, Konigsmark BW (eds): The Clinical Delineation of Birth Defects, Vol 10, The Endocrine System, pp 240–246, Baltimore, Williams & Wilkins, 1971

Peris-Menketa MD, Martin Caballero JM, Costa Guirao M, et al: Sindrome Facial-Digital-Genital de Aarskog. Presentation de un nuevo caso y revision de la literatura. Acta Pediatr Esp 43:26–32, 1985

AASE-SMITH

Synonyms. Anemia congenital–triphalangeal thumb; triphalangeal thumb.

Symptoms. Occur in males; present from birth. Delayed closure of fontanels. Pallor. Mild growth deficiency (third percentile). Triphalangeal thumbs; mild radial hypoplasia; narrow shoulders. Ventricular septal defect and others. Hepatosplenomegaly of variable degree. Cleft lip and palate reported.

Etiology. Autosomal recessive inheritance seems likely.

Pathology. Bone marrow. Hypoplasia.

Diagnostic Procedures. Blood. Anemia; variable leukopenia. X-ray of skeleton and chest. Bone marrow cultures.

---

*Good and poor results claimed by each of the three schools using procedures based on the etiologic hypothesis.

Fail to stimulate production of erythropoietic precursors. *Dermatoglyphics.* Help to distinguish whether a triphalangeal thumb is indeed a thumb or a duplicated index finger with absence of the thumb.

Therapy. The preferred treatment is frequent blood transfusions for the first 12 months of life. Iron overload is prevented by chelation therapy. The benefit of prednisone is not clear; its use should be avoided if possible during the first year of life because of the serious implications for growth and the developing brain. Bone marrow transplantation may be the ultimate treatment when other therapies fail.

Prognosis. Anemia tends to recede spontaneously with age.

BIBLIOGRAPHY. Aase JN, Smith DW: Congenital anemia and triphalangeal thumbs. J Pediatr 74:471–474, 1969
Pfeiffer RA, Ambs E: Das Aase-Syndrome: autosomal rezessive vererbte konnatal insuffiziente Erythropoese und Triphalangie der Daumen. Monatsschr Kinderheilk 131:235–237, 1983
Muis N, Beemer FA, Van Dijken P, Klep-de-Pater JM: The Aase syndrome: case report and review of the literature. Eur J Pediatr 145:153–157, 1986

ABDOMINAL ANGINA

Synonyms. Abdominal intermittent claudication; angina abdominalis; intestinal angina; visceral angina; chronic midgut ischemia; claudicatio intermittens abdominalis; intermittent anemic dysperistalsis; intermittent ischemia of mesenteric arteries; ischemic abdominal; mesenteric vascular insufficiency; vascular abdominal insufficiency; mesenteric arterial insufficiency.

Symptoms. Appear in middle and old age; prevalent in males. Cramping abdominal pain usually developing 15 to 30 minutes after a meal, and lasting 1 to 3 hours (direct correlation between amount of food, and intensity and duration of pain). Nausea, vomiting, diarrhea may occur. Weight loss. Clinical manifestation may be chronic and unremitting, recurrent with long remission, or transient.

Signs. Moderate abdominal distension during attacks. Occasionaly, systolic bruit in upper part of abdomen.

Etiology and Pathology. Arteriosclerotic narrowing and obliteration of ostia of gastrointestinal branches of the abdominal aorta, usually superior mesenteric artery involved. In intestine, there may be villose atrophy, ulcerations, or small infarctions.

Diagnostic Procedures. *Blood.* Anemia (malnutrition type); leukocytosis (occasional). *Stool.* Occult blood. *X-ray of abdomen.* Negative. *Angiography.* Exposure with patient in lateral position so that the obstruction is not obscured by the aorta.

Therapy. Elective surgical revascularization of superior mesenteric artery, celiac axis, or both. Endarterectomy, resection, replacement by graft, or bypass with a graft.

Prognosis. Eventual development of abdominal apoplexy syndrome (see).

BIBLIOGRAPHY. Schnitzler J: Zur Symptomatologie des Darmarterienverschulussen. Wien Med Wochenschr 51:505–509; 568–572, 1901
Jaxheimer EC, Jewell ER, Persson AU: Chronic intestinal ischemia: the Lahey Clinic approach to management. Surg Clin N Am 64:123–130, 1985

ABDOMINAL APOPLEXY

Synonyms. Massive intraperitoneal hemorrhage; intraabdominal apoplexy; mesenteric or subperitoneal hemorrhage.

Symptoms. Prevalent in arteriosclerotic hypertensive males. Sudden severe abdominal pain, restlessness, shock.

Signs. Peritoneal irritation.

Etiology and Pathology. Spontaneous rupture of intraabdominal vessel. Arteriosclerosis and hypertension in young patient; rupture of small localized aneurysm has been suggested. Rupture of superior mesenteric aneurysm mycotic (60% of cases), atherosclerotic (40%).

Diagnostic Procedures. *Blood.* Anemia; leukocytosis. *X-ray.* Flat abdominal plate to evaluate fluid level.

Therapy. Early surgery with suture of bleeding point; endoaneurysmorrhaphy; for branch aneurysms bowel resection.

Prognosis. Excellent if suture of bleeding point performed in time.

BIBLIOGRAPHY. Cushman GF, Kilgore AR: The syndrome of mesenteric or subperitoneal hemorrhage (abdominal apoplexy). Ann Surg 114:672–681, 1941
Wright CB, Schoepfle WJ, Kurtock SB, et al: Gastrointestinal bleeding and mycotic superior mesenteric aneurysm. Surgery 92:40–44, 1982

ABDOMINAL COCOON

Symptoms and Signs. Intestinal obstruction, mass of palpable bowel loops in the abdomen, in patients treated by LeVeen shunt.

Etiology. Unknown. Hypotheses include: subacute peritoneal infections, fibrin deposition from increased ascitic fluid turnover. Increased potential for intraperitoneal clotting of ascites caused by chronic disease.

Pathology. Large fibrotic sac wrapping the small bowel in the manner of a cocoon. The examination shows a fibrosing, nonspecific, chronic inflammatory process.

Diagnostic Procedures. *Plain X-ray of the abdomen.*

Therapy. Surgical lysis of the fibrous cocoon.

Prognosis. Depends on the hepatic disease.

BIBLIOGRAPHY. Cambria RP, Shamberger RC: Small bowel obstruction caused by the abdominal cocoon syndrome: possible association with the LeVeen shunt. Surgery 95:501–503, 1984

ABDOMINAL THORACIC

Synonyms. Thoracoabdominal. Includes all pathologic conditions in which thoracic pathology is manifested by abdominal symptoms and vice versa; for instance, symptoms of gastrointestinal type due to coronary artery sclerosis or pneumonia, and anginal type of pain due to gallbladder pathology.

Etiology. Interrelationship of nervous (spinal and autonomous system) reflexes between abdomen and chest.

Pathology. Varies according to lesions determining the reflex mechanism.

Diagnostic Procedures. *Laboratory.* May be useful (e.g., high leukocytosis in pneumonia with abdominal pathologic changes). *X-rays of chest and abdomen.* Detection of pneumonia or abdominal pathology. *Electrocardiography.* Diagnosis of coronary artery diseases.

Therapy. Of the underlying disorder.

Prognosis. According to etiology.

BIBLIOGRAPHY. Long WB, Cohen S: The digestive tract as a cause of chest pain. Am Heart J 100:567–572, 1980
Mellow MH: A gastroenterologist's view of chest pain. Curr Prob Cardiol 7:7–9, 1983

ABESHOUSE'S TRIAD

Synonyms. Adrenal cysts.

Symptoms. Flank discomfort; occasionally, gastrointestinal and renal symptoms.

Signs. Palpable mass in homolateral side; radiologically evident downward displacement of kidney.

Etiology. Congenital malformation, endothelial cysts and pseudocysts in the adrenal gland. In differential diagnosis, consider also parasites (*Echinococcus*) and neoplasia.

Pathology. Majority (39%) are endothelial (angiomatous) cysts and pseudocysts.

Diagnostic Procedures. *Echography and CT scan.*

Therapy. Surgical excision.

Prognosis. Lesions benign.

BIBLIOGRAPHY. Doran AG: Cystic tumour of the suprarenal body successfully removed by operation. Br Med J 1:1558–1563, 1908
Abeshouse GA, Goldenstein RB, Abeshouse BS: Adrenal cysts: review of the literature and report of three cases. J Urol 81:711–719, 1959
Incze JS, Lui MA, Merriam JC, et al: Morphology and pathogenesis of adrenal cysts. Am J Path 95:423–432, 1979
Copland PM: The incidentally discovered adrenal mass. Ann Int Med 98:940–948, 1983

ABLEPHARON-MACROSTOMIA

Synonyms. McCarthy-West; AMS.

Symptoms and Signs. Male children. Delayed physical and mental development. Absence of eyelids, eyebrows, and lashes; mouth defects; rudimentary ears: abnormal genitalia; dry, folded skin.

Etiology. Possibly autosomal recessive.

Therapy. Plastic and reconstructive surgery.

Prognosis. Poor.

BIBLIOGRAPHY. McCarthy GI, West CM: Ablepharon macrostomic syndrome. Develop Med Clin Neurol 19:659–672, 1978

ABRIKOSSOFF'S MYOBLASTOMA

Synonyms. Abrikossov's tumor; Abrikossoff's M and T; granular cell myoblastoma.

Symptoms. Onset between 30 and 50 years of age. Asymptomatic or paucisymptomatic.

Signs. Firm, round nodule, sessile or pedunculated, on skin or beneath tongue. Color varies from pink to grayish.

Rarely, skin over the tumor ulcerates. Frequently affected are oral tissue (lips; palate; uvula; tongue) and genital tract (vulva).

Etiology. Unknown.

Pathology. Pseudoepitheliomatous hyperplasia; large cells with acidophilic cytoplasm, small nucleus, large nucleolus, arranged in syncytium; fibers of striated muscle in layers; dyskeratosis.

Therapy. Excision.

Prognosis. Benign tumor of slow growth.

BIBLIOGRAPHY. Abrikossoff A: Ueber Myome, Ausgehend von der quergestreiften willkurlichen Musckulatur. Virchows Arch [Pathol Anat] 260:215–233, 1926
Rook A, Wilkinson DS, Ebling FJG, et al: Textbook of Dermatology. 4th ed, p 2475. Oxford, Blackwell Scientific Publications, 1986

ACANTHOSIS NIGRICANS, MALIGNANT

Synonyms. Keratosis nigricans, malignant; acanthosis nigricans paraneoplastic.

Symptoms and Signs. Both sexes affected. Lesions may appear at any age, preceding, accompanying, or following other symptoms of presence of malignancies such as adenocarcinoma or reticulosis. Frequently, pruritus. Pigmentation, dryness, roughness of skin, which assumes a gray-brown to black color; hyperkeratosis; papillomatous elevation. Mucosae involved in 50% of cases. Compared to benign form lesions are more copious, extended, and severe, and involve the extremities. Symptoms and signs of associated malignancy.

Etiology. Unknown; paraneoplastic syndrome. No genetic factor demonstrated.

Pathology. Hyperkeratosis; papillomatosis; acanthosis and pigmentation of variable degree even within single section. Occasionally, horny inclusion cysts.

Diagnostic Procedures. *Blood.* Glycemia (frequent association with lipodystophic diabetes). *Biopsy of skin.*

Therapy. Medical or surgical treatment of associated malignancy.

Prognosis. Occasionally, total or partial regression with removal of underlying tumor. Frequently, recurrence.

BIBLIOGRAPHY. Degas R: Dermatologie, p 636. Paris, Flammarion, 1964
Curth HO: How and why the skin reacts. Ann NY Acad Sci 230:435–442, 1974
Rook A, Wilkinson DS, Ebling FJG, et al: Textbook of Dermatology. 4th ed, p 1462–1464. Oxford, Blackwell Scientific Publications, 1986

ACANTHOSIS NIGRICANS SYNDROMES

1. Acanthosis nigricans, malignant (see).
2. Acanthosis nigricans, familial (benign); benign familial form, nonprogressive (see Acanthosis nigricans, malignant).
3. A. Acanthosis nigricans-insulin resistant (see Miescher's I).
   B. Acanthosis nigricans-insulin resistance-acral hypertrophy-muscle cramps (Flier). Two cases described.
   C. Acanthosis nigricans Leprechaunism insulin resistance (see Donohue).
   D. Acanthosis nigricans, pineal hyperplasia-insulin resistant diabetes-somatic abnormalities (see Mendenhall).
   E. Acanthosis nigricans-lipodystrophy-hyperlipemia-hepatosplenomegaly-insulin resistance (see Lawrence-Seip).
4. Pseudoacanthosis nigricans (see).
5. Gourgerot-Carteaud (see).

BIBLIOGRAPHY. Flier JS, Young JB, Landsberg L: Familial insulin resistance with acanthosis nigricans, acral hypertrophy and muscle cramps. New Eng J Med 303:970–973, 1980
Tasjian D, Jarratt M: Familiar acanthosis nigricans. Arch Derm 120:1351–1354, 1984

ACCIDENT-PRONE

Symptoms and Signs. Most common patients are males under age 21. Variable physical, mental, or emotional symptoms result in occurrence of accident. Occasionally, recurrent at same time (hours, weeks, months). More frequent in summer.

Etiology. The child's impulsivity and self-harm may be related to problems of parental marital discord or to the withdrawal or depression of a parent.

Therapy. Complete assessment of physical psychological, and developmental status, careful evaluation of family and especially of parental interactions.

Prognosis. Accidents usually decrease after age 21, but some people remain accident prone for life.

BIBLIOGRAPHY. Freedman AM, Kaplan HI, Sadok BJ: Comprehensive Textbook of Psychiatry, 2nd ed, pp 1708–1711. Baltimore, Williams & Wilkins, 1975
Behrman RE, Vaugham VC (eds): Nelson's Textbook of Pediatrics, 12th ed, Philadelphia, WB Saunders, 1983

ACCOMMODATIVE EFFORT

Symptoms. Blurring of images (asthenopia) with near vision appearing within few minutes after reading, sewing, or observing a near object.

Signs. Measurable abnormality of accommodative functions. Increased amplitude of accommodative adduction. Abnormal relaxation of accommodation induced by relative divergence at close distances. Latent convergence insufficiency.

Etiology. Accommodative fatigue; presbyopia; hyperopia; accommodative paralysis.

Pathology. Depends on etiology.

Diagnostic Procedures. Keep patient under observation until blurring of images appears. Then it is easy to observe typical findings.

Therapy. Correction of latent convergence insufficiency in addition to accommodative effort.

BIBLIOGRAPHY. Hill RV: Accommodative-effort syndrome: Pathologic physiology. Am J Opthalmol 34: 423–431, 1951

ACHARD'S

Synonyms. Marfan's variant.

Symptoms and Signs. Same as in Marfan's (see), plus mandibulofacialis dysostosis. Joint laxity limited to hands and feet.

Etiology. Autosomal dominant with incomplete expression (see Marfan's). Not recognized as an autonomous clinical entity by many authors.

BIBLIOGRAPHY. Achard C: Arachnodactylie. Bull Mem Soc Med Hôp Paris 19:834–840, 1902
McKusick VA: Mendelian Inheritance in Man, 7th ed, p 7. Baltimore, Johns Hopkins University Press, 1986

ACHARD-THIERS

Synonym. Diabetic bearded woman.

Symptoms. Voice changes; absent or sparse menstruation.

Signs. Hypertrichosis and acne of face; hypertrophy of clitoris; atrophy of breast; obesity; abdominal striae; increased blood pressure.

Etiology. Hyperplasia of adrenal cortex with increased production of androgens and 11-oxysteroids.

Pathology. Hyperplasia or adenoma of adrenal glands; atrophic or sclerotic ovaries; pancreatic changes consisting of increase of islet cells and pericanalicular sclerosis; liver cirrhosis; colloid changes of thyroid.

Diagnostic Procedures. *Urine.* Test for hyperglycemia; decreased sugar tolerance, increased excretion of steroids in urine following adrenocorticotropic hormone (ACTH) stimulation.

Therapy. Surgery of adrenal may be useful.

BIBLIOGRAPHY. Achard C, Thiers J: Le virilisme pilaire et son association a l'insuffisance glycolytique (diabete des femmes à barbe). Bull Acad Nat Med (Paris) 86:51–66, 1921
Rook A, Wilkinson DS, Ebling FJG, et al: Textbook of Dermatology. 4th ed, p 1968. Oxford, Blackwell Scientific Publications, 1986

ACHENBACH'S

Synonyms. Finger apoplexy; paroxysmal hand hematoma.

Symptoms. Appear in both sexes; more frequent in females. Spontaneous severe pain in the hands after strain or temperature changing (e.g., cooling).

Signs. Small, round hematoma with or without edema of affected hand.

Etiology. Unknown; postulated allergic-hyperergic mechanism, neurosympathetic reaction.

Pathology. Blood effusion without rupture of venous walls.

Diagnostic Procedures. *Coagulation test.* Negative. *Pinching test.* Positive (occasionally).

Prognosis. Spontaneous regression in days. Recurrence in the same or opposite hand. In some cases development of phlebectasia.

BIBLIOGRAPHY. Achenbach W: Ematomi parossistici della mano. Athena (Rome) 23:187–189, 1957

ACHONDROPLASIA

Synonyms. Chondrodystrophia fetalis; hypoplastic chondrodystrophy; achondroplastic dwarfism; Parrot's; rickets fetal; ACH.

Symptoms and Signs. Occur in both sexes. Dwarfed from birth. *Head.* Bulging; marked saddling of nose; "bulldog-face" appearance. *Extremities.* Absolute diminution in length; disproportionate proximal parts. Fingers pudgy; characteristic "trident hands." *Spine.* Seldom, kyphosis; paraplegia may develop in 2nd or 3rd decades. Mild hyptonia; delayed motor progress. Intelligence usually normal. Forme fruste exists where only x-ray findings demonstrate condition.

Etiology. Unknown; autosomal dominant inheritance (10%) or spontaneous mutation (90%).

Pathology. Tubular bones short and proportionally thick. Foramen magnum compressed and small internal hydrocephalus frequent. *Histology.* Epiphyseal line discloses shorter cartilage columns without usual linear arrangement; some cartilage cells show mucinoid derangement.

Diagnostic Procedures. *X-ray.* In infants, excessive separation in ossification centers of vertebrae; caudal narrowing; short iliac wings and changes in sacroiliac curve: ossification centers set into metaphyseal ends. *Blood.* Relative glucose intolerance.

Therapy. Orthopedic-neurologic follow-up. Relative intervention, if possible, deferred until full growth. Surgical therapy of some complications like hydrocephalus (which results from obstruction at the foramen magnum), dental malocculsion, strabismus (resulting from craniofacial dysmorphism), and spine deformities like kyphosis. Medical therapy for recurrent otitis media. Physiotherapy. Psychological counseling during childhood. Genetic counseling.

Prognosis. Dwarfism in majority of cases; serious neurologic complication in early adulthood in some cases. In the majority of cases, the life span is normal; the mean adult height 131.5 cm in men and 125 cm in women.

BIBLIOGRAPHY. von Soemmering JT: Abbildungen und Beschreibungen einiger Misgerburden die sich ecemals auf den anatomischen Theater zu Cassel befanden, p 30. Mainz, Kurfustlen privilegirten universitäts Buchhandlung, 1791

Parrot JMJ: Sur la malformation achondroplasique et le Dieu Phtah. Bull Soc Anthrop Paris I (3rd sers): 296–308, 1878

Fitzsimmons JS: Familial recurrence of achondroplasia. Am J Med Genet 22:609–613, 1985

ACHONDROPLASIA REGIONAL–DYSPLASIA ABDOMINAL MUSCLE

Insufficient evidence to substantiate diagnosis. This condition may represent other dwarfisms.

Symptoms and Signs. Regional achondroplasia of ribs and ilium associated with abdominal muscle weakness.

BIBLIOGRAPHY. Caffey J: Achondroplasia of pelvis and lumbosacral spine. Am J Roentgen 80:449–457, 1958

Shapira E, Fischel E, Moses S, et al: Syndrome of incomplete regional achondroplasia (ilium and ribs) with abdominal muscle dysplasia. Arch Dis Child 40:694–697, 1965

ACHOO

Synonyms. Peroutka's sneeze; helio-ophthalmic outburst; photic sneeze.

Symptoms. Very common phenomenon (circa 25% of population). In both sexes. Uncontrollable sneezing when passing from dark to bright light (usually sun); from 2 or 3 sneezes to 40 or more.

Etiology. Dominant inheritance. Poorly understood phenomenon. Photic reflex.

BIBLIOGRAPHY. Everett HC: Sneezing in response to light. Neurology 14:483–490, 1964

Peroutka SJ, Peroutka LA: Autosomal dominant transmission of the photic sneeze reflex. New Engl J Med 310:599–600, 1984

ACHROMATOPSIA

Synonyms. Total color blindness; congenital cone dysfunction; monochromasy; color blindness total; day blindness.

Symptoms. Both sexes affected; rare; evidence since childhood. Photophobia. All objects perceived as gray; subnormal visual acuity 20/50 to 20/200 or less. Scotopic vision.

Signs. Head posture against strong light. Undulatory nystagmus; absence of photopic flicker.

Etiology. Autosomal recessive inheritance; possibly, partial sex-linkage.

Pathology. Alterations of cone morphology in external area; depigmentation, degeneration, and normal number of cones in macular area.

Diagnostic Procedures. *Test pseudoisochromatic plates. Electroretinography.* Reduction of critical fusion frequencies; reduction of b wave and absence of a wave.

Therapy. None.

Prognosis. Nonprogressive permanent condition. Visual defects according to degree of involvement from total color blindness to ability to read when holding the book close and shaded from glare. Nystagmus diminishing in adult life.

BIBLIOGRAPHY. Larsen H: Demonstration mikrocopischer Präparate von einem monochromatischen. Augen Klin Monatsbl Augenheilk 72:1, 1924

Voke-Fletcher J: Congenital rod monochromatism in a brother and sister. Mod Probl Ophthal 19:236–237, 1978

ACHROMIC NEVI

Synonym. Amelanotic nevus, nevus anemicus.

Symptoms and Signs. Occur in both sexes; present since birth, or onset early in life. Unilateral or bilateral lack of pigment in a systematized distribution; no change in distribution throughout life; no alteration of texture or changes in sensation in affected areas; no pigmented border around achromic area (one case reported). No other cutaneous or systemic defect.

Etiology. Unknown; negative family history. Congenital mesenchymal alteration that inhibits migration of melanoblast precursor cell. Autosomal dominant familial form described.

Diagnostic Procedures. *Biopsy of skin.* Absence of melanophores.

Therapy. None.

Prognosis. Permanent condition.

BIBLIOGRAPHY. Lesser E. In Ziemssen HV: Handbook der Hautkrankeiten, Bd 2, p 183. Leipzig, Vogel, 1884

Coupe RL: Unilateral systematized achromic naevus. Dermatologica 134:19–35, 1967

Cardoso H, Vignale R, Abreu de Sastre H: Familial nevus anemicus. Am J Med Genet 27:24A, 1975

Rook A, Wilkinson DS, Ebling FJG, et al: Textbook of Dermatology, 4th ed, p 1589. Oxford, Blackwell Scientific Publications, 1986

ACID PHOSPHATASE DEFICIENCY

Synonyms. Nadler-Egan.

Symptoms and Signs. Vomiting; hypotonia; lethargy; opisthotonus; bleeding; recurrent infections.

Etiology. Autosomal recessive inheritance. Deficiency of acid phosphatase in all cell lines.

Diagnostic Procedures. *Assay acid phosphatase.* No activity.

Therapy. None.

Prognosis. Death a few days after birth.

BIBLIOGRAPHY. Nadler HL, Egan TJ: Deficiency of lysosomal acid phosphatase: a new familial metabolic disorder. New Engl J Med 282:303–307, 1970

ACKERMAN'S (J.L.)

Synonyms. Molar root (pyramidal)-juvenile glaucoma-upper lip deformity; Glaucoma, juvenile-upper lip deformity-dental roots.

Symptoms and Signs. Present from birth. Fused molar roots; single root canal (taurodontism); juvenile glaucoma; sparse body hair; full upper lip (absence of "cupid bow"); thick filtrum. Occasionally, syndactyly and hyperpigmentation of interphalangeal joints of fingers and clinodactyly of fifth finger.

Etiology. Unknown; has appeared in two generations of a family.

BIBLIOGRAPHY. Ackerman JL, Ackerman AL, Ackerman AB: Taurodont, pyramidal and fused molar roots associated with other anomalies in a kindred. Am J Phys Anthrop 38:681–694, 1973

ACRAL FIBROKERATOMA

Synonyms. Acquired digital fibrokeratoma.

Symptoms. Males more commonly affected than females; onset at any age from 17 but predominant in patients over 60 years of age.

Signs. Growth usually on fingers, with a slight or major resemblance to a rudimentary supernumerary digit. Occasionally, similar growth may appear also on palms or on soles.

Etiology. Unknown.

Pathology. Core of lesion formed by modified dermis, both reticular and papillary layer features included. Presence of elastic fibers (differential elements with true fibroma). Epithelial covering: acanthosis and hyperkeratosis.

Therapy. Excision.

Prognosis. After rather abrupt appearance a rapid growth follows until the final size is reached. Lesion remains at maximum size for months or years.

BIBLIOGRAPHY. Hare PJ: Rudimentary polydactyly. Br J Dermatol 66:402–408, 1954

Bart RS, Andrade R, Kopf AW, et al: Acquired digital fibrokeratomas. Arch Dermatol 97:120–129, 1968

Rook A, Wilkinson DS, Ebling FJG, et al: Textbook of Dermatology, 4th ed, p 2392. Oxford, Blackwell Scientific Publications, 1986

ACROCALLOSAL

Synonyms. Corpus callosum absence–hallux duplication–postaxial polydactyly.

Symptoms and Signs. From birth. Both sexes. Mental retardation; macrocephaly; hallux duplication, postaxial polydactyly.

Etiology. Sporadic cases. Proposed autosomal dominant mutation or autosomal recessive inheritance.

Pathology. Absence of corpus callosum.

Diagnostic Procedures. *CT brain scan.*

BIBLIOGRAPHY. Schinzel A: Post-axial polydactyly hallux duplication, absence of corpus callosum, macroencephaly and severe mental retardation: a new syndrome. Helv Pediatr Acta 34:141–146, 1979
Nelson MM, Thomson AJ: The acrocallosal syndrome. Am J Med Genet 12:195–199, 1982

ACROCEPHALOSYNDACTYLY II

Synonyms. ACS II; Apert-Crouzon; cephalosyndactyly; Vogt cephalodactyly.

Symptoms and Signs. Present from birth. Head and facial characteristic of Crouzon's syndrome (see); extremely hypoplastic maxilla associated with syndactyly (typical of Apert's—see—however, less severe).

Etiology. Autosomal inheritance, dominant or recessive type. Possibly equal to Apert's syndrome with unusually marked facial features.

BIBLIOGRAPHY. Vogt A: Dyskephalie (Dysostosis craniofacialis, Maladie de Crouzon 1921) und eine neuartige Kombination dieser Krankheit mit Syndaktylie der 4 Extremitaeten (Dyskephalodaktylie). Klin Monatsbl Augenheilkd 90:441–454, 1933
Temtamy SA, McKusick VA: The Genetics of Hand Malformation. New York, National Foundation March of Dimes, 1978

ACRODERMATITIS, PERSISTENT

Synonyms. Pustular recalcitrant acrodermatitis; acropustulosis acrodermatitis perstans; Andrew's; Hallopeau's; "Dermatite continue" dermatitis repens pustular acrodermatitis; acrodermatitis continua.

Symptoms and Signs. Both sexes affected; onset in middle age. Burning or itching. Starts on fingers or thumbs, frequently following minor trauma or infection. Skin surrounding nail usually first affected by vesicles, pustules, or erosions with hemorrhagic periphery. Then, lesions burst leaving exuding areas that evolve in crusts or eczematous scaling. New lesions appear on other fingers or palms and soles. Seldom, lesions extend to forearm or elbow.

Etiology. Unknown. Bacterial or infective origin excluded by negative cultures. Some patients later exhibit psoriasis.

Pathology. *Early lesions.* Wide range of histologic features resembling eczema, intraepithelial vesicles, or pustules. *Later lesions.* Resemble psoriasis, but without its typical features.

Diagnostic Procedures. *Biopsy.* Repeated in well-chosen sites.

Therapy. Corticosteroids, coal tar and salicylic acid of limited benefit. X-rays of marginal value. Prolonged courses of tetracycline, in low doses, beneficial in 30% of cases. Removal of foci. Etretinate of relative value because of relapse in course of treatment and local after effects (palmo or plantar skin painful).

Prognosis. Chronic, recurrent condition.

BIBLIOGRAPHY. Hallopeau H: Sur les acrodermatites (Polydactylites continues recidivantes). Ann Dermatol Syph 35:473–475, 1897
Andrew GC, Birkman FW, Kelly RJ, et al: Recalcitrant pustular eruptions of the palms and soles. Arch Dermatol Syph 29:548–563, 1934
Rook A, Wilkinson DS, Ebling FJG, et al: Textbook of Dermatology, 4th ed, pp 1521–1522. Oxford, Blackwell Scientific Publications, 1986

ACRODYSOSTOSIS

Synonyms. Acrodysplasia I; Arkless-Graham; Maroteaux-Malamut.

Symptoms and Signs. Both sexes affected; onset prenatal. Growth deficiency. Middle ear infections. Brachycephaly; flat nasal bridge; hypoplastic maxilla; prognathism. Shortness of extremities more pronounced in distal parts: hands short, broad; radius, ulna, and distal humerus deformed; cone-shaped epiphyses. Mental deficiency (90% of cases). Hypogonadism. Occasionally, several additional malformations are present: teeth, skin (hypopigmented ulcer), genital, skeletal.

Etiology. Unknown. Sporadic. Older parental age (suggesting autosomal dominant inheritance).

Prognosis. Deformities slowly progressing during growth period with restriction of joint mobility.

BIBLIOGRAPHY. Arkless R, Graham GB: An unusual case of brachydactyly. Am J Roentgen 99:724–739, 1967
Maroteaux P, Malamut G: L'acrodystose. Presse Med 76:2189–2192, 1968
Jones KL, Smith DW, Harvey MAS, et al: Old parental age and fresh gene mutation: data on additional disorders. J Pediatr 86:94–98, 1975

ACROKERATOELASTOIDOSIS

Synonyms. AKE; Costa's.

Symptoms and Signs. Appearance of yellow, nodular, hyperkeratotic lesions on the palms and soles, possibly extending to dorsum of hands and feet. Absence of systemic manifestations.

Etiology. Possible autosomal dominant inheritance.

Pathology. Hyperkeratosis and disorganization of elastic fibers.

Therapy. Vitamin A, topical and systemic.

BIBLIOGRAPHY. Costa OG: Acrokeratoelastoidosis: a hitherto undescribed skin disease. Dermatologica 107:164–167, 1953
Greiner J, Kruger J, Palden L, et al: A linkage study of acrokeratoelastoidosis: possible mapping to chromosome 2. Hum Genet 63:222–227, 1983

ACROMEGALOID FACIAL APPEARANCE

Synonyms. AFA; thick lips–oral mucosa.

Symptoms and Signs. From birth. Thickened lips, prominent rugae and phrenula of the intraoral mucosa. Blepharophimosis; highly arched eyebrows. Bulbous nose. Large hands.

Etiology. Proposed autosomal dominant inheritance.

BIBLIOGRAPHY. Hughes HE, McAlpine PJ, Cox DW, et al: An autosomal dominant syndrome with acromegaloid features and thickened oral mucosa. J Med Genet 22:119–125, 1985

ACRO-OSTEOLYSIS

Synonyms. Schinz's. See Nélaton's.

Symptoms and Signs. Both sexes. Onset at puberty. Recurrent ulcers of fingers and toes. Elimination of bone sequestra. Normal sensitivity.

Etiology. Acquired in workers with vinylchloride. Congenital; autosomal dominant inheritance.

Prognosis. Healing with loss of digits.

BIBLIOGRAPHY. Schinz HR, Baensch WE, Friedl E, et al: Roentgen-diagnostic, Vol. 1, pp. 734, 969. New York, Grune & Stratton, 1981
Ross JA: An unusual occupational bone change. In Jeliffe AM, Strickland B (eds): Symposium Ossium. London, Livingstone, 1970

ACROPARESTHESIA

Synonyms. Nocturnal arm dysesthesias; Nothnagel's; Putnam's; Schultze's; sciatic arm neuralgia; sleep tetany; tired arm; Wartenberg's.

Symptoms. Prevalent in women of middle age. Paresthesias, anesthesias, pain in the arm occurring exclusively while patient is lying down, involving first and primarily muscles innervated by the ulnar. Numbness develops also when sustained grip is used. It always affects the dominant arm. In the morning hand is stiff and can be used freely only after it is massaged.

Signs. Absence of objective signs, even after long duration of the symptoms.

Etiology. Idiopathic form is extremely rare, and direct causes such as compression and irritation, or indirect ones such as heart diseases must always be carefully sought, so that this will not become a diagnosis of escape. The syndrome is observed in rheumatoid arthritis myxedema, acromegaly, amyloidosis, mucopolysaccharidosis, myeloma multiple.

Pathology. None. See Etiology. Common finding: thickening of transverse carpal ligaments or synovia of flexor tendons and median nerve compression.

Diagnostic Procedures. *X-ray of cervical column and shoulder* in different projections. *Electrocardiography. Spinal tap. Electromyography.* See Etiology.

Therapy. Hydrocortisone beneath carpal ligaments and chlorothiazide or other diuretics. Section of transverse carpal ligaments final treatment.

Prognosis. If true form (extremely rare), recurrent pain without complication and self-limited.

BIBLIOGRAPHY. Nothnagel H: Zur Lehre von den vasomotorischen Neurosen. Dsch Arch Klin Med 2:173–191, 1867
Putnam JJ: A series of cases of paresthesia, mainly of the hands, of periodical recurrence, and possibly of vasomotor origin. Arch Med NY 4:147–162, 1880
Schultze F: Neber Akroparaesthesie Dsch Z Nervenh 3:300–318, 1893

Wartenberg R: Brachialgia statica paresthetica (nocturnal arm dysesthesias). J Nerv Ment Dis 99:877–887, 1944

Ford FR: The tired arm syndrome: a common condition manifest by nocturnal pain in the arm and numbness of the hand. Bull Johns Hopkins Hosp 98:464–466, 1956

Adams RD, Victor M: Principles of Neurology, 3rd ed, p 297. New York, McGraw-Hill, 1985

ACROPECTOROVERTEBRAL

Synonyms. F syndrome (initial of family name).

Symptoms and Signs. Broad, short thumbs with partial duplication of distal phalanx and webbing with index that shows radial deviation; webbing of toes; sternal deformity, spina bifida occulta (L5-S1).

Etiology. Autosomal dominant inheritance.

Diagnostic Procedures. *X-ray of hand.* Fusion of capitate and hammate and, occasionally, other carpal bones.

BIBLIOGRAPHY. Grosse FR, Hermann J, Opitz JM: The F-form of acropectorovertebral dysplasia: the F syndrome. Birth Defects Orig Art Ser V (3):48–63, 1969

ACRO-RENAL

Synonyms. Dicker-Opitz.

Symptoms and Signs. Male. Malformations of limbs and kidneys.

Etiology. Dominant inheritance. Not a casual entity but a nonspecific development field defect?

BIBLIOGRAPHY. Dicker H, Opitz JM: Associated acral and renal malformation. Birth Defects Orig Art Ser V (3):68–77, 1969

Curran AS, Curran JP: Associated acral and renal malformations: a new syndrome? Pediatrics 49:716–725, 1972

ACRO-RENAL-MANDIBULAR

Synonyms. Halal's; split hands and feet–mandibular hypoplasia.

Symptoms and Signs. In two female sibs. Split hands and feet, renal and genital malformations, severe mandibular hypoplasia.

Etiology. Recessive inheritance.

BIBLIOGRAPHY. Halal F, Desgranges M-F, Leduc B, et al: Acro-renal-mandibular syndrome. Clin Genet 5:277–284, 1980

ACRO-RENAL-OCULAR

Synonyms. Duane's with radial defect.

Symptoms and Signs. Both sexes. Variable ocular defects: Duane's anomaly (see); coloboma, ptosis. Variable degrees of hypoplasia of thumb, polydactyly, and reduction of mobility of interphalangeal joints. Variable renal anomalies: kidney malrotation, crossed renal ectopia, urinary tract anomalies.

Etiology. Autosomal dominant inheritance.

Diagnostic Procedures. *X-rays of skeleton; urography; dermatoglyphic pattern.* Abnormalities.

BIBLIOGRAPHY. Halal F, Homsy M, Perrault G: Acro-renal-ocular syndrome: autosomal dominant thumb hypoplasia, renal ectopia, and eye defect. Am J Med Genet 753–762, 1984

ACUTE TUBULAR INSUFFICIENCY

Synonyms. Acute tubular necrosis, ATN; acute renal failure, ARF; acute kidney tubular necrosis; acute renal tubular insufficiency.

Symptoms. Oliguria of variable degree (from 50 to 75 ml/day to 1000 ml/day or more) and according to severity of syndrome; anorexia; nausea; vomiting; dry mouth.

Signs. Facies drawn; postural hypotension in 25% of cases; cardiac arrhythmias; seizures; lethargy up to coma.

Etiology. Assumption of nephrotoxins: antibiotics; various drugs; organic solvents; radiographic contrast materials; metals. Ischemia; hypovolemia; shock; hemolytic crisis or crush syndrome (see Bywaters').

Pathology. In acute phase, large edematous kidney. Histologically uniform pattern with diffuse lesions of various degrees of severity up to necrosis, but intact basement membrane or "Patchy pattern" with proximal and distal tubular cell involvement associated with disruption of basement membrane. Glomeruli usually normal in appearance.

Diagnostic Procedures. *Urine.* Specific gravity lower than 1.020; osmolality 280 to 320 mOsm/kg water; sodium in excess of 20 mEq/liter. Renal failure index greater than 2 or 3. Fractional excretion Na (FENA). Proteinuria, red cells, hemoglobin, casts according to etiology. *Blood.* Metabolic acidosis; increase in blood urea nitrogen (BUN) and creatinine, potassium phosphate; decrease in sodium, calcium and carbon dioxide. *Electrocardiography.* Signs of hyperkalemia. In atypical cases consider renal biopsy and arteriography of renal and splanchnic vessels.

Therapy. *Prophylaxis.* Avoidance of use of (or prolonged therapy with) nephrotoxic agents; cure water balance when using radiographic contrast materials in particular pathologic conditions; rapid correction of hypovolemic conditions. Diuretics: mannitol, furosemide, and follow up with glucose-saline infusions; if they fail, establishment of fluid administration according to minimal balance and to provide caloric support (if gastrointestinal tract not usable). Dialysis. Antihypertensive agents. In diuretic phase follow water and electrolyte loss, and provide for caloric and plastic needs. Early diagnosis and treatment of infections.

Prognosis. According to determining causes. Posttraumatic 50–70% mortality; medical 25–30%. Nonoliguric cases 26%; oliguric cases 50%. Diffuse pattern: better prognosis than for patchy pattern. Recovery may be complete, or near normal renal function.

BIBLIOGRAPHY. Kanfer A, Kourilsky O, Sraer JD, et al: Acute renal failure. In Tinker J, Rapin M (eds): Care of the Critically Ill Patient, p 433. Berlin, Springer-Verlag. 1983
Brenner BN, Lazurus JM (eds): Acute renal failure. Philadelphia, WB Saunders, 1983
Meeks ACG, Sinus DG: Treatment of renal failure in neonates. Arch Dis Child 63:1372–1376, 1988

ACYL-CoA DEHYDROGENASE, LONG CHAIN, DEFICIENCY OF

Synonyms. Nonketotic hypoglycemia, dicarboxylic aciduria deficit in oxidation of fatty acids, Hale's.

Symptoms. From childhood. Hypoglycemia and respiratory arrest with fasting.

Signs. Cardiomegaly; hepatomegaly; hypotonia.

Etiology. Autosomal recessive inheritance. Deficiency of acyl-CoA dehydrogenase, which oxidizes long-chain fatty acids.

Diagnostic Procedures. *Blood.* Low plasma carnitine. *Urine.* No ketones at fasting; dicarboxylic acids; low hydroxy butyrate levels. *Assay for enzyme.* Activity absent.

Therapy. No fasting. Carnitine administration.

Prognosis. In some cases death.

BIBLIOGRAPHY. Naylor EW, Mosovich LL, Guthrie R, et al: Intermittent nonketotic dicarboxylic aciduria in two siblings with hypoglycemia: an apparent defect in beta-oxidation of fatty acids. J Inherit Metab Dis 3:19–24, 1980
Hale DE, Batshaw M-L, Coates PM, et al: Long chain acyl coenzyme A dehydrogenase deficiency: an inherited cause of non ketotic hypoglycemia. Pediatr Res 19:666–671, 1985

ACYL-CoA DEHYDROGENASE, MEDIUM CHAIN, DEFICIENCY OF

Synonyms. Nonketotic hypoglycemia; carnitine deficiency due to medium-chain acyl-CoA dehydrogenase deficiency; MCADH deficiency, dicarboxylic aciduria defect in beta oxidation of fatty acids.

Symptoms. In adolescence, hypoglycemia, lethargy, coma. Symptoms similar to Reye's (see).

Signs. Hepatomegaly.

Etiology. Autosomal recessive inheritance. Deficiency of MCADH that does not permit oxidation of medium-chain fatty acids.

Pathology. *Liver.* Peripheral lobular fatty changes; steatosis.

Diagnostic Procedures. *Blood.* Low serum carnitine. *Urine.* Dicarboxylic aciduria (C6–C14), no ketosis with fasting.

Therapy. Carnitine administration.

Prognosis. If identified, benign condition.

BIBLIOGRAPHY. Naylor EW, Mosovich LL, Guthrie, et al: Intermittent dicarboxylic aciduria and hypoglycemia in two siblings: apparent defect in beta oxidation of fatty acids. (Abst.) Am J Hum Genet 30:35A, 1978
Amendt BA, Rhead WJ: Catalytic defect of medium-chain acylcoenzyme A dehydrogenase deficiency: lack of both cofactor responsiveness and biochemical heterogeneity in eight patients. Clin Invest 76:963–969, 1985

ADAMANTIADES-BEHÇET

Synonyms. Behçet's; Gilbert's (W.); Halushi-Behçet; oculobuccogenital; Touraine's aphthosis; triple symptom complex of Behçet.

Symptoms. Prevalent in young males; more frequent in Mediterranean area. Recurrent every 2 to 3 months and lasting from 1 week to a month. Pain and irritation of eyes; disturbed vision (initially unilateral); pain in the mouth (98%) and dysphagia; considerable pain on walking because of painful lesions on scrotum or labia. Other manifestations include fever, arthralgia, malaise; gastrointestinal, lung, and neurologic manifestations (the latter appear between second to fifth year of disease); acute meningomyelitis; meningoencephalitis; dementia; erythema nodosum (80%); arthritis (30% to 60%); parkinsonism.

Signs. Iritis (first manifestation); hypopyon; conjunctivitis; keratitis; retinal hemorrhages. In mouth aphthae appearing in crops extending to pharynx. On genitals small papules that ulcerate.

Etiology. Unknown: virus (?); related to collagen diseases (?); possible autosomal dominant inheritance of autoimmune disorder.

Pathology. Nonspecific inflammation; perivascular lymphocytic infiltration of meninges, brain, spinal cord; cerebral edema; destruction ganglion cells; thrombophlebitis (25%); arterial aneurysm reported in some cases.

Diagnostic Procedures. *Blood.* Anemia; hypergammaglobulinemia; high sedimentation rate; high antiplasmin level. *Complement and immunoglobulin studies.*

Therapy. Adrenal steroids and antibiotics have doubtful benefits. Chlorambucil reported beneficial; levamisole helps for oral and genital ulcerations; corticosteroids and azathioprine used in relapses.

Prognosis. Poor; condition recurrent and progressive; vision impaired by recurrent attacks. Oral and genital lesions regress leaving scarring. Case history of 17 years' duration reported. Central nervous system involvement cause of death.

BIBLIOGRAPHY. Bluthe L; Zur Kenntnis des recidivirenden Hypopyons (thesis). Heidelberg, 1908
Adamantiades, B: Sur un cas d'iritis a hypopyon recidivant. Ann Ocul 168:271, 1931
Behçet H: Uber rezidivierende Aphthöse, durch ein Virus verursachte Geschwure am Mund, am Auge und an den Genitalien. Derm Wochenschr 105:1152–1157, 1937
Feigenbaum A: Description of Behçet's syndrome in Hippocratic third book of endemic diseases. Br J Ophthalmol 40:355–357, 1956
Shimizu K: Harada's, Behçet, Vogt-Koyanaga syndromes: Are they clinical entities? Trans Am Acad Ophthalmol Otolaryngol 77:281–290, 1973
Dundar SV, Gencalp V, Simsek H: Familial cases of Behçet's disease. Br Med J I:599, 1985
Benamour S, Benmimoun M, Zaoni A, et al: Behçet's disease: a review of 60 cases. Sem Hôp Paris 62:1317–1321, 1986

ADAMS-OLIVER

Synonyms. Absence defect of limbs, scalp, skull.

Symptoms and Signs. Both sexes. From birth. Absence of lower extremities and fingers of hands. Ulcerated area on vertex of scalp, bone defect underneath. Skin and skull lesions similar to those of aplasia cutis congenita (see).

Etiology. Dominant inheritance variable expressivity.

BIBLIOGRAPHY. Adams FH, Oliver CP: Hereditary deformities in man due to arrested development. J Hered 36:3–7, 1949
Bonafede RP, Beighton A: Autosomal dominant inheritance of scalp defects with ectrodactyly. Am J Med Genet 3:35–41, 1979

ADAMS-VICTOR-MANCALL

Synonym. Alcohol myelinolysis pontine; central pontine myelolysis; myelinolysis, central pontine.

Symptoms and Signs. Both sexes affected; onset usually in adulthood, in alcoholic or nutritionally deprived patients. Progressive facial and tongue weakness, speech and deglutition impairment. Occasionally, pseudobulbar phenomena: emotional lability. In some cases, quadriparesis at onset that results in flaccid and areflexic quadriplegia. Positive Babinski. Sensorial alteration frequently observed. Sphincters seldom affected.

Etiology. Alcoholism or nutritional deficiency. May be associated with various conditions such as Wilson's, Wernicke's, diabetes, amyloidosis, leukemia, infections, and kidney transplantation.

Pathology. Central pontine myelinolysis of variable extension involving center of basal portion of middle and upper pons. Nerve cells and blood vessels relatively unaffected.

Diagnostic Procedures. *Spinal fluid.* Normal. *Blood.* Anemia and other findings associated with nutritional deficiency; severe electrolyte changes. Reduced serum osmolality, P_{CO_2} increased. *CT brain scan and MRI.*

Therapy. Thiamine and other vitamins; dietary treatment. Electrolyte deficit correction.

Prognosis. Poor; rapid evolution in 2 to 3 weeks; coma and death. Some patients have survived with intensive treatment.

BIBLIOGRAPHY. Victor M, Adams RD: Effect of alcohol on nervous system. Res Publ Assoc Res Nerv Ment Dis 32:526–573, 1953

Adams RD, Victor M, Mancall EL: Central pontine myelosis. Arch Neurol Psychiatr 81:154–161, 1959

Dreyfus PM: Nutritional disorders of obscure etiology. Med Sci 17:44–48, 1966

Wiederholt WC, Kobayashi RM, Stockard JJ, et al: Central pontine myelolysis: A clinical reappraisal. Arch Neurol 34:220–227, 1977

Adams RD, Victor M: Principles of Neurology, 3rd ed, pp 778–780. New York, McGraw-Hill, 1985

ADDISONIAN SYNDROMES

Synonyms. Addison's disease; adrenal cortical insufficiency; melasma suprarenale. Adrenal cortical insufficiency clinically results in two types of syndromes: acute adrenal insufficiency and chronic adrenal insufficiency.

ACUTE ADRENAL INSUFFICIENCY

Synonyms. Addisonian crisis; adrenal crisis; Bernard-Sergent.

Symptoms. Dramatic appearance. Anorexia; nausea; vomiting; abdominal pain; cyanosis; mental torpor.

Signs. Weak pulse; extremely severe hypotension; heart sound weak and soft; dehydration; hypothermia. When treatment is started fever appears.

Etiology. Secretory failure of adrenals; hemorrhage into adrenals. Infections (Waterhouse-Friderichsen); trauma; tumor; vascular thrombosis. Bilateral adrenalectomy (occurrence not justifiable since must be prevented by proper medications); adrenal cortical atrophy and abrupt discontinuation of cortisone; cortisonelike therapy; stress of different nature with a decreased production of hormones and incapability to increase the production.

Pathology. Bilateral adrenal hemorrhage; atrophy induced by prolonged treatment with adrenal steroids (decreased weight; loss of lipid content of cells of both glomerular and fascicular zones).

Diagnostic Procedures. In such emergency, treat first, refine diagnosis later. *Blood.* Preliminary tests: blood sugar; sodium; potassium; blood urea nitrogen; plasma cortisol.

Therapy. Start immediately intravenous (IV) infusion 5% dextrose while waiting for other medications. Hydrocortisone (100–400 mg) added to dextrose and given in 2-hour period (repeated every 6 hours). After 24–36 hours, hydrocortisone (100 mg/day). Penicillin or other antibiotic (even if no sign of infection), plasma, or albumin to counteract shock. Catecholamine only with precaution (after some dextrose and hydrocortisone have been given).

Prognosis. Without treatment, rapidly fatal. With treatment, dramatic improvements. Continue treatment as long as necessary. Do not exceed 3000 ml of fluid a day especially if sodium-containing solutions are used. Once out of shock, the patient may be maintained on oral medication (prednisone 5 mg in the morning and 2.5 mg in the early evening).

CHRONIC ADRENAL INSUFFICIENCY

Synonym. Addison's disease.

Symptoms. Early emotional lability; irritability. The following symptoms appear: asthenia; weakness; easy fatigability (improving with rest and sleep); anorexia; nausea; vomiting; weight loss; abdominal pain; constipation or diarrhea; increase of emotional lability; salt craving; amenorrhea; loss of libido; impotence; muscle cramps; contractures.

Signs. Hypotension; hyperpigmentation of skin, patches of dark grayish pigmentation in mucosa of mouth, vagina, rectum; asymmetric areas of vitiligo; decrease of body hair; dehydration.

Etiology. Several mechanisms may induce adrenal insufficiency. They are subdivided as primary type and secondary type.

Primary type.

1. Primary atrophy (related to the development of autoantibodies). In this type, the frequent association with extraadrenal endocrine deficiencies (pancreatic, gonadal) has been interpreted as due to a generalized tendency toward endocrine organ failure with adrenal insufficiency as the most prominent component. (See Multiple endocrine deficiency syndrome.)

2. Infections: tuberculosis; viral, bacterial and mycotic diseases.

3. Infiltration by leukemia, reticuloendotheliosis, Hodgkin's disease, metastatic tumors, amyloidosis.

4. Hemorrhages: trauma; infections; anticoagulant treatment; thrombocytopenia; thrombosis.

5. Congenital familial form. Autosomal dominant, recessive and X-linked.

6. Induced by drugs that alter adrenal cortisol metabolism (Triparanol, amphenone 33bis4aminofenil2butanone 1,1-dichloro-2-(O-chlorophenyl)-2-(P-chlorophenyl) ethane).

Secondary type. Pituitary failure due to tumor; necrosis; iatrogenic (medicamental; surgical; radiologic); suppression of activity; hypothalamic failure to produce corticotropin-releasing factor (CRF).

Pathology. Lesions of adrenal or pituitary (or both) depending on etiology. Over 50% of patients show lymphocyte infiltration of adrenal cortex.

Diagnostic Procedures. Evidence of adrenal insufficiency may be gathered by direct and indirect tests of adrenal functions. *Adrenocorticotropic hormone (ACTH) stimulation.* The most reliable test for measuring adrenal function directly. Preferable is the IV 8-hour technique (administration of dexamethasone orally to protect from reactions), determination of urinary 17-hydroxysteroid, and 17-ketosteroid or plasma cortisol level or both, used as indexes of adrenal response.

Lack of increase is present in both primary and secondary (pituitary) insufficiencies. To differentiate the two forms, continue injection of ACTH for several days, and repeat determination. If levels increase, secondary type is indicated.

Determination of level of urinary 17-ketosteroid and 17-hydroxycorticosteroid and of plasma cortisol of relative value. *Other diagnostic procedures.* Indirect indications of adrenal insufficiency are given by a group of tests more economical and less complicated, although not very specific, than the previous ones: water load test; salt deprivation test; serum and salivary sodium potassium ratio; absolute number of circulating eosinophils; glucose tolerance test. Other findings in Addison's syndrome are normocytic, normochromic anemia, lymphocytosis presence of antiadrenal antibodies (in about 50% of cases). *X-ray of skull; of chest* (for heart size); *of abdomen* (adrenal calcification). *Electrocardiography.* Hypokalemia. *Electroencephalography.* Generalized theta activity; alpha rhythm suppressed; occasionally, delta activity.

For diagnosis of pituitary type, the frequent association of other endocrine defects is important: high cholesterol; low basal metabolic rate; urinary gonadotropins; oligospermia. Determination of ACTH; metyrapone test after prolonged ACTH administration.

Therapy. A combination of glucocorticoid, mineralocorticoid, and androgenic-anabolic agents. The combination cortisolfluohydrocortisone-fluor-oxymesterone is one of the more recommended.

Prognosis. With adequate treatment normal health may be maintained.

BIBLIOGRAPHY. Addison T: Diseases of suprarenal capsules. London Med Gaz O S 43(NS 8):517–518, 1849
Farwleg FF: Adrenal cortical insufficiency. In Eisenstein AB (ed): The Adrenal Cortex. Boston, Little Brown, 1967
Nelson DH: Diagnosis and treatment of Addison disease. In De Groot L, et al (eds): Endocrinology, p 1193. New York, Grune & Stratton, 1979
Chuandi L, Junquing C, Ruohua S, et al: Addison's disease of autosomal dominant inheritance: a report of 11 cases in one family. Kexue Tongbao 30:981–984, 1985

ADDISON-BIERMER

Synonyms. Biermer's. Addison's anemia; pernicious anemia.

Symptoms and Signs. Presenting complaints: symptoms of anemia (58% of cases); paresthesia (13%); gastrointestinal symptoms (11%; sore tongue or mouth (7%); weight loss (5%); difficulty in walking (3%). Long-term complication: carcinoma of the stomach.

Etiology. The disease occurs in two forms: an adult type (common) and a congenital variety (rare). In the first type, the lack of intrinsic factor (necessary for absorption of vitamin B_{12}) is associated with gastric atrophy and deficiency of many other gastric secretions (achylia gastrica). In the congenital form, only intrinsic factor is lacking, other components of gastric juice remaining normal. An autoimmune mechanism has been postulated.

Pathology. Skin pallor; yellowish hue. Heart dilated, flabby. Fatty changes in parenchymatous viscera, with generalized iron deposition. Extramedullary myeloid metaplasia. Tongue and gastric mucosa atrophic. Neurologic features (see Lichtheim's).

Diagnostic Procedures. *Blood.* Macrocytic anemia, poikilocytosis; mean corpuscular volume increased; hemoglobin content of red cell increased. Platelets slightly decreased. Slight to marked hyperbilirubinemia. High serum iron; low serum alkaline phosphatase; high lactic acid dehydrogenase. *Leukocytes.* Macropolycytes; some immature cells may be found. *Bone marrow.* Erythroid series; megaloblastosis; hyperplasia. Abnormal myelopoiesis; enlargement of elements, especially metamyelocytes; nuclear changes. *Gastric analysis.* Achlorhydria. *Biopsy of stomach mucosa.* Typical changes. *Schilling test.* Positive: antibodies against parietal cells of stomach.

Therapy. Vitamin B_{12} lifelong administration.

Prognosis. Good with treatment.

BIBLIOGRAPHY. Addison T: On the constitutional and local effects of disease of the suprarenal capsules. London, 1855
Biermer A: Form von progressiver pernicioser Anamie. Korresp Bl Schweiz Arzt 2:15–18, 1872
Wintrobe MM (ed): Clinical Hematology, 8th ed. Philadelphia, Lea & Febiger, 1981

ADDISON-SCHILDER

Synonym. Adrenoleukodystrophy, ALD; adrenomyeloneuropathy; Simerling-Creutzfeld; Addison-Scholz; Bronze; Schilder's; melanodermic leukodystrophy.

Symptoms and Signs. Only males affected. Symptoms and signs of adrenal insufficiency (see Addison's) precede neurologic ones (see Schilder's) that become evident between 5 and 14 years of age. Onset various ages, also advanced, reported.

Etiology. Sex-linked recessive inheritance. Strong suggestion that this syndrome is the result of two phenotypic expressions of a single complex genotype. In some families some subjects may present only symptoms of Addison's disease and others the combination of Addison's and neurologic signs. X-linked inheritance.

Pathology. *Brain.* Extensive demyelination or myelinoclastic diffuse sclerosis or both; cytoplasmatic inclusion bodies in the macrophages. *Adrenal cortex.* Nests of large eosinophilic cortical cells with hypochromatic nuclei.

Diagnostic Procedures. See Addison's. *Cerebrospinal fluid.* Protein elevated; IgG elevated. *CT brain scan.*

Therapy. Symptomatic.

Prognosis. Death from 6 months to 4 years from onset of neurologic signs.

BIBLIOGRAPHY. Scholz W: Klinische, pathologisch-anatomische underbiologische Undersuchungen bei familiarer, diffuser Hirnsklerose im Kindesalter: Ein Bertrag zur Lehr von den Heredodegenerationem. Z Ges Neurol Psychiatr 99:651–717, 1925

Fanconi A, Prader A, Isler W, et al: Morbus Addison mit Hirnsklerose im Kindersalter. Ein hereditaeres Syndrom mit X-chromosomaler Vererbung? Helv Paediat Acta 18:480–501, 1964

Moser HW, Moser AE, Singh I, et al: Adrenoleukodystrophy: survey of 303 cases: biochemistry, diagnosis and therapy. Am Neurol 16:628–641, 1984

ADDUCTED THUMB

Synonyms. Arthrogryposis–cleft palate–craniosynostosis; Christian-Andrews-Conneally; thumb, congenital clasped.

Symptoms and Signs. Both sexes affected; present from birth. Dysphagia; muscular fibrillation; craniosynostosis; microcephaly; prominent occiput; hypertelorism; antimongoloid slant; ophthalmoplegia; ear abnormalities; cleft palate. Camptodactyly; abducted thumbs; occasionally, reduced extension of elbow and knees.

Etiology. Autosomal recessive inheritance.

Pathology. See Symptoms and Signs. Laryngomalacia. Dysmyelinization and glial proliferation in white matter of brain.

BIBLIOGRAPHY. Christian JC, Andrews PA, Conneally PM, et al: The adducted thumb syndrome: An autosomal recessive disease with arthrogryphosis, dysmyelinization, craniostenosis and cleft palate. Clin Genet 2:95–103, 1971

Kunze J, Park W, Hansen KH, et al: Adducted thumb syndrome: Report of a new case and a diagnostic approach. Europ J Pediat 141:122–126, 1983

ADENINE PHOSPHORIBOSYLTRANSFERASE DEFICIENCY

Synonyms. 2,8-dihydroxyadenine lithiasis, (2,8-DHA); APRT deficiency.

Symptoms and Signs. From birth, variable expression from benign to severe. Colics; hematuria; urinary tract infection, dysuria, passage of gravel or stones. In some cases renal failure.

Etiology. Autosomal recessive inheritance. Deficiency of adenine phosphoribosyltransferase (chromosome 16)

Pathology. Stones composed of 2,8-DHA. Because of their radiolucency they often are confused with uric acid.

Diagnostic Procedures. *Blood.* Uric acid normal levels. *Urine.* Normal uric acid, excretion of abnormal adenine derivatives.

Therapy. Diet (purine restriction). Allopurinol. Avoid alkali.

Prognosis. Depends on degree of renal failure at moment of discovery.

BIBLIOGRAPHY. Cartier P, Hamet M: Une nouvelle maladie métabolique: le deficit complet en adénine-phosphorybosiltransférase avec lithiase de 2,8-dihydroxyadénine. CR Acad Sci (Paris) 279:883–886, 1974

Simmonds, HA, Van Acker KJ: Adenine phosphoribosyltransferase deficiency: 2,8-dihydroxyadenine lithiasis. In Stanbury JB, Wyngaarden JB, Fredrickson DS, et al: The Metabolic Basis of Inherited Disease, 5th ed, p 1144. New York, McGraw-Hill, 1983

Kishi T, Kidani K, Komazawa Y, et al: Complete deficiency of adenine phosphoribosyltransferase: a report of three cases and immunologic and phagocytic investigation. Pediatr Res 18:30–34, 1984

ADH-RESISTANT DIABETES INSIPIDUS

Includes all conditions where renal tubular inability to respond to antidiuretic hormone (ADH) predominates over other renal pathologic manifestations that may be present.

Synonyms. Nephrogenic diabetes insipidus; diabetes insipidus nephrogenic type II; vasopressin-resistant diabetes insipidus; water baby.

Etiology. *Congenital conditions.* (1) Hereditary nephrogenic diabetes insipidus syndrome, or water baby, is due to X-linked inheritance with variable degrees of manifestation in females. The defect resides (improbably) in the mobility of ADH to stimulate renal tubular cAMP (2) Associated with Fanconi's or Lightwood's syndromes (see).

Acquired Conditions. (1) Hypokalemia; (2) hypercalcemia; (3) Conn's syndrome; (4) drug-induced (demethylchlortetracycline, metoxyflurane, lithium); (5) in systemic diseases amiloidosis, Sjogren's.

Pathology. None.

Diagnostic Procedures. If diabetes insipidus, administration of ADH does not modify symptomatology.

Therapy. Proper fluid intake, hydrochlorothiazide 0.5–1.5 mg/kg/24 hr. in combination with a sodium intake of less than 1 mEq/kg/24 hr; potassium supplements if required. Indomethacin has been effective in some patients.

Prognosis. With early diagnosis and proper therapy, good.

BIBLIOGRAPHY. La Combe Lu: De la polydipsie. L'Experiance. J Med Chir 7:305, 1841
Weil A: Ueber die hereditare form des diabetes insipidus. Dtsch Arch Klin Med 93:180–290, 1908
Culpepper RM, Hebert SC, Andreoli TE: Nephrogenic diabetes insipidus. In Stanbury JB, Wyngaarden JB, Fredrickson DS: The Metabolic Basis of Inherited Disease, 5th ed, p 1867. New York, McGraw-Hill, 1983

ADIE-CRITCHLEY

Synonyms. Forced grasping and groping; Fulton's; premotor cortex.

Symptoms and Signs. *Grasping.* When an object is placed in one hand of patient, he grasps it, and it cannot be withdrawn because he involuntarily does not release it. Patient may also be unable to release object voluntarily and if he tries to throw it away, it remains firm in his hand. *Groping.* The affected hand goes after and attempts to grasp objects that touch it, or grasps other hand when it moves.

Etiology. Tumor of contralateral frontal lobe superior part of area 6. When syndrome affects both hands, localizing value is lost.

BIBLIOGRAPHY. Adie WJ, Critchley M: Forced grasping and groping. Brain 50:142–170, 1927
Walshe FMR: On the "Syndrome of the premotor cortex" (Fulton) and the definition of the terms "premotor" and "motor": With a consideration of Jackson's views on the cortical representation of movements. Brain 58:49–80, 1935
Grinker RR, Sahs AL: Neurology, 6th ed. Springfield, IN, CC Thomas, 1966

ADIE'S

Synonyms. Holmes-Adie; Holmes' G. III; Markus; Weill-Reys. When not associated with disturbed deep tendon reflexes: Adie's partial; Argyll-Robertson's nonluetic; Argyll-Robertson pupil with mydriasis.

This syndrome was fully described before Adie's publications (1931): Piltz J 1899; Strasburger J 1902; Saeger J 1902; Markus C 1905; Holmes D 1931.

See pupillotonic pseudotabes.

BIBLIOGRAPHY. Piltz J: Ueber neue Papillenphaenome. Neurol Zentralbl. 18:248–254, 1899
Strasburger J: Pupillentraegheit bei Accommodation und Convergenz. Neurol Zentralbl 21:738–740, 1902
Saeger J: Ueber die sogenaunte Myotonische Pupillenbenegung. Neurol Zentralbl 21:1000–1004, 1902
Markus C: Notes on a peculiar pupil phenomenon in two cases of partial iridoplegia. Lancet, 2:1257, 1905
Holmes G: Partial iridoplegia with symptoms of other diseases of nervous system. Trans Ophthalmol Soc UK 51:209–228, 1931
Adie WJ: Pseudo-Argyll-Robertson pupils with absent tendon reflexes, a benign disorder simulating tabes dorsalis. Br Med J 1:928–930, 1931

ADIPONECROSIS SUBCUTANEA NEONATORUM

Synonyms. Pseudosclerema; Haxthausenis II.

Symptoms and signs. Occur in healthy, well-nourished newborns; onset frequently after exposure to cool air. Formation of movable indurated subepidermal masses on the cheeks or other body areas (e.g., trunk; extremities).

Etiology. Unknown; possibly low content of olein in subcutaneous fat or secondary to traumatic injuries. Maternal preeclampsia, diabetes also have been considered.

Pathology. Necrosis of subcutaneous fat with perivascular inflammatory reaction. Giant cells containing needlelike crystals.

Diagnostic Procedures. *X-rays.* Occasionally, microcalcification lesions. *Blood.* Occasionally, hypercalcemia, thrombocytopenia.

Therapy. None. If hypercalcemia, calcium and vitamin D restriction, furosemide, corticosteroids.

Prognosis. Complete spontaneous resolution in 3 to 4 months. In rare cases, if visceral fat involved or severe hypercalcemia, may be fatal.

BIBLIOGRAPHY. Fabyan M: Disseminated fat necrosis occurring in an infant without other lesions. Bull Johns Hopkins Hosp 18:349, 1907
Haxthausen H: Adiponecrosis a frigore. Br J Dermatol 53:83–89, 1941
Chen TH, Shewmake SW, Hansen DD: Subcutaneous fat necrosis of the newborn: a case report. Arch Dermatol 117:36–37, 1981

ADRENAL HEMORRHAGE, NEONATAL

Synonyms. Neonatal adrenal.

Symptoms. Incidence over 1% of postmortem findings in newborn; onset between 2nd and 7th postnatal days. Occasionally, asymptomatic (and discovered as calcification and adrenal insufficiency in later life). High fever; tachypnea; convulsions; vomiting; collapse.

Signs. There may be a mass in the flank with overlying skin discoloration; jaundice may also develop. Pallor; cyanosis; skin rash; purpura.

Etiology. Stress and trauma at birth (leading cause). Physiologic involution of adrenals. Systemic diseases such as thrombocytopenia, syphilis.

Pathology. In 70% of cases, right adrenal involved; in 5 to 10% bilateral. From small hemorrhage to destruction of entire gland.

Diagnostic Procedures. *X-ray.* Lateral abdominal. Retroperitoneal mass. *Urography.* Kidney displacement. Calcification of adrenal sometimes as early as 12th day of life. Catecholamines, methoxyamines, and vanillylmandelic acid determination to rule out neuroblastoma. *Ultrasonography of abdomen.* May be very helpful.

Therapy. According to symptomatology. Exploration frequently indicated to differentiate from neuroblastoma. Transfusions; antibiotics; hormone replacement; fluid and electrolyte balance.

Prognosis. Depends on extension of lesion.

BIBLIOGRAPHY. Goldzieher MA, Gordon MD: Syndrome of adrenal hemorrhage in a newborn. Endocrinology 15:165–181, 1932
Behrman RE, Vaugham VC (eds): Nelson's Textbook of Pediatrics, 12th ed. Philadelphia, WB Saunders, 1983

ADRENOGENITAL SYNDROMES

Synonyms. Corticosexual; adrenal virilizing; adrenal feminizing; congenital adrenal hyperplasia; adrenal hyperplasia III.

Clinical findings and treatment vary according to etiology, which includes congenital adrenal hyperplasia, feminizing adrenal tumors, virilizing adrenal tumors, ill-defined group with hirsutism with or without menstrual disorders. (For last group see Hirsutism.)

A. CONGENITAL ADRENAL HYPERPLASIA

May be subdivided into four major subtypes: (1) Simple virilizing form; (2) sodium-losing form; (3) hypertensive form; (4) 17-hydroxylase deficiency; (5) 3-B-hydroxysteroid dehydrogenase defect.

SIMPLE VIRILIZING FORM
MALE

Symptoms. Infants a few months old exhibit frequent erections; from 1 to 5 years of age deepening of voice and marked muscular development occur.

Signs. Macrogenitosomia precox: at a few months of age, penis enlargement with normal small testis, pubic and axillary hair, increased pigmentation (Addison-like), seborrhea; between 1 and 5 years of age acne; at 8 to 10 years, fusion of epiphysis.

Etiology. Congenital familial condition; autosomal recessive mutant gene. Excessive secretion of adrenal androgens beginning during fetal life. Autosomal recessive inheritance. Deficiency of 21-hydroxylase. No production of cortisol, increase of ACTH, increased production of sex hormones and cortisol precursors.

Pathology. *Testis.* Biopsy shows small seminiferous tubules, no Leydig cells; occasionally, hyperplastic adrenal tissue; seldom, testicular maturity and spermatogenesis. *Adrenals.* Markedly enlarged. Not many studies done on this form of adrenal hyperplasia. In young children, glands brownish in color, irregular, cerebriform surface: In older patients, adenomas have been observed (see salt-losing form for description of microscopic changes).

Diagnostic Procedures. *Urine.* Increase in excretion of 11-oxysteroids and 17-ketosteroids and pregnanetriol; regression of size of testis with cortisone therapy. Cortisone and glucocorticoids decrease the excretion of 17-ketosteroids and pregnanetriol (last test differentiates this form from virilizing adrenal tumors). *Adrenocorticotropic hormone (ACTH) administration.* Markedly increases excretion of pregnanetriol and related steroids and causes a moderate rise of androgens and estrogens. Cortisol metabolites show absence of or insufficient response to ACTH (pathognomonic response). *Metyrapone administration.* Increases excretion of pregnanetriol and 17-ketosteroids.

Therapy. Cortisone or hydrocortisone intramuscularly (IM) at high dose (from 25 to 100 mg, according to age) regulated according to excretion of 17-ketosteroids. After 7 to 10 days of treatment, maintenance treatment: cortisone IM every third day, or per os daily, adjusting doses to requirement of individual patient.

Prognosis. Treatment started before age 2 years, normal development; if at later age, no changes in physical appearance or height, but fertility is restored.

FEMALE

Synonyms. De Crecchio; Apert-Gallais, pseudohermaphroditism, female.

Symptoms. Rapid and progressive virilization starting from birth; hypertrophic clitoris will have frequent erection. Voice deep; somatic growth accelerated. Pubic and then axillary hair appears between 6 months and 3 years of age. Acne develops early. Somatic growth accelerated. Thick muscles, heavy beard and body hair; no breast development; amenorrhea.

Signs. Diagnosis easier than in males since at birth various degrees of external genitalia abnormalities are present, resulting in pseudohermaphroditism. Changes may be minimal (simple enlargement of clitoris) to maximal (child is mistaken for a cryptorchid male).

Etiology. See Male.

Pathology. Pseudohermaphroditism with various degrees of abnormal evolution of external genitalia. Five types of abnormality differentiated by the degree of fusion of labial-scrotal folds, development of clitoris, closure of the urogenital sulcus. Ovaries polycystic with thick albuginea, similar to Stein-Leventhal (see). With time, disappearance of follicle and progressive follicular inactivity; cortex entirely stromatous. In rare cases, abnormal adrenal tissue found in the broad ligament. For adrenal changes, see Male.

Diagnostic Procedures. *Nuclear chromatin and chromosomal studies.* For sex determination. *Urethroscopic examination. X-ray vaginogram* (with injection of radiopaque material). *Hormonal excretion studies.* See Male.

Therapy. See Male. If condition discovered in early infancy, raise as a female and treat with cortisone. If mistake has been made and child raised as a male, after 3 years of age psychologic evaluation and advice. Hormonal therapy and surgery ideal between 1 and 3 years age. Correction of sex may be considered even in early adult life.

Prognosis. Excellent response. Correction dependent upon degree of abnormalities. Properly treated female may become pregnant. Marked tendency to abortion; in normal offspring adrenals function.

BIBLIOGRAPHY. DeCrecchio L: Sopra un caso di apparenza virile in una donna. II. Morgagni 7:151, 1865

Apert M: Dystrophies en relation avec les lésions des capsules surrénales. Bull Soc Pediatr Paris 12:501–518, 1910

Gallais A: Le Syndrome génito-surrénal; Etude anatomo clinique (thesis). Paris, 1912

Gordon MT, Conway DI, Anderson DC, et al: Genetics and biochemical variability of variants of 21-hydroxylase deficiency. J Med Genet 22:354–360, 1985

SODIUM-LOSING FORM

Synonyms. Debré-Fibiger; Fibiger-Debré-von Gierke; Pirie's; interrenal androgenic intoxication; salt-wasting CAH.

Symptoms and Signs. Appear at 5 to 10 days of age, or later in life if precipitated by infections. Acute adrenal crisis: apathy; anorexia; vomiting; diarrhea; abdominal pain; convulsion; circulatory collapse. In other cases, sudden death without dehydration and circulatory collapse. Severe dehydration; changes in skin color (dusky).

Etiology. Congenital, familial, adrenal hyperplasia with marked deficiency of 21-hydroxylase enzyme, with hypersecretion of aldosterone antagonists (progesterone and 17-hydroxyprogesterone); low cortisol secretion contributes to loss of salt.

Pathology. Marked enlargement of zona reticularis and zona fasciculata; atrophy of zona glomerulosa. The adrenal cells are hyperplastic, with eosinophilic cytoplasm, vesicular nuclei and large nucleoli. Among enlarged hyperpigmented cells, cells with granular cytoplasm and lipidic vacuoles, often in cordlike arrangements.

Diagnostic Procedures. *Blood.* Hematocrit. Electrolyte studies. High serum potassium appearing before low serum sodium; low bicarbonate. *Urine.* Increased excretion of 17-ketosteroids and pregnanetriol. *Electrocardiogram.* Hyperkalemia. *Weight determination. Blood pressure. Nuclear sex chromatin or chromosome studies.* In ambiguous sex.

Therapy. *In acute adrenal crisis.* (1) Sodium chloride IV (NaCl 0.9% solution) immediately (3 to 6 g NaCl in first 24 hours). (2) Desoxycorticosterone acetate 2 mg IM, if no response. (3) Hydrocortisone 25 mg added to NaCl infusion. *After crisis is over* (24 to 36 hours). (1) Resumption of oral feeding and 3 to 5 g NaCl a day. (2) Cortisone IM daily; high dose to reach maintenance dose. (3) Then deoxycorticosterone acetate 1 to 2 mg daily. *When patient is in good condition.* (1) Implantation of 125 mg deoxycorticosterone acetate pellets (effective for 8 to 12 months). *Further maintenance.* (1) Reimplantation of desoxycorticosterone acetate pellets, or 9-fluorocortisol 5 to 100 µg per day. *Mild case.* Salt addition to diet only.

BIBLIOGRAPHY. Debré R, Semelaigne G: Hypertrophie considérable des capsules surrénales chez un nourrison mort a 10 mois sans avoir augmente de poid depuis sa naissance. Bull Soc Pediatr Paris 23:270, 1925

HYPERTENSIVE FORM

Synonym. 11-B-hydroxylase deficiency; adrenal hyperplasia IV.

Symptoms and Signs. Moderate to severe hypertension in patient exhibiting symptoms and signs of simple virilizing form. Some patients have only minor signs of virilization.

Etiology. Congenital familial adrenal hyperplasia with severe 11-B-hydroxylase defect and excessive excretion of desoxycorticosterone and other cortisol precursors. Autosomal recessive inheritance. Deficiency of 11-B-hydroxylase which causes absent production of cortisol, increase in ACTH, excessive production of desoxycorticosterone and other cortisol precursors which may be the cause of hypertension.

Pathology. Markedly enlarged adrenals with hyperplastic zona glomerulosa.

Diagnostic Procedures. *Hypertension measurement.* Moderate to severe. *Biochemical and cytologic studies.* As above; pregnanetriol not as much increased.

Therapy. Cortisone, as outlined in treatment of simple adrenal hyperplasia of male. Blood pressure responds to treatment.

Prognosis. Good with adequate treatment.

BIBLIOGRAPHY. Birke G, Diczfalusy E, Plantin LO, et al: Familial congenital hyperplasia of the adrenal cortex. Acta Endocrinol (Copenh) 29:55–69, 1958
Hochberg Z, Schechter J, Benderly A, et al: Growth and puberal development in patients with congenital adrenal hyperplasia due to 11-B-hydroxylase deficiency. Am J Dis Child 139:771–776, 1985

17-HYDROXYLASE DEFICIENCY

See Biglieri's.

FORM WITH 3-B-HYDROXYSTEROID DEHYDROGENASE DEFICIENCY

Synonyms. Bongiovanni's; 3B-HSD deficiency; adrenal hyperplasia II.

Symptoms and Signs. *Female.* Fewer virilization signs than in other form (hypertrophy of clitoris; labial fusion; no displacement of urethral orifice). *Male.* Normal differentiation of external genitals incomplete (perineal hypospadias).

Etiology. Congenital adrenal hypertrophy with 3-B-hydroxysteroid dehydrogenase deficiency resulting in impaired production of testosterone and less androgenic activity. Small partial peripheral transformation of dehydroepiandrosterone (DHEA) to testosterone accounts for minor virilization in males and females.

Diagnostic Procedures. *Blood.* Low testosterone and high DHEA production.

Prognosis. Death in early infancy despite medical treatment. If partial deficiency, survival possible.

BIBLIOGRAPHY. Bongiovanni AM: Adrenogenital syndrome with deficiency of 3-B-hydroxysteroid dehydrogenase. J Clin Invest 41:2086–2092, 1962
Zachmann M, Forest MG, De Peretti E: 3-B-hydroxysteroid dehydrogenase deficiency: follow up study in a girl with pubertal bone age. Hormone Res 11:292–302, 1979

B. CONGENITAL LIPOID HYPERPLASIA OF ADRENAL GLANDS

Synonyms. Praeder-Gunter; cholesterol desmolase deficiency; 20-22 desmolase deficiency; P450 side chain cleavage enzyme; adrenal hyperplasia.

Symptoms and Signs. Weight loss; apathy; anorexia; vomiting; diarrhea. Skin pigmentation. *Male.* Testis in the abdomen or inguinal canal. *Female.* Complete or almost complete female appearance.

Etiology. Defect of 3-B-hydroxysteroid (Bongiovanni's syndrome) or altered transformation of cholesterol to pregnenolone. Autosomal recessive inheritance. Defect of 20-22 desmolase converting cholesterol to pregnenolone. Mild cases might be confused with 3-B-hydroxysteroid dehydrogenase deficiency.

Pathology. Enlarged, yellowish, nodular surface due to focal hyperplasia; cells distended by large deposit of lipoids, rich in cholesterol.

Diagnostic Procedures. Not well studied. *Urine.* 17-ketosteroid and 17-hydroxycorticosteroid low? *Nuclear sex chromatin and chromosome studies.*

Therapy. Cortisone and desoxycorticosterone acetate (temporary response).

Prognosis. Death before 8 months for adrenal insufficiency.

BIBLIOGRAPHY. Praeder A, Gunter HP: Das Syndrom des Pseudohermaphroditismus masculinus bei kongenitaler Nebennierenrindenhyperplasie ohne Androgenüberproduktion (adrenaler Pseudohermaphroditismus masculinus). Helvet Paediatr Acta 10:397–412, 1955
Praeder A, Anders GJ, Habich H: Zur Genetik des kongenitalen adrenogenitalen Syndroms (virilisierende nebennierenhyperplasia). Helvet Paediatr Acta 17:271–284, 1962
Miller WL, Chung DC, Matteson KJ: Molecular biology of steroid hormone synthesis. DNA 5:61, 1986

C. FEMINIZING ADRENAL TUMORS

Symptoms and Signs. *Young boy.* (Rare; three patients reported 5 to 7 years old). Gynecomastia; accelerated development of bones and musculature. *Young girl.* (Rare, two patients reported). Precocious puberty (3 and 4 years old); breast, pubic and axillary hair; vaginal bleeding; accelerated development of bones and musculature. *Adult male.* (Twenty-five to 66 years old).

Symptoms. Decreased libido and potency; pain at site of tumor.

Signs. Gynecomastia with or without tenderness, and atrophy of testis, areolar pigmentation and seldom secretion; prostate and penis seldom atrophic, generally normal; feminizing hair changes.

Etiology. Carcinomas or adenomas of adrenals.

Pathology. Difficult differentiation between benign and malignant tumors in the adrenal; most or all feminizing tumors believed malignant. Metastasis to lung, liver, local lymph nodes, brain, bones. Contralateral adrenal atrophy or normal atrophic changes in testis.

Diagnostic Procedures. *X-ray.* Perirenal air insufflation. *Urine.* Estrogens usually highly elevated; 17-ketosteroids increased in most cases; pregnanetriol and pregnanediol usually highly increased; 17-hydroxycorticosteroids in 50% of patients increased. ACTH stimulation negative; cortisone suppression negative.

Therapy. Surgical removal and x-ray after surgery. Cortisone therapy before and during operation.

Prognosis. Poor. Regression of symptoms and return of spermatogenesis after operation. After surgery frequent appearance of metastasis and death in one year, except in adenomas. In children, more favorable because of earlier diagnosis.

BIBLIOGRAPHY. Bittorf A: Nebennierentumor und Geschelchtsdrüsenausfall beim Manne. Klin Wochenschr 56:776, 1919
Wilkins L: Feminizing adrenal tumor causing gynecomastia in a boy of five years contrasted with virilizing tumor in five-year-old girl; classification of seventy cases of adrenal tumor in children according to their hormonal manifestations and review of eleven cases of feminizing adrenal tumor in adults. J Clin Endocrinol 8:111–132, 1948
Gabrilove JL, Shaima DC, Wotiz HH, et al: Feminizing adrenocortical tumors in the male. Medicine 44:37–53, 1965
Baulieu EE, Peillon F, Migeon CJ: Adrenogenital syndrome. In Eisenstein AB (ed): The Adrenal Cortex. Boston. Little, Brown, 1967

D. VIRILIZING ADRENAL TUMORS

Symptoms and Signs. *Prepuberal female.* From few months to puberal age. Hirsutism; clitoral hypertrophy; rapid bone and musculature development; no breast development; short stature; no menses at puberal age. *Prepuberal male.* Macrogenitosomia Precox. (For other symptoms and signs see Adrenogenital syndromes: con-

genital adrenal hyperplasia.) *Adult female.* Usually 30 to 40 years or later; also after menopause). Hirsutism (first sign) beard and mustache and head hair loss: acne; voice change; oligomenorrhea progressing to amenorrhea; clitoral hypertrophy; muscular hypertrophy; loss of fat deposit; breast atrophy; increased libido. *Adult male.* Chance discovery.

Etiology. Carcinomas and adenomas.

Pathology. *Carcinomas.* Usually round, large, localized in one pole of adrenal. Tumor often commixed with some normal tissue; left side more frequent; well vascularized on surface; cellular polymorphism and atypia. *Adenoma.* Normal cells; no mitosis; intact capsule. Difficult differential diagnosis between malignant and benign tumor; frequent metastasis from apparently benign tumor.

Diagnostic Procedures. *X-ray.* May show tumor; retrorectal gas insufflation. *Urine.* Increase of 17-ketosteroids (with DHEA more than 50% of 17-ketosteroids). *ACTH stimulation.* Negative. *Cortisone suppression.* Negative.

Therapy. Surgical removal.

Prognosis. Rapid regression of symptoms after surgery. Virilizing tumor grows slowly. Prognosis, however, depends on degree of malignancy, time of surgery, and presence of metastasis. In malignant type, 3 years survival 30%. In adenoma, much better.

BIBLIOGRAPHY. Baulieu EE, Peillon F, Migeon CJ: Adrenogenital syndrome. In Eisenstein AB (ed): The Adrenal Cortex. Boston, Little, Brown, 1967
Gabrilove TJ, Seman AT, Sabet R, et al: Virilizing adrenal adenoma with studies on the steroid content of the adrenal venous effluent and a review of the literature. Endocrine Rev 2:462–483, 1981

ADRENOGENITAL SYNDROMES WITH HIRSUTISM, NONTUMOR FORM

Affect mostly females. Rare cases reported in men.

FEMALE

Synonyms. 21-hydroxylase deficiency mild form; 21-hydroxylase deficiency nonclassical form; cryptic adrenal hyperplasia; simple virilizing adrenal hyperplasia.

Symptoms. Usually patients have normal puberty, menstruation may be normal or abnormal, and some patients become pregnant with normal offspring. Growth accelerated during childhood; premature closure of epiphyses leads to shortened adult stature.

Signs. Important to know date of onset of signs. Hirsutism of various degree alone or combined with various degrees of masculine habitus and acne.

Etiology. Unknown. Suggested for some cases: partial deficiency of 21-hydroxylase or defect of 11-B-hydroxylase or both. Both forms with and without demonstrated hormonal abnormalities are familial.

Pathology. In many cases mild form of congenital adrenal hyperplasia. In some cases polycystic ovaries have been found.

Diagnostic Procedures. *Urine.* Increased excretion of pregnanetriol (in 2–3% of total cases); moderate increase of 17-ketosteroids. *Adrenocorticotropic hormone* (ACTH). *Stimulation.* Increase of excretion of pregnanetriol and corticosteroids. *Cortisone suppression.* Decrease of pregnanetriol.

A subgroup may be recognized on the basis of the biochemical findings of increased urinary excretion of dehydroepiandrosterone (DHEA), and other androgenic steroids. An increased DHEA excretion combined with hirsutism and menstrual disorders may also be found in mild form of congenital adrenal hyperplasia, simple obesity, Cushing's, acromegaly, and mental disorders.

Therapy. Cortisone or synthetic glucocorticoid, prolonged treatment.

Prognosis. With prolonged treatment, decrease of virilization signs. Minor response of hirsutism in some cases; always improvement of menstrual cycles and often correction of sterility.

BIBLIOGRAPHY. Jayle MF, Malassis D, Pinaud H: Excretion de la dehydroepiandrosterone avant et après administration d'ACTH en pathologie surrenalienne. Acta Endocrinol (Copenh) 31:1–32, 1959

Decurt J, Jayle MF, Mauvais-Jarvis P: Virilisme surrenalien para ou post-pubertaire avec pregnanetriolurie. Rev Eur Endocrinol 1:17, 1964

Kutten F, Coulin P, Girard F, et al: Late onset adrenal hyperplasia in hirsutism. New Engl J Med 313:224–231, 1985

MALE

Symptoms. Asthenia; sterility.

Signs. Associated with increased hirsutism, gynecomastia.

Etiology. Moderate adrenal hyperplasia. May be partial defect of 21-hydroxylase (?).

Pathology. Adrenal hyperplasia; arrested spermatogenesis.

Diagnostic Procedures. *Sperm count.* Low. *Urine.* Increased 17-ketosteroid (DHEA++) and in some cases, estrogens. *Biopsy of testis.*

Therapy. Cortisone.

Prognosis. Spermatogenesis is resumed following cortisone administration.

BIBLIOGRAPHY. Perloff WW, Hadd HE: The adrenogenital syndrome "Virilizing Type" in an adult male: a case report. Am J Med Sci 234:441–443, 1957

Bigozzi U, Borghi A, Giusti C, et al: An unusual case of adrenal dysfunction in male. J Clin Endocrinol 19:1506–1510, 1959

New MI, Dupont B, Grumbach K, et al: Congenital adrenal hyperplasia and related conditions. In Stanbury JB, Wyngaarden JB, Fredrickson DS, et al: The Metabolic Basis of Inherited Disease, 5th ed, p 973. New York, McGraw-Hill, 1983

ADRENOLEUKODYSTROPHY, AUTOSOMAL NEONATAL

Synonyms. Neonatal adrenoleukodystrophy, NALD. (See Addison-Schilder and Zellweger's syndromes.)

Symptoms. Both sexes. From birth. Seizures; delayed neurological development; respiratory infections.

Signs. Dolicocephaly, prominent forehead, esotropia, epicanthic folds, broad nose, high arched palate, low-set ears, anteverted nostrils. Tanning of skin during first months of life.

Etiology. Recessive inheritance.

Pathology. Adrenal atrophy; degenerative changes of CNS white matter.

Diagnostic Procedures. *Blood.* Hyperpipecolicacidemia. See Addison's.

Therapy. Antibiotics. See Addison's.

Prognosis. Neurological deterioration begins at 1 year of age. Death in infancy.

BIBLIOGRAPHY. Benke PJ, Reye PF, Parker JC Jr: New form of a adrenoleukodystrophy. Hum Genet 58:204–208, 1981

ADVERSIVE

Synonym. Compulsory turning.

Symptoms and Signs. Homolateral miosis and turning of head in opposite direction; compulsive turning when patient attempts to progress forward; nystagmus.

Etiology. Following neurosurgery, after ablation of Brodmann area of one frontal lobe; stimulation of red nucleus: nitrogen mustard treatment; neoplastic, inflammatory, or vascular frontal lobe lesions.

Pathology. Ablation of Brodmann's area; posterior longitudinal fascicle destruction.

Therapy. Phenylhydantoin.

Prognosis. No recovery.

BIBLIOGRAPHY. Vick NA (ed): Grinker's Neurology, 7th ed. Springfield, Ill, CC Thomas, 1976

AFZELIUS' (A.)

Synonyms. Erythema chronicum migrans; Lipschutz's.

Symptoms and Signs. Both sexes affected; onset all ages. Eruption of single or multiple lesions of erythema annulare centrifugum, expanding to reach massive extension. Meningitic symptoms and signs in a number of cases.

Etiology. Tick (*Ixodes*) bite (?). Rickettsial or spirochetal infection (?).

Therapy. Penicillin.

Prognosis. Prompt response to treatment.

BIBLIOGRAPHY. Afzelius A: Erythema chronicum migrans. Acta Derm Venereol (Stockh) 2:120–125, 1921
Hellerström S: Erythema chronicum migrans Afzelli. Acta Derm Venereol (Stockh) 11:315–321, 1930
Rook A, Wilkinson DS, Ebling FJG, et al: Textbook of Dermatology, 4th ed, p 1090. Oxford, Blackwell Scientific Publications, 1986

AGAMMAGLOBULINEMIA

Synonym. Antibody deficiency.

CONGENITAL

See individual syndromes.

Symptoms and Signs. Normal at birth; onset at about ninth month of life. Increased susceptibility to infections due to pyogenic bacteria, controlled by antimicrobial chemotherapy. Manifestation of atopy. Failure to thrive as consequence of repeated infections, If surviving, chronic bronchiectasis, a condition similar to rheumatoid arthritis (may precede infection manifestation), and other collagenlike conditions may develop.

Etiology. See Immunologic deficiency syndromes.

ACQUIRED

Symptoms. Both sexes affected; onset in adulthood. Susceptibility to recurrent sinusitis, pneumonia, chronic progressive bronchiectasis. Spruelike syndrome. Protein-losing enteropathy. Arthritic manifestation (rare in this form). Exfoliative dermatitis; nephrotic syndrome (occasionally).

Signs. Hepatosplenomegaly (frequent); evidence of non-caseating granulomas in lungs, skin, liver, spleen (without particular microorganism involved).

Etiology. Associated, through unknown, mechanism, with lymphatic system malignancies, or other dysglobulinemic conditions (e.g., myoclonia). Possibility of a congenital type suggested by occurrence in relatives. See Immunologic deficiency syndromes (secondary).

BIBLIOGRAPHY. Rosen FS: Genetic defects in gammaglobulin synthesis. In Stanbury JB, Wyngaarden JB, Fredrickson DS, et al: The Metabolic Basis of Inherited Disease, 5th ed, p 1921. New York, McGraw-Hill, 1983

AGAMMAGLOBULINEMIA, X-LINKED, DERMATOMIOSITISLIKE

Synonyms. Bruton's–dermatomiositis-like. (See Bruton's.)

Symptoms and Signs. Appear in males; present from early age. Weakness; rash over extensor areas of joints; edema; induration of muscle; infections.

Etiology. See Bruton's. (This represents a variant.)

Pathology. See Bruton's. Also lymphorrhages (normal lymphocytes) around small blood vessels of skin and in the muscles and occasionally in the central nervous system.

Diagnostic Procedures. *Blood.* See Bruton's. *Biopsy of skin and muscle.* See Pathology.

Therapy. None. Steroids, antimetabolites, and gammaglobulins useless.

Prognosis. Fatal.

BIBLIOGRAPHY. Gitlin D, Janeway CA, Apt L, et al: Agammaglobulinemia in Cellular and Humoral Aspects of Hypersensitivity States: Symposium. New York, Hoeber-Harper, 1959
Pace AR, Hansen AE, Good RA: Occurrence of leukemia and lymphoma in patients with agammaglobulinemia. Blood 21:197–206, 1963
Rosen FS: Genetic defects in gammaglobulin synthesis. In Stanbury JB, Wyngaarden JB, Fredrickson DS, et al: The Metabolic Basis of Inherited Disease, 5th ed, p 1921. New York, McGraw-Hill, 1983

AGLOSSIA-ADACTYLIA

Synonyms. De Jussieu's; hypoglossia-hypodactyly; Meyer's; Hanhart's II.

Symptoms and Signs. Total or partial absence of tongue; underdeveloped mandible; enlargement of sublingual muscular ridges; hypertrophy of sublingual and submaxillary glands; cleft and high arched palate; lower lip defects; missing lower incisors; bony fusion of dental arches; intraoral bands. Hypoplasia of extremities: from complete peromelia to absence of distal digits; syndactylia; anonychia. Dextrocardia; transposed viscera.

Etiology. Unknown. Intrauterine environmental factors; expression of lack of genes responsible for growth of distal structures (?).

Pathology. See Symptoms and signs.

Diagnostic Procedures. *Chromosome studies.* Normal.

Therapy. Depending on manifestation, surgical or orthopedic corrections or both.

Prognosis. If intelligence not impaired and tongue not totally absent, speech not severely affected.

BIBLIOGRAPHY. De Jussieu M: Observation sur la manière dont une fille sans langue s'acquitte des fonctions qui dépendent de cet organe. Hist Acad Roy Sc Paris Mem, 6–14; 1718–1719
Meyer MW: Ueber die angeborenen Fehlen der Zunge und die dadurch bedingte Hinderung des Saugens. Jahrb Kinderhulkd 13:328–354, 1849
Hanhart E: Ueber die kombination von Peromelie mit Mickrognathie, ein neues Syndrom beim Menschen, entsprechend der Akroteriasis congenita von Wriedt und Mohr beim Rind. Arch Hlaus Stift Vererbungsforsch 25:531–543, 1950
Hall BD: Aglossia-Adactylia: A case report, review of the literature, and classification of closely related entities. Birth Defects 7:233–236, 1971
Tuncbilek E, Yalcin C, Atasu M: Aglossia adactilia syndrome (special emphasis on the inherited pattern). Clin Genet 11:421–423, 1977

AGRANULOCYTOSIS, CONGENITAL

Synonym. Congenital neutropenia.

Symptoms and Signs. The same as in infantile genetic agranulocytosis syndrome except for lack of evidence of familial occurrence.

Etiology. Unknown. Sporadic.

Diagnostic Procedures. *Blood.* Marked neutropenia, eosinophilia, and monocytosis. *Bone marrow.* Increased eosinophils that may or may not appear in the peripheral blood. Decreased numbers of mature neutrophilic precursors.

Therapy. No effective therapy. Hematinics, corticosteroids, and splenectomy produce no beneficial effect. Antibiotics may be of temporary value.

Prognosis. Death frequently occurs during infancy or the first year of life as a result of overwhelming sepsis.

BIBLIOGRAPHY. Krill CE, Mauer AM: Congenital agranulocytosis. J Pediatr 68:361–366, 1966
L'Esperance PL, Brunning R, Deinard AS, et al: Congenital neutropenia: Impaired maturation with diminished stem cell input. In Bergsma D (ed): Immunodeficiency in Man and Animals, pp 59–65. New York, National Foundation March of Dimes, 1975

AICARDI'S

Synonyms. Chorioretinal anomalies–corpus callosum agenesis–infantile spasms; corpus callosum (agenesis)-chorioretinal abnormality.

Symptoms. Appear in females only (males, intrauterine death). Infantile spasms, which may become manifest between 1 day and 4 months of age; epileptic attacks; mental abnormalities; hypotonia; delayed postural acquisition.

Signs. Microcephaly and head deformities: biparietal bossing; occipital flattening; plagiocephaly; facial asymmetry; low-set ears; microphthalmia. Cyanosis. Telangiectasia. Vertebral anomalies: hemivertebrae; fusion; spina bifida. Rib anomalies. Absence of pupillary reflexes. Specific diagnostic chorioretinopathy: multiple lacunae with the aspect of atrophic white-yellowish, round holes crossed over by vessels. Funnel-shaped disk.

Etiology. Possibly, single dominant gene of X-chromosome is determinant. Unknown. The current theories include congenital infection, an X-linked genetic defect, and an intrauterine environmental agent.

Pathology. See Signs. Agenesis of corpus callosum.

Diagnostic Procedures. *X-ray.* See Signs. *Pneumoencephalography.* Typical image of total agenesis of corpus callosum (in most cases) or, less evident, alteration of ventricle outlines. *CT brain scan. Electroencephalography.* Hypsarrhythmia; independent bioelectrical activity of the hemispheres. *Spinal fluid.* Normal. *Blood and urine.* Normal. *Dermatoglyphics.* High number of digital arches. *Chromosome studies.* Normal. *Ophthalmologic findings.* Microphtalmia, nystagmus, optic nerve colobomas, and pathognomonic chorioretinal lesions.

Therapy. Hydrocortisone; adrenocorticotropic hormone (ACTH); antiepileptic compounds.

Prognosis. Manifestations progress with age. Temporary improvement with treatment. High mortality for different causes. If onset of symptoms in adolescence period, greater life expectancy.

BIBLIOGRAPHY. Aicardi J, Chevrie JJ, Rousselie F: Le syndrome spasmes en flexion, agénesie calleuse, anomalies chorio-rétiniennes. Arch Fr Pediatr 26:1103–1120, 1969

Yamamoto N, Watanabe K, Negoro T, et al: Aicardi syndrome: Report of 6 cases and review of Japanese literature. Brain Devel 7:443–449, 1985

AIDS

Synonyms. Acquired immunodeficiency syndrome.

Symptoms and Signs. The full-blown syndrome can be preceded by a constellation of signs and symptoms: termed "the AIDS-related complex" or "ARC": fever, weight loss, diarrhea, fatigue, night sweats, lymphadenopathy. Patients can die from the ARC, or develop full-blown AIDS, that is: pneumocystic carinii pneumonia; cytomegalovirus infections; persistent diarrhea; acute or chronic meningitis; progressive dementia; hypercatabolic wasting syndrome; Kaposi's sarcoma, and other malignancies.

Etiology. Infection with the human retrovirus HTLV III/LAV.

Diagnostic Procedures and Pathology. Immunologic profile: lymphopenia with a selective deficiency of the T4 subset of lymphocytes; presence of antibodies to the retrovirus; isolation of the virus from peripheral blood lymphocytes or other body materials.

Therapy. Radiation therapy for the transient palliation of Kaposi's sarcoma; chemotherapy against the malignant diseases; antimicrobial agents for the various infections. Specific drugs against the virus have been tried, with variable success: DHPG; suramin; HPA-23; ribavirin; 3'-zido-3'-deoxythymidine. Immune reconstitution: bone marrow transplantation; infusion of histocompatible lymphocytes; IL-2; interferons.

Prognosis. Poor. Mortality is very likely to approach 100%.

BIBLIOGRAPHY. Fauci AS, Masur H, Gellmann EP, et al: The acquired immunodeficiency syndrome: an update. Ann Intern Med 102:800–813, 1985

Crumpacker C, Heagy W, Bubley G, et al: Ribavirin treatment of the acquired immunodeficiency syndrome (AIDS) and the acquired-immunodeficiency-syndrome-related complex (ARC). Ann Intern Med 107:664–674, 1987

Rosner F: Acquired immunodeficiency syndrome: ethical and psychosocial considerations. Bull Acad Med 63:123–133, 1987

Fauci A: AIDS: immunopathogenic mechanism and research strategies. Clin Res 35:503–510, 1987

Edelman AS, Zolla-Pazner S: AIDS: A syndrome of immune dysregulation, dysfunction and deficiency. Faseb J 3:22–30, 1989

AIDS EMBRYOPATHY

Symptoms and Signs. Growth failure; microcephaly; hypertelorism, marked prominence and boxlike appearance of the forehead; a flat nasal bridge that, because of the prominent forehead, appears "scooped out" in profile; mild upward or downward obliquity of the eyes; long palpebral fissures with blue sclerae; a short nose with flattening of the columella; a well-formed, triangular philtrum; markedly patulous lips.

Etiology. Dysmorphic syndrome associated with intrauterine HTLV III infection.

Diagnostic Procedures. *Blood.* Antibodies to HTVL-III measured by ELISA or western blot techniques; after the first 6 months of life immunologic aberrations: reverse T4 to T8 ratios, depressed lymphocyte mitogenic responses, hypergammaglobulinemia.

Therapy. None.

Prognosis. Unknown (recently described). Probably poor.

BIBLIOGRAPHY. Marion RW, Wiznia AA, Hutcheon G, Rubinstein A: Human T-cell lymphotropic virus type III (HTLV III) embryopathy. Am J Dis Child 140:638–640, 1986

Barbour SD: Acquired immunodeficiency syndrome of childhood. Pediatr Clin North Amer 34:247–268, 1987

AINHUM

Synonym. Dactylolysis spontanea.

Symptoms and Signs. Found mostly in black races in Africa, America, and the Panama Canal Zone. Cases in whites have been reported. Onset between 30 and 40 years of age. Some fingers and toes (usually only fingers or toes) completely encircled by tight constricting bands 0.5 to 1.0 cm wide. Frequently, there is associated hyperkeratosis of palms and soles, and thickening of skin with wart-like formation over joints (usually knee). Absence of systemic manifestations.

Etiology. Unknown in true ainhum. In pseudoainhum, associated with various neurologic and ectodermal dysplasias (see Vohwinkel's syndrome). Dominant inheritance also reported.

Pathology. Connective tissue constricting bands. Epidermal hypertrophy; wall of large arteries supplying involved fingers, thickened; bone resorption and skin ulceration of involved digits.

Diagnostic Procedures. *X-ray.* Absorption of the bones.

Therapy. Protection from trauma. Transverse incision of constricting bands.

Prognosis. Unsatisfactory results from surgery.

BIBLIOGRAPHY. Da Silva JF: On Ainhum. Arch Derm Syph 6:367–376, 1880
Horwitz MT, Tunick I: Ainhum: report of six cases in New York. Arch Derm Syph 36:1058–1063, 1937
Rook A, Wilkinson DS, Ebling FJG, et al: Textbook of Dermatology, 4th ed, p 1830. Oxford, Blackwell Scientific Publications, 1986

AKINETIC

Synonym. Hypokinetic.

Symptoms. Muscular rigidity associated with slight slowing of voluntary movement. Speech is slow and monotonous. Tremor may be present, mostly in upper extremity and usually hands and forearms; little movement. Disorder of station and gait. Face expression fixed, with infrequent blinking.

Signs. Cogwheel phenomenon; tendon reflexes normal; Babinski negative.

Etiology. Part of the paralysis agitans (Parkinson's) syndrome.

Pathology. Multiple lesions, now well defined, affecting the globus pallidus, substantia nigra and other parts of extrapyramidal system.

Diagnostic Procedures. *Neurologic examination.*

Therapy. Belladonna and derivatives; synthetic substance such as trihexyphenidyl hydrochloride (Artane); cyrimine hydrochloride (Pagitane); procyclidine hydrochloride (Kemadrine), levamphetamine, levodopa; amantadine hydrochloride, imipramine; amieziptyline. Neurosurgical procedures available.

Prognosis. Progressive condition, partially relieved by medical and surgical procedures.

BIBLIOGRAPHY. Grinker RR, Sahs AL: Neurology, 6th ed. Springfield, Ill, CC Thomas, 1966
Adams RD, Victor M: Principles of Neurology, 3rd ed, p 59. New York. McGraw-Hill, 1985

AKINETIC MUTISM

Synonyms. Cairn's syndrome.

Symptoms. Silent, brief immobility that characterizes certain subacute or chronic states of altered consciousness in which sleep-wake cycles have returned, but external evidence for mental activity remains almost entirely absent and spontaneous motor activity is lacking.

Etiology. Large bilateral frontal lobe lesions; bilateral diffuse destruction of the cerebral cortical mouth; bilateral hemispheric demyelinizations, hydrocephalus; large bilateral lesions of ganglia; paramedial lesions of the reticular formation of the midbrain.

Diagnostic Procedures. *CT brain scan. Electroencephalography. Sensory evoked potentials. Electroencephalographic brain mapping.*

Therapy. As in persistent vegetative state.

Prognosis. Poor.

BIBLIOGRAPHY. Cairns H: Disturbances of consciousness with lesions of the brainstem and diencephalon: 75–109, 1952
Plum F, Posner JB: Diagnosis of Stupor and Coma, 3rd ed, p 9. Philadelphia, FA Davis, 1982

ALACRIMA, CONGENITAL

Synonyms. Dry eye.

Symptoms and Signs. Deficient lacrimal secretion.

Etiology. Congenital form present in children; rare; unilateral form very rare. Reported cases may be classified into five categories: Persistence of normal lack of tears in newborn; neurogenic hyposecretion; absence or hypoplasia of lacrimal gland; associated Riley-Day syndrome; associated anhydrotic ectodermal dysplasia or in association with other nervous system anomalies, such as aplasia of cranial nerve nuclei.

Pathology. According to the above categories. Aplasia of gland, injury or aplasia of trigeminal (V), facial (VII) nerve, or respective nuclei, greater superficial petrosal nerve, sphenopalatine ganglion, geniculate ganglion.

Diagnostic Procedures. See associated syndromes.

Therapy. Protective ointment. In some cases occlusion of the lacrimal puncta is helpful. In severe cases tarsorraphy may be necessary to protect the cornea.

Prognosis. See associated syndromes.

BIBLIOGRAPHY. Thurnam J: Two cases in which the skin, hair, and teeth were very imperfectly developed. Med Chir Trans 31:71–82, 1848
Smith RS, Maddox SF, Collins BE: Congenital alacrima. Arch Ophthalmol 79:45–48, 1968

Mondino BJ, Brawn SI: Hereditary congenital alacrima. Arch Ophthalmol 94:1478–1480, 1976

ALACTASIA

Synonyms. Lactase deficiency in infancy; lactase isolated intolerance.

Symptoms and Signs. Both sexes affected; variable age of onset. Usually intolerance to milk, and other symptoms that appear in adolescence or young adult life, although the symptomatology may begin at 3 to 4 years of age. Quite rare in infants and young children (inherited or of transitory type). *In infants,* diarrhea, failure to thrive, dehydration. *At later age,* ill-defined complaint of milk intolerance.

Etiology. Variable: hereditary form autosomal recessive with onset of manifestation at various age; temporary deficiency related to various pathologic conditions; deficiency secondary to reduced mucosal contact time after surgery of gastrointestinal tract.

Pathology. No constant features. Possibly, blunting of duodenal and jejunal villi.

Diagnostic Procedures. *Intestinal biopsy.* Histologic and enzyme assays. *Oral lactose tolerance test.* Development of the syndrome. *C-lactose breath test. Hydrogen breath test. Urine.* Lactosuria.

Therapy. Elimination of lactose from diet.

Prognosis. Except in rare cases in infancy, usually a tolerable condition, which does not produce any severe complication.

BIBLIOGRAPHY. Durand P: Lattosuria idiopatica in una paziente con diarrea cronica ed acidosi. Minerva Pediatr 10:706–711, 1958
Milue MD: Hereditary abnormalities of intestinal adsorption. Br Med Bull 23:279–284, 1968
Gray GM: Intestinal disaccharidase deficiencies and glucose-galactose malabsorption. In Stanbury JB, Wyngaarden JB, Fredrickson DS: The Metabolic Basis of Inherited Disease, 5th ed, p 1729. New York, McGraw-Hill, 1983

ALAGILLE'S

Synonyms. Arteriohepatic dysplasia, AHD; cholestasis-peripheral pulmonary stenosis.

Symptoms. Both sexes affected. Neonatal jaundice; retarded physical, mental, and sexual development.

Signs. Broad forehead, pointed mandibula, bulbous nose, posterior embryotoxon, retinal pigmentary changes. Heart murmurs and other signs of pulmonar valve stenosis and peripheral arterial stenosis. Absence of deep tendon reflexes. Finger foreshortening.

Etiology. Autosomal dominant inheritance.

Pathology. Liver cholestasis and inflammation; Pulmonary valve and peripheral pulmonary arterial stenosis. *X-ray.* Abnormal vertebrae (butterfly). *Electroencephalogram. Echography. Blood.* Hyperbilirubinemia, serum glutamate pyruvate transaminase (SGPT) chronic elevation.

Therapy. Cardiosurgery may be considered according to conditions. Medical treatment of cholestasis.

Prognosis. Patients reach adult age.

BIBLIOGRAPHY. Alagille D, Odievre M, Gautier M, et al: Hepatic ductular hypoplasia associated with characteristic facies, vertebral malformations, retarded physical, mental and sexual development and cardiac murmur. J Pediatr 86:63–71, 1975
Shulman SA, Hyams JS, Gunta R, et al: Arteriohepatic dysplasia (Alagille syndrome). Am J Med Genet 19:325–332, 1984

ALAJOUANINE'S

Symptoms and Signs. Both sexes affected. In newborn, bilateral facial (VII) and external oculomotor (VI) paralysis; convergent strabismus. Talipes equinovarus.

Etiology. Unknown.

BIBLIOGRAPHY. Alajouanine T, Huc G, Gopcevitch M, et al: Quatre cas d'une affection congénitale caractérisée par une double pied bot, une double paralysie faciale et une double paralysie de la sixième paire. Rev Neurol (Paris) 2:501–511, 1930

ALBATROSS

See also Postgastrectomy.

Synonyms. Postgastrectomy–personality defect.

Symptoms. In patients with (1) history of antisocial behavior, (2) addiction to salicylates or other analgesics, (3) psychiatric illness or personality derangements, who have had any type of surgical treatment for peptic ulcer disease. Abdominal pain without demonstrable cause; intermittent nausea; vomiting; continuing dependency on analgesic drugs; severe nutritional deficiency.

Signs. Lack of correlation between objective signs and symptomatology. Weight loss and other signs of malnutrition.

Etiology. Psychologic derangement focusing its expression in an actual (iatrogenic) anatomic and physiologic defect. Syndrome named after the poem of Coleridge in which the sailor shot the albatross. When calamity followed, his shipmates hung the dead bird around his neck.

Pathology. Some patients had true ulcer; generally no ulcer found at surgery.

Diagnostic Procedures. *X-rays of gastrointestinal tract.*

Therapy. Prophylaxis very important; careful screening of patients with this type of psychologic derangement before surgery. Psychotherapy; correction of malnutrition.

Prognosis. Poor; recurrence of symptoms with request for continuous medical care.

BIBLIOGRAPHY. Johnstone FR, Holubitsky IB, Debas HT: Post-gastrectomy problems in patients with personality defects: the "albatross" syndrome. Can Med Assoc J 96:1559–1564, 1967

ALBERS-SCHÖNBERG'S I

Synonyms. Ivory bones; Henck-Assman; marble bones; generalized congenital osteosclerosis; osteosclerosis fragilis generalisata; osteopetrosis generalisata.

BENIGN DOMINANT FORM
Synonym. Henck-Assman.

Symptoms. Asymptomatic (50%); fractures (40%); osteomyelitis of mandible (10%); cranial nerve palsy (16%): optic (II), oculomotor (III), facial (VII) nerves optic atrophy. Bone pains most frequently in lumbar areas.

Signs. Nonspecific; frontal bossing (18%); exophthalmos (6%); no hepatosplenomegaly.

Etiology. Unknown; dominant inheritance with variable expression. Suggested abnormality of thyrocalcitonin.

Pathology. Absence or reduction of medullary cavity areas of hematopoiesis in enlarged haversian canals. Noncalcified hyaline cartilage remnants diffuse in the bones. Few fibrils in bone matrix and seldom cross between osteons. Remodeling of bone prominent.

Diagnostic Procedures. *Blood.* Normal, except for increase of acid phosphatase. *X-rays.* Required for diagnosis. Bones symmetrically involved by diffuse sclerotic process is early sign; increased density of diaphyseal region of growing bones.

Therapy. None.

Prognosis. Good; normal longevity may be expected with this form. Cranial nerve palsy may be incapacitating, but does not affect longevity.

MALIGNANT RECESSIVE FORM
Symptoms and Signs. Manifestation in childhood. Optic atrophy (78%); poor growth (36%); repeated fractures (28%); deafness (22%); mental retardation (22%); osteomyelitis (18%); facial palsy (10%). Splenomegaly (62%); hepatomegaly (48%); frontal bossing (34%); large head (22%); lymphoadenopathy (18%); genu valgum (16%); pectus deformities (8%).

Etiology. Unknown; recessive inheritance.

Pathology. See Benign form. Myeloid metaplasia in spleen and liver.

Diagnostic Procedures. *Blood.* Anemia; thrombocytopenia. Nucleated red cells and immature myeloid elements. Increased acid phosphatases.

Therapy. None.

Prognosis. Poor; no patient lived past 20 years of age. Usually death in infancy because of anemia or infections.

BIBLIOGRAPHY. Albers-Schönberg H: Roentgenbilder einer seltenen Knochenerkrankung. München Med Wochenschr 51:365, 1904
Key L, Carnes D, Cole S, et al: Treatment of congenital osteopetrosis with high-dose calcitriol. New Engl J Med 310:409–415, 1984

ALBERT'S

Synonyms. Achillodynia; Achilles tendon bursitis; hindfoot bursitis; calcaneal bursitis; Achilles tendinitis; Achillobursitis; Schanz's I.

Symptoms. Pain and difficulty in walking.

Signs. Swelling of different consistencies (from tense to bony) over posterior part of foot; frequently, hyperkeratosis of overlying skin; associated occasionally with infections.

Etiology. Chronic irritation from shoes; overprominent border of calcaneus; trauma.

Pathology. Bursitis in region of attachment of Achilles tendon. In some cases calcification in the bursae.

Diagnostic Procedures. *X-ray.*

Therapy. Reduction of pressure on inflamed area. Topical cortisone injection. Surgery seldom efficient.

Prognosis. Tendency to relapse.

BIBLIOGRAPHY. Albert E: Achillodynie. Wien Med Presse 34:41–43, 1893

Schanz A: Eine typische Erkrankung der Achilles. Schne Zbl Chir 32:1289–1291, 1905

Justis EJ: Nontraumatic disorders. In Crenshaw AH (ed): Campbell's Operative Orthopedics, 7th ed, pp 2252–2253. St. Louis, CV Mosby, 1987

ALBINISM-MICROCEPHALY-DIGITAL ANOMALIES

Synonyms. Microcephaly-albinism-digital anomalies.

Symptoms and Signs. Both sexes. Microcephaly, oculocutaneous albinism, hypoplasia of fingers and agenesis of the phallanx of toe.

Etiology. Autosomal recessive.

Therapy. Symptomatic. See Albinism, minimal pigment type.

Prognosis. Poor.

BIBLIOGRAPHY. Castro-Gago M, Pombo M, Novo I, et al: Syndrome familiar de microcefalia con albinism oculocutaneo y anomalias digitales. Ann Esp Pediatr 19:128–131, 1983

ALBINISM, MINIMAL PIGMENT TYPE

Synonyms. Type III albinism.

Symptoms and Signs. From birth. No pigment in skin and eyes, with hair, blue irides. Minimal amount of pigment develops in first decade.

Etiology. Autosomal recessive.

Therapy. Protection with a broad-spectrum sun screen preparation during exposure to sunlight.

Prognosis. Depends on the occurrence of skin cancer.

BIBLIOGRAPHY. King RA, Wirtsehafter JD, Olds Dl, et al: Minimal pigment: a new type of oculocutaneous albinism. Clin Genet 29:42–50, 1986

ALBINISM, OCULAR–LATE ONSET SENSINEURAL DEAFNESS

Synonyms. Ocular albinism–sensineural deafness, OASD; deafness–ocular albinism.

Symptoms and Signs. In male (Afrikaner). From birth. Typical ocular albinism. In middle age, develop moderate deafness.

Etiology. X-linked recessive inheritance. Differs from Margolis-Ziprkowski.

Pathology. Typicality of this albinism presence of numerous macromelanosomes on skin biopsy.

BIBLIOGRAPHY. Winship I, Gericke G, Beighton P: X linked inheritance of ocular albinism with late-onset sensorineural deafness. Am J Med Genet 19:797–803, 1984

ALBINISM, PARTIAL IMMUNODEFICIENCY

Synonyms. Griscelli's. See Chediack-Higashi.

Symptoms and Signs. From birth. Hair and eyelashes silver. Repeated infections. Hepatosplenomegaly.

Etiology. Autosomal recessive inheritance.

Diagnostic Procedures. *Blood.* Pancytopenia with recurrent episodes of hypofibrinemia.

Prognosis. Fair.

BIBLIOGRAPHY. Griscelli C, Durandy A, Guy-Grand D, et al: A syndrome associating partial albinism and immunodeficiency. Am J Med 65:691–702, 1978

ALBINISM, OCULAR, AUTOSOMAL RECESSIVE

Synonyms. Autosomal recessive ocular albinism, AROA.

Symptoms and Signs. Both sexes equally affected; onset from birth. Skin and hair color normal, with presence of pigmented nevi or freckles (or both) and without increased tendency to skin neoplasia. Eye color presents normal range. Nystagmus and photophobia are present in variable intensities; visual acuity shows moderate to severe decrease.

Etiology. Autosomal recessive inheritance.

Pathology. Melanosomes are normal.

Diagnostic Procedures. *Ophthalmoscopy.* Transillumination of iris shows cartwheel to diaphanus pattern; in males red reflex present; in both sexes the fundal pigment absent or reduced. *Blood.* Serum tyrosine and the beta melanocyte-stimulating hormone level are unknown. *Incubation of hair bulb.* In tyrosine: pigmentation.

Therapy. None.

Prognosis. Good.

BIBLIOGRAPHY. Witkop CR, Quevedo WC, Fitzpatrick TB: Albinism and other disorders of pigment metabolism. In Stanbury JB, Wyngaarden JB, Fredrickson DS: The Metabolic Basis of Inherited Disease, 5th ed, p 301. New York, McGraw-Hill, 1983

ALBINISM, TY-NEG

Synonyms. ATN; albinism I; Garrod's albinism; Oculocutaneous–Ty-neg albinism; OCA Ty-neg; tyrosine negative albinism; complete perfect albinism.

Symptoms and Signs. Both sexes affected; present from birth. Skin color pink to red; hair color white (for all of life); absence of pigmented nevi and freckles; high incidence of skin neoplasia. Eye color gray to blue; visual acuity progressively worsening (practically and legally blind). Marked nystagmus and photophobia.

Etiology. Autosomal recessive inheritance. Mutation of the tyrosinase locus.

Pathology. Melanosomes in hair bulb show only stage I and II.

Diagnostic Procedures. *Ophthalmoscopy.* Transillumination of iris shows no visible pigment; the red reflex is present; the fundal pigment absent. *Blood.* Serum tyrosinase and the beta melanocyte-stimulating hormone levels are normal. *Incubation of hair bulb.* In tyrosine: no pigment formation.

Therapy. None.

Prognosis. Blindness. High incidence of skin neoplasia.

BIBLIOGRAPHY. Wafer L: A new voyage and description of the isthmus of America, giving an account of the author's above, there: Collection of Voyages, 3rd ed, Vol 3, p 261–463. London, 1729
Garrod AE: Inborn errors of metabolism. (Croonian lectures. Lecture I.) Lancet 2:1–7, 1908
Witkop CJ, Quevedo WC, Fitzpatrick TB: Albinism and other disorders of pigment metabolism. In Stanbury JB, Wyngaarden JB, Fredrickson DS: The Metabolic Basis of Inherited Disease, 5th ed, p 301. New York, McGraw-Hill, 1983

ALBINISM, TY-POS

Synonyms. Albinism II; albinoidism; OCA Ty-pos; Oculocutaneous–Ty-pos albinism. Complete unperfect albinism.

Symptoms and Signs. Both sexes affected; present from birth. Skin from pink-white to cream color; pigmented nevi may be present; hair color white yellow reddish darkening with age. Eye color blue, yellow, or brown. Visual acuity defect severe in childhood; vision improving with age; nystagmus and photophobia not as severe as in albinism, Ty-neg (see).

Etiology. Autosomal recessive inheritance.

Pathology. Melanosomes in hair bulb to early stage III; polyphagosomes.

Diagnostic Procedures. *Ophthalmoscopy.* Transillumination of iris shows pigmented cartwheel at pupil and limbus; red reflex may be absent; fundal pigment in adult absent to reduced. *Blood.* Serum tyrosine level normal to reduced; beta melanocyto-stimulating hormone normal. *Incubation of hair bulb.* In tyrosine: pigmentation.

Therapy. None.

Prognosis. High incidence of skin neoplasia. Prognosis for vision better than for albinism I.

BIBLIOGRAPHY. Kugelman TP, Van Scott EJ: Tyrosinase activity in melanocytes of human albinos. J Invest Dermatol 37:73, 1961
Witkop CR Jr, Van Scott EJ, Jacoby GA: Evidence for two forms of autosomal recessive albinism in man. Proc II Int Congr Hum Genet, Institute G. Mendel, Rome 1064–1069, 1961
Witkop CJ, Quevedo WC, Fitzpatrick TB, Albinism and other disorders of pigment metabolism. In Stanbury JB, Wyngaarden JB, Fredrickson DS: The Metabolic Basis of Inherited Disease, 5th ed, p 301. New York, McGraw-Hill, 1983.

ALBINISM, YELLOW MUTANT

Synonyms. Amish albinism; oculocutaneous-albinism yellow mutant; OCA yellow mutant; xanthous albinism.

Symptoms and Signs. Both sexes affected; present from birth. Skin color pink-white to cream; pigmented nevi and freckles may be present and abundant; hair white at birth, by 6 months yellow reddish. Eyes blue in infancy, tendency to darken with age. Nystagmus of variable intensity; photophobia not extremely severe (+ to ++); reduced vision in infancy tends to improve with age.

Etiology. Autosomal recessive inheritance.

Pathology. Melanosomes in hair bulb to stage III; polyphagosomes.

Diagnostic Procedures. *Ophthalmoscopy.* Transillumination of iris shows, in adult, cartwheel effect; red reflex present; fundal pigment from absent to ++. *Blood.*

Serum tyrosinase level normal. *Incubation of hair bulb.* In tyrosine: pigmentation.

Therapy. None.

Prognosis. Fair. Improvement of vision; susceptibility to skin neoplasia unknown.

BIBLIOGRAPHY. Witkop CJ, Quevedo WC, Fitzpatrick TB: Albinism and other disorders of pigment metabolism. In Stanbury JB, Wyngaarden JB, Frederickson DS: The Metabolic Basis of Inherited Disease, 5th ed, p 301. New York, McGraw-Hill, 1983

ALBINOIDISM, DOMINANT

The term *albinoidism* is used to indicate the absence of photophobia and nystagmus.

Symptoms and Signs. Both sexes affected; present from birth. Skin color pink; presence of pigmented nevi or freckles unknown. Eye color blue. Absence of nystagmus and photophobia; vision normal to slightly reduced.

Etiology. Autosomal dominant inheritance.

Diagnostic Procedures. *Blood.* Serum tyrosine level and beta melanocyte-stimulating hormone levels unknown. *Ophthalmoscopy.* Transillumination of iris shows punctate pigmentation; red reflex present; fundus punctate pigmentation.

BIBLIOGRAPHY. Waardenberg PJ: Remarkable Fact in Human Albinism and Leukism. Nederlands, Van Gorkum Assen, 1970
Witkop CJ, Quevedo WC, Fitzpatrick JB: Albinism and disorders of pigment metabolism. In Stanbury JB, Wyngaarden JB, Frederickson DS: The Metabolic Basis of Inherited Disease, 5th ed, p 301. New York, McGraw-Hill, 1983

ALBRIGHT-HADORN

Eponym obsolete; used to indicate the occurrence of the hypokalemic periodic paralysis (see) in patients with renal tubular acidosis (see).

BIBLIOGRAPHY. Albright F: Osteomalacia and late rickets, the various etiologies met in the U.S. with emphasis on that resulting from aspecific form of renal acidosis, the therapeutical indications for each etiological subgroup, and the relationship between osteomalacia and Milkman's syndrome. Medicine 25:399–479, 1946
Hadorn W: Osteomalacie mit paroxysmaler hypokaliämisher. Muskellähmung; ein neues Syndrome. Schweiz Med Wochenschr 78:1238–1242, 1948

ALCOHOLIC CARDIOMEGALY-EMPHYSEMA

Symptoms and Signs. Exclusive in chronic alcoholic males. Chronic bronchitis; slow progressive cardiopulmonary insufficiency.

Etiology. Alcohol ingestion; secondary pulmonary infections as complicating factor.

Pathology. Cardiomegaly; chronic bronchitis; lung emphysema.

Diagnostic Procedures. *Blood.* Anemia; pyruvic acid level, liver function test. *Pulmonary function tests. Electrocardiography. X-ray of chest.*

Therapy. Discontinuation of alcohol intake. Thiamine and correction of diet. Antibiotics. Symptomatic for cardiac insufficiency.

Prognosis. Poor; high mortality between 55 to 70 years of age for cardiopulmonary insufficiency.

BIBLIOGRAPHY. Josserand A: Le syndrome gros coeur et emphyseme importante complications viscerale de l'alcoolisme et facteur de surmortalité masculine. Lyon Medical 189:42–44, 1953
Segel LD, Klausner SC, Gnadt JTH, et al: Alcohol and the heart. Med Clin N Am 68:147–161, 1984

ALCOHOLIC KETOACIDOSIS

Synonyms. Dillon's.

Symptoms and Signs. Occur in chronic alcoholics; onset after a binge of several days. Cessation of food intake and continuous alcohol consumption; persistent vomiting that causes patient to stop alcohol intake. After 12–96 hours; severe dehydration, mental obtundation, and specific metabolic changes. (See Diagnostic procedures.)

Etiology. Not clearly established. Consequence of alcohol withdrawal (see).

Diagnostic Procedures. *Blood.* Marked metabolic acidosis; hyperketonemia; moderate (and variable) elevation of plasma lactate; glucose normal or slightly elevated.

Therapy. Fluid and electrolyte balance as in diabetic ketoacidosis, prevention of shock and hypokalemia; acid-base derangement correction. Thiamine 50–100 mg; chlordiazepoxide.

Prognosis. Recurrent condition. Possibility of fatality.

BIBLIOGRAPHY. Dillon ES, Dyer WW, Smells LS: Ketone acidosis of nondiabetic adults. Med Clin North Am 24:1813–1822, 1940
Goldstein DB: Pharmacology of Alcohol. New York, Oxford University Press, 1983

ALCOHOLIC NEUROPATHY

Synonym. Alcoholic pseudotabes; neuropathic beriberi.

Symptoms and Signs. Onset subacute. Burning pain in the legs and feet; muscle tenderness; superficial hyperesthesia; paresthesia in the lower and upper extremities, predominant in the distal parts, progressing to decreased tactile and deep sensibility and paradoxical hyperalgesia, loss of sense of position at passive motion. Weakness of legs; ataxia; muscle weakening and atrophy with fasciculation. Temporary tendon hyperreflexia followed by areflexia. Ulcer and trophic changes of skin.

Etiology. Chronic alcohol intoxication plus nutritional deficiency.

Diagnostic Procedures. *Blood.* Anemia; liver function test. *Gastric.* Achlorhydria. Frequent. *Spinal fluid.* Normal. *Serology.* For syphilis.

Therapy. Withdrawal of alcohol; restoration of adequate diet, high caloric, high carbohydrates, vitamin B complex. Prevention of contraction.

Prognosis. Long period to recover. Because of alcohol addiction, possible relapses.

BIBLIOGRAPHY. Adams RD, Victor M: Principles of Neurology, 3rd ed, pp 768–770. New York, McGraw-Hill, 1985

ALCOHOLIC PARANOIA

See also Othello.

Symptoms and Signs. Usually occurs in males. Delusion of jealousy; suspicion and distrust; brutality to sexual partners. Alcohol-induced impotence; recurrent paniclike state.

Etiology. Impairment of personality development that leads to alcoholism and to paranoid state.

Therapy. Psychotherapy.

Prognosis. Poor. Patient feels better when hospitalized. Return to normal environment produces recurrences.

BIBLIOGRAPHY. Freedman AM, Kaplan HI, Sadock BJ: Comprehensive Textbook of Psychiatry, 2nd ed, p 1342. Baltimore, Williams & Wilkins, 1975

Adams RD, Victor M: Principles of Neurology, 3rd ed, p 821. New York, McGraw-Hill, 1985

ALCOHOLIC, REVERSIBLE ACUTE MUSCULAR

Synonym. Alcoholic muscular cramps.

Symptoms and Signs. Appear in chronic alcoholic patients; spontaneous onset or precipitated by exercise. Muscle aching or cramps; tenderness; weakness; myoglobinuria. Other symptoms and signs of chronic alcoholism. Red conjunctivae, flushing of skin, "whiskey nose"; edema of mucous membranes; characteristic hoarseness; vomiting, diarrhea; coarse tremor.

Etiology. Unknown; possible depression of glycolytic enzymes by ethanol or its metabolites. Secondary defects (e.g., thiamine, magnesium) may also be responsible. Intrinsic muscle defect; alcohol sensitivity (?).

Pathology. Muscles show histologic evidence of necrotic changes.

Diagnostic Procedures. *Blood.* Anemia; hyperkalemia, increased serum glumatic-oxalacetic transaminase (SGOT); *liver function test. Special studies.* Basal serum creatine phosphokinase activity elevated; ischemic exercise tests, lactic acid-marked rise with exercise. *Immunodiffusion studies.* Demonstration of antimyoglobin antibody. *Biopsy of muscle. Electromyography. Electrocardiography. Urine.* Myoglobin may be present. *X-ray of chest.* Frequently, cardiomegaly.

Therapy. Discontinuation of alcohol intake; thiamine and correction of diet.

Prognosis. Lesions reversible upon discontinuation of alcohol intake.

BIBLIOGRAPHY. Hed R, Larrson H, Wahlgren F: Acute myoglobinuria: report of a case with fatal outcome. Acta Med (Scand) 152:459–463, 1955
Perkoff GT, Hardy P, Valez-Garcia E: Reversible acute muscular syndrome in chronic alcoholism. New Engl J Med 274:1277–1285, 1966
Adams RD, Victor M: Principles of Neurology, 3rd ed, p 1042. New York, McGraw-Hill, 1985.

ALCOHOL WITHDRAWAL

Symptoms. In chronic alcoholics when they attempt to stop drinking (most severe symptoms in those who have been drinking the longest). Aggravation of tremulousness or "shakes"; severe anxiety; insomnia; inability to concentrate; feeling of unreality. In most severe cases truncal ataxia, nausea, vomiting, diarrhea, abdominal cramps.

Hallucination within 24 to 25 days after alcohol withdrawal (25%). Patients remain able to describe hallucinations and communicate coherently. "Rum fits" or grand mal seizures may be first symptom. Delirium tremens is a combination of severe tremulousness and hallucination in severe form.

Signs. Evidence of dehydration, tachycardia, dilation of pupils, profuse sweating. Increased temperature may be observed. Increased blood pressure.

Etiology. Alcohol withdrawal alone may precipitate syndrome; thiamine deficiency and other nutritional deficiencies concur in determining this syndrome.

Diagnostic Procedures. *Blood.* Liver function test, pyruvate serum level; pyruvate tolerance curve.

Therapy. Benzodiazepines; IV fluids with glucose, electrolytes, and vitamin B complex; complete diet reevaluation. Antiemetics; antacids; ataractics; anticonvulsants. Lofexidine, atenolol.

Prognosis. Often limited to 3 to 7 days. Delirium tremens mortality estimated between 2% and 12%. Repeated attacks following resumption and discontinuation or increasing or decreasing intake of alcohol. A delayed type of syndrome with milder symptoms is reported that may occur years after discontinuation of alcohol intake.

BIBLIOGRAPHY. Sutton T: Tracts on Delirium Tremens, on Peritonitis, on Some Other Internal Inflammatory Affections and on the Gout. London, Thomas Underwood, 1813

Blake A: A Practical Essay on the Disease Generally Known under the Denomination of Delirium Tremens. London, Burgess Hill, 1825

Brown CG: The alcohol withdrawal syndrome. Ann Emerg Med II:276–280, 1982

Lerner WD, Fallon HJ: The alcohol withdrawal syndrome. New Engl J Med 313:951–952, 1985

ALDER'S

Synonyms. Alder-Reilly anomaly.

Symptoms and Signs. No particular clinical feature attributable to the presence of anomaly (See Diagnostic procedures). However, found in association with many syndromes: Hurler's; Hunter's; Maroteaux-Lamy's; and other types of bone and cartilage abnormalities.

Etiology. Dominant inheritance. Incomplete degradation of protein-bound carbohydrate complexes because of enzymatic deficiencies.

Pathology. See Diagnostic Procedures.

Diagnostic Procedures. *Blood.* In leukocytes, presence of azurophil and basophil granulations, larger than normal; similar bodies may be present in lymphocytes and monocytes. Function of leukocytes normal. *Bone marrow.* Granulation presence more evident than in peripheral blood.

Therapy. None. That of associated syndrome.

Prognosis. Permanent characteristic.

BIBLIOGRAPHY. Alder A: Ueber konstitutionell bedingte Granulation-veraenderungen der Leukocyten. Dtsch Arch Klin Med 183:372–378, 1939

Reilly WA: Granules in leukocytes in gargoylism. Am J Dis Child 62:489–491, 1941

Wintrobe MM, et al: Clinical Hematology, 8th ed. Philadelphia, Lea & Febiger, 1981

ALEXANDER'S

Synonyms. Factor VII deficiency. Proconvertin deficiency. SPCA deficiency.

Symptoms and Signs. Frequency 1/500,000. From childhood or in adulthood life. Like hemophilia but less severe. Postoperative blood losses are not great. Thromboembolism is possible.

Etiology. Autosomal recessive. Heterozygotes sometimes have hemorrhagic manifestations.

Diagnostic Procedures. *Blood.* Quick time lengthened, prothrombin time normal, cephaline and Stypven time are normal (different from factor X deficiency; see Christmas').

Therapy. Plasma, concentrates of vitamin K dependent factors. Contraceptives to prevent menorrhagia.

Prognosis. Good.

BIBLIOGRAPHY. Alexander B, Goldstein R, Landwehr G, et al: Congenital SPCA deficiency: a hitherto unrecognised coagulation defect with hemorrhage rectified by serum and serum fractions. J Clin Invest 30:596, 1951

Jesty J: Coagulation factor VII. In Selogon D, Schmidt RM (eds): Handbook Series in Clinical Laboratory Science. Section I: Hematology, Vol 3, p 41. Boca Raton, Fla, CRC Press, 1980

ALEXANDER'S (W.S.)

Synonyms. Fibrinoid degeneration of astrocytes; dysmyelogenic leukodystrophy-megalobarencephaly; leukodystrophy-megalobarencephaly.

Symptoms and Signs. Prevalent in males, onset in infancy. Retardation of development and slow progressive enlargement of head. Frequently, seizures.

Etiology. Metabolic disorder of unknown nature that interferes with myelinization of white matter. Autosomal recessive inheritance.

Pathology. Megalencephaly; hydrocephalus. Eosinophilic deposit spreads along all interfaces of central nervous system, including pial-glial and perivascular tissue. Leukodystrophy prevalent in frontal lobe.

Diagnostic Procedures. *Blood and urine.* Normal. *Spinal tap.* Increased pressure. *Electroencephalography.* CT *brain scan.*

Therapy. Symptomatic.

Prognosis. Poor. Progressive condition; death within one to two years from onset. In exceptional cases, a few years of survival from onset.

BIBLIOGRAPHY. Alexander WS: Progressive fibrinoid degeneration of fibrillary astrocytes associated with mental retardation in a hydrocephalic infant. Brain 72:373–381, 1949

Herndon RN, Rubinstein LJ, Freeman JN, et al: Light and electron microscopic observations on Rosenthal fibers in Alexander's disease and in multiple sclerosis. Neuropath Exp Neurol 29:524–551, 1970

ALEZZANDRINI'S

Symptoms and Signs. Occur in adolescent and early adulthood. Unilateral impairment of vision and after months or years, facial vitiligo and poliosis appear on the same side. Bilateral perceptive deafness occasionally develops.

Etiology. Unknown.

Pathology. Degenerative retinitis.

BIBLIOGRAPHY. Alezzandrini AA: Manifestation unilaterale de degenerescence tapeto-retinienne, de vitiligo, de poliose, de cheveux blancs et d'hypoacousie. Ophthalmologica 147:409–419, 1964

ALIBERT-BAZIN

Synonyms. Auspitz's; Vidal-Brocq; Hallopeau-Besnier; mycosis fungoides; cutaneous T cell lymphoma, CTCL.

Symptoms. Rare, more frequent in males (2–1). Onset at any age after seventh year, usually in middle age. Pruritus, pain, insomnia.

Signs. Isolated nonspecific eczematosous lesions. In some cases at onset, they assume the aspect of generalized erythroderma (Hallopeau-Besnier syndrome). (See also Sézary's.) The lesions consist in extending patches of varying hues, which may present bizarre shapes; dry and moderate scaling; no spontaneous vesiculation. This stage lasts many years and lesions may simulate psoriasis, parapsoriasis, lichen, exfoliative dermatitis, and other conditions. In a second stage they may ulcerate (fungate). Lymphadenopathy may be present from onset or develop later.

Etiology. Unknown. Cutaneous lymphoma T cell type. Occasional familial occurence autosomal recessive.

Pathology. Skin lesions show histologic alterations that vary during course of disease. At onset, lesions may be nonspecific. With progression, superficial dermal infiltrates develop, especially perivascularly, formed by lymphocytes, histiocytes, reticular cells, neutrophils, eosinophils and plasma cells, and frequently also by fragmented nuclei. Mixed with these elements are a variable number of "mycosis cells" (characterized by a large, round, deeply stained nucleus, crenated at its margin). These cells, however, must not be considered specific for this condition. With progression, infiltration of the lower corium and subcutaneous layers. Tumor transformation implies a more monoformic pattern with or without predominance of mycosis or reticular cells, followed thinning and ulceration of epidermis.

Diagnostic Procedures. *Skin biopsy.* See Pathology. *Lymph node biopsy.* Seldom, pattern of lymphoma; frequently, signs of chronic inflammation. *Bone marrow.* Seldom, mycosis cells; increase of plasma cells. *Blood.* Anemic neutrophilic leukocytosis and eosinophilia (if lymphocytosis, consider Sézary's syndrome, see).

Therapy. At onset weak steroid cream, photochemotherapy (PUVA). Total lymphoid irradiation (TLI) (remission for months), corticosteroids, mechlorethamine, etretinate. Trials with cyclosporin and interferon.

Prognosis. Possible transformation to Sézary's (see). Median survival approximately five years.

BIBLIOGRAPHY. Alibert JL: Description des maladies de la peau observées à l'Hôpital Saint Louis et exposition des meilleures methodes survies pour leur traitment. Paris, Barrois L'Aîné, 1806

Bazin APE: Leçons théorique et cliniques sur les affections cutanée de nature arthritique et dartreuse, considérées en ellememes et dans leurs rapports avec les éruptions, scrofuleuses, parasitaires et syphilitiques. Paris, A Delahaye, 1860

Auspitz H: Ein Fall von Granuloma Fungoides. Urtljschr Dermatol 12: 123–143, 1885

Auspitz H, Shelley WB: Familial mycosis fungoides revisited. Arch Derm 116:1177–1178, 1980

Lamberg SI, Green SB, Byar DP, et al: Clinical staging for cutaneous cell lymphoma. Ann Intern Med 100:187–192, 1984

ALIBERT'S I

Synonyms. False keloid; cicatricial keloid; Hawkin's; posttraumatic keloid; scar hypertrophy; hypertrophic scars.

Symptoms. Black race particularly susceptible. Females more susceptible. May appear during pregnancy. Rare in infancy and old age. Maximum between puberty and age 30. Local pain; tenderness.

Signs. Three to 4 weeks after trauma, scar begins to thicken and form a reddish plaque, which may continue to grow forming a cordlike excrescence of a more or less bizarre configuration.

Etiology. To be differentiated from true keloid. Local factor or systemic factors (or both) have been called responsible. Both autosomal recessive and dominant inheritance reported.

Pathology. In early stages, impossible to differentiate between false and true keloids: both have perivascular cellular nodules of collagen fibers. Later, in false keloids, the bundles of fibers aggregate and shrink, while elastic fibers appear.

Diagnostic Procedures. *Biopsy.*

Therapy. Early treatment produces best results, radiotherapy; intralesion injection (preceded by liquid nitrogen spray application) or systemic administration of corticosteroids. Retinoic acid application (good results). Surgery as last resort, since spontaneous regression is frequent.

Prognosis. Good response to treatment; spontaneous regression in many cases.

BIBLIOGRAPHY. Alibert JL: Note sur la kéloide. J Univ Sci Med 2:207–216. 1816
Hawkins CH: On warty tumours in cicatrices. London Med Gaz 13:481–482, 1833
Rook A, Wilkinson DS, Ebling FJG, et al: Textbook of Dermatology, 4th ed, pp 1831–1833. Oxford, Blackwell Scientific Publications, 1986

ALIBERT'S II

Synonyms. Aleppo boil; Bagdad boil; Biskra button; Borovskii's; Chiclero ulcer; cutaneous leishmaniasis; Delhi sore; Kandahar sore; Lahore sore; leishmaniasis old world; oriental boil.

Symptoms. Endemic on the Mediterranean coasts and warm countries from Asia to South America. Both sexes and all ages can be affected. Incubation period 1 to 6 months. Malaise; pruritus.

Signs. *First stage.* Wet or early ulcerative form. Red nodules at site of inoculation, which ulcerate in the center and extend ulcerating edges. Occasionally, small secondary nodules around the main lesion. *Second stage.* Dry or late ulcerative form. Brown nodules extend into a plaque; after 6 months, ulcerate and, then, crust. Satellite nodules more frequent. *Third stage.* Leishmaniasis recidivans. Brown papules re-form around area of previous lesion, and slowly coalesce to form lupuslike plaques.

Etiology. *Leishmania tropica* parasite transmitted by sand fly.

Pathology. Preulceration, dermal infiltrate of histiocytes with Leishman-Donovan (L-D) bodies, surrounded by lymphocytes and plasma cells. After ulceration, large number of neutrophils and reduction of number of L-D bodies.

Diagnostic Procedures. *Biopsy.* From ulcer floor. Culture in NNM (Nicolle-Novy-MacNeal) medium and antibiotics. *Montenegro test.*

Therapy. Pentostam intramuscularly or intravenously and for local infiltration; mepacrine; glucantime IM.

Prognosis. *Wet form.* After 2 to 6 months, healing with residual scar. *Dry form.* After 8 to 12 months, regression with residual scar. *L. recidivans.* Exceedingly chronic course.

BIBLIOGRAPHY. Alibert JL: Note sur la pyrophlyctide endémique ou pustule d'Alep. Rev Med Franc et Etrang (Paris) 3:62–68, 1829
Karagezian LA, Kozhniilevshmanioz-Armenii. Vestn Dermatol Venerol 40:61–64, 1966
Rook A, Wilkinson DS, Ebling FJG, et al: Textbook of Dermatology, 4th ed, pp 1021–1024. Oxford Blackwell Scientific Publications, 1986

ALIBERT'S III

Synonyms. Barber's itch; sycosis vulgaris; coccogenic sycosis; ficosis; mentagra; sycosis simplex; tinea barbae.

Symptoms. Only adult males affected. Pruritus on the face.

Signs. Small annular, moderately scaly lesions on the beard area. Peripheral growth with central healing. May assume features of chronic bacterial folliculitis.

Etiology. *Trichophyton mentagrophytes; T. verrucosum; T. violaceum; T. schoenleini.*

Pathology. Chronic inflammatory lesions, pustules, or abscess with hyphae in follicles.

Diagnostic Procedures. *Mycologic examination.* Of infected hairs. *Cultures.*

Therapy. Scrubbing with soap and water. Fungistatic preparations for topical use. Griseofulvin orally.

Prognosis. Inflammatory lesions may clear spontaneously or persist for months.

BIBLIOGRAPHY. Alibert JL: Déscription Des Maladies de la Peau, Vol 2, p 214. Bruxelles, Wahlew, 1825
Rook A, Wilkinson DS, Ebling FJG, et al: Textbook of Dermatology, 4th ed, pp 741–742. Oxford, Blackwell Scientific Publications, 1986

ALICE IN WONDERLAND

Synonym. Todd's.

Symptoms. Bizarre disturbance of body image; feeling of levitation; alteration of sense of passage of time; depersonalization; doubling of personality.

Etiology. Migraine attack; epilepsy; hypnagogic states; schizophrenia; hallucinogenic drugs; various diseases of parietal lobe.

Therapy. Depending upon etiology.

BIBLIOGRAPHY. Todd J: Syndrome of Alice in Wonderland. Can Med Assoc J 73:701–704, 1955

ALIQUORRHEA

Synonyms. Cerebral ventricular collapse; spontaneous hypoliquorrhea.

Symptoms. Severe headache, increasing when the patient attempts to sit up or stand up; stiff neck; nausea; dizziness; buzzing of ears.

Signs. Bradycardia; Kernig's sign; optic disc normal; normal reflexes; no paresis or sensibility disturbance.

Etiology. Unknown. Spontaneous decrease of secretion of spinal fluid, establishing a negative pressure in the cerebrospinal cavity. In addition to rare condition, frequently observed after lumbar puncture, injury and operation of brain, chronic subdural hematomas, and in general dehydration.

Diagnostic Procedures. *Lumbar puncture.* Absent or low cerebrospinal pressure; very little or no fluid obtained; typical air suction through the needle with noise when the patient passes from a sitting position to lying down. Queckenstedt's increase in pressure. *Cerebrospinal fluid.* When obtained is blood-tinged or yellowish; protein increased; normal cells. *Blood.* Normal; in some cases, moderate increase of sedimentation rate.

Therapy. Injection of warm Ringer's solution into the spinal canal until normal pressure is reached; relieves all symptoms for a day or two.

Prognosis. All patients recovered.

BIBLIOGRAPHY. Ingvar S: Danger of leakage of cerebrospinal fluid after lumbar puncture. Acta Med Scand 58:67–101, 1923
Lindqvist T, Moberg E: Spontaneous hypoliquorrhea; report of a case. Acta Med Scand 132:556–561, 1949
Adams RD, Victor M: Principles of Neurology, 3rd ed, p 470. New York, McGraw-Hill, 1985

ALLAN-HERNDON-DUDLEY

Synonyms. Mental retardation (X-linked); hypotonia.

Symptoms and Signs. Male. Normal at birth but for hypotonia. At 6 months inability to hold up the head. Retarded motor development, muscular atrophy. At more advanced age, joint contractures and hyporeflexia.

Etiology. X-linked inheritance suggested.

Prognosis. Reach adult life.

BIBLIOGRAPHY. Allan W, Herndon CN, Dudley FC: Some examples of the inheritance of mental deficiency; apparently sex-linked idiocy and microcephaly. Am J Ment Defic 48:325–334, 1943–1944
Opitz JM, Sutherland GR: International workshop on the fragile X and X-linked mental retardation. Am J Med Genet 17:5–94, 1984

ALLEMANN'S

Symptoms and Signs. Club fingers (one element of syndrome). In some cases facial asymmetry and signs relative to degeneration of various motor branches of nerves present as well.

Etiology. Unknown.

Diagnostic Procedures. *Urography.* Duplication of the renal images (second element of syndrome).

BIBLIOGRAPHY. Allemann R: Die klinische Bedeutung familiarer Heredopatie und Mutation für die Urologie. Z Urol 80:641–649, 1936

ALLEN-HINES

Synonym. Lipedema legs.

Symptoms. Frequently, family history of big legs. Almost exclusively in women. Distress (emotional and physical because of the appearance of the leg). Increase of symptoms and signs with warm weather.

Signs. Gradual onset; bilateral enlargement of buttocks and legs. Fat and fluid accumulation; sensitivity to pressure; swelling soft; pitting edema minimal. Usually the fat accumulation limited to legs and the rest of body appears normal; occasionally accompanied by generalized obesity. Feet normal in size and configuration.

Etiology. Unknown; possibly constitutional hereditary character. Emotional reaction precipitated by the fact that "fat legs" are considered unattractive in modern societies. Older civilizations and Hottentots, for instance, consider them a sign of beauty.

Therapy. Nonspecific; bed rest induces moderate degree of decrease in size of legs.

Prognosis. Course progressive.

BIBLIOGRAPHY. Allen EV, Hines EA Jr: Lipedema of the legs: a syndrome characterized by fat legs and orthostatic edema. Proc Staff Meet Mayo Clinic 15:184–187, 1940
Wold LE, Hines EA, Allen EV: Lipedema of legs: a syndrome characterized by fat legs and edema. Ann Intern Med 34:1243–1250. 1951

ALLEN-MASTERS

Synonyms. Broad ligament laceration; laceration of uterine support; ligamentum latum laceration; Masters-Allen.

Symptoms. Occur mainly in multiparas. Pain in the pelvic region; dyspareunia; dysmenorrhea; backache; urinary frequency; rectal tenesmus.

Signs. Laceration of the posterior aspect of the broad ligament; angiomatous aspect of the blood vessels in broad ligament. Cervix may be moved in any direction with minimal or no movement of the uterus.

Etiology. Unknown. Surgical, traumatic, or precipitated delivery; criminal abortion, excessive packing.

Pathology. Nonspecific inflammatory infiltration; angiomatous aspect of the vessels; cellular necrosis. Endometriosis can often be demonstrated macroscopically and microscopically with the same frequency. Hyperplasia of the venous tissue and neuroma can be found.

Therapy. Suturing the rupture is not enough. It is recommended that after laparotomy the pelvic peritoneum be resected, with the exception of pouch of Douglas.

Prognosis. Good with treatment.

BIBLIOGRAPHY. Allen WM, Masters WH: Traumatic laceration of uterine support: The clinical syndrome and the operative treatment. Am J Obstet Gynecol 70:500–513, 1955
Bret AJ, Bardiaux M, de Brux J: Algies pelviennes d'origine genitale; La pelviperitonite chronique scleroinflammatoire. Etude clinique et histopathologique de 25 cas. A propos du syndrome d'Allen et Masters. Sem Hôp Paris 43:173–182, 1967
Philipp EE, Barnes J, Newton M: Obstetrics and Gynecology, 3rd ed, pp 93–94. William Heinemann Med Books Ltd, London, 1986

ALLERGIC ALVEOLITIS, EXTRINSIC

Clinical features depend on immunologic response of the patient, antigenicity of dust, and intensity and frequency of exposure. Manifestations are similar regardless of the organic dust inhaled.

Symptoms. Develop within 4 to 6 hours of exposure. Cough; dyspnea; chills, fever, malaise, myalgia.

Signs. Bibasilar moist rales; patient appears acutely ill and exhausted.

Etiology. Immunoreactions: type I (allergic reactions); type III (precipitin mediated); type IV (delayed hypersensitivity) involved. Very often serum precipitins against the offending antigen can be detected. Types of dusts responsible give the name to the syndromes.
1. *Bagassosis.* Dust from moldy sugar cane
2. *Bible printer's.* Moldy paper; solutions used for printing
3. *Cheese-washer's lung.* Dust from cheese particles
4. *Christmas tree allergy* (Variant of "wood-pulp worker's"). Dust from the bark of Christmas tree
5. *Coffee-roaster's lung.* Dust from green coffee
6. *Coptic* (Mummy disease). Dust from mummy bandage
7. *Dog house.* Dust from moldy straw mattresses used for dogs
8. *Farmer's lung.* Dust from grains and hay
9. *Humidistat* (Humidifier lung; air conditioner pneumonitis; heating system disease). Aerosol of microorganisms or dusts from contaminated heating or cooling system
10. *Malt worker's lung.* (Brewer's lung). Malt dust
11. *Maple bark.* Dust from moldy maple bark (see also wood-pulp)

12. *Mushroom worker's lung* (Mushroom picker's lung). Dust from cultivated mushrooms in mushroom-growing farms
13. *Paprika splitter's lung.* Paprika dust
14. *Pigeon breeder's* (Bird breeder's lung; bird fancier's lung). Dust from bird's excreta and plumage
15. *Pituitary snuff taker's lung.* Pituitary powder
16. *Research-assistant's lung.* Dust from rat's excreta; rat serum proteins
17. *Sequoiosis.* Redwood dust (see also "wood-pulp")
18. *Sisal-worker's disease.* Dust from *Agave sisalana* fibers
19. *Smallpox handler's lung.* Aerosol from smallpox lesions (affects medical and nursing staff dealing with smallpox patients).
20. *Suberosis.* Dust from moldy cork
21. *Tea-grower's lung.* Dust from moldy tea.
22. *Thatched roof disease* (Papuan lung; New Guinea lung). Dust from the thatched roof common in New Guinea houses
23. *Tobacco grower's lung.* Dust from moldy tobacco
24. *Wood-pulp worker's lung* (Papermill worker's disease). Dust from wood-pulp.
25. *Woolsorter's lung.* Dust from wool

Pathology. Infiltration of alveolar walls by lymphocytes, plasma cells, and histiocytes with foamy cytoplasm; infiltration of the interstitium with mononuclear cells; sometimes, giant cell granulomas.

Diagnostic Procedures. *Blood.* Leukocytosis. *Pulmonary function tests.* Decreased vital capacity; decreased pulmonary compliance. *X-ray of chest.* Fine nodular densities.

Therapy. Avoidance of offending antigen; appropriate ventilation of working areas. Corticosteroids; bronchodilators. Oxygen.

Prognosis. Good with prevention. Repeated episodes produce chronic pulmonary and cardiac damages.

BIBLIOGRAPHY. De Francisci G, Magalini SI, Scrascia E: Etiopatogenesi e problemi rianimativi nelle polmoniti da ipersensibilità. Rec Progr Med 66:541–552, 1979
De Francisci G, Magalini SI: Le pneumopatie interstiziali da farmaci. Rec Progr Med 68:65–76, 1980
Reed CE, De Shazo R: Immunologic aspect of granulomatous and interstitial lung diseases. JAMA 248:2683–2691, 1982

ALLERGIC CYSTITIS

Synonyms. Cystitis allergy; food allergy.

Symptoms. Strangury; pollakiuria.

Signs. Pain on palpation of suprapubic area.

Etiology. Allergy to specific foods or drugs.

Pathology. *Bladder wall.* Edema and infiltration with eosinophils and monocytic cells.

Diagnostic Procedures. *Urine.* Usually, absence of signs of infection (possibly secondary); occasionally, presence of eosinophils and red cells in sediment. *Cystoscopy.* (to be performed only after acute situation has subsided). Edema and congestion of bladder wall. *Allergy tests.*

Therapy. Identification of and abstention from ingestion of allergic food or drug. Epinephrine; ephedrine; antihistamines; corticosteroids (usually temporarily useful). Attempts at desensitization.

Prognosis. Tendency to become a chronic condition. Complication of infection frequent. May be cured by avoidance of offending agents or successful desensitization.

ALLERGIC GASTROENTERITIS

Synonyms. Allergic jejunitis; Quincke's edema; angioneurotic edema of gastrointestinal tract; eosinophilic gastroenteritis; gastrointestinal idiopathic eosinophilic infiltrations; granuloma eosinophilic stomach. (See also Loeffler's and Quincke's I.)

Symptoms and Signs. Nearly equal sex distribution; seen in all ages, but most common in the sixth decade. Symptomatology may vary in kind with the organ involved. However, common pattern may be observed: recurrent gastrointestinal disorders lasting many years; vomiting; flatulence; diarrhea; epigastric pain; cramps; heart burn (in class II pain and cramping more prolonged and not intermittent, see Pathology). In some cases also history of melena or hematemesis; pyloric obstruction; cholecystitis and cholelithiasis; history of allergy (in 50% of cases).

Etiology. Unknown. Allergic mechanism (hypersensitivity reaction) postulated for the diffused type (class I); local inciting agents for the circumscribed types (class II).

Pathology. Two classes appear not related. *Class I* (diffused type). (1) Polyenteric: more than one portion of intestine involved; antrum of the stomach characteristically affected with extension to jejunum and ileum. Areas affected are firm, with edematous appearance; omentum and mesentery may appear inflamed or fibrotic; pylorus usually narrowed. Diffuse inflammatory infiltration from submucosa (occasionally also serosa) by mature eosinophils, with rare macrophages and giant cells; occasionally, hyalinization or necrosis of muscles. Mucosa free of involvement. (2) Monoenteric: similar pattern of lesions limited to the stomach (3) Regional: similar pattern involving only a limited region: prepyloric and pyloric with borders not well defined. *Class II* (circumscribed type). (1) Regional: pseudotumors located at any site of the gastrointestinal tract; mucosa may be ulcerated; granuloma type of lesion, with rich reticular fibrillar and fibroblastic elements; varying numbers of blood vessels and inflammatory cells. Scarce eosinophilic infiltration; histiocytes rare. (2) Polypoid pedunculated polyps; microscopically same pattern as regional type.

Diagnostic Procedures. *X-ray.* Varying findings according to location and extension of lesions. In class I, usually smooth concentric narrowing of the antrum; absence of peristalsis in involved area; signs of pyloric obstruction; with bowel involvement, tubular segmental narrowings, alternating with dilated loops. *Blood.* Eosinophilia (up to 60%). *Bone marrow.* High percentage of eosinophils may be found. *Biopsy of lesion.* See Pathology.

Therapy. Conservative treatment with adrenocorticotropic hormone (ACTH) and corticosteroids usually brings prompt control of symptoms and of eosinophilia. When indicated, exploratory laparotomy and biopsy. According to location and extension of lesions, surgical intervention may be decided upon. Usually gastroenterostomy is adequate; in some cases subtotal gastrectomy and total gastrectomy have been performed. According to recent findings, surgery seems necessary only for control of bleeding.

Prognosis. Lesions do not recur after resection. If they recur after conservative treatment, response to successive steroid administrations is prompt.

BIBLIOGRAPHY. Konjetzny GE: Ueber Magenfibrome. Beitr Klin Chir 119:53, 1920

Barrie HJ, Anderson JC: Hypertrophy of pylorus in an adult with massive eosinophil infiltration and giant cell reaction. Lancet II:1007–1009, 1948

Lane RE: Eosinophilic gastroenteritis. Northwest Med 66:357–359, 1967

Schulze K, Mitros FA: Eosinophilic gastroenteritis involving the ileocecal area. Dis Colon Rectum 22:47–50, 1979

Kohler PF, Brown WR: Immunologic aspects of hepatic and gastrointestinal tract disease. JAMA 248:2704–2709, 1982

ALLERGIC RHINITIS

Synonyms. Bostocks; Engels atopic hypersensitivity autumnal catarrh; hay fever; immune reaction type 1; pollinosis; see Angelucci's and Besnier's prurigo.

Symptoms and Signs. Both sexes affected; first manifestation seldom observed before 2 months of age. Atopic infantile eczema frequently is early manifestation (see Unna's); allergic rhinitis develops in 30 to 50% of cases of infantile eczema. Accurate family anamnesis reveals history of typical skin or systemic disorders of allergic type. All year around or in particular seasons or special environments (indoor, open air, country, gardens, humid places) attacks of rhinitis, conjuntivitis occasionally followed by asthmatic attack.

Etiology. Interplay of genetic factors (of complex nature, both dominant and recessive reported) and precipitating factors (immunological contact of mucosae with allergens; psychological). Most frequent airborne allergens responsible: pollens, molds, types of dust, dermatophagoides (dust mites).

Pathology. Hypertrophy of nasal and first airway mucosae with eosinophilic infiltration. Frequent development of poliposis.

Diagnostic Procedures. *Blood.* IgE level increased (in 80% of cases); IgG, IgA, IgM usually normal. Eosinophilia; search for specific antibodies (RAST). *Skin tests and provocative tests* (inhalation).

Therapy. General allergic management. Avoid exposure to allergens. Specific treatment for desensitization: antihistaminics; corticosteroids; Cromolyn sodium.

Prognosis. With age, intensity of symptoms may decrease.

BIBLIOGRAPHY. Bias WB, Marshal DG, Platt-Mills TAE: Genetic control of factor involved in bronchial asthma, hay fever and other allergic states. In Litwin SD (ed): Genetic Determinants of Pulmonary Disease, pp 127–148. New York, M Dekker, 1978

Charpin J, Dry J, Michel FB: Desensibilization des maladies allergiques: allergenes nouveaux, vigilance accrue. La Presse Med 33:1754, 1985

ALLERGIC SEMINAL

Synonyms. Allergic vulvovaginitis.

Symptoms and Signs. Vaginal. Burning and pain during coitus or after ejaculation lasting from 2 to 70 hours. Erythema and edema, bullae on the labia.

Etiology. Family described (mother and four daughters) suggests autosomal dominant inheritance.

Diagnostic Procedures. *Skin test.* Reactivity to seminal fluid. *Blood.* No sperm agglutinating antibody detectable.

Therapy. Benadryl per os and/or topical.

BIBLIOGRAPHY. Chang T-W: Familial allergic seminal vulvovaginitis. Am J Obstet Gynecol 126:442–444, 1976

ALLGROVE'S

Synonyms. Achalasia-Addisonian; glucocorticoid deficiency—achalasia; Addisonian-achalasia; alacrima-achalasia-Addisonianism; triple A.

Symptoms. Both sexes. Defective tear formation at birth. Addisonian symptoms and achalasia may develop later in life.

Etiology. Recessive inheritance.

Pathology. Absence of the zona fasciculata and almost normal zona glomerulosa.

Diagnostic Procedures. See Addisonian syndromes (chronic adrenal insufficiency).

Therapy. See Addisonian syndromes (chronic adrenal insufficiency).

Prognosis. Death may be caused by adrenal crisis.

BIBLIOGRAPHY. Allgrove J, Clayden GS, Grant DB, et al: Familial glucocorticoid deficiency with achalasia of the cardias and deficient tear production. Lancet I:1284–1286, 1978
Lanes R, Platnick LP, Byunn TE, et al: Glucocorticoid and partial mineral corticoid deficiency associated with achalasia. J Clin Endoc Met 50:268–270, 1984

ALLISON'S

Synonyms. Astronaut bone demineralization; bone-demineralization; non-use bone atrophy.

Symptoms and Signs. Appear after periods of prolonged immobilization. From asymptomatic to generalized weakness and articular pain on motion.

Etiology. It has been observed that immobilization (in bed, casting, on orbital flights) produces significant bone demineralization. In astronauts the change has been related to the diet and the immobilization produced by the confinement in the capsule.

Therapy. Gradual exercise and diet rich in calcium may reduce the extent of calcium loss.

Prognosis. Usually good with treatment and return to normal life.

BIBLIOGRAPHY. Allison N, Brooks B: Bone atrophy: A clinical study of the changes in bone which result from non-use. Arch Surg 5:499–526, 1922
Mack PB, La Chance PA, Vose GP et al: Bone demineralization of foot and hand of Gemini-Titan IV, V, and VII astronauts during orbital flight. Am J Roentgenol 100:503–511, 1967

ALPERS'

Synonyms. Cerebral gray matter diffuse progressive degeneration; Christensen-Krabbe; poliodystrophia cerebri. See Wefring-Lamvik.

Symptoms and Signs. Convulsions; myoclonus, spasticity, choreoathetosis; dementia; cerebellar ataxia.

Etiology. Anoxia; postepileptic, sequelae of trauma mentioned among other etiologic factors.

Pathology. Degenerative changes in the middle layers of cerebral gray matter, may also be present in basal ganglia and cerebellar cortex.

Therapy. None.

Prognosis. Very poor. Status epilepticus often terminating event.

BIBLIOGRAPHY. Alpers BJ: Diffuse progressive degeneration of the gray matter of the cerebrum. Arch Neurol Psychiatr 25:469–505, 1931
Christensen E, Hojgaard K: Poliodystrophia cerebri progressiva infantilis. Acta Neurol Scand 40:21–40, 1964
Gabreels FJM, Prick MJJ, Reiner WO, et al: Progressive infantile poliodystrophy (Alper's disease) associated with disturbed NADH oxidation, lipid myopathy and abnormal muscle mitochondria. In Busch HFM (ed): Mitochondria and Muscular Disease, pp 165–171. Beetsterzwaag, The Netherlands, Mefar 1981

ALPHA-ANTITRYPSIN DEFICIENCY

Symptoms and Signs. Present from birth or early infancy. Cholestatic jaundice eventually remitting (leaving mild liver abnormalities) or progressing to ascites and hepatic failure or, later (in first decade or adolescence), to cirrhosis. Onset in early adulthood, frequently associated with pulmonary emphysema.

Etiology. Deficiency of $alpha_1$-antitrypsin (A-1-AT). Twenty-four different codominant alleles, each contributing to the measured antitryptic activity. Affected individual is (PiZZ) phenotype; heterozygous MZ(PiMZ) relatives are identified by typing (see Diagnostic Procedures). Autosomal recessive inheritance.

Pathology. *Liver.* Severe form micronodular portal cirrhosis; in PiZZ homozygous, presence of cytoplasmic granules in hepatocytes remain PAS positive after diastasis exposure. *Lung.* Panacinar form of emphysema.

Diagnostic Procedures. *Typing of Pi (protease inhibitor).* Polymorphic variants identified by letters (first alphabetical letters assigned to faster moving forms; slower designated PiZZ; PiMM = homozygous normal). Presence of slower form (PiZZ) responsible for low-serum antitrypsin level.

Therapy. Symptomatic. No response (release of A-1-AT) to phenobarbital, estrogen, steroid. Successful liver transplantation is followed by good life expectancy.

Prognosis. Variable, from no harmful effects to death in infancy or adult life. Pulmonary emphysema: danazole, stop smoking (concomitant aggravating factor); parenteral administration of synthetic analogs.

BIBLIOGRAPHY. Laurel CB, Erikson S: The electrophoretic alpha 1 globulin pattern of serum in alpha 1 antitrypsin deficiency. Scand J Clin Lab Invest 15:132–140, 1963
Gadek JE, Crystal RG: Alpha-1-antitrypsin deficiency. In Stanbury JB, Wyngaarden JB, Fredrickson DS, et al: The Metabolic Basis of Inherited Disease. 5th ed, p 1450. New York, McGraw–Hill, 1983

ALPHA₂-ANTIPLASMIN DEFICIENCY

Synonyms. Alpha$_2$-AP deficiency.

Symptoms and Signs. Rare. From birth, severe hemorrhages from umbilical cord and all other sites.

Etiology. Autosomal recessive.

Diagnostic Procedures. *Blood.* Shortening of time of lysis of clot. *Radioimmunoassay* of alpha$_2$-antiplasmin: reduced or absent.

Therapy. Antifibrinolytic agents: tranexamic acid.

BIBLIOGRAPHY. Kluft C, Vellenga E, Brommer EJP: Homozygous alpha-2-antiplasmin deficiency. Lancet II:206, 1979

ALPORT'S

Synonyms. Dickinson's; hereditary deafness nephropathy; hematuria-nephropathy-deafness; hemorrhagic familial nephritis.

Symptoms. Both sexes affected. Initially asymptomatic. Later progressive renal insufficiency; loss of hearing; reduced vision (in males).

Signs. In the female, hematuria often only manifestation; occasionally nerve deafness complication of renal insufficiency in pregnancy (hypertension edema). In the male, hematuria; albuminuria; cylindruria; recurrent pyelonephritis; usually deafness, auditory nerve or Corti's organ; occasionally congenital anomalies of the eyes (cataracts; spherophakia), including Alport's-like hereditary nephritis (NALD).

Etiology. Unknown; autosomal dominant inheritance (possibly modified by a sex-linked suppressor gene). Proposed also in some families is an X-linked inheritance.

Pathology. Chronic glomerulonephritis with interstitial renal foam cells.

Diagnostic Procedures. *Urine.* Hematuria; albuminuria; cylindruria; hyperaminoaciduria. *Blood.* Increased blood urea nitrogen and creatinine; anemia. *Ophthalmoscopy.* Fundus albipunctatus; lens alterations. *Audiometry.* Nerve deafness.

Therapy. Treatment of pyelonephritis. Kidney transplantation when indicated.

Prognosis. In the female, normal life span except for complications. In male renal failure by the 5th decade.

BIBLIOGRAPHY. Alport AC: Hereditary familial congenital hemorrhagic nephritis. Br Med J 1:504–506, 1927
Dickinson WH: Diseases of the kidney and urinary derangements, part 2:379. London, Longman, 1875
Di Bona GF: Alport's syndrome: a genetic defect in biochemical composition of basement membrane of glomerulus, lens and inner ear? J Lab Med 101:817–820, 1983
Hasstealt SJ, Atkin CL: X-linked inheritance in Alport syndrome, family P revisited. Am J Hum Genet 35:1241–1291, 1983

ALSTROEM'S

Synonyms. Retinitis pigmentosa–deafness–obesity–diabetes mellitus. See Laurence-Moon; Leber's II.

Symptoms and Signs. High incidence in Sweden and Holland. At birth, blindness or marked reduction of vision; neuropathic deafness; acanthosis nigricans; obesity; manifestations of nephropathy and hypogonadism. Absence of polydactyly and mental retardation.

Etiology. Autosomal recessive inheritance.

Pathology. Defect of cones.

Diagnostic Procedures. *Fundus oculi.* In childhood normal; in later life pigmentation or depigmentation; occasionally, narrowing vessels. *Blood.* Hyperuricemia; hypertriglyceridemia. Hyperglycemia (as result of resistance to insulin) hyperprebetalipoproteinemia. *Electroretinography.* Absence or reduction of electrical activity.

Therapy. Symptomatic.

Prognosis. Poor. Possible development of or association with, cataract, keratoconus, or progression of optic atrophy or both.

BIBLIOGRAPHY. Alstroem CH, Hallgren B, Nielson LB, et al: Retinal degeneration combined with obesity, diabetes mellitus and neurogenous deafness. A specific syndrome (not hitherto described) distinct from the Laurence-Moon-Biedl syndrome. A clinical endocrinological and genetic examination based on a large pedigree. Acta Psychiat Neurol Scand 34(suppl 129):1–35, 1959

Rudiger HW, Ahrens P, Dreyer M, et al: Impaired insulin-induced RNA synthesis secondary to a genetically defective insulin receptor. Hum Genet 69:76–78, 1985

ALTAMIRA

Synonyms. Altamira hemorrhagic.

Symptoms and Signs. Low-grade fever precedes hemorrhages of skin, followed by bleeding of the mucous membranes; asthenia. Hemorrhagic skin lesions caused by insect bites; traumatic hematomas; petecchiae and ecchymoses on the whole surface of the body, or restricted to face and extremities. Small and painless lymph nodes in groin and axillae; seldom, moderate hepatosplenomegaly.

Etiology. The disease is due to the bite of the black fly *Simulium*. Affected are immigrants living in an area called Altamira in a forest region of Brazil. No specific etiologic agent has been isolated. This hemorrhagic syndrome may be due to a hypersensitivity phenomenon or response to a toxin associated with intense black fly bites. Either a direct toxic effect or a hypersensitivity reaction could lead to an arrest of megakaryocyte maturation.

Pathology. Bone marrow biopsy shows increased number of megakaryocytes.

Diagnostic Procedures. *Blood.* Platelets below 100,000; anemia; white blood cells normal; plasma clotting factors normal.

Therapy. Intravenous glucose; prednisone (20 to 40 mg day until symptoms relieved). In severe cases, blood transfusions.

BIBLIOGRAPHY. Pinheiro FP, Bensabath G, Costa D, Jr, et al: Haemorrhagic syndrome of Altamira. Lancet I:639–642, 1974

Simpson DHI: Viral hemorrhagic fevers of man. Bull WHO 56:819, 838 1978

ALVEOLAR CAPILLARY BLOCK

Synonyms. Alveolar hypoventilation; interstitial diffuse pulmonary fibrosis. See Hamman-Rich's.

Symptoms. Dyspnea on effort; pleuritic pain.

Signs. Digital clubbing (may follow or precede dyspnea). Cyanosis; diffuse fine rales. Frequently, subcutaneous rheumatoid nodules.

Etiology. All conditions that reduce the total oxygen diffusing capacity of the lungs because of alteration of the pulmonary surface (alveolar-capillary block). Diseases of pulmonary interstitium: granulomatosis; scleroderma; rheumatoid arthritis.

Now it is known that the importance of alveolar-capillary block has been greatly exaggerated in the past, because arterial hypoxia in patients at rest with decreased diffusing capacities has been shown to be caused mainly by ventilation-perfusion inequalities and changes in pulmonary capillary blood volume and not by a simple reduction in the oxygen diffusing capacity.

Pathology. Initially, nonspecific interstitial pneumonia; then formation of mature fibrous tissue which evolves into "honeycomb lung"; bronchiectasis.

Diagnostic Procedures. *Blood.* Polycythemia. *X-rays of lung.* Early subacute stage, punctate nodular miliarylike pattern; later, medium to coarse reticulation. Occasionally, pleural effusion. *Pulmonary function test.* Restrictive; ventilatory defect; reduction of diffusing capacity.

Therapy. According to etiology. Adrenal steroid useful in collagen forms. Intensive care; ECG and pulse oxymetry monitoring; oxygen; in severe cases consider mechanical ventilation.

Prognosis. Evolving into congestive heart failure.

BIBLIOGRAPHY. Ellman P, Ball RE: "Rheumatoid disease" with joint and pulmonary manifestations. Br Med J 2:816–820, 1948

Fishman AP, Turino GM, Bergofsky EH: The syndrome of alveolar hypoventilation. Am J Med 23:333–339, 1957

Fraser RG, Paré JAP: Diagnoses of Diseases of the Chest, 2nd ed, p 1961. Philadelphia, WB Saunders, 1977

Murray JF: Respiratory structure and function. In Beeson PB, McDermott W: Cecil-Loeb Textbook of Medicine, p 339. Philadelphia, WB Saunders, 1982

Trulock EP, Schuster DP: Acute respiratory failure. In Orland MJ, Saltman RJ (eds): Manual of Medical Therapeutics, p 144. Boston, Little, Brown, 1986

ALZHEIMER'S

Synonyms. A D; Presenile dementia. See Pick's (A.) arteriopathic dementia; senile dementia.

Symptoms. Predominant in female; onset usually in fifth or sixth decades. Gradual loss of immediate memory; patient conscious of defect and initially worried about it. Slovenly in dress; speech dysarthric; change in behavior;

short temper or euphoria; disorientation in time and space; more need for sleep. Occasionally, hemiparesis; tremor; convulsions.

Signs. Focal signs of central nervous system defects. Hyperreflexia or hyporeflexia.

Etiology. Unknown; autosomal dominant inheritance reported and suggested for most cases.

Pathology. Shrinking of brain; thickening of pia; diffuse rarefaction of cortex, moderate glial reaction; large number of senile plaques. Neurofibrillar degeneration (dustlike argentophilic bodies or curled ends).

Diagnostic Procedures. *Electroencephalography.* Loss of frequencies; slow high voltage activity. *Pneumoencephalography.* Dilatation of ventricles and increased subarachnoid space. *Spinal fluid.* Normal or moderately increased protein.

Therapy. Symptomatic (anticonvulsant, if needed).

Prognosis. Death in 5 to 10 years.

BIBLIOGRAPHY. Alzheimer A: Ueber Einen Eigengartigen Schweren Krankheits: Prozess der Hirnrinde. Zentralbl Nerverkh 25:1134, 1906; 30:177–179, 1907
McKhann G, Drachman D, Folstein M, et al: Clinical diagnosis of Alzheimer's disease. Neurology 34:939–944, 1984
Cogan DG: Alzheimer syndromes. Am J Ophthalmol 104:183–184, 1987

AMAUROSIS FUGAX

Symptoms. Transient visual loss; continuous recurrence may result in complete blindness.

Signs. Depends on etiology. Blood hypertension; polycythemia.

Etiology. Tabagism; hypertension; polycythemia; reduction of cerebral flow, as part of carotid insufficiency syndrome indicating insufficiency of the ophthalmic artery. Microemboli of cholesterol arising from ulcerating arteriosclerotic placques that temporarily obstruct the retinal artery; as part of syncope, migraine, or insufficiency of the vertebral-basilar system.

Pathology. Depending on etiology. Vascular spasm, if recurrent, results in ischemic retinal necrosis.

Therapy. Application of cold or hot water is beneficial within minutes in recurrent attacks. Elimination or treatment of pathogenetic factors: tobacco; polycythemia; hypertension. Sympathectomy.

Prognosis. Varies according to etiology.

BIBLIOGRAPHY. Moore RF: Medical Ophthalmology. London, Churchill, 1922
Thorpe RM: Ocular signs in cerebral disease. In Gay JA, Burde RM (eds): Clinical Concept in Neuroophthalmology. Int Ophthalmol Clinics 7:707, 1967
Adams RD, Victor M: Principles of Neurology, 3rd ed, p 182. New York, McGraw-Hill, 1985

AMBLYOPIC SCHOOLGIRL

Synonyms. Hysterical amblyopia.

Symptoms and Signs. Amblyopia. Alterations of visual fields: variable abnormal dark adaptation curve. Ring scotomas; hemianopsias.

Etiology. Related directly or indirectly to psychological disturbances.

Therapy. Psychotherapy.

BIBLIOGRAPHY. Schlaegel TF, Jr, Quilala FV: Hysterical amblyopia. Arch Ophth 54:875–884, 1955
Manty Jarvi MI: The amblyopic school girl syndrome. J Ped Ophthal Strabys 18:30–33, 1981

AMENDOLA'S

Synonyms. Brazilian pemphigus; fogo selvagem; wildfire pemphigus.

Symptoms. Endemic in Brazil (state of São Paulo in particular). All ethnic groups and ages affected (benign course if onset before 30 years of age). Fever; chills; localized pain (enhanced by movements).

Signs. Bullae initiate on face, frequently affecting eyes (anterior pole cloudiness 5%) and chest; then become generalized and evolve into pustules, crusts, and exfoliate (pemphiguslike); Nikolsky's sign; mucosa not involved.

Etiology. Unknown; possibly an infectious condition associated with endocrine disorders. *Simulium pruinosum* suspected vector.

Pathology. In upper epidermis, acanthosis, derma infiltration. In older lesions, acanthosis, papillomatosis, hyperkeratosis.

Diagnostic Procedures. *Biopsy.* Indirect immunofluorescence specific antibodies.

Therapy. Symptomatic. Local and oral corticosteroids.

Prognosis. Evolution in 2 weeks to 1 year. Complications: ocular lesions; gonadal lesions; impotence. Possibly fatal.

BIBLIOGRAPHY. Amendola F: Cataracte no pemfigo fo-liáceo (nota previa). Rev Paul Med 26:286, 1945

Sevadjian C: Nosology of Brazilian pemphigus foliaceus. Int J Dermatol 18:781–786, 1979

Collins JF: Handbook of Clinical Ophthalmology. New York, Masson, 1982

AMENORRHEA-GALACTORRHEA-HYPOTHYROIDISM

Symptoms and Signs. Postpartum galactorrhea and amenorrhea, accompanied by all symptoms and signs of hypothyroidism.

Etiology. Unknown. See Multiple endocrine deficiency (acquired?).

Pathology. Unknown.

Diagnostic Procedures. *Thyroid function.* Hypothyroidism. *X-ray of skull.* Normal sella turcica. *Blood.* Increase in prolactin.

Therapy. Thyroid.

Prognosis. Amenorrhea and galactorrhea as well as hypothyroidism corrected by treatment.

BIBLIOGRAPHY. Ross F, Nusynowitz ML: A syndrome of primary hypothyroidism, amenorrhea, and galactorrhea. J Clin Endocrinol 28:591–595, 1968

Mazzaferri EL: The thyroid. In Mazzaferri EL (ed), Textbook of Endocrinology, p 212. New York, Medical Exam Publishing 1985

AMENORRHEA-GALACTORRHEA SYNDROME

Synonyms. Including: Ahumada-del Castillo (Argonz-del Castillo, galactorrhea-amenorrhea in nullipara); Chiari-Frommel (Chiari I, Frommel-Chiari; lactation uterus atrophy; galactorrhea-amenorrhea postpartum); Forbes-Albright (galactorrhea-amenorrhea pituitary enlargement); hyperprolactinemia.

Symptoms and Signs. Association of galactorrhea and amenorrhea concomitant or not with postpartum. Associated with neurological symptoms of pituitary tumor.

Etiology. Increase of prolactin secretion. Adenoma (prolactin secreting) of pituitary.

Diagnostic Procedures. *Blood.* Prolactin values raised; prolactin release test altered (TRH test particularly useful). *Computerized tomography scan of pituitary. MRI.* Pituitary enlargement.

Therapy. If tumor, hypophysectomy or radation. Bromocriptine, lergotrile mesylate.

Prognosis. Avoid pregnancy if pituitary tumor. Depends on stage of disease and treatment.

BIBLIOGRAPHY. Frommel R: Ueber puerperale Atrophie des Uterus. Z Geburtshilfe Gynak 7:305–313, 1882

Chiari JB, Braun C, Spaeth J: Report of diseases of women observed during the years 1848 to 1855, inclusive, in the Department of Gynecology (Municipal Clinic), Vienna Klin. Geburtsh V Gynak: 371, 1855

Ahumada JC, del Castillo EB: Sobre un caso de galactorrea y amenorrea. Bol Soc Obst Gin(Buenos Aires) 11:64–72, 1932

Krestin D: Spontaneous lactation associated with enlargement of pituitary, with report of 2 cases. Lancet 1, 928–930, 1932

Argonz J, del Castillo EB: A syndrome characterized by estrogenic insufficiency, galactorrhea and decreased urinary gonadotropin. J Clin Endocrinol 13:79–87, 1953

Forbes AP, Heunemann PH, Griswald GC, et al: Syndrome characterized by galactorrhea, amenorrhea and low urinary FSH: comparison with acromegaly and normal lactation. J Clin Endocrinol 14:265–271, 1954

Koppelman MCS: Hyperprolactinemia amenorrhea and galactorrhea. Ann Int Med 10:115–121, 1984

AMINOPTERIN

Synonyms. Fetal aminopterin.

Symptoms and Signs. Present at birth. Variable combination of the following: small body; microcephaly; hypoplasia of cranial bones; broad nasal bridge; prominent eyes; micrognathia; cleft palate; low-set ears; short limbs (particularly mesomelic); hypodactyly; talipes equinovarus; hydrocephalus; craniosynostosis.

Etiology. Teratogenic effect of aminopterin and derivatives.

Therapy. Neurosurgery (ventriculo-peritoneal shunt, correction of craniosynostosis).

Prognosis. Frequent fetal or early postnatal death; several patients have survived, with handicaps but normal intelligence.

BIBLIOGRAPHY. Thirsch JB: Therapeutic abortions with a folic acid antagonist: 4 aminopteroylglutamic acid (4 amino PGA) administered by the oral route. Am J Obstet Gynecol 63:1298–1309, 1952

Shaw EB, Steinbach HL: Aminopterin-induced fetal malformation. Am J Dis Child 115:477–482, 1968

Smith DW: Recognizable Patterns of Human Malformation, 3rd ed. Philadelphia, WB Saunders, 1982.

AMNESIA, GLOBAL TRANSIENT

Synonyms. Transient global amnesia; Fisher-Adams.

Symptoms. Occasionally, abrupt onset of profound memory loss and disorientation without consciousness change after sexual intercourse or, in some cases, also after fatigue. No evidence of aphasia or memory alterations.

Signs. Most patients have a history of arterial hypertension. Physical examination otherwise normal.

Etiology. Unknown. Suspected vascular basis, cerebral ischemia in distribution of posterior cerebral arteries supplying inferomedial parts of both temporal areas.

Diagnostic Procedures. *Electroencephalography and CT brain scan.* Negative.

Therapy. None. Treatment of hypertension.

Prognosis. Return of mental state to normality, usually, within 12 to 24 hours. Occurrence of single (usual) or repeated episodes; successive sexual relations could be asymptomatic.

BIBLIOGRAPHY. Fisher CM, Adams RD: Transient global amnesia. Acta Neurol Scand (suppl) 9:7–83, 1964
Matthew NT, Meyer JS: Pathogenesis and natural history of transient global amnesia. Stroke 5:303–311, 1974
Mayeux R: Sexual intercourse and transient global amnesia. Lancet 1:864, 1979
Adams RD, Victor M: Principles of Neurology, 3rd ed, p 319. New York, McGraw-Hill, 1985

AMNIOTIC BAND

Synonyms. Amnion adhesion fetus; Streeter's bands; Adam complex; amputation (congenital); constricting bands; terminal transverse defect of arms.

Symptoms and Signs. Uncommon anomaly, which, rarely, involves the head and, more frequently, the fetal limbs, producing peromelia.

Etiology. Unknown (controversial). Sporadic occurrence possible; genetic origin has been considered. (1) Primary lesion within developing limbs mesenchyme, external band or band only secondary (Streeter). (2) Primary abnormality of the amnion and amniotic bands encircling distal part of limbs (Ballantyne-Smith).

Pathology. Rupture of amnion, chorion intact; amniotic bands producing, on vascular basis, necrosis of fetal limbs.

Therapy. In some cases, surgical procedures to remove constricting band.

Prognosis. Permanent alteration.

BIBLIOGRAPHY. Ballantyne JW: Manual of Antenatal Pathology and Hygiene. The Foetus. Edinburgh, W Greene, 1902
Streeter GL: Focal deficiencies in fetal tissues and their relation to intra-uterine amputation. Contrib Embryol Carnegie Inst Washington 22(126):1–144, 1930
Fiedler JM, Phelan JP: The amniotic band syndrome in monozygotic twins. Am J Obstet Gynecol 146:864–865, 1983

AMNIOTIC FLUID

Synonym. Amniotic fluid embolism.

Symptoms. Sudden dyspnea; shock. Common in multiparas over 30, with history of hard labor or pitocin administration or both.

Signs. Tachypnea; percussion of lung areas obtuse; cyanosis; hypotension. Uterine relaxation followed by profuse vaginal bleeding.

Etiology. Embolism of amniotic fluid into the cardiovascular system causes pulmonary edema, embolic phenomena, depression of fibrinogen in circulation with resulting uncontrollable bleeding.

Pathology. Massive intravascular clotting. Emboli in pulmonary vessels of mucus, amniotic cells and debris; pulmonary edema.

Diagnostic Procedures. *Blood.* Hypofibrinogenemia; prolonged clotting time.

Therapy. Treatment of shock; care to prevent right heart insufficiency. Fibrinogen administration.

Prognosis. Usually fatal.

BIBLIOGRAPHY. Aguillon A, Andjus A, Grayson A, et al: Amniotic fluid embolism: A review. Obstet Gynecol Surv 17:619–636, 1962
Anonymous: Amniotic fluid embolism. Lancet II:398, 1979
Philipp EE, Barnes J, Newton M: Obstetrics and Gynecology, 3rd ed, p 360. London, William Heinemann, 1986

AMOK

Symptoms. Reported in the past in Malayan and African people. Occasionally seen in Western countries. Homicidal attack, preceded by period of depression; preoccupation. In an unprovoked outburst of rage patient runs about armed, usually with a knife, and attacks indiscriminately any person or animal that he encounters before he is overpowered or kills himself.

Etiology. Unknown; toxic or chronic psychotic condition; brain syndromes (see).

Therapy. Overpowering and physical restraint of patient. Then specific antitoxic and psychiatric assistance, removing underlying cause. Prevention through education.

BIBLIOGRAPHY. Westermeyer J: A comparison of amok and other homicide in Laos. Am J Psych 129:708–709, 1972

Murphy HBM: History and evolution of syndromes: The striking case of latah and amok. In Hammer M, Salzinger K, Sutton S (eds): Psychopathology: Contribution from the Social, Behavioral and Biological Sciences. New York, Wiley & Sons, 1973

AMORPHOSYNTHESIS

Symptoms. Both sexes affected; onset at all ages. Neglected extrapersonal or personal space. Usually, unawareness or neglect of left side of the body; inability to orientate to same side space. Patients do not integrate perceptions (hearing; visual) of the affected side in his total consciousness.

Etiology. Brain tumor.

BIBLIOGRAPHY. Denny-Brown D, Meyer JS, Horenstein S: The significance of perceptual rivalry resulting from parietal lesion. Brain 75:433–471, 1952

Adams RD, Victor M: Principles of Neurology, 3rd ed, p 340. New York, McGraw-Hill, 1985

Dimond SJ, Blizard DA: Evolution and lateralization of the brain. Ann NY Acad Sci 299:1–501, 1977

AMOTIVATIONAL

Synonyms. Marijuana toxicity.

Symptoms and Signs. In adolescent marijuana smokers. Energy loss, diminished attentiveness, harmed parental relationship, behavioral disruptions.

Etiology. Marijuana smoking. Many authors contest this syndrome.

BIBLIOGRAPHY. Beaubrun MH, Knight F: Psychiatric assessments of 30 chronic users of cannabis and 30 matched controls. Am J Psychiat 130:309–311, 1983

AMYLOIDOSIS III

Synonyms. Amyloid cardiomyopathy I; Denmark amyloid cardiomyopathy. Denmark type; Fredriksen's.

Symptoms and Signs. Both sexes affected; onset between 37 and 46 years of age. From dyspnea and rather rapidly progressing right heart failure to cachexia and anasarca. Marked splitting of second sound; extrasystoles.

Etiology. Unknown. Autosomal dominant.

Pathology. Thick-walled heart; amyloid infiltration in pericardium. Infiltration of gastrointestinal tract including tongue, peripheral nerves, and fat deposits; lack of infiltration of liver, brain, and skeletal muscles.

Diagnostic Procedures. *X-ray of chest.* Moderate cardiomegaly. *Electrocardiography.* Two categories: (1) right bundle block, left axis deviation, P-R prolonged; (2) left ventricular hypertrophy with left axis deviation or low voltage in peripheral leads. *Heart catheterization.* Low cardiac output; elevation of pulmonary wedge, right atrial, and pulmonary artery pressures.

Therapy. Diuretics give temporary benefit.

Prognosis. Duration of condition for 2 to 6 years from onset. In some cases sudden death or death from congestive heart failure.

BIBLIOGRAPHY. Fredriksen T, Gotzsche H, Harboe N, et al: Familial primary amyloidosis with severe amyloid heart disease. Am J Med 33:328–348, 1962

Husby G, Ranlov PJ, Sletter K, et al: The amyloid in familial amyloidotic cardiomyopathy of Danish origin is related to prealbumin. In Glenner GG: Proceedings of the IV International Symposium on Amyloidosis. Amsterdam, Excerpta Medica, 1985

AMYLOIDOSIS VII

Synonyms. Oculoleptomeningeal amyloidosis; Ohio amyloidosis.

Symptoms and Signs. Dementia, seizures, strokes, visual deterioration, coma; neurological dysfunctions are episodic.

Etiology. Possibly autosomal dominant.

Pathology. Severe diffuse amyloidosis of leptomeninges and subarachnoid vessels; patchy fibrosis and obliteration of subarachnoid space. Diffuse neuronal loss in brain and cerebellum. Occasional superficial brain infarction. Minimal amyloid deposits in other organs, except vitreous and retinal membranes and vessels.

BIBLIOGRAPHY. Goten H, Steinberg MC, Farboody GH: Familial oculoleptomeningeal amyloidosis. Brain 103: 473–495, 1980

AMYLOIDOSIS IX

Synonyms. Amyloidosis primary cutaneous, familial lichen amyloidosis, Lichen amyloidosis.

Symptoms and Signs. More frequent in South America and Asia. Onset at puberty. Intense pruritis, moderate lichenoid lesions. Absence of other signs. Scratching relieves pruritus by removing core of papules.

Etiology. Autosomal dominant inheritance.

BIBLIOGRAPHY. Issak L: Localized amyloid cutis associated with psoriasis in siblings. Arch Dermatol Syph 61:859–862, 1950
Sagher F, Shanon J: Amyloidosis cutis: familial occurrence in three generations. Arch Derm 87:171–175, 1963
Newton JA, Jagjvan A, Bhogal B, et al: Familial primary cutaneous amyloidosis. Br J Derm 112:201–208, 1985

ANALBUMINEMIA

Symptoms. Both sexes affected; present at birth. Asymptomatic or asthenia.

Signs. Mild persistent edema; occasionally, arterial hypotension and mild diarrhea.

Etiology. Defective synthesis of albumin. Likely autosomal recessive inheritance.

Pathology. Reported in some cases, but not likely related to the condition: aortic valve insufficiency; skin changes (angiomas; eczema; lipodystrophy); gynecomastia; rheumatoid arthritis. Related to the condition: high concentration of albumin in the tissue and early arteriosclerotic changes. Liver biopsy shows normal pattern and moderate increase of reticuloendothelial system.

Diagnostic Procedures. *Blood.* Protein electrophoresis shows absence of albumin band, increase of most globulin fractions; immunochemical quantitation confirms lack of or extremely low levels of albumin. IgG and IgM, fibrinogen, alpha₁-acidglycoprotein, alpha₁-antitrypsin, haptoglobulin, C-reactive protein, and prealbumin increased. Beta-lipoproteins, cholesterol, and esterified fatty acids are increased. Free fatty acids are normal. Erythrocyte sedimentation, rarely, increased. Serum osmolality reduced 50%. *Test with injection of albumin.* Marked by (55 days) prolonged survival (normal: 13–21 days).

Therapy. None, or repeated injection of albumin advisable in certain physiopathologic conditions (e.g., pregnancy, infections).

Prognosis. Excellent. No known impairment except from lack of albumin. Increased tendency to arteriosclerotic changes.

BISALBUMINEMIA
Symptoms and Signs. None.

Etiology. Unknown; co-dominant hereditary characteristic with normal and abnormal genes fully expressed.

Diagnostic Procedures. *Protein electrophoresis.* Shows the presence of an abnormal albumin in addition to the normal one.

Therapy. None.

ANOMALOUS ALBUMINEMIA
Congenital abnormality; possibly nonspecifically associated with syndrome of goiter and deafness.

BIBLIOGRAPHY. Bennhold H, Peters H, Roth E: Ueber einen Fall bon kompletter Analbuminaemie ohne wesentliche klinische Krankheitszeichen. Verh Dsch Ges Inn Med Kong 60:630–634, 1954
Scheurlen PG: Ueber Serumeiweissveranderungen beim Diabetes mellitus. Klin Wochenschr 33:198–205, 1955
Fraser GR, Harris H, Robson EB: A new genetically determined plasma-protein in man. Lancet J:1023–1024, 1959
Gitlin D, Schmid K, Earle DP, et al: Observations on double albumin. II. A peptide difference between two genetically determined human serum albumins. J Clin Invest 40:820–827, 1961
Dammacco F, Miglietta A, D'Addabbo A, et al: Analbuminemia: report of a case and review of the literature. Vox Sang 39:153–161, 1980

ANCELL'S

Synonyms. Ancell-Spiegler cylindromas; Brooke-Fordyce trichoepitheliomas; Spiegler's; turban tumors; cylindromatosis.

Symptoms and Signs. Prevalent in females (not definitely established); onset during late childhood or early adolescence. Presence of small scalp lesions (Ancell-Spiegler turban tumors) or facial skin lesions affecting especially nasolabial area (Brooke-Fordyce trichoepitheliomas) or both in the members of affected families. No systemic manifestations.

Etiology. Unknown; autosomal dominant inheritance. Some isolated cases reported (phenocopies).

Pathology. Scalp tumors with appearance of typical cylindromas. Epithelial cell islands surrounded by hyaline membrane. Face tumors, appearance of tricoepitheliomas, cystlike spaces, and horn cells.

Diagnostic Procedures. *Biopsy.*

Therapy. Surgical excision and skin graft. X-ray therapy (may cause chronic ulceration and risk of neoplastic changes).

Prognosis. Benign lesions; occasionally malignant changes (basal cell epithelioma) have been noted.

BIBLIOGRAPHY. Ancell H: History of a remarkable case of tumors, developed on the head and face. Med Chir Trans 25:227–246, 1842
Brooke HG: Epithelioma adenoides cysticum. Br J Dermatol 4:269–286, 1892
Fordyce JA: Multiple benign cystic epitheliomas of the skin. J Cut Dis 10:459–472, 1892
Spiegler E: Ueber Endothelioma der Haut. Arch Dermatol Syph 50:163, 1899
Harper PS: Turban tumors (cylindromatosis). Birth defect Orig Art Ser VII (8)338–341, 1971

ANDERMANN'S

Synonyms. Corpus callosum agenesis–neuropathy; Charlevoix's disease.

Symptoms and Signs. Both sexes. Mental and physical retardation, areflexia, paraparesis. Microcephaly, optic atrophy, seizures. Progressive motor neuropathy.

Etiology. Autosomal recessive inheritance.

Therapy. Orthopedic surgery when needed.

Prognosis. Motor neuropathy leads to loss of ambulation by adolescence and progressive scoliosis.

BIBLIOGRAPHY. Andermann F, Andermann E, Goubert M, et al: Familial agenesis of corpus callosum with anterior horn cell disease. Trans Am Neurol Assoc 97:242–244, 1972
Larbrisseau A, Vanasse M, Brochu P, et al: The Andermann syndrome. Canad J Neurol Sci 11:257–261, 1984

ANDERSEN'S II

Synonyms. Alpha 1,4 glucan: alpha 1,4 glucan 6-gluconyl transferase deficiency; brancher deficiency; amylopectinosis; cirrhosis liver-abnormal glycogen; Cori's type IV glycogenosis; glycogenosis type IV.

Symptoms. Very rare or difficult to identify. Onset in early infancy, full manifestation between 7th and 12th months. Poor development; repeated respiratory infections; hypotonia.

Signs. Marked hepatosplenomegaly with enlargement of abdomen; ascites.

Etiology. Autosomal recessive inheritance (suggested). Alpha 1,4 glucan: alpha 1,4-glucan 6-gluconyl transferase (brancher) deficiency.

Pathology. Liver cirrhosis; complete disruption of architecture; vacuolated cells containing described type of glycogen. Same material (in granular form) has been found in spleen, lymph nodes, lung macrophages, heart, and muscle fibers.

Diagnostic Procedures. *Blood.* Moderate anemia; diminished hyperglycemic response to epinephrine and glucagon. Initially, liver function test slightly impaired; then progressive deterioration and hyperbilirubinemia. *Electroencephalography.* Nonspecific abnormalities.

Therapy. Treatment for liver failure and ascites.

Prognosis. Very poor; invariably fatal. Terminal diarrhea; melena; hyperpyrexia. Older case died at 4 years of age.

BIBLIOGRAPHY. Andersen DH: Studies on glycogen disease with report of a case in which the glycogen was abnormal. In Najjar VA: Carbohydrate Metabolism, pp 28–42. Baltimore, Johns Hopkins University Press, 1952
Andersen DH: Familial cirrhosis of the liver with storage of abnormal glycogen. Lab Inv 5:11–20, 1956
Pearson CM: Glycogen metabolism and storage diseases of type III, IV, and V. Am J Clin Pathol 50:29–43, 1968
Howell RR, Williams SC: The glycogen storage diseases. In Stanbury JB, Wyngaarden JB, Fredrickson DS (eds): The Metabolic Basis of Inherited Disease, 5th ed, p 141. New York, McGraw-Hill, 1983

ANDERSON'S

Synonyms. Osteodysplasia familial.

Symptoms and Signs. Present from birth. Midfacial hypoplasia; mandibular prognathism; pointed chin; mandible with wide angle, increased length, reduced height, and reduced bigonial width. Large ears. Kyphoscoliosis. Hypertension.

Etiology. Unknown; Autosomal recessive inheritance.

Diagnostic Procedures. *X-rays.* Calvaria thinned; mastoid pointed; abnormal ribs; spinous process of cervical vertebra anomalies; superior pubic ramus thin. *Blood.* Hyperuricemia.

BIBLIOGRAPHY. Anderson LG, Cook AJ, Coccaro PJ, et al: Familial osteodysplasia. JAMA 220:1687–1693, 1972

Buchignani JS, Cook AJ, Anderson LG: Roentgenographic findings in familial osteodysplasia. Am J Roentgen 116:602–608, 1972

ANDOGSKY'S

Synonyms. Atopic cataract; cataracta dermatogenes; dermatitis lichenoides pruriens; dermatogenous cataract; nummular eczema; eczema plaques; lichen circumscriptus chronicus (Vidal); pruritus diathesique (Besnier).

Symptoms and Signs. Chronic eczematous skin lesions from childhood, and in third decade of life development of bilateral cataracts. Skin lesions produce lichenification of the skin in the neck, flexor surfaces of extremities, especially elbows and knees. Leonine facies may result from the skin lesions. Atopic keratoconjunctivitis; keratoconus; uveitis; asthma occasionally associated.

Etiology. Unknown; heredity reported in only one case. See Mesoectodermal dysplasia syndromes.

Diagnostic Procedures. *Blood.* Occasionally, eosinophilia.

Therapy. Symptomatic; cataract extraction.

Prognosis. Variable.

BIBLIOGRAPHY. Andogsky N: Cataracta dermatogenes. Klin Monatbl Augenheilk 52:824–831, 1914

Thannhauser SJ: Werner's syndrome (progeria of adult) and Tothmund's syndrome: Two types of closely related heredofamilial atrophic dermatosis with juvenile cataracts and endocrine features; a critical study with five new cases. Ann Intern Med 23:559–626, 1945

Reed CE, Friedlaender M: Immunologic aspects of disease of the eye. JAMA 248:2692–2699, 1982

ANDRADE'S

Synonyms. Transthyretin abnormality; TTR abnormality; prealbumin defect; amyloidosis I, amyloidosis neuropathic; Portuguese type amyloidosis (including Japanese, British, and Swedish types).

Symptoms. Both sexes affected; onset in second to fourth decades. Orthostatic hypotension precedes other symptoms. Insidious progression of initial peripheral symmetric paresthesias of lower extremities, slowly to motor weakness (difficulty in walking), and eventually spreading into upper extremities and trunk. Cyclic diarrhea and constipation; impotence. Heat intolerance; hoarseness (rare); occasional blurring of vision.

Signs. Pupils irregular and unequal; sluggish reaction to light. Dissociation of sensory impairment: pain and temperature affected, while vibration and position spared. Tendon reflexes gradually lost. Trophic ulcers on the legs. Muscle wasting not prominent. Occasionally, cardiomegaly. In some families vitreous opacity and exophthalmos may be associated.

Etiology. Unknown; autosomal dominant inheritance.

Pathology. Amyloid material infiltrating autonomic ganglia, spinal nerve roots and peripheral nerves between fibers and vessel walls. Brain and spinal cord not involved.

Diagnostic Procedures. *Blood.* Normal (occasionally, anemia). *Electrocardiography.* S-T and T wave changes. *Spinal fluid.* Moderate increase of protein. *Biopsy of nerve.* *X-ray.* Occasionally, osteoporosis of metatarsal and phalanges or circumscribed translucent areas.

Therapy. None.

Prognosis. Death occurs in approximately 10 years from cachexia, intercurrent infections, and other complications.

BIBLIOGRAPHY. De Bruyer RS, Stern RO: A case of progressive hypertrophic polyneuritis of Dejerine and Sottas with pathological examination. Brain 52:84–107, 1929

Andrade C: A peculiar form of peripheral neuronopathy: Familial typical generalized amyloidosis with special involvement of the peripheral nerves. Brain 75:408–427, 1952

Benson MD, Dwulet FE: Identification of carriers of variant plasma prealbumin (transthyretin) associated with familial amyloidotic polyneuropathy type I. J Clin Invest 75:71–75, 1985

ANEMIC-HEMATURIC

Synonyms. Hematuria-anemia.

Symptoms and Signs. Vary with season in which they occur. Constant asthenia; fever; tachycardia; anemia; vesiculoerythematous dermatitis may occur in either season. *Summer.* Anorexia; vomiting; gastralgia; diarrhea; jaundice; dehydration; nervousness. *Winter.* Edema; oliguria; hematuria; albuminuria; cylindruria; increase of anemia.

Etiology. Unknown. Epidemic in Argentina, in relation with a regional cattle disease.

Therapy. Symptomatic.

Prognosis. Long convalescence without complication.

BIBLIOGRAPHY. Villar JB: Epidemic anemic-hematuric syndrome. Rev Asoc Med Argent 62:649, 1948 (abst) JAMA 140:364, 1949

ANETODERMA, PERIFOLLICULAR

Symptoms. Appear in women of advanced age.

Signs. Bluish-reddish spots on internal side of thighs.

Etiology. Unknown. Endocrine factors (?); fat accumulation (?). Elastase-producing strains of *Staphylococcus* could be responsible.

Pathology. Thinning of epidermis; thickening of horny layer; widening of follicles; and formation of keratinized masses. In some cases, prolapse of fatty tissue toward epidermis.

Diagnostic Procedures. None, or *biopsy*.

Therapy. None. Penicillin topical and general in early stage.

Prognosis. Persistent asymptomatic condition.

BIBLIOGRAPHY. Rook A, Wilkinson DS, Ebling FJG, et al: Textbook of Dermatology, 4th ed, p 1805. Oxford, Blackwell Scientific Publications, 1986

ANEURYSM OF AORTA

Synonyms. Dissecting aortic hematoma; dissecting aortic aneurysm; abdominal aortic aneurysm, AAA; aortic aneurysm.

Symptoms. Appears mostly in young men; followed by equal incidence between two sexes; onset from 40 to 70 years of age. Severe anterior chest pain not responding to morphine or responding only to high doses. Strongest at onset (and not progressing as in myocardial infarction) radiating mostly to the back, to the abdomen, legs, neck, and head. Pain in some cases may be missing. Shock; coma; hemiplegia; confusion; weakness of legs.

Signs. Absent or unequal pulsations of carotid, brachial, femoral arteries occurring immediately or within a few hours of onset of pain. Pulsation of sternoclavicular joint. Distension of neck veins, heart systolic and diastolic murmur (10–15% of cases). Blood pressure high (contrasting with signs of shock, pallor, tachypnea).

Etiology. Dissecting aneurysm of the aorta usually found in association with cystic medial necrosis; in some cases, associated with pregnancy, coarctation of aorta, aortic stenosis, myxedma, atheromatous aortic lesion, aortic abscess. Reported familial autosomal inheritance of condition.

Pathology. Transverse tear of the intima a few cm from aortic valve. Intramural hematoma (sometimes blood re-enters aorta through another intimal lesion). Following De Bakey's nomenclature proximal dissection is type I and distal dissection is type III; in type II dissection is limited to the ascending aorta.

Diagnostic Procedures. *Electrocardiography.* Left ventricular hypertrophy; no specific changes; pericarditis. *X-ray.* Enlargement of aorta. *Blood.* Anemia; leukocytosis; increase of bilirubin. *Urine.* Red blood cell; albumin; casts. *Echocardiography, aortography, CT scan, and digital subtraction angiography.*

Therapy. Medical treatment only palliative effect and symptomatic. Surgery to create a reentry into the aorta, and suturing of the false lumen; when possible aortic replacement.

Prognosis. Usually fatal in hours or days; spontaneous reentry of blood into the aorta improves symptomatology and chance of survival. Surgical treatment mortality about 25%.

Subdivision of the clinical pattern of aneurysm of the aorta on the basis of the dominant clinical symptoms and signs gives five syndromes:

1. *Cardiovascular.* Hypertension, chest pain, cardiac failure dominate, making the differential diagnosis from that of myocardial infarction very difficult.
2. *Cerebral.* Neurologic findings with confusion and coma confuse the diagnosis with that of a vascular cerebral accident.
3. *Pulmonary.* Dyspnea, parenchymal changes, left hemothorax suggest the diagnosis of pneumonia.
4. *Abdominal.* Pain in the epigastrium is present in 60% of the cases in which pain is a symptom of dissecting aneurysm; hematemesis and melena and in some cases an abdominal mass may simulate intestinal bleeding from peptic ulcer or suggest the diagnosis of a tumor.
5. *Renal.* Involvement of the renal artery gives pain and hematuria as main symptoms, focusing the attention on the kidney rather than the aorta.

BIBLIOGRAPHY. Baer S, Goldburgh H: The varied clinical syndromes produced by dissecting aneurysm. Am Heart J 35:198–211, 1948
Hirst AE, Hohns VJ Jr, Kime SW Jr: Dissecting aneurysm of aorta: a review of 505 cases. Medicine 37:217–279, 1950
De Bakey ME, Henley WS, Cooley DA: Surgical management of dissecting aneurysms of aorta. J Thorac Cardiovasc Surg 49:130–149, 1965

Johnson G Jr, Avery A, McDougal EG, et al: Aneurysm of the abdominal aorta: incidence in blacks and whites in North Carolina. Arch Surg 120:1138–1140, 1985

ANGELUCCI'S

Synonyms. Critical allergic conjunctivitis; spring catarrah; periodic allergic conjunctivitis; vernal conjunctivitis.

Symptoms. Both sexes affected; onset at any age, but mainly in young adults: in patients with allergic condition in the family. Recurrence usually in the spring. Cutaneous or mucous itching with sudden onset and sudden termination. Reaction may always affect the same site or alternate. Lacrimation; photophobia; excitability.

Signs. Conjunctival congestion; generally watery discharge, which may become stringy secretion; granulations on upper tarsus or gelatinous perilimbic areas. Vasomotor lability; tachycardia.

Etiology. Unknown. In the group of allergic diseases.

Pathology. Large cobblestonelike tissue changes, known as giant papillae, most prominent on the upper palpebral conjunctiva. Local synthesis of IgE occurs in them. Histologically, high number of basophils, eosinophils and mast cells. White opacities (Trantas' dots), containing eosinophils, may be seen at the corneoscleral limbus. Their presence parallels the activity of the disease.

Diagnostic Procedures. *Blood.* Occasionally, eosinophilia. *Conjunctival smear.* Negative for bacteria; eosinophilic cells usually present. *Skin test.* Positive for several antigens, especially pollens. Most patients have elevated serum IgE levels and also elevated tear levels of IgE.

Therapy. Topical vasoconstrictors; cold compresses; moving to a cool climate or air-conditioning the patient's room can be useful. Topical corticosteroids may relieve symptoms but are not recommended for long-term use because of their ocular side effects (glaucoma, cataract formation, opportunistic infections). Specific treatment for desensitization.

Prognosis. The disease usually subsides with aging of the patient.

BIBLIOGRAPHY. Angelucci A: Di una sindrome sconosciuta negli infermi di catarro primaverile. Arch Ottol (Palermo) 5:270–276, 1897–98
Reed CE, Friedlander M: Immunologic aspects of diseases of the eye. JAMA 248:2692–2695, 1982
Feducowicz HB, Stetson S: External infections of the eye: bacterial, viral and mycotic, with noninfections and immunologic disease, 3rd ed. Norwalk, Conn, Appleton-Century-Croft, 1985

ANGIECTASIS PREGNANCY

Synonym. Hemangiomas in pregnancy.

Symptoms. Occur in less than 5% of pregnancies. Appearance of well-defined small areas, painful, with increased temperature on posterior side of legs during third month of pregnancy.

Signs. Intradermal, raised cluster of blood vessels in the back of legs.

Etiology. Relationship between lesion and female sex hormones has been postulated. More painful lesions observed with lower level of estrogen or pregnanediol.

Treatment. Estrogen administration.

Prognosis. May disappear spontaneously in a few weeks or persist during entire pregnancy. Pain disappears with estrogen administration.

BIBLIOGRAPHY. Rook A, Wilkinson DS, Ebling FJG, et al: Textbook of Dermatology, 4th ed, p. 275. Oxford, Blackwell Scientific Publications, 1986

ANGIOIMMUNOBLASTIC LYMPHADENOPATHY

Synonyms. Immunoblastic lymphadenopathy.

Symptoms. Fever; sweating; pruritus; rash; anorexia.

Signs. Weight loss; generalized lymphadenopathy.

Etiology. Unknown. Abnormal immune state. Aggressive lymphoma or nonneoplastic hyperimmune proliferation of B lymphocytes.

Pathology. *Lymph nodes.* Loss of architecture; lymphocyte depletion; pleomorphic infiltrate (histiocytes, plasma cells etc); vascular proliferation and infiltration by amorphous eosinophilic material.

Diagnostic Procedures. *Biopsy of lymph node.* See Pathology. *X-rays.* Lung initially has coarse, reticulonodular pattern, then consolidation; mediastinal lymph node enlargement. *Blood.* Hypergammaglobulinemia. Polyclonal hypergammaglobulinemia. Hemolytic anemia, positive Coombs' test.

Therapy. Corticosteroids and immunosuppressive agents.

Prognosis. Poor. Death in one year.

BIBLIOGRAPHY. Frizzera G, Moran EM, Rappaport H: Angio-immunoblastic lymphadenopathy with dysproteinemia. Lancet 1:1070–1073, 1974

Azevedo SJ, Yunis AA: Angioblastic lymphoadenopathy Am J Hematol 20:301–312, 1985

ANGIOMA, MULTIPLE PROGRESSIVE

Symptoms. Appear in both sexes; onset in infancy or adolescence.

Signs. Bluish, compressible nodules, scattered along the course of a vein appear on face or extremities or both, in the subcutaneous tissue.

Etiology. Possibly congenital malformation.

Pathology. Cavernous angioma.

Therapy. Surgical excision.

Prognosis. After months or years, spontaneous disappearance.

BIBLIOGRAPHY. Rook A, Wilkinson DS, Ebling FJG, et al: Textbook of Dermatology, 4th ed, p 2464. Oxford, Blackwell Scientific Publications, 1986

ANGIOMA NEUROCUTANEOUS, HEREDITARY

Symptoms and Signs. Both sexes. Presence of angiomas at various sites with wide distribution on the skin. Sudden hemiparesis or strokes. Absence of retinal angiomas or telengiectases.

Etiology. Autosomal dominant.

Pathology. Typical cavernous angiomas.

Therapy. Surgery.

Prognosis. Death at different ages due to strokes.

BIBLIOGRAPHY. Zaremba J, Stapien M, Jellowicka M, et al: Hereditary neurocutaneous angioma: a new genetic entity? J Med Genet 16: 443–447, 1979

ANGIONEUROTIC EDEMA, HEREDITARY

Synonym. Hereditary angioedema; angioedema hereditary; Hane; C1 esterase inhibitor deficiency; Osler (W)I; C1-INH.

Symptoms and Signs. Rare condition. Both sexes affected; onset in early childhood. Episodes may be elicited by traumas (especially dental). Nausea; vomiting; colics; painless swellings of skin and mucosae; itching. Circumscribed edema in various areas of skin and mucosae; in some cases, signs simulating acute abdomen; in other cases only edema of glottis.

Etiology. Unknown; autosomal dominant. Hereditary absence of C1 inhibitor causes excessive production and slow catabolism of activated C1 which increases permeability of vessels and starts complement cascade. Angioedema due to *acquired* C1-inhibitor deficiency can occur, as a consequence of B-cell lymphoproliferative disorders such as chronic lymphatic leukemia, multiple myeloma, or essential cryoglobulinemia. In this case the defect is due not to defective synthesis but to markedly increased catabolism of the C1-inhibitor protein.

Diagnostic Procedures. *Blood.* Decreased C2 and C4 component of complement. Measurements of C1-INH, reduction of serum levels of C1, C4, and C2.

Therapy. Prophylaxis of attacks by administration of inhibitors of the conversion of plasminogen to plasmin: anabolic steroids. During attacks plasma transfusions. Infusion of fresh plasma; danazol and stanozolol (nonvirilizing androgen). Tried also epsilon-aminocaproic acid and tranexamic acid.

Prognosis. Response to treatment generally poor; over 20% die of laryngeal obstruction before early middle age.

BIBLIOGRAPHY. Osler W: Hereditary angio-neurotic oedema. Am J Med Sci 95:362–367, 1888
Hartmann L: L'oedemic angioneurotique hereditaire a propos de 185 malades et 40 families. Bull Acad Nat Med 167:343–351, 1983

ANIRIDIA

Synonyms. Iridemia.

Symptoms and Signs. Frequency in general population 1:50,000 to 1:100,000. Present from birth; usually bilateral (hereditary); or later in any period of life (traumatic). Impaired vision. Vestigial iris; various deformities of anterior eye.

Etiology. (1) Dominant type; (2) recessive (two-thirds of cases): sporadic, frequently associated with various conditions (cerebellar ataxia; mental retardation with microcephaly; Wilms' tumor, Marinesco's; Sjögren's syndromes). (3) Trauma.

Pathology. Various aspects (see Diagnostic procedures).

Diagnostic Procedures. *Ophthalmoscopy.* (1) Hereditary dominant: thin iris margin associated or not associated with cataract or glaucoma. (2) Hereditary recessive: macula normal aspect. (3) Traumatic: iridodialysis; iris contracted or sinking (or both); partial inversion; hyphemia; partial dislocation of lens. Sporadic aniridia is associated with an increased incidence of Wilms' tumor;

periodic abdominal examination, supplemented by ultrasound examination or intravenous pyelography is advised in all children with sporadic aniridia.

Therapy. Hereditary form: none. Traumatic form: cold applications; silk anchoring suture of periphery of iris.

Prognosis. Hereditary: poor. Traumatic: variable according to lesions and time of repair.

BIBLIOGRAPHY. Mollenbach CJ: Congenital defects in internal membrane of the eye. Clinical and genetic aspects. In Opera ex Domo Biologiae Heriditariae Humanae Universitatis Hafniensis, Vol 15, p 152. Copenhagen, Munksgaard (ed), 1947

Shaw MW, Falls HF, Neel JV: Congenital aniridia. Am J Hum Genet 12:389–415, 1960

François J, Coucke D, Coppieters R: Aniridia Wilms' tumor syndrome. Ophthalmologica 174:35–39, 1977

ANKYLOBLEFARON FILIFORME ADENATUM–CLEFT PALATE

Symptoms and Signs. At birth oval facies, broadened nasal bridge, maxillary hypoplasia, cleft lip, cleft palate, widely spaced teeth, hypodontia, ankyloblepharon filiforme adnatum, palmar plantar keratoma, partial anhydrosis, hyperpigmentation, alopecia. Normal intelligence. Occasionally: deafness, cup-shaped auricles, lacrimal duct atresia, supernumerary nipples, syndactyly. Rarely: heart defects.

Etiology. Autosomal dominant.

Therapy. Surgical excision of ankyloblepharon, surgical closure of facial clefting.

Prognosis. Good *quoad vitam.*

BIBLIOGRAPHY. Khama N: Ankyloblepharon filiforme adenatum. Am J Ophthalmol 43:774–777, 1957

Akkermans CH, Skern LM: Ankyloblepharon filiforme adenatum. Br J Ophthalmol 63:129–131, 1979

ANKYLOSING SPONDYLITIS–AORTIC INSUFFICIENCY

Symptoms and Signs. Two percent present aortic regurgitation at 10 years, 30 years later up to 10%. Aortic insufficiency initially silent course, then becomes manifest.

Etiology and Pathology. Inflammatory process extended immediately above and below aortic valve causing aortic insufficiency.

Therapy. That of ankylosing spondylitis. When aortic insufficiency becomes manifest, valve replacement may be considered.

Prognosis. Not particularly severe.

BIBLIOGRAPHY. Graham DC, Smythe HA: The carditis and aortitis of ankylosing spondylitis. Bull Rheumat Dis 9:171–174, 1958

Roberts WC, Hollingsworth JF, Bulkley BH: Combined mitral and aortic regurgitation in ankylosing spondylitis. Am J Med 56:237–243, 1974

ANORECTAL

See Janbon's and see pseudomembranous enterocolitis.

Symptoms. Burning, anal pruritus, sometimes diarrhea, appearing after administration of large spectrum antibiotic.

Signs. Redness around the anus.

Etiology. Antibiotic modification of intestinal flora.

Therapy. Discontinuation of antibiotic. Symptomatic: cortisone ointment or suppository.

Prognosis. Recovery in a few days except for possible further development and evolution into Pseudomembranous Enterocolitis (see).

BIBLIOGRAPHY. Borriello SP (ed): Antibiotic-associated diarrhea and colitis. Amsterdam, Martinus Nijhoff, 1984

ANOREXIA NERVOSA

Synonym. Apepsia hysterica; Magersucht.

Symptoms. Occur in young girls from adolescence to early adulthood. Not eating and other disturbances of eating function because of morbid aversion to food. Occasionally, vomiting, abdominal symptoms (belching; sensation of fullness; dull pain; nausea); usually, constipation, occasionally diarrhea. Depression and other neurotic symptoms. Continuing vigorous activity despite rapidly increasing cachexia. Closely bound with parents, but with underlying hostility against one or both of them. Lack of sexual adjustment. Weight loss; menstrual disturbance. Seldom observed in adolescent boys.

Signs. Severe cachexia, absence of hair.

Etiology. Unknown. Compulsive neurosis with a pattern fixed on refusal to eat.

Pathology. Loss of fat deposits; severe generalized cachexia; osteoporosis.

Diagnostic Procedures. *Urine.* Determination of follicle-stimulating hormone (FSH), 17-ketosteroids. *X-ray of skull and chest. Blood.* Normal serum protein; anemia, leukopenia; bone marrow hypoplasia.

Therapy. Psychiatric care; if no response, hospitalization and tube feeding.

Prognosis. Symptomatic recovery or chronic course with fluctuations of symptoms for many years. Mortality from 4% to 30% (inanition or infections).

Therapy. Imipramine. In the male antidepressant medication alone is frequently adequate.

BIBLIOGRAPHY. Morton R: Phisiologia or a Treatise of Consumptions. London, 1689
Gull WW: Address in medicine. Lancet II:171–176, 1868
Nemiah JC: Anorexia nervosa: Clinical psychiatric study. Medicine 29:225–268, 1950
Browning CH, Miller SI; Anorexia nervosa: a study in prognosis and management. Am J Psychiatr 124:1128–1132, 1968
Adams RD, Victor M: Principles of Neurology, 3rd ed, pp 1131–1133. New York, McGraw-Hill, 1985

ANOSOGNOSIA

Synonyms. Asomatognosia. See Anton-Babinski and Gerstmann's.

Symptoms. Inability of the patient to recognize a body or functional defect such as the existence of hemiparesis; blindness (see Anton's); postoperative states; vomiting; sphincter incontinence. Denies the existence of the condition and attempts to disprove it by going through psychic process that lets him convince himself that what is said by the physician is false.

Etiology. Organic brain diseases; increased intracranial pressure; bleeding; tumor.

Therapy. Depending upon etiology.

Prognosis. Some cases may respond to treatment.

BIBLIOGRAPHY. Adams RD, Victor M: Principles of Neurology, 3rd ed, pp 339–340. New York, McGraw-Hill, 1985

ANOXIC OVERWEAR

Synonyms. Contact lens reaction; pupillary conjunctivitis.

Symptoms and Signs. Refractive error, corneal neovascularization, papillary conjunctivitis.

Etiology. Hydrogel lens reaction due to reduction in oxygen supply. Allergic or toxic reaction to cleaning and preservative liquids.

Pathology. Endothelial cell changes.

Prognosis. Good with substitution to eyeglasses.

BIBLIOGRAPHY. Binder PS: The physiologic effects of extended wear of soft contact lenses. Ophthalmology 87:745–749, 1980

ANTERIOR ABDOMINAL WALL

Symptoms. Two subtypes according to localization of pain: (1) *Lower quadrant area* right or left; (2) *superior margins of upper quadrant.* Pain: continuous; sometimes in relation with motion; no relation with food ingestion or evacuation.

Signs. With patient lying on his back, firmly compress with single finger or thumb the painful area and ask the patient to raise both legs a few inches. If pain increases because of the contraction of muscles, it is of abdominal wall origin; if decreased, it is of visceral origin.

Etiology. Unknown. It may be associated with, but independent from gastrointestinal disorders.

Pathology. No specific changes of muscles.

Diagnostic Procedures. Tests for differential diagnosis of gastrointestinal diseases.

Therapy. Infiltration of various abdominal layers with hydrocortisone.

BIBLIOGRAPHY. Long C: Myofascial pain syndromes. Henry Ford Hosp Med Bull 4:102–106, 1956
Steinheber FV: Medical conditions mimicking the acute surgical abdomen. Med Clin N Am 57:1559–1567, 1973
Wilson DH, Wilson PD, Walmsley RJ, et al: Diagnosis of acute abdominal pain in the accident and emergency department. Br J Surg 64:250–254, 1977

ANTERIOR CERVICAL CORD

Synonyms. Cervical cord, anterior.

Symptoms and Signs. Complete motor loss of pain and temperature differentiation below level of injury with spared deep touch, position, and vibratory sensation.

Etiology. Direct trauma from spinal hyperextension, hyperflexion extrusion of intervertebral disc, or secondary to lesion of anterior spinal artery system.

Therapy. Trial with corticosteroid immediately after trauma or surgery.

Prognosis. Complete paralysis and absolute loss of pain and temperature sensation lasts usually 48 hours but sensation is never recovered completely below the affected level.

BIBLIOGRAPHY. Schneider RC, Kaln EA: Chronic neurological sequelae of acute trauma to the spine and spinal cord. Part II: The syndrome of chronic anterior spinal cord injury or compression: herniated intervertebral discs. J Bone Joint Surg 41 A:449–456, 1959

ANTERIOR CHEST WALL SYNDROMES

Synonyms. Costal margin; costochondral junction; inframammary; pectoralis major; xiphoid process; chest wall pain.

Symptoms and Signs. Pain of somatic structures of anterior chest wall associated with marked tenderness on fingertip pressure; not relieved by rest, food, or nitroglycerine. According to localization, five subtypes have been recognized.
1. *Pectoralis major syndrome.* More frequent on left side. Pain present in the upper half of chest, second and third costal region; on occasion pain may radiate to arm. It may exist in association with cardiac disease. Responds to specific treatment (see).
2. *Inframammary syndrome.* More frequent in women on the left side. Pain present under the breast in the midclavicular line sixth-seventh costal region. It may coexist with gastrointestinal pathology. Responds to specific treatment and when associated with an antispastic and antacids.
3. *Coastal margin syndrome.* Both sides of chest. Pain localized on the margins of the eighth, ninth, and tenth ribs at their conjunction. Responds to specific treatment.
4. *Costochondral junction syndrome.* Tietze's syndrome (see). Pain in the upper chest at the costochondral junctions. Responds to specific treatment.
5. *Xiphoid process syndrome* (see).

Etiology. Unknown.

Pathology. Finding inconsistent; occasionally, lymphocytic infiltration of connective tissue; muscle degeneration. In Tietze syndrome, osteochondritis.

Therapy. Injections of corticosteroid on the trigger points rapidly relieve the symptoms. If area of pain too extensive, adrenal steroid or derivatives orally, or local ethyl chloride spray.

Prognosis. Good or depending on possible coexisting associations.

BIBLIOGRAPHY. Prinzmetal M, Massumi R: The anterior chest wall syndrome—chest pain resembling pain of cardiac origin. JAMA 159:177–184, 1955
Long C: Myofascial pain syndromes. Henry Ford Hosp Med Bull 4:102–106, 1956
Hurst JW: The Heart, 6th ed, p 918. New York, McGraw-Hill, 1986

ANTERIOR CHOROIDAL ARTERY

Synonyms. Von Monakow's; Monakow's.

Symptoms and Signs. Hemiplegia; hemianesthesia, hemianopia; contralateral to lesion. Actual clinical pattern rather variable and the hemianesthesia and hemianopia may be partial.

Etiology. Rupture or thrombosis of antieror choroidal artery; aneurysm; or tumor.

Pathology. Softening and hemorrhage on posterior part of internal capsule; globus pallidus; lateral geniculate body; and area of origin of optic nerve.

Diagnostic Procedures. *Spinal tap. Angiography. CT brain scan.*

Therapy. Symptomatic, or surgery if indicated.

Prognosis. Poor, depending on site of occlusion.

BIBLIOGRAPHY. Kolinsko A: Ueber die Beziehung der Arteria choroidea anterior zum hinteren Schenkel der inneren Kapsul des Genhirnes. Vienna, 1891
Steegmann AT, Roberts DJ: The syndrome of the anterior choroidal artery. JAMA 104:1695–1697, 1935
Masson M, Decroix JP, Henin D, et al: Syndrome de l'artère choroidienne antérieure. Rev Neurol 139:547–552, 1983

ANTERIOR CORNUAL

Synonyms. Anterior spinal; anterior myelopathy.

Symptoms. Motor disturbance due to muscular atrophy and paralysis of different muscles of extremities or trunk or both, in combination or affecting single muscles; urinary disturbances if bladder is affected.

Signs. Fasciculation and finally after weeks or months, paralysis and atrophy of single (occasional) or group of muscles, loss of reflexes, sensorium intact or temporarily mildly affected. Electric reaction of degeneration can be demonstrated in denervated muscles. Trophic changes of the overlying skin, which appears cyanotic and cold.

Etiology. Degenerative lesions of nervous tissue selectively involving anterior cornua of spinal cord. Progressive muscular atrophy; poliomyelitis; amyotrophic lateral sclerosis; syphilis.

Pathology. Varies according to etiology. Initial hyperemia of pia vessels and affected gray matter; later edema and yellow-gray color and softening of gray matter. Microscopically, degenerative and necrotic changes.

Diagnostic Procedures. Findings vary according to etiology. *Blood.* Leukocytosis in poliomyelitis. *Cerebrospinal fluid.* Various changes according to stages.

Therapy. Depends upon etiology.

Prognosis. Depends upon etiology.

BIBLIOGRAPHY. Adams RD, Victor M: Principles of Neurology, 3rd ed, p 126. New York, McGraw-Hill, 1985

ANTERIOR ETHMOIDAL NERVE

Symptoms. Bilateral intense continuous pain over frontal, parietal, occipital, and vertical areas; recurrent aching and stiffness of neck, lasting one or more days.

Signs. Hypersensitive areas around the anterior ethmoidal foramen and over the path of nasal nerves.

Etiology and Pathology. Hypersensitivity reaction due to surface or intratissue (or both) pressure at the anterior ethmoidal foramen and the foramen of the middle turbinate body causing interference with normal conduction of the action current.

Diagnostic Procedures. Touching the area around the anterior ethmoidal foramen lightly with an applicator causes sharp intense pain. Epinephrine solution 3% applied to the area reduces the symptoms effectively, but temporarily.

Therapy. Epinephrine application; in severe cases resection of the anterior ethmoidal nerves.

Prognosis. Recovery with surgery; improvement with medical treatment.

BIBLIOGRAPHY. Burnham HH: Anterior ethmoidal nerve syndrome: Referred pain and headache from lateral nasal wall. Arch Otolaryngol 50:640–646, 1949

ANTERIOR INTEROSSEUS

Symptoms and Signs. Pain in the proximal forearm lasting hours. Weakness or paralysis of flexor pollicis longus, flexor digitorum profundus (to index and long fingers) and pronator quadratus. Pinching is impossible. Variation or pattern according to abnormal innervation.

Etiology. Trauma or nerve entrapment of medium nerve by tendons, arteries; thrombosis of vessels; Volkmann's (see) contracture.

Diagnostic Procedures. *Electromyography. Triketohydrindene hydrate test.*

Therapy. Surgery to free the nerve in all cases if traumatic nature; and in spontaneous cases, when there is no improvement after 12 weeks.

Prognosis. Good with proper treatment.

BIBLIOGRAPHY. Wright P: Peripheral nerve injury. In Crenshaw AH (ed): Campbell's Operative Orthopedics, 7th ed, pp 2824–2827. St. Louis, CV Mosby, 1987

ANTERIOR TIBIAL COMPARTMENT

See Overuse syndromes.

Synonyms. March; March gangrene.

Symptoms. Pain of muscles of anterior tibial region; sensory loss in foot and leg. Pretibial exercise pain in chronic states.

Signs. Redness, swelling, tenderness in anterior tibial region.

Etiology. Injury of muscle or overstraining causes compression of tibial arteries and lymphatics. Anterior tibial nerve lesion (?); spasm, or thrombosis or embolism of anterior tibial artery (?); accumulation of fluid in the anterior tibial compartment.

Pathology. Biopsy of muscle shows various degrees of necrosis. In chronic stage, possible tendonitis.

Therapy. Bed rest; analgesic; fasciotomy in refractory cases.

Prognosis. If fasciotomy performed in time, good recovery; if excessively delayed, irreversible changes and persistent neuromyopathy.

BIBLIOGRAPHY. Bhild CG: Noninfective gangrene following fractures of lower leg. Ann Surg 116:721–728, 1942

Vogt PR: Ischemic necrosis of anterior crurual muscles. Read at Oregon Med Soc, Sept 4, 1943

Justis EJ: Traumatic disorders. In AH Crenshaw (ed): Campbell's Operative Orthopedics. 7th ed, pp 2223–2225. St Louis, CV Mosby, 1987

ANTIMONGOLISM

Synonyms. Chromosome 21 partial deletion; G-deletion; long arm 21 deletion; monosomy-21 partial; 21g-. See G-deletion syndromes.

Symptoms and Signs. Mental retardation; muscle hypertonia; downward slope of eyes (antimongoloid); blepharochalasis; occasional cataracts; large external ear; wide external auditory canal; prominent nasal bridge; micrognathia; systolic murmur; pyloric stenosis; cryptorchidism; hypospadias; skeletal system shows retarded growth and various defects; nails dystrophic; normal palmar folds.

Etiology. Deletion of a part of a G-group chromosome, possibly 21 or 22.

Pathology. See Signs.

Diagnostic Procedures. *Chromosome studies. Blood.* Thrombocytopenia; eosinophilia; normal or elevated leukocyte alkaline phosphatase.

Therapy. None.

BIBLIOGRAPHY. Lejeune J, Berger R, Rethore MO, et al: Monosomie partielle pour un petit acrocentrique. CR Acad Sci (Paris) 259:4187–4190, 1964

Greenwood RD, Sommer A: Monosomy G: Case report and review of literature. J Med Genet 8:496–500, 1971

Fryns JP, D'Hondt F, Goddeeris P, et al: Full monosomy 21: a clinically recognizable syndrome? Hum Genet 37:155–159, 1977

ANTITHROMBIN III DEFICIENCY

Synonyms. Hereditary antithrombin III deficiency.

Symptoms and Signs. Both sexes. From teenage: thromboembolic disease, ulcers of lower part of legs.

Etiology. Autosomal dominant.

Diagnostic Procedures. *Blood antithrombin III assay.* Antithrombin III may be greatly reduced or normal (inactive protein).

Therapy. Coumarin anticoagulants.

Prognosis. Depends on severity of thrombosis.

BIBLIOGRAPHY. Marcinia KE, Farley CH, De Simone PA: Familial thrombosis due to antithrombin III deficiency. Blood 43:219, 1974

Sas G, Peto I, Banhegyi D, et al: Heterogeneity of the classical antithrombin III deficiency. Thromb Haemost 44:133, 1980

ANTLEY-BLIXER

Synonyms. Trapezoidocephaly-synostosis; multisynostotic osteodysgenesis–long bone fractures; osteodysgenesis-multisynostosis-fractures, long bones.

Symptoms and Signs. From birth. Both sexes. Midface hypoplasia, trapezoidocephaly; humeroradialsynostosis; femoral bowing; easy bone fractures (frequently connatal).

Etiology. Sporadic and autosomal recessive inheritance.

Pathology. Associated possible heart and kidney malformations.

Prognosis. Poor. Respiratory failure as possible cause of death.

BIBLIOGRAPHY. Antley RM, Blixen D: Trapezoidocephaly, midface hypoplasia and cartilage abnormalities with multiple synostosis and skeletal fractures. Birth Def Orig Art Ser XI(2):397–401, 1975

Antley RM, Bixler D: Development in trapezoidocephaly–multiple synostosis syndrome. Am J Med Genet 14:149–150, 1983

ANTON-BABINSKI

Synonyms. Asomatoagnosia unilateral.

Symptoms and Signs. In patient with dense left hemiplegia. Conceptual negation of paralysis anosognosia: unawareness or indifference toward the condition expressed by denial of it, admission of weakness, justification by pain that prevents movements, denial of the left part of body as if not belonging and relative neglect of it (dressing apraxia).

Frequently associated: mental derangements, blunted emotivity, illusions, hallucinations of movements, allocheiria, disturbed perception of space.

Etiology and Pathology. Lesion of the cortex, and white matter of the superior parietal lobule. Its variable extension into post-central gyrus, frontal motor areas, and temporal and occipital lobes explains the possible associated anomalies. In right hemiplegia symptoms obscured by concurrent aphasia.

BIBLIOGRAPHY. Anton G: Ueber die Selbstwahrnehmung der Herderkrankungen des Gehinrs durch den Krauken bei Rindenblindheit und Rindentaubheit. Arch Psychiat Nervenkr 32:86, 1899

Adams RD, Victor M: Principles of Neurology, 3rd ed, p 342. New York, McGraw-Hill, 1985

ANTON'S

Synonyms. Denial–visual hallucination; visual anosognosia.

Symptoms. Denial of blindness (the objects described as seen must be regarded as hallucinations); confabulation; allocheiria (reference of sensation to opposite site from stimulus application).

Signs. Blindness.

Etiology. Not well established. Tumor; neurosurgery; arteriosclerosis; bilateral obstruction of occipital region arteries; lesion of calcar or thalamic connections.

Pathology. See Etiology.

Therapy. None.

Prognosis. Poor *quoad vitam.*

BIBLIOGRAPHY. Anton G: Ueber die Selbstwahrnehmung der Herderkrankungen des Gehirns durch den Kranken bie Rindenblindheit und Rindentaubheit. Arch Psychiatr Nervenkr 32:86, 1899
Adam RD, Victor M: Principles of Neurology, 3rd ed, p 342. New York, McGraw-Hill, 1985

ANTON-VOGT

Synonyms. Double athetosis; congenital chorea; Hammond's athetoid; infantile partial striatal sclerosis; status marmoratus; Vogt and Vogt. See Little's (W.J.).

Symptoms. Premature infants frequently affected; onset months after birth when complex motor activity develops, such as sitting, standing, and walking. Purposeless, involuntary, slow, sinuous movements of face, neck, trunk, and extremities, exaggerated by activity and excitement. Dysarthria; association with mental and emotional disturbances; convulsions.

Etiology. Not clear; related to asphyxial disturbances or fetal encephalitis. Autosomal inheritance reported of both dominant and recessive type.

Pathology. Striatum shrunken; ganglion cells absent; structure invaded by thin myelinated fibers (status marmoratus). Findings observed only in some patients.

Diagnostic Procedures. *Electroencephalography. Spinal tap.*

Therapy. In severe cases, section of central portion of cerebral peduncle. Sedative and antispasmodic agents.

Prognosis. Disease static. Manifestations depending on cerebral defects. Mental deficiency of variable degree. Long survival possible (60-year-old reported).

BIBLIOGRAPHY. Oppenheim H, Vogt C: Wesen und Localisation der kongennitalen und infantilen Pseudobulbärparalyse. J Psychol Neurol 18:293–308, 1911
Athetosis. Medical Times Gaz London 2:747–748, 1871
Anton G: Ueber die Beteiligung der grossen basalen Gehirnganglien bei Bewegungstörungen and Inshesondere. Chorea Jahrh J Psychiatr Neurol 14:141–147, 1896
Vogt C: Quelques considerations générales á propos du syndrome due Corps strié. J Psychiat Neurol 18:479–492, 1911
Vogt C, Vogt O: Zur Lehre der Ezkrankungen des Striäten Systems. J Psychol Neurol 25:627–846, 1920
Adams RD, Victor M: Principles of Neurology, 3rd ed, pp 925–926. New York, McGraw-Hill, 1985

ANUS, IMPERFORATE

Symptoms and Signs. Occur in males; present from birth. Absence of communication between rectal sections; anal membranes intact. Absence of emission of meconium. After two to three days, abdominal distension. If the point of obstruction is low, digital exploration may reveal defect.

Etiology. Hereditary malformation of sex-linked recessive type.

Pathology. Anal membrane preventing communication of intestinal lumen. Frequently associated with other malformations of lower intestinal tract (e.g., rectoperineal, rectovesical, rectourethral).

Diagnostic Procedures. *X-ray.* With infant head-down, an opaque object inserted in anus: gas level separated from object by a membrane.

Therapy. Excision of membrane. If underweight (in case of associated anomalies), temporary colostomy to precede more complex intervention.

Prognosis. Good with intervention. In some cases rupture of cecum in labor; fecal impaction and megacolon; residual constipation.

BIBLIOGRAPHY. Weinstein ED: Sex-linked imperforate anus. Pediatrics 35:715–717, 1965
Winkler JM, Weinstein ED: Imperforate anus and heredity. J Ped Surg 5:555–558, 1970

ANXIETY-TENSION

Synonym. Anxiety neurosis.

Symptoms. Anxiety manifested by tension in the voice, anxious look; patient characteristically sits on the edge of chair, wipes wet palms. Concern often oriented not to mental reactions, but to the somatic manifestations consisting of muscular hypertension, headache, tight throat, dizziness, blurred vision, precordial distress, rapid heart, spastic colon, diarrhea or constipation, flushing and all symptoms that are found in the psychologic "alarm reaction." Fatigue-blueness may appear in advanced stages of the condition. Persons physically well-endowed, intelligent, perfectionists, hard-driving, economically and socially successful, not complacent about their situation and symptoms, as opposed to "neurotics," who instead appears complacent, inadequate socially and economically, not equally intelligent.

Signs. Objective changes; gastrointestinal; cardiovascular, and others, corresponding to somatic symptoms.

Etiology and Pathology. Chronic "alarm reaction" with shifting of attention from tangible obstacle to feelings and person himself.

Therapy. Mild sedative. Psychiatric explanation of mechanism of symptoms and training in relaxation. Rhythmic exercises. Vitamins and a combination of betaine hydrochloride and glycocyamine useful in advance states with fatigue symptoms.

Prognosis. Excellent with adequate treatment.

BIBLIOGRAPHY. Dixon HH, et al: Therapy in anxiety states and anxiety complicated by depression. West J Surg 62:338–341, 1954

Freud S: Mourning and melancholia. In The Complete Psychological Works of Sigmund Freud, Vol 14, pp 237–258. London, Hogarth, 1957

Freedman AM, Kaplan HI, Sadock BJ: Comprehensive Textbook of Psychiatry, 2nd ed, p 1199. Baltimore, Williams & Wilkins, 1975

Adams RD, Victor M: Principles of Neurology, 3rd ed, pp 1108–1110. New York, McGraw-Hill, 1985

AORTA COARCTATION

Synonyms. Coarctation of aorta.

Symptoms. Predominant in males (isthmus) or equal sex distribution (abdominal); onset in two periods: early infancy (dyspnea) and between 20 and 30 years of age. Usually, initially asymptomatic. Constant onset of symptoms in second period. *Minor.* Headache, spontaneous epistaxes; leg fatigue; claudication of leg (abdominal coarctation); dysphagia; ache in the shoulders, tinnitus. *Major.* Symptoms related to congestive heart failure; rupture of anterior aneurysm; endocarditis; and cerebral hemorrhage.

Signs. Physical appearance usually normal; at times athletic (broad chest and shoulders, thin hips and legs). Typical signs: hypertension (systolic) in arms (if proximal to obstruction); hypotension (systolic) in the legs or absence of pulse. Search for collateral vessels (seldom obvious). Forceful pulses in the neck and supraclavicular regions. Systolic murmur (posterior chest interscapular auscultation) over constricted zone.

Etiology. Abnormality of development in embryonal life. Sometimes hereditary.

Pathology. Deformity composed of medial tissue and shown by localized thickening, infolding of aortic wall, which reduces the lumen at arch-descending aorta junction. Bulging above and below constricted segment. Frequent association with other cardiac malformation. *Infantile type.* Aortic isthmus, or proximal involvement. *Adult type.* At or below obliterated ductus insertion distal to isthmus.

Diagnostic Procedures. *Electrocardiography.* Ventricular hypertrophy; left bundle branch block. *X-rays.* Normal to pathognomonic. Signs usually present after 2 years of age: ribs notching posterior at inferior margin (at 6 years of age); left subclavian and descending aortic shadows classic features in isthmus coarctation; deformity of barium-filled esophagus. *Echocardiogram. Cardiac catheterization.*

Therapy. *Medical.* According to heart failure (digitalis, or, diuretics, IV sedation), prostaglandin E, to give relief and allow further assessment and surgery. *Surgical.* Prompt correction in infants who do not respond to medical management, or with other associated defects. Elective correction between 4 and 6 years of age to prevent relatively high occurence of recoarctation.

Prognosis. Those who survive hazard of infancy reach early adulthood; 25% die before age 20; 50% before 30; 75% before 50. Good results with surgery.

BIBLIOGRAPHY. Jarcho S: Coarctation of the aorta. Am J Cardiol 7:844–851, 1961

Smallborn JF, Huhta JC, Adams PA, et al: Cross-sectional echocardiographic assessment of coarctation in the sick neonate and infant. Br Heart J 50:349–361, 1984

Hurst JW: The Heart, 6th ed, pp 627–634. New York, McGraw-Hill, 1986

AORTIC ARCH

This syndrome includes: (1) Carotid artery occlusion syndrome; (2) vertebral-basilar artery occlusive syndrome; (3) subclavian artery occlusive syndrome, and subclavian steal syndrome.

Symptoms and Signs. Although each of the syndromes shows a particular pattern of symptoms and signs, there is a variable degree of overlapping; lesions of more than one artery, and congenital anatomic variation will further confuse differentiation. In the tables below, Jones and colleagues have attempted differentiation of symptoms and signs.

Symptoms Associated with Artery Involved

Symptoms	Artery		
	Innominate	Vertebral	Subclavian
Motor-sensory impairment	×		
Seizures	×		
Visual impairment	×		
Diplopia	×		
Aphasia-dysphasia		×	
Syncope	×	×	
Memory change	×	×	
Lightheadedness	×	×	×
Vertigo		×	×
Arm			×
None			×

Physical Findings Associated with Artery Involved

Findings	Artery		
	Innominate	Vertebral	Subclavian
Blood pressure			
Reduction (arm) 160 to 30 mm Hg	×		×
Pulse change			
Arm	×		×
Neck	×		
Bruit neck	×		×
Neurologic deficits	×		
Ischemic changes			
Hand			×
Subclavian steal	×		×
			(66.7%)

Jones TW, Thomas GI, Edmark KW: Thoracocervical occlusive disease. Am Surg 33:535–541, 1967

Etiology. Atherosclerosis (in majority of cases); nonspecific arthritis (16%, this last group form the Takayasu's syndrome, see; trauma; embolization).

Pathology. Atherosclerotic changes of the arterial walls, thrombosis and neurologic alterations according to artery affected.

Diagnostic Procedures. *Four-vessel arteriography. Non-*

invasive techniques: Doppler, ocular pneumoplethysmography.

Therapy. Surgical reconstruction procedures.

Prognosis. According to degree and time of occlusion and variations in surgical possibilities and skill, death due to cerebral vascular insufficiency.

BIBLIOGRAPHY. Broadbent WH: On ingravescent apoplexy. Med Chir Soc London 8:103–108, 1876
Ross RR, McKusick VA: Aortic arch syndromes, diminished or absent pulses in arteries arising from arch of aorta. Arch Intern Med 92:701–740, 1953
Bustamante RA, Milanes B, Casas R, et al: Chronic subclavian-carotid obstruction syndrome (pulseless disease). Angiology 5:479–485, 1954
Davis JB, Grove WJ, Julian OC: Thrombotic occlusion of the branches of the aortic arch, Martorell's syndrome: Report of a case treated surgically. Ann Surg 144:124–126, 1956
Weir AM Jr, Kyle JW: Reversed coarctation, review of pulseless disease and report of a case. Ann Intern Med 45:681–691, 1956
Jones TW, Thomas GI, Edmark KW: Thoracocervical occlusive disease. Amer Surg 3:535–541, 1967
Hurst JW: The Heart, 6th ed, pp 622, 1334. New York, McGraw-Hill, 1986

AORTIC ARCH HYPOPLASIA

Symptoms. Both sexes affected; normal at birth. Onset before 6 weeks of age. Intensity of symptoms according to degree of lesion. Dyspnea; feeding difficulty; failure to thrive. Possibly, development of progressive cardiac failure.

Signs. Cyanosis: mild and involving primarily lower extremities. Acyanosis if associated with large ventricular septal defect. Murmurs absent or minor; seldom, left parasternal systolic murmurs (of associated ventricular septal defect), or midsystolic.

Etiology. Congenital defect.

Pathology. Uniform tubular narrowing of ascending part and arch of aorta. Seldom present as isolated defect; frequently associated with ventricular septal defect, patent ductus arteriosus, or other malformations.

Diagnostic Procedures. *Electrocardiography.* Right atrium and ventricle hypertrophy. *X-ray.* Normal pattern to marked cardiac enlargement and pulmonary venous congestion. *Cardiac catheterization.*

Therapy. Corrective plastic surgery.

Prognosis. Variable according to degree of lesion. Amenable to surgical repair. Recoarctation is common and often necessitates a second operation.

BIBLIOGRAPHY. Lev M: Pathologic anatomy and interrelationship of hypoplasia of the aortic arch complex. Lab Invest 1:61–70, 1952

Perloff JK: The Clinical Recognition of Congenital Heart Disease, 2nd ed, p 736. Philadelphia, WB Saunders, 1978

Braunwald E: Heart disease, Vol 2, pp 1003–1004. Philadelphia, WB Saunders, 1980

AORTIC ATRESIA

Synonyms. Aortic valve atresia.

Symptoms. Predominant in males; at birth may appear normal, but symptoms develop within first few days of life. Critical illness; listlessness; tachypnea.

Signs. Severe pallor; mild to intense cyanosis; edema; absent or diminished arterial pulses; signs of severe pulmonary hypertension; absent heart murmurs; sternal lift. Later, hepatomegaly.

Etiology. Congenital malformation.

Pathology. Complete closure of aortic orifice by fibrous membrane. Hypoplasia of ascending aorta. Mitral valve hypoplasic or atresic. Patent ductus arteriosus.

Diagnostic Procedures. *Electrocardiography.* Right ventricular hypertrophy; right atrial P waves. *X-ray.* Cardiomegaly; absence of aortic shadow; pulmonary venous congestion. *M-mode and two-dimensional echocardiography. Cardiac catheterization.*

Therapy. Intravenous prostaglandin E infusion (to maintain ductal patency prior to catheterization and surgery). Palliative surgery; emotional support, genetic counseling for parents.

Prognosis. Fatal within first week. A few children survive a few months (optimal interatrial communication).

BIBLIOGRAPHY. Norwood WJ, Lange P, Hansen DD: Physiologic repair of aortic atresia–hypoplastic: Left heart syndrome. New Engl J Med 308:23–26, 1983

Hurst JW: The Heart, 6th ed, pp 645–647. New York, McGraw-Hill, 1986

AORTIC–LEFT VENTRICULAR TUNNEL

The tunnel begins in the ascending aorta, lies on the anterior wall, proceeds into the epicardium, penetrates the ventricular septum and empties in subaortic zone of left ventricle.

Symptoms. Very rare: early birth or early infancy. Mild symptoms. Few present congestive heart failure, others dyspnea, fatigue, growth failure in weeks or months.

Signs. Bounding arterial pulses, wide pulse pressure, hyperdynamic left ventricular lift. To and from murmur, diastolic sound louder.

Etiology. Unknown.

Diagnostic Procedures. *Cardiac catheterization. Echocardiography. X-ray.*

Therapy. Medical and early surgical management. Progressive also when mild initial symptoms.

Prognosis. Rapid onset of congestive failure and death if surgery is not performed (80.9% survive surgery).

BIBLIOGRAPHY. Levy MJ, Schachner A, Blieden LC: Aortic–left ventricular tunnel: collective review. J Thorac Cardiovasc Surg 84:102–109, 1982

AORTICOPULMONARY WINDOW

Synonyms. Aorticopulmonary septal defect; Elliotson's; aortopulmonary fistula.

Symptoms and Signs. Both sexes affected; present from birth. Acyanosis; physical underdevelopment. Clinical signs suggest patent ductus arteriosus (see); systolic murmur maximum in third intercostal space. Wide and bounding pulse.

Etiology. Embryological fault resulting in persistence of a round or oval window communication between ascending aorta and pulmonary trunk.

Diagnostic Procedures. *Electrocardiography.* Ventricular hypertrophy with diastolic overload of left heart. *X-rays.* Pattern similar to large patent ductus (left-to-right shunt) and pulmonary hypertension.

Therapy. Cardiosurgery.

Prognosis. Early death.

BIBLIOGRAPHY. Elliotson J: Case of malformation of the pulmonary artery and aorta. Lancet I:247–248, 1830

Doty DB, Richardson JV, Falkovsky GE, et al: Aortopulmonary septal defect: hemodynamic angiography and operation. Ann Thorac Surg 32:244–250, 1981

Hurst JW: The Heart, 6th ed, pp 618–619. New York, McGraw-Hill, 1986

AORTOCAVAL FISTULA

A. SPONTANEOUS

Symptoms. Predominant in males (no cases reported in females); onset between 40 and 78 years of age. Pain in the back or abdomen, or both; occasionally, radiation to legs. Dyspnea; anorexia; nausea; vomiting; restlessness; confusion; lethargy; stupor; oliguria; shock.

Signs. Palpable aneurysm; abdominal bruit usually systolic and diastolic, seldom only systolic; cardiomegaly; edema of legs; pulsating vein; ascites; hepatomegaly. Blood pressure: low diastolic; wide pulse pressure.

Etiology. Rupture of aortic aneurysm (usually arteriosclerotic; seldom syphilis; Marfan's; mycosis).

Pathology. Fistula of aorta into vena cava; fluid retention (10–15 kg) in legs, abdomen.

Diagnostic Procedures. *Venous pressure.* In legs markedly increased. *Urine.* Hematuria. *Stool.* Presence of blood. *Blood.* Hyperazotemia. *Aortography.*

Therapy. Treatment of shock. Surgical interruption of fistula.

Prognosis. Without operation, survival from 1 hour to 47 days. Cause of death congestive heart failure, shock, rectal hemorrhage, cerebral insufficiency, anuria.

B. TRAUMATIC

Symptoms. Pain in the back or abdomen, occasionally, radiation to legs. Dyspnea; oliguria; anorexia; nausea; vomiting.

Signs. Palpable aneurysm; systolic and diastolic bruit; pulmonary rales; cardiomegaly; edema; ascites; hepatomegaly.

Etiology. Trauma.

Pathology. Formation of fistula between aorta and vena cava.

Diagnostic Procedures. *X-ray. Aortography.*

Therapy. Surgery.

Prognosis. Traumatic form is relatively benign since systemic arterial insufficiency and regional venous hypertension are, if at all, exceptional complications. Without surgery, survival may go for years (mean 5.3 years).

BIBLIOGRAPHY. Syme J: Case XV—Case of spontaneous varicose aneurysm. Edinb Med Surg J 36:105, 1931
Nennhaus HP, Javid H: The distinct syndrome of spontaneous abdominal aortocaval fistula. Am J Med 44:464–473, 1968
Pardue GD, Smith RB III: Diseases in the peripheral veins and the venae cavae. In Hurst JW (ed): The Heart, 6th ed. New York, McGraw-Hill, 1986

APATHETIC THYROTOXIC STORM

Synonyms. Lahey's II; Lahey's apathetic form; Zondek's comatose form; thyrotoxic storm, apathetic.

Symptoms and Signs. Occur in hyperthyroidal patients. Extreme weakness; emotional apathy; usually, normal or slight elevation of temperature. Absence of delirium and agitation typical of thyrotoxic storm (see Waldenström's II). Signs of decompensation of various organs and systems.

Etiology. See Waldenström's II.

BIBLIOGRAPHY. Lahey EH: The crisis of exophthalmic goiter. New Engl J Med 199:255–257, 1928
Toft AD (ed): Hyperthyroidism (Symposium). Clin Endocrinol Metab 14:(whole issue), 1985

APERT-GALLAIS

Synonyms. Cooke-Apert's; Gallais'; genito-surrenal; suprarenal genital; suprarenal pseudohermaphroditism—virilism—hirsutism.

French designation of the congenital adrenal hyperplasia syndrome in females (see Adrenogenital syndromes). See also Achard-Thiers, Pellizzi's, Cushing's, and Hirsutism.

BIBLIOGRAPHY. Apert M: Dystrophies en relation avec les lésions de capsules surrénales, hirsutisme et progeria. Bull Soc Pediat 12:501–518, 1910
Gallais A: La Syndrome Génito-Surrénale: Étude Anatomo-Clinique (thesis). Paris, 1912

APERT'S

Synonyms. Acrocephalosyndactyly I; syndactylic oxycephaly; ACS I.

Symptoms. Headache; visual loss.

Signs. Acrocephaly (head pointed in region of anterior fontanelle); beak-shaped nose; hypoplastic maxilla; occasionally associated with exophthalmos and visual loss. Mental retardation. Cases with normal intelligence reported. Syndactylism of various types, partial or total fusion or webbing of fingers and toes. Other skeletal deformities.

Etiology. Most cases sporadic. Autosomal dominant and recessive cases reported. Old paternal age.

Pathology. Premature fusion of cranial bone; synostosis and synarthrosis; agenesis of bones.

Diagnostic Procedures. *X-ray.*

Therapy. Orthopedic or surgical correction when feasible. Craniectomy early in life.

BIBLIOGRAPHY. Wheaton SW: Two specimens of congenital cranial deformity in infants associated with fusion of the fingers and toes. Trans Path Soc London 45:238, 1894

Apert E: De l'acrocephalosyndactyly. Bull Soc Med Hôp Paris 23:1310–1330, 1906

Leonard CO, Daikoku NH, Winn K: Prenatal photoscopic diagnosis of the Apert's syndrome. Am J Med Genet 11:5–9, 1982

APLASIA CUTIS CONGENITA

Synonyms. Skull-scalp defect, congenital; scalp defect congenital, including: parietal foramina; Catlin marks.

Symptoms and Signs. Lesion(s) present at birth; one (more frequently) or multiple sharply marginated lesions with red glistening base of variable shape. Usually on the scalp (⅔) (may be taken as forceps injuries), frequently close to the midline, less frequently on limbs (¼), seldom on trunks. Infection possible; meningitis in case of deep lesions reported. Possible associated lesions: limbs ring constriction or anomalies; congenital heart defects; thracheoesophageal fistula; cleft lip-palate; uterus and cervix duplication; cerebral malformations; mental retardation.

Etiology. Unknown. Most cases sporadic. Autosomal dominant and recessive forms reported (in form involving the scalp)

Pathology. Absence of epidermis and occasionally of dermis and subcutaneous fat; if reepithelization absence of epidermal appendices and possible hypertrophic scar.

Diagnostic Procedures. *Biopsy of skin.*

Therapy. Prevention of infection; larger lesion: early grafting.

Prognosis. Excellent in absence of complication and for shallow lesions.

BIBLIOGRAPHY. Hoffman E: Wien Med Presse 18:552, 1885

Dubusson JD, Schneider P: Manifestation familiale d'une aplasie cutanée circonscrite du vertex (ACCV) associée dans un cas a une malformation cardiaque. J Genet Hum 26:351–356, 1978

APOLIPOPROTEIN DEFICIENCY, FAMILIAL

Synonyms. Apo C-II deficiency.

Symptoms and Signs. Detection in adulthood. Recurrent abdominal pain due to pancreatitis, which may lead to diabetes and its symptoms and signs. No xantomas or hepatomegaly (see LPL deficiency). Anemia.

Etiology. Autosomal recessive inheritance. Absence of apolipoprotein C-II, which is essential for lipoproteinlipase clearance of chylomicron and VLDL from plasma.

Pathology. *Pancreas.* Acute pancreatitis typical signs. *Blood.* Anemia probably hemolytic. *Lipids.* Elevated fasting plasma triglycerides mostly of chylomicrons but also of VLDL; cholesterol high, in VLDL low in LDL and HDL; plasma apolipoprotein A-1 reduced. The lipid pattern may be classified as type 1 or type 5.

Therapy. Restriction of fats in diet. Plasma transfusions (containing Apo C-II) cause immediate decrease of plasma triglycerides.

BIBLIOGRAPHY. Breckenridge WC, Little JA, Steiner G, et al: Hypertriglyceridemia associated with deficiency of apolipoprotein C-II. New Engl J Med 298:1265, 1978

Nikkila EA: Familial lipoprotein lipase deficiency and related disorders of chylomicron metabolism. In Stanbury JB, Wyngaarden JB, Fredrickson DS, et al (eds): The Metabolic Basis of Inherited Disease, 5th ed, p. 1385. New York, McGraw-Hill, 1983

APOPLEXIA UTERI

Synonyms. Hemorrhagic necrosis senile endometrium.

Symptoms. Vaginal bleeding; symptoms of cardiac decompensation such as cough, dyspnea, chest pain, edema of lower extremities. Symptoms of bleeding in gastrointestinal tract: vomiting of blood; passage of dark stool.

Signs. Signs of cardiac failure; tachycardia; enlargement of heart; enlarged, tender liver; edema of lower extremities. Postmenopausal bleeding with normal pelvic findings.

Etiology. Necrosis of the endometrium.

Pathology. Findings at autopsy: severe generalized and uterine arteriosclerosis. Some form of cardiovascular disease associated with a variable degree of circulatory decompensation.

Therapy. Curettage to rule out endometrial carcinoma. Treatment of the symptoms and of the arteriosclerosis.

Prognosis. Postmenopausal bleeding of this kind has some prognostic significance. Thus, if vaginal bleeding develops in a postmenopausal female with cardiovascular decompensation, it should prompt the consideration of endometrial ischemia as a likely cause. Though of relatively little consequence in itself, this occurrence should alert the physician to the possibility of coincidental or subsequent development of the far more important and severe hemorrhagic necrosis of the bowel.

BIBLIOGRAPHY. Novak ER, Woodruff JD: Gynecologic and Obstetric Pathology with Clinical and Endocrine Relations, 6th ed. Philadelphia, WB Saunders, 1967

Daly JJ, Balogh K Jr.: Hemorrhagic necrosis of the senile endometrium ("apoplexia uteri"): relation to superficial hemorrhagic necrosis of the bowel. New Engl J Med 278:709–711, 1968

Gompel C, Silverberg SG: Pathology, Gynecology and Obstetrics, 3rd ed, pp 194–197. Philadelphia, JB Lippincott, 1985

APPLE PEEL

Synonyms. Jejunal atresia.

Symptoms. At birth. Vomiting of bile, abdominal distension, failure to pass meconium.

Signs. At surgery, the distal small bowel comes straight off the cecum and twists around the marginal artery like an apple peel.

Etiology. Autosomal recessive inheritance.

Pathology. Jejunal atresia. Obliteration of superior mesenteric artery may underlie the malformation.

Diagnostic Procedures. *X-ray, plain abdominal. Barium enema.*

Therapy. Surgery.

Prognosis. Good with surgery.

BIBLIOGRAPHY. Mishalany HG, Najjar FB: Familial jejunal atresia: three cases in one family. J Pediat 73:753–755, 1968

Blyth HM, Dikson JAS: Apple peel syndrome (congenital intestinal atresia): a family study of seven index patients. J Med Genet 6:275–277, 1969

Rickham PP, Karplus M: Familial hereditary intestinal atresia. Helv Ped Acta 26:561–564, 1971

Haller JA Jr: Intestinal atresia: correct concepts of pathogenesis pathophysiology and operative management. Ann Surg 49:385–395, 1983

APRACTOGNOSIA

Synonyms. Minor parietal, right parieto-occipital.

Symptoms and Signs. Body scheme disturbances: denial of left hemiplegia hemiagnosia; motor hemispontaneity. Apraxia for dressing: difficulty in recognizing the relationship between clothes and body, especially the right-left relation (particularly in difficult maneuver that requires left-right manual performance, such as tightening shoelace and necktie). Vasoconstrictive disabilities: inability to draw a three-dimensional pattern or a complex figure (attempt to reproduce a bicycle or a man is a good test.) Disorders of "spatial thought": unilateral spatial agnosia; disturbed orientation resulting in the inability of the patient to find his way, since he turns constantly to the right. Disturbance of calculation and counting. Opticovestibular disturbances: sensation of vertigo; distortion of subjective horizontal and vertical lines.

Etiology and Pathology. Lesions of the minor (nondominant) cerebral hemisphere, which includes the supramarginal gyrus and part of the angular gyrus, and the posterior part of the first temporal convolution. Surgical excision of the area; vascular, traumatic, neoplastic lesions.

Prognosis. In past surgical cases, improvements of various symptoms.

BIBLIOGRAPHY. Hecaen H, Penfield W, Bertrand C, et al: The syndrome of apractognosia due to lesions of the minor cerebral hemisphere. AMA Arch Neurol Psychiatr 75:400–434, 1956

ARAN-DUCHENNE

Synonyms. Charcot's amyotrophic lateral sclerosis; motor neuron system; progressive spinal muscular atrophy; amyotrophic lateral sclerosis.

Symptoms. Predominant in males; onset in the 4th to 6th decades of life. Symmetric weakness in small hand muscles, particularly interossei, thenar, and hypothenar. Fibrillation and atrophy that rapidly appear. Atrophy gradually and progressively extends, involving muscles of arms, shoulders, and trunk.

Signs. Fasciculation and atrophy of affected muscles.

Etiology. Unknown; possibly inherited; toxic (?); nutritional and metabolic (?); pancreatic adenoma.

Pathology. Anterior cell of spinal tract affected by degenerative changes; muscle shows typical changes from damaged innervation; connective tissue replacement of muscle fibers.

Diagnostic Procedures. *Blood and urine.* Negative. *Cerebrospinal fluid.* Normal.

Therapy. Symptomatic; avoidance of contractures.

Prognosis. Progressive without remissions; death in 3 years.

BIBLIOGRAPHY. Aran FA: Recherches sur une maladie non encour décrit du système musculaire (atrophie musculaire progressive). Arch Gen Med (Paris) 24:172–214, 1850

Duchenne, GB: Etude comparée des lésions anatomique dans l'atrophie musculaire progressive et dans la paralysie générale. Union Med Prat Fr 7:202, 1853

Adams RD, Victor M: Principles of Neurology, 3rd ed, p 830. New York, McGraw-Hill, 1985

ARCHER'S

Synonym. Uncomplicated supraclavicular aortic stenosis. See hypercalcemia, infantile and Williams-Beuren syndromes; supravalvular aortic stenosis, SVAS.

Symptoms and Signs. More frequent in males. History of cyanosis in infancy; inequality between right and left arm and neck pulses; high basal systolic murmur; no systolic click or aortic diastolic murmur. Normal facies and intelligence. Congestive failure may develop.

Etiology. Congenital malformation: (1) Nonfamilial sporadic occurrence; (2) autosomal dominant; (3) incomplete form of infantile hypercalcemia (see).

Pathology. Most frequent lesion shelflike thickening or ridge at upper border of Valsalva sinuses; circular narrowing of aorta or long stenotic segment of aorta; fibrous bands from aortic cusps to ridge.

Diagnostic Procedures. *X-ray of chest. Angiocardiography. Electrocardiography. Echocardiography.*

Therapy. Surgical correction; complete correction impossible in some cases.

Prognosis. Reduced longevity.

BIBLIOGRAPHY. Archer RS: Note on a congenital band stretching across the origin of the aorta. Dublin J Med Sci 65:405–406, 1878

Logan WF, Jones EW, Walker E, et al: Familial supravalvular aortic stenosis. Br Heart J 27:547–559, 1956

Antia AU, Wiltse HE, Rowe RD, et al: Pathogenesis of the supravalvular aortic stenosis syndrome. J Pediatr 71:431–441, 1967

Johnson LW, Fishman RA, Schneider B, et al: Familial supravalvular aortic stenosis: report of a large family and review of literature. Chest 70:494–500, 1976

ARDS: ADULT RESPIRATORY DISTRESS

Synonyms. Congestive atelectasis; noncardiogenic pulmonary edema; push-pull pump; septic lung; shock lung; wet lung; white lung; capillary leak.

Symptoms and Signs. Onset of respiratory symptoms occurs after 24–48 hours from the initial insult. Tachypnea; labored breathing followed by cyanosis.

Etiology. Tissue damage caused by vasoactive substances released by neutrophils, platelets, and complement activation. Associated with a variety of conditions that may directly or indirectly damage the pulmonary capillary endothelium. Direct damage includes trauma, infections, aspiration, fat embolism. Indirect damage mediated by humoral factors includes sepsis, pancreatitis, shock, DIC, drugs.

Pathology. Pulmonary capillary damage with interstitial damage followed by alveolar edema. Later extensive pulmonary fibrosis.

Diagnostic Procedures. *Blood.* Findings of hypoxemia at gas analysis. *X-ray.* Diffuse pulmonary infiltrates. Reduced lung compliance. Increased shunt fraction and dead space ventilation.

Therapy. Increased inspired oxygen tension. Mechanical ventilation and positive end expiratory pressure (PEEP). Extracorporeal CO_2 elimination. Prostaglandins (PGE1) under investigation. Cardiovascular support with dopamine.

Prognosis. About 50% mortality. Good recovery for people who survive.

BIBLIOGRAPHY. Ashbaug MDG, Bigelow DB, Petty TL, Levine BE: Acute respiratory distress syndrome in adults. Lancet II: 319–323, 1967

Robin ED, Carey LC, Grenvik A, et al: Capillary leak syndrome with pulmonary edema. Arch Int Med 130:66–71, 1972

Zapol WM, Trelstad RL, Snider MT, et al: Pathophysiologic pathways of the adult respiratory distress syndrome. In Tinker J, Rapin M (eds): Care of the Critically Ill Patient, p 341. Berlin, Springer-Verlag, 1983

ARGINASE DEFICIENCY

Synonyms. Hyperargininemia; Terheggen's; argininemia; hyperargininemia.

Symptoms and Signs. Rare. Onset in neonatal period. Spastic diplegia; mental retardation; seizures.

Etiology. Autosomal recessive trait (?). Arginase deficiency. Autosomal recessive. Arginase deficiency.

Diagnostic Procedures. *Blood, urine, cerebrospinal fluid.* Hyperargininemia; chromatographic amino acid screening. Confirmation by determination of arginase activity in red cells or liver tissue. Variable abnormalities of blood ammonia.

Therapy. Low-protein diet.

Prognosis. Mental and physical retardation.

BIBLIOGRAPHY. Peralta Serrano A: Argininuria, convulsiones y oligofrenia; un nuevo error innato del metabolismo? Rev Clin Esp 97:176–183, 1965.

Walser M: Urea cycle disorders and other hereditary hyperammonemic syndromes. In Stanbury JB, Wyngaarden JB, Fredrickson DS (eds): The Metabolic Basis of Inherited Disease, 5th ed, p 408. New York, McGraw-Hill, 1983

ARGININOSUCCINATE LYASE DEFICIENCY

Synonyms. Allan's; argininosuccinase aciduria; ASase aciduria; Allan's argininosuccinase aciduria; ASAL (argininosuccinate lyase) deficiency.

Symptoms and Signs. Both sexes affected; prevalent in females (2 : 1). Three types according to time of onset:
1. *Neonatal* (soon after birth). Poor feeding; lethargy; tachypnea; seizures and coma.
2. *Subacute*. Early infancy feeding difficulties; failure to thrive; seizures; delayed mental milestones; hepatomegaly; friable tufted hair (trichorrhexis nodosa).
3. *Late onset*. Mental retardation becomes evident in second year of life; history of feeding troubles, vomiting, irritability; intelligence quotient between 30 and 60 seizures; hair changes (see above) in 50% of cases.

Etiology. Autosomal recessive inheritance. Deficiency of argininosuccinase (ASase) activity. Autosomal recessive inheritance. Deficiency of ASAL activity (chromosome 7).

Pathology. Nonspecific. Multiple necrotic foci. *Kidney.* Degenerative alterations; tubular casts. *Myocardium.* Extensive necrosis. *Brain.* Spongy alteration of gray and white matter; demyelinization.

Diagnostic Procedures. *Urine.* Arginosuccinic acid (ASA) in great quantity. *Blood.* Increase of ASA, increase of transaminases and alkaline phosphatases. *Cerebrospinal fluid.* Higher increase of ASA (compared with blood).

Therapy. Symptomatic. Selective diet (low-protein diet and in small feedings).

Prognosis. *Neonatal type.* Death in the first days. *Subacute type.* Unknown. *Late onset type.* From severe mental disorder to asymptomatic evolution.

BIBLIOGRAPHY. Walser M: Urea cycle disorders and other hereditary hyperammonemic syndromes. In Stanbury JB, Wyngaarden JB, Fredrickson DS (eds): The Metabolic Basis of Inherited Disease, 5th ed, p 408. New York, McGraw-Hill, 1983

ARGYLL ROBERTSON'S

Synonyms. Reflex iridoplegia; Argyll Robertson's pupil; Robertson's spinal miosis.

Symptoms and Signs. Vision not significantly affected; associated with various symptoms of syphilis of central nervous system: general paresis, tabes dorsalis. Unilateral or bilateral small pupils that do not react to light but react to accommodation and convergence; dilate poorly or not at all with mydriatic. Usually, unequal and irregular.

Etiology. Syphilis (tabes; meningovascular); alcoholic midbrain changes; diabetes; general paresis; Wernicke's syndrome; arteriosclerosis; posttraumatic.

Pathology. Not exactly determined. Lesions of pretectal region to oculomotor nucleus (?), iris (more likely), ciliary ganglion (?). Lesions of axons of ciliary ganglion have been demonstrated.

Diagnostic Procedures. *Light and convergence accommodation. Blood and spinal fluid.* For syphilis.

Therapy. None.

Prognosis. Depends upon etiology.

BIBLIOGRAPHY. Robertson DA: On an interesting series of eye-symptoms in a case of spinal disease: with remarks on the action of Belladonna on the iris, etc. Edinb Med J 14:696–708, 1869; Med Classics 1:851–868, 1937

Lebensohn JE: Centenary of the Horner and Argyll Robertson pupillar syndromes. Proc Inst Med Chic 28:65, 1970

Adams RD, Victor M: Principles of Neurology, 3rd ed, p 209. New York, McGraw-Hill, 1985

ARHINENCEPHALIA

Synonyms. Holoprosencephaly; familial Alobar.

Symptoms and Signs. Four types of facial anomalies are associated with this type of single malformation: cyclopia (see); ethmocephaly (see); cebocephaly (see); and holoprosencephaly (see).

Etiology. Variable; most cases undetermined. Varying degrees of deficit of midline facies development and incomplete morphogenesis of brain, depending on prochordal mesoderm defect. In some cases, chromosomal defects.

Pathology. According to mentioned varieties.

Therapy. Limited to medical assistance to survival measures.

Prognosis. Poor *quoad vitam*.

BIBLIOGRAPHY. De Myer W, Zeman W, Palmer CG: The face predicts the brain: diagnostic significance of median facial anomalies for holoprosencephaly (arhinencephaly). Pediatrics 34:256–263, 1964
Ellis R: On a rare form of twin monstrosity. Trans Obstet Soc 7:160–164, 1965
Seidlitz G, Kadow I, Theel L, et al: Genetische Aspekte und umangenetische Beratung der Holoprosencephalic. Dtsch Gesundh-Wessen 38:665–669, 1983

ARIAS'

Synonyms. Crigler-Najjar type 2; hyperbilirubinemia, intermediate degree; bilirubin defect; partial defect conjugation; hyperbilirubinemia congenital type II.

Symptoms. Onset from first year of life or later (at 4 to 30 years of age). Asymptomatic; only occasionally instances of neurologic manifestations.

Signs. Generalized jaundice. Gallstones sometimes present (coincidental?).

Etiology. Genetic disorders of type not yet established; suggested: autosomal dominant with uncomplete penetrance or recessive type. Depression of glucuronide formation and absence, or great reduction of bilirubin conjugates.

Pathology. Extrahepatic ducts patent; no histologic abnormalities, except for hypertrophy-hyperplasia of smooth endoplasmic reticulum and Golgi's apparatus. In limited cases, brain abnormalities.

Diagnostic Procedures. *Blood.* Serum bilirubin (unconjugated type) increased (6–20 mg/100 ml); fasting (24 hours); elevation of bilirubin. *Duodenal aspiration.* Bile pigment hourly output of bilirubin below calculated production rate. Most pigment in form of monoglucuronide. *Menthol and salicylamide tests.* Abnormal.

Therapy. Phenobarbital (60–180 mg daily); dichlorodiphenyl trichloroethane (chlorophenothane).

Prognosis. Benign disorder; good response to treatment.

BIBLIOGRAPHY. Arias IM: Chronic unconjugated hyperbilirubinemia without overt signs of hemolysis in adolescents and adults. J Clin Invest 41:2233–2245, 1962
Wolkoff AW, Chowdhury JR, Arias IM: Hereditary jaundice and disorders of bilirubin metabolism. In Stanbury JB, Wyngaarden JB, Fredrickson DS, et al (eds): The Metabolic Basis of Inherited Disease, 5th ed, p 1385. New York, McGraw-Hill, 1983

ARLT-DAVIDSEN

Eponym (obsolete) used to indicate the association: lamellar cataract, brown hypoplasia of the teeth, and epilepsy.

BIBLIOGRAPHY. Moortgat P: Syndromes á noms propres. Paris J Prélat, 1966

ARLT'S

Synonyms. Egyptian ophthalmia; chronic follicular keratoconjunctivitis; granular conjunctivitis; trachoma. Chlamydial keratoconjunctivitis.

Symptoms. Both sexes affected; onset variable insidious or acute. Initially, photophobia, tears, blepharospasm.

Signs. Swollen eyelids; mucopurulent discharge; preauricular lymph nodes; conjunctival blebs. Later, scarring, lacrimal dysfunction, and corneal opacities.

Etiology. Infection due to a *Bartonella* (psittacosis), *Lymphogranuloma venereum,* transmitted by contact. Infection due to *Chlamydia trachomatis* transmitted by contact.

Pathology. Papillary hypertrophy of conjunctiva; corneal invasion by dense fibrous tissue, lymphocyte infiltration. Necrosis of conjunctival follicles followed by scarring (Herbert's pits).

Diagnostic Procedures. *Agent isolation.* Inclusion bodies in epithelial cells.

Therapy. Local and systemic antibiotics (tetracycline per os).

Prognosis. According to treatment. Possible complications: entropion; ectropion; symblepharon; xerosis; blindness. Corneal transplantation if severe scarring.

BIBLIOGRAPHY. Arlt CF, von: Die Kranheiten des Auges. Praga, Credner & Kleinbub, 1851
Persson K, Rönnesiam R, Svanberg L, et al: Neonatal chlamydial eye infection: an epidemiological and clinical study. Br J Ophthalmol 67:700–704, 1983
Feducowiez HB, Stetson S: External Infections of the Eye: Bacterial, Viral, and Mycotic, with Noninfectious and Immunologic Diseases, 3rd ed. Norwalk, Conn, Appleton-Century-Croft, 1985

ARMENDARES'

Synonyms. Craniosynostosis-dwarfism-retinitis pigmentosa.

Symptoms and Signs. Present from birth. Microcephaly; craniosynostosis; cranial asymmetry; small face; short nose; micrognathia; high palate; scanty eyebrows; ptosis eyelids; epicanthal fold; retinitis pigmentosa; ear malformation.

Etiology. Unestablished inheritance; X-linked or autosomal recessive.

BIBLIOGRAPHY. Armendares S, Antillon F, Del Castillo V: A newly recognized inherited syndrome of dwarfism, craniosynostosis, retinitis pigmentosa and multiple congenital malformation. J Pediatr 85:872–873, 1974

ARNASON'S

Synonyms. Amyloid cerebral deposits; hereditary cerebral hemorrhage; Iceland hereditary cerebral hemorrhage; amyloidosis VI: HCHWA (hereditary cerebral hemorrhage with amyloidosis); gammatrace, defect of; cerebral amyloid angiopathy.

Symptoms and Signs. In Icelandic families. Both sexes affected; onset of cerebral hemorrhages at young age (in one family, at 44 years in first generation; at 30 years in second generation; at 22.5 years in third generation).

Etiology. Autosomal dominant inheritance.

Pathology. Amyloid deposits in the walls of cerebral vessels. Absence of senile plaques. Absence of amyloid infiltration in brain or other visceral parenchyma.

Prognosis. Death on first episode or survival of variable duration; up to 13 years in one case.

BIBLIOGRAPHY. Árnason Á: Apoplexie und ihre Vererbung. Acta Psychiatr Neurol (suppl) 7:1–180, 1935
Cosgrove GR, Leblanc R, Meagher-Villemure K, et al: Cerebral amyloid angiopathy. Neurology 35:625–639, 1985.

ARNDT-GOTTRON

Synonyms. Lichen myxedematous variant papular mucinosis; papular myxedema; scleromyxedema; lichen fibromucinodosis.

Symptoms and Signs. Appear in 3rd to 5th decades. Diffuse thickening of skin underlying lichenoid papular eruption, often in linear patterns, approximately of uniform size. Infiltrations involve the greater part of the body. Distortion of facial features and limitation of finger movements. Lassitude and muscular weakness may be present.

Etiology. Unknown.

Pathology. Proliferation of fibroblasts and deposition of acid mucopolysaccharides in upper section of dermis. Muscles may be infiltrated with lymphocytes.

Diagnostic Procedures. *Biopsy of skin. Blood.* Presence of a paraprotein of the IgG class. *Bone Marrow.* Mild plasma cell infiltration.

Therapy. None. Melphalan or cyclophosphamide (attention to toxicity). Corticosteroids useless; dermabrasion of some help.

Prognosis. Poor; no spontaneous resolution; with melphalan, gradual resolution of skin lesions within 3 months.

BIBLIOGRAPHY. Gottron HA: Skleromyxeodem (eine eigenartige Erscheinungsform von Myxothesaurodermie). Arch Dermatol Syph 199:71–91, 1954
Rook A, Wilkinson DS, Ebling FJG, et al: Textbook of Dermatology, 4th ed, pp 2296–2297. Oxford, Blackwell Scientific Publications, 1986

ARNETH'S

Not a syndrome but the combination of auscultory sounds modification induced by lung hepatization: bronchial murmur; bronchophony; whispering pectoriloqui.

BIBLIOGRAPHY. Minerbi C: La "sindrome polmonitica di Arneth." La vera natura fisica del fremito vocale tattile. Atti Accad Sc Med Ferrara 3–4:47–49, 1928

ARNOLD-CHIARI

Synonyms. Basilar impression; Celand-Arnold-Chiari; cerebello medullary malformation; platybasia.

Symptoms. Both sexes affected; onset usually in 3rd or 4th decade; symptoms may appear in childhood. Headache; vomiting; visual disturbances; diplopia; mental dullness; paralysis of extremities; ataxia. Respiratory complications can consist of abnormal control of breathing, upper airway-dysfunction, aspiration pneumonia and cor pulmonale. Particularly, abnormalities in control of ventilation are manifested by hypoventilation, sleep apnea, and prolonged breath-holding spells. Milder forms (adult): dizziness; weakness of extremities.

Signs. Hydrocephalus; spinal fluid block; papilledema; nystagmus; paresthesias (transient), glossopharyngeal (IX), vagus (X), spinal accessory (XI), and hypoglossal

(XII) nerve palsies; posterior and lateral column nerve palsies; cerebellar ataxia.

Etiology. Unknown. Congenital malformation of occipital bone and proximal end of cervical spine, determining herniation and molding of brainstem and cerebellum into the foramen magnum.

Pathology. Deformity of occipital bone (platybasia) and proximal end of cervical spine; displacement of cerebellum and medulla oblongata; hydrocephalus; structural derangement in the pontomedullary respiratory controller or in its afferent and efferent pathways. Association with spina bifida, meningocele common.

Diagnostic Procedures. *X-ray.* Platybasia; narrowing of foramen magnum. *Encephalography.* Herniation of cerebral tonsils. *Spinal fluid.* Increased pressure and proteins. *Volume of ventricular system and rate of disappearance of radioiodinated serum albumin. CT brain scan.*

Therapy. Condition may be corrected by neurosurgical procedures. Ventriculoatrial shunting. Early and prolonged ventilatory support can result in favorable outcome.

Prognosis. Differs according to the degree of alterations. In children, extensive deformity, death during first year of life.

BIBLIOGRAPHY. Arnold J: Myelocyste, Transposition von Gewebskeimen und Sympodie. Beitr Path Anat Allg Path 16:1–28, 1894
Chiari H: Ueber Veränderungen des Kleinhirns infolge von Hydrocephalie des Grosshirns. Dtsche Med Wochenschr 17:1172–1175, 1891
Oren J, Kelly DH, Todres ID, Shannon D: Respiratory complication in patients with myelodysplasia and Arnold-Chiari malformation. Am J Dis Child 140:221–224, 1986
Dong ML: Arnold-Chiari malformation type I appearing after tonsillectomy. Anesthesiology 67:120–122, 1987

ARNOLD'S NERVE COUGH

Synonyms. Arnold's neuralgia; vagus auricular branch neuralgia.

Symptoms. Reflex cough, caused by friction from clotting, temperature changes; associated with attack of suboccipital stabbing or burning pain, shifting to neck occasionally and to shoulder. Auricular neuralgia may be present. During remission of pain, tenderness and paresthesias of area.

Signs. Pain on pressure on the area posterior to ear.

Etiology. Irritation of auricular branch of vagus (X) nerve.

Pathology. Neuritis, or compression of nervous branch by different pathologic process.

Therapy. Removal of cause of irritation when identified. Trial with phenytoin or carbamazepine, analgesics, anti-inflammatories, local anesthetics. In refractory cases: surgical interruption of nerve seldom successful and may cause "anesthesia dolorosa".

Prognosis. Depends upon etiology.

BIBLIOGRAPHY. Alayza Escardo F: Arnold's neuralgia. JAMA 161:391, 1956
Vick NA: Grinker's Neurology, 7th ed. Springfield, Ill, CC Thomas, 1976
Adams RD, Victor M: Principles of Neurology, 3rd ed, p 146. New York, McGraw-Hill, 1985

ARRHYTHMOGENIC RIGHT VENTRICULAR DYSPLASIA

Synonyms. See dilated myocardiopathy.

Symptoms and Signs. Right ventricular type, with ventricular arrhythmias of dilated myocardiopathy (see).

BIBLIOGRAPHY. Pietras RJ, Lam W, Bauernfiend R, et al: Chronic recurrent right ventricular tachycardia in a patient without ischemic heart disease: clinical hemodynamic and angiographic findings. Am Heart J:105:357–366, 1983

ARTERIAL VARICES

Synonyms. Arteriovenous aneurysm; arteriovenous anastomosis; arteriovenous fistula.

Symptoms. Onset usually at puberty or after straining activities; usually occur in young persons. Enlargement of the vessels of the lateral side of legs noted; increase in skin temperature may be experienced.

Signs. Enlarged vessels with pulsation synchronous with cardiac pulsation; bruit and thrill may be detected. Arterial-type bleeding.

Etiology. Congenital; arteriovenous connections; familial occurrence.

Diagnostic Procedures. *Elevation.* Veins remain filled; after pressure rapid refilling. Introduction of needle shows pulsation of syringe barrel. Oxygen saturation higher than recorded in blood from other veins of patient. *Angiography.* Useful on confirming the diagnosis.

Therapy. Surgical excision.

Prognosis. Recurrence after surgery. Repeated interventions.

BIBLIOGRAPHY. Pratt FH: Arterial varices syndrome. Am J Surg 77:456–460, 1949

Szilagyi DE, Smith RF, Elliot JP, Hageman JH: Congenital arteriovenous anomalies of the limbs. Arch Surg 111:423–429, 1976

Braundwald E: Heart Disease, Vol 2, p 286. Philadelphia, WB Saunders, 1980

ARTERIOSCLEROSIS OF SPINAL VESSELS

Symptoms. Appear in middle to late age; onset insidious. Weakness starting in one leg, and extending then to the other; intermittent claudication. Urinary urgency, retention, incontinence.

Signs. Hyperreflexion of lower extremities; positive Babinski sign.

Etiology. Arteriosclerotic degeneration of spinal arteries. Arteritis of spinal vessel (syphilis).

Pathology. Nonspecific occlusive arteritis and secondary ischemic atrophy of dorsolumbar cord.

Diagnostic Procedures. *Spinal fluid. Arteriography. Blood serology.*

Therapy. Nonspecific.

Prognosis. Slow or rapid evolution to spastic paraplegia.

BIBLIOGRAPHY. Keschner M, Davison C: Myelytic and myelopathic lesions: arteriosclerotic and arteritic myelopathy. Arch Neurol Psychiatr 29:702–725, 1933

Vick NA: Grinker's Neurology, 7th ed. Springfield, Ill, CC Thomas, 1976

ARTERIOVENOUS FISTULA OF CORONARY ARTERY

Synonym. Coronary arteriosystemic fistula.

Symptoms. Both sexes equally affected. Usually, asymptomatic. Growth and development not compromised.

Signs. Continuous, relatively soft murmur that does not peak on second heart sound and that usually becomes evident only after neonatal fall in pulmonary vascular resistance. Increased frequency of respiratory infections. Heart failure may develop after fourth decade.

Etiology. Defective embryogenesis of coronary artery entering right heart chambers, pulmonary artery, or left chambers (coronary arterosystemic fistula) due to persistence of primitive intramyocardial sinusoids or faulty development of distal branches.

Pathology. Usually solitary, rarely multiple. A saccular aneurysm may develop expecially in adult and shows calcification.

Diagnostic Procedures. *Electrocardiography.* Usually normal. *X-ray.* Normal to variable, according to volume of fistula. *Arterial pulse.* Normal; pulse pressure increased. Selective *cardiac catheterization* or *aortography.*

Therapy. *Medical.* Prevention of complication (thrombosis, myocardial ischemia, infective endocarditis, rupture). *Surgical.* Recommended because it is simple, safe, effective.

Prognosis. Good. Heart failure may develop after age 40. Good with surgery.

BIBLIOGRAPHY. Krause W: Ueber den Ursprung einer accessorishen A coronaria cordis aus der A pulmonalis. Med 24:225–227, 1865

Liberthson RR, Jagar K, Berkoben JP, et al: Congenital coronary arteriovenous fistula: report of 13 patients, review of the literature and delineation of management. Circulation 59:849–854, 1979.

Hurst JW: The Heart, 6th ed, pp 707–708. New York, McGraw-Hill, 1986

ARTHROGRYPOSIS

Synonyms. Amyoplasia congenita, AMC; arthrogryposis multiplex congenita; arthromyodysplasia; Guérin-Stern; myodystrophy fetal deformans; Otto's; Rocher-Sheldon; Rossi's. See Gordon (H.).

Symptoms. Both sexes equally affected. Limited motion of all joints with the exception of mandibular and spinal. Occasional paralysis of different muscles. Reduced facial gesticulation confers a melancholic aspect.

Signs. Osteoarticular deformity with enlargement of joints, hypoplasia of attached muscles, and zones of thickening of the overlying skin (cardboard aspect), alternated with atrophic tracts. *Arms.* Rotated inward; cylindrical elbows; flexed wrists and fingers. *Leg.* Thighs rotated outward; dislocated hip; extended knees; clubfoot; absence of the fibula (occasional). *Skull.* Premature synostosis; palate defect. *Spine.* Absence of sacrum (occasional). No specific dermatoglyphic alterations.

Etiology. Unknown. Congenital neuromuscular disorder; osteoarticular deformities seem to be secondary to muscular atrophy. Lower motor neuron deficiency present in high proportion of cases.

Pathology. Degeneration of some muscle fibers dispersed among normal ones, with fibrotic changes, and fatty infiltration. Inelastic articular capsules; atrophy of the bone. Degeneration of motor neurons of spinal cord.

Diagnostic Procedures. *Muscle biopsy. X-ray.* Bone atrophy. *Electromyography.*

Therapy. Surgical mobilization partly successful.

Prognosis. Situation not progressive. Mortality 10% at early age; infections and visceral malformations are the leading causes.

BIBLIOGRAPHY. Paré A: Monstre et prodiges. In Malgaigue JF: Oevres Completes Revues et Collationnees 3rd ed, p 25. Paris, JB Baillieres, 1573

Otto AW: Monstrorum sexcentorum descriptio anatomica. Bratislava, 1841

Guérin JR: Recherches sur les deformités congénitales chez les monstres. Paris, 1880

Rocher HL: Les raideursarticulaires congénitales multiples. J Med Bordeaux 4:772–780, 1913

Stern WG: Arthrogryposis multiplex congenita. JAMA 81:1507–1510, 1923

Scheldon W: Amyoplasia congenita (multiple congenital articular rigidity, arthrogryposis multiplex congenita) Arch Dis Child (London) 7:117–136, 1932

Rossi E: Le syndrome arthromyodysplasique congénital. Helv Paediatr Acta 2:82–97, 1947

Hall JG, Reed SD, Driscoll EP: Part I Amyoplasia: a common sporadic condition with congenital contractures. Am J Med Gent 15:571–590, 1983

Herring JA: Instructional case: Arthrogryposis. J Pediatr Orthoped 8:353–355, 1988

ARTHROGRYPOSIS, DISTAL TYPE

TYPE I

Symptoms and Signs. From birth. Involvement of hands and feet. See arthrogryposis; variable contraction of other joints.

Etiology. Autosomal dominant inheritance.

Prognosis. Good response to physiotherapy.

TYPE II

Symptoms and Signs. Major involvement of hands and feet associated with other defects: fused cervical vertebrae; cervical pterygia; scoliosis; congenital hip dislocation; contractures of other joints.

Etiology. Autosomal dominant.

Prognosis. Moderate response to physiotherapy.

BIBLIOGRAPHY. Lin P, Hall J, Grever R, et al: A new familial arthrogryposis with autosomal dominant type of inheritance. West Pediatr Clin Res Meeting, Carmel, Calif, 1977

Kawira EL, Bender HA: An unusual distal arthrogryposis. Am J Med Genet 20:425–429, 1985

ARTHROGRYPOSIS MULTIPLEX CONGENITA, DISTAL, X-LINKED

Three distinctive types or X-linked AMC have been reported with variable manifestations, ranging from mild and moderate to lethal forms.

BIBLIOGRAPHY. Hall JG, Reed SD, Scott CI, et al: Three distinct types of X-linked arthrogryposis seen in six families. Clin Genet 21:81–97, 1982

ARTHROGRYPOSIS MULTIPLEX CONGENITA–RENAL HEPATIC ABNORMALITIES

Symptoms and Signs. Males. See Arthrogryposis multiplex congenita, distal, X-linked. Jaundice. Renal impairment.

Etiology. X-linked inheritance.

Pathology. *Kidney.* Tubular cell degeneration and nephrocalcinosis. *Liver.* Black color due to pigmentary deposits.

Prognosis. Death at birth or within first months.

BIBLIOGRAPHY. Nezelof C, Dupart MC, Joubert F, et al: A lethal familial syndrome associating arthrogryposis multiplex congenita, renal dysfunction and a cholestatic and pigmentary liver disease. J Pediat 94:258–260, 1979

ARTHROGRYPOSIS, NEUROGENIC

Synonyms. Arthrogryposis multiplex neurogenic.

Symptoms and Signs. Arthrogryposis-like lesions with primary neurologic lesions.

Etiology. Possibly autosomal recessive inheritance.

BIBLIOGRAPHY. Frischknecht W, Branchi L, Pilleri G: Familiaere arthrogryposis multiplex congenita. Helv Paediat Acta 15:259–279, 1960

ARTICHOKE, MODIFICATION OF TASTE BY

Symptoms. Eating an artichoke (*Cymara scolymus*) makes water taste sweet in some subjects.

Etiology. Temporary alteration in the tongue. Genetic basis unknown.

Pathology. None.

Therapy. None.

BIBLIOGRAPHY. Blakeslee AF: A dinner demonstration of threshold differences in taste and smell. Science 81:504–507, 1935
Bartoshuk LM, Lee CH, Scarpellino R: Sweet taste induced by artichoke. Science 178:988–989, 1972
McKusick V: Mendelian Inheritance in Man. Baltimore, Johns Hopkins University Press, 1986

ASA TRIAD

Synonym. Asthma–nasal polyps–aspirin intolerance.

Symptoms and Signs. Both sexes. Early or late onset in life of asthmatic attacks, nasal polyposis, and aspirin intolerance. Cases with incomplete triad.

Etiology. Recessive inheritance, also dominant reported; possible importance of environmental factors. Probably due to aspirin inhibition of cyclooxygenase pathway.

BIBLIOGRAPHY. Miller FF: Aspirin-induced bronchial asthma in sisters. Am Allergy 29:263–265, 1971
Von Maur K, Adkinson NF, Jr, Van Metre TE, Jr, et al: Aspirin intolerance in a family. J Allergy Clin Immun 54:380–395, 1974

ASBOE-HANSEN

See Bloch-Sulzberger. Considered by the authors as the initial phase of the Bloch-Sulzberger syndrome. There is no reason for autonomy as an entity.

BIBLIOGRAPHY. Asboe-Hansen G: Bullous keratogenous and pigmentary dermatitis with blood eosinophilia in newborn girls: report of four cases. Arch Dermatol Syph 67:152–157, 1953

ASCHER'S

Synonyms. Blepharochalasis-thyroid; struma–double lips; Laffer-Ascher; blepharochalasis–double lips.

Symptoms and Signs. *Eyes.* Blepharochalasis fundamental sign (see Fuch's syndrome for description). Two phases as in Fuch's: (1) Recurrent edemas; (2) atrophy of skin and subcutaneous tissue of eyelids, and prolapse of orbital cavity contents. *Mouth.* Thickening of lips and gums; mucosa gives the aspect of double lips. *Thyroid.* Enlargement (occasional).

Etiology. Unknown. Localized cutaneous atrophy. This syndrome needs a modern evaluation with new techniques of endocrine studies. Autosomal dominant.

Pathology. Early localized edema of eyelids and lips. Later, atrophy of skin; subcutaneous with progressive degeneration; disappearance of elastic fibers. In early stages, perivascular lymphocytic infiltration that tends to disappear with progress of the disease has also been noticed. Thyroid alteration not described.

Diagnostic Procedures. *Blood and urine.* Normal. *Basal metabolism rate.* Usually normal; occasionally slightly elevated.

Therapy. Some improvements in cases have been obtained with the use of thyroid extract. Plastic surgery for correction of skin defect.

Prognosis. Good result obtainable by plastic correction of defect. Otherwise, progressive condition.

BIBLIOGRAPHY. Ascher KW: Blepharochalasis mit Struma und Doppellippe. Klin Monatsbl Augenheilkd 65:86, 1920
Segal P, Joblonska S: Le syndrome d'Ascher. Ann Oculist 194:511–526, 1961
McKusick VA: Heritable Disorders of Connective Tissue, 4th ed. St Louis, CV Mosby, 1972

ASEPTIC MENINGITIS

Synonyms. Acute benign choriomeningitis.

Symptoms. Headache; mild stiffness of neck and back; anorexia; nausea; vomiting.

Signs. Fever; convulsions; papilledema occasionally; absence of normal reflexes; positive Kerning's and Brudzinsky's signs. Sensory disturbances.

Etiology. Polio, echo, mumps, measles, rubella, coxsackie virus. Leptospirosis; spirochetosis; toxoplasmosis; tuberculosis; trichinosis; cysticercosis cerebri. Serum sickness; vaccines; toxic substances; pyogenic infections contiguous to meninges not adequately treated. (See Benign intracranial hypertension.)

Pathology. Lymphocytic leptomeningeal choroid plexus; ependyma infiltrations; inclusion body in viral etiology.

Diagnostic Procedures. *Cerebrospinal fluid.* Increased in pressure; clear becoming turbid with progression of disease. Sugar, proteins normal or slightly increased, presence of mononuclear cells, usually negative cultures, titer of viral antibodies rising (when virus infection causative). *Blood.* White blood cells; lymphocytosis (virus); polymorphs (bacteria); eosinophils (parasites). *Urine cultures. X-rays of skull.*

Therapy. Depends on etiology.

Prognosis. In aseptic viral meningitis, usually, symptoms and signs subsiding in 7 days; residual fatigue. If other agents responsible, may be extremely severe and fatal if not promptly diagnosed and treated.

BIBLIOGRAPHY. Wallgren A: Une nouvelle maladie infectieuse du systeme nerveux central. Acta Paediatr (Belge) 4:158–182, 1925
Rosenthal MS: Viral infections of the central nervous system. Med Clin N Am 58:593–603, 1974
Adams RD, Victor M: Principles of Neurology, 3rd ed, 553–556. New York. McGraw-Hill, 1985

ASHERMAN'S

Synonyms. Traumatic uterine adhesions; traumatic amenorrhea.

Symptoms. Amenorrhea (traumatic amenorrhea); repeated abortions; impaired fertility or hypomenorrhea.

Signs. Cervix uteri occluded; uterine probe cannot be passed into the cervical canal.

Etiology. Dilatation and curettage of a puerperal uterus. According to Asherman: "Most prone to damage, however, are the succulent and hyperemic walls of the puerperal uterus."

Pathology. Two varieties are known: (1) Cervical adhesions giving rise to the amenorrhea; (2) corporeal adhesions, repeated abortions, impaired fertility, and hypomenorrhea. Adhesions in the corpus uteri are either endometrial or, most often, consist of fibromuscular bands.

Diagnostic Procedures. *Hysterography.* Stable filling defects.

Differential Diagnosis. Other causes of amenorrhea; intrauterine polyps.

Therapy. For the cervical type, adequate dilatation of the cervical canal. For the corporeal type, therapy only indicated if symptomatic. It consists of instrumental separation of the adhesions. Prophylaxis, though, is the best way to treat the condition. Postpartum curettage should be avoided.

Prognosis. Good, once condition is recognized and treated.

BIBLIOGRAPHY. Asherman JG: Amenorrhea traumatica (atretica). J Obstet Gynaecol Br Emp 25–30, 1948; Traumatic intrauterine adhesions. J Obstet Gynaecol Br Emp 57:892–896, 1950
Dalsace J, Musset R, Netter A, et al: Les synechies uterines. Proceedings XVII Congres Fed Soc Gyn et Obst Langue Francoise, pp 196–252. Marseille, 9–12, 1957. Paris, Masson
Wilson JR, Carrington ER (eds): Obstetrics and Gynecology, 8th ed, p 101. St Louis, CV Mosby, 1987

ASHERSON'S

Synonyms. Cricopharyngeal achalasia sphincter.

Symptoms and Signs. Dysphagia (of all degrees of severity), followed immediately by episodes of coughing (mild or in severe paroxysms). There is a hold-up of swallowed contents in the hypopharynx detectable on a pharyngoscopic mirror, or demonstrable on x-ray, after a radiopaque material is swallowed. In cricopharyngeal achalasia the dysphagia is most noticeable when liquids are swallowed; when there is a "spill-over" into the air passage, producing paroxysms of coughing; and when, in extreme cases, the inhaled contents produce pneumonia.

Etiology. The causes are many, but the syndrome is seen at its most extreme in certain cases of sudden bilateral recurrent laryngeal paralysis, and in poliomyelitis with pharyngeal paralysis. It is due to a neuromuscular incoordination, with failure of relaxation of the cricopharyngeal muscle.

Diagnostic Procedures. *X-ray.* Diagnosis confirmed after a radiopaque swallow.

Therapy. In mild cases, dilatation of the cricopharyngeal sphincter; in severe cases, myotomy of the cricopharyngeal muscle.

BIBLIOGRAPHY. Asherson N: Achalasia of the cricopharyngeal sphincter. J Laryngol Otol 64:747–758, 1950

Bonavina L, Khan MA, De Meester TR: Pharyngoesophageal dysfunction: the role of crycopharyngeal myotomy. Arch Surg 120:541–549, 1985

aminuria. In Stanbury JB, Wyngaarden JB, Fredrickson DS, et al (eds): The Metabolic Basis of Inherited Disease, 5th ed, p 788. New York, McGraw-Hill, 1983

ASPARAGUS, URINARY EXCRETION OF ODORIFEROUS COMPONENT OF

Symptoms and Signs. After eating asparagus, urinary excretion of an odoriferous substance, called methanethiol. A subject who is a nonexcretor may become an excretor during pregnancy; the child to be born will probably be an excretor.

Therapy. None. The syndrome does not have any pathological significance.

BIBLIOGRAPHY. Allison AC, McWhinter KG: Two unifactorial characters for which man is polymorphic. Nature 178:748–749, 1956
McKusick V: Mendelian Inheritance in Man. Baltimore, Johns Hopkins University Press, 1985

ASPARTYLGLYCOSAMINURIA

Symptoms and Signs. Predominant in females. Normal at birth, then recurrent infections, diarrhea, hernias. Failure to thrive and hepatomegaly. By first decade coarsening of facies, increased acne and photophobia, joint laxity, macroglossia, brachycephaly. Mental deterioration between age 6 and 15. Latter hypotonia or spasticity.

Etiology. Autosomal genetic disorder, probably recessive defect of aspartylglycosaminidase.

Pathology. *Blood.* Vacuolated lymphocytes (not always present). *Other tissues.* Vacuolated cells. *Urine.* Aspartylglycosamine.

Diagnostic Procedures. *Fibroblast cultures.* Defect of metabolism of aspartylglycosamine.

Therapy. None.

Prognosis. Mental deterioration. No reduced life expectancy.

BIBLIOGRAPHY. Antio S: Aspartylglycosaminuria: analysis of thirty-four patients. J Ment Defic Res Monogr Ser 1:1, 1972
Beaudet AL: Disorders of glycoprotein degradation mannosidosis, glucosidosis, sialidosis and aspartylglycos-

ÅSTRÖM-MANCALL-RICHARDSON

Synonym. Multifocal progressive leukoencephalopathy, PML.

Symptoms. Both sexes affected; onset insidious, usually, after 40 years of age. Unilateral weakness; dysphagia; visual impairment up to blindness; aphasia; alteration of consciousness up to dementia.

Signs. Hemiparesis; homonymous hemianopia; and other signs associated to myeloproliferative or lymphoproliferative syndromes (see); Besnier-Boeck-Shaumann (see); tuberculosis; primary hypersplenism; Whipple's syndrome (see) carcinomatosis; blue sea histiocyte.

Etiology. Viral infection (papovavirus SV 40 and more frequently JC type) in patients with impaired immunologic response due frequently to myeloproliferative, neoplastic, infective, chronic granulomatosis conditions.

Pathology. Wide demyelinization (central and peripheral) in perivascular foci, with sparing of axis cylinders; variable cytologic reactions, occasionally, presence of inclusion bodies formed by crystalline arrays of particles similar to papoviruses.

Diagnostic Procedures. Diagnosis of associated condition. *Spinal fluid.* Pressure normal or slightly elevated; pleocytosis, protein elevated; search for serological evidence of presence of papoviruses. *Electroencephalography.* Slow wave, diffuse activity; alteration according to localization and extension of lesions.

Therapy. That of associated conditions. Trials with cytosine arabinoside and vidarabine usually without success.

Prognosis. Poor; remission or improvement may follow the treatment of associated condition. Progressive deterioration. Death usually within 3–20 months of onset.

BIBLIOGRAPHY. Åström K, Mancall EL, Richardson EP Jr: Progressive multifocal leukoencephalopathy: A hitherto unrecognized complication of chronic lymphatic leukemia and Hodgkin's disease. Brain 81:93–111, 1958
Richardson EP Jr: Our evolving understanding of progressive multifocal leukoencephalopathy. Ann NY Acad Sci 230:358–364, 1974
Adams RD, Victor M: Principles of Neurology, 3rd ed, pp 563–564. New York, McGraw-Hill, 1985

ATHEROSCLEROSIS OBLITERANS

Synonyms. Arteriosclerosis obliterans; arterial insufficiency of common iliac artery. Arterial insufficiency; atherosclerotic occlusive; obliterative arteriosclerosis; peripheral arterial. See also Moenckeberg's.

Symptoms. Occur in patients over 40 years of age; 75% are male. Resulting from sudden arterial occlusion or more frequently of slow, insidious progression. Most important symptoms: pain; tightness; cramps that develop while walking and subside with rest, most frequently in the calf, but may occur as well in the foot, thigh, and buttocks (intermittent claudication). With progression of the disease, rest pain (pretrophic) may be present, mostly in the foot and occurring at night; sensory symptoms may also be experienced; hyperesthesia.

Signs. Pallor; cyanosis; trophic changes of the skin; ulcer and gangrene in advanced stage precipitated by trauma; decrease of skin temperature; decrease or absence of arterial pulsations; atrophy of muscle. Elevation pallor and dependent rubor. Later sign: hyporeflexia.

Etiology. Unknown. Risk factors for arteriosclerosis: smoking, diabetes mellitus, hyperlipemia hypertension, obesity.

Pathology. Arteries thrombosed by occluding masses; atheromatous changes of arterial wall; calcareous deposits.

Diagnostic Procedures. *Blood.* Hyperlipemia. *Arterial pulse. Angiography.* Shows site and nature of lesion (calcifications). *Noninvasive diagnostic techniques: Doppler ultrasonic velocity detector segmental plethysmography.*

Therapy. Conservative; some cases benefit from thromboarteriectomy, vascular graft, and sympathectomy. Protect leg and foot from injuries. Control associated pathologies; diet; walking; refrain from smoking; pain treatment; thromboembolytic therapy.

Prognosis. Progressive.

BIBLIOGRAPHY. Imparato AM, Kim G, Davidson T, et al: Intermittent claudication: its natural course. Surgery 78:795, 1975
Risins B, Zelch MC, Graor RA, et al: Catheter-directed low dose streptokinase infusion: a preliminary experience. Radiology 150:349–353, 1984
Bergan JJ, Flinn WR, Yao JST: Operative therapy of peripheral vascular disease. Progr Cardiovasc Dis 26:273–294, 1984

ATHROMBIA

Synonyms. Factor 3 platelet deficiency; PF3; platelet factor 3 deficiency (possibly the same syndrome); thrombopathia.

Symptoms. Bleeding tendency.

Etiology. Unknown. Deficient platelet adhesion to collagen fibers. Autosomal recessive or X-linked inheritance discussed.

Diagnostic Procedures. *Coagulation tests.* Platelets do not spread or agglutinate normally on slide. In presence of added adenosine diphosphate (ADP) platelet adhesiveness, aggregation, and factor 3 release becomes normal (differentiates this form from Glanzmann's). *Type I.* Prolonged bleeding time, normal clot retraction, defective Salzman test in presence of PF3. *Type II.* Altered interaction between platelets and collagen with normal ADP and adrenalin induced aggregation and normal Salzman test.

BIBLIOGRAPHY. Inceman S, Ucar S, Ulutin ON: Athrombia thrombocytopathica. Thromb Diath Haemorrh 4:234–243, 1960
Weiss HJ: Platelet aggregation, adhesion and adenosine diphosphate release in thrombopathia (platelet factor 3 deficiency): a comparison with Glanzmann's thrombasthenia and von Willebrand's disease. Am J Med 43:570–578, 1967
Goldman BA, Aledort LA: Essential athrombia: a family study. Ann Intern Med 76:269–273, 1981

ATHYROTIC HYPOTHYROIDISM

Synonym. Agoitrous hypothyroidism; cretinism, athyrotic; thyroid dysgenesis.

Symptoms. Present at birth. Feeding problems; decreased activity. Severe damage on morphogenesis and function of brain.

Signs. At birth only minor signs of hypothyroidism (see), which become in time progressively more evident. Constipation; jaundice; cold and dry skin; mottling, large tongue; umbilical hernia.

Etiology. Unknown. Simple development defect of sporadic occurrence.

Pathology. Absence of small nonfunctional residue of thyroid gland.

Diagnostic Procedures. See Gull's.

Therapy. Thyroid hormone given as soon as possible.

Prognosis. According to time of onset of thyroid hormone administration. Variable grades of brain function impairment.

BIBLIOGRAPHY. Ainger LE, Kelly VC: Familial athyrotic cretinism: report of 3 cases. J Clin Endocr 15:469–475, 1955

Winkins L: The Diagnosis and Treatment of Endocrine Disorders in Childhood and Adolescence. Springfield, Ill, CC Thomas, 1965

Smith DW: Recognizable patterns of human malformations. Philadelphia, WB Saunders, 1982

ATLANTOAXIAL SPINE DISLOCATION

Synonyms. Cervical spine dislocation; odontoid dysplasia; atlantoaxial spine subluxation.

Symptoms and Signs. One of the most important clinical manifestations in short stature syndromes. Progressive neuromuscular disturbances ranging from a decrease of physical endurance to paraplegia or sudden death (particularly under anesthesia).

Etiology. Two factors necessary to cause atlantoaxial instability and secondary myelopathy: odontoid hypoplasia or aplasia and ligamentous laxity.

Pathology. Variable degree of odontoid dysgenesis and ligamentous laxity, plus thick wad of soft tissue posterior to the dysplastic odontoid process; spinal cord compression and displacement to one side of the canal.

Diagnostic Procedures. *X-ray. Gas myelography. CT brain scan.*

Therapy. Surgical stabilization of involved area; posterior cervical fusion.

Prognosis. After successful stabilization, improvement of neurologic symptoms (increase in strength and physical endurance) within 2 years. If not treated, possibility of sudden death.

BIBLIOGRAPHY. Bailey JA: Disproportionate Short Stature: Diagnosis and Management. Philadelphia, WB Saunders, 1973

Williams JP, Somerville G, Miner ME, Reilly D: Atlantoaxial subluxation and trisomy 21: another perioperative complication. Anesthesiology 67:253–254, 1987

Wood GN: Other disorders of the spine. In Crenshaw AH (ed): Campbell's Operative Orthopedics, 7th ed, pp 3354–3355. St Louis, CV Mosby, 1987

ATRIAL SEPTAL DEFECT–ATRIOVENTRICULAR CONDUCTION, PROLONGED

Symptoms and Signs. Complete form in addition to symptoms of atrial septal defect–persistent ostium secundum (see); prolongation of PR interval. Incomplete forms in members of same family (atrial septal defect only or PR prolongation).

Etiology. Non-sex-linked autosomal dominant inheritance.

Diagnostic Procedures. See Atrial septal defect–persistent ostium secundum. *Electrocardiography.* PR interval ranging between 0.22 and 0.56 sec; left axis deviation. *Clinical examination of family members of suspected cases.* Biochemical marker for the mutant gene.

Therapy. Symptomatic.

Prognosis. Possibility of sudden death.

BIBLIOGRAPHY. Kahler RL, Braunwald E, Plauth WH Jr, et al: Familial congenital heart disease. Am J Med 40:384–399, 1966

Bizarro RO, Callahan JA, Feldt RH, et al: Familial atrial defect with prolonged atrioventricular conduction. Circulation 41:677–683, 1970

Pease WE, Mordenberg A, Ladda RL: Familial atrial septal defect with prolonged atrioventricular conduction. Circulation 53:759–762, 1976

Braunwald E: Heart Disease, Vol 2, p 1695. Philadelphia, WB Saunders, 1980

ATRIAL SEPTAL DEFECT–PERSISTENT OSTIUM PRIMUM

Symptoms and Signs. Pure form is not different from atrial septal defect–persistent ostium secundum (see). For complicated form see Endocardial cushion defect. Mitral stenosis and mitral valve prolapse are unusual but important associated defects.

ATRIAL SEPTAL DEFECT–PERSISTENT OSTIUM SECUNDUM

Synonym. Sinus venous defect.

Symptoms and Signs. Ostium secundum: female-male ratio 1.5 to 3.5 : 1. Usually not detected for years. Children delicate, frail, underweight, normal height. Growth retardation if large left-to-right shunts. Possible recurrent respiratory infections. First sound may be split at left sternal margin and tip; second component is loud. Soft midsystolic murmur after first sound. Conspicuous thrust of right ventricle on left sternal edge.

Etiology. Autosomal dominant or recessive inheritance. Most common congenital condition in adults.

Pathology. *Atrial septal defect.* In the region of the fossa ovalis; inferior to the fossa or in the upper part of atrium septum (sinus venous variety).

Diagnostic Procedures. *Arterial pulse.* Within normal limit. *Jugular venous pulse.* Usually normal. *Echocardiography.* Findings characteristic of right ventricular volume overload: (1) increased right ventricular end-diastolic dimension, (2) abnormal motion of the ventricular septum, (3) real-time two-dimensional scans from the apical position to identify the location and size of the atrial defect. *Phonocardiography. Electrocardiography.* P wave normal or peaked; small q waves in II, III, and aVF leads. *X-ray.* Pulmonary arterial plethora; small aorta; conspicuous pulmonary artery; dilatation of right heart. *Cardiac catheterization.* The oxygen content of blood from the right atrium is much higher than that from the superior vena cava.

Therapy. Surgical treatment according to pulmonary systemic blood flow ratio. For asymptomatic infants and children, surgery is recommended prior to entry into school.

Prognosis. Pulmonary hypertension begins to appear in the early 20s. Passage of time, after adolescence, is associated with an increase in the frequency and severity of symptoms; congestive failure is the most common cause of death in unoperated atrial septal defects.

BIBLIOGRAPHY. Rokitansky CF: Die Defecte der Scheidewände des Herzens Braumüller. Wien, 1875

Bedford DE, Papp C, Parkinson J: Atrial septal defect. Br Heart J 3:37–60, 1941

Haworth SG: Pulmonary vascular disease in secundum atrial septal defect in childhood. Am J Cardiol 51:265–278, 1983

Hurst JW: The Heart, 6th ed, pp 597–603. New York, McGraw-Hill, 1986

ATRIOVENTRICULAR BLOCK, HIGH DEGREE, CONGENITAL

Synonyms. Atrioventricular block, congenital; Morquio's I.

Symptoms and Signs. Present at birth. Frequently asymptomatic may be detected in young age. Isolated anomaly. Ventricular rate between 40 and 90 beats. In some cases severe ventricular tachyarrhythmias and Morgagni-Adams-Stokes (see) attacks.

Etiology. Unknown.

Diagnostic Procedures. *Electrocardiography, Electrophysiological studies. Outpatient monitoring.*

Therapy. Pacing indicated in all cases where monitoring reveals additional unstable ventricular ectopic foci.

Prognosis. Good. True incidence of sudden death difficult to establish.

BIBLIOGRAPHY. Morquio L: Sur une maladie infantile et familial caracterisée par des modifications permanentes du pouls, des attaques syncopales et epileptiformes et la mort subite. Arch Méd Enf 4:467, 1912

Hurst JW: The Heart, 6th ed, pp 488–489. New York, McGraw-Hill, 1986

ATRIOVENTRICULAR CONGENITAL HEART BLOCK

Symptoms. Incidence 1 : 10,000 to 1 : 20,000. Appear in children. Both sexes affected; onset from fetal life to adult life. (The later discovered, the less probability of congenital origin.) Asymptomatic. Exercise tolerance normal or slightly reduced. In low percentage poor tolerance to stress or continuous febrile illnesses. Complaints from mild dizziness to frank syncope and convulsions.

Signs. Normal growth, development, and physical aspect. Seldom, cyanosis. Arterial pulse slow; resting rate above 40 beats/min (inappropriate to patient age). Acceleration of 10 to 20 beats/min after exercise. Waterhammer pulse. Heart area palpation: left ventricular impulse prominent. Auscultation: slow rate and regular variation of rhythm; variation in intensity of first sound; grade 2 to 3 midsystolic murmur; normal respiratory splitting of second sound; third heart sound common. Systolic hypertension. Irregular jugular pulsation.

Etiology. Congenital defect in the main stem of the bundle of His.

Pathology. Seventy percent of cases have no other evidence of heart disease; the most frequently associated cardiac malformations are "corrected" transposition of the great arteries (ventricular inversion), single ventricle, and patent ductus arteriosus.

Diagnostic Procedures. *Arterial pulse.* Low rate; pulse pressure; wide arterial upstroke brisk; arterial waves abnormalities. *Venous pulse.* Intermittent common waves; abnormalities of a wave. *Electrocardiography.* Inconstant ratio between P waves. *X-ray.* Normal heart size to moderate increase.

Therapy. Implantation of a permanent pacemaker.

Prognosis. Generally good. In some cases heart may be unable to respond to increased circulation demands, and congestive heart failure and death, especially in neonatal period, may occur.

BIBLIOGRAPHY. Morquio L: Sur une maladie infantile et familiale characterisée par des modifications permanentes du pouls, des attaques syncopales et epileptiforme et la mort subite. Arch Med Enf 4:467–475, 1901
Hurst JW: The Heart, 6th ed, pp 488–489. New York, McGraw-Hill, 1986

ATROPHY-DEAFNESS NEUROGENIC-AMYOTHROPHY

Synonyms. Iwashita's;   Rosenberg-Chutorian.   See Treft's.

Symptoms and Signs. Both sexes. From birth. Progressive polyneuropathy (similar to Charcot-Marie-Tooth, see); deafness and visual loss.

Etiology. Not established if autosomal dominant, recessive, or X-linked disorder (possible cluster of syndromes).

Pathology. Degeneration of acoustic and optic peripheral nerves.

Prognosis. Progressive disorder. Visual loss in 4th decade.

BIBLIOGRAPHY. Iwashita H, Inone N, Araki S, et al: Optic atrophy, neural deafness and distal neurogenic amyothrophy: report of a family with two affected siblings. Arch Neurol 22:357–364, 1970
Rosenberg RN, Chutorian A: Familial opticoacoustic nerve degeneration and polyneuropathy. Neurology 17:827–832, 1967
Treft RL: Unique hereditary syndrome found involves vision and hearing loss. Ophthal Times, July:12–13, 1983

ATYPICAL FACIAL NEURALGIA

Symptoms. Prevalent in young or middle-aged women. Long history of attacks of pain in the face, neck, or head persisting or remitting; not confined to territorial distribution of cranial nerves.

Etiology. Conversion hysteria; hypochondrias; vascular pathology.

Diagnostic Procedures. *X-rays of teeth, sinuses, cervical column.*

Therapy. Antidepressant and antianxiety medication. Only a few cases responded to ergotamine tartrate. Analgesic (addiction frequent); psychotherapy. Refrain from alcohol injection or neurosurgery.

Prognosis. Difficult to cure.

BIBLIOGRAPHY. Harris W: Neuritis and Neuralgia. London, Oxford, 1926
Harris W: An analysis of 1,433 cases of paroxysmal trigeminal neuralgia (trigeminal-tic) and end-results of gasserian alcohol injection. Brain 63:209–224, 1940
Adams RD, Victor M: Principles of Neurology, 3rd ed, p 147. New York, McGraw-Hill, 1985

AUSTRIAN

Eponym to indicate the triad; alcoholic debilitation, pneumococcal pneumonia, and pneumococcal meningitis.

Prognosis. Poor.

BIBLIOGRAPHY. Strauss AL, Hamburger M: Pneumococcal endocarditis in the penicillin era. Arch Intern Med 118:190–198, 1966

AUTONOMIC SPINAL

Lesions of the autonomic fibers connected with the spinal cord result in different syndromes according to the level of the lesions.

1. C8–T1 (ciliospinal reflex center): pupillary miosis; enophthalmos; ptosis (Horner's syndrome).
2. T1 segment: dilatation of pupil; exophthalmos; upper eyelid elevation; cervical sympathetic chain (Claude Bernard syndrome); perspiration; and vasoconstriction.
3. T1–T6 spinal cord; T1–T4 sympathetic ganglia: tachycardia.
4. T4–T7 (?) spinal cord: inhibition of bronchiolar constriction; upper thoracic sympathetic chain.
5. T2–T9: perspiration and vasoconstriction; upper extremity piloerection; cervical sympathetic chain.
6. T10–L4: perspiration; vasoconstriction, lower extremity piloerection.
7. T5–L4: perspiration; vasoconstriction; thoracic wall and abdomen piloerection.
8. T5–T9: inhibition of gastric muscles and contraction of sphincter.
9. Thoracolumbar ganglionated chain; celiac ganglion, superior mesenteric ganglia; splanchnic nerve: visceral vasoconstriction; inhibition of intestinal wall; contraction of ileocecal sphincter.
10. L1–L2 inferior mesenteric ganglion: vasoconstriction in kidney; constriction of rectal sphincter.

11. L1–L3 inferior mesenteric ganglion: inhibition of detrusor (?) plus constriction of internal sphincter (?) of bladder.
12. S1–S3 and pelvic nerves: contraction of detrusor; relaxation of rectal and vesical sphincters; muscles; erection.

BIBLIOGRAPHY. Vick NA: Grinker's Neurology, 7th ed. Springfield, IL, CC Thomas, 1976

AUTOSCOPIC

Synonyms. Lukianowicz's; mirror image. See also Capgras' syndrome.

Symptoms and Signs. Occur in patients suffering from depression, migraine, epilepsy, schizophrenia: delusion of suddenly experiencing of seeing double (not in color, but as a white or grayish image).

Etiology. Delusional dislocation of body image in the visual sphere. Well-known psychic phenomenon cited in history and literature.

Therapy. That of the basic neurologic psychotic condition.

BIBLIOGRAPHY. Critchley M: Neurological aspects of visual and auditory hallucinations. Br Med J 2:634–639, 1939
Lukianowicz N: Autoscopic phenomena. AMA Arch Neurol Psychiatr 80:199–220, 1958

AVELLIS'

Synonyms. Ambiguospinothalamic paralysis; Avellis-Longhi; Avellis' hemiplegia; palatopharyngeal paralysis; spinothalamic tract–nucleus ambiguous.

Symptoms. Dysphagia; dysphoria; unilateral loss of pain and temperature to trunk and limbs; Horner's syndrome may be associated.

Signs. Paralysis of soft palate and larynx controlateral to the pain and temperature loss.

Etiology. Vascular or inflammatory or neoplastic lesions involving the nucleus ambiguous and the vagus (X) and accessory nerves, and spinothalamic tract.

Pathology. See Etiology. Lesion localized in the medulla or near the jugular foramen.

Therapy. Depends upon etiology.

Prognosis. As above.

BIBLIOGRAPHY. Avellis G: Klinicshe Beitrage zur halbseitigen Kehlkopflähmung. Berl Klin 40:1–26, 1891
Fox SL, West GB, Jr: Syndrome of Avellis; review of literature and report of one case. Arch Otolaryngol 46:773–778, 1947
Adams RD, Victor M: Principles of Neurology, 3rd ed, p 1010. New York, McGraw-Hill, 1985

AXENFELD'S

Synonyms. Arcus juvenilis; posterior embryotoxon; Hagedoom's syndromes. See Rieger's and Reese-Ellsworth.

Signs. Posterior corneal embryotoxon; increased visibility of the Schwalbe line. When associated with other anterior segment disturbances and juvenile glaucoma, the complex is called Reiger's. The eponym Axenfeld's is also used as synonym for Reiger's, and Hagedoom's mesostromal dysgenesia. This syndrome is often a component of the more complex syndromes that involve oculodentodigital systems, or associated with other diseases and developmental anomalies (Marfan's syndrome; dystrophia myotonica; facial deformities).

Etiology. Unknown. Developmental arrest with persistence of deficient absorption and atrophy of mesodermal uveal tissue in the angle of anterior chamber (Reiger). Developmental arrest of anterior vitreous body (mesostrom anterior; Hagedoom).

BIBLIOGRAPHY. Axenfeld T: Embryotoxon corneae posterius. Ber Dtsch Ophthalmol Ges 42:301, 1920
Rieger HV: Über Subconjunctivitis epibulbous metastatica bei Parotitis epidemica. Arch Ophthalmol 133:505–507, 1935
Hagedoom A: Congenital anomalies of the anterior segment of the eye. Arch Ophthalmol 17:223–227, 1937
Montes JG, Montes JCG: Syndrome de Rieger, anomalie de Axenfeld con glaucoma juvenil familiar. Arch Soc Ophth Hisp Am 27:93–99, 1967

AXENFELD-SCHÜRENBERG

Synonyms. Congenital cyclic oculomotor paralysis.

Symptoms and Signs. Congenital or appear during first year of life. Unilateral oculomotor (III) nerve paralysis, upper lid ptosis, eye abduction, and midriasis (relaxed phase), alternating with the paralysis of automatic contraction (lasting 30 seconds to 1 minute) of the muscle innervated by the oculomotor (III) nerve, with resulting lifting of upper lid, myosis, and deviation of the eye (spastic phase).

Etiology and Pathology. Unknown; possibly congenital. One case reported after trauma.

BIBLIOGRAPHY. Axenfeld T, Schürenberg E: Zur Kenntniss der angeborenen Beweglichkeitdefekete der Augen. Klin Monatsb Augenhleilkd 39:64; 844, 1901
Latorre-Morasso S, Agular J: Enfermedad de Axenfeld-Schürenberg. Arch Soc Oftal Hispano Am 1:625–632, 1942
Susac JO, Smith JL: Cyclic oculomotor paralysis. Neurology 24:24–27, 1974
Leigh RJ, Zee DS: The Neurology of Eye Movements. Philadelphia, FA Davis, 1983

AYERZA-ARRILAGA

Eponym obsolete. Used to indicate a variety of Ayerza's syndrome (see), when due to chronic bronchopulmonary syphilis and to a syphilitic obliterans sclerosis of the pulmonary artery.

BIBLIOGRAPHY. Arrilaga RC: Esclerosis secundaria de la arteria pulmonary y su quadro clinico (cardiacos negros). Buenos Aires, 1912
Garnier M, Delamare V: Dizionario dei termini tecnici e medicina, 19th ed. Rome, DEMI, 1974

AYERZA'S

Synonyms. Cardiac block; cardiopathy nigra; pulmonary arteriosclerosis; pulmonary arteritis.

Symptoms and Signs. Gradual onset in 5th decade of life in patients with preceding bronchopulmonary symptomatology. Respiratory insufficiency with severe dyspnea; marked cyanosis of face, hands, and feet. Signs of pulmonary emphysema and right ventricular hypertrophy. Digital clubbing. Occasionally, splenomegaly. Passive congestion of liver.

Etiology. Unknown; associated with diseases of pulmonary artery such as atherosclerosis, syphilis.

Pathology. Hypertrophy of right ventricle; sclerosis with intimal thickening; atheroma formation; loss of elastic fibers with resulting generalized (arterial and arteriolar) narrowing of vascular bed; pulmonary emphysema.

Diagnostic Procedures. *Blood.* Polycythemia. *Pulmonary function tests. X-ray of chest.*

Therapy. Control of secondary polycythemia, congestive failure, and other symptomatic treatments.

Prognosis. Poor.

BIBLIOGRAPHY. Ayerza L: Unpublished clinical lecture at National University of Buenos Aires, 1901
Arrilaga FC: Esclerosis secundaria de la arteria pulmonary su cuadro clinico (Cardiacos negros). Buenos Aires, 1912
Wintrobe MM (ed): Clinical Hematology, 8th ed. Philadelphia, Lea & Febiger, 1981

AZOREAN NEUROLOGIC

Synonyms. Machado-Joseph; Joseph's; spinopontine atrophy.

Symptoms and Signs. Both sexes. Onset in 4th decade. In family prevalently descendant from Azores inhabitants, also reported in Japan, the U.S., Europe. Variable clinical features. Four phenotypic variations tentatively identified (variation even occur in the same family): (1) cerebellar ataxia, external ophthalmoplegia, pyramidal signs; extrapyramidal signs; (2) same as variation 1 without extrapyramidal signs; (3) same as 1 plus distal muscular atrophy; (4) same as 1 plus neuropathy and parkinsonism.

Etiology. Unknown. Autosomal dominant inheritance.

Pathology. Loss of neurons and gliosis in substantia nigra, nuclei pontis, vestibular nuclei, cranial nerves. Clarke columns and anterior horns.

Diagnostic Procedures. *Pneumoencephalography.* Presence of air in the posterior fossa. *CT brain scan. Electroencephalography. Electromyography. Cerebrospinal fluid. Blood.* Frequent hyperglycemia.

Prognosis. Progressive condition of ataxia, parkinsonism; limited eye movements, muscle fasciculation, reflex loss in lower limbs, nystagmus, cerebellar tumor, and Babinski sign.

BIBLIOGRAPHY. Boyer SH, Christholm AW, McKusick VA: Cardiac aspect of Friedreich's ataxia. Circulation 25:493–505, 1962
Nakano KK, Dawson DM, Spence A: Machado disease: a hereditary ataxia in Portuguese immigrants to Massachusetts. Neurology 22:49–55, 1972
Barbeau A, Roy M, Cunha L, et al: The natural history of Machado-Joseph disease: an analysis of 138 personally examined cases. Can J Neurol Sci 11:510–525, 1984

BAASTRUP'S

Synonyms. Kissing osteophytes; Michotte's.

Signs. Radiologic syndrome: formation of bridges between closely approximated adjacent osteophytes observed in degenerative joint disease—to be differentiated from other types of senescent vertebral ankylosis (see Forestier-Rotes-Querol and von Bekhterer-Strüpell). Contact of spinus process has to be considered among the many mechanisms determining nerve root compression. Cervical thoracic or lumbar vertebrae may be involved.

Diagnostic Procedure. *Roentgenograms.* Necessary to differentiate pathogenic mechanism responsible for the syndromes deriving from the compression.

BIBLIOGRAPHY. Baastrup CJ: Proc Spin Vert lumb unter einige zwischen diesen liegende Gelenkbildunger mit pathologischen Prozzessen in dieser Region. Rortsch Röntger 48:430–435, 1933
Michotte LJ: Le syndrome des épineuses. Rev Rheum 16:249–258, 1949

BABINSKI-NAGEOTTE

Synonyms. Dorsolateral oblongata; hemibulbar; medullary tegmental paralysis. See also Céstan-Chenais and Wallenberg's.

Symptoms and Signs. On one side; hemiparesis; sensibility alteration. On the other; cerebellar hemiataxia. Ocular findings: enophthalmus; ptosis; nystagmus; miosis (see Bernard-Horner syndrome). Occasionally, analgesia of hemiface, vocal cord, and soft palate and adiadochokinesia, lateral pulsion; dysmetria.

Etiology. Neoplasia; vascular.

Pathology. Lesion of pontobulbar or medullobulbar regions.

Therapy. According to lesion.

Prognosis. Poor.

BIBLIOGRAPHY. Babinski J, Nageotte J: Hémisynergie, latéropulsion et miosis bulbaire. Nouv Icon Salpétrière Paris: 1902, 492
Bogorodinski DK, Pojarisski KM, Rasorenova RA, et al: The Babinski-Nageotte syndrome (pathogenesis and correlation with other alternate syndromes). Rev Neurol (Paris) 119:505–512, 1968

Biemond A: Brain diseases, p 159. Amsterdam, Elsevier Pub Co., 1970

BAELZ'S

Synonyms. Cheilitis glandularis apostematosa; myxodermatitis labialis; Puente's disease; Volkmann's cheilitis.

Symptoms. Onset in childhood or early adolescence. Suppurative form, (Volkmann's): pain and tenderness of lower lip.

Signs. Lower lip slightly enlarged; on the internal aspect small orifices from which saliva can be easily squeezed. In the Volkmann's variety, crusts and scales cover the orifices.

Etiology. Unknown; developmental defect (?). Frequent association with Ascher's.

Pathology. *Simple form.* Sclerosis around hyperplastic salivary glands. *Suppurative form.* Inflammatory infiltration.

Diagnostic Procedures. None.

Therapy. Plastic excision of tissue presenting hyperplastic glands.

Prognosis. Both forms may persist for life; in some cases complicated by squamous cell carcinoma.

BIBLIOGRAPHY. Unna PG: Ueber Erkrankungen der Scheimdruesen der Mundes. Mhefte Prackt Dermatal 11:317–321, 1890
Puente JJ, Acevedo A: Quelitis glandularis. Rev Med Lat Am 22:671–679, 1927
Michalowski R: Cheilite glandulaire suppurée en surface au maladie de Baelz. Acta Derm Venereol 27:31–38, 1946
Rook A, Wilkinson DS, Ebling FJG, et al: Textbook of Dermatology, 4th ed, p 2126. Oxford, Blackwell Scientific Publications, 1986

BAGASSE WORKER'S

Synonyms. Bagassosis. See also allergic alveolitis, extrinsic.

Symptoms. In person working with bagasse, a residue of sugar cane. May be acute, subacute, or chronic. Onset insidious or sudden after exposure to dust from bagasse. Fever, chills, sweat, malaise; dry cough; anorexia, weight loss; aches in the chest, backache; occasionally, hemoptysis.

Signs. Tachypnea; tachycardia; hypoxemic signs; fine inspiratory rales in the chest.

Etiology. Hypersensitivity to moldy bagasse.

Pathology. Interstitial pneumonitis.

Diagnostic Procedures. *X-ray of chest.* Fine reticular or nodular opacities. *Blood.* Moderate anemia; no eosinophilia; monocytes may be increased. *Skin test.* Positive reaction against specific antigen.

Therapy. Corticosteroids; removal from exposure.

Prognosis. Good if further exposure is prevented; otherwise, chronic pulmonary condition.

BIBLIOGRAPHY. Jamison SC, Hopkins J: Bagassosis, a fungus disease of the lung: Case report. New Orleans Med Surg J 93:580–582, 1941

Nicholson DP: Bagasse worker's lung. Am Rev Respir Dis 97:546–560, 1968

BAILEY-CUSHING

Synonyms. Cerebellar midline; archicerebellum; flocculonodular lobe; vermis; medulloblastoma (misnomer). See fourth ventricle.

Symptoms. Both sexes affected; male-to-female ratio 3 : 2 or 3 : 1; most common in childhood. Unsteadiness in balance, disturbed coordination of the body in space, without appreciable ataxia; walking very poor; good coordination when lying or with body well braced. Headache and vomiting; marked anorexia and weight loss frequent findings.

Etiology. Midline cerebellar tumor, medulloblastoma, other tumors; vascular lesions; idiopathic atrophies seldom affect this part of cerebellum.

Pathology. Medulloblastoma most frequent type of neoplastic lesion.

Diagnostic Procedures. *CT brain scan. Arteriography. Spinal tap.*

Therapy. Surgery; radiotherapy.

Prognosis. Very poor; survival from months to 2 to 3 years; 5 years survival with therapy in 60% of cases.

BIBLIOGRAPHY. Bailey P, Cushing H: Medulloblastoma cerebelli: a common type of midcerebellar glioma of childhood. Arch Neurol Psychiatr 14:192–224, 1925

Adams RD, Victor M: Principles of Neurology. 3rd ed, pp 491–492. New York, McGraw-Hill, 1985

BAKER'S CYSTS

Synonyms. Popliteal bursitis; popliteal hernia; popliteal cysts.

Symptoms. Occur at any age; more frequent in males (15 to 30 years of age). Mild aching and stiffness of knee, usually unilateral.

Signs. Fluctuating in size; swelling in popliteal space, 10 by 5 cm approximate size; enlargement extends toward Achilles tendon. Limited extension of knee. Transillumination reveals cystic nature of lesion.

Etiology. Unknown; trauma (?). All causes increasing synovial fluid tension. Autosomal inheritance reported in a family.

Pathology. Posterior herniation of capsule of knee or herniation of superior tibiofibular articulation; enlarged semimembranous bursa. Escape of synovial fluid from knee into one of posterior bursae. Moderate inflammatory changes.

Diagnostic Procedures. *Transillumination.* Pneumography contraindicated.

Therapy. Surgical dissection and binding of peduncle. Conservative treatment only temporary effect.

Prognosis. Good if dissection complete; otherwise recurrences.

BIBLIOGRAPHY. Baker WM: Baker's cyst: formation of abnormal synovial cysts in connection with joints. Med Classics 5:805–820, 1941

Toyama WM: Familial popliteal cysts in children. Am J Dis Child 124:486–587, 1972

BALINT'S

Synonym. Psychic paralysis of visual fixation. Few observations of complete form (major syndrome); the minor form presents the same symptoms, but they are inconspicuous and transitory.

Symptoms and Signs. Inability of the patient to look toward a point that is in his peripheral visual field; inability to move eyes to command and follow objects in motion; inability to estimate distance between two objects standing in different relationships to patient (can see only one at a time). "Optic ataxia": inability to execute voluntary movement in response to visual stimuli. The patient tries to grasp an object, extending his hand in the wrong direction, and reaches the object by chance after repeated attempts. "Disturbed attention": normal attention for all nonvisual stimuli; patient does not turn his head to a sudden light on the side. When walking, bumps against obstacles; cannot find his way although he knows and can describe the route. The symptoms are lateralized and more noticeable on one side. Concomitant symptomatology is represented by some language difficulty, agraphia, and ideomotor apraxia. Tonic and motor phenomena of arms and loss of coordination of two parts of the body. Stereoscopic vision, gnosis, visual memory are preserved.

Etiology and Pathology. Bilateral parietooccipital lesions. In major syndrome very large lesion involving both occipital and frontal areas. Frontal lesion anatomic or functional (?). Neoplastic; vascular.

Diagnostic Procedures. *CT brain scan. Brain mapping.* Diffuse cortical atrophy. *Electroencephalography. Spinal fluid. Ophthalmologic examination. Evoked visual potentials.*

Therapy. Depends upon etiology.

Prognosis. Depends upon etiology.

BIBLIOGRAPHY. Balint R: Seelenlähmung des "Schauens", optische Ataxia, räumliche Störung der Aufmerksamkeit. Mschr Psychiar Neurol 25:51–81, 1909

Hecaen H, DeAjuriaguerra J: Balint's syndrome (psychic paralysis of visual fixation and its minor forms). Brain 77:373–400, 1954

Stieglmayr FS: Balint's syndrome. New Engl J Med 277:660, 1967

Adams RD, Victor M: Principles of Neurology, 3rd ed, pp 345–346. New York, McGraw–Hill, 1985

BALKAN NEPHRITIS

Synonyms. Yugoslavian chronic endemic nephropathy; southeastern Europe endemic nephropathy; Danubian endemic familial nephropathy, DEFN.

Symptoms. None; negative history of edema; hematuria; upper respiratory infection.

Signs. Usually normal blood pressure; occasionally, hypertension.

Etiology. Unknown. Condition affects one-third of population in endemic areas (small villages along rivers in Yugoslavia, Bulgaria, Romania). People who move out do not develop the disease; people who move in develop the disease in approximately 10 years.

Pathology. With advanced form; small kidney of about 50 g atrophy of surface of cortex, deeper portion spared; interstitial fibrosis affecting tubules that are hyperplastic with mitotic figures; glomerular lesions seem secondary to tubular lesions. Histology of kidney consistent with primary amyloidosis.

Diagnostic Procedures. *Urine.* Proteinuria, not over 1 g/day; few leukocytes; occasionally, casts. *Blood.* Hyperazotemia (occurring in patients older than 30 to 40 years); hyperchloremic acidosis.

Therapy. Symptomatic and kidney transplantation.

Prognosis. Slow progression of renal insufficiency over 5 to 10 years to death.

BIBLIOGRAPHY. Hall PW, Dammin GJ, Griggs RC, et al: Investigation of chronic endemic nephropathy in Yugoslavia. Am J Med 39:210–217, 1965

Cracium EC, Rosculescu I: On Danubian endemic familial nephropathy. Am J Med 49:774–779, 1970

Brenner BM, Rector FC: The Kidney, 3rd ed, pp 1166–1167. Philadelphia, WB Saunders, 1986

BALLANTYNE'S

Synonyms. Clifford's; gestation prolonged I; placental dysfunction I; postmaturity; prolonged gestation; Runge's; yellow vernix. See Placental insufficiency.

Symptoms and Signs. Gestation exceeding the date of delivery by 3 weeks. Arrest of increase in weight of fetus. At birth, low weight and alertness of newborn; absence of vernix; skin: dry, colloidlike, and desquamating; umbilical cord, nails, and occasionally all skin stained yellow or greenish. Frequently, respiratory distress.

Etiology. Unknown; attributed to placental insufficiency.

Pathology. Placenta shows avascular chorionic villi. Newborn may exhibit amniotic fluid inhalation.

Diagnostic Procedures. *Umbilical vein blood.* Low PO_2; high: hemoglobin, blood urea nitrogen, and bilirubin.

BIBLIOGRAPHY. Ballantyne JW: The problem of the postmature infant. J Obstet Gynaecol Br Emp 2:512–554, 1902

Runge H: Ueber einige besondere Merkmale der weber fragener Frucht. Zentralbl Gynaekol 66:1202–1206, 1942

Clifford SM: Postmaturity. Adv Pediatr 9:1957

BALLARD'S

Synonyms. Mu chain; heavy chain (μ); μ HCD.

Symptoms and Signs. Both sexes affected. Hepatomegaly; splenomegaly; pathologic fractures.

Etiology. Unknown. See Pathology. Possibly autoimmune disorder.

Pathology. Infiltration of visceral organs (liver, spleen, lymph nodes) by lymphocytes, plasma cells, reticular cells. Most patients exhibit associated chronic lymphocytic leukemia or non-Hodgkin's lymphoma.

Diagnostic Procedures. *Blood.* Hypogammaglobulinemia; presence of a rapidly migrating protein (μ). *Bone marrow.* Presence of vacuolated plasma cells.

Therapy. That of the associated condition. Cyclophosphamide and chlorambucil.

Prognosis. That of the associated condition.

BIBLIOGRAPHY. Ballard HS, Hamilton LM, Mazcus AJ: A new variant of heavy chain disease (μ chain disease). New Engl J Med 282:1060–1062, 1970
Brouet JC: Le maladies des chaines lourdes. In Encycl Med Chir, Paris Sang, 13013 F10, 1980

BALLER-GEROLD

Synonym. Craniosynostosis–radial aplasia.

Symptoms and Signs. *Head and facies.* Turribrachycephaly; steep forehead; ocular hypertelorism; high nasal bridge; low philtrum; occasionally, epicanthic folds, dysplastic ears. *Extremitis.* Radius hypoplastic or absent; ulna short and bowed; carpal bones missing or fused; thumb hypoplastic or missing; knee ankylosis; hip dislocation; varus feet; hypoplasia of 3th and 4th toe. Cryptorchidism. Normal intelligence, occasionally mental retardation.

Etiology. Autosomal recessive inheritance.

Diagnostic Procedures. *X-ray.* See Symptoms and signs; craniosynostosis involving coronal suture.

BIBLIOGRAPHY. Baller F: Radiusaplasie und Inzucht. Z Menschl Vererb Kostit Lehre 29:782–790, 1950
Gerold M: Frankturheilung bei einen seltenenen Fall Kongenitaler Anomalie der oberen Gliedmassen. Zentralbl Chir 84:831–843, 1959
Pelias MZ, Superneau DW, Thurmon TF: A sixth report (eighth case) of craniosynostosis-radial aplasia (Baller-Gerold) syndrome. Am J Med Genet 10:133–139, 1981

BALÓ'S

Synonyms. Concentric sclerosis; encephalitis periaxialis concentrica.

Symptoms and Signs. Both sexes affected; onset in childhood. Progressive, spastic paralysis, and symptoms and signs of neurologic disorders according to areas of brain affected.

Etiology. Unknown. Possibly a variety of Schilder's (see).

Pathology. Central nervous system: diffuse areas of demyelinization arranged concentrically.

Diagnostic Procedures. *Electroencephalography. Pneumoencephalography. CT brain scan. Spinal tap. Serology.*

Therapy. Symptomatic.

Prognosis. Death in weeks or in 2 to 3 years.

BIBLIOGRAPHY. Baló J: Encephalitis periaxialis concentrica. Arch Neurol Psychiatr 19:242–264, 1928
Courville CB: Concentric sclerosis. In Vinken PJ, Bruyer GW: Handbook of Clinical Neurology, Vol 9, p 437. Amsterdam, North Holland, 1970
Adams RD, Victor M: Principles of Neurology, 3rd ed, p 712. New York, McGraw-Hill, 1985

BALSER-FITZ

Synonyms. Balser's; Fitz's; hemorrhagic pancreatitis; acute pancreatitis.

Symptoms. Occurs at any age; slightly higher incidence in female (see Etiology). Unbearably epigastric pain, radiating over large areas, especially on the back, many times may not even be alleviated by opiates; sitting and bending forward partially relieves the intensity of pain, which is usually steady, occasionally colicky. Nausea, vomiting, constipation; shock.

Signs. Fever; tachycardia; weak pulse; hypotension. *Skin.* Cold, clammy and jaundiced. *Abdomen.* Seldom, skin discoloration 7 days after onset of pain due to ecchymosis; Grey-Turner signs (on the loin); Cullen's sign (around the umbilicus); tenderness; muscle guarding; ausculatory peristalsis usually normal. *Chest.* Presence of fluid or atelectasis or pneumonia, especially left lower side (30% of patients).

Etiology. In children, mumps infection or idiopathic. In adults (usually in 5th decade), chronic alcoholism. In adults in 6th decade, biliary tract diseases. Other causes of pancreatitis: parasitic infestation; adrenal steroid administration; hyperparathyroidism; metabolic disorders; trauma; hereditary; allergy.

Pathology. Pancreas edematous, friable, hemorrhagic (in some cases this feature may be completely absent); fatty necrosis. Microscopically, acinar necrosis, edema, polymorphonuclear infiltration. In cases of some duration, abscess may develop. Fat necrosis is also observed in mesentery, omentum, and peritoneum. Associated pathology may be found in hepatobiliary tract, spleen, thrombosis, thrombophlebitic legs.

Diagnostic Procedures. *Blood.* Leukocytosis; anemia (not constant); bilirubin elevated; alkaline serum phosphatase elevated; hypocalcemia (confirmatory of diagnosis second day from onset); hyperglycemia (occasionally); plasma antithrombin titer elevated (?); serum amylase high values (immediate rise); serum lipase high values (later rise but longer lasting). *Urine.* Amylase and lipase high values. *Abdominal and thoracic paracentesis.* Fluids show high values of amylase and lipase. *Echosonography. CT scan.*

Therapy. Immediate medical management of shock, pain, prevention of infection, neutralization of the enzymes. Gastric suction; anticholinergic drugs; antibiotics. Surgery only in case when diagnosis in doubt, or if present biliary tract infection (cholangitis). Peritoneal washout. With trasylol and cimetidine increased occurrence of complications.

Prognosis. Much improved with modern medical treatment, but still very severe. Mortality about 30% with hemorrhagic type and 5% with acute edematous type.

BIBLIOGRAPHY. Balser W: Ueber Fattenneckrose eine zuwellen toedliche Krankheit des Menschen. Arch Pathol Anat 90:520–535, 1882
Fitz R: Acute pancreatitis: A consideration of pancreatic haemorrhage, hemorrhagic, suppurative and gangrenous pancreatitis and disseminated fat-necrosis. Boston Med Surg J 120:181–187; 205–207, 1889
Sleisenger MH, Fordtran JS: Gastrointestinal Disease, p 1409. Philadelphia, WB Saunders, 1978
De Francisci G, Magalini SI, Sollazzi L, et al: Le pancreatiti da farmaci. Etiopatogenesi e problemi rianimativi. Rec Progr Med 72:201–212, 1982
Gullo L, Durbee JP: Epidemiology and etiology of pancreatitis. In Gyr KE, Singer MV, Sarles H (eds): Pancreatitis: Concepts and Classification, pp 371–376. Excerpta Medica International Congress Series 1984

BAMATTER'S

Synonyms. Hereditary geroderma osteoplastic; osteoplastic geroderma; geroderma osteodysplastic; Walt Disney dwarfism.

Symptoms and Signs. Rare. Full syndrome from early childhood: stunted growth; senile changes in skin; normal scalp hair; microcornea; corneal opacities; articular hyperthrophy; multiple fractures and bone malformations.

Forme fruste: partial forms presenting geroderma, osteodysplasia, microphthalmia, glaucoma without dwarfism.

Etiology. Unknown; hereditary X-linked or autosomal recessive. Less severe in female heterozygotes.

Pathology. Osteoporosis. Senile changes in skin.

Diagnostic Procedures. *Hormonal studies. X-ray of skeleton. Biopsy of skin.*

Therapy. None.

Prognosis. Variable according to degree. Generally resulting in dwarfism.

BIBLIOGRAPHY. Bamatter F: Gérodermie osthéodysplastique heréditaire (Un noveau biotype de la progeria). Ann Paediatr 174:126–127, 1950
Lisker R, Hernandez A, Martin-Lavin M, et al: Gerodermia osteodysplastica hereditaria: report of three affected brothers and literature review. Am J Med Genet 3:389–395, 1978
Hall BD: Gerodermia osteodysplastica. Proc Greenwood Genet Center 2:101–102, 1983

BAMBERG'S I

Synonyms. Palmus; saltatory spasm.

Symptoms and Signs. Ambulation jumpy or springy owing to clonic spasms of muscles.

Etiology. Irritation of motor cells of spinal cord.

BIBLIOGRAPHY. Bamberg H: Saltatorischer Reflekskampf, eine merkwür dige Form von Spinal-Irritation. Wein Med Wochenschr 9:49–53, 1859

BAMBERG'S II

Synonyms. Concato's; chronic polyserositis.

Symptoms and Signs. Those relative to the formation and progression of effusion in the pleural and peritoneal cavities.

Etiology. In majority of cases, tubercular disease; in remaining cases, idiopathic.

BIBLIOGRAPHY. Bamberg H: Ueber zwei selrene Herzaffktionen usw. Wien Med Wochenschr 14–25, 1872
Concato L: Sulla poliomenorrea scrofolosa o tisi delle sierose. Gior Intern Sc Med 3:1037–1053, 1881

BANKI'S

Symptoms and Signs. Hungarian family (3 generations). Fusion of lunate and cuneiform bones, clinodactyly, brachymetacarpy, and thin diaphysis.

Etiology. Autosomal dominant inheritance.

BIBLIOGRAPHY. Banki Z: Kombination erblicher Gelenk und Knochenanomalien an der Hand. Fortschr Roentgenstr 103:588–604, 1965

BANNAYAN-ZONANA

Synonym. Macrocephaly–multiple lipomas–hemangiomata.

Symptoms and Signs. Subcutaneous predominantly hemangiomata on the trunk and at proximal multiple cutaneous lipomata; macrocephaly; large intra-abdominal masses (angiomata) and abdominal swelling. Normal neurological and intellectual development.

Etiology. Autosomal dominant inheritance.

Pathology. Cavernous angiomatous nevi. Absence of hydrocephalus.

Prognosis. Tendency to spontaneous resolution.

BIBLIOGRAPHY. Bannayan GA: Lipomatosis, angiomatosis and macrocephalia: a previously undescribed congenital syndrome. Arch Path 92:1–5, 1971
Miles JH, Zonana J, McFarlane J, et al: Macrocephaly with hamartomas: Bannayan-Zonana syndrome. Am J Med Genet 19:225–234, 1984

BANNWART'S

Synonym. Facial palsy in lymphocytic choriomeningitis.

Symptoms. Facial palsy (see Bell's) occurring during subacute or chronic lymphocytic choriomeningitis.

BIBLIOGRAPHY. Bannwarth A: Chronische lymphocytaere Meningitis, extzuendliche Polyneuritis und "Rheumatismus." Ein Beitrag zum Problem "Allergie und Nervensystem." Arch Psychiatr 113:284–376, 1941

BANTI'S

Synonyms. Nonfamilial splenic anemia; chronic congestive splenomegaly; fibrocongestive splenomegaly; hepatolienal fibrosis; splenic anemia.

Symptoms. Most frequently occur in patients under 35 years of age; insidious or sudden onset. Vomiting of blood; melena; weakness; flatulence; diarrhea, vague indigestion; abdominal pain or distress; epistaxis (30% of cases).

Signs. Pallor and occasionally mild jaundice, or sallow brown pigmentation of skin; liver slightly enlarged; remarkable splenomegaly.

Etiology. Portal hypertension, intrahepastic (e.g., cirrhosis, schistosoma) extrahepatic (e.g., portal vein thrombosis compression; aneurysm).

Pathology. Spleen weight up to 600–1200 g or more. Capsule thickened and occasionally adherent to adjacent organs. Pulp firm, grayish red; histologically, fibrosis, dilatation of the sinuses, hyaline degenerative changes of the malpighian bodies. Periarterial hemorrhages; periarteriolar siderotic nodules. Liver cirrhosis may not be grossly evident but is found on microscopic examination.

Diagnostic Procedures. *Blood.* Normocytic anemia; leukopenia; thrombocytopenia. *Bone marrow.* Myeloid hyperplasia; maturation arrest of myeloid and megakaryocytic series; later erythroid series arrest. *X-rays of upper gastrointestinal tract.* Esophageal varices; sodium sulfobromophthalein excretion. *Portal venography and pressure. Spleen scan.* After administration of chromium-tagged red cells.

Therapy. Splenectomy (to relieve leukopenia and thrombocytopenia) not useful, however, for reduction in portal hypertension. Splenectomy plus venovenous anastomosis provides a better shunt. Portacaval shunt and side-to-side portacaval anastomosis have reduced operative mortality and prolonged survival. Supradiaphragmatic splenic-transplantation is other good technique to reduce portal hypertension.

Prognosis. Slowly evolving course. Hemorrhage may precipitate the situation.

BIBLIOGRAPHY. Banti G: Dell' Anemia splenica. Arch Scuola Anat Patol (Firenze) 2:53–122, 1883
Wintrobe MM: Clinical Hematology, 8th ed. Philadelphia, Lea & Febiger, 1981

BARAKAT'S

Synonym. Nephrosis-deafness-hypoparathyroidism.

Symptoms and Signs. Deafness, hypoparathyroidism manifestations. Nephrosis, steroid resistant. Renal failure.

Etiology. Autosomal recessive inheritance.

Prognosis. Death within a few months.

BIBLIOGRAPHY. Barakat AY, D'Albora JB, Martin MM, et al: Familial nephrosis, nerve deafness and hypoparathyroidism. J Pediatr 91:61–64, 1977

BARANY'S

Synonyms. Paroxysmal, positional vertigo; vertigo, paroxysmal, positional.

Symptoms and Signs. Periodic recurrences for days or months. When the patient is moved from sitting position to recumbency with the head straight or tilted backward and laterally, after a few seconds paroxysm of vertigo and fright occur that cause him to attempt to sit up and induce nystagmus (vertical-torsional) lasting for 10–15 seconds. From recumbency to sitting same phenomenon reversed. Repeating the maneuver several times brings reduction then disappearance of phenomenon. It returns after a protracted period of rest. Absence of abnormalities in hearing or of vestibular paresis.

Etiology. Possibly due to cuprolythiasis of the posterior semicircular canal and to their free movement with change of the position.

Therapy. In a few patients section of the nerve of the ampulla of the canal has been reported as curative.

Prognosis. Benign condition. Danger of possible cranial trauma due to fall.

BIBLIOGRAPHY. Barany R: Vestibularapparat und Centralnerven System. Med Klin 7:1818–1821, 1911
Adam RD, Victor M: Principles of Neurology. 3rd ed, p 226–227. New York, McGraw-Hill, 1985

BARBER'S (H.W.)

Synonyms. Abortive acrodermatitis; palmoplantar pustolosis; pustular bacterid; pustolosis palmplantaris. See acrodermatitis, persistent.

Symptoms. Rare. Moderate prevalence in females; onset at any age; more frequent between 40 and 60 years of age. Itching (occasionally, severe at night). Bilateral lesions start and remain on thenar eminences and on the heels: areas glazed and reddish, with scaling and numerous pustules in various stages of evolution.

Etiology. Unknown. Psoriatic or eczematoid origin debated. Considered by some authors to be due to a secondary (vasculitic) reaction to foci.

Pathology. Early lesions show hyperkeratosis, parakeratosis, and scarce or absent spongiosis. On pustule area and periphery, granular layer intact, among invading leukocytes lymphocytes predominate. Later, scaling of the pustules with return of the underlying epidermis to normal.

Therapy. Removal of foci occasionally effective. Corticosteroids, coal tar, salicylic acid, roentgen treatment, and prolonged courses of tetracycline of partial benefit.

Prognosis. Protracted course. Remission and relapses.

BIBLIOGRAPHY. Audry C: Les phlycténose récidivantes des extremités (acrodermatites continues de Hallopeau). Ann Dermatol Syph 2:913–928, 1901
Barber HW: Pustular psoriasis of the extremities. Guy's Hosp Rep 86:108–119, 1936
Rook A, Wilkinson DS, Ebling FJG, et al: Textbook of Dermatology, 4th ed, p 1521. Oxford, Blackwell Scientific Publications, 1986

BARDET-BIEDL

Synonyms. Biedl-Bardet: incorrectly called, Laurence-Moon-Bardet-Biedl; see Laurence-Moon. See also Biemond's II and Alstroem's.

Symptoms. Both sexes. From birth. Mental retardation. Vision loss progressing to blindness. Absence of paraplegia (to distinguish it from Laurence-Moon).

Signs. Obesity; polydactyly; hypogenitalism.

Etiology. Unknown. Autosomal recessive inheritance.

Pathology. *Eyes.* Retinitis pigmentosa. *Kidney.* Renal abnormalities (chronic glomerulonephritis or hydronephrosis) *Liver.* Frequently fibrosis. *Pituitary and gonads.* Abnormalities or features of secondary hypogenitalism.

Diagnostic Procedures. *Electroretinography. Hormonal studies. Chromosomal studies.*

Therapy. Symptomatic.

Prognosis. Usually fatal at early age from infections renal and/or liver insufficiency. If adulthood reached, blindness at 20 years of age (27%); other features stationary.

BIBLIOGRAPHY. Bardet G: Sur une syndrome d'obesité infantile avec polydactylie et retinité pigmentaire (contribution a l'etude des formes cliniques de l'obesité hypophysaire). Thesis Paris, n 479, 1920
Biedl A: Ein Geschwisterpaar mit adiposo-genitaler Distrophie. Dtsch Med Wschr 48:1630, 1922
Schachat AP, Mannence IH: The Bardet-Biedl syndrome and related disorders. Arch Ophthalm 100:285–288, 1982

BARD-PIC (PICK)

Obsolete eponym to indicate symptoms and signs associated with pancreatic carcinoma.

BIBLIOGRAPHY. Bard L, Pic A: Contribution a l'étude clinique et anatomo-pathologique du Cancer primitif du pancreas. Rev Med Par 8:257–282; 363–405, 1888

BARD'S

Eponym to indicate pulmonary metastasis from stomach carcinoma.

BIBLIOGRAPHY. Samson M, et al: Syndrom de Bard. Carcinomatose miliaire polmonaire sécondaire à une neoplasie gastrique. Laval Med 33:106–110, 1962

BARE LYMPHOCYTE

Symptoms and Signs. Both sexes. First symptoms at 3 to 4 months of age. Persistent diarrhea, malabsorption, mucocutaneous candidiasis, bacterial infections of upper and lower respiratory tract.

Etiology. Autosomal recessive inheritance. Part of the class of combined immunodeficiency. Lack of expression of HLA antigen on some hematopoietic cells.

Diagnostic Procedures. *Blood.* Lymphocytes lack HLA-A, B, C antigens and beta 2 microglobulin.

Prognosis. Most cases died in infancy.

BIBLIOGRAPHY. Touraine JL, Betuel H, Souillet G, et al: Combined immunodeficiency disease associated with absence of cell-surface HLA-A and B antigens. Lancet I:319–320, 1978
Mercadet A, Cohen D, Dausset J, et al: Genotyping with DNA probes in combined immunodeficiency syndrome with defective expression of HLA. New Engl J Med 312:1287–1292, 1985

BARLOW'S

Barlow originally described a case exhibiting a combination of scurvy and rickets. Today Barlow's syndrome is used as eponym for infantile scurvy.

Synonyms. Ascorbic acid deficiency; Cheadle-Moeller-Barlow; Moeller-Barlow; sea scurvy; scorbutus; scurvy; subperiosteal hematoma.

Symptoms. Tenderness of legs and pseudoparalysis; irritability; anorexia; diarrhea; hemorrhagic gums.

Signs. Hemorrhagic skin changes (4%); fever (19%); swelling over long bone (14%). Costochondral beading.

Etiology. Vitamin C deficiency.

Pathology. Ecchymotic lesions on gums, skin, mucosae due to capillary fragility and traumas. Heart enlarged. Lack of osteoid formation, thickening of calcification zones. Cartilage shows spiculae of calcified matrix disarrayed and fractures at the chondro-osteal conjunction. Only some degree of healing at the fracture site. Bone cortex thinned and subperiosteal dissecting hemorrhages present along the shaft of long bones up to the epiphysis.

Diagnostic Procedures. *Blood.* Anemia microcytic, occasionally, macrocytic; low vitamin C level. *Urine.* No excretion of vitamin C after intravenous injection of 200 mg. *X-rays.* Bone cortex appears as "ground glass" dense line at the end of shaft; proximal zone of rarefaction at corners of tibia, radius.

Therapy. Vitamin C.

Prognosis. Very good with specific treatment; some bone changes remain radiologically evident after cure.

BIBLIOGRAPHY. Barlow T: On cases described as "acute rickets" which are probably a combination of scurvy and rickets, the scurvy being an essential, and the rickets a variable element. Med Chir Trans 66:159–220, 1883
Woodruff C: Infantile scurvy, the increasing incidence of scurvy in the Nashville area. JAMA 161:448–456, 1956
Reuler JB, Broudy VC, Cooney TG: Adult scurvy. JAMA 253:805–807, 1985

BARNARD-SCHOLZ

Synonyms. Ophthalmoplegia-retinal degeneration; oculopharyngeal muscular dystrophy. See also Kearns-Sayre.

Symptoms and Signs. Both sexes affected; onset at all ages. Unilateral or bilateral progressive weakness of muscles of eyelids, up to severe ptosis; progressive ocular myopathy up to complete ophthalmoplegia. Retinitis pigmentosa. Occasionally present, weakness of facies, neck, and shoulder muscles; hearing defects and heart block.

Etiology. Variable; considered nuclear ophthalmoplegia; ocular myopathy. Autosomal dominant inheritance; recessive also reported.

Therapy. None.

Prognosis. Progressive condition.

BIBLIOGRAPHY. Barnard RI, Scholz RO: Ophthalmoplegia and retinal degeneration. Am J Ophthalmol 27:621–624, 1944

Kiloh LG, Nevin S: Progressive dystrophy of the external ocular muscles (ocular myopathy). Brain 74:115–143, 1951

Knoblauch A, Koppel M: Die okulopharingeale Muskeldystrophie. Schweiz Med Wschr 114:557–561, 1984

BARNES'

Synonyms. Muscular dystrophy, Barnes'.

Symptoms and Signs. Protean myopathy: predominantly hypertrophic, pseudohypertrophic, peroneal atrophy; myotonia of some thigh muscles; affecting 6 generations of same family.

Etiology. Autosomal dominant inheritance.

BIBLIOGRAPHY. Barnes S: Myopathic family, with hypertrophic, pseudohypertrophic, atrophic and terminal (distal in upper extremities) stages. Brain 55:1–46, 1932

BARRÉ-LIÉOU

Synonyms. Bartschi-Rochain's; chronic cervical arthritis; sympathetic posterior cervical; sympathetic cervical.

Symptoms. Both sexes affected; onset usually after middle life. Headache; pain in eyes; recurrent disturbed vision; pain in the ears; tinnitus and vertigo; vasomotor disturbance of face; occasionally swallowing and phonation may be affected. Pain in cervical region with neck movements; impaired memory and thinking; anxiety and depression.

Signs. Hypoesthesia of cornea; recurrent small ulcers on palpebral fissure (in chronic cervical arthritis).

Etiology and Pathology. Arthritis of 3rd and 4th cervical vertebra; trauma; cervical disc causing irritation of trigeminal (V) and vestibulocochlear (VIII) nerves.

Diagnostic Procedures. *Audiologic evaluation; caloric stimulation; electronystagmography; CT brain scan; brainstem auditory evoked potentials; X-ray of cervical spine.*

Therapy. Traction; ultrasound; deep x-rays; thermal; antiflammatory therapy. Meclizine, cyclizine, diazepam, scopolamine.

Prognosis. Chronic condition responding to treatment.

BIBLIOGRAPHY. Barré JA: Sur un syndrome sympathique cervical postérieur et sa cause frequente, l'artrite cervicale. Rev Neurol (Paris) 1:1246–1248, 1926

Liéou YC: Syndrome sympathique cervical postérieur et arthrite cervicale chronique. Étude clinique et radiologique (thesis). Strasbourg, 1928

Brandt T, Dazoff RB: The multisensory physiological and pathological vertigo syndromes. Ann Neurol 7:195–203, 1980

BARRÉ-MASSON

Synonyms. Angiomyoneuroma; glomangioma; glomus tumor; multiple.

Symptoms. Intense pain at sites of lesion.

Signs. Round, firm, red blue neoformation on skin of distal parts of limbs. Hemorrhagic foci under fingers and toenails. Tumors are present at birth or appear within 20 years. Isolated tumors may appear also later (33 years average age).

Etiology. Unknown. Usually sporadic. Familial occurrence (autosomal dominant) reported.

Pathology. Well-defined masses of vascular channels in association with aggregates of glomus cells.

Therapy. Excision.

Pathogenesis. Responding to treatment; no recurrences after removal.

BIBLIOGRAPHY. Masson P: Le glomus neuromyoartériel des régions tactiles et ses tumeurs. Lyon Chir 21:247–280, 1924

Barré JA, Masson P: Étude anatomo-clinique de certaines tumeurs sous-unguéales douloureuses (tumeurs du glomus neuro-myo-artériel des extrémitiés). Bull Soc Fr Dermatol Syph RS 31:148–159, 1924

Rycroft RJG, Meuter MA, Sharvill DE, et al: Hereditary multiple glomus tumors: report of four families and review of literature. Trans St John Hosp Derm Soc 61:70–81, 1975

BARRETT'S

Synonyms. Esophagitis-peptic ulcer; Barrett's ulcer; gastroesophageal reflux, GER.

Symptoms. Occur in middle-aged or elderly people. Recurrent low retrosternal pain and heartburn; pain may radiate to the neck, scapular region, or both arms, especially after eating acid or hot or cold food, or while lying down; in later cases, dysphagia; vomiting; melena; hematemesis.

Etiology. Chronic peptic ulcer of the esophagus. Autosomal dominant inheritance also reported.

Pathology. Peptic ulcer in association with esophagitis. When ulcer penetrates through walls of esophagus mediastinal tissue shows fibrosis and inflammatory adenitis; if blood vessel perforates; hemorrhage, mediastinal and pleural suppuration. *Microscopically.* Developmental, anomalous lining of mucosa with atypical columnar epithelium.

Diagnostic Procedures. *X-ray.* Discrete crater or niche on the esophagus wall, with absence of or atypical rugae distal to the crater; spasm above the lesion; stricture due to edema. *Esophagoscopy.* Crater; poorly developed rugae, edema; inflammation; hemorrhage; leukoplakia. *Exfoliative cytology.* Negative for malignancy.

Therapy. Frequently, surgery is required.

Pathogenesis. Ulcer penetrates, perforates, or bleeds.

BIBLIOGRAPHY. Barrett NR: Chronic peptic ulcer of the oesophagus and oesophagitis. Br J Surg 38:175–182, 1950

Crabb DW, Berk MA, Hall TR, et al: Familial gastroesophageal reflux and development of Barrett's esophagus. Am Int Med 103:52–54, 1985

Saubier EC, Gouillat C, Samaniego C, et al: Adenocarcinoma in columnar lined Barrett's esophagus: analysis of 13 esophagectomies. Am J Surg 150: 365–369, 1985

Heading RC: Barrett's oesophagus. Br Med J 294:461–462, 1987

BARR-SHAVER-CARR

Synonyms. 48(XXXY); XXY.

Symptoms. Males affected; present from birth. Mental retardation; delayed growth.

Signs. Flat nasal bridge; epicanthal folds; mild prognathism; radioulnar synostosis; hypogonadism.

Etiology. XXXY.

Diagnostic Procedures. *Chromosome studies. Urine.* Increased gonadotropins.

Prognosis. Good *quoad vitam.*

BIBLIOGRAPHY. Barr ML, Shaver EL, Carr BH, et al: An unusual sex chromatin pattern in three mentally deficient subjects. J Ment Defic Res 3:78–87, 1963

Theilgaard A: A psychological study of the personalities of XYY and XXY men. Acta Psychiatr Scand 69 (suppl 315):106–109, 1984

BARRY-PERKINS-YOUNG

Synonyms. Young's; azoospermia, obstructive, sinopulmonary infections; sinusitis-infertility.

Symptoms and Signs. History of bronchitis and chronic sinusitis from childhood; infertility.

Etiology. Autosomal recessive inheritance postulated.

Pathology. Sinusitis; bronchiectasis. *Testis.* Failure of the vasa efferentia to join together in the epidymis.

Diagnostic Procedures. *X-ray of chest. Bronchography. Sperm analysis.*

Therapy. Microsurgery of efferents may restore fertility.

BIBLIOGRAPHY. Young D: Surgical treatment of male infertility. J Reprod Fertility 23:541–542, 1970

Handelsman DJ, Conway AJ, Boylan LM; et al: Young's syndrome: obstructive azoospermia in chronic sinopulmonary infections. New Engl J Med 310:3–9, 1984

BAR'S

Synonym. Colibacillosis in pregnancy. Eponym used to indicate the manifestations of abdominal pain (gallbladder; ureters; appendix), hyperthermia, and presence of bacteria in the urine during pregnancy.

BIBLIOGRAPHY. Editorial: Bar's syndrome or colibacillosis gravidique. JAMA 128:244, 1948

BARTON'S

See Colles' and Smith fractures, distinct in dorsal Barton's, which has a dorsal marginal fracture, and volar Barton's, which has a volar one.

Etiology. Trauma.

Therapy. These fractures may be reduced by closed reduction and cast. If unstable, open reduction is needed.

BIBLIOGRAPHY. Sisk FD: Fractures of shoulder girdle and upper extremities. In Crenshaw AH (ed): Campbell's Operative Orthopedics, 7th ed, pp 1827–1828. St Louis, CV Mosby, 1987

BART'S

Synonyms. Epidermolysis bullosa–skin absence; dysonychia; epidermolysis bullosa dystrophica (Bart type).

Symptoms and Signs. Congenital absence of skin over lower extremities and of nails (or their deformities); blistering of skin and mucosae.

Etiology. Unknown. Sporadic or autosomal dominant inheritance. Congenital absence of skin may represent "intrauterine" blistering.

Therapy. Protection from trauma. Antibiotics, corticosteroids.

BIBLIOGRAPHY. Bart BJ, Gorlin RJ, Anderson VE; et al: Congenital localized absence of skin and associated abnormalities resembling epidermolysis bullosa: a new syndrome. Arch Derm 93:296–304, 1966
Stokoven I, Drzewiechi KT: Congenital localized skin defect and epidermolysis bullosa hereditaria fetalis. Arch Dermavenerol 59:533–537, 1979

BARTSOCAS-PAPAS'

Synonym. Popliteal pterygium lethal type.

Symptoms and Signs. At birth. Both sexes. Those of popliteal pterygium (see), plus synostosis of hand and foot bone, digital hypoplasia and syndactly.

Etiology. Autosomal recessive inheritance.

BIBLIOGRAPHY. Bartsocas CS, Papas CV: Popliteal pterygium syndrome: evidence for a severe autosomal recessive form. J Med Genet 9:222–226, 1972
Hall JG: The lethal multiple pterygium syndromes. Am J Med Genet 17:803–807, 1984

BARTTER'S

Synonyms. Aldosteronism–normal blood pressure; hyperaldosteronism without hypertension; juxtaglomerular complex hyperplasia–hypoaldosteronism–hypokalemic alkalosis.

Symptoms. Mental retardation; slow growth or dwarfism, weakness; polydipsia; polyuria; episodes of cramps in legs and arms; convulsive seizures (disappearing after potassium administration).

Signs. Chvostek's, Trousseau's signs; physical and neurologic examination otherwise noncontributory. Normal blood pressure or hypertension.

Etiology. Hyperplasia and hypertrophy of juxtaglomerular apparatus and primary hyperaldosteronism with hypokalemic alkalosis and normal blood pressure. Possibly, aldosteronism and juxtaglomerular abnormalities stem from unknown cause. Prostaglandins appear to be mediators of renin release in this syndrome. Suggestion that renal lesion responsible for the adrenal one. Recessive cases of inheritance reported.

Pathology. *Adrenal tissue.* Hypertrophy of zona glomerulosa. *Kidney tissue.* Hyperplasia of juxtaglomerular vessel; basement membrane continuous throughout length of afferent arteriole, obstructing space normally present between juxtaglomerular wall and macula densa; atrophy of glomeruli.

Diagnostic Procedures. *Blood.* Hypokalemic alkalosis; serum angiotensin II increased. *Urine.* Loss of potassium is in excess of intake. Potassium loss prevented by infusion of albumin and by treatment with aldosterone antagonists, but not prevented by restriction of dietary sodium, or treatment with alkalis. Increased aldosterone excretion. Resistance to pressor effect of angiotensin. II. ADH-resistant renal concentrating defect. *Electrocardiography.* Pattern of hypokalemia. *Electroencephalography.* Diffuse dysrhythmia.

Therapy. Partial adrenalectomy; aldosterone antagonists. Acetylsalicylic acid; indomethacin plus spironolactone, or dyrenium.

Prognosis. Good response and fast improvement with treatment.

BIBLIOGRAPHY. Pronove P, MacCardle RC, Bartter FC: Aldosteronism, hypokalemia, and a unique renal lesion in a five year old boy. Acta Endocrinol (suppl 6) (Copenh) 51:167, 1960
Bartter FC, Pronove P, Gill JR: Hyperplasia of the juxtaglomerular complex with hyperaldosteronism and hypokalemic alkalosis. Am J Med 33:811–828, 1962
Brackett NC, Koppel M, Randall RE, et al: Hyperplasia of the juxtaglomerular complex with secondary aldosteronism without hypertension (Bartter's syndrome). Am J Med 44:803–819, 1968
Rodriguez Pereira R, Van Wersch J: Inheritance of Bartter's syndrome. Am J Med Gen 15:79–84, 1983
Brenner BM, Rector FC: The Kidney, 3rd ed, pp 525–527. Philadelphia, WB Saunders, 1986

BASAN'S

Synonyms. Epidermolysis bullosa–skin absence; dysonychia; epidermolysis bullosa dystrophica (Bart type).

Symptoms and Signs. Both sexes. Congenital milia on the chin, ruptured bullae on hands and feet, tapering of fingertips, bilateral simian creases, absence of dermatoglyphic patterns.

Etiology. Autosomal dominant inheritance.

BIBLIOGRAPHY. Basan M: Ektodermale dysplasie, fehlendes Papillarmuscler. Nagelveraenderungen und Vierfingerfurche. Arch Klin Exp Derm 222:546–557, 1965

BASILAR ARTERY MIGRAINE

Synonym. Premenstrual tension headache. Bickerstaff's; vertebrobasilar migraine. See also Migraine.

Symptoms. Occur in girls and young women; associated with menstrual periods. Prodromal visual loss and scintillation in both halves of visual field, followed by dysarthria, ataxia, vertigo, tinnitus, paresthesia of fingers and toes. Consciousness disturbances occasionally associated. Attack of severe throbbing, occipital headache, and vomiting occurs within few (up to 45) minutes. No symptoms during intervals between attacks.

Etiology. Circulatory disorder of basilar artery; transitory constriction of main trunk or branches.

Diagnostic Procedures. *Angiography.* Negative. *Electroencephalography. CT brain scan. Cochlear and vestibular functional studies.* Normal.

Therapy. Symptomatic; diuretics of some benefit.

Prognosis. As patient grows older this syndrome is replaced by "classic" or "common" migraine syndrome (see).

BIBLIOGRAPHY. Bickerstaff ER: Basilar artery migraine. Lancet I:15–17, 1961

Friedman AP: The migraine syndrome. Bull NY Acad Med 44:45–62, 1968

Adams RD, Victor M: Principles of Neurology, 3rd ed, p 136. New York, McGraw-Hill, 1985

BASS'

Synonym. Brachymesodactylia–nail dysplasia; brachydactyly type A5–nail dysplasia.

Symptoms and Signs. Both sexes affected; present at birth. Brachydactyly; hypoplastic fingers and toenails; absent middle phalanges in the fingers and lateral four toes; duplicated distal phalanges of thumbs. Hypoplasia of aricular cartilage.

Etiology. Autosomal dominant inheritance.

BIBLIOGRAPHY. Bass HN: Familial absence of middle phalanges with nail dyplasia: a new syndrome. Pediatrics 42:318–323, 1968

BASSEN-KORNZWEIG

Synonyms. Abetalipoproteinemia; acanthocytosis; betalipoprotein deficiency; lipoprotein deficiency, low-density.

Symptoms. Predominant in males (71%); appear in infancy. The patients are normal at birth but usually fail to thrive during the 1st year; fatty diarrhea; intellectual development slightly retarded; eye trouble (retinitis) that progresses eventually to blindness; ataxia; intentional tremor; slurred speech; muscular weakness; athetoid movements (occasionally); kyphosis; lordosis.

Signs. Height and weight of kyphotic, lordotic infant and child in the lowest percentile. Retinitis pigmentosa; muscular atrophy; signs of malabsorption. Neuropathy involvement signs; ataxia; absence of deep reflexes.

Etiology. Autosomal recessive inheritance. Altered synthesis of ApoB or altered intracellular conjunction of ApoB with lipid.

Pathology. Intestinal mucosa normal length and shape; many lipid droplets in the cells; no lipid in submucosa and lamina propria. Liver fatty infiltration without hepatomegaly; loss of myelin in the nerves. (All data obtained from biopsies.)

Diagnostic Procedures. *Blood.* Appearance and composition of red cells are part of the characteristic of this syndrome. Red cells thorny (acanthocyte); look like crenated cells. Increased susceptibility to mechanical trauma, increased rate of destruction in lysolecithin test. Normal serum does not modify their shape and normal cells are not affected by patient's serum. With Twin solution 80% of the cells revert to normal aspect. Abnormal biochemical composition of their membrane. *Blood lipids.* Beta-lipoprotein absent; cholesterol low; triglycerides low, total phospholipids low; lecithin and sphingomyelin increased. No chylomicrons, VLDL and LDL. *Stool.* High content of fat; ^{131}I Triolein study shows decreased absorption; normal xylose, and B_{12} absorption tests. *X-ray.* Usually not diagnostic; from normal to gross alterations. *Biopsy of jejunum.* See Pathology (pathognomonic).

Therapy. Specific therapy is not available; large supplements of vitamins A, D, E, and K are advised. Massive doses of vitamin E (100 mg/kg/24 hr) arrest neurological degeneration. Long-chain fat intake must be eliminated; medium-chain triglycerides can be used in the diet.

Prognosis. Progression of neurologic and ophthalmic symptoms.

BIBLIOGRAPHY. Bassen FA, Kornzweig AL: Malformation of erythrocytes in a case of atypical retinitis pigmentosa. Blood 5:381–387, 1950

Herbert PN, Assmann G, Gotto AH Jr, Fredrickson DS: Familial lipoprotein deficiency: abetalipoproteinemia, hypobetalipoproteinemia, and Tangier disease. In Stanbury JB, Wyngaarden JB, Fredrickson DS: The Metabolic Basis of Inherited Disease, 5th ed, p 589. New York, McGraw-Hill, 1983

BATEMAN'S

Synonyms. Corticosteroid purpura; cushingoid purpura; death blossoms; cachectic purpura; purpura senilis; steroid purpura.

Symptoms and Signs. In old (Bateman's) or debilitated (cachectica) people, after prolonged corticosteroid administration, or in person with Cushing's syndrome (steroid). Small petecchiae and hematomas, especially on forearm and back of hands (1–4 cm in diameter).

Etiology. Shearing injury of dermal vessels from hypermobility, due to lack of fixation by tissues, especially in areas of prolonged actinic exposure.

Pathology. Atrophy of skin; lack of subcutaneous fat; petecchieae and hematomas.

Diagnostic Procedures. *Blood.* Clotting normal; platelets normal.

Therapy. None of proven value.

Prognosis. Hematomas persist for weeks and leave brown pigmentation.

BIBLIOGRAPHY. Bateman T: Delineations of Cutaneous Disease Exhibiting the Characteristic Appearances of the Principle Genera and Species Comprised in the Classification of the Late Dr. Willan, and Completing the Series of Engravings Begun by that Author. London, Longman, 1817

Rook A, Wilkinson DS, Ebling FJG, et al: Textbook of Dermatology, 4th ed, pp 1113–1114. Oxford, Blackwell Scientific Publications, 1986

BATTEN'S

Synonyms. Neuronal ceroid-lipofuscinosis; amaurotic family juvenile idiocy; Vogt-Spielmeyer; Spielmeyer-Vogt. See also Pelizaeus-Merzbacher; Jansky-Bielkoschowsky; Spielmeyer's; Kufs', Santavuori's, and Tay-Sachs.

Symptoms. Both sexes equally affected; onset at 5 to 10 years of age. Rapid deterioration of vision and intelligence; later seizures and psychotic behavior.

Signs. Spastic weakness; rigidity; athetosis or dystonia; ataxia.

Etiology. Autosomal dominant inheritance. Cerebral degeneration with storage of ceroid lipofuscin. To be distinguished from disorders of sphingolipid metabolism. No enzyme deficiency has been yet demonstrated.

Pathology. Deposits of autoflourescent lipopigments in all tissues, predominant in the brain. *Brain.* Small, loss of nerve cells and status spongiosus; various sizes and structures of lipopigment deposits (lamellar, granular, "fingerprint" aspect), with acid phosphatase activity. *Retina.* Loss of cones and rods; degeneration of epithelial cells; lipoid pigment accumulation.

Diagnostic Procedures. *Bone marrow and other tissue biopsy.* Presence of lipopigments. *Urine.* Presence of lipopigments in sediment. *Blood.* Lipopigments in lymphocytes; azurophilic hypergranulation in neutrophils and lymphocyte vacuolization (only in homozygotes). *Electroencephalography.* Various abnormalities.

Therapy. None.

Prognosis. Variable according to onset. Early form more rapid evolution. Death 1 year to 10 years from onset.

BIBLIOGRAPHY. Batten FE: Cerebral degeneration with symmetrical changes in the maculae in two members of a family. Trans Opthalmol Soc UK 23:386–390, 1902

Vogt H: Ueber familiäre amaurotische Idiotie und verwandte Krankheitsbilder. Mschr Psychiat 18:161–71, 310–57, 1905

Spielmeyer W: Klinische und anatomische Untersuchungen über einen besonderen Fall von amaurotischer Idiotie. Nissle Beitr Nerv Geistes Krh, Berlin 1908

Burrig KF, Schwendemann G, Lohler J: Lack of structural abnormalities in lymphocytes from heterozygotes of juvenile type of generalized ceroid-lipofuscinosis: a light and electron microscopic study. Neuropediatrics 13:216–218, 1982

BATTEN-TURNER

Synonyms. BTMD; benign congenital muscular dystrophy.

Symptoms. Onset in both sexes in early childhood. Floppiness and frequent falling and stumbling. Slight delay on reaching milestones or early motor development; normal walking; somewhat handicapped in physical exercises.

Signs. Mild weakness of muscles more pronounced on pelvic girdle, neck flexors, and shoulder girdle; absence of contractures and pseudohypertrophy.

Etiology. Unknown; hereditary transmission compatible with autosomal recessive pattern; no definite conclusion has been reached, however.

Pathology. Muscle biopsy shows dystrophic changes that differ from more common type of muscular dystrophy with respect to endomysial fibrosis, degeneration, and regeneration.

Diagnostic Procedures. *Electromyography. Blood.* Serum glutamic-oxaloacetic transaminase (SGOT); creatine kinase; lactic dehydrogenase; aldolase markedly increased. *Biopsy of muscle.*

Therapy. None.

Prognosis. Very good; muscular deficiency minimal; stationary and frequently well compensated.

BIBLIOGRAPHY. Batten FE: Three cases of myopathy, infantile type. Brain 26:147–148, 1903
Turner JWA: On amyotonia congenita. Brain 72:25–34, 1949
Zellweger H, Afifi A, McCormick WF, et al: Benign congenital muscular dystrophy: a special form of congenital hypotonia. Clin Pediatr (Phila) 6:655–663, 1967
Adams RD, Denny-Brown D, Pearson CM: Disease of the Muscle. 3rd ed, p 272. New York, Harper & Row, 1986

BATTERED BUTTOCK

Synonyms. Fat fracture; traumatic lipoma. See Cluneal nerve.

Symptoms and Signs. Rare. Reported only in females. Aching and tenderness occurring early, or late in areas of the buttocks after blunt trauma. Local deformity with a swelling or retraction.

Etiology. Trauma of the buttocks, following different types of accidents.

Pathology. The fat compartments are burst open, with rupture of the septa and shearing off of the anchorage between the skin and deep fascia. Local vascular damage; varying amount of bruising and different sizes of hematoma. Traumatic lipoma formation, after retraction, of detached subcutaneous tissue into the buttock or thigh. Tissue defect above reabsorbed hematoma, and fat swelling below.

Diagnostic Procedures. *Biopsy.*

Therapy. Surgical repair or excision.

Prognosis. In children, swelling may recede with general body growth. In adults, deformity is permanent. Correction of deformity by wide excision gives good results with complete relief of tenderness and pain.

BIBLIOGRAPHY. Meggitt BF, Wilson JN: The battered buttock syndrome—fat fractures. Br J Surg 59:165–169, 1972

BATTERED CHILD

Synonyms. Child abuse; maltreatment of children.

Symptoms and Signs. Bruises confined to the buttocks and lower back; lash marks; traumatic alopecia; bruises and scars, at various stages of healing, over the foreminences; petechiae; burns; subdural hematoma leading to coma, convulsions and increased intracranial pressure; intraabdominal injuries, most commonly ruptured liver or spleen.

Etiology. Maltreatment of children by their parents, guardians, or other caretakers.

Pathology. Hematomas, scars, burns, welts.

Diagnostic Procedures. *X-rays.* Fractures, cortical thickening; subperiosteal ossification.

Therapy. Institutionalization of the child; proper therapy of the various lesions; psychological help to the family.

Prognosis. The family can be rehabilitated to adequate care of the child only with intensive and comprehensive treatment.

BIBLIOGRAPHY. Nelson Textbook of Pediatrics. Philadelphia, WB Saunders, 1983
Green AH: Child maltreatment: recent studies and future directions. J Child. Psychiatr 23:675–678, 1984

BAUER'S

Synonyms. Brachydactyly type A3; brachydactyly-clinodactyly; brachymesophalangy V.

Symptoms and Signs. More frequent in females. Shortening of the middle phalanx of fifth finger with clinodactyly.

Etiology. Autosomal dominant inheritance.

BIBLIOGRAPHY. Bauer B: Eine bischer nicht beobachtete kongenitale, hereditaere Anomalie des Fingerskelettes. Dtsch Z kir 86:252–259, 1907
Herzog KP: Shortened fifth medial phalanges. Am J Phys Anthrop 27:113–118, 1967

BAYFORD-AUTENRIETH

Synonyms. Arkin's; dysphagia lusoria.

Symptoms and Signs. Appear in newborn or in infants. Difficulty in swallowing.

Etiology. Abnormal right subclavian artery pressing on the esophagus.

Therapy. Surgery.

Prognosis. Good.

BIBLIOGRAPHY. Bayford D: An account on a singular case of obstructed deglutition. Mem Med Soc London 2:271–282, 1789
Autenrieth, Pfleiderer: De Dysphagia lusoria. Arch Physiol Halle 7:145–188, 1807
Mok CK, Cheung KL, Kong SM, et al: Translocating the aberrant right subclavian artery in dysphagia lusoria. Br J Surg 66:113–116, 1979
Hurst J: The Heart, 6th ed, p 622. New York, McGraw-Hill, 1986

BAZELON'S

Synonyms. Lesch-Nyhan variant.

Symptoms and Signs. Females affected. Mental retardation; mutilation of lips and hands; absence of choreoathetosis; spasticity or severe growth retardation.

Etiology. Unknown.

Diagnostic Procedures. *Blood.* Hyperuricemia. Erythrocytes: hypoxanthine-guanine-phosphoribosyl tranferase (HGPRT) normal. *Urine.* Normal uric acid excretion.

Prognosis. Unknown.

BIBLIOGRAPHY. Bazelon M, Stevens H, Davis M, et al: Mental retardation, self mutilation and hyperuricemia in female. Trans Am Neurol Assoc 93:187–188, 1968

BAZEX-GRIFFITH

Synonyms. Bazex's II; Acrokeratosis paraneoplastica.

Symptoms and Signs. In men (except in one case). Hyperkeratotic psoriasisform plaques on hand, feet, nose, ears. Nail thick and fragile, lesions may spread to proximal upper respiratory limbs and the trunk. Associated neoplasia of upper respiratory tract. Enlargement of nodes in cervical and submaxillary areas.

Etiology. In the spectra of paraneoplastic syndromes.

Pathology. Dermatitis with inflammatory changes, hyper and parakeratosis.

Therapy. That of primary malignancy.

Prognosis. That of primary malignancy.

BIBLIOGRAPHY. Barriere H: Les dermatoses para-neoplastiques. Ann Med Interne (Paris) 126:177–181, 1979.
Bazex A, Griffith WA: Acrokeratosis paraneoplastica: new cutaneous marker of malignancy. Br J Dermatol. 103:301–306, 1980
Pecora AL, Landsman L, Imgrund SP, et al: Acrokeratosis paraneoplastica (Bazex's syndrome): report of a case and review of literature. Arch Dermatol 119:820–826, 1983

BAZEX'S I

Synonyms. Follicular atrophoderma; basal cell carcinoma.

Symptoms and Signs. Present from birth. Both sexes. Occasionally facial eczema shortly after birth. Follicular atrophoderma affecting dorsa of hands and feet ("multiple ice pick marks"), occasionally affecting also the exterior surfaces of the lower back. From adolescence multiple basal cell carcinoma of the face. Occasionally associated hypohidrosis (facial or generalized); sparse hair.

Etiology. Unknown. Autosomal dominant inheritance. Possibility of X-linked inheritance reported in one family.

Pathology. *Skin biopsy.* No true atrophy, but deep and lax follicular hostia of follicles. Basal cells carcinoma resembles melanocitic nevi.

BIBLIOGRAPHY. Bazex A, Dupe A, Chirstol B: Genodermatose complexe de type indetermine associant une hypothricose un etat atrophodermique generalisé et des degenerescences cutanées multiples (epitheliomas-baso-cellulaires). Bull Soc Fr Derm Syph 71:206, 1964
Rook A, Wilkinson DS, Ebling FJG, et al: Textbook of Dermatology, 4th ed, p 129. Oxford, Blackwell Scientific Publications, 1986

BAZIN'S

Synonyms. Erythema induratum; nodular vasculitis; see Whitfield's.

Symptoms and Signs. Predominant in women. Chronic and persistent nodular and indurative lesions evolving with the formation of deep ulcers. Affects calves of legs (rather than lower parts, as in Pernio syndrome) during winter months. Lesion may also be observed in arms and breasts. Usually lesions improve, but do not clear completely, during the summer.

Etiology. Tuberculid that affects the backs of legs with perniotic circulation.

Pathology. Nonspecific granuloma, as well as tubercular granuloma with caseation and varying degree of vasculitis and foregin body giant cells reaction. Fibrosis at later stage. Vascular changes may dominate with the exclusion of granulomatous lesions.

Diagnostic Procedures. *Biopsy. Tuberculin skin test. X-ray of thorax.*

Therapy. If tuberculosis or other etiology proved, specific treatment.

Prognosis. Chronic persistent condition. Spontaneous remissions and relapses frequent.

BIBLIOGRAPHY. Bazin APE: Leçons théoriques et cliniques sur la scrofule, considérée en ellemême et dans ses rapports avec la syphilis, la dartre et l'arthritis, 2nd ed, p 668. Paris, A Delahaye, 1861
Rook A, Wilkinson DS, Ebling FJG, et al: Textbook of Dermatology, 4th ed, p 1168. Oxford, Blackwell Scientific Publications, 1986

BAZZANA'S

Synonyms. Ophthalmoauricular angiospastic.

Symptoms. Otosclerosis with progressive deafness. In early stage, attacks of visual field defect; then permanent concentric contraction.

Signs. Trophic alteration of auditory meatus; vasospasm of retina vessels (during attacks).

Etiology. Unknown.

Prognosis. Progressive deafness and visual field contraction.

BIBLIOGRAPHY. Bazzana EC, Lombardo LE, Montanelli M: Otosclerosi e campo visivo. Arch Ital Otol Rinol Lar 61:620–628, 1950
Roy FH: Ocular Syndromes and Systemic Diseases. Grune & Stratton, Orlando, 1985

BEALS' I

Synonym. Auriculo-osteodysplasia.

Symptoms. Both sexes affected. Slight limitation of elbow motion. In some patients, limping.

Signs. Elbow dysplasia (characteristic): from mild dysplasia to dislocation, either anterior or posterior. Bilateral, often asymmetric. Hip dysplasia (occasional): bilateral only in female member of affected family. Other skeletal features: torso of masculine appearance; broad shoulders; wide muscular base of the neck; horizontal clavicles; scapular prominence; short metacarpals in some

patients. Nails, teeth, and hair normal. Auricular dysplasia; elongation of lobe accompanied by a small posterior lobule. Short stature (consistently) below 50th percentile in height.

Etiology. Unknown; autosomal dominant inheritance.

Pathology. Chrondroectodermal dysplasia.

Therapy. Intermittent bracing in extension and supination to prevent posterior dislocation.

Prognosis. Good; posterior dislocation results in major disability; anterior dislocation in a minor degree of disability.

BIBLIOGRAPHY. Beals RK: Auriculo-osteodysplasia, a syndrome of multiple osseous dysplasia, ear anomaly, and short stature. J Bone Joint Surg [AM] 49:1541–1550, 1967
McKusick VA: Mendelian Inheritance in Man, 7th ed. Baltimore, John Hopkins University Press 1986

BEALS-HECHT

Synonyms. Beal's arachnodactyly; Beals' II; contractural arachnodactyly.

Symptoms and Signs. Both sexes affected, present from birth. *Facies.* Micrognathia. Ears: "crumpled," poor conchae; prominent crura. Short neck. *Extremities.* Long; arachnodactyly; joint contractures. Kyphoscoliosis.

Etiology. Autosomal dominant inheritance.

Therapy. Orthopedic.

Prognosis. Spontaneous gradual improvement of articular limitation. Kyphoscoliosis usually progressive.

BIBLIOGRAPHY. Beals RK, Hecht F: Delineation of another heritable disorder of connective tissue. J Bone Joint Surg 53:987–993, 1971
Hecht F, Beals RK: "New" syndrome of congenital contractural arachnodactyly originally described by Marfan in 1896. Pediatrics 49:574–579, 1972
Ramos Arroyo MA, Weaver DD, Beals RK: Congenital contractural arachnodactyly: report of four additional families and review of literature. Clin Genet 27:570–581, 1985

BEAN'S

Synonym. Blue rubber bleb nevus.

Symptoms and Signs. Both sexes affected; onset in early childhood. Appearance of one or many (hundreds) blue, small, rubbery subcutaneous nodules. Easily compressible and promptly refilling after compression. They vary in color, size, shape, and number and may be tender. Recurrent melena; pallor. Nocturnal pain and regional hyperhidrosis. Subconjunctival hemangioma with overlying fibrosis; hemorrhagic lesion near macula.

Etiology. Unknown; autosomal dominant inheritance.

Pathology. Cavernous type hemangioma in the skin (legs and trunk most affected areas) and intestinal wall (small intestine more affected than distal; then colon). Occasionally present in spleen, liver, and central nervous system.

Diagnostic Procedures. *X-ray. Blood.* Anemia when bleeding occurs.

Therapy. Symptomatic; correction of anemia. Surgery with resection of intestine in repeated or uncontrollable bleeding. Some severe cases required amputation of limbs affected by angiomatous gigantism.

BIBLIOGRAPHY. Bean WW: Vascular Spiders and Related Lesions of the Skin. Springfield, Ill, CC Thomas, 1958
Walshe MM, Evans CD, Warin RP: Blue rubber bleb nevus. Br Med J 2:931–932, 1966
Munkvad M: Blue rubber bleb nevus syndrome. Dermatologica 167:307–309, 1983

BEARD'S

Synonym. Neuroasthenic neurosis.

Symptoms. Both sexes affected, predominant in women especially, in 4th or 5th decade (information to be reconsidered with modern change in life and modern version of this neurosis). Onset gradual or sudden. Precipitating factors frequently reported by the patient as overwork, emotional strain, progressive infection or other pathologic conditions. Beard reports 50 symptoms and signs that have been grouped in the following categories: variable muscular spasms and body aches; autonomic nervous system involvement (discharge); heavy limbs and tiredness; phobic neurosis; hopelessness; insomnia; group of miscellaneous complaints, which may represent the temporary or permanent focus of distress (ie, dyspepsia; impotence). Patients appear tired, apathetic; accomplish all movements with great effort and keep seeking relief from symptoms.

Etiology. Unknown. Various hypotheses according to schools of psychiatry.

Therapy. Psychological evaluation to establish the need for mental manipulation. Dexedrine.

Prognosis. Episodic recurrence or unremitting long period or chronic status.

BIBLIOGRAPHY. Beard GM: Neuroasthenia or nervous exhaustion. Boston Med Surg J 80:217–221, 1869

Freedman AM, Kaplan HI, Sadock BJ: Comprehensive Textbook of Psychiatry, 2nd ed, p 1264. Baltimore, Williams & Wilkins, 1975
Adams RD, Victor M: Principles of Neurology, 3rd ed, p 372. New York, McGraw-Hill, 1985

BEARN-KÜNKEL-SLATER

Synonyms. CALH; chronic active lupoid hepatitis; lupoid hepatitis; hypergammaglobulinemic hepatitis; Künkel's; plasma cell hepatitis.

Symptoms. Occur in women, insidious onset at puberty; may however affect anyone from childhood to old age. Asthenia; amenorrhea or menstrual irregularities; epistaxis and gingivorrhagia; hepatalgia; arthralgia; recurrent idiopathic fever episodes; respiratory distress. later, hematemesis.

Signs. Hirsutism; acne; striae; spider telangiectases; moon facies; obesity; hepatosplenomegaly; jaundice. Later, ascites.

Etiology. Unknown; autoimmmunity (?); variant of lupus erythematosis (?). Immune complex formation and deposition in tissues.

Pathology. Hepatomegaly; nodular cirrhosis; marked plasma cells infiltration.

Diagnostic Procedures. *Blood.* Hypergammaglobulinemia (IgG markedly increased); biologic fixative reaction for rheumatoid arthritis (25%); presence of antinuclear antibodies (75%); positive latex reaction for smooth muscle IgG antibodies (90%). *Biopsy of liver.* See Pathology. *Sodium sulfobromophthalein retention.*

Therapy. Trials with steroids and immunosuppressants. If indicated, liver transplantation.

Prognosis. Within 10 years of onset, liver insufficiency, bleeding esophageal varices, coma, death.

BIBLIOGRAPHY. Bearn AG, Künkel HG, Slater RJ: The problem of chronic liver disease in young women. Am J Med 21:3–15, 1956
Wright R, Alberti KGMM, Karran S, et al: Liver and Biliary Disease, p 189. London, WB Saunders, 1979

BEAT KNEE

Synonyms. Prepatellar bursitis; carpet layer's; coal miner's. See also Housemaid's knee.

Symptoms and Signs. (1) *Acute.* Local pain, swelling, tenderness. (2) *Chronic.* Chronic distention of one of the prepatellar bursae, usually the one over tibial tubercle. (3) *Infective.* Local wound, abrasion, or swelling (secondary infection of preexisting bursitis) with all signs of infection.

Etiology. (1)Unaccustomed work involving kneeling or trauma. (2) Long period of kneeling. (3) Direct or indirect infection of bursa.

Pathology. (1) Effusion of serous fluid. (2) Chronic effusion; hemorrhages; loose bodies; adhesions; calcifications. (3) Formation of pus.

Diagnostic Procedures. *X-ray of knee. Prepatellar tap.*

Therapy. (1) Elastic compression; if great pain, aspirate. (2) Use of protecting knee pads; in some cases surgery. (3) Bed rest; systemic antibiotics or injection into bursa. If suppuration, establish drainage. Fibrosis and synovial thickening with painful nodules do not respond to treatment: excision of the bursae.

Prognosis. Varies according to extent of lesion and prevention of further damage.

BIBLIOGRAPHY. Smillie LS: Injuries of the Knee Joint, 4th ed. Baltimore, Williams & Wilkins, 1962
Pinals RS: Traumatic arthritis and allied conditions. In Hollander JL, McCarty DJ (eds): Arthritis and Allied Conditions, 8th ed, p 1403. Philadelphia, Lea & Febiger, 1978
Justis EJ: Nontraumatic disorders. In Crenshaw AH (ed): Campbell's Operative Orthopedics, 7th ed, pp 2253–2254. St Louis, CV Mosby, 1987

BECKER-REUTER

Symptoms. Reported in females; appear in early infancy. Asymptomatic.

Signs. On the neck and forearms, presence of discrete or confluent brown macules. Absence of telangiectasias and atrophic changes.

Etiology. Unknown.

BIBLIOGRAPHY. Becker S, Reuter MJ: Familial pigmentary anomaly. Arch Dermatol Syph 40:987–998, 1939
Rook A, Wilkinson DS, Ebling FJG, et al: Textbook of Dermatology, 4th ed, p 1564. Oxford, Blackwell Scientific Publications, 1986

BECKER'S (P.E.)

Synonyms. Duchenne's late type; benign Duchenne's muscular dystrophy, BMD; pseudohypertrophic muscular hypertrophy; muscular dystrophy, progressive, tardive.

Symptoms and Signs. Those of Duchenne's muscular dystrophy syndrome with later onset, and slower rate of progression; greater enlargement of calves during adolescence or young adulthood. Frequently associated with color blindness.

Etiology. Unknown; sex-linked recessive inheritance.

Pathology. See Duchenne's.

Diagnostic Procedures. See Duchenne's.

Therapy. See Duchenne's.

Prognosis. Longer survival and less impairment than Duchenne's. Same cause of death; cardiac failure and skeletal disease.

BIBLIOGRAPHY. Becker PE: Neue Ergebnisse der Genetik der Muskeldystrophien. Acta Genet 7:303–310, 1957
Zundel WS, Tyler FH: The muscular dystrophies. New Engl J Med 273:537–543; 596–601, 1965
Adams RD, Denny-Brown D, Pearson CM: Diseases of the Muscle. 3rd ed, p 272. New York, Harper & Row, 1975
Grimm T: Genetic counseling in Becker type X-linked muscular dystrophy II: practical considerations. Am J Med Genet 18:719–723, 1984

BECKER'S (S.W.)

Synonym. Pigmented hairy epidermal nevus.

Symptoms. Common condition. All races, both sexes affected; prevalent in young men. May become evident or conspicuous on exposure to sunlight.

Signs. Appearance of irregular pigmentation on shoulder, chest, less frequently in other areas, which spreads to the size of about 20 cm in diameter by confluence of irregular spots, assuming a geographic map aspect. Dark heavy hairs may grow in and around the pigmented area 1 or 2 years later.

Etiology. Unknown.

Pathology. Minimal changes from normal skin pattern. Central area of lesion may show thickening and elongation of ridges and dermal papillae.

Therapy. None. Cosmetic masking.

Prognosis. Benign lesion.

BIBLIOGRAPHY. Becker SW: Diagnosis and treatment of pigmented nevi. Arch Dermatol Syph 60:44–65, 1949
Rook A, Wilkinson DS, Ebling FJG, et al: Textbook of Dermatology, 4th ed, p 186. Oxford, Blackwell Scientific Publications, 1986

BECK-IBRAHIM

Synonyms. Candidiasis; moniliasis; cutaneous anergy. including familial, chronic, mucocutaneous candidiasis, dominant and recessive type. See also Multiple Endocrine Deficiency.

Symptoms. Cutaneous anergy. Symmetric crusted lesions of skin about the mouth, nose, neck, ears, perineum, buttocks, groin.

Signs. Paronychia with redness and swelling at the base of fingernails and toes. Arrested growth; change of color of hair to white, then alopecia; thrush of mouth. Normal appetite; no diarrhea. Chronic cutaneous fungal infection.

Etiology. Unknown. 1) Late onset form nongenetic type. 2) Early infancy a) recessive inheritance: relationship to ferritin and/or myeloperoxidase alteration, b) Autosomal dominant: immunodeficiencies (see Diagnostic Procedures).

Diagnostic Procedures. *Cultures from mouth and stool.* For fungi. *Monilia, Candida intradermal skin tests.* Markedly decreased. *Contact sensitization.* 2,4-dinitro-1-chlorobenzene (DNCB); 2,4-dinitro-1-fluorobenzene (DNFB) markedly decreased; sensitization by transfer of lymphocytes: absent. *Lymphocytic stimulation with phytohemagglutinin.* Positive; normal lymphocyte count. *Rejection of skin homografts.* Decreased. *Circulating antibody level.* Normal. *Resistance to systemic infection.* Normal. In autosomal dominant form: candida skin test positive and lymphocyte transformation normal under 2 years of age; negative at older age.

Therapy. Nystatin, flucytosine, ketoconazole. Topical application of alkaline and gentian violet solutions.

Prognosis. Recurrence of skin lesions and alopecia with intermittent regrowth of hair. Dwarfism.

BIBLIOGRAPHY. Beck SC: Ueber das Erythema mycoticum infantile. Derm Stud Unna Ftschr 1:494, 1910

Ibrahim J: Ueber eine Soormykose der Haut im fruhen Saeugligsalter. Arch Kinderheilkcl 55:91–101, 1911

Schultz FW: Two cases of thrush with unusual symptoms and skin manifestations. Am J Dis Child 29:283, 1925

Wells RS, Higgs JM, McDonald A, et al: Familial chronic mucocutaneous candidiasis. J Med Genet 9:302–310, 1972.

Sams WM Jr, Jorisso JL, Snyderman R, et al: Chronic mucocutaneous candidiasis: immunologic studies of three generations of a single family. Am J Med 67:948–959, 1979

Canton P, Dupont B, May T: Nouveaux aspects des candidioses systemiques. Med Mal Infec 14:582–588, 1984

BECK'S

Synonyms. Anterior spinal artery occlusion; Davison's; hemianesthetic hemiplegia; medullary; myelomalacia.

Symptoms. Syndrome may follow trauma. Onset sudden, apoplectiform; sometimes symptoms preceded by pain and paresthesias. Vary according to site of lesion.
1. Occlusion of anterior spinal artery of medulla oblongata (Davison's): flaccid quadriplegia, loss of discriminative sensation below level of lesion.
2. Occlusion of branches that supply paramedian area of medulla: homolateral paralysis of tongue and contralateral paralysis of arm and leg with altered tactile sensation.
3. Occlusion at thoracolumbar level: muscular atrophy (segmental) and spastic paralysis of legs; occasionally unilateral with contralateral sensory loss; dissociated sensory loss below the lesion.
4. Occlusion of lower spinal cord: flaccid paralysis of legs with dissociated sensory changes.

Signs. Abolished reflexes of part involved; sensory changes; vibratory and position sense conserved; coldness of skin.

Etiology. Thrombosis (most frequent); neoplastic or other cause occluding vessel; infection; syphilis; atherosclerosis; coarctation of aorta; trauma.

Pathology. Occlusion of artery; softening of spinal cord in zones on anterior horns, anterior half of cord, pyramidal tract, and spinothalamic tracts; myelomalacia and little glial reaction of zone involved.

Diagnostic Procedures. *Cerebrospinal fluid.* Normal or slightly xanthochromic; proteins may be increased.

Therapy. Anticoagulants or as indicated by etiology. Control of infections and rehabilitation of bladder.

Prognosis. Variable.

BIBLIOGRAPHY. Spiller WG: Thrombosis of the cervical anterior median spinal artery; syphilitic acute anterior polymyelitis. J Nerv Ment Dis 36:601–613, 1909

Beck K: Das Syndrom des Verschusses der verderen Spinalarterie. Dtsch Z Nervenh 167:164–186, 1951–52

Peterman AF, Yoss RE, Corbin KB: The syndrome of occlusion of the anterior spinal artery. Proc Mayo Clin 33:31–37, 1958

Walman L, Bradshaw P: Spinal cord embolism. J Neurol Neurosurg Psychiatry 30:446–454, 1967

Johnson JR, Leatherman KD, Holt RT: Anterior decompression of the spinal cord for neurologic deficit. Spine 8:396–405, 1983

BECKWITH-WIEDEMANN

Synonyms. BWS; exomphalos-macroglossia-gigantism, EMG; neonatal hypoglycemia-visceromegaly-macroglossia-microcephaly, Wiedemann-Beckwith.

Symptoms. Occur in newborn; 60% females. Lethargy and poor feeding developing within the first 2 or 3 days after birth; clonic seizures (controlled by intravenous injection of glucose). Elements of congestive heart failure.

Signs. Somatic gigantism at birth or developing postnatally; macroglossia; mild microcephaly; hepatomegaly (not essential feature); omphalocele or umbilical hernia; bilateral noncystic renal hyperplasia; cryptorchidism.

Etiology. Unknown. Sporadic; autosomal dominant inheritance reported.

Pathology. *Kidney.* Immaturity of renal tubules; glomeruli closely packed and normal maturity for infant age. *Liver and muscle.* Biopsy normal. *Pancreas.* Hypertrophy. *Bone marrow.* Normal. *Gonads.* Interstitial cell hyperplasia. *Pituitary.* Amphophilic hyperplasia. *Suprarenals.* Fetal adrenocortical cytomegaly.

Diagnostic Procedures. *Blood.* Hypoglycemia; normal galactose tolerance test; polycythemia (nonspecific, perhaps secondary to hypoglycemia). *X-ray.* Accelerated bone maturation; metaphysical flaring and overconstriction of diaphyses.

Therapy. Zinc glucagon; cortisone; diazoxide useful to relieve hypoglycemia.

Prognosis. Normal growth. Unknown beyond childhood. Normal growth. Frequent association with various neoplasias.

BIBLIOGRAPHY. Beckwith JB, Wang CI, Donnell GN, et al: Hyperplastic fetal visceromegaly with macroglossia, omphalocele, cytomegaly of adrenal fetal cortex, postnatal somatic gigantism and other abnormalities: Newly recognized syndrome (Abst no 41). Proc Am Pediatr Soc, Seattle, June 16–18, 1964

Wiedemann, HR: Complexe malformatif familial avec hernie ombelicale et macroglossiè—un syndrome nouveau. J Genet Hum 13:223–363, 1964

Best LG, Hoeckstra RE: Wiedemann-Beckwich syndrome autosomal-dominant inheritance in a family. Am J Med Genet 9:291–299, 1981

Bose B, Wilkie RA, Malden M, Forsyth JS, Faed MJW: Wiedmann-Beckwith syndrome in one of monozygotic twins. Arch Dis Child 60:1191, 1985

BEEMER'S

Synonyms. Hydrocephalus; cardiac malformation; dense bone.

Symptoms and Signs. From birth. Hydrocephalus, unusual facies: bulbous nose, broad nasal bridge; ambiguous genitalia. Heart signs related to double-outlet right ventricle.

Etiology. Unknown. Autosomic recessive inheritance.

Diagnostic Procedures. *Blood.* Thromocytopenia. *X-ray.* Dense bone.

Prognosis. Lethal condition.

BIBLIOGRAPHY. Beemer FA, Ertbruggen I: Peculiar facial appearence, hydrocephalus, double-outlet right ventricle, genital anomalies and dense bones with lethal outcome. Am J Med Genet 19:391–394, 1984

BEER AND COBALT

Synonym. Beer drinker's.

Symptoms. Occur usually in person with no history of heart disease. Severe dyspnea; abdominal pain; edema.

Signs. Cyanosis; enlargement of heart; venous distension; tachycardia; gallop rhythm; hepatomegaly; edema (in some cases massive); Hypotension.

Etiology. Occurs in beer drinkers (average 6–12 bottles a day for years). Possibly beer containing cobalt (added to enrich flavor by manufacturers). No new cases after removing beer containing cobalt from the market.

Pathology. *Heart.* Pale; soft; increase in weight; interstitial edema; enlargement of myofibrils and necrosis. *Liver.* Centrilobular necrosis.

Diagnostic Procedures. *Electrocardiography.* Low voltage; enlargement of P waves; flattened T waves; right axis deviation. *Blood.* Electrolyte study, metabolic acidosis; enzyme studies, lactic dehydrogenase (LDH) and serum glutamic-oxaloacetic transaminase (SGOT) very high level; hematocrit high (58–60%).

Therapy. Treatment of heart failure; thiamine.

Prognosis. Death 50%.

BIBLIOGRAPHY. McDermott PH: Nutritional deficiency in myocardiopathy. Am J Clin Nutr 18:313, 1966

McDermott PH, Delaney RL, Egan JD, et al: Myocardosis and cardiac failure in men. JAMA 198:253–256, 1966

Sullivan J, Parker M, Carson SB: Tissue cobalt content in "beer drinkers' myocardiopathy." J Lab Clin Med 71:893–911, 1968

Regan TJ: The heart, alcoholism and nutritional disease. In Hurst JW: The Heart, 6th ed, p 1446–1451. New York, McGraw-Hill, 1986

BEHR'S I

Synonym. Optic atrophyataxia.

Symptoms. Both sexes affected, optical atrophy prevalent in males. In infants, disturbed vision, disturbed coordination with ataxia; urinary sphincter weakness, mental deficiency. *Forme fruste* described with only slight optical atrophies developing later in life in members of affected families.

Signs. Temporal atrophy of optic nerve. Nystagmus; tendon hyperreflexia; positive Babinski. Clubfoot.

Etiology. Autosomal recessive inheritance.

Pathology. Bilateral optic atrophy (mainly papillomacular bundles); slight affection of pyramidal bundles, posterior cords, and spinocerebellar pathways.

Therapy. None.

Prognosis. In full syndrome, death may occur in first or second decade. In *forme fruste,* normal life with only minor visual impairment.

BIBLIOGRAPHY. Behr C: Die komplizierte, hereditärfamiliäre Optikusatrophie des Kindesalters; ein bisher nicht beschriebener Symptomkomplex. Klin Monatsbl Augenheilkd 47:138–160, 1909

van Leeuwen A, Babel J, Van Bogaert L, et al: Heredoataxies par degenereescence spino-ponto-cerebelleuse; Leurs manifestations retiniennes, optiques et cochleaires. Rev Otoneuroophtalmol 20:1–226, 1948

Thomas PK, Workman JM, Thage O: Behr's syndrome: a family exhibiting pseudodominant inheritance. J Neural Sci 64:137–148, 1984

BEHR'S II

Synonyms. Macula lutea retinae adult degeneration: (1) macula lutea retinae presenile degeneration, (2) macular senile degeneration.

Symptoms. (1) Onset about 20 years of age. (2) Onset between 40 and 90 years of age. Impairment of central vision.

Signs. Central atrophic degeneration with pigmentary changes in and around macula.

Etiology. Unknown; Autosomal dominant or recessive inheritance.

Therapy. Symptomatic.

Prognosis. Progressive condition.

BIBLIOGRAPHY. Behr C: Die Heredodegeneration der Makula. Klin Monatsbl Augenheilkd 69:469–505, 1920

Bradley AE: Dystrophy of the macula. Am J Ophthalmol 61:1–24, 1966

BEIGHTON'S

Synonyms. Osteogenesis imperfecta; opalescent teeth-blue sclerae–Wormian bones–absent fractures. See Osteogenesis imperfecta.

Symptoms and Signs. Those of osteogenesis with moderate osteoporosis. Absence of joint hyperextensibility.

Etiology. Autosomal dominant. Possibly the same as osteogenesis imperfecta type I.

Diagnostic Procedures. X-ray. In older patients, mild flattening and biconcavity of vertebrae. Wormian bones.

Prognosis. Good.

BIBLIOGRAPHY. Beighton P: Familial dentinogenesis imperfecta, blue sclerae and Wormian bones without fractures: another type of osteogenesis imperfecta? J Med Genet 18:124–128, 1981

BELL'S

Synonyms. Facial nerve palsy; refrigeration palsy; Facial paralysis.

Symptoms. Both sexes (equal distribution) all ages and all times of year, higher incidence in diabetic patients. Sometimes following exposure to cold or draft; most cases begin without apparent reason. Onset (usually) slight fever; pain behind ear; stiffness of neck followed by stiffness of one side of face; homolateral lacrimation; difficulty with speech; occasionally, peculiar taste in the mouth or loss of taste in ipsilateral side of tongue. Hyperacousis may occur. Bilateral palsy occasionally occurs.

Signs. Forehead cannot be wrinkled; upper eyelids close slowly or partially and eyeballs roll upward and outward when attempting to close the eyes. Change of voice; inability to whistle.

Etiology. Unknown; familial cases reported. Virus suspected but not proved.

Pathology. (Presumed) swelling and hyperemia of nerve sheath or periostium with compression of facial nerve in the facial canal.

Therapy. Thiamine; adrenal corticoids; protection of eyes; massage. In permanent paralysis; anastomosis of end of peripheral nerve with spinal accessory (X) or hypoglossal (XII) nerve to restore tone of facial muscles and allow closure of eyes.

Prognosis. Usually, recovery in 1 or 2 months. In some cases, permanent paralysis.

BIBLIOGRAPHY. Bell C: On the nerves of the face; being a second paper on that subject (reprint). Med Classics 1:155–169, 1936
Vick NA: Grinker's Neurology, 7th ed. Springfield, Ill, CC Thomas, 1976
Adams RD, Victor M: Principles of Neurology, 3rd ed, p 1012. New York, McGraw-Hill, 1985

BENCZE'S

Synonyms. Hemifacial hyperplasia–strabismus; facial asymmetry; dental articulation derangement. See Plagiocephaly.

Symptoms and Signs. Both sexes. Facial asymmetry; amblyopia; strabismus; submucous cleft palate.

Etiology. Autosomal dominant inheritance.

BIBLIOGRAPHY. Bencze J, Schmitzler A, Nalawska J: Dominant inheritance of hemifacial hyperplasia associated with strabismus. Oral Surg 35:489–500, 1973
Kurnit D, Hall JG, Schurtleff DB, et al: An autosomal dominant inherited syndrome of facial asymmetry, esotropia, amblyopia and submucous cleft palate (Bencze syndrome). Clin Genet 16:301–304, 1979

BENEDIKT'S

Synonyms. Mesencephalic tegmental paralysis; tegmentum.

Symptoms. Disturbed vision due to complete oculomotor paralysis of the affected side; involuntary movements; coarse tremor at rest, increasing amplitude under emotion and motion, so that the latter may not be controlled. The tremor paresis, and hypoesthesia, as well as hemichorea, are contralateral to ocular paralysis, arm alone, or both arm and leg.

Signs. Complete (upward, downward, inward) oculomotor paralysis; ptosis; external strabismus; loss of reflex to light and accommodation. Tremor and hemichorea.

Etiology. Arteriosclerosis, syphilis, or neoplasm occluding vessels and resulting in softening of side of tegmentum with involvement of afferent fibers of cerebellum pedunculus cerebellaris superior as they pass through the red nucleus on the way to the thalamus.

Diagnostic Procedures. *Neurologic, opthalmologic examinations. Serology. Electroencephalography.*

Therapy. Symptomatic and etiologic.

Prognosis. Reserved.

BIBLIOGRAPHY. Benedikt M: Tremblement avec paralysie croisée du moteur oculaire commun. Bull Med Paris 3:547–548, 1889
Adams RD, Victor M: Principles of Neurology, 3rd ed, p 1010. New York, McGraw-Hill, 1985

BENNETT'S

Synonyms. Boxer fracture; carpometacarpal thumb ray fracture; thumb fracture-dislocation; stave of thumb.

Symptom. Extreme pain at base of thumb.

Signs. Tenderness, swelling at base of thumb.

Etiology. Forced metacarpal flexion with fracture of anterior lip over carpal bone and backward dislocation of metacarpal.

Therapy. Prompt reduction; if dislocation persists, application of traction, surgical fixation, and protective strapping.

Prognosis. Possible correction of deformity by prompt fixation. If orthopedic intervention, healing in 6 weeks. Residual pain, subluxation, arthropathic degeneration possible.

BIBLIOGRAPHY. Bennett EH: Fractures of the metacarpal bones of the thumb. Dublin J Med Sci 73:72, 1882
Canale ST: Fractures and dislocations in children. In Crenshaw AH (ed): Campbell's Operative Orthopedics, 7th ed, p 1844. St Louis, CV Mosby, 1987

BENSON'S

Synonyms. Asteroid hyalitis; scintillatio albescens.

Symptoms. Occur in people of advanced age. Asymptomatic or slight impairment of vision.

Signs. On simple inspection, vitreous appears normal. Slit-lamp examination shows presence of small, variously shaped bodies irregularly distributed. On ophthalmoscopy, bodies appear shiny and cream colored.

Etiology. Unknown.

Pathology. Crystal of calcium polynitrate or stearate (or both) deposited in the vitreous.

Therapy. None.

BIBLIOGRAPHY. Benson AH: A case of "monocular asteroid hyalitis." Trans Ophthalmol Soc UK 14:101–104, 1894
Gartner J: Whipple disease of the central nervous system associated with ophthalmoplegia externa and severe asteroid hyalitis: a clinicopathological study. Doc Ophthal 49:155–187, 1980

BERDON'S

Synonyms. Megacystis-microcolon-intestinal hypoperistalsis, MM1H. See Megaduodenum-megacystis.

Symptoms and Signs. Prevalent in females. Onset from early age or later. Intestinal hypoperistalsis symptoms (achalasia), constipation and urinary retention.

Etiology. Unknown. Familial cases reported.

Pathology. Degeneration of smooth intestinal muscles and neuronal abnormalities.

Diagnostic Procedures. *Sonography. X-ray. Biopsy.*

BIBLIOGRAPHY. Berdon WE, Baker DH, Blan WA, et al: Megacystis-microcolon-intestinal hypoperistalsis syndrome: a new case of intestinal obstruction in a newborn: report of radiologic findings in five newborn girls. Am J Roentgen 126:957–964, 1976
Redeman JF, Jemenez JF, Golladay ES, et al: Megacystis-microcolon-intestinal hypoperistalsis syndrome: case report and review of literature. J Urol 131:981–983, 1984

BERENDES-BRIDGE-GOOD

Synonyms. Chronic granulomatous disease, CGD; congenital dysphagocytosis; familial granulomatosis; septic progressive granulomatosis.

Symptoms and Signs. Prevalence in males. From birth, susceptibility to infection. Development of inflammatory masses of characteristic pathology which compress vital organs. Failure to thrive, reticuloendothelial hyperplasia, hypergammaglobulinemia, anemia. Infections more frequent from *Staphylococcus aureus* and enteric bacteria, *Candida albicans,* aspergillus on skin, mucosae, intestinal tract, *Candida esophagitis* (with stenosis), chronic enteritis and colics, diarrhea, intestinal obstruction from inflammatory masses (especially gastric antrum) hepatosplenomegaly, suppurative lymphadenitis, hepatic and perihepatic abscesses, osteomyelitis of metacarpals and metatarsals common (*Serratia marcescens*), pneumonia, granulomatous cystitis, pyelonephritis, renal abscesses, meningitis, salmonella septicemia.

Etiology. Failure of respiratory burst of phagocytes. Two inheritance patterns: (1) X-linked (majority of cases) and (2) autosomal recessive. The defect consists in the incapacity of neutrophils to be activated to respiratory burst by normal stimuli.

Pathology. Hyperplastic, with chronic inflammation with granulocytes. Histiocytes containing pigmented lipid material. Masses consist of granulomatous tissue. *Lymph nodes.* Macrophages containing bacteria.

Diagnostic Procedures. *Blood.* Mild anemia, neutrophils increased or normal. Normal B- and T-lymphocyte functions. Serum Ig elevated. Neutrophil chemotaxis, degranulation, and phagocytosis are normal. Abnormalities of bacterial killing action.

Therapy. Supportive. Antibiotics and corticoids of some symptomatic value. Surgical intervention for complications. Bone marrow transplantation.

Prognosis. From rapidly fatal to compatible with life until middle age.

BIBLIOGRAPHY. Johnston RB Jr, Newman SL: Chronic granulomatous disease. Pediatr Clin N Am 24:365–376, 1977
Babior BM, Crowley CA: Chronic granulomatous disease and other disorders of oxidative killing by phagocytes. In Stanbury JB, Wyngaarden JB, Fredrickson DS: The Metabolic Basis of Inherited Disease, 5th ed, p 1956. New York, McGraw-Hill, 1983

BERGER-HINGLAIS

Synonyms. IgA nephropathy; mesangial IgA/IgG nephropathy. See Hematuria, essential.

Symptoms and Signs. Prevalent in male; mean age of onset 28 years. Recurrent episodes of gross hematuria, following respiratory infections or associated with diarrhea or strenuous exercises. Mild hypertension.

Etiology. Unknown. Entrapment of IgA in glomerular mesangium and activation of complement (spontaneous or consequent to systemic infection?). Autosomal dominant inheritance reported in some families.

Pathology. Focal segmental proliferative glomerulanephritis; glomerular deposits of IgA in mesangial areas, associated with IgG and C_3 and fibrin-related antigens. IgA may also be found around skin capillaries.

Diagnostic Procedures. *Urine.* Hematuria with minimal proteinuria. *Renal function.* Normal. *Blood.* Serum

IgA levels elevated (not constant) serum complement components normal. *Biopsy of kidney. Immunofluorescent stain.* (See Pathology.)

Therapy. No therapy has been shown to influence the natural history of the disease. Intermittent steroid and antibiotic therapy has been used. When indicated, kidney transplantation.

Prognosis. Slow progression. Fifty percent of patients develop end-stage renal failure within 25 years of the time of diagnosis.

BIBLIOGRAPHY. Berger J, Hinglais N: Les dépôts intercapillaires d'IgA-IgG. J Urol Nephrol (Paris) 74:694–695, 1968

Berger J: IgA glomerular deposits in renal disease. Transplant Proc 1:939–944, 1969

Culpepper RM, Andreoli TE: The pathophysiology of the glomerulopathies. Adv Intern Med 28:161–206, 1983

Julian BA, Quiggins PA, Thompson JS, et al: Familial IgA nephropathy: evidence of inherited mechanism of the disease. New Engl J Med. 312:202–208, 1985

BERGER'S

Synonym. Eponym obsolete.

Symptoms. Weakness and paresthesia of lower limbs without any objective evidence of pathology or associated condition.

Etiology. Unknown.

BIBLIOGRAPHY. Berger O: Ueber eine eigenthümliche Form von Paraesthesie. Bresl Arztl 1:60–61, 1879

BERGSTRAND'S

Synonym. Osteoid osteoma.

Symptoms. Both sexes affected, onset at 10 to 25 years of age. Localized pain, exacerbated at night, corresponding to bone location of lesion. Pain worse at night and relieved by aspirin.

Signs. May affect all bones; most frequently involved are tibia and femur, usually in the metaphyseal-epiphyseal region. Tenderness. Localized swelling seldom evident.

Etiology. Neoplastic theory (Jaffe, et al) supported by the almost constant sterility of lesion and type of histologic changes; inflammatory theory (Brailsford, Ottolenghi, and others) supported by the occasional presence of hyperthermia. A familial (autosomal dominant) form reported.

Pathology. When process terminates its evolution, lesion appears as round bone nodule more or less vascularized, isolated from adjacent tissue. *Histology.* Nidus formed by highly vascular cellular connective tissue without any inflammatory feature and surrounded by osteoid or partially calcified trabeculae, which project toward periphery.

Diagnostic Procedures. *Blood and urine.* Normal. *X-ray.* Image of round intracortical or extracortical rarefied nucleus of variable dimension (2–3 mm to 1–2 cm) with one or more zones of increased density. *CT scan.*

Therapy. Excision.

Prognosis. If entire lesion removed, relapses do not occur and symptoms disappear completely.

BIBLIOGRAPHY. Bergstrand H: Ueber eine eigenartige, wahrseheinlich bisher nicht beschriebene osteoblastiehe Krankheit in den dangen Knochen der Hand in des Fusses. Acta Radiol (Stockh) 11:596–613, 1930

Kaye JJ, Arnold WD: Osteoid osteoma in siblings. Clin Orthoped 126:273–275, 1977

Carnesale PG: Benign tumor of bone. In Crenshaw AH (ed): Campbell's Operative Orthopedics, 7th ed. St Louis, CV Mosby, 1987

BERLIN'S (C.I.)

Synonym. Leukomelanoderma–infantilism–mental retardation–hypodontia–hypotrichosis. See Christ-Siemens-Touraine and Naegeli's.

Symptoms and Signs. Both sexes (two males and two females). Physical and mental development retarded. Eruption of teeth delayed. Facies similar to anhydrotic ectodermal dysplasia, with generalized mottled pigmentation of the skin, thickening of palms and soles; body hair sparse or absent; reduced sweating.

Etiology. Unknown; autosomal recessive inheritance.

BIBLIOGRAPHY. Berlin CI: Congenital generalized melanoleucoderma associated with hypodontia, hypotrichosis, stunted growth, and mental retardation occurring in two brothers and two sisters. Dermatologica 123:227–243, 1961

Rook A, Wilkinson DS, Ebling FJG, et al: Textbook of Dermatology, 4th ed, p 141. Oxford, Blackwell Scientific Publications, 1986

BERLIN'S I (R.)

Synonyms. Commotio retinae; traumatic retinal edema.

Symptoms. In some cases, gradual loss of central vision and, usually, successive return of it.

Signs. None.

Etiology. Trauma to eye.

Pathology. Retinal edema; cones in fovea destroyed.

Diagnostic Procedures. *Ophthalmoscopy.* Cloudiness of retina; macula appears bright reddish in contrast.

Therapy. Antiedema treatment: corticosteroids; diuretics. Vitamin A.

Prognosis. Usually good recovery.

BIBLIOGRAPHY. Berlin R: Zur sagenarnten Commotio Retinae. Klin Monatsbl Augenheilkd 11:42–78, 1873

BERLIN'S II (R.)

Synonym. Canalis opticus.

Symptoms. After head trauma without direct involvement of eye. Unilateral or bilateral amaurosis.

Signs. In case of complete blindness, absence of pupillary reflexes.

Etiology. Trauma directly or indirectly producing necrosis of ocular nerve fibers.

Pathology. Necrosis of nerve fibers on border of intracanalicular or intracranial segment (or both) of optic (II) nerve. Fractures of optic canal; dislocation or compression of optic nerves are not necessary components of the syndrome.

Therapy. Attempt to relieve pressure useless.

Prognosis. Variable from reversible to irreversible blindness.

BIBLIOGRAPHY. Berlin R: Ueber Sehstörungen nach Verletzung durch stumpfe Gewalt. Klin Monatsbl Augenheilkd 17:1878
Seitz R: Canalis-opticus-syndrome. Ophthalmologica Ann 158:318–324, 1969

BERLOQUE

Synonyms. Berlock; berloque dermatitis; contact photosensitization. See Civatte's, light eruption, polymorphous and Richl's.

Symptoms and Signs. Occur only in susceptible individuals. Exposure to the light after application of perfumes. Deep brown pigmentation in wide stripes and in pattern formed by trickle of droplets on face, neck, or other areas.

Etiology. Stimulated melanogenesis by light and by furocoumarins of bergamot, lemon oils, and orange peels, usually contained in eau de cologne (offensive agent = psoralens).

Diagnostic Procedure. *Patch tests.* Open (light exposed) and closed dressing with suspected perfume.

Therapy. None.

Prognosis. Fading of discoloration after weeks or months.

BIBLIOGRAPHY. Freund E: Ueber bisher noch nicht beschriebene künstliche Hautverfarbungen. Derm Wschr 63:931–936, 1916
Harber LC: Berloque dermatitis. Arch Dermatol 90:572–576, 1964
Rook A, Wilkinson DS, Ebling FJG, et al: Textbook of Dermatology, 4th ed, p 513. Oxford, Blackwell Scientific Publications, 1986

BERNARD'S

Synonyms. Claude Bernard's; cervical sympathetic irritation. See also Horner's.

Symptoms and Signs. Midriasis; eyelid lag; diminished blinking; retraction of upper and, occasionally, of lower, lids; relative enophthalmos. Ipsilateral side of face: vasoconstriction; decreased local temperature; increased sweating; increased lacrimation.

Etiology and Pathology. Irritative lesions of cervical sympathetic system; tumors; aneurysm; infection or any cause of mechanical compression in any location of path of this system mediastinal; cervical; medullar; midbrain.

Diagnostic Procedures. *X-rays of chest, neck, skull. Angiography. CT brain scan.*

Therapy. Depends upon etiology.

Prognosis. Depends upon etiology.

BIBLIOGRAPHY. Bernard C: Recherches expérimentales sur le grand sympathique et spécialement sur l'influence que le section de ce nerf exerce sur la chaleur animal. CR Soc Biol (Paris) 5:77, 1853
Shafar J: The syndromes of the third neuron of the cervical sympathetic system. Am J Med 40:97–109, 1966

BERNARD-SOULIER

Synonyms. Hemorrhagic dystrophic thrombocytopenia; thromboasthenia-thrombocytopenia (autosomal recessive).

Symptoms and Signs. Both sexes affected; present from infancy. Moderate to severe purpura; epistaxis; menorrhagia.

Etiology. Autosomal recessive inheritance. Autosomal recessive. Absence of platelet membrane glycoprotein Ib. (receptor for plasma Von Willebrand factor).

Diagnostic Procedures. *Blood.* Giant platelets (up to 8 μm diameter); mild thrombocytopenia; variable abnormalities in PF-3 activity: platelet aggregation by bovine fibrinogen deficient. *Clotting test.* Bleeding time prolonged; clot retraction and platelet aggregation by adenosine triphosphate (ATP) normal. *Bone marrow.* Megakaryocytes normal or increased in number.

Therapy. None. Splenectomy ineffective. Supportive. Splenectomy and corticosteroids ineffective.

Prognosis. Variable according to intensity of hemorrhagic manifestations.

BIBLIOGRAPHY. Bernard J, Soulier JP: Sur une nouvelle variété de dystrophie thrombocytaire hémorrhagipare congénitale Bull Mem Soc Med Hôp 64:969–974, 1948
McEver RP, Majerus PW: Inherited disorders of platelets. In Stanbury JB, Wyngaarden JB, Fredrickson DS: The Metabolic Basis of Inherited Disease, 5th ed, p 1561. New York, McGraw-Hill, 1983

BERNHARDT-ROTH

Synonyms. Bernhardt's; cutaneous neuritis; meralgia paresthetica; lateral femoral paresthesia; Roth's; Rot's.

Symptoms. Paresthesia and numbing in affected leg; burning pain after a long period of standing or walking.

Signs. Decreased objective sensation to touch; pain; temperature (not constant) in the anterolateral surface of thigh.

Etiology. Compression and irritation of lateral femoral cutaneous nerve by clothing or infectious process. Frequent in obesity and diabetes. Postsurgical etiology in several cases, secondary to retroperitoneal tumor. Familial occurrence autosomal dominant has also been reported.

Pathology. Compression neuritis; proliferation of interstitial tissue.

Therapy. Relief of pressure; if symptoms persist, surgical decompression or nerve resection.

Prognosis. Spontaneous remission in few months, occasionally longer (years); good response to treatment.

BIBLIOGRAPHY. Hager W: Neuralgia femoris. Resection des Nerv. Cutan. Femoria Anterior externus Heilung. Dtsch Med Wochenschr 11:218, 1885
Bernhardt M: Ueber isoliert im Gebiete des N. cutaneus femoris externus vorkommende Parästhesien Neurol Centralbl 14:242–244, 1895
Flowers RS: Meralgia paresthetica. A clue to retroperitoneal malignant tumor. Am J Surg 116:89–92, 1968
Massey EW: Familial occurrence of meralgia paresthetica. Arch Neurol 35:182, 1987

BERNHEIM'S

Synonyms. Right ventricle failure; right ventricle obstruction-failure.

Symptoms. Two stages: (1) Few or no clinical symptoms; (2a) dyspnea may be absent; (2b) total heart failure, dyspnea, orthopnea, and other symptoms.

Signs. Two stages: (1) Enlargement of right atrium; distension of cervical veins; increased venous pressure; normal circulation time. (2a) Systemic venous enlargement; lungs clear to percussion and ausculation; hepatic enlargement; dependent edema; possibly ascites. Circulation time normal or slightly increased. (2b) Total heart failure.

Etiology. Left ventricular hypertrophy and enlargement, bulging of septum into the right ventricle and obstruction of the blood flow from right atrium. Existence of syndrome denied by some cardiologists (White, Evans), accepted by others (Russek, Zohman, Drago).

Pathology. *First stage.* Left ventricle hypertrophy. *Second stage.* Heart enlargement; left atrium normal size; right atrium dilated; left ventricle enlarged and bulging on the right. Liver markedly congested, enlarged; cardiac cirrhosis. Lung congestion, infarction, and atelectasis from compression of the enlarged heart.

Diagnostic Procedures. *Electrocardiography. Circulation time. X-ray of chest. Fluoroscopy. Cardiac catheterization.*

Therapy. Treatment of hypertension and heart failure.

Prognosis. That of heart failure, modified by treatment.

BIBLIOGRAPHY. Bernheim P: De l' Asistolie Veineuse dans l'hypertrophie du coeur gauche par stenose concomitante du ventricule droit. Rev Med (Paris) 30:785–800, 1910
Drago EE, Aquilina JT: Bernheim's syndrome. Am J Cardiol 14:568–572, 1964
Hurst JW: The Heart, 6th ed, p 322. New York, McGraw-Hill, 1986

BERNUTH'S

Synonyms. Hemophilia sporadica; von Bernuth. Eponym indicates sporadic hemophilia. See Hemophilia.

BIBLIOGRAPHY. von Bernuth F: Ueber Kapillarbeobachtungen bei Hämophilie und anderen hämorrhagischen Diathesen. Dtsch Arch Klin Med 152:321–330, 1926

BERTOLOTTI'S

Synonym. Sacralization-scoliosis-sciatica. See also Cotugno's.

Symptoms. Numbness; hypersensitivity or pain along the course of sciatic nerve; low back pain; morning stiffness.

Signs. Scoliosis.

Etiology. Sacralization of lumbar vertebrae.

Diagnostic Procedures. *X-ray of spine.* Sacralization of 5th lumbar vertebra. *CT scan. Myelography.*

Therapy. Special postural exercises. Salicylates or other analgesic and anti-inflammatory agents. Deep radiation; thermotherapy.

Prognosis. Insidious progression.

BIBLIOGRAPHY. Bertolotti M: Contributo alla conoscenza dei vizi di differenzazione regionale del rachide con speciale riguardo all' assimilazione sacrale della V lombare. Radiol Med (Torino) 4:113–144, 1917
Bertolotti M: Les syndromes lombo-ischialgiques d'origine vertébrale. Rev Neurol (Paris) 29:1112–1125, 1922

BESNIER-BOECK-SCHAUMANN

Synonyms. Boeck sarcoid; Hutchinson-Boeck; lupus pernio; benign lymphogranulomatosis; Jungling's; Mortimer's; sarcoidosis; Schaumann's.

Symptoms. More frequent in females 20 to 30 years of age. *Early stages.* Often asymptomatic; fatigue; moderate cough; mild weight loss; vague chest pains. (In Scandinavian countries and Great Britain, acute symptoms of fever, arthralgia, erythema nodosum more frequently observed.) *Later stages.* Expectoration; hemoptysis; cyanosis; dyspnea; difficulty in vision; blindness; Bell's palsy.

Signs. *Early stage.* Physical examination negative; minor pulmonary changes; rales. *Later stage.* Adenopathy; cutaneous polymorphic lesions; hepatosplenomegaly (20–25%); iridocyclitis; scleral nodules; chorioretinitis; acute migratory monoarthritis or polyarthritis; fever.

Etiology. Unknown.

Pathology. Granulomatous lesions formed by concentric arrangement of elongated epithelioid cells, giant cells of Langerhans or foreign body type, inclusion body, fibroblasts surrounding lesions; absence of caseation; later, necrosis and fibrosis with formation of scar. Nodules may be found in all involved organs: liver; lung; kidney; heart; central nervous system; skin; lymph nodes; eyes.

Diagnostic Procedures. *Biopsy.* Kveim test positive; Mantoux test negative. *Blood.* High sedimentation rate, high alpha and gamma globulins; high alkaline phosphatases; high calcium; anemia; moderate leukopenia; eosinophilia; thrombocytopenia (when splenic involvement). *Urine.* Hypercalciuria. *Liver biopsy.* See Pathology. *X-ray.* Hilar or paratracheal lymphoadenopathy; later stage, pulmonary parenchymal nodular involvement, then fibrosis. Bone involvement 10%, affecting mostly bones of the hands.

Therapy. Patients with hypercalcemia can be managed with a low calcium diet. Local steroid therapy for ocular sarcoidosis; intradermal steroids for cutaneous lesions. Indications for systemic corticosteroid therapy include progressive pulmonary impairment or respiratory symptoms, ocular involvement, myocardial and central nervous system involvement, disfiguring cutaneous lesions, persistent hypercalcemia or hypercalciuria with renal involvement. The disease is characterized by frequent spontaneous remissions.

Prognosis. Remissions and relapses frequent, with gradual progression. Average survival 10 years. Fatal outcome in about 20% at earlier phases. In North American patients more benign prognosis; symptoms subside and disappear in 2 years in 9 of 10 patients.

BIBLIOGRAPHY. Besnier E: Lupus pernio de la face; synovites fongueuses (scrofulo-tuberculeuses) symétriques des extrémités superieures. Ann Dermat Syph 10:333–336, 1889
Boeck C: Multiple benign sarcoid of the skin. J Cutan Genito Urin Dis 17:543–550, 1889
Schaumann, J: Sur une forme érythrodermique du lymphogranulome bénin. Ann Dermatol Syph 1:561–574, 1920
Silzbach LE (ed): Seventh International Conference on Sarcoidosis and other Granulomatous Disorders. Ann NY Acad Sci 278:1–751, 1976
Reed CE, de Shazo R: Immunological aspects of granulomatous and interstitial lung diseases. JAMA 248:2683–2691, 1982

BESNIER'S PRURIGO

Synonyms. Atopic dermatitis; neurodermatitis disseminated; exudative eczema; diathesic prurigo.

Symptoms. Usually follows (also years later) infantile atopic dermatitis. Pruritus on localized lesion (see Signs) often associated with asthma; exacerbations of asthmatic attack and prurigo alternate.

Signs. Patches of lichenized papules most frequently on bend of knees, elbows, face, and wrists.

Etiology. Unknown. Interplay of genetic factors (of complex nature, dominant inheritance or recessive reported) and precipitating factors (immunological, climatic, and psychological). Inherent itchiness of the skin (?).

Pathology. Scratching lesions and lichenification (not constant).

Diagnostic Procedures. *Blood.* IgE increased (80% of cases). IgG, IgA, and IgM usually normal except severe eczema; presence of specific antibodies (RAST). *Skin reactivity.* To allergens, physical (cold, pressure) and pharmacological agents (histamine, nicotine acid esters, acetylcholine).

Therapy. General allergic management (avoid injection and contact with suspected antigens). Specific desensitizations (effective only in few cases); antipruritic agents (antihistamines), hydroxyzine hydrochloride, cortisone (for acute phase), antibiotic (if infection); topical treatment: ointment, with or diluted corticosteroids, zinc, coal tar, ultraviolet light (caution: may have opposite effect). In the author's experience, lactic acid-producing organisms and S-adenosyl L-methionine (200 mg daily) have been useful.

Prognosis. Recurrences, sometimes throughout life.

BIBLIOGRAPHY. Besnier E: Première note et observation preliminaire pour servir d'introduction à l'étude des prurigos diasthesiques. Ann Dermatol Syph 3:634–648, 1892
French H: French's Index of Differential Diagnosis, 9th ed. Baltimore, Williams & Wilkins, 1967
Rook A, Wilkinson DS, Ebling FJG, et al: Textbook of Dermatology, 4th ed, pp 419–434. Oxford, Blackwell Scientific Publications, 1986

BETA-KETOTHIOLASE DEFICIENCY

Synonym. Ketotic hyperglycinemia.

Symptoms and Signs. In children, episodic ketoacidosis with seizures and hyperammoniemia or psychomotor retardation.

Etiology. Autosomal recessive inheritance. Deficiency of beta-ketothiolase.

Diagnostic Procedures. *Blood.* Hypoglycinemia, hyperammonemia. *Urine.* Hyperglycinuria, 2-methyl-3-hydroxybutyrate, 2-methylacetoacetate and butanone (gas chromatographic analysis).

Therapy. Control of ketoacidosis.

Prognosis. Ranging from early death to normal development.

BIBLIOGRAPHY. Daum RS, Lamm PH, Mamer OA, et al: A new disorder of isoleucine catabolism. Lancet II: 1289–1290, 1971
Hillman RE, Keating JP: Beta-ketothiolase deficiency as a cause of the ketotic hyperglycinemia syndrome. Pediatrics 53:221–225, 1974
Bennett MJ, Littlewood JM, McDonald A, et al: A case of beta-ketothiolase deficiency. J Inherit Metab Dis 6:157, 1983

BETA-METHYLCROTONYL CoA CARBOXYLASE DEFICIENCY

Synonym. 3-methyl-crotonic aciduria.

Symptoms and Signs. Rare. Clinical picture of Werding-Hoffman (see). Peculiar "tomcat odor" of urine.

Etiology. Unknown. Deficiency of 3-methylcrotonyl CoA carboxylase.

Diagnostic Procedures. *Urine.* Increased 3-hydroxyisovaleric acid and 3-methylcrotonylglycine.

Therapy. None.

Prognosis. Death at an early age.

BIBLIOGRAPHY. Eldjarn L, Jellum E, Stokke O, et al: Beta hydroxyisovaleric aciduria and beta-methylcrotonyl-glycinuria: a new error of metabolism. Lancet II:521–522, 1970
Wolf B, Feldman GL: The biotin dependent carboxylase deficiencies. Am J Hum Genet 34:699–716, 1982

BETA-THALASSEMIA INTERMEDIA

Symptoms. Intermediate between thalassemia minor and Cooley's syndrome.

Etiology. Due to different genetic interactions:
1. Homozygosity for two mild beta thalassemia genes or double heterozygosity for one mild and one unusually severe gene;

2. Homozygosity or double heterozygosity for beta thalassemia genes of unusual severity, but with coinheritance of a modifying factor;
3. Heterozygous beta thalassemia of unusual severity.

BIBLIOGRAPHY. Bunn HF, Forget BG: Hemoglobin: molecular genetic and clinical aspects, p 340. Philadelphia, WB Saunders, 1986

BETA-THALASSEMIA MINIMA

Synonyms. Microcythemia minima; heterozygous beta thalassemia.

Symptoms. Asymptomatic. See Silvestroni-Bianco.

Etiology. Variable patterns of inheritance.

BIBLIOGRAPHY. Bunn HF, Forget BG: Hemoglobin: molecular genetic and clinical aspects, p 333. Philadelphia: WB Saunders, 1986

BETTLEY'S

Synonyms. Fetal cutaneointestinal; cutaneous-intestinal-oropharyngeal ulceration. See also Koehlmeir-Degos.

BIBLIOGRAPHY. Binswanger O: Die angrenzung der allgemeinen, progressiven Paralyse. Berl Klin Wochenschr 31:1103–1105, 1894
Freedman AM, Kaplan HI, Sadock BJ: Comprehensive Textbook of Psychiatry, 2nd ed, p 1075. Baltimore, Williams & Wilkins, 1975
De Reuck J, Crevits L, De Coster W, et al: Pathogenesis of Binswanger chronic progressive subcortical encephalopathy. Neurology 30:920, 1980

BEZOLD'S

Synonyms. Bezold abscess; temporal bone subperiosteal abscess.

Symptoms. Severe pain in perimastoidal region; difficulty of swallowing; sore throat; difficulty in breathing; nuchal rigidity; fever.

Signs. Swelling in the area between the tip of mastoid process and mandible; otorrhea.

Etiology. Otitis media with rupture of tympanic membrane; infiltration of pus into neck musculature.

Pathology. Perforation of inner surface of mastoid into digastric fossa; abscess extending behind sternocleidomastoid muscle, less frequently reaching perivertebral region or thoracic cavity.

Diagnostic Procedures. *Culture of pus. Blood and urine. X-ray of head and neck.*

Therapy. Sinus opening from mastoid process to neck and drainage. Antibiotics.

Prognosis. Recovery following surgery.

BIBLIOGRAPHY. Bezold F: Ein neuer Weg fur Ausbreitung eitriger Entzündung aus den Räumen des Mittelohrs auf die Nachbarschaft und die in diesem Falle einzuschlagende Therapie. Dtsch Med Wochenschr, 7:381–385, 1885

BHATTACHARYYA-CONNOR

Synonyms. Sitosterolemia-xanthomatosis; phytosterolemia.

Symptoms and Signs. Rare defect. From childhood, tendon xanthomas, xanthelasma: atherosclerosis of coronaries and large vessels, hemolytic anemia, platelet abnormalities; arthralgia and arthritis.

Etiology. Autosomal recessive inheritance. Increased absorption of sitosterol and defective turnover with accumulation in tissues.

Pathology. Xanthomas similar to those of hypercholesterolemia and cerebrotendinous xanthomatosis.

Diagnostic Procedures. *Blood.* High concentrations of sitosterol and compesterol. Hemolytic anemia. Platelets: functional defects.

Therapy. Diet low in plant sterols. Cholestyramine.

Prognosis. Fair. Death by coronary heart disease possible at early age.

BIBLIOGRAPHY. Bhattacharyya AK, Connor WE: Sitosterolemia and xanthamatosis: a newly described lipid storage disease in two sisters. J Clin Invest 53:1033–1043, 1974
Salen G, Shefer S, Berginer VM: Familial diseases with storage of sterols other than cholesterol: cerebrotendinous xanthomatosis and sitosterolemia with xanthomatosis. In Stanbury JB, Wyngaarden JB, Fredrickson DS, et al: The Metabolic Basis of Inherited Disease, 5th ed, p 713. New York, McGraw-Hill, 1983

BIANCHI'S

Synonym. Alexia-aphasia-apraxia; parietal. See Head-Holmes; Anton-Babinski; Gerstmann's; Pick's (A).

Symptoms and Signs. Expressive alexia; contralateral to lesion, hemianesthesia with tactile agnosia of corresponding hand and foot. Transient hemiplegia.

Etiology and Pathology. Usually, lesion of left parietal lobe.

BIBLIOGRAPHY. Bianchi L: La sindrome parietale. Med Ital (Napoli) 9:187, 243, 333, 1911

Adams RD, Victor M: Principles of Neurology, 3rd ed, pp 338–341. New York, McGraw-Hill, 1985

BIBER-HAAB-DIMMER

Synonyms. Buckler's III; corneal lattice dystrophy; Haab-Dimmer; lattice corneal dystrophy, LCD; Reis-Buckler.

Symptoms. Both sexes affected; onset early in life (20–30 years of age). Progressive vision reduction.

Signs. Corneal grayish lines, translucent cottonlike threads, mostly limited to a zone between center of cornea and periphery, not reaching limbus. Dots with distinct borders scattered all over. Cornea clear between opacities.

Etiology. Unknown; autosomal dominant inheritance.

Pathology. Hyaline degeneration involving stromal lamellae without mucopolysaccharide accumulation.

Diagnostic Procedures. *Biopsy of cornea.*

BIBLIOGRAPHY. Biber H: Ueber einige seltenere Hornhauterkrankungen. Inaugural Dissertation, Zurich, 1890 (cited by Haab O: Die gittrige Keratitis. Z Augenheilkd 2:235–246, 1899)

Kivlin JD, Lovrien EW, Maumenee IH, et al: Linkage analysis in lattice corneal dystrophy. Am J Med Genet 19:387–390, 1984

BICARBONATE DEFICIT

Symptoms and Signs. Weakness; malaise; headache; nausea; vomiting; abdominal pain; Kussmaul's breathing. If condition progresses, respiratory depression develops. Associated clinical manifestation of basic disease: diabetes; uremia; congestive heart failure.

Etiology. Excess of organic or inorganic acid in the body. *Excessive production of acids.* (1) Diabetic acidosis; (2) starvation; (3) high fever; (4) thyrotoxicosis; (5) violent exercise; (6) shock. *Excessive intake of acid.* Administration of sodium, calcium, or ammonium chlorides, or of carbonic anhydrase inhibitors; or cation exchange resins, salicylate poisoning (see); methyl alcohol intoxication. *Acid retentions.* In renal diseases. *Loss of bases.* Diarrhea; fistulas; Lightwood's (see); in ureteroenterostomy patients.

Pathology. Depends upon etiology.

Diagnostic Procedures. *Blood.* Leukocytosis (occasional). (1) Uncompensated metabolic acidosis: blood pH low; P_{CO_2} normal, CO_2 capacity low; bicarbonate low; chloride increased; sodium low; normal or high according to etiology. (2) Compensated metabolic acidosis: pH low or normal; P_{CO_2} low; CO_2 capacity normal; bicarbonate low; chloride low, normal, or high; sodium low or normal; potassium high. *Urine.* Acid; very high ammonia (in renal disease normal pH).

Therapy. Correct causes (see Etiology); correct electrolyte balance.

Prognosis. Depends upon etiology. In chronic cases, defect persists for years. In acute, may result in death if treatment not adequate.

BIBLIOGRAPHY. Goldberger E: A Primer of Water, Electrolyte, and Acid-base Syndromes, 3rd ed. Philadelphia, Lea & Febiger, 1965

Schade DS (ed): Metabolic acidosis. Clin Endocrinol Metab 12:265, 1983

BICIPITAL SYNDROME

Synonym. Gilcreest's.

Symptoms and Signs. Bicipital tendon dislocation.

Etiology. Trauma.

Diagnostic Procedures. *Specific test.* Dumbbell in each hand (2–3 kg), extension of arms, lifting to the overhead position in external rotation. Examiner's finger on tendon of long head of the biceps; as the patient lowers the outstretched arms, at 90–100 degree angle a sharp pain occurs and a snap is palpable and audible.

Therapy. Surgery.

BIBLIOGRAPHY. Gilcreest EL: The common syndrome of rupture, dislocation and elongation of the long head of the biceps brachii: analysis of 100 cases. Surg Gynecol Obstet 58:322–340, 1934

Justis EJ Jr: Traumatic disorders. In Crenshaw, AH (ed): Campbell's Operative Orthopedics, 7th ed, pp 2242–2243. St Louis, CV Mosby, 1987

BICIPITAL TENOSYNOVITIS

Synonym. Shoulder tendonitis.

Symptoms. Prevalent in females; onset gradual or abrupt. Especially disturbing during night when resting on affected shoulder. Pain of various degrees; disability (abduction and internal rotation limited).

Signs. Tenderness on anterior area of humeral head over bicipital groove, Yergason's sign positive in 50% of cases.

Etiology. Trauma; strain; temperature change; humidity; idiopathic.

Pathology. Inflammatory changes of synovia of bicipital tendon; serofibrinous exudate. According to stage, various degrees of adhesion and involvement of surrounding tissues.

Therapy. X-ray treatment; systemic corticosteroid; local injection of procaine or hydrocortisone; physical therapy. Exploratory surgery: transplantation of tendon to coracoid process or to floor of bicipital groove.

Prognosis. Acute, subacute, chronic types are known to evolve from one stage to another, or start directly as subacute or chronic. Chronic stage lasts weeks or months. Atrophy of biceps and shoulder muscles may develop.

BIBLIOGRAPHY. Pasteur F: Les algies de l'épaule et la physiothérapie la téno-bursite bicipitale. J Radiol Electrol 16:419–426, 1932
Steinbrocker O: The painful shoulder. In Hollander JL, McCarty DJ (eds): Arthritis and Allied Conditions, 8th ed, p 1477. Philadelphia, Lea & Febiger, 1978
Justis EJ Jr: New traumatic disorders. In Crenshaw AH (ed): Campbell's Operative Orthopedics, 7th ed, p 2259–2260. St. Louis, CV Mosby, 1987

BICKERS-ADAMS

Synonyms. X-linked hydrocephalus; hydrocephalus X-linked; aqueductal stenosis.

Symptoms and Signs. Males affected; females carriers (dull intelligence); present from birth. Spasticity, especially lower extremities. Mental deficiency (IQ in the range of 30); hydrocephalus or narrow scaphocephalic cranium. Flexed thumb over palm; short first metacarpal. Occasionally asymmetric and course facies; seizures.

Etiology. X-linked recessive inheritance.

Pathology. Aqueductal stenosis and hydrocephalus. Occasionally, various brain defects.

Diagnostic Procedures. *Electroencephalography.* Diffuse abnormalities. *CT brain scan. X-ray.*

Therapy. Neurosurgical.

Prognosis. Poor.

BIBLIOGRAPHY. Bickers DS, Adams RD: Hereditary stenosis of the aqueduct of Sylvius as a cause of congenital hydrocephalus. Brain 72:246–262, 1949
Wiliamson RA, Schauberger CW, Warner MW, et al: Heterogeneity of prenatal onset hydrocephalus: management and counseling implications. Am J Genet 17:497–508, 1984

BIELSCHOWSKY-LUTZ-COGAN

Synonyms. Lhermitte's; medial longitudinal fasciculus, MLF; internuclear ophthalmoplegia.

Symptoms. Unilateral or bilateral palsy on conjugate lateral gaze; recognized various possibilities (1) paresis of convergence and paresis of homolateral internal rectus muscle on lateral gaze; (2) homolateral internal rectus muscle paralysis on lateral gaze without alteration of convergence. With maximal abduction elicited a dissociated nystagmus of contralateral eye.

Etiology. Any lesion (hemorrhagic, neoplastic, traumatic) that affects the medial longitudinal fasciculus, interconnecting 3rd and 4th and 6th nuclei. (1) Anterior internuclear ophthalmoplegia. (2) Posterior internuclear ophthalmoplegia.

Therapy. According to etiology.

Prognosis. According to etiology.

BIBLIOGRAPHY. Bielschowsky A: Die Innervation der musculi recti interni als Seitenwaender. Ber Zusammenkunft Dtsch Ophthalmol Ges 30:164–171, 1902
Lutz, A: Ueber einseitige Ophthalmoplegia. Internuclearis anterior. Graefes Arch Ophthalmol 115:692–717, 1924
Cogan DG, Kubik CS, Smith L: Unilateral internuclear ophthalmoplegia: report of eight clinical cases with one postmortem study. Arch Ophthalmol 44:783–796, 1950
Stroud MH, Newman NM, Keltner JL, Gay AJ: Abducting nystagmus in the medial longitudinal fasciculus (MLF) Syndrome-internuclear ophthalmoplegia (INO) Arch Ophthalmol 92:2–5, 1974
Adams RD, Victor M: Principles of Neurology, 3rd ed, pp 203–204. New York, McGraw-Hill, 1985

BIELSKOWSKY'S

Synonyms. Bernheimer-Seitelberger; GM_2 gangliosidosis type 3; juvenile GM_2 gangliosidosis.

Symptoms. Both sexes affected; onset between 2 and 6 years of age. Locomotor ataxia. *Initial manifestation.* The illness often starts with progressive loss of vision. Progressive spasticity; athetosis; loss of speech; minor convulsions. *Later.* Blindness; frequent respiratory infections. Clinically similar to Batten's (see) with which it can be easily confused.

Signs. Facies normal. Absence of hepatosplenomegaly and of the macular cherry-red spot.

Etiology. Autosomal recessive inheritance. Severe or partial deficiency of hexosaminidase A.

Pathology. Prominent neuronal lipoidosis. Neurons are distended with material that has the staining characteristics of lipofuscin. Particularly affected are the cells in the anterior horn of the spinal cord and in the peripheral autonomic ganglia. Pathologic pattern exhibiting features common to both Tay-Sachs and Sandhoff's. Lipofuscinlike material also accumulates in other organs, particularly thyroid gland and sweat glands.

Diagnostic Procedures. *Blood-urine-spinal fluid, tissue and cell cultures.* Assay of hexosaminidases. *X-rays.* Absence of bone changes. *Bone marrow.* Absence of foamy cells. *Ophthalmologic changes.* Retinitis pigmentosa, pigmentary degeneration of the macular region, or simple optic atrophy. *Biopsy of muscle or sweat glands.* Electron-dense bodies similar to those found in neurons.

Prognosis. Death between 5 and 15 years of age.

BIBLIOGRAPHY. Bielskowsky M: Ueber spatinfantile familiaere amaurotische Idiotie mit Kleinhirnsymptomen. Dtsch Z Nervenheilk 50:7–29, 1914

O'Brien JS: The gangliosidoses. In Stanbury JB, Wyngaarden JB, Fredrickson DS, et al: The Metabolic Basis Inherited Disease, 5th ed, p 945. New York, McGraw-Hill, 1983

BIEMOND'S I

Synonyms. Brachydactyly-nystagmus; cerebellar ataxia; cerebellar ataxia–nystagmus–brachydactyly.

Symptoms and Signs. Mental deficiency; cerebellar ataxia; strabismus, nystagmus; and one short metacarpal and one short metatarsal. Not all members of family present the full syndrome.

Etiology. Possibly autosomal dominant inheritance.

BIBLIOGRAPHY. Biemond A: Brachydactylie, Nystagmus en cerebellaire Ataxie als familiair Syndroom. Nederl T Geneesk 78:1423–1431, 1934

BIEMOND'S II

Synonym. See Laurence-Moon-Biedl.

Symptoms and Signs. Pituitary dwarfism; mental retardation; iris coloboma; obesity; secondary hypogenitalism; postaxial polydactyly; hydrocephalus; hypospadias.

Etiology. Irregular autosomal dominant inheritance.

BIBLIOGRAPHY. Biemond A: Het syndroom van Laurence-Biedl en een aarverwant nieuw syndroom. Nederl T Geneesk 78:1801–1814, 1934

Blumel J, Kniker WT: Laurence-Moon-Bardet-Biedel syndrome: review of the literature and a report of five cases, including a family group with three affected males. Texas Rep Biol Med 17:391–410, 1959

BIEMOND'S III

Synonyms. Spinothalamic ataxia; congenital pain indifference; analgia congenital; familial analgia; spinothalamic ataxia; pain indifference congenital; Dearborn's.

Symptoms. Both sexes affected; normal at birth. Failure to register pain. Usually, normal physical and mental development; occasionally associated with oligophrenia, convulsions; aphasia (auditory).

Signs. Evidence of repeated injuries both to soft and hard tissues: scars; fractures; joints with Charchot's jointlike (see) lesions. Nail is thickened and deformed. Irregular dentition with vertical grooves on teeth. Deep tendon reflexes diminished or absent. Corneal reflexes diminished. Absence of sympathetic reaction to pain. Frequent oral mutilation.

Etiology. Unknown; autosomal recessive inheritance.

Pathology. Cholinesterase-positive nerves present only around eccrine sweat gland. Spinothalamic tract and/or posterior ascending tract occasionally absent. Hypoplasia of pyramidal tracts. Cutaneous nerves reveal only non-myelinated fibers. Reduction of neurons in autonomic and sensory ganglia.

Therapy. Symptomatic.

Prognosis. Severe, up to total incapacitation.

BIBLIOGRAPHY. Dearborn G: A case of congenital pure analgesia. J Nerv Ment Dis 75:612–615, 1932

Biemond A: Investigation of the brain in a case of congenital and familial analgia. Proc XI Intern Cong Neuropath, London, 1955

BIETTI'S I

Synonyms. Marginal corneal dystrophy; dystrophia marginalis cristallinea cornae; crystalline retinopathy; tapetoretinal degeneration.

Symptoms. Relatively common in China. Both sexes equal incidence. Onset in middle to advanced age (average age 30 years). Asymptomatic.

Signs. Recurrent irritation; inflammation. Progressive night blindness, reduction of visual fields. In some families chronic changes may be absent.

Etiology. Unknown. Autosomal recessive trait.

Pathology. Marginal corneal dystrophy with loose connective tissue replacing stroma; limbal area thinned; Descemet's membrane bulging; Bowman's capsule degenerated. Retinal degeneration, sclerosis of choroidal.

Diagnostic Procedures. *Ophthalmoscopy.* Numerous glistening intraretinal dots over the fundus.

Therapy. Symptomatic.

Prognosis. Slow progression. Seldom, eyeball rupture.

BIBLIOGRAPHY. Bietti G: Ueber familiäres Vorkommen von "Retinitis punctata albescens" (verbunden mit "Dystrophia marginalis cristallinea corneae"). Glitzern des Glaskörpers und anderen degenerativen Augenveränderungen. Klin Monatsbl Augenheilkd 99:937–956, 1937

Hayasake S, Okuyama S: Crystalline retinopathy. Retina 4:177–181, 1984

BIGLIERI'S

Synonyms. Adrenal and gonadal-17-hydroxylase deficiency; hypogonadism–mineral corticoid excess; 17-hydroxylase deficiency, adrenal hyperplasia V. See Adrenogenital syndromes.

Symptoms. Genotype female adults. Primary amenorrhea; lack of secondary sexual development; fatigue; episodes of marked muscle weakness; numbness and tingling in extremities; episodes of partial hair loss.

Signs. Undeveloped breasts; scanty body hair; infantile uterus; small ovaries (on palpation). Wrinkling and premature aging of facial skin. Hypertension.

Etiology. Congenital defect of 17-hydroxylase activity resulting in decreased synthesis of cortisol, estrogens, and androgens.

Pathology. Unknown.

Diagnostic Procedures. *Blood.* Hypokalemia; alkalosis; low secretion rate of cortisol. Injection of adenocorticotropic hormone (ACTH) fails to increase secretion of cortisol. Androsterone and testosterone essentially undetectable. Plasma ACTH markedly increased. *Urine.* Increased 11-oxycorticosteroids; pregnanetriol markedly decreased, 17-ketosteroid apparently normal (no detectable dehydroisoandrosterone and very low conjugated androsterone and etiocholanolone). Excretion of estrone and estradiol low; increase of urinary gonadotropin, increased production of desoxycorticosterone, corticosterone, progesterone, and aldosterone. *Electrocardiography.* Signs of hypokalemia.

Therapy. Dexamethasone 0.5 mg three times a day.

Prognosis. Optimal response to treatment.

BIBLIOGRAPHY. Biglieri EG, Herron MA, Brust N: 17-hydroxylation deficiency in man. J Clin Invest 45:1946–1954, 1966

Goldsmith O, Solomon DH, Horton R: Hypogonadism and mineralocorticoid excess: the 17-Hydroxylase deficiency syndrome. New Engl J Med 277:673–677, 1967

Miller WL, Chung B-C, Matteson KJ, et al: Molecular biology of steroid hormone synthesis. DNA 5:61, 1986

BILE REFLUX

Symptoms and Signs. Usually after gastric surgery or cholecystectomy, occasionally only with no prior surgery. Substernal distress, anorexia, nausea and vomiting of bile-stained fluid.

Etiology. Reflux of bile into stomach.

Therapy. *Medical.* Unsatisfactory. *Surgical.* Roux-en-Y anastomosis.

Prognosis. Good with surgery.

BIBLIOGRAPHY. Buxbaum KL: Bile gastritis occurring after cholecystectomy. Am J Gastroenterol 77:305, 1982

BILGINTURAN'S

Synonym. Brachydactyly-hypertension.

Symptoms and Signs. Short phalanges and metacarpals. Arterial hypertension.

Etiology. Autosomal dominant inheritance.

BIBLIOGRAPHY. Bilginturan N, Zileli S, Karacadag S, et al: Hereditary brachydactyly associated with hypertension. J Med Genet 10:253–259, 1973

BILLROTH'S

Synonyms. Traumatic cephalohydrocele; spurious meningocele.

Symptoms and Signs. Appear in children with history of head trauma. Fluid accumulation under scalp.

Etiology. Trauma, with skull fracture and tear of arachnoid.

Diagnostic Procedures. *X-rays. Cerebral CT scan.* Differentiation from hematoma, abscess, meningocele.

Therapy. Usually conservative.

Prognosis. Good, if infection prevented and according to other consequence of trauma.

BIBLIOGRAPHY. Billroth T: Ein Fall von Meningocele spuria cum Fistula ventriculi cerebri. Arch Klin Chir 3:398–412, 1862

Adams RD, Victor M: Principles of Neurology, 3rd ed, p 648. New York. McGraw-Hill, 1985

BINDER'S

Synonym. Maxillonasal dysplasia. See Villaret-Desoilles.

Signs. Present from birth. Flat vertical nose; absence of nasofrontal angle; nasal hypoplasia and flat alae and tip; nostrils crescent-shaped; normal sense of smell. Upper lip convex and poorly developed philtrum; hypoplasia of premaxillary area, flattening of maxillary base and short dental arch; increased gonial angle and flat chin; relative mandibular prognathism.

Etiology. Unknown. Sporadic; possibly, inherited cases.

Diagnostic Procedures. *X-rays.* Hypoplasia of anterior nasal spine and of frontal sinuses. Thickness reduction of labial plate of alveolar bone over upper incisors.

BIBLIOGRAPHY. Noyes FB: Case report. Angle Orthodon 9:160–165, 1939

Binder KH: Dysostosis maxillo-nasalis: ein arhinencephaler Missbildungkomplex. Dtsch Zahnalrztl Z 17:438–444, 1962

Gorlin RJ, Pindborg JJ, Cohen MM: Syndromes of the Head and Neck, 2nd ed. New York, McGraw-Hill, 1976

BING-NEEL

Synonym. Macroglobulinemic neuropsychiatric. See Waldenström's.

Symptoms. Anorexia; pronounced weight loss; slight elevation of temperature. After variable length of time with these symptoms: In one case, sudden paralysis of arms, legs, whole body, vomiting, headache, no pains, no paresthesia. In a second case, vomiting, dizziness, loss of feeling at end of fingers. In a third case, psychic changes, pain in arm and legs, deep asthenia of arms without paralysis; deep asthenia of legs with probable paresis. In all cases, symptomatology cannot be attributed to any localized process and appears as due to disseminated lesions resulting in irregular generalized neurologic patterns.

Signs. Pallor; generalized mild muscular asthenia; decreased fat; patient looks older than chronologic age; lymphadenopathy. Neurologic examination reveals irregular reflexes, alteration paralysis as due to disseminated spinal lesions.

Etiology. See Waldenström's.

Pathology. Widespread alteration of nervous system, especially cauda equina, spinal cord, pons, optic nerves, representing the picture of a toxicoinfectious radiculo-meningomyeloencephalopathy. Irregular alteration of other organs, no evidence of multiple myeloma.

Diagnostic Procedures. *Blood.* Anemia; marked increase of sedimentation rate; normal white blood cells with prevalence of lymphocytic elements; hyperproteinemia, with hyperglobulinemia; positive test for coloidal lability (Formol gel, Sia's test). bone marrow hyperplastic in only one case; no evidence of myeloma or leukosis. *Urine.* Albuminuria; casts.

Therapy. No therapeutic attempt is reported in the presentation of the original cases. Since this condition seems to be a complication of macroglobulinemic syndromes, for treatment, see Waldenström's.

Prognosis. Death follows within 6 to 12 months from start of neurologic symptomatology.

BIBLIOGRAPHY. Bing J, Neel AV: Two cases of hyperglobulinemia with affection of central nervous system on a toxi-infectious basis. Acta Med Scand 88:492–506, 1936

Bing J, Fog M, Neel AV: Reports of a third case of hyperglobulinemia with affection of central nervous system on toxi-infectious basis. Acta Med Scand 41:409–426, 1937

Voigt AE, Frick PG: Macroglobulinemia of Waldenström: a review of literature and presentation of a case. Ann Intern Med 44:419–425, 1956

Edgar R, Dutcher TF: Histopathology of the Bing-Neel syndrome. Neurology 11:239–245, 1961

Wintrobe MM (ed): Clinical Hematology, 8th ed. Philadelphia, Lea Febiger, 1981

BINSWANGER'S

Synonym. Subcortical arteriosclerotic encephalopathy, SAE. See also Senile dementia.

Symptoms and Signs. Onset between 50 and 60 years of age. Progressive dementia associated with variable signs of focal cerebral diseases.

Etiology. Arteriosclerosis. Considered as form with no essential difference from the lacunar syndrome (see).

Pathology. Subcortical demyelinization associated with arteriopathy of small arteries of white matter.

Diagnostic Procedures. *Electroencephalography. Angiography. CT brain scan. Cerebrospinal fluid.* Normal pressure, protein slight increase.

Therapy. Symptomatic.

Prognosis. Slowly progressing condition alternating with periods of stabilization lasting months or years.

BIBLIOGRAPHY. Binswanger O: Die angrenzung der allgemeinen, progressiven Paralyse. Berl Klin Wochenschr 31:1103–1105, 1894

Freedman AM, Kaplan HI, Sadock BJ: Comprehensive Textbook of Psychiatry, 2nd ed, p 1075, Baltimore, Williams & Wilkins, 1975

De Reuck J, Crevits L, De Coster W, et al: Pathogenesis of Binswanger chronic progressive subcortical encephalopathy. Neurology 30:920, 1980

BIORKMAN-DACIE

Synonyms. Anemia refractaria sideroblastica; ineffective idiopathic erythropoiesis; IRSA; primary acquired refractory sideroblastic anemia; refractory normoblastic anemia.

Symptoms. Occurs in old adults (average age 66); very seldom in people younger than 50. Onset insidious. Asthenia.

Signs. Mild pallor; modest hepatosplenomegaly (40%).

Etiology. Unknown, acquired condition. Impairment of heme synthetase reaction. Possibly, neoplasia, drug or toxic hypersensitivity reactions, somatic mutation. X-linked inheritance reported.

Pathology. *Liver.* Marked deposition of iron. *Blood.* Moderate anemia, normocytic or macrocytic type; occasionally, hypochromic; heavily stippled cells, moderate leukothrombocytopenia; leukocyte alkaline phosphatase reduced in 90% of cases; transferrin increased, modest hyperbilirubinemia. *Bone marrow.* Erythroid hyperplasia; lack of PAS positivity in normoblast; megaloblastic changes (20%); increased hemosiderin; ringed sideroblasts (45–90% of normoblasts).

Therapy. Pyridoxine 50 to 200 mg per day (usually ineffective). Some patients who did not respond to pyridoxine were able to respond to pyridoxal phosphate, the coenzyme form of the vitamin. Transfusion of packed cells (minimal benefit). Androgens.

Prognosis. About half of the patients are not severely incapacitated by their anemia, which does not progress for many years. In these cases no treatment is required. In cases with significant cardiovascular symptoms: transfuse with packed red cells. Number of transfusions should be kept to a minimum because of iron overload. Some patients respond to large doses of androgens (50–100 mg of oxymetholone per day). Some patients develop leukemia and acute myelofibrosis.

BIBLIOGRAPHY. Biorkman S: Chronic refractory anemia with sideroblastic bone marrow. Blood 11:250–259, 1956

Dacie JV: Refractory normoblastic anemia. Br J Haematol 5:245–256, 1959

Wintrobe MM (ed): Clinical Hematology, 8th ed. Philadelphia, Lea & Febiger, 1981

BIRD-HEADED DWARFISM, MONTREAL TYPE

Synonym. See Seckel's.

Symptoms. Both sexes. Normal weight at birth. Mental retardation.

Signs. Ptosis. Premature graying and baldness; redundant, wrinkled skin of palms; cryptorchidism.

Etiology. Autosomal recessive inheritance postulated.

BIBLIOGRAPHY. Fitch N, Pinsky L, Lachance RC: A rare form of bird-headed dwarfism with features of premature senility. Am J Dis Child 120:260–264, 1970

McKusick VA: Mendelian Inheritance in Man, 7th ed. Baltimore: Johns Hopkins University Press, 1986

BIRNBAUM'S

Eponym used to indicate a combination of Huntington's (see) with cerebellar atrophy.

Synonyms. Progressive chorea–cerebellar atrophy.

BIBLIOGRAPHY. Birnbaum G: Chronisch-progressive Chorea mit Kleinhirnatrophie. Arch Psychiat 114:160–182, 1941

BIRSCH-HIRSCHFIELD

Symptoms and Signs. Onset in old age. Idiopathic hypertrophic parotitis.

BIBLIOGRAPHY. Moortgat P: Syndromes à noms propres. Paris, J Prélat 1966

BIVENTRICULAR TRANSPOSED AORTA AND LEFT VENTRICULAR STENOTIC PULMONARY ARTERY

Symptoms and Signs. Early deep cyanosis with physical endurance not markedly decreased; apical systolic murmur (grade 1); accentuation of second pulmonary sound; left-sided enlargement of the heart; clubbing of fingers and toes.

Etiology. Unknown; congenital malformation.

Pathology. Biventricular transposed aorta and left stenotic pulmonary artery.

Diagnostic Procedures. *X-rays of chest.* Frontal view, concave middle segment; oblique view, concavity disappears and is replaced by prominence of a vessel whose anterior contour is tangent to anterior border of underlying ventricle. Left-sided enlargement of heart chambers. *Simultaneous catheterization and angiocardiography. Electrocardiography.*

Therapy. None.

Prognosis. In these cases, in contrast with cases with transposition of great vessels with or without pulmonary stenosis, life is prolonged for unusual length of time (second decade).

BIBLIOGRAPHY. De la Cruz MV, da Rocha JP: An ontogenetic theory for the explanation of congenital malformations involving the truncus and conus. Am Heart J 51:782–805, 1956
De la Cruz MV, Espino-Vela J, Anselmi G: Biventricular transposed aorta and left ventricular stenotic pulmonary artery: an embryologic and pathologic account of a new syndrome whose existence was previously theoretically predicted. Am Heart J 59:902–912, 1960
Perloff JK: The Clinical Recognition of Congenital Heart Disease, 2nd ed, p 445. Philadelphia, WB Saunders, 1978

BIXLER-ANTLEY

Symptoms and Signs. Those of Gsell-Erdheim (see) associated with ectopia of the pigment layer of the iris into anterior surface of iris.

BIBLIOGRAPHY. Bixler D, Antley RM: Familial aortic dissection with iris anomalies: a new connective tissue disease syndrome? Birth Defects Orig Art XII (5):229–234, 1976

BJORNSTAD'S

Synonym. Deafness–pili torti; pili torti deafness. See Ronchese.

Symptoms. Both sexes affected; manifested since early infancy. Sensory neuronal hearing loss occurring as a significant association with pili torti (see).

Etiology. Unknown; autosomal recessive inheritance.

BIBLIOGRAPHY. Bjornstad R: Pili torti and sensory loss of hearing. Proc Fermo Scand Assoc Dermatol 3, 1965
Cremers CWJ, Geerts SJ: Sensoneural hearing loss and pili torti. Am Otal Rhinol Laryng 88:100–104, 1979

BLACKFAN-DIAMOND

Synonyms. Hypoplastic congenital anemia; primary red cell asplasia; congenital aregenerative anemia; idiopathic erythroblastopenia; erythrogenesis imperfecta; erythrophthisis; Josephs-Diamond-Blackfan; Kaznelson's I.

Symptoms. Noted at birth or recognized within first 6 months. Growth retardation; failure of sexual maturation; seldom, dyspnea; decrease of activity. Recently two adults with the syndrome have been described.

Signs. Weight at birth lower than normal; pallor; no jaundice. Presence of minor congenital anomalies (occasionally, hepatomegaly; rare, splenomegaly) which initially regress after blood transfusion.

Etiology. Unknown; familial incidence in some cases (genetically determined?). Abnormalities of tryptophan metabolism in some cases. In one case, association with chromosome abnormality. Spectrum of various conditions characterized by pure erythroid deficiency.

Pathology. Pallor; underdevelopment; failure of sexual maturation. Hemosiderosis (secondary to blood transfusion); cirrhosis. Portal hypertension. Osteoporosis.

Diagnostic Procedures. *Blood.* Normocytic, normochromic anemia; reticulocytes (less than 1%); normoblasts; leukocytes and platelets normal. Hypocalcemia. *Bone marrow.* Erythroid deficiency. *Other series.* Normal.

Therapy. Blood transfusion. Adrenal cortical steroid results in hematologic repair. Splenectomy is of doubtful utility.

Prognosis. Course insidious and progressive; spontaneous remissions (permanent or temporary) reported.

BIBLIOGRAPHY. Diamond LK, Blackfan KD: Hypoplastic anemia. Am J Dis Child 56:464–467, 1938

Bernard J, Seligmann M, Chassigneux J, et al: Anemie de Blackfan-Diamond. Nouv Rev Fr Hematatol 2:721–739, 1962

Josephs HW: Anemia of infancy and early childhood. Medicine 15:307–451, 1936

Balaban EP, Buchanan GR, Graham M, Frenkel EP: Diamond-Blackfan syndrome in adult patients. Am J Med 78:533–538, 1985

BLACK HEEL

Synonyms. Talon noir; calcaneal petechiae; purpura traumatica pedis.

Symptoms and Signs. Boys predominantly affected, especially if athletically active; usually epidemic occurrence, seldom sporadic. Blackish discoloration in isolated or aggregated specks in horny layer of back or side of heels; seldom in the forefoot (metatarsal area).

Etiology. Unknown; blood extravasion. Reason for epidemic outbreak unknown.

Therapy. Not needed. Felt pad in the shoes may help.

Prognosis. Spontaneous regression at the end of athletic season.

BIBLIOGRAPHY. Bazex A, Salvador R, Dupre A: Plantar chromhidrosis. Bull Soc Fr Dermatol Syph 69:489–490, 1962

Rook A, Wilkinson DS, Ebling FJG, et al: Textbook of Dermatology, 4th ed, pp 606–607. Oxford, Blackwell Scientific Publications, 1986

BLACKOUT

Synonyms. Hydrostatic pressure; negative acceleration.

Symptoms. In passengers in vehicles (especially airplanes) subjected to rapid acceleration or deceleration. Rise of visual threshold; altered perception of intensity of lights and colors, up to complete loss of consciousness.

Signs. Moderate mydriasis; periorbital edema; subconjunctival hemorrhages.

Etiology. Reduction of retinal arterial pressure.

Pathology. Retinal hemorrhages.

Diagnostic Procedures. *Ophthalmoscopy.* Retinal arterial collapse.

Prognosis. Good. Vision restored after cessation of cause.

BIBLIOGRAPHY. Stokes WH: Unusual retinal vascular changes in traumatic injury to the chest. Arch Ophthalmol 7:101–108, 1932

Lyle DJ, Stapp JP, Button RR: Ophthalmological hydrostatic pressure syndrome. Trans Am Ophthalmol Soc 54:121–128, 1956

BLACK WIDOW SPIDER BITE

Synonyms. Arachnidism; araneism; *Latrodectus mactans* bite; latrodectism.

Symptoms. *Local.* Unnoticed or pain. *Systemic.* In the regional lymphatic nodes spreading to the lumbar region, the abdomen, the waist, the thighs, and the whole lower extremities. Muscular pain, cramps, tremors, athralgias, fever (maximum intensity for 20 hr). Photophobia. Exocrine secretion (eye, nose, mouth, and skin).

Signs. *Local.* A red, gooseflesh area of 0.5 cm in diameter, increasing in size and intensity. Then a pallid area up to 5 cm in diameter delimited by a reddish, bluish circular border; anesthesia dolorosa. *Cardiovascular.* First tachycardia then bradycardia, cardiac failure; extrasystole, first hypotension then hypertension. *Respiratory.* Tachypnea followed by bradypnea, increased bronchial secretion, bronchoconstriction. *Abdomen.* Rigidity of the abdominal wall; liver enlargement or subicterus. *Urogenital.* Oliguria or anuria during the first 12 hr.

Etiology and Pathology. Bite by female black widow spider (13 mm long, completely black with clepsydralike red marking on the ventral side).

Diagnostic Procedures. Observation of lesion and progression of muscle involvement to differentiate from acute abdomen. *Blood.* Leukocytosis, neutrophilia, lymphopenia, increased erythrocyte sedimentation rate, decrease of sodium and chlorides, increased blood urea nitrogen. *Urine.* Albuminuria; sediment RBC, WBC, and casts.

Therapy. Calcium gluconate (10%) 10 ml intravenously, specific antivenim when available. Hot bath and analgesic (careful with respiratory depression), neostigmine for muscle spasm. Corticosteroid for fast relief.

Prognosis. Rapid recovery, but in children may be fatal.

BIBLIOGRAPHY. Brown HW: Venenating arthropods (centipedes, scorpions, spiders, ticks, wasps, ants, blister beetles, caterpillars). In Beeson PB, McDermott W (eds): Cecil-Loeb Textbook of Medicine, 12th ed, pp 418–419. Philadelphia, WB Saunders, 1967

Bettini S: Arthropod Venoms. Berlin, Springer-Verlag, 1978

BLADDER NECK

Synonym. See Marion's.

Symptoms. Initial urinary hesitancy; weak stream; terminal dribbling. Urinary infection.

Signs. Increasing volume of residual urine and large decompensated bladder with cellules and diverticula.

Etiology. Narrowing of bladder outlet (congenital); dysfunction of vesical neck sphincteral muscles; acquired: bladder neck operation or chronic infections and fibrosis of bladder neck. To be differentiated from pseudobladder neck syndrome where the compression is extrinsic (pelvic tumors; pregnancy).

Pathology. See Etiology.

Diagnostic Procedures. *Determination of residual urine volumes. Cystograms. Cystourethrography. Cystoendoscopy. Neurologic examination.* To exclude neurogenic bladder. *Calibration of bladder neck.*

Therapy. Conservative or surgical according to etiology and degree of involvement.

Prognosis. Good with adequate treatment.

BIBLIOGRAPHY. Ward JN, Lavengood RW J, Draper JW: Pseudo bladder neck syndrome in women. J Urol 99:65–68, 1968
Waterhouse K, Langani G, Patil V: The surgical repair of membranous urethral stricture: experience with 105 consecutive cases. J Urol 123:500–505, 1980
Older RA: Urinary tract obstruction: current methods of evaluation. JAMA 245:1854–1856, 1981

BLAND-GARLAND-WHITE

Synonyms. Coronary left artery of anomalous origin.

Symptoms. Onset in first month of life; occasionally, later. Dyspnea; tachypnea; failure to thrive. Attacks of precordial pain: sweating; increased dyspnea; pallor; crying following exertion or feeding.

Signs. Enlarged heart mostly left ventricle; usually, no murmur or apical holosystolic murmur.

Etiology. Congenital anomaly with origin of left coronary artery from pulmonary artery.

Pathology. Necrosis and fibrosis of left ventricle especially subdendocardial and of papillary muscles. Thrombosis of small arteries and arterioles.

Diagnostic Procedures. *Electrocardiography.* Inversion T_1, T_2, deep Q_1. *Retrograde aortography.* Diagnostic. *Cardiac cathererization.*

Therapy. Surgery to provide anastomotic channel to supply blood to left ventricle and ligation of aberrant coronary artery.

Prognosis. Usually death before 2 years of age; occasionally, asymptomatic or paucisymptomatic cases may reach adolescence or adulthood.

BIBLIOGRAPHY. Brooks HS Jr: Two cases of an abnormal coronary artery arising from the pulmonary artery. J Anat Physiol 20:26, 1886
Abrikossoff A: Aneurysma des linken Harzventrikels mit abnormer abgangstelle der linken Koronararterie von der Pulmonalis bei einem funsononatlichen Kinde. Virchow's Arch [Pathol Anat] 203:413–420, 1911
Bland EF et al: Congenital anomalies of the coronary arteries, report of an unusual case associated with cardiac hypertrophy. Am Heart J 8:787–801, 1932–33
Perloff JK: The Clinical Recognition of Congenital Heart Disease, 2nd ed, pp 561–573. Philadelphia, WB Saunders, 1978
Hurst J: The Heart, 6th ed, pp 708–710. New York, McGraw-Hill, 1986

BLAST

Synonym. Blast injury.

Symptoms. Dyspnea; pain in ears; partial or complete deafness; pain in the chest or other regions. (See Blast scrotum.)

Signs. Shock, loss of consciousness; bradycardia; signs of injury in lung, heart, abdominal organs; abdominal distension; petecchiae in eardrum.

Etiology. Phase of overpressure and underpressure after detonation.

Pathology. Hemorrhages in lung parenchyma; arterial embolizations; pneumothorax.

Diagnostic Procedures. *Electrocardiography.* Atrial flutter; fibrillation. *Blood.* Hematocrit, electrolytes. *X-ray of chest.* Increased or decreased transparency.

Therapy. According to type and degree of lesions. Tracheal intubation and mechanical ventilation frequently required.

Prognosis. Variable.

BIBLIOGRAPHY. De Candole CA: Blast injury. Can Med Assoc J 96:207–214, 1967
Fishman AP, Pietra GG: Stretched pores, blast injury and neurohemodynamic pulmonary edema. Physiologist 23:53–56, 1980

BLAST SCROTUM

Symptoms. See Blast; pain in the scrotum.

Signs. See Blast; unilateral swelling of testis and epididymis.

Etiology and Pathology. Pressure from blast increases tension on the external inguinal ring preventing circulatory return.

Therapy. Cold packs.

Prognosis. Recovery.

BIBLIOGRAPHY. Swersie AK: Unilateral scrotal swelling following blast injury: a syndrome. Urology 55:292–294, 1946
Cass AS: Testicular trauma. J Urol 129:299–300, 1983

BLATIN'S

Synonym. Hydatid fremitis. Eponym used to indicate the sign yielded by a hydatis cyst under tension; the hydatid thrill or vibratory sensation is felt on the palm of the hand when this lies flat over the tumor and a finger is percussed. This sign may be elicited, however, with other types of cyst as well.

BIBLIOGRAPHY. MacLaurin C: The symptoms of liver hydatid. Aust Med Gaz 28:295–300, 1909
Barnett LE: Hydatid thrill: its rarity, physical explanation and diagnostic value. N Z Med J 20:277–285, 1921

BLATT'S

Synonyms. Craniooculoorbital dysrhaphia-meningocele; oculocranioorbital dysraphia-meningocele; orbitocranioocular dysraphia-meningocele.

Symptoms and Signs. Both sexes affected; present from birth. Anisometropia; meningocele or meningoencephalocele; cranial deformities; facial bone malformation; hypertelorism; microphthalmus; distichiasis; meibonian glands absent.

Etiology. Unknown, autosomal dominant inheritance.

BIBLIOGRAPHY. Blatt N: Cranio-orbito-ocular dysraphia and meningocele. Rev Otoneurophthalmol 33:185–232, 1961
Tessier P: Surgical treatment of genetically caused eyelid and orbitofacial deformities. Buech Augenarzt 50:82–121, 1968

BLEGVAD-HAXTHAUSEN

Synonyms. Anetoderma–osteogenesis imperfecta; osteogenesis imperfecta (see).

Symptoms and Signs. Both sexes affected. Skin appears thin, translucent, slackening, and shows well-defined round or oval areas of variable size (from milia to coin) of grayish color. Grosser anomalies of skin usually absent, but described in some cases. Eye: blue sclerae: zonal cataract. Partial or total deafness. Multiple bone fractures from minor traumas. Wounds heal slowly, with ample scars. Vascular fragility with easily forming hematomas. Reported associated defects include those of Ehler-Danlos syndrome.

Etiology. Generalized defect in collagen maturation; autosomal dominant heredity. Identical to Ekman's. The macular atrophy of the skin described represents one of the nonconstant signs of the osteogenesis imperfecta.

Pathology. *Dermis.* Thin, increase of argentophil and elastic fibers; immaturity and swelling of collagenous fiber. *Bones.* Osteogenesis imperfecta (see).

Diagnostic Procedures. *Biopsy of skin. X-ray.* Skeletal survey.

Therapy. Symptomatic.

Prognosis. Osteogenesis imperfecta (see).

BIBLIOGRAPHY. Blegvad O, Haxthausen H: Blaa sclerae og tendens til knoglebrud med pletformet hudatrofi og zonulaer catarat. Hospitalstidende 64:609–616, 1921

BLENCKE'S

Synonym. Calcaneus metaepiphyseal osteodystrophy.

Symptoms and Signs. Pain on the calcaneal region; increased by walking.

Etiology. See Epiphyseal ischemic necrosis.

BIBLIOGRAPHY. Toniolo G: Perchè non può esistere una osteodistrofia metafisaria del calcagno. Radiol Clin Basel 19:81–94, 1950

BLEPHARONASOFACIAL

Synonym. Pashayan-Putterman.

Symptoms and Signs. Both sexes affected; present from birth. *Facies.* Masklike; telecanthus; lateral displacement and stenosis of lacrimal puncta; nose bulky; broad bridge, midfacial hypoplasia; horizontal cheek furrows; trapezoidal upper lip. *Extremities.* Soft tissue syndactyly. *Joints.* Hyperextensibility. *Nervous system.* Poor coordination; torsion distonia; positive Babinski sign.

Etiology. Autosomal dominant inheritance.

BIBLIOGRAPHY. Pashayan H, Pruzansky S, Putterman A: A family with blepharo-naso-facial malformation. Am J Dis Child 125:389–393, 1973

Putterman AM, Pashayan H, Pruzansky S: Eye findings in the blepharo-naso-facial malformation syndrome. Am J Ophthalmol 76:825–831, 1973

BLESSIC-IWANOFF

Synonyms. Iwanoff's; retinal cystoid degeneration; retinoschisis.

Symptoms and Signs. Both sexes affected; onset after 50 years of age. Asymptomatic or sudden impairment of vision.

Etiology. Unknown.

Pathology. Retinal cyst located primarily in nuclear layers; later, all layers involved; cystic areas coalescence with adjacent areas; splitting of retina in two layers with eventual detachment.

Diagnostic Procedures. *Ophthalmoscopy.* In retinal periphery small translucent areas or branching channels.

Therapy. None specific.

Prognosis. Variable according to evolution. Usually favorable, but detachment of retina may follow.

BIBLIOGRAPHY. Hogn MJ, Zimmerman LE: Ophthalmic Pathology. Philadelphia, WB Saunders, 1962

BLIND LOOP

Synonyms. Afferent loop; gastrojejunal loop obstruction; stagnant loop.

Symptoms. Anorexia; nausea; diarrhea; postprandial fullness, and pain in upper abdomen, followed by vomiting bile, no food (only violent retching induces food vomiting). Fatty foods precipitate vomiting.

Signs. Pallor. Lichtheim's syndrome signs (see); abdominal distension; palpable mass.

Etiology. Obstruction of gastrojejunal loop following subtotal gastrectomy. In patients with Billroth II.

Pathology. Afferent loop of anastomosis may present partial volvulus, herniation, adhesion or simply be too short or too long, signs of inflammation, necrosis, perforation with leakage may be present.

Diagnostic Procedures. *X-ray. Blood.* Megaloblastic type of anemia. *Bone marrow. Schilling's test.*

Therapy. Surgery to remove obstruction. Broad spectrum antibiotic may correct the anemia. If surgery not feasible, administration of antibiotics for 2 weeks every month.

Prognosis. Chronic and recurrent condition until surgically corrected.

BIBLIOGRAPHY. Tabaqchali S, Hatzioannou J, Booth CC: Bile salt deconjugation and steatorrhea in patients with the stagnant-loop syndrome. Lancet II:12–16, 1968

Lewis B, Panveliwalla D, Tabaqchali S, Wootton IDP: Serumile-acids in the stagnant-loop syndrome. Lancet I:219–220, 1969

Baker WH, Hummel LE: Macrocytic anemia in association with intestinal structures and anastomoses. Bull Johns Hopkins Hosp 64:215–256, 1939

Meyer JH: Chronic morbidity after ulcer surgery. In Sleisenger MH, Fordtran JS (eds): Gastrointestinal disease: Pathophysiology: Diagnosis and Management, 3rd ed, pp 757–779. Philadelphia, WB Saunders, 1983

BLINDNESS, TRANSIENT POSTRAUMATIC

Synonym. Transient postictal hemianopsia.

Symptoms. Usually, bilateral total or partial blindness of few minutes or many hour duration; occasionally, only whitish, foggy aspect of visual field; headache; drowsiness; restlessness; agitation.

Signs. Normal pupillary reaction to light or fixed pupils. Fundus oculi normal.

Etiology. Head trauma, especially of parietooccipital regions causing vasospasm, edema.

Diagnostic Procedures. *Electroencephalography.* In early period, slowing of occipital pattern.

Therapy. None; diuretics.

Prognosis. Good. Complete recovery usually within 24 hours. Recurrences possible.

BIBLIOGRAPHY. Walsh FB: Clinical Neurophthalmology, 2nd ed, Baltimore, Williams & Wilkins, 1957

Ropper AH, Kennedy SK, Zervas NT (eds): Neurological and Neurosurgical Intensive Care. Baltimore, University Park Press, 1983

BLIND POUCH

Symptoms. Usually appear years after surgery with side-to-side intestinal anastomosis. Weakness; failure to gain weight; intermittent diarrhea; cramping abdominal pain. Symptoms in combination or alone. Complication or hemorrhage and perforation possible.

Signs. Pallor; abdominal scar. Tenderness on abdominal palpation. Sometimes soft tissue mass is palpable.

Etiology. Dilated blind ends of small intestine after side-to-side intestinal anastomosis; not to be confused with "blind loop syndrome," which has different clinical, laboratory, and anatomic abnormalities.

Pathology. Dilation of afferent and efferent blind pouches; hypertrophy; edema; ulceration of mucosa.

Diagnostic Procedures. *Blood.* Macrocytic or microcytic anemia (in blind loop usually macrocytic anemia). *X-rays.* Demonstration of blind ileal pouch.

Therapy. Surgical correction. End-to-end anastomosis of normal intestine.

Prognosis. Excellent after surgical correction.

BIBLIOGRAPHY. Brief DK, Botsford TW: Primary bleeding from the small intestine in adults: the surgical management. JAMA 184:18–22, 1963
Botsford TW, Gazzaniga AB: Blind pouch syndrome: a complication of side to side intestinal anastomosis. Am J Surg 113:486–490, 1967

BLOCH-SULZBERGER

Synonyms. Block-Siemens; incontinentia pigmenti, cutaneous lineal melanoblastosis. See also Asboe-Hansen.

Symptoms and Signs. Appear at birth or within one or two years; females affected 10 times more frequently than males. Recurrent inflammatory lesions (papules, vesicles, bullae) initially localized, then spreading in configurate bizarre patterns. Lesions subside after weeks or months and either pass through papillary or warty stages or directly develop into pigmentary macules. Distribution of lesions highly irregular, not corresponding to blood vessels and nerve dermatomes. Resulting macules chocolate, grayish in color, persisting or fading or disappearing or leaving atrophic areas. Localized atrophic alopecia of scalp; dystrophic nails; keratotic areas. Associated abnormalities present in two-thirds of patients: dental anomalies; strabismus; cataracts; optic atrophy; retinal abnor-malities; nervous system disorders; spastic paralysis; epilepsy; microcephaly; mental retardation; deafness; osseous changes with retarded growth; and abnormal development; heart malformation.

Etiology. Unknown; congenital familial condition; anomalies of ectomesodermal development; viruses, Herpes simplex? Pedigree patterns in a family suggest X-linked dominance of autosome X translocation with lethality in the male.

Pathology. Deposit of melanin inside and outside melanophores in pigmented area. Other abnormalities described in symptoms.

Diagnostic Procedures. Vesicle fluid contains eosinophils (95%). *Blood.* Eosinophilia (30% to 50%). *X-rays.* Tooth abnormalities.

Therapy. Corticosteroid perhaps beneficial on vesicular stage.

Prognosis. According to severity of form and organ involvement. Cutaneous involvement without other abnormalities, normal life.

BIBLIOGRAPHY. Garrod AE: Peculiar pigmentation of the skin in an infant. Trans Clin Soc London 39:216, 1906
Bardach M: Systematisierte Naevusbildunger dei einem cineügen Zwillingspaar. Ein Beitrag zur Naevusaetiologie. Z Kinderheilkd 39:542, 1925
Bloch B: Eigentümliche bisher nicht beschriebene Pigmentaffektion (Incontinentia pigmenti). Schweiz Med Wochensch 56:404–405, 1926
Sulzberger MB: Ueber eine bisher nicht beschriebene congenitale Pigmentanomalie (Incontinentia pigmenti). Arch Dermatol Syph 154:19–32, 1928
Hodgson SV, Neville B, Jones RWA, et al: Two cases of X autosome translocation in females with incontinentia pigmenti. Hum Genet 71:231–234, 1985

BLOODGOOD'S

Synonyms. Blue dome; cystic breast; Cheatle's; Cooper's I; fibrocystic; chronic cystic mastitis; mastopathia chronica cystica; Reclus' I; Schimmelbusch's syndromes; Tillaux-Phocas.

Symptoms. Occurs in women; onset between 45 and 55 years of age. Usually, asymptomatic or pain in the breast, especially premenstrually; receding after onset.

Signs. Bilateral masses in the breasts; round, smooth, tense, mobile, not adherent to skin.

Etiology. Unknown; possible hormonal imbalance.

Pathology. Mammary ducts dilatation; blue brownish cysts filled by turbid fluid; papillary formation inside the cysts.

Diagnostic Procedures. *Mammography. Xerography. Thermography. Biopsy. Hormonal study. Echography.*

Therapy. Vitamin A. Surgery. Danazol for severe pain. Stop coffee, tea, and chocolate (reported improvement). Bromocryptine.

Prognosis. Malignancy transformation (1–6%).

BIBLIOGRAPHY. Cooper A: Illustrations of the Diseases of the Breast. London, Longmans, 1829
Reclus P: La maladie kystique des mamelles. Bull Soc Anat Paris 8:428–433, 1883
Bloodgood JC: The pathology of chronic cystic mastitis of the female breast, with special consideration of the blue-dome cyst. Arch Surg 3:442–445, 1921
Dupont WD, Page DL: Risk factors for breast cancer in women with proliferative breast disease. N Engl J Med 312:146–151, 1985
Hutter RUP: Goodbye to 'fibrocystic disease.' New Engl J Med 312:179–181, 1985
Vorherr H: Fibrocystic breast disease: pathophysiology, pathomorphology, clinical picture and management. Am J Obstet Gynecol 154:161–179, 1986

BLOOM'S

Synonyms. Bloom-Torre-Mackacek; Levi's type dwarfism; telangiectasis facial dwarfism.

Symptoms and Signs. Males preponderant. Usually, low birth weight following full-term gestation; facial rash, discoid lupus erythematouslike hypersensitivity to sun, skin manifestations in other parts of body, erythematous type, areas of increased and decreased pigmentation, hypersensitivity to light; failure to grow. Microcephaly variable; dolichocephaly, with zygomatic hypoplasia, with or without small nose. Occasionally associated, various abnormalities of eyes, ears, extremities, digits.

Etiology. Autosomal recessive inheritance.

Pathology. *Skin lesions.* Moderate parakeratosis; absence of granular layer; thin rete of Malpighi; moderate intercellular edema; corium with capillary and perivascular telengiectasis; lymphocytic infiltrates; hyalinized material in superficial corium; eosinophilic stain.

Diagnostic Procedures. *Blood.* Occasionally, immunoglobulin deficiency (IgA, IgM). *Urine.* Normal porphyrin excretion. *X-ray.* Retarded bone growth. *Chromosome study.* Tendency to chromosomal breakage in vitro.

Prognosis. Except for failure to grow, early development appears normal. Possibilities of malignancies (leukemia, gastrointestinal).

BIBLIOGRAPHY. Bloom D: Congenital telangiectatic erythema resembling lupus erythematosus in dwarfs. Am J Dis Child 88:754–758, 1954
German J, Bloom D, Parsage E: Bloom's syndrome: XI progress report for 1983. Clin Genet 25:166–174, 1984
Gretzula JC, Hevia O, Weber PJ: Bloom's syndrome. J Am Acad Dermatol 17:479–488, 1987

BLOUNT-BARBER

Synonyms. Tibia Blount's; bowlegs; Erlacher-Blount; osteochondrosis deformans tibiae; tibia vara. See also Fairbank's and Conradi's.

Symptoms. *Infantile type.* Appears at 1 or 2 years of age; usually in overweight children. Gradual increasing of leg bowing without apparent cause. Usually bilateral; occasionally unilateral. (Limp in unilateral; waddle in bilateral.) Pain from strain in the knee or foot observed sometimes. *Adolescent type.* Same symptoms appear at 6 to 12 years of age; usually unilaterally. Higher frequency in Blacks.

Signs. Shortening (1–2 cm) of the leg(s) affected. Abrupt angulation with the apex laterally below the knee joint; bulbous enlargement of medial condyle; internal rotation of tibia; abnormal mobility of knee. All other general physical findings are normal.

Etiology. Unknown. Rickets, tuberculosis, syphilis excluded. Faulty growth of epiphyseal cartilage and delayed ossification of the medial or lateral (?) portion of proximal tibial epiphysis. Multifactorial inheritance proposed.

Pathology. In the beaklike prominence, under the epiphysis are islands of hyaline cartilage, with cells in irregular disposition instead of columnar. In adolescent type, arrest of epiphyseal growth rather than dysplasia.

Diagnostic Procedures. *X-ray.* Irregularity of contour of the proximal tibial epiphyseal line. Areas of rarefaction observed in enlarged metaphysis.

Therapy. In infantile type, progressive correction with conservative measures; if severe deformity, osteotomy required. In adolescent type, osteotomy usually required.

Prognosis. Good with adequate correction.

BIBLIOGRAPHY. Blount WP: Tibia vara, osteochondrosis deformans tibiae. Am J Bone Joint Surg 19:1–29, 1937
Enklaar JE: Osteochondrosis deformans (Blount) bij kinderen. Monatschr Kindergeneesk 23:235–238, 1955

Duncan PA, Shapiro LR, Brust MB, et al: Heterogeneity of the Blount's disease. Proc Greenwood Genet Center 2:106–107, 1983

BLUE COLOR BLINDNESS

Synonyms. Tritanopsia; color blindness tritanopsia.

Symptoms and Signs. Retain red or green, lack blue and yellow color vision.

Etiology. Autosomal dominant inheritance.

BIBLIOGRAPHY. Went LN, Pronk N: The genetics of tritan disturbances. Human Genet 69:255–262, 1985

BLUE VELVET

Symptoms. Follow repeated intravenous injections of strong analgesics with talcum filler. Euphoria, excitement, or depression.

Signs. Apical thrust; tachycardia; systolic murmur; pulmonary rales; hepatomegaly; ankle edema.

Etiology. Intravenous injection of paregoric-triphenamine hydrochloride plus talcum filler.

Pathology. Hypertrophy of muscle cells of heart ventricles; pulmonary subedema; centrilobular hepatic necrosis with hemosiderin deposits and talc crystal in lungs and other tissues.

Diagnostic Procedures. *Blood.* Leukocytosis; hypoalbuminemia.

Therapy. Symptomatic.

Prognosis. Poor. Sudden death may follow the injection.

BIBLIOGRAPHY. Gordon BL, Barclay WR, Rogers HC (eds): Current Medical Information and Terminology, 4th ed. Chicago, American Medical Association, 1971

BOBBLE-HEAD DOLL

Symptoms. Appears in childhood. Continuous bobbing of head (3 sec periods); rhythmical extension and flexion of head and arms. The bobbing may be stopped voluntarily, and ceases during sleep and intentional movements. Generalized fine tremor; hypersensitivity to cutaneous stimuli. Mental retardation; impaired vision.

Signs. Moderate hydrocephalus; obesity.

Etiology. Cyst in region of third ventricle.

Pathology. Large cyst in region of third ventricle with thin wall of fibrous tissue; astroglia of blood vessels; no epithelial lining.

Diagnostic Procedures. *Pneumoencephalography. Echoencephalography. CT brain scan. Spinal tap. Aspiration of fluid from cyst.*

Therapy. Aspiration of fluid in the cyst and possible removal. Ventriculo-peritoneal shunt.

Prognosis. After surgery, bobbing stops. Hydrocephalus, diabetes insipidus, and other diencephalic disturbances may persist or stop.

BIBLIOGRAPHY. Benton JW, Nellhaus G, Huttenlocher PR, et al: The bobble-head doll syndrome: report of a unique truncal tremor associated with third ventricular cyst and hydrocephalus in children. Neurology 16:725–729, 1966
Adams RD, Victor M: Principles of Neurology, 3rd ed, pp 494–495. New York, McGraw-Hill, 1985

BODY OF LUYS

Synonyms. Ballism; corpus Luysii; hemiballism subthalamic nucleus.

Symptoms and Signs. Appears in early or adult life. Violent involuntary movements of one or both body sides; movements greater in the proximal portions; more pronounced on arm than leg; intensity so strong as to bruise tissue or break bones. Movements subside during sleep.

Etiology. Lesion of contralateral body of Luys (hemorrhage; softening; tumor; granulomas; trauma; hereditary degenerative disorders). In cases in which the body of Luys has been found intact, lesions of afferent and efferent fibers are suspected to be involved.

Therapy. Nursing; sedatives; chlorpromazine. Neurosurgery; section of cerebral peduncle, incision of precental gyrus, section of anterior or posterolateral columns of spinal cord.

Prognosis. If progressive, patient dies from exhaustive cardiac insufficiency in a few weeks. If patient survives acute stage, disease may go into remission or symptoms disappear altogether.

BIBLIOGRAPHY. Fisher O: Zur Frage der anatomischen Grundlage der Athetose double und der posthemiplegischen Bewegungsstörung überhaupt. Z Ges Neurol Psychiar 7:463, 1911
Denny-Brown D: The Basal Ganglia. London, Oxford University Press, 1962
Adams RD, Victor M: Principles of Neurology, 3rd ed, p 64. New York, McGraw-Hill, 1985

BOERHAAVE'S

Synonym. Esophagus laceration spontaneous. See Mallory-Weiss syndrome.

Symptoms. Prevalent in males (5:1), more common in 5th and 6th decades. While straining violently to vomit and retching, excrutiating pain in the chest, dyspnea, small amount of blood appears in the vomitus, significant hematemesis rare, shock.

Signs. Subcutaneous emphysema, tachycardia.

Etiology. Laceration of esophagus.

Pathology. Laceration linear and longitudinal (usually posterior) of lower part of esophagus, hydrothorax, and pneumothorax.

Diagnostic Procedures. *X-rays of chest. Blood and electrolyte work-up.*

Therapy. Emergency blood replacement. Treatment of shock. Surgical repair of rupture. Antibiotics.

Prognosis. If untreated, death within 24 hours (50% of cases) or 48 hours (90%), or in a few days (100%). Treated, the mortality is 35%.

BIBLIOGRAPHY. Boerhaave H: Atrocis, nec descripti prius, morbi historia. Secundum medicae artis leges conscripta. Lugduni Batavorum, Boutesteniana, 1724
Bruno MS, Grier WR, Ober WB: Spontaneous laceration and rupture of esophagus and stomach; Mallory-Weiss syndrome, Boerhaave syndrome, and their variants. Arch Int Med 112:574–583, 1963
Walker WS, Cameron EW, Walbaum PR: Diagnosis and management of spontaneous transmural rupture of esophagus (Boerhaave's syndrome). Br J Surg 72:204–207, 1985

BORJESON-FORSSMAN-LEHMANN

Synonyms. Mental deficiency–epilepsy–endocrine disorders. See Coffin-Lowry, Bardet-Biedl, Prader-Willi.

Symptoms. Appears in males in complete form, onset in childhood. Epilepsy; mental retardation.

Signs. Obesity; genital infantilism; myxedema.

Etiology. Autosomal recessive inheritance. X-linked inheritance.

BIBLIOGRAPHY. Borjeson M, Forssman H, Lehmann O: Zusammentreffen von'Idiotie, Epilepsie, Zwergewuchs, Keimdruesen Unterfunktion, myxoedem und morphologischen Besonderheiten als rezessiv-erbliches Syndrom. II. Inter Kong Psych Entwichg Kind Wien, 1961
Robinson LK, Jones KL, Culler F, et al: The Borjeson-Forssmann-Lehmann syndrome. Am J Genet 15:457–468, 1983
Flannery DB, Piussan C, Wright LE: Dermatoglyphics in Borjeson-Forssmann-Lehmann syndrome. Am J Med Genet 21 401–404, 1985

BOGORAD'S

Synonyms. Crocodile tears; gustatory lacrimation.

Symptoms. Unilateral lacrimation on chewing on introduction of strongly flavored food into the mouth.

Signs. Mechanical stimulation and chewing without food do not produce lacrimation.

Etiology and Pathology. Sequela of facial paralysis, faulty regeneration of facial nerve fibers where the salivary fibers are directed along the path of lacrimal nerve.

BIBLIOGRAPHY. Bogorad FA: Symptom of crocodile tears. Vrach Delo 11:1328–1330, 1928
Chorobski J: The syndrome of crocodile tears. Arch Neurol Psychiatry 65:299–318, 1951
Gorlin RJ, Pindborg JJ, Cohen MM: Syndromes of the Head and Neck, 2nd ed. New York, McGraw-Hill, 1976
Adams RD, Victor M: Principles of Neurology, 3rd ed, p. 406. New York, McGraw-Hill, 1985

BONHOEFFER'S

Synonyms. Bonhoeffer's chorea; Claude's; midbrain tremor; nucleus ruber inferior; rubral tremor; rubrospinal cerebellar peduncle; Souquez-Bertrand.

Symptoms and Signs. Hemianesthesia and, occasionally hemiataxia with paralysis of contralateral eye muscles innervated by oculomotor and trochlear nerves.

Etiology and Pathology. Occlusion (thrombosis, neoplasia) of terminal branches of paramedian artery of inferior part of red nucleus.

Diagnostic Procedures. *Angiography. CT brain scan.*

Therapy. Anticoagulant; surgery if indicated.

Prognosis. Poor.

BIBLIOGRAPHY. Bonhoeffer K: Ein Beitrag zur Lokalisation der choreatsichen Bewegungen. Mschr Psychiatr Neurol 1:6–41, 1987
Claude H: Syndrome péducolaire de la région du noyau rouge. Rev Neurol 23:311–313, 1912
Hiller F: Vascular syndromes of basilar and veretebral arteries and their branches. J Nerv Ment Dis 116:988–1016, 1952

Denny-Brown D: The Basal Ganglia and Their Relation to Disorders of Movement. London, Oxford University Press, 1962

Vick NA: Grinker's Neurology, 7th ed. Springfield, Ill, CC Thomas, 1976

BONNET-DECHAUME-BLANC

Synonyms. Neuroretinal angiomatosis; cerebroretinal arteriovenous aneurysm. See Wyburn-Mason.

Symptoms. Hemiplegia appearing in early childhood; mental deterioration.

Signs. Babinski positive; abdominal reflexes absent. Auscultation of skull: systolic murmur synchronous with heart beat. Ophthalmologic examination: unilateral exophthalmia not pulsating, with dilatation of conjunctival vessels; strabimus; nystagmus; absent reflex to light and accommodation. Fundus oculi examination shows diffuse aneurysm, which makes it impossible to differentiate arteries from veins. *Heart.* Left hypertrophy.

Etiology and Pathology. Congenital nonmalignant aneurysms of retina, thalamus, and mesencephalus.

Diagnostic Procedures. *X-rays of cervical column, skull. Angiography: carotid or vertebral. Phlebography. Orbit. CT brain scan.* See Signs.

Prognosis. According to entity of lesions; blindness of one eye; mental deterioration.

BIBLIOGRAPHY. Bonnet P, Dechaume J, Blanc E: L'anéurysme cirsoïde de la rétine (anéurysme racemeux). Ses relations avec l'aneurysme cirsoïde de la face et avec l'aneurysme cirsoïde du cerveau. J Med Lyon 18:163–178, 1937

Fischgold H, Bregeat P, Le Besnerais Y, et al: Iconographie de l'angiomatose neuroretinene (syndrome de Bonnet, Dechaume et Blanc). Presse Med 60:1790–1792, 1952

Chomette G, Aurial M: Classification des angiodysplasies et tumeurs vasculaires. Rev Stom Clin Maxillofac 87:1–5, 1986

BONNET'S (C.)

Synonym. Charles Bonnet.

Symptoms. Appear in aged blind or partially blind persons not exhibiting other mental disorders. Vivid, polychromic visual hallucinations, which the patient generally recognizes as such, and discusses as a curiosity, without emotional involvement.

Etiology. See Cerebral, chronic. If lesion can be identified, it usually is situated in occipital lobe or posterior part of temporal lobe.

BIBLIOGRAPHY. Bonnet C: Essai Analytique sur les Facultés de l'Ame, vol 2, pp 176–178. Copenhagen, 1769

de Morsier G: Le syndrome de Charles Bonnet: Hallucinations visuelles des Veillards, sans déficience mentale. Ann Med Psychol (Paris) 2:678–702, 1967

Adams RD, Victor M: Principles of Neurology, 3rd ed, p 343. New York, McGraw-Hill, 1985

BONNET'S (P.)

Synonyms. Trigeminosympathetic; trigemino sympaneuralgia. See Orbital apex.

Symptoms and Signs. Those of Fothergill's (see), associated with those of Bernard's (see).

BIBLIOGRAPHY. Bonnet P: Les syndromes trigéminosympathiques. Arch Ophthalmol 16:361–379, 1956

Adams RD, Victor M: Principles of Neurology, 3rd ed, p 503. New York, McGraw-Hill, 1985

BONNIER'S

Synonym. Deiters' nucleus.

Symptoms. Apprehension; somnolence; weakness of limbs; trigeminal neuralgia; oculomotor manifestations. Vertigo and deafness may be associated.

Etiology. Neoplastic; vascular lesion of lateral nucleus of vestibular nerve (Deiters) or vestibular tract.

Pathology. See Etiology.

Diagnostic Procedures. *Audiography. Electroencephalography. Angiography. CT brain scan.*

Therapy. Surgery if feasible.

Prognosis. Possible improvement.

BIBLIOGRAPHY. Bonnier P: Syndrome du noyau de Deiters. C R Soc Biol Paris 4:1525–1528, 1902

BÖÖK'S

Synonyms. Premature hereditary canities; hereditary premature graying hair. PHC.

Symptoms and Signs. Premature canities; palmoplantar hyperhidrosis; hypodontia of premolars with bicuspid partially or completely lacking.

Etiology. Unknown; autosomal dominant inheritance.

BIBLIOGRAPHY. Böök JA: Clinical and genetical studies of hypodontia; premolar aplasia, hyperhidrosis, and canities prematuria; new hereditary syndrome in man. Am J Hum Genet 2:240–263, 1950

BORDERLINE

Symptoms. Chief complaint: attention provoking histrionic episodes. No delusion or paranoid symptoms. Five subgroups may be delineated: (1) Expresses anger as main emotion; has no capacity for affection; depressive loneliness. (2) Attempts to relate but reacts with anger (psychotic borderline). (3) Attempts and persists in seeking relation, but reacts with "repulsion." (4) Reacts with anger to most people, but seeks a mother figure and, failing, becomes depressed (neurotic borderline). (5) Reacts to anger and loneliness; takes a passive attitude awaiting signs as to how to react (as in type of borderline syndrome).

Etiology. Disturbance of ego function.

Therapy. Persistent psychotherapeutic attempts.

Prognosis. Only some patients may respond to treatment.

BIBLIOGRAPHY. Grinker RR, Werble B, Drye C: The Borderline Syndrome: A Behavioral Study of Ego Functions. New York, Basic Books, 1968
Vick NA: Grinker's Neurology, 7th ed. Springfield, Ill, CC Thomas, 1976

BORNHOLM

Synonyms. Dabney's grip; devil's grip; myalgia endemic; myalgia epidemic; pleurodynia epidemic, Sylvest's.

Symptoms. Epidemic occurrence in summer and early autumn; person-to-person contact; incubation 3 to 5 days. Affects both sexes in all age groups; prevalent in children and young adults. Recurrent episodes of sudden excruciating pain in abdominal or thoracic regions, increased by movement and respiration. Headache, malaise, sore throat, vomiting (especially in early phase of disease) may be present. In infants, convulsions during attacks.

Signs. During attacks, shallow tachypulse and fever. During remissions of attacks, mild tenderness in affected areas, with minor muscle swelling, hyperestesia, and altered reflexes. Pleural rubs may be present.

Etiology. Coxsackie viruses B3 and B5. Other viruses that can be associated with epidemic disease are Coxsackie virus B1 and B2 and echoviruses 1 and 6.

Pathology. No specific changes.

Diagnostic Procedures. *Throat swabs and stool swabs.* Coxsackie B virus. *X-ray of chest.* Negative. *Blood.* Normal findings; increase of neutralizing antibodies against Coxsackie B type.

Treatment. Nonspecific. Analgesic and antipyretics. Bed rest.

Prognosis. Attacks persist for a few days. Patient afraid and usually remains in bed for several days. After apparent recovery, relapses may occur for about 1 month. Complications include orchitis (common, lasting 3 to 7 days); fibrinous pleurisy (common); aseptic meningitis (rare); pericarditis (in adults); myocarditis (in newborn). Long-lasting immunity.

BIBLIOGRAPHY. Dabney WC: Account of an epidemic resembling dengue which occurred in and around Charlottesville and the University of Virginia in June 1888. Am J Med Sci 96:488–495, 1888
Sylvest E: En Bornholmsk epidemi–Myositis epidemica. Ugeskr Laeger 92:798–801, 1930
Behrman R, Vaughan V (eds): Nelson Textbook of Pediatrics. Philadelphia, WB Saunders, 1983

BOUILLAUD'S

Synonyms. Rheumatic fever, Sokolskii-Bouillaud. First report of the triad: endocarditis, pericarditis, and acute inflammation of joints.

BIBLIOGRAPHY. Bouillaud JB: Traité Clinique des Maladies due Coeur, précédé de recherches nouvelles sur l'anatomie et la physiologie de cet organe, Vol 2, pp 170–192. 1835
Sokolskii GI: O reumatizme myshechnai tkani serdtsa (rheumatismus cordis). Uchen Zap Imp Mosk Univ 12:568, 1838

BOURNEVILLE'S

Synonyms. Adenoma sebaceum (misnomer); Bourneville-Brissaud; Bourneville-Pringle; epiloia; Bourneville's phakomatosis; tuberous sclerosis. See Pringle-Bourneville.

Symptoms and Signs. Clinically characterized triad: (1) mental and physical retardation; (2) epileptic seizures; (3) sebaceous adenomas of skin and warts, polyps, nevi, usually butterfly distribution on the nose bridge and cheeks.

Retinal and other tumors in different organs coexist. Involuntary movements; local paresis.

Etiology. Congenital hereditary dominant malformations of neuroectodermal system. About 50% of cases appears to be new mutations.

Pathology. *Skin.* Hyperplastic connective or muscular tissue; neurofibromatatype (sebaceous adenoma a misnomer). *Retina.* Small, round growths (phakomas). *Brain.* Many nodules on surfax of cortex and ventricular surfaces (pearly white); microgyri or macrogyria. Disturbed cytoarchitecture of brain and localized neoplastic formation (various types of gliomas). Pathologic changes may be found in heart, lung, and kidney as well.

Diagnostic Procedures. *X-ray.* Multiple intracranial calcification; osteoporosis of skull and other bones. *CT brain scan.* Characteristic calcifications. *Electroencephalography.* Abnormal in 87% of cases; grossly disorganized hypsarrhythmic pattern.

Therapy. Treatment of seizures; assessment of intellectual function; control of hyperactivity in children can be achieved with methylphenidate or dextroamphetamine. Surgical excision of tumors only if they are symptomatic. Genetic counseling.

Prognosis. Extremely variable. Patients with mild involvement may have a good prognosis. Death may be due to status epilepticus, brain tumor, renal failure; or rhabdomyoma of the heart.

BIBLIOGRAPHY. Bourneville DM, Brissaud E: Encéphalite ou sclérose tubéreuse des circonvolutions cérébrales. Arch Neurol (Paris) 1:397–412, 1880–1881
Gomez MR: Tuberous Sclerosis. New York, Raven Press, 1979
Sugita K, Itoh K, Tekeuchi Y, et al: Tuberous sclerosis: report of two cases studied by computer assisted cranial tomography within one week after birth. Brain Dev 7:438–443, 1985

BOUVERET'S

Synonyms. Idiopathic auricular paroxysmal tachycardia; paroxysmal atrial tachycardia.

Symptoms. Onset in any age; more frequent in 2nd to 4th decades. In childhood, affects boys almost exclusively. Onset sudden, without warning, occasionally precipitated by emotion or rapid change in position. Sudden thump in the chest; apparent stopping of the heart; precordial discomfort, then palpitation. Occasionally, (1) pain sensation on throat, pulsation in the neck; (2) anxiety, generalized weakness, cold, or sweating may accompany attack; (3) gastrointestinal symptoms, epigastric discomfort, abdominal distention, burping, nausea, vomiting; (4) polyuria during or at termination of attack.

Signs. Tachycardia. Only with prolonged attack or in presence of underlying disease, signs of congestive failure may appear. Pulse rapid and small. Blood pressure may drop (especially systolic with resultant decrease of pulse pressure).

Etiology. Obscure; occasionally associated with biliary tract diseases; in patient with Wolf-Parkinson-White syndrome; a congenital type is known.

Pathology. None; except of associated diseases.

Diagnostic Procedures. *Electrocardiography.* Rapid regular ventricular complex T waves that are frequently difficult to identify and slightly modified by fusion with P waves.

Therapy. Reassurance; Valsalva's maneuver; Müller's maneuver; inducing vomiting; carotid sinus stimulation (unilateral). Sedatives; intravenous digitalis, phenylephrine ajmalinum; levarterenol. Prevention: avoid precipitating causes, if known: mild sedatives, quinidine.

Prognosis. Attacks usually terminate spontaneously, or with maneuvers or medication. Occasionally, prolonged attacks may induce cardiac failure.

BIBLIOGRAPHY. Bouveret L: De la tachycardie essentielle paroxystique. Rev Mid 9:753–793; 837–855, 1889
Hurst JW: The Heart, 6th ed, pp 413–420. New York, McGraw-Hill, 1986

BOWEN'S (D.A.L.)

Synonym. Tracheobronchopathia osteochondroplastica.

Symptoms and Signs. Predominantly in men over 50 years of age. Dyspnea; hoarseness; cough; expectoration; wheezing; hemoptysis.

Etiology. Unknown. In several cases established relation with amyloidosis.

Pathology. In majority of cases, diagnosis at autopsy. Subcutaneous nodules, usually confined to portion of the trachea and bronchial wall containing cartilage which produce sessile and polypoid growth; seldom, ulcerating.

Diagnostic Procedures. *Bronchoscopy.* Beaded appearance. *Pulmonary function tests.* Variable degree of alterations. *X-rays.* Variable findings. Bronchial obstruction; evidence of bone formations on lateral and anterior walls of trachea.

Therapy. Symptomatic.

Prognosis. Poor.

BIBLIOGRAPHY. Bowen DAL: Thacheopathia osteoplastica. J Clin Pathol 12:435–439, 1959

Whitehouse G: Tracheopathia osteoplastica: case report. Br J Radiol 41:701–703, 1968
Fraser RG, Paré JAP: Diagnosis of Diseases of the Chest, p 1323. Philadelphia, WB Saunders, 1977

BOWEN'S (J.F.)

Synonyms. Intradermal carcinoma epidermoid; precancerous dermatosis.

Symptoms. Severe local pruritis (not constant).

Signs. Appear anywhere on skin or mucosal surfaces. Formation of a limited, reddish, scaly area, which progressively enlarges. The whitish scales remove with difficulty and leave red, granular surface without bleeding. Lesions are slightly raised. Crusting and hyperkeratosis follow and after years, ulceration. Other lesions may form and frequently become confluent.

Etiology. Various theories: considered associated to exposure to trivalent arsenic compounds or to light, or as manifestation of systemic carcinomatosis.

Pathology. Atypical squamous cell proliferation through the entire epidermis. Acanthosis of variable degree. Cells have large hyperchromatic nuclei; frequently, mitosis. Disorganized epidermal structure. Various degrees of inflammatory changes.

Diagnostic Procedures. *Biopsy.*

Therapy. Destruction by freezing, cauterization, or diathermy. Surgical excision preferred.

Prognosis. Recurrences not infrequent. It represents a precancerous lesion; 42.6% develop premalignant or malignant lesion of skin within 6 to 7 years; 25% show primary systemic cancer within 5 years.

BIBLIOGRAPHY. Bowen JF: Precancerous dermatoses: a study of 2 cases of chronic atypical epithelial proliferation. J Cutan Dis 30:241–255, 1912
Rook A, Wilkinson DS, Ebling FJG, et al: Textbook of Dermatology, 4th ed, pp 2448–2249. Oxford, Blackwell Scientific Publications, 1986

BOWEN'S (P.)

Synonym. Pulmonary faciocamptodactyly ankyloses. See Fraser's. Maybe not to be considered a syndrome. Probably the one family described had cerebrohepatorenal syndrome

Symptoms and Signs. Appear in both sexes during intrauterine life. Small birth weight and reduced length. Respiratory insufficiency. *Facies.* Ear malformation; hypertelorism; depressed nose tip; micrognathia. *Extremi-*

ties. Camptodactyly of fingers; talipes equinovarus; ankylosis of knees, fixed in extension, and of hips in semiflexion.

Etiology. Autosomal recessive inheritance.

Pathology. See signs; plus pulmonary hypoplasia; cardiac defects; in males, cryptorchidism; in females, clitoral hypertrophy. Occasionally, agenesis of corpus callosum, arhinencephalia, cerebellar hypoplasia.

Prognosis. Death in perinatal period.

BIBLIOGRAPHY. Bowen P, Lee C, Zeliweger N, et al: A familial syndrome of multiple congenital defects. Johns Hopkins Hosp Bull 114:402–414, 1964

BOYD-STEARNS

Obsolete eponym to indicate a Fanconi like syndrome: dwarfism; rickets; hypophosphatemia; vitamin D resistant; glycosuria; acidosis and hypochloremia. See Prader's.

BIBLIOGRAPHY. Boyd JD, Stearns G: Late rickets resembling the Fanconi syndrome. Am J Dis Child 61:1012–1022, 1941
McKusick VA: Heritable Disorders of Connective Tissue, 4th ed, p 749. St. Louis, CV Mosby, 1972

BRACHYDACTYLY TYPE B

Synonym. Symbrachydactyly.

Symptoms and Signs. Short middle phalanges. Absence or rudimentary distal phalanges of fingers and toes. Thumb and hallux often involved. Symphalangism and mild syndactyly may be present.

Etiology. Autosomal dominant inheritance.

Prognosis. The most disabling of brachydactylies.

BIBLIOGRAPHY. McKender D: Deficiency of fingers transmitted through six generations. Br Med J 1:845–846, 1857
McArthur JW, McCullough E: Atypical dystrophy as inherited defect of hands and feet. Hum Biol 4:179–207, 1932

BRACHYDACTYLY TYPE C

Symptoms and Signs. Frequent in Mormon families. Various and variable anomalies of digits: brachymetapody, hyperphalangy, symphalangy, brachydactyly of middle phalanx of index and middle finger; triangulation of fifth middle phalanx.

Etiology. Autosomal dominant inheritance (?).

BIBLIOGRAPHY. Pol D: Brachydactylie "Klinodaktylie" hyperphalangie und ihre Grundlagen. Vichow Arch Pat Anat 229:388–530, 1921

Baraitser M, Burn J: Recessively inherited brachydactyly type C. J Med Genet 20:128–129, 1983

BRACHYDACTYLY TYPE E

Synonym. Dwarfism-brachydactyly, type E. See pseudopseudohypoparathyroidism, Biemond's I, and Gorlin-Sedano.

Symptoms and Signs. Prevalent in females; present from birth. Dwarfism; short limbs, metacarpals, metatarsals, and some phalanges; cone epiphyses. Considered by same authors are distinguishing features. Cases have been described with associated multiple impacted teeth (cryptodontic metacarpalia–Gorlin-Sedano).

Etiology. Autosomal dominant inheritance.

Prognosis. Benign condition.

BIBLIOGRAPHY. Bell J: On brachydactyly and symphalangism. In Treasury of Human Inheritance, vol 5, pp 1–31. London, Cambridge University Press, 1951

Riccardi WM, Holmes LB: Brachydactyly, type E. J Pediatr 84:251–254, 1974

Bale AE, Ludwig IH, Heffron LA, et al: Linkage between the genes for Wolfram syndrome and brachydactyly E. Am J Med Genet 20:733–734, 1985

BRADBURY-EGGLESTON

Synonyms. Idiopathic orthostatic hypotension, IOH. See Orthostatic hypotension and Shy-Dragger.

Symptoms and Signs. In middle age. Prevalent in male. Gradual onset postural hypotension with fixed heart rate; heat intolerance; anhidrosis; nocturnal polyuria; deterioration of abdominal, urinary, and anal sphincter functions; impotency.

Etiology. Unknown. Chronic autonomic failure.

Pathology. Degeneration of efferent sympathetic pathway.

Diagnostic Procedures. *Blood.* Low level of epinephrine, that is not modified by change in position or exercise. Low level of plasma dopamine hydrolase. *Metabolic studies.* Absence of vasoconstriction to intraarterial administration of tyramine; exaggerated response to norepinephrine. *Urine.* Decreased excretion of metabolites of norepinephrine. *Histochemical studies.* In perivascular nerve fibers absence of catecholamine-specific flourescence.

Therapy. *Mechanical measures.* Volume expanders; pharmacological agents (sympathomimetics, vasoconstrictors, beta receptor blockers, alpha-2 receptor agonists; prostaglandin synthesis inhibitors, antiserotonergics, MAO inhibitors, vasopressin. Atrial tachypacing (100 rate).

Prognosis. Less severe than in Shy-Dragger. General debilitation and complications.

BIBLIOGRAPHY. Bradbury S, Eggleston C: Postural hypotension: report of three cases. Am Heart J 1:73–86, 1925

Kopin IJ, Polinsky RJ, Oliver JA, et al: Urinary catecholamine metabolites distinguish different types of sympathetic neuronal dysfunction in patients with orthostatic hypotension. J Clin Endocrinol Metab 57:632, 1983

BRADBURY-EGGLESTON TRIAD

1. Orthostatic hypotension
2. Impotence
3. Anhidrosis

Considered as one of the two conditions repsonsible for primary hypotension, orthostatic (see).

Etiology. Attributed to lesions involving mainly the post-ganglionic sympathetic neurons and sparing of the parasympathetic system.

BIBLIOGRAPHY. Bradbury S, Eggleston C: Postural hypotension: report of three cases. Am Heart J 1:73–86, 1925

Adams RD, Victor M: Principles of Neurology, 3rd ed, p 404. New York, McGraw-Hill, 1985

BRADLEY'S

Synonyms. Epidemic collapse; epidemic vomiting; Goodall's; hyperemesis hiemis; intestinal grippe; nausea epidemica; nonbacterial gastroenteritis; Spencer's; winter vomiting.

Symptoms. Both sexes affected; onset at all ages. Onset usually in winter months and early spring. Sudden and explosive epidemic of profuse vomiting, usually beginning in early morning, associated with severe headache, muscular pains, sweating. Fever may be absent (probably in previously exposed subjects) or very high (first episode) but usually is short-lasting (24–48 hours). Diarrhea in some epidemics, or only in some subjects.

Etiology. Viral condition: Norwalk agent; Haway agent; human reoviruslike agent. Rule out epidemic food poisoning; mass hysteria.

Diagnostic Procedures. Usually none necessary.

Therapy. Symptomatic.

Prognosis. Short-lasting condition (2–3 days), occasionally up to 10 days. Within 3 weeks relapses may occur and bronchopulmonar manifestations complicate the relapsing episode.

BIBLIOGRAPHY. Bradley WH: Epidemic nausea and vomiting. Br Med J 1:309–312, 1943

Goodall JF: The winter vomiting disease: a report from general practice. Br Med J 1:197–198, 1954. Epidemic vomiting. Br Med J 2:327–328, 1969

Kapikian AZ, Kim HW, Wyatt RG, et al: Human reoviruslike agent as the major pathogen associated with "winter" gastroenteritis in hospitalized infants and young children. New Engl J Med 294:969–972, 1976

BRAILSFORD'S

Synonyms. Acrodysplasia II; peripheral dysostosis.

Symptoms and Signs. Present from birth. Reduced height and weight; short tubular bones of hands and feet; loose skin around fingers. Slow in learning to walk and talk. Frequent respiratory, cutaneous, and ear infections.

Etiology. Autosomal dominant inheritance. Autosomal recessive form reported also by Goodman.

Diagnostic Procedures. *X-rays.* Shortening of metacarpals and metatarsals; all peripheral bones underdeveloped; absent or minor skeletal changes.

Therapy. Treatment of infection.

Prognosis. Infections frequently cause of death. Final height variable from short to normal; normal mental development.

BIBLIOGRAPHY. Brailsford JF: The Radiology of Bones and Joints, 4th ed, p 33. Baltimore, Williams & Wilkins, 1948

Singleton EB, Siggers DC: Peripheral dysostosis. In Bergsma D (ed): Skeletal dysplasias. Amsterdam Excerpta Medica, pp 510–517, 1974.

Goodman RM, Weinberg U, Hertz M, et al: Peripheral dysostosis: an autosomal recessive form. Birth defects Org Art Ser 10(12):137–146, 1974

BRAIN, ACUTE

Synonyms. Delirium; toxic psychosis.

Symptoms. Disordered thoughts and behavior; restlessness; stimuli reach mind, but there is lack of recognition and integration; hallucination.

Signs. Confusion; disorientation; rapidly changing behavioral pattern and reactions to stimuli and surroundings; deterioration of conscious motor activity (e.g., dressing, eating). Incontinence of sphincters. Findings depending on specific etiology.

Etiology. Diffuse brain tissue impairment from many causes: toxemia from general infections, exogenous poisons, and drugs; endogenous intoxication; sudden cessation of drugs; infection of nervous system; noninfective cerebral diseases, cerebral anemia; heat stroke; trauma; hypertension.

Pathology. Depends on etiology.

Diagnostic Procedures. *Electroencephalography.* Slowing of activity.

Therapy. Correction of medical or surgical (hypertension) conditions; sedatives (phenothyazine; chlordiazepoxide); hypnotic (chloral hydrate).

Prognosis. Good response with proper treatment. Depending on etiology, permanent impairment of cerebral functions in some cases.

BIBLIOGRAPHY. Hirsch CJ, Caulfield PA: The acute brain syndrome: early recognition and management. G P 35:87–94, 1967

Freedman AM, Kaplan HI, Sadock BJ: Comprehensive Textbook of Psychiatry, 2nd ed, p 1062. Baltimore, Williams & Wilkins, 1975

Adams RD, Victor M: Principles of Neurology, 3rd ed, pp 309–310. New York, McGraw-Hill, 1985

BRAIN-BONE-FAT

Synonyms. Dementia   progressive–lipomembranous polycystic osteodysplasia; Hakola's. See Alzheimer's.

Symptoms. Most cases in Finland and Japan. Onset in 3rd decade. Following minor accidents or strain: pain and swelling of wrist or ankle. In 4th decade loss of inhibitions; impotency or frigidity. Intestinal motility disorders.

Signs. Tendon reflexes accentuated, pathologic reflexes; myoclonias, seizures. Development of cysts on hand and foot bones and ends of long bones.

Etiology. Unknown. Autosomal dominant inheritance. Defective development of vascular bed considered as primary.

Pathology. *Cysts.* Contain jellylike material; membranous-lamellar structure interposed between fat and collagen tissue. *Brain.* Narrowing of small vessels; calcification of basal ganglia, glyosis and demyelinization of white matter, senile plaques and neurofibrillar nests.

Diagnostic Procedures. *X-ray of skeleton.* Typical cysts. *Electroencephalography.* Typical changes. *Biopsy. Blood.* Occasionally leukemia. *CT brain scan.* Dilated ventricles and cortical atrophy.

Therapy. None.

Prognosis. Progressing condition leading to death.

BIBLIOGRAPHY. Hakola HPA: Neuropsychiatric and genetic aspects a new hereditary disease characterized by progressive dementia and lipomembranous polycystic osteodysplasia. Acta Psychiatr Neurol Scand 232 (suppl):1–173, 1972

Bird TD, Koerker RM, Leaird BJ, et al: Lipomembranous polycystic osteodysplasia (brain, bone and fat disease): a genetic cause of presenile dementia. Neurology 33:81–86, 1983

BRAIN, CHRONIC

Synonyms. Dementia; feeblemindedness; mental retardation.

Symptoms and Signs. Failure of memory, particularly for recent events, is presenting symptom. Decline in work efficiency, with or without anxiety and depression; loss of emotional balance; irritability; sometimes rush of sexual feeling. Hygiene and appearance deteriorated; dysarthria; aphasia.

Etiology and Pathogenesis. Idiopathic degenerative diseases; endocrine-metabolic conditions; vascular insufficiency; nutritional deficiency; intoxication; encephalitis-meningitis; tumor.

Pathology. Related to etiology; destruction of nerve cells and fiber of cortex and diencephalon.

Diagnostic Procedures. Search for etiology.

Therapy. According to etiology; general care; in depression or anxiety, specific agents.

Prognosis. Depends on etiology; usually progressive.

BIBLIOGRAPHY. Busse EW: Geriatrics today—an overview. Am J Psychiatr 123:1226–1233, 1967

Freedman AM., Kaplan HI, Sadock BJ: Comprehensive Textbook of Psychiatry, 2nd ed, p 1062. Baltimore, Williams & Wilkins, 1975

Adams RD, Victor M: Principles of Neurology, 3rd ed, pp 302–321. New York, McGraw-Hill, 1985

BRAIN PURPURA

Synonym. Pericapillary encephalorrhagia.

Symptoms and Signs. Suddenly the patient (of various ages) becomes stuporous or comatose without focal neurological signs.

Etiology. Unknown. It may complicate viral pneumonia and some intoxication (arsenic) or be sporadic.

Pathology. Small hemorrhagic pericapillary lesions (1–2mm) in the white matter, corpus callosum, centrum ovale, or cerebellar peduncles. Destruction of adjacent myelin and axis cylinders. Absence of inflammatory changes.

Diagnostic Procedures. *Cerebral spinal fluid.* Normal or moderate increase of proteins. *Electroencephalography. CT brain scan.*

Therapy. None specific.

Prognosis. Variable.

BIBLIOGRAPHY. Adams RD, Victor M: Principles of Neurology, 3rd ed, p 716. New York, McGraw-Hill, 1985

BRAIN'S

Synonyms. Exophthalmic ophthalmoplegia; orbit pseudo-tumor; superior orbital fissure.

Symptoms. Prevalent in males: later age of onset compared to exophthalmic goiter. Onset gradual. Both eyes may be involved or one eye's exophthalmos may precede that in the other by months. Pain; ophthalmoplegia; vision not affected (usually); no sensory disturbances of first branch of trigeminal (V) nerve.

Signs. Exophthalmos; edema of eyelid; chemosis.

Etiology. It may develop in patient with or without hyperthyroidism. Unknown; possibly low grade infection.

Pathology. Inflammatory mass in ocular muscles.

Diagnostic Procedures. *X-ray of skull. Angiography.*

Therapy. Steroids; antibiotics. Partial suture of the lids to protect eyes. Seldom needed, removal of roof or orbit and canal of optic nerve through anterior craniotomy.

Prognosis. Good response to treatment with improvement of vision. Usually progression spontaneously steps.

BIBLIOGRAPHY. Brain WR: Exophthalmic ophthalmoplegie. Q J Med 7:293, 1938.

Ingalls RG: Tumor of the Orbit and Allied Pseudotumors. Springfield, Ill, CC Thomas, 1953

Lakke JPWF: Superior orbital fissure syndrome. Arch Neurol 7:289–300, 1962

Adams RD, Victor M: Principles of Neurology, 3rd ed, pp 1059–1060. New York, McGraw-Hill, 1985

BRAIN TUMOR–NEUROASTHENIA

Synonym. Pseudoneurotic brain tumor. See also Amorphosynthesis; organic brain.

Symptoms. Fatigue; weight loss; vague headache; slow speech; depression and emotional instability (irritability, fits of anger or depression, insomnia, decrease or loss of libido and potency).

Etiology. Initial stage precedes objective signs of brain tumor.

Pathology. Brain tumors (neoplastic aneurysm).

Diagnostic Procedures. *CT brain scan. X-ray of skull. Angiography. Electroencephalography. Spinal fluid.*

Therapy. Surgery when feasible.

Prognosis. Early diagnosis important because psychotic symptoms may mask organic disease and make the prognosis unfavorable because of the delayed treatment.

BIBLIOGRAPHY. Horenstein S: Effects of cerebrovascular disease on personality and emtionality. In Benton AL (ed): Behavioral Changes in Cerebrovascular Disease, p 171. New York, Harper & Row, 1970

BRANDT'S

Synonyms. Acrodermatitis enteropathica; Danbolt-Closs.

Symptoms. Appear in both sexes; onset in early infancy. Gastrointestinal troubles with intermittent diarrhea. In acute phase, psychic disturbances of schizoid type. Retarded growth rate; photophobia.

Signs. Symmetric rash involving face, ears, back of scalp, buttocks, elbows and knees, and hands and feet, starting as vesiculobullous, then drying to erythematosquamous type. Paronychia and dysonychia; alopecia; loss of eyebrows and eyelashes; conjunctivitis; blepharitis; scattered superficial opacities of cornea.

Etiology. Autosomal recessive inheritance (?). Possibly a defect of zinc absorption at jejunal level.

Pathology. Histopathologic changes in the skin and gastrointestinal tract are nonspecific; a cytoplasmic inclusion body has been noted in the Paneth cells.

Diagnostic Procedures. *Biopsy of skin. Study of digestive enzymes. Blood.* Low serum zinc.

Therapy. Oral therapy with zinc compounds: 50 mg of zinc sulfate, acetate, or gluconate daily for infants and up to 150 mg daily for children. Plasma zinc levels should be monitored.

Prognosis. Without treatment, fatal within 10 years of onset. With treatment, disease kept under control until puberty. Long remission often occurs, including remission of corneal opacities.

BIBLIOGRAPHY. Brandt T: Dermatitis in children with disturbances of the general condition and the absorption of food elements. Acta Dermatol Venereol 17:513–546, 1936

Danbolt N, Closs K: Akrodermatitis enteropathica. Acta Dermatol Vernereol 23:127–169, 1942

BRANDYWINE DENTINOGENESIS IMPERFECTION

Synonyms. Dentinogenesis imperfecta; Shields III.

Symptoms and Signs. Found in southern Maryland. Crown of both deciduous and permanent teeth eroded and pulp exposed. Dentin color amber and smooth. No stigmata or osteogenesis imperfecta.

Etiology. Autosomal dominant inheritance. May be same entity or separate mutation of Capdepont's (see).

Diagnostic Procedures. *X-ray of teeth.* Large pulp chambers and root canals, which become reduced with age.

BIBLIOGRAPHY. Schimmelpfennig CB, McDonald RE: Enamel and dentine aplasia. Oral Surg 6:1444–1449, 1953

Hursey RJ, Witkop CJ Jr, Miklashek D, et al: Dentinogenesis imperfecta in a racial isolate with multiple hereditary defects. Oral Surg 9:641–658, 1956

BRAUER'S

Synonyms. See Hidrotic ectodermal dysplasia, and Tylosis; focal facial dermal dysplasia; forceps marks.

Symptoms and Signs. Both sexes affected; present from birth. Scarlike defects at the temporal regions (similar to forceps lesions). Median furrow on the chin; scarlike lesion. Eyebrows slanted up and outward; eyelashes absent or multiple in upper and absent in lower lids. Protuberant nose.

Etiology. Unknown; autosomal dominant inheritance.

Pathology. *Skin.* Mesodermal dysplasia with absence of subcutaneous fat and contiguity of muscles and skin.

BIBLIOGRAPHY. Brauer A: Heréditarer symmetrischer systematisierter Naevus aplasticus bei 38 Personen. Derm Wochschr 89:1163–1168, 1929
McGeoch AH, Reed WB: Familial focal facial dermal dysplasia. Arch Derm 107:591–596, 1973

BRAUN-FALCO'S

Synonym. Circumscribed cutis laxa.

Symptoms and Signs. Present from birth. Presence of cutis laxa lesions on thorax and anterior abdominal muscles; thorax deformity; mediastinal hernia.

Etiology. Unknown. See Cutis laxa syndromes.

Pathology. See Cutis laxa syndromes.

BIBLIOGRAPHY. Braun-Falco O: Angeborene Dermatochalasis als Leitsymptom eines Symptomkomplexes. Arch Klin Exp Dermatol 220:166–182, 1964

BRAZILIAN PURPURIC FEVER

Symptoms and Signs. Occurs in children 3 months to 8 years old. Fever, vomiting, and abdominal pain, followed by purpura and death. The initial symptom is often a purulent conjunctivitis. The illness is often complicated by disseminated intravascular coagulation (DIC).

Etiology. Infection with *Haemophilus influenzae* type B. Cases have been described in Brazil town of Promissao, (São Paulo state) and in Central Australia.

Pathology. Ischemia of upper and lower limbs in cases of DIC.

Diagnostic Procedures. *Blood cultures.*

Therapy. Symptomatic treatment of shock: antibiotics as suggested by blood cultures. Usually the *Haemophilus* is susceptible to ampicillin, cefotaxime, chloramphenicol, and co-trimoxaxole.

Prognosis. Poor.

BIBLIOGRAPHY. Centers for Disease Control. CDC preliminary report: epidemic purpuric fever among children—Brazil. MMWR 34:217–219, 1985

McIntyre P, Wheaton G, Erlich J, Hansman D: Brasilian purpuric fever in central Australia. Lancet II:112, 1987

BREGEAT'S

Synonym. Oculo-orbital-thalamo-encephalic angiomatosis.

Symptoms and Signs. From birth. Angiomatosis of eye and orbit, controlateral forehead. Variable neurological signs according to extension of thalamoencephalic angioma.

Etiology. Unknown. Sporadic.

Pathology. Angioma in thalamus extending to choroidal plexus.

Diagnostic Procedures. *CT brain scan.*

Therapy. Evaluation for possible neurosurgery.

Prognosis. Variable.

BIBLIOGRAPHY. Brégeat P, Juge P, Pouliquen Y, et al: A propos d'une angiomatose orbitothalancéphalique. Bull Mem Soc Franc Ophthalm 71:581–594, 1958
Chonnette G, Auriel M: Classification de angiodysplasies et tumeurs vasculaires. Rev Stom Clin Maxillo Fac 87:1–5, 1986

BRENNEMANN'S

Synonyms. Mesenteric lymphadenitis–upper respiratory; mesenteric lymphadenitis; pseudotuberculous mesenteric; Brennemann's retroperitoneal.

Symptoms. Abdominal pain; nausea; vomiting; fever; following upper respiratory tract infection (usually in children under 15 years of age).

Signs. Pain in lower abdominal quadrant; rebound tenderness; not as severe as in appendicitis. Upper tract respiratory inflammation.

Etiology. Viral infections (adenovirus and others).

Pathology. Mesenteric and retroperitoneal adenitis.

Diagnostic Procedures. Leukocytosis; occasionally, increase of lymphomonocytic elements (virocytes).

Therapy. It is good to operate because of the almost impossible differential diagnosis with acute appendicitis. If diagnosed, treatment is supportive. Specific vaccines are being tested.

Prognosis. Spontaneous recovery. In some young children the occurrence of intussusception has been reported.

BIBLIOGRAPHY. Brenneman J: The abdominal pain of throat infection. Am J Dis Child 22:493–499, 1921

Fox JP, Hall CE, Cooney MK: The Seattle virus Watch VII. Observations of adenovirus infections. Am J Epidemiol 10:362–386, 1977

BRENNER'S

Synonym. Ovarean fibroepithelioma ovary.

Symptoms. Appear in elderly women. Asymptomatic or postmenopausal recurrent bleeding.

Signs. Possibly, adnexal mass on palpation.

Etiology. Unknown (obsolete entity).

Pathology. Benign ovarian tumor: small, well-capsulated, usually unilateral, seldom estrogenic.

Diagnostic Procedure. *Ultrasonography* or *CT scanning*. Surgical exploration.

Therapy. Removal.

Prognosis. Good.

BIBLIOGRAPHY. Brenner F: Das Ophoroma folliculare. Frankf Zschr Pathol 1:150–171, 1907

Lawson TL, Albarelli JN: Diagnosis of gynecologic pelvic masses by gray scale ultrasonography: analysis of specificity and accuracy. Am J Roentgen 128:1003–1006, 1977

Scully RE: Tumors of the ovary and maldeveloped gonads. Armed Forces Inst Path Fasc 16, 1979

BRETT'S

Synonym. Janus.

Eponym used to indicate an occasional radiologic finding: clear lung on one side and opaque shadow on the other side. This aspect is observed in Fallot's tetralogy (see) with atresia of a branch of pulmonary artery or in case of truncus ateriosus with solitary pulmonary artery.

BIBLIOGRAPHY. Bret J: Le syndrome de Janus. Arch Mal Coeur 49:468–472, 1956

Perloff JK: The Clinical Recognition of Congenital Heart Disease. Philadelphia, WB Saunders, 1978

BRIDGE JUMPING

Symptoms. Prevalent in white males, age 25 to 34. Repeated episodes common; exacerbated by media publicity, which leads to clusters; usually, occurrence affected by season, holiday, and weather; predilection for particular bridges.

Etiology. Variable, but common psychological characteristics. Exhibitionist personality; depression associated with stress. Frequently also association with alcohol or drug ingestion.

Therapy. Prevention at different level when "on site" and have identified the intention: establish communication; stabilize environment; coordinate harbor patrol; if possible, physically prevent jump or fall in water.

Prognosis. Variable. Often unsuccessful in suicide attempts.

BIBLIOGRAPHY. Pascarelli EF, Katz IB, Nolte C: The epidemiology of bridge jumping. Presented at the 32nd Conference Internationale Médicine Catastrophe, Monte Carlo, April 6–9, 1979

BRIESKY'S

Synonyms. Leukokraurosis vulvae; kraurosis vulvae; senile genital atrophy; vulvae senile atrophy.

Symptoms. Pruritus (mild and inconstant); dyspareunia; easy traumatism.

Signs. Gradual shrinkage of labia, clitoris, and frenulum. Dryness of mucosa. Leukoplakia may be associated. Vaginitis frequent (responsible for symptoms).

Etiology. Postmenopausal or postovariectomy hormonal deficiencies; or loss of response to hormone (Seabright-Bantam type, see). Obsolete since the older classification of senile atrophy and primary vulvar atrophy relate both to physiological effects of aging and "do not indicate to a specific form of disease." The syndrome today has been subdivided in the following conditions: benign dermatoses of the vulva (lichenification, psoriasis, Lichen planus, seborrheic dermatitis, eczematous dermatitis); vulvar epithelial hyperplasia (with and without atypia); lichen sclerosus; leucoderma; infections; Bowen's (see) and Paget's (see).

Pathology. Thinning of epithelium; hyperkeratinization; elastic tissue altered; collagenous tissue increased. Associated inflammatory feature. See Etiology.

Therapy. Estrogens (particularly useful for vaginitis, less for atrophy). Local estrogen cream. For benign dermatoses antibiotics and antimycotic topical.

Prognosis. Frequent exacerbation. Irreversible condition.

BIBLIOGRAPHY. Briesky A: Die Krankheiten der Vagina Hand. Allerg Spec Chir 4:1–256, 1879

Rook A, Wilkinson DS, Ebling FJG, et al: Textbook of Dermatology, 4th ed, pp 2221–2226. Oxford, Blackwell Scientific Publications, 1986

BRIGHT'S

Synonyms. Acute nephritic; acute glomerulonephritis; acute nephritis; postinfective glomerulonephritis; poststreptococcal glomerulonephritis, PSGN.

Symptoms. Prevalent in males; onset at any age; highest incidence between 3 and 7 years of age. Ten days after airway infection: fatigue; anorexia; cephalalgia; backache; abdominal pain; vomiting; somnolence; dyspnea; oliguria; hematuria.

Signs. Edema of face, less frequently of legs; tachycardia; hypertension; basal rales; moderate temperature elevation.

Etiology. Streptococcal infection by nephrogenic strains (type 4–12 in respiratory infection and a type 49 in impetigo) or other infection (staphylococcal; pneumococcal; viral) causing glomerular damage through the following pathogenetic mechanisms: immunologic reactions; vascular diseases; abnormalities of coagulation; and metabolic defects. In some cases mechanism remains unknown. (type 1–12; 18, 25, 49, 55, 57, 60) suspected (31, 52, 56, 59, 61); group C streptococcus pathogenetic mechanisms: immune complex (IgG and C3).

Pathology. *Kidney.* Enlarged, edematous, pale, with punctate hemorrhages or grey spot on surface. Capsule tense; cortex smooth; medulla congested. Glomeruli swollen, filled with cells covering the tuft network. Immunoflourescence reveals granular pattern.

Diagnostic Procedures. *Blood.* Elevated blood urea nitrogen; occasionally, anemia; leukocytosis. Antistreptolysin, antistaphylolysin (and others) titers increased. Increased red cell sedimentation rate. *Urine.* Red blood cells; casts of various type (RBC, epithelial, granular); proteinuria (lower than 2 g/day); decreased sodium excretion. *Renal function tests.* Abnormal in 50% of cases. *Renal biopsy:* See Pathology. *Light microscopy.* Enlarged glomeruli capillary lumen occluded by mesangial and endothelial cells and infiltrated by leukocytes. Few crescents. *Electron microscopy.* Electron-dense deposits (lumps) on the endothelial side of basement membrane. *Immunofluorescence.* Three patterns: starry sky, mesangial, and garland, which are deposits of IgG and C3.

Therapy. Bed rest; low protein and low sodium diet; antihypertensive agents; antibiotics.

Prognosis. More intense and severe onset implies a more guarded prognosis. A few deaths from pulmonary edema, hypertensive encephalopathy, or infection; 1% fatality for renal failure. Some patients exhibit proteinuria and hematuria for weeks or months and finally recover; some may develop a chronic condition; 90% of children are finally completely cured; 50% of adults develop chronic glomerular disease.

BIBLIOGRAPHY. Bright R: Cases and observations illustrative of renal disease accompanied with the secretion of albuminous urine. Guy's Hosp Rep London 1:338–400, 1836

Brenner BM, Rector FC: The Kidneys, 3rd ed, p 292. Philadelphia, WB Saunders, 1986

BRILL-SYMMERS

Synonyms. Brill-Boehr-Rosenthal; macrofollicular lymphoblastoma; giant follicular lymphoma; giant cell lymphosarcoma; Symmers'; nodular lymphosarcoma.

Eponym denotes a "clinicohistologic" entity, which is no longer considered distinct but is classified into the broader category of non-Hodgkins lymphomas. The clinical element was (and it is believed by many authors) a distinctly superior survival and the histologic feature of a well-differentiated lymphocytic-follicular pattern as compared with other follicular varieties of lymphomas. In later stages 50% lose the follicular pattern and presents unstructured cellular infiltration, modifications that usually precede the fatal outcome.

BIBLIOGRAPHY. Brill NE, Boehr G, Rosenthal N: Generalized giant follicle hyperplasia of lymph nodes and spleen: a hitherto undescribed type. JAMA 84:668–671, 1925

Symmers D: Follicular lymphadenopathy with splenomegaly: A newly recognized disease of the lymphatic system. Arch Pathol 3:816–820, 1927

Dumont J: La maladie de Brill-Symmers. Concours Med 103:2437–2453, 1981

BRIQUET'S

Synonyms. Conversion reaction; hysteria conversion; hysterical neurosis.

Symptoms. Prevalent in females; caution for diagnosis in men (rare). Onset in adolescence or later. Prodromal manifestation at earlier age frequent; lack of energy; laziness; somatic symptoms recorded in 30% of cases; flirtatiousness of female; juvenile sexual offense. In women, high incidence of polysurgery. In men, history of criminal acts and drinking. Anxious impulse converted to functional symptoms: motor and sensory disturbances not related to neural pathway but to anatomic distribution (e.g., glove, stocking areas) hemiplegia, paraplegia, disorders of phonation, hearing, sight. Frequently, symptoms arise when patient tries to evade an unpleasant situation.

Etiology. Psychiatric disorder related (not invariably, however) to sexual dysfunction. Use of sexual signals to convey nonsexual messages (placate agression?). Association with antisocial personality.

Therapy. Psychotherapy.

Prognosis. Tendency to convert to new symptoms; better prognosis for monosymptomatic hysteria of adult life.

BIBLIOGRAPHY. Briquet P: Traité clinique et thérapeutique de l'hysterie. Paris, Bailliere, 1859
Freedman AM, Kaplan HI, Sadock BJ: Comprehensive Textbook of Psychiatry, 2nd ed, p 1505. Baltimore, Williams & Wilkins, 1975.
Adams RD, Victor M: Principles of Neurology, 3rd ed, p 1113–1117. New York, McGraw-Hill, 1985

BRISSAUD-MARIE

Synonyms. Conversion reaction; conversion hysteria; hysterical neurosis. See also Briquet's.

Symptoms. Glossolabial hemispasm.

Etiology. Hysteria.

BIBLIOGRAPHY. Brissaud E, Marie P: De la déviation faciale dans l'hémiplégie hystérique. Pro Med, 5:84, 1887

BRISSAUD'S I

Synonyms. Habit spasm; psychogenic tic; spasmodic tic; tic nondouloureux.

Symptoms. Appear in active children between 5 and 10 years of age. Sudden, brief, recurrent movements or series of movements. Patient claims that he cannot prevent them. Aggravated by tension. Facial muscles most frequently affected; neck and extremities occasionally involved.

Etiology. Unknown; psychogenic tension in predisposed individual. Tics may also appear after encephalitis.

Therapy. Psychotherapy. Calm environment; sedatives, some of ataraxic drugs.

Prognosis. Good, if early treatment instituted.

BIBLIOGRAPHY. Trousseau A: Clinique médicale de L'Hôtel-Dieu de Paris, Vol 1, p 855. 1873
Brissaud E: La chorée variable des dégénerés. Rev Neur (Paris) 4:417–431, 1896
Adams RD, Victor M: Principles of Neurology, 3rd ed, pp 86–87. New York, McGraw-Hill, 1985

BRISSAUD-SICARD

Synonym. Brissaud's IV.

Symptoms and Signs. Unilateral facial spasm with contralateral paralysis of limbs.

Etiology and Pathology. Irritative lesion of the pons.

BIBLIOGRAPHY. Brissaud EA, Sicard J: Type special de syndrome alterne. Rev Neurol (Paris) 16:86, 1908

BRISTOWE'S

Synonym. Corpus callosum tumor.

Symptoms. Not distinctive; more marked form of mental changes seen from involvement of one of frontal lobes; difficulty in concentration; personality changes; memory disturbances; psychoses; negativism and disregard of requests and commands. Apraxia of left hand (in tumor affecting anterior portion of corpus collosum).

Diagnostic Procedures. *Cerebrospinal fluid.* Xanthochromia; pleocytosis. *CT brain scan.* Distortion of one or both lateral ventricles and third ventricle.

Prognosis. Progressive: stupor; coma; death.

BIBLIOGRAPHY. Bristowe JS: Cases of tumour of the corpus callosum. Brain 7:315–333, 1884
Ironside R, Guttmacher M: The corpus callosum and its tumors. Brain 52:442–483, 1929
Alpers BJ, Grant FC: The clinical syndrome of corpus callosum. Arch Neurol Psychiatr 25:67–86, 1931
Adams RD, Victor M: Principles of Neurology, 3rd ed, p 344. New York, McGraw-Hill, 1985

BROADBENT'S

Synonyms. Ingravescent apoplexy; intraventricular brain hemorrhage.

Symptoms and Signs. Sudden loss of consciousness (from stupor to deep coma) preceded, usually, by severe headache or vomiting or both; Cheyne-Stokes respiration or other breathing abnormalities; generalized flaccidity or focal signs; cerebral shock or diaschisis (loss of functional continuity among various centers of neural pathways). Blood hypertension.

Etiology. Primary subarachnoid hemorrhage with sudden and imposing invasion of blood into ventricular system. Hypertension; trauma.

Pathology. Subarachnoid hemorrhage.

Diagnostic Procedures. *Spinal fluid. Blood. Electroencephalography. Angiography. CT brain scan.*

Therapy. Intensive care; antiedema treatment (with caution).

Prognosis. Severe.

BIBLIOGRAPHY. Broadbent WH: On ingravescent apoplexy. Med Chir Soc London 8:103–108, 1876
Adams RD, Victor M: Principles of Neurology, 3rd ed, p 570–575. New York, McGraw-Hill, 1985

BROCA'S APHASIA

Synonyms. Expressive aphasia; motor aphasia; verbal aphasia.

Symptoms. Predominant impairment of expressive speech; preserved ability to think in abstraction; some minor difficulty in understanding, resulting in inability to find words that express thoughts. In Broca's aphasia, the patient may say a few words but cannot write. This differs from other forms of aphasia.

Etiology. Lesions of the posterior part of third frontal convolution and lower part of precentral convolution of dominant hemisphere.

Prognosis. A certain degree of recovery sometimes occurs as other hemisphere asserts itself.

BIBLIOGRAPHY. Broca P: Sur le siège de la faculté du language articulé, avec deux observations d'aphémie. Bull Soc Anat (Paris) 36:330–357, 1861
Adams RD, Victor M: Principles of Neurology, 3rd ed, pp 355–357. New York, McGraw-Hill, 1985

BROCK'S

Synonyms. Graham-Burford-Mayer; lung, middle lobe; middle lobe.

Symptoms. Can be observed at any age; onset acute febrile episode. Recurrent hemoptysis and pneumonitis. In interval between episodes, chronic cough and fatigability.

Signs. During acute episodes, signs of peneumonia; in interval, signs of bronchiectasis or chronic suppuration.

Etiology. No single factor responsible; any inflammatory process that results in hilar lymphadenopathy and compression of middle lobe (right) or lingula (left) bronchus, with consequent atelectasis and pneumonitis.

Pathology. Enlargement of peribronchial lymph nodes that encircle the bronchus of middle lobe; obstructive pneumonitis of the middle lobe; bronchiectasis and destruction of lung parenchyma.

Diagnostic Procedures. *X-ray of chest. Bronchoscopy. Bronchography.*

Therapy. Surgical extirpation of affected lobe. Antibiotics only induce remission. Responds well to antibiotics. Surgery rarely required.

Prognosis. Good after surgery.

BIBLIOGRAPHY. Brock RC, Cann RJ, Dickinson JR: Tuberculous mediastinal lymphadenitis in childhood: secondary effects on lungs. Guy's Hosp Rep London 97:295–317, 1937
Graham EA, Burford TH, Mayer JH: Middle lobe syndrome. Postgrad Med 4:29–34, 1948
Wagner RB, Johnson MR: Middle lobe syndrome. Ann Thorac Surg 35:679–686, 1983

BROCQ-PAUTRIER

Synonyms. Median rhomboid glossitis, glossite losangique médiane.

Symptoms and Signs. Present in 0.3% of population. Syndrome becomes clinically manifest in 3rd or 4th decade or later. Asymptomatic or burning while eating spicy foods and dryness of mouth. Accidental notice of area on the midline of base of tongue, smooth and devoid of papillae, or elevated and nodular.

Etiology. Considered a developmental defect; persistency of tuberculum impar.

Pathology. Epithelial thickening; acanthosis; slight hyperkeratosis; fibrosis extending into muscular layer.

Diagnostic Procedures. In case of doubt, biopsy (seldom required).

Therapy. None.

Prognosis. Harmless anomaly.

BIBLIOGRAPHY. Brocq L, Pautrier LM: Glossite losangique médiane de la face dorsale de la langue. Ann Dermatol Syph 5:1–18, 1914
Rook A, Wilkinson DS, Ebling FJG, et al: Textbook of Dermatology, 4th ed, pp 2117–2118. Oxford, Blackwell Scientific Publications, 1986

BRODIE'S I

Synonyms. Brodie's abscess; suppurative focal osteomyelitis.

Symptoms. Initially asymptomatic (for years). Intermittent pain at end of a long bone (e.g., tibia); possible fever.

Signs. Initially none. Then edema and erythema of skin of painful zone; fusiform swelling of affected bone; localized bone tenderness.

Etiology. Chronic bone abscess where necrotic debris and infective agents have usually been walled off; 50% *Staphylococcus aureus*, 20% culture negative. Some surgeons call any bone abscess "Brodie abscess."

Pathology. Ulceration of head of bone; encapsulated abscess included in sclerosed bone.

Diagnostic Procedures. *Blood.* Occasionally, leucocytosis. *X-rays.* Bone area rarefied in metaphysis, well demarcated. *Biopsy.*

Therapy. Drilling and evacuation (Brodie), or excision (preferred).

Prognosis. Excellent with excision. Otherwise, spontaneous remission and possible relapses.

BIBLIOGRAPHY. Brodie BC: An account of some cases of chronic abscess of the tibia. Med Chir Tr London 17:239–249, 1832
Carnesale PG: General principles of infection. In Crenshaw AH (ed): Campbell's Operative Orthopedics, 7th ed, p 663. St Louis, CV Mosby, 1987

BRODIE'S II

Synonyms. Breast adenofibroma; breast cystosarcoma phylloides.

Symptoms. Pain in the breast.

Signs. Usually absent; or distortion of breast contour; nipple flattened; no retraction.

Etiology. Unknown.

Pathology. Benign tumor; nodular, gray-white color. Fibroblastic proliferation, stroma rich cellularity; epithelial growth not prominent; intracanalicular invasion.

Diagnostic Procedures. *Mammography. Ultrasonography. Thermography.*

Therapy. Surgical excision.

Prognosis. Benign; seldom metastasis.

BIBLIOGRAPHY. Brodie BC: Lectures on serocystic tumors of the breast. Lond Med Gaz 25:808–814, 1939
Briggs RM, Walter M, Rosenthal D: Cystosarcoma phylloides in adolescent female patients. Am J Surg 146:712–714, 1983

BRODIN'S

Synonym. Appendicitis–duodenal stenosis.

Symptoms. Double symptomatology related to duodenal stenosis and appendicitislike condition.

Etiology. Mesenteric lymphadenitis.

BIBLIOGRAPHY. Brodin M: L'appendice cronique. Son diagnostic par la palpation abdominale en position verticale et son retentissement duodénal avec arrêt en "genu inferius" mis en évidence par l'étude radiologique de la traversée digestive. Presse Med 49:619–621, 1941

BROMHIDROSIS

Synonym. Osmidrosis.

Symptoms. Malodorous sweating. (Marked individual and racial variations in social acceptability.)

Signs. Generalized and, frequently, associated with hyperhidrosis. Localized forms (axillae, feet, genitalia).

Etiology. Eccrine secretion per se is odorless; however various substances may be excreted with it (garlic; onions; arsenic; sulfinylidric compounds). Bacterial decomposition liberates fatty acids with characteristic odor in gout, diabetes, scurvy, and typhoid.

Therapy. Omission of particular foods from diet. Washing of involved areas and application of antibacterial agents. Agents to control hyperhidrosis such as aluminum salts and anticholinergic drugs of little benefit.

Prognosis. Good response to treatment.

BIBLIOGRAPHY. Hurley HJ, Shelley WB: The Human Apocrine Sweat Gland in Health and Disease. Springfield, Ill, CC Thomas, 1960
Smith M, Smith LG, Levinson B: The use of smell in differential diagnosis. Lancet II: 1452, 1982

BROWN OCULOCUTANEOUS ALBINISM

Synonym. Albinism, moderate pigment reduction.

Symptoms and Signs. In Africans and New Guineans. Medium brown hair, light brown skin, hazel eyes; moderate nystagmus, photophobia; pachidermia and keratoses.

Etiology. Autosomal recessive. Defect of pigment accumulation.

Pathology. *Hair bulbs.* Melanosomes in all stages but slight pigment accumulation.

Diagnostic Procedures. *Ophthalmoscopy.* Light retinal pigmentation. *Incubation of hair bulb.* Low tyrosine incorporation.

Therapy. None.

Prognosis. Low accumulation of pigment, with age.

BIBLIOGRAPHY. King RA, Creel D, Cervanka J, et al: Albinism in Nigeria with delineation of new recessive oculocutaneous type. Clin Genet 17:259–262, 1980

BROWN RECLUSE SPIDER BITE

Synonyms. Arachnidism; araneism; *Loxosceles reclusa.*

Symptoms. Stinging sensation, not too painful; pain follows within 2 to 8 hours accompanied by nausea, arthralgia, abdominal cramps, and fever, vomiting, delirium.

Signs. Blister on the skin with surrounding area of hemorrhage, which subsequently ulcerates and may become gangrenous. Occasionally, morbilliform, petechial rash appearing within 24 to 48 hours of bite.

Etiology. Venom from bite by a spider (brown recluse; fiddler spider; *Loxosceles reclusa*) native to the Central and Southern states of the United States.

Pathology. Ischemic hemorrhagic necrosis from one to several centimeters in diameter. Dermoepidermal separation, clots occluding small arterioles; moderate inflammatory infiltrate.

Diagnostic Procedures. *Blood.* May show hemolytic anemia and thrombocytopenia, especially in children; leukocytosis *Urine.* Proteinuria; hemoglobinuria.

Therapy. Corticosteroids (prompt administration) good to prevent necrosis and systemic effect of venom. Skin graft for large lesion, poor take.

Prognosis. In children (if not treated), severe. Death may follow. Healing time of lesion proportional to size.

BIBLIOGRAPHY. Atkins JA, Wingo CW, Sodeman WA: Probable cause of necrotic spider bite in midwest. Science 126:73, 1957
Dillaha CJ, Jansen GT, Honeycutt WM, et al: North American loxoscelism: necrotic bite of the brown recluse spider. JAMA 188:33–36, 1964

BROWN'S

Synonyms. Superior oblique tendon sheath; tendon sheath adherence.

Symptoms. Both sexes affected; present from birth. Congenital strabismus; bilateral ptosis; backward head tilt. Palpebral fissure may widen when attempting upward gaze. Adduction and abduction restricted or abolished. Associated choroidal coloboma.

Etiology. Unknown.

Pathology. Shortening of sheath of superior oblique muscle and attachment to the troclea. Decreased elasticity of conjunctiva.

Diagnostic Procedure. *CT brain scan.*

Therapy. Surgery.

BIBLIOGRAPHY. Brown HW: Congenital structural motor anomalies. In Allen JH (ed): Strabismus. Ophthalmic Symposium. St Louis, CV Mosby, 1950
Goldhammer J, Smith JL: Acquired intermittent Brown's syndrome. Neurology 24:666–668, 1974
Crawford JS: Surgical treatment of true Brown's syndrome. Am J Ophthal 81:289–295, 1976
Sprague Eustis H, O'Reilly C, Crawford JS: Management of superior oblique palsy after surgery for true Brown's syndrome. J Pediatr Ophthalmol Strabismus 24:10–16, 1987

BROWN-SEQUARD'S

Synonyms. Hemiparaplegic; spastic spinal monoplegia.

Symptoms. Unilateral paralysis of voluntary motion below the level of lesion; segmental atrophy and sensory loss at the level of lesion; contralateral analgesia and thermanesthesia few segments below the lesion; sphincteral disturbances.

Signs. At the side of lesion, increase in muscle tone; increase in deep reflexes; clonus and Babinski sign.

Etiology. Lesion of one lateral half of spinal cord. Hemisection from wound; localized pressure from vertebral, meningeal, neoplastic, degenerative, infectious diseases. Pure forms are rare; lesions can spare part of the one half or extend to other side.

Pathology. Depends upon etiology.

Diagnostic Procedures. *Cerebrospinal fluid.* Increase in protein. *X-ray. Myelogram.*

Therapy. In case of trauma, avoid manipulation and use care in transporting of patient. Avoid overdistension of bladder and prevent infection. General hygienic care of patient, avoiding soiling and decubitus ulcers; fluid intake and metabolic status care. Early activity to avoid osteoporosis and hypercalcemia. Surgery if indicated.

Prognosis. *Quoad vitam* good with proper care. In case of compression or partial lesion, good degree of functional recovery.

BIBLIOGRAPHY. Brown-Sequard CE: De la transmission par la moelle épinière. C R Soc Biol (Paris) 2:33–34, 1850

Brody IA, Wilkins RH: Brown-Sequard syndrome. Arch Neurol 19:347, 1968

Freeman BL III: Fractures, dislocations and fracture-dislocation of spine. In Crenshaw AH (ed): Campbell's Operative Orthopedics, 7th ed, p 3112. St Louis, CV Mosby, 1987

BROWN-VIALETTO-VAN LAERE

Synonyms. Bulbar palsy; perceptive deafness; pontobulbar palsy–deafness.

Symptoms and Signs. Most cases female. Onset in childhood. Irregularly progressive. Multiple cranial nerves (usually VII, IX, X, XI, XII; seldom III, V, VI) and spinal nerve palsies.

Etiology. Autosomal recessive inheritance or sporadic cases.

BIBLIOGRAPHY. Brown CH: Infantile amyotrophic lateral sclerosis of the family type. J Nerve Ment Dis 21:707–716, 1984

Van Laere J: Paralysie bulbo-pontine chronique progressive familial avec surdité: un cas de syndrome de Klippel-Trenaunay de la même fatric (problems diagnostiques et genetiques). Rev Neurol 115:289–295, 1966

Gallai V, Hockaday JM, Hughes JT, et al: Ponto-bulbar palsy with deafness (Brown-Vialetto-Van Laere syndrome): a report of three cases. J Neurol Sci 50:259–275, 1981

BRUCK-DE LANGE

Synonyms. Cornelia De Lange II; De Lange's II; extrapyramidal-muscular hypertrophy; Lange's II; mental deficiency–muscular hypertrophy; muscular hypertrophy, cerebral.

Symptoms and Signs. Present from birth. All muscles, or only selected muscle groups, larger and firmer than normal (athletic look). Head may be small and deformed.

Muscle rigidity (extrapyramidal type); tendon reflexes normal. Mental deficiency.

Etiology. Unknown.

Pathology. Muscle not studied. *Brain.* Numerous cavities in white matter, thalami, microgyria, and polygyria.

Diagnostic Procedures. *X-rays of skull. Electroencephalography. CT brain scan. Serum enzymes. Electromyography.*

Therapy. None.

Prognosis. Poor; all patients died within a few months.

BIBLIOGRAPHY. Bruck F: Ueber einen Fall von congenitaler Makroglossie, combiniert mit allgemeiner wahrer Muskelhypertrophie und Idiotie. Dtsch Med Wochenschr 15:229–232, 1889

De Lange C: Congenital hypertrophy of muscles, extrapyramidal motor disturbances and mental deficiency. Am J Dis Child 48:243–268, 1934

Adams RD, Victor M: Principles of Neurology, 3rd ed, p 1096. New York, McGraw-Hill, 1985

BRUNAUER'S

Synonyms. Keratoderma palmoplantaris striata; palmoplatar keratoderma striatum; Furs'.

Symptoms and Signs. Various patterns. Both sexes. Onset 2nd or 3rd decade. Diffuse striate thickening of palms and soles and islands of keratoderma at pressure points. Occasionally associated corneal opacities, pilitorti, sensorineural hearing loss, hypohidrosis, dental abnormalities.

Etiology. Autosomal dominant inheritance.

Therapy. Trials with retinoic acid.

Prognosis. Benign condition.

BIBLIOGRAPHY. Brunauer SR: Zur Symptomatologie und Histologie der kongenitalen Dyskeratosen. Dermatol Z 42:6–26, 1925

Rook A, Wilkinson DS, Ebling FJG, et al: Textbook of Dermatology, 4th ed, p 1457. Oxford, Blackwell Scientific Publications, 1986

BRUNS'

Synonym. Postural change.

Symptoms. Sudden development of attacks of vertigo, headache, and vomiting on change of posture of head (extension more than flexion). Freedom from symptoms between attacks. Amaurosis; flashes of light; irregular breathing; occasionally, syncope with apnea.

Signs. Constant anterior flexion of head at midline or with lateral flexion. Neck muscles contracted firmly. Tachycardia.

Etiology. Organic lesion of 4th ventricle or adjacent structures. Tumor, cysticercosis, colloid cyst. Obstruction of flow of cerebrospinal fluid or disturbance of vestibular mechanism or both.

Pathology. See Etiology.

Diagnostic Procedures. *X-ray of skull. Angiography. Electroencephalography. Spinal tap* (with caution). *CT brain scan.*

Therapy. Neurosurgery if feasible.

Prognosis. Depends on etiology.

BIBLIOGRAPHY. Bruns O: Neuropathologische Demonstrationen. Neurol Centrabl 21:561–567, 1902

Alpers BJ, Yaskin HE: The Bruns' syndrome. J Nerv Ment Dis 100:115–134, 1944

Grinker RR, Sahs AL: Neurology, 6th ed, p 592. Springfield, Ill, CC Thomas, 1966

BRUSA-TORRICELLI

Synonyms. Aniridia-Wilms' tumor; Miller's. See also Beckwith-Wiedemann.

Symptoms and Signs. Both sexes affected; more frequent in males. Congenital sporadic aniridia (see). Nephroblastoma, which develops before the age of 3 years. Associated frequently: cataract and glaucoma; mental retardation; microcephaly; growth retardation; genitourinary anomalies (hypospadias, cryptorchidism); external ear malformation; Seldom; facial dysmorphism; umbilical and inguinal hernias.

Etiology. Unknown. Aniridia always sporadic (with rare exception). Wilms' tumor (40% congenital; 60% sporadic). The association is probably genetic, of autosomal dominant type or dependent from chromosomal deletion (11 p 13). Environmental factors can not be excluded in initiating germinal and the postzygotic mutations.

Pathology. See Aniridia. *Nephroblastoma.* Cells and tissue suggesting abortive renal elements of mesoderm origin.

Diagnostic Procedures. See Aniridia. *X-rays of abdomen. Retrograde pyelogram. Kidney scan.*

Therapy. Surgery. Chemotherapy.

Prognosis. Poor.

BIBLIOGRAPHY. Brusa P, Torricelli C: Nefroblastoma di Wilms ed affezioni renali congenite nelle casistiche dell' IIPAI di Milano. Minerva Pediatr 5:457–463, 1953

Miller RW, Fraumeni JF, Manning MD: Association of Wilm's tumor with aniridia, hemihypertrophy and other congenital malformation. New Eng J Med 270:922–927, 1964

François J, Concke D, Coppieters R: Aniridia Wilm's tumor syndrome. Ophthalmologica 174:35–39, 1977

Riccardi VM, Hittner HM, Strong LC, et al: Wilm's tumor with aniridia/iris dysplasia and apparently normal chromosomes. J Pediatr 100:574–577, 1982

Turleau C, De Grouchy J, Nihoul-Fekete C, et al: Del 11 p 13 nephroblastoma without aniridia. Hum Genet 67:455–456, 1984

BRUSHFIELD-WYATT

Symptoms and Signs. Trigeminal port-wine lesion with calcified angioma in cerebral hemisphere. See Wyburn-Mason's.

BIBLIOGRAPHY. Brushfield T, Wyatt W: Hemiplegie associated with extensive naevus and mental defect. Br J Child Dis 24:98–106, 1927

Brinton BD: Brushfield-Wyatt syndrome. Proc R Soc Med 26:846–847, 1933

BRUTON'S

Synonyms. Sex-linked agammaglobulinemia; X-linked agammaglobulinemia.

Symptoms and Signs. Appear only in males; appear at 5 to 6 months of age. Severe infections. In about 50% rheumatoid arthritislike manifestation (large joints). High frequency of atopic eczema; poisoning; allergic rhinitis; asthenia.

Etiology. Unknown; sex-linked recessive inheritance.

Pathology. Thymus normal; plasma cells absent; lack of tonsils, appendix, and Peyer's patches.

Diagnostic Procedures. *Blood.* Complete absence of all types of immunoglobin; normal cellular immunity.

Therapy. Antibiotic and gammaglobulin (monthly intervals).

Prognosis. Death delayed by treatment, but inevitable in late infancy, early childhood usually by pulmonary infection.

BIBLIOGRAPHY. Lederman HM, Winkelstein JA: X-linked agammaglobulinemia: an analysis of 96 patients. Medicine 64:145–156, 1985

Bruton OC: Agammaglobulinemia. Pediatrics 9:722–728, 1952

Rosen FS: Genetic defects in gamma globulin synthesis. In Stanbury JB, Wyngaarden JB, Fredrickson DS, et al: The Metabolic Basis of Inherited Disease, 5th ed, p 1921. New York, McGraw-Hill, 1983

BUCCOLINGUAL MASTICATORY

Synonyms. Tardive dyskinesia.

Symptoms and Signs. In patients (0.5–40%) assuming neuroleptics from youth. Stereotyped involuntary tongue protrusion, lip smacking, puckering, and chewing. Associated can be chorea, athetosis, dystonia, myoclonus, tics, and facial grimacing. Movements are accentuated in stress and disappear during sleep.

Etiology. Extrapyramidal effects of neuroleptics. Dopamine receptor hypersensitivity.

Therapy. Withdrawal of neuroleptic.

Prognosis. Variable. Slow remission of signs or permanent tardive dyskinesia.

BIBLIOGRAPHY. Jeste D, Plotking SG, Sinha S, et al: Tardive dyskinesia: reversible and persistent. Arch Gen Psychiatr 36:585–590, 1979

Burke RE: Tardive dyskinesia: current clinical issue. Neurology 34:1348–1353, 1984

BUCHANAN'S

Synonym. Truncus arteriosus.

Symptoms. Slight male predominance; onset in first week of life or early infancy. Dyspnea; recurrent respiratory infections; failure to thrive.

Signs. Normal birth weight. Cyanosis or dusky hue on crying or during efforts (nonconstant). Murmur (becomes evident with onset of syptomatology) harsh, systolic, at the base and left sternal edge; over upper sternum continuous bruit; clear and loud second sound; thrill maximal over base.

Etiology. Congential heart malformation, possibly viral etiology; some familiar cases reported.

Pathology. Unique great artery originating from the base of the heart and providing the systemic, pulmonary, and coronary circulation. Three varieties distinguished: (1) undivided aorta and pulmonary trunk with a single valve; (2) aortic trunk without pulmonary valve, main pulmonary artery, or branches; (3) undivided aorta and pulmonary trunk with two normal semilunar valves.

Diagnostic Procedures. *Blood.* Polycythemia *Electrocardiography.* Right axis deviation. *X-rays.* Cardiomegaly; concave shadow at left of sternum; absence of pulmonary conus; increase in pulmonary vascularization. *Angiography.* See Pathology. *Catheterization.* Shunt at aortic, pulmonary areas. *Two-dimensional echocardiography.*

Therapy. Surgical correction.

Prognosis. Mortality 25%. Average survival poor when large pulmonary arterial branches originate from short main pulmonary artery. Longevity if pulmonary arteries are small. If pulmonary circulation regulated, occasionally, survival into 3rd or 4th decade.

BIBLIOGRAPHY. Buchanan G: Malformation of the heart; undivided truncus arteriosus; heart otherwise troubled. Trans Pathol Soc Lond 15:89–91 1864

Ebert PA: Truncus arteriosus in Glenn WL, Banc AE, Geha AS, et al: Thoracic and Cariovascular Surgery, p 785. Appleton-Century-Crofts, Norwalk, Conn, 1983

Hurst J: The Heart, 6th ed, p 671. New York, McGraw-Hill, 1986

BUCKEY'S

Synonym. Hyperimmunoglobulinemia E.

Symptoms. From birth. Eczema with staphylococcal infection. Respiratory distress. Bronchopneumopathies. Suppurating lymphoadenopathies.

Etiology. Unknown.

Pathology. Pulmonary abscesses. Mycotic or staphyloccocal.

Diagnostic Procedures. *Blood.* IgE over 5000 Ul/ml. Eosinophilia. Neutrophils increased. Polynucleates: defect of chemotaxis.

Therapy. Antibiotics. Antimycotics.

Prognosis. Poor. Repeated infections.

BIBLIOGRAPHY. Buckley RH, Wrag BB, Belmaker EZ: Extreme hyperimmunoglobulinemia E and undue susceptibility to infections. Pediatrics 49:59–70, 1972

Buckey RH, Sampsom HA: The hyperimmunoglobulinemia E syndrome. In Franklin EC (ed): Clinical Immunology Update, pp 147–162. Edinburgh, Churchill Livingston, 1981

BUCKLED INNOMINATE ARTERY

Synonyms. Innominate artery kinking; kinked innominate artery; innominate artery buckling.

Symptoms. Occur usually in middle-aged, obese women with hypertension. Painless; occasionally intermittent swelling on left side of neck. Swelling and gurgling sensation in the left side of neck occasionally are also observed.

Etiology. Buckling of innominate artery that compresses the left innominate vein against sternum.

Pathology. Loss of elasticity of artery, and buckling of innominate artery.

Diagnostic Procedures. *Angiography.* To differentiate from arteriovenous fistula, cervical pseudoaneurysm, superior vena cava syndrome, subclavian, and axillary vein thrombosis. *Ultrasound techniques and arteriography employing digital subtraction imaging.*

Therapy. Surgery not necessary.

Prognosis. Good.

BIBLIOGRAPHY. Smith KS: The kinked innominate vein. Br Heart J 22:110–116, 1960
Coppola ED, Seller R: Isolated distention of the left external jugular vein; a clinical sign of the syndrome of the buckled innominate artery. Ann Surg 167:586–589, 1968
Smith RB, Perdue GD Jr: Aortic arch syndromes. In Lindsay J Jr, Hurst JW: The Aorta, p 225. New York, Grune & Stratton, 1979

BUDD-CHIARI

Synonyms. Chiari's II: hepatic vein thrombosis; liver veins occlusion; Rokitansky's; hepatic veins thrombosis von Rokitansky's I.

Symptoms. More common in males. *Acute.* Sudden abdominal epigastric pain with nausea and vomiting. *Chronic.* Gradual and intermittent symptomatology and signs.

Signs. Progessive tender hepatomegaly; ascites; edema of legs; abdominal collateral vein distentions; mild splenomegaly. Occasionally jaundice and hermorrhages from esophageal varices.

Etiology. Acute or chronic obstruction of major hepatic veins by thrombus or tumor. Reported after taking oral contraceptives or pyrrolizidine alkaloid (selzer). Role of congenital malformation discussed. In two-thirds of patients, etiology unknown.

Pathology. Hepatomegaly; smooth, cirrhotic liver; with irregular fatty degeneration; centrilobular atrophy, hepatic veins closed; ascites; congestive splenomegaly.

Diagnostic Procedures. *Liver function tests.* Moderate increase of bilirubin; alkaline phosphates high. *Biopsy of liver.* Portal pressure measurement. *Isotope liver scan. Arteriography and venography.* Selective.

Therapy. Surgery when indicated. Fibrinolytic agents, anticoagulants, diuretics. Peritoneovenous shunt. Liver transplantation when indicated.

Prognosis. *Acute.* Death possibly in few days. *Chronic.* Survivial for months, possibly years.

BIBLIOGRAPHY. Budd G: On Diseases of the Liver. London, Churchill, 1852
Chiari H: Ueber dei selbstandige Phlebitis obliterans der Haupstamme der Venae hepaticae als Todesurasche. Beitr Pathol Anat 26:1–8, 1899
Selzer G, Parker RGF: Senecio poisoning exhibiting as Chiari's syndrome: a report of 12 cases. Am J Path 27:885–907, 1951
Perdue GD, Smith RB III: Diseases in the peripheral veins and the venae cavae. In Hurst J (ed): The Heart, 6th ed. New York, McGraw-Hill, 1986

BUERGER'S

Synonyms. Endarteritis obliterans; presenile gangrene; thromboangiitis obliterans; Winiwarter-Manteuffel-Buerger.

Symptoms. Occur almost exclusively in males; larger incidence between 28 and 50 years of age. Severe pain of extremities at rest (first symptom in four-fifths of cases), resembling that of intermittent claudication, which usually causes insomnia. Vasomotor manifestations frequent: cold sensation at extremities; cold hypersensibility; sudden sweating; dyshidrosis, occasionally, Raynaud's phenomenon (see).

Signs. At onset, discrepancy between intensity of symptoms and scarse physical signs; occasionally, however, these signs may represent the first manifestation: trophic changes, ulcerations, and gangrene. It is interesting that the course is represented by progression and regression of signs. Frequent migratory phlebitis, preceding or accompanying arterial disease. Absence or decreased dorsal pedal or posterior dorsal pulse or both; normal proximal pulse.

Etiology. Unknown. Several hypothesis considered: (1) Tobacco intoxication (2) cold; (3) malnutrition; (4) traumas (to be considered aggravating or favoring agents); (5) infections; (6) collagen disorder; (7) atherosclerosis.

Pathology. Nonsuppurative segmental perivascular reaction, which joins artery, vein, and nerve bundle and
makes their separation difficult. High frequency of involvement of superficial veins; scarce involvement of
deep veins. Segmental red thrombi; frequently, integrity
of inner elastic wall; moderate interstitial fibrosis of the
media; constantly present, adventitous sclerosis.

Diagnostic Procedures. *Blood.* Usually, normal value
of glycemia and of lipidic pattern; frequently increased
viscosity and platelet number *X-rays.* Occasionally, osteoporosis and osteomyelitis of phalanges. *Angiography.*
Site of lesion always distal, bilateral but not symmetric;
great arterial trunks normal; absence of image of arteriovenous shunts; reduction of arterial caliber. *Vasodilation
tests.* Vasospasm. *Doppler.*

Therapy. Antibiotics (in case of positive direct or indirect demonstration of infections); fibrinolytic and anti-
clotting agents; cortisone or anti-inflammatory agents or
both; local treatment of infections and gangrene; analgesics. Surgery: sympathectomy; arterial reconstructive surgery may be attempted with uncertain results.

Prognosis. Little response to any kinds of treatment except occasionally to the tobacco abstinence, which may
induce remission. Increased incidence of myocardial infarction.

BIBLIOGRAPHY. Buerger L: Thromboangitis obliterans: A
    study of the vascular lesions leading to presenile spon-
    taneous gangrene. Ann J Med Soc 136:567–580, 1908
Young JR: Diseases of peripheral arteries. In Hurst JW
    (ed): The Heart, 6th ed. New York, McGraw-Hill,
    1986

BULLDOG

Synonym. Simpson's dysmorphia.

Symptoms. In males. *Facies.* Large protruding jaw,
wide nasal bridge, upturned nose tip, macroglossia.
Limbs. Broad, short hands and fingers. Broad stocky
body. Normal intelligence.

Etiology. Unknown. X-linked inheritance.

Prognosis. When patients reach adulthood (usual
height above average), they lose some of the clumsiness
and general distinguishing features become less apparent.

BIBLIOGRAPHY. Simpson JL, New M, Laudey S, et al: A
    previously unrecognized X-linked syndrome of dys-
    morphia. Birth Defect Org Art Ser XI (2):18–24, 1973
Behmel A, Plochl E, Rosenkranz W: A new X-linked
    dysplasia gigantism syndrome: identical with the Simp-
    son dysplasia syndrome? Hum Genet 67:409–413,
    1984

BULLOUS ICHTHYOSIFORM HYPERKERATOSIS

Synonyms. Brocq's; ichthyosiform erythroderma (bullous form). See also During-Brocq; epidermolysis hyperkeratosis.

Symptoms and Signs. Both sexes affected; normal at
birth; onset within first 7 days. Rapid repeated eruptions
of bullae, associated with erythema and scaling. From 3rd
month, appearance of hyperkeratotic lesions that become
more evident around third to fourth year, in the form of
warty streaks in flexure zones. Nails and hair normal.
General good health usually preserved.

Etiology. Unknown; autosomal dominant inheritance.

Pathology. Hyperkeratosis and acanthosis. Granular
layer and stratum Malpighii show marked intracellular
and intercellular edema; nuclear pyknosis; perivascular
inflammatory infiltrate in dermis. *Electromicroscopy.* Concentric unbroken shells of abnormal tonofilaments around
the nucleus.

Therapy. Symptomatic.

Prognosis. Seldom, death in infancy from very severe
forms. Generally, good health and normal development.
Bullous eruptions become less and less frequent and stop
in 80% of cases before adult life. Hyperkeratotic lesions
persist for life.

BIBLIOGRAPHY. Brocq L: Erythrodermie congenitale ich-
    thyosiform avec hyperepidermotrophie. Ann Dermatol
    Syph 3:1, 1902
Golbus MS, Sagebiel RW, Filly RA, et al: Prenatal diag-
    nosis of congenital bullous ichthyosiform erythroderma
    (epidermolytic hyperkeratosis) by fetal skin biopsy.
    New Engl J Med 302:93–95, 1980

BUREAU-BARRIERE

Synonyms. Acquired perforating foot ulcer; acquired
sensory radicular neuropathy. See Nelaton's, Morvan's,
Trophic ulcer foot.

Symptoms and Signs. Prevalent in males (almost exclusively); onset in adulthood. Usually, in people with
chronic malnutrition; frequently, in alcoholics, Physical
trauma to feet frequently contributory factor. Transient
bullous lesion resulting in single or multiple perforating
indolent ulcer of soles. Floor of ulcer granulating and
crusting. Progressive deformity of foot with shortening
and broadening to assume a cuboid shape. Cyanosis and
hyperhidrosis of affected foot. Sensory changes: socklike
distribution, loss of temperature sensibility; touch and

pain usually only partly affected. Deep sense preserved. Tendon and plantar reflexes normal.

Etiology. Peripheral trophic changes of nervous origin; protein deficiency; alcoholism.

Pathology. *Spinal cord.* Absence of syringomyelia *Peripheral nerves.* Posterior roots and sciatic trunk degenerative changes.

Diagnostic Procedures. *X-ray of foot.* Early arthritis of interphalangeal or metatarsal phalangeal joint; later absorption of bone; partial dislocation. *Oscillometry. Arteriography. Blood.* Possible positivity of liver function test. *Spinal fluid.* Normal. *Nonpictorial tracer techniques, Doppler, thermography.*

Therapy. Protection from shearing forces: plaster cast or "Scotchcast Boot."* Surgical intervention (increases deformity); sympathectomy; diet; vitamins.

Prognosis. Chronic course; increasing deformity, bouts of inflammation; elimination of bone sequestra. Good response to sympathectomy.

BIBLIOGRAPHY. Bureau Y, Barriére H: Ulcerating and multilating trophic lesions of the lower limbs. Br J Dermatol 70:372–377, 1958

Burden AC, Jones GR, Jones R, Blandford RL: Use of the "Scotchcast Boot" in treating diabetic foot ulcers. Br Med J 286:1555–1557, 1983

BURGER-GRUTZ

Synonyms. Familial lipoprotein lipase deficiency; lipoid hepatosplenomegalia; essential hyperlipemia; fat-induced hyperlipemia; familial hyperchylomicronemia; hyperlipoproteinemia type I; LPL.

Symptoms. Both sexes affected; age of detection usually early childhood; onset as soon as child begins intake of fat. Attacks of abdominal pain; malaise and anorexia; no nausea or vomiting. Fever may occur with attacks.

Signs. Appearance of xanthomas (30%) of eruptive type at any site including mucous membranes—yellow nodules on erythematous base. Fading and completely disappearing in a few weeks. Signs of peritoneal irritation. Hepatosplenomegaly, tenderness in splenic region. Lipemia retinalis. Heterozygotes only have recurrent acute pancreatitis episodes.

Etiology. Autosomal recessive inheritance. Decreased activity of lipoprotein lipase causing a defect of removal of chylomicrons from circulation. Autosomal recessive inheritance. Absence (homozygotes) or decreased activity

(heterozygotes) of lipoprotein lipase which clears chylomicrons from plasma.

Pathology. Skin xanthomas; foam cells found in all tissues rich in reticulum cells (e.g., bone marrow; spleen; liver). Pancreatitis.

Diagnostic Procedures. *Blood.* Characteristic aspect (white-cap top; clear below) of plasma when blood left at 4°C. Type I hyperlipoproteinemia. Very low-density lipoproteins (VLDL), low-density lipoproteins (LDL)(?), high-density lipoproteins (HDL) normal or decreased; cholesterol increased; tryglycerides increased. Attacks reproduced by ingestion of fat. Leukocytosis during attacks *Liver function test and glucose tolerance tests.* Normal.

Therapy. Decrease fat intake to 20 to 25% of caloric intake. Glycerides of medium-chain fatty acids available to substitute for regular fat.

Prognosis. This group of patients seems to be remarkably immune to atheromatous complications when compared with other types of hyperlipemia groups. Particular danger due to repeated pancreatitis.

BIBLIOGRAPHY. Bürger M, Grütz O: Ueber hepatosplenomegale Lipoidose mit xanthomatsen Veränderungen in Haut und Schleimhaut. Arch Dermatol Syph 166:542–575, 1932

Fredrickson DS, Goldstein JL, Brown MS: The familial hyperlipoproteinemias. In Stanbury JB, Wyngaarden JB, Fredrickson DS: The Metabolic Basis of Inherited Disease, 4th ed, p 608. New York, McGraw-Hill, 1978.

Nikka EA: Familial lipoprotein lipase deficiency and related disorders of chylomicron metabolism. In Stanbury JB, Wyngaarden JB, Fredrickson DS, et al: The Metabolic Basis of Inherited Disease, 5th ed, p 622. New York, McGraw-Hill, 1983

BURKE'S (R.M.)

Synonyms. De Martini-Balestra; lobar lung atrophy; progressive pulmonary dystrophy. See also Vanishing lung syndromes.

Symptoms. Onset slow or rapid, and symptoms related to rapidity of progression. Cough; dyspnea; pain in the chest (if rapid evolution).

Signs. Reduction or absence of breath sound over involved areas. Wheezing; diaphragmatic depression.

Etiology. Formation or expansion of blebs or bullae in lungs. Various degree of obstruction causing pulmonary emphysema.

Pathology. Pulmonary emphysema; presence of blebs or bullae or both.

---

*3M UK-Ltd, Lughborough, Leichestershire, UK

Diagnostic Procedures. *X-rays.* Considered a radiologic syndrome and represented by progressive decrease of pulmonary density, compression or fanning out of bronchi.

Therapy. If localized bullae, consider resection.

Prognosis. Generally poor.

BIBLIOGRAPHY. Burke RM: Vanishing lungs: a case reported of bullous emphysema. Radiology 28:367–371, 1937
Martini A de, Balestra G: Sindromi di rarefazione polmonare con particolare riguardo alla atrofia polmonare idiopatica. Minerva Med 2:917–926, 1951
Fraser RG: Diagnosis of Diseases of the Chest, p 541. Philadelphia, WB Saunders, 1977

BURKITT'S

Synonyms. African lymphoma; maxillary lymphosarcoma; nonleukemic lymphoma.

Symptoms and Signs. Slightly prevalent in males. Present in central equatorial Africa, cases reported from other non-African areas (United States, Colombia, India). Onset in infancy to adolescence.

Tumor mass of jaw (approximately 50%), salivary glands, cervical lymph nodes, or abdomen. In Africa, facial bone involvement prevalent. (In other countries, abdominal tumors predominate.)

Etiology. It is not established if this syndrome represents a different pathologic entity from conventional lymphosarcoma. Causally related to Epstein-Barr virus (mechanism still unknown). Chromosomal alterations reported (8, 2, 14, 22).

Pathology. Jaw; liver; mostly visceral lymph nodes. Microscopically, lymphoblastic neoplastic cells and actively phagocyting histiocytes. Absence of leukemia. Criteria for classification of this form are: (1) histology as described; (2) clinical presentation and tumor localization similar to that reported for African cases.

Diagnostic Procedures. *Biopsy of tumor; bone marrow. Blood.* Negative for leukemia. In Africans, levels of IgG increased and IgM decreased. In Americans, IgG normal or decreased and IgM normal.

Therapy. X-rays and antiblastic chemotherapeutic agents. Particularly responsive to cyclophosphamide alone or in combination (vincristine, methotrexate and cytosine arabinoside).

Prognosis. More than 50% complete remission after first dose of cyclophosphamide. Dissemination does not exclude a good prognosis. Spontaneous remission also reported.

BIBLIOGRAPHY. Burkitt D: A sarcoma involving the jaws in African children. Br J Surg 46:218–223, 1958
Burkitt DP: The discovery of Burkitt's lymphoma. Cancer 51:1777–1786, 1983

BURNETT'S

Synonyms. Milk-alkali; milk drinker's; milk poisoning.

Symptoms. Weakness; headache; dizziness; depression; nausea; vomiting; anorexia.

Signs. Conjunctivitis; ocular band keratitis; mental confusion or psychosis.

Etiology. Excessive intake of milk or soluble alkali as in therapy for peptic ulcer.

Pathology. Nephrocalcinosis; deposit of calcium in different tissues.

Diagnostic Procedures. *Blood.* Hypercalcemia; hyperazotemia; milk alkalosis; alkaline phosphatases normal or slightly elevated *Urine.* Calcium and phosphates within normal ranges *X-ray.* Nephrocalcinosis; calcification periarticular and in other tissues.

Therapy. Discontinuation of milk and alkali; intravenous administration of sodium chloride.

Prognosis. Recovery with treatment.

BIBLIOGRAPHY. Burnett C, Commons RR, Albright F, et al: Hypercalcemia without hypercalcuria or hypophosphatemia, calcinosis and renal insufficiency: a syndrome following prolonged intake of milk and alkali. New Engl J Med 240:787–794, 1949
Cameron AJ, Spence MP: Chronic milk-alkali syndrome after prolonged excessive intake of antacid tablets. Br Med J 3:656–657, 1967
Bockus HL: The therapy of peptic ulcer. In Bockus HL: Gastroenterology, 3rd ed, vol I, p 687. Philadelphia, WB Saunders, 1974

BURNING TONGUE

Synonym. Glossodynia.

Symptoms. Prevalent in middle-aged or elderly women. Especially when tired or promoted by eating hot or spicy foods. Patients complain of spontaneous intense burning pain of tongue. Occasionally also report unpleasant taste. Cancerphobia.

Signs. None.

Etiology. Psychological origin. Neurologic disorder (?).

Pathology. None.

Diagnostic Procedures. *Blood test. X-ray.* Gastrointestinal. To rule out reflux from hiatus hernia.

Therapy. Medical measures useless. If severe symptoms, psychiatric help.

Prognosis. Persistence of symptoms in spite of reassurance and treatment.

BIBLIOGRAPHY. Ziskin DE, Moulton R: Glossodynia: study of idiopathic orolingual pain. J Am Dent Assoc 33:1422–1432, 1946
Karshan M: Studies in etiology of idiopathic orolingual paresthesias. Am J Dig Dis 19:341–344, 1952
Rook A, Wilkinson DS, Ebling FJG, et al: Textbook of Dermatology, 4th ed, p 2120. Oxford, Blackwell Scientific Publications, 1986

BURNOUT

Synonym. Chronic stress syndrome.

Symptoms and Signs. Impairment of short-term memory, decreased memory storage, decreased attention span, tendency to view minor problems as major, racing thoughts, negative thoughts that stick in the mind, rigid and stubborn positions, feelings of being victimized, loss of sense of humor, demanding behavior; increased muscular tension, tremulousness, palpitations, a feeling of pulsation in the body, epigastric gnawing, retrosternal oppression; self-medication, sometimes drug addiction.

Etiology. Chronic stress that stems from various factors such as low pay, long hours, dead-end career, too much paperwork, inadequate training, no appreciation by clients or by supervisors, powerlessness.

Therapy. Psychiatric counseling; taking the person out of the environment (forced vacation); restructuring the life-style to reduce stress to tolerable levels; marital, family, recreational, economic, and work adjustments.

Prognosis. Good.

BIBLIOGRAPHY. Freundenberger HJ: The staff burnout syndrome in alternative institutions. Psychother Res Pract 12:73–82, 1975
Wilson WP: Burnout and other stress syndromes. South Med J 79:1327–1330, 1986

BUSCHKE-FISHER-BRAUER

Synonym. Keratosis palmoplantaris papulosa. See Greither's.

Symptoms and Signs. Both sexes. Female less severe manifestations. Keratosis on palms and plants with papular aspect.

Etiology. Autosomal dominant inheritance.

BIBLIOGRAPHY. Schirren V, Dinger R: Untersuchungen ber keratosis palmoplantaris papulosa. Arch Klin Exp Derm 221:481–495, 1965
Salomon T, Stalic V, Lazovic-Tepavac O, et al: Peculiar findings in a family with keratoderma palmo-plantaris papulosa, Buschke-Fisher-Brauer. Hum Genet 60:314–319, 1982

BUSCHKE-OLLENDORFF

Synonyms. Curth's; dermatofibrosis lenticularis disseminata (Schreus'); osteopoikilosis; dermo-osteopoikilosis; osteopathia condensans disseminata; Albers-Schönberg's II.

Symptoms. Both sexes affected. Cutaneous signs may appear from the second decade, but, usually, become incidentally evident in adult life. Asymptomatic.

Signs. Firm, small, skin-colored or yellowish nodules (less than 1 cm in diameter) located on posterior aspect of thighs and buttocks, occasionally on arms and trunk, never on the face. They are usually arranged in streaks, not in constant relation with distribution of bone lesions. (See Osteodermopoikilosis.) Keloids occur with high intensity.

Etiology. Hyperplasia of collagen in the corium. Autosomal dominant heredity. This syndrome represents one manifestation of osteodermopoikilosis where both the components, skin lesions (Schreus') and bone lesions (Albers-Schönberg's I, see), are evident.

Pathology. Skin patterns varying from disordered arrangement of fibroblasts and collagen fibers to histocytoma characteristics.

Diagnostic Procedures. *Biopsy of skin. X-ray.* Skeletal survey. For differential diagnosis of osteoblastic metastasis of skeleton.

Therapy. None.

Prognosis. Benign; once complete development reached no further changes.

BIBLIOGRAPHY. Buschke A, Ollendorff H: Ein Fall von Dermatosfibrosis lenticularis disseminata und Osteopathia condensans disseminata. Dermatol Wochenschr 86:257–262, 1928
Albers-Schönberg H: Eine seltene, bisher nicht bekannte Strukturanomalie des Skelettes. Fortsch Geb Roentgenstrahlen 23:174, 1915
Stieda A: Ueber umschriebene Knochenverdichtungen im Bereich der substantia spongiosa im Röntgenbilde Beitr Z Klin Chir 45:700–703, 1905

Young LW, Gershman I, Simon PR: Osteopoikilosis: familial documentation. Am J Dis Child 134:415–416, 1980

BUSCHKE'S I

Synonym. Scleredema adultorum.

Symptoms and Signs. Prevalent in females, onset at all ages (29% before 10, 22% between 10 and 20 years of age). History of preceding infection (days or weeks before). Moderate fever, malaise, myalgia, and arthralgia. Appearance of symmetric skin induration, nonpitting with sharp outline that separates it from normal skin on neck or face, difficulty in opening mouth; occasionally difficulty in swallowing. Skin induration later involves shoulders, arms, trunk, seldom other areas. Occasionally, pleuropericardial effusion; eyes and parotid involvement.

Etiology. Unknown; possibly lymphatic channel obstruction or hormone (estrogen) derangement.

Pathology. Epidermis normal. Dermal swelling and degenerative changes of collagen, spaces, and fenestration; metachromatic stain; increase in mast cells.

Diagnostic Procedures. *Biopsy. Blood.* Normal, except moderate increase of sedimentation rate. Lupus erythematosis (LE) IgA, IgG paraprotein reported; antistreptolysin O titer increased. *Electrocardiography.* Negative. Reversible changes.

Therapy. Trial with cortical steroids, thyroid hormone.

Prognosis. Usually, spontaneous remission in a few months, occasionally persistence for years.

BIBLIOGRAPHY. Piffard HG: An Elementary Treatise on Diseases of the Skin, for the Use of Students and Practitioners. London, Macmillan, 1876
Buschke A: Ueber Scleroedem. Berl Klin Wockensckr 39:955–957, 1902
Rook A, Wilkinson DS, Ebling FJG, et al: Textbook of Dermatology, 4th ed, pp 1374–1376. Oxford, Blackwell Scientific Publications, 1986

BUSQUET'S

Synonyms. Metatarsal periostitis; osteoperiostitis ossificans metatarsal. See Epiphyseal syndromes.

Symptoms and Signs. Pain in foot enhanced by walking.

Etiology. Unknown.

Pathology. Osteoperiostitis of metatarsal bones and exostosis.

BIBLIOGRAPHY. Busquet B: L'Ostéo-périostite ossifiante des metatarsiens. Rev Chir 17:1065–1099, 1897

BUSSIERE-ESCOBAR

Synonyms. Obsolete. Multiple pterygium; Escobar. See also Arthrogryposis.

Symptoms and Signs. Small stature; ptosis of eyelids, canthal folds, micrognathia; pterygia of neck, axillae, elbows, and knees; camptodactyly, syndactyly. *Feet.* Equinovarus or rocker bottom. Cryptorchidism; absence of labia major. Anomalies of vertebra or limbs.

Etiology. Autosomal recessive.

Therapy. Surgical.

Prognosis. Good *quoad vitam*.

BIBLIOGRAPHY. Escobar V, Bixler D, Gleiser S, et al: Multiple pterygium syndrome. Am J Dis Child 132:609–611, 1978

BYLER'S

Synonyms. Fatal familial, intrahepatic cholestasis; familial intrahepatic jaundice cholestasis.

Symptoms. Both sexes affected in members of an Amish family (named Byler; other ethnic origins reported); present from early infancy. Recurrent bouts of jaundice often associated with infection episodes. Epistaxis; pruritus, foul-smelling stools. Stunted growth.

Signs. Icterus; protuberant abdomen; appearance of chronic illness. Hepatosplenomegaly.

Etiology. Congenital biochemical abnormality with recurrent cholestasis due to defect of excretion of conjugated bile salts. Autosomal recessive inheritance.

Pathology. Liver cirrhosis.

Diagnostic Procedures. *Blood.* Hyperbilirubinemia; high serum alkaline phosphatase; normal or low serum cholesterol; hypoprothrombinemia *Stool.* Light color; steatorrhea. *Urine.* Dark; hyperbilirubinuria.

Therapy. Symptomatic phenobarbital, cholestyramine, and medium triglyceride formula. Vitamin E. Liver transplantation when indicated.

Prognosis. Symptomatic improvement with treatment, but no effect on progressive nature of disease. Death at ages varying between 17 months and 8 years.

BIBLIOGRAPHY. Clayton RJ, Iber FL, Buebner BH: Byler's disease: fatal familial intrahepatic cholestasis in an Amish kindred (abst). J Pediatr 67:1025–1028, 1965

Sokol RJ, Guggenheim MA, Iannaccone ST, et al: Improved neurologic function after long-term correction of vitamin E deficiency in children with chronic familial intrahepatic cholestasis. Acta Neuropath 58:187–192, 1985

BYWATERS'

Synonyms. Muscular necrosis compression; ischemic muscular necrosis; crush.

Symptoms. Pain where trauma has occurred; thirst; nausea; oliguria; anuria; shock.

Signs. Signs of injury; hypertension; signs of moderate or severe shock.

Etiology. Extensive trauma of soft tissue; prolonged tissue ischemia (as from use of parachute harness).

Pathology. Injured muscles; loss of pigments. Kidney pigmentary casts occluding tubules with degeneration of tubular epithelium.

Diagnostic Procedures. *Blood.* Hyperkalemia; hyponatremia; hyperazotemia (maximum between 6th and 9th day following injury). *Urine.* Myoglobinuria; hematuria; proteinuria; glucosuria; pigmentary and granular casts. *Electrocardiography.* Signs of hyperkalemia.

Therapy. Fluid balance and liquid diet, with minimum protein and potassium. If hyperkalemia present, intravenous calcium indicated (better to use cation exchange enemas). If transfusion indicated, drain plasma to remove potassium. If acidosis symptoms are present; small amount of sodium bicarbonate. Hemodialysis with artificial kidney often indicated. When the patient resumes diuresis, liberal amounts of fluid and control of electrolyte balance.

Prognosis. Less severe than in the past because of medical management and prevention of complication; infection; lung edema; cardiac insufficiency.

BIBLIOGRAPHY. Bywaters EGL, Beall D: Crush injuries with impairment of renal function. Br Med J 1:427–432, 1941

Paxson NF, Golub LJ, Hunter RM: The crush syndrome in obstetrics and gynecology. JAMA 131:500–504, 1946

Zuidema GB, Rutherford RB, Balliger WF (eds): The management of trauma, 4th ed. Philadelphia, WB Saunders, 1985

Knochel JP: Rhabdomyolysis and myoglobinuria. Ann Rev Med 33:435–443, 1982

BYWATERS' LESIONS

Symptoms and Signs. Small, painless reddish-brown infarcts on nail folds or maculopapular, hemorrhagic, painful lesions on digital pads.

Etiology. Necrotizing angiitis observed primarily in rheumatoid disease and in many other vasculites.

Therapy. That of the basic disorders. Role of penicillamine to be evaluated.

Prognosis. Lesions first darken, then are extruded. Pitted scarring may result.

BIBLIOGRAPHY. Bywaters ECL: Peripheral vascular obstruction in rheumatoid arthritis and its relationship to other vascular lesions. Ann Rheumat Dis 16:84–103, 1957

C

C-TRIGONOCEPHALY

Synonyms. C syndrome, MCA/MR syndrome; Opitz J.M.

Symptoms and Signs. Anomaly of the anterior cranium and frontal cortex (trigonocephaly), the root of the nose (broad nasal bridge, epicanthus, and short nose), and palate (thick anterior alveolar ridges); abnormalities of the limbs (polysyndactyly, bridged palmar creases, short limbs, and joint dislocations and or contractures); visceral defects (congenital heart defects, cryptorchidism, and abnormal lobulations of the lungs and kidneys). Auricular, mandibular, skin, and genital abnormalities can occur, as well as hypotonia, strabismus, and psychomotor retardation.

Etiology. Autosomal recessive inheritance.

Pathology. In autopsied cases, there has been a suggestion of defective central nervous system myelination.

Diagnostic Procedures. *Chromosome study.* Normal. *X-ray and CT scan.* Anomalies of the skull and face.

Therapy. Neurosurgery; other type of surgery when indicated.

Prognosis. About one half of the cases have died within the first year. All survivors have mental retardation.

BIBLIOGRAPHY. Opitz JM, Johnson RC, McCreadie SR, Smith DW: The C syndrome of multiple congenital anomalies. Birth Defects V (2):161–166, 1969
Opitz JM: C syndrome. Birth Defects Compendium, 2nd ed, pp 160–161. New York, Alan R. Liss, 1979
Antley RM, Sung Hwang D, Theopold W, et al: Further delineation of the C (trigonocephaly) syndrome. Am J Med Genet 9:147–163, 1981

CACCHI-RICCI

Synonyms. Medullary sponge kidney; nephrospongiosis (inaccurate term); precaliceal diffuse canalicular ectasia; sponge kidney (inaccurate term); See Polycystic disease.

Symptoms. Both sexes equally affected; onset of detection from 3 weeks of age to 71 years. Uncomplicated form usually asymptomatic. Pain in loin (38%); colic (28%); nocturnal polyuria (28%); occasional polydipsia.

Signs. Seldom, enlargement of kidneys (observed mostly in children).

Etiology. Unknown; frequently, congenital and familial. Dysembryoplastic origin, comparable to that responsible for polycystic disease (see), or secondary to neonatal obstruction; progressive dystrophy in the collective tubules, analogous to cystic degeneration of mucous membranes. Families reported with autosomal dominant inheritance.

Pathology. Few reports. Precaliceal canalicular ectasia; enlarged medulla and integrity and normal dimension of cortex. Histologic findings in the medulla: cystic tubular dilatation alternated with areas of normal tissue; cysts communicating with excretory tract; basement membrane of ectasic area is thinned.

Diagnostic Procedures. *Blood.* Protein level occasionally elevated; uric acid level increased (in 50% of cases); serum alkaline phosphatase often moderately increased; calcium normal. *Urine.* Proteinuria (50%); blood usually absent, leukocyturia (50%). *Renal function tests.* Usually normal, except for presence of manifest defect in concentrating ability. *X-ray of kidneys.* "Bunches of flowers prolonging the calices." The precaliceal canalicular ectasia defines the condition.

Therapy. Symptomatic. Prevention of urinary infection and dehydration.

Prognosis. Benign clinical course.

BIBLIOGRAPHY. Lenarduzzi G: Reperto pielografico poco comune (dilatazione della vie urinarie intrarenali). Radiol Med (Torino) 26:346, 1939
Cacchi R, Ricci V: Sopra una rara et forse ancora non descritta affezione cistica della piramidi renali (rene a spugna). Atti Soc Ital Urol 21:59, 1948
Litwak A, Hartel-Ulkowska N: La maladie kystique des pyramides rénales (rein en éponge). J Urol Nephrol 70:95–106, 1964
Chamberlin BC, Hagge WW, Stickler GB: Juvenile nephronophthysis and medullary cystic disease. Mayo Clin Proc 52:485–491, 1977

CAFFEY-SILVERMAN

Synonyms. Infantile cortical hyperostoses, Caffey-Smith; DeToni-Silverman-Caffey; hyperplastic hyperostosis; Hyperplastic periostosis; Roske-DeToni-Caffey; Smith-Caffey.

Symptoms. Prevalent in females. Onset in early infancy (less than 5 mo); occasionally, lesion of bone observed radiographically prenatally. Sudden onset; irritability; fever; conjunctivitis; swelling of bones; tenderness and movement limitation of affected parts.

Signs. Sudden swelling of jaw and face (occasionally, swelling starts in extremities and only after a few days involves the face) and other parts of the body. No discoloration, edema, or increase of temperature of skin overlying bone swellings; no lymphadenopathy.

Etiology. Unknown; autosomal dominant inheritance. Collagen disease (?); virus infection (?).

Pathology. Cortical thickening due to normal but immature lamellar bone. No inflammatory changes. In acute stage, periosteum is loose. A gelatinous alteration is present with mitotic figures and mucinous changes extending to neighboring tendons and fascias. Later, muscular necrosis and fibrous change.

Diagnostic Procedures. *Blood.* Moderate anemia; moderate increase of neutrophils; increase in sedimentation rate and of serum phosphatase. *Urine and cerebrospinal fluid.* Normal. *X-ray.* Thickening of cortex of bones involved; thickening or patchy sclerosis remains after remission of acute stage.

Therapy. Symptomatic.

Prognosis. Variable course from complete disappearance of swelling in a few weeks, with or without local relapse or involvement of other bones for months or years, to fatality (rare).

BIBLIOGRAPHY. Caffey J, Silverman WA: Infantile cortical hyperostoses: Preliminary report on a new syndrome. Am J Roentgen 54:1–16, 1945
Caffey J: Infantile cortical hyperostoses: A review of the clinical and radiographic features. Proc R Soc Med 50:347–354, 1956
Emmery L, Timmermans J, Christens J, et al: Familial infantile cortical hyperostosis. Eur J Pediatr 141:56–58, 1983

CAIRNS'

Synonym. Tubercular arachnoiditis–hydrocephalus.

Symptoms and Signs. Occur in children who have survived meningitis. Symptomatology similar to that caused by a posterior fossa neoplasm; communicating or noncommunicating hydrocephalus; occasionally, impaired vision and presence of visual field defects (chiasma lesions); focal symptoms (cerebral cortex lesions).

Etiology. Chronic arachnoiditis following tubercular meningitis (may occur also after other types of meningitis

or spontaneous subarachnoid hemorrhage) caused by intracranial adhesions of leptomeninges.

Pathology. Adhesive leptomeningitis over posterior fossa and chiasma or less frequently involving the cortex. Thick arachnoid with chronic inflammatory cell reaction.

Diagnostic Procedures. *Pneumoencephalography* or *ventriculography* (or both), and *CT brain scan.*

Therapy. Surgery when lesion localized.

Prognosis. Fair with modern medical and surgical methods.

BIBLIOGRAPHY. Cairns H: Surgical aspects of meningitis. Br Med J 1:969–976, 1949
Adams RD, Victor M: Principles of Neurology, 3rd ed, p 512. New York, McGraw-Hill, 1985

CAISSON

Synonyms. Aerobullosis; aeroembolism; bends; chokes; decompression sickness; diver.

Symptoms. Occur in SCUBA divers (and workers in caissons and tunnels) working under high pressures, when brought back without slow decompression to atmospheric pressure; onset possibly hours after decompression. Headache; weakness; nausea; vomiting; vertigo with tinnitus; dyspnea; chokes; nonproductive cough; occasionally paraplegia with paralysis of bladder and bowel; hemiplegia; shock; convulsions; back and articular pains (bends); abdominal pain; pruritus.

Signs. Tachypnea with shallow respiration; shock, hypotension; bradycardia.

Etiology. Bubbles of nitrogen released in the blood and migrating into different tissues.

Pathology. Infarctions of the brain, spinal cord, and other tissues.

Therapy. Prevention by slow decompression. When symptoms occur, rapid recompression followed by slow decompression. Administration of antiaggregating drugs (e.g., acetylsalicylic acid) and corticosteroids.

BIBLIOGRAPHY. Bassoe P: The late manifestations of compressed air disease. Am J Med Sci 165:526–542, 1913
Cockett AT, Pauley SM, Zehl DM, et al: Pathophysiology of bends and decompression sickness: An overview with emphasis on treatment. Arch Surg 114:296–301, 1979
Mebane GY, Dick A, Miller J (eds): Underwater Diving Accident Manual. National Diving Accident Network, Durham (North Carolina), 1981

CALCAREOUS TENDONITIS

Symptoms. Occur in sedentary workers; prevalent in males; age of onset between 35 to 60 years old, right shoulder affected twice as frequently as left shoulder. Pain, tenderness, and limited mobility of shoulder, of different intensities and degrees. Fever only occasionally (in acute attacks).

Signs. Arm voluntarily fixed, adducted to side; forearm flexed, impaired movement of abduction and external rotation in particular. Tenderness on lateral area of humeral head, above insertion of deltoid.

Etiology. Trauma; idiopathic.

Pathology. Inflammation of one or more of rotator tendons with deposition of calcium around the tendon. Supraspinatus most frequently involved.

Diagnostic Procedures. *X-ray*. Calcific deposit in area of tendon involved. *Blood*. Leukocytosis and elevated erythrosedimentation rate only in acute attacks.

Therapy. Rest; analgesics; physical therapy; x-ray therapy; injection of procain or steroids; washing out bursa with saline injection. Treatment has to be conducted according to symptomatology, stressing the simple, conservative measures whenever possible.

Prognosis. Acute symptoms may persist for days. Spontaneous remission (abrupt or gradual) frequent. Subacute and chronic forms may persist longer.

BIBLIOGRAPHY. Justis EJ, Jr: Traumatic disorders. In Crenshaw AH (ed): Campbell's Operative Orthopedics, 7th ed, pp 2250–2252. St. Louis, CV Mosby, 1987

CALCINOSIS UNIVERSALIS

Synonyms. Interstitial calcinosis; metabolic calcinosis; myositis ossificans, progressive; Teutschlaender's.

Symptoms. Both sexes affected (mostly girls); onset during first 2 decades of life. Varies according to extent of abnormal calcium deposition in the skin, subcutaneous tissues, fascia, muscles, nerve sheaths, tendons, and visceral organs (seldom). Vague history of nonspecific fever; weakness; painful, stiff joints.

Signs. Irregularly shaped plaques palpable beneath the skin and in deeper tissues. Most frequently in periarticular locations; seldom involving the joints directly. At first, painless, and overlying skin freely movable and normal; then pain and tenderness develop; finally, necrosis and ulceration of skin with discharge of chalklike material. Sinus tract difficult to heal. Superimposed infections.

Etiology. Unknown; possibly mucopolysaccharides disorder. Reported associated with numerous collagen disorders: scleroderma, dermatomyositis; lupus erythematosus; rheumatoid arthritis; myositis ossificans.

Pathology. Granular deposits of mineral material (apatite crystals) with fibrous reaction of connective tissue; occasional giant cells.

Diagnostic Procedures. *X-ray*. Calcific deposits of various size and shape, mostly as dense lines along course of muscles, tendons, and nerves. *Blood*. Normal. *Urine*. Normal. Differential diagnosis includes studies for parasitic infestations, renal insufficiency, vitamin D intoxication, hyperparathyroidism, hypoparathyroidism, pseudohypoparathyroidism, Burnett's.

Therapy. No specific treatment. Various trials including adrenal steroids, edetate (EDTA), cellulose phosphate, and low calcium diet. Results vary, but usually poor.

Prognosis. Calcium deposits may disappear spontaneously and return in years. Chronic course. Septicemia frequently develops when ulcerations occur.

BIBLIOGRAPHY. Teissier LL: Du diabete phosphatique; recherches et variations des phosphates dans les urines (thesis), p 439. Paris, 1876
Teutschlaender O: Ueber progressive lipogranulomatose der Muskulatur. Klin Wochenschr 14:451–453, 1935
Leistyna JA, Hassan AH: Interstitial calcinosis: Report of a case and a review of the literature. Am J Dis Child 107:96–101, 1964
Rook A, Wilkinson DS, Ebling FJG, et al: Textbook of Dermatology, 4th ed, p 2332. Oxford, Blackwell Scientific Publications, 1986

CAMERA'S

Synonyms. Osteopathic lumbosciatalgia; neuralgic osteopathy.

Symptoms. Occur in middle-aged patients. Pain that may affect practically any bone; intermittent and progressively increasing, sudden onset without apparent cause or following trauma. Difficulty of precise localization because of the diffuse character of pain or of its occasional radiation. Typical exacerbation during night. Contraction of neighboring muscles. Loss of weight. Lack of response to any medical, orthopedic, or physical treatment.

Signs. Absence of bone swelling and change in temperature of overlying skin. Presence of trigger point not larger than 1 cm over affected bone that can be found with the finger tip and better localized with a needle.

Etiology. Localized bone fibrosis and hyperemia.

Pathology. Partial marrow fibrosis; increased number of osteocytes; bone hyperemia.

Diagnostic Procedures. *X-ray.* Negative. Localization of trigger point.

Therapy. Removal of trigger zone of the bone.

Prognosis. Good results with treatment in about 80% of cases.

BIBLIOGRAPHY. Bertola L, Pedrocca A: Osteopatie nevralgiformi lombosciatalgiche a localizzazioni vertebrali e paravertebrali (Sindrome del Camera). Minerva Ortop 4:215–218, 1953

CAMPAILLA-MARTINELLI

Synonym. Acromesomelic dwarfism.

Symptoms and Signs. Normal at birth. Growth deficiences during first year. Frontal prominence, short nose, short distal limbs, coned epiphyses, limited elbow extension. Lower thoracic kyphosis. Large great toe, corneal clouding. Intelligence normal.

Etiology. Autosomal recessive.

BIBLIOGRAPHY. Maroteaux P, Martinelli B, Campailla E: Le nanisme acromesomelique. Presse Med 79:1839–1842, 1971
Campailla E, Martinelli B: Deficit staturale con micromesomelia. Minerva Ortop 22:180–184, 1971
Langer LO, et al: Acromesomelic dwarfism manifestations in childhood. Am J Med Genet 1:87–100, 1977

CAMPTOCORMIA

Synonym. Hysterical back pain.

Symptom. Pain in lumbar area.

Signs. Extreme flexion of spine; normal orthopedic and neurologic findings. Correction of posture on recumbency or by suggestion.

Etiology. Psychological.

BIBLIOGRAPHY. Rockwood CA, Eilert RE: Camptocormia. J Bone Joint Surg 51:553–556, 1969

CAMPTODACTYLY–CLEFT PALATE–CLUB FOOT

Synonyms. Arthrogryposis multiplex congenita, distal, type IIa; Gordon's (H.); Moldenhauer's; Nielson's.

Symptoms and Signs. Both sexes. Camptodactyly, cleft palate, and club foot or minor anomalies of foot. Usually all three anomalies present or one of them can be missing in some members of the families (cleft palate most frequently missing).

Etiology. Unknown. Autosomal dominant inheritance. Penetrance reduced more in females than in males.

BIBLIOGRAPHY. Moldenhauer E: Zur Klinik des Nielsensyndromes. Derm Wschir 150:594–611, 1964
Gordon H, Davies D, Berman MM: Camptodactyly, cleft palate and club foot syndrome showing the autosomal dominant pattern of inheritance. J Med Genet 6:266–279, 1969
Hall JC, Reed SD, Greene G: The distal arthrogryphosis: Delineation of new entities: Review and nosologic discussion. Ann J Med Genet 11:185–239, 1982

CAMPTOMELIC DYSPLASIA I

Synonyms. CMD I; Camptomelic dwarfism.

Symptoms. Both sexes affected; present from birth. Frequent respiratory insufficiency; feeding problems; failure to thrive; severe cerebral deficiency.

Signs. At birth, length reduced; subcutaneous fat scarce. Micromelia; bowed tibiae and femora; cutaneous dimple over tibial bend; fibular hypoplasia; foot deformities. Flat facies; hypertelorism; micrognathia; cleft palate. Thorax narrow; scoliosis. Frequently sexual characteristics abnormal.

Etiology. Unknown; most cases sporadic; autosomal recessive inheritance.

Pathology. Tracheomalacia; various degrees of cerebral malformations.

Diagnostic Procedures. *X-rays.* Skeletal survey. Numerous skeletal malformations of long and flat bones.

Therapy. Generally medical.

Prognosis. Extremely poor. Most patients die from respiratory conditions within the first few weeks of life.

BIBLIOGRAPHY. Bound JP, Finaly HVL, Rose FC: Congenital anterior angulation of the tibia. Arch Dis Child 27:179–184, 1952

Môroteaux P, Spranger JW, Opitz JM, et al: Le syndrome camptomelique. Presse Med 22:1157–1162, 1971

Cooke CT, Mulcahy MT, Cullity GJ, et al: Camptomelic dysplasia with sex reversal: Morphological and cytogenetic studies of a case. Pathology 17:526–529, 1985

CAMPTOMELIC DYSPLASIA II

Synonyms. CMD II, camptomelic–long-limb type.

Symptoms and Signs. See Camptomelic Dysplasia I except for long limbs.

Etiology. May be autosomal recessive. Effect of drugs on embryo. Questioned the difference from CMD I.

BIBLIOGRAPHY. Khajavi A, Lachman R, Rimoin D, et al: Heterogeneity in the camptomelic syndromes: Long and short varieties. Radiology 120:641–647, 1976

Spranger J: Advances in bone dysplasia. Sixth Int Congr Hum Genet, Jerusalem, 1981

CAMURATI-ENGELMANN'S

Synonyms. Progressive diaphyseal dysplasia; Engelmann's; osteopathia hyperostotica multiplex infantilis; Ribbing's; multiple epiphyseal dysplasia tarda (type Ic); Lehman-Ribbing-Mueller; MEDT (Ic); Mueller-Ribbing-Clémant.

Symptoms. Both sexes affected. Manifestation onset before age 30, often before age 10. Severe bone pain in the legs. Delayed walking; failure to gain weight; anorexia; headaches; deafness; diplopia; pain; weakness of legs; widebased gait.

Signs. Underdevelopment; elongation of legs; atrophy of muscles; bilateral symmetric fusiform enlargement of diaphyses of long bones; genu varum; genu valgum; coxa valga; scoliosis. Hypogonadism; hepatosplenomegaly; various ocular findings (exophthalmos; hypertelorism; cataract; papilledema). Less frequently, changes also in flat bones, ribs, and pelvis. Face bones unaffected. (See Craniodiaphyseal dysostosis).

Etiology. Unknown; autosomal dominant inheritance with wide variance in expression.

Pathology. Subcortical hyperostosis; simple thickening of lamellae of compact bones. Muscular atrophy.

Diagnostic Procedures. *Blood.* Normal calcium, potassium, and alkaline phosphatase. *X-ray.* Cortical thickening; fusiform osteosclerotic enlargement of diaphyses of tubular bones; normal epiphyses and metaphyses.

Therapy. Cortisone treatment beneficial for pain and reduction of bone changes; if optic nerve compression neurosurgical intervention.

Prognosis. Progressive condition, but not affecting life expectancy, and not too disabling.

BIBLIOGRAPHY. Cockayne EA: Case for diagnosis. Proc R Soc Med 13:132–136, 1920

Camurati M: Di un raro caso di osteite simmetrica ereditaria degli arti inferiori. Chir Organi Mov 6:662–665, 1922

Engelmann G: Ein Fall von Osteopathia hyperostotica (sclerotisans), multiplex infantilis. Fortschr Geb Röntgehstr 39:1101–1106, 1929

Ribbing S: Studien ueber heriditaere multiple epiphysenstoerungen. Acta Radiol [Suppl] (Stockh) 34:1–105, 1937

Mueller W: Das Bildung der multiplen erblichen Stoerungen der Epiphysenverknoecherung. Z Orthop 69:257, 1939

Ribbing S: Hereditary multiple diaphyseal sclerosis. Acta Radiol 31:522–536, 1949

Crisp AJ, Brenton DP: Engelmann's disease of bone. A systemic disorder? Ann Rheum Dis 41:183–188, 1982

CANAVAN-VAN BOGAERT-BERTRAND

Synonyms. Spongy degeneration of white matter; Van Bogaert-Bertrand.

Symptoms: Both sexes affected; onset in infancy (third to ninth mo). Spastic paralysis, blindness; occasionally, deafness.

Signs. Enlargement of head; separation of sutures. Neurologic signs of spastic paralysis; pathologic reflexes.

Etiology. Unknown; autosomal recessive inheritance.

Pathology. Small cystic spaces in white matter, basal ganglia, and cerebellum; diffuse demyelinization.

Therapy. Symptomatic.

Prognosis. Death in weeks or months.

BIBLIOGRAPHY. Canavan MM: Schilder's encephalitis periaxialis diffusa, report of a case in a child aged sixteen and one-half months. Arch Neurol Psychiat 25:299–308, 1931

Van Bogaert L: Familial spongy degeneration of brain (Complementary study of family R). Acta Psychiat Neurol Scand 39:107–113, 1963

Ungar M, Goodman RM: Spongy degeneration of brain in Israel: A retrospective study. Clin Genet 23:23–29, 1983

CANINE TOOTH

Synonym. Superior oblique palsy Class VII.

Symptoms and Signs. Brown's syndrome (see). Restriction of the upward gaze.

Etiology. Trauma to the trochlear area. Strengthening (with or without residual palsy) of the superior oblique, and underaction of the inferior oblique of the same side; or combination of trauma to the trochlea and closed head trauma producing a fourth nerve palsy.

BIBLIOGRAPHY. Ellis FH, Helveston EM: Superior oblique palsy: Diagnosis and classification. Int Ophthal Clin 16:127–135, 1976
Fraunfelder FT, Roy FH: Current Ocular Therapy, 2nd ed. Philadelphia, WB Saunders, 1984

CANNON-DE LA PAZ

Synonyms. Cannon's reflex; Cannon's (W.B.)

Symptoms. Flushing, hot skin; tachycardia; increased sweating.

Etiology. Emotional stress. Increase of epinephrine secretion.

BIBLIOGRAPHY. Cannon WB, De la Paz D: Emotional stimulation of adrenal secretion. Am J Physiol 28:64–70, 1911

CANNON'S (A.B.)

Synonyms. White folded gingivostomatitis; nevus spongiosus albus mucosae; white sponge nevus mucosae.

Symptoms. Both sexes affected; onset at any age. Asymptomatic.

Signs. Oral and labial mucosae exhibit white, thickened, folded, spongy lesions. Occasionally, same lesions in anal and vaginal mucosae.

Etiology. Unknown; autosomal dominant inheritance.

Pathology. Acanthosis; parakeratosis; hyperkeratosis; vacuolated cells.

Diagnostic Procedures. *Biopsy.*

Therapy. None.

Prognosis. Chronic benign condition.

BIBLIOGRAPHY. Cannon AB: White sponge nevus of mucosa (naevus spongiosus albus mucosae). Arch Dermatol Syph 31:365–370, 1935
Witkop CJ, Shankle CH, Graham JB, et al: Hereditary benign intraepithelial dyskeratosis; II. Oral manifestations and hereditary transmission. Arch Pathol 70:696–711, 1960
Rook A, Wilkinson DS, Ebling FJG, et al: Textbook of Dermatology, 4th ed, pp 2078–2079. Oxford, Blackwell Scientific Publications, 1986

CANTRELL'S PENTALOGY

Symptoms and Signs. Midline supraumbilical abdominal wall defect; defect of lower sternum; deficiency of anterior diaphragmatic pericardium; congenital intracardiac malformation (80% ventricular septal defect). Two thirds of patients also have muscular diverticulum of the apical portion of left ventricle.

BIBLIOGRAPHY. Cantrell JR, Haller JA, Ravitch MM: A syndrome of congenital defects involving the abdominal wall, sternum, diaphragm, pericardium and heart. Surg Gynecol Obstet 107:602–614, 1958
Van Praagh R, Weinberg PM, Matsuoka R, et al: Malposition of the heart. In Adams FH, Emmanoulides GC (eds): Moss' Heart Disease in Infants, Children and Adolescents, p 422. Baltimore, William & Wilkins, 1983

CANTU'S

Symptoms and Signs. Mild mental retardation; short stature; macrocranium; prominent forehead; hypertelorism; exophthalmos; cardiac anomalies; cutis laxa; wrinkled palms and soles; joint hyperextensibility; wide ribs; and small vertebral bodies.

Etiology. Probable autosomal dominant mutation. The father's age in each case was advanced (45–55).

Therapy. Symptomatic.

Prognosis. Good if successful treatment of cardiac anomalies. Mental retardation.

BIBLIOGRAPHY. Cantu JM, Sanchez-Corona J, Hernandes A, Mazara Z, Garcia-Cruz D: Individualization of a syndrome with mental deficiency, macrocranium, peculiar facies, and cardiac and skeletal anomalies. Clin Genet 22:172–179, 1982
McKusick V: Mendelian Inheritance in Man. Baltimore, Johns Hopkins Univ Press, 1986

CAPDEPONT'S

Synonyms. Brown teeth; dentinogenesis imperfecta; opalescent dentin; Stainton's; hypoplastic tooth enamel; pitted teeth; DGI_1, Shields II.

Signs. Both sexes affected. Teeth smaller than normal; color orange, slightly translucent; all or most of teeth become progressively worn down to gum level. Same appearance and wearing occur in deciduous and permanent teeth.

Etiology. Unknown; autosomal dominant inheritance. If coexistence with osteogenesis imperfecta, is called Shields II.

Pathology. Tooth roots slender; pulp chambers small, cavities uncommon. Dentinal structure disrupted with typical histologic features. Decreased hardness with non-tubular character of dentin.

Diagnostic Procedures. *Blood.* Normal; serum phosphate high in some cases. *X-ray of teeth and skeletal survey.*

Therapy. Removal of teeth; prosthesis.

Prognosis. Edentia.

BIBLIOGRAPHY. Stainton CW: Crownless teeth. Dental Cosmos 24:972, 1892

Capdepont C: Kysté du maxillaire superieur presentant un signe clinique rare. Rev Stomatol 12:18–20, 1905

Zellner R: Die Klinik und Morphologie der capdepontischen Erkrankung. Denth Zahnaarzt Stschr 15:479–486, 1960

Schields ED, Bixler D, El-Kafrawy AM: A proposed classification for hereditable human dentine defect with a description of a new entity. Arch Oral Biol 18:543–553, 1973

Corney G, Ball S, Noades JE: Linkage studies on dentinogenesis imperfecta DGI_1. Cytogenet Cell Genet 37:439, 1984

CAPGRAS'

Synonyms. Illusion of doubles; phantom double.

Symptoms. Prevalent in women. Patient with otherwise clear consciousness believes that a double has replaced another person, who, as a rule, is a key figure for the patient at time of onset of symptoms (if married, always the husband or wife accordingly). Patient continues to be firmly convinced of this, despite all evidence presented to the contrary. Admits a strong resemblance, but denies the person's identity.

Etiology. Unknown; complex psychopathologic characteristic clinical pattern, associated with paranoid psychosis of schizophrenic or affective type and other psychiatric conditions. No organic basis to the condition, but rather functional condition.

Therapy. No treatment for the syndrome. Treatment of associated psychotic symptoms.

Prognosis. Psychosis may respond to treatment and the illusion of double persist, or vice versa. Changing the attitude of object of delusion toward the patient may improve response.

BIBLIOGRAPHY. Capgras J, Reboul-Lachaux J: Illusion des sosies dans un délire systématisé chronique. Bull Soc Clin Méd Ment 11:6, 1923

Enoch MO, Trethowan WH, Barker JC: Some Uncommon Psychiatric Syndromes, Baltimore, Williams & Wilkins, 1967

Freedman AM, Kaplan HI, Sadock BJ: Comprehensive Textbook of Psychiatry, 2nd ed, p 995. Baltimore, Williams & Wilkins, 1975

CAPLAN'S

Synonyms. Colinet-Caplan; rheumatoid lung silicosis; rheumatoid arthritis–pneumoconiosis; silicoarthritis.

Symptoms and Signs. Usually in patient exposed to fibrogenic dust. Migratory painful joint swelling and other symptoms of rheumatoid arthritis preceding or following pulmonary pathology (cough; mild dyspnea; hemoptysis) with typical chest radiologic pattern.

Etiology. Rheumatoid arthritis or rheumatoid state, plus exposure to fibrogenic dust (as in miner, quarryworker, grinder, wheel worker). Whether exposure to dust plays a role in enhancing or determining the rheumatoid conditions is under discussion.

Pathology. Thickened alveolar septa, and patches of fibrosis. Granulomas with central necrosis with epithelioid cells and giant cells; coalescence of several nodules with necrotic center and formation of cavitations. Rheumatoid endoarteritis.

Diagnostic Procedures. *Blood.* Elevated sedimentation rate; positive latex and Waaler-Rose tests. *X-ray.* Typical alteration of joints and of chest showing multiple and bilateral lung nodules (0.5–5.0 cm in size), frequently peripheral. Negative search for tubercle, bacillus fungi, and negative skin tests for those diseases. *Pulmonary function tests.*

Therapy. Steroid affecting the lung lesions; chloroquine.

Prognosis. The same as rheumatoid arthritis; spontaneous remission of pulmonary lesions make the evaluation of treatment difficult.

BIBLIOGRAPHY. Caplan A: Certain unusual radiological appearances in chest of coalminers suffering from rheumatoid arthritis. Thorax 8:29–37, 1953
Colinet E: Polyarthite chronique evolutive et silicose pulmonaire. Acta Physiother Rheum Belg 8:37–41, 1953
Caplan A, Payne RB, Withey JL: A broader concept of Caplan's syndrome related to rheumatoid factors. Thorax 17:205–212, 1962
Ramirez RJ, Lopez-Majano V, Schultze G: Caplan's syndrome, a clinicopathologic study. Am J Med 27:643–652, 1964
Naeye RL: Types of fibrosis in coal workers pneumoconiosis. NY Acad Sci 200:381–400, 1972

CAPSULAR THROMBOSIS

Symptoms. Complete paralysis involving face, arms, and legs; contractures; occasionally hemianopsia; aphasia (if lesion on dominant side).

Signs. Exaggerated deep reflexes; positive Babinski.

Etiology. Thrombosis or other cause of occlusion of perforating branches alone.

Pathology. Thrombosis of perforating arteries; edema of perfused zone including lenticular nucleus and extrapyramidal pathway (spastic component of syndrome).

Diagnostic Procedures. *Neurologic examination. Arteriography. Electroencephalography. Cerebrospinal fluid. CT brain scan.*

Therapy. Anticoagulant.

Prognosis. Hemiplegia recedes as innervation from ipsilateral hemisphere asserts itself; recovery more marked on leg than arm.

BIBLIOGRAPHY. Vick NA: Grinker's Neurology, 7th ed. Springfield, CC Thomas, 1976
Fisher CM: Capsular infarct: The underlying vascular lesions. Arch Neurol 36:65–73, 1979

CAPSULOTHALAMIC (OBSOLETE)

See Capsular thrombosis syndrome.

Symptoms and Signs. Homolateral hemiplegia and hemianesthesia; emotional lability.

Etiology. Lesion (tumor) of internal capsule and thalamus or thalamic sensory fibers.

CARBAMYL PHOSPHATE

Synonyms. CPS deficiency; hyperammonemia, type I; synthetase deficiency.

Symptoms. Heterogeneous features reported. Both sexes affected; onset in first days or weeks of life. Vomiting; lethargy; dehydration after onset of feeding.

Etiology. Deficiency of carbamyl phosphate synthetase; possibility of other underlying enzyme defects has been considered. Autosomal recessive inheritance.

Diagnostic Procedures. *Blood.* Hyperammonemia (in absence of specific amino acid abnormalities), metabolic acidosis; leukocytes show deficiency of carbamyl synthetase (CBS). *Enzyme studies. Liver biopsy.*

Therapy. Subtraction of protein from diet; correction of acidosis.

Prognosis. Frequently, death in neonatal age. Patients surviving longer are severely retarded and have neuronal deficits.

BIBLIOGRAPHY. Freeman JM, Micholson JF, Masland WS, et al: Ammonia intoxication due to a congenital defect in urea synthesis. J Pediatr 65:1039–1040, 1964
Walser M: Urea cycle disorders and other hereditary hyperammonemic syndromes. In Stanbury JB, Wyngaarden JB, Fredrickson DS, et al: The Metabolic Basis of Inherited Disease. 5th ed, p 402, New York, McGraw-Hill, 1983

CARBON DIOXIDE NARCOSIS

Synonyms. Anoxic encephalopathy; hypoventilation; hypoxic encephalopathy; pulmonary insufficiency. See Ondine's curse.

Symptoms. *Minor.* Headache; nausea; anorexia. *Severe.* Delirium (see Brain, acute). If patient is anoxic, pallor, cyanosis, or shock. Delirium may persist after hypoxia is no longer present.

Signs. Decreased respiratory rate and depth. Patients with ineffective lungs are tachypnoic, but practically hypoventilating. Papilledema. Insufficient ventilatory drive in patient with normal lungs.

Etiology and Pathology. Respiratory acidosis; metabolic alkalosis; bicarbonate ingestion alkalosis; hypokalemic alkalosis; depressant drug poisoning; head trauma;

pickwickian syndrome, heart disease; diuretic therapy; Cushing's syndromes; Conn's syndrome; myxedema-coma syndrome.

Diagnostic Procedures. *Blood.* Serum *p*H; serum bicarbonates; electrolytes determination; arterial blood oxygen tension; hemoglobin; glucose level. *Spinal fluid.* Increased pressure.

Therapy. If patient is delirious and awake, keep in quiet, isolated surroundings with light on; small dose of paraldehyde; avoid other sedatives; oxygen at reduced concentration, intermittent positive-pressure breathing. If anemia present, blood transfusion; electrolyte and fluid balance.

Prognosis. Correction of systemic disorder produces remission of symptoms; encephalopathy, when present, improves more slowly than systemic illness. Severe hypoxia may result in death or leave permanent neurologic sequelae. See posthypoxic syndromes.

BIBLIOGRAPHY. Miller A, Bader RA, Bader M: The neurologic syndrome due to marked hypercapnia with papilledema. Am J Med 33:309–318, 1962

Adams RD, Victor M: Principles of Neurology, 3rd ed, p 790. New York, McGraw-Hill, 1985

CARBONIC ANHYDRASE II DEFICIENCY

Synonyms. Recessive osteopetrosis–renal tubular acidosis–cerebral calcification, marble brain.

Symptoms and Signs. Prevalent in families of Saudi Arabian descent. From birth. Osteopetrosis; renal tubular acidosis both proximal and distal; cerebral calcification; mental retardation; growth failure; typical facial features: broad head, prominent forehead, prominent narrow nose, slight epicanthal folds, small philtrum, micrognathia, teeth abnormalities. Moderate to severe lung disease.

Etiology. Autosomal recessive inheritance.

Diagnostic Procedures. *Radiology.* Intracranial calcifications. *EEG.* Abnormal for age. *Urine.* Alkaline, *p*H > 6.0. *Blood.* Metabolic acidosis, hyperchloremia, normal anion gap. Low carbonic anhydrase II in red cell hemolysate.

Therapy. Symptomatic.

Prognosis. Death in early childhood or adolescence.

BIBLIOGRAPHY. Sly WS, Lange R, Avidi L, et al: Recessive osteopetrosis: A new chemical phenotype abstracted. Am J Hum Genet 24:34a, 1972

CARCINOID

Synonyms. Argentaffinoma; Bjoerck's; carcinoid major; flush; Hedlinger's; Scholte's; Thorson-Bjoerck; Cassidy's.

Symptoms. Slight prevalence in males; age of presentation in males 18 to 80 years, in females 33 to 80 years. Intermittent diarrhea; abdominal pain; cutaneous flushing; asthmatic attacks; weight loss. Arthralgias.

Signs. Cutaneous rash (resembling pellagra); telangiectasis; precordial murmur. A precordial lift (right ventricular type) and systolic thrill palpable. Distention of jugular veins in upright position; hepatomegaly (occasionally, pulsating liver). Occasionally, peripheral edema and ascites.

Etiology. Tumors derived from the APUD cells (amine precursor uptake and decarboxylation). The syndrome is usually determined by metastatic carcinoid tumor. The pathogenesis of different symptoms and pathologic findings of this syndrome are not yet definitely assessed. Excessive production of either serotonin, bradykinin, histamine, or catecholamines has been considered as responsible for the symptoms. Possibly, different biologically active substances are elaborated and released in different combination, thus explaining also the variability of the clinical symptoms that have been described in patients with carcinoid tumor in different organs (*e.g.*, bronchial, gastric).

Pathology. Primary tumor may originate in any part of the epithelium of gastrointestinal tract from cardias to anus, and in the epithelium of biliary and pancreatic ducts. In addition, it may (although rarely) originate in the bronchial epithelium. Metastasis to liver, lymph nodes, lungs, and bones. Fibrous valve formation on both tricuspid and pulmonary valves of heart. Occasionally, involvement of one gland more extensive than the other; systemic veins may also be involved. Involvement of left side rare. At microscopy with staining methods argyrophil reaction in those containing serotonin.

Diagnostic Procedures. *Urine.* Excretion of high amount of 5-hydroxy-3-indol-acetic acid (5HIAA). *Plasma.* 5HIAA; serotonin. *X-ray of chest, gastrointestinal tract, and bones. Biopsy. Electrocardiography. Liver ultrasonography. CT scan. Celiac angiography.*

Therapy. Surgical removal of primary lesions (*e.g.*, bronchi, ovaries) leads to cure. Embolization of hepatic artery. For liver metastasis, removal for cure or improvement with cytotoxic drugs. Pharmacologic treatment to inhibit synthesis of 5-HT, parachlorophenylalanine, alphamethyldopa, or kallikrein and bradykinin, aprotinin (Trasylol).

To prevent release of active substances, alpha adrenergic blocking agents. To inhibit action of active substances, methysergide. Somatostatin and analogs (SMS 201-995) inhibit hormone secretion.

Prognosis. Ileal tumor (primary and metastasis) growth is very slow; bronchial and pancreatic faster. Extremely variable prognosis; cardiac and metabolic features severe aggravating factors.

BIBLIOGRAPHY. Lubarsch O: Über den primaren Krebs des Ileum nebst Bernerkungen über das gleichzeitige Vorkom men von Kiebs und tuberkulose. Virchow Arch (A) 3:280–317, 1888

Oberndorfer S: Karcinoide Tumoren des Dünndarms. Frank F. Z Pathol 1:426–29, 1907

Cassidy MA: Abdominal carcinomatosis with probable adrenal involvement. Proc R Soc Med London 24:139, 1930–31

Biörck G, Axén O, Thorson A: Unusual cyanosis in a boy with congenital pulmonary stenosis and tricuspid insufficiency: Fatal outcome after angiocardiography. Am Heart J 44:143–148, 1952

Pernow B, Wöldenström J: Paroxysmal flushing and other symptoms caused by 5-hydroxytriptamine and histamine in patients with malignant tumors. Lancet 11:951, 1954

Creutzfeldt W, Stöckmann F: Carcinoids and the carcinoid syndrome. Am J Med 82(Suppl 5B):4–16, 1987

CARDIAC RADIATION

High doses of x-ray radiation damage the heart and pericardium following radiotherapy for thoracic cancer. A spectrum of syndromes is observed which, however, cannot be differentiated clinically, from others, without recognizing different etiologic agents.
1. Acute pericarditis
   a. During radiation
   b. Delayed
2. Chronic pericarditis
   a. Effusion
   b. Constrictive, associated with myocardial fibrosis and endocardial fibroelastosis.
3. Coronary artery disease with myocardial infarction.
4. Mitral insufficiency and myocardial disease.

BIBLIOGRAPHY. Stewart JR, Cohn KE, Fajardo LF, et al: Radiation induced heart disease: A study of twenty-five patients. Radiology 89:302–310, 1967

McKenna G, Glatstein E: When radiation therapy causes heart disease. J Respir Dis 5:96, 1984

CARDIOMEGALY, FAMILIAL

Synonyms. Cardiomyopathy, familial idiopathic; see Dilated myocardiopathy; Evans W.

Symptoms and Signs. Various clinical patterns. "Hypertrophic congestive" types with various clinical course from extremely severe (death in first day) to survival.

Etiology. Various inherited traits; autosomal dominant and recessive types described.

BIBLIOGRAPHY. Evans W: Familial cardiomegaly. Br Heart J 11:68–82, 1949

Whitfield AGW: Familial cardiomyopathy. Q J Med 30:119–134, 1961

Ibsen HHW, Baandrup V, Simousen EE: Familial right ventricular dilated cardiomyopathy. Br Heart J 54:156–159, 1985

CARDIOMEGALY, IDIOPATHIC

Synonyms. Abramo-Fiedler's; Fiedler's; Becker's; Meadow's (see); adult fibroelastosis; alcoholic heart; cardiac hypertrophy (unknown etiology); cardiovascular collagenosis; pernicious myocarditis; noncoronary cardiomyopathy; nutrition heart; obscure cardiopathy; South African cardiomyopathy.

Cluster of syndromes today subdivided in three major groups.
1. Dilated myocardiopathy (see).
2. Hypertrophic cardiomegaly (see Idiopathic hypertrophic subaortic stenosis).
3. Restrictive/obliterative cardiomegaly (see Davies')

BIBLIOGRAPHY. Uber akute interstitielle Myokarditis in Festschrift zur Feier des funfzigjahrigen Bestehens des Stadkrankenhauses zu Dresden-Friedrichstadt Dresden W. Baensch 1899, pp 1–20

Becker BJP, Chatgidakis CB, Van Lingen B: Cardiovascular collagenosis with parietal endocardial thrombosis: A clinical pathologic study of forty cases. Circulation 7:345–356, 1953

Kass Wenger N, Goodwin JF, Roberts WC: Cardiomyopathy and myocardial involvement in systemic disease. In Hurst JW: The Heart, 6th ed, pp 1181–1248. New York, McGraw-Hill, 1986

CARINI'S

Synonyms: Alligator baby; collodion baby; lamellar ichthyosis; lamellar exfoliation; newborn desquamation; Seeligman's.

Symptoms and Signs. Infant bright red with generalized or partial shiny collodionlike covering that after a few days dries and peels off in large sheets, but may repeatedly re-form. Manifestation of underlying diseases (see Etiology) eventually appear.

Etiology. *Mild.* In normal infant. *Moderate.* Lamellar ichthyosis. *Severe.* Ichthyosiform erythroderma. Ichthyosis vulgaris and sex-linked ichthyosis.

Pathology. Parakeratotic horny layer shedding and that of underlying condition.

Therapy. Usually none. In severe forms, that of underlying disease.

Prognosis. Depends on underlying disease.

BIBLIOGRAPHY. Seeligman E: De Epidermis, Imprimis neonatorum desquamatione (inaugural dissertation). Berlin, 1841
Carini A: Di una forma attenuata della cosidetta "ittiosi sebacea". Gior Ital Mal Venereol 36:82–88, 1895
Rook A, Wilkinson DS, Ebling FJG, et al: Textbook of Dermatology, 4th ed, pp 237–1420. Oxford, Blackwell Scientific Publications, 1986

CARL SMITH'S

Synonyms. Lymphocytosis, acute infectious.

Symptoms and Signs. Most frequent in children, occasionally in young adults. Incubation 2 to 3 weeks. Frequently asymptomatic or seldom nonspecific signs. Fever: moderate; morbilliform eruption, pharyngeal exanthema; diarrhea, abdominal distension; latent meningeal reaction; cervical or generalized adenopathy; moderate splenomegaly.

Etiology. Infective agent suggested by epidemiology, but not clearly assessed; possibly more than one type of enterovirus could be responsible.

Pathology. Lymph nodes: nondiagnostic degeneration of follicles and sinus reticuloendothelial proliferation.

Diagnostic Procedures. *Blood.* Normal except for hyperlymphocytosis (population T-CD4) over 20,000 up to 120,000, early onset and returning to normal value in 3 to 6 weeks. Occasionally moderate eosinophilia, Paul Bunnuel negative. *Bone marrow.* Normal except for lymphocytosis (30–40%). *Cerebrospinal fluid.* Occasionally lymphocytosis.

Therapy. Symptomatic.

Prognosis. Spontaneous recovery.

BIBLIOGRAPHY. Smith CH: Acute infectious lymphocytosis: A specific infection. JAMA 125:342, 1944

Leborrier M: Lymphocytose infecteuse (Maladie de Carl Smith). Encycl Med Chir (Paris) Sang 13009 B10–2, 1988

CARNI'S

Synonyms. Aplasia cutis; gastrointestinal atresia.

Symptoms and Signs. Both sexes. From birth. Aplasia cutis usually involving predominantly the scalp. Difficulty in feeding from atresia in variable localization (pyloric, esophageal). Occasionally associated: lid ectropion, axillary pterygia.

Etiology. Unknown. Autosomal recessive inheritance.

Diagnostic Procedures. In gestational period high alpha protein in amniotic fluid. *X-ray of digestive tract. Skin biopsy.*

BIBLIOGRAPHY. Leschot NJ, Treffers PE, Beckel-Bloenkolk MJ, et al: Severe congenital skin defects in a newborn: Case report and relevance of several obstetrical parameters. Eur J Obstet Gynecol Reprod Biol 10:381–388, 1980
Carni S, Sofer S, Karplus M, et al: Aplasia cutis congenita in two sibs discordant for pyloric atresia. Am J Med Genet 11:319–328, 1982
Toriello HG, Higgins JV, Waterman DF: Autosomal recessive aplasia cutis congenita: Report of two affected sibs. Am J Med Genet 15:153–156, 1983

CARNITINE DEFICIENCY

Synonyms. Cardiomyopathic carnitine deficiency, systemic cardiomyopathic carnitine deficiency.

Symptoms and Signs. Rare condition, affects families of Germanic origin. Early onset skeletal muscle weakness, ECG alterations.

Etiology. Various causes: biosynthetic defects, defects in transport of carnitine.

Diagnostic Procedures. *ECG.* High theta waves in mid precordial leads.

Therapy. Carnitine administration intravenously.

Prognosis. Good with early therapy.

BIBLIOGRAPHY. Hart ZH, Chang CH, Di Mauro S, et al: Muscle carnitine deficiency and fatal cardiomyopathy. Neurology 28:147, 1978
Waber LJ, Valle D, Neill C, et al: Carnitine deficiency presenting as familial cardiomyopathy: A treatable defect in carnitine transport. J Pediatr 101:700, 1982

CARNOSINASE DEFICIENCY

Synonyms. Carnosinemia, hyper-β-carnosinemia.

Symptoms and Signs. Appear in first month of life. Myoclonic and grand mal seizures. Severe psychomotor retardation.

Etiology. Probably autosomal, but X-linked type cannot be excluded. Lack of degradation of carnosine in serum due to deficient carnosinase.

Diagnostic Procedures. *Blood. Plasma.* Carnosinemia increased at least twice normal range (also when on a protein-free diet). Serum carnosinase activity lacking. *Spinal fluid.* High concentration of homocarnosine. *Urine.* Excretion of carnosine. *Electroencephalography.*

Therapy. Trial with low-protein diet. Intravenous carnosinase replacement.

Prognosis. Poor.

BIBLIOGRAPHY. Perry TL, Hansen S, Tischler B, et al: Carnosinemia: A new metabolic disorder associated with neurologic disease and mental defect. N Engl J Med 277:1219–1227, 1967
Scriver CR, Perry TL, Nutzenadel W: Disorders of β-alanine, carnosine and homocarnosine metabolism. *In* Stanbury JB, Wyngaarden JB, Fredrickson DS, et al (eds): The Metabolic Basis of Inherited Disease, 5th ed, p 570. New York, McGraw-Hill, 1983

CAROLI'S

Synonym. Congenital biliary ectasias.

Symptoms. Both sexes affected; onset in first years of life or later (frequently around 35 yr of age). Nausea; vomiting; gastralgia; fever.

Signs. Hepatomegaly. Occasionally, jaundice or subicterus.

Etiology. Unknown; probably autosomal recessive inheritance. Defect of proliferation of some tracts of epithelium, which gives origin to biliary tracts, with resulting intrahepatic cysts. Frequent association with polycystic kidney, infantile type (see).

Pathology. *Pure form.* Congenital, sectorial, round, oval, or digitate dilatations of intrahepatic biliary tracts (rare). Normal epithelium with tendency to pseudopapillomatosis. Normal hepatic parenchyma. In 66% of cases, associated dilatations of extrahepatic biliary tract; occasionally, association with Cacchi-Ricci syndrome (see). *Fibrocholangiomatosis form.* Associated with the above features, diffuse hepatic fibrosis, and portal hypertension

(form more frequent, especially in children). Fibrocirrhosis. Splenomegaly. Lithiasis frequently associated with both forms.

Diagnostic Procedures. *X-ray. Cholangiography.* Integrated with *tomography,* and *selective angiography. CT scan. Blood and urine.* Changes secondary to lithiasic obstruction, portal hypertension and infections.

Therapy. According to localization, surgery or symptomatic medical treatment. Liver transplantation good results.

Prognosis. Of variable severity according to extension and forms of the condition.

BIBLIOGRAPHY. Caroli J, Couinaud C: Une affection nouvelle, sans doute congénitale, des voies biliaires: La dilatation kystique unilobulaire des canaux hépatiques. Sem Hop Paris 34:496–502, 1958
Bernstein J, Viranuvatti V, Boyer JL: What is Caroli disease? Gastroenterology 63:417–419, 1975
Paris JC, Quandalle P et al: Un cas de maladie de Caroli associée à un kyste congénital du cholédoque et compliquée d'une lithiase biliaire intra-hépatique. Lille Med 22:226–228, 1977
Nagasue N: Successful treatment of Caroli's disease by hepatic resection. Report of six patients. Ann Surg 200:718–724, 1984

CAROTID ARTERY ANEURYSM

Synonym. Internal carotid artery aneurysm.

Symptoms and Signs. Unilateral oculomotor paralysis; loss of pupillary reflexes of light and accommodation (occasionally, pupillary escape); ptosis; pain in the eye or face, or both (trigeminal ganglion compression). Occasionally, homonymous hemianopia, unilateral blindness, optic atrophy; scotoma, headache, attacks of migraine.

Etiology and Pathology. Aneurysm of internal carotid artery. Congenital defect of tunica media, atherosclerosis, trauma, and inflammations usual contributory factors. Twenty-seven percent of all cerebral aneurysms affect this artery.

Diagnostic Procedures. *Angiography. X-ray of skull. CT brain scan.*

Therapy. Surgical intervention.

Prognosis. Variable.

BIBLIOGRAPHY. Dailey EJ, Holloway JA, Murto RE, et al: Evaluation of ocular signs and symptoms in cerebral aneurysms. Arch Ophthalmol 71:463–474, 1964
Pia HW, Laugmaid C, Zierski J: Cerebral Aneurysms. Berlin, Springer-Verlag, 1979

Ojemann RG, Crowell RM: Surgical Management of Cerebrovascular Disease. Baltimore, William & Wilkins, 1983

CAROTID ARTERY–CAVERNOUS SINUS FISTULA

Symptoms. Prodromata of headache and vertigo prior to rupture (rare). Sudden, sharp pain in the eye and headache; seldom, loss of consciousness. Slowly progressing exophthalmos; bruit or thrill, synchronous with heart beat, heard by the patient and described as "buzzing" or "sawing."

Signs. Edema of soft tissues of orbit; superficial vein of eyelid and forehead dilated; partial or total ophthalmoplegia of affected eye. Compression of homolateral common carotid artery suppresses or decreases bruit.

Etiology. Spontaneous or traumatic formation of arteriovenous fistula between internal carotid artery and cavernous sinus.

Diagnostic Procedures. *Ophthalmoscopy.* Pulsation of retinal veins; elevation of optic disk; retinal edema; occasionally, hemorrhages. *X-ray.* (Later). Erosion of sella and sphenoid orbital walls. *Arteriography.* Shows fistula.

Therapy. Ligation of common or internal carotid (possible hemiplegia). Better result obtained by ligating the carotid intracranially above the cavernous sinus. Direct attack on fistula.

Prognosis. Infrequent remission due to formation of thrombus; possible recurrence from recanalization. Good results with surgery.

BIBLIOGRAPHY. Travers B: A case of aneurysm by anastomosis in the orbit, cured by ligation of common carotid artery. Med Chir Trans 2:1–16, 1817
Troost TB, Glaser JS: Aneurysms, arteriovenous communications and related vascular malformations. In Duane TD (ed): Clinical Ophthalmology, Vol II, p 16–18. Philadelphia, Harper & Row, 1982

CAROTID BODY TUMOR

Synonyms. Chemodectoma; nonchromaffin paraganglioma; paragangliomata; glomus jugulare tumor. See also Carotid sinus.

Symptoms. Equal sex distribution; age at onset ranges from second to seventh decades, average age 45 years. Average duration of symptoms before diagnosis, 2.1 years. Frequently asymptomatic. Hoarseness; vertigo; facial nerve palsy; vocal cord palsy.

Signs. Cervical mass that can be moved laterally but not vertically. Hypopharyngeal mass; majority of cervical masses pulsatile; bruit only occasionally; very seldom metastasis.

Etiology. Sporadic; rare familial occurrence with autosomal dominant inheritance.

Pathology. Circumscribed tumor 3 to 6 cm in diameter, with partial sort of capsule formed by compressed connective tissue arising at the bifurcation of one of carotid arteries. Red brown color; focal hemorrhage; very vascular, cells arranged in nest with vascular fibrous septa. Frequently, extension into adventitia.

Diagnostic Procedures. *Angiography of carotid.*

Therapy. Surgical excision.

Prognosis. Usually cured by surgery. Local recurrences; development of second primary; neoplastic spreading rare.

BIBLIOGRAPHY. Chase WH: Familial and bilateral tumors of carotid body. J Path Bact 36:1–12, 1933
Lattes R: Nonchromaffin paraganglioma of ganglion nodosum, carotid body, and aortic arch bodies. Cancer 3:667–694, 1950
Oberman HA, Holtz F, Sheffer LA, et al: Chemodectomas (nonchromaffin paraganglioma) of the head and neck. Cancer 21:838–851, 1968
Van Baars FM, Cremers CNRJ, Van Den Broeck P, et al: Familial non-chromaffinic paragangliomas (glomus tumors): Clinical and genetic aspects. Acta Otolaryngol 91:589–593, 1981

CAROTID SINUS

Synonyms. Cardioinhibitory carotid sinus; tight-collar; vagal syncope; Weiss-Baker syndromes; Charcot-Weiss-Baker.

Symptoms. More frequent in males over 45 years of age; sudden onset. Headache; transient attack of dizziness; vertigo; fainting; loss of consciousness; convulsions. Unilateral paresthesia; slurred speech.

Signs. Homonymous hemianopia; hemiplegia; bradycardia; drop of blood pressure during attack. Three types of carotid sinus syndrome may be recognized: (1) Vagal type with bradycardia, heart block, or asystole; (2) Depressor type with extensive peripheral dilatation. (3) Type without heart rate and pressure changes (see Weiss-Baker).

Etiology and Pathology. Hypersensitivity of carotid sinus from pressure, tight collar, turning head, shaving, swallowing, or emotion, or may be spontaneous. Atheromatous narrowing of opposite sinus or basilar artery.

Diagnostic Procedures. *Electroencephalography.* Diffuse slow waves. Moderate pressure over carotid sinus reproduces the attack.

Therapy. Prevention by eliminating pressure on the neck (*e.g.*, loose collar). In the depressive type, amphetamine sulfate. In vagal type, atropine sulfate. Surgical denervation of sinus in cases refractory to medical treatment. Ventricular demand pacemaker application.

Prognosis. In simple sensitivity, attack lasts a few minutes. If associated with atheromatous narrowing, serious prognosis.

BIBLIOGRAPHY. Waller A: Experimental researches on the functions of the vagus and the cervical sympathetic nerves in man. Proc R Soc Med 11:302–315, 1862

Charcot JM: Leçons sur les Maladies du Système Nerveux Faites à la Salpétrière. Paris, 1872–1873

Weiss S, Baker JP: The carotid sinus reflex in health and disease. Its role in the causation of fainting and convulsions. Medicine 12:297–354, 1933

Hurst JW: The Heart, 6th ed, p 514. New York, McGraw-Hill, 1986

CAROTID SYSTEM ISCHEMIA

Synonyms. Carotid artery insufficiency; carotid artery system ischemia; carotid artery occlusion; transient ischemic carotid insufficiency included. See Determann's.

Symptoms. Usually appear in adult males. More frequently on left side. Digital compression of carotid bulb in patient with partial or complete obstructive disease may cause syncope. Onset could be intermittent, gradual, or apoplectiform. Intermittent: repetitive with full recovery between attacks; episodes lasting less than 1 hour (rule out hypotension or heart conditions, vertigo, vertebral-basilar ischemia); pain on affected side (inconstant); episodes of temporary homolateral blindness or contralateral hemiplegia or both.

Signs. Absence of pulsation on affected side; bruits over carotid occasionally present; blood pressure determination on both arms to detect differences.

Etiology. Atherosclerosis (leading cause); complication of angiography; closed trauma; digital compression of artery; congenital kinking; hypoplasia of internal carotid artery (see also Fibromuscular dysplasia).

Pathology. Bifurcation of carotid predisposes site of obstruction; atherosclerotic changes; thrombosis.

Diagnostic Procedures. *Angiography.* In high risk group; absence of total agreement on using this test. *Electroencephalography.* 11% of low-voltage, electroencephalogram fast.

Therapy. Variable, from sympathectomy to endoarterectomy or transposed graft. Anticoagulants.

Prognosis. *Quoad vitam* fair; various types of residual incapacity.

BIBLIOGRAPHY. Fisher RG, Friedmann KR: Carotid artery thrombosis in persons fifteen years of age or younger. JAMA 170:1918, 1959

Persson AV, Robichaux WT, Silverman M: The natural history of carotid plaque development. Arch Surg 118:1048–1052, 1983

Whisnant JP, Sandok BA, Sundt TM: Carotid endarterectomy for unilateral carotid system transient cerebral ischemia. Mayo Clin Proc 58:171–175, 1983

CARPAL TUNNEL

Synonyms. Median neuropathy; median neuritis; tardy median palsy; tenosynovitis stenosans–carpal tunnel; thenar amyotrophy, carpal; constrictive median neuropathy.

Symptoms. Prevalent in women; fairly common complaint during pregnancy and in menopause. Numbness, paresthesia, burning pain on index finger, middle finger, or medial half of ring finger, occurring mostly at night and waking the patient. Weakness of thumb.

Signs. Anesthesia of thumb and mentioned fingers. Atrophy of thenar eminence; weakness of abductor pollicis and opponens pollicis; thickening and tenderness of flexor tendons; pain increased by flexing wrist to extreme degree; flexion of wrist aggravates symptoms; occasionally, extension does also.

Etiology. Most common cause is nonspecific synovitis involving the flexor synovia in carpal tunnel and compressing the median nerve. Precipitating factor may be traumas or disorders such as acromegaly. May be observed in amyloidosis, mucopolysaccharidoses and mucolipidoses. Autosomal dominant inheritance reported (male-to-male transmission).

Pathology. Fibrous proliferation with chronic inflammation and edema of synovial sheaths; fatty or mixedematous fibrous tissue.

Diagnostic Procedures. *Electromyography.* Slow conduction of median nerve and atrophy of muscles. *X-ray of cervical spine* to rule out herniated disc. Syringomyelia and muscular atrophy to be considered in differential diagnosis. *Biopsy.* Flexor synovia.

Therapy. Wrist splint for mild symptoms. Better results obtained with surgery sectioning transverse carpal tunnel.

Prognosis. When occurring in pregnancy 85% of cases recover spontaneously, 15% require surgery, and all obtain complete relief. In about 10%, recurrence of the syndrome with subsequent pregnancies.

BIBLIOGRAPHY. Marie P, Foix C: Atrophie isolée de l'éminence thénar d'origine névritique, rôle du ligament anulaire antérior du carpe dans la pathogénie de la lésion. Rev Neurol (Paris) 26:647–649, 1913
Serratrice G, Roger J, Guastalla B, et al: Amyotrophies thenariennes familiales d'origine carpienne. Rev Neurol (Paris) 141:746–749, 1985

CARPENTER'S

Synonyms. Acrocephalopolysyndactyly; acrocephalopolysyndactyly II; ACPS II.

Symptoms and Signs. Mental retardation; acrocephaly; peculiar facies; syndactyly (mainly third and fourth fingers); brachymesophalangia; preaxial polydactyly with syndactyly of toes; coxa valga; pes varus. Mild obesity; congenital heart disease; hypogenitalism.

Etiology. Unknown; rare autosomal recessive disorder. Development related to, but genetically distinct from, Apert's and the Laurence-Moon-Biedl.

Pathology. See Signs.

Therapy. Surgical correction and orthopedic measures when feasible.

BIBLIOGRAPHY. Carpenter G: Two sisters showing malformation of the skull and other congenital abnormalities. Rep Soc Study Dis Child (London) 1:110–118, 1901
Robinson LK, James HE, Maburak SJ, et al: Carpenter's syndrome: Natural history and clinical spectrum. Am J Med Genet 20:461–469, 1985

CARR-BARR-PLUNKETT

Synonyms. 48 XXXX; tetra-X; XXXX.

Symptoms and Signs. Variable features. Mental retardation (IQ average 55). Midfacial hypoplasia; hypertelorism; micrognathia. Clinodactyly of fifth finger; radial synostosis. Narrow shoulders; web neck. Irregular menstrual cycles.

Etiology. XXXX.

Diagnostic Procedures. *Chromosome studies.* In 6 to 9% of cells, three-X chromatin bodies.

Prognosis. Mental deficiency and behavioral problems.

BIBLIOGRAPHY. Carr DH, Barr ML, Plunkett ER: A XXXX sex chromosome complex in two mentally defective females. Can Med Assoc J 84:133–137, 1961
Jones KL: Smith's recognizable patterns of human malformations, p 72. Philadelphia, WB Saunders, 1988

CARRINGTON-LIEBOW

Synonym. Wegener's limited form. See also Liebow-Carrington.

Symptoms and Signs. Limited form of Wegener's granulomatosis (see) with prevalent pulmonary (with or without limited extrapulmonary) lesions, but without nephritis.

Therapy. Effectiveness of prednisone uncertain.

Prognosis. Better than in patients with classic symptoms triad of Wegener's.

BIBLIOGRAPHY. Carrington CB, Liebow AA: Limited forms of angiitis and granulomatosis of Wegener's type. Am J Med 41:497–527, 1966
Fraser RG, Pare JAP: Diagnosis of Diseases of the Chest, 2nd ed, p 917. Philadelphia, WB Saunders, 1978
Fauci AS, Haynes BF, Katz P, et al: Wegener's granulomatosis. Prospective clinical and therapeutical experience with 85 patients for 21 years. Ann Intern Med 98:76–85, 1983

CARSON-NEILL

Synonyms. Homocystinuria; cystathionine β-synthase deficiency; CBS deficiency. See also Pyridoxyne deficiency syndromes.

Symptoms. Both sexes equally affected. Normal parents. Infant appears entirely normal at birth. At 5 to 6 months may develop seizures followed by paralysis. At 3 to 5 years, develops dislocation of lenses, mental deficiency, delayed speech development, dyslalia, clumsiness, droolings, and thromboembolic accidents.

Signs. In early childhood development of skeletal abnormalities; genu valgum; pes cavus; pectus excavatum or carinatum; kyphoscoliosis; arachnodactyly. Occasionally, also characterized by fine, fair hair, malar flush, livedo reticularis.

Etiology. Autosomal recessive condition characterized by a deficiency of the enzyme cystathionine β-synthetase, which leads to accumulation of homocystine and methionine in blood and spinal fluid, increasing blood coagulation, vascular degeneration, and brain degeneration.

Pathology. In brain, mild diffuse neuronal rarefaction of cortex, hippocampus, basal ganglia; venous infarction and arterial thrombosis. Vessels, medial degeneration of aorta and other elastic arteries. Thrombus formation. Skeletal deformities.

Diagnostic Procedures. *Urine screening test.* Positive cyanide nitroprusside reaction. Confirmatory amino acid chromatography shows presence of homocystine and increased methionine. *Blood.* Increased coagulability; increased platelet adhesiveness; increased level of homocystine and methionine. *Spinal fluid.* Presence of homocystine. *Electroencephalography.* Alteration.

Therapy. Low methionine diet supplemented by L-cystine and pyridoxine, folic acid, anticoagulants, and platelet antiaggregating agents (results of such treatment still unknown).

Prognosis. Death from thrombosis, cerebral and other organ infarctions. Different response to pyridoxine allows the separation of this syndrome into at least two varieties.

BIBLIOGRAPHY. Carson NAJ, Neill DW: Metabolic abnormalities detected in a survey of mentally backward individuals in Northern Ireland. Arch Dis Child 37:505–513, 1962

Skovby F: Homocystinuria: Clinical biochemical and genetic aspects of cystathionine β-synthetase and its deficiency in man. Acta Paediat Scand 321 (Suppl):1–21, 1985

CARTILAGE-HAIR HYPOPLASIA-DWARFISM

Synonyms. CHH; McKusick's metaphyseal chondrodysplasia; metaphyseal dysplasia type A II.

Symptoms. Both sexes affected; disproportionate number of females; onset at birth. Motor milestones normal; frequent infections (bacterial, viral), malabsorption syndrome. Severe myopia. Normal intelligence.

Signs. At birth, short limbs; final height less than 150 cm. Head normal; hair sparse, silky, fine, brittle, short; in males thin silky beard; eyebrows and eyelashes sparse. Joint hypermobility with inability to fully extend elbow; fingernails short and wide. Foot may be inverted because of overlong fibula. Chest deformity. Abdomen protuberant with prominent veins. High pitched voice in males; delayed hair development in females.

Etiology. Unknown; autosomal recessive inheritance with reduced penetrance.

Pathology. Biopsy of costochondral junction shows achondroplasticlike changes. Lack of pigmented core in hair. Congenital megacolon. Signs of chronic otitis and pulmonary infections. Occasionally, avascular necrosis of femoral head.

Diagnostic Procedures. *Blood.* Normal; neutropenia and abnormal cellular immunity reported in some cases. *X-ray.* In younger patients metaphyseal changes of long bones (irregular sclerosis and cysts; femoral bowing).

Therapy. Medical (antibiotics and treatment of malabsorption) and orthopedic. Leukocyte interferon.

Prognosis. Life span reduced.

BIBLIOGRAPHY. Maroteaux P, Savart P, Lefebre J, et al: Le formes partielles de la dysostose metaphysaire. Presse Med 71:1523–1526, 1963

McKusick VA, Eldridge R, Hastetler, JA, et al: Dwarfism in the Amish. II. Cartilage-hair hypoplasia. Bull Johns Hopkins Hosp 116:285–326, 1965

Pierce GF, Polmar SH: Lymphocyte dysfunction in cartilage-hair hypoplasia: Evidence for an intrinsic defect in cellular proliferation. J Immunol 129:570–575, 1982

CASSIRER'S

Synonyms. Acroasphyxia; acrocyanosis; Crocq's; Curtius II.

Symptoms. Prevalent in females; onset in peripuberal age. Asymptomatic, or cold or sweating (or both) of extremities, aggravated or caused by cold exposure, emotions. Occasionally relieved by warmth. Paresthesias frequently accompany other symptoms. In some cases, instead of paresthesias, hypoesthesia (anesthetic form) is present.

Signs. Persistent dusky, mottled blue or reddish discoloration of hands and feet, occasionally of ears and nose. Lifting the extremities reduces the cyanosis; absence of frank edema; presence of tissue succulence.

Etiology. Unknown; family history frequently reported. Venular atonia, accompanied by arteriolar hypertony. Cold, humidity, emotion considered as causes. Neurovegetative disturbance, hormonal imbalance have also been considered but not proved.

Pathology. Functional condition. Increase in interstitial fluid. In prolonged chronic cases, possible muscular atrophy and connective tissue proliferation.

Diagnostic Procedures. *Diaphragmatic irides test.* Pressure on acrocyanosis zone causes anemia, which regresses slowly and progressively from the edges as a closing diaphragm, as opposed to normal tissue where color returns to entire area at the same time.

Therapy. Protection from cold. No curative treatment.

Prognosis. Spontaneous remission around the age of 20 to 25 years; seldom, persistence to advanced age; first pregnancy frequently causes disappearance or marked improvement.

BIBLIOGRAPHY. Cassirer R: Die Vasomotorischtrophiscen. Neurosen Berlin Karger, 1901

Curtius F, Kruger KH: Das vegetativendoktrine Syndrom der Frau. München, Urban et Schwarzenberg, 1952

Spittle JA Jr: Raynaud's phenomenon and allied vasospastic disorders. In Juergens JJ, Spittle JA Jr (eds): Allen-Barker-Hines: Peripheral vascular disease. Philadelphia, WB Saunders, 1980

CASTELLANI'S

Synonyms. Dermatosis papulosa nigra.

Symptoms and Signs. In blacks (Jamaica and Central America). At time of puberty, more frequent in black or dark brown females. Papules of the face on both malar regions, sparing lower face and chin.

Etiology. Unknown. Autosomal dominant inheritance considered as a variant of seborrheic keratoses.

BIBLIOGRAPHY. Castellani A: Observations on some diseases of Central America. J Trop Med Hyg 28:1–14, 1925

Rook A, Wilkinson DS, Ebling FJG, et al: Textbook of Dermatology, 4th ed. Oxford, Blackwell Scientific Publications, 1986

CATAPLEXY

Synonyms. Tonelessness. Henneberg's.

Symptoms. Both sexes affected; onset all ages. Following strong emotions (laughter, fright, anger), sudden brief attacks of severe muscle weakness and tone loss; consciousness retained; light attacks may be limited to leg weakness; in severe form, total inability to move and total helplessness. Absence of jerking or twitching.

Signs. Skin color, eye and tendon reflexes normal.

Etiology. Unknown. Frequent association with narcolepsy (see Gelineau's).

Prognosis. Spontaneous resolution within one to a few minutes.

BIBLIOGRAPHY. Westphal C: Eigetuemlizhe mit Einschlafen verbundene Anfaelle. Arch Psychiat Nervenkr 7:631–635, 1877

Passonant P: The history of narcolepsy. In Guilleminault C, Dement WC, Passonant P (eds): Narcolepsy, p 3–13. New York, Spectrum, 1976

Merritt HH: A Textbook of Neurology, 6th ed, p 890. Philadelphia, Lea & Febiger, 1979

CAT CRY

Synonyms. B_1 deletion; *Cri du chat*; chromosome 5 short arm deletion; Lejeune's; 5p; 46XX.

Symptoms. Strange high-pitched plaintive cry by an infant, similar to the cry of a cat. Growth retardation; mental retardation.

Signs. Microcephaly; oblique palpebral fissures; epicanthus; moon facies; low-set ears; abnormal palmar dermatoglyphs. Occasionally, micrognathia and strabismus; laryngeal abnormalities (small larynx, small epiglottis). Variable congenital heart disease.

Etiology. Congenital abnormality; deletion of a portion of short arm of chromosome number 5 (group B).

Diagnostic Procedures. *Chromosome study.* Of patient and parents. *Dermatoglyphics.*

Prognosis. Compatible with life. Mental retardation is invariably severe; speech development is slow. The IQ is most commonly in the 20 to 30 range. Most patients remain short and underweight, and almost all are microcephalic.

BIBLIOGRAPHY. LeJeune J, Lafourcade J, Berger R et al: Trois cas de délétion partielle du bras court d'un chromosome 5. C R Acad Sci [D] Paris 257:3098–3102, 1963

MacIntyre MN, Staples WI, Lapolla J, et al: The "cat cry" syndrome. Am J Dis Child 108:538–542, 1964

Niebuhr E: The cri-du-chat syndrome. Epidemiology, cytogenetics and clinical features. Hum Genet 44:227–275, 1978b

Wilkins LE, Brown JA, Wolf B: Psychomotor development in 65 home-reared children with cri-du-chat syndrome. J Pediatr 97:401–405, 1980

CAT-EYE

Synonyms. Anal atresia–coloboma iris; partial G-trisomy; Schachenmann's; Schmid-Fraccaro; ocular coloboma–imperforate anus; CES.

Symptoms and Signs. Present from birth. Variable growth deficiency. Mild mental deficiency. Mild hypertelorism; microphthalmos; antimongoloid slant of palpebrae; inferior strabismus; vertical iris coloboma (cat-eye gives the name to the syndrome); cataract; choroidal coloboma. Bilateral prearicular fistulas; umbilical hernia. Anal atresia; occasionally, retrovestibular fistula. Occasionally, heart and kidney malformations.

Etiology. Presence of one extra chromosome acrocentric about the half of a G group autosome 22 g$^+$. Autosomal dominant inheritance (?).

BIBLIOGRAPHY. Schachenmann G, Schmid W, Fraccaro M et al: Chromosomes in coloboma and anal atresia. Lancet 2:290, 1965
Schmid W, Fraccaro M: The cat eye syndrome. Presented at 4th Conference of Mammalian Cytology and Somatic Cell Genetics, Williamsburg, VA, 1969
Schinzel A, Schmid W, Fraccaro M, et al: The "Cat-eye syndrome:" Dicentric small marker chromosome probably derived from a No 22 (tetrasomy 22pter q 11) associated with a characteristic phenotype. Report of 11 patients and delineation of clinical picture. Hum Genet 57:148–158, 1981
Verma RS, Babu KA, Rosenfeld W, et al: Marker chromosome in cat-eye syndrome. Clin Genet 27:526–528, 1985

CAUDA EQUINA

Synonyms. Chronic arachnoiditis–cauda equina; claudication of cauda equina; filum terminale–cauda equina; pseudoclaudication; Verbiest's; conus medullaris; anogenital-vesicle; sacral.

Symptoms and Signs. Intense pain in small of back, sciatic region, or perineum. Pain may be unilateral at first (hemicaudal syndrome), but becomes bilateral soon (bilateral sciatica diagnostic of spinal tumor). Sphincter disorders (see Neurogenic bladder syndromes). Flaccid paralysis of gluteal and leg muscles; eventually atrophy and fibrillation. Achilles tendon reflex absent. Occasionally, vascular malformation or lymphosarcoma may infiltrate the region without giving neurologic symptoms but only spasm and shortening of hamstring muscles. A particular variety of this syndrome is represented by the intermittent claudication of the cauda equina (Verbiest's), symptoms appearing after walking and usually due to protrusion of lumbar disc.

Etiology. Tumors or other causes (trauma) compressing or infiltrating cauda equina region.

Pathology. See Signs and Etiology.

Diagnostic Procedures. *X-ray. Myelography. Cystometrogram. CT scan..*

Therapy. Surgical decompression.

Prognosis. Depends upon etiology.

BIBLIOGRAPHY. Dejerine J: La claudication intermittente de la moelle épinière. Presse Med 2:981–984, 1911
Roussy G, Lhermitte J: Le Blesseurs de la Moelle et de la Queue de Cheval. Paris, 1918

Verbiest H: A radicular syndrome from developmental narrowing of the lumbar vertebral canal. J Bone Joint Surg [Br]: 36:230–237, 1954
Spanos NC, Andrew J: Intermittent claudication and lateral lumbar disc protrusions. J Neurol Neurosurg Psychiatr 29:273–277, 1966
Kavanaugh GJ, Svien HJ, Holman CB, et al: "Pseudoclaudication" syndrome produced by compression of the cauda equina. JAMA 206:2477–2481, 1968
Wood GW: Other disorders of spine. In Crenshaw AH (ed): Campbell's Operative Orthopedics, 7th ed, pp 3347–3353. St. Louis, CV Mosby, 1987

CAUHEPE-FIEUX

Symptoms. Functional lateral deviation of the jaw.

Etiology. Persistence of infantile type of deglutition.

BIBLIOGRAPHY. Moortgat P: Syndromes a Noms Propres. Paris, J Prélat, 1966

CAUSALGIA

Synonym. Traumatic erythromelalgia. See also Mitchell's I syndrome.

Symptoms. Complication in 3% of cases of major nerve injuries. Paroxysmal severe burning pain may localize and especially affect palm of hand or sole of foot. Aggravated by physical and emotional stimuli, cold and dryness; relieved by warmth and humidity.

Signs. Skin hyperesthetic, often hypoalgesic when tested, cold, smooth, devoid of hairs, discolored, flossy edematous, hyperhydrotic. Trophic changes on nails, curved at the end, brittle. Stiffness of joints.

Etiology. Incomplete lesions of nerve, usually median and sciatic (60%). Irritation of unsevered sensory fibers; neuritis of periarterial sympathetic fibers.

Pathology. Incomplete lesion of nerve; atrophied muscles of affected part; atrophy of small bones.

Diagnostic Procedures. *X-ray.* Atrophy of small bones. *Electromyography. Nerve conduction studies. Tinel sign. Sweat test. Skin resistance test. Electrical stimulation.*

Therapy. Wet dressing for symptomatic relief. Sympathetic ganglia block with procain for temporary relief. Sympathectomy in cases that respond to block.

BIBLIOGRAPHY. Mitchell SW, Morehouse GR, Keen WW: Gunshot Wounds and Other Injuries of the Nerves. Philadelphia, JB Lippincott, 1864
Wright PE: Peripheral nerve injuries. In Crenshaw AH (ed): Campbell's Operative Orthopedics, 7th ed, pp 2791–2792. St. Louis, CV Mosby, 1987

CAYLER'S

Synonyms. Asymmetric crying facies–cardiac defect; cardiofacial defect; crying facies–cardiac defect; depression anguli oris muscle.

Symptoms and Signs. Appear in both sexes; present at birth. Asymmetric crying facies (especially right side); symptoms and signs of cardiac defect (especially ventricular septal type) associated more or less with variable other anomalies (vertebral; renal; limb).

Etiology. Unknown. It seems that right-sided asymmetric crying facies is associated with cardiac defect; in left-sided form the association is much less frequent, although left-sided form is much more frequent.

Pathology. Facial asymmetry due to partial agenesis of depressor anguli oris muscle. Cardiac defects.

BIBLIOGRAPHY. Cayler GG: Cardiofacial syndrome. Congenital heart disease and facial weakness, a hitherto unrecognized association. Arch Dis Child 44:69–75, 1969
Perlman M, Reisner SH: Asymmetric crying facies and congenital anomalies. Arch Dis Child 48:627–629, 1973
Singhi S, Singhi P, Lall KB: Congenital asymmetrical crying facies. Clin Pediat 19:673–678, 1980

CEBOCEPHALY

Term derived from name of Cebus monkey. See Arhinencephalia.

Symptoms and Signs. Hypotelorism; flat incomplete nose; full cheeks; median nostrils; no palate or cleft lips; upper lip forming semicircle with insufficiently developed philtrum and labial tubercle.

Etiology. See Arhinencephaly.

Pathology. Usually halobaroprosencephaly.

BIBLIOGRAPHY. Klopstock A: Familiaerws Vorkommen von Cyklopie und Arrhinencephalie. Mschr Geburtsh Gynaek 56:59–71, 1921
Aita JA: Congenital Facial Anomalies with Neurologic Defects. Springfield, CC Thomas, 1969
Cohen MM Jr: Haloprosencephaly revisited. Am J Dis Child 127:597, 1974

CEELEN-GELLERSTEDT

Synonyms. Brown pulmonary induration; pulmonary idiopathic hemosiderosis; IPH; essential brown induration lung. See also Goodpasture's.

Symptoms. Prevalent in males; occurs mostly in childhood; onset sudden. Recurrent episodes of cough, dyspnea, hemoptysis; occasionally, recurrent fever, and abdominal pain.

Signs. Skin pale; sometimes jaundice, and cyanosis. Occasionally, clubbing of fingers and enlargement of spleen.

Etiology. Unknown; recurrent lung hemorrhages; possibly immune reaction. Considered a variety of Goodpasture's syndrome, especially in adult form.

Pathology. Hemorrhages and fibrosiderosis of lungs; no generalized hemosiderosis. Lymphoreticular system: changes compatible with immunodeficiency.

Diagnostic Procedures. *Blood.* Hypochromic anemia; bilirubin increased; normal clotting tests; late secondary polycythemia, decreased gamma-A globulin. *X-ray of lung.* Ill-defined opacities rapidly changing; later diffuse reticulonodular pattern.

Therapy. Steroids of relative benefit in acute episode. Splenectomy has no significant effect.

Prognosis. Death in 3 years from hemorrhage or right heart failure.

BIBLIOGRAPHY. Ceelen W: Die Kreislaufstoerungen der Lungen. In Henke F, Lubarsch O: Handbuch der Speziellen pathologischen Anatomie und Histologie, vol 3, p 10. Berlin, Springer, 1931
Gellerstedt N: Uber die essentielle anaemisierende Form der braunen Lungeninduration. Acta Pathol Microbiol Scand [A] 16:386–400, 1939
Soergel KH, Sommers SC: Idiopathic pulmonary hemosiderosis and related syndrome. Am J Med 32:499–511, 1962
Fraser RG, Paré JAP: Diagnosis of Disease of the Chest, 2nd ed, p 886. Philadelphia, WB Saunders, 1977

CEREBELLAR ATAXIA— HYPOGONADISM

Synonyms. Hypogonadotropic hypogonadism–cerebellar ataxia; LHRH deficiency–ataxia; Holms (G.) I.

Symptoms and Signs. Association of cerebellar syndrome (Marie's ataxia, Friedreich's ataxia, or neocerebellar) with primary hypogonadism. Partial or total failure of pituitary to stimulate gonadal development at puberty.

Etiology. Syndrome does not represent a homogeneous group. Not known if nervous and endocrine disorders are genetically determined or only fortuitously linked or if pituitary insufficiency is due to primary dysgenesis or secondary to failure of gonadotropin excretion. Genetic determination of autosomal recessive type shown in some families.

Pathology. See Etiology.

Diagnostic Procedures. *Urine.* Gonodotropin excretion low; increased steroid excretion of a single fraction of adrenal origin reported in some cases. *CT brain scan.* Cerebellar and brain stem atrophy.

Therapy. Hormonal treatment.

Prognosis. Depends on severity of cerebellar syndrome.

BIBLIOGRAPHY. Holmes G: A form of familial degeneration of the cerebellum. Brain 30:466–488, 1907

Matthews WB, Rundle AT: Familial cerebellar ataxia and hypogonadism. Brain 87:463–468, 1964

Bercino J, Amado JA, Freijanes J, et al: Familial cerebellar ataxia and hypogonadotropic hypogonadism: Evidence for hypothalamic LHRH deficiency. J Neurol Neurosurg Psychiat 45:747–751, 1982

CEREBELLAR CATALEPSY

Symptoms. Those of cerebellar lesions.

Signs. With patient lying on his back, flex lower extremities at both hips and knees, lift lower extremities from bed and separate the feet. Initially, oscillation of trunk and legs, which later become abnormally fixed.

Etiology. Lesion of cerebellum.

BIBLIOGRAPHY. Babinski J: De l'equilibre volitionnel statique et de l'equilibre volitionnel cinetique. Rev Neurol (Paris) 10:470–474, 1902

Dow RS, Moruzzi G: Physiology and Pathology of the Cerebellum. Minneapolis, University of Minnesota Press, 1958

Adams RD, Victor M: Principles of Neurology, 3rd ed, pp 71–75. New York, McGraw-Hill, 1984

CEREBELLAR SUPERIOR PEDUNCLE

Synonym. Anterosuperior cerebellar artery.

Symptoms and Signs. Sudden onset without loss of consciousness. Homolateral hypotonia; asthenia; severe difficulty in walking (after ability is regained, leg placed unsteadily in abduction). Contralateral loss of sensibility to pain and temperature, including in head. Occasionally, contralateral loss of hearing. Hyperkinetic movements; palatal myoclonus may be observed occasionally. Horner's syndrome occasionally observed. Normal findings: normal swallowing; no palatal weakness or anesthesia in glossopharyngeal zone of distribution; no aphonia; no pyramidal tract signs.

Etiology. Obstruction of anterosuperior cerebellar artery; thrombosis; less frequently, embolism. Neoplasia; inflammation.

Pathology. Gross softening of cerebellum on side affected or lesion of superior cerebellar peduncle (or both).

Diagnostic Procedures. *Arteriography. CT brain scan. Spinal tap.*

Therapy. Acute stage not major problem since swallowing not problem. Rehabilitation to overcome cerebellar deficiency. Surgery when indicated.

Prognosis. Variable according to extension and nature of lesions. Fair recovery frequent.

BIBLIOGRAPHY. Porot A: Hémorragie limitée du pédoncle cérébelleux superiéur droit; hémisyndrome cérébelleux direct. Lyon Méd 106:1137–1141, 1906

Dow RS, Moruzzi G: The Physiology and Pathology of the Cerebellum. Minneapolis, University of Minnesota Press, 1958

Adams RD, Victor M: Principles of Neurology, 3rd ed, p 588. New York, McGraw-Hill, 1985

CEREBRAL CONCUSSION

Synonym. Brain concussion; brain cerebral contusion, and Homen's.

Symptoms. Period of unconsciousness or disturbance in consciousness (confusion; dazing; stunning) usually lasting less than 5 minutes; and seldom more than 10, following a cerebral concussion. Complete recovery; amnesia consistent accompaniment.

Signs. None, or ecchymosis or discoloration at place of trauma; pallor; superficial respiration; mydriasis; loss of light reflexes; loss of cutaneous and tendon reflexes; hypotension; muscle flaccidity.

Etiology. Injury to head not associated with cerebral lesions such as hemorrhage, contusion, lacerations, or cerebral edema.

Pathology. No gross or microscopic evidence of injury to nervous tissue; small areas of cell loss in cortical areas; or nuclear masses of brain stem.

Diagnostic Procedures. *X-ray of skull. Spinal fluid. Electroencephalography.* Slow, decreased amplitude; occasionally, spikes. *CT brain scan.*

Therapy. Observation (2–3 days); respiratory assistance. According to symptoms, antiedema treatment (diuretics; corticosteroids; barbiturates).

Prognosis. Usually, complete recovery. Repeated concussion, however, results in the Homen's syndrome (see); or if a subacute type of encephalitis develops, the sequelae named Friedmann's syndrome. In children, after minor head injury, it is possible to have a lucid interval with vomiting and mild shock, followed by stupor and recovery in 24 hours. This condition has to be differentiated from the extradural hematoma.

BIBLIOGRAPHY. Gilbert MM: Etiology and treatment of postconcussion syndrome. Headache 8:57–61, 1968
Walt AJ, Wilson RF: Management of Trauma. Philadelphia, Lea & Febiger, 1975
Gennarem TA: Cerebral concussion and diffuse brain injury. In Cooper PR (ed): Head Injury, pp 108–124. Baltimore, Williams & Wilkins, 1987

CEREBRAL CONTUSION

Synonym. Brain contusion. See also Homen's and Brain.

Symptoms and Signs. *Mild form.* Loss of consciousness followed by drowsiness; headache; vertigo. *Severe form.* Loss of consciousness; hypotension; hypothermia; shallow breathing; arrhythmias; loss of reflexes; pupils unequal; ocular palsies. Later, delirium. Associated with fracture or laceration or both: paraplegia; focal signs; seizures; respiratory arrest.

Etiology. Direct head trauma or rebound.

Pathology. Brain edema from capillary oozing to intracerebral hemorrhages.

Therapy. Corticosteroids; diuretics (glycerol; mannitol); fluid restriction; if needed, respiratory assistance; if needed, intracranial pressure monitoring and surgery.

Prognosis. Variable according to extent of lesions.

BIBLIOGRAPHY. Graham DI, Adams JH, Gennarem TA: Pathology of brain damage in head injury. In Cooper PR (ed): Head Injury, pp 72–88. Baltimore, Williams & Wilkins, 1987

CEREBRAL MALARIA

Many clinical varieties of this syndrome may be recognized; they may simulate many different conditions.

Symptoms and Signs. According to different types:
1. Meningitic
2. Monoplegic and hemiplegic
3. Myelitic
4. Ataxic
5. Disseminated sclerotic
6. Bulbar
7. Cerebellar
8. Polyneuritic
9. Korsakoff's
10. Aphasic
11. Acute personality change

Etiology. *Plasmodium falciparum.*

Pathology. Cerebral edema; perivascular hemorrhages. Thrombosis of intracerebral vessels by pigment and clumped erythrocytes and endothelial proliferation (actual vessel occlusion denied by some authors).

Diagnostic Procedures. *Blood.* Demonstration of parasites. *Spinal tap.* Completely normal or slight increase in pressure. In some cases pleocytosis and protein increase.

Therapy. Quinine sulfate; pyrimethamine; sulfadiazine. If patient is comatose or vomiting, quinine intramuscularly and pyrimethamine and sulfadiazine by nasogastric tube. Diphenylhydantoin and sedative. Fluid balance. Relief of CSF increased pressure (diuetics, glycerol, mannitol, barbiturates, phenylhydantoin).

Prognosis. Severe. With early treatment, good. Usually, recovery without permanent neurologic sequelae.

BIBLIOGRAPHY. Brill NQ, Pellicano VL: Estivoautumnal malaria with frontal lobe syndrome. JAMA 121:1150–1152, 1943
Daroff RB, Deller JJ, Kastl AJ, et al: Cerebral malaria. JAMA 121:1150–1152, 1943
Scrascia E, Magalini SI: Trattamento rianimativo nelle sindromi renali e cerebrali da infestazione malarica. Minerva Anestesiol 38:329–334, 1972
De Francisci G, Magalini SI: Terapia intensiva nella malaria cerebrale. Rec Prog Med 74:873–874, 1983
Adams RD, Victor M: Principles of Neurology, 3rd ed, p 540. New York, McGraw-Hill, 1985

CEREBRAL RADIATION

Synonym. Brain radiation necrosis. See also Postirradiation vascular insufficiency.

Symptoms and Signs. Usually in patient with acromegaly resistant to radiation treatment, which is treated with heavy dose or multiple courses of ionizing radiation. Syndrome develops 7 to 12 months after last treatment. Variable symptomatology: headache; convulsions; paresis; impairment of memory; emotional lability; aphasia; stupor.

Etiology. Degenerative process of nervous cells due to direct effect of radiation and, at least in part, to ischemic origin from postirradiation vascularity.

Pathology. Marked damage to neurons; glial degeneration and delayed reparative glial response. Proliferation of collagen; vascular endothelial proliferation; thrombosis; hyalinization of basement membranes.

Diagnostic Procedures. *Arteriography. Pneumoencephalography. CT brain scan. Spinal fluid.*

Therapy. Anticoagulants; craniotomy; removal of gliomatous tissue when feasible.

Prognosis. Progressive, often fatal condition.

BIBLIOGRAPHY. Fisher AW, Holfelder H: Lakales Amyloid im Gehirn eine Spätfolge von Rontgenbestrahlungen. Dtsch Z Chir 227:475–483, 1930
Peck FC, Jr, McGovern ER: Radiation necrosis of the brain in acromegaly. J Neurosurg 25:536–542, 1966
AMA: A guide to the hospital management to injury arising from exposure to or involving ionizing radiation. AMA 1985

CERVICAL AORTA

Symptoms. Vascular ring, dysphagia, dyspnea, stridor, brassy cough, usually occurring at the end of childhood or adolescent period.

Signs. Pulsatile mass on the right side of neck above the clavicle; murmur and thrill over the mass; compression of pulsatile mass produces marked diminution or obliteration of femoral pulses.

Etiology. Aortic arch anomaly.

Pathology. Right aortic arch retained in cervical region; retroesophageal course; left common carotid artery originates from ascending aorta; right subclavian artery originates directly or through a common duct with right common carotid artery near apex of aorta arch; left subclavian artery originates distally to retroesophageal segments of aorta.

Diagnostic Procedures. *Esophagography. Angiography.* Seldom necessary.

Therapy. Removal of first rib on the right to make room for aortic growth and prevention of vascular symptoms and degenerative phenomena. Consider aortic resection and intrathoracic graft.

Prognosis. If not relieved, early degenerative phenomena of aorta wall, erosion, and possibly rupture.

BIBLIOGRAPHY. Beaven TED, Fatti L: Ligature of aortic arch in the neck. Br J Surg 34:414–416, 1946
Massumi R, Wiener L, Charif P: The syndrome of cervical aorta; report of a case and review of the previous cases. Am J Cardiol 11:678–685, 1963
McCue CM, Mauck HP Jr, Tingelstad JB, et al: Cervical aortic arch. Am J Dis Child 125:738–742, 1973

CERVICAL RIB

Synonym. First thoracic rib. See Thoracic outlet syndromes.

Symptoms. Usually appear in adult life after trauma to the shoulder, stretching of the arm, pregnancy. Usually unilateral (although supernumerary ribs may be bilateral) and more frequent in female patients. Pain on the ulnar border increased by movement; weakness of hand, arm, shoulder; numbness, tingling, and sensory loss on the same ulnar distribution.

Signs. Cyanosis; edema; coolness; spastic vasomotor; muscular atrophy; pulse weak on affected side; occasionally, bony mass palpable in supraclavicular fossa.

Etiology. Supernumerary cervical rib arising from seventh cervical vertebra, irritating the brachial plexus, restricting it between the rib and the scalenus anticus muscle. Autosomal dominant inheritance reported.

Pathology. Neuritis; atrophy of muscles involved.

Diagnostic Procedures. *Adson's test.* Positive (costoclavicular and hyperadduction maneuvers). *X-ray.* Shows the supernumerary cervical rib(s).

Therapy. Proper support of shoulder with pillows may relieve syndrome without surgery. Surgery: section or removal inferior part of scalenus anticus. Differential diagnosis with cervical disk that may produce same syndrome.

Prognosis. Recovery with removal of compression.

BIBLIOGRAPHY. Willshire: Supernumerary first rib. Lancet 2:633, 1860
Murphy T: Brachial neuritis caused by pressure of first rib. Aust Med J 15:582–585, 1910
Weston WJ: Genetically determined cervical ribs: A family study. Brit J Radiol 29:455–456, 1956
Holst S: Cervical rib and associated vascular complications. J Oslo City Hosp 13:173–182, 1963
Roos DB: The place for scalenectomy and first rib resection in thoracic outlet syndrome. Surgery 93:1077–1085, 1982

CERVIX, ANNULAR DETACHMENT OF

Synonym. Traumatic avulsion of cervix uteri.

Symptoms and Signs. Unusual bleeding after delivery of child. Detached cervix may be covering the head of the child: cardinal's sign. On inspection of the cervix, might see the partial circular tearing: bucket-handle detachment. Often on inspection, cervix is hanging by a strand of tissue.

Etiology. Predisposing factors are prolonged labor, cervical dystocia, more prevalent in primiparas, cephalopelvic disproportion, length of cervix (an unusually long cervix prevents the external os from opening in normal manner).

Pathology. The detachment of cervix may result in partial circular tearing, a bucket-handle detachment; the detached portion may be closely applied to child's head like a cardinal's cap, or may be found hanging by a strand of tissue after child's birth. *Microscopic picture.* Acute congestion; hemorrhage; edema; necrosis.

Therapy. *Prevention.* Early recognition and treatment of cervical dystocia. *Treatment after detachment.* If incomplete, pedicle divided between clamps and base transfixed. Culture from the vaginal vault, and prophylactic chemotherapy. In management of future pregnancies, elective cesarean section indicated.

Prognosis. *Mother.* Hemorrhage uncommon; puerperal sepsis responsible for a high maternal mortality. *Fetus.* Fetal mortality 30 to 40% primarily due to failure of recognition of the cervical dystocia.

BIBLIOGRAPHY. Ingraham CB, Taylor ES: Spontaneous annular detachment of the cervix during labor. Am J Obstet Gynecol 53:873–877, 1947
Fliegner JR: Spontaneous annular detachment of the cervix. Med J Aust 1:438–441, 1968

CESTAN-CHENAIS

Synonym. Cestan's II. Represents a combination of Avellis' and Babinski-Nageotte.

Symptoms and Signs. Pharyngolaryngeal or glossopharyngeal paralysis (Avellis'). Contralateral cerebellar hemiataxia; sensibility alterations; ipsilateral enophthalmos; ptosis, nystagmus; miosis (Babinski-Nageotte).

Etiology. Thrombosis; inflammation; neoplasia producing vertebral artery lesion (medially to posterior inferior cerebellar arteries and anterior spinal branches).

Pathology. Infarct lesion of lateral portion of medulla oblongata. See Etiology.

Diagnostic Procedures. *Arteriography. CT brain scan.*

Therapy. Depends upon etiology.

Prognosis. Depends upon etiology.

BIBLIOGRAPHY. Cestan RJ, Chenais J: Du myosis dans certaines lésions bulbaires en foyer (hémiplégie du type

Avellis associée au syndrome oculaire sympathique). Gaz d Hôp 76:1229–1233, 1903
Geeraets WJ: Ocular Syndromes, 3rd ed. Philadelphia, Lea & Febiger, 1976

CHANARIN-DORFMAN

Synonyms. Triglyceride storage–impaired long-chain fatty acid oxidation; ichthyotic–neutral lipid storage; ichthyosiform erythroderma–leukocyte vacuolization.

Symptoms and Signs. Both sexes. From infancy. Ichthyosis, hepatosplenomegaly. In some cases delayed development (in middle age) of cataracts, nystagmus, deafness, ataxia, areflexia.

Etiology. Multisystem nonlysosomal triglyceride storage, decreased oxidation of oleate. Possibly autosomal recessive inheritance.

Pathology. Triglyceride intracellular infiltration (not membrane enclosed) in many organs: liver, spleen, muscle, central nervous system, intestine leukocytes.

Diagnostic Procedures. *Blood.* Hypertriglyceridemia; leukocytes: vacuolated. Absence of ketone bodies on fasting. *Cerebrospinal fluid.* After onset of neurologic manifestation: increased protein. *Electromyography.* Mild primary myopathy.

Therapy. Diet with medium-chain triglycerides.

Prognosis. Diet reverses hepatosplenomegaly. Survival into adulthood with development of quoted manifestations.

BIBLIOGRAPHY. Chanarin I, Patel A, Slavin G, et al: Neutral lipid storage disease: A new disorder with impaired long-chain fatty oxidation. Ann Neurol 7:5–10, 1980
Dorfman ML, Hershko C, Eisenberg S, et al: Ichthyosiform dermatosis with systemic lipidosis. Arch Dermatol 110:261–266, 1974
Williams ML, Koch TK, O'Donnell JJ, et al: Ichthyosis and neutral lipid storage disease. Am J Med Genet 20:711–726, 1985

CHANDLER'S (P.A.)

Symptoms and Signs. Glaucoma from occlusion of angle by anterior peripheral synechiae. Atrophy of iris; eccentric pupil; corneal dystrophy and edema.

Etiology. Unknown.

BIBLIOGRAPHY. Chandler PA: Atrophy of the stroma of iris, endothelial dystrophy, corneal edema and glaucoma. Am J Ophthamol 41:607–615, 1956

Gasset AR, Worthen DM: Keratonus and Chandler's syndrome. Ann Ophthalmol 6:819–821, 1974

CHANDLER'S (S.A.)

Synonyms. Femoral head idiopathic necrosis; hip osteochondritis dissecans. See Epiphyseal ischemic necrosis, Koenig's (F.), and observation hip.

Symptoms and Signs. Male predominance; onset in middle age. Unilateral or symmetric pain of the hip and occasionally of the knee.

Etiology. See Epiphyseal ischemic necrosis.

BIBLIOGRAPHY. Chandler SA: Aseptic necrosis of the head of the femur. Wisc Med J 35:583–618, 1936

CHANDRA-KHETARPAL

Synonym. Levocardia–bronchiectasis–sinus abnormality. See Kartagener's.

Symptoms and Signs. Present from infancy. Repeated fever episodes with symptoms and signs of bronchiectasis. Evidence at physical examination of levocardia.

Etiology. Unknown; congenital malformation.

Pathology. Levocardia; bronchiectasis; paranasal sinus not developed.

Diagnostic Procedures. *X-ray of chest and skull. Bronchoscopy. Bronchiography. Electrocardiography. Sputum culture.*

Therapy. Antibiotics. If feasible, surgery to excise part of the lung with bronchiectasis.

Prognosis. Repeated infectious episodes.

BIBLIOGRAPHY. Chandra RK, Khetarpal SK: Levocardia with bronchiectasis and paranasal sinus abnormalities. Indian J Pediar 30:78–80, 1963
Datta P: Chandra's syndrome. Lancet 2:1350–1351, 1968

CHARCOT-MARIE-TOOTH

Synonyms. Charcot-Marie-Tooth-Hoffman; peroneal muscular atrophy; progressive neural muscular atrophy; Tooth's. Motor sensory neuropathy, hereditary; HMSN.

Symptoms. Begins in puberty or early adult life. Foot drop or clubfoot; weakness, paresthesia in legs; later weakness and atrophy of hands, then arms. Occasionally sensory changes.

Signs. Atrophy progressing slowly from peroneal to other muscles of legs (stork legs). Atrophy progressing from hands to arms. Shoulders, hips, trunk well developed. Loss of deep sensibility and reflexes of parts affected; sloping gait.

Etiology. Unknown; hereditary (dominant or recessive, sex-linked inheritance). Siblings may show abortive form of the disease.

Pathology. Demyelinization of peripheral nerves (*e.g.*, peroneal, tibial); degenerative changes of anterior horn cells, dorsal columns; myopathic changes may be present.

Diagnostic Procedures. *Electromyography. Nerve conduction. Spinal fluid.* Normal; occasionally, slight increase in proteins.

Therapy. Orthopedic support.

Prognosis. Very slow progression; seldom totally incapacitating; frequently becomes stationary.

BIBLIOGRAPHY. Charcot JM, Marie P: Sur une forme particulière d'atrophie musculaire progressive, souvent familaire débutant pas les pieds les jambes et atteignant plus tard les mains. Rev Med 6:97–138, 1886
Tooth HH: The Peroneal Type of Progressive Muscular Atrophy. London, Lewis, 1886
Bird TD, Ott J, Gibblett ER, et al: Genetic linkage evidence for heterogeneity in Charcot-Marie-Tooth neuropathy (HMSN type I). Ann Neurol 14:679–684, 1983
Phillips LH II, Kelly TE, Schnatterly P, et al: Hereditary motor-sensory neuropathy (HMSN): Possible X-linked dominant inheritance. Neurology 35:498–502, 1985

CHARCOT'S ANGINA CRURIS

Synonyms. Obsolete. Angina cruris; angiosclerotic paroxystic myasthenia; intermittent claudication.

Symptoms and Signs. Observed usually in elderly persons. Pain, cramps, tension, weakness and temperature reduction of upper and, more frequently, lower extremities, which occurs after exercise and recedes after rest.

Etiology. Reduced vascular bed and blood supply not adequate to metabolic needs of tissues. Atherosclerosis; Moenckberg's (see); Buerger's (see); other vasculopathic processes.

Diagnostic Procedures. *Angiography. Doppler.*

Therapy. Thrombolytic, acetylsalicylic acid. Vasodilators of doubtful benefit. According to the etiology; sympathectomy, bypass, arterial grafts.

Prognosis. Improved by treatment.

BIBLIOGRAPHY. Charcot JM: Sur la claudication intermittente observée dans un cas d'oblitération de l'une des artères iliaques primitives. C R Soc Biol (Paris) 5:225–258, 1858

CHARCOT'S INTERMITTENT BILIARY FEVER

Synonyms. Intermittent biliary fever; secondary cholangitis. See Hanot-Roessle's.

Symptoms. More frequent in females; onset in middle age. Recurrent episodes of dull or colicky pains in right hypochondrium radiating to the back, accompanied by chills and hyperthermia; nausea, vomiting, anorexia.

Signs. Weight loss; hepatomegaly, hepatalgia. Occasionally, subicterus.

Etiology. Infection of various extrahepatic ducts, enhanced by mechanical or functional obstruction.

Pathology. Purulent (or nonpurulent) inflammation of intrahepatic and extrahepatic ducts; dilatation above obstruction and bile stasis; variable hepatic cell damage.

Diagnostic Procedures. *Blood.* Acute stage leukocytosis; positive culture; hyperbilirubinemia; increased alkaline phosphatase and other enzymes. *Urine.* Bilirubinemia. *X-ray.* Cholangiography; splenic portography; angiography. *Liver scan. Ultrasonography.*

Therapy. Antibiotics; antispastics; surgery indispensable.

Prognosis. Spontaneous temporary remissions may characterize course according to degree of obstruction. Variability depends on treatment. In some cases, once hepatic damage has developed, it may tend to progress slowly, even after obstruction is removed and the infection cured.

BIBLIOGRAPHY. Slesinger MH, Fordtran JS: Gastrointestinal Disease, p 1314. Philadelphia, WB Saunders, 1978
Fox MS, Wilk PJ, Weissmann HS, et al: Acute acalculous cholecystitis. Surg Gynecol Obstet 159:13–16, 1984
Dawson SL, Mueller PR: Nonoperative management of biliary obstruction. Ann Rev Med 36:1–11, 1985

CHARCOT'S JOINTS

Synonyms. Neurogenic arthropathy; tabetic osteoarthropathy.

Symptoms. Prevalent in males; onset usually after 40 years of age; usually, insidious onset. Painful joint swelling (degree of discomfort disproportionally milder than degree of swelling). Other signs of neurologic abnormalities from basic condition frequently not reported by patient.

Signs. Joint (single or groups) swelling with effusion; initially, hypermobility, warmth, tenderness; followed by deformity, instability, coarse crepitation. On palpation, "bag of nuts."

Etiology. Initially associated with tabes dorsalis of syphilitic origin; other conditions responsible are diabetic neuropathy, syringomyelia, myelomeningocele, and various spontaneous or traumatic central and peripheral nervous system pathologies.

Pathology. Combination of destructive and hypertrophic changes; erosion of cartilage; destruction of menisci; loose body formation and osteophyte growth, which may extend to shaft of bone or into ligaments and muscle. Subluxation. Effusion frequently hemorrhagic; synovial inflammatory reaction.

Diagnostic Procedures. *X-ray.* See Pathology. *Blood, spinal fluid.* Identification of primary pathology. See Etiology.

Therapy. Immobilization and reduction of patient's weight. Surgical and orthopedic measures in accord with nature of basic condition and degree of lesion.

Prognosis. Usually, progressive condition; poorly responsive to specific and general types of treatment.

BIBLIOGRAPHY. Charcot JM: Sur quelques arthropathies qui paraissent dépendre d'une lésion du cerveau ou de la moelle épinère. Arch Physiol 1:161–178; 370–400, 1868
Richardson EG: Miscellaneous nontraumatic disorders. In Crenshaw AH (ed): Campbell's Operative Orthopedics, 7th ed, p 1060. St. Louis, CV Mosby, 1987

CHARCOT'S TRIAD

The triad consists of (1) nystagmus; (2) scanning speech; (3) intention tremor. This syndrome was considered pathognomonic for multiple sclerosis; however, it is seen only occasionally and in advanced cases of long duration.

BIBLIOGRAPHY. Charcot JM: Diagnostic des formes frustes de la sclérose en plaques. Prog Med 7:97–99, 1879

CHARCOT-WILBRAND

Symptoms. Visual agnosia; agraphia; associated occasionally with Gerstmann's (see).

Etiology. Lesion of the artery of the angular gyrus of dominant side.

BIBLIOGRAPHY. Charcot JM: Sur un Cas de Ceocite' Verbales. Ouvres Completes de Charcot. Paris, Delahaye Lecrosnier, 1887

Tyler HR: Cerebral disorders of vision. In Smith JL (ed): Neuro-Ophthalmology, vol 4. St Louis, CV Mosby, 1968

CHARLIN'S

Synonyms. Nasal nerve; nasociliaris nerve. Identical to cluster headache with the difference that inflammatory changes of eyes are more severe (pseudopurulent conjunctivitis; keratitis; corneal ulcers, iritis). See also Anterior ethmoidal nerve.

Therapy. Cocaine applications in the anterior part of nasal fossa give rapid relief of ocular symptoms.

Prognosis. Very painful, recurrent episodes may induce suicide.

BIBLIOGRAPHY. Charlin C: Sindrome del nervio nasal. Dia Méd 2:839, 1930

Pan H: Differential Diagnosis of Eye Diseases, p 98. Philadelphia, WB Saunders, 1978

CHASSAIGNAC'S

Symptoms and Signs. Appear in infants. Pain in the arms preventing movements and thus simulating a paralytic condition.

Etiology. Referred to excessive muscle stretching.

BIBLIOGRAPHY. Chassaignac PME: De la paralysie douloureus de jeunes enfants. Arch Gen Med 7:653–669, 1856

CHATTLE'S

Synonym. Laryngeal nerve duosyndrome.

Symptoms and Signs. Appear in newborn. Weakness or unilateral palsy of facial muscles; weakness or palsy of vocal cords or of muscles (or both) of deglutition on contralateral side.

Etiology. Forced flexed lateral position in utero, which causes compression of laryngeal nerve between the thyroid cartilage and the thyroid or cricoid cartilage.

Therapy. B complex vitamins.

Prognosis. According to degree of nerve lesion and possibility of functional restoration.

BIBLIOGRAPHY. Chattle CC: A duosyndrome of the laryngeal nerve. Am J Dis Child 91:14–18, 1956

CHAVANY-BRUNHES

Synonyms. Falx calcification; Fritzsche's. See Fahr's.

Symptoms and Signs. Variable degree of psychoneurotic manifestations; cephalalgic attacks following stress, fatigue or keeping the head in a fixed position for a prolonged period of time. Oligophrenia in some cases (Fritzsche's).

Etiology. Unknown; may be familial (autosomal recessive trait).

Diagnostic Procedures. *X-ray of skull.* Calcification of falx, or other areas of scattered calcification (Fritzsche).

Therapy. Analgesic.

Prognosis. Variable.

BIBLIOGRAPHY. Chavany JA, Brunhes J: Syndromes céphalgique et psychonévrotique avec calcification de la faux du cerveau. Rev Neurol (Paris) 69:113–131, 1938

Fritzsche R: Eine familiar auftretende Form von Oligophrenia mit röntgenolish machwzisbaren symmetrischen Kalkablagerungen in Gehirn, besonders in den Stammganglien. Schweiz Arch Neurol Neurochir Psychiatr 35:1, 1935

Adams RD, Victor M: Principles of Neurology, 3rd ed, p 746. New York, McGraw–Hill, 1985

CHEDIAK-HIGASHI

Synonyms. Oculocutaneous albinism; Bégnez-César's; Chediak-Steinbrinck-Higashi; leukocytic anomaly–albinism. Gigantism peroxidase granules-granulation; anomaly leucocytes: gigantism of cytoplasmic organelles.

Symptoms. Photophobia; shifting nystagmus on exposure to light. Weakness; fever not related to infections; cerebellar tremor; dysmetria may be present as well as paralysis. Progressive peripheral neuropathy.

Signs. Decreased pigmentation of skin, hair, and eyes. Red, tender nodules, pustules and crusted ulcers of the skin may occasionally be found. Underdevelopment; moderate hepatomegaly; occasionally, splenomegaly and lymphadenopathy.

Etiology. Unknown; autosomal recessive inheritance.

Pathology. Hepatosplenomegaly; lymphoadenopathy; bone changes. Often associated with lymphomas. Histiocytic infiltration of brain and other tissue.

Diagnostic Procedures. *Blood.* Typical abnormalities in the granulation and nuclear structure of all types of leukocytes: gigantic, monstrous peroxidase-positive granules; cytoplasmic inclusion and Döhle bodies. Anemia;

thrombocytopenia. *Bone marrow.* Large eosinophilic inclusion bodies in myeloblasts and promyelocytes.

Therapy. None; prevention of infection. Long-term treatment with ascorbic acid.

Prognosis. Poor; high susceptibility to infection (not related to deficient antibody production). Lymphomas and hemorrhage (because of thrombocytopenia) are usually cause of death.

BIBLIOGRAPHY. Chédiak M: Nouvelle anomalie leucocytaire de caractère constitutionel et familial. Rev Hématol 7:362–367, 1952
César AB: Neutropenia crònica maligna familiar con granulaciones atipic de los leucocites. Bol Soc Cub Ped 15:900–910, 1953
Higashi O: Congenital gigantism of peroxidase granules; first case ever reported of qualitative abnormality of peroxidase. Tohoku J Exp Med 59:315–332, 1954
Witkop CJ, Queredo WC, Fitzpatrick TB: Albinism and other disorders of pigment metabolism. In Stanbury JB, Wyngaarden JB, Fredrickson DS, et al: The Metabolic Basis of Inherited Disease, 5th ed, p 301. New York, McGraw-Hill, 1983

CHERRY RED SPOT MYOCLONUS

Symptoms and Signs. Cherry red spot in the macula present before the patient is 10 years old; myoclonus, which is precipitated by voluntary movement, the thought of movement, light touch, passive joint movement and sound, but not by light. Insidious visual loss.

Etiology. Storage of sialidated glycopeptides and glycolipids in the brain and liver due to the deficiency of a neuroaminidase.

Pathology. Morphologic changes reflect a storage process in lysosomes of retinal ganglion cells, cortical neurons, neurons of the myenteric plexus, hepatocytes, and Kupffer cells.

Diagnostic Procedures. *Electroencephalography. Electromyography. Liver biopsy.*

Therapy. None of the drugs used was successful in controlling the myoclonus.

Prognosis. Myoclonus and visual loss can be very crippling.

BIBLIOGRAPHY. Rapin I, Goldfischer S, Katzman R, et al: The cherry red spot–myoclonus syndrome. Ann Neurol 3:234–242, 1978
Engel J, Jr, Rapin I, Giblin DR: Electrophysiological studies in two patients with cherry red spot–myoclonus syndrome. Epilepsia 18:73–87, 1977

CHESHIRE CAT

Synonym. Lanthanic. Refers to no specific disease complex, but to the two following possible categories embracing all diseases:
1. Patients showing all symptoms and signs of a well-defined entity, which the pathology findings fail to confirm.
2. Patients with a lanthanic condition (presence of the disease but no symptoms or signs, or awareness of them by the patient, so that medical help is not sought), or patients who do not show the entire diagnostic spectrum of the condition (*formes frustes*).

   This term, proposed by Bywaters to describe the syndrome, is taken from *Alice in Wonderland* in which Alice saw the grin without the cat, and because of its lack of ears she feels it useless to attempt to speak to it. This situation exemplifies the difficulty encountered by the physician in dealing with pathologic entities unexpressed or not fully expressed.

BIBLIOGRAPHY. Feinstein AR: Clinical Judgment. Baltimore, Williams & Wilkins, 1967
Bywaters EGL: The Cheshire cat syndrome. Postgrad Med J 44:19–22, 1968

CHILAIDITI'S

Synonym. Wanderleber.

Symptoms. In adults, very often asymptomatic; in children, symptomatology is instead well evident. Abdominal pain frequently associated with vomiting, occurring typically at the end of day when maximum distention occurs; pain relieved by lying down. Less frequent symptoms; anorexia; constipation and passage of flatus; air swallowing.

Signs. Abdominal distention; liver dullness absent; liver edge results at palpation significantly lowered.

Etiology. Altered relationship of liver, colon, and diaphragm, where the colon interposes itself between liver and diaphragm. Intestinal distention; paralysis of diaphragm; abnormalities of liver ligaments. In children, aerophagia and abdominal distention seem to be among the main causes.

Pathology. See Etiology.

Diagnostic Procedures. *X-ray.* Colon partially or totally interposed between liver and diaphragm.

Therapy. Lying down relieves most of the symptoms. Avoiding gassy foods and aerophagy, abdominal belt. Surgery has been suggested, but seems a too drastic procedure for a usually rather mild situation.

Prognosis. Improvement of symptoms with age has been reported.

BIBLIOGRAPHY. Chilaiditi D: Zur Frage der Hepatoptose und Ptose im allgemeinem im Anschluss an drei Fälle von temporären, partieller Leberverlagerunz. Fortschr Rontgenstr Berl 16:173–208, 1910
Jackson ADM, Hodson CJ: Interposition of the colon between liver and diaphragm (Chilaiditi's syndrome) in children. Arch Dis Child 32:151–158, 1957

CHINESE RESTAURANT

Synonyms. Glutamic acid toxicity; post-sino-cibal; sin-cib-sin. Food migraine, hot-dog headache.

Symptoms. Onset within 15 to 25 minutes of an abundant meal in a Chinese restaurant. Burning sensation in the back of the neck. Followed by burning over forearms and anterior chest and substernal discomfort. Followed by infraorbital pressure and tightness.

Signs. None; no erythema or sign of muscular contraction in areas of burning or constriction.

Etiology. In susceptible person, monosodium glutamate (5 g) used in Chinese cooking. Nonsusceptible person will have no reaction with even 25 g. Inborn error of metabolism. Autosomal recessive.

Pathology. None.

Diagnostic Procedures. None.

Therapy. None.

Prognosis. As many as eight episodes a day can be survived, as proved by the personal experience of a dedicated physician.

BIBLIOGRAPHY. Kwok RHM: Chinese restaurant syndrome. New Engl J Med 278:1122, 1968
Reif–Lehrer L: Possible significance of adverse reaction to glutamate in humans. Fed Proc 35:2205–2212, 1976
De Francisci G, Parisi N, Magalini: SI: La sindrome del ristorante Cinese. Rec Prog Med 70:353–357, 1981

CHIN QUIVERING

Synonyms. Frey's (E.); mentalis muscle tremor; trembling chin.

Symptoms and Signs. Both sexes affected; present from birth. Chin quivering (fine, transitory tremor) caused by emotion or activities that require concentration. Tremor stops during sleep. Possible interference with speech and occasional association with nystagmus. Reported also, nocturnal myoclonus and tongue biting.

Etiology. Autosomal dominant inheritance with complete penetrance.

Prognosis. Attacks decreasing in frequency with age.

BIBLIOGRAPHY. Frey E: Ein streng dominant aeribiches Kirmmuskelzittern. Dtsch Z Nervenheilk 115:9–26, 1930
Gorlin JK, Pinborg JJ, Cohen MM Jr: Syndromes of the Head and Neck, 2nd ed. New York, McGraw-Hill, 1976

CHIRAY'S

Synonyms. Biliary atony; biliary hypotonic; cholecystic atony; lazy gallbladder.

Symptoms. Dyspepsia; anorexia; nausea; intolerance to fatty foods; attack of pain in right hypochondrium frequently radiating to the back; headache; nervous depression.

Signs. Pain on palpation of right hypochondrium.

Etiology. Motor disorder of gallbladder; atonic state that determines full capacity of distention so that any sudden increase in pressure results in pain. Other motor disorders such as spasmodic gallbladder or hypertension produce exactly the same symptomatology; secondary to impaired flow, because of sphincter of Oddi spasm or organic impediment.

Pathology. Gallbladder is flaccid; neck poorly visualized. Secondary inflammation of bile ducts and gallbladder may be present.

Diagnostic Procedures. *Cholecystography. Timed biliary drainage.*

Therapy. Stimulation of gallbladder contraction with cholecystokinetic foods plus biliary salts. In hyperkinetic conditions, opposite diet has to be used. Vitamin B complex; exercises. Relief of tension and fatigue; psychotherapy.

Prognosis. Good with adequate treatment.

BIBLIOGRAPHY. Galen, 131–201, AD
Chiray M: Etat actuel de le cholecystoatonic. In Albot e Poilleux: Les Voies Biliares. Paris, Masson, 1953
Blumgart LH (ed): The Biliary Tract. New York, Churchill Livingstone, 1982

CHLOASMA

Synonyms. Liver spot; melasma.

Symptoms. Frequent in women during the entire reproductive period and/or in menopause; considered physiological during pregnancy; rarely occurring in men. Asymptomatic.

Signs. Symmetric brown masklike patches involving cheeks and forehead, sometimes also genitalia and breast.

Etiology. Unknown; attributed to endocrine mechanism (in some cases, produced by progestional steroids or hydantoin).

Pathology. Increased deposition of melanin in skin basal layer.

Diagnostic Procedures. *Pregnancy test. Hormonal studies.*

Therapy. All treatment attempts generally useless. Recommended for trial: hydroquinone agents.

Prognosis. After pregnancy usually fades; it may, however, persist or recur.

BIBLIOGRAPHY. Newcomber VD, Lindberg HC, Sternberg, TH: A melanosis of the face ("chloasma"). AMA Arch Dermatol 83:284–299, 1961
Rook A, Wilkinson DS, Ebling FJG, et al: Textbook of Dermatology, 4th ed, p 1578. Oxford, Blackwell Scientific Publications, 1986

CHOLANGITIS, PRIMARY SCLEROSING

Synonyms. Fibrosing cholangitis; chronic obliterative cholangitis; primary sclerosing cholangitis.

Symptoms. More frequent in males; onset middle age. Pruritus; dragging or pain in right upper abdominal quadrant; anorexia, nausea and vomiting; occasionally chills.

Signs. Jaundice (after week of discomfort or pain); occasionally hepatomegaly, weight loss.

Etiology. Unknown. Stenosing inflammatory process of bile ducts. Frequently associated with ulcerative colitis, less frequently with Crohn's, Ormond's, mediastinal fibrosis or retroorbital tumor.

Pathology. Thickening of entire system of extrahepatic bile ducts and occasionally edema of adjacent tissues. Collagen scar with few inflammatory cells. Seldom, involvement of intrahepatic ducts. Lymph nodes enlarged.

Diagnostic Procedures. *Blood.* White blood cells increase; eosinophilia; hyperbilirubinemia. Antimitochondrial antibodies usually absent. An increased level of alkaline phosphatase in a young man, particularly if affected by ulcerative colitis strongly suggestive for this syndrome. *Intravenous and oral cholangiography.* Failure of ducts to become opaque. *Retrograde and transhepatic*

cholangiography. Good diagnostic results. *Biopsy of liver.* Bile stasis; periportal fibrosis.

Therapy. Surgery. Ductal dilatation and insertion of T or V tubes (left for 6 mos or longer). Systematic corticosteroids. If necessary, liver transplantation.

Prognosis. Outcome unpredictable; from complete recovery to secondary biliary cirrhosis or related to associated conditions.

BIBLIOGRAPHY. Schwartz SI: Primary sclerosing cholangitis. Surg Clin North Am 53:1161–1167, 1973
Javitt NB: Hyperbilirubinemic and cholestatic syndromes. Postgrad Med 65:120–130, 1979
La Russo NF, Wiesner RH, Ludwig J, et al: Primary sclerosing cholangitis. N Engl J Med 310:899–903, 1984

CHOLERRHEIC ENTEROPATHY

Synonym. Interrupted enterohepatic circulation.

Symptoms. Occur in patients with ileal disease or ileal resection. Diarrhea; steatorrhea; weight loss.

Etiology. Interrupted enterohepatic circulation of bile salt due to pathology of ileum (site of reabsorption of bile salts); ulcerative colitis with ileal involvement; regional ileitis; or resection of ileum; conceivably virus enteritis. Increase of turnover rate and synthesis rate of bile salts due to lack of bile return.

Pathology. See Etiology.

Diagnostic Procedures. *Stool.* Determination of cumulative fecal excretion of labeled bile acid. Determination of rate of absorption of fat, cholesterol, carotene, vitamins D, E, and K.

Therapy. Dilemma: administration of bile salts corrects the malabsorption, but worsens diarrhea. In three patients, however, it increased absorption of lipids and corrected diarrhea. Cholestyramine reduces diarrhea, but increases steatorrhea.

Prognosis. Natural history of this recently established syndrome is unknown. It is thought that with time liver may stop compensatory hyperproduction of bile and upper intestine or large intestine may develop ability to absorb bile, and finally large intestine may become refractory to the cathartic effects of bile salts.

BIBLIOGRAPHY. Hofmann AF: The syndrome of ileal disease and the broken enterohepatic circulation: Cholerrheic enteropathy. Gastroenterology 52:752–757, 1967
Blumgart LH (ed): The Biliary Tract. New York, Churchill Livingstone, 1982

CHOLESTEROL PERICARDITIS

Synonym. Alexander's (J.S.).

Symptoms and Signs. Both sexes. In all ages from adolescence. Symptomatic, recurrent pericardial effusions that eventually lead to constricting calcific pericarditis.

Etiology. Unknown. A familial occurrence also reported (autosomal recessive?)

Diagnostic Procedures. *Chest X-rays. Electrocardiography. Echocardiography. Pericardial tapping.* Fluid with abundant cholesterol crystals (gold-paint aspect).

Therapy. Symptomatic.

Prognosis. Cardiac failure.

BIBLIOGRAPHY. Alexander JS: A pericardial effusion of gold paint appearance due to the presence of cholesterin. Brit Med J 2:463, 1919
Stanley RJ, Subramanian R, Lie JT: Cholesterol pericarditis terminating as constrictive calcific pericarditis; follow-up study of patient with 40 years history of disease. Am J Cardiol 46:511–514, 1980

CHOLESTERYL ESTER HYDROLASE DEFICIENCY

Synonyms. CESD; hepatic cholesteryl storage; polycorie cholestérolique. See also Wolman's. Cholesteryl ester storage disease.

Symptoms. Both sexes affected; prevalent in females; detection between 2 and 23 years. Hepatomegaly (constant sign) may be present at birth, or become evident later; splenomegaly is frequently present. Absence of jaundice, signs of malabsorption and of neurologic involvement.

Etiology. Deficiency of acid cholesteryl ester hydrolase. Genetic pattern of inheritance not assessed. Autosomal recessive (?).

Pathology. Three categories of findings respectively related to (1) intralysosomal storage of lipids; (2) portal hypertension; (3) atherosclerosis. *Liver.* Prominent lipid accumulation; enlarged, orange color; septal fibrosis (or cirrhosis); focal periportal accumulation of lymphocytes, plasma cells, and foamy macrocytes. *Spleen.* May be similarly infiltrated. *Intestine.* May show infiltration with extracellular lipids and foamy cells.

Diagnostic Procedures. *Blood.* Hyperbetalipoproteinemia; cholesterol and cholesteryl ester markedly increased; total lipids normal. Anemia. *Biopsy of liver.* See Pathology. *Bone marrow.* Foamy cells or normal. *Fibroblast cul-*ture. Demonstration of cholesteryl ester hydrolase deficiency.

Therapy. None.

Prognosis. Patients survive into adulthood, reported to live past 40 years of age.

BIBLIOGRAPHY. Fredrickson DS: Newly recognized disorders of cholesterol metabolism. Ann Intern Med 58:718–719, 1963
Assmann G, Fredrickson DS: Acid lipase deficiency: Wolman's disease and cholesteryl ester storage disease. In Stanbury JB, Wyngaarden JB, Fredrickson DS, et al: The Metabolic Basis of Inherited Disease, 5th ed, p 803. New York, McGraw-Hill, 1983

CHONDRODYSPLASIA PUNCTATA—X-LINKED

Synonyms. CDPX, CPX.

Symptoms and Signs. Males homozygous usually die; females survive. Similar to Conradi's (see) and as distinctive features: pigmentary lesions of the skin (whorled or linear) that evolve toward ichthyosis, follicular atrophoderma, cicatrical alopecia and hypoplasia of distal phalanges. Cerebral involvement, asymmetric cataracts.

Etiology. X-linked dominant.

Prognosis. Fatal or extremely severe in males.

BIBLIOGRAPHY. Spranger JW, Opitz JM, Bibber V: Heterogeneity of chondrodysplasia punctata. Hum Genet 11:190–212, 1971
Apple R: X-linked dominant chondrodysplasia punctata. Review of the literature and report of a case. Hum Genet 53:65–73, 1979

CHONDROMALACIA PATELLAE

Synonym. Aleman's.

Symptoms and Signs. Prevalent in middle aged women; early onset possible due to recurrent patellar subluxation or dislocation. Frequently bilateral; crepitus on knee extension; then pain, snapping and catching and, finally, extensive effusion.

Etiology. Friction of patellofemoral joint aggravated by excessive mobility (subluxation).

Diagnostic Procedures. *X-rays.*

Therapy. *Preventive.* Medial transfer of patellar tendon insertion; plication of medial capsule and alignment correction. *Curative.* Strain relief or, in severe case, patellectomy.

Prognosis. According to efficiency of treatment. Patellectomy restores function.

BIBLIOGRAPHY. Aleman O: Chondromalacia posttraumatic patellae. Acta Chir Scand 63:149–152, 1928
Bronitsky JB: Chondromalacia patellae. J Bone and Joint Surg 29:931–945, 1947
Sisk TD: Arthroscopy of knee and ankle. In Crenshaw AH (ed): Campbell's Operative Orthopedics, 7th ed, pp 2601–2602. St. Louis, CV Mosby, 1987

CHOREA GRAVIDARUM

Symptoms. Choreiform movement occurring during pregnancy, usually starting in first trimester. In young primiparas, occasionally recurrent in successive pregnancies.

Therapy. Only if very severe case, termination of pregnancy.

Prognosis. After termination of pregnancy, further attacks may recur years later in about 30% of cases.

BIBLIOGRAPHY. Adams RD, Victor M: Principles of Neurology, 3rd ed, p 61. New York, McGraw-Hill, 1985

CHOREA, SENILE

Synonym. Chronic progressive nonhereditary chorea.

Symptoms. Sudden onset after 50 years of age. The same symptoms as in other forms of chorea; rarely, mental deterioration; only changes in emotion and memory.

Etiology. Brain changes secondary to vascular pathology.

Pathology. Degenerative lesion of large and small cells of putamen and corpus striatum. Atherosclerotic vascular changes.

Prognosis. Slowly progressing disability.

BIBLIOGRAPHY. Alcock NS: Note on pathology of senile chorea (nonhereditary). Brain 59:376–387, 1936
Adams RD, Victor M: Principles of Neurology, 3rd ed, p 872. New York, McGraw-Hill, 1985

CHOREIFORM

Different pathologic entities that have in common the symptoms of choreiform movements. Four distinct nosographical entities may be differentiated with different etiology, therapy, and prognosis:
1. Acute chorea, which includes chorea gravidarum
2. Chronic, progressive, hereditary chorea
3. Chronic, progressive, nonhereditary, senile chorea
4. Wespthal-Leyden ataxia.
   Other forms such as Dubini's, Henoch's I, Bergeron's, Morvan's and Muratow's are rare and only of historical interest. Choreiform movements are also present in congenital defects of the corpus striatum (nonprogressive).

BIBLIOGRAPHY. Dubini A: Primi cenni sulla corea elettrica. Ann Univ Med (Milano), 117:5–50, 1846
Henoch E: Beitrage zur Kinderheilkunde. Berlin, A Hirschwald, 1861
Huntington G: On chorea. Med Surg Reporter 26:317–321, 1872
Berland, R: Traitement par le tartre stibié d'une forme de la chorée dite électrique. Poitiers, 1880
Morvan AM: De la chorée fibrillaire. Gaz Hebd Méd 27:173–176, 1890
Muratow W: Zur Pathogenese der Hemichorea postapoplectica. Monatsschr Psychiatr Neurol 5:180–192, 1899
Bremme H: Ein Beitrag zur Bindearmchorea. Monatsschr Psychiat Neurol Berl 45:107–120, 1919
Tsiminakis Y: Zur Localisation der Hemichorea. Arb Neurol Wien Univ 35:57–75, 1933
Wolff PH, Hurnitz I: The choreiform syndrome. Dev Med Child Neurol 8:160–165, 1966
Adams RD, Victor M: Principles of Neurology, 3rd ed, pp 744–745. New York, McGraw-Hill, 1985

CHORIOCARCINOMA

Synonyms. Chorioepithelioma; syncytioma malignum.

Symptoms. Choriocarcinoma nearly always follows hydatidiform mole, abortion, or term pregnancy. Bleeding from the uterus during pregnancy in the second trimester of pregnancy. Very often, however, first symptoms and signs are related to metastases to lungs, liver, brain, or other areas.

Etiology. Unknown.

Pathology. Composed of both syncytial and cytotrophoblastic cells that do not form chorionic villi, but grow and destroy the uterine muscle.

Therapy. Hysterectomy and excision of all localized and accessible metastases. In advanced cases chemotherapy (*e.g.,* methotrexate).

Prognosis. Very poor; few cures on record.

BIBLIOGRAPHY. Lurain JR, Brewer JI, Torok EE, et al: Natural history of hydatidiform mole after primary evacuation. Am J Obstet Gynecol 145:591–595, 1983
Szulman AE: Syndromes of hydatidiform moles. Partial versus complete. J Reprod Med 29:788–791, 1984

CHORIOCARCINOMA, INFANTILE

Symptoms. Both sexes affected; onset between 5 weeks to 7 months. Anemia; hemophthysis; hematemesis; hematuria or melena.

Signs. Hepatomegaly; breast enlargement; growth of pubic hair; abdominal mass may be palpated.

Etiology. Choriocarcinoma metastasized from placenta during intrauterine life.

Pathology. Choriocarcinoma in lung, liver, occasionally subcutaneous, adrenals, brain.

Diagnostic Procedures. *X-ray.* Presence of mass in lung. *Urine.* Chorionic gonadotropin marked elevation.

Therapy. Methotrexate.

Prognosis. Death is usually rapid. Early recognition important because it will lead to diagnosis and treatment of mother.

BIBLIOGRAPHY. Emery JL: Chorionepithelioma in a newborn male child with hyperplasia of the interstitial cells of the testis. J Pathol Bacteriol 64:735–739, 1952
Witzleben CL, Bruninga, G: Infantile choriocarcinoma: A characteristic syndrome. J Pediatr 73:374–378, 1968
Voûte PA, Barrett A, Bloom HJC, Lemerle J., Neidhardt NK (eds): Cancer in Children: Clinical Management. Springer Verlag, 1986

CHRISTIAN (J.C.)

Synonyms. Brachydactyly, preaxial. Hallux varus–thumb abduction.

Symptoms and Signs. Both sexes affected to similar degree. Short thumbs and halluxes with varism. Metacarpal, metatarsal, and distal phalanges short, proximal and medial phalanges normal.

Etiology. Autosomal dominant inheritance.

BIBLIOGRAPHY. Christian JC, Chu KS, Franken EA, et al: Dominant preaxial brachydactyly with hallux varus and thumb abduction. Am J Hum Genet 24:694–701, 1972

CHRISTMAS

Synonyms. Factor IX deficiency; hemophilia B; plasma thromboplastin component; PTC deficiency.

Symptoms and Signs. Virtually limited to males. Almost identical with those of hemophilia, classic (see).

Usually milder; variation of severity correlated with degree of deficiency of plasma thromboplastin component.

Etiology. Congenital deficiency of factor IX. X-linked recessive type of inheritance. Seldom observed in females. See Hemophilia, classic, for explanation. Several factor IX variants have been recognized.

Diagnostic Procedures. *Blood.* Normal bleeding time; normal or prolonged clotting time; usually abnormal thromboplastin generation test; abnormal absorbed plasma reagent in factor IX deficiency; abnormal serum reagent in factor IX deficiency; normal or abnormal prothombin consumption test; factor IX assay diagnostic; normal one stage prothrombin time.

Therapy. As in hemophilia, stored plasma may be used, or combination of lyophilized factor IX–X–prothrombin commercially available (Bebulin).

Prognosis. Prognosis depends on severity of defect; grossly like classic hemophilia.

BIBLIOGRAPHY. Aggler PM, et al: Plasma thromboplastin component (PTC) deficiency; a new disease resembling hemophilia. Proc Soc Exp Biol Med 79:692–694, 1962
Biggs R, Douglas AS, MacFarlane RG. Christmas disease: a condition previously mistaken for haemophilia. Br Med J 2:1378–1382, 1952
Schulman I, Smith CH: Hemorrhagic disease in an infant due to deficiency of a previously undescribed clotting factor. Blood 7:794–807, 1952
Roberts HR, Chung KS, Goldsmith JC: Mutant forms of factor IX. Thromb Haemost 38:338, 1977
Usharani P, Warn-Cramer BJ, Kasper CK, et al: Characterization of three abnormal factor IX variants (Bm Lake Elsinore, Long Beach, and Los Angeles) of hemophilia B. J Clin Invest 73:76–83, 1985

CHRIST-SIEMENS

Synonyms. Anhidrotic-ectodermal dysplasia; congenital ectodermal defect; Guilford's; Siemens; Thurman's; Wedderhorn's; Weech's. See Jacquet's and Rapp-Hodgkin. Christ-Siemens-Touraine.

Symptoms. Prevalent in males; onset from birth. Temperature disturbances due to reduced or absent perspiration. Increased respiratory infections; dysphagia; poor physical and mental development. Some cases with signs of adrenal medullary insufficiency (see Addison's).

Signs. Hypotrichosis and partial or total anodontia (characteristic features). Various degrees of intensity of manifestations. Complete form: smooth, soft, dry skin; prominent frontal ridges and chin; sunken cheeks; thick lips; large ears; saddle nose; defects of nails; occasionally, congenital cataract.

Etiology. Unknown; autosomal dominant (mild), recessive X-linked inheritance (severe) with different penetrance and occasionally some manifestation in female carriers.

Pathology. Exocrine sweat glands absent or rudimentary; apocrine glands, hair follicles and sebaceous glands may be normal, hypoplastic, or absent.

Diagnostic Procedures. *Sweat tests. Biopsy of skin. Blood.* In some cases protein-bound serum thyroxine is increased.

Therapy. Avoidance of exposure to hot environment.

Prognosis. Incurable condition.

BIBLIOGRAPHY. Darwin CH: The Variation of Animals and Plants under Domestication, (2nd ed), London, John Murray, 1875
Christ J: Uber die Kongenit ectodermalen Defeckte und ihre Beziehungen zu einanden; vikariirendes Pigment fuer Haarbildung. Arch Dermatol Syph 116:685–703, 1913
Week AA: Hereditary ectodermal dysplasia (congenital ectodermal defect). A report of two cases. Am J Dis Child 7:766–790, 1929
Siemens HW: Studien ueber Veredung von Hautkrankheiten. XII Anhidrosis hipotrichotica Arch Dermatol Syph 175:567–577, 1937
Thurman J: Two cases in which the skin, hair and teeth were imperfectly developed. Proc R Med Clin Soc (London) 31:71–82, 1948
Touraine A: L'Anidrose avec hypotricose et anodontic Polydysplasie ectodérmique héréditaire. Presse Med 44:145–149, 1946
Soderholm A-L, Kaitila I: Expression of X-linked hypohidrotic ectodermal dysplasia in six males and in their mothers. Clin Genet 28:136–144, 1985

CHROMHIDROSIS

See Pseudochromhydrosis.

Symptoms and Signs. Rare in recognizable form. Slightly colored sweat (yellow, blue, or green) seen in 10% of population. May become manifested continuously or intermittently. Both sexes affected; prevalent in females of any age. Site most frequently involved is face (lower eyelids); less frequently, axillae, groin, breast, and hands. Colors can be black, violet, blue, brown, yellow, green, and seldom, red.

Etiology. Granules of lipofuscin in apocrine glands. Commonest cause is ingested drugs or dyes.

Pathology. Large amount of lipofuscin in apocrine glands.

Diagnostic Procedures. *Sweat tests.* Examination with ultraviolet light and chromatography.

Therapy. Surgical: excision of sweat gland involved.

Prognosis. Persistent condition. Good response to surgery.

BIBLIOGRAPHY. Le Roy de Méricourt H: Chromidrose rose. Azch Gen de Med, Nov 1857. Bull Acad Med 13:425–428, 1884
Hurley HJ, Shelley WB: The human apocrine sweat gland in health and disease. Springfield, CC Thomas, 1960
Stewart WM: Physiologie and physiopathologie de la sécrétion sudorale eccrine. Encycl Méd Chir (Paris). Dermatologie 12230 A 10, 1978

CHROMOSOME 1, PARTIAL TRISOMY

Symptoms and Signs. Facial dysmorphisms: triangular shape with synophrys, beaked nose, midfacial hypoplasia, long philtrum, thick lips, short mandible, prenatal and postnatal growth retardation; microcephaly; heart defects, gastrointestinal tract stenoses, cleft palate, corneal opacities, and microphthalmia.

Etiology. Partial trisomy of chromosome.

Prognosis. Many of the patients described died early after birth. All survivors were severely mentally retarded.

BIBLIOGRAPHY. Rehder H, Friedrich U: Partial trisomy 1q syndrome. Clin Genet 15:534–540, 1979
Serena Lungarotti M, Falorni A, Calabro A, et al: De novo duplication 1q 32-q42: Variability of phenotypic features in partial trisomics. J Med Genet 17:398–402, 1980

CHROMOSOME 1, PROXIMAL DELETION

Symptoms and Signs. Severe intrauterine and postnatal growth retardation, microbrachycephaly, profound mental deficiency; round facies with frontal bossing, sparse eyebrows, small mandible, small and dysplastic earlobes; inguinal hernias; hypoplastic genitalia; short and broad hands and feet.

Etiology. Interstitial deletion of the long arm of chromosome 1.

Prognosis. Poor.

BIBLIOGRAPHY. Taysi K, Sekhon GS, Hillman RE: A new syndrome of proximal deletion of chromosome 1: 1q, 21-23-24-25. Am J Med Genet 13:423–430, 1982

CHROMOSOME 1,
TERMINAL DELETION

Symptoms and Signs. Mild intrauterine growth deficiency; severe postnatal growth deficiency; microcephaly; profound mental retardation with muscular hypotonia and seizures; facial dysmorphisms: inner epicanthic folds, upslanting palpebral fissures, bulbous nose with flat bridge; scoliosis; genital ambiguity; minor skeletal anomalies.

Etiology. Terminal deletion of the long arm of chromosome 1.

BIBLIOGRAPHY. Juberg RC, Haney NR, Stallard R: New deletion syndrome: 1q 42. Am J Hum Genet 33:455–463, 1981
Zabel BU, Baumann WA: 1q deletion syndrome. Clin Genet 19:544–545, 1981

CHROMOSOME 2,
PARTIAL TRISOMY

Symptoms and Signs. Short stature, microcephaly, mental retardation; facial dysmorphisms: high forehead, frontal bossing, hypertelorism, epicanthic folds, ptosis and strabismus, nasolacrimal duct obstruction, narrow and high palate, small and pointed chin; scoliosis; cryptorchidism, hypospadia; aortic stenosis.

Etiology. Partial duplication of the short arm of chromosome 2.

Prognosis. Poor; death in the first months or years of life or severe mental deficiency.

BIBLIOGRAPHY. Cassidy SB, Heller RM, Chazen EM, et al: The chromosome 2 distal short arm trisomy syndrome. J Paediatr 91:934–938, 1977
Rosenfeld W, Verma RS, Jhaveri R, et al: Partial duplication for the short arm of chromosome 2: The 2p 23 syndrome. Am Genet (Paris) 25:28–31, 1982

CHROMOSOME 3,
PARTIAL DELETION

Symptoms and Signs. Asymmetry of the skull and facies, low frontal and nuchal hairline, hypertelorism, synophrys, upslanting palpebral fissures, epicanthic folds, ptosis, strabismus, narrow nose with prominent bridge, long philtrum, small and protruding ears; scoliosis; small fingers and toes; pre and postnatal growth retardation and delayed bone maturation; mental retardation.

Etiology. Partial deletion of the short arm of chromosome 3.

Prognosis. Mental retardation.

BIBLIOGRAPHY. Fineman RM, Hecht F, Ablow RC, et al: Chromosome 3 duplication q/deletion p syndrome. Pediatrics 61:611–618, 1978
Merrild U, Berggreen S, Hansen L, et al: Partial deletion of the short arm of chromosome 3. Eur J Pediatr 136:211–216, 1981

CHROMOSOME 3,
PARTIAL TRISOMY

Symptoms and Signs. Facial clefts; heart malformations; renal anomalies; syndactyly of fingers; choanal atresia; microphthalmia; accessory nipples; esophageal atresia; atresia of colon and rectum; genital anomalies; mental deficiency.

Etiology. Trisomy for the distal end of the short arm of chromosome 3.

Prognosis. High incidence of early death.

BIBLIOGRAPHY. Yunis JJ: Trisomy for the distal end of the short arm of chromosome 3. A syndrome. Am J Dis Child 132:30–33, 1978
Braga S, Schmidt A: Clinical and cytogenetic spectrum of duplication 3p. Eur J Pediatr 138:195–197, 1982

CHROMOSOME 5,
PARTIAL TRISOMY

Symptoms and Signs. Cerebral malformations; coloboma of the iris with or without microphtalmia; hiatal or other hernias; congenital heart defects; anal atresia; malformations of gut and kidneys.

Etiology. Complete or partial trisomy for chromosome 5.

Prognosis. High frequency of early death caused by fatal infections. Mental retardation in the survivors.

BIBLIOGRAPHY. Briblecombe FSW, Lewis FJ, Vowles M: Complete 5p trisomy: 1 case and 1q translocations in 6 generations. J Med Genet 14:271–274, 1977
Leschot NJ, Lim KS: Complete trisomy 5p; de novo translocation (2;5) (q36;p11) with isochromosome 5p. Case report and review of the literature. Hum Genet 46:271–278, 1979

CHROMOSOME 8, PARTIAL DELETION (SHORT ARM)

Symptoms and Signs. Pre- and postnatal growth retardation; microcephaly and moderate to severe mental retardation; congenital nystagmus, short nose, long upper lip; barrel chest with widely spaced nipples; hypospadias and cryptorchidism; congenital heart defects; inguinal hernias; vertebral anomalies.

Etiology. Deletion of short arm of chromosome 8.

Prognosis. Depends on heart defects; mild mental retardation in the survivors.

BIBLIOGRAPHY. Orye E, Craen M: A new chromosome deletion syndrome. Report of a patient with 46 XY, 8p- chromosome constitution. Clin Genet 9:289–301, 1976
Reiss JA, Brenes PM, Chamberlin J, et al: The 8p- syndrome. Hum Genet 47:135–140, 1979

CHROMOSOME 9, PARTIAL DELETION (SHORT ARM)

Symptoms and Signs. Trigonocephaly with a prominent metopica and depressed temples, synophrys and bushy eyebrows, upslanting palpebral fissures, mild hypertelorism, pseudoexophthalmos, midface hypoplasia with short nose and depressed nasal bridge and anteverted nares; small mandible, irregular teeth, high and narrow palate; small posteriorly rotated ears with hypoplastic, adherent lobules and prominent anthelices, and a short and broad neck; wide-set nipples, hernias, scoliosis, diastasis recti, genital anomalies, foot position anomalies; mental retardation is frequent, as well as seizure disorders. Rarely: cardiac defects.

Etiology. Deletion of the short arm of chromosome 9.

Prognosis. Many adult patients have been reported. Mental disorders are frequent in the survivors.

BIBLIOGRAPHY. Alfi O, Donnell GN, Grandall BF, et al: Deletion of the short arm of chromosome 9 (46, 9p-): A new deletion syndrome. Ann Genet (Paris) 16:17–22, 1973
Funderburk SJ, Sparkes RS, Klisak I: The 9p- syndrome. J Med Genet 16:75–79, 1979
Wishiewski L, Szymanska J, Niezabitowska A, et al: Two new cases of 9p- syndrome. Klin Paediatr 192:270–274, 1980

CHROMOSOME 10, PARTIAL DELETION (SHORT ARM)

Symptoms and Signs. Newborns are moderately underweight with widely open fontanels, square-shaped face with high forehead, down slanting palpebral fissures, ptosis of the upper eyelids, short nose with anteverted nostrils and broad and flat bridge, receding mandible, posteriorly rotated and mishaped ears; genital anomalies. Frequently babies present feeding difficulties and infections.

Etiology. Deletion of the short arm of chromosome 10.

Prognosis. Many patients die early in life. The survivors are growth retarded, with moderate to severe mental retardation and seizures.

BIBLIOGRAPHY. Berger R, Laroche JC, Toubas PL: Deletion of the short arm of chromosome 10. Acta Paediatr Scand 66:659–662, 1977
Klep-de-Pater JM, Bijllsma JP, Alkema FMJ: Partial monosomy 10p syndrome. Eur J Pediatr 137:243–246, 1981

CHROMOSOME 11, PARTIAL DELETION (LONG ARM)

Synonym. Monosomy 11q.

Symptoms and Signs. Trigonocephaly, upslanting palpebral fissures, inner epicanthic folds, ptosis of the upper lids, depressed bridge and short tip of the nose with anteverted nares, cup-shaped upper lip, and receding mandible; heart malformations: single ventricle with or hypoplasia of the left ventricle with or without atresia of the mitral valve; coloboma of the iris, optic atrophy; pyloric stenosis; anal stenosis; hydronephrosis, cystic kidneys and duplication of kidneys.

Etiology. Deletion of the long arm of chromosome 11.

Prognosis. 25% of the patients described died within the first days to months of life, from cardiac and respiratory failure. Survivors were short, microcephalic, and often affected by mental retardation.

BIBLIOGRAPHY. Turleau C, Chavin-Colin F, Robin M, et al: Monosomic partielle 11q et trigonocephalie. un nouveau syndrome. Ann Genet (Paris) 18:257–260, 1975
Lee ML, Sciorra LJ: Partial monosomy of the long arm of chromosome 11 in a severely affected child. Ann Genet (Paris) 24:51–53, 1981

CHROMOSOME 13, PARTIAL DELETION (LONG ARM)

Synonyms. Lele's; 13q.

Symptoms. Variable pattern of features present in about 50% of cases. Prenatal onset. Growth deficiency. At birth; muscle hypotony, reduced vision. *Head.* Microcephaly; tendency to trigonocephaly and other severe skull-brain defects (holoprosencephaly); hypertelorism; ptosis; lid antimongoloid slant; microphthalmia, coloboma; nasal bridge and maxilla prominence; micrognathia; delayed and abnormal dentition. *Ears.* Low set and large. *Neck.* Short and webbed. *Hands.* Thumbs absent or small; fifth finger brachyphalangia. *Feet.* Short, large toe; pes equinovarus. *Genitalia.* Hypospadias; cryptorchidism. Cardiac defect. Retinoblastoma occasional finding that seems related to the genetic condition.

Etiology. Partial deletion of the long arm of chromosome 13. No hereditary factor.

Diagnostic Procedures. *Chromosome studies. X-rays.* Dilated cerebral ventricles and cisterna cerebellomedullaris; poroencephalia.

Prognosis. *Quoad vitam*, variable survival into adulthood. Severe mental retardation.

BIBLIOGRAPHY. Lele KP, Penrose LS, Stallarf HB: Chromosome deletion in a case of retinoblastoma. Ann Hum Genet 27:171–174, 1963

Schmidt A, Passarge E: Variable mental development associated with deletion of the short arm of chromosome 18. Clin Genet 20:390–391, 1981

CHROMOSOME 18, LONG ARM DELETION

Synonyms. De Grouchy II; 18q.

Symptoms and Signs. Both sexes affected. Gross mental retardation, growth deficiency, hypotonic, poor coordination nystagmus, conductive deafness, microcephaly; talipes equinovarus; skin nodules in nasal folds; tapering fingers, widely separated nipples. In males, minute penis, cryptorchidism. In females, hypoplastic labia minora. Congenital cardiac defects.

Etiology. Deficiency of the long arm of chromosome 18.

Diagnostic Procedures. *Chromosome studies. Blood.* Occasionally, absence of IgA globulin.

Therapy. None.

Prognosis. From severe handicap to fair prognosis.

BIBLIOGRAPHY. De Grouchy J, Royer P, Salmon CH, et al: Deletion partielle des bras longs du chromosome 18. Pathol Biol 12:5–79, 1964

Insley J: Syndrome associated with a deficiency of part of the long arm of chromosome no. 18. Arch Dis Child 42:140–146, 1967

Wilson MG, Towner JW, Forsman I, et al: Syndromes associated with deletion of the long arm of chromosome 18 (del) (18 q). Am J Med Genet 3:155–174, 1979

CHROMOSOME 18, SHORT ARM DELETION

Synonyms. Short arm partial deletion of chromosome 18p; monosomy-18 partial short arm; De Grouchy-Lamy-Thieffry.

Symptoms and Signs. Present from birth. Variable pattern of features: dysphagia; mental retardation; delayed speech (until 9 yrs of age); oliguria; rheumatoidlike manifestations (rare). *Head.* Microcephaly; moon facies; hypertelorism; flat bridge of nose; eye lid ptosis; epicanthal folds; mongolism or antimongolian slant; strabismus; nystagmus (rare); cataract; wide mouth; micrognathia; large ears. *Extremities.* Small hands and feet. *Skin.* Alopecia (rare); depigmentation (rare); haloprosencephaly-arhinencephalia defects (rare).

Etiology. Deletion of short arm of chromosome 18 (clinically similar to cat cry, see).

Diagnostic Procedures. *Chromosome studies.*

Prognosis. *Quoad vitam* good (except for cases with haloprosencephaly). Reproduction possible. Mild to severe mental deficiency.

BIBLIOGRAPHY. DeGrouchy J, Lamy M, Thieffry S, et al: Dysmorphie complexe avec des oligophrenie: deletion des bras courts d'un chromosome 17-18. Ct R Acad Sc 256:1028, 1963

Migeon BR: Short arm deletions in group E and chromosomal "deletion" syndromes. J Pediatr 69:432–438, 1966

Gorlin RJ, Yunis J: Short arm deletion of chromosome 18 in cebocephaly. Am J Dis Child 115:473–476, 1968

Levenson JE, Crandall BF, and Sparkes RS: Partial deletion syndromes of chromosome 18. Ann Ophthalmol 3:756–760, 1971

CHRONIC FATIGUE*

Synonyms. Akureyri's; chronic EBV; Epstein-Barr virus reactivation, CFS; mononucleosislike, chronic neuromyasthenia; postinfectious neuromyasthenia; epidemic neuromyasthenia; neuromyasthenia, sporadic; asthenia, chronic; yuppie disease; Iceland disease; viral chronic hyperfatigability; chronic spasmophilia; low NK cell; myalgic encephalomyelitis; Royal Free disease; see Beard's and Burnout.

Symptoms. Affects people of all ages, races, and classes. Prevalence in young Caucasian women. Sometimes symptoms follow EBV infections. Onset sudden, not alarming headache, sore throat, low-grade fever, fatigue, weakness, arthralgia, inability to concentrate, paresthesias, paresis, anorexia, nausea, vomiting, diarrhea, depression, crying. Feeling of tiredness enhanced by physical or emotional stress, persisting for at least 6 months to years.

Signs. Onset tenderness of lymph nodes and other signs mimicking those of flu. In the second phase absence of physical findings.

Some authors consider for diagnosis major and minor criteria.

Major criteria.
1. New onset of persisting or relapsing severe fatigue (over 50% impairment of activity) lasting 6 months or longer
2. Absence of other illnesses

Minor criteria.
1. Mild fever
2. Sore throat
3. Painful lymph nodes
4. Generalized muscle weakness and myalgia
5. Headache
6. Migratory arthralgia
7. Neuropsychologic complaints: photophobia, transient scotomas, forgetfulness, irritability, confusion, inability to concentrate, depression, sleep disturbances.

Etiology. Still debated. Previously considered anemia, hypoglycemia, allergy, candidiosis; more recently considered chronic virus infection (Epstein-Barr virus, human herpes virus). Other possible causes are immune system dysfunctions; alteration of cytokine release (overproduction of IL-1, IL-2 and interferons).

Pathology. Unknown.

Diagnostic Procedures. Nonspecific. *Blood.* High antibody levels against any virus (CMV, HS1 measles); abnormal production of interferon or abnormality of 2,5-oligoadenylate synthetase, lack of antibodies to some protein components of EBV, abnormal NK cell function.

Therapy. No treatment proved effective. Antivirals, antidepressants, immunomodulation tried.

Prognosis. Nonprogressive disease. Symptoms reach stable state early in the course and thereafter wax and wane. Some cases of spontaneous recovery reported.

BIBLIOGRAPHY. Albrecht R, Oliver VL, Poskanzer DC: Epidemic neuroasthenia: Outbreak in a convent in New York State. JAMA 187:904–907, 1964

Holmes GP, Kaplan JE, Gantz NM, et al: Chronic fatigue syndrome: A working case definition. Ann Intern Med 108:387–389, 1988

CINDERELLA

Synonyms. Ashy dermatosis; dermatosis cenicienta; erythema dyschromicum perstans; erythema chromicum-figuratum-melanodermicum; Ramirez's.

Symptoms and Signs. Both sexes affected; onset from childhood to adulthood. No systemic symptoms or internal manifestations. Disseminated macular lesions "ash gray" in color appearing in the trunk, arms, and face, in both exposed and unexposed areas, sparing palms, soles, and scalp. Various lesions enlarge with coalescence and form bizarre patterns. Early lesions slightly elevated; zone of pigmentation and hypopigmentation may be observed on the same lesion.

Etiology. Unknown.

Pathology. *Active phase.* Malpighian layer vacuolization of cells; edema of dermal papillae; moderate perivasculitis in upper third of cutis; infiltrate consisting of histiocytes; small round cells and macrophages containing melanin granules. *Inactive phase.* Histologic pattern resembling incontinentia pigmenti.

Diagnostic Procedures. *Biopsy of skin. Serology.* To exclude pinta.

Therapy. None.

Prognosis. Good.

BIBLIOGRAPHY. Ramirez CO: Los cenicientos: problema clinico. Proc I Cent Amer Cong Derm San Salvadore, Dec. 5–8; 122–130, 1952

Knox JM, Dodge BG, Freeman RG: Erythema dyschromicum perstans. Arch Dermatol 97:262–272, 1968

Novick NL, Phelps R: Erythema dyschromicum persistans. Int J Dermatol 24:630–633, 1985

---

* To request written information, including information on CFS support groups, contact Chronic Fatigue Syndrome Society, Inc, PO Box 230108, Portland, OR 97223, 503-684-5261.

CITELLI'S

Synonym. Aprosexia.

Symptoms and Signs. Occur in children. Loss of power of concentration; insomnia or drowsiness; mental retardation. Facial changes due to respiratory obstruction may develop.

Etiology. Large adenoids or chronic severe sinus infection.

Therapy. Medical or surgical.

BIBLIOGRAPHY. Citelli S: Vegetazioni adenoidi e sordomutismo. Boll Mal Orecchio Gola Naso 22:141–150, 1904

CITRULLINEMIA

Synonyms. Argininosuccinate synthetase deficiency; ASA synthetase deficiency.

Symptoms and Signs. Prevalent in Japanese males. Four types have been identified:
1. *Neonatal.* Normal at birth; onset after first days of life. Vomiting; irritability; lethargy; hypotonia or hypertonia of muscles; tachypnea; convulsions; coma.
2. *Subacute.* Initially, normal physical and mental development; onset insidious. Poor feeding and attacks of vomiting followed by tremor, ataxia, convulsions, and delayed physical and mental development. Occasionally, hepatomegaly.
3. *Asymptomatic or mild.* Asymptomatic.
4. *Atypical.* Recurrent episodes of irritability, insomnia, visual alterations, delirium. Normal physical and mental development.

Etiology. Genetic inheritance not assessed, may be due to an autosomal recessive deficiency of argininosuccinate (ASA) synthetase in the liver.

Pathology. *Liver.* Nonspecific signs of fatty degeneration. *Brain.* Edema, degeneration of neurons and myelin; presence of enlarged glial cells with lipoid accumulation.

Diagnostic Procedures. *Blood, urine, spinal fluid.* High level of citrulline; hyperammonemia.
1. *Neonatal.* Hyperammonemia after infections; metabolic acidosis; hypoglycemia, hypocalcemia; serum glutamic-pyruvic transaminase (SGPT) increased.
2. *Subacute.* SGOT increased; deficiency of plasma thromboplastin component; blood urea nitrogen low. *Electroencephalography.* Abnormal. *Pneumoencephalography.* Cortical atrophy.

Therapy. Nonspecific. Low-protein diet.

Prognosis.
1. *Neonatal.* Death in first weeks or months of life.
2. *Subacute.* Physical and mental development delayed.
3. *Asymptomatic.* Development within normal range.
4. *Atypical.* After long period of normal life, spastic paraparesis.

BIBLIOGRAPHY. McMurray WC, Rathbun JC, Mohynddin F, et al: Citrullinemia. Pediatrics 32:347–357, 1963
Walser M: Urea cycle disorders and other hereditary hyperammoniemic syndromes. In Stanbury JB, Wyngaarden JB, Fredrickson DS et al: The Metabolic Basis of Inherited Disease, 5th ed, p 408. New York, McGraw-Hill, 1983

CIVATTE'S

Synonyms. Civatte's poikiloderma. See also Riehl's and Berloque.

Symptoms and Signs. Relatively common, especially in the mild form; occurs in middle-aged women. Pruritus; erythema; edema; followed by reticulated reddish brown pigmentation and telangiectasia, forming irregular, generally symmetric patches on the cheeks and sides of neck but sparing areas not exposed to light.

Etiology. Unknown. Attributed to photodynamic substances in cosmetics. Probably identical to Riehl's.

Pathology. Atrophic macules on skin, covered by white adherent scales.

Therapy. Avoidance of use of cosmetics and protection of skin from actinic exposure.

Prognosis. Irregular development with remissions or relapses, in some cases progressing to reticular atrophy.

BIBLIOGRAPHY. Civatte A: Poikilodermie réticulée pigmentaire du visage et du cou. Ann Dermatol Syph 4:605–620, 1923
Rook A, Wilkinson DS, Ebling FJG, et al: Textbook of Dermatology, 4th ed, p 1579. Oxford, Blackwell Scientific Publications, 1986

CLAM DIGGER'S ITCH

Synonyms. Dermatitis schistosomiasis; cutaneous schistosomiasis; swimmer's itch; marine dermatitis; sea bather eruption.

Symptoms and Signs. Appears in clam diggers and sea bathers on east and west coasts of United States, after few minutes of penetration of cercariae (see Etiology).

Intense itching lasting half an hour and leaving small macules; hours later, macules become papules; some pustules accompanied by local edema and severe itching (scratching lesions). Symptoms reach their peak in 3 days and subside in 7 days.

Etiology. Cercarial dermatitis: Penetration in the skin by cercariae of different types of schistosomes, avian or mammalian. Adult worms carried mostly by migratory birds and transmitted to sea snails who transmit them to bathers. Marine dermatitis: salt water and other agents frequently not identifiable.

Pathology. Cercariae in the skin with inflammatory reaction.

Diagnostic Procedures. Identification of infesting agent.

Therapy. Antipruritic and antihistamine topical application. For prevention, destruction of snails on beaches (copper sulfate), and in the water (copper carbonate 2½ lbs/1,000 sq ft of bottom of sea along beaches). Drying skin after swimming reduces the infestation remarkably.

Prognosis. Spontaneous recovery in 7 days; repeated infestation more severe.

BIBLIOGRAPHY. Cort WW: Studies on schistosome dermatitis: Status of knowledge after more than 22 years. Am J Hyg 52:251–307, 1950

Rook A, Wilkinson DS, Ebling FJG, et al: Textbook of Dermatology, 4th ed, p 1008. Oxford, Blackwell Scientific Publications, 1986

CLARKE-HADEFIELD

Synonyms. Andersen's I; pancreas hypoplasia; pancreatic infantilism. See cystic fibrosis. Obsolete entity.

Symptoms and Signs. Both sexes affected; onset at early age. Delayed growth and development; poor muscles; lack of subcutaneous fat; digestive troubles comparable with mucoviscidosis (see). Usually, absence of respiratory complication. Occasionally, associated with hematologic alterations (see Shwachman's).

Etiology. Unknown; congenital exocrine hypoplasia of pancreas on genetic basis.

Pathology. Atrophic pancreas; hepatomegaly.

Diagnostic Procedures. *Stool.* Bulky, fatty. *Pancreatic enzymes determination.* In duodenal secretion, blood, urine, stools. *Biopsy of pancreas.* (No danger of fistula because of lack of enzymes). *Sweat test.* Normal.

Therapy. Pancreatic enzymes administration.

Prognosis. Better than in mucoviscidosis syndrome.

BIBLIOGRAPHY. Clarke C, Hadefield G: Congenital pancreatic disease with infantilism. J Med 17:358–364, 1924

Andersen DH: Cystic fibrosis of the pancreas and its relation to celiac disease. Am J Dis Child 56:344–399, 1938

Bodian M, Sheldon W, Lightwood R: Congenital hypoplasia of the exocrine pancreas. Acta Paediatr Scand (Stockh) 53:282–293, 1964

CLIVUS EDGE

Synonyms. See Foix-Jefferson and Orbital apex.

Symptoms and Signs. Myosis followed by mydriasis and sluggish pupil reaction; paresis of extraocular muscles.

Etiology. Rise in intracranial pressure on the roots of oculomotor nerve against bone at the entrance into cavernous sinus.

Pathology. Subdural hematoma, temporal bone tumor. Supraclinoid aneurysm.

BIBLIOGRAPHY. Fischer-Brugge E: Anatomische Ursachen functionaler kreislangstoerungen des Gehirns und am N. Oculomotorius. Bruns' Beitrage Klin Chir 181:323–336, 1951

Roy A: Ocular Syndromes and Systemic Disease, Orlando (Florida), Grune & Stratton, 1985

CLOUGH-RICHTER

Synonym. Erythrocyte autoagglutination. Of historical interest; one of the first reports of red cell autoagglutination.

BIBLIOGRAPHY. Clough MC, Richter IM: A study of an autoagglutinin occurring in a human serum. Bull Johns Hopkins Hosp 29:86–93, 1918

CLOUSTON'S

Synonyms. Hidrotic ectodermal dysplasia; ectodermal dysplasia, hidrotic.

Symptoms and Signs. Both sexes affected; present from infancy. Dystrophy of nails; thickened; striated; discolored or thin; short and brittle (may be the only manifestation). Repeated paronychial infections. Skin on edges of nail, finger joints, knuckles, knees, elbows may occasionally be thickened. Hyperkeratosis of palms and soles. In complete form, hair fine, sparse, or absent; usually hair defect develops at puberty. Normal sweating; normal teeth; physical development normal or slightly impaired. Mental development normal or retarded. Strabismus.

Etiology. Unknown; autosomal dominant inheritance.

Pathology. Hyperkeratosis.

Diagnostic Procedures. *Biopsy of skin.*

Therapy. None.

Prognosis. Sexual development normal. Life expectancy not affected, except in some homozygous state, where it may be fatal.

BIBLIOGRAPHY. Clouston HR: A hereditary ectodermal dystrophy. Can Med Assoc J 21:18–31, 1929
Escobar V, Goldblatt LI, Bixler D et al: Clouston syndrome: An ultrastructural study. J Clin Genet 24:140–146, 1983

CLOVERLEAF SKULL

Synonyms. Gruber's; hydrocephalus chondrodystrophicus congenitum; Kleeblattschaedel anomaly; trefoil skull.

Symptoms and Signs. Both sexes affected. Almost all affected children are born dead. Reported in two adults. Grotesque trilobed skull; downward displacement of the ears; exophthalmos; beak nose with deeply recessed nasal root; prognathism. In the majority of cases, associated deformities of bones (achondroplasia); seldom, ankylosis of elbows have been observed.

Etiology. Unknown. Abnormality of ossification resulting in intrauterine synostosis of coronal and lambdoid sutures with hydrocephalus. May be considered, according to recent view, more a sign than a syndrome. It may be observed as isolated anomaly or associated with various pathologic conditions such as Crouzon's (see); thanatophoric dwarfism (see); limb bony ankylosing; Carpenters's (see); Pfeiffer's.

Pathology. Characteristic skull deformity and musculoskeletal alteration (see Signs).

Prognosis. Poor.

BIBLIOGRAPHY. Gruber GB: Veber einen akrocephalen Reliefschaedel. Ein Beitrag zur Frage der partiellen Chondrodystrophie. Beitr Path Anat 97:9–12, 1936
Holtermüeller K, Wiedemann HR: Kleeblattschädel syndrome. Med Wockenschr 14:439–446, 1960
Angle CR, McIntire MS, Moore RC: Cloverleaf skull: Kleeblattschädel deformity syndrome. Am J Dis Child 114:198–202, 1967
Hall BD, Smith DW, Schiller JG: Kleeblattschaedel (Cloverleaf syndrome): Severe form of Crouzon's disease. J Pediatr 80:526–527, 1972

Cohen MM: The Kleeblattschaedel phenomenon sign or syndrome? Am J Dis Child 124:944, 1972
Aksu F, Mietens C: Kleeblattschaedel syndrome. Klein Paediat 191:418–428, 1979

CLUNEAL NERVE

Synonyms. Episacroiliac lipoma; gluteal. See also Battered buttock.

Symptoms. Low back pain from mild to extremely severe radiation of pain along the distribution of cluneal nerves (buttock; back of hip) occasionally referred pain in the groins or extremities (burning; aching; rarely, sharp or stabbing). Various postures and actions aggravate pain such as sitting, bending, lying, or walking.

Signs. Localized tender area 2 cm in diameter in low lumbar or episacroiliac areas; injection over the deep fascia in trigger point must relieve the symptomatology for longer than half an hour. Occasionally, fatty nodules are observed at the site of trigger zone; restriction of spinal mobility is observed in 62% of cases.

Etiology. Establishment of trigger zone by a violent or minor trauma that initiates degenerative changes of subcutaneous tissue, increase of fibrous stroma, and hypersensitization of sensory nerves to mechanical stimuli (tension).

Pathology. No definite pathology has been observed.

Diagnostic Procedures. See Signs.

Therapy. Surgical differentation of trigger area of tenderness or cluneal neurectomy.

Prognosis. With surgery, 79% excellent results, 11% good results, the remaining recurrent cluneal nerve syndrome.

BIBLIOGRAPHY. Strong EK, Davila JC: The cluneal nerve syndrome. 26:417–429, 1957

CLUSTER HEADACHE

Synonyms. Horton's II; Bing Horton; histamine cephalalgia; paroxysmal cephalalgia, nocturnal orbital; ciliary neuralgia; Charlin's; erythroprosopalgia; Harris; vascular headache; periodic migrainous neuralgia; Vallery-Radot's.

Symptoms. Affect men 30 to 40 years old; rare in females. No prodromes. Severe, unilateral aching pain beginning in the infraorbital area, and spreading, increasing in intensity on homolateral side of head and neck. Symptoms appear usually during the night at the same time, regularly several times a day for days or weeks (cluster) followed by remission of days or years. Precipitated occasionally by alcohol or heat; cold brings relief. Pain reaches peak in 10 minutes, attack lasts 1 to 3 hours; no sequelae. Nostril of same side usually feels obstructed and may have watery discharge. Repeated sweating same side of face also reported. No nausea or vomiting. Recurrences occasionally seasonal.

Signs. Flushing of affected side of face; conjunctiva congested. Occasionally, Horner's sign and bradycardia.

Etiology. Unknown; allergy excluded by all tests or at least not confirmed. Possibly, basic psychological disturbance.

Diagnostic Procedures. *Thermography.* Unique spotted pattern of hypothermia in 66% of patients which does not change in presence or absence of attacks or vasoactive drugs.

Therapy. All failed including psychotherapy. Ergotamine tartrate intramuscularly seems to bring some symptomatic relief.

BIBLIOGRAPHY. Harris BT: Neuritis and Neuralgia. London, 1926
Bing R: Ueber traumatische Erythromelalgia und Erythroprasopalgie. Nervenarzt 3:506–512, 1930
Vallery-Radot P, Blamoutier P: Syndrome de vasodilation hemicephalique d'origine sympathique (hemicranie, hemihydrorrhea, hemilarmoiement). Bull Mem Soc Med Hop Paris 49:1488–1493, 1925
Charlin C: La sindrome del nervo nasale. Boll Ocul (Firenze) 10:921–936, 1931
Horton BT: The use of histamine in the treatment of specific types of headaches. JAMA 116:377–383, 1941
Friedman AP: The migraine syndrome. Bull NY Acad Med 44:45–62, 1968
Adams RD, Victor M: Principles of Neurology, 3rd ed, pp 138–139. New York, McGraw-Hill, 1985

CLUTTON'S

Synonym. Syphilitic knee synovitis.

Symptoms and Signs. Usually, an insidious onset between 6 to 16 years of age. Symmetric, indolent, chronic swelling of joints (knee 85%); occasionally recurrent. In few cases, acute or subacute. Periarticular redness, pain, limitation of motion; fever; systemic manifestations. Seldom, polyarticular involvement.

Etiology. Congenital syphilis. Difficult differential diagnosis when not associated with other manifestations of congenital syphilis.

Pathology. Chronic hydrarthrosis; no damage to joints; involves soft tissues exclusively.

Diagnostic Procedures. *Serology. Synovial fluid aspiration.* Rich in lymphocytes. *Biopsy of joint. X-rays.* Negative except for presence of fluid.

Therapy. No response to antibiotics.

Prognosis. Good response to conservative treatment and complete recovery.

BIBLIOGRAPHY. Clutton HH: Symmetrical synovitis of the knee in hereditary syphilis. Lancet 1:391–393, 1886
Clark JM: Syphilitic joint disease. In Hollander JL, McCarty DJ: Arthritis and Allied Conditions, 6th ed, p 1256. Philadelphia, Lea & Febiger, 1972

COAL MINER ELBOW

Synonyms. Olecranon bursitis; student's elbow.

Symptoms. Pain in the elbow.

Signs. Tenderness; swelling of elbow; limitation of movement.

Etiology. Trauma by repeated jolts (*e.g.,* with pneumatic hammer) or frictions; associated with elbow disease, gout, arthritis, or unknown causes.

Pathology. Bursitis; degeneration of lining of bursa; adhesion and thickening of wall, villi with intraarticular calcifications.

Diagnostic Procedures. *X-ray.* Intraarticular calcification.

Therapy. Rest and physical therapy (heat); deep x-ray if not responsive; or infiltration with procain or hydrocortisone for acute pain. When indicated excision of the bursa.

Prognosis. Good if traumatic causes removed. The progression of condition may result in atrophy of the joint.

BIBLIOGRAPHY. Justis EJ: Nontraumatic disorders. In Crenshaw AH (ed): Campbell's Operative Orthopedics, 7th ed, p 22. St. Louis, CV Mosby, 1987

COATS'

Synonyms. Exudative retinitis. Leber's miliary aneurysma + retinal teleangiectasia.

Symptoms. Prevalent in male children or adolescents (juvenile form). For adult form see Hyperlipemic retinitis. Development of photophobia with cloudy vision, usually unilateral.

Signs. *Group I.* Presence of deep, yellowish, massive exudate in and under external retina, producing localized solid elevation of the retina. No evidence of hemorrhage or vascular changes. *Group II.* Marked changes of small retinal arterioles, fresh hemorrhages; plus above-mentioned retinal findings. *Group III.* Reported association with hearing loss, muscular weakness, and mental retardation.

Etiology. Unknown; in juvenile form, supposed intermediary tissue factor that precipitates cholesterol. In adult form, chronic inflammation and hypercholesterolemia as trigger mechanism. Toxoplasmosis may in some cases be responsible; in group III possible autosomal recessive inheritance.

Pathology. Massive exudate formed primarily by free cholesterol esters in external retina and subretinal space, containing foam cells and hemosiderin pigment. Minor inflammatory changes of nongranulomatous type and adhesion between choroid and subretinal organized mass. Same findings in juvenile and adult forms.

Diagnostic Procedures. *Blood.* In juvenile form, blood lipids are normal; in adult form, blood lipids are elevated (cholesterol in particular). *Sabin-Feldman dye test.* Positive in some patients.

Therapy. Diathermy; corticosteroids have limited efficacy.

Prognosis. Progressive loss of visual acuity.

BIBLIOGRAPHY. Coats G: Forms of retinal disease with massive exudation. R London Ophthalmol Hosp Rep 17:440–525, 1908
Small RG: Coats' disease and muscular dystrophy. Trans Am Acad Ophthal Otolaryngol 72:225–231, 1968
Collins JF: Handbook of Clinical Ophthalmology, p 307. New York, Masson, 1982
Chang M, McLean IW, Merritt JC: Coats' disease: A study of 62 histologically confirmed cases. J Pediatr Ophthalmol Strabismus 21:163–168, 1984

COBB'S

Synonyms. Cutomucomeningospinal angiomatosis. Angiomatosis, cutaneomeningospinal. See Sturge-Weber.

Symptoms and Signs. From birth: port wine or angiokeratomatous lesion in dermatomal distribution on trunk or extremities. In childhood or adolescence spastic paralysis of one or both extremities and sensory loss below level of spinal lesion.

Etiology. Unknown. Reported possible autosomal dominant inheritance.

Pathology. Angioma of spinal cord.

Diagnostic Procedures. *CT scan. Angiography. Myelography.*

Therapy. Neurosurgery.

Prognosis. Good with early treatment.

BIBLIOGRAPHY. Cobb S: Hemangioma of the spinal cord associated with skin naevi of these same metamers. Am Surg 62:641–649, 1915
Chometta G, Auriol M: Classification des angiodysplagies et tumeurs vasculaires. Rev Stomatol Clin Maxillofac 87:1–5, 1986

COCHRANE'S

Synonym. Leucine-sensitive hypoglycemia.

Symptoms and Signs. Occur in children. Following ingestion of protein, a hypoglycemic crisis (see Hypoglycemic syndromes in newborn). In adulthood, usually asymptomatic; ingestion of a test dose of leucine or prolonged fasting induces hypoglycemic crisis.

Etiology. Unknown. In adult: (1) Idiopathic; familial condition; (2) associated with islet cell adenoma; (3) following treatment with chlorpropamide.

Diagnostic Procedures. *Blood.* Fasting hypoglycemia (very frequently); postprandial hypoglycemia. *Leucine tolerance test.*

Therapy. Low leucine diet.

Prognosis. Marked improvement with diet; loss of irritability; increased alertness; no hypoglycemic attacks.

BIBLIOGRAPHY. Cochrane WA, Payne WW, Simpkiss MJ et al: Familial hypoglycemia precipitated by amino acids. J Clin Invest 35:411–422, 1956
Ebbin AJ, Huntley C, Tranquada RE: Symptomatic leucine sensitivity in mother and daughter. Metabolism 16:926–932, 1967

COCKAYNE'S

Synonyms. Deafness–dwarfism–retinal atrophy; progeroid nanism; Neill-Dingwall. See Blooms.

Symptoms. Onset in second year of life after normal infancy. Cutaneus photosensitivity with pigmentation and scars; decrease of vision; progressive deafness; mental deficiency; unsteady gait.

Signs. Dwarfism with long extremities and large hands and feet. Musculoskeletal abnormalities: flexion deformities of extremities; kyphosis; thickened skull: loss of subcutaneous fat. Senile face; sunken eyes; thin nose; prognathism. Optic atrophy with retinal pigmentation; poor pupillary response to mydriatics; cataracts. Hepatosplenomegaly in some cases; older patients sexually underdeveloped.

Etiology. Unknown; hereditary disorders (autosomal recessive type). Trisomy in group 19–20. In other cases, normal karyotype.

Pathology. Microcephaly. Cerebral cortex and cerebrum atrophic. Patchy or tigroid demyelinization greatest in occipital lobe. Pericapillary calcification in the cortex, basal ganglia, and cerebellum; larger artery and arteriole mineralization.

Diagnostic Procedures. *Chromosome study. X-rays of skull and extremities.* Intracranial calcification; marble epiphyses in some digits. The ultraviolet (UV) sensitivity of cultured fibroblast cells derived from patients with this syndrome has been studied. The depression of RNA synthesis after UV irradiation is variable among the individual patients, and the level of UV sensitivity does not parallel the severity of the clinical manifestations.

Therapy. None.

Prognosis. Progressive deterioration to blindness, deafness, paralysis, inanition, and death in adolescence or early adulthood. Aspiration pneumonia constitutes a leading cause of death.

BIBLIOGRAPHY. Cockayne EA: Dwarfism with retinal atrophy and deafness. Arch Dis Child 11:1–8, 1936
Moossy J: The neuropathology of Cockayne's syndrome. J Neuropathol Exp Neurol 26:654–660, 1967
Sugita K, Suzukin R, Kojima T, Tanabe Y, Nakajima H, Hayashi A, Arima M: Cockayne syndrome with delayed recovery of RNA synthesis after ultra-violet irradiation but normal ultraviolet survival. Pediatr Res 21:34–37, 1986

COCKAYNE-TOURAINE

Synonyms. Hyperplastic epidermolysis bullosa. Epidermolysis bullosa, hyperplastic; Weber-Cockayne; hyperplastic epidermolysis bullosa.

Symptoms and Signs. Both sexes affected, onset in early infancy or later (also in adulthood). Appearance of bullae, usually after trauma, also spontaneous. Head and limbs mostly affected; scarring and occasionally mutilation results. Normal mental and physical development. Frequent association with ichthyosis, keratosis pilaris, tylosis with hyperhydrosis, and dystrophic nails; hypertrichosis. Involvement of mucosa 20%.

Etiology. Unknown; autosomal dominant inheritance.

Therapy. Symptomatic; antibiotics; corticosteroids. Protection from trauma. Prevention of bullae: frictioning with ice water.

Prognosis. According to severity of form and age of onset.

BIBLIOGRAPHY. Elliot GT: Two cases of epidermolysis bullosa. J Cutan Genitourin Dis 13:10–18, 1895
Weber FP: Recurrent bullous eruptions of the feet in a child. Proc R Soc Med 19:72, 1938
Cockayne EA: Recurrent bullous eruption of the feet. Brit J Dermatol Syph 50:358–362, 1938
Touraine A: L'heredité en Medicine. Paris, Mason, 1955
Mulley JC, Turner T, Nicholls C et al: Genetic linkage analysis of epidermolysis bullosa dystrophica Cockayne-Touraine type. Clin Genet 28:31–35, 1985

COCKTAIL PARTY

Synonyms. Chronic brain–hydrocephalus; chatter-box; hyperactivity. See Strawpeter.

Symptoms. Occur in children with arrested hydrocephalus (either spontaneous or therapeutic). Characteristic behavior pattern consisting of high sociability, pseudobrightness, excessive talkativeness without complete understanding what they are talking about. Characteristic scanning speech due to a combination of moderate dysrhythmia and altered intonation pattern. This syndrome is associated, more or less, with the neurologic symptoms and signs related to chronic infantile hydrocephalus.

Etiology. Infantile hydrocephalus.

Prognosis. Educational ability of these patients is relatively poor compared with their conversational ability.

BIBLIOGRAPHY. Ingram TT, Naughton JA: Paediatric and psychological aspects of cerebral palsy associated with hydrocephalus. Dev Med Child Neurol 4:287–292, 1962
Hagberg B, Sjorgen I: The chronic brain syndrome of infantile hydrocephalus; a follow-up study of 63 spontaneously arrested cases. Am J Dis Child 112:189–196, 1966
Adams RD, Victor M: Principles of Neurology, 3rd ed, pp 444–445. New York, McGraw-Hill, 1985

CODMAN'S

Synonym. Benign chondroblastoma.

Symptoms. 400 cases well documented. Prevalent in males; onset usually in adolescence or young adult age. Localized pain and limited motion of contiguous joint.

Signs. Swelling and tenderness at epiphyseal extremities of long bones (femur, tibia, and radius in particular); overlying skin is warmer and local muscles show atrophy.

Etiology. Unknown.

Pathology. Foci of necrosis; inflammatory changes; hemorrhages; fibrous scarring and presence of spindle cells; scattered multinucleated giant and polyhedral cells with large central nuclei.

Diagnostic Procedures. *X-ray.* Well-defined area of rarefaction with surrounding thin zone of denser bone; periosteal thickening.

Therapy. Excision.

Prognosis. Seldom, malignant transformation. Possibility of pathologic fractures.

BIBLIOGRAPHY. Codman EA: Epiphyseal chondromatous giant cell tumours of the upper end of the humerus. Surg Gynecol Obstet 32:543–548, 1931

Carnesale PG: Sometime malignant tumors of the bone. In Crenshaw AH (ed): Campbell's Operative Orthopedics, 7th ed, p 765. St. Louis, CV Mosby, 1987

COFFIN-LOWRY

Symptoms. Occur in males (females carriers): onset in postnatal period. Mild growth deficiency; severe mental deficiency; muscle weakness. No speech capability.

Signs. In males. *Head.* Mild hypertelorism; downslanting palpebrae; prominent brows; maxillar hypoplasia; thick alae and nasal septum. *Extremities.* Hands large and soft; fingers tapering; clubbing of the distal phalanges (Hippocratism); accessory thenar crease; flat feet; lax ligaments. *Trunk.* Pectus carinatum and short bifid sternum; vertebral defects; thoracolumbar scoliosis. In females. Milder features. Anomalies of the genitourinary tract have been reported; congenital microureteral junction; vesicoureteral reflux; absence of one kidney; massive hydronephrosis.

Etiology. X-linked semidominant inheritance. Autosomal recessive inheritance has been proposed.

Diagnostic Procedures. *X-rays.* Intravenous pyelography.

Therapy. None.

Prognosis. In males, severe mental deficiency. Stooped posture; muscular weakness.

BIBLIOGRAPHY. Coffin GS, Siris E, Wegienke LC: Mental retardation with osteocartilagenous anomalies. Am J Dis Child 112:205–213, 1966

Lowry RB, Miller JR and Fraser FC: A New dominant gene mental retardation syndrome: associated with small stature, tapering fingers, chracteristic facies, and possible hydrocephalus. Am J Dis Child 121:496–500, 1971

Mattei JF, Laframboise R, Rouault F, Giraud F: Brief clinical report: Coffin-Lowry syndrome in sibs. Am J Clin Genet 8:315–319, 1981

COFFIN'S

Synonym. Lean spastic dwarfism.

Symptoms and Signs. Both sexes affected. Low birth weight; neonatal cyanosis and respiratory infections. Retarded motor development; sitting at age 3 or later; unable to stand or speak; low IQ; retarded dental development; convulsions; frequent respiratory infections. *Appearance.* Helpless; speechless; slender; dwarfism; brachycephaly. *Face.* Prominent forehead and eyes; exotropia; small upturned nose; external ears large; low, single, helix or anthelix poorly developed. *Chest.* Anteroposterior thickening. *Back.* Bifid sacrum; coccygeal pit. *Extremities.* Slender fingers; lax joints; flaccid muscle; spasticity at passive motion; pes cavus.

Etiology. Unknown; no family history. Possibly, drugs taken during pregnancy.

Pathology. See Signs.

Diagnostic Procedures. *X-ray.* Slender bones; retarded bone age; brachycephaly; underdeveloped distal phalanges; short forearm. *Blood, urine, endocrinologic, amino acid, chromosomal studies.* Normal.

Therapy. Symptomatic.

Prognosis. Unknown.

BIBLIOGRAPHY. Coffin GS: A syndrome of retarded development with characteristic appearance. Am J Dis Child, 115:698–702, 1968

COFFIN-SIRIS

Synonyms. Dwarfism-onychodysplasia; fifth digit. See also Meadow's and Senior's.

Symptoms. Both sexes affected (F/M 4:1); present from birth. Feeding problems; recurrent respiratory infections; mental deficiency; hypertonia (from mild to severe).

Signs. Growth deficiency. Hirsutism; sparse scalp hair. Microcephaly; full lips. Fifth finger hypoplastic or absent. Toenails hypoplastic or absent. Lax joints (elbow dislocation); small patellae. Occasionally, variable skin, skeletal, genital cardiac defects and Dandy-Walker (see).

Etiology. Unknown. Sporadic, possibly autosomal recessive inheritance.

BIBLIOGRAPHY. Coffin GS, Siris E: Mental retardation with absent fifth fingernail and terminal phalanx. Am J Dis Child 119:433–439, 1970

Weissvasser WH, Hall BD, Delevan GW et al: Coffin-Siris syndrome: Two new cases. Am J Dis Child 125:838–860, 1973

Haspeslagh M, Fryns JP, van den Berghe H: The Coffin-Siris syndrome: Report of a family and further delineation. Clin Genet 26:374–378, 1984

COGAN'S I

Synonyms. Keratitis-deafness; interstitial nonsyphilitic keratitis; nonsyphilitic keratitis; vestibulo-auditory keratitis.

Symptoms. Occur in young adults; occasionally in old people; sudden onset. Unilateral or bilateral blurring of vision; pain in the eye; lacrimation; blepharospasm; nausea; vomiting; tinnitus; vertigo; rapid development of deafness. Convulsive seizures have also been reported.

Signs. Congestive conjunctivitis with hemorrhages.

Etiology. Unknown. Manifestations associated with polyarteritis nodosa.

Pathology. In eyes; patchy granular infiltration, in mainly posterior half of cornea.

Diagnostic Procedures. *Blood.* Leukocytosis and mild eosinophilia.

Therapy. Adrenal corticosteroid, topical and systemic; adrenocorticotropic hormone (ACTH).

Prognosis. Chronic course with relapse affecting both eyes or alternating. With increasing deafness vertigo symptomatology decreases in intensity.

BIBLIOGRAPHY. Cogan DG: Syndrome of nonsyphilitic interstital keratitis and vestibuloauditory symptoms. Arch Ophthalmol 33:144–149, 1945
Fisher ER, Hellstrom HR: Cogan's syndrome and systemic vascular disease; Analysis of pathologic features with reference to its relationship to thromboangitis obliterans (Buerger). Arch Pathol 72:572–592, 1961
Vollertsen RS, McDonald TJ, Younge BR et al: Cogan's syndrome: 18 cases and a review of the literature. Mayo Clin Proc 61:344–361, 1986

COGAN'S II

Synonyms. Oculomotor apraxia.

Symptoms and Signs. Observed only in children, prevalent in males. Patient unable to turn eyes quickly when asked to look at an object while he is lying on his side, or when his attention is suddenly attracted. To compensate he turns his head, but in doing so, the eyes deviate to the opposite side because of the vestibular reflex. To focus on the object he has to turn his head farther; in this way, he can fixate on the object. The entire cycle occurs in less than 1 second, with a jerky movement of the head. He may carry out such movement when free from stimulus. The mechanism of oculomotor apraxia is the opposite of what occurs in normal person, who moves first the eyes and then the head.

Etiology. Unknown; congenital condition (in one case carbon monoxide intoxication of mother in second month of pregnancy, and the condition associated with extrapyramidal disease). Possibly also autosomal recessive inheritance.

Therapy. None.

Prognosis. Unknown; condition not handicapping except for difficulty in reading and making quick turns.

BIBLIOGRAPHY. Wilson SAK: A contribution to the study of apraxia: With a review of the literature. Brain 31:164–216, 1908
Cogan DG: Type of congenital ocular motor apraxia presenting jerky head movement. Jackson Memorial Lecture Trans Am Acad Ophthalmol 56:853–862, 1952
Vassella F, Lutschh J, Mumenthaler, M: Cogan's congenital oculomotor apraxia in two successive generations. Dev Med Child Neurol 14:788–796, 1972

COGAN'S III

Synonyms. Corneal dystrophy, epithelial basement membrane; corneal dystrophy, map-dot-fingerprint type; corneal dystrophy microcystic.

Symptoms and Signs. Eyes (on slit-lamp examination): gray, course epithelial lines (geographic pattern map) and whitish refractile lines (fingerprints)

Etiology. Unknown. Autosomal dominant inheritance.

BIBLIOGRAPHY. Cogan DG, Donaldson DD, Kuwabara I et al: Microcystic dystrophy of the corneal epithelium. Trans Am Ophthalmol Soc 62:213–225, 1964
Brodick JD, Dark AJ, Peace GN: Fingerprint dystrophy of the cornea: A histologic study. Arch Ophthalmol 92:483–489, 1974

COHEN'S

Synonyms. Cerebral-obesity-ocular-skeletal; hypotonia-obesity-cerebral-skeletal; Pepper's (family name).

Symptoms and Signs. Onset from birth. *Craniofacial anomalies.* Microcephaly; microphthalmia; antimongoloid slant of lids; strabismus; myopia; micrognathia; narrow, high-arched palate; short filtrum. *Skeletal abnormalities.* Tapering extremities; simian creases; syndactyly; joint hyperextensibility; cubitus valgus; genus varus; scoliosis; lordosis. Muscle hypotonia. Mental retardation. Obesity (onset in middle childhood). Periureteric obstruction. Seizures (possibly new features).

Etiology. Unknown; possibly, autosomal recessive inheritance with variable expressivity. This syndrome presents characteristics in common with Prader-Willi (see) and Laurence-Moon-Biedl (see).

Diagnostic Procedures. *Chromosome studies.* Normal. *Electroencephalography.* Diffuse, high-voltage spikes and wave discharge.

BIBLIOGRAPHY. Cohen MM: A new syndrome with hypotonia, obesity, mental deficiency, and facial, oral, ocular and limb anomalies. J Pediatr 83:280–284, 1973

Hall BD, Smith DW: Prader-Willi syndrome. J Pediatr 81:286–293, 1972

Gorlin RJ, Pindborg JJ, Cohen MM: Syndromes of the Head and Neck, 2nd ed. New York, McGraw-Hill, 1976

North C, Patton MA, Baraitser M et al: The clinical features of the Cohen's syndrome: Further case reports. J Med Genet 22:131–134, 1985

COINDET'S

Synonyms. Iodide-induced thyrotoxicosis. Job Basedow (misnomer).

Symptoms and Signs. After administration of pharmacologic doses of iodine the following complications may develop:
1. Iodide-induced thyroiditis
2. Iodide-induced thyrotoxicosis
3. Iodide goiter with or without hypothyroidism (see Iatrogenic hypothyroidism).
Acute painful thyroid enlargement that recedes with discontinuation of treatment. Male : female ratio 1 : 3; exophthalmos absent; goiter; symptoms and signs of hyperthyroidism (see Flajani's).

Etiology. In subject with preexisting or with absent thyroid disease immediately or even years after following administration of: amiodarone; KJ; benzidiazone; radiographic contrast; iodochlorohydroxyquinoline; seaweed; topical application of I preparation.

Pathology. Thyroid gland usually nodular.

Diagnostic Procedures. *Blood.* Hyperthyroxinemia (100%); hypertriiodothyroninemia (79%); antithyroid antibodies absent.

Therapy. Response to antithyroid agents 60%.

Prognosis. Self-limited course in about 40% of cases.

BIBLIOGRAPHY. Coindet JR: Nouvelle recherches sur les effect de l'iode. Am Chim Phys 16:252, 1821

Fradkin JE, Wolff J: Iodide-induced thyrotoxicosis. Medicine 62:1–20, 1983

COLCOTT-FOX

Synonyms. Cutaneous abscesses infantilis; impetigo contagiosa streptogenes; impetigo simplex; porrigo. Tilbury Fox.

Symptoms and Signs. Occur in feeble and debilitated infants. Development of multiple abscesses of skin following infection of sweat glands (periporitis).

Etiology. Staphylococcal infection. Two forms recognized. Nonbullous impetigo (*Staphylococcus aureus* or *Streptococcus* or both); bullus impetigo (staphylococcal).

Pathology. That of subcutaneous abscess.

Diagnostic Procedures. *Culture of pus. Bacteriologic examination.*

Therapy. Care of environmental factors (temperature and humidity); nutritional and fluid balance. Antibiotics.

Prognosis. Good.

BIBLIOGRAPHY. Fox WT: On impetigo contagiosa or porrigo. Br Med J 1:467–469, 495–496; 607–609, 1864

Rook A, Wilkinson DS, Ebling FJG, et al: Textbook of Dermatology, 4th ed, pp 734–737. Oxford, Blackwell Scientific Publications, 1986

COLD HYPERSENSITIVITY

Symptoms. Disturbing reactions experienced when immersed in water.

Signs. Failure to decrease heart rate when immersed in water below body temperature.

Etiology. Lack of emotional adjustment (fear) or failure to compensate physiologically (hypersensitivity to cold). Body immersion normally produces bradycardia that is enhanced by immersion of head.

Diagnostic Procedures. *Heart rate.* Determination of variation of heart rate according to temperature of water in which immersed. *Ice-cube test.* Ice cube held in contact with forearm of a person for 3 minutes. A wheal, slightly raised with erythematous peripheral reaction, appears in persons hypersensitive to cold.

BIBLIOGRAPHY. Horton BT, Gabrielson MA: Hypersensitivity to cold: A condition dangerous to swimmers. Res Q 11:119–126, 1940

Tuttle WW, Templin JL: Study of normal cardiac response to water below body temperature with special reference to submersion syndrome. J Lab Clin Med 28:271–276, 1942

COLD PANNICULITIS (CHILDREN)

Synonym. Subcutaneous fat necrosis.

Symptoms and Signs. In children exposed to cold weather. Development of tender, well-demarcated, reddish induration in submental region.

Etiology. Immaturity of subcutaneous fat (excessive saturated fatty acids with high solidification point) exposed to cold.

Pathology. Panniculitis.

Therapy. None.

Prognosis. Spontaneous resolution in 2 to 3 weeks.

BIBLIOGRAPHY. Hochsinger C: Ueber eine akute kongelative Zellgewebsverhartung in der submental Regionen bei Kinder. Monatsschr Kinderheilk 1:323–327, 1902
Lowe LB: Cold panniculitis in children. Am J Dis Child 115:709–713, 1968
Rook A, Wilkinson DS, Ebling FJG, et al: Textbook of Dermatology, 4th ed, p 254. Oxford, Blackwell Scientific Publications, 1986

COLD URTICARIA (FAMILIAL)

Synonyms. Cold hypersensitivity. See Mucke-Wells.

Symptoms and Signs. In area exposed to cold: skin wheals, pain and swelling of joint; chills and fever.

Etiology. Autosomal dominant inheritance; systemic amyloidosis may be observed in cases with cold urticaria.

Diagnostic Procedures. Leukocytosis during attacks.

Therapy. Symptomatic; avoid unprotected exposure to cold.

Prognosis. Good.

BIBLIOGRAPHY. Kile RL, Rush HA: A case of cold urticaria with unusual family history. JAMA 114:1067–1068, 1940
Witherspoon FG, White CB, Bazemore JM et al: Familial urticaria due to cold. Arch Dermatol Syph 58:52–55, 1948
Mathews KP: Exploiting the cold-urticaria. Model. N Engl J Med 305:1090–1091, 1981

COLEMAN-MEREDITH

Symptoms and Signs. Combination of symptoms and signs related to one lesion (or multiple) of the occipital-cervical shoulder girdle associated with those relative to cord injury.

BIBLIOGRAPHY. Coleman CC, Meredith JM: Treatment of fracture dislocation of the spine associated with cord injury. JAMA 11:2168–2172, 1938
Freemann BL III: Fractures dislocation and fracture dislocation of spine. In Crenshaw AH (ed): Campbell's Operative Orthopedics, 7th ed, pp 3109–3142. St. Louis, CV Mosby, 1987

COLLAGENOMA, CUTANEOUS FAMILIAL

Synonyms. Cardiomyopathy-hypogonadism-collagenoma.

Symptoms and Signs. Both sexes. In postpuberal period, appearance of multiple cutaneous nodules, movable with the skin, on trunk and proximal arms. Possibly, association with disease of other organs; no common denominator, however, in organ system involvement, including signs related to moderate myocardiopathy, hypogonadism, eye and sensorineural ear trouble, recurrent vasculitis.

Etiology. Autosomal dominant inheritance.

Pathology. Localized thickening of the dermis due to increased collagen.

Therapy. Symptomatic.

Prognosis. All patients reached adulthood.

BIBLIOGRAPHY. Henderson RR, Wheeler CE, Abele DC, et al: Familial cutaneous collagenoma. Arch Dermatol 98:23–27, 1968
Sacks HN, Crawley IS, Ward JA et al: Familial cardiomyopathy hypogonadism and collagenoma. Ann Intern Med 93:813–817, 1980

COLLAGENOSIS, FAMILIAL REACTIVE PERFORATING

Synonyms. PC, Mehregan's.

Symptoms and Signs. Both sexes. Onset in early childhood. Recurrent umbilicated papules on the skin that resolve spontaneously in 2 months.

Etiology. Autosomal recessive inheritance. Trauma and cold are triggering factors.

Pathology. Extrusion of collagen fibers through epidermis.

BIBLIOGRAPHY. Mehregan AH, Schwartz OD, Livingood CS: Reactive perforating collagenosis. Arch Dermatol 96:277–282, 1967
Poliak SC, Lebwhol MC, Parris A et al: Reactive perforating collagenosis associated with diabetes mellitus. N Engl J Med 306:81–84, 1982

COLLES'

Synonym. Hyperextension fracture.

Symptoms. Occurs usually in elderly persons. Pain in the wrist; numbness in the fingers; reduced radioulnar motion.

Signs. Tenderness at the lower end of radius; swelling and ecchymosis; distal fragment displaced backward; mass over dorsal aspect of wrist; deformity at "silver fork."

Pathology. Nonarticular fracture of distal radius with volar angulation and dorsal displacement.

Etiology. Extension, compression (indirect) trauma as in falling on outstretched hand.

Therapy. May successfully be treated nonoperatively. Open reduction and internal fixation are needed when radial shortening in young patients or marked crushing.

BIBLIOGRAPHY. Colles A: On the fractures of the carpal extremity of the radius. Edinburgh Med Surg J 10:182–186, 1814
Sisk FD: Fractures of shoulder girdle and upper extremities. In Crenshaw AH (ed): Campbell's Operative Orthopedics, 7th ed, p 1825–1826. St. Louis, CV Mosby, 1987

COLLET-SICARD

Synonyms. Condyloposterior lacerated foramen; glossolaryngoscapulopharyngeal hemiplegia; pharyngeal paralysis; posterior laterocondylar space; retroparotid space; Sicard's. See Villaret's. Vernet-Sargnon.

Symptoms and Signs. Difficulty in swallowing; nasal regurgitation; loss of sensation over posterior third of tongue; hoarseness; paralysis of sternocleidomastoid and trapezius muscles; hemiatrophy of tongue.

Etiology and Pathology. Lesions of the last four cranial nerves (glossopharyngeal; vagus; spinal accessory; hypoglossal) by tumor, adenopathies, aneurysm, penetrating injuries, infections.

BIBLIOGRAPHY. Collet FJ: Sur un nouveau syndrome paralytique pharyngo-laryngé par blessure de guerre (hémiplégie glosso-laryngoscapulo-pharyngée). Lyon Méd 124:121–129, 1916
Sicard JA: Syndrome du carrefour condylo-déchiré postérieur (type pur de paralysie des quatre derniers nerfs craniens). Marseilles Méd 53:385–397, 1916–17
Svien HJ, Baker HL, Rivers MH: Jugular foramen syndrome and allied syndromes. Neurology 13:797–809, 1963
Adams RD, Victor M: Principles of Neurology, 3rd ed, p 504. New York, McGraw-Hill, 1985

COLOR BLINDNESS, BLUE-MONOCONE-MONOCHROMATE TYPE

Synonyms. CBBM, partial color blindness, achromatopsia incomplete.

Symptoms and Signs. Defective vision of blue color which worsens with age.

Etiology. X-linked. Progressive abiotrophy.

Diagnostic Procedures. Pseudoisochromatic plates. (Ishihara plates). *Electroretinography.* Fundus: young age normal; at 50 to 60 years, macular scarring.

Prognosis. Progressive anomaly.

BIBLIOGRAPHY. Sloan LL: Congenital achromatopsia. J Ophthalmol Soc Am 44:117–128, 1954
Fleischman JA, O'Donnel FE: Congenital X-linked incomplete achromatopsia. Arch Ophthalmol 99:468–471, 1981

COLOR BLINDNESS, PARTIAL DEUTAN SERIES

Synonyms. CBD, DCB, deuteranopia, daltonism.

Symptoms and Signs. Predominant in males, but also possible in women. From birth defective vision of colors blue and green.

Etiology. X-linked.

Diagnostic Procedures. Holmgren's test; Ishihara plates.

Prognosis. Traffic light problems.

BIBLIOGRAPHY. Dalton J: Extraordinary facts relating to the vision colours, with observation. Mem Literary Philos Soc: Manchester 5:28–45, 1798

Purrello M, Nussbaum R, Rinaldi A, et al: Old and new genetics help ordering loci at the telomere of the human X-chromosome long arm. Hum Genet 65:295–299, 1984

COLOR BLINDNESS, PARTIAL PROTEAN SERIES

Synonyms. CBP, protanopia.

Symptoms and Signs. From birth. Defective vision of color red.

Etiology. Unknown.

Diagnostic Procedures. Holmgren's test; Ishihara tables.

BIBLIOGRAPHY. Waaler GH: Uber die Erblichkeitsvethaeltnisse der verscheidenen Arten von angeborener Rotgruenblindheit. Z Induckt Abstammungs Vererbungse 45:279–333, 1927

Emerson BT, Thompson L, Wallace DC, et al: Absence of measurable linkage between the loci for hypoxanthine-guanine phosphoryl transferase and deutan color blindness. Am J Hum Genet 26:78–82, 1974

COLOR BLINDNESS, PARTIAL TRITANOMALY

Synonym. Tritanomalous color blindness.

Symptoms and Signs. In males. Patients retain red and green, and lack blue and yellow sensory mechanisms.

Etiology. X-linked.

Diagnostic Procedures. Holmgren's test; Ishihara plates.

BIBLIOGRAPHY. Kalmus H: Diagnosis and Genetics of Defective Color Vision, p 59. Oxford, Pergamon Press, 1965

COMBETTE'S

Synonyms. Cerebellar aplasia; congenital cerebellar; Nonne's; Nonne-Marie.

Symptoms and Signs. Both sexes affected; onset from neonatal period. Delayed growth; poor mental development, speech, and walking; frequent falling; severe weakness. Convulsions. In some cases, continuous masturbation. Indifference to environment; sensation normal.

Etiology. Unknown.

Pathology. Absence of development, or small, rudimentary cerebellum.

Diagnostic Procedures. *X-rays. CT brain scan.*

Therapy. None.

Prognosis. Death usually during first decade. Cases with small rudimentary cerebellum reported with fair prognosis for survival and adjustment to a life limited by poor mental development.

BIBLIOGRAPHY. Combette: Absence complete du cervelet, des pedoncules postérieurs et de la protuberance cerebrale chez une jeune fille morte dans sa onzieme annee. Bull Soc Anat Paris 5:148–157, 1831

Dow RS, Moruzzi G: The Physiology and Pathology of the Cerebellum. Minneapolis, University of Minnesota Press, 1958

COMFORT-STEINBERG

Synonyms. Recidivant pancreatitis; hereditary pancreatitis; pancreatitis, hereditary.

Symptoms and Signs. Onset in childhood or adolescence (4–15 yr old); no sex prevalence. May begin in an acute or chronic form. Recurrent episodes of abdominal pain with repeated episodes of Balser-Fitz's syndrome. Several years later, development of diabetes mellitus symptoms. In some members of the family, diabetes not preceded by pain. In two of three families reported, episodes of hemorrhagic pleural or ascitic effusions.

Etiology. Unknown; genetic transmission, of autosomal dominant type. Suggestion that hypotrophy of Oddi's sphincter could be due to an inherited factor.

Pathology. Progressive destruction of pancreas; each acute relapse leaves increased damage in the gland. Fibroblastic proliferation and fibrosis; infiltration with lymphocytes, plasma cells; atrophy of acinar cells; frequently, calcium deposit.

Diagnostic Procedures. *X-ray:* Calcification in the pancreas. *Pancreas scan with isotopes. Blood.* Glucose. *Stool.* Steatorrhea and determination of pancreatic enzymes. *Urine.* Glucose; no aminoaciduria (except in one family, where this finding was reported, resembling recessive type of cystinuria); urinary amylase increased during episodes of pain. *Duodenal fluid.* Determination of enzymes.

Therapy. Symptomatic: pancreatic enzymes. Trial with steroids. In one family, surgical procedures to drain pancreatic ducts relieved symptoms. In another family, no benefit from surgery.

Prognosis. Chronic relapsing condition with progressive functional and anatomic damage. To be differentiated from acute relapsing pancreatitis where pancreas recovers completely between attacks. Increased incidence of pancreatic carcinoma possible; insufficient data, however, to incriminate genetic relationship for this association.

BIBLIOGRAPHY. Comfort MW, Gambill EE, Baggenstoss AH: Chronic relapsing pancreatitis: A study of 29 cases without associated disease of biliary or gastrointestinal tract. Gastroenterology 6:239–285, 1946

Comfort MW, Steinberg AG: Pedigree of family with hereditary chronic relapsing pancreatitis. Gastroenterology 21:54–63, 1952

Makela P, Aarimaa M: Pancreatography in a family with hereditary pancreatitis. Acta Radiol 26:63–66, 1985

COMLY'S

Synonyms. Acquired methemoglobinemia; well methemoglobinemia. See also Stakis-Talma.

Symptoms and Signs. Usually observed in children living in rural environment or in zone not served by aqueduct. Cyanosis of mucosae and skin (occasionally, misdiagnosis of congenital heart disease). According to the entity of intoxication, metabolic and respiratory symptoms may become associated.

Etiology. Nitrates present in well water inducing formation of methemoglobin.

Pathology. Absence of typical findings, except the cyanotic hue of skin.

Diagnostic Procedures. *Blood.* Pressure of methemoglobin; absence of other alteration. *Electrocardiography.* Normal (see Symptoms).

Therapy. Stop ingestion of contaminated water. In severe case methylene blue, 1 mg/kg body weight in a 1 g/dl solution given intravenously over 5 minutes. A second dose of 2 mg/kg can be given if cyanosis has not cleared within an hour. Doses exceeding 7 mg/kg can be toxic. Ascorbic acid (300–500 mg daily orally) can be useful but its action is slow. Therapy with methylene blue is very dangerous in patients with G6PD deficiency (may trigger hemolytic episodes). The only way to treat these patients is by exchange transfusion.

Prognosis. Good.

BIBLIOGRAPHY. Comly HH: Cyanosis in infants caused by nitrates in well water. JAMA 129:112–116, 1945

Wintrobe MM (ed): Clinical Hematology, 8th ed. Philadelphia, Lea & Febiger, 1981

Kaplan JC, Labie D: Les méthémoglobinémies. Encycl Med Chir, Paris Sang 13007 D10, 1983

CONDORELLI'S

Synonyms. Mediastinal obesity. See also Pickwickian.

Symptoms. Occur in obese people. Slight cyanosis of the face, which becomes more marked on recumbency; episodes of tonicoclonic muscular contractions; alterations of the sleeping rhythm, and alteration of frequency and rhythm of breathing when lying down.

Signs. Diffuse obesity; lack of edema; cyanosis of face; turgor and lack of pulsation of external jugular veins; spasm of vessels on funduscopic examination.

Etiology. Fat infiltration in the mediastinum and water-salt retention.

Pathology. Generalized obesity and mediastinal fat infiltration that constricts the venous margin of the heart and the vascular stem.

Diagnostic Procedures. *Venous pressure.* Markedly increased (diagnostic). *X-ray. Radiochymography. Electrocardiography. Echocardiography. Electroencephalography.*

Therapy. Strict diet; nicotinic acid (when vasospasm predominates); digitalis (if cardiovascular failure); thyroid (if hypothyroidism).

Prognosis. Regression of symptoms immediately follows weight loss.

BIBLIOGRAPHY. Condorelli L: Fisiopatologia clinica del mediastino (sistemazione su base anatomo-fisiologica delle sindromi mediastiniche sensu strictiori). Cong Soc Ital Med Int 48:1–163, 1947

Marrazza P, Zilli E: La sindrome venosa degli adiposi di Condorelli, contributo casistico. Policlinico Sez Part 61:12–22, 1954

CONE-ROD DYSTROPHY

Synonym. CDH.

Symptoms and Signs. Both sexes, onset from childhood in the first decade. Progressive constriction of peripheral visual fields.

Etiology. Autosomal dominant.

Pathology. Eye: dystrophy of retinal photoreceptors and pigment epithelium; abiotrophic degeneration of rods and cones.

Prognosis. Inexorable progression to blindness.

BIBLIOGRAPHY. Hittner HM, Murphree AL, Garcia CA, et al: Dominant cone-rod dystrophy. Docum Ophthal 39:29–52, 1975
Heckenlively JR, Rosales I, Martin D: Optic nerve changes in dominant cone-rod dystrophy. Doc Ophthalmol Proc Ser 27:183–192, 1981

CONGENITAL EYELID

Synonym. Epicanthus inversus–blepharophimosis–ptosis.

Signs. Bilateral ptosis; epicanthus inversus with telecanthus; palpebral phimosis; or blepharophimosis; deficiency of upper and lower eyelid tissue; elevation of eyebrows; absent supraorbital rims; poorly developed nasal bridge.

Etiology. Unknown; definite hereditary influence of autosomal dominant type demonstrated in many cases.

Therapy. Canthoplasty and correction of ptosis, implantation of inert materials for reconstruction of supraorbital region and nasoglabellar angle.

Prognosis. Good cosmetic and functional results obtained by adequate surgical treatment.

BIBLIOGRAPHY. Blair VP, Brown JB, Hamn WG: Correction of ptosis and epicanthus. Arch Ophthalmol 7:831–846, 1932
Lewis SR, Arons MS, Lynch JB, Blocker TG: The congenital eyelid syndrome. Plast Reconst Surg 39:271–277, 1967

CONN'S

Synonyms. Aldosterone-producing adenoma; Conn-Louis.

Symptoms. More common in women, usually in patients 30 to 50 years of age. Central or frontal headache; nicturia; or return to diurnal urinary excretion when patient lying in bed during the day; polydipsia and polyuria (over 2.5 liter in 50% of cases); mild asthenia (early); muscle weakness or paralysis (in advanced cases).

Signs. Arterial hypertension; optic fundi may show narrow tortuous arteries (no marked vasospasm or papilledema). Heart normal size; later may enlarge. Loss of deep tendon reflexes (late sign; edema rare).

Etiology. Primary aldosteronism due to a solitary adrenocortical adenoma, producing inappropriate amount of aldosterone partially under the effect of normal adrenocorticotropic (ACTH) response. A serotonin-mediated mechanism could be responsible for the bilateral hyperplasia.

Pathology. Small adrenal adenoma (66% of cases), more frequently on left adrenal. If near surface, evident; if in the gland, enlargement and increased consistency of gland. Bilateral hyperplasia of zona glomerulosa (33% of cases).

Diagnostic Procedures. *Blood.* Increased aldosterone concentration; low or hyporesponsive renin activity; low potassium level; study of potassium balance by administering potassium salt; of sodium balance, reduction of sodium intake results in a rise of serum potassium. Serum sodium concentration and carbon dioxide-combining power increased (in advanced cases.) *Urine.* Increased potassium excretion; increased aldosterone excretion. With administration of spironolactone, increased sodium excretion and decreased potassium excretion. *Plasma renin.* Diminished. *Electrocardiography.* Sagging ST segments; inverted T waves; large U waves and prolonged ST interval (changes reverting to normal after spironolactone administration or potassium replacement). Administration of thiazide, or other diuretics, reveals in early cases the latent potassium-wasting tendency. Tetany may be elicited by hyperventilation or by compression of artery (Trousseau maneuver). *CT scan.*

Therapy. Unilateral adrenalectomy after preparation with spironolactone if unilateral adenoma. If bilateral hyperplasia: long-term high-dose spironolactone (side-effects: malaise, gynecomastia, impotence) and eventually surgery.

Prognosis. With surgery in unilateral cases cure in 90% of cases; in bilateral cases: reversion of electrolytes disorder, but frequently blood pressure does not normalize.

BIBLIOGRAPHY. Conn JW: Primary aldosteronism: A new clinical syndrome. J Lab Clin Med 45:3–17, 1955
Conn JW: Aldosteronism in men. JAMA 183:871–878, 1963
Grekin R: The adrenal gland. In Mazzaferri EL (ed): Textbook of Endocrinology, 3rd ed, pp 278–381. New York Med Exam Rev Pub, 1985

CONRADI'S

Synonyms. Chondrodystrophia calcificans congenita; dyplasia epiphysialis punctata; stippled epiphyses; Huenermann's; koala bear dominant.

Symptoms and Signs. Occur in infancy. Approximately 25% of patients have a distinctive ichthyosiform eruption at birth; thick, yellow, tightly adherent keratinized plaques are distributed in a whorled pattern over the entire body, which may be intensely erythematous. Slow growth, absent cataracts, muscle contractures. Visual trouble; shortening of proximal long bones; scoliosis. Other skeletal abnormalities including macrocephaly or microcephaly; hypertelorism; syndactyly; club foot. Mild mental deficiency. Congenital vascular defects, like severe pulmonary arterial stenoses, may be present.

Etiology. Unknown; autosomal dominant disorder or fresh gene mutation affecting bones and ectodermal structures. May be considered a form of multiple epiphyseal dysplasia.

Pathology. Calcific areas in epiphyses of hips, knees, shoulder, wrists. Other malformations (see Symptoms and Signs). The histologic changes include hyperkeratosis that penetrates to the depths of the hair follicles.

Diagnostic Procedures. *X-ray.* Characteristic presence of multiple punctate calcific deposits in epiphyses during infancy. Various skeletal abnormalities (see Signs). In patients who survive, epiphysis calcifications disappear between first and third years of life. *Chromosome studies.* Normal. *Urine.* Moderate nonspecific aminoaciduria. *Echocardiography:* Dilatation of the right ventricle; signs of pulmonary hypertension.

Therapy. Symptomatic. Orthopedic.

Prognosis. Infants with full syndrome usually die during the first year of life. Survivors exhibit multiple skeletal, ocular, and mental (more or less) debilitating defects. Abnormal calcification disappears by age 1 to 4 years.

BIBLIOGRAPHY. Conradi E: Vorzeitiges Auftreten von Kochen und eigenartigen Verkalkungskernen bei Chondrodystrophia fötalis hypoplastica, Histologische und Röntgenuntersuchungen. J Kinderheilk 80:86–97, 1914
Huenermann C: Chondrodystrophia calcificans congenita als abortive Form der Chondrodystrophye. Kinderheilk 51:1–19, 1931
Trowitzsch E, Richter R, Eisenberg W, Kallfelz HC: Severe pulmonary arterial stenoses in Conradi-Hünermann disease. Eur J Pediatr 145:116–118, 1986

CONSCIOUS IMMOBILITY

Synonyms. Night nurse's paralysis. Writer's cramp, loss of lip (in instrumentalists), occupational neurosis, focal dystonia.

Symptoms and Signs. Affects nurses of both sexes (60% according to one author); also reported in people driving cars or engaged in navigation or engaged in other skilled motor acts as piano playing, etc. Occur at any time of day or night and lasts a few seconds. Brief transient disability of voluntary muscles with full awareness of it and inability to terminate it; speech impossible. Not associated with other symptoms.

Etiology. Some features are in common with cataplexy; psychogenic conversion discussed. Probably an intention spasm, where discrete movements are impaired by spreading innervation of unneeded muscles.

BIBLIOGRAPHY. Rudolf G de M: A Conscious Immobility. Bristol, J Wright, 1969
Adams RD, Victor M: Principles of Neurology 3rd ed, pp 87–89. New York, McGraw-Hill, 1985

CONVISART'S

Eponym used to indicate Fallot's syndrome (see) with dextroposed aorta.

BIBLIOGRAPHY. Convisart JN: Traité des mal du coeur, Vol II. Paris, 1814
Perloff JK: The Clinical Recognition of Congenital Heart Disease, 2nd ed, p 445. Philadelphia, WB Saunders, 1978

COOPERMAN-MIURA

Synonym. Uvula tongue malposture.

Symptoms. Respiratory disorders; headache; facial pain, often of an intensity suggesting trifacial neuralgia; temporomandibular disarticulations.

Signs. Various degrees of irritation of the covering tissues of the dorsum of the tongue and uvula. Mandibular retrusion. Narrowing of respiratory and alimentary pathways. Abnormalities of the dental plane of occlusion.

Etiology. Underlying cause of irritative phenomena is postural. Mandibular protrusion as seen in Stone Age skulls was a protective mechanism that functioned to preserve head, neck, and throat physiology.

Pathology. Possible presence of potential lesions in such specialized fields of neuropathy, otitis, sinusitis, allergic hypersensity, and asthma.

Diagnostic Procedures. Visual examination of uvula tongue malposture during mandibular opening. Noting abnormalities of orthopedic gait of the mandible. Observing nasal breathing. Interpretation of dental plane of occlusion.

Therapy. Mechanical correction of uvula tongue malposture. Intervention by metal or nonmetal oropharyngeal wedges.

Prognosis. Favorable by oral wedge intervention restoring anatomic and physiologic derangements.

BIBLIOGRAPHY. Cooperman HN: New approaches to establishing the plane of occlusion and freeway space in dentures. Dent Dig 71:202, 1965

Cooperman HN, Miura N, Vanhakendover S, Rich H: Uvula tongue malposture. A new approach to Costen's syndrome. Dent Diamond (Japan) 2:127–129, 1977

Miura N, Ueno K, Karasawa J: Dental technology of myodontics. Quintessence, Tokyo, 1987

COOPER'S I

Synonyms. Breast fibrosis; irritable breast; mastodynia; mammary neuralgia.

Symptoms. Occur in women; onset between 30 and 35 years of age. Mammary pain; menometrorrhagia.

Signs. In mammary tissue (usually unilaterally) in upper external quadrant presence of palpable, indurated, mass; process not well defined.

Etiology. Unknown. Considered excessive internal secretion of estriol.

Pathology. Mass formed by whitish, homogeneous tissue, which includes and compresses epithelial structures; atrophy of the latter.

Diagnostic Procedures. *Mammography*: may show calcification. *Echo, Xerography, Thermography.*

Therapy. Vitamin A. Surgery. Bromocryptine or danazol (in cyclic mastalgia). Excision of wedge of the areola (painful nipple).

BIBLIOGRAPHY. Cooper A: Illustration of the Diseases of the Breast. London, Longman, 1829

Rook A, Wilkinson DS, Ebling FJG, et al: Textbook of Dermatology, 4th ed, p 2179. Oxford, Blackwell Scientific Publications, 1986

COOPER'S II

Synonyms. Genitofemoral causalgia; Lyon's; testis neuralgia; pudendal neuralgia; Zuelzer's.

Symptoms. Recurrent annoying pain of testis.

Etiology. Unknown. May be considered a form of psychalgias when organic cause cannot be found. May be considered as part of the pudendal neuralgia (Zuelzer) or genitofemoral causalgia (Lyon).

Therapy. Mild analgesic; psychotherapy if indicated.

Prognosis. Possible conversion to other symptoms.

BIBLIOGRAPHY. Cooper A: Observations on the Structures and Diseases of the Testis. London, Longman, 1830

Vick NA: Grinker's Neurology, 7th ed. Springfield, CC Thomas, 1976

CORDS'

Synonym. Angiopathia retinae juvenilis.

Symptoms. Occur in adolescents or young adults. Reduction of visual fields with possible progression to total blindness.

Etiology. Phlebitis or thrombosis of the central vein of retina caused by a tubercular infection.

Pathology. Wall of vein shows infiltration by lymphocytes; thrombosis; edema of adjacent tissues; optic nerve atrophy. Retina shows edema, congestion or degenerative changes.

Therapy. Specific. Anticoagulants.

Prognosis. Variable according to degree reached by condition before the treatment.

BIBLIOGRAPHY. Cords R: Papillitis und Glaukom zugleich ein Beitrang zur juvenilen Phlebitis der zentral Vein. Graefes Arch Ophthalmol 105:916–963, 1931

CORK WORKER'S

Synonyms. Maple-bark worker's suberosis. See Allergic alveolitis, extrinsic .

Symptoms. Occur in person working with cork; onset insidious. Cough; malaise; weight loss; or sudden fever, dry cough.

Signs. Diffuse fine rales over both sides of chest.

Etiology. Hypersensitivity to moldy cork dust.

Pathology. Interstitial pneumonitis; eosinophil cell infiltration; fibrosis.

Diagnostic Procedures. *Blood*. Eosinophilia. Presence of specific serum precipitin against moldy cork dust. *X-ray*. Increased bronchovascular maskings; diffuse nodular, reticular infiltration. In acute phase, patchy densities.

Therapy. Corticosteroids.

Prognosis. Acute attacks resolve spontaneously in 24 to 48 hours after removal from exposure. Recurrences on reexposure. Chronic pulmonary fibrosis if reexposure not prevented.

BIBLIOGRAPHY. Emanuel DA, Lawton BR, Wensel FJ: Maple-bark disease, pneumoconiosis due to coniosporum corticale. New Engl J Med 266:333–337, 1962
Avila R, Villar TG: Suberosis-respiratory disease in cork workers. Lancet 1:620–621, 1968

CORNEAL DERMOIDS–SHORT STATURE

Symptoms and Signs. Corneal opacities, short stature.

Etiology. Autosomal recessive trait.

Pathology. Cornea: abnormal mesoblastic tissue covered by epithelium.

Diagnostic Procedures. *Slit-lamp examination.* Corneas with superficial and vascularized tissue. *Corneal biopsy.* See Pathology.

Therapy. In severe cases, corneal transplantation.

Prognosis. It depends on the extent of corneal involvement.

BIBLIOGRAPHY. Guizar-Vazquez J, Luengas-Munoz FS, Antillon F: Brief clinical report: Corneal dermoids and short stature in brother and sister. A new syndrome? Am J Med Genet 8:229–234, 1981

CORNEAL DYSTROPHY, POLYMORPHOUS POSTERIOR

Synonyms. Hereditary nonprogressive corneal dystrophy; PPCD; posterior polymorphous corneal dystrophy.

Symptoms. Both sexes affected. Minor or no decrease of visual acuity. Nonprogressive or extremely slowly progressive; rarely may be associated with glaucoma.

Signs. Faint haze in corneas.

Etiology. Unknown; autosomal dominant inheritance.

Pathology. Lesion limited to Descemet's membrane and endothelium. Multiple small nodular and larger vesicle excrescences of Descemet's membrane, some protruding into anterior chamber, equally distributed all over the membrane. Descemet's membrane shows faint cloudiness between lesions.

Diagnostic Procedures. *Slit lamp examination.*

Prognosis. Nonprogressive; seldom associated with rupture of Descemet's membrane and glaucoma.

BIBLIOGRAPHY. Koeppe L: Klinische Beobachtungen mit der Nernstspalmlampe und dem Hornhautmikroscop. Graefe Arch Klin Exp Ophthalmol 91:363–379, 1916

Rodriguez MM, Sun T-T, Krachmer J, et al: Posterior polymorphous corneal dystrophy recent development. Birth Defect Orig Art Ser 18(6):476–491, 1982

CORONARY ARTERY STEAL

See Intramural coronary artery aneurysm and left coronary artery arising from pulmonary artery (IV phase).

Symptoms. Onset in childhood shortly after adequate collateral circulation has developed or when a communication between coronary arteries and heart chambers or intramural coronary aneurysm steals blood from coronary circulation. Onset in later life, in cases of abnormal origin of left coronary artery from pulmonary artery. Angina; dyspnea; fatigue on exertion.

Signs. Harsh systolic and diastolic murmur along left sternal border and on apex.

Etiology. See Symptoms.

Pathology. See Symptoms.

Diagnostic Procedures. *Electrocardiography. Cardiac catheterization. Cinecardioangiography.* Blood from coronary artery flows in retrograde direction. *X-ray of chest.*

Therapy. If evidence of adequate collateral circulation, ligation of anomalous arteries at their origins. If intramural coronary aneurysm, closure of aneurysmal neck and approximation of walls.

Prognosis. Good when surgery indicated and performed.

BIBLIOGRAPHY. Bane AE, Baum S, Blakemore WS et al: A later stage of anomalous coronary circulation with origin of the left coronary artery from the pulmonary artery. Circulation 36:878–885, 1967
Perloff JK: The Clinical Recognition of Congenital Heart Disease, 2nd ed, p 576. Philadelphia, WB Saunders, 1978

CORPUS CALLOSUM AGENESIS

Synonym. See Andermann's.

Symptoms and Signs. Rare condition with variable clinical findings. None, or convulsions and mental deficiencies. Macrocephaly or microcephaly. Lack of neuropathy (see Andermann's).

Etiology. Unknown. Many genetic causes. Autosomal recessive. For partial agenesis reported X-linked inheritance.

Pathology. Corpus callosum agenesis with frequent association of other developmental defects: absent septum pellucidum; microgyria; arteriovenous malformations.

Diagnostic Procedures. *CT brain scan.* Third ventricle extending between lateral ventricles.

Prognosis. According to associated defects; various degrees of mental retardation, but normal mental development and normal life are possible.

BIBLIOGRAPHY. Alpers BJ, Grant FC: The clinical syndrome of the corpus callosum. Arch Neurol Psychiat 25:67–86, 1931

Kaplan P: X-linked recessive inheritance of agenesis of the corpus callosum. J Med Genet 20:122–124, 1983

Young ID, Trounce JQ et al: Agenesis of the corpus callosum and macrocephaly in siblings. Clin Genet 28:225–230, 1985

CORPUS LUTEUM INSUFFICIENCY

Synonym. Inadequate luteal phase.

Symptoms. History of abortion, particularly habitual abortion.

Etiology. Poor endogenous secretion of progesterone hormone during the luteal phase of menstrual cycle.

Diagnostic Procedures. *Blood.* Low level of pregnanediol excretion during the initial phase of menstrual cycle. *Biopsy of endometrium on 24th day of cycle.* Poor secretory response; lowered cell storage of glucose, alkaline phosphatase, and other enzymes. Documentation in two cycles.

Therapy. Once diagnosis is established by history and endometrial biopsy, a plan should be set to treat this syndrome during (1) preconceptional period; (2) implantation period; (3) postconceptional period.
1. *During the preconceptional period.* Progesterone intramuscular (IM) vaginal suppository daily during luteal phase, or daily injection of progesterone in oil starting at the rise of basic body temperature until onset of menses. Use of clomiphene citrate or human chorionic gonadotropin (hCG) every other day in luteal phase have also been proposed.
2. *If pregnancy occurs.* Long-acting progestational agents, (*e.g.,* Delalutin) until week 28. If spotting occurs, dosage increase.

Prognosis. Good for successful pregnancy with adequate treatment.

BIBLIOGRAPHY. Kupperman HS: Treatment of endocrine causes of sterility in the female. Clin Obstet Gynecol 2:808–825, 1959

Davajan V, Israel R: Infertility causes, evaluation and treatment. In De Groot LJ, Cahill GH Jr, Odell WD (eds): Endocrinology, p 1470. New York, Grune & Stratton, 1979

Yen SSC, Jaffe RB (eds) Reproductive Endocrinology, 2nd ed. Philadelphia, WB Saunders, 1986

CORRIGAN'S

Synonyms. Congenital aortic regurgitation; congenital aortic valve insufficiency; congenital regurgitation.

Symptoms. Great prevalence in males. Usually asymptomatic for long period of life span. Then, weakness; inappropriate diaphoresis; lethargy; awareness of neck pulsations or heart contractions; vascular pain on carotid, subclavian, or thoracic and abdominal aorta; exertional dyspnea. In some cases, sudden intractable cardiac failure.

Signs. Rapid pulse rise and collapse (Corrigan's pulse); high blood pressure with high pulse pressure; Quincke's pulse; anteroposterior head shaking; chest palpation (apex heart heaving); displaced left and downward; high-pitched diastolic murmur; blowing decrescendo (best heard with patient sitting or standing and leaning forward); Austin-Flint murmur.

Etiology. Congenital malformation; most commonly bicuspid aortic valve.

Pathology. Hypertrophy of left ventricle. Several possible defects and associations: unicuspid, unicommisural aortic valve; bicuspid, tricuspid, quadricuspid valves; associated with subvalvular aortic stenosis (see), supravalvular aortic stenosis (see) or ventricular septal defect.

Diagnostic Procedures. *Electrocardiography.* In mild form, normal. In severe form, R waves tall in left precordium; S waves deep in right precordium; depression of ST segment; T wave inversion in DI, aVL, V_5, V_6 leads. *X-ray.* Enlargement of left ventricle; dilatation of ascending aorta. *Echocardiography. Cardiac catheterization. Radionuclide angiography.*

Therapy. Prevention of bacterial endocarditis. Eventually, consideration for surgery. Ideally surgery should be performed before clinical symptoms of heart failure develop.

Prognosis. Normal life and insidious progression of condition and sudden manifestation in young adults. Acute form may present a much faster evolution and a stormy course. All forms eventually lead to cardiac failure. For valve replacement the early mortality is approximately 2 to 3%; late results are mostly related to the junctional status of the left ventricle.

BIBLIOGRAPHY. Corrigan DJ: On permanent patency of the mouth of the aorta or inadequacy of the aortic valves. Edinburgh Med Surg J 37:225–245, 1832
Perloff JK: The Clinical Recognition of Congenital Heart disease, 2nd ed, p 113. Philadelphia, WB Saunders, 1978
Hurst JW: The Heart, 6th ed, pp 739–751. New York, McGraw-Hill, 1986

COR TRIATRIATUM

Synonym. Stenosis of common pulmonary vein.

Symptoms. Both sexes affected; onset in early age (not in newborn; occasionally in adolescence or in adulthood). Seldom completely asymptomatic (mild obstruction). Cyanosis; failure to thrive; exertional dyspnea; tachypnea; orthopnea; cough; irritability. With later onset; exertional dyspnea, then episodes of pulmonary edema. Recurrent hemophthysis.

Signs. Normal or growth retardation and aspects of chronic illness. On auscultation, first sound normal or loud and snapping; second sound loud pulmonic component. Murmurs may be absent or systolic, diastolic, or continuous types may be present.

Etiology. Congenital malformation.

Pathology. Drainage of pulmonary vein into an accessory left atrial chamber proximal to left atrium.

Diagnostic Procedures. *Electrocardiography.* P waves peaked (right atrial involvement); right axis deviation and variable right ventricle hypertrophy. *X-ray.* Pulmonary venous congestion; ground glass aspect; acute pulmonary edema (on attacks). Heart size normal or marked cardiomegaly. *Two-dimensional echocardiography. Cardiac catheterization.*

Therapy. Medical management. Treatment of intercurrent infections: (Congestive failure and bacterial endocarditis). If symptoms appear, surgical removal of diaphragm is indicated.

Prognosis. Interval between onset of symptoms and death usually short. Extremely variable survival according to degree of lesions, from death in early infancy to survival in the fourth decade without symptoms. Progressive pulmonary venous hypertension and congestion with right-sided heart failure.

BIBLIOGRAPHY. Andral G: Précis d'Anatomie Pathologique, Paris Vol II, p 313. Gaben, 1829
Borst M: Ein Cor triatriatum. Verh Dtsch Ges Pathol 178–192, 1905
Ostman-Smith I, Silverman NH, Oldershaw P, et al: Cor triatriatum sinistrum. Diagnostic features on cross-sectional echocardiography. Br Heart J 54:211–219, 1984

Williams RG, Bierman F, Sanders SP: Echocardiographic diagnosis of cardiac malformations. 1st ed, p 118. Boston, Little Brown & Co, 1986
Hurst JW: The Heart, 6th ed, pp 651–652. New York, McGraw-Hill, 1986

COSSIO-BERCONSKY

Eponym used to indicate the association of interatrial communication and Pick's (F.) (see).

BIBLIOGRAPHY. Cossio P, Berconsky I: Communication interauricolar y sinfisis pericardica. Rev Argent Cardiol 3:360–366, 1936

COSTELLO-DENT

Synonyms. Hypohyperparathyroidism.
Eponym used to indicate a clinical syndrome represented by the combination of mild tetany (attributed to hypothyroidism) and osteitis fibrosa generalisata.

BIBLIOGRAPHY. Costello JM, Dent CE: Hypohyperparathyroidism. Arch Dis Child 38:397–407, 1963

COSTEN'S

Synonym. Temporomandibular joint.

Symptoms. Headache; facial pain; stuffy sensations in the ears; tinnitus; earache; impaired hearing; dizziness; nystagmus, burning throat, mouth, and tongue.

Signs. Herpes in external auditory canal.

Etiology. Overaction of jaw joint, followed by development of a loose joint produced by absorption of meniscus, condyles, and bone (Costen). Myofascial trigger zone that produces, through an unknown mechanism, all symptoms when the area is stimulated by various stimuli such as heat, cold, pressure, needling (Freese).

Pathology. Erosion of glenoid or mandibular fossa with impaction of the condyles.

Diagnostic Procedures. *X-ray of jaw.*

Therapy. Dental correction of malocclusions; injection of corticosteroids in temporomandibular joint.

BIBLIOGRAPHY. Costen JB: A syndrome of ear and sinus symptoms dependent upon disturbed function of the temporomandibular joint. Ann Otol Rhinol Laryngol 43:1–15, 1934

Costen JB: Classification and treatment of temporomandibular joint problems. J Michigan Med Soc 55:673–677, 1956

Freese AS: Costen's syndrome: A reinterpretation. Arch Otolaryngol 70:309–314, 1959

Adams RD, Victor M: Principles of Neurology, 3rd ed, p 147. New York, McGraw-Hill, 1985

COTARD'S

Synonym. Delirium of total negation.

Symptoms. Patient complains of having lost everything: possessions; strength; part of (blood; heart; intestine) or entire body. Also, world does not exist for him anymore, and paradoxically he feels that he has become immortal. Other megalomelancholic ideas may be present.

Etiology. Unknown. Seen especially in manic-depressive patients or in certain brain syndromes.

Therapy. Acute syndrome lasts only a few days or weeks. Responds to treatment of basic disorder.

BIBLIOGRAPHY. Cotard J: Du délire des negations. Arch Neurol 4:152–282, 1882

Freedman AM, Kaplan HI: Comprehensive Textbook of Psychiatry, 2nd ed. Baltimore, Williams & Wilkins, 1975

COT-SIDES

Symptoms and Signs. Falling out of a bed with its cot-sides up. Loss of consciousness. It occurs in brain-damaged patients (trauma, cerebral vascular accidents, neoplasms).

Pathology. Those of the original injury or illness, plus signs of recent contusion or generalized brain edema.

Diagnostic Procedures. *CT brain scan.*

Therapy. Surgical intervention when indicated. Prevention: strapping in, or heavy sedation, or both, in brain-damaged person who can climb out of bed and fall.

Prognosis. Poor. In most of the patients described, coma persisted until death in a few days.

BIBLIOGRAPHY. Crompton R: Cot-sides syndrome, medico-legal entity. Lancet 1:1278–1279, 1985

COTTLE'S

Synonym. Wide nose.

Symptoms. Occur at any age; more common in older people, and in females, especially after menopause. Exac-erbated in spring and fall and in winter when going into the cold from a warm room. Tearing; sensation of dryness in the eyes and nasal mucosa; nasal mucosal crusting.

Signs. Keratoconjunctivitis sicca and rhinitis sicca. Epiphora; nasal index and tip index disproportion.

Etiology. Failure in the conduction of tears, without organic obstruction of drainage passage. Hypertrophy of inferior turbinate, occluding Hasner's valve; insufficiency of buffer system of nasal vestibule on expiration and nasal valve in inspiration.

Diagnostic Procedures. *Schirmer's test.* Positive. *Cotton test.*

Therapy. Small cotton ball placed in the vestibule (of such size as not to constitute an obstruction) and determined if less effort needed in breathing. Usually beneficial within 5 minutes: decrease of lacrimation, and conjunctiva and nasal mucosa become moist. Initially, cotton ball worn continuously; then when needed.

Prognosis. Wearing cotton ball permits healing; and size of lobule may be considerably reduced.

BIBLIOGRAPHY. Cottle MH: Structure and function of nasal vestibule. Arch Otolaryngol 62:173–181, 1955

Gunderson HC: The wide nose. Presented at the American Rhinological Society, Chicago, Oct. 11, 1956

Gaynon IE: Lacrimal insufficiency, keratoconjunctivitis sicca and malfunction of the inferior turbinate in the wide nose or open nasal space syndrome (Cottle). Am J Ophthalmol 53:614–618, 1962

COTTON-BERG

Synonyms. Proximal end tibia fracture; fender fracture. Eponym used to indicate a fracture of the external side of tibial head resulting from a violent abduction and the consequent impact against the external condyle of the femur.

BIBLIOGRAPHY. Cotton FJ, Berg R: Fender fracture of the tibia and the knee. N Engl J Med 201:989–995, 1929

Sisk TD: Fractures of lower extremities. In Crenshaw AH (ed): Campbell's Operative Orthopedics, 7th ed, pp 1637–1653. St. Louis, CV Mosby, 1987

COTUGNO'S

Synonyms. Sciatic neuritis; sciatica. See also Facets and Putti-Chavany.

Symptoms. Occur most often in males, onset usually abrupt. Unilateral pain in posterior portions of thighs and back of leg, worsened by movement, sneezing, coughing.

Signs. Weakness of leg involved, especially below knee; ankle jerk absent; sensory impairment. Tenderness on palpation along course of sciatic nerve; loss of lumbar curve. Gaenslen's sign; Patrick's sign; straight-leg raising test; Lasègue's sign; Ober's test.

Etiology and Pathology. *Most frequent.* Radicular compression and neuritis of L4-5 interspace by herniation of intervertebral disk. *Other causes.* Tumor (primary or metastatic); infection; arthritic changes; fractures of spine; pelvic conditions compressing the nerve (*e.g.,* pregnancy; neoplasm; abscess).

Diagnostic Procedures. *X-ray of spine. Spinal tap.* Increase of total protein.

Therapy. Rest; analgesic; antiinflammatory agent; vitamin B_{12}; physiotherapy. According to etiology, surgery or antibiotics.

Prognosis. Usually subacute or chronic course. Increasing in days to a maximum, then receding gradually.

BIBLIOGRAPHY. Cotugno D: De ischiade nervosa commentarius. Napoli Frates Simonis 1764; Vienna, Gräffer, 1770
Cotugno D: A Treatise of the Nervous Sciatica, or Nervous Hip Gout. London, Wilkie, 1775

COUGH SYNCOPE

Synonyms. Charcot's vertigo; laryngeal epilepsy; posttussive; tussive syncope; laryngeal vertigo.

Symptoms. Occur most frequently in middle-aged men who excessively indulge in tobacco, alcohol, and food. Following cough attack (dry, unproductive, paroxysmal, with intense muscular effort); burning or tingling of larynx may precede cough. Sudden syncope (occurs within seconds; no sequelae; frequently no memory of consciousness loss).

Signs. Usually pyknic, slightly obese patient. Frequent signs of respiratory tract infections, emphysema, or bronchial asthma. During syncope, complete muscle relaxation, and patient falls or slumps. Face congested, then pale; diaphoresis frequent; convulsion rare (10%).

Etiology. Not clearly defined. Relation to epilepsy, and narcolepsy-cataplexy (Gelineau's, see) has been discussed, but elements of differentiation exist to establish this syndrome as an autonomous clinical entity.

Diagnostic Procedures. *Serology.* To differentiate from laryngeal crisis of tabes dorsalis. *Electroencephalography.* To differentiate from epilepsy. *X-ray of chest.*

Therapy. No treatment during attack. Treatment of underlying respiratory condition. Procaine block of superior laryngeal nerve in refractory cases. Change in diet and smoking habits.

Prognosis. Attacks generally benign and of little consequence; death, however, may occur. Cure of respiratory condition prevents recurrences of attacks.

BIBLIOGRAPHY. Charcot JM: Seance du 19 Novembre 1876. Gaz Med Paris 5:588–589, 1876
Weissler AM, Warren JU: Syncope: Pathophysiology and differential diagnosis. In Hurst JW: The Heart, 6th ed, p 517. New York, McGraw-Hill, 1986

COUNTER-DISASTER

See Disaster.

Symptoms and Signs. Psychological state that drives uninjured or slightly injured people to volunteer after the disaster to participate in extremely vigorous rescue activity. They become physically overexerted and perform with poor efficiency. Danger of becoming careless, especially in applying first aid measures.

Therapy. Education and training.

BIBLIOGRAPHY. Garb S, Eng E: Disaster Handbook. New York, Springer, 1964

COURVOISIER-TERRIER

Synonym. Ampulla of Vater obstruction.

Signs. Courvoisier's law: Palpable distended gallbladder indicates a neoplasm as cause of obstructive jaundice. Important sign, but not invariably present; gallbladder may be distended, but not palpable.

BIBLIOGRAPHY. Courvoisier LG: Casuistischstatistische Beiträge zur Pathologie und Chirurgie der Gallenwege, pp 57–58. Leipzig, Vogel, 1890

COUVADE

Synonym. Male pseudopregnancy.

Symptoms. Occur in men whose wives are pregnant; usually symptoms start in third month of wife's pregnancy. Mostly gastrointestinal symptoms: appetite loss; toothache; nausea; vomiting; morning sickness; constipation; diarrhea. Abdominal swelling rare (see Simpson's). Tension and anxiety may be present or absent. Different from delusion of pregnancy: patient with couvade syndrome never has the idea of being pregnant.

Etiology. Unknown; this neurotic development appears equivalent to the couvade ritual, which was practiced since antiquity and is still practiced in different parts of the world by many races. It consists of the father retiring at time of wife's labor, mimicking labor pain, receiving the attention due to the parturient woman.

Therapy. None; symptoms disappear with termination of wife's pregnancy.

Prognosis. Self-limited, very benign neurosis. In some cases, recurrence on successive pregnancies of wife.

BIBLIOGRAPHY. Taylor EB: Research into the Early History of Mankind and the Development of Civilization, 2nd ed, p 301. London, Murray, 1865

Enoch MO, Trethowan WH, Barker JC: Some Uncommon Psychiatric Syndromes. Baltimore, Williams & Wilkins, 1967

Bogren LY: The couvade syndrome: Background variables. Acta Psychiatr Scand 70:316–320, 1984

COUVELAIRE'S

Synonyms. Uteroplacental apoplexy; Couvelaire's premature separation of placenta. Abruptio placentae. (See Defibrinating.)

Symptoms. Vaginal bleeding, and shock out of proportion to external bleeding; local pain and tenderness.

Signs. Tender and firm uterus; rapid enlargement of uterus. Fetal signs: sudden, violent movement of the fetus; changes in rate and quality of heart sounds.

Etiology. By definition, placental detachment after the 24th week. Cause unknown. Predisposing factors: toxemia; hypertension; chronic glomerulonephritis; trauma; chronic vascular disease.

Pathology. Retroplacental hematoma occurring between basal decidua and myometrium; rupture into amniotic sac. In severe cases, extensive hemorrhagic infiltration occurs between muscle bundles producing bluish mottling of uterus, broad ligaments, tubes, and ovaries— "Couvelaire uterus." Complication of separation: hypofibrinogenemia (see Defibrinating syndrome); acute renal failure.

Diagnostic Procedures. *Ultrasound examination.*

Therapy. Depends on stage of labor, efficiency of uterine contractions, period of gestation, and actual or potential infection. (1) Watchful expectancy; (2) rupture of membranes; (3) cesarean section. Cesarean section limited to (1) severe detachment seen early and fetus living, (2) patients in whom cervix is uneffaced, and undilated, (3) those showing no progress in labor after rupture. Replacement of blood; intravenous (IV) infusion of fibrinogen; IV infusion of epsilon-aminocaproic acid. Occasion-ally a cesarean hysterectomy is necessary if bleeding is uncontrollable.

Prognosis. Fetal mortality around 40%; maternal mortality under 1%.

BIBLIOGRAPHY. Couvelaire A: Traitment chirurgical des hémorrhagies utero-placentaires avec décollement du placenta normalment inséré. Ann Gynecol Obstet (Paris) 8:591–608, 1911

De Lee JB: A case of fatal hemorrhagic diathesis, with premature detachment of the placenta. Am J Obstet 44:785–792, 1901

Novak ER, Woodruff JD: Novak's Gynecologic and Obstetric Pathology, 8th ed, p 621. Philadelphia, WB Saunders, 1979

Monteiro AA, Inocencio AC, Jorge CS: Placental abruption with disseminated intravascular coagulopathy in the second trimester of pregnancy with fetal survival. Br J Obstet Gynecol 94:811–812, 1987

COWDEN'S*

Synonyms. Multiple hamartoma; Lloyd-Dennis.

Symptoms. Both sexes. Recurrent diarrhea (in some cases). Virginal hypertrophy of breasts; birdlike facies; hypoplastic mandible and maxilla, high-arched palate; scrotal tongue; papillomatosis of lips and oral mucosa. Also, frequent multiple thyroid adenomas, scoliosis, and pectus excavatum. Skin biopsy: trichillemomas, oral mucosa: fibromas. Hands-feet: benign keratosis.

Etiology. Autosomal dominant inheritance.

Pathology. Hamartomatous polyps of intestine in some cases.

Therapy. Surgery.

Prognosis. Fair; one case developed acute myelogenous leukemia.

BIBLIOGRAPHY. Lloyd KM, II, Dennis M: Cowden's disease, a possible new symptom complex with multiple system involvement. Ann Intern Med 58:136–142, 1963

Thyresson HN, Doyle JA: Cowden's disease (multiple hamartoma syndrome). Mayo Clin Proc 56:179–184, 1981

Ruschak PJ, Kauh YC, Luscombe HA: Cowden's disease associated with immunodeficiency. Arch Dermatol 117:573–575, 1981

---

* Name of family affected members.

CRAIN'S

Synonym. Erosive osteoarthritis.

Symptoms and Signs. Predominantly affects women; onset in middle age or postmenopause. Episodes of painful inflammations of distal interphalangeal joints, followed by proximal joint involvement. Recurrent for years, with long intermittent periods of complete remission (up to 10 yr). Presence of mucous cysts over affected joints (to be differentiated from Heberden's nodes, see).

Etiology. Unknown; hereditary condition or sporadic.

Pathology. Bony ankylosis; juxtaarticular bone erosions; proliferative synovitis.

Diagnostic Procedures. *Blood.* Sedimentation rate normal; rheumatoid factor normal. *X-rays.* Cartilage loss; osteophyte formation; subchondral sclerosis; juxtaarticular bone erosion. Absence of findings of generalized osteoarthritis.

Therapy. Corticosteroids and antiinflammatory agents during attacks.

Prognosis. Evolution toward severe functional impairment.

BIBLIOGRAPHY. Crain DG: Interphalangeal osteoarthritis. JAMA 175:1049–1053, 1961
Moskowitz RW: Clinical and laboratory findings in osteoarthritis. In Hollander JL, McCarty DJ: Arthritis and Allied Conditions, 8th ed, p 1047. Philadelphia, Lea & Febiger, 1972

CRANIODIAPHYSEAL DYSOSTOSIS

Synonym. See Craniometaphyseal dysplasia and Camurati-Engelmann's.

Symptoms. Both sexes affected; present from infancy, becoming symptomatic within first few years. Nasal obstruction; anorexia; vomiting; blindness; deafness; mental retardation.

Signs. Marked facial distortion; widened ribs; clavicles thickened in midportions.

Etiology. Unknown; autosomal recessive trait.

Pathology. Sclerosis of skull bones; paranasal sinuses overgrown. In long bones thin-cortex, uniform thickness of shafts; in metacarpals and metatarsals, some degree of ballooning in midportions with thin cortex.

Diagnostic Procedures. *Blood.* Normal calcium, phosphorus, and alkaline phosphatase. *X-rays of bones.*

Therapy. Surgical correction of nerve compression.

Prognosis. Poor; condition more severe than Pyle's. Faster progression to blindness and death.

BIBLIOGRAPHY. De Souza O: Leontiasis ossea. Porto Alegre (Brazil) Faculdade de Med Rev Dos Cursos 13:47–54, 1927
Halliday J: A rare case of bone dystrophy. Br J Surg 37:52–63, 1949
Gorlin RJ, Sedano H: Craniometaphyseal dysostosis. Mod Med 36:154–155, 1968
Macpherson RI: Craniodiaphyseal dysplasia, a disease or group of diseases? J Can Assoc Radiol 25:22–23, 1974

CRANIOMETAPHYSEAL DYSPLASIA

Synonym. See Craniodiaphyseal dysostosis and Pyle's.

Symptoms and Signs. Both sexes affected; onset from infancy. Deafness; blindness; facial paralysis; multiple involvement of cranial nerves. Normal intelligence. Leonine facies; complete nasal obstruction (in recessive form).

Etiology. Both autosomal recessive and dominant inheritance.

Pathology. Hyperostosis of cranial and facial bones with compression of cranial nerves at foramina. Metaphyseal changes of long bones (clublike rather than like Erlenmeyer's flask, flask shape is more typical of Pyle's, see).

Diagnostic Procedures. *X-rays.* See Pathology.

Therapy. Surgical decompression of nerves.

Prognosis. Recessive form more severe. Without treatment, extremely severe incapacitation.

BIBLIOGRAPHY. Spranger JW, Paulsen K, Lehmann W: Die kraniometaphysare Dysplasia. Z Kinderheilk 93:64–79, 1965
Penchaszadeh VB, Gutierriz ER, Gigueroa EP: Autosomal recessive craniometaphyseal dysplasia. Am J Med Genet 5:45–55, 1980
Carnevale A, Grether P, Castillo V et al: Autosomal dominant craniometaphyseal dysplasia: Clinical variability. Clin Genet 23:17–22, 1983

CRETINISM, SPORADIC

Synonyms. Congenital hypothyroidism. Includes endemic cretinism. See Kocher-Debre-Semelaigne.

Symptoms and Signs. Both sexes affected at birth; overweight; lethargy; facies with heavy expression; eyes piglike; nystagmus; large tongue; mouth open; latter, drooling and delayed dentition; yellow tint on cheek; hypothermia; altered tone of voice; persistent neonatal jaundice; protuberant belly; umbilical hernia; skin dry, flabby, and cold; hair coarse. Failure to thrive; poor appetite; constipation. Cardiomegaly (occasionally); slow pulse. In endemic cretinism, frequently deafness. In 50% of cases; ataxia, muscular hypotonia, diplegia. Clumsy gait. Delayed sexual development. Mental development retarded. Final result dwarfism and imbecility. Occasionally goiter.

Etiology. Variable. Usually autosomal recessive in all types of syndromes described. Can be due to complete lack (athyreosis), to reduced thyroid function because of enzyme defects; impaired thyroid response to thyrotropin, thyroid stimulating hormone (TSH) defective production, failure of iodide transport, failure to form organic iodine, defect of peroxidase, failure of coupling of iodotyrosines. Endemic in particular areas (Creta, Beotia, Alpine Valleys). Failure of iodotyrosine deiodinase activity, altered thyroglobulin synthesis, deficiency of TBG.

Pathology. Many features of delayed development (cerebral, skeletal). Generally, marked hypertrophy of pituitary.

Diagnostic Procedures. *Blood.* Free thyroxine (FT_4), total thyroxine (TT_4) decreased; TSH increased. *X-ray of knee.* Absent calcification of epipheses. Numerous other signs of delayed skeletal growth.

The different forms described require for the diagnosis complex thyroid stimulating and inhibiting tests that distinguish the various enzymatic defects.

Therapy. Thyroid hormone started as soon as possible and maintained at adequate levels.

Prognosis. Strictly correlated with time of onset and adequacy and maintenance of therapy. Normal physical and mental development possible with correct treatment.

BIBLIOGRAPHY. Stanbury JB, Dumont JE: Familial goiter and related disorders. In Stanbury JB, Wyngaarden JB, Fredrickson DS, et al: The Metabolic Basis of Inherited Disease, 5th ed, p 231. New York, McGraw-Hill, 1983

CREUTZFELDT-JAKOB

Synonyms. Corticostriatal spinal degeneration; Jakob-Creutzfeldt; spastic pseudosclerosis.

Symptoms. Both sexes affected; onset between the fifth and sixth decades of life. Some affected patients in their 20s have been reported. Prodromic symptoms: vague psychic disturbances that progress within a few months to dementia. Neurasthenia followed by confusion; disorientation; weakness; stiffness of limbs; choreoathetoid movements; dysarthria; cortical blindness.

Signs. Spastic weakness of extremities; unsteady ataxic gait; nystagmus; rigidity; tremor; athetosis; localized amyotrophies; decreased abdominal and increased tendon reflexes; occasionally, positive Babinski.

Etiology. The syndrome is transmitted by a virus that withstands usual methods of sterilization. (Equipment that has come in contact with tissue or blood from these patients should be autoclaved for 1 hr.) The natural route of transmission of this disease is unknown. Because it occurs both in a sporadic and familial form, in some families there is a genetic susceptibility to the infection.

Pathology. Diffuse neuronal degeneration of cerebral cortex (deeper layers), basal ganglia, descending corticospinal tracts; status spongiosus, neuroglial reaction.

Therapy. None.

Prognosis. Rapid course; death in 12 to 16 months.

BIBLIOGRAPHY. Creutzfeldt HG: Uber eine eigenartige herdformige Erkrankung des Zentralnervensystems. In Nissl F, Alzheimer A: Histologie und Histopathologie. Jena, Fischer, Arbeit Erganzungband, 1921
Jacob A: Ueber eigenartige Erktrankungen des Zentralnerven-systems mit bemerken wertem anatomischen Befunde (Spatische Pseudoslerose-Encephalomuelopathic mit disseminierten Degenerationherden) Zschr Ges Neurol Psychiat 64:147–228, 1921
Brown P, Coker-Vann M, Pomeroy K, Franko M, Asher DM, Gibbs CJ, Gajdusek DC: Diagnosis of Creutzfeldt-Jakob disease by Western-blot: identification of marker protein in human brain tissue. N Engl J Med 314:547–551, 1986

CREYX-LEVY

Synonyms. Ophthalmorhinostomato hygrosi; Sjögren's reverse (see).

Symptoms and Signs. Generalized hypersecretions (lacrimal; nasal; oral; gastric). Cervical arthritis.

Etiology. Unknown.

Diagnostic Procedures. *Blood.* In some cases, leukopenia, eosinophilia and thrombocytopenia; increase of erythrocyte sedimentation rate; hypochloremia. *Gastric juice.* Hyperchlorhydria. *X-ray of skeleton.* Calcification of cervical vertebrae, ligaments and cervical lymph nodes. *Sialography.* Schitzmer's test.

Therapy. Hypersecretion is not affected by atropine and derivates. Trials with corticosteroids.

Prognosis. Chronic condition responding poorly to treatment.

BIBLIOGRAPHY. Creyx M, Lévy J: Syndrome d'opthalmo-rhino-stomatoxérose, dit des "Gougerot-Sjoegren", sindrome d'opththalmo-rhino-stomato-hygrose. Bull Soc Med Hop 64:1123–1128, 1948

CRIGLER-NAJJAR TYPE I

Synonyms. Congenital hyperbilirubinemia; congenital familial nonhemolytic jaundice.

Symptoms and Signs. Both sexes affected. Jaundice appears in first few days after birth. Majority of cases develop central nervous system symptomatology resembling kernicterus (see). Recurrent fever; no hepatomegaly or splenomegaly.

Etiology. Congenital absence (or marked reduction?) of glucoronyl transferase activity resulting in the lack of conjugation of bilirubin with gluconuride and high level of indirect bilirubin in blood and brain damage (kernicterus). Autosomal recessive inheritance.

Pathology. *Liver.* Normal parenchymal cells; bilirubin in hepatic canaliculi. *Brain.* Basal nuclei stained with bile.

Diagnostic Procedures. *Blood.* High level of indirect bilirubin with considerable fluctuation; absence of incompatibility of blood group. Failure to respond to phenobarbital treatment. *Liver function test.* Normal. *Urine.* Absence of bilirubin; urobilinogenuria. *Stool.* Reduced fecal urobilinogen. *Cholangiography.* Patency of extrahepatic bile duct. *Biopsy of liver.*

Therapy. Continuous extracorporeal perfusion; plasmapheresis; peritoneal dialysis with albumin; cholestyramine orally; phototherapy.

Prognosis. Fatal in early infancy, amount of brain damage determining prognosis. Patients without brain involvement survive. Patients without early brain involvement survive but may have kernicterus at later age.

BIBLIOGRAPHY. Crigler JF, Najjar V: A congenital familial non-hemolytic jaundice with kernicterus. Pediatrics 10:169–179, 1952

Wolkoff AW, Chowdhury JR, Arias IH: Hereditary jaundice and disorders of bilirubin metabolism. In Stanbury JB, Wyngaarden JB, Fredrickson DS et al: The Metabolic Basis of Inherited Disease, 5th ed, p 1385. New York, McGraw-Hill, 1983

CRISSCROSS HEART

Synonyms. Upstairs-downstairs heart, superoinferior heart.

Symptoms and Signs. Rare. Cyanosis or heart failure or both.

Etiology. Unknown. Congenital condition.

Pathology. Atrioventricular spatial relation that places each ventricle in a contralateral position to its associated atrium.

Diagnostic Procedures. *Cardiac catherization. Angiography.*

Therapy. Palliative surgery in infancy.

Prognosis. Poor.

BIBLIOGRAPHY. Vaan Praagh S, La Corte M, Falows KE, et al: Superoinferior ventricles: Anatomic and angiographic findings in ten post-mortem cases. In Van Praagh R, Takao A (eds): Etiology and Morphogenesis of Congenital Heart Disease. Mount Kisco, NY, Futura Publishing, 1980

Attie F, Munoz-Castellanos L, Ovseyevitz J, et al: Crossed atrioventricular connections. Am Heart J 99:163–172, 1980

Hurst JW: The Heart, 6th ed, p 706. New York, McGraw-Hill, 1986

CROHN'S

Synonyms. Crohn-Lesniowsky; regional enteritis.

Symptoms. Slight prevalence in males; Jewish people most frequently affected; onset at any age; average 25 years. Symptoms variable according to anatomic location and amount of involvement. Onset usually mild, insidious symptoms: borborygmus; bloating; flatulence; mild abdominal cramps and mild diarrhea; occasional temperature elevation. Slow progression to more severe symptoms: (1) Pain (85% of patients), peristaltic type with or without diarrhea; cramps usually do not subside following defecation; with more advanced disease pain becomes constant. Initially pain localized in periumbilical region; may mimic "acute appendicitis"; later corresponds to site of the lesion. (2) Diarrhea (90%), soft or semiliquid, seldom liquid; tenesmus rare, except if perineal lesions have developed. (3) Fever (33%), not accompanied by chills. (4) Perianal-perirectal fistulas (20%). (5) Symptoms of bowel obstruction or perforation in stomach or duodenal localization; nausea, vomiting, ulcerlike pain dominant symptoms. (6) Melena (4%). Systemic manifestation: fever; weight loss; polyarthritis (5%); rarely, erythema nodosum; pyoderma gangrenosum; nervousness; tension; depression. When condition begins in childhood, growth retardation and delayed maturation are observed.

Signs. Abdominal distention; tenderness on palpation of abdomen in region corresponding to areas of involvement. Mass in right lower quadrant frequently may be palpated.

Etiology. Unknown; possibly included in the autoimmune group of diseases. Familial cases reported (10% of cases).

Pathology. Lesion may occur in any part of intestine, from stomach to rectum. Terminal ileum involved in 75% of cases. Areas of lesions alternated with normal areas. Affected tract appears rigid, thickened. Serosa covered by mesenteric fat and fibrostenotic exudate; chronic subserous inflammation. Mesentery edematous, rubbery, with several enlarged lymph nodes. (When fistulas have developed, matting of intestinal loops.) Marked narrowing of intestinal lumen; mucosal ulcerations and nodularity; frequently, lesions stop abruptly at ileocecal junction; however, in some cases may continue into proximal colon. *Histology.* Mucosa inflamed, ulcerated, or atrophic. Submucosa thickened, with granulomatous formations, with or without giant cells. Granulomas are also found in subserosa and lymph nodes. Muscular coat normal. Marked fibrotic changes in submucosa and subserosa.

Diagnostic Procedures. *Blood.* Moderate anemia; leukocytosis; hypoproteinemia; hypoprothrombinemia (frequent); electrolyte alterations; hypocalcemia. *X-ray.* Early, blunting, flattening, thickening of plical circulares; lumen and contour irregularities. Later, longitudinal ulcerations; finally; uniform, rigid tube with disappearance of mucosal pattern and various degree of narrowing of the lumen (initially spastic; later stenotic, Kantors sign), alternated with skipped areas of normal intestine are characteristic features.

Therapy. *Medical.* Diet; correction of anemia; rest; psychotherapy; anticholinergic drugs; sedatives; salicylazosulfapyridine (most effective antibacterial); adrenal steroids, nitrogen mustard, Azathioprine (Imuran®). *Surgical.* Resection of affected tracts.

Prognosis. More severe in young people; milder in old-age onset. Frequent remission and relapses. Relapses after surgical procedures frequent. With treatment, patients may have relatively good health most of the time.

BIBLIOGRAPHY. Leśniowski A: Przyczynek Do Chirurgii Kiszek. Medycyna 31:460–464, 483–489, 514–518, 1903
Crohn BB, Ginzburg L, Oppenheimer GD: Regional ileitis. JAMA 99:1323–1329, 1932
Gronhagen-Riska C, Fyhrquist F, Hortling L et al: Familial occurrence of sarcoidosis and Crohn's disease. Lancet I:1287–1288, 1983
Harper PH, Fazio VW, Lavery IC, et al: The long-term outcome in Crohn's disease. Dis Colon Rectum 30:174–179, 1987

CRONKHITE-CANADA

Synonyms. Alopecia–polyposis–skin pigmentation–onychotrophia.

Symptoms and Signs. Prevalent in females. Diffuse brownish pigmentation of skin (more intense at body folds); alopecia, onychotrophia. These changes may precede or follow gastrointestinal complaints: nausea; vomiting; diarrhea.

Etiology. Unknown; nonfamilial form of generalized gastrointestinal polyposis.

Pathology. Benign adenomatous polyps affecting practically the entire gastrointestinal mucosa.

Diagnostic Procedures. *X-rays of gastrointestinal tract. Biopsy.*

Therapy. In some patients, malabsorption is partly corrected by removal of polyps. Endoscopic resection. Gastrectomy, hemicolectomy according to prevalence of polyps in different regions.

Prognosis. Usually fatal within 18 months from onset of diarrhea. Some patients may have a long survival time.

BIBLIOGRAPHY. Cronkhite LW, Canada WJ: Generalized gastrointestinal polyposis. New Engl J Med 252:1011–1015, 1955
Cunliffe WJ, Anderson J: Case of Cronkhite-Canada syndrome with associated jejunal diverticulosis. Br Med J 4:601–602, 1967
Gardner AJ et al: Gastrointestinal polyposis syndromes and genetic mechanisms. West J Med 132:488–499, 1980

CROSS'

Synonyms. Gingival fibromatosis–hypopigmentation–microphthalmia–oligophrenia–athetosis. Hypopigmentation-oculocerebral.

Symptoms and Signs. Rare. Four cases described; present from birth. Skin pink with presence of pigmented nevi and freckles; hair white to light blond. Eye color gray blue; microphthalmia, cataracts. Nystagmus very marked; blindness; oligophrenia; athetosis; gingival fibromatosis.

Etiology. Autosomal recessive inheritance.

Pathology. Melanosomes in hair bulb scanty, from stage III to IV.

Diagnostic Procedures. *Blood.* Serum tyrosine levels normal; beta melanocyte-stimulating hormone level unknown. *Incubation of hair with tyrosine.* Pigmentation.

Therapy. Symptomatic.

Prognosis. Poor.

BIBLIOGRAPHY. Cross HE, McKusick VA, Breen W: A new oculocerebral syndrome with hypopigmentation. J Pediatr 70:398–406, 1967

Witkop CJ, Queredo WC, Fitzpatrick TB: Albinism and other disorders of pigment metabolism. In Stanbury JB, Wyngaarden JB, Fredrickson DS, et al: The Metabolic Basis of Inherited Disease, 5th ed, p 301. New York, McGraw-Hill, 1983

CROSTI'S

Synonym. Reticulohistiocytoma.

Symptoms and Signs. Tumorous infiltrations of the back.

Etiology. Unknown; to be differentiated clinically from multiple reticulohistiocytoma syndrome (see). To be included in the spectrum of T cell lympho-proliferative syndromes.

Pathology. Tumors containing hystiocytes and large xanthomatous cells.

Diagnostic Procedures. *Biopsy.*

Therapy. Radiotherapy; cortisone.

Prognosis. Good.

BIBLIOGRAPHY. Crosti A: Mycosis fongoide et rèticulo-histiocytome cutanè malin. Minerva Dermatol 26:3–11, 1951

Toonstra J, Van Der Putte SC, Kalsbeek GL: Multilo-bated cutaneous T cell lymphoma. Report of two cases resembling Crosti's reticulosis. Dermatologica 166(3):128–135, 1983

CROUZON'S

Synonyms. Apert-Crouzon; craniofacial dysostosis; oxycephaly-acrocephaly; Virchow's oxycephaly; Vogt's cephalosyndactyly; pseudo-Crouzon (Franceschetti's).

Symptoms. More frequent in males; present at birth. Headache, subnormal mental development; moderate hearing loss; progressive visual loss. In mild cases, vision may not be severely affected.

Signs. Exophthalmos (possible luxation of globe); bluish sclerae; widely separated eyes (hypertelorism); obliquity of palpebral fissure; outer canthus slanting downwards; nystagmus; divergent strabismus; papilledema. Beak-shaped nose; hypoplastic maxilla; short upper lip, and protruding lower lip; head pointed in region of anterior fontanelle.

Etiology. Premature closure of cranial bones; transmitted as dominant trait.

Pathology. Premature closure of cranial bones with secondary brain damage due to intracranial hypertension.

Diagnostic Procedures. *Spinal fluid.* Increased pressure. *X-ray.* Facial-cranial abnormalities.

Therapy. Open affected sutures widely and prevent closure by interposition of polyethylene; if marked exophthalmos, orbital decompression.

Prognosis. Good with surgery.

BIBLIOGRAPHY. Crouzon MO: Dysostose craniofaciale héréditaire. Presse Med 20:737–739, 1912

Vogt A: Dyskephalie (Dysostosis Craniofacialis, Maladie de Crouzon 1921) und neuartige Kombination dieser Kraukheit mit Sybdaktylie der 4 Extremitaeten (Dyskephalodakttylie). Klin Monatsbl Augenheilkd 90:441–454, 1933

Kreilborg S, Jensen BL: Variable expressivity of Crouzon's syndrome within a family. Scand J Dent Res 85:175–184, 1977

CROW-FUKASE

Synonyms. PEP, POEMS, Takatsuki's, Shimpo's.

Symptoms and Signs. Chronic progressive peripheral sensorimotor polyneuropathy; skin changes: diffuse hyperpigmentation, hypertrichosis, and hair thickening; anasarca-pitting edema on the lower extremities, ascites and pleural effusion; gynecomastia and impotence in men and amenorrhea in women; hepatosplenomegaly and generalized lymphadenopathy; papilledema; fever; hyperhidrosis and finger clubbing.

Etiology. Abnormal proliferation of plasma cells that presumably secrete a substance that is toxic for many organs.

Pathology. Nerve biopsy: axonal degeneration and segmental demyelination. Lymph node biopsy: capillary proliferation and sheets of mature plasma cells in the interfollicular tissue.

Diagnostic Procedures. *Nerve conduction velocities* (motor and sensory). Slow. *Cerebrospinal fluid.* Elevated protein level. *X-rays.* Skeletal sclerotic and lytic lesions.

Therapy. Prednisone; cyclophosphamide; radiation therapy.

Prognosis. Transient improvement with therapy. Death in a few years.

BIBLIOGRAPHY. Saikawa S: On the etiology of "PEP syndrome" (a peculiar progressive polyneuritis associated with pigmentation, edema, plasma cell dyscrasia). Med J Kagoshima Univ 32:219–243, 1980

Bardwick PA, Zvaifler NJ, Gill GN et al: Plasma cell neoplasia with polyneuropathy, organomegaly, endocrinopathy, M protein and skin changes: The POEMS syndrome. Report on two cases and a review of the literature. Medicine (Baltimore) 59:311–322, 1980

Takanishi T, Sobue I, Toyokura Y: The Crow-Fukase syndrome: A study of 102 cases in Japan. Neurology (Cleveland) 34:712–720, 1984

CRST SYNDROME

Synonyms. Calcinosis–Raynaud's phenomenon–sclerodactyly–telangiectasis; Thibierge-Weissenbach. See Calcinosis universalis; Profichet's, including CREST (E for esophageal involvement).

Symptoms. Prevalent in females; condition at an average age of 45 years. Reported only in whites. No family history of telangiectasia. First symptoms referable to hands. Bleeding manifestations rare (epistaxis; melena; or from cutaneous telangiectasis). Raynaud's phenomenon; dysphagia.

Signs. Placques of calcinosis on different subcutaneous locations; hands usually involved. Sclerodactyly, telangiectasia on different cutaneous locations (face and hands involved). Mucosae occasionally involved.

Etiology. Unknown; belongs in the group of collagen disorders. Relation with scleroderma not clearly defined (different prognosis). Possible relation with Rendu-Osler-Weber syndrome; several criteria for differential diagnosis: lack of familial occurrence; prevalence in female.

Pathology. Dilated capillaries and venules; absence of muscular and elastic tissue, covered by thinned epithelium. Skin in sclerodermatoid lesion compatible with but not typical of scleroderma.

Diagnostic Procedures. *X-ray.* Subcutaneous calcinosis. *Esophageal studies.* Abnormal pattern compatible with scleroderma. *Blood.* Normal calcium, phosphorus and alkaline phosphatases; total protein and electrophoresis. L.E. test negative. No anemia or white blood cell abnormalities. *Renal and liver tests.* Usually normal. *Urine.* Normal.

Therapy. Sympathectomy for Raynaud's phenomenon. Corticosteroids, prostacyclin, dextran dipenicillamine, plasmapheresis, azathioprine.

Prognosis. Slow progressive evolution even in presence of systemic manifestations. Average follow-up of 15 years. (In scleroderma, 5 yr survival about 50%).

BIBLIOGRAPHY. Thibierge G, Weissenbach RJ: Concrétions calcaires sous-cutanées at sclérodermie. Ann Dermatol Syph 2:129–155, 1911

Dellipiani AW, George M: Syndrome of sclerodactyly, calcinosis, Raynaud's phenomenon, and telangiectasia. Br Med J 4:334–335, 1967

Shuck JW, Oetgen WJ, Tesaz JT: Pulmonary vascular response during Raynaud phenomenon in progressive systemic sclerosis. Am J Med 78:221–227, 1985

CRUVEILHIER-BAUMGARTEN

Synonym. Baumgarten's portal hypertension variant.

Symptoms. Digestive troubles; hematemesis.

Signs. Abdominal distention; prominent periumbilical and thoracoabdominal veins; continuous venus hum and thrill on the periumbilical region; small liver; splenomegaly.

Etiology. Failure of obliteration of umbilical vein; cirrhosis without ascites.

Pathology. Liver cirrhosis; congestive splenomegaly; development of collateral circulation including esophageal varices.

Diagnostic Procedures. *Liver function test.* Altered. *Blood.* Anemia; leukopenia; thrombocytopenia (in hypersplenism). *Abdominal phlebography.* Determination of portal hypertension.

Therapy. Portacaval shunt or splenectomy and splenorenal anastomosis.

BIBLIOGRAPHY. Cruveilhier J: Maladies des veines. In Anatomie Pathologique du Corps Humain, Vol 1 p 16. Paris, Baillière, 1829–1835

Von Baumgarten P: Ueber vollstandiges Offenbleiben der Vena umbilicalis; zugleich ein Beitrag zur Frage des Morbus Banti, p 6; Baumgartens, Arbeiten, 1908, Arb Geb Path Anat Inst Tubing 6:93, 1907

Abraham AS, Atkinson M: The disappearance of ascites in alcoholic cirrhosis with the development of the Cruveilheir-Baumgarten syndrome. Ann Intern Med 62:1045–1049, 1965

Way LW: Liver. In Way LW (ed): Current Surgical Diagnosis and Treatment, 7th ed, p 471. Los Altos, California, Lange Med Pub 1983

CRYPTORCHIDISM

Synonym. Testicular ectopia.

Symptoms and Signs. Disturbed testicular descent, so that testis remains in the inguinal canal or migrates in suprapubic, femoral, or perineal area. At birth, incidence of this abnormality is 10%. Associated renal anomalies possible (in inherited cases).

Etiology. Unclear; anatomic factors (preventing migration) seem predominant, but concurrence of genetic factors seems possible. Autosomal recessive inheritance. Pituitary hypogonadism in mother seems a predisposing factor.

Pathology. Dislocation of testis (see Symptoms). Possible abnormality of germinal epithelium.

Diagnostic Procedures. *Endocrine and cytogenetic studies, testicular biopsy* (at time or during surgery). To rule out possibility of genetic disorders. *Blood.* Testosterone level increase follows administration of human chorionic gonadotropins (hCG).

Therapy. *Medical.* Human chorionic gonadotropin 2000 IU three times a week for 6 weeks; if needed the cycle may be repeated once. *Surgical.* Positioning of testis into scrotum.

Prognosis. In 96%, spontaneous descent of testis in correct position. In cryptic testes increased incidence of neoplasia (40%).

BIBLIOGRAPHY. Corbus BC, O'Connor VJ: The familial occurrence of undescended testis. Report in six brothers with testicular anomalies. Surg Gynecol Obstet 34:237–240, 1922
Steinberg E: Disorders of testicular function (male hypogonadism). In De Groot LJ, Cahill GF Jr, Odell WD (eds): Endocrinology, p 1554. New York, Grune & Stratton, 1979
Czeiler A, Erodi A, Toth J: Genetics of undescended testis. J Urol 126:528–529, 1981

CRYPTOTHYROIDISM

Indicates the presence of an arrested development and descent of the thyroid primordiun, which does not hypertrophy to meet increased demands in juvenile period of development and results clinically in the juvenile myxedema syndrome (see).

BIBLIOGRAPHY. McGirr EM, Hutchinson JH: Dysgenesis of the thyroid gland as a cause of cretinism and juvenile myxedema. J Clin Endocrinol Metab 15:668–679, 1955
Fisher BA, Klein AH: Thyroid development and disorders of thyroid function in the newborn. New Engl J Med 304:702–712, 1981

CURLING'S ULCER

Synonym. Gastrointestinal postburn ulcer. See von-Rokitanski-Cushing.

Symptoms and Signs. Clinical onset at various times after burns; serious bleeding begins usually between 4th and 10th day. Repeated, severe rectal bleeding, occurring after severe burning. Gastrointestinal perforation with peritonitis may occur. The full-blown episode of severe gastrointestinal bleeding after burning is relatively rare (2–4%). Moderate gastrointestinal bleeding, however, seems to be much more frequent (58%). Hematemesis and melena occur with equal frequency.

Etiology. Unknown. Curling's ulcer (active gastrointestinal hemorrhage) represents the end point of common, usually concealed, gastrointestinal ulceration with microscopic hemorrhages.

Pathology. Ulceration may be found in any part of the gastrointestinal tract from esophagus to terminal ileum (posterior duodenum more frequent location).

Diagnostic Procedures. *Stool.* Blood determination.

Therapy. Intense antacid program as soon as burned patient able to take fluid. Cimetidine (800 mg to 2g/day intravenously or orally) and pirenzepine bichloridrate (75–125 mg/day) have been suggested as prophylactic measures. Initial treatment: gastric lavage with chilled solutions and systemic antibiotics (if sepsis). Infusion of vasopressin into left gastric artery through a placed catheter. Blood replacement. Surgery with same principles of therapy for treatment of gastrointestinal hemorrhages.

Prognosis. Very severe if massive bleeding unless rapid treatment is instituted.

BIBLIOGRAPHY. Curling TB: On acute ulceration of the duodenum in cases of burn. Medico-Chir Trans (London) 25:260–281, 1942
Ousterhout DK, Feller I: Occult gastrointestinal hemorrhages in burned patients. Arch Surg 96:420–422, 1968
Croker JR: Acute gastro-intestinal bleeding in the critically ill patients. Int Care Med 5:1–4, 1979
Ivarsson L, Sjodahl R, Haglund U (eds): Proceeding from a symposium: Acute mucosal damage to the stomach. Scand J Gastroenterol (suppl 105):5 (all issue) 1984

CURRACINO-SILVERMAN

Synonyms. Pigeon breast; pectus carinatum; Silverman's II.

Symptoms. Both sexes affected; onset from infancy. Asymptomatic; occasionally, dyspnea.

Signs. Projection of sternum outward. Thoracic antero-posterior diameter increased and lateral decreased.

Etiology. Variable. (1) Hereditary form; autosomal dominant; (2) rickets; (3) secondary; other conditions (see Marfan's).

Pathology. Accelerated obliteration of sutures, which causes the pectus carinatum; secondary excessive growth of ribs. Hypertrophy of posterolateral section of diaphragm; hypotrophy of ventral part.

Therapy. Surgery.

Prognosis. Stable condition. Good esthetic and functional results with surgical correction.

BIBLIOGRAPHY. Curracino F, Silverman FN: Premature obliteration of the sternal sutures and pigeon breast deformity. Radiology 70:532–540, 1958
Pickard LR, Tepas JJ, Shermeta DW, et al: Pectus carinatum. Results of surgical therapy. J Pediatr Surg 14:228–230, 1979

CURTIUS' I

Synonyms. Ectodermal dysplasia–ocular malformation; Friedreich's; Steiner's. Hemifacial microsomic–radial defects. See also Hemihypertrophy, First arch and Goldenhar's.

Symptoms. Males more frequently affected; onset from birth, but may become accentuated at puberty. Asymptomatic or variable according to signs. Frequently, ambliopia, reduced capacity to thermal regulation, mental retardation (15–20%).

Signs. Abnormalities may be segmented, unilateral, or crossed. Frequently, ichthyosis vulgaris (see). Hypertelorism; telangiectasia; absent or sparse eyebrows and eyelashes; decreased tear secretion; congenital cataract; coloboma, hypodontia and unilateral tooth enlargment; occasionally: dyscephaly; tongue enlarged and thicker on involved side. Associated defects of limbs (unilateral macrodactyly; polydactyly; syndactlyly; clubfoot; and long bone enlargement) may be present.

Etiology. Unknown; occasionally, familial occurrence. Uncertain classification. Eponym obsolete. Autosomal dominant inheritance. Suggested to be form of Goldenhar's.

Pathology. Only a limited number of autopsies. Nonspecific pathologic changes. Frequent enlargement of kidney and adrenal gland.

Diagnostic Procedures. *Dental X-ray.* Abnormalities; greater diameter of canine early diagnostic sign.

Therapy. Symptomatic; plastic reconstruction of structures involved after completion of maturation.

Prognosis. Variable according to degree of involvement of neurologic structures.

BIBLIOGRAPHY. Barwell R: Case of unilateral hypertrophy of the head and face involving bones and soft parts. Trans Pathol Soc Lond 32:282–284, 1881
Meckel JF: Ueber die seitliche Asymmetrie im teirischen Korper, anatomische physiologisches Beobachtungen und Untersuchungen, p 147. Halle, Renger, 1822
Curtius F: Kongenitaler partieller Piesenwuchs mit endocrien Stoerungen. Dtsch Arch Klin Med 147:310–319, 1925
Hanley FJ, Floyd E, Parker D: Congenital partial hemihypertrophy of the face. J Oral Surg 26:136–141, 1968
Berch V: Genetic aspects of hemifacial microsomic. Hum Genet 64:291–296, 1983

CUSHING'S I

Synonyms. Acoustic neuroma; angle tumor; cerebellopontine angle; pontocerebellar angle tumor.

Symptoms and Signs. Prevalent in females (3 : 1); onset of acoustic neuroma in majority of cases between third and sixth decades; onset of glioma before age 20. Chronology of onset of symptoms is of utmost importance for differential diagnosis. Headache; vomiting; vertigo; tinnitus; dimness of vision. Cranial nerve involvement, particularly trigeminal (V), abducens (VI), facial (VII), and acoustic (VIII) (more frequent in extracerebral lesions), with relative symptomatology. Cerebellar symptoms include ataxia of extremities; lower extremities more affected than upper ones; adiadochokinesia; spontaneous nystagmus; pyramidal tract signs may be present. Later, with increasing intracranial pressure, other symptoms, such as olfactory loss, may also occur. Bilateral forms also described.

Etiology. Neoplastic or vascular (less frequently) pontine angle lesion. Brain stem may be primary or secondary site of involvement. Extracerebral lesions may also induce the syndrome. Bilateral forms are hereditary with autosomal dominant transmission.

Pathology. Acoustic neuroma originates in peripheral part of vestibular division of acoustic (VIII) nerve. Oval and well circumscribed; adapt to the wall of posterior fossa and stretches and compresses adjacent nerves and brain stem.

Diagnostic Procedures. *Pneumoencephalography. Arteriography. CT brain scan. Spinal tap.*

Therapy. Surgery if feasible.

Prognosis. Poor; average life expectancy of untreated patients is 3.5 to 5 years after diagnosis. Good results with surgery.

BIBLIOGRAPHY. Wishart JH: Case of tumours in skull dura mater and brain. Edinburgh Med Surg J 18:393, 1822

Cushing HW: Tumors of the nervus acusticus and the Syndrome of the Cerebello Pontine Angle. Philadelphia, WB Saunders, 1917

Keschner M, Grossman M: Cerebellar symptomatology evaluation on the basis of intracerebellar and extracerebellar lesions. Arch Neurol Psychiatr 19:78–94, 1928

Eldridge R: Central neurofibromatosis with bilateral acoustic neuroma. Adv Neurol 29:57–65, 1981

CUSHING'S II

Synonyms. Chiasmal; suprasellar meningioma. Optic tract; upper omonymous quadrantanopia.

Symptoms. Usually occur in adults. Characterized by three elements. Initial decrease of lateral or central vision: (1) bitemporal field defects, usually progressive; (2) primary optic atrophy, total blindness may result; (3) essentially normal sella turcica (see Diagnostic Procedures).

Etiology. Usually a suprasellar meningioma (Cushing's original description), other space-occupying lesions in the region of optic chiasm, such as craniopharyngiomas, pituitary adenoma, giant aneurysm, chiasmal glioma, nasopharyngeal carcinoma, colloid cyst of third ventricle, or remote lesions that produce dilatation of third ventricle and secondary chiasm compression.

Diagnostic Procedures. *X-ray of skull.* Essentially normal sella turcica. With modern technique it is possible, however, to detect bone reaction in the area of tuberculum sellae. Occasionally, calcification may be present in suprasellar meningioma. *Pneumoencephalography. CT brain scan. Angiography.*

Therapy. Surgery.

Prognosis. Depends on etiology and extent of lesions.

BIBLIOGRAPHY. Cushing H: Chiasmal syndrome of primary optic atrophy and bitemporal field defects in adults with normal sella turcica. Arch Ophthalmol 3:505–551, 1930

Bebin J, Knighton RS: Chiasmatic syndrome. Henry Ford Hosp Med J 16:223–233, 1968

Waller RR, Riley FC, Sundt TM: A rare cause of the chiasmal syndrome. Arch Ophthalmol 88:269–272, 1972

Adams RD, Victor M: Principles of Neurology, 3rd ed, p 192. New York, McGraw-Hill, 1985

CUSHING'S III

Synonyms. Adrenal cortex adenoma; adrenal cortex carcinoma; pituitary basophilism. Three clinical forms may be recognized: (1) adrenal neoplasm; (2) Cushing's disease; (3) ectopic ACTH syndrome (see).

CUSHING'S SYNDROME DUE TO BENIGN OR MALIGNANT NEOPLASM OF THE ADRENALS

Symptoms. Weakness; fatigability; oligomenorrhea; backache; loss of libido; loss of potency in man; mental aberrations from simple irritability to schizophrenia.

Signs. Obesity of face, neck, trunk, or generalized plethoric face; purple striae of abdomen and legs; ecchymosis; peripheral edema; hirsutism; hypertension; enlarged heart.

Etiology. Neoplasm of adrenal that secretes cortisol autonomously, not dependent on adrenocorticotropic hormone (ACTH) stimulation, with suppression of ACTH production and atrophy of normal adrenal tissue.

Pathology. Carcinoma or benign adenoma of adrenals; atrophy of normal adrenal tissue. Heart enlarged; obesity generalized or with typical distribution; osteoporosis; atrophy of muscles; nephrosclerosis and nephrocalcinosis; hyperplasia of islet of pancreas; atrophy of pituitary.

Diagnostic Procedures. *Urine.* Increased urinary 17-ketosteroids; 17-hydroxy-corticoids; glycosuria. *Blood.* Decreased plasma ACTH level; increased plasma 17-hydroxycorticoid; decreased lymphocytes and eosinophils; increased neutrophils and red cells; increased sugar and cholesterol. *ACTH stimulation.* Lack of response with malignant tumor; normal response in benign adenoma. *Metyrapone responsiveness.* Failure to respond; response in benign adenoma. *Dexamethasone suppression.* Lack of response; response in benign adenoma. *X-ray.* Osteoporosis; pyelogram possibly showing adrenal tumor; nephrocalcinosis.

Therapy. Surgical removal of tumor; adequate coverage with cortisol for acute adrenal insufficiency. After surgery, administration of cortisol for 1 year or longer, plus ACTH to stimulate atrophic tissue. If tumor can not be removed, admission of 2, 2'-bis-(2-chlorophenyl, 4-chlorophenyl)-1, 1-dichloroethane (o, p' DDD) or Metyrapone.

Prognosis. Good in benign adenoma, good if malignant tumor removed in time and no metastasis has occurred.

CUSHING'S DISEASE

Symptoms and Signs. See Cushing's syndrome due to benign or malignant neoplasm of the adrenal.

Etiology. Inappropriate levels of ACTH produced by pituitary, resulting in adrenal hyperplasia.

Pathology. Pituitary adenoma or hyperfunction; bilateral adrenal hyperplasia; other organs and tissue involved (see Pathology of Cushing's syndrome).

Diagnostic Procedures. *Blood.* Increase of plasma ACTH or prolonged secretion during the day. Increased 17-hydroxycorticoids. Hematologic and biochemical changes (see Diagnostic Procedures of Cushing's syndrome). *Urine.* Some changes as in Cushing's syndrome. *ACTH stimulation.* Threefold to 5-fold increase of urinary 17-hydroxycorticoids. *Metyrapone responsiveness.* Qualitatively normal. *Dexamethasone suppression.* Response only to high doses.

Therapy. If pituitary tumor with sellar enlargement, ablation of pituitary; if no enlargement, choice of adrenal ablation or pituitary ablation. Radiation of pituitary gland when partially removed or not neurologically aggressive. Implantation of ^{90}yttrium rods in the pituitary gland. If adrenal ablation (fastest method to control severe hypercortisonism), substitutive therapy has to be instituted and followed for life. Good results also with pharmacologic treatment: cyproheptadine; bromocriptine; aminoglutethimide or o,p'DDD.

Prognosis. Good result with adequate treatment. If patient is not treated, death in 5 years.

ECTOPIC ACTH SYNDROME

Listed separately under Ectopic ACTH.

BIBLIOGRAPHY. Cushing H: The basophil adenomas of the pituitary body and their clinical manifestations (pituitary basophilism). Bull Johns Hopkins Hosp 50:137–195, 1932
Liddle GW: Cushing's Syndrome. In Eisenstein AB (ed): The Adrenal Cortex. Boston, Little Brown, 1967
Hardy JD, Moore DO, Lanford HG: Cushing's disease today: Late follow-up of 17 adrenalectomy patients with emphasis on eight with adrenal autotransplants. Ann Surg 201:595–603, 1985
Grekin R: The adrenal gland. In Mazzaferri EL (ed): Textbook of Endocrinology, 3rd ed. New York, Med Exam Publishing, 1985

CUSHING'S SYMPHALANGISM

Synonyms. Symphalangism, proximal; Vessel's.

Symptoms and Signs. Symphalangism. Fusion of carpal and tarsal bones. Conductive deafness frequent association. Strabismus.

Etiology. Unknown. Autosomal dominant inheritance.

Therapy. Surgical approach to correct symphalangism unsuccessful.

BIBLIOGRAPHY. Cushing H: Hereditary ankylosis of proximal phalanges joints (symphalangism). Genetics 1:90–106, 1916
Vessel ES: Symphalangism, strabismus and hearing loss in mother and daughter. N Engl J Med 263:839–842, 1960
Cremer C, Theunissen E, Kuijpers W: Proximal symphalangy and stages ankylosis. Arch Otolaryngol 111:765–767, 1985

CUTIS LAXA SYNDROMES

Synonyms. Chalasodermia; dermatochalasia; dermatolysis, dermatomegaly.

CONGENITAL

Symptoms and Signs. Present at birth or noticed within first months of life, frequently after episodes of edema. Loss of elasticity of skin; formation of skin folds, particularly noticeable on face and trunk, progressing during infancy and becoming less evident after puberty. Many infants have a hoarse cry, probably due to laxity of the vocal cords. Adult males exhibit infantile genitalia and impotence. General development is normal. Frequently respiratory insufficiency due to emphysema and resulting in cor pulmonale. Occasionally, symptoms and signs related to presence of esophagus, duodenum, ileum, and bladder diverticula.

Etiology. Autosomal dominant, autosomal recessive, and X-linked inheritance described. Deficiency of lysyloxidase activity, low levels of copper (disorder of copper metabolism?).

Pathology. Skin thickness normal. Elastic fibers reduced, shortened, and degenerated. Increase of mucopolysaccharides. Other tissues may show similar changes. Tortuous artery; pulmonary stenosis; aortic dilatation.

Diagnostic Procedures. *Biopsy of skin.* See Pathology. *Blood and other fluids.* Normal if not affected by respiratory or gastrointestinal complications. *Pulmonary function tests. X-ray of chest and gastrointestinal tract.* Differential diagnosis with Ehlers-Danlos, Grönblad-Stranberg-Touraine; von Recklinghausen's II; Donahue's; Debré-Fittke.

Therapy. Plastic surgery sometimes useful.

Prognosis. Patients with forms without emphysema have normal life expectancy; otherwise early death. Recessive inheritance more severe (lethal). Dominant inheritance milder course; frequently only cosmetic problem.

ACQUIRED

Symptoms and Signs. Appear at puberty or later, preceded by episodes of angioedema or inflammatory process.

Slow development of skin changes represented by folding, generalized or limited to face, body, or neck. Vascular fragility and purpura. Occasionally respiratory insufficiency due to emphysema or gastroenteric manifestation.

Etiology. Unknown.

Pathology. See Congenital form.

Therapy. See Congenital form.

Prognosis. Determined by intensity, progression, and pulmonary complications.

BIBLIOGRAPHY. Variot G, Cailliau F: Peau ridée sénile chez un enfant de deaux ans. Agénesie de réseux élastique du derme. Bull Soc Méd Hôp (Paris) 43:989–994, 1919
Vaglio R: Un caso di cutis laxa. Pediatria (Napoli) 31:321–323, 1923
Weber FP: Chalasodermia or "loose skin" and its relationship to subcutaneous fibroids or calcareous nodules, etc. Urol Cutan Rev 27:407–409, 1923
McKusick VA: Heritable Disorders of Connective Tissue, 4th ed, p 371. St Louis, CV Mosby, 1972
Behrman RE, Vaugham VC: Nelson's Textbook of Pediatrics, p 1701–1702, WB Saunders, Philadelphia, 1983

CUTIS MARMORATA

Synonyms. Marble skin. See also Livedo reticularis and Van Lohuizen; telangioectasia congenita. CMTC, included cutis marmorata.

Symptoms. None.

Signs. Manifested especially in children (50% of cases) less frequently in adults and young women. With cold exposure bluish red mottling of skin, which subsides in warm environment. Areas more affected are extremities and pectoral region. Frequently associated with Cassirer's (see), Pernio (see) and erythrocyanosis. In some cases association with telangiactasis and superficial erosions.

Etiology. Unknown. Considered a physiologic reflex. Could be a mild form of Livedo reticularis (see).

Pathology. Spasmodic narrowing of arterioles with dilatation of capillaries and venules.

Diagnostic Procedures. For severe form see Livedo reticularis.

Therapy. None.

Prognosis. Benign (physiologic condition); in majority of cases it may evolve into Livedo reticularis.

BIBLIOGRAPHY. Van Lohuizen CHJ: Uber eine seltene angeborene Haut-anomalie. (Cutis marmorata te-

langectatica congenita). Acta Dermatol Venerol 3:202–211, 1922
Champion RH: Livedo reticularis; A review. Br J Dermatol 77:167–179, 1965
Kurczynski TW: Hereditary cutis marmorata telangectatica congenita. Pediatrics 70:52–53, 1982

CUTIS VERTICIS GYRATA

Synonyms. Bulldog scalp; gyrate scalp; washboard scalp. See Rosenthal-Kloepfer.

Symptoms and Signs. Both sexes affected, onset at all ages. Presence of folds and furrows of scalp and face, imparting to scalp a corrugated or gyrate appearance. Isolated sign or component of other syndromes: (1) Touraine-Salente-Golé; (2) Marie's; (3) microcephalic idiocy; (4) myxedema; (5) local inflammatory or traumatic causes; (6) melanocytic nevi. Frequently associated with mental deficiencies; in one family thyroid aplasia reported.

Etiology. Autosomal inheritance.

Pathology. Hypertrophy of cutis; according to etiology.

Therapy. None. In nevoid form, plastic surgery.

BIBLIOGRAPHY. Robert A: Journal de Chirurgie par Malgaigne Paris 1:125–126, 1843
McDowall TW: Case of abnormal development of the scalp. J Ment Sci 39:62–64, 1893
Akesson HO: Cutis verticis gyrata and mental deficiencies in Sweden I. Epidemiological and clinical aspects. Acta Med Scand 175:115–127, 1964

CYCLICAL EDEMA

Synonyms. Cyclic idiopathic edema. See also Angioneurotic edema, hereditary, Periodic edema and Leg stasis.

Symptoms. In women edema begins to collect mostly in legs when they assume the standing position. In many cases edema disappears when patient is lying down; in some cases recumbency does not help, and the edema becomes generalized. In the premenstrual period symptom may be aggravated. Many patients appear emotionally disturbed, hysterical, or psychotic.

Signs. Edema that recedes with bed rest.

Etiology. Unknown; possibly aldosterone hypersecretion or increased permeability of capillaries of legs.

Diagnostic Procedures. Useful to exclude other causes of edema; diseases of heart, liver, kidneys, veins, thyroid; and simple water and sodium retention.

Therapy. Bed rest; elastic stockings. Diuretic; low-salt diet; aldosterone antagonists, vasopressor agents. In some cases refractory to above treatment, exploration and excision of adenomas or hyperplastic adrenal tissue if found.

BIBLIOGRAPHY. Mach RS, Fabre J, Muller, AF et al: Idiopathique edeme par retention sodique avec hyperaldosteronurie. Bull Mem Soc Med Hop (Paris) 71:726–732, 1955

Leutscher JA, Dowdy, AJ, Arustein AR et al: Idiopathic oedema and increased aldosterone excretion. In Balien E (ed.): C.I.O.M.S. Symposium on Aldosterone. Oxford, Blackwell, 1964

Luetscher JA: Disorders associated with altered secretion of aldosterone. In Eisenstein AB (ed): The Adrenal Cortex. Boston, Little Brown & Co, 1967

CYCLIC NEUTROPENIA

Synonyms. Cyclic agranulocytosis; myelocytic periodic; cyclic leukopenia; periodic neutropenia. Periodemitis mucosa necrotica, recurrent I. Neutropenia, cyclic.

Symptoms. Most cases from infancy present cyclic (21 day) recurrence of fever, malaise, and ulcer in the oral mucous membranes associated with recurrent neutropenia. Occasionally associated are arthralgia, abdominal pain, conjunctivitis, sore throat, headache, lymphadenitis, skin ulcers, ischiorectal and vaginal infections, and mental depression.

Signs. Splenomegaly and the recurrent lesions mentioned above.

Etiology. Unknown; recurrent deficit of myelopoiesis at primitive cell level; occasionally, autosomal dominant inheritance.

Pathology. Spleen shows different degree of vascular and perivascular hyalinization.

Diagnostic Procedures. *Blood.* Leukopenia; recurrent depression of neutrophils. *Bone marrow.* Maturation arrest of myeloid series during cycle.

Therapy. *Splenectomy.* Has some effect on number of neutrophils; recurrent symptoms persist. Corticosteroid. Have some symptomatic effect on lesions and fever while administered.

Prognosis. Persistence of recurrent manifestation despite any known treatment.

BIBLIOGRAPHY. Leale M: Recurrent furunculosis in an infant showing an unusual blood picture. JAMA 54:1854, 1910

Rutledge BH, Hansen-Prüss OC, Thayer WS: Recurrent agranulocytosis. Bull Johns Hopkins Hosp 46:369–389, 1930

Thompson WP: Observations on possible relationship between agranulocytosis and menstruation with further studies on a case of cyclic neutropenia. N Engl J Med 210:176–178, 1934

Wright DG, Dale DC, Fauci AS et al: Human cyclic neutropenia: Clinical review and long-term follow-up of patients. Medicine 60:1–13, 1981

CYCLIC STRABISMUS

Synonyms. Periodic esotrophia, alternate-day squint.

Symptoms and Signs. Both sexes from infancy. Cycles of 24 hours with eyes alternatively straight and crossed. Frequent strabismus in the other members of the family.

Etiology. Unknown. Autosomal dominant trait.

BIBLIOGRAPHY. Richter CP: Clock-mechanism esotrophia in children (alternate-day squint). John Hopkins Med J 122:218–223, 1968

Friendly DS, Manson RA, Albert DG: Cyclic strabismus. A case study. Doc Ophthalmol 34:189–202, 1973

CYCLOPIA

Synonyms. Synopsy. Fraser's syndrome.

Symptoms and Signs. The most extreme form of holoprosencephaly. Single eye globe with varying degrees of doubling of intrinsic ocular structures, arhinia and a blind-ending proboscis located under the median eye.

Etiology. Inherited condition due to deletion of a small chromosomal segment.

Diagnostic Procedures. *Karyogram.* Reveals presence of a missing third chromosome and a supplementary chromosome in C group. Same karyogram noted in healthy relatives.

BIBLIOGRAPHY. Ellis R: On a rare form of twin monstrosity. Trans Obstet Soc 7:160–164, 1865

Pfitzer P, Muntefering H: Cyclopism as an hereditary malformation. Nature 217:1071–1072, 1968

Gorlin RJ, Pindborg JJ, Cohen MM Jr: Syndromes of the Head and Neck, 2nd ed, p 179. New York, McGraw-Hill, 1976

CYRIAX'S

Synonyms. Davies-Colley; slipping rib. See Anterior chest wall.

Symptoms. Pain in the chest, which may be dull and recurrent or very sharp and associated with symptoms of shock. It may be elicited by sneezing, deep inspiration, movement of arm. Occasionally, patient feels a snapping, "slipping of something" just before the onset of pain.

Signs. Compression of cartilage of rib involved always reproduces symptomatology.

Etiology and Pathology. Injury of the interchondral synovial membrane of the first three false ribs (8th, 9th, and 10th) that allows the anterior end of the rib to curl under the cartilage and compress the intercostal nerve and sympathetic fibers. Trauma direct or indirect (false movements) or idiopathic.

Therapy. Surgical or conservative. The three principal methods of treatment are reassurance, injection of the affected area with local anesthetic, and surgical excision of the affected cartilage (in few cases, two or more cartilages).

Prognosis. Complete recovery. Diagnosis of this condition may prevent useless abdominal surgery or wrong treatment for nonexistent heart conditions.

BIBLIOGRAPHY. Cyriax EJ: On various conditions that may simulate referred pain of visceral disease. Practitioner 102:314–322, 1919
Telford KM: The slipping rib syndrome. Can Med Assoc J 62:463–465, 1950
Porter GE: Slipping rib syndrome: An infrequently recognized entity in children: A report of three cases and review of the literature. Pediatrics, 76:810–813, 1985

CYSTATHIONINURIA

Synonyms. Cystathionase deficiency; CTH deficiency.

Symptoms and Signs. Rare condition. No clinical abnormalities are characteristically associated with this enzyme deficiency, but the following have been encountered: congenital defects (*e.g.*, club foot, small ears); acromegaly; motor and mental retardation; cataract; diabetes mellitus and insipidus.

Etiology. Gamma cystathionase deficiency. Genetic heterogeneity; autosomal inheritance. Relatives of those patients also had increased cystathionine level; however, they were asymptomatic. The relationship between metabolic defect and malformations may be coincidental.

Pathology. *Brain.* Diffuse atrophy. *Liver.* Smaller than normal; pale; fibrotic. *Heart.* Fatty degeneration (data based only on one autopsy).

Diagnostic Procedures. *Plasma, cerebrospinal fluid, and urine.* Marked increases of cystathionine.

Therapy. Pyridoxine reduces concentration of cystathionine. Only in some patients (expression of genetic heterogeneity). Low methionine diet.

Prognosis. Relatives of patients with the metabolic defect remained completely asymptomatic. Both patients reached advanced age despite mental and physical defects.

BIBLIOGRAPHY. Harris H, Penrose LS, Thomas DHH: Cystathioninuria. Ann Hum Genet 23:442, 1959
Mudd SH, Levy HL: Disorders of transsulfuration. In Stanbury JB, Wyngaarden JB, Fredrickson DS, et al: The Metabolic Basis of Inherited Disease, 5th ed, p 522. New York, McGraw-Hill, 1983

CYSTIC DUCT

Synonyms. Infundibulocystic; organic gallbladder siphopathy; gallbladder stasis; precholecystectomy.

Symptoms. Prevalent in women with numerous pregnancies. Sharp pain in the area of gallbladder, sometimes radiating to the back following fatty food ingestion.

Signs. Tenderness over gallbladder region; gallbladder may be palpated. Minimal jaundice.

Etiology. Mechanical, noncalculous, partial obstruction of the cystic duct. Forceful contraction of gallbladder to overcome resistance to bile flow.

Pathology. Constrictive bands, adhesions, kinking of cystic duct; adherence of gallbladder with resulting angulation of infundibulocystic junction. Congenital or acquired cystic stenosis. All are possible findings. Gallbladder normal or slightly inflamed.

Diagnostic Procedures. *Cholecystography.* Determination of biliary drainage by serial cholecystography or cholecystokinin cholecystography.

Therapy. Surgical.

Prognosis. Following surgery, complete and lasting recovery.

BIBLIOGRAPHY. Schieden V: Uber die "Stauungsgallenblase." Zentralbl Chir 41:1257, 1920
Camishion RC, Goldstein F: Partial noncalculous cystic duct obstruction (cystic duct syndrome). Surg Clin North Am 47:1107–1114, 1967
Bode WE, Aust JB: Isolated cystic dilatation of the cystic duct. Am J Surg 145:828–829, 1983

CYSTIC DUCT STUMP

Synonyms. Reformed gallbladder; cystic duct remnant; Oddi's.

Symptoms. Appear a few months or years after cholecystectomy. Pain in right epichondrium; radiation to right shoulder. Nausea; vomiting; chills and fever (rare).

Signs. Jaundice in high percentage of cases. Pain on Murphy's maneuver.

Etiology. Formation of a pouch or sac on stump of gall bladder or behind the common duct below the junction of left and right hepatic ducts.

Pathology. Cystic formation containing concentrated bile and occasionally calculi; choledochitis.

Diagnostic Procedures. *Intravenous cholangiography.*

Therapy. Surgery.

Prognosis. Good.

BIBLIOGRAPHY. Oddi R: Effetti dell' estirpazione della cistifellea. Bull Sci Med di Bologna 21: 194–202, 1888
Peterson FR: Re-formed gallbladder review of 27 cases. Tr West SA 51:203–220, 1942
Brown MJ: Diseased cystic duct remnant. AMA Arch Surg 79:304–310, 1959
Hopkins SF: The problem of the cystic duct remnant. Surg Gynecol Ostet 148:531–533, 1979

CYSTIC FIBROSIS

Synonyms. CF; fibrocystic, meconium ileus (see), mucoviscidosis, Clarke-Hadefield (see). Generalized defect of exocrine glands. Thick mucous secretions in many organs cause clinical manifestations of (1) chronic obstructive lung disease with recurrent infections, accompanied by cor pulmonale; (2) exocrine pancreatic insufficiency with steatorrhea and azotorrhea; (3) intestinal obstruction in neonatal period (see Meconium ileus) or adult life; (4) cirrhosis of liver due to focal biliary involvement; (5) infertility in males; (6) high sodium chloride in sweat.

Symptoms and Signs. Prevalence of 1:2000 live births. May start from birth with meconium ileus (see). Pulmonary involvement starts in childhood with obstruction of small airways, recurrent infection, bronchiolitis, barrel chest deformity, growth retardation, cyanosis, digital clubbing. More frequent infections with *Staphylococcus aureus* and *Pseudomonas aeruginosa*. Cor pulmonale in late phases of disease. Later in life obstruction of pancreatic ducts and loss of pancreatic enzyme activity with progressive absent weight gain, abdominal distention, frequent evacuation with bulky, oily stool and rectal prolapse. Pancreatitis is not frequent. A meconium ileus equivalent of adulthood may appear in 21% of patients with intestinal obstruction. Focal biliary cirrhosis is present in 25% of patients and can present itself as a persistent neonatal icterus. In later life this can evolve (2–3%) in partial hypertension and splenomegaly. Liver complications are seen only in patients with pancreatic insufficiency. Adult males are infertile in 98% of cases due to mechanical obstruction of vas deferens. In females

delayed puberty and various gynecologic malformations; pregnancy is possible. Visual defects, venous engorgement of retinal veins and blurring of the optic nerve head are possible. Salivary glands are enlarged. Sweat is rich in Na^+ and Cl^- due to decreased transductal reabsorption.

Etiology. Autosomal recessive either single mutant allele or genetic hetereogenicity. CF has coincidental occurrence with other congenital diseases (Down, cri-duchat, agammaglobulinemia, Wiskott-Aldrich).

Diagnostic Procedures. Sweat test method of Gibson-Cooke with quantitative pilocarpine ionophoresis: chloride concentration above 60 mEq/liter is consistent with diagnosis of CF. Anamnesis with characteristic symptoms and signs.

Therapy. Psychosocial support and qualified long-term medical assistance. Surgery for intestinal obstruction often needed. Adequate nutritional support, prevention of pulmonary infections.

Prognosis. Variable. Prognosis is determined by degree of pulmonary involvement. Prognosis has improved in the last three decades. Mean age 21 years in 1978.

BIBLIOGRAPHY. Fanconi G, Uehlinger E, Knaunuer C: Das coeliakiesyndrom be: Angeborener zystischer pankreas fibromatose und bronkiektasien. Wien Med Wockenschr 86:753, 1936
Andersen DH: Cystic fibrosis of pancreas and its relation to celiac disease: Clinical and pathological study. Am J Dis Child 56:344–399, 1938
Di Santa Agnese P, Blanc W: A distinctive type of biliary cirrhosis of the liver associated with cystic fibrosis of the pancreas. Pediatrics 18:387–408, 1956
Talamo RC, Rosenstein BS, Berninger RW: Cystic fibrosis. In Stanbury JB, Wyngaarden JB, Fredrickson DS et al: The Metabolic Basis of Inherited Disease, 5th ed, p 1889. New York, McGraw-Hill, 1983

CYSTINOSIS

Synonyms. Cystindiathesis, Abderhalden-Kaufman-Lignac-Fanconi-Debré.
Metabolic disorder characterized biochemically by an abnormally high intracellular content of free cystine. There are 3 forms of the disease:
1. Infantile nephropathic (see also Fanconi's)
2. Benign
3. Intermediate

INFANTILE NEPHROPATHIC
Synonyms. Fanconi-De Toni, cystinosis, early onset.

Symptoms and Signs. Onset at 6 months. Polyuria, polydipsia, recurrent fever, growth retardation, rickets, acidosis, clinical picture of Fanconi-De Toni syndrome (see). Mentally normal, hydrocephalus. Blond hair, fair complexion, severe photophobia.

Etiology. Autosomal recessive. Impaired cystine transport across lysosomal membrane.

Diagnostic Procedures. *Urine analysis.* Glycosuria, organic aciduria, aminoaciduria, proteinuria. *Eye transillumination.* Homogenously dispersed tinsellike refractile opacities, cornea and conjunctiva. *Bone marrow.* Presence of cystine crystals.

Pathology. Specific lesion deposition of cystine crystals in all organs (not brain and muscle). Kidney: characteristic "swan neck" deformity of tubule, cystine crystals in cornea and conjunctiva. Peripheral retinopathy.

Therapy. Symptomatic, vitamin D, penicillamin, dithiothreitol (DTT), cysteamine, ascorbic acid, diet, renal transplantation.

Prognosis. Poor *quoad vitam.* Better with kidney transplantation but death in second decade.

BENIGN

Synonyms. Cystinosis. Adult nonnephropathic type.

Symptoms and Signs. Both sexes affected. Detection at various ages, childhood asymptomatic: normal growth, absence of skin pigmentation, rickets, retinopathy. Incidental discovery during routine ophthalmic examination.

Diagnostic Procedures. *Slit-light transillumination.*

Pathology. Cystine deposits in cornea.

Prognosis. Good.

INTERMEDIATE

Synonyms. Late-onset cystinosis, adolescent cystinosis, nephropathic.

Symptoms and Signs. Late onset in adolescence. No complete Fanconi syndrome. Same as infantile form but less severe. Photophobia, chronic headaches.

Etiology. Either double heterozygotes with one gene of infantile form and one benign form or genetic compounds.

Pathology. Renal biopsy: glomerular changes.

BIBLIOGRAPHY. Abderhalden F: Familiare cystindiathese. Z Physiol Chem (Strassb) 38:557–561, 1903
Garrod AE: Inborn error of metabolism. Lancet Z Lecture I, p 1; Lecture II, p 73; lecture III, p 142; lecture IV, p 214, 1908
Schneider JA, Schulman JD: Cystinosis. In Stanbury JB, Wyngaarden JB, Fredrickson DS et al: The Metabolic Basis of Inherited Disease, 5th ed, p 1844. New York, McGraw-Hill, 1983

CYSTINURIA

Symptoms and Signs. Males affected more seriously than females. Formation of renal stones by the age of 30 in 50% of cases, with typical clinical manifestation (*e.g.,* pain, hematuria). The majority of these patients are of small stature (because of malabsorption and loss of the essential amino acid, lysine). Prevalence 1 : 7000.

Etiology. Inherited condition. Characterized by altered transepithelial transport mechanism of the amino acid, expressed primarily in kidney and intestine, as excessive urinary excretion of cystine, lysine, arginine, and ornithine. Two forms of inheritance patterns: (1) Autosomal recessive (with heterozygote with normal urine); (2) incomplete recessive (with heterozygote with some amount of mentioned amino acids in the urine). This syndrome is not to be confused with Abderhalden-Kaufaman-Lignac and Lignac-Debré-Fanconi (see), and with other syndromes where cystinuria occurs as part of general aminoaciduria (*e.g.,* Fanconi-De Toni syndrome, Wilson's syndrome).

Pathology. Renal calculosis with secondary inflammatory and fibrotic changes of kidney parenchyma.

Diagnostic Procedures. *Urine.* Excessive excretion of amino acids mentioned in etiology; passage of cystine stone; hematuria; proteinuria. *X-ray.* Intravenous pyelogram.

Therapy. Diet with reduced methionine (maintains urine alkalinity) and abundant in volume.

Prognosis. Except for formation of stone and small stature, would be a benign disorder. Kidney complication leads patients to death at the end of the fourth decade.

BIBLIOGRAPHY. Garrod AE: The Croonian lectures on inborn errors of metabolism. Lancet 2: Lecture I, p 1; Lecture II, p 73; Lecture III, p 142; Lecture IV, p 214, 1908
Segal S, Thier SO: Cystinuria. In Stanbury JB, Wyngaarden JB, Fredrickson DS, et al: The Metabolic Basis of Inherited Disease, 5th ed, p 1774. New York, McGraw-Hill, 1983

CYSTITIS, IRRADIATION

Synonym. Radiation cystitis.

Symptoms. Both sexes affected, onset at least 1 year to 10 years after radiation treatment. Pollakiuria; stranguria, incontinence; hematuria.

Signs. Pain at palpation over bladder.

Etiology. X-ray; radium treatment of pelvic condition.

Pathology. *Mild.* Mild mucosal inflammatory edematous changes; dilation of submucosal vessels and increased vascularization. *Severe.* Ulcerative necrotic generalized lesions. *Chronic.* Defined lesions; bulbous edema; ulcerative necrotic lesions.

Diagnostic Procedures. *Urine.* Proteinuria; hematuria; presence of white blood cells and cellular debris.

Therapy. Antinflammatory agents. Antibiotics.

Prognosis. Generally, remission; in severe cases, fibrosis and reduction of bladder capacity and formation of fistulas.

D'ACOSTA'S

Synonyms. Acosta's; acute mountain sickness; altitude anoxia; altitude sickness; hypobarism—acute mountain sickness; See Monge's syndrome.

Symptoms and Signs. Occur from 4 to 6 hours after reaching high altitude, or later (96 hr). Variability in intensity of symptoms, according to altitude. Pulsatile headache; nausea; vomiting; anorexia; insomnia; irritability. In some cases, symptoms may progress to confusion, coma, and death. Signs of pulmonary edema may also develop.

Etiology. Hypoxia; inappropriate secretion of antidiuretic and corticoadrenal hormones; fluid retention; hypervolemia. Increase in ventilation stimulated by hypoxia and resulting in hypocapnia and respiratory alkalosis.

Pathology. Cerebral and pulmonary edema.

Therapy. Diuretics. Acetazolamide, 250 mg every 8 hours prior to and during the ascent to altitude. (The drug acts by increasing renal excretion of bicarbonate and reducing the extent of the respiratory alkalosis). In severe cases, prompt transfer to lower altitude. Oxygen and cardiopulmonary resuscitation in cases of pulmonary edema.

Prognosis. Minor symptoms disappear after 4 to 8 days of acclimatization. In severe case, without treatment death can occur. The return at lower altitude immediately improves the clinical manifestations.

BIBLIOGRAPHY. D'Acosta J: Efecto estraño que hace en ciertas terras de Indias el aire, coviento que corre. Nella sua Historia Natural y Moral de las Indias Forms, Vol 3, Chap 9. Sevilla, Juan de Leon, 1950

Blume FD, Boyers SJ, Braverman LE, et al: Impaired osmoregulation at high altitudes. Studies on Mt Everest. JAMA 252:524–526, 1984

DA COSTA'S (J.M.)

Synonyms. Neurocirculatory asthenia, cardiac neurosis; effort syndrome (misnomer); nervous heart; soldier heart. See Orthostatic. The designation "effort syndrome" has been dropped since symptoms and signs of this syndrome closely resemble those of emotion and fear, rather than those of "effort" in normal subject, and depend on central stimulation.

BIBLIOGRAPHY. DaCosta JM: On irritable heart: A clinical study of a form of functional cardiac disorder and its consequences. Am J Med Sci 61:17–52, 1871

Hurst JW: The Heart, 6th ed, p 1526. New York, McGraw-Hill, 1986

DAENTAL'S

Synonym. Femoral-facial.

Symptoms and Signs. Full syndrome only in females. Facies: upslanting of palpebral fissures; nose short and broad-tipped, long filtrum, thin upper lip, micrognathia and cleft palate. Femoral hypoplasia; foot deformities.

Etiology. Unknown. Sporadic occurrence. Autosomal dominant inheritance advanced.

BIBLIOGRAPHY. Daentl DL, Smith DW, Scott CI et al: Femoral hypoplasia-unusual facies syndrome. J Pediatr 86:107–111, 1975

Burch U, Riebel T, Held KR et al: Bilateral femoral dysgenesis with micrognathia, cleft palate, anomalies of the spine and pelvis and foot deformities. Helv Paediatr Acta 36:473–482, 1981

DAHLBERG'S

Synonyms. Lymphedema-hypoparathyroidism; Hypoparathyroidism-lymphedema.

Symptoms and Signs. Broad nasal bridge, displacement of inner canthi, noted after birth. Described in two brothers. Congenital lymphedema; signs of hypoparathyroidism (see Hypoparathyroidism syndromes) nephropathy, mitral valve prolapse, and brachytelephalangy, bilateral cataract (in one case developed at age 19 yr).

Etiology. Unknown. Possibly autosomal recessive or X-linked inheritance.

Diagnostic Procedures. *Blood.* See hypoparathyroidism plus evidence of renal failure (slowly developing). *X-Ray.* Suspect pulmonary lymphagiectases. *Electrocardiography.*

Therapy. Symptomatic; in one case needed kidney transplant.

Prognosis. Both cases were recognized in adult life.

BIBLIOGRAPHY. Dahlberg PJ, Borer WZ, Newcomer KL, et al: Autosomal or X-linked recessive syndrome of congenital lymphedema, hypoparathyroidism, nephropathy, prolapsing mitral valve and brachytelephalangy. Ann J Med Genet 16:99–104, 1983

DANA'S I

Synonyms. Benign essential tremor; hereditary benign tremor; presenile tremor; tremor, benign hereditary.

Symptoms. Both sexes affected; on the average onset at 50 years of age and later in women than men, extending progressively. More or less rhythmic, fine, or coarse tremor (rate 4–12/sec). Present when there is increase in muscle tone (static tremor), and in movement (kinetic or intentional). Enhanced by emotion, fatigue, and cold; relieved by rest, sedation, and sleep. Affects mostly hands, arms, neck, and head; trunk may occasionally be involved.

Signs. Lack of parkinsonian signs (rigidity; postural flexion; mask face). No deficit of reflexes or sensations; no pathologic reflexes; good coordination. Mild extrapyramidal symptoms.

Etiology. Unknown; autosomal dominant inheritance. Earlier appearance in subsequent generation noted.

Pathology. Not contributory to interpret nature of disorder.

Diagnostic Procedures. *Thyroid function studies.* Negative. *Electromyography.* Negative. *Spinal fluid.* Negative.

Therapy. Nonspecific; some benefit from sedatives.

Prognosis. Benign course. After more or less rapid progression, the situation becomes stabilized, and patients are not incapacitated.

BIBLIOGRAPHY. Dana CL: Hereditary tremor; A hitherto undescribed form of motor neurosis. Am J Med Sci 94:386–393, 1887
Critchley M: Observation on essential (heredofamilial) tremor. Brain 72:113–139, 1949
Murray TJ: Essential tremor. Can Med Assoc J 124:1559–1565, 1981

DANDY-WALKER

Synonyms. Obstructed Sylvius aqueduct; Luschka-Magendie foramina atresia; internal hydrocephalus; noncommunicating hydrocephalus; see also Arnold-Chiari.

Symptoms. Vomiting, hyperirritability, convulsions.

Signs. Progressive enlargement of the head; congested veins in the scalp; bulging of anterior fontanelle; separated cranial sutures; papilledema, bradycardia; bradypnea.

Etiology. Internal hydrocephalus developing *in utero* and other unidentified primitive factors responsible for the development of following malformations: complete or partial obstruction of foramina of Luschka and Magendie due to a noninvolution of posterior medullary velum of fourth ventricle, which persists as a thick membrane, and other midline malformations (e.g., agenesis of corpus callosum). In some cases, occurrence of the syndrome in siblings suggests a recessive inheritance.

Pathology. Dolichocephaly; thinning of occipital squama; high insertion of tentorium and lateral sinuses; dilatation of fourth ventricle; cerebellum displaced by the cystlike dilatation and consequent partial or complete aplasia of the vermis. Additional midline malformations may occasionally be present. Brain and cerebellar cortex affected first; white matter contains fat from distruction of myelin. Proliferation of glia.

Diagnostic Procedures. Fetal hydrocephalus diagnosed by antenatal ultrasound examination; postnatally: computed tomography and ultrasonic examination.

Therapy. Surgical treatment during the first week of life: simultaneous shunting of both the ventricles and the cyst through the same valve in the peritoneum.

Prognosis. Poor.

BIBLIOGRAPHY. Dandy WE, Blackfan KD: Internal hydrocephalus: An experimental clinical and pathological study. Am J Dis Child 8:406–485, 1914
Dandy WE: The diagnosis and treatment of hydrocephalus due to occlusion of the formina of Magendie and Luschka. Surg Gynecol Obstet 32:112–124, 1921
Taggart JK, Walker AE: Congenital atresia of the foramina of Luschka and Magendie. Arch Neurol Psychiatr 48:583–612, 1942
Walker AE: A case of congenital atresia of the foramina of Luschka and Magendie: Surgical cure. J Neuropathol Exp Neurol 3:368–373, 1944
Serlo W, Kirkinen P, Heikkinen E, Jouppila P: Ante and postnatal evaluation of the Dandy-Walker syndrome. Child's Nerv Syst 1:148–151, 1985

DARIER-FERRAND

Synonyms. Dermatofibroma; progressive recurrent dermatofibrosarcoma; protuberans dermatofibroma.

Symptoms and Signs. Rare. Equal incidence in both sexes in adult life. Small, hard nodules infiltrating the skin that may enlarge to form freely movable plaques or may become pedunculated. They appear mostly in the trunk and flexural regions. Later they become painful, fixate to the underlying structure, ulcerate and discharge.

Etiology. Unknown. Nodules may appear in area previously traumatized. Malignant tumor.

Pathology. Well-differentiated fibrosarcoma. Uniform fibroblasts extending up to dermoepithelial junction and down to subcutaneous fat; peripherally, they blend into normal dermis. Occasionally, modest, mitotic activity. The arrangement is that of spokes of a wheel. Blood vessels scarse and difficult to identify. Older lesions show mucoid degeneration.

Diagnostic Procedures. *Biopsy.*

Therapy. Surgical excision providing large margin of healthy tissue to prevent recurrence.

Prognosis. Slow growth over periods of months or years. Metastasis and spread to lymph nodes very rare. Recurrence after excision 20% (due to inadequate removal of tissue.)

BIBLIOGRAPHY. Darier J, Ferrand M: Dermatofibromes progressive et récidivante ou fibro-sarcomes de la peau. Ann Dermatol Syph 5:45–62, 1924
Burkhardt BR, Soule EH, Winkelmann RK et al: Dermatofibrosarcoma protuberans. Study of fifty-six cases. Am J Surg 111:638–644, 1966
Rook A, Wilkinson DS, Ebling FJG, et al: Textbook of Dermatology, 4th ed, p 2461. Oxford, Blackwell Scientific Publications, 1986

DARIER-ROUSSY

Synonym. Subcutaneous sarcoidosis.

Symptoms and Signs. Subcutaneous nodules on the trunk, thighs, shoulders, symmetric distribution, skin-colored or bluish red, slowly evolving without ulceration.

Etiology. Sarcoidosis; possibly other causes. See Besnier-Boeck-Schaumann.

Pathology. See Besnier-Boeck-Schaumann.

BIBLIOGRAPHY. Darier J, Roussy G: Des sarcoides soubcutanees; contribution à l'étude des tuberculides ou tuberculose atténuees de l'hypoderme. Arch Méd Exp Anat 18:1–50, 1906
Rook A, Wilkinson DS, Ebling FJG et al: Textbook of Dermatology, 4th ed, p 1772. Oxford, Blackwell Scientific Publications, 1986

DARIER-WHITE

Synonyms. Darier's I; dyskeratosis follicularis vegetans; keratosis follicularis; psorospermosis; White's. See Hopf's and Gougerot-Hailey-Hailey.

Symptoms and Signs. Both sexes affected; onset in childhood. Many confluent flesh-colored keratotic papules forming greasy crusted areas, vegetating and malodorous, on the skin of head, neck, back, abdomen, and groin. Seldom, hair loss. Punctate keratosis on palms and soles. Palmoplantar keratoderma (10%). Seldom, hemorrhagic macules in hands and feet. Occasionally (10%), lesions are in zosteriform pattern and limited to one half of body. Mucosae of mouth, esophagus, genitals, and anus may exhibit white umbilicate papules; hypertrophy of gums may also occur. Onychodystrophy. Small stature; low intelligence; genital hypoplasia.

Etiology. Unknown; autosomal dominant inheritance. Defect in synthesis, organization, maturation of tonofilament-desmosome complex. Considered as a variant of Hopf's (see).

Pathology. Early, fissures above basal layer, later extending through Malpighian layer. Around lacunae small separated groups of cells enlarged with dark nuclei, clear cytoplasm, and glistening ring (partial keratosis). Hyperkeratosis; parakeratosis; acanthosis of different degrees.

Diagnostic Procedures. *Biopsy of skin. Blood.* Low vitamin A level. *X-ray of chest.* Diffuse fibrosis with nodulation mainly affecting lower lobes. Occasionally, cystic changes in the bones.

Therapy. In adult, high doses of vitamin A (for 2 mo); maintenance with smaller doses. In children, consider the possibility of hyperostosis. Keratolytic ointments.

Prognosis. Chronic benign condition. Treatment may give excellent, moderate, or no improvement. Relapses when treatment is discontinued. Degree of mental retardation variable from institutional care required to fairly normal life.

BIBLIOGRAPHY. Darier J: Psorospermose folliculaire vegetante. Ann Dermatol Syph 10:597–612, 1889
White JC: A case of keratosis (ichthyosis) follicularis. J Cutan Genitourin Dis 7:201–209, 1889
Witkop, CJ Jr, and Gorlin RJ: Four hereditary mucosal syndromes. Arch Derm 84:762–771, 1961
Matsuoka LY, Wortsman J, McConnachie P: Renal and testicular agenesis in a patient with Darier's disease. Am J Med 78:873–877, 1985

DAVID'S (W.)

Synonym. Purpura feminarum typica.

Symptoms and Signs. Occur in women during reproductive period. Hemorrhages from gums and other mucosal areas periodically recurring usually during menstrual periods.

Etiology. David believes that a deficit of ovarian hormones is the cause of the syndrome.

Diagnostic Procedures. *Blood.* Complete clotting studies; evaluation of hormonal activities. *Evaluation of psychic balance.* See Psychogenic purpura.

BIBLIOGRAPHY. Hyde JH: A contribution to the study of bleeding stigmata. J Cutan Dis 15:557, 1897
David W: Ueber Purpura—Erkrankungen bei Frauen. Med Klin 22:1755–1756, 1926
Agle DP, Ratnoff OD: Purpura as a psychosomatic entity. Arch Intern Med 109:685–694, 1962

DAVID-STICKLER

Synonyms. Progressive arthrootoophthalmopathy; Stickler's. See Marshall's, Weissbacher-Zweymuller and Nance-Insley.

Symptoms. Both sexes affected; onset at birth. Congenital progressive myopia, astygmatism, blindness. Hypermobility of joints; in childhood, onset of stiffness and articular pain. Progressive deafness (sensorineural type).

Signs. Nasal bridge depressed; maxillar hypoplasia; philtrum prolonged; occasionally, cleft palate. Arthropathy primarily affected knees, hips, and spine; less severely, wrists, elbows, and ankles. Articular bony enlargement and hypermobility and then deforming changes (third and fourth decades). Phthisical or glaucomatous blind eyes; chronic uveitis; keropathy; chorioretinal degeneration; total retinal detachment (during first decade). Skeletal abnormalities.

Etiology. Autosomal dominant inheritance. Included by David in mucopolysaccharidosis group (not confirmed by other authors). Abnormal development of epiphyseal plate. Confused relationship with Marshall's and Weissbacher-Zweymuller syndromes.

Pathology. See Signs.

Diagnostic Procedures. *X-Rays of Skeleton.* Eccentroorthochondrodysplasia (Morquio's). *Ophthalmoscopy. Audiography. Blood and urine.* Normal.

Therapy. Orthopedic.

Prognosis. Blindness during first decade. Severe arthropathy by third or fourth decade.

BIBLIOGRAPHY. David B: Ueber einen dominanten Erbgang beieiner polyopen enchondralen Dysostose typ Pfaundler-Hurler. Z Orthop 84:657–660, 1953
Strickler GB, Pugh DG: Hereditary progressive arthroophthalmopathy: II. Additional observations of vertebral abnormalities, a hearing defect, and a report of a similar case. Mayo Clin Proc 42:495–500, 1967
Ayme S, Preus M: The Marshall and Stickler syndromes: Objective rejection of lumping. J Med Genet 21:34–38, 1984

DAVIES'

Synonyms. Endomyocardial fibrosis; EMF; mural endomyocardial fibrosis. Loeffer endomyocardial; tropical endomyocardial fibrosis; eosinophilic endomyocardial.

Symptoms. Reported mostly in Uganda; cases in Ceylon, South America, and other African countries. No sex or racial predominance; onset before adolescence. Dyspnea; palpitation; cough; occasionally, chest pains. Fever in initial period then usually subsiding, in some cases prolonged.

Signs. Peripheral edemas. Digital clubbing; cyanosis; jaundice. Early apical systolic murmur, and S_3 opening snap (after S_2). Diminution of cardiac pulsation (constrictive, pericarditislike).

Etiology. Unknown. Primary myocardial condition with thrombosis and endocardial disease. Considered as possible causes; excessive serotonin; malnutrition; parasites; viruses; anemia; hypersensitivity. Suggested infective origin.

Pathology. *Early stage.* Endocardial and inner myocardial cells of connective tissue are swollen with mucopolysaccharides and covered by fibrin; thrombus formation followed by fibroblastic proliferation. *Late stage.* Extensive, white, endocardial thickening mostly at left ventricular apex; right ventricle similarly thickened, but less extensively affected.

Diagnostic Procedures. *Electrocardiography.* No consistent pattern. *X-rays.* Massive pericardial effusion; right atrial dilatation; dilatation right infundibular vestibulum. Pulmonary hypertension; enlargement of main pulmonary artery. *Blood.* Eosinophilia (occasional). *Biopsy of endocardium by right heart catheterization.* See pathology. *Angiography. Echography. Radionuclide imaging.*

Therapy. Symptomatic. Corticosteroids. Surgical treatment useful on short term.

Prognosis. Survival 1 to 2 years from onset of symptoms; longer survival (8–12 yr) occasionally possible.

BIBLIOGRAPHY. Davies JPN: Endocardial fibrosis in Africans. East Afr Med J 25:10–14, 1948

Davies JPN, Cales RM: Some considerations regarding obscure diseases affecting the mural endocardium. Am Heart J 59:600–631, 1960

Kass Wengen N, Goodwin JF, Roberts WC: Cardiomyopathy and myocardial involvement in systemic disease. In Hurst JW: The Heart, 6th ed, pp 1208–1213. New York, McGraw-Hill, 1986

DAVIS' (J.A.)

Synonyms. Achondroplasia–Swiss type agammaglobulinemia. Dysplasia metaphyseal (type B-III); metaphyseal dysostosis (type B-III); thymolymphopenia–metaphyseal dysostosis. See Swiss type agammaglobulinemia.

Symptoms. Both sexes affected; present from birth. High susceptibility to infections.

Signs. Absence of hair and eyebrows; ichthyosiform lesions; erythoderma; cutis laxa; short limb dwarfism.

Etiology. Unknown; autosomal recessive inheritance (probably).

Diagnostic Procedures. *Blood.* See Swiss type agammaglobulinemia. *X-rays of long bones.* Short (femora more so than humeri); metaphyseal widening; irregularity of growth plates; pelvic abnormalities; hands, skull, fibula normal.

Therapy. Antibiotics; immunoglobulins; blood transfusion (with caution and preferably after removal of white cells and injection of blood older than 21 days).

Prognosis. Poor. Death frequently before reaching first year.

BIBLIOGRAPHY. Davis JA: A case of Swiss type agammaglobulinemia and achondroplasia. Br Med J 2:1371, 1966

Ammann AJ, Sutliff W, Nillinchick E: Antibody-mediated immunodeficiency in short limbed dwarfism. J Pediatr 84:200–203, 1974

DAVIS' (M.D.)

Synonym. Rheumatoid arthritis–uveitis.

Symptoms. Most frequent in children, but occur at all ages. Symptoms of rheumatoid arthritis, trouble with vision; pain; lacrimation; photophobia.

Signs. Those of rheumatoid arthritis. Uveitis; iridocyclitis; less frequently, scleritis; secondary formation of band-shaped keratopathy; choroidal inflammation. Occasionally, hepatosplenomegaly.

Etiology. Unknown; possibly, collagen disorder or autoimmune condition.

Pathology. See Signs.

Diagnostic Procedures. *Blood.* Sedimentation rate; R. A. test.

Therapy. Systemic and topical (eye) corticosteroids.

Prognosis. Often poor.

BIBLIOGRAPHY. Davis MD: Endogenous uveitis in children: Associated band-shaped keratopathy and rheumatoid arthritis. Arch Ophthalmol 50:443–454, 1953

Smith RE, Nozik RM: Uveitis: A Clinical Approach to Diagnosis and Management. Baltimore, Williams & Wilkins, 1983

DAWSON'S

Synonyms. Inclusion body encephalitis; subacute sclerosing leukoencephalitis.

Symptoms. History of measles, before 2 years of age; for 6 to 8 years asymptomatic then gradual onset. Predominant in children younger than 12 years of age. *Early.* Intellectual deterioration; jerky movements of trunk and extremities. *Later.* Bilateral spasticity; decerebrate rigidity; cachexia and dementia. Possibly, cranial nerve palsies; vision and hearing usually spared until last stage.

Etiology. Unknown. Delay in the development of immune response, unable to clear the infection. Failure of the brain cells to synthesize 'M' protein and lack of protection from seeding of virus in the brain during first infection in early age.

Pathology. *Brain.* Fibrillary gliosis; infiltration by lymphocytes and plasma cells. Inclusion bodies in neurons.

Diagnostic Procedures. *Cerebrospinal fluid.* Pressure and cells normal; gammaglobulins increased, measles-virus specific antibodies. *Electroencephalography.* High-voltage slow complexes; initial spike or sharp wave.

Therapy. Measles vaccination has reduced the incidence. Amantadine or inosiplex may prolong survival.

Prognosis. In younger children, death within months. In adolescents, from many months' to years' survival.

BIBLIOGRAPHY. Dawson JR Jr: Cellular inclusions in cerebral lesions of lethargic encephalitis. Am J Pathol 9:7–16, 1933

Dawson JR Jr: Cellular inclusions in cerebral lesions of epidemic encephalitis. Arch Neurol Psychiatr 31:685–700, 1934

Adam RD, Victor M: Principles of Neurology, 3rd ed, pp 562–563. New York, McGraw-Hill, 1985

DEAD FETUS

Synonyms. Macerated fetus; macerated stillborn.

Symptoms and Signs. Diagnosis may be based on clinical manifestation of hemorrhages, or (better) on fibrinogen determination on patients who are known or suspected to be carrying a dead fetus in uterus. The latter method allows recognition of three grades of the syndrome.

1. *Potential.* No hemorrhages; fibrinogen declining to or below 150 mg/100 dl with or without evidence of fibrinolysis.
2. *Occult.* No hemorrhages; fibrinogen below 90 mg/100 dl, or fibrinolytic activity high.
3. *Overt.* Hemorrhages of unclottable blood because of hypofibrinogenemia and hyperfibrinolysis.

Etiology. Death of fetus after 4 to 5 weeks of retention. Maternal absorption into the circulation of products of pregnancy (amniotic fluid and products of autolysis of fetus) and activation of fibrinolytic mechanism resulting in slow defibrination of blood.

Pathology. Fetus dead; sign of intravascular coagulation and fibrinolysis of the clots.

Diagnostic Procedures. *Serial determination of fibrinogen levels. X-ray.* To demonstrate death of fetus.

Therapy. Rupture of membranes early in labor. A traumatic delivery, administration of fibrinogen, antifibrinolytic agents and heparin as indicated.

Prognosis. Enormously improved with recognition and adequate treatment.

BIBLIOGRAPHY. Weiner AE, Reid DE, Roby CC et al: Coagulation defects with intrauterine death from Rh sensitization. Am J Obstet Gynecol 60:1015–1022, 1950

Hodgkinson CP, Thompson RJ, Hodari AA: Dead fetus syndrome. Clin Obstet Gynecol 7:349–360, 1964

Pilipp EE, Barnes J, Newton M: Obstetrics and Gynecology, 3rd ed, p 360. London, William Heinemann, 1986

DEAFNESS, CONGENITAL AND OTITIC MENINGITIS

Synonym. Cerebrospinal otorrhea meningitis–congenital deafness.

Symptoms. Congenital unilateral deafness. Otorrhea without history of trauma. Recurrent episodes of meningitis.

Etiology. Unknown (possibly virus infection or trauma). Congenital malformation of inner ear with communication of middle ear and encephalic cavity through the vestibule of the labyrinth.

Pathology. See Etiology.

Diagnostic Procedures. *X-ray.* Basal cisternography. *CT brain scan.*

Therapy. Surgical correction through direct transaural approach.

Prognosis. Good when corrected.

BIBLIOGRAPHY. Neuzelius C: Spontaneous cerebrospinal fluid otorrhea due to congenital malformation. Acta Otolaryngol (Stockh) 39:314, 1951

Barr B, Wersall J: Cerebrospinal otorrhea with meningitis in congenital deafness. Arch Otolaryngol 81:26–28, 1965

Stool S, Leeds NE, Shulman K: The syndrome of congenital deafness and otitic meningitis: Diagnosis and management. J Pediatr 71:547–552, 1967

DEAFNESS, OPTIC ATROPHY

Synonym. Gernet's.

Symptoms and Signs. Both sexes. Congenital deafness. Late in life progressive optic atrophy leading to mild visual impairment.

Etiology. Unknown. Autosomal dominant transmission.

BIBLIOGRAPHY. Gernet H: Kombination mit Tanbheit. Dtsch Ophthalmol Ges 65:545–547, 1964

Konigsmark BK, Knox DL, Husserl IE et al: Dominant congenital deafness and progressive optic nerve atrophy. Arch Ophthalmol 91:99–103, 1974

DEAN-BARNES

Synonyms. Porphyria cutanea tarda hereditaria; mixed hepatic porphyria, porphyria variegate; South African genetic porphyria. Royal malady (because members of British royalty suffered from it).

Symptoms. Both sexes affected. In women milder manifestations; may be more pronounced during pregnancy. In South Africa Afrikaaners 3 : 1000 incidence. Clinical onset difficult to determine because of variability of intensity and type of skin lesions. Usually noticed in third decade of life. (1) Skin manifestation (in 50% of patients, the only finding): increased sensitivity to light and minor mechanical traumas; erythema; edema; bullae healing with moderate scarring; hyperpigmentation or atrophic depigmented areas. (2) Abdominal and neurologic symptoms and signs identical with those observed in Swedish type of porphyria (see). These are usually precipitated by ingestion of barbiturates and other drugs.

Etiology. Unknown; autosomal dominant inheritance. Either deficiency of protoporphyrinogen oxidase or defect in ferrochelatase different from that of erythroid protoporphyria (see Magnus). Metabolic derangement of porphyrin synthesis, defect very likely limited to liver.

Pathology. Absence of particular findings with the exception of high concentration of porphyrin precursors in the liver.

Diagnostic Procedures. Increased concentration of protoporphyrin and coproporphyrin in the feces of all patients (also in asymptomatic or paucisymptomatic). During attacks, larger amounts of aminolevulinic acid and porphobilinogen and porphyrins in the urine. Electrolytes imbalance (excessive vomiting; fluid loss).

Therapy. Symptomatic. See Swedish type protoporphyria.

Prognosis. During acute attack of abdominal pain, 25% mortality. Overall mortality not significantly increased, however, because many patients never have acute attacks, but only skin manifestations.

BIBLIOGRAPHY. Barnes, HD: Further South African cases of porphyrinuria. S Afr J Clin Sci 2:117–169, 1951
Dean G: Porphyria. Br Med J 2:1291–1294, 1953
Kappas A, Sassa S, Anderson KE: The porphyrias. In Stanbury JB, Wyngaarden JB, Fredrickson DS, et al: The Metabolic Basis of Inherited Disease, 5th ed, p 1301. New York, McGraw-Hill, 1983

DE BARSEY'S

Synonyms. Cutis laxa-corneal clouding-mental retardation; Progeroid De Barsey's.

Symptoms and Signs. Both sexes. From birth. Cutis laxa (see). Cloudy corneas. Delayed psychomotor development and hypotonic dwarfism. Facies progerialike, normal hair.

Etiology. Unknown. All cases sporadic.

Pathology. Skin. Sparse dermal elastin. Cornea degeneration of Bowman membrane.

BIBLIOGRAPHY. De Barsey AM, Moens E, Dierckx L: Dwarfism, oligophrenia and degeneration of the elastic tissue in skin and cornea. A new syndrome? Helv Paediatr Acta 23:305–313, 1968
Kunze J, Majewski F, Montgomery P et al: De Barsey syndrome—An autosomal recessive progeroid syndrome. Eur J Pediatr 144:384–394, 1985

DEBRE-FITTKE

Synonym. Cutis laxa–dysostosis.

Symptoms and Signs. *Skin and viscera.* Those described in cutis laxa congenital form (see). Associated from birth with persistent fontanelles, moderate oxycephaly, hip dislocation. Isolated features of pigeon breast, flat feet, scoliosis. Weak joints may also be present in relatives of patients.

Etiology. Probably autosomal recessive inheritance.

Pathology. See Cutis laxa congenital form.

Therapy. See Cutis laxa congenital form.

Prognosis. Good *quoad vitam.*

BIBLIOGRAPHY. Debré R, Marie J, Seringe P: "Cutis laxa" avec dystrophies osseuses. Bull Soc Méd Hôp 53:1038–1039, 1937
Fittke H: Ueber eine ungewöhliche Form "multipler Erbubartung" (Chalodermie und Dysostose). Z Kinderheilk 63:510–523. 1942
Fitzsimmonds JS, Fitzsimmonds EM, Guibert PR et al: Variable clinical presentation of cutis laxa. Clin Genet 28:284–295, 1985

DE CLERAMBAULT'S

Synonyms. Clerambault's I; pure erotomania.

Symptoms. Generally occur in women. Sudden onset in a state of clear consciousness. Delusional belief that a man is profoundly in love with the patient. Person selected is usually a prominent public figure, older than the patient or her husband, with whom only a brief acquaintance exists. Other features that usually coexist are her interpretations of his reaction to her approaches expressing, not rejection, but a form of love, and belief that presents received from husband or other friends are secretly sent by him. Attempts with sexual intent, or actual assaults on the object of affection frequently occur.

Etiology. Unknown; erotomania may exist as autonomous entity or be premonitory syndrome of other psychosis, or occasionally just a symptom of psychosis of a paranoid type. This psychiatric entity rests upon a basis of unsatisfied affection associated with a rebellious tendency.

Therapy. Hospitalization frequently necessary, especially if patient becomes actively aggressive.

Prognosis. Pure form chronic, stable, and persistently vehement. Persists usually for many years. When their approaches have been rejected, patients may become aggressive against victim or relatives.

BIBLIOGRAPHY. De Clérambault GG: Les Psychoses Passionelles; Oevre psychiatrique. Paris, Presses Universitaires, 1942

Enoch MO, Trethowan WH, Barker JC: Some Uncommon Psychiatric Syndromes. Baltimore, Williams & Wilkins, 1967

DEFECATION SYNCOPE

Symptoms and Signs. In elderly. Usually after arising from bed at night or during disimpaction. Frequently associated AV block, sinus bradycardia.

Etiology. Sudden decompression of rectum.

Diagnostic Procedures. *Electrocardiography. Valsalva maneuver.* May reproduce syncope. *X-ray of chest* (to exclude pulmonary embolism).

Prognosis. Good. Related to basic condition.

BIBLIOGRAPHY. Pathy MS: Defecation syncope. Age Ageing 7:233–238, 1978

DEFIBRINATING

Synonyms. Consumption coagulopathy; defibrination; disseminated intravascular coagulation. Compared with congenital hypofibrinogenemia or afibrinogenemia, deficiency of fibrinogen may develop in many pathologic conditions. The hemorrhages and bleeding tendency becoming a dramatic feature of the following conditions:
1. High hematocrit and inadequate fibrinogen to form good clot
   Cyanotic congenital heart disease
   Vaquez-Osler
2. Impaired synthesis of fibrinogen
   Hepatic diseases (rare)
   Amyloidosis
3. Excessive utilization and secondary general deficiency
   Massive venous thrombosis

De Gimard's
Moschcowitz's
Waterhouse-Friderichsen
Giant cavernous hemangioma
Incompatible blood administration
Abruptio placenta
Dead fetus
Septic abortion
Amniotic fluid
Neoplastic diseases—hypofibrinogenemia
Extracorporeal circulation
4. Fibrinolysis
   Primary form (hyperplasminemia)
   Iatrogenic (administration of plasminogen activator). Endogenous release (surgery of lung; prostate; brain, neoplasm)
   Deficiency inhibitors (liver disease)
   Other proteolytic enzymes (leukemias)
   Secondary (association of defibrination and fibrinolysis)
   Placenta previa
   Dead fetus
   Amniotic fluid
   De Gimard's
   Lymphomas
   Leukemias
   Kasabach-Merritt
   Waterhouse-Friderichsen
   Overwhelming infections
See individual syndromes for symptoms, signs, and therapy.

BIBLIOGRAPHY. Fletcher AP, Alkjaersig N, Sherry S: Pathogenesis of the coagulation defect developing during pathological plasma proteolytic (fibrinolytic) states. I. The significance of fibrinogen proteolysis and circulating fibrinogen breakdown products. J Clin Invest 41:896–916, 1962

Sharp AA: Pathological fibrinolysis. Br Med Bull 20:240–245, 1964

Wintrobe MM (ed): Clinical Hematology, 8th ed. Philadelphia, Lea & Febiger, 1981

DE GIMARD'S

Synonyms. De Gimard's; purpura gangrenosa hemorrhagica; purpura fulminans; Sheldon's.

Symptoms and Signs. Appear most often in children, in association with various infections (viral, streptococcal) or with pregnancy; sudden onset. Fever; prostration; diffuse skin ecchymosis; no involvement of mucosae; gangrene may rapidly occur. In childhood gangrene and auto amputation of distal extremities, bleeding (gastrointestinal and CNS).

Etiology. *Neisseria meningitidis* infection in children with immature protein C and S systems that causes dermal microvascular thrombosis.

Pathology. In addition to hemorrhagic manifestation (Schwartzmann type reaction in the skin), extensive intravascular thrombosis may occur.

Diagnostic Procedures. *Blood.* Usually, no abnormal coagulation; however, in some cases, deficiency of factor V, excess antithrombin, hypofibrinogenemia.

Therapy. Treatment of infection; general supportive treatment; heparin; fibrinogen; hyperbaric oxygenation.

Prognosis. Rapid, fatal course of 1 to 4 days.

BIBLIOGRAPHY. De Gimard M: Purpura hemorrhagique primitif au purpura infectieux primitif (thesis). Paris, 1844

Sheldon JH: Purpura neonatica. A possible clinical application of the Schwartzman phenomenon. Arch Dis Child 22:7–13, 1947

Marcinia KE, Wilson HD, Marlar RA: Neonatal purpura fulminans: A genetic disorder related to the absence of protein C in blood. Blood 65:15–20, 1985

DEGOS' ACANTHOMA

Synonym. Clear cell acanthoma.

Symptoms and Signs. Both sexes affected; onset from middle age. Single or multiple lesions formed by brown plaques, marginated, reddish, scaly, occurring mostly on limbs.

Etiology. Unknown.

Pathology. Acanthosis and papillomatosis with cells with clear cytoplasm and infiltration by granulocytes.

Diagnostic Procedures. *Biopsy.*

Therapy. Excision.

Prognosis. No recurrence after excision.

BIBLIOGRAPHY. Degos R, Dehort J, Civatte J, et al: Epidermal tumour with an usual appearance: Clear cell acanthoma. Ann Dermatol Syph 9:361–371, 1962

Rook A, Wilkinson DS, Ebling FJG, et al: Textbook of Dermatology, 4th ed, pp 2393–2395. Oxford, Blackwell Scientific Publications, 1986

DEJANS'

Synonym. Orbital floor.

Symptoms and Signs. Intense pain in superior maxillary region; hypoesthesia and paresthesia in area of first and second branch of trigeminal (V) nerve; exophthalmos; diploplia.

Etiology. Any lesion (*e.g.,* infection; tumor) involving floor of orbit.

Pathology. See Etiology.

Diagnostic Procedures. *X-ray of skull. Cultures.*

Therapy. Depends on etiology.

Prognosis. Extension of lesion to cranial cavity may occur.

BIBLIOGRAPHY. DeJans MC: Le syndrome du plancher de l'orbite. Bull Mem Soc Fr Ophthalmol 48:473–485, 1935

Adams RD, Victor M: Principles of Neurology, 3rd ed, p 503. New York, McGraw-Hill, 1985

DEJERINE-KLUMPKE'S

Synonyms. Brachial plexus neuritis; lower radicular; Klumpke's; paralysis brachial plexus.

Symptoms. Pain; hyperesthesia or lack of sensation on medial side of arm; weakness and then paralysis of hand. Disturbed vision.

Signs. Atrophy of interossei, thenar, hypothenar, flexor carpi ulnaris, flexor digitorum muscles; sensory changes ulnar side of arm. Enophthalmos; myosis, narrowed palpebral fissure; hemifacial sweating (Horner's).

Etiology. Lesion affecting inner cord of brachial plexus (eighth cervical to first thoracic) and sympathetic fibers. Infection and tumor (50%); trauma (50%).

Therapy. Depends on etiology.

Prognosis. Depends on etiology.

BIBLIOGRAPHY. Klumpke A: Contribution à l'étude des paralysies radiculaires du plexus brachial; paralysies radiculaires totales; paralysies radiculaires inférieures; de la participation des filets sympathiques oculopupillaires dans ces paralysies. Rev Med (Paris) 5:591–616; 739–790, 1885

Bauer J: Letter-Augusta Dejerine-Klumpke (Historical review). Ann Intern Med 81:128, 1974

Adams RD, Victor M: Principles of Neurology, 3rd ed, p 995. New York, McGraw-Hill, 1985

DEJERINE'S "ONION PEEL SENSORY LOSS"

Symptoms. Sensory loss starting from mouth and nose and extending concentrically outward: "onion peel distribution."

Etiology. Lesions of medulla oblongata affecting the trigeminal (V) nerve centers.

BIBLIOGRAPHY. Déjérine J: Semiologie des Affections du Systeme Nerveux. Paris, Masson, 1914

DEJERINE'S RADICULAR

Eponym indicating the radicular pain and motor, sensorial, and trophic changes in areas of distribution of nerves compressed or irritated by any cause, mechanical (see Discogenic syndromes) or inflammatory, at nerve root site within dural cavity. To be differentiated from peripheral neuritis.

BIBLIOGRAPHY. Déjérine J: Semiologie des Affections du Systeme Nerveux. Paris, Masson, 1914

DEJERINE-ROUSSY

Synonyms. Thalamic hyperesthetic anesthesia; posterior thalamic; retrolenticular; thalamic.

Symptoms and Signs. Complete hemianesthesia (contralateral to site of lesion), involving superficial, deep, and stereognostic sensations (face often spared). Threshold for stimuli raised considerably, but when sensation is elicited, intense and unpleasant reaction. Cold in particular elicits strong reaction, often accompanied by violent motor reaction. Passive movements and position apperception decreased or absent. Thalamic hyperpathia or phenomenon of central pain due to unappreciated stimuli or central thalamic lesions. Occasionally, temporary flaccid hemiplegia or hemiparesis; hemitaxia with choreoathetoid movements and dysarthria; emotional overreactions.

Etiology. Thrombosis of thalamogeniculate artery, neoplastic lesion affecting nucleus ventralis posterolateralis of thalamus. May occur also with lesion of the white matter of parietal lobe.

Pathology. Edema; hemorrhagic softening of thalamus unilateral.

Therapy. General; symptomatic care. Amitriptyline, imipramine, thioridazine, fluphenazine. Surgery last resort since increases the sensory defect.

Prognosis. Progressive to complete loss of position hemibody. Relieved occasionally by surgery of frontal lobe.

BIBLIOGRAPHY. Déjérine J, Roussy G: Le syndrome thalamique. Rev Neurol (Paris) 14:521–532, 1906
Adams RD, Victor M: Principles of Neurology, 3rd ed, pp 110–111. New York, McGraw-Hill, 1985

DEJERINE-SOTTAS

Synonyms. Gombault's; interstitial hypertrophic radiculoneuropathy; hypertrophic interstitial infantile neuritis; hypertrophic interstitial neuritis. Hypertrophic neuropathy Déjérine-Thomas. See Roussy-Levy; Charcot-Marie-Tooth, Roussy-Cornie.

Symptoms. Onset in infancy or early adolescence. Weakness and atrophy beginning in lower extremities and later spreading to upper ones (resembling Charchot-Marie-Tooth). Marked sensory loss in all four extremities; incoordination of arms.

Signs. Kyphoscoliosis; clubfoot; fasciculation; areflexia; Romberg's sign; miosis; nystagmus; increase in size of nerve trunks.

Etiology. Unknown; possibly includes different entities; considerable difference in inheritance reported in various groups. Recessive and dominant types. Autosomal dominant inheritance.

Pathology. Hypertrophic neuropathy (onion bulb formation in histology).

Diagnostic Procedures. *Laboratory.* Negative. *Spinal fluid.* (In some groups of patients, increase of protein.) *Biopsy of nerve.* See Pathology. *Electromyography.*

Therapy. None.

Prognosis. Progressive condition; death from complication in third to fourth decade.

BIBLIOGRAPHY. Déjérine J, Sottas S: Sur la névrite interstitielle, hypertrophique et progressive de l'enfant. CR Soc Biol 2:43–53, 1890
Mongia SK, Ghanem Q, Preston D et al: Dominantly inherited hypertrophic neuropathy. J Can Sci Neurol 5:239–246, 1978

DEJERINE-THOMAS

Synonyms. Presenile ataxia; olivopontocerebellar; pontooliivocerebellar. See Friedreich's ataxia and Menzel's.

Symptoms. Onset in middle life or later. Progressive ataxia of extremity and trunk. Dysarthria; oscillation of head and body. Mental deterioration. Later sphincters affected.

Signs. Wavering gait; rigidity and extrapyramidal signs; nystagmus; deep reflexes exaggerated; Babinski sign.

Etiology. Unknown.

Pathology. Atrophy of cortex of cerebellum, olivary, pontine, and arcuate nuclei, middle cerebellar peduncle.

Diagnostic Procedures. *Cerebrospinal fluid.* Increase in pressure.

Therapy. Symptomatic.

Prognosis. Progression in 5 to 10 years to total incapacitation. Death from intercurrent diseases.

BIBLIOGRAPHY. Déjérine J, Thomas A: L'atrophie olivo-ponto-cérébelleuse. Nov Iconog Salpêt 13:330–370, 1900

Geary JR, Earll KM, Rose AS: Olivopontocerebellar atrophy. Neurology 6:218–224, 1956

Adams RD, Victor M: Principles of Neurology, 3rd ed, p 988. New York, McGraw-Hill, 1985

DE LANGE'S I

Synonyms. Amstelodamensis typus degenerativus; Amsterdam dwarfism; Brachmann-de Lange; Cornelia De Lange's I.

Symptoms and Signs. *Skin.* Hirsutism of face; forehead; back cutis marmorata; perioral pale cyanosis. *Head.* Brachycephaly or microbrachycephaly. *Eyebrows.* Long, usually meeting on midline. *Eyes.* Extropia, usually alternating. *Ears.* Low set. *Nose.* Small, upturned. *Mouth.* Widely spaced teeth; upper lip small midline beak; lower lip corresponding notch, angles downward. *Arms.* Limited extension at the elbow. *Hands.* Simian crease; thumb proximally inserted or absent; fingers small, incurved; some rudimentary or absent. Difference between two hands. *Feet.* Syndactyly, partial or total. *Other.* Mental retardation, limited vocabulary or no speech. Walking possible with assistance or alone. Development and weight gain markedly impaired. Epilepsy (20%). Congenital heart defect (17%).

Etiology. Unknown; discussed genetic basis probably autosomal dominant inheritance. (In some cases chromosomal abnormalities have been reported: apparent translocation of major portion of one chromosome of G group to chromosome A_3 and other group alterations.) Environmental damage during gestation excluded.

Pathology. See Signs. Developmental anomalies of brain; microcephaly and convolutional distortion; abnormality of gastrointestinal system; occasionally, cardiac malformations.

Diagnostic Procedures. *Chromosome study. Blood, urine, and cerebrospinal fluid.* Usually normal. *Nitrogen balance study, basal metabolic rate.* Usually normal; paradoxically with the severe growth failure. *Endocrinologic studies.* For possible associated defect and differential diagnosis.

Therapy. Symptomatic.

Prognosis. Progressive condition. Intestinal obstruction, infections, complication often cause of death.

BIBLIOGRAPHY. De Lange C: Sur un type nouveau de dégénération (typus Amstelodamensis). Arch Med Enfant 36:713–719, 1933

Hawley PP, Jackson LG, Kurnit DM: Sixty-four patients with Brachmann-De Lange syndrome: A survey. Am J Med Genet 20:453–459, 1985

DE LANGE'S III

Synonyms. Muscular dystrophy, congenital, rapid progression. See Bruck-De Lange, floppy infant, and Oppenheim's.

Symptoms. Both sexes affected; present at birth. Muscular weakness involving arms and legs equally; neck muscle most severely affected so that patients cannot raise head. Weakness also involves facial, extraocular, and oropharyngeal muscles. Contractures develop readily.

Signs. Tendon reflexes decreased or absent. Severe muscle wasting. No neurologic defect or pseudohypertrophy.

Etiology. Unknown; autosomal recessive inheritance.

Pathology. In muscle, variation in fiber size, central nuclei; nuclear proliferation; phagocytosis; degeneration of fibers; no attempt to regeneration; marked fibrosis.

Diagnostic Procedures. *Blood.* Slight to moderate elevation in serum aldolase, creatin phosphokinase; serum glutamic-oxaloacetic transaminase (SGOT), lactic dehydrogenase (LDH). *Biopsy of muscle. Electromyography.*

Therapy. None.

Prognosis. Stationary course. All patients reported died (a few months after birth to 13 yr), generally from respiratory infections.

BIBLIOGRAPHY. De Lange C: Studien uber angeborene Lähmungen bzw. Angeborene Hypotonie. Acta Paediatr (Scand) 20:1–51, 1937

Zellweger H, Afifi A, McCormick WF: Severe congenital muscular dystrophy. Am J Dis Child 114:591–602, 1967

DEL CASTILLO'S

Synonyms. Germinal aplasia; testicular dysgenesis; Sertoli cell only. See Male pseudohermaphrodism, incomplete hereditary (Type I).

Symptoms. Sterility; normal libido and erection.

Signs. Normally developed man with all secondary sexual characteristics; testis small or normal.

Etiology. Either X-linked inheritance or male limited autosomal dominant or recessive inheritance has been proposed. The same findings observed after exposure to radiation.

Pathology. Seminiferous tubules with Sertoli cells; little or absent tubular fibrosis; no germinal cells. Leydig cells normal.

Diagnostic Procedures. *Sperm count.* Low. *Urine.* Decreased 17-ketosteroids; normal FSH hormone.

Therapy. None.

Prognosis. When due to radiation, damage may be reversible.

BIBLIOGRAPHY. Del Castillo E, Trabucco A, de la Balze FA: Syndrome produced by absence of germinal epithelium without impairment of Sertoli or Leydig cells. J Clin Endocrinol 7:493–502, 1947

Chaganti RSK, Jhanwar SC, Ehrenbard LT, et al: Genetically determined asynapsis, spermatogenic degeneration and infertility in men. Am J Hum Genet 32:833–848, 1980

DEMARQUAY'S

Synonyms. Demarquay-Richet; cleft lip–palate; lip pit–cleft palate; Van der Woude's.

Symptoms and Signs. No sex predominance or limitation; very rare (1 : 75,000–1 : 100,000). Fistulas of lower lip appearing as pits or humps on vermillion part of lip, usually equidistant from midline, or, occasionally, with different degrees of asymmetry. Different depths of depression; usually asymptomatic or secreting small amount of saliva. All types of clefts. Some members of family may have double lower lip only. Association with other malformations found: anomalies of extremities; popliteal pterygia; anomalies of genitourinary tract.

Etiology. Unknown; autosomal dominant inheritance with variable expressivity of the trait; high degree of penetrance (80%). Pits expressed more frequently than clefts.

Pathology. Fistula lined by stratified squamous epithelium; large epithelial cells with small nuclei also found. Serous acini and mucous acini may be present.

Therapy. Surgical excision; correction of cleft.

BIBLIOGRAPHY. Demarquay JN: Quelques considerations sur le bec-de-lievre. Gaz Med Paris 13:52–54, 1845

Van der Woude A: Fistula labii inferioris congenita and its association with cleft lip and palate. Am J Hum Genet 6:244–256, 1954

Burdick AB, Bixler D, Puckett CL: Genetic analysis in families with Van der Woude syndrome. J Craniofac Genet Dev Biol 5:181–208, 1985

DEMENTIA PARALYTICA

Synonyms. General paralysis of the insane; paretic neurosyphilis; general paresis; syphilitic paresis.

Symptoms. Combination of psychotic and neurologic symptoms: *Psychotic.* Demented; expansive; agitated; depressive, with possible variation and interlacing of manifestations in same individual. First symptoms, usually, impairment of efficiency and disorientation, memory failure, dreamlike activity, delusional states, emotional changes, defect in judgment. Patient usually does not worry over his condition. *Neurologic.* Headache; body pains; vague muscle weakness; hyporeactive midriasis or Argyll Robertson's (see); variable reflex changes; slurred speech; tremor; Lissauer's paralysis (see).

Etiology. Late form of syphilis.

Pathology. Leptomeninges cloudy, thickened, arachnoid adherent to pia; atrophy of brain with hydrocephalus *ex vacuo;* infiltration of leptomeninx greatest at frontal pole, extending into cortex and into adventitial spaces; increased iron content of brain; involvement of ganglion cells (degeneration); glia increased; presence of free spirochetes.

Diagnostic Procedures. *Spinal fluid.* Positive serologic tests; increased (monocytic) cells and proteins. *Blood.* Serologic tests. *CT brain scan.* Brain shrinkage.

Therapy. Penicillin. Symptomatic and nursing care.

Prognosis. Progressive course. Death in 3 years; delayed by prompt and full treatment.

BIBLIOGRAPHY. Adams RD, Victor M: Principles of Neurology, 3rd ed, pp 532–533. New York, McGraw-Hill, 1985

DE MORGAN'S

Synonyms. Capillary angioma; senile angioma; cayenne pepper spots; rub spots; papillary varix. Teleagiectasias, spider angiomas.

Symptoms and Signs. Elderly persons affected; occasionally appear in younger people. Predominantly affect face and ears. Small, red masses, not branching, of dilated vascular loops.

Etiology. Unknown; immunologic reaction considered. Dilatation of venules.

Pathology. Dilated, thin-walled venules, without vascular tissue proliferation; decrease of elastic tissue in layers of corium.

Therapy. None.

Prognosis. Persistent and progressive condition.

BIBLIOGRAPHY. De Morgan C: The Origin of Cancer. Considered with Reference to the Treatment of the Disease. London, Churchill, 1872
Bean WB: Vascular Spiders and Related Lesions of the Skin. Springfield, CC Thomas, 1958

DE MORSIER'S I

Synonyms. Acromegalo-epileptic; epiletic-endocrine; Morsier I.

Symptoms. Appear in first decade of life. Seizures or other epileptic manifestations (spasm, myoclonus). Mental deterioration; precocious puberty.

Signs. Accelerated growth and weight increase; acromegalic aspect in some cases. All signs of precocious sexual development.

Etiology and Pathology. Possible causes: infundibular, mammilary, or epiphyseal tumors, inflammatory lesions with meningoencephalitis; traumatic lesions.

Diagnostic Procedures. *Electroencephalography.* Pattern consistent with subcortical deep lesion. *CT brain scan. Pituitary hormonal excretion studies.*

Therapy. That of the type of epilepsy.

Prognosis. Poor; mental deterioration constant feature.

BIBLIOGRAPHY. De Morsier G: Pathologie du diencéphale. Les syndromes psicologiques et syndromes sensorio-moteurs. Schweiz Arch Neurol Psychiatr 54:161–226, 1944
Bondin G, Barbizet J: D'association epilepsieendocrinopathie. Rev Neurol (Paris) 91:330–347, 1954
De Morsier G: Contribution à l'étude clinique des altérations de la formation réticulée: Le syndrome sensoriomoteur et psychologique. J Neurol Sci 4:15–49, 1966
Kohler MC: L'association comitialité, croissance excessive et puberté précoce, arrieration mentale, une forme particuliere de séquelles d'encéphalopathies ou d'encéphalite infantile. J Med Lyon 48:1437–1530, 1967

DENIAL

Symptoms. Patient denies objective deficits, such as blindness, paralysis, speech defects (see Anton's and Cotard's). When confronted with evidence, vigorously denies that affected part (*e.g.*, extremities) belongs to him.

Etiology. Disturbed psychology related to personality changes, usually due to structural brain damage.

DENNIE-MARFAN

Synonyms. Paralysis, congenital syphilitic; juvenile paresis; syphilitic congenital paralysis. See Hutchinson's triad.

Symptoms and Signs. Both sexes affected; onset insidious or acute in infancy or childhood. Acute vomiting; fever; convulsions; loss of consciousness; spastic or flaccid tetraplegia; development of mental retardation. Insidious, slow progression from weakness to tetraparesis.

Etiology. Congenital syphilitic infection.

Pathology. Diffuse syphilitic lesions in brain, cerebellum, and spinal cord.

Diagnostic Procedures. *Blood. Spinal fluid. Serology. Electroencephalography.*

Therapy. Penicillin.

Prognosis. Locomotor symptoms recede with treatment. Mental retardation remains.

BIBLIOGRAPHY. Dennie C: Partial paralysis of the lower extremities in children accompanied by backward mental development. Am J Syph 13:157–163, 1929
Vick NA: Grinker's Neurology, 7th ed. Springfield, CC Thomas, 1976

DENNY-BROWN'S I

Synonyms. Carcinomatous neuromyopathy; myopathy–sensorial paraneoplastic neuropathy; paraneoplastic neuromyopathy.

Symptoms and Signs. Many neurologic syndromes (seldom in the pure form; usually in variable combinations) occur in patients with neoplastic diseases. Peripheral neuropathies; radiculopathies; posterior root degeneration; myelopathies; cerebellar degeneration; dementia. These syndromes can cause disability that is out of proportion to the neoplastic condition and thus dominates the clinical aspect. In addition, neuromuscular involvement may precede the discovery of tumor.

Etiology. Unknown. Most tumors may be associated with these manifestations.

Therapy. Early surgery of neoplasia.

Prognosis. Early surgery may be extremely rewarding for the control of the paraneoplastic syndromes.

BIBLIOGRAPHY. Denny-Brown N: Primary sensory neuropathy with muscular changes by carcinoma. J Neurol 2:73–87, 1948
Tyler HR: Paraneoplastic syndromes of nerve, muscle and neuromuscular junction. NY Acad Sci 230:348–357, 1974
Adams RD, Victor M: Principles of Neurology, 3rd ed, p 980. New York, McGraw-Hill, 1985

DE QUERVAIN'S I

Synonyms. Congenital clasped thumb; flexor pollicis longus–stenosing tendovaginitis; pollex varus; Quervain's I; snapping thumb; trigger thumb.

Symptoms. More frequent in adults (prevalent in females) than in children (equal sex distribution); insidious onset. In adults, in addition to the thumb, other fingers may be involved; in children, limited to the thumb. Adult reports a snapping phenomenon in the distal interphalangeal joint. In children, mother reports that child has the thumb in fixed flexion.

Signs. Small nontender mass palpable at metacarpophalangeal articulation. Frequently, both thumbs present nodule also, if snapping phenomenon is present in only one hand.

Etiology. Congenital, traumatic, or both. Snapping caused by the passage of the bulbous tendon through narrowed sheath both in extension and flexion.

Pathology. Local thickening of tendon sheath. Microscopic inflammatory changes according to duration of condition.

Therapy. Surgery.

Prognosis. Complete correction by surgery.

BIBLIOGRAPHY. De Quervain F: Ueber eine Form von chronischer Tendovaginitis. Cor Bl Schweiz Arzte (Basel) 25:389–394, 1895
Hauck G: Ueber eine Tendovaginitis stenosans der Beugeschnenscheide mit dem Phanomen des schnellende Finger. Arch Klin Chir 123:233–258, 1923
Bollinger JA, Fahey JJ: Snapping thumb in infants and children. J Pediat 41:445–450, 1952

Weckesser EC, Reed JR, Heiple KG: Congenital clasped thumb (congenital flexion-adduction deformity of the thumb): A syndrome, not a specific entity. J Bone Joint Surg [Am] 50:1417–1428, 1968
Milford L: Carpal tunnel and ulnar tunnel syndrome. In Crenshaw AH (ed): Campbell's Operative Orthopedics, 7th ed, pp 462–463. St. Louis, CV Mosby, 1987

DE QUERVAIN'S II

Synonyms. Giant cell thyroiditis; granulomatous thyroiditis; pseudotuberculous thyroiditis; acute nonsuppurative thyroiditis; subacute thyroiditis; Quervain's.

Symptoms. More common in middle-aged women; onset dramatic, often after infection of respiratory tract. Hyperthermia; sweating; malaise; agitation; diffuse myalgia; cephalalgia; pain in thyroid area radiating to ear or face; dysphagia.

Signs. Moderate enlargement and tenderness of thyroid. Tachycardia.

Etiology. Unknown. Viral infection and autoimmune nature considered possibilities.

Pathology. Thyroid enlarged, firm, pale; capsule not involved. *Histology.* Inflammatory changes, fibrous scarring. Presence of pseudotubercles (clusters of fibroblasts, lymphocyte macrophages, plasma cells, arranged around giant cells) among normal tissue.

Diagnostic Procedures. *Blood.* Leukocytosis or normal white blood cell count; increased erythrocyte sedimentation rate; moderate increase of protein-bound iodine level. *Basal metabolic rate.* Normal. *Thyroid scan.* Typical reduction of iodine uptake. *Biopsy.* See Pathology. *Fine needle aspiration.*

Therapy. Rest. Analgesics and anti-inflammatory agents. For severe symptoms, short trials with corticosteroid (3 wk). For refractory form roentgen treatment of thyroid area (300–400 r) advised by some authors.

Prognosis. Usually, spontaneous regression with possible relapses of decreasing intensity.

BIBLIOGRAPHY. De Quervain F: Ueber acute, nicht eiterige Thyroiditis. Arch Klin Chir 67:706–714, 1902
Magalini SI, Pericoli F: La tiroidite subacuta: Osservazione su alcuni aspetti ematochimici e coagulativi. Minerva Med 2:2–16, 1955
Hamburger JI: The various presentation of thyroiditis: Diagnostic considerations. Ann Intern Med 104:219–221, 1986

DERCUM'S

Synonyms. Anders'; adiposis dolorosa; fibrolipomatosis dolorosa; lipalgia; lipomatosis dolorosa.

Symptoms. Prevalent in women 40 to 60 years of age. Pain in part of body where localized accumulation of fat occurs. Asthenia; headache; frequently amenorrhea and ecchymoses; diminution of sweating; terminally, mental depression and deterioration.

Signs. Subcutaneous accumulation of elevated, dry, reddish or bluish fat; anesthesia and diminished cutaneous sensibility.

Etiology. Unknown; autonomous existence of clinical entity is doubted. Considered as part of generalized obesity.

Pathology. Multiple, nodular subcutaneous fat accumulation and degeneration.

Diagnostic Procedures. Nonspecific.

Therapy. Weight reduction, excision of tumors, lidocaine intravenously.

Prognosis. Long progressive course. Cardiac failure often terminal episode.

BIBLIOGRAPHY. Dercum FX: Three cases of an hitherto unclassified affection resembling in its grosser aspects obesity, but associated with special nervous symptoms, adiposis dolorosa. Am J Med Sci 104:521–535, 1892
Joseph HL: Adiposis dolorosa (Dercum's disease). Arch Dermatol 74:332, 1956
Rook A, Wilkinson DS, Ebling FJG, et al: Textbook of Dermatology, 4th ed, p 1872. Oxford, Blackwell Scientific Publications, 1986

DERMAL ERYTHROPOIESIS

Synonyms. Erythropoiesis, dermic; dermic erythropoiesis.

Symptoms and Signs. Appear in newborn. Generalized hemorrhagic-purpuric rash. Individual lesions 2 to 7 mm in diameter, raised dark blue magenta, slowly regressing and disappearing in 3 to 4 weeks. Hepatomegaly; splenomegaly; jaundice (not constant); lymphadenopathy.

Etiology. Associated with intrauterine viral infections; cytomegalovirus demonstrated in some cases; rubella strongly considered in other cases.

Pathology. *Skin.* Poorly delimited aggregates of large nucleated cells; erythroblasts in different stages of maturation from normoblast to orthochromatic erythroblast, and nonnucleated erythrocytes. Absence of myeloid elements, megakaryocytes, and lymphocytes. Erythroblast plaques present exclusively in extravascular sites. Other pathologic findings consistent with cytomegalic infections or other virus infection. (*e.g.,* hepatitis, encephalitis). Various congenital malformations.

Diagnostic Procedures. *Blood.* Anemia; reticulocytosis; thrombocytopenia; hyperbilirubinemia. *Virus cultures. Biopsy of liver by needle.*

Therapy. Symptomatic.

Prognosis. Rash completely disappears in 3 to 4 weeks. Life expectancy depends on associated pathologic involvement and malformations.

BIBLIOGRAPHY. Dieterich H: Studien uber extramedullare Blutbildung bei chirugichen Erkrankungen. Arch Klin Chir 134:166–175, 1925
Brough AJ, Jones D, Page RH, et al: Dermal erythropoiesis in neonatal infants. Pediatrics 40:627–635, 1967

DERMATITIS ARTEFACTA

Synonyms. Factitial dermatitis; neurotic excoriation. See Purpura, psychogenic.

Symptoms. Prevalent in adolescent women or young adults; rare in children, except if mental retardation is present; connected with malingering for reluctant induction in armed services or for insurance claims. Peculiar patient demeanor. Strong denial of self-infliction of lesions and display of ingenuity and cunning. Complaint of unusual sensation in the skin.

Signs. Cutaneous lesions that widely vary in configuration and distribution, usually localized in areas easily reached by patient's hands. Pattern of lesion does not conform with known pathologic process.

Etiology. Hysterical derangement; calls attention to patient or compensates for psychological disturbance, inferiority complex, lack of sexual satisfaction, or malingering.

Pathology. Acute or chronic inflammation resulting from nail, glass fragments or knife scratching, caustic application, cigarette burning.

Diagnostic Procedures. Differential diagnosis with polyarteritis nodosa (see) and porphyria tarda (see). Once nature of lesions is suspected, firm dressing and supervision.

Therapy. Psychiatric treatment.

Prognosis. In cases where the simple basic emotional problem is identified the situation can be cured. Generally expression of deep disturbance bodes poor prognosis.

BIBLIOGRAPHY. Freedman AM, Kaplan HI, Sadock BJ: Comprehensive Textbook of Psychiatry, 2nd ed. Baltimore, Williams & Wilkins, 1975

Rook A, Wilkinson DS, Ebling FJG, et al: Textbook of Dermatology, 4th ed, pp 2262–2264. Oxford, Blackwell Scientific Publications, 1986

DERMATITIS, RADIATION

Synonyms. Radiodermatitis; roentgen poikiloderma; roentgen atrophy. Two forms are recognized: Acute form and chronic form.

ACUTE
Symptoms and Signs. The course is divided into four phases:
1. Erythema and edema of exposed areas that progress for 48 hours and then rapidly subside.
2. Absence of symptoms and signs for 1 to 4 days.
3. Erythema with occasional blood extravasation into involved areas; progressive formation of vesicles and bullae; after third week after exposure bullae dessicate and desquamate.
4. Regression of signs; however, areas greatly injured do not heal.

Etiology. Exposure to roentgen rays.

Pathology. In acute stage, hydropic alterations in epidermis. In dermis, inflammatory infiltrates, edema, homogenization of collagen bundles.

Therapy. Corticosteroids for topical and systemic use.

Prognosis. According to intensity of exposure.

CHRONIC
Symptoms and Signs. Slow progressive formation of telangiectasis, pigmentation, atrophy, and finally ulceration of areas exposed.

Etiology. Repeated, small doses of x-rays.

Pathology. Atrophy, hyperplasia, and finally neoplasia, involving all skin components.

Therapy. Small areas can be excised and grafts applied.

Prognosis. Malignant incidence between 10% and 28%.

BIBLIOGRAPHY. Rook A, Wilkinson DS, Ebling FJG, et al: Textbook of Dermatology, 4th ed, pp 653–654. Oxford, Blackwell Scientific Publications, 1986

DERRY'S

Synonyms. Generalized gangliosidosis type 2; gangliosidosis type 2 GM1; juvenile GM gangliosidosis type 2.

Symptoms. Both sexes affected; onset in early infancy (at 6–20 mo). Locomotor ataxia present from 1 year of age. Internal strabismus; loss of coordinated movements and speech; weakness of extremities, then spasticity; mental and motor deterioration up to lethargy; startle response to sound; seizures; late blindness; recurrent respiratory infections.

Signs. Normal facies. Macrocephaly. This type of gangliosidosis does *not* have facial and peripheral edema, hepatosplenomegaly, macular cherry spot, and macroglossia.

Etiology. Autosomal recessive inheritance. Enzyme defect: acid beta galactosidase deficiency; difference in residual enzyme activity could explain the phenotypic difference between types 1 and 2, rate of storage in type 2 being slower. Defect on chromosome 3.

Pathology. Neuronal lipoidosis and renal epithelial ballooning similar to type 1; visceral histocytosis not as pronounced.

Diagnostic Procedures. *Blood.* Vacuolated lymphocytes. *Bone marrow.* Foamy cells and vacuolated lymphocytes. *Urine.* Moderate amount of mucopolysaccharide; assay of beta-galactosidase. *X-rays.* Mild changes of long bones; vertebral beaking; modeling deformity of pelvis. *Fibroblast culture.* Assay of beta-galactosidase.

Therapy. None.

Prognosis. Death at 3 to 10 years of age, usually from overwhelming infection.

BIBLIOGRAPHY. Derry DM: Late infantile systemic lipidosis: Delineation of two types. Neurology 18:340–348, 1968

O'Brien JS: The Gangliosidosis. In Stanbury JB, Wyngaarden JB, Fredrickson DS, et al: The Metabolic Basis of Inherited Disease, 5th ed, p 945. New York, McGraw-Hill, 1983

DE SANCTIS-CACCHIONE

Synonyms. Xerodermic idiocy; xeroderma pigmentosum–idiocy. Xeroderma pigmentosum types A, B, D, and G. See Kaposi's II.

Symptoms and Signs. Both sexes affected; onset in infancy or early childhood. *Dermatologic.* Lentigines and areas of pigmentation. Manifestations of xeroderma pigmentosum are dependent on age and environment (sun sensitivity). Skin tumor, usually basal and squamous cell carcinoma and, less frequently, malignant melanoma. *Neurologic.* Microcephaly; speech disorders; mental deficiency; spastic paralysis; convulsions. *Ocular.* Photophobia; keratitis; ectropion. *Endocrine.* Stunted growth; gonadal hypoplasia. *TYPE A.* Classical form of the syndrome with all the above described characteristics. *TYPE B.* Symptoms of XP and Cockayne's syndrome (see). *TYPE D.* Neurologic symptoms develop in later life than in group A. *TYPE G.* All signs but no development of tumors.

Etiology. Autosomal recessive inheritance. Affected children are unable to repair DNA damaged by ultraviolet light and are sensitive to light in the wavelength range of 280 to 310 nm (UVB). Defective capacity of performing excision repair of damaged DNA at pyrimidine dimers because of enzyme deficiencies. The various forms all have different enzymatic alterations in that fibroblasts from one group of patients may correct defects of another group of patients when hybridized.

Pathology. Disturbances of pigmentation and maturation of epidermal cells, resulting eventually in malignant transformation, basal and squamous cell, and melanoma. Small brain; gliosis; loss of neurons.

Diagnostic Procedures. *Biopsy of skin. Electroencephalography.* Abnormalities. *X-ray of skull.* Extremely small sella turcica. *Urine.* Occasionally, porphyrinuria. *Cell culture study. CT brain scan.*

Therapy. Surgical excision of lesions that show neoplastic changes. Grafting of skin from non-light-exposed areas; topical antimitotic agents (5-fluorouracil).

Prognosis. When the condition shows the neoplastic tendency, poor. Affected families should have genetic counseling. The defect is detectable in cells cultured from amniotic fluid, so amniocentesis can provide an early diagnosis during pregnancy.

BIBLIOGRAPHY. Pick FJ: Ueber Melanosis lenticularis progressiva. Vschratol Derm Syph 11:3–32, 1884

DeSanctis C, Cacchione A: L'idiozia xerodermica. Riv Sper Freniat 56:269–292, 1932

Robbins JH, Kraemer KH, Lutzner MA et al: Xeroderma pigmentosum: An inherited disease with sun sensitivity, multiple cutaneous neoplasms and abnormal DNA repair. Ann Intern Med 80:221–248, 1974

Cleaver JE: Xeroderma pigmentosum. In Stanbury JB, Wyngaarden JB, Fredrickson DS, et al: The Metabolic Basis of Inherited Disease, 5th ed, p 1227. New York, McGraw-Hill, 1983

DE SOUZA'S

Synonym. Amyloidosis, cutaneous bullous.

Symptoms and Signs. One family reported. One male, three females. Onset between 10 and 13 years. Bullous lesions mainly around the joints.

Etiology. Autosomal recessive.

BIBLIOGRAPHY. De Souza AR: Amyloidoise cutanea bulhosa familial: Observacao de 4 casos. Rev Hosp Clin Fac Med Sao Paulo 18:413–417, 1963

DESQUAMATIVE INTERSTITIAL PNEUMONIA

Synonyms. DIP. See "Usual" interstitial pneumonia.

Symptoms. Prevalent in adults. In 50% of cases preceded by a nonspecific upper respiratory infection. Gradual onset of dypsnea, dry cough, weight loss, anorexia, and fatigability. Arthralgia and myalgia may be present.

Signs. Cyanosis (in half of adult patients); finger clubbing. Physical examination unrevealing.

Etiology. Unknown. Response to a variety of insults (*e.g.*, infections, drugs, and toxic agents). DIP is probably an early stage in the development of the more commonly observed UIP (Usual interstitial pneumonitis).

Pathology. Lungs diffusely nodular and stiff. Diffuse massive proliferation of alveolar lining cells; cell masses well preserved; some mitotic figures. Some containing PAS-positive, iron negative, golden brown pigment granules. Minimal interstitial inflammation; moderate thickening of alveolar septa; absence of necrosis; bronchioles normal. At the periphery of lung, small lymphoid center.

Diagnostic Procedures. *X-ray of chest.* Ground glass wedge-shaped opacity at the bases, radiating from hilus. Hilar adenopathy may be present. *Electrocardiography.* Right ventricular predominance. *Pulmonary function.* Hyperventilation; decreased arterial oxygen tension; elevated alveolar arterial oxygen gradient. *Biopsy of lung.* See Pathology.

Therapy. Corticosteroids.

Prognosis. Dramatic response to steroid treatment. Relapses follow withdrawal of treatment. Process generally irreversible, but more benign course than other chronic interstitial pneumonias. Over a period of 10 years after diagnosis, 16% mortality. In some cases, cure with complete reversibility and no sequelae.

BIBLIOGRAPHY. Liebow AA, Steer A, Billingsley JG: Desquamative interstitial pneumonia. Am J Med 39:369–404, 1965

Schneider RM, Nevius DB, Brown HZ: Desquamative interstitial pneumonia in a four-year-old child. N Engl J Med 277:1056–1058, 1967

Fraser RG, Paré JAP: Diagnosis of Diseases of the Chest, 2nd ed, p. 1695. Philadelphia, WB Saunders, 1977

DETERMANN'S

Synonyms. Angiosclerotic intermittent akinesia; angiosclerotic intermittent dyskinesia; angiosclerotic paroxysmal myasthenia. See Carotid system ischemia.

Symptoms. Transitory attacks of akinesia.

Etiology. Atherosclerosis. See Carotid artery system ischemia.

BIBLIOGRAPHY. Determann H: "Intermittierendes Hinken" eines Armes, der Zunge und der Beine (Dyskinesia intermittens angiosclerotica). Dtsch Z Nervenb 29:152–162, 1905

Vick NA: Grinker's Neurology, 7th ed. Springfield, CC Thomas, 1976

DEUTSCHLAENDER'S

Synonyms. March foot; march fracture.

Symptoms. Slow onset of mild, persistent pain in the foot while walking.

Signs. Tenderness on dorsum of foot; lump palpable in region of second or third metatarsal.

Etiology. Prolonged and repeated marches; inadequate footwear.

Pathology. Fracture of second or third metatarsal; formation of bone callus around fracture.

Diagnostic Procedures. *X-ray.* See Pathology.

Therapy. Rest. Change of footwear.

Prognosis. Good, if adequate treatment and possible avoidance of determining cause.

BIBLIOGRAPHY. Deutschlaender CW: Ueber entzuendliche Mittel-fussgeschmieleste. Arch Klin Chir 118:530–548, 1921

DE VAAL'S

Synonyms. Congenital aleukia; reticular dysgenesis; panaleukia. Hematopoietic hypoplasia.

Symptoms and Signs. Severe intractable infections in first few days of life.

Etiology. Unknown. Autosomal recessive inheritance proposed.

Pathology. *Thymus.* Represented by few immature lobules and fibrous connective tissue; absence of small lymphocytes; presence of so-called large lymphocytes, reticular cells; no differentiation between cortex and medulla in the lobules; Hassell's body absent. *Lymph nodes.* Slightly enlarged; formed by cells similar to the ones seen in the thymus and cells resembling plasma cells; few lymphocytes scattered at the periphery of nodes; no primary follicles and germinal centers. *Spleen.* Normal size; substitution of Malpighi's follicles by clear zones of reticular cells and plasma cell–like cells. Groups of cocci; absence of granulocytes. *Intestinal mucosa.* Accumulation of similar cells; small lymphocytes practically absent; granulocytes absent despite zones of ulcerations and erosion. *Bone marrow.* Complete absence of myeloid series; normal erythroid series and megakaryocytes; rarely, monocytes. *Other tissues.* Focal necrosis; groups of cocci, lack of granulocytes close to bacterial colonies.

Diagnostic Procedures. *Blood.* Complete agranulocytosis; only few large lymphocytes and monocytes.

Therapy. Antibiotics and symptomatic. Bone marrow transplantation.

Prognosis. Death within a few days after birth.

BIBLIOGRAPHY. De Vaal OM, Seynhaeve V: Reticular dysgenesia. Lancet 2:1123–1125, 1959

Gitlin D, Vawter G, Craig JM: Thymic alymphoplasia and congenital aleukocytosis. Pediatrics 33:184–192, 1964

Roper M, Parmley RT, Crist WM, et al: Severe congenital leukopenia (reticular dysgenesis): Immunologic and morphologic characterization of leukocytes. Am J Dis Child 138:832–835, 1985

DEVERGIE'S

Synonyms. Hebra's; Kaposi's IV; lichen ruber acuminatus; pityriasis rubra pilaris; Tarral-Besnier.

Symptoms. Both sexes affected; onset at any age. At onset, slight pruritus.

Signs. When it begins in early infancy, insidious appearance of signs; scaling of scalp and face; generalized erythema; reddening, thickening, and scaling of palms and soles; follicular papules firm and red, presenting a horny cap, especially on proximal phalanges, knees, and elbows, rare on limbs, and still less frequently on trunk; lesions may group into plaques. Almost all cases, however, begin after 15 years of age. Same signs as above, developing rapidly (in days) into follicular plaques (in weeks). Milder forms are common both in children and adults.

Etiology. *Infantile form.* Autosomal dominant heredity suggested. *Adult form.* No demonstration of genetic factors.

Pathology. The histologic changes are not characteristic: acanthosis; hyperkeratosis; cellular perinuclear vacuolization; mild secondary inflammatory alterations.

Diagnostic Procedures. *Biopsy of cutaneous lesions. Blood.* Decrease of vitamin A level (frequent). *Liver function tests.* Altered (in adult form).

Therapy. In adult form, recommended high doses of vitamin A for 2 months; if good results, continue administration. Addition of corticosteroids accelerates remission, especially of erythrodermic phase. Folic acid antagonists produce a temporary improvement; in mild cases, recommended topical application of vitamin A and keratolytic agents. In congenital forms, all therapeutic trials have little effect.

Prognosis. Course is variable. Hereditary type is less severe and manifestation may last for entire life; the acquired type is more severe; however, in some cases, complete remission may occur within months. Association with neuromuscular diseases has been reported. Severe forms may be associated with very low intelligence, requiring institutional care.

BIBLIOGRAPHY. Devergie MG: Pityriasis pilaris, maladie de la peau non décrite par les dermatologistes. Gaz Hebd Méd 3:197–201, 1856
Kaposi M: Lichen ruber acuminatus und Lichen ruber planus. Arch Dermatol Syph 31:1–32, 1895
Rook A, Wilkinson DS, Ebling FJG, et al: Textbook of Dermatology, 4th ed, pp 1445–1449. Oxford, Blackwell Scientific Publications, 1986

DEVIC'S

Synonyms. Devic-Gauld; optic myelitis neuritis; optic neuromyelitis; optic neuritis; ophthalmoneuromyelitis; ophthalmoencephalomyelitis, neuromyelytis optica.

Symptoms. Occur at any age; more common between 20 and 50 years of age. Nonspecific upper respiratory infection may precede neurologic manifestations. Acute loss of vision with central scotoma; rapidly progressing ascending myelitis with loss of sphincter control. Headache, consciousness changes, convulsion.

Etiology. Unknown; considered by some authors as manifestation of multiple sclerosis. Familial cases reported. Considered also as a particular clinical variation of Leber's I.

Pathology. Areas of softening in both white and grey matter in brain and spinal cord; axis cylinders destroyed; microglial response; mild leptomeningeal reaction. Complete necrosis and cavitation may be observed. Neuritis in optic nerve.

Diagnostic Procedures. *Cerebrospinal fluid.* Normal or protein elevation; increased lymphocytes; occasionally, spinal block. *Ophthalmoscopy.* Bilateral optic neuritis; from mild edema of optic disk to optic atrophy.

Therapy. General care; prevention of infection.

Prognosis. Variable from complete remission to repeated attacks with finally paraplegia and blindness, or vision recovery in about 50%, with variable impairment. Mortality 50%.

BIBLIOGRAPHY. Devic ME: Myélite subaigue compliquée de nérvite optique. Bull Med Par 8:1033, 1894
Gault F: De la neuromyélite optique aiguë (Thesis). Lyon, 1894
Lees, F, McDonald AME, Turner JWA: Leber's disease with symptoms resembling disseminated sclerosis. J Neurol Neurosurg Psychiatry 27:415–421, 1964
Chusid MJ, Williamson SJ, Murphy JV, et al: Neuromyelitis optica (Devic's disease) following varicella infection. J Pediatr 95:737–738, 1979

DIABETES, CHEMICAL

Absence of clinical findings of diabetes mellitus in patients who show altered glucose tolerance test, tolbutamide test, and other tests showing faulty insulin production or utilization.

DIABETES INSIPIDUS, NEUROHYPOPHYSEAL

Synonym. Neurohypophyseal diabetes insipidus.

Symptoms. Prevalent in males; onset usually at young age. Insatiable polydipsia; polyuria; pale urine, occasionally up to 15 to 30 liters a day. Dehydration; constipation.

Signs. Dryness of skin and mucosae.

Etiology. Lesion damaging structure of hypothalamic-neurohypophyseal tract; trauma; surgery; tumor; granulomas. Two inherited forms known: a sex-linked recessive and an autosomal dominant.

Pathology. Pathologic lesion according to cause (see Etiology). Secondary dilatation and hypertrophy of bladder with megaloureter.

Diagnostic Procedures. *Urine.* Low specific gravity. *X-ray of skull. CT brain scan. Spinal tap. Secretory function test.* Nicotine; hypertonic saline solution; vasopressin.

Therapy. Correction of determining cause, if possible. Replacement treatment with vasopressin (nasal insufflation, or intramuscular administration). Chlorothiazide or hydrochlorothiazide with vasopressin. Desaminocys-D-arginine-vasopressin (DDAVP).

Prognosis. Usually, condition lasts for life. Transient forms with spontaneous recovery are sometimes observed after trauma or neurosurgery. Development of resistance or allergy to vasopressin complicates treatment.

BIBLIOGRAPHY. Weil A: Veber die hereditaere Form des Diabetes insipidus. Virchows Arch Pathol Anat 95:70–95, 1884

Forssman H: On hereditary diabetes insipidus with special reference to a sex-linked form. Acta Med Scand 159(suppl)1–196, 1945

Pedersen EB, Lamm LU, Albertsen K, et al: Familial cranial diabetes insipidus: A report of five families: Genetic, diagnostic and therapeutical aspects. Q J Med 57:883–896, 1985

DIABETES MELLITUS

Symptoms. Both sexes affected; onset at all ages. Polyuria; thirst; enuresis; increased appetite and loss of weight (in children more than in adults); pruritus (vulvae; generalized); premature loosening of the teeth; asthenia; somnolence; impotence; history of delivering large babies and hydramnios.

Signs. *Ocular.* Premature cataract; retinopathy; microaneurysms; vitreous and retinal hemorrhages. *Dermal.* Mycotic infections (*Candida albicans*); xanthochromia; xanthomatous tumors. *Cardiovascular.* Atherosclerotic vascular occlusion; nonhealing leg ulcers with gangrene; edema; heart failure. *Renal.* Kimmelstiel-Wilson syndrome; nephrosclerosis; chronic pyelonephritis; papillary necrosis. *Neurologic.* Peripheral neuritis; areflexia; loss of vibration sense; neurogenic bladder; nocturnal diarrhea; coma.

Etiology. *Type I.* (Insulin-dependent diabetes mellitus) is strongly associated with certain HLA antigens—B8, BW 15, DW 3, and DW 4—and with islet cell antibodies. Likely, type I diabetes results from an infection or

toxic environmental insult to pancreatic B cells of genetically predisposed individuals. In this form, circulating insulin is absent. *Type II.* (Non-insulin-dependent diabetes mellitus) is transmitted as an autosomal dominant trait on chromosome 11. In this type, circulating insulin is sufficient to avoid ketosis, but inadequate in the face of increased needs due to tissue insensitivity.

Diagnostic Procedures. *Urine.* Glycosuria; ketonuria. *Blood.* Hyperglycemia; ketosis; hypercholesterolemia. *Glucose tolerance test. Insulin tolerance test. Ornithene test.* For insulin reserve. Good to detect a latent diabetic state. *Cortisone test.* Decreased glucose tolerance after cortisone therapy. *Insulin antibodies demonstration.* In blood or tissues. *Biopsy of skin and muscles. X-ray of abdomen.* Calcification of aorta.

Differential Diagnosis. To differentiate from pentosuria and fructosuria, use Tes-tape (specific for glucose). DeToni-Fanconi syndrome; renal glycosuria; alimentary hyperglycemia (*e.g.,* dumping syndrome; starvation; liver disease).

Complications. *Acute.* Ketosis; acidosis; coma (see Diabetic Ketoacidosis); insulin allergy (local, usually). *Chronic.* Premature arteriosclerosis with leg ulcers; neuropathy; ocular disorders, Kimmelstiel-Wilson (intracapillary glomerulosclerosis; hypertension; proteinuria; edema); pyelonephritis; papillary necrosis; skin lesions; xanthomas; chronic pyogenic infections; increased incidence of tuberculosis; insulin resistance.

Therapy. Correct diet and avoid obesity. Vitamin B complex. *Insulin therapy.* Indications: (1) diabetes mellitus, especially in older and obese; (2) pancreatectomy; (3) diabetic coma. *Crystalline insulin.* Short acting (6–8 hr); used most frequently in (1) diabetic coma, (2) postprandial blood sugar elevation, (3) after surgical operations. *Protamine zinc insulin (PZI).* Long-acting (up to 40 hr); used in very mild forms of hyperglycemia. *Intermediate.* Neutral protamine Hagedorn (NPH) globin insulin, zinc insulin (lente, semilente). *Mixtures.* Most commonly used are 2 : 1 and 3 : 1 crystalline: PZI; 2 : 1 and 3 : 1 NPH: crystalline. *Toxicity.* Iatrogenic hypoglycemic syndrome (hypoglycemia, especially if the patient fails to eat or after long exercise, manifested by weakness, hunger, sweating, irritability, faintness, tremors, convulsions.) If patient is conscious, give orange juice and sugar. If the patient is unconscious, administer: (1) 20 to 30 ml of 50% glucose intravenously (IV) (treatment of choice); (2) epinephrine 0.5 ml subcutaneously; (3) glucagone 1 mg IV. Insulin allergic reactions are rare. Frequent instead is lipoatrophy (atrophy of subcutaneous fat at the site of injection). *Oral hypoglycemic agents.* Indications: (1) adult type diabetes; (2) mild degree diabetes without complications; (3) good responsiveness (fall of blood sugar to 110 mg in 4 hr after administration of 3.0 mg of these drugs); (4) insulin-resistant diabetes. Contraindicated in juvenile diabetes and in diabetes with complications (ketosis; infections). *Sulfonylurea.* Tolbutamide (Orinase); chlorpropamide (Diabinese), acetohexamide (Dymelor). *Dosage.* Chlorpropamide: 0.5 g per os daily initially, then 0.1 g daily. Tolbutamide: 1 g three times a day. Acetohexamide: 250 mg initially. *Biguanides.* Indications: (1) may replace insulin therapy or sulfonylurea; (2) in combination with insulin in some juvenile diabetes. Dosage: Phenformin (DBI): 25 mg three times a day per os initially, increasing slowly. Long acting (DBI-TD): 50 mg daily. Pancreas transplantation.

Prognosis. The outlook for the juvenile diabetic is not so favorable as compared to the adult diabetic who is adequately treated. Factors affecting the prognosis: pregnancy (increased mortality rate of babies; hydramnios; toxemia; edema; prolonged gestation; atherosclerosis; trauma; infections; emotional stress (often precipitate the disease in susceptible persons). Periods of insulin resistance (treated with corticosteroids). Periods of increased sensitivity to insulin with hypoglycemia. Central and peripheral nervous degeneration. Prophylaxis: No marriage between diabetics. Individual with family history of diabetes should not marry with members of similar families. Avoidance of obesity.

BIBLIOGRAPHY. Fajans SS: Diabetes mellitus: Description etiology and pathogenesis natural history and testing procedures. In De Groot L, Cahill GF Jr, Odell WD, et al (eds): Endocrinology, p. 1007. New York, Grune & Stratton, 1979
Various authors: The diabetes annual/3—Edited by Alberti KGMM, Krall LP. Amsterdam, Elsevier, 1987
Bajal JS: New WHO classifications and diagnostic criteria of diabetes mellitus. IFD Bulletin 32:165, 1987

DIABETES MELLITUS, TRANSIENT NEONATAL

Synonym. Transient neonatal diabetes.

Symptoms and Signs. Babies usually born at term; emaciation and underweight; absence of subcutaneous fat; skin not dry or wrinkled. Poor weight gain; polyuria; polydipsia. Frequent development of infections; abscess; fever.

Etiology. Hypoplastic pancreatic islets unable to produce adequate insulin. Mother with low blood sugar (alimentary; overproduction of insulin) or placental disease that prevents normal transport of sugar from mother to fetus, or primary delayed maturation of islet cells.

Pathology. Dehydration; absence of subcutaneous fat.

Diagnostic Procedures. *Blood.* High fasting blood sugar; diabetic glucose tolerance curve. *Urine.* Glycosuria; absence of ketonuria.

Therapy. Insulin; adequate formula; antibiotic for infections.

Prognosis. Self-correcting condition between 7 days to 18 months. Child blood sugar and glucose tolerance curve normal. In cases not detected, death may occur from inanition, marasmas. Mental retardation may also be observed in some cases.

BIBLIOGRAPHY. Gerrard JW, Chin W: The syndrome of transient diabetes. J Pediatr 61:89–93, 1962

DIABETES, TRANSITORY– MENINGITIS

Symptoms and Signs. Those of meningitis (see). This syndrome may be observed in about 25% of meningococcal meningitis as well as in tuberculous meningitis.

Etiology. Etiologic agents of meningitis (*Mycobacterium tuberculosis; meningococcus*) affect endocrine regulation of carbohydrate metabolism through damage of thalamus, hypothalamus, pituitary, adrenals, pancreas, liver.

Pathology. *Central nervous system.* Basilar accumulation of exudate and changes typical of meningitis. Prominent microscopic changes limited to pituitary and adrenals, with various degrees of cellular swelling and degeneration. *Pancreas.* No definite changes.

Diagnostic Procedures. *Blood.* Hyperglycemia and acidosis. *Urine.* Glycosuria and acetone. *Spinal tap.* Findings of meningitis (diagnosis may be impeded if diabetic acidosis only considered).

Therapy. Treat meningitis and do not be misled by the diabetic findings.

Prognosis. That of meningitis. The diabetic findings are transitory and disappear at time of convalescence from meningitis.

BIBLIOGRAPHY. Loeb M: Ein erklarungs Versuch der verschiedenartigen Temperaturverhaltnisse bei der tuberculosen Basilarmeningitis. Dsch Arch Klin Med 34:433, 1883–1884
Fox MJ, Kuzma JF, Washam WT: Transitory diabetic syndrome associated with meningococcic meningitis. Arch Intern Med 79:614–621, 1947
Edwards MS, Baker CJ: Complications and sequelae of meningococcal infections in children. J Pediatr 99:540–545, 1981

DIABETES, TRUE RENAL

Synonyms. Renal glycosuria. Glycosuria renal.

Symptoms and Signs. Both sexes affected. Asymptomatic (in pregnancy or starvation). Constant glycosuria of variable severity, from 10 to 100 g/25 hour; dehydration and ketosis without hyperglycemia; independent of diet.

Etiology. A group of different genetic abnormalities. One group identified as autosomal dominant inheritance; another, recessive type. Relationship with diabetes mellitus not clear; many patients belong to diabetic families.

Pathology. In some patients, structural defects of proximal convoluted tubules have been shown.

Diagnostic Procedures. *Urine.* Glycosuria. *Blood.* Normal glycemia. *Glucose tolerance test.* Flat; decrease in maximal glucose reabsorptive capacity (Tmg).

Therapy. None.

Prognosis. Excellent. Normal life and survival; usually patients do not develop diabetes mellitus.

BIBLIOGRAPHY. Hjärne UA: Study of orthoglycaemic glycosuria with particular reference to its hereditability. Acta Med Scand 67:422–495, 1927
Brenner BM, Rector FC (eds): The Kidney, 3rd ed, pp 1314–1318. Philadelphia, WB Saunders, 1986

DIABETIC KETOACIDOSIS

Symptoms. Occur more frequently in juvenile diabetes. *Ketosis.* Mild nausea; thirst; malaise. *Acidosis.* Vomiting; drowsiness; hyperpnea.

Signs. Skin and mucosa dry; eyeball soft; fruity odor to breath; deep breathing (Kussmaul); fever; coma.

Etiology. Precipitating factors: infections; vomiting; diarrhea; circulatory failure; in patient with diabetes (see Diabetes Mellitus).

Diagnostic Procedures. *Urine.* Sugar increased; acetone increased. *Blood.* Acetone increased. Test at the bedside and start treatment without waiting for the rest of chemistry. Differential diagnosis with hypoglycemic coma solved by the response to glucose intravenous (IV) injection. Blood sugar increased, blood urea nitrogen (BUN) increased, sodium decreased, potassium increased. *Electrocardiography. X-ray. Cultures. Sensitivity test.* In infections.

Therapy. *Simple ketosis.* Hospitalization indicated. Start treatment of infection, circulatory or other complications. Diet (three main meals, three light). Short-acting insulin after every meal. *Acidosis.* Hospitalization. Insulin (liberal and repeated use of short-acting insulin): (1) In severe cases, 100 to 200 IU (half IV, half subcutaneously (SC)); every 2 hours additional 50 IU until ketonuria disappears. (2) If no change in 6 hours increase insulin (sign of insulin resistance requiring massive dose). *Fluid and electrolytes.* (1) Initial isotonic or slightly hypotonic fluid, 2 to 3 liters given rapidly; sodium chloride plus sodium lactate or sodium chloride plus sodium bicarbonate. (3) After improvement in blood sugar, start glucose 5% in hypotonic multiple electrolytes (sodium 40 mEq/liter; potassium 30–40 mEq/liter). Correction of precipitating and complicating factors (infection; circulatory failure; renal disease; pancreatitis; surgical abdomen). If coma results, hospitalization. If differential diagnosis requires, start glucose 5% IV and watch for response. If shock occurs, plasma, vasopressor, insulin as outlined for acidosis; fluid as outlined for acidosis. *Follow-up.* Electrocardiography; electrolyte studies. As soon as patient is conscious, 200 ml of fruit juice. As soon as ketonuria is disappearing, 200 ml of milk every 3 to 4 hours and insulin (25–35 IU).

Prognosis. When severe, death if adequate treatment not instituted at once.

BIBLIOGRAPHY. Winegrad AI, Morrison AD: Diabetic ketosis, non ketotic hyperosmolar coma and lactic acidosis. In De Groot LJ, Cahill GF Jr, Odell WD, et al (ed): Endocrinology, p 1025. New York, Grune & Stratton, 1979
Skillman TG: Diabetes mellitus. In Mazzaferri EL (ed): Textbook of Endocrinology, 3rd ed, pp 627–635. New York Med Exam Publishing Co., 1985

DIABETIC MYELOPATHY

Synonyms. Diabetic amyotrophy; diabetic myelopathy. See Diabetic pseudotabes. Diabetic neuropathy; mononeuropathy multiplex.

Symptoms. Both sexes affected; diabetic patients in the fifth to seventh decades. Pain in the leg, severe, asymmetric, occasionally unilateral, maximal in hip and thigh.

Signs. Asymmetric wasting of muscles, and loss of tendon reflexes. Fasciculation. Lack of objective sensory disturbances; tenderness; ulcers. Normal vibration sense at the ankles; Babinski extensor response.

Etiology. Diabetes (doubtful if this condition exists as a separate entity). Part of radicular lesions of diabetes. This syndrome is, according to the authors, mainly motor as contrasted with the diabetic pseudotabes, which is mainly sensory. Actually several clinical syndromes may go under this denomination: acute mononeuropathy; mononeuropathy multiplex; symmetric motor and sensorial loss with subacute or chronic evolution.

Pathology. Not reported, indirect indication of cord lesion.

Diagnostic Procedures. *Spinal fluid.* High protein level. *Electromyography.* Partial denervation of leg muscles; no fibrillation activity. *Blood.* Enzymes.

Therapy. Diet; insulin; vitamin B complex; physical therapy.

Prognosis. Variable form, rapid improvement with treatment. Unremitting course, possibly, spontaneous improvement.

BIBLIOGRAPHY. Bruns L: Ueber neuritische Lähmungen beim Diabetes mellitus. Berl Klin Wochenschr 27:509–515, 1890
Garland H, Taverner D: Diabetic myelopathy. Br Med J 1:1405–1408, 1953
Adams RD, Victor M: Principles of Neurology, 3rd ed, p 976. New York, McGraw-Hill, 1985

DIABETIC PSEUDOTABES

See Pseudotabetic and Diabetic myelopathy.

Symptoms and Signs. In diabetic patients, shooting pain, more intense at night; cutaneous hyperesthesia. Charcot's joints, impotence, neurogenic bladder may be associated.

Etiology. Diabetes; radicular and peripheral neuropathy rather than myelopathy. Clinically the following syndromes may be distinguished frequently overlapping with those indicated in diabetic myelopathy: (1) symmetric primary sensory polyneuropathy affecting mainly feet and legs slowly progressing; (2) autonomic neuropathy involving bowel, bladder, and circulation; (3) painful thoracoabdominal radiculopathy.

Diagnostic Procedures. *Blood.* Demonstration of diabetes mellitus. *Serology.* Negative for syphilis. *Spinal tap.* Normal or slight increase in protein.

Therapy. That of diabetes, plus vitamin B complex.

Prognosis. Variable, occasionally good response to treatment.

BIBLIOGRAPHY. Gowers WR: Diseases of Nervous System. London, Churchill-Livingston, 1938
Adams RD, Victor M: Principles of Neurology, 3rd ed, p 976. New York, McGraw-Hill, 1985

DIALLINAS-AMALRIC

Synonyms. Amalric's; deaf muteness–macular dystrophy.

Symptoms. Both sexes affected; onset early infancy (in acquired type, from birth; in inherited type, at 5 yr). Partial deafness (50–60%); minor troubles of vision with normal visual fields, dark vision, and color vision.

Signs. Reddish fovea in marked contrast with deep grayish background; occasionally, pigmentation extends in streak to the periphery, usually bilateral. Heterochromic iridis.

Etiology. Unknown; hereditary (autosomal recessive) or embryopathic; postnatal infections.

Pathology. In most cases, labyrinthal changes; in inherited cases, cochlear involvement.

Diagnostic Procedures. *Electroretinography.* Normal.

Therapy. None.

Prognosis. No progressive macular degeneration. Deafness progressive in hereditary cases; nonprogressive in acquired type.

BIBLIOGRAPHY. Diallinas NP: Les altérations oculaires chez les sourdsmuets. J Genet Hum 8:225–262, 1959
Amalric P: A new type of tapetoretinal degeneration in the course of deaf-mutism. Bull Soc Ophthalmol Fr 73:196–212, 1960
Remky H, Klier A, Kobor J: Maculadystrophie bei Taubstummheit (syndrom von Amalric). Klin Monatsbl Augenheilkd 114:180–187, 1964
Charamis J, Tsamparlakis J, Palimeris G et al: Deaf-mutism and ophthalmic lesions. J Pediatr Ophthalmol 5:230, 1968
Konigsmark BW, Knox DL, Husserls IE et al: Dominant congenital deafness and progressive optic nerve atrophy. Arch Ophthalmol 91:99–103, 1974

DIAPHRAGM, CONGENITAL ABSENCE

Synonyms. Lewis-Besant. Diaphragm unilateral agenesis.

Symptoms and Signs. Both sexes affected. Respiratory insufficiency and then heart failure and death.

Etiology. Congenital absence of diaphragm (often associated with other muscle defects: pectoralis; abdominal) causing a displacement of abdominal viscera into thoracic cavity and determining lung collapse. Multifactorial inheritance.

Therapy. Plastic surgery. Intensive care; mechanical ventilation. In severe cases, extracorporeal membrane oxygenation (ECMO).

Prognosis. Poor.

BIBLIOGRAPHY. Lewis AJ, Besant DF: Muscular dystrophy in infancy. J Pediatr 60:376–384, 1962
Wolff G: Familial congenital diaphragmatic defect: Review and conclusions. Hum Genet 54:1–5, 1980
Czeizel A, Kovacs M: A family study of congenital diaphragmatic defects. Am J Med Genet 21:105–115, 1985
Ortiz RM, Cilley RE, Bartlett RH: Extracorporeal membrane oxygenation in pediatric respiratory failure. Pediatr Clin N Am 34:39–46, 1987

DIAPHRAGM EVENTRATIO

Symptoms. Asymptomatic or minor symptoms (postprandial fullness; eructation; dyspnea).

Signs. In recumbent position, peristaltic sounds in the chest.

Etiology. Congenital. Atrophy or relaxation (hemilateral or total) of diaphragm, without phrenic nerve deficit.

Pathology. Involved part of diaphragm thinner, with muscle degeneration; atelectasia, or aplasia of part of compressed lung. Displacement of mediastinum.

Diagnostic Procedures. *X-ray of chest and abdomen. Pulmonary function test.*

Therapy. If needed to improve ventilation, surgery to strengthen diaphragm through plication.

Prognosis. Good.

BIBLIOGRAPHY. Norio R, Kaariainen H, Rapala J, et al: Familial congenital diaphragmatic defects: Aspects of etiology, prenatal diagnosis and treatment. Am J Med Genet 17:417–483, 1984

DIAPHRAGM RUPTURE

Symptoms. Intense dyspnea; sharp pain in abdominal region and shoulder; vomiting.

Signs. Reduced expansion of inferior edge of lung. Distant respiratory sounds; rales.

Etiology. Trauma (*e.g.*, car accident, surgery). Complication of abdominal or thoracic conditions.

Pathology. Diaphragmatic laceration; possibly, herniation of intestinal loop or omentum into thorax.

Diagnostic Procedures. *X-ray of chest and abdomen.*

Therapy. If shock occurs, control of evolution and indicated treatment. Plastic surgery.

Prognosis. Generally good, determined by associated lesions. Possibly development of diaphragmatic hernia.

BIBLIOGRAPHY. Cox EF: Blunt abdominal trauma: A 5-year analysis of 870 patients requiring celiotomy. Ann Surg 199:467–474, 1984

DIAPHYSEAL ACLASIS

Synonyms. Exostosis, multiple hereditary; external chondromatosis; multiple exostosis.

Symptoms and Signs. Both sexes. From birth to early childhood: diaphyseal-juxtaepiphyseal outgrowths leading to various types of deformity. The growth of the exostosis slows down at adolescence. Area most frequently affected: knees, pelvis, ribs. Shortness of stature variable.

Etiology. Autosomal dominant.

Pathology. Exostosis capped by hyaline cartilage.

Therapy. When needed orthopedic procedures.

Prognosis. No new growths occur in adult life; 2 to 10% incidence of sarcoma only in adulthood.

BIBLIOGRAPHY. Solomon L: Hereditary multiple exostosis. J Bone Joint Surg 45B:292–304, 1963
Solomon L: Hereditary multiple exostosis. Am J Hum Genet 16:351, 1964
Hall JG, Wilson RD, Kalonsek D, et al: Familial multiple exostosis—No chromosome 8 deletion observed. Am J Med Genet 22:640, 1985

DIASTROPHIC DWARFISM

Synonyms. Diastrophic dysplasia; DD.

Symptoms. Both sexes affected; present from birth. Frequent respiratory infection. Severe functional impairment of hand and foot functions. Delayed motor milestones.

Signs. At birth, weight normal, length reduced. Micromelia: forearms and legs more involved than distal parts of limbs. Stiff fingers, "hitch-hiker" thumb; club foot. Joint contractures. Scoliosis. Variable webbing at joints. Ear lobe deformities with hypertrophic cartilages (86%); cleft palate (common). Facies normal; however, occasionally, beaking of nose; broad nasal bridge; midface hemangiomas.

Etiology. Autosomal recessive.

Pathology. Cartilaginous deformities and muscle contraction leading to the severe joint stiffness. Irregular arrangement of cartilage cells and capillaries in the epiphyses.

Diagnostic Procedures. *X-ray of skeleton.* Multiple joint deformities especially of hands and feet; long bone deviation; bowing of large metaphyses; scoliosis or kyphoscoliosis (66%).

Therapy. Orthopedic treatment; deformities are prone to early recurrences after correction.

Prognosis. Mortality rate high, especially in neonatal and early infancy periods, generally from respiratory infections. In survivors, good general health; normal mental development; severe orthopedic problems.

BIBLIOGRAPHY. Lamy M, Maroteaux P: Le nanisme diastrophique. Paris, Presse Med 68:1977–1980, 1960
Gustavson K-H, Holmgren G, Jagell S et al: Lethal and non-lethal diastrophic dysplasia: A study of 14 Swedish cases. Clin Genet 28:321–334, 1985

DIBASIC AMINOACIDURIA I

Symptoms and Signs. Generally Finnish population, rare in other populations. Asymptomatic. Possible mild intestinal malabsorption; mental retardation.

Etiology. Autosomal recessive inheritance.

Diagnostic Procedures. *Urine.* High excretion of lysine, ornithine, and arginine. *Blood.* Normal plasma level of said amino acids. Impaired intestinal absorption of L-cystine. Homozygotes, protein intolerance. Heterozygotes, normal or protein intolerance.

BIBLIOGRAPHY. Whilar DT, Scriver CR: Hyperbasicaminoaciduria: An inherited disorder of amino acid transport. Pediatr Res 2:525–534, 1968

DIETLEN'S

Synonym. Pericardial diaphragmatic adhesion.

Symptoms and Signs. During inspiration, tachycardia and feeling of epicardial tension.

Etiology. Complication of pericarditis, pleurisy, or diaphragmatitis, with formation of adhesions between pericardium and diaphragm.

Pathology. See Etiology.

Diagnostic Procedures. *Electrocardiography.* Flutter during inspiration. *X-ray and Kinocardiography of chest to demonstrate adhesions.*

Therapy. If needed, surgery.

Prognosis. Good.

BIBLIOGRAPHY. Dietlen H: Herz und Gefaesse im Roentgenbild. Ein Lehrbuch. Leipzig, Barth, 1923.

DIETL'S

Synonyms. Floating kidney; movable kidney; nephroptosis; ren mobilis.

Symptoms. More frequent in older, thin females. When standing, acute pain in lumbar area, possible radiation to genitals; nausea and vomiting and feeling of general prostration. Oliguria. When lying down, symptoms subside.

Signs. Palpable movable kidney.

Etiology. Loss of perirenal fat and defective renal fascia. Frequently follows a rapid loss of weight. Associated with visceroptosis.

Pathology. Reduction of fat in perirenal tissue.

Diagnostic Procedures. *X-rays.* Pyelogram shows kidney mobility.

Therapy. Weight gain; proper posture; exercises to strengthen muscle; surgery.

Prognosis. Good with treatment or various complications may arise (*e.g.*, kinking of ureters; hydronephrosis).

BIBLIOGRAPHY. Dietl J: Merki wedrujace i ich uwiezquienie. Przegl Lek 3:225–227, 1864
Kissane JN: Congenital malformation. In Heptinstall RH: Pathology of the Kidney, 3rd ed, p 83. Boston, Little, Brown & Co, 1983

DIETRICH'S

Synonyms. Dysplasia, epiphyseal-metacarpal Type III b; metacarpal epiphyseal necrosis; MEDT type III b; multiple epiphyseal dysplasia type III b. See also Multiple epiphyseal dysplasias.

Symptoms. Both sexes affected; onset in infancy and up to 18 years of age. Pain and limitation of movements in toe joints.

Signs. Fusiform enlargement of proximal interphalangeal joints, especially of second and third metatarsal bones, less frequently of other digits. Later, possible digital shortening.

Etiology. Unknown; in some cases proven autosomal dominant; in other cases, suspected recessive-type inheritance.

Pathology. Avascular osteolysis in epiphyseal-diaphyseal zone of digits.

Diagnostic Procedures. *X-rays of hands and feet.* Destruction of cartilages; lacunae of bone reabsorption; hazy outline; shortening of phalangeal epiphyses.

Therapy. Symptomatic.

Prognosis. Severe deformities. Spontaneous arrest after closure of epiphyses. Eventual regeneration of cartilage.

BIBLIOGRAPHY. Odman P: Hereditary enchondral dysostosis: Twelve cases in three generations mainly with peripheral location. Acta Radiol 52:97–113, 1959

DI FERRANTE'S

Synonyms. Mucopolysaccharidosis VIII; glucosamine-6-sulfate-sulfatase deficiency.

Symptoms and Signs. Only one case described. Male, dwarfism, mental retardation, abundant coarse hair, hepatomegaly, minor dysostosis multiplex.

Etiology. Autosomal recessive inheritance. The syndrome is not confirmed and quoted only because number VIII was attributed to it.

BIBLIOGRAPHY. Ginsburg LC, Di Ferrante DT, Caskey CT et al: Glucosamine-6-SO₄ sulfatase deficiency: A new mucopolysaccharidosis. Clin Res 25:471A, 1977
McKusick VA: Mendelian inheritance in man, 7th ed. Baltimore, Johns Hopkins Press, 1986

DI GEORGE'S

Synonyms. Parathyroid-thymic aplasia; pharyngeal (3-4) pouch.

Symptoms and Signs. Both sexes affected (male predominance 2:1); early onset. Severe infection; diarrhea; tetany; Chostek's, Trousseau's signs. Dehydration; pulmonary and mucosal infections. Several malformations: microcephaly, hypertelorism; down slanting palpebral fissures; ear anomalies. Aortic arch anomalies; ventricular septal defects and other congenital cardiac defects.

Pathology. Congenital absence, hypoplasia, ectopia of parathyroid; absence of thymus.

Etiology. Unknown; sporadic.

Diagnostic Procedures. *Blood.* Anemia; progressive lymphopenia; hypocalcemia; high phosphorus; hypoglobulinemia; normal immunoglobulins. *Cellular immunity.* Diminished.

Therapy. Calcium; parathormone; antibiotics; thymus transplant. Bone marrow transplant should be considered, especially when a fetal thymus is unobtainable and an HLA-matched sibling is available.

Prognosis. Very poor; death from infections, cardiovascular defects, or seizures within the first month or second year of life.

BIBLIOGRAPHY. Lobdell, DH: Congenital absence of parathyroid glands. Arch Pathol 67:412–415, 1959
Di George AM (moderator): New concept of cellular basis of immunity. (Discussion of Cooper MD, Peterson RDA, Good RA.) J Pediatr 67:907–908, 1965
Kretschmer R, Say B, Brown D, et al: Congenital aplasia of the thymus gland (Di George's syndrome). New Engl J Med 279:1295–1301, 1968
Fudenberg HH, Stites DP, Caldwell JC, et al: Basic and Clinical Immunology. Los Altos, Lange Medical Publishers, 1976
Goldsobel AB, Haas A, Stiehm ER: Bone marrow transplantation in Di George syndrome. J Pediatr 111:40–44, 1987

DIGITOTALAR DYSMORPHA

Synonyms. Ulnar drift. See arthrogryposis multiplex congenita, distal type.

Symptoms and Signs. Ulnar deviation of fingers. Adduction and flexor deformity of thumbs, bilateral vertical talus and rockerbottom feet. Mild reduction of stature.

Etiology. Autosomal dominant inheritance.

BIBLIOGRAPHY. Sallis JG, Beighton P: Dominantly inherited digitotalar dysmorphism. J Bone Joint Surg 54:509–515, 1972
Dhaliwal AS, Myeres TL: Digitotalar dysmorphism. Orthopedic Rev 14:90–94, 1985

DI GUGLIELMO'S I

Synonyms. Erythremia; erythroblastomatosis; erythroleukemia; erythromyelosis; Helmeyer-Schoener; Guglielmo's I.

ACUTE

Three types of disorders may be distinguished: (1) pure form, (2) mixed form, (3) transient (see table).

Symptoms. Tiredness; shortness of breath on exertion; occasionally, early bruising; bleeding from gums; fever.

Signs. Pallor; occasionally, petechiae and ecchymosis; hepatosplenomegaly; moderate irregular lymphadenopathy.

Polyphasic Myeloproliferative Diseases

→Pure forms (permanent)

Pure erythromyelosis

→Pure erythromyelosis——→erythroleukemia

→Polyphasic forms →Pure erythromyelosis——→erythroleukemia——→pure leukemia

→Pure erythromyelosis——→erythroleukemia——→pure leukemia

↘——→reticulosis

→Pure forms (permanent)

Erythroleukemia

→Erythroleukemia——→leukemia

→Polyphasic forms →Erythroleukemia——→erythromyelosis

→Erythroleukemia——→leukemia——→myelofibrosis

Magalini SI, Ahstrom L: J Pediatr 52:501–530, 1958

Etiology. Unknown. Familial cases with autosomal dominant inheritance have been reported.

Pathology. Hepatomegaly; splenomegaly; lymphadenopathy. Infiltration with pathologic erythroid elements in spleen, lymph nodes, liver, heart, skin, muscle, esophagus, stomach, adrenal, kidney, and gonads. Focal necrosis of spleen. Frequently, superimposed fungi (*Candida; Mucor*) growth. Some cases, end with total bone marrow aplasia and metaplastic infiltration of different organs.

Diagnostic Procedures. *Blood.* Presence of nucleated red cells in different stages of maturation with numerous pathologic features. *Bone marrow.* Prevalence of erythroid elements with anaplastic, dysplastic changes. Decreased number of megakaryocytes.

Therapy. Blood transfusion and symptomatic. Most of these cases are completely refractory to steroids and chemotherapy. Transient forms and mixed form may respond with partial or total remission to cortiocosteroids and chemotherapy.

BIBLIOGRAPHY. Copelli M: Di una emopatia sistemizzata rappresentata da una iperplasia eritoblastica. Pathologica 4:460–465, 1912
Di Guglielmo G: Un caso di eritroleucemia. Folia Med 3:319, 1917
Di Guglielmo G: Eritremie acute. Rel 29th Congr di Med Int Roma, 1923
Peterson HR Jr, Bowlds CF, Yam LT: Familial DiGuglielmo syndrome. Cancer 54:932–938, 1984.

CHRONIC

Symptoms and Signs. Weakness; chronic refractory anemia; splenomegaly usually treated for years before gradual appearance of nucleated red cells in peripheral blood.

Etiology. Unknown; similar or identical with refractory normoblastic anemia (possibly preleukemic phase).

Pathology. See Acute form.

Diagnostic Procedures. *Blood.* Anemia; anisocytosis; poikilocytosis; siderocytes; scarce reticulocytosis. *Bone marrow.* Hyperplastic erythroid series; frequently, megaloblastic features; increased mitosis; bizarre erythrocyte morphology; erythrophagocytosis.

Therapy. Symptomatic; megaloblastic changes not affected by vitamin B_{12} or folic acid.

Prognosis. Progressive deterioration with increasing number of circulating nucleated red cells. Evolution into aplastic phase; blastic crisis (sudden increase of nucleolar cells in peripheral blood) may precede death that occurs within 2 to 5 years from first appearance of nucleated cells in circulation.

BIBLIOGRAPHY. Baldini M, Fudenberg HH, Fukutake K, et al: The anemia of the Di Guglielmo syndrome. Blood 14:334–366, 1959
Thurm RH, Casey MJ, Emerson CP: Chronic Di Guglielmo syndrome. Am J Med Sci 44:399–405, 1967
Wintrobe MM (ed): Clinical Hematology, 8th ed, pp 1543–1544. Philadelphia, Lea & Febiger, 1981

DILATED MYOCARDIOPATHY

Synonyms. Abramo-Fiedler's; adult fibroelastosis; alcoholic heart disease; Becker's; cardiac hypertrophy–unknown etiology; cardiovascular collagenosis; chronic pernicious myocarditis; endocardial fibrosis; Fiedler's; Meadow's; noncoronary cardiomyopathy; nutritional heart disease; obscure cardiopathy; subendocardial fibroelastosis; South African cardiomyopathy. Including Keshan. See Cardiomegaly, idiopathic.

Symptoms. Prevalent in males (78%); mean age of clinical onset 34 years. Easy fatigability; exertional dyspnea;

palpitations; ankle swelling (in late afternoon); progressing to orthopnea, paroxysmal nocturnal dyspnea, effort syncope, right upper abdominal quadrant pain.

Signs. Cardiac enlargement: first sound normal; pulmonic component of second sound accentuated (when other signs of congestion develop); pathologic third sound; occasionally, murmurs of secondary mitral or tricuspid insufficiency. Hepatomegaly; positive liver-jugular sign.

Etiology. Spectrum of conditions includes alcohol abuse, systemic arterial hypertension, pregnancy (see Meadow's), genetic factors, microvascular spasm, infectious and immunologic derangements, toxic cobalt (see Beer and cobalt), selenium deficiency (Keshan disease), Catecholamine increase and autonomic function derangements, thyroid hormone.

Pathology. Massive increase in heart size up to 1000 g. Chronic inflammatory change; fibroplastic proliferation of myocardium, of endocardium, thickened in patchy fashion, and occasionally also of pericardium. Passive congestion of liver.

Diagnostic Procedures. *X-Ray of chest.* Cardiomegaly, both ventricles dilated; occasionally also atria, right more than left one; pleural effusion occasionally present. *Electrocardiography. Phonocardiogram. Echocardiogram. Radionuclide imaging. Angiocardiogram. Endomyocardial biopsy.*

Therapy. Symptomatic; diuretics.

Prognosis. Unexpected death may occur from myocardial irritability or embolic phenomena, hemoptysis, hemiplegia.

BIBLIOGRAPHY. Fiedler A: Ueber akute interstitielle Myokarditis. In Festschrift zur Feier des fünfzigjährigen Bestehens des Stadtkrankenhauses zu Dresden-Friedrichstadt, pp 1–20. Dresden, W Baensch, 1899
Sanders V: Idiopathic disease of myocardium. Arch Intern Med 112:661–676, 1963
Wenger NK, Goodwin JF, Roberts WC: Cardiomyopathy and myocardial involvement in systemic disease. In Hurst JW: The Heart, 6th ed, pp 1181–1193. New York, McGraw-Hill, 1986

DI MAURO-HARTLAGE

Synonym. Muscle phosphorylase deficiency type I.

Symptoms and Signs. Three cases described. From birth generalized, rapidly progressive muscle weakness.

Etiology. No detectable phosphorylase activity in muscle.

Diagnostic Procedures. See McArdle.

Pathology. Muscle histology: disorganization of myofibrils by excesses of glycogen in intermyofibrillar space.

Therapy. None.

Prognosis. Poor. Death in a few weeks from respiratory failure.

BIBLIOGRAPHY. Di Mauro S, Hartlage PL: Fatal infantile form of muscle phosphorylase deficiency. Neurology 28:1124–1129, 1978
De La Marza M, Patten BM, Williams JC, Chambers JP: Myophosphorylase deficiency: A new cause of infantile hypotonia simulating infantile muscular atrophy. Neurology 30:402, 1980

DIMMER'S

Synonym. Keratitis nummularis.

Symptoms. Onset after minor ocular trauma. Ocular pain; photophobia; excessive lacrimation.

Signs. Diskoid infiltration of superficial layers of cornea without consensual conjunctivitis.

Etiology. Trauma.

Therapy. Topical application of analgesic and antibiotics.

Prognosis. Slow progression and then healing.

BIBLIOGRAPHY. Dimmer F: Ueber eine der Keratitis nummularis mahestehende Hirnhutentzuendung. Augenheilkd 13:621–635, 1905

DI SAIA'S

Synonyms. Coumadin; fetal warfarin.

Symptoms. Both sexes affected; present from birth. Poor feeding; variable degree of mental deficiency; hypotonia; seizures; visual impairment to blindness; respiratory infections.

Signs. Nose hypoplasia, low bridge; mild ocular hypertelorism; short neck; brachydactyly.

Etiology. Warfarin taken by mother during pregnancy. The critical period of exposure is between 6 and 9 weeks' gestation. Most of the effects on bones are secondary to the inhibition of gamma-carboxylation of glutamyl residues of osteocalcins in the developing bone. Central nervous system abnormalities are associated with exposure in the second or third trimester and are related to hemorrhage in the nervous tissues of the fetus.

Diagnostic Procedures. *X-ray.* Stippled mineralization in vertebrae, epiphyses, cartilage.

Prognosis. For CNS manifestations, poor.

BIBLIOGRAPHY. Di Saia PJ: Pregnancy and delivery of a patient with Stan-Edwards mitral valve prosthesis. Report of a case. Obstet Gynecol 28:469–471, 1966
Shaul WL, Emery H, Hall JC: Chondrodysplasia punctate and maternal warfarin use during pregnancy. Am J Dis Child 129:360–362, 1975
Smith DW: Recognizable Patterns of Human Malformation. Philadelphia, WB Saunders, 1982

DISASTER

Symptoms. Response of person involved in disaster, injured or not. (Does not apply to person who arrives at site of disaster later.) Four stages may be distinguished:
1. *Few minutes to hours.* Stunned; apathetic; not responding to directions; disorganized behavior regarding injury or priority of activities.
2. *Several days.* Suggestibility; tries to be helpful with reduced efficiency; minimizes his need of care. Onset of guilty feeling because he survived and could not help others.
3. *Few weeks.* Mild euphoria; enthusiasm for rebuilding and repairing damages; feeling of identification with community.
4. *Eventually fading and disappearing into normality.* Hypercriticism; annoyance.

BIBLIOGRAPHY. Garb S, Garb E: Disaster Handbook. New York, Springer-Verlag, 1964
Stutman RK, Bliss EL: Posttraumatic stress disorder, hypnotizability, and imagery. Am J Psychiatry 142:741–743, 1985
Manni C, Magalini SI (eds): Emergency and Disaster Medicine. Heidelberg, Berlin, Springer-Verlag, 1985

DISCOGENIC

Syndromes due to nerve root or spinal cord compression by herniation of nucleus pulposus or narrowing of intervertebral disks with reduction of space. Local and radicular pain.

BIBLIOGRAPHY. Schmorl G: Die pathogische Anatomie der Wirbelsäule. Verh Dtsh Orthop Ges 21:3–41, 1927
Schmorl G: Ueber die an den Wirbelbandscheiben vorkommenden Ausdehnughs-und Zerresisungsvorgänge und die dadurch an ihnen und der Wirbelspongiosa hervorgerufenen Veränderungen. Verh Dtsch Pathol Ges 22:250–262, 1927

Wood GN: Lower back pain and disorders of intervertebral disc. In Crenshaw AH (ed): Campbell's Operative Orthopedics, 7th ed, pp 3255–3321. St. Louis, CV Mosby, 1987

DISTICHIASIS–HEART AND VASCULATURE ANOMALIES

Symptoms and Signs. Recently reported combination of distichiasis and variable heart (ventricular septal defect, patent ductus arteriosus, sinus bradycardia, wandering atrial pacemaker) and vasculature (edema, varicosities, arterial disease of legs) in members of both sexes of a family.

Etiology. Autosomal dominant.

BIBLIOGRAPHY. Goldstein S, Qazi QM, Fitzgerald J, et al: Distichiasis, congenital heart defects and mixed peripheral vascular anomalies. Am J Med Genet 20:283–294, 1985

DISTICHIASIS-LYMPHEDEMA

Synonym. Lymphedema-distichiasis.

Symptoms and Signs. Both sexes affected. Extra eyelashes that cause eye irritation. Lymphedema of limbs, especially below knees, that becomes manifest at adolescence. Occasionally, epidural spinal cysts and vertebral anomalies.

Etiology. Autosomal dominant inheritance.

Therapy. Eyelash removal and surgery for lymphedema has little effectiveness; frequent recurrences.

BIBLIOGRAPHY. Falls HS, Dertesz ED: A new syndrome combining pterygium colli with developmental anomalies of the eyelids and lymphatics of the lower extremities. Trans Am Ophthalmol Soc 62:248–275. 1964
Pap Z, Biro T, Szabo L et al: Syndrome of lymphedema and distichiasis. Hum Genet 53:309–310, 1980

DIVER'S SYNCOPE

Symptoms and Signs. Loss of consciousness (even sudden death) during underwater diving.

Etiology. Poorly understood. Several factors in combination may be responsible: age, hypoxia, "diving reflex", cold hypersensitivity (see).

Prognosis. "Per se" fair.

BIBLIOGRAPHY. Weisler AM, Warren JV: Syncope: Pathophysiology and differential diagnosis. In Hurst JW: The Heart, 6th ed, p 518. New York, McGraw-Hill, 1986

DIVRY-VAN BOGAERT

Synonyms. Angiomatosis, diffuse corticomeningeal; diffuse corticomeningeal angiomatosis; Bogaert-Divy; Van Bogaert-Divry.

Symptoms. Present from infancy. Spastic diplegia; seizures; physical and mental developmental retardation.

Signs. Cutis marmorata; generalized acrocyanosis; trophic changes of nails; occasionally, hypertricosis.

Etiology. Unknown; autosomal recessive inheritance.

Pathology. Angiomatosis of cortex and meninges (not calcific); diffuse sclerosis.

Therapy. None.

Prognosis. Poor.

BIBLIOGRAPHY. Divry P, Van Bogaert L: Une maladie familiale caractérisée par une angiomatose diffuse corticomeningée non calcifiante et une démyélinisation progressive de la substance blanche. J Neurol Neurosurg Psychiatry 19:41–54, 1946
Martin JJ, Navarro C, Roussel JM et al: Familial capillaro-venous leptomeningeal angiomatosis. Eur Neurol 9:202–215, 1973

DNA AUTOSENSITIVITY

Synonyms. Autosensitization DNA; purpura, DNA sensitivity.

Symptoms and Signs. All female patients in good health. Painful spot in the extremities preceding appearance of wheal or tender nodules. In 2 to 48 hours, wheals or red nodules evolve into hematomas that spread circumferentially with a diameter of 10 to 12 cm, sometimes from midthigh to ankle or from elbow to fingertips. Lesions appear in crops at intervals of 2 to 4 weeks.

Etiology. Unknown; autosensitization to deoxyribonucleic acid (DNA) limited to extremities.

Pathology. *Biopsy of skin.* Feulgen-positive masses resembling hematoxylin bodies in lesions 20 to 72 hours old. In older lesions, infiltration with mature lymphocytes in the adventitia of small dermal vessels.

Diagnostic Procedures. Injection of DNA preparation in the skin of extremities reproduces the specific lesions. Injection in the skin of trunk gives a negative result. For differential diagnosis: *Injection of red cell membranes.* Negative result (see Gardener-Diamond). *Injection of histamine.* Negative. *Lupus erythematosus test.* Negative. *Coagulation studies.* Negative.

Therapy. Dramatic result with administration of chloroquine or primaquine, complete cessation of pain and tenderness; immediate recurrence of symptoms when therapy is stopped.

Prognosis. Chronic recurrent condition.

BIBLIOGRAPHY. Levin MB, Pinkus H: Autosensitivity to deoxyribonucleic acid (DNA). Report of a case with inflammatory skin lesions controlled by chloroquine. New Engl J Med 264:533–537, 1961
Little, AS, Bell HE: Painful subcutaneous hemorrhages of the extremities with unusual reactions to injected deoxyribonucleic acid. Ann Intern Med 60:886–891, 1964
Wintrobe MM (ed): Clinical Hematology, 8th ed. Philadelphia, Lea & Febiger, 1981

DOAN-WISEMAN

Synonyms. Splenic neutropenia (primary); splenic panhematopenia; Wiseman-Doan. See Neutropenic.

Symptoms. Fever; pain on left hypochondrium.

Signs. Various degrees of splenomegaly.

Etiology. Unknown; splenic selective dysfunction with trapping and destruction of granulocytes. Often associated with other features of hypersplenism, anemia, thrombocytopenia (see Doan-Wright).

Pathology. Spleen enlarged; active phagocytosis of granulocytes. In bone marrow, normal cellularity or slight decrease of mature granulocytes.

Diagnostic Procedures. *Blood.* Marked neutropenia. *Spleen scan. Bone marrow. Search for leukocytes antibodies.*

Therapy. Splenectomy.

Prognosis. Normalization of granulocyte count.

BIBLIOGRAPHY. Wiseman BK, Doan CA: Primary splenic neutropenia. A newly recognized syndrome closely related to congenital hemolytic icterus and essential thrombocytopenic purpura. Ann Intern Med 16:1097–1117, 1942
Doan CA, Wright CS: Primary congenital and secondary acquired splenic panhematopenia. Blood 1:10–26, 1946
Wintrobe MM (ed): Clinical Hematology, 8th ed. Philadelphia, Lea & Febiger, 1981

DOAN-WRIGHT

Synonyms. Splenic neutropenia (acquired); splenic panhematopenia; Wright-Doan. See Neutropenic.

Symptoms and Signs. Both sexes affected; onset at all ages; acute or gradual onset. All clinical manifestations of anemia, thrombocytopenia, neutropenia. Splenomegaly; no lymphadenopathy.

Etiology. Unknown.

Pathology. *Spleen.* Congestion; erythrophagocytosis; granulocyte phagocytosis; megakaryocytosis. *Bone marrow.* Hyperplasia of all series of production; erythrocytic; myelocytic; megakaryocytic.

Diagnostic Procedures. *Blood.* Anemia; variable reticulocytosis; neutropenia; thrombocytopenia; variable hyperbilirubinemia. *Coomb's and agglutination tests.* Negative. *Spleen scan.*

Therapy. Splenectomy.

Prognosis. Condition may be present for weeks or years; periodic recurrences with spontaneous return to normal values reported. Splenectomy is followed by return of blood elements to normal values.

BIBLIOGRAPHY. Doan CA, Wright CS: Primary congenital and secondarily acquired splenic panhematopenia. Blood 1:10–26, 1946
Wintrobe MM (ed): Clinical Hematology, 8th ed. Philadelphia, Lea & Febiger, 1981

DOBRINER'S

Synonyms. Berger-Goldberg; hereditary coproporphyria; HCP; porphyria hepatica II; Watson's.

Symptoms and Signs. Both sexes affected; onset at various ages. From completely asymptomatic form to intermittent attacks of abdominal pain and neurologic and psychiatric manifestations (usually associated with signs of hepatic insufficiency). Acute attacks may be precipitated by drugs.

Etiology. Autosomal dominant inheritance; 50% deficiency of coproporphyrin oxidase. Primary partial block in conversion of coproporphyrinogen III to protoporphyrinogen IX.

Pathology. Absence of particular findings.

Diagnostic Procedures. *Stool.* Increased excretion of coproporphyrin III (95% isomer III); increase of coproporphyrin, ALA and PBG.

Therapy. See Swedish type porphyria.

Prognosis. From asymptomatic to fatal attacks.

BIBLIOGRAPHY. Dobriner K: Simultaneous excretion of coproporphyrin I and III in a case of chronic porphyria. Proc Soc Exp Biol Med 35:175–176, 1936
Watson CJ, Schwartz S, Schulze W et al: Studies on coproporphyrin III. Idiopathic coproporphyrinuria a hitherto unrecognized form characterized by lack of symptoms in spite of the excretion of large amounts of coproporphyrin. J Clin Invest 28:465–468, 1949
Berger H, Golderg A: Hereditary coproporphyria. Br Med J 2:85–88, 1955
Kappas A, Sassa S, Anderson KE: The porphyrias. In Stanbury JB, Wyngaarden JB, Fredrickson DS, et al: The Metabolic Basis of Inherited Disease, 5th ed, p 1301. New York, McGraw-Hill, 1983

DOCKHORN'S

Synonyms. Alport's syndrome variant; hereditary nephropathy without deafness. Alport's syndrome features without associated deafness.

BIBLIOGRAPHY. Dockhorn RJ: Hereditary nephropathy without deafness. Am J Dis Child 114:135–138, 1967

DOEHLE-HELLER

Synonyms. Syphilitic aorta; cardiovascular syphilis.

Symptoms. Both sexes affected but more prevalent in males; average age at onset was 35 to 55 years (today higher, 60–65 yr). In untreated cases of syphilis, present in 75% of cases. Clinically manifested in only 10% of affected individuals. Symptoms related to complications: coronary ostial stenosis; aortic insufficiency; aneurysm.

Signs. Described as a characteristic "loud bell-like or tamborlike second aortic sound"; however, this sign is not specific for this condition. A rough aortic systolic murmur of some significance. (Both signs assume high suggestive value if associated with positive serology for syphilis, in patients over 40 years of age, and in absence of hypertension.)

Etiology. Infection by *Treponema pallidum*. This syndrome usually develops 10 to 25 years after onset of primary syphilitic infection. Inadequacy of early antisyphilitic therapy to be considered among etiologic factors.

Pathology. The lesions are those of syphilitic infection, originating in the aorta or myocardium. Distinctive features: intimal bluish gray plaques; wrinkling of inner aspects of aorta, radial or parallel grooves; sharp demarcation between lesions and healthy areas. Most severe lesions usually located in the ascending aorta above sinus aorta. The histologic changes affect adventia, media (productive mesoarteritis), and intima, with specific inflammatory changes and scarring.

Diagnostic Procedures. *Blood. Serology. Electrocardiography. X-ray of chest. Angiocardiography.*

Therapy. Penicillin and other antibiotics. Surgical treatment.

Prognosis. Condition most frequently diagnosed at autopsy. Uncomplicated forms, relatively benign prognosis. Asymptomatic phase lasts an average of 6 years. Symptomatic phase, formerly considered ominous prognostic sign, today ascertained to last an average of 6.5 years. If heart failure occurs, prognosis becomes very doubtful.

BIBLIOGRAPHY. Döhle KG: Ein Fall von eigentümlicher Aortener-Krankung bei einem Syphilitischen. Kiel, Lipsius und Tischer, 1885
Heller AL: Ueber die syphilitische Aortitis und ihre Bedeutung für die Entstehung von Aneurysmen. Verh Dtsch Pathol Ges p. 346, 1900
O'Neal H, Bulkey BH: Syphilis and the cardiovascular system. In Hurst JW: The Heart, 6th ed, pp 1314–1320. New York, McGraw-Hill, 1986

DOHI'S

Synonyms. Dohi's acropigmentation; symmetric dyschromatosis extremitis.

Symptoms. Relatively frequent in Japan; described also in Europe. Both sexes affected; onset in infancy or early childhood. Asymptomatic.

Signs. Mottled pigmentation and depigmentation on back of hands and feet, occasionally, on upper and lower limbs: Face not affected, except for few small maculae.

Etiology. Unknown. Autosomal dominant inheritance.

BIBLIOGRAPHY. Komaya G: Symmetrische Pigmentanomalie der Extremitaeten. Arch Dermatol Syph 147:389–393, 1924
Gartmann H: Dermatol Wochenschr 125:532, 1952
Siemens HW: Acromelanosis albo-punctate. Dermatologica 128:86–87, 1964
Ortonne JP: "Dyschromies" Encycl Mé Chir Paris 5-1978 Dermatologie 12280 A 10, 1978

DONOHUE'S

Synonym. Leprechaunism.

Symptoms. Prevalent (possibly exclusively) in females, some cases reported in males; rejected by other authors;

present at birth. Failure to thrive; mental retardation; retarded osseous development; sexual precocity.

Signs. *Body.* Hirsutism. Broad nose; hypertelorism; large ears. Lack of adipose tissue. Nipples are hypertrophic; hypertrophy of external genitals.

Etiology. Unknown; familial condition; possibly, recessive inheritance; frequently demonstrated in consanguinity of parents; absence of chromosomal defect. Pathogenetic mechanism: intrauterine follicular maturation.

Pathology. Morphologic changes described. *Pituitary.* Prevalence of chromophobe cells. *Ovary.* Premature follicular maturation with no evidence of luteinization. *Pancreas.* Hyperplasia of islet of Langerhans. *Kidney.* Calcium deposit in collecting tubules. *Liver.* Hemosiderosis. Generalized lymphocyte depletion. *Bones.* Delayed growth.

Diagnostic Procedures. *Blood.* Hypoglycemia. *Urine.* Low gonadotropin excretion; high 17-ketosteroid excretion.

Prognosis. Frequently, death at early age.

BIBLIOGRAPHY. Donohue, WL: Dysendocrinism. J Pediatr 32:739–748, 1948
Frindik JP, Kemp SF, Fiser RH, Schedewie H, Elders JM: Phenotypic expression in Donohue syndrome (leprechaunism): A role for epidermal growth factor. J Pediatr 107:428–429, 1985

DOOR

Synonyms. Deafness, congenital onychoosteodystrophy, recessive; see Robinson's G.C.).

Symptoms and Signs. Both sexes. Mental retardation, seizures, sensorineuronal deafness, onycodystrophy, triphalangeal thumbs, abnormal dermatoglyphics.

Etiology. Autosomal recessive inheritance.

Diagnostic Procedures. *Blood and urine.* Increased organic acid 2-oxoglutarate.

BIBLIOGRAPHY. Walbaum R, Fontaine G, Lienhardt J, et al: Surdite familiale avec osteo-onyco dysplasie. J Genet Hum 18:101–108, 1970
Patton MA, Winter RM, Krywawych S, et al: Raised 2-oxoglutarate in the DOOR syndrome. J Med Genet 22:139, 1985

DORMANDY-PORTER

Synonyms. Fructose-galactose. See Fructose intolerance, hereditary.

BIBLIOGRAPHY. Dormandy TL, Porter RJ: Familial fructose and galactose intolerance. Lancet 1:1189–1194, 1961

Gitzelmann R, Steinman B, Van den Berghe G: Essential fructosuria, hereditary fructose intolerance, and fructose-1,6-diphosphatase deficiency. In Stanbury JB, Wyngaarden JB, Fredrickson DS, et al: The Metabolic Basis of Inherited Disease, 5th ed, p 118. New York, McGraw-Hill, 1983

DORPH'S

Synonym. Cast, acute form.

Symptoms and Signs. Occur in patients wearing body casts for orthopedic reason. Prolonged nausea; repeated vomiting.

Etiology and Pathology. Mechanical compression of fourth portion of duodenum by superior mesenteric artery, resulting in gastric and duodenal dilatation. Intermittent symptoms due to the fact that flatus intermittently passes.

Diagnostic Procedures. *Blood.* Hypokalemic alkalosis; hypovolemia. *Electrocardiography. X-ray.* Dilated duodenum; linear obstruction at the level of duodenal crossing of superior mesenteric vessels. Presence of a long air-fluid level.

Therapy. Removal of cast; surgical duodenal decompression. Early nasogastric suction.

Prognosis. If adequate treatment not instituted when condition becomes manifest, death from hypovolemia and hypokalemic alkalosis may result.

BIBLIOGRAPHY. Dorph MH: The cast syndrome: Review of literature and report of a case. New Eng J Med 243:440–442, 1950

Nelson JP, Ferris DO, Ivins JC: The cast syndrome: Case report. Postgrad Med 42:457–461, 1967

Edmond AS: Scoliosis. In Crenshaw AH (ed): Campbell's Operative Orthopedics, 7th ed, pp 3212–3215. St. Louis, CV Mosby, 1987

DOUBLE OUTLET–LEFT VENTRICLE

Symptoms. Extremely rare. Majority cyanosis; clinical manifestation similar to tricuspid atresia, tetralogy of Fallot, or transposition of great arteries with ventricular septal defect.

Etiology. Unknown.

Pathology. Both great vessels arise above morphologic left ventricle. Ventricular septal defect, pulmonary stenosis. Tricuspid valve abnormalities and right ventricular hypoplasia are frequently associated.

Diagnostic Procedures. *Biplane angiography.*

Therapy. Surgical.

Prognosis. Therapy of palliative value.

BIBLIOGRAPHY. Sakakiara S, Takao A, Arai T et al: Both great vessels arising from left ventricle. Bull Heart Inst J 66, 1967

Van Praagh R, Weinberg PM: Double-outlet left ventricle. In Adams FH, Emmanoulides C (eds): Moss' Heart Disease in Infants, Children and Adolescents, p 370. Baltimore, Williams & Wilkins, 1983

DOUBLE OUTLET–RIGHT VENTRICLE I

Synonym. Right ventricular origin of both great arteries—without pulmonic stenosis. Clinically and hemodynamically not easily distinguished from Tausig-Bing complex (see).

BIBLIOGRAPHY. Perloff JK: The Clinical Recognition of Congenital Heart Disease, 2nd ed, p 496. Philadelphia, WB Saunders, 1978

DOUBLE OUTLET–RIGHT VENTRICLE II

Synonyms. Right ventricle origin of both great arteries—infracristae ventricular septal defect-absence of pulmonic stenosis.

Symptoms and Signs. Both sexes equally affected; present from birth. Initially, cyanosis and digital clubbing mild or absent; later both may appear. Retarded growth; frequent respiratory infections; early congestive heart failure; overactive bulging precordium; both right and left systolic impulses; murmur of ventricular septal defect; loud pulmonic component of second sound.

Etiology. Congenital malformation.

Pathology. Right ventricular origin of both great arteries with infracristal ventricular septal defect and no pulmonic stenosis.

Diagnostic Procedures. *Electrocardiography.* Right ventricular hypertrophy; biatrial P waves. *X-ray.* Cardiomegaly; pulmonary congestion. *Echocardiography. Cardiac catheterization.*

Therapy. Surgical correction.

Prognosis. According to degree of defects. Chronic heart failure.

BIBLIOGRAPHY. Perloff JK: The Clinical Recognition of Congenital Heart Disease, 2nd ed, p 501. Philadelphia, WB Saunders, 1978

DOUBLE OUTLET–RIGHT VENTRICLE IV

Synonyms. Right ventricular origin of both great arteries–pulmonic stenosis.

Symptoms and Signs. Both sexes affected. Cyanosis early sign; initially intermittent or delayed. Other symptoms and signs similar to Fallot's tetralogy (see), including squatting. Symptoms may vary from mild to very severe (complete pulmonary atresia). Signs that differenciate this diagnosis from Fallott's are palpable left ventricular impulse with fourth heart sound and a holosystolic murmur at lower sternal left edge.

Etiology. Congenital malformation.

Pathology. Ventricular origin of both great arteries from right ventricle; ventricular septal defect located below crista supraventricularis (rarely above) and variable degree of pulmonic stenosis.

Diagnostic Procedures. *Electrocardiography.* Left axis deviation; counterclockwise depolarization. *X-ray.* Rounded cardiac apex (in Fallott's tetralogy, bootshaped). *Selective angiocardiography. Echocardiography. Cardiac catheterization.*

Therapy. Surgical correction.

Prognosis. According to degree of defects and treatment.

BIBLIOGRAPHY. Braun K, De Vries A, Feingold DS, et al: Complete dextroposition of aorta, pulmonary stenosis, interventricular septal defect, and patent foramen ovale. Am Heart J 43:773–780, 1952
Perloff JK: The Clinical Recognition of Congenital Heart Disease, 2nd ed, p 154. Philadelphia, WB Saunders, 1978
Hurst JW: The Heart, 6th ed, pp 696–699. New York, McGraw-Hill, 1985
Williams RG, Bierman FZ, Sanders SP: Echocardiographic Diagnosis of Cardiac Malformations, pp 178–183. Boston, Little, Brown & Co, 1986

DOUBLE WHAMMY

Synonym. Voluntary eye propulsion.

Symptoms. Ability to voluntarily propel and retract one or both eyes.

Etiology. Phenomenon produced by contracting superior and inferior obliques while relaxing all rectus muscles, and successive moderate contraction of orbicularis muscle.

Pathology. After years of propulsion, no apparent damage to eyeballs and optic nerve.

BIBLIOGRAPHY. Friedenwald H: Luxation and avulsion of eyeball during birth. Am J Ophthalmol 1:9–12, 1918
Ferrer H: Voluntary propulsion of both eyeballs. Am J Ophthalmol 11:833–855, 1928
Walsh TJ, Gilman M: Voluntary propulsion of the eyes. Am J Ophthalmol 67:583–585, 1960

DOWLING-MEARA

Synonyms. Epidermolysis, herpetiform simple; herpetiform simple epidermolysis bullosa.

Symptoms and Signs. In infancy. Severe and extensive blistering, occasionally involving also mucosae, spontaneous herpetiform blistering of trunks (distinctive feature).

Etiology. Unknown.

Pathology. Initial blister initiating in the basal cells; cytolysis followed by inflammation.

Therapy. Prolonged warm saline soaks. Fever may induce remission.

Prognosis. Condition improving with age.

BIBLIOGRAPHY. Dowling GB, Meara RH: Epidermolysis bullosa resembling juvenile dermatitis herpetiformis. Br J Dermatol 66:139–143, 1954
Rook A, Wilkinson DS, Ebling FJG, et al: Textbook of Dermatology, 4th ed. Oxford, Blackwell Scientific Publications, 1986

DOWN'S

Synonyms. Mongolian idiocy; mongolism; trisomy 21; trisomy 22; trisomy G_1.

Symptoms. Both sexes, all races affected. Incidence related to maternal age. Twenty-five-year-old mother: 1:2000; 35-year-old mother: 1:200; over 40-year-old mother: 1:40 or higher incidence. Two populations: one with high mortality in first year of life or stillborn and another that survives infancy. Mental retardation (IQ 20–60) becoming evident to parent at end of first year of life. Usually, child is happy, affable, and affectionate; walking, speech, and toilet training delayed until 2 to 3 years of age. Generalized hypotonia. Persistent infection and obstructive symptoms of nose. Delayed puberty. In female, early menopause.

Signs. Newborn small, remaining short of stature; tendency to overweight. *Extremities.* Short limbs, hands square; fingers short and stubby; feet short with poorly developed arch. *Dermatoglyphic.* Changes of dermal ridge pattern allows objective diagnosis. *Pelvis.* Iliac wing wide and flat, small iliac angle. *Head.* Small; occiput flat; neck short and thick. *Eyes.* Hypotelorism; small orbital sockets; upper outward slant of palpebral fissures. Iris usually blue or grey, small whitish speckles (Brusfield's spots). Squint common; later in life cataracts frequent. *Nose.* Small; hypoplasia of maxilla; protrusion of tongue; thickened, fissured (scrotal) lower lip may enlarge and hang down in later life. *Teeth.* Malocclusion. Signs of congenital heart defects (in 50% of cases). In neonatal period in some cases, atresia of duodenum. *Genitals.* In male, genitalia undescended and small penis. In female, genitalia show large labia majora and small labia minora. Occasional abnormalities: seizures; strabismus; nystagmus; keratoconus; cataract; low placement of ears; web neck; funnel or pigeon breast; tracheoesophageal fistula; duodenal atresia. The incidence of leukemia is about 1 : 95, or close to 1%.

Etiology. Chromosomal anomalies: (1) Non-disjunction trisomy 21 "regular mongol" (most usual variety); (2) "de novo" translocation (relatively rare); (3) inherited translocation (very rare); (4) mongol mosaicism. Full trisomy 21 94%; 21 trisomy/normal mosaicism 2.4%; translocation cases (equal D/G and G/G) 3.3%.

Pathology. See Signs. In 50%, congenital heart malformations: large cushion septal defect; atrioventricularis communis (most common); frequently tetralogy of Fallot and other types. Fatty metamorphosis in liver (69%); portal tract abnormalities (96%); amyloidosis (8%). Testis frequently undescended; azospermia; absence of part or all of epididymis.

Diagnostic Procedures. *Dermatoglyphic* and *chromosome studies.* See Etiology. *Blood.* Acute leukemia three times more common than in comparable age group. Alkaline phosphatase of leukocytes increased. A number of enzymes are also increased.

Therapy. No cure; help family to adjust to situation. Treat repeated respiratory infections and heart conditions when present.

Prognosis. Fifty percent die within first year. Average life span of survivors around 30 years. Female may be fertile; male infertile.

BIBLIOGRAPHY. Down JLH: Observations on an ethnic classification of idiots. Clin Lect Rep London Hosp 3:259–262, 1866
Roberts DF, Callow MH: Origin of the additional chromosome in Down's syndrome: A study of 20 families. J Med Genet 17:363–367, 1980
Trisomy 21: An International Symposium. Hum Gen Suppl 2, Heidelberg, Springer, 1981
Hartley XY: A summary of recent research into the development of children with Down's syndrome. J Ment Defic Res 30:1–14, 1986
Gath A, Gumley D: Behavior problems in retarded children with special reference to Down's syndrome. Br J Psychiatry 149:156–161, 1986

DOW-VAN BOGAERT

Synonym. See Choreiform syndromes.

BIBLIOGRAPHY. Dow RS, Van Bogaert L: On complex involuntary movements appearing late following the resection of a cerebellar hemisphere. J Belge de Neurol Psychiat 38:803–807, 1938

DOYNE'S

Synonyms. Honey-comb retinal degeneration. Halt House–Batten. See Retina posterior pole colloidal degeneration.

Symptoms and Signs. Both sexes affected; onset in third decade. Formation of white spots in peripapillary areas, and usually in the macular area as well. Between fourth and fifth decades lesions multiply; finally, white bodies become confluent to produce a white confluent atrophic area. Visual deterioration progressive in 75% of cases (white bodies on nasal side of optic disk pathognomonic of this form).

Etiology. Unknown; autosomal dominant transmission.

Pathology. Nodular thickening of Bruch's membrane; choroid normal; evolution to homogeneous atrophy involving optic disk and macular area.

Diagnostic Procedures. *Ophthalmologic examination.*

Prognosis. Progressive visual deterioration. Absence of lesion in macular area in a 35-year-old patient can be regarded as a favorable prognostic sign.

BIBLIOGRAPHY. Doyne RW: Peculiar condition of choroiditis occurring in several members of the same family. Trans Ophthamol Soc UK 19:71, 1899
Pearce WG: Doyne's honey-comb retinal degeneration. Br J Ophthalmol 52:73–78, 1968

DREIFUSS-EMERY

Synonyms. Emery-Dreifuss (X-linked); muscular dystrophy, tardive; rigid spine.

Symptoms and Signs. Males. Onset 4 to 5 years of age. Muscle weakness, initially involving the lower extremities (tendency to walk on tip-toes, followed in the early teens by waddling gait), then by marked weakness of shoulder girdle muscles. Increase lumbar lordosis, flexion deformities of elbows. Mild pectus excavatum, cardiac involvement and absence of muscular pseudohypertrophy. Mental retardation.

Etiology. Unknown. X-linked inheritance. An autosomal dominant form identified with various clinical differences. See Emery-Dreifuss, autosomal dominant.

BIBLIOGRAPHY. Cestan R, LeJonne NI: Une myopathy avec retractions familiales. Nous. Iconog. Salpetriere 15:38–52, 1902

Dreiffus FE, Hogan GR: Survival in X-linked chromosomal muscular dystrophy. Neurology 11:734–737, 1961

Emery AEH, Dreifuss FE: Unusual type of benign X-linked muscular dystrophy. J Neurol Neurosurg Psychiatry 29:338–342, 1966

Thomas PK, Petty RKH: Emery–Dreifuss muscular dystrophy. J Med Genet 22:138–139, 1985

DRESBACH'S

Synonyms. Hemolytic elliptocytic anemia, hereditary ovalocytosis, hereditary elliptocytosis (HE), hereditary pyropoikilocytosis (HPP) which probably represents a more severe form of the same disease. Five clinical phenotypes have been described.

1. MILD HE

Symptoms and Signs. All races, no anemia or splenomegaly, mild hemolysis. Elliptocytosis is a morphologic curiosity except in cases (5–20%) in which cirrhosis, infectious mononucleosis or malaria decompensate the disease. Cases of mild HE with abnormal erythropoiesis are described in southern Italians.

Etiology. Autosomal dominant.

Diagnostic Procedures. *Blood smear.* More than 30% of RBC are elliptocytes.

Therapy. When necessary, splenectomy.

Prognosis. Good.

2. MILD HE WITH POIKILOCYTOSIS IN INFANCY

Symptoms and Signs. Neonatal jaundice, hemolytic anemia in childhood. Predominant in blacks. In adult life only mild HE.

Etiology. Autosomal dominant.

Diagnostic Procedures. *Blood smear of parents.* One will have mild HE. *Blood smear.* Poikilocytes or elliptocytes.

Therapy. Splenectomy usually not necessary.

Prognosis. Good.

3. SPHEROCYTIC HE

Symptoms and Signs. Families of European descent. Hemolysis always present. Splenomegaly.

Etiology. Autosomal dominant.

Diagnostic Procedures. *Blood smear.* Elliptocytosis and spherocytosis.

Therapy. Splenectomy often necessary.

Prognosis. Good.

4. STOMATOCYTIC HE

Symptoms and Signs. Only in aborigines of Melanesia. Mild hemolysis.

Etiology. Autosomal recessive.

Diagnostic Procedures. *Blood smear.* Roundish elliptocytes traversed by one or two traverse bars (appearance of double stomatocytes).

Therapy. None.

Prognosis. Good.

5. HEREDITARY PYROPOIKILOCYTOSIS (HPP)

Symptoms and Signs. In blacks. In childhood severe hemolytic anemia with complications, growth retardation, frontal bossing.

Etiology. Unknown. Maybe autosomal recessive.

Diagnostic Procedures. *Blood smear.* Extreme poikilocytosis with spherocytes, elliptocytes, triangulocytes. Abnormal thermal sensitivity of blood.

Therapy. Splenectomy.

Prognosis. Severe.

BIBLIOGRAPHY. Dresbach M: Elliptical human red corpuscles. Science 19:469–470, 1904

Bunn HF, Forget BG: Hemoglobin: Molecular, Genetic and Clinical Aspects. Philadelphia, WB Saunders, 1986

DRESSLER'S (D.)

Synonyms. Donath-Landsteiner; Harley's; paroxysmal cold hemoglobinuria. See Hemolytic anemia of newborn.

Symptoms. Both sexes affected; onset at all ages (syphilitic type onset in young group). Paroxysmal attacks of hemoglobinuria; in some patients frequent episodes induced by minor cold exposure; in others, rare attacks induced by exposure to very low temperature. From a few minutes to hours after exposure to cold (also limited to an area of the body) pains in the back and legs, abdominal cramps, headache, shaking chills, hyperpyrexia and hemoglobinuria lasting a few hours; temporary enlargement of spleen and jaundice with each attack. Abortive attacks may occur with simple hemoglobinuria without systemic manifestations. Vasomotor phenomena. Paresthesias; urticaria; cyanosis; Raynaud's phenomena with or without gangrene observed in several cases.

Etiology. Congenital syphilis (chronic type), idiopathic (acute transient type and chronic type), or associated with cold agglutinin.

Pathology. That of congenital syphilis when it is the cause.

Diagnostic Procedures. *Blood.* Anemia after attack; all findings of hemolytic crisis; leukopenia followed by neutrophilic leukocytosis; erythrophagocytosis. *Donath-Landsteiner antibody test.* Positive, "biphasic test." *Rosenbach's test* (immersion of extremity in cold water induces hemolytic crisis). *Erlich's test* (ligature around finger). Immersion in icy water: demonstration of local hemoglobinemia. *Serology.* For syphilis. *Coomb's test* (and other studies). For differential diagnosis of other hemolytic anemias. *Urine.* Presence of hemoglobin and methemoglobin.

Therapy. Antisyphilitic treatment (when syphilis demonstrated). In idiopathic case, no specific treatment. Adrenocorticotropic hormone (ACTH) and steroid reported beneficial. Avoidance of exposure to cold.

Prognosis. Usually chronic, relatively benign condition; seldom cause of severe anemia or death. Great variability of clinical manifestations, from simple, minimal hemoglobinuria after exposure to intense cold to repeated attacks with minimal temperature variations.

BIBLIOGRAPHY. Elliotson J: Diseases of the heart united with ague. Lancet 1:500–501, 1832
Dressler DR: Ein Fall von intermittirender Albuminurie und Chromaturie. Arch Pathol Anat Physiol 6:264–266, 1853
Donath J, Landsteiner K: Ueber paroxysmale Hämoglobinurie. Münch Med Wochenschr 51:1590–1593, 1904
Wintrobe MM (ed): Clinical Hematology, 8th ed. Philadelphia, Lea & Febiger, 1981

DRESSLER'S (W.)

Synonym. Postmyocardial infarction.

Symptoms and Signs. Develops after 2 to 10 weeks in 3% to 4% of cases of recent myocardial infarction. Fever; chest pain; symptoms and signs of pericarditis, pleurisy, and pneumonitis; tendency to recurrences, although the full picture (including pericarditis and pneumonia) is not always present.

Etiology. Unknown. Some evidence has been found that an antigen produced by myocardial necrosis may induce the formation of autoantibodies.

Pathology. That of myocardial infarction, pleurisy, pneumonia.

Diagnostic Procedures. *Blood.* Increase of sedimentation rate and leukocytosis; demonstration of heart autoantibodies. *Blood Cultures. X-ray of chest. Electrocardiography.*

Therapy. Corticosteroids, indomethacin, aspirin.

Prognosis. Good response to corticosteroids. Danger of cardiac tamponade, especially with patients on anticoagulant. Repeated episodes last for a week or two (exceptionally, 3–6 weeks); recurrences may occur up to 12 months.

BIBLIOGRAPHY. Dressler W: A complication of myocardial infarction resembling idiopathic recurrent benign pericarditis. Circulation 12:697, 1955
Markoff R: Klinische Bedeutung des Dressler-Syndroms. Dtsch Med Wochenschr 93:627–633, 1968
Hurst JW: The Heart, 6th ed, p 987. New York, McGraw-Hill, 1986

DREUW'S

Synonym. Alopecia parvimaculata.

Symptoms and Signs. Both sexes affected; onset at all ages. Usually, epidemic outbreaks. Rapid development of several small, irregular patches of alopecia.

Etiology. Unknown.

Pathology. Lymphocytic infiltration around hair follicle, sparing the bulbs, followed by atrophic, sclerotic changes. Sebaceous glands and hair follicles disappear; sweat glands remain.

Therapy. None.

Prognosis. The hair may regrow or permanent bald scars remain.

BIBLIOGRAPHY. Dreuw M: Ueber epidemische Alopecia; Vorlaufige Mitteilung. Monatsschr Prakt Dermatol 51:18–22, 1910
Hofer W: Sporadisches Auftreten von Alopecia parvimaculata. Dermatol Wochenschr 149:381–386, 1964

DREYFUS'

Synonym. Platyspondylisis (Obsolete).

Symptoms. Short neck; slow development of kyphoscoliosis; joint laxity; muscle weakness; batracian (froglike) abdomen; short stature.

Etiology. Unknown. Not a clear entity. Individual manifestations and their associations are present in many syndromes.

BIBLIOGRAPHY. Dreyfus JR: Ueber ein neues mit allgemeiner wahrer oder scheinbarer Breitwirbligkeit (Platyspondylia vera aut spuria generalisata) ein hergehends Syndrom. Jahr Kinderheilkd 150:42–54, 1938

DROBIN'S

Synonym. Renal-ocular.

Symptoms. Fever, myalgias, conjunctival/scleral injection of eyes, enlargement of lymph nodes.

Signs. Ophthalmologic examination: acute iritis. Blood tests: abnormal renal function.

Etiology. Unknown; probably it is a virallike illness.

Pathology. Renal biopsy: acute interstitial nephritis that can be mononuclear or eosinophilic; bone marrow, lymph nodes: granulomas.

Diagnostic Procedures. Blood screening for kidney function; renal biopsy; lymph node or bone marrow biopsies.

Differential Diagnosis. Tuberculosis, sarcoidosis, Wegener's granulomatosis, collagen vascular disorder, Behcet's disease, syphilis, toxoplasmosis, cytomegalovirus infection, leprosy, *Chlamydia psittaci* infection, herpes simplex infection.

Therapy. Steroids, *e.g.*, prednisone, 60 mg/day, tapered after 1 month to 30 mg/day. Topical steroids and atropine on the affected eye.

Prognosis. Good.

BIBLIOGRAPHY. Drobin RS, Vernier RL, Fish AL: Acute eosinophilic interstitial nephritis and renal failure with bone marrow-lymph node granulomas and anterior uveitis. A new syndrome. Am J Med 59:325–333, 1975
Steinman TI, Silva P: Acute interstitial nephritis and iritis. Renal-ocular syndrome. Am J Med 77:189–191, 1984

DRUMMOND'S

Synonyms. Blue diaper; hypercalcemia-nephrocalcinosis-indicanuria.

Symptoms. Both sexes affected; onset during first year of life. Anorexia; vomiting; constipation; irritability; failure to thrive; fever and recurrent infections; renal failure; reduced visual acuity.

Signs. Pallor; dwarfism; depressed nose bridge; prominent epicanthal folds; nystagmus; strabismus; papilledema; optic atrophy. Bluish discoloration of diaper.

Etiology. Metabolic defect, possibly familial; defective transport of tryptophan (which produces increased indole and indicanuria: thus blue diaper). Reported cases from vitamin D intoxication.

Pathology. See Signs. Occasionally, sclerosis of optic foramina. Peripheral retinal atrophy and optic atrophy. Osteosclerosis. Nephrocalcinosis in the cortex; granuloma formation in medulla; periglomerular fibrosis.

Diagnostic Procedures. *Urine.* Indicanuria and other indole derivatives. Reduced inulin and para-aminohippuric acid (PAH) clearances; increased phosphorus excretion. *Stool.* Increase of tryptophan and derivatives. *Blood.* Hypercalciuria; hyperazotemia; hypercreatinemia

Therapy. Reduction of calcium intake. Corticosteroids.

Prognosis. Poor for function and *quoad vitam.*

BIBLIOGRAPHY. Drummond KN, Michael AF, Ulstrom RA, et al: The blue diaper syndrome: Familial hypercalcemia with nephrocalcinosis and indicanuria. A new familial disease, with definition of the metabolic abnormality. Am J Med 37:928–948, 1964

DUANE'S

Synonyms. Eye retraction; retraction; Stilling's; Stilling-Türk-Duane; Türk-Stilling.

Symptoms and Signs. Prevalent in females; onset from birth. Deficiency of convergence and occasionally up or down deviation on adduction. Reduction or loss of abduction of the globe; retraction on adduction with occasional limitation of this movement; narrowing of palpebral fissure in adduction and widening in attempts of abduction. Pupillary changes; heterochromia iridis. Frequently associated, Klippel-Feil (see) and various malformations of face, ears, and teeth.

Etiology. Congenital defect; central nervous system probably supranuclear lesion determining a paradoxical synergism of the external and internal rectus muscles instead of the usual antagonism. This etiologic hypothesis is based on characteristic electromyographic response; histologic evidence still not provided.

Pathology. Alteration of external rectus muscle occasionally observed. Pathologic changes may be central (supra-nuclear lesion); aberrant innervation affects oculomotor (III) and facial (VII) nerves. The syndrome has been described in association with cerebral arteriovenous malformation and with other associated malformations that have been simplified into four categories: skeletal, auricular, ocular, and neural.

Diagnostic Procedures. *Electromyography.* Pattern of eye muscles. *CT brain scan. Cerebral arteriography.* When indicated.

Therapy. When electromyography shows paradoxical innervation, surgery for correction is contraindicated. Surgical correction of associated anomalies.

BIBLIOGRAPHY. Türk S: Ueber Retractions-bewegungen der Augen. Dsch Med Wochenschr 22:199, 1896
Duane A: Congenital deficiency of abduction, associated with impairment of adduction, retraction movements, contraction of palpebral fissure and oblique movements of the eye. Arch Ophthalmol 34:133–159, 1905
Blodi FC, Van Allen MW, Yarbrough JC: Duane's syndrome: A brain stem lesion. Arch Ophthalmol 72:171–177, 1964
Singh P, Patnaik B: Heredity in Duane's syndrome. Acta Ophthalmol (Copen) 49:103–110, 1971
Sachdev JS, Harrington JL: Duane's retraction syndrome associated with cerebral arteriovenous malformation. South Med J 79:623–625, 1986

DUBIN-JOHNSON

Synonyms. Black liver–jaundice; Dubin-Sprinz; icterus–hepatic pigmentation; chronic idiopathic jaundice; Sprinz-Nelson.

Symptoms. Both sexes affected; onset in childhood or adult life. In women, occasionally unmasked by contraceptive pills or pregnancy. Intermittent episodes of jaundice associated with mild pain in right hypochondrium. Absence of pruritus. Occasionally weakness, fatigue. Frequent occurrence in Persian Jews associated with factor VII deficiency.

Signs. Mild enlargement of liver and tenderness.

Etiology. Autosomal recessive inheritance. Primary defect in secretion of conjugated bilirubin and other organic anions.

Pathology. *Liver.* Black color; deposit of melaninlike pigment in parenchymal cells; especially centrilobular ar-

eas; normal bile canaliculi, no fibrosis or inflammation; Kupffer's cells no pigment.

Diagnostic Procedures. *Blood.* Increased conjugated bilirubin; serum alkaline phosphatases normal; sodium sulfobromophthalein level increased. *Urine.* Bilirubinuria; abnormal distribution of coproporphyrin isomer I and III (pathognomonic). *Cholecystography.* Often, lack of visualization of biliary system. *Biopsy of liver.* Diagnostic (see Pathology).

Therapy. None; advise the patient about congenital nature of condition and reassure about benign nature and no need for unnecessary surgery.

Prognosis. Good; no limitation on normal life.

BIBLIOGRAPHY. Dubin IN, Johnson FB: Chronic idiopathic jaundice with unidentified pigment in liver cells: New clinicopathologic entity with report of 12 cases. Medicine 33:155–197, 1954
Sprinz H, Nelson RS: Persistent non-hemolytic hyperbilirubinemia associated with lipochrome-like pigment in liver cells: Report of 4 cases. Ann Intern Med 41:952–962, 1954
Wolkoff AW, Chowdbury JR, Arias IM: Hereditary jaundice and disorders of bilirubin metabolism. In Stanbury JB, Wyngaarden JB, Fredrickson DS, et al: The Metabolic Basis of Inherited Disease, 5th ed, p 1385. New York, McGraw-Hill, 1983

DUBOWITZ'S

Synonyms. Dwarfism, eczema, peculiar facies.

Symptoms. Both sexes affected; present from birth. Mental deficiencies mild to moderate; hyperactivity; stubborness; shyness; high-pitched cry. Feeding difficulties; diarrhea; rhinorrhea; otitis.

Signs. Low birth weight. *Head.* Microcephaly (mild); small facies; shallow supraorbital ridge; hypertelorism, short palpebral fissures; lateral telecanthus; palpebral ptosis; micrognathia; caries. *Face and flexural areas.* Eczema; scarce hair; missing or reduced lateral eyebrows. Occasionally cleft palate, pes planus, cryptorchidism, hypospadia. *Vascular (arterial) abnormalities.* Right internal carotid artery occlusion; aberrant right subclavian artery; coarctation of the aorta.

Etiology. Autosomal recessive (?) inheritance.

Therapy. Surgical correction of vascular abnormalities.

Prognosis. Eczema recedes between second and fourth year of age. Lack of speech development. Proportioned dwarfism.

BIBLIOGRAPHY. Dubowitz V: Familial low birth weight dwarfism with unusual facies and a skin eruption. J Med Genet 2:12–17, 1969

Bailey JA: Congenital facial anomalies with neurological defects. Springfield, CC Thomas, 1969

Smith DW: Recognizable patterns of Human Malformation. Philadelphia, WB Saunders, 1976

Orrison WW, Schnitzler ER, Chun RWM: The Dubowitz syndrome. Further observations. Am J Genet 7:155–170, 1980

Shuper A, Merlob P, Weitz R, et al: The diagnosis of Dubowitz syndrome in the neonatal period—A case report. Eur J Pediatr 145:151–152, 1986

DUCHENNE'S I

Synonyms. Progressive bulbar palsy; labioglossolaryngeal paralysis.

Symptoms. Onset between 50 and 60 years of age. Progressive speech defect, from minor defect in articulation to the production of incomprehensible sound (laryngeal). Mastication and deglutition defect with occasional nasal regurgitation; drooling; gait and movement affected by spasticity of extremities; occasionally ophthalmoplegia. Loss of emotional control with episodes of sudden laughing and crying.

Signs. Weakness of facial muscles; spasticity of extremity muscles; hyperreflexia.

Etiology. Degeneration of the bulbar nuclei of trigeminal (V), facial (VII), glossopharyngeal (IX), vagus (X), and hypoglossal (XII) nerves, in association with other degenerative disorders, or primary. Considered as a variant of amyotrophic lateral sclerosis (see Aran-Duchenne).

Pathology. Degeneration of mentioned nuclei and corticobulbar tracts. Atrophic changes and glial reaction.

Therapy. None.

Prognosis. Poor; involvement of respiratory centers cause of death.

BIBLIOGRAPHY. Duchenne G: Paralysie musculaire progressive de la langue, du voile du palais et des lèvres: Affection non encore décrite comme espéche morbide distincte. Arch Gen Med 16:283–296, 1860

Adams RD, Victor M: Principles of Neurology, 3rd ed, p 830. New York, McGraw-Hill, 1985

DUCHENNE'S II

Synonyms. Duchenne-Griesinger; pseudohypertrophic muscular dystrophy; Landouzy-Duchenne. Muscular dystrophy, pseudohypertrophic, progressive; DMD.

Symptoms. Affects only males (see Duchenne's dystrophy in females); onset between first and sixth years. Waddling gait; frequent falling; clumsiness. Gower's maneuver to arise when lying on the floor. Axial and proximal girdle muscles of lower and then upper extremities involved before distal girdle muscles. Eventually, patient becomes confined to wheelchair and contractures develop. Frequent respiratory infections.

Signs. Pseudohypertrophy of calves and occasionally of deltoid triceps and other muscles. Palpation reveals doughy consistence. Scoliosis, muscular atrophy, and contractures develop when patient can no longer walk. Cardiac enlargement and sinus tachycardia.

Etiology. Unknown; sex-linked recessive inheritance. Sporadic cases also reported. Possibility of a group with autosomal recessive type has been discussed.

Pathology. Muscle pale; fishlike, abnormal fibers surrounded by fat and fibrous tissue.

Diagnostic Procedures. *Blood.* Aldolase; creatine phosphatase, serum glutamic-oxaloacetic transaminase (SGOT), glutamic-pyruvic transaminase (GPT), lactic dehydrogenase, increased during course of disease; in advanced disease revert to normal or remain only slightly elevated. *Electroencephalography. Electromyography:* Abnormalities of conduction. *Biopsy of muscle.*

Therapy. Exercise and activity to limit of tolerance. Bracing, surgery (in young patients, fasciotomy), and orthopedic measures prolong self-sufficiency.

Prognosis. Confinement to wheelchair usually at 9 to 12 years of age. Velocity of progression of disease grossly inversely proportional to age of onset; 75% of patients die by the age of 20. Mortality rate drops sharply after that age; 5% remain alive at age 50. Sudden death from myocardial failure, respiratory infections.

BIBLIOGRAPHY. Duchenne GB: Recherches sur la paralysie musculaire pseudohypertrophique, ou paralysie myosclérosique. Arch Gen Med 11:5–25, 179–209; 305–321; 421–443, 552–588, 1868

Dubowitz V: Involvement of the nervous system in muscular dystrophy in man. NY Acad Sci 317:431–439, 1979

Moser H: Duchenne muscular dystrophy: Pathogenetic aspects and genetic prevention. Hum Genet 66:17–40, 1984

DUCHENNE'S DYSTROPHY IN FEMALES

Symptoms and Signs. Only females are carriers of the condition, since it has a recessive sex-linked type of transmission. Carrier without clinical manifestations may be identified in approximately 80% of cases by biochemical studies: increase of creatine phosphokinase. Occasionally, female may present typical clinical symptoms of Duchenne's syndrome. The course is usually mild and slowly evolving.

Etiology. Unknown. Occurrence of clinical form of syndrome in female difficult to explain because of inheritance type of pattern. The following possibilities considered: (1) chromosomal mosaicism; (2) possible existence of an autosomal type of transmission; (3) Lyon hypothesis.

BIBLIOGRAPHY. Pearson CM, Fowler WM, Wright SW: X-chromosome mosaicism in females with muscular dystrophy. Proc Nat Acad Sci USA 50:24, 1963

Verellen–Dumolin C, Freund M, De Meyer R, et al: Expression of X-linked muscular dystrophy in a female due to translocation involving X p21 and non-random inactivation of the normal X-chromosome. Hum Genet 67:115–119, 1984

DUCKERT'S

Synonyms. Factor XIII deficiency; fibrinase deficiency; fibrin stabilizing factor; FSF deficiency; LL factor; Laki-Lorand.

Symptoms and Signs. Prevalent in males. After birth bleeding from umbilicus. Usually after injury episode of serious bleeding. Wounds heal slowly and may break repeatedly. Hematomas; hematuria.

Etiology. Possibly autosomal recessive inheritance or X-linked (evidence lacking).

Diagnostic Procedures. *Blood.* Clotting tests normal. Fibrin prepared from patient soluble in 5 molor urea or 1% monoacetic acid.

Therapy. Transfusion of small amount of plasma (also stored) controls bleeding. Fibrin life (3–5 days).

Prognosis. Intracranial bleeding frequent cause of death. Good response to treatment; long survival possible.

BIBLIOGRAPHY. Duckert I, Jung E, Shmerling DH: A hitherto undescribed congenital haemorrhagic diathesis probably due to fibrin stabilizing factor deficiency. Thromb Diath Haemorrh 5:179–186, 1961

Kitchen CS, Newcomb TF: Factor XIII. Medicine 58:413, 1979

DUCTUS ARTERIOSUS, PATENT

Synonyms. Patent ductus arteriosus.

Symptoms. Symptoms are usually restricted to patients with large shunts that produce heart failure. Prevalent in

females (3 : 1). In most cases, asymptomatic, in few cases exertional dyspnea, palpitation, fatigability. Occasionally, physical underdevelopment. Cardiac failure sooner or later. Frequent complication; bacterial endocarditis.

Signs. Pallor; habitus gracilis. *Heart.* Typical Gibson's murmur; machinerylike occupying most of systole and diastole, with characteristic crescendo-systolic thrill over site of maximal intensity of sound. Second pulmonic sound accentuated; high pulse pressure; occasionally, a Corrigan pulse; capillary pulsation; pistol-shot femoral pulse and radial pulses may be unequal.

Etiology. Unknown; reported as inherited recessive characteristic, or autosomal dominant inheritance. Maternal rubella complication.

Pathology. Patency of ductus arteriosus, uncomplicated or associated with other cardiac anomalies. In uncomplicated cases, pulmonary artery and branches become dilated, as well as both ventricles, which also show different degree of hypertrophy.

Diagnostic Procedures. *H-mode echocardiography. Pulsed Doppler ultrasonography. X-ray.* Prominence of pulmonic arc in left upper portion of heart silhouette. *Angiocardiography. Electrocardiography. Cardiac catheterization.*

Therapy. Surgical (closure of ductus) and medical (Indomethacin).

Prognosis. Excellent; complete recovery with surgery in uncomplicated cases. If not treated, cardiac failure and endocarditis cause death.

BIBLIOGRAPHY. Wells HG: Persistent patency of the ductus arteriosus. Am J Med Sci 136:381, 1908

Perloff JK: The Clinical Recognition of Congenital Heart Disease, 2nd ed, p 524. Philadelphia, WB Saunders, 1978

Keith JD, Rowe RD, Vlad P: Heart Disease in Infancy and Childhood, 3rd ed. New York, Macmillan, 1978

Hurst JW: The Heart, 6th ed, pp 614–618. New York, McGraw-Hill, 1986

DUCTUS ARTERIOSUS, PATENT REVERSED FLOW

Symptoms. Usually present at birth. Exertional dyspnea; squatting occasionally present. Patent ductus is more common in the premature infant, especially those with birth asphyxia or respiratory distress syndrome.

Signs. Cyanosis (increasing with exercise) more intense in lower half of the body and in left hand rather than right. Clubbing may involve only lower extremities. Only a faint systolic murmur in third left interspace or no murmur. Seldom, diastolic murmur on left sternal border, loud with diastolic thrill.

Etiology. Unknown; patent ductus arteriosus with high pulmonary vascular resistance and reversed flow from pulmonary artery to aorta.

Pathology. Patency of ductus arteriosus. Hypertrophy of right ventricle. Pulmonary arteries normal or with occlusive lesions.

Diagnostic Procedures. *X-ray.* Prominence of pulmonary artery and its branches; sharp cut off of small peripheral pulmonary artery. *Angiocardiography. Electrocardiography. Cardiac catheterization. Pressure determination. Oximetry. H-mode echocardiography. Pulsed Doppler ultrasonography.*

Therapy. Surgery usually contraindicated when pulmonary pressure very high and with shunt reversal. When transient (exertional) reversal of flow, surgery may be highly beneficial.

Prognosis. Smaller degree of myocardial insufficiency than in simple patent ductus arteriosus. High incidence of bacterial endocarditis. Patient may live for many years.

BIBLIOGRAPHY. Perloff JK: The Clinical Recognition of Congenital Heart Disease, 2nd ed, p 524. Philadelphia, WB Saunders, 1978

Keith JD, Rowe RD, Vland P: Heart Disease in Infancy and Childhood, 3rd ed. New York, Macmillan, 1978

Braunwald E: Heart Disease, vol 2, pp 994–996. Philadelphia, WB Saunders, 1980

Hurst JW: The Heart, 6th ed, pp 614–618. New York, McGraw-Hill, 1986

DUDLEY-KLINGENSTEIN

Synonyms. Jejunum neoplasm. See Peutz-Jeghers and Gardner's.

Symptoms. Combination of melena and abdominal pain, simulating a gastroduodenal lesion.

Signs. Pallor; tachycardia; abdominal distention.

Etiology. Benign or malignant lesion of jejunum.

Diagnostic Procedures. *X-ray of gastrointestinal tract.* Negative for gastroduodenal ulcer (pyloric spasm may occasionally be observed); jejunum shows filling defect. *Gastric fluid.* Usually, normal or low values of chlorhydric acid. *Blood.* Posthemorrhagic anemia.

Therapy. Surgery.

Prognosis. Depends on nature of lesion.

BIBLIOGRAPHY. Dudley HD: Vascular tumors of the small intestine with symptoms simulating peptic ulcer. Surg Clin North Am 14:1331–1337, 1934

Klingenstein P: Benign neoplasms of the small intestine complicated by severe hemorrhage: Report of two cases operative intervention and recovery. J Mt Sinai Hosp 4:972–979, 1938

Garvin PJ: Benign and malignant tumors of the small intestine. Curr Prob Cancer 3:1 (all issue), 1979

Perzin KH, Bridge MF: Adenomas of the small intestine: A clinicopathologic review of 51 cases and a study of their relationship to carcinoma. Cancer 48:799–819, 1981

DUHRING'S

Synonyms. Brocq-Duhring; dermatitis herpetiformis; dermatitis multiformis.

Symptoms and Signs. Prevalent in males (2 : 1); onset usually between 20 to 55 years of age; occasionally, in child over 5 years of age. Onset acute or gradual. Pruritus; pleomorphic, symmetric skin eruptions: erythematous, urticarial, papular, vesicular or bullous that excoriate easily (small papules without blistering also seen); eczematous, exudative; or lichenified. Progressive pigmentation at site of lesion (in 50% of cases). Lesion affects extensor aspects of extremities, especially knee and elbows, and buttocks. Also frequently involved, axillary folds, shoulders, trunk, and face. Seldom, mucosal lesions. Occasionally, laryngeal involvement. Majority of patients: asymptomatic gluten enteropathy.

Etiology. Unknown. Role of gluten not yet clearly established.

Pathology. Accumulation of neutrophils and eosinophils within dermal papillae; in vicinity of early blisters, formation of subepidermal vesicles. No advanced acantholysis.

Diagnostic Procedures. *Biopsy. Blood.* Occasionally, increase of circulating eosinophils. A variety of antibodies in some patients (antithyroid, antireticulin, antigluten, and antigliadin); IgA-containing immune complexes in 25% of patients, more rarely IgG or IgM complexes.

Therapy. Prolonged treatment with maintenance doses of dapsone. Sulfapyridine better tolerated by some patients. Topical application of corticosteroids (symptomatic).

Prognosis. Long course, remissions and relapses; 20 to 30% with permanent or prolonged remission.

BIBLIOGRAPHY. Duhring LA: Dermatitis herpetiformis. JAMA 3:325–329, 1884

Brocq L: De la dermatite Herpetiforme de Duhring. Ann Dermatol Syph 9:1–20, 1888

Duhring LA: Selected Monographs on Dermatology. London, New Sydenham Soc, 1893

Rook A, Wilkinson DS, Ebling FJG, et al: Textbook of Dermatology, 4th ed, p 1651. Oxford, Blackwell Scientific Publications, 1986

DUPLAY'S

Synonyms. Subacromial bursitis; scapulohumeral bursitis; subdeltoid bursitis; frozen shoulder; periarticular fibrositis shoulder; scapulohumeral periarthritis; shoulder adhesive capsulitis.

Symptoms. Occur after 40 years of age; prevalent in women (seldom before menopause); in older men, and in sedentary workers. Gradually increasing pain in the shoulder during abduction and internal rotation, up to severe debilitating pain. Pain radiates to the arm and forearm, occasionally to scapular area.

Signs. Scapulohumeral fixation; arm adducted. Tenderness on palpation in various areas of shoulder.

Etiology. Trauma (15%); idiopathic (85%); frequently observed after periods of inactivity; muscle spasm in anxiety and depression; associated with some visceral diseases.

Pathology. Adhesive capsulitis arising from joint lining and spreading to it from other extrarticular joint structures.

Diagnostic Procedures. *X-ray.* Negative. After 2 to 3 months, demineralization of upper humerus.

Therapy. Moderate exercise initially; treatment of emotional aspects. In chronic cases; x-ray treatment, systemic corticosteroids, hydrocortisone injections. Surgery: closed or open manipulation.

Prognosis. Chronic course and prolonged disability frequent. Response to treatment not as good as in calcareous tendonitis.

BIBLIOGRAPHY. Duplay ES: De la peri-arthrite scapulo-humerale et des raideurs de l'épaule qui en sont la conséquence. Arch Gen Med 20:513–542, 1872
Richardson EG: Miscellaneous nontramatic disorders. In Crenshaw AH (ed): Campbell's Operative Orthopedics, 7th ed, pp 1016–1017, 2258. St Louis, CV Mosby, 1987

DUPRE'S

Synonym. Meningism.

Symptoms. Occurs mostly in infancy and childhood. Suddenly during the onset of an acute febrile disease: headache; neck stiffness; occasionally, convulsion and coma.

Signs. Positive Kernig's sign.

Etiology. Increase in pressure of spinal fluid during the onset of acute febrile disease due to relative hemodilution and filtration through choroid plexus.

Diagnostic Procedures. *Cerebrospinal fluid.* Increased pressure; increased proteins; negative bacteriologic studies; negative virus studies.

Therapy. Diuretics and control of pressure.

Prognosis. Spontaneous recovery within a few days.

BIBLIOGRAPHY. Dupré E: Le méningisme. Cong Fr Med 1:411–423, 1895
Adams RD, Victor M: Principles of Neurology, 3rd ed, pp 463–469. New York, McGraw–Hill, 1985

DUPUYTREN'S

Synonym. Palmo-plantar fibromatosis.

Symptoms. Prevalent in males (6:1); high familial incidence; gradual increase of incidence with age, especially after 40 years of age. Unilateral or bilateral involvement. Right hand more frequently affected. Fingers affected in the following order: little, middle, index. Pain on the palm of hands. Progressive loss of function of hand due to inability to extend fingers.

Signs. Small nodular thickening of palmar connective tissue, especially over fourth and fifth fingers. Puckering of palmar skin. Various degrees of flexion contracture of fingers.

Etiology. Unknown; hereditary (observed in several generations of same family). Associated with many different pathologic conditions: epilepsy; pulmonary tuberculosis; chronic alcoholism; Steinbrocker's; Peyronie's.

Pathology. Small nodules or thickening of palmar connective tissues overlying tendons of fingers; adherence between fascia and skin, successive appearance of fibrous bands from nodules to base of fingers.

Therapy. For pain (in nodular stage) reassurance of benign nature of pain. Ultrasound; heat; exercises; local injection of steroids (in early phase). Surgery after contracture begins according to degree of involvement; best results after active phase has subsided.

Prognosis. Different degrees and speeds of evolution in different patients. Chronic benign condition that leads, however, to severe incapacitation. In some patients, fibrosis may remain nonprogressive for years.

BIBLIOGRAPHY. Dupuytren G: Permanent retraction of the fingers, produced by an affection of the palmar fascia. Lancet 2:222, 1833–34

Bazin S, Lehous M, Duance VC et al: Biochemistry and histology of the connective tissue of Dupuytren's disease lesions. Eur J Clin Invest 10:9–16, 1980

DURAL SINUS THROMBOSIS

Symptoms. Often occur in debilitated children or in postpartum period. Headache; nausea; vomiting; chills; remittent fever; tachycardia; convulsions; stupor and variable symptoms according to localization and eventual embolization.

Signs. Swelling of optic disks; engorgement of scalp veins; palpation of thrombosed vessel when extended to jugular vein.

Etiology. Noninfective: malnutrition; heart conditions; trauma; postpartum; tumor; polycythemia. Infective: all kinds of infection spreading from middle ear and mastoid.

Pathology. Occlusion of the vessel by thrombus, bacteria, fibrin leukocytes; secondary thrombosis of almost all cortical veins; some of them rupture and cause hemorrhages, cerebral softening, edema, and abscess.

Diagnostic Procedures. *CT brain scan. Spinal fluid.* Leukocytosis; pressure and protein increased. *Blood.* Leukocytosis.

Therapy. Antibiotics; thrombolytics; anticoagulants.

Prognosis. Poor.

BIBLIOGRAPHY. Smith JC: Primary cerebral thrombophlebitis. JAMA 148:613–616, 1952

DURAND'S

Synonyms. Alpha-fucosidase acid deficiency; alpha-fucosidase deficiency; fucosidosis.

Symptoms. Both sexes affected; normal at birth. Psychomotor retardation becoming evident by 12 to 15 months of age. Different degrees of severity. Progressive deterioration. Spasticity; tremor; loss of contact with environment; frequent infections.

Signs. Facies becoming coarse; development of spondyloepiphyseal dysplasia; kyphoscoliosis; cornea clear and fundus normal; angiokeratoma corposis diffusum (see Fabry's). Vessels of the gums may be dilated and tongue large.

Etiology. Autosomal recessive inheritance; lack of acid alpha-fucosidase. Genetic polymorphism or heterogeneity may explain different clinical patterns (see Prognosis). Enzyme defect on chromosome 1.

Pathology. *Liver.* Abnormal lysosomes; vacuoles resembling those of Hurler's syndrome, or containing stocks of circular lamellae. *Brain.* Half-empty vacuoles (without Zebra's bodies). *Skin.* Full-blown angiokeratoma diffusum to minor vascular lesions.

Diagnostic Procedures. *Blood.* Vacuolization of lymphocytes. Deficient activity of lysosomal enzyme alpha-fucosidase in all cells and tissues, serum, and urine. *X-ray.* Minor skeletal alterations.

Therapy. None.

Prognosis. Two types clearly distinguishable: (1) death before sixth year of life; (2) death in early adulthood (with more marked clinical signs).

BIBLIOGRAPHY. Durand P: A new mucopolysaccharide lipid storage disease. Lancet 2:1313–1314, 1966
Beaudet AL: Disorders of glycoprotein degradation: Mannosidosis, fucosidosis, sialidosis, and aspartyl-glycosaminuria. In Stanbury JB, Wyngaarden JB, Fredrickson DS, et al: The Metabolic Basis of Inherited Disease, 5th ed, p 788. New York, McGraw-Hill, 1983

DUVERNOY'S

Synonyms. Abdominal gas cyst; bullous intestinal emphysema; cystic lymphopneumatosis; emphysema intestinalis; intestine gas cyst; peritoneal pneumatosis; pneumatosis cystoides intestinalis.

Symptoms. Present in both sexes; onset at all ages (greatest incidence in males between 30 and 50 yr of age and females between 60 and 70). Nonspecific. Alternating diarrhea and stypsis; abdominal distention; vague pains; rectal bleeding; partial or complete (rare) intestinal obstruction.

Signs. Crepitant, nontender, abdominal masses, plus signs of various complications, when occurring.

Etiology. Unknown (primary), (15%) or as complication, through unknown pathogenic mechanism of other intestinal conditions (see Pathology). In infants, consequences of bacterial invasion.

Pathology. Multiple gas-filled cysts in gastrointestinal tract and occasionally in other organs of abdominal cavity. Size of cysts variable from microscopic to many centimeters in diameter. Cysts (thin-walled) break easily. Small bowel most frequent site. Other pathology of gastrointestinal tract frequently associated: pyloric stenosis; appendicitis; regional enteritis; ulcerative colitis; tubercular enteritis.

Diagnostic Procedures. *X-ray of intestine.* Clusters of radiolucent areas following course of bowel; pneumoperitoneum (occasionally); Chilaiditi's (see). *Sigmoidoscopy* (when sigmoid involved). Submucosal cystic lesions.

Therapy. Secondary forms: treat underlying condition. In both primary and secondary forms: hyperbaric O_2 treatment, or let the patient breath O_2 by mask for several days. Dietary adjustment, antibiotics to modify intestinal flora. Surgery seldom needed except in secondary forms.

Prognosis. That of underlying condition. Cysts may disappear spontaneously or persist for a long time without serious symptoms.

BIBLIOGRAPHY. Combalusier: Pneumopathologie ou traité de maladies venteuses, vol 1, p 19. Paris, 1745

Bang, BLF: Luftholdige kyster i väggen af ileum og i nydannet bindeväv på sammes serosa. Nord Med Ark, 8:1–15, 1876

Koss LG: Abdominal gas cysts (pneumatosis cystoides intestinorum hominis). Arch Path 53:523–549, 1952

Stone HH, Alan WB, Smith RB, et al: Infantile pneumatosis intestinalis. J Surg Res 8:301–307, 1968

Miralbes M, Hinojosa J, Alonzo J, et al: Oxygen therapy in pneumatosis coli: What is the minimum oxygen requirement? Dis Colon Rectum 26:458–460, 1983

DWARFISM, ENVIRONMENTAL

Synonyms. Deprivation dwarfism; emotional dwarfism; environmental failure to thrive; growth failure–maternal deprivation; maternal deprivation; sensory deprivation.

Symptoms. Appear in infants or children. Failure to thrive; height-growth failure with subsequent correction in presence of appropriate nurturing. Mental retardation with subsequent acceleration when environment is changed. Apathy; intense irritability; withdrawal and defense against any kind of approach. May be present: vomiting; diarrhea; acute or chronic respiratory infections; anemia; neuromuscular disorders; signs of traumas (see Battered child syndrome). In some instances, failure to thrive may be observed in presence of a voracious appetite.

Etiology. Neglect or physical abuse or both. In the family, psychosocial factors, financial deprivation, sexual incompatibility or promiscuity in parents, familial illness, physical abuse, inexperience in mothering, unwanted pregnancy.

Pathology. Weight below third percentile; height below normal; signs of physical abuse.

Diagnostic Procedures. Evaluation of familial psychosocial factors. *X-ray. Blood. Urine.* Endocrine studies.

Therapy. Removal from environment or correction of negative environmental factors.

Prognosis. Good if adequate treatment possible.

BIBLIOGRAPHY. Talbot NB, Sobel EH, Burke BS, et al: Dwarfism in healthy children: Its possible relation to emotional, nutritional, and endocrine disturbances. New Engl J Med 236:783–793, 1947

Barbero GJ, Shaheen E: Environmental failure to thrive: A clinical view. J Pediatr 71:639–644, 1967

Freedman AM, Kaplan HI, Sadock BJ: Comprehensive Textbook of Psychiatry, 2nd ed. Baltimore, Williams & Wilkins, 1975

DWARFISM-IMMUNOPATHY-ASTHMA

Synonym. Asthma–dwarfism–high IgA.

Symptoms. Both sexes affected; onset from age 4 to 5 months. Recurrent attacks of asthma; between attacks, no respiratory symptoms. Four to 5 years later, seasonal episodes of nasal congestion, sneezing, nasal itching.

Signs. Shortness of stature.

Etiology. Unknown; genetically related defect of not yet established type.

Diagnostic Procedures. *Blood.* Great elevation of IgA globulin; depressed IgM concentrations.

Therapy. Asthma and atopic allergy respond well to sympatholytic and prednisone.

Prognosis. Persistent condition; mild; usually not requiring hospitalization.

BIBLIOGRAPHY. Huntley CC, Johnson HW, Lyerly AD: Asthma, short stature and elevated gamma IgA globulins. Am J Dis Child 109:353–358, 1965

Sly RM, Heimlich EM: Identical twins with short stature elevated IgA and asthma. Ann Allerg 25:578–586, 1967

DYGGVE-MELCHIOR-CLAUSEN

Synonyms. Dyggve-Melchior-Clausen dwarfism.

Symptoms and Signs. Mental retardation. Short trunk dwarfism. Exaggerated lordosis. Fingers clawed and with limited extension.

Etiology. Autosomal recessive inheritance. Erroneously interpreted as a mucopolysaccharidosis; the alleged lysosomal storage has not been demonstrated.

Pathology. Presence of focal nests of few (2 to 20) necrotic cells scattered into resting cartilage, surrounded by calcified fibrotic rings.

Diagnostic Procedures. *X-ray.* Skeletal survey. Spine with generalized platyspondylisis; irregularity of iliac crest (lace-bordered); flaring of metaphyses. *Urine.* Search for and eventual identification of mucopolysaccharides type.

Therapy. None.

Prognosis. See Symptoms and Signs.

BIBLIOGRAPHY. Dyggve HV, Melchior JC, Clausen J: Morquio-Ulrich's disease; An inborn error of metabolism? Arch Dis Child 37:525–534, 1962
Schlaepfer R, Rampini S, Wiesmann U: Das Dyggve-Melchior-Clausen-Syndrome: Fallbeschreibung und Literaturnebersicht. Helv Paediatr Acta 36:543–559, 1981

DYKE-DAVIDOFF-MASSON

Synonyms. Cerebral hemiatrophy; DDM.

Symptoms and Signs. Both sexes affected; present from birth. Cerebral hemiatrophy with homolateral skull and sinus hypertrophy. Mental retardation; seizures; difficulty and impairment of speech development.

Etiology. Unknown. Normal chromosomal pattern.

Diagnostic Procedures. *X-rays of skull.* Hemihypotrophy of skull and sinuses. *CT brain scan.* Hemireduction of brain size. *Electroencephalography.* Abnormal. *Dermatoglyphic pattern.* Normal. *Urine.* Amino acid excretion normal or increased.

Therapy. Anticonvulsants.

Prognosis. Not adequately known.

BIBLIOGRAPHY. Dyke CG, Davidoff LM, Masson CB: Cerebral hemiatrophy with homolateral hypertrophy of the skull and sinuses. Surg Gynecol Obstet 57:588–600, 1933
Parker CE, Harris N, Mavalwala J: Dyke-Davidoff-Masson syndrome; five cases: Studies and deductions from dermatoglyphics. Clin Pediatr 11:228–292, 1972

DYSBARISM

Gas nitrogen and fat embolism occurring in fliers who rapidly reach high altitude. Symptomatology, signs, etiology, pathology see Caisson.

BIBLIOGRAPHY. Niess OK, Stonehill RR: Dysbarism: A jet age problem of all physicians. Dis Chest 44:121-125, 1963
Vick NA: Grinker's Neurology, 7th ed. Springfield, CC Thomas, 1976

DYSCHROMATOSIS UNIVERSALIS HEREDITARIA

Synonym. See Dohi's (probably same condition).

Symptoms and Signs. Both sexes. Only in Japanese. Onset first or second year of life. Pigmented flecks and spots over all the body, varying in size, shape, and color, sparing frequently the face and concentrating on the abdomen. No associated defects.

Etiology. Autosomal recessive (quasi-dominant) difficult to assess because of frequent consanguineous marriages in the family.

BIBLIOGRAPHY. Suenaga M: Genetical studies on skin disease, VII. Dyschromatosis universalis hereditaria in five generations. Tohoku J Exp Med 55:373–376, 1952
Westerhoff W, Beeher FA, Cormane RM, Delleman JW, Faber WR, De Jong JG, Van der Schaar WW: Hereditary congenital hypopigmented and hyperpigmented macules. Arch Dermatol 114:931–936, 1978

DYSFIBRINOGENEMIA, HEREDITARY

Symptoms and Signs. Usually, asymptomatic or minor bleeding problems.

Etiology. Functionally defective fibrinogen. Twenty different types of abnormal fibrinogen have been identified; they are designated by the name of where discovered (e.g., Paris I, Baltimore, Detroit). Incomplete dominant autosomal inheritance.

Diagnostic Procedures. *Blood.* Usually clot forms, but at abnormally slow rate.

Therapy. None.

Prognosis. Good.

BIBLIOGRAPHY. Samama M, Soria J, Soria C: Congenital and acquired dysfibrinogenemia. In Polleor L (ed): Recent Advances in Blood Coagulation, p 313. New York, Churchill Livingstone, 1977.
Rupp C, Beck EA: Congenital dysfibrinogenemia. In Beck EA, Furlour M (eds): Varians of Human Fibrinogen. Berne, Hans Huber, 1984

DYSGAMMAGLOBULINEMIA

Synonyms. Hyperimmunoglobulin M immunodeficiency; hyper-IgM dysgammaglobulinemia.

Symptoms and Signs. From birth frequent various infective episodes.

Etiology. Sex-linked. Unknown. Considered impaired transformation of IgM in IgG, IgA, IgE.

Pathology. Frequent development of lymphomas.

Diagnostic Procedures. *Blood.* Normal lymphocytes B and T; IgM and IgD increased; IgG, IgA decreased.

Therapy. Immunoglobulin IgG.

Prognosis. Frequent development of lymphoma.

BIBLIOGRAPHY. Goldman AS, Ritzniann SE, Houston EW et al: Dysgammaglobulinemic antibodies deficiency syndrome increased gamma M-globulin and decreased gamma-G and gamma-A globulins. J Pediatr 70:16–27, 1967
Schwaber JF, Lazarus H, Rosen FS: Ig M-restricted production of immunoglobulin by lymphoid cell lines from patients with immunodeficiency with hyper IgM (Dysgammaglobulinemia). Clin Immunol Immunopathol 19:91–97, 1981

DYSTOCIA-DYSTROPHIA

Synonyms. Bradytocia; dyspituitaric dystocia.

Symptoms and Signs. Occur in females who are of stocky build, somewhat bull-necked with broad shoulders, short thighs, and tendency to obesity. May have male distribution of hair; hands are stubby with middle three fingers of approximately same length. Bony structure of pelvis: android type giving rise to deep transverse arrest and difficulties of delivery at the outlet. The cervix is small and dimensions of vagina are skimpy. These patients are rather subfertile. Spasmodic dysmenorrhea is very common, have tendency to abortion, incidence of eclampsia is high. Labor starts with fetal head often high and in majority cases occiput posterior; membranes rupture early in labor.

Etiology. Unknown.

Pathology. Nothing unusual, except the android type of pelvis.

Therapy. Close observation during labor, and recourse to cesarean section if necessary.

Prognosis. Good if carefully observed during antepartum period and intrapartum period.

BIBLIOGRAPHY. Horner DA: Bradytocia; a study based on 500 cases in the Chicago Lying-In Hospital. Surg Gynecol Obstet 44:194–201, 1927
Williams B: Dystocia dystrophia syndrome. J Obstet Gynecol Br Emp 49:412–425, 1942

DYSTONIA-DEAFNESS

Synonym. Scribanu's.

Symptoms and Signs. In male deafness onset in infancy; in childhood: dysartria, bizarre posture of head and neck, hyperactivity progressive symptoms that lead to inability to walk and talk.

Etiology. X-linked inheritance.

Pathology. Neuronal loss and gliosis of basal ganglia.

Prognosis. Death in the second decade. Forme fruste (only deafness, 1 case), survival into adulthood.

BIBLIOGRAPHY. Scribanu N, Kennedy C: Familial syndrome with dystonia, neuronal deafness and possibly intellectual impairment: Clinical course and pathologic findings. Neurol 14:235–243, 1976

DYSURIA-PYURIA

Synonyms. Acute urethral; see Honeymoon cystitis.

Symptoms and Signs. Most frequent in young women, acute dysuria and pollakiuria.

Etiology. In 88% lower urinary tract infection with coliforms or staphylococci or *Chlamydia trachomatis;* in other cases unknown.

Diagnostic Procedures. *Urine.* Culture.

Therapy. Antibiotics. Good results with doxycycline.

Prognosis. In cases with infections prompt remission. In the others prolonged condition.

BIBLIOGRAPHY. Komaroff AL, Friedland G: The dysuria-piuria syndrome. N Engl J Med 303:452–454, 1980
Stamm WE et al: Treatment of the acute urethral syndrome. N Engl J Med 304:956–958, 1981

DZIERSZYNSKY'S

Synonyms. Hyperplastic periosteal dystrophy; eponym obsolete. See also Van Buchem's. Eponym used to indicate a generalized hyperosteosis particularly affecting cranium, clavicles, sternum and phalanges. Hereditary condition.

BIBLIOGRAPHY. Dzierszynsky W: Dystrophia Periostalis, hyperplastica Familiaris. Zentralbl Ges Neurol 20:547, 1913

E-FEROL

Symptoms and Signs. In low-birth-weight infants. Progressive clinical deterioration, thrombocytopenia, renal dysfunction, cholestasis, ascites.

Etiology. Total parenteral nutrition, infants whose birth weight was less than 1500 g, supplemented with E-ferol, an intravenous vitamin E preparation.

Diagnostic Procedures. *Blood chemistry.*

Pathology. Progressive hepatic injury characterized initially by Kupffer's cell exfoliation, central lobular accumulation of cellular debris, and centrally accentuated panlobular congestion. Late stage: progressive intralobular cholestasis, inflammation of hepatic venules, and extensive sinusoidal venoocclusion by fibrosis.

Therapy. Symptomatic.

Prognosis. Poor.

BIBLIOGRAPHY. Bove KE, Kosmetatos N, Wedig KE, et al: Vasculopathic hepatotoxicity associated with E-ferol syndrome in low-birth weight infants. JAMA 254:2422–2430, 1985

EALES'

Synonyms. Periphlebitis retinae; retinal periphlebitis; retinal vasculitis; vasculitis retinae.

Symptoms and Signs. Prevalent in males; affects young adults. Occur in stress situation, after trauma, or after awakening. Sudden loss of vision usually in one eye, or vision impairment (scotoma; floating spots); occasionally associated with ataxia; paresthesias; speech disorders.

Etiology. Variable. Infective: tuberculosis; focal infection (dental; tonsillar; sinus); syphilis. Multiple sclerosis. Hemopathies: hemoglobin anomalies; Bassen-Kornzweig; Buerger's.

Pathology. Retina vasculitis. The primary form originates in venules; the secondary, after uveitis process. Retinal hemorrhages; detachment of retina.

Diagnostic Procedures. *Ophthalmoscopy.* See Pathology.

Therapy. Topical atropine, hydrocortisone. Photocoagulation of aneurysms and neovascularization.

Prognosis. Progressive condition with improvements and recurrences. Tendency to involvement of both eyes.

BIBLIOGRAPHY. Eales H: Cases of retinal haemorrhage associated with epistaxis and constipation. Birmingham Med Rev 9:262–273, 1880
Duane TD (ed): Clinical Ophthalmology, vol 3, pp 1–6. Philadelphia, Harper & Row, 1982

EAR CHOLESTEATOMA

Synonyms. Aural cholesteroeosis; cholesteatoma.

Symptoms. Onset in childhood or adolescence. Gradual onset of facial paralysis; homolateral deafness; tinnitus.

Signs. Loss of vestibular caloric response.

Etiology. Epidermoid theory; traumatic theory; metaplastic theory; inflammation theory.

Pathology. Cholesteatoma occupying antrum, usually unilateral with or without attic perforation.

Diagnostic Procedures. *X-rays. Otoscopy. Exploration.*

Therapy. Surgery.

Prognosis. Patient with family history followed, and if lesion is discovered, prophylactic treatment before it becomes secondarily infected. Facial paralysis does not show complete recovery after surgery when chronic infection has supervened.

BIBLIOGRAPHY. Cushing H: A large epidermal cholesteatoma. Surg Gynecol Obstet 51:334, 1928
Brosnan ML: Primary cholesteatomas of temporal bone. Arch Otolaryngol 86:363–366, 1967

EATON-LAMBERT

Synonyms. Bronchial carcinoma-myasthenia; Lambert-Eaton; See Erb-Goldflam and Paraneoplastic.

Symptoms and Signs. Onset in middle life. Those of Erb-Goldflam (see), plus muscular pain and tenderness, depression of tendon reflexes.

Etiology. Bronchial carcinoma.

Pathology. Bronchial carcinoma (oat cell or anaplastic).

Diagnostic Procedures. *Neostigmine (Prostigmin and edrophonuim chloride (Tensilon) tests.* Negative or feebly positive. *X-ray of chest. Bronchography. Bronchoscopy.*

Therapy. High voltage radiation, chemotherapy for carcinoma or both; or surgery if feasible. Treatment of Erb-Goldflam (see). Response to intravenous neostigmine usually slight or moderate.

Prognosis. According to degree of diffusion or metastasis of carcinoma. Usually, rapid deterioration and death.

BIBLIOGRAPHY. Anderson JH, Churchill-Davidson HD, Richardson AT: Bronchial neoplasm with myasthenia. Lancet 2:1291–1293, 1953

Lambert EH, Eaton LM, Rooke ED: Defect of neuromuscular conduction associated with malignant neoplasm. Am J Physiol 187:612–613, 1956

Adams RD, Victor M: Principles of Neurology, 3rd ed, p 1083. New York, McGraw-Hill, 1985

EBSTEIN'S

Synonym. Tricuspid valve anomaly.

Symptoms. Both sexes equally affected. Asymptomatic for years or dyspnea and fatigability; squatting unusual.

Signs. Cyanosis at birth or delayed, or recurrent with increasing severity. Moderate clubbing of fingers and toes. Paroxysmal arrhythmias; heart markedly enlarged; characteristic triple or quadruple rhythm; systolic murmur on left border of sternum, at apex. In many cases apical diastolic murmur as well.

Etiology. Congenital heart defect, with downward displacement of tricuspid valve into right ventricle, and deformation of valve leaflets.

Pathology. As described above, with atrialization of right ventricle above the valve. Right ventricle decreased in volume. Patency of foramen ovale in many cases and interatrial septal defect. Association with other cardiac anomalies frequent.

Diagnostic Procedures. *Electrocardiography.* Right bundle branch block and prolonged P-R interval; tall P waves; atrial tachycardia; premature beats and flutter frequent. *Two-dimensional echocardiography. Fluoroscopy and x-ray.* Enlargement of right atrium; small pulmonary artery; oligemic lung fields. *Angiocardiography.* Enormous right atrium. *Catheterization.* Right atrium increased pressure; evidence of right-to-left left-to-right shunts.

Therapy. Surgery produces variable results. Medical (symptomatic).

Prognosis. Variable; patient may survive to middle life. Average life span 22 years. Arrhythmias cause of sudden death.

BIBLIOGRAPHY. Ebstein W: Ueber einen sehr seltenen Fall von Insufficenz der Valvula tricuspidalis, bedingt durch eine angeborene hochgradige Missbildung derselben. Arch Anat Physiol 238–254, 1866

Danielson GK: Ebstein's anomaly: Editorial comments and personal observations. Ann Thorac Surg 34:396–400, 1982

Hurst JW: The Heart, 6th ed, pp 677–680. New York, McGraw-Hill, 1986

ECTOPIC ACTH

Synonyms. ACTH ectopic secretion. See Cushing's.

Symptoms. Weakness; fatigability; in women, oligomenorrhea. Symptoms due to the adrenocorticotropic hormone (ACTH) producing tumor (e.g., lung; pancreas).

Signs. Ecchymosis; edema. Most of the signs of classic Cushing's do not have time to develop because of the fast course of the disease; typical obesity usually does not develop; hypertension has been observed only in some cases.

Etiology. Tumors of lung (most frequent), pancreas, breast, prostate, parathyroid, thyroid, ovary, sympathicoblasts, and thymus producing ACTH, which induces adrenal hyperplasia.

Pathology. Lung tumor; oat cell carcinoma. Carcinomas of various endocrine glands mentioned. Early features of Cushing's.

Diagnostic Procedures. *Blood.* High level of plasma ACTH; increased cortisol. *Urine.* Increased 17-ketosteroids and 17-hydroxycorticoids; other typical changes due to excessive cortisol production and changes due to primary tumor. *ACTH stimulation.* Varying responses according to level of circulating ACTH. *Metyrapone responsiveness.* Varies according to level of circulating cortisol. *Dexamethazone suppression.* Negative response also with high doses.

Therapy. Usually inoperable at time of discovery; some cases operated in time have been cured.

Prognosis. Poor, death due to primary tumor and metastasis.

BIBLIOGRAPHY. Brown WH: A case of pluriglandular syndrome. Lancet 2:1022–1023, 1928

Strott CA, Nugent CA, Tyler FH: Cushing's syndrome caused by bronchial adenomas. Am J Med 44:97–104, 1968

George JM: Ectopic hormone syndromes. In Mazzaferri EL (ed): Textbook of Endocrinology, 3rd ed, pp 578–580. New York Med Exam Publishing Co, 1985

ECTOPIC PREGNANCY

Symptoms. Incidence 1 : 300 pregnancies. Precipitating incidents leading to rupture are straining at stool, coitus, or bimanual pelvic examination. Irregular bleeding; usually skipping of one period, then vaginal bleeding coming on one day or more later. Dull aching pain most common symptom. Referred shoulder pain when free intraperitoneal bleeding. Fainting and shock when massive intraperitoneal bleeding.

Signs. Palpable tender mass at the time of the examination. Sometimes signs of pelvic irritation. Bluish discoloration around the umbilicus (Cullen's sign).

Etiology. Chronic pelvic inflammatory disease, especially gonorrhea affecting the endosalpinx. Endometriosis; genital tuberculosis; congenital factors.

Pathology. Any fertilized ovum implanting outside the uterine cavity is called ectopic. Varieties: tubal pregnancy (most common); interstitial pregnancy; ampullar pregnancy; cornual pregnancy; cervical pregnancy; ovarian pregnancy; abdominal pregnancy (primary and secondary); intraligamentary pregnancy. Fate of the implanted fertilized ovum: rupture with blood loss into peritoneal cavity; rupture between the two leaves of the broad ligament; abortion via the fimbriated end of the fallopian tube; or abdominal pregnancy, secondary variety.

Diagnostic Procedures. In addition to the history and physical examination: *Culdocentesis* (tapping of cul-de-sac). *Pregnancy test. Colpotomy.* The important point is to have a "high index of suspicion" every time a woman in the reproductive period of her life gives a history of amenorrhea or pelvic pain.

Therapy. Surgical; exploratory laparotomy and removal of the affected tube. In some rare cases, salpingostomy, removal of the implanted ovum, and preservation of the affected tube.

Prognosis. Good if treatment is instituted as soon as diagnosis is made.

BIBLIOGRAPHY. Pritchard-McDonald-Gant: Williams Obstetrics, 17th ed, pp 423–438. Norwalk (Conn), Appleton-Century-Crofts, 1985

ECTRODACTYLY

Synonyms. Birch-Jensen; split-hand deformity. Radial defects. See Aase-Smith; Gross-Groh-Weippl; Holt-Oram; Roberts'.

Symptoms and Signs. *Skin.* Macular, blistering, crusting lesions. *Oropharynx.* Ulceration. *Intestine.* Perforation.

Etiology. Unknown.

Pathology. *Skin.* Edema basal layer; inflammatory reaction of dermis and subcutis. *Intestine.* Ulceration with fibrinoid necrosis of arterioles in floor of ulcers.

Therapy. Trial with corticosteroids. Surgery for perforation. Antibiotics.

Prognosis. Poor.

BIBLIOGRAPHY. Bettley FR: A fetal cutaneointestinal syndrome. Br J Derm 72:423–426, 1960
Rook A, Wilkinson DS, Ebling FJG, et al: Textbook of Dermatology. 4th ed, p 1178. Oxford, Blackwell Scientific Publications, 1986

EDELMANN'S

Synonyms. Pancreatohepatic; hepatopancreatic. A rather poorly defined syndrome. This designation has been used to indicate an atrophic or hypotrophic pancreatitis with fatty liver infiltration. The liver infiltration considered secondary to the pancreatic insufficiency.

BIBLIOGRAPHY. Edelmann A: Ueber eine bisher nicht beachtetes panchreo-hepatisches Syndrome. Wien Klin Wochenschr 49:1336–1339, 1936
Snell AM, Comfort MW: Hepatic lesions presumably secondary to pancreatic lithiasis and atrophy. Am J Dig Dis 4:217, 1937
Cole WH, Howe JS: The pancreaticohepatic syndrome. Surgery 8:19–33, 1940
Kessel L: Acute transient hyperlipemia due to hepatopancreatic damage in chronic alcoholics (Zieve's syndrome). Am J Med 32:747–757, 1962

EDEMA BLUE

Synonym. Charcot's edema syndromes. Eponym used to indicate the whitish blue hue, usually associated with the edema, that occurs in the limbs in hysterical palsy.

BIBLIOGRAPHY. Guinon G: L'oedème bleu de l'hystériques. Prog Med. 12:259–264, 1890

EDWARDS'

Synonyms. Trisomy E; trisomy 16-18; trisomy 18.

Symptoms. Prevalent in females; paternal and maternal age above normal; onset from fetal life. Babies thin, frail; failure to thrive; difficulty in feeding; generalized hypertonicity with rigidity in flexion of the limbs. Mental retardation.

Signs. Prominent occiput; low-set and malformed ears; receding chin; protruding eyes. Frequently, umbilical and inguinal hernias. Characteristic: tight flexion of fingers across the palm; index finger overlapping over third digit; occasionally syndactyly; fingers cannot be extended. Convex sole of foot ("rocker-bottom feet"); no hyperreflexia.

Etiology. Trisomy in group E chromosomes (18 possibly the deviant pair). Nondisjunction of maternal gamete or possibly balanced translocation-carrier in either parents or mosaicism.

Pathology. Frequently; abnormalities of cerebral or cerebellar development. Spina bifida; meningomyelocele; high incidence of Meckel's diverticulum; esophageal atresia; heterotopic pancreatic tissue; atresia of extrahepatic biliary tree; malrotation of colon; several cardiovascular abnormalities; radial malformation.

Diagnostic Procedures. *Chromosome study.* Trisomy E group. *Dermatoglyphics.* Transversal palmar crease present with greater frequency than in normal. *Blood.* Congenital thrombocytopenia in some cases.

Therapy. None.

Prognosis. Mean survival time in male patient, 58.5 days; in females, 282 days. Seldom survival to second year.

BIBLIOGRAPHY. Edwards JH, Harnden DG, Cameron AH, et al: A new trisomic syndrome. Lancet 1:787–790, 1960
Rabinowitz JG, Moseley JE, Mitty HA, et al: Trisomy 18, esophageal atresia, anomalies of the radius, and congenital hypoplastic thrombocytopenia. Radiology 89:488–491, 1967
Moerman P, Fryns JP, Goddeeris P, et al: Spectrum of clinical and autopsy findings in trisomy 18 syndrome. J Genet Hum 30:17–38, 1982

EHLERS-DANLOS

Synonyms. Arthrochalasis-dermatorrhexis-dermatochalasis; cutis hyperelastica; Danlos'; E-D; fibrodysplasia elastica generalisata; India rubber skin; Meekeren-Ehlers-Danlos; rubber man; Sack's; Sack-Barabas; Van Meekerent's I.

Symptoms. Described primarily in people of European ancestry. Both sexes affected (some authors report male prevalence); recognized from birth. Several clinical forms have been outlined: *ED I (gravis type).* Frequently, prematurity; skin hyperextensible, marked bruisability; severe and generalized joint hypermobility. Delayed sitting and walking; unsteadiness with falling and fractures. *ED II (mitis type).* Milder manifestations; joint hypermobility may be limited to hands and feet. *ED III (benign hypermobile type).* Minimal skin involvement; maximal joint hypermobility and sequelae. *ED IV (ecchymotic; Sack's type; Sack-Barabas syndrome).* Minimal skin involvement; moderate or minimal joint involvement; marked bruisability; extensive ecchymosis; pigmented scar over bony prominences. Frequently, visceral rupture. It has been divided in three forms according to etiology. *Type A:* autosomal dominant. *Type B:* autosomal recessive in which the biochemical defect is diminished type III collagen synthesis. *Type C:* of unknown etiology in which there is an intracellular accumulation of type III collagen. It has been divided in two forms. In subtype A, lysyl oxidase is deficient, and in subtype B, the biochemical defect is unknown. Frequently, visceral rupture. *ED V (X-linked form).* Marked skin hyperextensibility; moderate joint hypermobility; moderate vascular fragility. *ED VI (Hydroxylysine-deficient collagen or ocular type, autosomal recessive type).* Predominance of ocular abnormalities over other features. Biochemical diagnosis: low hydroxylysine residue from collagen. Two types have been described: one with autosomal recessive inheritance and procollagen aminoprotease deficiency, and one of sporadic occurrence with a structural mutation of proα₂ (I). *ED VII (procollagen-persistent type).* Floppiness in infancy; moderate skin and vascular abnormalities; marked joint hypermobility. Dwarfism. Autosomal recessive inheritance (?). *ED VIII (periodontitis type).* Autosomal dominant. Mild skin hyperelasticity, joint hypermobility and bruisability, moderate cutaneous fragility, and severe periodontitis leading to premature loss of teeth and alveolar bone absorption. *ED IX (mental retardation)* with mental retardation, hernias, protuberant ears, and fragile skin.

Etiology. Various types of inheritance. First four varieties mentioned above are autosomal dominant. Collagen theory: defect of collagen fibers, which allows hyperextensibility of skin, joints, and vessel walls.

Pathology. Debated, no consistent findings. Loose fragmented elastic tissue observed in some cases in the skin ligaments, joint capsules (whether result of trauma or primary abnormality not established). Pseudotumors formed by noncapsulated fat, with calcification of connective tissue, vascular proliferation, and cystic formation. Organization of collagen bundles into an intermeshing network. *ED I, II, and III:* increased collagen fibril diameter. *ED IV, C:* small collagen fibril diameter with dilatation of rough endoplasmic reticulum. *ED V B:* increased collagen fibril diameter. *ED VI:* small fibril diameter.

Diagnostic Procedures. See individual types for biochemical defects.

Therapy. Avoidance of traumas; drainage of big hematomas. Orthopedic measures sometimes necessary. Surgical procedures, with caution because of eventual dehiscence.

Prognosis. Good *quoad vitam.* According to intensity of manifestations, joint hypermobility reduces with age. Complication from visceral malformation occasionally is cause of death.

BIBLIOGRAPHY. Van Meekeren JA: De dilatabilitata extraordinaria cutis. In: Observations Medico-Chirurgicales. Amsterdam, 1682.
Tschernogobow A: Cutis laxa. Mhft Prokt Derm 14:76, 1892
Ehlers E: Cutis laxa, Neigung zu Haemorrhagien in der Haut lockerung mehrerer Artikulationen. Dermatol Z 8:173–174, 1901
Danlos H: Un cas de cutis laxa avec tumeurs par contusion chronique des coudes et des genoux. Bull Soc Fr Dermatol Syph 19:70–72, 1908
Pinnel SR, Murad S: Disorders of collagen. In Stanbury JB, Wyngaarden JB, Fredrickson DS, et al: The Metabolic Basis of Inherited Disease. 5th ed, p 1425. New York, McGraw-Hill, 1983

EHRENFRIED'S

Synonyms. Diaphyseal aclasis; metaphyseal aclasis; hereditary deforming chondrodysplasia; chondromatosis externa; hereditary deforming dyschondroplasia; multiple hereditary exostosis; multiple osteochondromatosis, exostoses, multiple.

Symptoms and Signs. Deformity of extremities, including hands (short metacarpal); short stature; excrescence at diaphyseal end of bones; ribs and scapula also involved, never the skull. Neurologic complication from nerve or spinal cord compression.

Etiology. Unknown; autosomal dominant inheritance.

Pathology. Cartilage excrescences. Sarcomatous transformation frequent.

Diagnostic Procedures. *X-ray. Blood.* Normal.

Therapy. Decompression if indicated.

Prognosis. Consider possible malignant transformation.

BIBLIOGRAPHY. Ehrenfried A: Multiple cartilaginous exostoses hereditary deforming chondrodysplasia. A brief report on a little known disease. JAMA 64:1642–1646, 1915
Jaffe HL: Hereditary multiple exostosis. Arch Pathol 36:335–337, 1943
Shapiro F, Simon S, Glimcher MJ: Hereditary multiple exostoses: Anthropometric, roentgenographic and clinical aspects. J Bone Joint Surg 61A:815–824, 1979

EHRET'S

Synonyms. Postantalgic posture atrophia; postantalgic atrophy.

Symptoms. Pain, reduced functional capacities of involved muscle groups.

Signs. Muscle contracture and atrophy.

Etiology. After period of immobilization of muscle groups due to painful stimuli.

Therapy. Gradual physical therapy.

Prognosis. Good for anatomic and functional recovery.

BIBLIOGRAPHY. Ehret H: Ueber eine functionelle Lähmungsform der peronealmuskel traumatischen Ursprunges. Arch Unfall 2:32–56, 1898

18-DEHYDROGENASE OF 18-HYDROXYCORTICOSTERONE DEFICIENCY

See Ulick's.

18-HYDROXYLASE DEFICIENCY

See Visser's.

18p-SYNDROME

See page 1.

18q-SYNDROME

See page 1.

EISENLOHR'S

Synonym. Bulbar paralysis variant.

BIBLIOGRAPHY. Eisenlohr C: Ueber Abscesse in der Medulla oblungata. Dtsch Med Wochenschr 19:111–113, 1892

EISENMENGER'S COMPLEX

Symptoms. Both sexes equally affected. Exertional dyspnea. Delayed physical development; repeated pulmonary infections with occasional hemophtysis. Cough may be the dominant symptom in later life.

Signs. *Infancy.* Moderate cardiomegaly; thrill on left sternal border; systolic murmur; diastolic rumble. *Adolescence, early adult life.* Cyanosis; clubbing of fingers and toes.

Etiology. Congenital heart defect. Left-to-right shunt (ventricular, occasionally also atrial) reverted to right-to-left by pulmonary hypertension.

Pathology. Ventricular septal defect, patent ductus arteriosus or atrial septal defect. Hypertrophy of both ventricles. Pulmonary artery dilated. Lung fibrosis.

Diagnostic Procedures. *Electrocardiography.* Left axis deviation in infants; right axis deviation in older children. Short circulation time. Two-dimensional echocardiography. *Pulmonary function tests.* Oxygen saturation decreased in older children. *X-ray.* Enlargement of right ventricle, prominent main pulmonary artery and central branches with cutoff of peripheral branches. *Catheterization.* Increased pressure in pulmonary artery; increased oxygen in right ventricle. *Blood.* Increased number of red blood cells.

Therapy. Symptomatic. Surgical intervention is generally felt to be contraindicated because elevated pulmonary vascular resistance persists or increases after surgical closure of the defect.

Prognosis. Most patients die from heart failure, thrombosis, or endocarditis before reaching 30 years of age.

BIBLIOGRAPHY. Eisenmenger V: Die angeborenen Defekte der Kommerscheidewand des Herzens. Z Klin Med (suppl) 32:1–28, 1897
Graham TP Jr: The Eisenmenger reaction and its management. In Roberts WC (ed): Congenital Heart Disease in Adults, p 531. Philadelphia, FA Davis, 1979
Alpert BS, Cook DH, Vargese PJ, et al: Spontaneous closure of small ventricular defects: 10 years follow-up. Pediatrics 63:204–206, 1979

Brandwald E: Heart Disease, vol 2, pp 994–996. Philadelphia, WB Saunders, 1980
Hurst JW: The Heart, 6th ed, pp 590–596. New York, McGraw-Hill, 1986

EKMAN-LOBSTEIN

Synonyms. OI type IV. See Osteogenesis imperfecta with normal sclerae and absence of deafness.

Etiology. Autosomal dominant.

Diagnostic Procedures. See OI.

Pathology. See OI.

BIBLIOGRAPHY. Ekman OJ: Dissertation medica. Descriptionem et casus aliquot osteomalaciae Sistens. Upsala 1788
Lobstein JG CFM: Lehrbuch der patologischen Anatomie. Stuttgart vol II, p 179, 1835
Sillence DO, Jenn A, Danks DM: Genetic hetereogeneity in osteogenesis imperfecta. J Med Genet 16:101–116, 1979

ELBOW-KNEE MEDT

Synonyms. Multiple epiphyseal dysplasia; MEDT type III C.

Symptoms and Signs. Limitation of elbow movements; occasionally also of knees, and development of osteochondromas.

Etiology. Unknown. Autosomal dominant inheritance.

BIBLIOGRAPHY. Maroteaux P: Spondyloepiphyseal dysplasias and metatropic dwarfism. Birth Defects 9:35–41, 1969

ELECTROSHOCK-INDUCED PSYCHOTIC

Synonym. Postelectroshock psychosis.

Symptoms. Occur in some patients who undergo electroconvulsive treatment. Intellectual changes of memory impairment; emotional, organic changes; euphoria or complete affective dullness; hallucination may occur.

Etiology. Intensity of these symptoms depends (not constantly) on number and spacing of the treatments.

Therapy. When in excitement state, barbiturate intravenously.

Prognosis. Acute psychotic symptoms disappear in 1 week or 2; memory defect may persist longer.

BIBLIOGRAPHY. Freedman AM, Kaplan HI, Sadock BJ: Comprehensive Textbook of Psychiatry, 2nd ed. Baltimore, Williams & Wilkins, 1975

ELIAKIM'S

Synonym. Granulomatous hepatitis.

Symptoms. Both sexes affected. Polymyalgialike illness; hyperthermia; hepatomegaly. Those of the underlying disorder.

Etiology. A wide variety of infectious diseases: bacterial, mycobacterial, spirochetal, viral, rickettsial, fungal, parasitic. Hepatobiliary disorders. Systemic disorders: sarcoidosis; Wegener's granulomatosis; inflammatory bowel disease; chronic granulomatous disease; granulomatous arteritis; melanoma; Hodgkin's disease. Drugs and other exogenous agents.

Pathology. Compact collection of mature mononuclear phagocytes. Epithelioid cells. Giant cells and necrosis.

Diagnostic Procedures. *Biopsy of liver.* Granulomas. *Blood.* Mild abnormalities of liver test (particularly of alkaline phosphatase). Hyperbilirubinemia (25% of cases).

Therapy. Moderate doses of corticosteroids. Antibiotics of no use. Treatment of the underlying disorder.

Prognosis. When the underlying disorder can be successfully treated or an offending exogenous agent eliminated, liver dysfunction disappears. Granulomas may persist for a variable length of time.

BIBLIOGRAPHY. Eliakim M, Eisenberg S, Levij I, et al: Granulomatous hepatitis accompanying a self limited febrile illness. Lancet 1:1348–1352, 1968
Cecil Textbook of Medicine. Philadelphia, WB Saunders, 1982
Timbrell JA: Drug hepatotoxicity (review). Br J Clin Pharmacol 15:3–14, 1983

ELLIS—VAN CREVELD

Synonyms. Acrodysplasia III; chondroectodermal dysplasia; mesoectodermal dysplasia.

Symptoms and Signs. Polydactyly, especially hands; dysplasia of nails and teeth; dwarfism; shortening of extremities; mostly proximal (contrast with achondroplasia). Fusion of metacarpal bones; knock-knees due to defect of proximal tibia. Features of congenital heart defects often associated (mostly atrial septal defect). Small thorax; genital anomalies; mental retardation (30%).

Etiology. Unknown; autosomal recessive inheritance. Occurs in the Amish group in Pennsylvania (5:1000 births).

Pathology. Ectodermal, chondral dysplasia. Failure of epiphysis to produce columnar cartilage. Deformity of proximal metaphyses of the tibia; accelerated maturation of bones and fusion in hands and feet.

Therapy. Cardiac surgery. Orthopedic and orthodontic procedures.

Prognosis. Thirty percent die in first 2 weeks of life. Dwarfism in those who survive. Heart failure frequent cause of death.

BIBLIOGRAPHY. Ellis RWB, Van Creveld S: A syndrome characterized by ectodermal dysplasia, polydactyly; chondrodysplasia, and congenital morbus cordis: Report of three cases. Arch Dis Child 15:65–84, 1940
McKusick VA, Egeland JA, Eldridge R, et al: Dwarfism in the Amish: The Ellis-Van Creveld syndrome. Bull Johns Hopkins Hosp 115:306–336, 1964
Taylor GA, Jordan CE, Dorst SK, et al: Polycarpaly and other abnormalities of the wrist in chondroectodermal dysplasia: The Ellis-Van Creveld syndrome. Radiology 151:393–396, 1984

ELPENOR'S

Synonyms. Dipsomania; alcoholic hallucinosis; postalcoholic behavior. See Alcoholic syndromes.

Symptoms. After abuse of alcohol, sedative drugs, or hallucinogens, when awakening in unknown surroundings and still partially or totally without contact with consciousness, patient behaves abnormally, antisocially, endangering himself or others.

Etiology and Pathology. Intoxication. Complication of alcoholism or drug use. The name of the syndrome is taken from mythologic character, Elpenor, described by Homer in the Odyssey: "The youngest man among us, Elpenor, a lad / Not any too brave or bright, had gone apart / From his friends in the hallowed halls of Circe, seeking / Fresh air. Heavy with wine, he went to sleep. Then hearing the noise and bustle of his comrades / Stirring about, he sprang up, but forgot the long / Ladder by which he came up and proceeded to fall / Headlong from the roof, breaking his neck / His Soul went down to Hades."

BIBLIOGRAPHY. Carrot E, Velluz J, Rigal: Syndrome d'Elpenor. Press Med 55:573, 1947

Rees Ennis: The Odyssey of Homer [Newly Translated for the Modern Reader], p 171. New York, Random House, 1960

Walin SJ, Mello MK: The effects of alcohol on dreams and hallucinations in alcohol addicts. Ann NY Acad Sci 215:266–302, 1973

ELSAHY-WATERS

Synonyms. Branchioskeletogenital; BSG.

Symptoms. Reported in three male siblings. Seizures; mental retardation.

Signs. Pectus excavatum; penoscrotal hypospadias. Facies: brachycephaly; midfacial hypoplasia. *Eyes.* Hypertelorism; strabismus; nystagmus; mild ptosis. *Nose.* Broad bridge; wide tip. *Mouth.* Submucous palatal cleft; multiple jaw cysts; dysplastic dentin.

Etiology. Autosomal recessive(?), X-linked(?) inheritance.

BIBLIOGRAPHY: Elsahy NI, Waters WR: The branchio-skeleto-genital syndrome. Plast Reconstr Surg 48:542–550, 1971

ELSCHINIG'S I

Synonym. Meibonian conjunctivitis.

Symptoms. Smarting of eyes; ocular scratching sensation; photophobia; minimal visual impairment.

Signs. Conjunctivitis. Foamy secretion.

Etiology. Chronic inflammation.

Pathology. Chronic conjunctivitis with hyperplasia of tarsal glands.

Therapy. Topical antiinflammatory agents; antibiotics.

Prognosis. Benign.

BIBLIOGRAPHY. Elsching A: Beitrag zur Aetiologie und Therapie der chronischen Conjunctivitis. Dtsch Med Wochenshr 34:1133–1135, 1908

ELSCHNIG'S II

Symptoms and Signs. Present from birth. Palpebral fissures extending laterally; lateral canthus displaced out and downward; lower eyelids ectropion; hypertelorism; frequently, cleft palate and lip.

BIBLIOGRAPHY. Elschnig A: Zur Kenntnis der Anomalien der Lidspaltenform. Klin Monatsbl Augenheilkd 50:17–30, 1912

EMBOLISM, ATHEROMATOUS

Synonyms. Cholesterol embolization; livedo reticularis-digital infarct.

Symptoms and Signs. Polymorphous and highly variable, reminiscent of those of collagen diseases (in particular periarteritis nodosa). Involvement of kidney most frequent (75%), with resulting hypertension and symptoms of renal failure; pancreas, with symptoms and signs of acute pancreatitis; central nervous system (less frequently observed), with manifestations of focal lesions; gastrointestinal tract, the gastroduodenal ulcer of the aged sometimes results of this pathogenesis; obstruction of various arteries, mesenteric with acute abdominal manifestations; lower extremities with resulting livedo reticularis and occlusion of digital arteries.

Etiology. Embolization of atheromatous material in various areas of body; spontaneous or following trauma or surgery.

Pathology. Changes in small and medium-sized arteries of various organs (kidney; pancreas; thyroid) containing cholesterol crystals.

Therapy. Symptomatic; resistent to anticoagulants and vasodilators. If feasible, removal of diseased tissue that is source of the embolic material.

Prognosis. Poor.

BIBLIOGRAPHY. Panum PL: Untersuchungen über den plötzlich Tod durch Embolie mittelst der durch dieselbe gesetzten Unterbrechung des Blutstromes. Arch Pathol Anat Berl 25:310–338, 1862; Die Embolie der Arterien des grossen Kresilaufes. Arch Pathol Anat Berl 25:488–530, 1862

Kazmier FJ, Sheps SG, Bernatz PE, et al: Livedo reticularis and digital infarcts: A syndrome due to cholesterol emboli arising from atheromatous abdominal aortic aneurysms. Vasc Dis 3:12–24, 1966

Rook A, Wilkinson DS, Ebling FJG, et al: Textbook of Dermatology, 4th ed, pp 627–630. Oxford, Blackwell Scientific Publications, 1986

EMBOLISM, PARADOXICAL

Synonym. Cardiac anomaly–cerebral abscess.

Symptoms. May occur at any age. Patients with cardiac anomaly with right-to-left shunt; headache; stiff neck; drowsiness; fever, indicating a possible protective role of the pulmonary capillary bed in removing bacteria from blood.

Signs. Hemiplegia; aphasia; jacksonian convulsion, coma. Other signs of expanding intracranial lesions or meningitis.

Etiology. Acute infective process of central nervous system in patients with congenital cardiac anomaly.

Pathology. Patient with right-to-left cardiac shunt. Usually, single abscess in central nervous system. Occasionally, meningitis.

Diagnostic Procedures. *Blood.* Polycythemia; leukocytosis. *Cerebrospinal fluid.* Increased pressure; increased proteins. (If meningitis, increased leukocytes.) *X-ray of skull. Angiography. CT brain and vertebrae scan.*

Therapy. Antibiotics; surgery if lesions are localized.

Prognosis. Guarded.

BIBLIOGRAPHY. Farre JR: Pathological Researches. Essay I. On malformations of the human heart; illustrated by numerous cases, and preceded by some observations on the method of improving the diagnostic part of medicine. London, Longman, 1814

Gintrac E: Observations et recherches sur la cyanose ou maladie bleue. Paris, Pinard, 1824

Ballet G: Des abscès du cerveau consécutifs à certaines malformations cardiaques. Arch Gen Med 145:659–667, 1880

Chambers WR: Brain abscess associated with pulmonary arteriovenous fistula. Ann Surg 141:276–277, 1955

Hurst JW: The Heart, 6th ed, pp 1109–1362. New York, McGraw-Hill, 1986

EMERY-DREIFUSS

Symptoms and Signs. Onset in the first decade. Toe walking, partial flexion of the elbows, inability to fully flex the neck and spine. Absence of major muscle weakness and of hypertrophy. In early adulthood emerges the final component of the clinical syndrome: atrial conduction abnormalities, with chest pain and recurrent syncope. The cardiac arrhythmia, however, may be seen in childhood, or not appear until the sixth decade, or may be seen without muscle weakness.

Etiology. X-linked inheritance.

Pathology. Muscle biopsies: predominance of type II fibers; changes suggesting dystrophy, including fibrosis, necrosis, and marked variation in fiber size.

Diagnostic Procedure. Serum creatine kinase activity elevated (3–10 times; in Duchenne dystrophy it is elevated 50–200 times). The EMG pattern is myopathic,

with motor unit potentials of short duration and reduced amplitude.

Therapy. Pacemaker, if severe conduction defects are present.

Prognosis. Most children tolerate their undiagnosed disorder through the first 10 years because of the slow insidious progression and resultant mild disability. The rhythm disturbance, if untreated, proves fatal by mid-adulthood.

BIBLIOGRAPHY. Emery A, Dreifuss F: Unusual type of benign X-linked muscular dystrophy. J Neurol Neurosurg Psychiatry 29:338–342, 1966

Dickey R, Ziter F, Smith R: Emery-Dreifuss muscular dystrophy. J Pediatr 104:555–559, 1984

EMERY-DREIFUSS, AUTOSOMAL DOMINANT

Synonyms. Scapuloilioperoneal atrophy. Cardiopathy. See Kaeser's and Dreifuss-Emery.

Symptoms and Signs. Both sexes. Onset myopathy between 17 to 42 years of age, cardiac signs later. Muscle contractures, neck stiffness slowly progressing; weakness of humeral and peroneal muscles, pelvic involvement, tendon areflexia. Atrial fibrillation, heart block, heart failure.

Etiology. Unknown. Autosomal dominant inheritance. Clinically overlapping with Charcot-Marie-Tooth and Kungelberg-Welander and other X-linked scapuloperoneal conditions.

Pathology. Muscle: inflammatory changes, perivascular cuffing.

Diagnostic Procedures. *Electromyography.*

Therapy. None. Cardiac pacemaker (when indicated).

Prognosis. Progressive condition.

BIBLIOGRAPHY. Miller RG, Layzer RB, Mellenthin MA, et al: Emery-Dreifuss muscular dystrophy with autosomal dominant transmission. Neurology 35:1230–1233, 1985

EMERY-NELSON

Synonym. Hand–foot–flat facies.

Symptoms and Signs. Both sexes affected; present from birth. Unusual facies; long philtrum; flatness, flexion and extension deformities of hands; clawed toes. Retarded physical and mental development.

Etiology. Unknown. Autosomal dominant (?) inheritance.

BIBLIOGRAPHY. Emery AEH, Nelson MM: A familial syndrome of short stature, deformities of hands and feet and an unusual facies. J Med Genet 7:379–382, 1970
Gorlin RJ, Pindborg JJ, Cohen MM, Jr: Syndromes of the Head and Neck, 2nd ed. New York, McGraw-Hill, 1976

EMPTY SELLA, ACQUIRED

Symptoms. Occur after treatment of pituitary tumors by surgery, isotopes, x-ray. Reduced visual acuity that in some cases, can evolve into blindness. Hemianopia; top quadrantanopsia; central scotoma (occasionally).

Signs. Irregular visual field defects; pale optic disks. Acromegaly or other manifestations due to the tumor do not belong to the syndrome.

Etiology. X-ray damage and secondary atrophy or scar with mechanical action altering chiasm, optic nerve, or vascular tree.

Pathology. Empty and enlarged sella. See Etiology.

Diagnostic Procedures. Exclude recurrence of tumor (with similar symptomatology). *X-ray.* Enlarged sella. *Pneumoencephalography.* May reveal air in the sella. *CT brain scan.*

Therapy. None.

Prognosis. Poor.

BIBLIOGRAPHY. Colby MY Jr, Kearns TP: Radiation therapy of pituitary adenomas with associated visual impairment. Proc Staff Meet Mayo Clin 37:15–24, 1962
Lee WM, Adams JE: The empty sella syndrome. J Neurosurg 28:351–356, 1968
Barbarino A, De Marinis L, Mancini A et al: Prolactin dynamics in normoprolactinemic primary empty sella: Correlation with intracranial pressure. Hormone Res 27:141–151, 1987

EMPTY SELLA, PRIMARY

Symptoms and Signs. In absence of surgery or radiotherapy. Familial form. Finding of empty sella turcica (radiologically) associated to osteosclerosis, meningoceles (thoracic or lumbar), wormian bones, moderate dwarfism, facial structure abnormalities. Sporadic cases in obese, middle-aged women with normal pituitary function.

Diagnostic Procedures. See Empty sella, acquired.

BIBLIOGRAPHY. Lehman RAW, Stearns JC, Wesenberg RL, et al: Familial osteosclerosis with abnormalities of the nervous system and meninges. J Pediatr 90:49–54, 1977

ENCEPHALITIC PARKINSONISM

See Parkinson's syndrome.

Symptoms and Signs. Onset at any age from childhood. Onset gradual; development rapid. Involvement frequently limited; seldom generalized. Rigidity symptoms and signs prevalent over tremor component. Ptyalism almost constant; pupillary reaction often impaired. Face and scalp covered with greasy secretion. Frequently associated with other sequelae of encephalitis: tics; spasms; behavioral changes; respiratory disorders.

Etiology. Complication of von Economo type of encephalitis. Exposure to certain toxins (manganese dust, carbon disulfide); severe CO poisoning and some drugs: neuroleptic, reserpine, metoclopramide.

Pathology. Lesions of substantia nigra and globus pallidus.

Diagnostic Procedures. See Parkinson's.

Therapy. See Parkinson's.

Prognosis. See Parkinson's.

BIBLIOGRAPHY. Current concepts and controversies in Parkinson's disease (editorial). Can J Neurol Sci 11 (Suppl), 1984

ENCEPHALOMYELITIS, DISSEMINATED ACUTE

Synonyms. Acute perivascular myelinoclasis; postinfective encephalomyelitis; postexanthematous encephalomyelitis; postvaccinal encephalomyelitis.

Symptoms and Signs. Occur in both sexes; onset at all ages; associated with virus infection (e.g. measles or after vaccination), basal infection, or without recognizable preceding illness. Onset explosive. Cranial palsies; optic neuritis; vertigo; nausea; vomiting. Then development of paraplegia, hemiplegia, diffuse brain stem signs, and slight fever.

Etiology. Unknown; possibly allergic reaction. Relationship with multiple sclerosis (see) in idiopathic cases not established, but clinically the two conditions are undistinguishable.

Pathology. Similar to multiple sclerosis syndrome (see). In acute cases, marked lymphocytic infiltration.

Diagnostic Procedures. *Blood.* Leukocytosis. *Spinal fluid.* Moderate pleocytosis.

Therapy. In acute form (not postinfective) some benefit from adrenocorticotropic hormone (ACTH) and cortical steroids. Symptomatic.

Prognosis. Variable; from rapid steady progression with groups of symptoms appearing and receding, to sequelae or complete recovery.

BIBLIOGRAPHY. Greenfield JG: Acute disseminated encephalomyelitis as a sequel to influenza. J Pathol Bacteriol 33:453, 1930
Miller HG, Evans MJ: Prognosis in acute disseminated encephalomyelitis, with a note on neuromyelitis optica. J Med 87:347–379, 1953
Adams RD, Victor M: Principles of Neurology, 3rd ed, pp 712–713. New York, McGraw-Hill, 1985

ENCEPHALOPATHY, HYPERTENSIVE

See Hypothalamic carrefour and Page's.

Symptoms. Intermittent, often transient headache; apathy; anorexia; vomiting; generalized weakness; temporary amaurosis. Convulsion and transient paralysis also frequently seen.

Signs. Marked elevation of blood pressure; hypertensive retinopathy; enlarged heart.

Etiology. Essential hypertension (malignant phase) or secondary hypertension to glomerulonephritis; eclampsia; pheochromocytoma; Cushing's; hyperaldosteronism.

Pathology. Vasculocerebral alteration with subintimal hyalinization; hypertrophy of media; cerebral hemorrhage; thrombosis; edema.

Diagnostic Procedures. To determine etiology of blood hypertension. *Blood: Blood urea nitrogen. Urine, renography, urography, hormonal studies. Spinal fluid.* Increased pressure, increased proteins. *Ophthalmoscopy.* Retinal hemorrhages; bilateral papilledema. *Electrocardiography.* Left ventricular hypertrophy.

Therapy. That of hypertension.

Prognosis. Usually a bad prognostic sign in essential malignant hypertension. In secondary correctable hypertension, good response to treatment.

BIBLIOGRAPHY. Vick NA: Grinker's Neurology, 7th ed. Springfield, CC Thomas, 1976
Adams RD, Victor M: Principles of Neurology, 3rd ed, p 625. New York, McGraw-Hill, 1985

ENDOCARDIAL CUSHION MALFORMATIONS

Synonyms. Atrioventricular defect–persistent A-V ostium; ostium atrioventricularis communis; persistent common A-V canal.

Symptoms and Signs. Female slightly predominant in incomplete form; equal sex ratio in complete form. *Complete form.* High incidence in Down's syndrome (see). Onset in early infancy. Recurrent respiratory infections; failure to thrive; dyspnea; orthopnea; signs of congestive heart failure. Absent or slight cyanosis accompanying crying or strains. First heart sound single; soft prominent systolic murmur with first sound. At site of left ventricular impulse, murmur of mitral regurgitation radiating toward sternum, becoming evident after a few weeks. At lower left sternal margin, murmur of ventricular septal defect. Second sound shows constant splitting with loud second component. *Incomplete form.* Onset in childhood according to extent and combination of malformations. Relatively asymptomatic or several symptoms. Murmur of mitral regurgitation or ventricular septal defect. Arrhythmias increasing with age.

Etiology. Defects (singly or in association) of atrial septum, ventricular septum, atrioventricular (A-V) valves, and A-V conduction system.

Diagnostic Procedures. *Electrocardiography.* Sinus rhythm; prolonged P-R; P wave direction normal peaked and of increased amplitude; QRS left axis deviation and distinctive vectocardiographic patterns. *X-ray.* Pulmonary plethora; cardiomegaly. *M-mode and two-dimensional echocardiography. Cardiac catheterization. Aortography.*

Therapy. Symptomatic. Cardiac surgery.

Prognosis. *Complete form.* Death usually in early infancy; some patients may reach childhood. *Incomplete form.* If surviving childhood; symptoms will be delayed to first or second decades; arrhythmias to complete heart block; susceptibility to infective endocarditis.

BIBLIOGRAPHY. Perloff JK: The Clinical Recognition of Congenital Heart Disease, 2nd ed, p 344. Philadelphia, WB Saunders, 1978
Becker AE, Anderson RH: Atrioventricular septal defects: What's in a name? J Thorac Cardiovasc Surg 83:461–469, 1982
Hurst JW: The Heart, 6th ed, pp 605–612. New York, McGraw-Hill, 1986
Williams RG, Bierman FZ, Sanders SP: Echocardiographic diagnosis of cardiac malformations, pp 63–70. Boston, Little, Brown & Co, 1986

ENDOCARDIAL FIBROELASTOSIS, SECONDARY

See Weinberg-Himmelfarb.

Symptoms and Signs. Onset at same age as primary form (see Weinberg-Himmelfarb) or later; in adult life after myocardial infarction. Symptoms and signs of Weinberg-Himmelfarb, plus those of associated malformation or pathology: aortic stenosis; coarctation of aorta; anomalous origin of left coronary artery from pulmonary trunk; hypoplastic left heart (see); generalized glycogenosis and others. Respiratory distress, mostly rales in the lung fields, enlarged heart, gallop rhythm, no significant murmur early in the illness.

Diagnostic Procedures. *X-ray.* Heart massively enlarged with left atrial dilatation; left lower lobe atelectasis. *Electrocardiography.* Left ventricular and left atrial hypertrophy. *M-mode echocardiography. Cardiac catheterization.*

Therapy. Medical treatment of heart failure (digitalis and diuretics), L-carnitine if carnitine levels (plasma, muscle) are reduced; restriction of activity. Cardiac transplant attempted.

BIBLIOGRAPHY. Perloff JK: The Clinical Recognition of Congenital Heart Disease, 2nd ed, p 174. Philadelphia, WB Saunders, 1978
Hurst JW: The Heart, 6th ed, pp 653–654. New York, McGraw-Hill, 1986

ENDOMETRIOSIS

Symptoms. Found most frequently among women in the higher socioeconomic group; median age 37 years. Characteristics of patient with endometriosis: underweight; overanxious; intelligent and perfectionist; marriage and childbearing are deferred for prolonged periods. Disease occurs only after the female begins to menstruate and regresses after menopause. Rarely seen in women with anovulatory cycles, but common in those who have uninterrupted cyclic menstruation. Endometriosis improves during pregnancy and during artificially induced anovulation. Frequent pregnancies seem to prevent the disease. Endometriosis is associated with infertility. Progressive, severe suprapubic pain during menstruation or just before menstruation; dyspareunia; painful defecation; premenstrual staining; hypermenorrhea; dysuria; hematuria.

Etiology. Unknown, but numerous theories. Sampson theory: viable endometrial fragments are regurgitated with menstrual blood into peritoneal cavity with subsequent implantation. Meyer theory: peritoneal mesothelium possessed totipotency and therefore, may be converted into endometrial tissue. Hertig theory: formation of a fibrinopurulent exudate; organization by endometrial stroma; formation of glandlike spaces. Familial occurrence reported (autosomal dominant).

Diagnostic Procedures. *Pelvic examination. Culdoscopy. Laparotomy.* Differential diagnosis: adenomyosis uteri, pelvic inflammatory disease, nonspecific adhesions; ovarian carcinoma.

Pathology. Commonest site is ovary; other areas include uterosacral ligaments, rectovaginal septum, sigmoid colon, lower genital tract, round ligaments, pelvic peritoneum, small intestine, umbilicus, laparotomy scars, bladder, ureter, breasts, pleura, lung. *Microscopically.* Endometrial epithelium, glands or glandlike structures, stroma, hemorrhage.

Therapy. The aims of therapy: observation and analgesia; suppression of ovulation; conservative operation; radical operation.

1. Observation and analgesia is beneficial to those patients having only minimal involvement.
2. Ovulation may be suppressed by danazol or estrogens and progestins or medroxyprogesterone acetate (Depoprovera). Pseudopregnancy should be continued for a minimum of 9 months, and if extensive endometriosis, should be extended to 12 to 24 months.
3. Conservative surgery includes lysis of adhesions, removal of endometrial implants and endometrial cysts of ovary, presacral neurectomy, uterine suspension.
4. Radical surgery consists of total hysterectomy and bilateral salpingo oophorectomy.

BIBLIOGRAPHY. Novak ER, Woodruf JD: Novak's Gynecologic and Obstetric Pathology, 8th ed. Philadelphia, WB Saunders, 1979
Hinson JM Jr, Brigham KL, Danieli J: Catamenial pneumothorax in sisters. Chest 80:633–635, 1981

ENGEL-ARING

Synonym. Periodic hypothalamic discharge. See Grahmann's and Transient Cushing's.

Symptoms. Recurrent at intervals of weeks or 2 to 3 months, or sporadic episodes lasting 3 to 5 days. Nausea, vomiting, thirst, fever, mental depression and withdrawal; weight loss. In intervals; weight regained and normal life. Rapid weight gain precedes attacks.

Signs. Obesity; centripetal distribution; no "buffalo hump"; purple striae on abdomen and buttocks. Blood hypertension and tachycardia during attacks. Neurologic and ophthalmologic examination may be normal or abnormal.

Etiology and Pathology. Unknown; trauma or infection of central nervous system determining alteration of thermoregulatory mechanism and intermittent type of hyperadrenocorticism. Cystic soft degeneration of lateral thalamus and dorsomedial nucleus (in one case hypothalamus not involved).

Diagnostic Procedures. *Blood.* During attacks leukocytosis (up to 20,000); neutrophilia; sedimentation rate slightly increased; fall of potassium, normal sodium and chloride; rise of cholesterol. *Urine.* Normal during interval. During attacks, abrupt increase of 17-ketosteroids and 17-hydroxycorticoid excretion. *Electrocardiography.* Normal. *X-ray of chest and skull. Of gastrointestinal tract:* stomach dilatation; spasm of pylorus during attacks (normal in interval).

Therapy. Dexamethasone prevents attacks.

Prognosis. Recurrence with temporary remission with treatment.

BIBLIOGRAPHY. Engel GL, Aring CD: Hypothalamic attacks with thalamic lesion. Arch Neurol Psychiatr 54:37–50, 1945
Wolff SM, Adler RC, Buskirk ER, et al: A syndrome of periodic hypothalamic discharge. Am J Med 36:956–967, 1964.
Adams RD, Victor M: Principles of Neurology, 3rd ed, p 413. New York, McGraw-Hill, 1985

ENGEL-VON RECKLINGHAUSEN'S

Synonyms. Osteitis fibrosa generalisata; parathyroid osteitis; Recklinghausen's; von Recklinghausen's II; renal osteodystrophy; glomerular rickets.

Symptoms. Manifestations of nephritis or primary or secondary hyperparathyroidism. Arthralgia; fractures.

Signs. Bowing of long bones; spinal and chest deformities.

Etiology. Various conditions may cause this syndrome: (1) chronic nephritis; (2) primary and secondary hyperparathyroidism.

Pathology. That of underlying disease. *Bone.* Increased osteoblastic-osteoclastic activity. Formation of cysts in rarefied bones. Fibrous replacement of bone marrow cavities. *Kidney.* Renal calculi.

Diagnostic Procedures. *X-ray.* Typical findings.

Therapy and Prognosis. According to etiology.

	Hyperpara-thyroidism	Acidosis
Blood		
Calcium	Increased	Normal or decreased
Phosphorus	Decreased	Increased
Alkaline phosphatase	Increased	Normal
Urine		
Calcium	Decreased	Decreased
Phosphorus	Increased or Normal	Decreased
(NPN)*	Increased (late)	Increased

*nonprotein nitrogen

BIBLIOGRAPHY. von Recklinghausen F: Untersuchungen über Rachitis und Osteomalacie. Jena, G Fisher, 1910
Engel G: Ueber einen Fall cystoider Entartung des gesamten Skeletts. Giessen, 1864
Brenner BM, Rector FC: The Kidney, 3rd ed, p 1675. Philadelphia, WB Saunders, 1986

ENTEROPATHIC ARTHRITIS

Synonyms. Acute toxic arthritis–ulcerative colitis; colitic-arthritis. Dermatosis-arthritis-bowel.

Symptoms and Signs. Same sex incidence than that of Crohn's (see) and ulcerative colitis; onset at all ages; more common between 25 and 45 years of age. Bouts of arthritic manifestation associated with enteric symptoms, usually initially involving only a few joints and frequently migrating to others. Prevalence of distal extremity joint involvement and big articulations over hands and feet.

Etiology. Controversial entity. Some authors consider the arthritic condition to be a complication of chronic ulcerative colitis, regional enteritis, and Whipple's disease; 15% of patients with jejunal bypass develop symmetric polyarticular inflammation. Many others distinguish this entity as an autonomous association. The form is recognized by the American Rheumatism Association.

Pathology. That of Crohn's or ulcerative colitis and arthritis (indistinguishable from that of rheumatoid arthritis).

Diagnostic Procedures. *Blood.* Leukocytosis; high sedimentation rate; hemoglobin reduced. *X-ray.* Nonspecific and minor alterations; usually rheumatoid factor absent. *Synovial fluid.* Total leukocytes from 4000 to 40,000, polymorphs 75% to 98%; increased viscosity.

Therapy. Corticosteroids for treatment of enteritis, secondarily benefiting arthritis. Indomethacin contraindicated.

Prognosis. In 50% of cases, attack lasts less than 1 month; in 10% more than 1 year. One or two attacks for a year or less. Final outcome is determined by the evolution of enteric manifestation.

BIBLIOGRAPHY. Hench PS: Nelson's Loose-Leaf Surgery, p 104. New York. Nelson & Son, 1935
Jorizzo JL: Bowel associated dermatosis-arthritis syndrome. Arch Intern Med 144:738–740, 1984

ENTHESITIS

Synonym. Myoenthesitis syndromes (enthesis-insertion). Includes all syndromes deriving from lesions of the so-called myoenthesic apparatus, the anatomicofunctional structural complex that is interposed between muscles and bones or joint structures. Lesions resulting from microtrauma or macrotrauma. See Overuse syndromes.

BIBLIOGRAPHY. La Cava G: Apparato musculo tendineo e sport. Minerva Med 55:461–463, 1964

ENTRAPMENT

Synonym. Entrapment neuropathy.

Symptoms. Pain of muscle groups, occasionally more severe at rest and during the night; hypoesthesia; paresthesia; muscular weakness.

Signs. Tenderness; muscle atrophy. Pressure on trigger point elicits localized pain in affected areas.

Etiology. Anatomic constriction of peripheral nerve. These are the most frequent sites of entrapment:

Spinoglenoid notch—median

Carpal tunnel—median

Bicipital groove—ulnar

Cubital tunnel—ulnar

Palmar fascia—pisiform bone—ulnar

Heads on pronator muscle—anterior interosseous

Inguinal ligament—lateral femoral cutaneous

Obturator canal—obturator

Tarsal tunnel—posterior tibial

Plantar fascia: heads of IV-IV metatarsal—plantar

See individual syndromes.

ENURESIS

Synonyms. Bed wetting; primary enuresis; secondary enuresis.

Symptoms and Signs. Between 4 and 5 years of age 10% to 15% of children continue to wet the bed. In adulthood symptoms present in 1% to 3%. *Primary enuresis.* No intercurrent episodes of dryness. *Secondary enuresis.* Periods of dry months and relapses. Episode usually occurs in first third of night.

Etiology. *Primary form.* Family history; organic conditions (*e.g.,* urologic obstruction, epispadias). *Secondary form.* Psychologic factors (relapses caused also by organic factors, *i.e.,* intercurring diseases).

Diagnostic Procedures. Rule out organic conditions. Assess psychologic status. *Sleep study.* Enuresis episodes usually in N REM (rapid eye movement) sleep; follows a burst of K complex waves and body movements.

Therapy. Correct organic conditions. Parent and child education. Imipramine.

Prognosis. Variable according to nature of condition and treatment. Suspension of imipramine causes relapses. Most children outgrow syndrome.

BIBLIOGRAPHY. Gastant H, Broughton R: A clinical and polygraphic study of episodic phenomena during sleep. Recent Adv Biol Psychiatr 7:197–223, 1969
Starfield B: Enuresis: Its pathogenesis and management. Clin Pediatr 11:343–350, 1972
Adams RD, Victor M: Principles of Neurology, 3rd ed, p 446–447. New York, McGraw-Hill, 1985

ENZYMOPATHIES OF ANAEROBIC GLYCOLYSIS

These syndromes are described together because of their similarity and rarity. They represent deficiencies of the six enzymes of the Embden-Meyerhof pathway and have the same symptoms and signs of pyruvate kinase deficiency.

HEXOKINASE DEFICIENCY
Synonym. HK deficiency.

Symptoms and Signs. Only 12 cases described. See PK deficiency.

Etiology. Autosomal recessive.

GLUCOSEPHOSPHATE ISOMERASE DEFICIENCY

PHOSPHOFRUCTOKINASE DEFICIENCY

Synonym. PFK deficiency.

Symptoms and Signs. Only 12 cases described. In some cases hemolytic anemia is associated with myopathy.

Etiology. Autosomal recessive.

ALDOLASE DEFICIENCY

Synonym. AL deficiency.

Symptoms and Signs. One case described with hemolysis and mental retardation.

Etiology. Autosomal recessive.

TRIOSEPHOSPHATE ISOMERASE

Synonym. TPI deficiency.

Symptoms and Signs. Hemolysis accompanied by progressive neurologic deficit from first month of life.

Etiology. Autosomal recessive.

Prognosis. Death in childhood.

PHOSPHOGLYCERATE KINASE DEFICIENCY

Synonym. PGK deficiency.

Symptoms and Signs. In males severe hemolytic anemia; mild mental retardation, neurologic aberrations. In females less evident traits.

Etiology. X-linked.

BIBLIOGRAPHY. Valentine WN, Tanaka KR, Paglia DE: Pyruvate kinase and other enzyme deficiency disorders of the erythrocyte. In Stanbury JB, Wyngaarden JB, Fredrickson DS: The Metabolic Basis of Inherited Disease, 5th ed, p 1606. New York, McGraw-Hill, 1983

EOSINOPHIL LUNG, SECONDARY

Synonym. Secondary pulmonary eosinophilic infiltrate.

Symptoms and Signs. Same clinical findings as in Loeffler's. Occasionally, recurrent episodes.

Etiology. *Parasites.* Ascaris; trichina; entamoeba; hookworms; filaria; toxocara; schistosomes; lung fluke; strongyloides; trichuris; liver fluke; tapeworms; echinococcus. *Infections.* Tuberculosis; coccidiomycosis; brucellosis; viral and bacterial pneumonia; bronchiectasis. *Neoplastic.* Hodgkin's disease; eosinophilic granuloma, eosinophilic leukemia. *Collagen diseases.* Periarteritis; rheumatoid arthritis; rheumatic fever. *Allergic.* Asthma; hay fever; eczema; serum sickness; Dressler's syndrome;

drugs. *Others.* Fat embolism, aspiration pneumonia; idiopathic familial eosinophilia with pneumonia.

Pathology. Pulmonary eosinophilic infiltrates plus specific findings according to etiology.

Diagnostic Procedures. *Blood.* Eosinophilia. *Sputum.* Eosinophilia. *X-ray of chest.* Pulmonary infiltrates plus specific findings according to etiology.

Therapy. Corticosteroids highly effective, except when contraindicated by particular etiology. Specific treatment according to etiology.

Prognosis. Good response to steroids; possible recurrences. Depends on etiology.

BIBLIOGRAPHY. Reeder WH, Goodrich BE: Pulmonary infiltration with eosinophilia, (P.I.E. syndrome). Ann Int Med 36:1217–1240, 1952
Hall JW, Kozak M, Spink WW: Pulmonary infiltrates, pericarditis and eosinophilia. Am J Med 36:135–143, 1964
Fraser RG, Paré JAP: Diagnosis of Diseases of the Chest 2nd ed, p 906. Philadelphia, WB Saunders, 1977

EPIDERMAL NEVUS

Synonyms. Schimmelpeming's; Feuerstein-Mims; including comedo cataract.

Symptoms and Signs. Any association of epidermal nevi (sebaceous, verrucus, linear inflammatory, comedo, syringocystadenomatosus papilliferus) with any significant *skeletal* (cystic, hypertrophy, and atrophy), *neurologic* (50% of patients): mental retardation (40%), epilepsy (30%), spastic emiparesis (20%), cerebral angiomata, atrophy, hydrocephalus palsies, *ocular* (33% circa eyelid or conjunctive) abnormalities, colobomata, corneal opacity. Association with various types of malignancy reported.

Etiology. Unknown. Usually sporadic. Few instances of inheritance, autosomal dominant.

BIBLIOGRAPHY. Feuerstein RC, Mims LC: Linear nevus sebaceous with convulsion and mental retardation. Am J Dis Child 104:675–679, 1962
Popou L, Boinaov L: Undescribed congenital cutaneo ocular syndrome (congenital cataract-comedo syndrome). Surv Med (Sofiia) 13:49–50, 1962
Solomon LL, Freizin DF, Dewald RL: The epidermal nevus syndrome. Arch Dermatol 97:273–285, 1968
Rook A, Wilkinson DS, Ebling FJG et al: Textbook of Dermatology, 4th ed. Oxford, Blackwell Scientific Publications, 1986

EPIDERMOLYSIS BULLOSA, SIMPLE OGUA*

Synonyms. Gedde-Dahl's.

Symptoms and Signs. From infancy, both sexes. Traumatic seasonal blistering of palms and soles and seldom other places, generalized bruising tendency, onychogryphotic big toe nails.

Etiology. Autosomal dominant inheritance. Linkage to erythrocyte glutamic pyruvic transaminase focus.

BIBLIOGRAPHY. Gedde-Dahl T: Epidermolysis bullosa. Baltimore, Johns Hopkins Press, 1971

EPILEPTIC AUTOMATISM

After an attack of grand mal or more frequently in psychomotor amnesic epilepsy, patient may wander, avoiding danger; talks and acts without memory of happenings after he comes out of the state and finds himself in strange surroundings (sometimes in another town).

BIBLIOGRAPHY. Jackson JH: Contribution to the comparative study of convulsions. Brain 9:1–23, 1886
Unvericht H: Die Myoclonie. Berlin, Franz Dentiche, 1918
Temkin O: The Falling Sickness: A History of Epilepsy from the Greeks to the Beginning of Modern Neurology. Baltimore, Johns Hopkins Press, 1945
Freedman AM, Kaplan HI, Sadock BJ: Comprehensive Textbook of Psychiatry, 2nd ed. Baltimore, Williams & Wilkins, 1975

EPIPHYSEAL DYSPLASIA, MULTIPLE

Synonyms. MEDT Type III D; microepiphyseal dysplasia tarda of hips; microepiphyseal dysplasia of hips; Elsbach's; Watt's. See Fairbank's (possibly same condition).

Symptoms and Signs. Present from birth. Growth deficit of epiphyses of femur, humerus, and hands. Precocious osteoarthritis.

Etiology. Autosomal dominant inheritance.

BIBLIOGRAPHY. Watt JK: Multiple epiphyseal dysplasia: Report of four cases. Brit J Surg 39:533–535, 1952
Elsbach L: Bilateral hereditary microepiphyseal dysplasia of hips. J Bone Joint Surg [Br] 41:514–523, 1959

Lic SO, Siggers DC, Dorst JP, et al: Unusual multiple epiphyseal dysplasias. Birth Defects Orig Art Ser 10(12):165–185, 1974

EPIPHYSEAL ISCHEMIC NECROSIS

Synonyms. Epiphyseal aseptic necrosis; epiphyseal osteochondritis; osteochondritis deformans juvenilis.

Symptoms. Prevalent in males (4:1, except in some forms. See individual syndromes); onset at young age, mostly in childhood, some varieties in adolescence or adult life. Pain corresponding to affected bone, primary epiphyses or secondary epiphyses. According to bone affected designated by various eponyms:

1. Blencke's (see)
2. Chandler's S.A. (see)
3. Dietrich's (see)
4. Kienboeck's (see)
5. Köhler's I (see)
6. Köhler's II (see)
7. Legg-Calvé-Perthes (see)
8. Osgood-Slatter (see)
9. Panner's (see)
10. Preiser's (see)
11. Scheuermann's (see)
12. Sever's (see)
13. Thiemann's (see)

Signs. At site involved, tenderness or palpation, skin changes, swelling, redness, occasionally, thickening.

Etiology. Degeneration and eventual replacement of the osseous nucleus of an epiphysis, due to interference with its blood supply: trauma(?); congenital hereditary factors(?); infection and endocrine disturbances(?).

Pathology. Scanty reports. Osseous nucleus: necrotic; fragmented and compressed; there may be evidence of hemorrhage, cystic degeneration and fibrosis. Enchondral plate may be softened and distorted. Histologic changes variable according to the phase in which the analysis is carried out.

Diagnostic Procedures. X-ray. Similar changes for all types of bones affected. In first stage, scanty modification (bulging of joint capsule; slight displacement of affected bone) followed by osseous manifestations (lucent crescent or other images); later the affected center becomes opaque. Demineralization in surrounding area. In second stage; opacity, fragmentation and flattening of epiphyseal center. In third stage; healing through new bone formation.

Therapy. Symptomatic. Analgesic. Avoidance of weight bearing.

---

* Name of village in Norway.

Prognosis. Spontaneous recovery in month or years. Complete normal restoration of morphology and function, or, in cases, persistent malformation due to irreversible anatomic changes during or following the acute stage.

BIBLIOGRAPHY. Canale ST: Osteochondrosis or epiphisitis. In Crenshaw AH (ed): Campbell's Operative Orthopedics, 7th ed, pp 989–1003. St. Louis, CV Mosby, 1987

EPSTEIN'S (A.A.)

Synonyms. Idiopathic nephrotic syndrome. INS. Includes various basic pathologic lesions which may represent different diseases. The classification adopted today is based on histopathology. But the clinical entity is approximately the same. Minimal change disease (see). Mesangial proliferative glomerulonephritis (see). Focal glomerular sclerosis (see). Diffuse glomerular sclerosis Membranous glomerulonephritis (see). Mesangiocapillary glomerulonephritis types I, II, III (see).

Symptoms and Signs. Insidious onset. Edema (legs and face), hematuria, hypertension. Oliguria, anuria possible. Malnutrition. Increased susceptibility to infections. Frequent cardiovascular symptoms and signs. Thromboembolism. Renal vein thrombosis.

Etiology. See individual syndromes.

Diagnostic Procedures. *Urine.* Proteinuria (more than 3.5 g/day), hematuria macroscopic or microscopic. *Blood.* Creatinine and BUN above normal ranges, hypoalbuminemia, electrophoretic alterations (alpha 1 and beta increased). Hyperlipidemia (LDL, VLDL).

Therapy. See individual syndromes.

Prognosis. See individual syndromes.

BIBLIOGRAPHY. Epstein AA: Concerning the causation of edema in chronic parenchymatous nephritis: Methods for its alleviation. Am J Med Sci 154:638–647, 1917
Glassock RJ: The nephrotic syndrome. In Brenner Z, Rector FC Jr (eds): The Kidney, 3rd ed, p 1351. Philadelphia, WB Saunders 1986
Schnaper HP, Robson AM: Nephrotic syndrome: minimal change disease, focal glomerulosclerosis, and related disorders. In Schreier RW and Gotteshalk CW (eds): Disease of the kidney, pp 1949–2004, 1988

EPSTEIN'S (C.J.)

Synonym. Macrothrombocytopenia-nephritis-deafness.

Symptoms and Signs. Both sexes. Nephropathy. More in females. Hearing loss and nephropathy symptoms identical with those of Alport's (see). Hemorrhagic tendency.

Etiology. Unknown. Possibly autosomal dominant trait.

Diagnostic Procedures. *Blood.* Giant thrombocytes, impaired aggregation with collagen and epinephrine, lack of release of factor III, and adherence to glass. Bleeding time prolonged.

BIBLIOGRAPHY. Epstein CJ, Sahud MA, Piel CF et al: Hereditary macrothrombocytopenia nephritis and deafness. Ann J Med 52:299–310, 1972
Hansen MS, Behnke O, Pedersen NT, et al: Megathrombocytopenia associated with glomerulonephritis, deafness and aortic cystic media necrosis. Scand J Hemat 21:197–205, 1978

ERB-CHARCOT

Synonyms. Erb's IV spastic spinal syphilitic paralysis; Struempel's.

Symptoms. Prevalent in males; onset 2 to 10 years after infection. Tiredness and stiffness of legs. Dragging feet; urgency and increased frequency of urination; gradual progression to paraplegia; minor sensory changes occur at later stage.

Signs. *Early.* Increase in muscular tone and in deep reflexes; ankle clonus; Babinski positive; abdominal reflexes abolished. *Later.* Minor defects in tactile and proprioceptive spheres.

Etiology. Rare form of spinal syphilis, occurring several years after primary infection.

Pathology. Mild endoarteritis of vessel of spinal cord causing degeneration of lateral column.

Diagnostic Procedures. *Blood and spinal fluid.* Serology to demonstrate syphilitic infections. Differentiate from other numerous causes of spastic paraplegia.

Therapy. Intense antisyphilitic therapy.

Prognosis. Poor; the form does not respond well to treatment.

BIBLIOGRAPHY. Erb, WH: Ueber syphilitische Spinalparalyse. Neurol Centralbl Leipz 11:161–168, 1892
Adams RD, Victor M: Principles of Neurology, 3rd ed, pp 534–535. New York, McGraw-Hill, 1985

ERB-DUCHENNE

Synonyms. Brachial plexus paralysis. Duchenne-Erb; Erb's I; upper brachial plexus paralysis.

Symptoms and Signs. Arm and forearm adducted and internally rotated and forearm extended and pronated. Flaccid paralysis and wasting of arm and shoulder muscles. No sensation loss, or loss of sensation in a small area on the lower border of deltoid.

Etiology. Lesion occurs during birth when traction of the head or arm is applied, or in twisting arm or shoulder down and backward; or vascular, infective, neoplastic lesion involving the fifth and sixth cervical roots with resulting paralysis of the shoulder and arm muscles.

Therapy. Immobilization of arm to relieve the brachial plexus.

Prognosis. Fair to good in neonatal paralysis; poor in other conditions.

BIBLIOGRAPHY. Duchenne GB: De L'eléctrisation localisée et de son application á la pathologie et á la therapeutique. Paris, Baillière, 1855
Erb W: Ueber eine eigenthümliche Localisation von Lähmungen im Plexus branchialis. Verh Naturh Med 2:130–137, 1874
Adams RD, Victor M: Principles of Neurology, 3rd ed, p 955. New York, McGraw-Hill, 1985

ERB-GOLDFLAM

Synonyms. Erb's II; Hoppe-Goldflam; myasthenia gravis.

Symptoms. Occur at any age; more frequent between 20 and 40 years; females more frequently affected earlier than males. Excessive fatigability of the musculature, resulting in extreme weakness after use; rapid recovery with rest. Especially in early stages, patient is normal after night rest; symptoms appear and increase as the day goes on. Muscles innervated by cranial nerves earlier and more severely involved. At onset, transient diplopia, progressive difficulty in chewing and talking, dyspnea, nasal regurgitation.

Signs. Expressionless face; ptosis of upper eyelids; sagging of jaw; manifestation changing during the day, becoming more severe with progression of disease. Reflexes decrease and return to normal after muscle groups rested.

Etiology. Unknown; acetylcholine mechanism of muscle contraction altered. Autoimmune disorder related somehow to thymus and lymphathic system. Possible autosomal recessive inheritance.

Pathology. No specific alteration in muscle. Presence of lymphorrhages (accumulation of perimysial lymphocytes). Thymus hyperplastic; thymoma occasionally present.

Diagnostic Procedures. *X-ray of chest.* May show thymoma. *Electromyography. Neostigmine test. Edrophonium test. Tubocurarine test. Immunofluorescent technique.* For antiskeletal muscle globulins.

Therapy. Neostigmine bromide. Edrophonium (Tensilon); pyridostigmine (Mestinon); ambenonium (Mytelase); ephedrine. Respiratory assistance (when needed). Thymectomy (remission 17%; marked improvement 29%). The latter procedure gives best results in young women with disease of short duration. X-ray therapy of thymus (3000 r). Corticosteroids; adrenocorticotropic hormone (ACTH); immunosuppressive agents; plasmapheresis.

Prognosis. Usually progressive; spontaneous remission possible; remission occasionally during pregnancy. Sudden death (myocardial involvement) or death from exhaustion, malnutrition, respiratory insufficiency, and complications.

BIBLIOGRAPHY. Willis T: Anima brutorum, pp 404–406. Oxford Theatro Sheldoniano, Oxford, 1672
Erb W: Zur Casuistick der bulbären Lähmungen. Arch Psychiatr Nervenkr 9:325–350, 1879
Goldflam S: Ueber einen scheinbar heilbaren bulbärparalytischen Symptomcomplex mit Betheiligung der Extremitäten. Dsch Z Nerven 4:312–352, 1893
Behan PO, Shakir RA, Simpson JA, et al: Plasma-exchange combined with immunosuppressive therapy in myasthenia gravis. Lancet 2:438–440, 1979
Grob O (ed): Myasthenia gravis: Pathophysiology and management. An NY Acad Sci 377, 1981
Allen N, Kissel P, Pietrasink D et al: Myasthenia gravis in monozygotic twins. Clinical follow-up nine years after thymectomy. Arch Neurol 41:994–996, 1984

ERB'S III

Synonyms. Juvenile muscular dystrophy; superior limb-girdle dystrophy; scapulohumeral muscular dystrophy; scapulohumeral dystrophy. Muscular dystrophy I; pelvofemoral muscular dystrophy, see Leyden-Moebius.

Symptoms. Both sexes equally affected; onset at any age from first to sixth decade, but usually between 20 and 30 years of age. Proximal muscle of arms first involved (Erb type) or more rarely of lumbosacral region (Leyden-Moebius type). Successive involvement of lumbosacral in the first type and of scapulohumeral in the second one, usually occurring within 20 years of the onset. Symptoms: see Duchenne's muscular dystrophy (pseudohypertrophy only in few cases) and Landouzy-Déjerine. Involvement of facial muscle as a late event differentiates it from Landouzy-Déjerine (see).

Etiology. Unknown; more than one genetic trait may be involved. Family with autosomal recessive type well demonstrated. Under this and the other various eponyms have been described many conditions all resulting in similar clustering of symptoms (syndrome).

Pathology. Muscle fiber degeneration. Fibrosis notable feature. Less fat than in Duchenne's type.

Diagnostic Procedures. *Serum enzymes.* Aldolase, creatine phosphokinase, serum glutamic-oxaloacetic transaminase (SGOT), variable elevation, higher value at early stage, normal or slight elevation later. *Electroencephalography.* Seldom abnormal.

Therapy. Exercise, bracing, surgery.

Prognosis. Contracture develops rapidly only after patient becomes immobilized. Very slow progression. Life span shortened.

BIBLIOGRAPHY. Erb WH: Ueber die "juvenil Form" der progressiven Muskelatrophie ihre Beziehungen zur sogneannten Pseudohypertrophie der Muskeln. Isch Arch Klin Med 34:467–519, 1884
Zundel WS, Tyler FH: The muscular dystrophies. New Engl J Med 273:537–542; 596–601, 1965
Adams RD, Denny-Brown D, Pearson CM: Disease of the Muscle, 3rd ed, p 265. New York, Harper & Row, 1976
Yates JRW, Emery AEH: A population study of adult onset limb-girdle muscular dystrophy. J Med Genet 22:250–257, 1985

ERDHEIM'S I

Synonyms. Aorta idiopathic necrosis; Erdheim's cystic necrosis of aorta. Gsell-Erdheim.

Symptoms and Signs. Frequently asymptomatic; or dramatic sequence of aortic rupture. In many cases, associated with various manifestations of Marfan's syndrome.

Etiology. Developmental factor or associated with Marfan's syndrome (genetic factor); metabolic and toxic factors also considered. Familial occurrence reported (autosomal dominant trait).

Pathology. Wall of aorta separates easily into two layers. Mucoid medial degeneration: loss of muscle and elastic fibers; diffuse ground substance among residual fibers positive for mucopolysaccharide stain.

Therapy. None. *Cardiosurgery.* Problems related to inconsistency and difficult healing of scar.

Prognosis. Variable.

BIBLIOGRAPHY. Gsell O: Wandnekrosen der Aorta als selbstaendige Erkrankung und ihre Beziehung zur Spontanruptur. Virchows Arch [Pathol] 270:1–36, 1928
Erdheim J: Medionecrosis aortae idiopathica. Virchows Arch [Pathol] 273:454–479, 1929

Anderson WA, Kissane JM: Pathology. St Louis, CV Mosby, 1977

ERDHEIM'S II

Synonyms. Acromegalic macrospondylitis; Scaglietti-Dagnini. Eponyms used to indicate a particular form of acromegaly, where the bone hypertrophy primarily affects the clavicles, vertebrae, and intervertebral disks causing kyphosis, movement impairment, and pain.

BIBLIOGRAPHY. Erdheim J: Ueber Wirbersaeulenveraen—derungen bei Akromegalie. Virchows Arch [Pathol Anat] 281:197–296, 1931
Scaglietti O, Dagnini G: Sul quadro radiografico delle alterazioni acromegaliche dei corpi vertebrali secondo Erdheim. Radiol Fis Med (Bologna) 2:251–264, 1939

ERNSTER-LUFT

Synonyms. Hypermetabolic mitochondrial; Luft's.

Symptoms and Signs. Onset in childhood. Profuse perspiration; polydipsia without polyuria; slenderness despite polyphagia; progressive weakness and hypotonia; tachycardia; elevation of body temperature up to 38.4°C. Tendon reflexes absent.

Etiology. Unknown; hypermetabolism caused by abnormal quantity and type of mitochondria.

Pathology. Increased number of mitochondria in subsarcolemmic areas with or without inclusions. Thyroid normal.

Diagnostic Procedures. *Basal metabolic rate.* Highly increased (+140 to +210); not changed by antithyroid treatment and by thyroidectomy. *Thyroid function study.* Normal. *Urine.* Creatinuria. *Electromyography.* Myopathic pattern.

Therapy. None.

Prognosis. Progressive weakness.

BIBLIOGRAPHY. Ernster L, Ikkos D, Luft R: Enzymic activities of human skeletal muscle mitochondria: A tool in clinical metabolic research. Nature 184:1851–1854, 1959
Luft R, Ikkos D, Palmieri G, et al: A case of severe hypermetabolism of nonthyroid origin with a defect in the maintenance of mitochondrial respiratory control. J Clin Invest 41:1776–1804, 1962

Shy GM, Gonatas NK, Perez MC: Two childhood myopathies with abnormal mitochondria. Brain 89:133–
158, 1966

Morgan-Hughes JA, Darveniza P, Kahn SN, et al: A
mitochondrial myopathy characterized by a deficiency
in reducible cytochrome B. Brain 100:617–640, 1977

ERYSIPELOID

Synonyms. Klauder's (diffuse septicemic variety); Rosenbach's (mild form); seal fingers; Baker-Rosenbach.

Symptoms. Appear in workers in contact with live infected animals or animal carcasses. High incidence in
summer and fall. Three days after inoculation a local
dusky erythema develops on upper extremities and extends centrifugally for about 10 cm. Fever (10%). Seldom, severe systemic involvement (form of Klauder) with
numerous bullae and plaques; weight loss; arthralgias.

Etiology. Acute (seldom chronic) infection with *Erysip-
elothrix rhusiopathiae;* gram-positive bacillus causative
agents of animal (swine) erysipelas and present also in the
skin of birds, fish.

Diagnostic Procedures. *Culture (in vitro) of biopsy material.*

Therapy. Penicillin; tetracyclines; erythromycin.

Prognosis. Resolution in 3 to 4 days with treatment; in
2 weeks spontaneously; occasionally, protracted with remission and relapses of systemic manifestations.

BIBLIOGRAPHY. Klauder JV: Erysipeloid and swine erysip-
elas in man. A clinical and bacteriological review:
Swine erysipelas in the United States. JAMA 86:536–
541, 1926
Rook A, Wilkinson DS, Ebling FJG, et al: Textbook of
Dermatology, 4th ed, p 763–764. Oxford, Blackwell
Scientific Publications, 1986

ERYTHEMA ELEVATUM DIUTINUM

Synonyms. Bury's, Crocker-Williams; erythema multiforme variant; cutaneous vasculitis.

Symptoms and Signs. Prevalent in males; onset in middle age. Slow, usually symmetric eruption of papulae or
nodules on back of hands aggravated by cold. Occasionally, extensor area of kness, elbows, wrists, ankles, or
buttocks may be involved. Plaques of irregular shape initially soft, then harden. Polyarthritis may be associated.

Etiology. Unknown; belongs to the group of cutaneous
vasculitis.

Pathology. Pericapillary hyaline degeneration; endothelial swelling; inflammatory infiltrate with leukocytoclasis;
lymphocytes; histiocytes; few eosinophils; and plasma
cells. Fibrosis supervenes at later stage.

Diagnostic Procedures. *Biopsy.*

Therapy. Nonspecific; moderate reduction of lesion by
topical injection with steroids. Dapsone may produce
very good remission.

Prognosis. After years, lesions may clear spontaneously.

BIBLIOGRAPHY. Bury SJ: A case of erythema with remark-
able nodular thickening and induration of the skin as-
sociated with intermittent albuminuria. Illus Med
Neur (London) 2:145–148, 1889
Crocker HR, William C: Erythema elevatum diutinum
Br J Dermatol 6:33, 1894
Rook A, Wilkinson DS, Ebling FJG, et al: Textbook of
Dermatology, 4th ed, pp 1151–1154. Oxford, Black-
well Scientific Publications, 1986

ERYTHEMA GYRATUM REPENS

See Paraneoplastic syndromes.

Signs. Erythematous lesions spread over the body resembling grain of wood (cypress burl).

Etiology. Associated with visceral malignant tumor.

Diagnostic Procedures. Search for malignancy.

Therapy. That of malignancy.

Prognosis. Poor; skin lesions disappear if tumor cured.

BIBLIOGRAPHY. Rothman S: Ueber Hauterscheinungen
bei bosartigen Geschwulsten innerer Organe. Arch
Dermatol U. Syph. 149:99–123, 1925
Curth HO: How and why the skin reacts. Ann NY Acad
Sci 230:435–442, 1974
Rook A, Wilkinson DS, Ebling FJG, et al: Textbook of
Dermatology, 4th ed, p 1091. Oxford, Blackwell Scien-
tific Publications, 1986

ERYTHEMA MULTIFORME

Synonyms. Dermatostomatitis; ectodermosis erosiva
pluriorificialis; erythema papulosum rheumaticum; ery-
théme polymorphe; herpes iris. See also Stevens-Johnson.
At least three major clinical patterns can be recognized:
(1) papular or simplex; (2) vesiculobullous; (3) Stevens-
Johnson. Atypical cases have also been reported.

PAPULAR OR SIMPLEX

Symptoms. All ages, both sexes affected; male-to-female ratio 3 : 1. Moderate malaise; discomfort; myalgia; pruritus; occasionally, mucosal erosions.

Signs. Maculopapules flat, red, increasing in 48 hours to 1 to 2 cm, assuming (because of change in color in the center) a target pattern. Successive formation at various intervals of crops of new lesions. Limbs generally affected.

VESICULOBULLOUS

Symptoms. More common in children and young adults. Same as above, but of greater intensity and with constant mucosal involvement.

Signs. Erythematous plaque with central bulla and ring of vesicles. Vesicles less abundant than in the papular form.

STEVENS-JOHNSON (SEE)

Etiology. Unknown. Attacks usually precipitated by a pathologic agent: viral, bacterial, or mycotic infections; neoplasia; collagen diseases; pregnancy; drugs or x-ray exposure. In many cases, however, no correlated condition could be found.

Pathology. *Upper dermis.* Edema; vasodilatation; polymorphs and then lymphohistiocyte infiltration, degenerative changes of small blood vessels and collagen. Absence of acantholysis.

Diagnostic Procedures. Identification of preceding or concomitant pathologic event.

Therapy. *Papular.* Symptomatic. *Vesiculobullous.* Corticosteroids for symptomatic relief, plus systemic antibiotics to prevent secondary infections.

Prognosis. Attacks usually of self-limited duration (1–4 wk). Tendency to recur.

BIBLIOGRAPHY. Ashby DW, Lazar T: Erythema multiforme exudativum major (Stevens-Johnson syndrome). Lancet 1:1091–1095, 1951
Rook A, Wilkinson DS, Ebling FJG, et al: Textbook of Dermatology, 4th ed, pp 1085–1086. Oxford, Blackwell Scientific Publications, 1986

ERYTHEMA NODOSUM

Synonym. Dermatitis contusiformis. See Loefgren's.

Symptoms. Occur at any age (max frequency from 20–30 yr) (rare in children and old people); most common in females (6.7 : 1). Majority of cases observed from January to June. Painful nodules on pretibial surface, anterior thigh, extensor side of forearms, back of arm, and face. Occasionally, feverishness, malaise, and arthralgia.

Signs. Crops of few or several lesions (2–5 cm in diameter) red, hot; as they involute, changes in color—darker red, greenish, yellow (bruiselike)—disappearing in a few days to 3 weeks. Cervical lymphadenopathy frequently associated.

Etiology. Unknown; hypersensitivity reaction. Secondary to numerous viral, bacterial, fungal infections, and drugs. Streptococcal infections and sarcoidosis most important in the United States.

Pathology. Perivascular polymorphonuclear infiltration of nodules; dilatation of blood vessel; edema.

Diagnostic Procedures. Search for primary disease. *Blood culture. Skin sensitivity tests. Blood.* Mild anemia, albuminuria; increased sedimentation rate may be present. *X-ray.* Association with hilar lymphadenopathy frequent.

Therapy. That of primary condition. Symptomatic (rest; analgesics). Corticosteroid with caution only when symptoms are severe and when underlying disease does not contraindicate.

Prognosis. Self-resolving in 3 to 6 weeks. Recurrences possible.

BIBLIOGRAPHY. Willan R: On cutaneous diseases. London, Johnson, 1798
Wilson E: A practical and theoretical treatise on the diagnosis, pathology and treatment of diseases of the skin. London, Churchill, 1842
Rook A, Wilkinson DS, Ebling FJG, et al: Textbook of Dermatology, 4th ed, pp 1156–1164. Oxford, Blackwell Scientific Publications, 1986

ERYTHROCYTOSIS, BENIGN FAMILIAL

Synonyms. Benign familial erythrocythemic; familial erythrocytosis; polycythemia, benign familial.

Symptoms. No sex predominance; usually discovered in childhood. Asymptomatic or paucisymptomatic. No thrombotic or hemorrhagic manifestations.

Signs. Splenomegaly of moderate degree in 50% of cases. Congenital disorders may be associated.

Etiology. Autosomal dominant inheritance associated with hemoglobinopathy and other varieties of dominant and recessive type. In some cases (recessive type), consequence of erythopoietin or precursor defect of regulation.

Diagnostic Procedures. *Blood.* Variable degree of erythocytosis; higher in recessive form hematocrit (Hmt greater than 0.1) and lower in dominant (Hmt 0.45–0.60). Studies of hemoglobin type, diphosphoglycerate

(DPG) defect. Leukocytes and platelets always within normal limit. Low plasma erythropoietin activity.

Therapy. None.

Prognosis. Good; many years survival without clinical manifestations.

BIBLIOGRAPHY. Bernstein J: Three cases of polycythemia rubra. West London Med J 19:207–208, 1914

Davey MG, Lawrence JR, Lander H, et al: Familial erythrocytosis; A report of two cases and a review. Acta Haematol (Basel) 39:65–74, 1968

Wintrobe MM (ed): Clinical Hematology, 7th ed, p 988. Philadelphia, Lea & Febiger, 1974

Ly B, Meberg A, Kannelonning K, et al: Dominant familial erythrocytosis with low plasma erythropoietin activity: Studies of four cases. Scand J Haemat 30 (Suppl) 39:11–17, 1983

ERYTHROCYTOSIS, SPORADIC

Synonym. Primary erythrocytosis. See Erythocytosis, benign familial. Two subgroups are recognized in this condition, which is characterized by an isolated increase of red cell mass, without any abnormality, known to cause secondary erythrocytosis and lack of familial type of transmission; although possible traits cannot always be excluded.
1. Cases with pure erythrocytosis without associated abnormalities of growth. Normal leukocytes and platelets; occasionally, slight splenomegaly.
2. Cases with pure erythrocytosis and complex abnormalities of growth and endocrine development. This group may be identical with the cases with diencephalic lesion and erythrocytosis.

BIBLIOGRAPHY. Hottinger A: Beitrage zur Kenntnis der Kindlichen Polycythämie. Klin. Unytersuchungen und hämatolg Studien. Z Kinderheilk 44:61–86, 1927

Nathan M: Erythrémies protopathiques et diencéphale. Presse Med 39:403–404, 1931

Davey MG, Lawrence JR, Langer H, et al: Familial erythrocytosis; A report of two cases and a review. Acta Haematol (Basel) 39:65–74, 1968

Distelhorst CW, Wagner DS, Goldwesser E, et al: Autosomal dominant familial erythrocytosis due to autonomous erythropoietin production. Blood 58:1155–1158, 1981

ESCAMILLA-LISSER

Synonym. Internal myxedema.
This case was reported to draw the attention to viceral manifestations in hypothyroidism with minor external classical manifestations. The so-called internal myxedema, according to these authors, presents ascites, atony of bladder, cardiac atony, intestinal atony, anemia, menorrhagia. All those manifestations respond to specific treatment. Evans first reported the occurrence of ascites and visceral atony in hypothyroidism.

BIBLIOGRAPHY. Evans W: Case of myxedema with ascites and atony of bladder. Endocrinology 26:409–416, 1932

Escamilla RF, Lisser H, Shepardson HC: Interna myxedema: Report of a case showing ascites, cardiac, intestinal and bladder atony, menorrhagia secondary anemia and associated carotinemia. Ann Intern Med 9:297–316, 1935

ESCHELER'S

Symptoms and Signs. Lateral deviation of moderate amplitude of movements. Difference in muscle tone and bone asymmetry.

Etiology. Congenital asymmetry of tonus and function of propulsive muscles.

BIBLIOGRAPHY. Moortgat P: Syndromes a noms propres. Paris, Prelat, 1966

ESOPHAGUS, ACHALASIA

Synonyms. Achalasia; cardiospasm; esophageal dystonia; esophageal dyssynergia; functional hiatal stenosis; megaesophagus.

Symptoms. Onset at any age; maximal incidence between fourth and sixth decades; equal incidence in both sexes. Onset of acute symptomatology usually abrupt, preceded however by minor swallowing abnormalities for years. Feeling of obstruction at the level of xiphoid cartilage. Pain or distress when ingesting food. Intermittent episodes at the beginning; controllable by eating slowly or drinking frequently during meal. Later, symptomatology at any meal plus, occasionally, sensation of fullness behind the sternum. Severe pain substernal may be observed after meal (in Pathology, see type 2). Regurgitation brings relief of symptoms. Regurgitation without nausea of sour or fetid odor, rich in mucous (advanced condition). Weight loss.

Signs. Scanty; determination of swallowing time with stethoscope applied to the xiphoid. In some cases, dilation of veins of neck and face, and cyanosis after meal (relieved by regurgitation); pallor.

Etiology. Unknown; neuromuscular dysfunction of entire esophagus; particularly defect of cholinergic innervation; psychogenic component.

Pathology. Dilatation of esophagus; esophagitis. *Type 1.* Enormous dilatation and thin-walled atrophic vestibule. *Type 2.* Moderate dilatation; hypertrophic wall vestibule, marked muscular hypertrophy.

Diagnostic Procedures. *X-ray of esophagus. Esophagoscopy.* Hypersensitive response to methacholine during fluoroscopy and pressure measurements of esophageal motility.

Therapy. Dilatation of vestibule. Surgery indicated in about 20% of patients. Correction of malnutrition before surgery. Nifedipine, isosorbide dinitrate (modest results).

Prognosis. Good response to treatment. Dilation may be repeated several times with good results.

BIBLIOGRAPHY. Hurst AF: Some disorders of the esophagus. JAMA 102:582–586, 1943
Van Trappen G, Janssens J: To dilate or to operate? That is the question. Gut 24:1013–1027, 1983
Traube M, Hongo M, Magyar L, McCallum RW et al: Effects of nifedipine in achalasia and in patients with high amplitude peristaltic esophageal contractions. JAMA 252:1733–1736, 1984

ESOPHAGUS, APOPLEXY

See also Boerhaave's and Mallory-Weiss.

Symptoms. Prevalent in later life in females. Severe retrosternal pain that spreads to the lower chest posteriorly.

Signs. Pallor; general distress; shock.

Etiology. Mucosal tear of the lower esophagus; modest blood loss into the lumen. Dissection by blood in the plane of submucosa of the lower esophagus, while the surrounding muscle remains intact. The disorder is often associated with dysfunction of the cardias.

Pathology. See Etiology.

Diagnostic Procedures. *Blood.* Anemia; white blood cells increased. *X-ray of chest with gastrography* shows filling defect of the esophagus with the appearance of intramural lesion. *Esophagoscopy.*

Therapy. Nasogastric aspiration; parenteral nutrition; conservative treatment.

Prognosis. Guarded.

BIBLIOGRAPHY. Clark DH, Tankel HT: Pressure rupture and spontaneous perforation of the esophagus. Gut 5:86–89, 1964
Thompson NW, Ernst CB, Fry WJ: The spectrum of emetogenic injury to the esophagus and stomach. Am J Surg 113:13–26, 1967
Marks IN, Keet AD: Intramural rupture of the oesophagus. Br Med J 3:536–537, 1968

Smith G, Brunnen PL, Gillanders LA et al: Oesophageal apoplexy. Lancet 1:390–392, 1974
Castell DO, Johnson LF: Esophageal function in health and disease. New York, Elsevier, 1980

ESOPHAGUS, CHALASIA

Synonyms. Cardiac sphincter chalasia; cardioesophageal relaxation. Gastroesophageal reflux.

Symptoms and Signs. Both sexes affected; onset usually in infancy; (few days after birth). After abdominal constriction by the holding arm and when child is positioned horizontally; vomiting; excessive regurgitation; failure to thrive; danger of aspiration.

Etiology. Unknown. Transitory motor disorder of esophagus with lack of closure of gastroesophageal junction after passage of food.

Diagnostic Procedures. *Fluoroscopy.* Retrograde filling of esophagus in inspiration and with increase of intraabdominal pressure.

Therapy. Keeping the infant in orthostatic position during and after feeding. For 1 hour in mild form up to 24 hours in severe form. Betanechol and antacids prior to meals and thickened food may improve situation in lack of response after 6 weeks' surgery.

Prognosis. Variable according to severity of form.

BIBLIOGRAPHY. Behrman RE, Vaughan VC. Nelson Textbook of Pediatrics, p 896. Philadelphia, WB Saunders, 1983

ESOPHAGUS SPASM, DIFFUSE

Differential diagnosis with esophagus achalasia and esophagus, vigorous achalasia (see). See Intestinal idiopathic pseudoobstruction.

Symptoms and Signs	Achalasia	Diffuse Spasm	Vigorous Achalasia
Pain	±	+++	++
Obstruction	+++	±	+++
Regurgitation	++	±	+++
Retention	+++	−	+++
Nervousness	±	+++	+
X-ray findings			
Diffuse dilatation	++	−	±
Segmental spasms	±	+++	++

Therapy. Nifedipine, isosorbide dinitrate (modest results).

BIBLIOGRAPHY. Sanderson DR, Ellis FH, Schlager JF, et al: Syndrome of vigorous achalasia: Clinical and physiological observations. Dis Chest 52:508–517, 1967
Richter JE, Castell DO: Diffuse esophageal spasm: A reappraisal. Ann Intern Med 100:242–245, 1984

ESOPHAGUS, VIGOROUS ACHALASIA

Synonyms. Esophageal dyschalasia.

Symptoms. No sex dominance; mean age of onset 51 years (range from 12 to 79 years). Marked or moderate obstruction to swallowing; dysphagia; regurgitation, especially in recumbent position. Pain (very distressing) in anterior part of chest or back, associated with meals and swallowing, or independent; lasting a few minutes to hours, passing spontaneously. Loss of weight; nervousness and psychiatric disorders in some cases.

Signs. See Diagnostic procedures.

Etiology. Unknown; represents or is a combination of esophagus, achalasia (see) and esophagus spasm, diffuse (see).

Pathology. Esophageal dilatation close to the stomach. Absence of ganglion cell from Aeurerbach's plexus (not constant).

Diagnostic Procedures. *X-ray of esophagus.* Cardiospasm; usually marked or moderate dilatation; diffuse spasm; occasionally, diaphragmatic hernia; strictures; abnormal motor pattern. *Esophageal motility studies.* Poor or absent relaxation after swallowing; premature contraction of the sphincter; amplitude of contractions greater than 50 cm of water pressure; methacholine test usually positive. *Endoscopy.* Achalasia with dilatation (30%); hiatal hernia (15%); esophagitis (12%); spasm of distal esophagus (10%); normal (24%).

Therapy. Simple dilatation; hydrostatic dilatation. Surgery (modified Heller myotomy) offers better results. Nifedipine, isosorbide dinitrate (modest results).

Prognosis. Marked improvement (in 95% of cases) with treatment (especially Heller myotomy offers better results).

BIBLIOGRAPHY. Moersch HJ, Code CF, Olsen AM: Dyschalasia of the esophagus. Coll Papers Mayo Clin 49:19, 1957
Sanderson DR, Ellis FH Jr, Schlegel JF, et al: Syndrome of vigorous achalasia: Clinical and physiologic observations. Dis Chest 52:508–517, 1967
Castell DO, Johnson LF: Esophageal Function in Health and Disease, New York, Elsevier, 1982

Traube M, Hongo M, Magyar L, McCallum RW: Effects of nifedipine in achalasia and in patients with high amplitude peristaltic esophageal contractions. JAMA 252:1733–1736, 1984
Skinner DB, Myotomy and achalasia. Ann Thorac Surg 37:183–197, 1984

ESPILDORA-LUQUE

Synonyms. Amaurosis-hemiplegia; ophthalmic sylvian.

Symptoms and Signs. Unilateral blindness; temporary contralateral hemiplegia.

Etiology. Embolus in ophthalmic artery and reflex spasm of middle cerebral artery.

Pathology. See Etiology.

Therapy. None.

Prognosis. Hemiparesis is temporary.

BIBLIOGRAPHY. Espildora-Luque C: Sindrome oftálmico-silviano. Arch Ophthal Hispano-Am 34:616–621, 1934
Geeraets WS: Ocular Syndromes, 3rd ed. Philadelphia, Lea & Febiger, 1976

ESTREN-DAMESHEK

Synonym. Fanconi I without congenital defect.

Symptoms. Early childhood appearance; weakness; epistaxis; easy bruising; poor development.

Signs. Pallor; ecchymosis; petechiae. Liver, spleen, and lymph node not palpable.

Etiology. Autosomal recessive inheritance. Familial bone marrow hypoplasia without other congenital defects. See Fanconi's I.

Pathology. In bone marrow, quantitative hypoplasia with normal qualitative development of cells. A certain degree of functional hypersplenism postulated.

Diagnostic Procedures. *Blood.* Anemia; leukopenia; thrombocytopenia; high reticulocyte count.

Therapy. Periodic blood transfusions. Testosterone; corticoids. Some cases benefit symptomatically from splenectomy. Bone marrow transplantation attempted with partial results.

Prognosis. Discontinuation of blood transfusions results in death. Conversion into leukemia.

BIBLIOGRAPHY. Estren S, Dameshek W: Familial hypoplastic anemia of childhood. Am J Dis Child 73:671–687, 1947

Nowell P, Bergman G, Besa E, et al: Progressive pre-leukemia with chromosomally abnormal clone in a kindred with Estren-Dameshek variant of Fanconi's anemia. Blood 64:1135–1138, 1984

ETHANOLAMINOSIS

Symptoms and Signs. From birth. Cardiomegaly, generalized muscular hypotonia, cerebral dysfunction, failure to thrive, early death.

Etiology. Deficiency of ethanolaminokinase.

Pathology. Deposition of ethanolamine (PAS +) in all tissues.

BIBLIOGRAPHY. Victor KW, Harsteien B, Harms D, Busse H, et al: Ethanolaminosis: A newly recognized, generalized storage disease with cardiomegaly, cerebral dysfunction and early death. Eur J Pediatr 126:61–75, 1977

ETHMOCEPHALUS

See Arhinencephalia.

Symptoms and Signs. Extreme hypotelorism; absent nose with proboscis; no palate or cleft lips.

Etiology. See Arhinencephalia.

BIBLIOGRAPHY. Aita JA: Congenital Facial Anomalies with Neurologic Defects. Springfield, CC Thomas, 1969

ETIOCHOLANOLONE FEVER

Symptoms and Signs. Attacks of periodic fever. This syndrome can be subdivided into three groups: (1) group with adrenogenital syndrome; (2) group with familial Mediterranean fever syndrome (see); (3) miscellaneous group with hypothalamic damage, impaired liver function (Hodgkin's granulomas; cirrhosis).

Etiology. Tendency to produce excessive etiocholanolone and retarded plasma clearance of unconjugated etiocholanolone. Reported families with lifelong persistent fever (102°F) (autosomal recessive inheritance). Alteration of β-glucuronidase metabolism suggested as responsible.

Pathology. See Symptoms and signs.

Diagnostic Procedures. *Blood.* Determination of plasma etiocholanolone. *Liver function tests. Studies for adrenogenital syndromes, granulomas.*

Therapy. Cortisol. Dexamethasone and uronic acids.

Prognosis. Attacks of fever aborted by administration of adrenal corticoids. Recurrences in milder form. Etiocholanolone fever associated with adrenocortical syndrome and Mediterranean fever type have benign prognosis and no complications. In miscellaneous group, prognosis determined by underlying cause.

BIBLIOGRAPHY. Bondy PK, Chon GL, Castiglione C: Etiocholanolone fever: A clinical study. Trans Assoc Am Physicians 73:186–196, 1960
Herman RH, Overholt EL, Hagler L: Familial life-long persistent fever of unknown origin responding to dexamethasone and uronic acids. Am J Med 46:142–153, 1969
Harrison's Principles of Internal Medicine. 8th ed, p 1124. New York, McGraw-Hill, 1977

EVANS'

The association of idiopathic hemolytic anemia with thrombocytopenia with or without purpuric manifestation, occurring concomitantly or in succession, in absence of any etiologic factors and with demonstrable autoimmune process affecting both red cells and platelets.

BIBLIOGRAPHY. Evans R, Takahashi K, Duane RT et al: Primary thrombocytopenic purpura and acquired hemolytic anemia. Arch Intern Med 87:48–65, 1951
Silverstein MN, Aaro LA, Kempers RD: Evans' syndrome and pregnancy. Am J Med Sci 252:106–111, 1966
Wintrobe MM (ed): Clinical Hematology, 8th ed, p 1181. Philadelphia, Lea & Febiger, 1981
Cartron J, Muller JY: Immunologiè de leucocytes et des plaquettes 13000 M52(4-1986). In Encyclopedie Medico-Chirurgicale Sang, Edit Techniques, Paris

EWING'S

Synonyms. Diffuse bone endothelioma; endothelial myeloma; Ewing's sarcoma.

Symptoms. Onset before 30 years of age (80%); prevalent in males. Intermittent pain in any bone, most frequently shafts of long bone and pelvis, increasing with progress of disease. Slight fever.

Signs. Palpation may reveal swelling and increased temperature of overlying skin. Marked pain on pressure.

Etiology. Unknown. Neoplastic proliferation of endothelial cells probably derived by reticular cells of bone marrow.

Pathology. Bone porous, with localized reabsorptions. Tumor found under displaced periostium and within the bone, soft and friable; gray white areas of necrosis and hemorrhage. New bone formation as a reaction (not by the tumor). Microscopically; small round cells in sheets growing between compartment of well-vascularized connective tissue. Nuclei prominent; little cytoplasm. Mitotic figures.

Diagnostic Procedures. *X-ray.* Periosteal irregularity; areas of different densities of bone marrow; tumor extension parallel to long axis of bone. *Isotope bone scan. Biopsy of bone marrow. Blood.* Leukocytosis; high sedimentation rate. *Electron microscopy.* Helpful in differential diagnosis.

Therapy. X-ray, supervoltage radiation; chemotherapy (cyclophosphamide; methotrexate). Avoid useless surgery.

Prognosis. Five-year survival (10–24%).

BIBLIOGRAPHY. Ewing J: Review and classification of bone sarcomas. Arch Surg 4:485–533, 1922
Carnesale PG: Malignant tumor of bone. In Crenshaw AH (ed): Campbell's Operative Orthopedics, 7th ed, p 797. St. Louis, CV Mosby, 1987

F

FABER'S

Synonyms. Achylic chloroanemia; hypochromic chronic anemia; Hayem-Faber; idiopathic hypochromic anemia; Kaznelson's II; Knud Faber's; Witt's.

Symptoms. Occur in women between 30 and 60 years of age; seldom (4%) in men; frequently in low-income class. In convalescence after pregnancy. Menstrual disorders; tiredness; weakness; exertional dyspnea.

Signs. Pallor. In some patients, same constitutional features of pernicious anemia. Light colored eyes; moderate hypertelorism; premature gray hair; nail brittleness.

Etiology. Menstrual disorders; uterine fibroids; hemorrhoids; peptic ulcer; hernia at esophageal hiatus; recurrent epistaxes; hereditary telangiectasia; other causes of chronic blood loss. With present knowledge this syndrome has become obsolete except as a term for the association of hypochromic anemia and achlorhydria and not as a separate entity.

Pathology. According to etiology. In chronic form of anemia, fatty degeneration of myocardium ("tigroid pattern"), cardiac hypertrophy and dilatation.

Diagnostic Procedures. *Blood.* Hemoglobin determination; red cell indices; serum iron low; iron binding capacity high. *Gastric secretion analysis.* Stool. Occult blood.

Therapy. Iron administration orally, intramuscularly, or intravenously.

Prognosis. Good with treatment and according to etiology.

BIBLIOGRAPHY. Faber K: Achylia gastrica mit Anaemie. Med Klin 5:1310–1312, 1909
Faber K: Om anaemiske Tilstande ved Achylia gastrica. Berl Klin 50:958–962, 1913
Wintrobe MM (ed): Clinical Hematology, 8th ed. Philadelphia, Lea & Febiger, 1981

FABRY'S

Synonyms. Alpha galactosidase A deficiency; GLA; ceramide trihexosidase deficiency; ACD; Anderson-Fabry; angiokeratoma corporis diffusum; glycolipid lipidosis; hemorrhagic-nodular; hemorrhagic nodular-glycolipid lipidosis; hereditary dystopic lipidosis; Ruiter-Pompen; Sweeley-Klionsky.

Symptoms. Prevalent in males, who present full-blown syndrome; females may present a partial form. Symptoms start in childhood or at puberty. Family history. Paresthesia of distal part of extremities with burning pain. Fever precipitated occasionally by variation in temperature or exertion. Frequently, concomitant with the attacks are nausea, vomiting, abdominal pain, dizziness, headache, and generalized weakness.

Signs. Increasing with progression of the disease. Typical cutaneous lesions: telangiectasis of various sizes clustering in areas such as periumbilical, genitals, buttocks, and thighs; bright red or bluish, nonpulsating, partially bleached by pressure. Lack of development of beard and body hair. Edema. Eyes show dilated venules in conjunctiva and retina. Frequent corneal and lens opacity. Later, hypertension and signs of cardiovascular disease; renal failure.

Etiology. Unknown; sex-linked, incompletely recessive inheritance. Female carrier asymptomatic. Derangement of glycolipid metabolism caused by alpha galactosidase A deficiency. Accumulation of globotrialosylceramide and galabiosylceramide in all tissues.

Pathology. Skin shows telangiectasis or dilated intraepidermal spaces filled with blood; vessel wall in nontelangiectatic zones shows infiltration with glycolipids (ceramide trihexoside) deposited in the endothelial cells and smooth muscles. Identical deposits are observed in the heart, muscles, renal tubules and glomeruli, central nervous system, spleen, liver, bone marrow, lymph nodes, cornea.

Diagnostic Procedures. *Urine.* Albuminuria (early finding); vacuolated cells containing glycolipids. Later, casts, hematuria, isosthenuria. *Blood.* Later, anemia; hyperazotemia. *Bone marrow.* Typical cells. *Ophthalmologic examination.* Slit-lamp shows characteristic findings.

Therapy. Symptomatic; dexamethazone may help relieve acute symptoms. Low doses of diphenylhydantoin or carbamazepin to relieve discomfort. Plasma exchange. Kidney transplantation.

Prognosis. Recurrent progressive attacks, eventually leading to renal failure and hypertension and cardiovascular disease. Death between 40 and 50 years of age. Females with milder form do not show decreased survival time.

BIBLIOGRAPHY. Fabry J: Ein Beitrag zur Kenntniss der Purpura haemorrhagica nodularis (purpura papulosa haemorrhagica Hebrae). Arch Dermatol Syph 43:187–200, 1898

Anderson W: A case of angiokeratoma. Br J Dermatol 10:113–117, 1898

Desnick RJ, Sweeley CC: Fabry disease: α-galactosidase A deficiency. In Stanbury JB, Wyngaarden JB, Fredrickson DS, et al: The Metabolic Basis of Inherited Disease, 5th ed, p. 906. New York, McGraw-Hill, 1983

FACETS

Synonyms. Articular facets; vertebrae; osteoarthritis; spinal osteophytosis.

Symptoms. Vertebral column or radiated pains, usually sciatic; static in type (relieved by certain postures and aggravated by other postures).

Signs. Sciatic scoliosis, homolateral, contralateral, or alternating; muscle spasm.

Etiology. Unknown.

Pathology. Osteoarthritic process with main involvement of vertebral articular facets. Cartilage degeneration, and subluxation of one or both articular processes; muscle spasm; nerve root compression.

Diagnostic Procedures. *X-ray of spine* in different projections. Local injection of the joint as a diagnostic as well as therapeutic procedure.

Therapy. Conservative measures; physical therapy or in rare cases surgical treatment. Lumbosacral ankylosis by bone graft or fusion or removal of the facets.

Prognosis. Recurrent progressive symptomatology responds fairly well to medical treatment or surgical intervention.

BIBLIOGRAPHY. Gormley RK: Low back pain with special reference to the articular facets with presentation of an operative procedure. Coll Papers Mayo Clinic 25:813–823, 1933

Wood GW: Lower back pain and disorders of intervertebral disc. In Crenshaw AH (ed): Campbell's Operative Orthopedics, 7th ed, pp 3268–3269. St. Louis, CV Mosby, 1987

FACTITIOUS PURPURA

Synonyms. Devil's pinches; simple easy bruising. Purpura psychogenic.

Symptoms and Signs. Recurrent painful bruises.

Etiology. Self-inflicted (consciously or unconsciously) bruises.

Pathology. On biopsy; hematoma without evidence of vasculitis.

Diagnostic Procedures. Protection of a designated part with plaster cast (bruises do not appear in protected part). For differential diagnosis see purpura of psychogenic origin and autosensitization purpura.

Therapy. Psychotherapy.

Prognosis. Difficult treatment; occasionally, conversion to other hysterical manifestations.

BIBLIOGRAPHY. Davidson E: Factitious purpura presenting as autoerythrocyte sensitization. Br Med J 1:104, 1964

Rook A, Wilkinson DS, Ebling FJG, et al: Textbook of Dermatology, 4th ed, p 2262. Oxford, Blackwell Scientific Publications, 1986

FAHR'S

Synonyms. Cerebral symmetric calcification. Striopalliododentate calcinosis; SPD calcinosis; ferrocalcinosis cerebrovascular.

Symptoms. Asymptomatic in many cases. Extrapyramidal disorder of different degree from simple generalized rigidity, athetosis, dystonia to full Parkinson's. The extrapyramidal disorder may be progressive and reach full expression in middle life, or occasionally is present from infancy accompanied or not accompanied by mental retardation.

Signs. Small and round head. Optic atrophy.

Etiology. Unknown; associated occasionally with hypoparathyroidism or pseudohypoparathyroidism. Possibly due to altered vascular permeability. Familial occurrence reported; autosomal recessive.

Pathology. Deposit of calcific material in basal ganglia. Usually, initial absence or loss of nerve cell fibers and ground substance. "Mulberry bodies" associated with capillary walls. When there is calcification of capillary walls, extensive rarefaction of cerebral tissue occurs.

Diagnostic Procedures. *X-rays of skull.* Demonstration of basal ganglia calcification. *CT brain scan.*

Therapy. None; orthopedic procedures if necessary.

Prognosis. Usually, slowly progressive condition in infantile form; poor for mental retardation and spastic features.

BIBLIOGRAPHY. Virchow R: Kalk-Metastasen. Virchows Arch Pathol Anat 8:103–113, 1855

Fahr T: Idiopathische Verkalkung der Hirngefasse Z Allg Pathol Anat 50:129–133, 1930

Smits MG, Gabreels FJM, Thijssen HOM, et al: Progressive idiopathic striopallidodentate calcinosis (Fahr's disease) with autosomal recessive inheritance: Report of three siblings. Eur Neurol 22:58–64, 1983

FAHR-VOLHARD

Synonyms. Arteriolar hyperplastic nephrosclerosis; malignant nephrosclerosis.

Symptoms. Both sexes affected; onset in males 44 years of age, in females 36 years of age. Abrupt onset of intermittent or constant headache; weight loss; followed by dyspnea; impairment of vision (sometimes preceeding other symptoms); abdominal pain.

Signs. Blood hypertension (diastolic greater than 130 mm Hg); cardiomegaly; edema; occasionally associated, papilledema, retinopathy (cotton wool exudates and hemorrhages), neurologic abnormalities.

Etiology. Unknown. Associated with malignant hypertension following benign nephrosclerosis or other kidney diseases. Considered as pathogenetic mechanisms: immunologic; derangement in renin, angiotensin, and aldosterone production; disseminated intravascular coagulation.

Pathology. Fibrinoid necrosis of kidney arterioles; endothelial proliferation of afferent arterioles and interlobular arteries.

Diagnostic Procedures. *Urine.* Proteinuria; frequently hematuria (25%); presence of red cell casts. *Blood.* Increased red cell sedimentation rate; in second phase, increased blood urea nitrogen BUN and creatinine. *Spinal fluid.* Increased pressure (86%) and protein concentration.

Therapy. Antihypertensive agents; management of renal failure, including dialysis. Kidney transplantation.

Prognosis. Without treatment, death in 15 months. With treatment, mortality at this time reduced to 10 to 20%; life can be prolonged 5 to 7 years.

BIBLIOGRAPHY. Fahr G: Hypertension heart, most common form of so-called chronic myocarditis. JAMA 80:981–984, 1924
Fahr G: Hypertension heart. Am J Med Sci 175:453–472, 1928
Papper S: Clinical Nephrology, 2nd ed, p 310. Boston, Little Brown, 1978
Kuruvila C, Schrier R: Chronic renal failure. Int Anesth Clin 22:101–117, 1984

FAIRBANK'S

Synonyms. Epiphyseal dysplasia mutiplex tarda; MEDT type Ia; megalia ossium cutis; multiple epiphyseal dysplasia (type Ia). See Conradi's and Blount-Barber.

Symptoms. Evident at 5 to 10 years of age. None or pain and difficulty in walking (coxa vara; genu valgum). Patients remain below average height (152 cm). Absence of disability.

Signs. Lesions bilateral and almost symmetric; after puberty some alterations of epiphyseal shape or joint angulation. Hands are typically short and stubby, with narrow, thick nails.

Etiology. Unknown; dominant genetic autosomal inheritance. Rare, autosomal recessive inheritance.

Pathology. Chondrodystrophy affecting only cartilaginous epiphyses. Cartilage hyaline softer, more mucinous than normal. Multiple centers of ossification may develop at different times in same epiphysis.

Diagnostic Procedures. *X-ray of skeleton.* Multiple ossification centers in epiphyses; epiphyseal union delayed. After puberty, epiphyseal changes. Bone of good structure and well ossified. Occasionally, double patella (seen on lateral views).

Therapy. Physical therapy to provide relief and prevent disability. Surgery to correct deformities delayed.

Prognosis. After puberty, no progression. Possibly, residual deformities may be cured by osteotomy. The patient will be short.

BIBLIOGRAPHY. Barrington-Ward LE: Double coxa vara with other deformities occurring in brother and sister. Lancet 1:157–159, 1913
Fairbank T: An Atlas of General Affections of the Skeleton. Baltimore, Williams & Wilkins, 1951
Jackson WPU, Hanelin J, Albright F: Metaphyseal dysplasia, epiphyseal dysplasia, diaphyseal dysplasia, and related conditions. Arch Intern Med 94:886–901, 1954
McKusick VA: Mendelian Inheritance in Man, 7th ed, p 233. Baltimore, Johns Hopkins Univ Press, 1986

FALLOT'S

Synonyms. Pulmonic stenosis-ventricular septal defect; Fallot's tetralogy.

Symptoms. Both sexes affected; slight male prevalence. Detected weeks or months after birth. Difficulty in feeding; failure to gain weight; poor development. Dyspnea or fatigability on exertion. Orthostatic dyspnea. After a few months of life, paroxysmal attacks of hyperpnea, "hypoxic spell" with increasing cyanosis (alarming manifestation), which disappear before 6 years of age. Characteristic "squatting" when tired or dyspnoic to relieve the symptoms.

Signs. Cyanosis from infancy; at first only when crying or exerting, then persistent. Clubbing of fingers and toes. Heart systolic murmur to the left of sternum (second-third space); systolic thrill. Second sound single for absence of the pulmonic elements. No diastolic murmur. Premedial systolic pulsation may be observed in the second-third interspace.

Etiology. Congenital heart multiple defect. Ventricular septal defect; pulmonic stenosis; dextroposition of aorta and right ventricular hypertrophy. The condition most commonly associated with tetralogy of Fallot is right aortic arch (about 30%).

Diagnostic Procedures. *X-ray.* Heart apex elevated; left lower margin prominent; diminution of pulmonary vessels; lack of pulsation of hilar pulmonary vessels. *Angiocardiography.* Provides information for location of defects. *Electrocardiography.* Right axis deviation; RS-T depression and inverted T in leads II and III. *Cardiac catheterization.* Right ventricular increased pressure; decrease of pulmonary artery pressure, and oxygen concentration alterations in the various cavities. *Circulation time.* Arm-to-tongue time and right ventricle-to-ear time remarkably shortened. *Blood.* Polycythemia. *M-mode echocardiography.*

Therapy. Palliative operation: Blalock-Taussig operation and aortic-pulmonary shunt. Open intracardiac repair: valvotomy or infundibular resection. Intracardiac surgical correction in extracorporal circulation. For the severely cyanotic newborn, prostaglandin administration may be of benefit, to open the ductus until surgery can be performed.

Prognosis. Majority of patients die before 20 years of age from complications. Some patients reach adult life with few symptoms.

BIBLIOGRAPHY. Fallot A: Contribution à l'anatomie pathologique de la maladie bleue (cyanose cardiaque). Marseille Med 25:77, 138; 207; 210; 341; 403, 1888
Hurst JW: The Heart, 6th ed, pp 662–664. New York, McGraw-Hill, 1986
Williams RG, Bierman FZ, Sanders SP: Echocardiographic Diagnosis of Cardiac Malformations, pp 155–161. Boston, Little, Brown & Co, 1986

FALLOT'S TETRALOGY– BALANCED SHUNT

Symptoms and Signs. Both sexes affected; detected weeks or months after birth. Spells of intermittent cyanosis; hyperpnea and syncope less frequent than in classic form. Physical development normal. Pulmonic murmur longer and louder, frequently with thrill. Soft pulmonic component of second sound.

Etiology. See Fallot's, with left-to-right functional shunt.

Diagnostic Procedures. *Electrocardiography.* Well-developed R waves; small Q in precordial leads. *X-rays.* Normal vascularity of lung; less prominence of the aortic arch; rounded heart apex. *Cardiac catheterization. Echocardiography.*

Therapy. See Fallot's.

Prognosis. Better than that for classic form.

BIBLIOGRAPHY. Perloff JK: The Clinical Recognition of Congenital Heart Disease, 2nd ed, p 485. Philadelphia, WB Saunders, 1978
Hurst JW: The Heart, 6th ed, pp 662–667. New York, McGraw-Hill, 1986

FALRET'S

Synonyms. Cyclothymia; folie circulaire; maniac-depressive.

Symptoms. In this disorder, there is at least one episode of mania (hypomania; acute delirious mania) and one of depression (simple retardation or acute depression). A brief period of normality may be present between the two states, but in the majority of cases transition is direct.

Etiology. Unknown; considered; hereditary, constitutional, biologic (psychobiologic; metabolic, and from antidepressant drugs), psychologic, and psychodynamic factors.

Therapy. Prevention of suicide attempt (higher risk in moments of transition between the two stages). Assessment of situation and decision to treat at home or to hospitalize. Treatment according to severity of form includes electroconvulsive therapy, drugs, psychotherapy.

Prognosis. States may last days or months. After 45 years of age, shorter periods. Five percent attempt suicide. Long-term prognosis poor.

BIBLIOGRAPHY. Falret JP: Mémoire sur la folie circulaire, forme de la maladie mentale caractérisée par la reproduction successive et régulière de l'état maniaque, de l'état mélancolique, et d'un intervalle lucide plus ou moins prolongé. Bull Acad Imp Med 19:382–400, 1854

Kraepelin E: Maniac-Depressive Insanity and Paranoia. Robertson GM (ed). Edinburgh, Livingstone, 1921

Freedman AM, Kaplan HI, Sadock BJ: Comprehensive Textbook of Psychiatry, 2nd ed, p 1012. Baltimore, Williams & Wilkins, 1975

FANCONI-DE TONI

Synonyms. Aminoaciduria-osteomalacia-hyperphosphaturia; de Toni-Debré-Fanconi; Fanconi's II; Fanconi-de Toni-Debré, nephrotic glycosuric-dwarfism-rickets hypophosphatemic. See cystinosis, benign.

Symptoms. Both sexes affected, normal at birth and during postnatal period; usual onset at 4 to 6 months of age. Failure to thrive; attacks of vomiting; unexplained fever; polyuria; dehydration.

Signs. Rickets.

Etiology. Multiple etiology. Hereditary basis (cystinosis, Lowe's, tyrosinemia type I; nephrosis familial, galactosemia, glycogen storage disease; hereditary fructose intolerance; Wilson's disease) and acquired as secondary to numerous conditions (myeloma; malignancies; various amino acid metabolism inherited syndromes). Common denominator renal tubular injury, with anatomic and functional derangement of excretion of amino acid, glucose, and phosphate.

Pathology. Cystine deposits in the tissues found only in some cases. Osteomalacia. In kidney (microdissection technique), characteristic lesions affecting nephrons; "swan neck" deformity; shortening of whole proximal convoluted tubule and other aspecific lesions. Pyelonephritis; vacuolization; fibrosis. Frequently, cirrhosis of liver.

Diagnostic Procedures. *Blood.* Chronic acidosis; glucose normal. Phosphate level low initially; with progression of the disease comes back to normal level. Calcium normal; alkaline phosphatase high, hypokalemia. *Urine.* Glycosuria; phosphaturia; generalized aminoaciduria. *X-ray.* Skeletal rickets.

Therapy. Rickets is resistant to vitamin D administration; however, some improvements may be obtained by large doses of this vitamin and supplements of phosphorus. Calcium may also be given with caution (if vitamin D is also given). Shohl's solution to control acidosis. Potassium supplement also necessary. Specific drugs [dithiothreitol (DTT), mercaptoethylamine (MEA), ascorbic acid still to be assessed]. Dietary measures and renal transplant.

Prognosis. Condition shows a slow progression leading ultimately to death from renal insufficiency and uremia. With treatment, immediate prognosis good.

BIBLIOGRAPHY. Fanconi G: Die nicht diabetishen Glykosurien und Hyperglykamien des älteren Kindes. Jahrb Kinderheilk 133:257–300, 1931

de Toni G: Remarks on the relations between renal rickets (renal dwarfism) and renal diabetes. Acta Paediatr Scand 16:479–484, 1933

Debré R, Marie J, Cleret F, et al: Rachitisme tardif coexistent avec une néphrite chronique et une glycosurie. Arch Med Enf 37:597–606, 1934

Morris RC, Jr, Sebastian A: Renal tubular acidosis and Fanconi syndrome. In Stanbury JB, Wyngaarden JB, Fredrickson DS, et al: The Metabolic Basis of Inherited Disease, 5th ed, p 1808. New York, McGraw-Hill, 1983

FANCONI-HEGGLIN

This eponym has been used to designate a nonspecific positive serology for syphilis in cases of viral pneumonias.

BIBLIOGRAPHY. Fanconi G: Die pseudoluetische, subakute hilifugale Bronchopneumonie des heruntergekommenen Kindes. Schweiz Med Wochenschr 66:821–826, 1936

Hegglin R: Das Wassermann positive Lungeninfiltrat. Hel R Med Acta 7:497–527, 1941

FANCONI'S (ADULT FORM)

Synonym. Luder-Sheldon included.

Symptoms and Signs. Onset in adulthood. Same features as infantile form (Fanconi-de Toni, see). Osteomalacia; fractures and pseudofractures; pain; deformity.

Etiology. In some cases, may possibly represent a delayed clinical onset of the congenital form (autosomal dominant trait). More frequently, secondary to heavy metal intoxication, malignancy, or myeloma.

Pathology. See Fanconi-de Toni; no cystinosis reported in adult form.

Diagnostic Procedures. See Fanconi-de Toni.

Therapy. See Fanconi-de Toni.

Prognosis. Depends on etiology. If etiologic agent is toxin (or other curable cause), complete recovery may be obtained with treatment of primary condition.

BIBLIOGRAPHY. Luder J, Sheldon W: Familial tubular absorption defect of glucose and amino acids. Arch Dis Child 30:160–164, 1955

Wilson DR, Yendt ER: Treatment of the adult Fanconi syndrome with oral phosphate supplements and alkali. Am J Med 35:487–511, 1963

Harrison JF, Blainey JD: Adult Fanconi syndrome with monoclonal abnormality of immunoglobulin light chain. J Clin Pathol 20:42–48, 1967

Brenton DP, Isenberg DA, Cusworth DC, et al: The adult presenting idiopathic Fanconi syndrome. J Inherited Metab Dis 4:211–215, 1981

Patrick A, Cameron JS, Ogg CS: A family with a dominant form of idiopathic Fanconi syndrome leading to renal failure in adult life. Clin Nephrol 16:189–292, 1981

FANCONI'S I

Synonyms. Aplastic anemia-congenital anomalies; congenital pancytopenia; Fanconi's panmyelopathy; infantile familial pernicious-like anemia. Fanconi anemia type 1 and type 2.

Symptoms. More common in males (high incidence in siblings); onset in first 8 years of life; tiredness; fatigue; pallor. Recurrent infections; easy bruising; prolonged bleeding, mental retardation; growth retardation.

Signs. Brown, patchy pigmentation of skin; various combinations of congenital abnormalities: microcephaly; microphthalmia; strabismus, deafness; dwarfism; hypogenitalism; hyperreflexia.

Etiology. Defect in the passage of DNA repair-related enzymes from site of synthesis in cytoplasm to the nucleus. Autosomal recessive inheritance. The existence of at least two separate loci has been demonstrated (type 1 and type 2 of the condition).

Pathology. Bone marrow hypoplasia; occasionally, normocellular; rarely, hypercellular. Spleen atrophy (common). Cardiovascular and kidney abnormalities.

Diagnostic Procedures. *Blood.* Pancytopenia; normochromic anemia; macrocytes and target cells observed. Reticulocytes may be slightly increased; white blood cells; usually, neutropenia; immature forms may be noticed. Bilirubin normal; Coomb's test negative. Hexokinase lacking in red cells. *Chromosome studies. Bone marrow.* Hyperplasia; inhibition of maturation; definite megaloblastosis, megakaryocytes decreased; increased deposition of hemosiderin; with progress of disease, cellular hypoplasia. *Urine.* Aminoaciduria reported in some patients.

Therapy. *Blood transfusion.* Testosterone and corticosteroids of some use. Surgical or orthopedic correction when indicated. *Splenectomy.* Sometimes moderately beneficial. Bone marrow transplantation with partial results.

Prognosis. High incidence of leukemia in family. Death relatively early after diagnosis (2–4 yr) from infections or hemorrhages.

BIBLIOGRAPHY. Fanconi G: Familiare infantile, perniciöseähnliche Anämie (perniziöses Blutbild und Konstitution). Jahrb Kinderheilk 117:257–280, 1927

Deeg HJ, Storb R, Thomas ED, et al: Fanconi's anemia treated by allogenic marrow transplantation. Blood 61:954–959, 1983

Duckworth-Rysiecki G, Cornish K, et al: Identification of two complementation groups in Fanconi anemia. Somatic Cell Mol Genet 11:35–41, 1985

Auerbach AD, Sagi M, Adler B: Fanconi anemia: Prenatal diagnosis in 30 fetuses at risk. Pediatrics 76:794–800, 1985

FANCONI-TUERLER

Synonym. Ataxic diplegia. See also Cerebellar syndromes (obsolete).

Symptoms and Signs. Both sexes equally affected (reported, one family with only boy involved); onset at birth. Cerebellar ataxia; spastic paresis; nystagmus; dysmetria; uncoordinated ocular movements. Mental deficiency.

Etiology. Unknown. Developmental abnormality of oculomotor (III) nerve. Both autosomal dominant and sex-linked inheritances have been reported.

BIBLIOGRAPHY. Fanconi G, Tuerler U: Congenitale Keinhirnatrophie mit supranuclearen Storungen der Motilitat der Augenmusklen. Helv Paediatr Acta 6:479–483, 1951

Pfeiffer RA, Palm D, Junemann G, et al: Nosology of congenital nonprogressive cerebellar ataxia: Report of six cases in three families. Neuropaediatrie 5:91–102, 1974

FARABEE'S

Synonym. Brachydactyly type A1.

Symptoms and Signs. Proximal phalanges of digits short, middle phalanges rudimentary or fused; short stature. Occasional mental retardation and ankylosis of thumbs.

Etiology. Autosomal dominant inheritance.

BIBLIOGRAPHY. Farabee WC: Hereditary and sexual influence in meristic variation: A study of digital malformations in man. PhD thesis Harvard Univ, 1903

Pussan C, Lanaerts C, Mathieu M, et al: Dominance reguliere d'une ankylose des pouches avec retard mental se trasmettant sur trois generations. J Genet Hum 31:107–114, 1983

FARBER'S

Synonyms. Ceramidase deficiency; Farber-Uzman; disseminated lipogranulomatosis.

Symptoms and Signs. Onset early months of life. Hoarse cry; laryngeal stridor; swelling of joints of extremities. Skin infiltrative lesions. Hepatomegaly; physical and mental development retardation. Diagnostic triad: arthritis, subcutaneous nodules, laryngeal involvement.

Etiology. Unknown; possibly autosomal recessive inheritance. Deficiency of lysosomal acid ceramidase.

Pathology. *Skin.* Tumefaction, tubular and nodular (yellowish, firm, 1–2 cm in diameter) in periarticular soft tissues, in other areas of pressure zones in the skin, and in subcutaneous tissues. Oily, yellowish plaques on parietal and visceral serosae. *Histology.* Early: infiltration with sheets of large histiocytes and scattered lymphocytes and plasma cells. Later: histiocyte cytoplasm becomes basophilic, granular, or foamy first, and then vacuolar and necrotic. Fibrosis gradually develops. *Larynx.* Lesions similar to the one described. *Heart.* Valves also similarly involved. *Reticular endothelial system.* Scarcely involved (bone marrow; spleen; lymph nodes). *Liver.* Enlarged but not involved. *Central nervous system.* Ballooning of large neurons and glial cells with stored materials, with the characteristics of a nonsulfonated acid mucopolysaccharide: accumulation of ceramide or deficiency of acid ceramidase or both have been demonstrated.

Diagnostic Procedures. *Biopsy of skin.* See Pathology. *Blood.* Moderate leukocytosis (15,000–20,000); anemia; normal cholesterol and total lipids. *X-ray.* Osteoporosis; destructive changes in joints and periarticular calcifications. *Bone marrow.* Occasionally, vacuolated histiocytes. *Biopsy of liver.* Normal. *Urine.* Increased mucopolysaccharide, especially ceramide. Determination of acid ceramidase activity and ceramide.

Therapy. Trial with steroids, methotrexate, chlorambucil, and other chemotherapeutic agents.

Prognosis. Progressive course; death within 2 years. Few patients survived into second decade with neurologic problems.

BIBLIOGRAPHY. Farber S: A lipid metabolic disorder—"disseminated lipogranulomatosis." A syndrome with similarity to and important differences from Niemann-

Pick and Hand Schüller-Christian disease (abstr). Am J Dis Child 84:499–500, 1952
Moser HW, Chen WW: Ceramidase deficiency: Farber's lipogranulomatosis. In Stanbury JB, Wyngaarden JB, Fredrickson DS, et al: The Metabolic Basis of Inherited Disease, 5th ed, p 820. New York, McGraw-Hill, 1983

FARMER-MUSTIAN

Synonym. Vestibulocerebellar ataxia. Ataxia periodic vestibulocerebellar.

Symptoms and Signs. Both sexes affected; onset in childhood or early adulthood. Episodic attacks of vertigo, diplopia, and ataxia, followed by progressive cerebellar disease.

Etiology. Autosomal dominant inheritance.

Therapy. Attacks of dizziness may be relieved by acetazolamide.

Prognosis. In one family slowly progressive cerebellar ataxia developed, in another one no permanent or progressive cerebellar abnormalities were found.

BIBLIOGRAPHY. Farmer TW, Mustian WM: Vestibulocerebellar ataxia. A new defined hereditary syndrome with periodic manifestations. Arch Neurol 8:471–480, 1963
Vance JM, Pericak-Vance MA, Payne CS, et al: Linkage and genetic analysis in adult onset periodic vestibulocerebellar ataxia: Report of a new family. Am J Hum Genet 36:785, 1984

FARMER'S LUNG

Synonyms. Harvester lung; thresher lung. See Allergic alveolitis, extrinsic.

Symptoms. Usually occur between October and May in male farmers exposed to moldy hay or crops. Cough; dyspnea; malaise; fever a few hours after exposure.

Signs. Cyanosis; diffuse rales on both lung fields.

Etiology. Hypersensitivity to a glycopeptide antigen produced by different fungi (thermopolyspora, polyspora, and others) from grains, hay, and other stored vegetable products.

Pathology. Inflammatory granulomatous reaction; frequently, foreign body material in lung parenchyma with secondary bronchopneumonia. In chronic cases, secondary fibrosis and organized endobronchial exudates.

Diagnostic Procedures. *Blood.* Moderate leukocytosis with moderate eosinophilia. *Pulmonary function tests.* X-ray *of chest.* Fine nodular density measuring 3 to 5 mm; occasionally, pneumonitis. *Immunologic studies.* In agar gel; precipitins.

Therapy. Excellent results with corticosteriods, removal from exposure.

Prognosis. Attack lasts a few days; occasionally, weeks. Repeated exposure leads to further attacks and development of pulmonary fibrosis, emphysema, chronic bronchitis; may become fatal because of pulmonary insufficiency and cor pulmonale.

BIBLIOGRAPHY. Campbell JM: Acute symptoms following work with hay. Br Med J 2:1143–1144, 1932
Emanuel DA, Wensel FJ, Bowerman CI, Lawton BR: Farmer's lung. Am J Med 37:392–401, 1964
De Francisci G, Magalini SI, Scrascia E: Etiopatogenesi e problemi rianimativi nelle polmoniti da ipersensibilità. Rec Prog Med 66:541–552, 1979
Reed E, de Shazo RD: Immunologic aspects of granulomatous and interstitial lung diseases. JAMA 248:2683–2691, 1982

FAVRE–RACOUCHOT

Synonym. Nodular elastoidosis.

Symptoms and Signs. Occur in people who are chronically exposed to sun. Usually becoming apparent in fourth or fifth decade. Yellowish thickening of skin, with comedones and follicular cysts, especially around the orbits, occasionally in the neck and behind the ears.

Etiology. Reaction to sun.

Pathology. Elastotic degeneration of collagen.

Diagnostic Procedures. *Biopsy.* Of skin.

Therapy. None. Sunscreens.

Prognosis. Permanent; slowly progressive condition.

BIBLIOGRAPHY. Favre M: Sur une affection kystique des appareils pilo-sebaces localisee a certaines regions de la face. Bull Soc Fr Dermatol Syph 39:93–96, 1932
Favre M, Racouchot J: L'elastéidose cutanée nodulaire a kystes et á comédons. Ann Dermatol Syph 78:681–702, 1951
Rook A, Wilkinson DS, Ebling FJG, et al: Textbook of Dermatology, 4th ed, p 1848. Oxford, Blackwell Scientific Publications, 1986

FAVRE'S

Synonyms. Acroangiodermatitis; dermite ochre; Favre-Chaix stasis purpura; gravitational purpura.

Symptoms and Signs. Prevalent in males. Small macules coalesce to form plaques along venous vessels; usually, in lower legs, extending to feet and upward. Varying shades of yellowish color (ochre).

Etiology. Stasis; venous insufficiency.

Pathology. Skin normal or with mild eczematoid changes. Association with signs of venous stasis, ulceration.

Therapy. Rest; elevation of legs; elastic stockings.

Prognosis. Chronic individual lesions persisting for months or years.

BIBLIOGRAPHY. Favre M: Nouvelle Pratique Dermatologie, Vol 5, p 113. Paris, Masson, 1936
Rook A, Wilkinson DS, Ebling FJG, et al: Textbook of Dermatology, 4th ed, pp 1118–1119. Oxford, Blackwell Scientific Publications, 1986

FAZIO-LONDE

Synonyms. Bulbar palsy progressive, infantilis. Londe's.

Symptoms. Both sexes. From infancy. Difficulty swallowing, absent gag reflex, respiratory difficulty.

Signs. Bilateral ptosis, facial weakness, generalized hyporeflexia. Decreased diaphragm motility.

Etiology. Autosomal recessive inheritance.

Prognosis. Death within 1 to 2 years of age.

BIBLIOGRAPHY. Londe P: Paralysis bulbaire progressive, infantile et familiale. Rev Med 14:212–254, 1894
Gomez MR, Clearmont V, Bernstein J: Progressive bulbar paralysis in childhood (Fazio-Londe's disease). Report of a case with pathologic evidence of nuclear atrophy. Arch Neurol 6:317–323, 1962
Benjamins D: Progressive bulbar palsy of childhood in siblings. Ann Neurol 8:203, 1980

FEER'S

Synonyms. Acrodynia; dermatopolyneuritis; erythredema polyneuropathy; pink disease; Selter's; Swift's.

Symptoms. Both sexes affected; onset in infancy or early childhood (4 mo to 4 yr). Restlessness; sleeplessness; hyperhidrosis continua; tremor; muscle flabbiness.

Signs. Cyanosis of fingers, toes, nose; ulcers and gangrene of fingers; ulcer of mucous membranes; loss of healthy teeth; rectal prolapse; exanthemata of palms and soles with exfoliation of large flaps of skin. Muscle hypotonia; tachycardia; blood hypertension; hypertrichosis. Moderate limb hypertrichosis; in some severe cases, may develop on limb, face, or trunk. Fifty percent of cases present ocular findings: proptosis; lacrimation; photophobia; conjunctival itching and injection; midriasis; seldom, keratitis; papilledema; mild optic neuritis.

Etiology. Unknown; possibly allergic reaction to mercury, infections.

Pathology. *Skin.* In spinous and basal cell layers: acanthosis; papillomatosis; parakeratosis; and necrobiotic changes. *Spinal cord and nerve roots.* Chronic inflammatory changes.

Diagnostic Procedures. *Urine.* Increased excretion of mercury (in some cases).

Therapy. Corticosteroids; dimercaprol in full dosage in severe reaction.

Prognosis. Mortality 10%. Complete recovery in months, occasionally years, with recurrences.

BIBLIOGRAPHY. Feer E: Eine eigenartige Neurase des vegetativen systems beim Kleinkinde. Ergeb Inn Med 24:100–122, 1923
Spencer PS, Schaumburg HH (eds): Experimental and Clinical Neurotoxicology. Baltimore, Williams & Wilkins, 1980
Dinehart SM, Dillard R, Raimer SS, et al: Cutaneous manifestations of acrodynia (pink disease). Arch Dermatol 124:107–109, 1988

FEGELER'S

Synonyms. Posttraumatic nevus flammeus; posttraumatic nevus. See Nevus flammeus.

Symptoms and Signs. Development of nevus flammeus in the area of the trigeminal (V) nerve; homolateral limb weakness and hyperesthesia.

Etiology. Unknown. Ascribed in the past to birth trauma.

Therapy. Nevus can be treated (see Nevus flammeus).

BIBLIOGRAPHY. Fegeler F: Naevus flammeus im Trigeminusgebiet nach Trauma im Rahmen. Eines posttraumatische-vegetativen syndrome. Arch Dermatol Syph 188:416–422, 1949

FELDAKER'S

Synonym. Livedo-ulceration. See also Leg stasis. Livedo vasculitis; recently grouped with Milian's II (see).

Symptoms and Signs. Occur in middle-aged obese and, frequently, hypertensive women; onset usually during summer. Attacks of edema and aching of legs (occasionally, other sites also), followed by appearance of patches of purplish color or purpura, which ulcerate and produce intense pain, especially at night.

Etiology. Unknown. Combination of various factors: edema; stasis; fibrosis.

Pathology. Mild vasculitis; necrosis of veins and arterioles; vascular walls with cellular infiltrates.

Therapy. Bed rest. Elastic stockings. Treatment of basic conditions: hypertension and obesity.

Prognosis. Protracted course, increasing intensity of manifestations every year. Good quoad vitam.

BIBLIOGRAPHY. Feldaker M, Hines EA Jr, Kierland RR: Livedo reticularis with summer ulcerations. Arch Dermatol 72:31–42, 1955
Rook A, Wilkinson DS, Ebling FJG, et al: Textbook of Dermatology, 4th ed, p 1171. Oxford, Blackwell Scientific Publications, 1986

FELTY'S

Synonyms. Rheumatoid arthritis-splenomegaly; neutropenic hypersplenism-arthritis. See Still's.

Symptoms. Malaise, fatigability; anorexia; weight loss; joint pains and deformity; recurrent infections, especially oral mucosa; sinusitis; bronchitis; furunculosis; leg ulcers refractory to antibiotic treatment. Occasionally, dragging sensation or pain in left upper quadrant of abdomen.

Signs. Joints with typical alterations of rheumatoid arthritis; spleen enlarged; mild hepatomegaly; generalized lymphadenopathy. Pallor; occasionally, brown pigmentation on exposed surface of extremities.

Etiology. Unknown; variant of rheumatoid arthritis in which there is unusual reticuloendothelial system stimulation with hypersplenism and neutropenia.

Pathology. Joints show typical changes of rheumatoid arthritis in different stages of evolution. Spleen enlarged (from 240–2400 g). Nonspecific changes, malphighian corpuscles with large germinative center, hyperplasia, reticulum endothelial cells, plasma cells, dilated venus sinuses. Liver within normal limits.

Diagnostic Procedures. *Bone marrow.* Moderate erythroid hyperplasia; marked myeloid hyperplasia with maturation arrest at metamyelocyte level. *Blood.* Moderate hypochromic anemia; moderate thrombocytopenia; marked neutropenia. Latex fixation test often positive; LE test negative; Coomb's test negative.

Therapy. Splenectomy beneficial for neutropenia and recurrent infections in most cases.

Prognosis. Progression of rheumatoid arthritis disease. The rheumatoid arthritis often precedes the hypersplenism, and neutropenia occasionally appears at the same time, or follows.

BIBLIOGRAPHY. Felty AR: Chronic arthritis in the adult, associated with splenomegaly and leukopenia: A report of five cases of an unusual clinical syndrome. Bull John Hopkins Hosp 35:16–20, 1924
Spivak JL: Felty's syndrome: An analytical review. Johns Hopkins Med J 141:156–162, 1977
Clinicopathologic Conference: Rheumatoid arthritis with Felty's syndrome, hyperviscosity and immunologic hyperactivity. Am J Med 70:89–100, 1981

FEMORAL-FACIAL

Symptoms and Signs. Both sexes affected, present from birth. Normal intelligence. *Facies.* Palpebral fissures upslanted; short nose; hypoplastic ala nasi; thin upper lip; cleft palate; micrognathia. *Legs.* Short; hypoplasia or absence of femur and fibula; club foot. *Arms.* Hypoplasia of humerus; reduced elbow movements. Lower spine anomalies and variable alteration of pelvis.

Etiology. Unknown. Sporadic. With a single exception of father-to-daughter transmission.

Prognosis. Normal intelligence. Ambulatory.

BIBLIOGRAPHY. Franz CH, O'Rahilly R: Congenital skeletal limb deficiencies. J Bone Joint Surg 43:1202–1224, 1961
Daentl DL, Smith DW, Scott CI, et al: Femoral hypoplasia–unusual facies syndrome. J Paediatr 86:107–111, 1975
Burk, U, Riebel T, Held KR, et al: Bilateral femoral dysgenesis with micrognathia, cleft palate, anomalies of the spine and pelvis and foot deformities. Helv Paediatr Acta 36:473–482, 1981

FETAL ALCOHOL

Symptoms. Both sexes affected; onset from birth. Poor sucking; mild to moderate mental retardation; poor coordination; irritability, apparent hyperacusia; hyperactivity.

Signs. Muscle hypotonia. Growth deficiencies; cerebral nervous system dysfunctions. Microcephaly. Almost pathognomonic are the facial abnormalities: short palpebral fissures; short upturned nose; hypoplastic philtrum; hypoplastic maxilla; thinned upper vermilion. Occasionally; malformations of eyes, ears, and cardiac, urogenital, cutaneous, and skeletal systems.

Etiology. Teratogenic effect of alcohol intake. The evidence to date suggests that chronic consumption of 90 ml of absolute alcohol or more per day; (the equivalent of about six "hard" drinks) constitutes a major risk to the fetus. However, no absolutely safe level of ethanol consumption has yet been established.

Pathology. Prenatal insult to cell proliferation leads to diminished fetal cell numbers and limitation of size. In particular, the following effects on the central nervous system are observed: failure or interruption in neuronal and glial migrations; cerebellar dysplasias; heterotopic cell clusters, especially on the brain surface; subsensorial anomalies leading to hydrocephalus.

Diagnostic Procedures. Tests of mental performances; careful clinical examination for detection of characteristic facial anomalies.

Therapy. None.

Prognosis. Poor.

BIBLIOGRAPHY. Ullaland CN: The offspring of alcoholic mothers. Ann NY Acad Sci 197:167–169, 1972
Clarren SK, Smith DW: The fetal alcohol syndrome. New Engl J Med 298:1063–1067, 1978
Rosenlicht J: Fetal alcohol syndrome. Oral Surg Oral Med Oral Pathol 47:8–10, 1979
Adams RD, Victor M: Principles of Neurology, 3rd ed, pp 881–882. New York, McGraw-Hill, 1985
Spohr HL, Steinhausen HC: Follow-up studies of children with fetal alcohol syndrome. Neuropediatrics 18:13–17, 1987

FETAL DISTRESS

Synonyms. Fetal asphyxia; asphyxia pallida of newborn; intrauterine hypoxia.

Symptoms and Signs. Change in the fetal heart rate and rhythm above 160 or below 100 beats/min, calculated in between uterine contractions. Bradycardia is more significant than fetal tachycardia. Passage of meconium or staining of amniotic fluid with meconium in a cephalic presentation. Changes in acid–base balance of blood detected by using scalp fetal blood.

Etiology. Predisposing factors are prematurity, toxemia of pregnancy, antepartum uterine infection or bleeding, diabetes mellitus, hypertensive disease during pregnancy. Rh isoimmunization, other complications during labor and delivery.

Pathology. At autopsy, usually evidence of anoxia.

Diagnostic Procedures. Detection of the cardiac arrhythmia either clinically or through the fetal electrocardiogram. Detection of the acidosis through fetal blood examination. Detection of meconium in cephalic presentation.

Therapy. A pediatrician should be available if possible. In cases of asphyxia (absence of respiration) due to excessive narcotics, an antidote should be given: nalorphine hydrochloride (5–10 mg intravenously) to mother for 5 to 15 minutes before delivery or 0.2 mg nalorphine or (better) naloxone hydrochloride (0.005–0.01 mg/kg) injected into the umbilical vein of the newborn. Respiratory stimulants, such as nikethamide (Coramine) or picrotoxin, have no place in the resuscitation of the newborn. As a general rule, if the newborn at the end of first minute fails to start breathing spontaneously, he is in danger. Without losing any time the trachea must be sucked clear of mucus, endotracheal intubation performed, and artificial respiration started. It can be started with gentle puffs from the mouth at a rate of 16/min, enriched with oxygen. As long as the heart is beating, this should be continued. If the heart stops, external cardiac massage should be started at once, at a rate of 60 to 80/min. As soon as the newborn starts spontaneous effort for respiration, the endotracheal cannula should be removed. Sodium bicarbonate should not be given unless the infant is being ventilated satisfactorily. Very often the low *p*H will correct itself with adequate ventilation, restoration of blood volume, and glucose infusion. In any case, the bicarbonate solution should be highly diluted; dilution and slow injection minimize the hazard of acute hyperosmolarity. No time must be wasted on such procedures as slapping of the buttocks of the baby, dilatation of the sphincter ani with finger, immersion of the baby in cold then hot water. Nothing is more harmful to the already handicapped baby.

Prognosis. Depends on the cause of the fetal distress and how rapidly measures for resuscitation are instituted after the diagnosis of the condition.

BIBLIOGRAPHY. Hampton LJ: Resuscitation of the newborn. Clin Obstet Gynecol 3:951–970, 1960
Sunshine P, Benitz WE: Neonatal resuscitation. In Nelson NM (ed): Current Therapy in Neonatal-Perinatal Medicine. Burlington, Ontario, BC Decker, 1986

FIBRINOID

Symptoms and Signs. In patients with long-standing diabetes. Postvitrectomy (2–14 days) appearance of white gray criss-cross layers of fibrin over retina and behind plane of iris. Visual impairment, rubeosis iris.

Pathology. Retinal detachment. Neovascular glaucoma.

Etiology. Unknown.

BIBLIOGRAPHY. Schepens CL: Clinical and research aspects of subtotal open-sky vitrectomy, 37 ed. Jackson Memorial Lecture. Am J Ophthalmol 92:143–171, 1981
Sebestren JG: Fibrinoid syndrome: A severe complication of vitrectomy surgery in diabetes. Ann Ophthalmol 14:853–856, 1982

FIBROMATOSIS, CONGENITAL–GENERALIZED

Synonyms. Including myofibromatosis juvenile. See Ollier's.

Symptoms and Signs. Onset present at birth or developing during first weeks. Multiple fibroblastic tumors in the skin, muscles, bones, and viscera. Absence of pigmentary skin changes. According to visceral organs involved.

Etiology. Unknown. Familial cases reported (autosomal recessive inheritance).

Pathology. Tumors of fibrous tissue containing also smooth muscle cells and vascular channels (Hamartoma type).

Diagnostic Procedures. *Biopsy.*

Prognosis. From spontaneous remission (rare) to death within 4 months (80%). Internal organs involvement poor prognostic factor.

BIBLIOGRAPHY. Touraine A, Ruel H: La polyfibromatose hereditaire. Am Derm Syph 29:1–5, 1945
Stont AP: Juvenile fibromatoses. Cancer 7:953–978, 1954
Altemani AM, Amstalden EI, Fihlo JM: Congenital generalized fibromatosis causing spinal cord compression. Hum Pathol 16:1063–1065, 1985

FIBROMATOSIS, GINGIVAL–HANDS, NOSE, AND EARS ABNORMALITIES–SPLENOMEGALY

Symptoms and Signs. Gingival fibromatosis (see Fibromatosis gingival-hypertrichosis) associated with large soft ears and nose, "whittling" of phalanges, atrophy or dysplasia of nails, hypermobility of joints, hepato or splenomegaly. Skeletal abnormalities.

Etiology. Autosomal dominant inheritance.

BIBLIOGRAPHY. Laband PF, Habib G, Humphreys GS: Hereditary gingival fibromatosis. Report of an affected family with associated splenomegaly and skeletal and soft tissue abnormalities. Oral Surg 17:339–351, 1964

FIBROMATOSIS, GINGIVAL–HYPERTRICHOSIS

Synonyms. Gingival fibromatosis–hypertrichosis.

Symptoms and Signs. Both sexes affected; onset from infancy to ninth year. Progressive growth of gingiva (especially anterior upper region of jaw), eventually to cover teeth completely, sometimes to such extent that lips may not be closed. (This may be the only manifestation.) Marked hypertrichosis, progressive from infancy. Mental retardation; cranial deformities; gynecomastia (not constant features).

Etiology. Unknown; autosomal dominant inheritance, and recessive forms with generalized and focal types.

Pathology. Hyperplasia of gingiva with thick bundles of hyalinized collagen; few fibroblasts; little or no inflammatory changes (except when secondary).

Therapy. Surgery.

Prognosis. Recurrences also after extensive surgery.

BIBLIOGRAPHY. Weski H: Elephantiasis gingival hereditaria. Dtsch Mschr Zahnheilk 38:557–584, 1920
Horning GM, Fisher JG, Barker BF, et al: Gingival fibromatosis with hypertrichosis: A case report. J Periodontol 56:344–347, 1985

FIBROMATOSIS, GINGIVAL–PROGRESSIVE DEAFNESS

Synonyms. Gingival fibromatosis-sensorineural deafness.

Symptoms and Signs. Gingival fibromatosis (see Fibromatosis gingival-hypertrichosis), progressive sensineural deafness.

Etiology. Autosomal dominant inheritance.

BIBLIOGRAPHY. Jones G, Wilroy RS, Jr, McHaney V: Familial fibromatosis associated with progressive deafness in five generations in a family. Birth Defects Org Art Ser XIII (3B) 195–201, 1977
Hartfield JK, Jr, Bixler D, Hazen RH: Gingival fibromatosis with sensineural hearing loss: An autosomal dominant trait. Am J Med Genet 22:623–627, 1985

FIBROMATOSIS, JUVENILE–HYALINE

Synonyms. Juvenile hyaline fibromatosis; hyalinosis systemic; Murray's.

Symptoms and Signs. Both sexes. Lesions present at birth or appearing first in childhood. Face and neck particularly affected. Small pearly papules or nodules and subcutaneous nodules of variable consistency and degree of mobility. Possible ulcerations. Commonly: genus hypertrophy: flexure contraction of joints. Poor muscle development.

Etiology. Altered glycosaminoglycan synthesis. Sporadic. Familial occurence reported.

Pathology. Lesions contain "chondroid cells" in eosinophilic ground substance in the dermis. Dermal collagen and fibrils decreased. In muscle and bone, presence of hyaline materials.

Diagnostic Procedures. *Biopsy. X-ray skeleton.* Osteolytic lesions (possible).

Therapy. Lesions unresponsive to treatment (including radiotherapy); joint contracture may benefit from steroids.

Prognosis. Persisting in adult life, disabling from joint contractures.

BIBLIOGRAPHY. Whitfield A, Robinson AH: A further report on the remarkable series of cases of molluscum fibrosum in children. Communicated to the Society by Dr. John Murray in 1873. Med Chir Trans London 86:293, 1903
Rook A, Wilkinson DS, Ebling FJG, et al: Textbook of Dermatology, 4th ed. Oxford, Blackwell Scientific Publications, 1986

FIBROMUSCULAR DYSPLASIA

Synonym. FMD.

Symptoms and Signs. Prevalent in females; onset from childhood to middle and later age. Extremely variable manifestations, including blood hypertension, stroke, claudication, myocardial infarction shortly after onset of manifestations.

Etiology. Unknown. Consistent with autosomal dominant inheritance.

Pathology. Small and medium-sized arterial lesions presenting as multiple, small, saccular, dilatations with areas of destruction and fragmentation of the media, alternated with rings of hyperplasia of muscular and fibrous elements of arterial wall. Carotid, cerebral, renal, mesenteric coronary, and iliac arteries may be affected.

Diagnostic Procedures. *Artery biopsy.* See Pathology. According to symptoms.

Therapy. None.

Prognosis. Early death.

BIBLIOGRAPHY. Hunt JC, Harrison EG, Jr, Kincaid OW, et al: Idiopathic fibrous and fibromuscular stenosis of the renal arteries associated with hypertension. Mayo Clin Proc 37:181–216, 1962
Sandok BA, Houser OW, Baka HL Jr, et al: Fibromuscular dysplasia: Neurologic disorders associated with diseases involving the great vessels of the neck. Arch Neurol 24:462–466, 1971
Rushton AR: The genetics of fibromuscular dysplasia. Arch Intern Med 140:233–236, 1980

FIBROSIS, MEDIASTINAL IDIOPATHIC

Synonym. Sclerosing mediastinitis.

Symptoms. Onset in middle life or later. Dyspnea; cephalalgia; tinnitus; disturbed sensorium; nosebleed and hemophtysis. Occasionally, intermittent claudication.

Signs. Facial edema and dusky color; superior vena cava obstruction. Frequent association with retroperitoneal fibrosis (see Ormond's). Pseudotumor orbit; Riedel's (see).

Etiology. Multiple. In most cases, end stage of chronic granulomatous conditions (e.g, histoplasmosis, tuberculosis). Other causes: collagenopathies; methysergide treatment. Autosomal recessive inheritance reported in some families.

Pathology. Mass or plaque of fibrous tissue located in the anterior area of upper mediastinum. Various structures in the area can be compressed: superior vena cava; innominate veins; aorta; pulmonary vessels; esophagus. Dense collagen tissue with variable infiltration of plasma cells, eosinophils.

Diagnostic Procedures. *X-ray.* Widening of upper part of mediastinum. *Biopsy.* See Pathology.

Therapy. For methysergide-induced type, discontinuation of drug. Corticosteroids, surgery.

Prognosis. Progressive condition evolving over years.

BIBLIOGRAPHY. Barrett NR: Idiopathic mediastinal fibrosis. Br J Surg 46:207–218, 1958
Feigin DS, Eggleston JC Siegelman SS: The multiple roentgen manifestations of sclerosing mediastinitis. Johns Hopkins Med J 144:1–8 1979
Goldbach P, Mohsenifar Z, Salik AI: Familial mediastinal fibrosis associated with seronegative spondylarthropathy. Arthritis Rheum 26:221–225, 1983

FIBROSITIS

Synonyms. Fibromyositis; rheumatoid myositis; periarticular fibrositis, nonarticular rheumatism.

Symptoms. Pain; stiffness; soreness, especially neck, shoulders, chest, and lower back muscles, with shifting pattern over years, and never uniform over an entire segment. No evidence of associated articular diseases, muscular weakness, atrophy, or neurologic symptoms. Usually accompanied by increased fatigability. All symptoms are worse in morning, relieved by activity, enhanced by cold, dampness, or emotional factors.

Signs. All objective signs are absent except the possible presence of "trigger point," especially painful subcutaneous nodules and spasm of muscles, or segment of muscles.

Etiology. Two types of this syndrome may be recognized: (1) primary type (or true fibrositis) without any underlying systemic disease: (2) secondary type to rheumatic, infective, bone diseases. For the primary type various hypotheses postulated but not completely satisfactory: (1) local pathology "trigger point"; (2) referred pain from minor and not directly expressed pathologic conditions; (3) psychosomatic. Each of these factors may play a role in this syndrome and often more than one at the same time. (See Polymyalgia.)

Pathology. No pathologic findings have been definitely demonstrated. Some differences have been observed, however, between a control group and fibrositic patients. Fat droplets in muscle fibers; increase of intestinal connective tissue nuclei; lymphocytes and plasma cell infiltrates in painful regions.

Diagnostic Procedures. *Laboratory tests.* All negative. *X-ray.* Negative.

Therapy. Reassurance of the patient on the benign nature of the disease, with explanation of its nature and psychological treatment of tension and other psychic factors (primary or superimposed). Analgesic and anti-spasmodic treatment; systemic or topical; salicylates and anesthetic; heat; message.

BIBLIOGRAPHY. Gowers WR: A lecture on lumbago: Its lessons and analogues. Br Med J 1:117–121, 1904
Stockman R: Rheumatism and Arthritis. Edinburgh, Livingstone 1920
Campbell SM, Clark S, Tindall EA, et al: Clinical characteristics of fibrositis. 1. A "blinded" controlled study of symptoms and tender points. Arthritis Rheum 26:817–824, 1983

FICKLER-WINKLER

Synonyms. Olivopontocerebellar II. See Dejerine-Thomas.

Symptoms and Signs. Onset at about 50 years of age. Those of Menzel's (see) differing from it in lack of involuntary movements and of sensory changes. In one of the families reported albinism.

Etiology. Autosomal recessive inheritance or pleiotropism.

BIBLIOGRAPHY. Fickler A: Klinische und pathologish-anatomische. Beitraege zu den Erkrankungeer des Kleinhirns. Dtsch Z Nervenheilk 41:306–375, 1911
Winkler C: A case of olivopontine cerebellar atrophy and our conceptions of neo- and pale-cerebellum. Schweiz Arch Neurol Psychiat 13:196–204, 1923
Skre H, Berg K: Cerebellar ataxia and total albinism: A kindred suggesting pleiotropism or linkage. Clin Genet 5:194–204, 1974

FILATOV-DUKES

Synonyms. Exanthem subitum; Dukes'; fourth disease; pseudorubella; roseola infantum; rose rash.

Symptoms. Onset usually in spring, autumn in children under 2 years of age. Symptoms present in 30% of affected. Mostly sporadic, occasionally limited, epidemic. Incubation period 10 to 15 days. High temperature (39.5–40 C) lasting 3 to 4 days without systemic symptoms, except in some cases with convulsions.

Signs. During fever fall or immediately after, rash of pink macular papule arising first on neck and trunk and spreading to face and limbs. Rash lasts 1 to 2 days. Cervical adenopathy.

Etiology. Rotavirus have been implicated.

Diagnostic Procedures. *Blood.* First 2 days leukocytosis; then leukopenia with relative lymphocytosis.

Therapy. Symptomatic. Soothing bath.

Prognosis. Benign form, completely cured; rare cases of encephalitis.

BIBLIOGRAPHY. Filatov N: Lektsii ob ostrykh infektsionnykh bolezniakh detei, p 113. Moskva, 1887
Dukes C: On the confusion of two different diseases under the name of rubeola (rose-rash) Lancet 2:89–94, 1900
Rook A, Wilkinson DS, Ebling FJG, et al: Textbook of Dermatology, 4th ed, p 706. Oxford, Blackwell Scientific Publications, 1986

FINNISH NEPHROSIS

Synonym. Congenital nephrotic.

Symptoms. High incidence in Finland or in people of Finnish extraction. High frequency of maternal toxemia. Onset in first days or weeks of life. Clinical manifestations identical with those of Epstein's (nephrosis) that never are evident before the age of 18 months.

Etiology. Autosomal recessive. Absence of heparin sulfate anionic sites in glomerular basement membrane. Disturbed metabolism of type IV collagen.

Pathology. *Renal biopsy.* Microcystic cortex and renal tubules.

Diagnostic Procedures. *Prenatal diagnosis.* High α-fetoprotein in amniotic fluid. The chemical changes identical with Epstein's.

Therapy. Steroids and immunosuppressive drugs ineffective.

Prognosis. Death usually before 1 year of age.

BIBLIOGRAPHY. Hallmann N, Hjelt L, Ahvenainen EK: Nephrotic syndrome in newborn and young infants. Ann Paediatr Fenn 2:227–241, 1956
Vernier RL, Klein DJ, Sisson SP, et al: Heparin sulfate-rich anionic sites in human glomerular basement membrane. N Engl J Med 309:1001–1009, 1983

FIRST ARCH SYNDROME(S)

This is used as an all-inclusive title to embrace numerous developmental errors of facial bones that have been described under different names. This grouping is justified since all these syndromes are considered as variable manifestations of one basic development error, a faulty vascularization of the first arch during embryonal life (abnormalities of stapedial artery). The different manifestations of the various syndromes depend on the speed with which collateral circulation develops and more or less compensates for this defect.

Etiology. Unknown; a common genetic defect, dominant with variable penetrance will be at the basis of all those syndromes, and the compensatory mechanism (anastomosis) determines its degree of penetrance and consequently the various clinical aspects.
1. Treacher–Collins
2. Pierre Robin
3. Franceschetti–Klein
4. Hypertelorism
5. Goldenhar's (?)
6. Cleft lip and cleft palate
7. Some deformities of external and middle ear including deafness
  The last two may also occur as a result of environmental agents and various recognized chromosomal disorders, and such cases must not be included in the first arch syndrome.

BIBLIOGRAPHY. McKenzie J: The first arch syndrome. Arch Dis Child 33:477–486, 1958
McKenzie J: The first arch syndrome. Dev Med Child Neurol 8:55–66, 1966
Forfar SC, Arneil GC: Textbook of Pediatrics, 2nd ed. Edinburgh, Churchill-Livingstone, 1978

FISHER'S

Synonyms. Ophthalmoplegia–ataxia–areflexia; disseminated encephalomyeloradiculopathy; Guillain–Barré variant; Miller–Fisher; Bickerstaff's; brain stem areflexia.

Symptoms. Reported in male patients between 38 and 65 years of age. Starting as a respiratory complaint (sore throat; tightness in the chest; pneumonitis; fever; severe headache); after 3 to 4 days; external ophthalmoplegia usually total; diplopia; unilateral or bilateral facial paralysis; cerebellar ataxia; migratory paresthesias of trunk and arms. No mental changes or sensory impairment (or the latter may be minimal); no motor weakness of extremities. Condition may evolve into apneic coma and complete paralysis of motor function of cranial nerves.

Signs. Tendon reflexes abolished; pupillary reflexes sluggish; sensory changes minimal or absent.

Etiology. Viral infection with hypersensitivity (?) of nervous system. May be considered a variant or an atypical form of the Guillain–Barré syndrome.

Pathology. None reported.

Diagnostic Procedures. *Spinal fluid.* Marked albumincytologic dissociation. *Electroencephalography.* CT brain scan (to rule out hemorrhage). *Acoustic evoked responses.* Preserved. *Motor and sensory nerve conduction studies and EMG.* Electrodiagnostic abnormalities characteristic of an axonal neuropathy or a neuronopathy with predominant sensory nerve changes in the limbs and motor damage in the cranial nerves. The pattern of abnormalities is distinct from the usual features seen in the Guillain–Barré.

Therapy. Cortisone may reduce the acute symptoms.

Prognosis. Self-limited disease of 10 to 12 weeks', duration with neurologic recovery complete or residual minor paresthesias and horizontal diplopia for some time after recovery.

BIBLIOGRAPHY. Fisher M: An unusual variant of acute idiopathic polyneuritis (syndrome of ophthalmoplegia, ataxia, and areflexia). N Engl J Med 255:57–65, 1956
Bickerstaff ER: Brain stem encephalitis (Bickerstaff's encephalitis). In Vinken PJ, Branyn GN (eds): Handbook of Clinical Neurology, Vol 34, pp 605–609. Amsterdam, North Holland Publishing, 1978
Al-Din ASN, Jamil A, Shakir R: Coma and brain stem areflexia in brain stem areflexia (Fisher's syndrome) Br Med J 291:535–536, 1985
Weiss JA, White JC: Correlation of 1A afferent conduction with the ataxia of Fisher syndrome. Muscle Nerve 9:327–332, 1986
Fross RD, Daube JR: Neuropathy in the Miller-Fisher syndrome: Clinical and electrophysiologic findings. Neurology 37:1493–1498, 1987

FISHER'S (C.M.)

Synonyms. One and a half.

Symptoms and Signs. Both sexes. Onset usually after 20 years of age. Presenting symptoms: vertigo, diplopia, dizziness, difficulty in walking, slurred speech. Development of lateral gaze palsy in one direction with internuclear ophthalmoplegia (INO) in the other direction. In the complete form: one eye fixed at the midline for all lateral movements; the other can only abduct and shows horizontal jerk nystagmus in abduction. Possibly associated other numerous ocular and neurologic signs.

Etiology. Brain stem infarction, multiple sclerosis, pontine glioma-arteriovenous malformation, pontine hemorrhage, basilar artery aneurysm, neoplasia, or metastasis.

Pathology. Unilateral lesion of lower part of dorsal pontine tegmentum affecting ipsilateral paramedian pontine reticular formation, abducens nucleus and internuclear fibers of ipsilateral medial longitudinal fasciculus.

BIBLIOGRAPHY. Bender MG, Weinstein EA: Dissociated monocular nystagmus with paresis of horizontal ocular movements. Arch Ophthamol 21:266–272, 1939
Fisher CM: Some neuro-ophthalmological observations: J Neurol Neurosurg Psychiatry 30:383–392, 1967
Wall M, Vray SH: The one and a half syndrome: A unilateral disorder of the pontine tegmentum. A study of 20 cases and review of the literature. Neurology 33:971, 1983

FISHER–VOLAVSEK

Synonyms. Palmo-plantaris keratoma syringomyelia; onychogryphosis syringomyelia.

Symptoms. Both sexes affected, present from birth. Congenital malformations (see Signs). Later, developing symptoms of syringomyelia.

Signs. Onychogryphosis; sparse hair of scalp, brows, and lashes. Thickening of terminal digits.

Etiology. Unknown; autosomal dominant inheritance.

BIBLIOGRAPHY. Fisher H: Familiär hereditares Vorkommen von Keratoma Palmare et Plantare. Nagelveranderungen, Haaranomalien und Verdickung der Endglieder der Finger und Zehen in 5 Generationen. Dermatol Z 32:114–142, 1921
Volavsek W: Zur Klinik der Nagelveränderungen und Palmarkeratozen bei Syringomyelie. Arch Dermatol Syph 182:52–57, 1941
Gorlin RJ, Sedano H, Anderson VE: The syndrome of palmar-plantar prekeratosis and premature periodontal destruction of the teeth. J Pediatr 65:895–908, 1964

FISH EYE

Synonyms. Corneal opacities–dyslipoproteinemia. Lipoproteinemia (dys)–Corneal opacities. See Tangier's and Hyperlipoproteinemia. Carlson's.

Symptoms. Described in a Swedish family (man and three daughters). Visual impairment.

Signs. Marked corneal opacities.

Etiology. Unknown. Probably autosomal dominant inheritance.

Diagnostic Procedures. *Blood.* Cholesterol and percentage of cholesterol esters normal, HDL cholesterol reduced. Triglycerides elevated: VLDL and LDH triglycerides very high. Lecithincholesterol acyltransferase (LCAT) activity normal; lipoprotein and hepatic lipases normal; very-low density triglycerides and cholesterol raised.

Prognosis. Unknown. Except for visual impairment general condition good.

BIBLIOGRAPHY. Carlson LA, Philipson B: Fish eye disease: A new familial condition with massive corneal opacities and dyslipoproteinaemia. Lancet 2:921–923, 1979
Rees J, Stocks J, Schoulders C, et al: Restriction enzyme analysis of the apolipoprotein A-1 gene in fish eye disease and Tangier disease. Acta Med Scand 215:235–237, 1984

FITZGERALD-WILLIAMS-FLAUJEAC TRAIT

Synonym. High molecular weight kininogen deficiency.

Symptoms and Signs. Laboratory curiosity.

Etiology. Autosomal recessive.

Diagnostic Procedures. *Blood.* Prolonged clotting time and partial thromboplastin time. Patient's plasma corrects defects in plasma deficient in high molecular weight kininogen.

Therapy. None.

Prognosis. Good.

BIBLIOGRAPHY. Waldman R, Abrahazam J: Fitzgerald Factor: A heretofore unrecognized coagulation factor. Blood 46:761, 1975
Colman RW, Bagdasarian A, Talamo RC, et al: William's trait: Human kininogen deficiency with diminished levels of plasminogen proactivator and prekallikrein associated with abnormalities of the Hageman factor-dependent pathways. J Clin Invest 56:1650, 1975
Wuepper KD, Miller DR, LaCombe MJ: Flaujeac trait deficiency of human plasma kininogen. J Clin Invest 56:1663, 1975

FITZ-HUGH AND CURTIS

Synonyms. Gonococcal perihepatitis; Stajano's; subcostal. Curtis.

Symptoms. Onset in young women between 20 and 30 years of age. Fever may be present. Right upper abdominal pain. Vaginal discharge may be present or absent, as well as pelvic pain.

Signs. Friction rub of hepatic region may be present. Pelvic inflammation and discharge; bartholinitis may be present or minimal. Jaundice (rare).

Etiology. Gonococcal perihepatitis.

Pathology. Adhesion of the liver and abdominal wall. In one case, necrosis of the liver cells, but few detailed reports of pathologic changes.

Diagnostic Procedures. *Vaginal smear.* For identification of gonococcus. *Culture. X-ray Gallbladder studies.* Normal gallbladder, occasionally pericholecystitis.

Therapy. Penicillin.

Prognosis. Excellent with treatment.

BIBLIOGRAPHY. Stajano C: La reaction frenica en ginecologia. Sem Med Buenos Aires 27:243–248, 1920
Curtis AH: Cause of adhesions in right upper quadrant. JAMA 94:1221–1222, 1930
Fitz-Hugh T Jr: Acute gonococcic peritonitis of right upper quadrant in women. JAMA 102:2094–2906, 1934
Vickers FN, Maloney PJ: Gonococcal perihepatitis: Report of three cases with comment on diagnosis and treatment. Arch Intern Med 114:120–123, 1964

5-OXOPROLINURIA

See section A.

FLAJANI'S

Synonyms. Basedow's; Bergie's; exophthalmic goiter; Graves'; hyperthyroidism; March's; Parry's; thyrotoxicosis; von Basedow's.

Symptoms. Female predominance, ratio 4:1; onset in third to fifth decade of life. Emotional instability; nervousness; palpitation; intolerance to heat; incessant sweating; occasionally, anorexia; nausea; vomiting; diarrhea; later, dyspnea.

Signs. Skin warm and moist; hyperpigmentation. Bilateral (seldom unilateral) exophthalmos; infrequent blinking (Stillwag's sign); absence of brow wrinkling when looking up (Joffroy's sign); lid lag (Graefe's sign); lack of convergence (Moebius's sign); thyroid enlarged bilaterally, soft and margins indistinct. Increased cardiac rate; enlargement of heart; hyperreflexia. Pretibial myxedema (rare). Acropachy (rare).

Etiology. Autosomal recessive inheritance with relative sex limitation to female. Primary thyroid hyperplasia, occasionally precipitated or initiated by trauma or stress. Metabolic; immunologic, toxic disorders.

Pathology. Thyroid enlarged, smooth, elastic, friable; deep fissure in sulci giving nodular aspect. Hyperplasia and hypertrophy of acinar cells; vesicular nuclei; depletion of colloid; enlarged intrafollicular spaces; increased lymph follicles.

Diagnostic Procedures. *Basal metabolic rate.* Increased. *Blood.* Increased protein-bound iodine; increased butanol-extracted iodine fraction; serum T_4, T_3, (T_4-binding globulin) levels, and antithyroid antibodies, lymphocytosis, occasionally macrocytic anemia. *Scan.* Increased uptake or radioactive iodine, and T_3; repeat scanning after thyroid-stimulating hormone (TSH).

Therapy. Radioactive iodine; antithyroid drugs; X-ray treatment; surgery.

Prognosis. If untreated, progression of symptoms to cardiac failure, through remission and relapses, spontaneous cure possible. Good results with treatment.

BIBLIOGRAPHY. Flajani G: Osservazione LXVII: Sopra un tumor freddo nell'anterior parte del dotto detto broncocele. In Collezione d'Osservazioni e Riflessioni di Chirugia, G. Flajani, Vol. 3, Rome, p 270. S. Michele A. Ripa Presso Lino Contedini, 1802
Parry CH: Collections from the Unpublished Papers of the Late Caleb Hillier Parry, Vol 2, pp 11–28. London, 1825
Graves RJ: Clinical lectures. London Med Surg J 7:516, 1835
von Basedow CA: Exophthalmos durch Hypertrophie des Zellgewebes in der Augenhohle. Wochenschr ges Heilkunde 13:197–204; 220–228, 1840
Toft AD (ed): Hyperthyroidism (Symposium). Clin Endocrinol Metab 14 (all issue), 1985

FLECKED RETINA

See Kandori's.

Symptoms and Signs. Normal peripheral visual fields. Slightly abnormal dark adaptation. Abnormal electrooculogram. High incidence of macular abnormalities. Stationary status of minor abnormalities of peripheral retina function. Similar fluorescein staining patterns (fluorescein angiography).

Etiology. Includes three ophthalmoscopically distinct entities: (1) fundus flavimaculatus (suggested autosomal recessive type of inheritance); (2) fundus colloid bodies or drusen (possibly familial congenital condition); (3) fundus albipunctatus (possibly familial congenital condition).

Pathology. Fundus flavimaculatus: distinctive changes in the pigmented epithelium; normal neuroepithelium, Bruch's membrane, and choroid. Lesion represented by deposition of acid mucopolysaccharides. Fundus colloid bodies: round or oval lesions of various sizes frequently with calcification and found in far periphery. They may be confluent and form different conglomerate patterns. Fundus albipunctatus: Uniform, dotlike lesion never confluent.

BIBLIOGRAPHY. Krill AE, Klien BA: Flecked retina syndrome. Arch Ophthalmol 74:496–508, 1965
Klien BA, Krill AE: Fundus flavimaculatus. Am J Ophthalmol 64:3–23, 1967

FLEGEL'S

Synonym. Hyperkeratosis-lenticularis perstans. See Kyrle's.

Symptoms and Signs. Both sexes. Onset after 30 years of age. Starts on dorsa of feet and in some cases successively involves the legs, thighs, arms, and dorsum of hands and seldom the trunk. Pink, reddish brown scaly papules (1–5 mm).

Etiology. Autosomal dominant inheritance.

Pathology. Parakeratotic hyperkeratosis over a flattened epidermis. Lymphocytic infiltration only sub papulae. Lack of Odlan bodies in affected epidermis.

Prognosis. In some families reported high incidence of skin tumors (squamous, basal cell carcinoma) in nonaffected areas.

BIBLIOGRAPHY. Flegel H: Hyperkeratosis lenticularis perstans. Hautarzt 9:362–364, 1958
Beau SF: The genetics of hyperkeratosis lenticularis perstans. Arch Dermatol 106:102, 1982
Rook A, Wilkinson DS, Ebling FJG, et al: Textbook of Dermatology, 4th ed, p 1451. Oxford, Blackwell Scientific Publications, 1986

FLEISCHNER'S

Synonyms. Disc-like atelectasis; reflex atelectasis. Eponym used to indicate not a syndrome but the radiologic linear or discoid shadow located in the lower third of one lung or both lungs. Shadow indicates the presence of atelectasis due to hypomobility of diaphragm because of thoracic or abdominal disease.

BIBLIOGRAPHY. Fleischner F: Plattenförmige Atelecthasen in der Unterlappen der Lunge. Fortschr Geb Roentgen 54:315–321, 1936

FLETCHER'S TRAIT

Synonym. Prekallikrein deficiency.

Symptoms and Signs. Laboratory curiosity.

Etiology. Autosomal recessive.

Diagnostic Procedures. *Blood.* Clotting time and partial thromboplastin time prolonged, corrected by preincubation with kaolin and phospholipid.

Prognosis. Good.

BIBLIOGRAPHY. Wuepper KD: Prekallikrein deficiency in man. J Exp Med 138:1345, 1973

FLOPPY INFANT SYNDROMES

1. Myelopathic and neuropathic causes
   Werding-Hoffmann
   Oppenheim's
   Walton's
   Guillain-Barré
   Poliomyelitis
   Spinal tumors
   Transverse myelopathy, traumatic or of different nature
2. Encephalopathic causes
   Mental deficiency (especially Down's)
   Progressive encephalopathy (especially Tay-Sachs)
   Brain tumors
   Riley-Day
   Cerebral palsies
3. Neuromuscular transmission
   Erb-Goldflam's
   Abnormal neuromuscular junctions
4. Myopathic causes
   Infantile muscular dystrophies
   Polymyositis syndrome
   Glycogen storage
   Shy-Magee
   Universal muscular hypoplasias
5. Tendons and ligaments syndromes
   Ehlers-Danlos syndrome
   Arachnodactyly
   Congenital laxity of ligaments
   Arthrogryposis
6. Osteogenic causes
   Osteogenesis imperfecta syndrome
   Rickets
   Barlow's
   Parrot's
7. Nonmuscular causes
   Malnutrition
   Vitamin deficiencies
   Chronic diseases
   Acute illness or infections
   Endocrinopathies (especially hypothyroidism and hypopituitarism)
   Metabolic syndromes

BIBLIOGRAPHY. Paine RS: The future of the "Floppy Infant." A follow-up study of 133 patients. Dev Med Child 5:115–124, 1963

FLOPPY VALVE

Synonyms. Mid-systolic click–late systolic murmur; click murmur; billowing mitral valve. See Marfan's.

Symptoms. Chest pain, nonexertional and sometimes prolonged; weakness, fatigue, palpitations, light headedness, dyspnea. Sometimes symptoms are vague or absent.

Signs. One or more mid-systolic clicks, which generally occur 0.1 second or more after the first heart sound; late systolic murmur.

Etiology/Pathology. Myxomatous degeneration of the mitral valve. Often the syndrome is associated with Marfan's syndrome, osteogenesis imperfecta, and other connective tissue diseases.

Diagnostic Procedures. *Electrocardiogram.* T wave inversions in leads II, III, and aVF and occasionally in V5 and V6; ventricular ectopic beats; supraventricular tachycardia. *Echocardiography.* Typical findings. *Cardiac catheterization.* Abnormalities in left ventriculography studies. Evaluation for presence of bacterial endocarditis.

Therapy. 24-hour ECG monitoring; β-adrenergic blockade; antiarrhythmic therapy; prophylaxis against endocarditis at the time of dental or surgical procedures. Drugs that may cause tachycardia, a reduction in peripheral vascular resistance, or a reduction in venous return can increase the prolapse. Progressive mitral regurgitation requiring valve replacement rarely appears.

Prognosis. In most patients the clinical course is benign. The incidence of complications is around 15%. These include progressive mitral regurgitation, bacterial endocarditis, ventricular arrhythmias.

BIBLIOGRAPHY. Jeresaty RM: Mitral Valve Prolapse. Raven Press, New York, 1979
Berry FA, Lake CL, Johns RA, Rogers BM: Mitral valve prolapse—Another cause of intraoperative dysrhythmias in the pediatric patient. Anesthesiology 62:662–664, 1985
Casthely PA, Dluzneski J, Resurreccion MA, et al: Ventricular fibrillation during general anaesthesia in a seven-year old patient with mitral valve prolapse. Can Anesth Soc J 33:795–798, 1986
Hurst JW: The Heart, 6th ed, p 184. New York, McGraw-Hill, 1986

FLUCKIGER'S

Synonym. Cyanosis–digital clubbing–hepatopathy.

Symptoms. Both sexes, all ages affected; most frequent in children. Cyanosis with or without dyspnea; clubbing of fingers develops after initiation of hepatic cirrhosis.

Etiology. The possible development of arteriovenous fistulas in the lungs due to release of a humoral substance from diseased liver (ferritin?) in susceptible individuals (familial trend?) has been proposed as mechanism to explain this syndrome. Possibly autosomal recessive inheritance.

Pathology. Liver cirrhosis. Microvenoarteriolar fistulas in lung.

Diagnostic Procedures. *Blood.* Secondary polycythemia; changes found in liver cirrhosis; arterial oxygen desaturation. *Dye dilution studies.* Indirect evidence of lung arteriovenous shunt. *X-rays.* Do not reveal lung alteration.

Therapy. None or portal shunt to decrease hypertension.

Prognosis. Poor; that of liver cirrhosis. Cyanosis and clubbing progressive.

BIBLIOGRAPHY. Fluckiger M: Vorkommen von trommelschlagel-förmigen Fingerendphalangen ohne chronische Veränderungen an den Lungen oder am Herzen. Wein Med 34:1457, 1884
Silverman A, Cooper MD, Moller JH, et al: Syndrome of cyanosis, digital clubbing, and hepatic disease in siblings. J Pediatr 72:70–80, 1968

FLYNN–AIRD

Synonyms. See Werner's, Refsum's, Cockayne's.

Symptoms and Signs. Both sexes. From birth. Blindness. *Eye.* Cataracts, atypical retinitis pigmentosa, myopia. *Teeth.* Marked caries. *Ear.* (At age 7 yr) progressive sensineural deafness. Skin atrophy, chronic ulcers. Dementia, ataxia, peripheral neuritis, epilepsy. Joint stiffness.

Etiology. Unknown. Autosomal dominant inheritance.

Diagnostic Procedures. *X-ray skeleton.* Cyst changes. *Cerebrospinal fluid.* Increased proteins.

BIBLIOGRAPHY. Flynn P, Aird RB: A neuroectodermal syndrome of dominant inheritance. J Neurol Sci 2:161–182, 1969
Konigsmark BW, Gorlin RJ: Genetic and Metabolic Deafness. Philadelphia, WB Saunders, 1976

FOCAL GLOMERULAR SCLEROSIS

Synonyms. Lohlein. Maybe it is only a superimposed lesion on minimal change disease or on minimal proliferative glomerulonephritis.

Symptoms and Signs. Those of idiopathic nephrotic syndrome.

Etiology. Unknown. Probably, immune complex disease.

Pathology. *Light microscopy.* Segmental sclerosis of glomeruli due to increased mesangial matrix and basement membrane. Tubular changes. *Electron microscopy.* Foot process alterations, mesangial cell hyperplasia. *Immunofluorescence.* IgM, C1q, C3 irregular granular distribution.

Therapy. Corticosteroids.

Prognosis. Rapid progression to renal failure. Recurrence of disease in grafts.

BIBLIOGRAPHY. Lohlein MH: Uber die entzundlichen Veranderungen der Glomeruli der menschliehen Nieren und ihre Bedeutung für die Nephritis. Leipzig, Hirzel, 1907

Rich AR: A hitherto unrecognized vulnerability of the juxta medullary glomeruli in lipoid nephrosis. Bull Johns Hopkins Hosp 100:A3, 1957

Brenner-Rector: The Kidney, 3rd ed, p 974. Philadelphia, WB Saunders, 1986

FOERSTER'S

Synonym. Atonic-astatic Foerster's; atonic congenital diplegia; atonic-astatic; cerebral diplegia; see "Floppy infant" syndrome.

Symptoms. Present at birth. Marked muscular hypotony; hypermobility of joints; severe mental defect; dysarthria. Absence of paresis; convulsions; sphincter incontinency.

Signs. Normal deep and superficial reflexes; absence of muscular atrophy; occasionally, strabismus. When the child is kept in standing position all body muscles may temporarily become hypertonic.

Etiology. Unknown; only in some cases positive serology for syphilis. Familial cases reported. Clinical features in common with both Creutzfeld-Jakob and dystrophia myotonica. Consanguinity described suggests autosomal recessive inheritance.

Pathology. Sclerotic lesions of frontal lobes involving the motor centers.

Diagnostic Procedures. *Blood. Serology. Cerebrospinal fluid. Electroencephalography. Electromyography.*

Therapy. Nonspecific.

Prognosis. Improvement of muscular hypotonia observed, and in some cases it becomes possible to sit, and also walk with support; mental deterioration does not improve, and language usually does not develop.

BIBLIOGRAPHY. Foerster O: Der atonisch-astatische Typus der infantilen Cerebrallähmung, Arch Klin Med 48:216–244, 1909

Floris V, Angelini C, Strazzeri, R: Sindrome di Foester in gemelle monocoriali. Riv Neurol 24:442–448, 1954

Van Rossum A: Foerster's atonic-astatic syndrome. Recent Neurological Research, Elsevier, 1959

Denny-Brown D: The Basal Ganglia. London, Oxford University Press, 1962

FOIX-ALAJOUANINE

Synonyms. Spinal cord hemangioma necrotizing subacute myelitis.

Symptoms. Spastic paraplegia; then flaccid amyotrophia; sensory loss first dissociated then complete. Sphincters involved.

Signs. Tendon reflexes abolished.

Etiology. Foix, et al: proliferative endomeso-vasculitis. Moersh, et al: vascular lesions. Neubuerger, et al: hyperplasia and hyalinosis of vascular walls.

Circulation of spinal cord may also be compromised by aorta operations or aortography.

Pathology. Necrosis of spinal cord without inflammation; amyotrophy. Dysgenesis of spinal vessels with hyperplasia and hyalinosis of walls.

Diagnostic Procedures. *Cerebrospinal fluid.* Protein increased. *X-ray.* Myelography.

Therapy. None.

Prognosis. Subacute course; death in 1 or 2 years.

BIBLIOGRAPHY. Foix C, Alajouanine T: La myelite necrotique subaique. Rev Neurol 2:1, 1926

Neuberger KT, Freed CG, Denst J: Vasal component in syndrome of Foix and Alajouanine: "subacute necrotizing myelitis." Arch Path 55:73–83, 1953

Adams RD, Victor M: Principles of Neurology, 3rd ed, p 677. New York, McGraw-Hill, 1985

FOIX-JEFFERSON

Synonyms. Cavernous sinus; Godtfredsen's; hypophyseal-sphenoidal; lateral wall cavernous sinus; ophthalmoneurologic-nasopharyngeal; cavernous sinus thrombosis. See Orbital Apex.

Symptoms. Development of orbital and supraorbital pain. Involvement of oculomotor (III), trochlear (IV), trigeminal (V) (limited to ophthalmic branch), and abducens (VI) nerves. Paralysis usually unilateral; if bilateral, asymmetric. Association with chiasma syndrome (later) relatively frequent.

Etiology and Pathology. Pituitary tumors (chromophobe more frequent association; eosinophil more absolute incidence); fibrosarcoma of sphenoid bone; aneurysms of cavernous sinus (symptoms acute); metastatic carcinoma; cavernous sinus thrombophlebitis.

Diagnostic Procedures. *X-ray of skull. Angiography. Pneumoencephalography. Electroencephalography. Hormonal studies.* For pituitary function.

Therapy. Depends on etiology: surgery; antibiotics.

Prognosis. According to etiology.

BIBLIOGRAPHY. Bartholow R: Aneurysms of the arteries at the base of the brain, their symptomatology, diagnosis, and treatment. Am J Med Sci 64:373–386, 1872
Foix C: Sindrome de la paroi externe du sinus cavernous. Rev Neurol (Paris) 37, 38:827–832, 1922
Godtfredsen E: Ophthalmoneurological symptoms in malignant nasopharyngeal tumors. Br J Ophthalmol 31:78–100, 1947
Nelson DA, Holloway WJ, Kara-Eneff SC, et al: Neurological syndrome produced by sphenoid sinus abscess, with neuroradiologic review of pituitary abscess. Neurology 17:981–987, 1967

FOIX'S

Synonym. Red nucleus.

Symptoms and Signs. Cerebellar ataxia; usually associated with hyperkinesia; without oculomotor paralysis.

Etiology. Lesion limited to the anterior portion of red nucleus (the oculomotor roots pass through the posterior part of the nucleus).

BIBLIOGRAPHY. Foix C: Le syndromes de la region thalamique. Presse Med 33:113–117, 1925
Hiller F: The vascular syndromes of the basilar and vertebral arteries and their branches. J Nerv Ment Dis 116:988–1016, 1952
Adams RD, Victor M: Principles of Neurology, 3rd ed, p503. New York, McGraw-Hill, 1985

FOLATE METABOLISM, INBORN ERRORS

Synonyms. Methylmalonic acidemia-homocystinuria; vitamin B_{12} defect.

1. Congenital defects of absorption

Synonyms. Luhby's, Lanzkowsky's, Santiago–Borrero's. Few cases described that share as symptoms and signs megaloblastic anemia and mental retardation.

2. Dihydrofolate reductase deficiency

Synonyms. DHFR deficiency; Walter. Three cases described that share as symptoms and signs megaloblastic anemia and early death.

3. Formiminotransferase deficiencies

Synonyms. FIGLU urics; Arakawa I. Mental and physical retardation, cortical atrophy, increased urinary FIGLU excretion in urine, megaloblastic anemia. Niederweiser-Perry: only slight mental retardation. FIGLU excretion in urine.

4. Methylene THE reductase deficiency

Synonyms. Mudd's. Differences in prognosis may be due to type of therapy used. Varying degrees of mental retardation and neurologic abnormalities. Moderate homocystinuria with homocystinemia. Three groups are distinguished according to time of onset; neonatal, childhood, and mild form.

5. Tetrahydrofolate methyl transferase deficiency

Synonyms. Arakawa's II. From birth; diarrhea, vomiting, megaloblastic anemia, delay of mental development. May be autosomal dominant.

Etiology. All these syndromes appear to have an autosomal recessive inheritance, except the fifth, which may be dominant.

BIBLIOGRAPHY. Luhby AL, Cooperman JM, Pesci Bourel A: A new born error of metabolism: folic acid responsive megaloblastic anemia, ataxia, mental retardation and convulsions. J Pediat 67:1052, 1965
Lanzkowsky P: Congenital malabsorption of folate. Am J Med 48:580–583, 1970
Santiago-Borrero PJ, Santini R Jr, Perez-Santiago E, et al: Congenital isolated defect of folic acid absorption. J Pediatr 82:450–455, 1973
Walters TR: Congenital megaloblastic anemia responsive to N5 formyltetrahydrofolic acid administration. J Pediatr 82:450–455, 1972
Arakawa T, Ohara K, Kudo Z, et al: Hyperfolic acidemia with formiminoglutamic aciduria, following histidine loading. Suggested for a case of congenital deficiency in formiminotransferase. Tohoku J Exp Med 80:370–382, 1963
Arakawa T, Narisawa K, Tanno K, et al: Megaloblastic anemia and mental retardation associated with hyperfolicacidemia. Probably due to N5 methyltetrahydrofolate transferase deficiency. Tohoku J Exp Med 93:1–22, 1967

Mudd SH, Uhlendorf BW, Freeman JM, et al: Homocystinuria associated with decreased methylenetetrahydrofolate reductase activity. Biochem Biophys Res Commun 46:909–912, 1972

Rowe PB: Inherited disorders of folate metabolism. In Stanbury JB, Wyngaarden JB, Fredrickson DS (eds): The Metabolic Basis of Inherited Disease, 5th ed, p 498. New York, McGraw-Hill, 1983

FOLLING'S

Synonyms. Hyperphenylalanine type I; idiotia phenylketonuria; phenylpyruvic oligophrenia; classic phenylketonuria; classic PKU.

Symptoms. Both sexes equally affected; normal at birth. Developmental landmarks reached at normal age or delayed. Frequent vomiting in early infancy (50%). Seizures developing in first 18 months of life and stopping spontaneously before adulthood (in about 25%). Marked irritability; hyperactivity almost constant. Severe mental defect. Inability to talk; inability to walk (associated with incontinence).

Signs. In children, height and weight below normal; microcephaly (68%); skin deficient pigmentation; blond hair; blue eyes. Stance and gait often "stooping," "stamping." Muscular hypertonicity; tendon hyperreflexia; abnormal, voluntary, purposeless body movements; tremor.

Etiology. Autosomal recessive inheritance. Phenylalanine hydroxylase deficiency. Impaired conversion of phenylalanine to tyrosine in the liver.

Pathology. *Brain.* Weight two thirds of normal; deficient myelinization (not constant); normally pigmented brain areas may lack pigmentation.

Diagnostic Procedures. *Blood, urine.* High level of phenylalanine. Peculiar "musty" odor of urine; positive ferric chloride and Phenistix tests. *Postprandial determination.* Of phenylalanine tyrosine radiodiagnostic aid to recognize types I (classic) and II. Nine types of hyperphenylalaninemia have been identified with variable clinical and etiologic characteristics (see Hyperphenylalaninemia syndromes). *Electroencephalography. Pneumoencephalography.*

Therapy. Diet with phenylalanine limitation to minimal amount necessary for growth and repair. Preliminary trials with 5-hydroxytryptophan and L-dopa promising.

Prognosis. Poor. Treatment started as early as possible prevents or ameliorates development of expected defects.

BIBLIOGRAPHY. Folling A: Uber Ausscheidung von Phenylbrenztraubensäure in den Harn als Stoffwechselanomalie in Verbindung mit Imbezillität. Z Physio Chem 227:169–176, 1934

Thourain AY, Sidbury JB: Phenylketonuria. In Stanbury JB, Wyngaarden JB, Fredrickson DS: The Metabolic Basis of Inherited Disease, 4th ed, p 240. New York, McGraw-Hill, 1978

FORBES'

Synonyms. Amylo-1-6-glucosidase deficiency; Cori's type III glycogenosis, debrancher deficiency; glycogenosis type III limit dextrinosis.

Symptoms. Frequent in Israel. Both sexes affected; clinical onset in early childhood. Desire for sweets and carbohydrates; mild mental retardation; mild muscular weakness; Harris' (see).

Signs. Doll's facial features; marked hepatomegaly that recedes as the child grows (after about 4 yrs). Occasionally, moderate splenomegaly.

Etiology. Amylo-1-6-glucosidase (debrancher) deficiency leading to increase of glycogen in the liver, muscle, heart. Autosomal recessive inheritance.

Pathology. In early stage, large accumulation of glycogen in liver and only a moderate accumulation in heart and muscle fibers. Later random scarring of liver and early cirrhosis.

Diagnostic Procedures. *Blood.* Deficiency of amylo-1-6-glucosidase in leukocytes and erythrocytes; hypoglycemia; acetonemia; hyperlipemia. *Biopsy.* Of liver and muscle. Increased glycogen, absent amylo-1-6-glucosidase activity. *Electrocardiography, electromyography.* Usually normal.

Therapy. Diet rich in protein, protection from hypoglycemic crisis; trial with glucagon.

Prognosis. At adolescence, patient has regained normal growth, hepatomegaly decreased, no hypoglycemia. Persistence of altered glucose tolerance test and biochemical defect.

BIBLIOGRAPHY. Forbes GB: Glycogen storage disease: Report of a case with abnormal glycogen structure in liver and skeletal muscle. J Pediatr 42:645–653, 1953

Howell RR, Williams JC: The glycogen storage disease. In Stanbury JB, Wyngaarden JB, Fredrickson DS, et al: The Metabolic Basis of Inherited Disease, 5th ed, p 141. New York, McGraw-Hill, 1983

FORDYCE'S

Synonyms. Pseudocolloid lip mucous membrane sebaceous milia; See also Steatocystoma multiplex.

Symptoms. Asymptomatic.

Signs. Small yellowish papules, distributed on oral mucosa, lips, occasionally, genital region and breast.

Etiology. Unknown.

Pathology. Hypertrophic sebaceous glands free or connected by true sebaceous ducts.

Therapy. None.

Prognosis. Good.

BIBLIOGRAPHY. Fordyce J: A peculiar affection of the mucous membrane of the lips and oral cavity. J Cutan Dis NY 16:413–419, 1896

Rook A, Wilkinson DS, Ebling FJG, et al: Textbook of Dermatology, 4th ed, pp 1930, 2079, 2185. Oxford, Blackwell Scientific Publications, 1986

FORESTIER-ROTES-QUEROL

Synonyms. Hyperostosic spondylosis; senile ankylosing–vertebral hyperostosis; spondylorheostosis.

Symptoms and Signs. Occur in elderly people. Symptoms related to spine ossification of anterior ligaments. Degenerative changes of intervertebral disks (see Pulposus) and marginal osteophytosis leading to ankylosing.

Etiology. Unknown. It may represent a severe spondylosis (see Marie-Strumpell).

Pathology. See Symptoms. The cortex of vertebrae adjacent to ligaments ossified shows destructive changes.

Therapy. Physical therapy. Calcium; vitamin D; testosterone derivatives.

Prognosis. Progressing condition leading to ankylosing.

BIBLIOGRAPHY. Forestier J, Rotés Querol J: Senile ankylosing hyperostosis of the spine. Ann Rheum Dis 9:321–330, 1950

Clinical pathologic osteoarthritis workshop. (Queen's University, Kinston Ontario Canada). J Rheumatol 10 (suppl 9):1 (all issue), 1983

FORSIUS-ERIKSSON

Synonyms. Åland (refers to the island where the syndrome was discovered among natives); retina tapetal degeneration; tapetoretinal degeneration; 0A2.

Symptoms. Affects only males; females are carriers, usually asymptomatic, but may have, in some cases, slight latent nystagmus. Prematurity; mental retardation; epileptic attacks; impaired hearing; poor vision (myopia); defect in dark adaptation; dyschromatopsia.

Signs. Microphthalmia. Irregular latent nystagmus; astigmatism; tapetoretinal degeneration; localized pigment deficiency around macula and disk.

Etiology. X-chromosomal dominant type of inheritance or X-chromosomal recessive inheritance.

BIBLIOGRAPHY. Forsius H, Eriksson W: Ein neues Augensyndrome mit X-Chromosomaler Transmission. Eine Sippe mit Fundus Albinismus, Foveahypoplasie, Nystagmus, Myopie, Astigmatismus und Dyschromatopsie. Klin Monatsbl Augenheilkd 114:447–457, 1964

Witkop CJ, Quevedo WC, Fitzpatrick TB: Albinism and other disorders of pigment metabolism. In Stanbury JB, Wyngaarden JB, Fredrickson DS, et al: The Metabolic Basis of Inherited Disease, 5th ed, p 301. New York, McGraw-Hill, 1983

FORSSELL'S

Synonyms. Nephrogenic erythrocytosis; nephrogenic polycythemia.

Symptoms and Signs. Increase of red cell mass, with or without other features of polycythemia vera (see Vaquez-Osler).

Etiology. Renal pathology of various type, most frequently hypernephroma, followed by (in order) cystic disease, hydronephrosis, carcinoma, other tumors, and renal ischemia due to a disease of extrarenal vasculature. The association between renal pathology and erythrocytosis is inconsistent. The erythrocytosis seems to depend on the incretion of erythropoietin or a precursor formed by the tumor on the adjacent tissues compressed by it.

Pathology. See Vaquez–Osler and Etiology.

Diagnostic Procedures. *Blood and bone marrow.* Exclusion of polycythemia vera. *X-ray of kidney.*

Therapy. Removal of kidney lesions.

Prognosis. With removal of kidney lesions, cessation of erythrocytosis. With recurrence of lesion, recurrence of increased red cell production.

BIBLIOGRAPHY. Forssell J: Polycytemic vid hypernefrom. Nord Med 30:1415–1419, 1946

Wintrobe MM (ed): Clinical Hematology, 8th ed. Philadelphia, Lea & Febiger, 1981

FOSTER KENNEDY'S

Synonyms. Basofrontal; Gowers-Paton-Kennedy; Kennedy's

Symptoms. Reduction in visual acuity; headache; dizziness; vertigo; occasionally; forceful vomiting; psychic changes (moria); memory loss.

Signs. Papilledema of one eye; optical atrophy of the other, with central scotoma.

Etiology. Frontal lobe tumor or abscess producing homolateral optic atrophy and contralateral papilledema.

Pathology. Tumor (e.g., gliomas) or abscess of frontal lobe determining retrobulbar neuritis and increased intracranial pressure.

Diagnostic Procedures. *X-ray of skull. Angiography. Pneumoencephalography. Brain isotope scan. Electroencephalography. Spinal tap. CT brain scan.*

Therapy. If amenable to surgery, simple decompression (therapeutic or tapping) may partially relieve the symptomatology.

Prognosis. Poor, except if surgery is feasible.

BIBLIOGRAPHY. Kennedy F: Retrobulbar neuritis as an exact diagnostic sign of certain tumors and abscesses in the frontal lobes. Am J Med Sci 142:355–368, 1911
Vick NA: Grinker's Neurology, 7th ed. Springfield, CC Thomas, 1976

FOTHERGILL'S

Synonyms. Trigeminal neuralgia; tic douloureux trifacial neuralgic.

Symptoms. Prevalent in females; onset usually after 45 years of age. Any division of trigeminal (V) nerve involved singly or in combination. Paroxystic attack of short, shooting pain, usually starting at a constant point (trigger point on the cheek, near lips or gums, side of tongue; and other locations) and diffusing to involve all territory of branch or branches affected. Ophthalmic branch less frequently involved. Peripheral stimulation of trigger point usually initiates attack. To avoid them, patient may not eat or drink and may become emaciated and dehydrated, or grow beard, and may not clean affected side. Usually, no night attacks, and little interference with sleep.

Etiology. Unknown; multiple types of sclerosis irritation around Gasser's ganglion may produce attacks. Autosomal dominant inheritance reported in some kindred.

Pathology. No specific findings of Gasser's ganglion.

Diagnostic Procedures. *X-rays of teeth, sinuses, skull. Angiography. Brain scan.*

Therapy. Vitamin B_{12}; hydantoin; carbamazepine (Tegretol); alcohol infiltration; retrogasserian neurotomy. Other neurosurgical procedures in particular cases.

Prognosis. Attacks last a few moments, stop spontaneously. Paroxysmal attacks recur frequently with intermission of weeks or years.

BIBLIOGRAPHY. Fothergill J: Of a painful affection of the face. Med Obs Ing 5:129, 1773
Herzberg L: Familial trigeminal neuralgia. Arch Neurol 37:285–286, 1980

FOURTH VENTRICLE

Synonyms. Cerebellar line median; vermis.

Symptoms and Signs. Both sexes, all ages affected. Severe trunk ataxia; bilateral choked disks; coarse horizontal nystagmus in lateral terminal positions. Variable signs of fourth ventricle nuclei involvement: facial palsy; diminished corneal reflex; ocular dysmetria; vomiting; stiffness, and pain in neck and shoulders.

Etiology. Lesions of fourth venricle.

Pathology. Neoplastic, vascular, or inflammatory lesion of floor of fourth ventricle, usually involving nuclei of trigeminal (V), abducens (VI), and facial (VII) nerves and medial longitudinal fasciculus.

Diagnostic Procedures. *CT brain scan. Pneumoencephalography. Angiography. Spinal tap.*

Therapy. According to etiology.

Prognosis. Depends on etiology.

BIBLIOGRAPHY. van Bogaert L, Marlin P: Les tumeurs du quatrième venricule et le syndrome cérébelleux de la ligne médiane. Rev Neurol 2:431–483, 1928
Acers TE, Tenney R: Ocular symptomatology of posterior fossa tumors. Am J Ophthalmol 65:872–876, 1968

FOVILLE'S I

Synonyms. Alternating inferior hemiplegia; Foville's peduncular.

Symptoms and Signs. Hemiplegia; deviation of eye opposite side or paralysis of lateral gaze, in irritative lesions deviation toward hemiplegic side. Ipsilateral nuclear facial paralysis.

Etiology. Neoplastic, hemorrhagic, infective, degenerative lesions of pons involving longitudinal fasciculus.

Pathology. See Etiology.

Therapy. Conservative or surgical if indicated.

Prognosis. Depends on etiology.

BIBLIOGRAPHY. Foville A: Note sur une paralysie peu connue de certain muscles de l'oeil, et sa liaison avec quelques points de l'anatomie et la physiologie la protubérance annulaire. Bull Soc Anat 33:394–414, 1858
Vick NA: Grinker's Neurology, 7th ed. Springfield, CC Thomas, 1976

FOVILLE'S II

Synonyms. Alternating inferior hemiplegia; pontine Foville's.

Symptoms and Signs. Same symptoms and signs as in Foville's I, but without facial nerve involvement.

BIBLIOGRAPHY. Foville A: Note sur une paralysie peu connue de certain muscles de l'oeil, et sa liasion avec quelques points de l'anatomie et la physiologie la protubérance annulaire. Gaz Hebd Med 6:146, 1859
Vick NA: Grinker's Neurology, 7th ed. Springfield, CC Thomas, 1976

FOVILLE-WILSON

Symptoms and Signs. Impairment of lateral convergence of different degree in the two eyes; paralysis of adduction; abduction insufficient. Abducted eye: ample horizontal nystagmus, but the other eye does not adduct, does not show nystagmus, or shows only irregular, exhaustible jerks. Preservation of convergence.

Etiology. See Multiple sclerosis.

Pathology. See Multiple sclerosis.

Therapy. See Multiple sclerosis.

Prognosis. See Multiple sclerosis.

BIBLIOGRAPHY. Foville A: Note sure une paralysie peu connue de certain muscles de l'oeil, et sa liasion avec quelques points de l'anatomie et la physiologie de la protubérance annulaire. Bull Soc Anat 33:394–414, 1858
Wilson SAK: Case of disseminated sclerosis with weakness of each internal rectus et nystagmus. Brain 29:298, 1906
Spaccarelli G: Sindrome di Foville-Wilson e paralisi internucleare posteriore. Boll Ocul 27:228–245, 1948

FOX-FORDYCE

Synonym. Apocrine miliaris.

Symptoms. Onset after puberty; prevalent almost exclusively in women. Males and children less frequently affected. Recurrent episodes of severe pruritus.

Signs. Skin hyperpigmentation in the axillae, pubis, sternum, and nipples areolae; presence of dry papulae. Broken hair.

Etiology. Obstruction of sweat glands pori; rupture of duct and escape of the sweat into epidermis. Emotional factors precipitating the attack.

Pathology. Formation of vesicle around duct of sweat glands; dilatation and rupture of the ducts.

Therapy. Topical and systemic hormonal treatment; (testosterone). Roentgen irradiation in epilation dose. Topical retinoic acid. Contraceptive agents.

Prognosis. Recurrence; possible remission during pregnancy; spontaneous remission after menopause. Encephalitis possible complication.

BIBLIOGRAPHY. Fox G, Fordyce J: Two cases of a rare papular disease affecting the axillary region. J Cutan Dis 20:1–5, 1902
Rook A, Wilkinson DS, Ebling FJG, et al: Textbook of Dermatology, 4th ed, pp 1895–1896. Oxford, Blackwell Scientific Publications, 1986

FOX'S

Obsolete term. Comprises both Weber-Cockaine (see) and Goldscheider's (see).

BIBLIOGRAPHY. Fox T: Notes on unusual or rare forms of skin disease. IV. Congenital ulceration of skin (two cases) with pemphigus eruption and arrest of development generally. Lancet 1:766–767, 1879

FRAGA'S

See Addisonian syndromes. Chronic or acute Addison's syndrome due to malaria.

BIBLIOGRAPHY. Fraga A: Supra-renalite aguda no impaludismo. Brazil Med 31:349, 1917
Fraga C: La forma suprarenal del paludismo. Rev Iber Am Cien Med 40:9–19, 1918

FRAGILE X

Synonyms. Martin-Bell; FRAXA.

Symptoms and Signs. Appears in boys (homozygous in the first year of life). Long face and large prominent ears; macroorchidism; prognathism, large head circumference in early childhood; hyperextensible finger joints, mitral valve prolapse, aortic dilation, pectus excavatum, high-arched palate, myopia, flat feet, abnormal dermatoglyphics. Behavioral features: hand stereotypes; cluttered speech; hyperactivity; autism. Heterozygous females have a broad range of dysfunction: normal, mildly affected, or severely autistic.

Etiology. A specific region on the X chromosome fails to condense normally during mitosis and is characterized by a nonstaining gap or constriction.

Diagnostic Procedures. *Lymphocyte cultures.* Affected patients demonstrate the defect in 5 to 50% (average 20%) of cells.

Therapy. Early speech and language therapy, occupational therapy, and special education assistance. Medical therapy: central nervous system stimulants, folic acid, and phenothiazines. Trimethoprim may lead to exacerbation of behavior problems, and this drug should be avoided.

Prognosis. With proper treatment decrease in the frequency and severity of autistic features and improvement in development performance.

BIBLIOGRAPHY. Martin JP, Bell J: A pedigree of mental defect showing sex-linkage. J Neurol Neurosurg Psychiatry 6:154–156, 1943
Mixon JC, Dev VG: Understanding the fragile X syndrome. Ala J Med Sci 21:284–286, 1984
Chludley AE, Hageiman RJ: Fragile X syndrome. J Paediatr 110:821–831, 1987

FRAME'S

Synonym. Axial osteomalacia.

Symptoms. Both sexes. Caucasian and black. Diagnosed in middle age. Presenting symptoms: vague chronic axial pain, followed by back pain, fatigue in the extremities.

Signs. Mild tenderness to percussion over lumbar spine, no paravertebral muscle spasm, limited spinal range of motion possibly associated with polycystic kidney and liver disease.

Etiology. Unknown. Bone cells enzyme defect leading to impaired bone formation. Disorder of vitamin D action (?). Autosomal dominant inheritance.

Pathology. Bone mean cortical width and cortical porosity increased; in medullary space: trabecular bone varies in thickness and forms a complicated branching network.

Diagnostic Procedures. *Blood.* Normal or negative results. Creatine phosphokinase increased; alkaline phosphatase activity increased. *Urine.* Normal. *X-rays.* From early adulthood. Coarsening of trabecular bone pattern of the axial, but not appendicular, skeleton. *Bone biopsy.* Osteomalacia of rib or iliac crest. Tetracycline labelling to assess rate of bone formation.

Therapy. Vitamin D + Ca: decreases unmineralized osteoid but no effect on symptoms.

Prognosis. Benign clinical course.

BIBLIOGRAPHY. Frame B, Frost HM, Ormond RS, et al: Atypical osteomalacia involving the axial skeleton. Ann Intern Med 55:632–639, 1961
White MP, Fallon MD, Murphy WA, et al: Axial osteomalacia: Clinical, laboratory and genetic investigation of an affected mother and son. Am J Med 71: 1041–1049, 1981

FRANCESCHETTI-KAUFMAN

Synonyms. Franceschetti's dystrophy; Kaufman's; metaherpetic keratitis; posttraumatic keratitis; corneal erosion recurring; keratitis fugax hereditaria; Valle's.

Symptoms. Pain when opening the eyes in the morning; diminishing as the day progresses. Mild fever.

Signs. Nondendritic corneal ulcer and stromal edema.

Etiology. Previous corneal trauma (virus; chemical; foreign bodies) that has damaged the epithelial basis. Or hereditary familial form autosomal dominant.

Pathology. Ovoid nondendritic ulcer due to poor attachment of new epithelial regrowth and accumulation of fluid in the stroma and corneal epithelium.

Diagnostic Procedures. *Virus culture.* Negative. Defects stain positively with fluorescein.

Therapy. Emollients and corticosteroids; not affected by chemical cautery or antiviral agents.

Prognosis. Good with proper treatment; improving with age.

BIBLIOGRAPHY. Franceschetti A: Hereditäre Rezidivierende. Erosion der Hornhaut. Z Augenheilkd 66:309–316, 1928
Kaufman HE: Epithelial erosion syndrome: Metaherpetic keratitis. Am J Ophthalmol 57:983–987, 1964
Valle O: Keratitis fugax hereditarie. Duodecim 80:659–664, 1964

FRANCESCHETTI-KLEIN

Synonyms. Berry-Franceschetti-Klein; mandibulofacial dysostosis; Franceschetti-Zwahlen-Klein; Treacher Collins-Franceschetti. See Pierre Robin and Treacher Collins.

Symptoms and Signs. Evident at birth. Difficulty in sucking and swallowing; excessive mucus in mouth; cyanotic spells. Complete form includes antimongoloid obliquity of palpebral fissures, notching of lower eyelids, flattening of molar bones (Treacher Collins), small mandible, receding chin, considerable overbite, high arched palate, macrostomia, malformation of ears. Atypical hair growth. Incomplete, abortive, and unilateral forms described.

Etiology. See First arch syndrome. Autosomal dominant inheritance.

Pathology. Faulty development of multiple elements of first arch.

Diagnostic Procedures. *Chromosome studies.* Normal. *X-ray. Audiography.*

Therapy. Feeding major problem, use of feeder or gavage. If cyanosis attacks frequent, immobilization of tongue by stitching it to lower jaw.

Prognosis. Feeding trouble and cyanosis attacks disappear in a few weeks or months. The other congenital defects affect life and development according to severity.

BIBLIOGRAPHY. Berry GA: Note of congenital defect (coloboma) of lower lid. London Ophthalmol Hosp Rep 12:255–277, 1889
Collins ET: Cases with symmetrical congenital notches in the outer part of each lower lid and defective development of the molar bones. Trans Ophthalmol Soc UK 20:190–192, 1933
Franceschetti A: Un syndrome nouveau; La dysostose mandibulofaciale. Bull Schweiz Akad Med Wiss 1:60–66, 1944
Franceschetti A, Klein D: The mandibulofacial dysostosis, a new hereditary syndrome. Acta Ophthalmol (Copenh) 27:143–224, 1949
Balestrazzi P, Baeteman MA, Mattei MG, et al: Franceschetti syndrome in a child with a de novo balanced translocation (5 : 13) (q11 : p11) and significant decrease of hexosaminidase B. Hum Genet 64:305–308, 1983

FRANCESCHETTI'S

Synonyms. Fundus flavimaculatus. FF; see Stargardt's.

Symptoms. Both sexes affected; onset between 10 and 25 years of age. Impairment of central vision with intact peripheral retinal function.

Signs. Irregular yellowish deposits in and around macula lutea forming a "garland."

Etiology. Unknown; autosomal recessive inheritance.

Diagnostic Procedures. *Electroretinography.* Normal.

Therapy. None.

BIBLIOGRAPHY. Franceschetti A, François J, Babel J: Les Hérédo-Dégénérescences chorio-rétiniennes, Vol 1. Paris, 1963

Isashiki Y, Ohba N: Fundus flavimaculatus: Polymorphic retinal change in siblings. Br J Ophthalmol 69:522–524, 1985

FRANCESCHETTI-THIER

Symptoms and Signs. Mental retardation; multiple lipomas; corneal dystrophy.

Etiology. Unknown; autosomal recessive inheritance.

BIBLIOGRAPHY. Franceschetti A, Thier CJ: Hornhautdystrophien bei Genodermatosen unter besonderen Berucksichtingung der Palmoplantarkeratosen. Albrecht von Graefes Arch Ophthalmol 162:610–670, 1961
Der Koloustian VM, Jarudi NI, Khoury MJ, et al: Familial spinocerebellar degeneration with corneal atrophy. Am J Med Genet 20:325–339, 1985

FRANÇOIS' I

Synonyms. Chondrodermal corneal dystrophy; corneal-chondrodermal dystrophy; dermochondrocorneal dystrophy; Jensen's.

Symptoms and Signs. Both sexes affected; normal at birth, onset at 1 to 2 years of age. Osteochondral deformities of hands and feet; subluxation and tendinous contractures may develop; concomitant development of xanthomalike, small, yellowish, hard nodules in the skin. Later, appearance of bilateral peripheral or central corneal opacities and seizures.

Etiology. Unknown; possibly autosomal recessive inheritance. Related to lipid storage and possibly to mucopolysaccharidosis (not studied) disorders.

Pathology. *Skin.* Corium with large, round or elongated cells with vacuolated cytoplasm (no lipids), dense connective tissue with some lymphatic space. Similar cells in the cornea. *Bone.* Defective endochrondral ossification involving short and long bones.

Diagnostic Procedures. *Blood.* Possibly, a hypercholesterolemic phase. *X-ray.* Skeleton survey. *Electroencephalography.* Abnormalities.

Therapy. Orthopedic correction.

Prognosis. Chronic progression.

BIBLIOGRAPHY. François J: Dystrophie dermochondrocornéene familiale. Ann Ocul 182:409–422, 1949
Jensen E: Retino-choroiditis justapa pillaris. Abrecht Von Graefes Arch Ophthalmol 69:41–48, 1909
Reigin RD, Caplan DB: Corneal opacities in infancy and childhood. J Pediatr 69:383–392, 1966

McKusick VA: Heritable Disorders of Connective Tissue. St Louis, CV Mosby, 1972
Caputo R, Sambvani N, Monti M, et al: Dermochondrocorneal dystrophy (François syndrome). Arch Dermatol 124:424–428, 1988

FRANCOIS-EVENS

Synonym. Annular dystrophy of corneal endothelium.

Symptoms. Occur at different ages. Vision and corneal sensitivity normal. Small flat granular opacity ring shaped at the level of corneal endothelium, peripheral zone of posterior side.

Etiology. Unknown.

Prognosis. Benign, nonprogressive condition.

BIBLIOGRAPHY. François J, Evens A: Hérédodystrophie anulaire de l'endothelium cornéen. Atti Congr Soc Oftalm Ital 18:352, 1959
Goldberg MF: Genetic and Metabolic Eye Disease, p 308. Boston, Little, Brown & Co, 1974

FRANÇOIS-HAUSTRATE

Synonym. Otomandibular dysostosis.

Symptoms and Signs. Hemifacial microsomia; microphthalmia, coloboma of uveal tract and optic disk.

Etiology. Consider a variant of hemifacial microsomia. (see).

BIBLIOGRAPHY. François J, Haustrate L: Anomalies colobomatuses de globe oculaire et syndrome du prémièr arc. Ann Ocul 187:340–368, 1954

FRANÇOIS-NEETENS

Synonyms. Corneal dystrophy speckled, corneal dystrophy flecked; François dystrophy I; corneal dystrophy cloudy.

Symptoms. Both sexes affected; identified from 2 years of age or later. Vision normal; corneal sensation normal.

Signs. In the corneal stroma presence of small, semiopaque, flat opacities involving the centrum and the periphery. Opacities show a granular or homogeneous gray color and are neatly separated from each other by clear cornea.

Etiology. Autosomal dominant inheritance.

Diagnostic Procedures. *Corneal reflexes.* May be depressed. *Retroillumination.* Shows opacities and their distribution, which does not involve Bowman's layer and Descemet's membrane.

Therapy. None.

Prognosis. Static disorders.

BIBLIOGRAPHY. François J, Neetens A: Nouvelle dystrophie hérédofamiliale du parenchyme cornéen (hérédodystrophie monchetée). Bull Soc Belg Ophthalmol 114:641–646, 1957
Nicholson DH, Green WR, Cross HE, et al: A clinical and histopathological study of François–Neetens speckled corneal dystrophy. Am J Ophthalmol 83:554–560, 1977

FRANKL-HOCHWART'S

Synonyms. Ophthalmic-neuropineal; von Frankl-Hochwart's

Symptoms and Signs. Bilateral deafness; ataxia; headache; vomiting; according to age of onset, various manifestation of hypopituitarism. Limitation of upward gaze; constriction of visual fields; choked disk; papilledema.

Etiology and Pathology. Tumor of pineal gland.

Diagnostic Procedures. *X-ray of skull. Pneumoencephalography. Angiography. CT brain scan. Blood and urine.* Demonstrate hypopituitarism. (See Simmond's).

Therapy. Surgery and x-ray treatment.

Prognosis. Poor.

BIBLIOGRAPHY. von Frankl–Hochwart L: Ueber Diagnose der Zirbeldrüsetumoren. Dtsch Z Nervenh 37:455, 1909; 38:309, 1910
Tassman I: The Eye Manifestations of Internal Disease, 3rd ed. St. Louis, CV Mosby, 1951
Roy FH: Ocular Syndromes and Systemic Diseases. Orlando, Grune & Stratton, 1985

FRANKLIN'S

Synonyms. Heavy chain (gamma); gamma heavy chain; gamma HCD.

Symptoms and Signs. Occur in both sexes (slight male predominance); onset in middle age. Abrupt onset of lymphadenopathy without fever. Edema and erythema of uvula and soft palate occasionally noticed. Spleen enlargement sometimes during course of disease; hepatomegaly not constantly. Spontaneous regression of lymphadenopathy after some time. Pallor. Frequently associated with various conditions; lupus erythematosus; rheumatoid arthritis; Sjögren's; Erb-Goldflam; hemolytic anemia.

Etiology. Unknown. Possible autoimmune disorder.

Pathology. *Lymph node.* Atypical and immature plasma cells; reticulum cells, atypical lymphocytes, eosinophils, and cells not easily classifiable. Lymph node pattern may suggest Hodgkin's disease. *Bone marrow.* Similar cells to these described in lymph nodes. Erythroid hyperplasia. Liver biopsy normal.

Diagnostic Procedures. *Blood.* Normochromic anemia; hyperuricemia. Presence in the serum of large amount of IgG fragment. Abnormal and incomplete production of antibodies. *Urine.* Presence of IgG fragment. *X-ray.* Chest lymphadenopathy; normal skeleton. *Bone marrow.* Normal or increased plasma cells, lymphocytes, reticular cells; eosinophilia. *Biopsy.* Of lymph node. Similar type of cells as those mentioned in bone marrow.

Therapy. Trial with chemotherapy; corticosteroids. Alkylating agents; corticosteroids; combination chemotherapy with MOPP. Radiotherapy not recommended.

Prognosis. Poor. Supervening infection is frequent cause of death. Some patients have survived for 5 years or longer.

BIBLIOGRAPHY. Franklin EC, Lowenstein J, Bigelow B, et al: Heavy chain disease: A new disorder of serum gamma globulins. Report of the first case. Am J Med 37:332–350, 1964

Osserman EF, Takatsuki K: Clinical and immunochemical studies of four cases of heavy (Hτ 2) chain disease. Am J Med 37:351–373, 1964

Brouet JC: Les Maladies des chaines lourdes. In Encycl Med Chir, Paris Sang 13013 F10, 1980

FRANZ'S

Indicates the cessation of the thrill that is observed after the proximal venous section of an arterovenous fistula.

BIBLIOGRAPHY. Franz CA: Klinische und experimentelle Beigrage betreffend das Aneurysma arteriovenosum. Arch Klin Chir 75:572–623, 1905

FRASER'S

Synonyms. Cryptophthalmos syndactyly; Meyers-Schwickerath; Ullrich-Feichtiger. See Cyclopia.

Symptoms and Signs. Both sexes affected. Occasionally, stillborn. Cryptophthalmos (hidden eye), complete failure in development of lid folds, or subsequent destruction and absorption of lids. May be bilateral, monolateral, or cryptophthalmos on one side and microphthalmos on the other side. Associated defects: middle and external ear malformation; high or cleft palate; deformity of larynx; hoarse voice; wide separation of symphysis pubis; displacement of umbilicus and nipples; various digital malformations; meningoencephaloceles; anal stenosis; congenital cardiac malformation; renal hypoplasia or agenesis. Masculinization of external genitalia in females. Cryptorchidism, small penis, hypospadias in males.

Etiology. Unknown; autosomal recessive inheritance(?). Possibility of altered sex chromosomal pattern.

Pathology. Eye enophthalmos or various alteration; buphophthalmos; absence of trabeculae, Schlemm canal, and ciliary muscles; abnormal lens. See Signs.

Diagnostic Procedures. *Chromosome study. Endocrine studies.*

Therapy. Early surgical intervention may help in preserving adequate visual perception.

Prognosis. Survival depends on renal involvement and other malformations.

BIBLIOGRAPHY. Zehender W: Eine Missgeburt mit hautüberwachsenen Augen oder Kryptophthalmus. Klin Monatsbl Augenheilkd 10:225, 1872

Gupta SP, Saxena RC: Cryptophthalmos. Brit J Ophthalmol 46:629–632, 1962

Fraser CR: Our genetic "load" A review of some aspects of genetical variation. Ann Hum Genet 25:387, 1962

Mortimer G, McEwans HP, Yates JRW: Fraser syndrome presenting as monozygotic twins with bilateral renal agenesis. J Med Genet 22:76–78, 1985

FREEMAN–SHELDON

Synonyms. Craniocarpotarsal dystrophy; whistling face. Windmill vane hand.

Symptoms. Present from birth. Prematurity. Vomiting; feeding difficulties; failure to thrive (secondary to feeding difficulties). Normal mental development. Nasal speech.

Signs. *Facies.* Masklike; small mouth; whistling aspect; H-shaped dimple of chin. *Eyes.* Deep set. Epicanthus. *Nose.* Small; broad bridge; hypoplastic alae; long philtrum. *Mouth.* Small tongue; high palate. *Hands.* Ulnar deviation; thickening of skin of flexor aspect of proximal phalanges. *Feet.* Equinovarus. Associated abnormalities: small stature; scoliosis; strabismus; blepharophimosis. Generalized myopathy that is associated with the later development of kyphoscoliosis. In addition to intercostal myopathy, this can lead to restrictive lung disease.

Etiology. Sporadic, or autosomal dominant inheritance.

Diagnostic Procedures. *X-ray.* Skeletal survey. *Blood.* Normal. *Chromosome studies. Electromyography. Muscle biopsy.*

Therapy. Treatment consists of correcting malnutrition of the infant combined with corrective surgery in the child and adult for the wide range of musculoskeletal deformities, especially scoliosis.

Prognosis. Occasionally, failure to thrive. Normal intelligence. Possible reproduction. Early corrective surgery of the deformities can result in the patient leading a normal life with normal expectancy.

BIBLIOGRAPHY. Freeman EA, Sheldon JH: Cranio-carpo-tarsal dystrophy. An undescribed congenital formation. Arch Dis Child 13:277–283, 1938
Laishley RS, Roy WL: Freeman–Sheldon syndrome: Report of three cases and the anaesthetic implications. Can Anaesth Soc J 33:388–393, 1986

FREIBERG'S INFRACTION

Synonyms. Freiberg's; metatarsal head osteochondritis. See Epiphyseal ischemic necrosis.

Symptoms and Signs. Dull pain in anterior part of foot induced by walking. Swelling of metatarsal-phalangeal joint; overlying skin red.

Etiology. Epiphyseal ischemic necrosis of 4th or 5th metatarsal head.

Therapy. In acute stage, antiflammatory agents. Later if pain, deformity, or disability, surgery.

BIBLIOGRAPHY. Köhler A: Eine typische Erkrankung des 2 Metatarso-phalangeal-gealaelenkes. MMW 67:1289–1290, 1920
Freiberg AH: The so-called infraction of the second metatarsal bone. J Bone Joint Surg. 8:257–261, 1926
Richardson EG: The foot in adolescents and adults. In Crenshaw AH (ed), Campbell's Operative Orthopedics, pp 959–960. 7th ed, St Louis, CV Mosby, 1987

FRENKEL'S

Synonyms. Eyeball contusion; ocular contusion, anterior segment traumatic.

Symptoms. History of trauma of the anterior segment of eye. Visual disturbances.

Signs. D-shaped mydriasis (chord replacing the arc in a sector) observed in 85% of cases; single or multiple iris dehiscences (50%); lens lesions (opacities and sublux-ation) (60%); retrolenticular pigment particles (56%). Posterior segment lesions may also coexist.

Etiology. The syndrome consists of the variable sequelae observed after the trauma (sometimes months or, occasionally, years later).

Pathology. See Signs.

Diagnostic Procedures. *Slit lamp microscopic examination. Transillumination of iris.*

Therapy. As indicated by type of lesions.

Prognosis. Guarded.

BIBLIOGRAPHY. Frenkel H: Sur la valeur médicolégale du syndrome traumatique du segment antéreur. Arch Ophthalmol 48:5–27, 1931
Paton D, Goldberg MF: Injuries of the lids and the orbit: Diagnosis and Management. Philadelphia, WB Saunders, 1976

FREY'S (L.)

Synonyms. Auriculotemporal; Baillarger's; Dupuy's; salivosudoriparous; sweating gustatory; von Frey's.

Symptoms and Signs. Unilateral localized flushing and hyperhydrosis of the pinna of ear and cheek, when eating hot, bitter, spicy substances or chocolate, or rinsing mouth, especially with acid substances; decreased sensitivity to the heat in the involved area. Flushing prevalent in females; sweating in males.

Etiology. Following injury or surgery of the parotid gland, or associated with infection of the gland in response to ingestion of acid food. Related to one of these mechanisms: regeneration of salivary fibers into sweat fiber; hypersensitivity of denervated sweat fibers.

Pathology. See Etiology.

Diagnostic Procedures. *Starch-iodine test.* Test the reflex with acid and substance on posterior third of tongue.

Therapy. Procaine injection of auriculotemporal nerve at the tragus level. Resection of parasympathetic tympanic plexus. Tympanic plexus resection.

Prognosis. Possible extension of area of involvement. In most patients symptoms tolerated; 10% require surgery.

BIBLIOGRAPHY. Frey L: Le syndrome du nerf auricolotemporal. Rev Neurol (Paris) 2:97–104, 1923
Daly RF: New observations regarding the auriculotemporal syndrome. Neurology 17:1159–1168, 1967
Ven Dishoeck HAE: The auriculo-temporal or Frey syndrome and tympanic neurectomy. Laryngoscope 78:122–131, 1968

Rook A, Wilkinson DS, Ebling FJG, et al: Textbook of Dermatology, 4th ed, p 1890. Oxford, Blackwell Scientific Publications, 1986

FRIEDREICH–AUERBACH

Synonym. Hypertrophic myopathy.

Symptoms. Prevalent in males; onset usually in childhood, adolescence, or early adult life. Vague onset. Occasionally, poorly localized, vague, painful sensation in muscles affected.

Signs. Slow enlargement of the muscles of limbs more frequently than trunk. Any muscle of the body however may be affected, including tongue. Different muscles may be involved at same time or successively. Strength of affected muscle usually increased. Myotonic phenomenon in 50% of cases. Reflexes normal. Hyperhidrosis of limb or side involved frequently observed. No visceral or skeletal involvement.

Etiology. Unknown.

Pathology. Enlargement of muscle fibers. Nuclei may be found in central part of fibers; occasionally, vascular wall slightly thickened.

Diagnostic Procedures. *Electromyography.* Normal.

Therapy. None.

Prognosis. Spontaneous arrest.

BIBLIOGRAPHY. Auerbach L: Ein Fall von Waher Muskelhypertrophie. Virchows Arch [Pathol Anat] 53:397–417, 1817
Friedriech N: Ueber congenitale halbseitige Kopfhypertrophie. Virchows Arch [Pathol Anat] 28:474–481, 1963
Adams RD, Denny–Brown D, Pearson CM: Diseases of the Muscle, 3rd ed, p 536. New York, Harper & Row, 1975

FRIEDREICH'S

Synonyms. Essential myoclonia; paramyoclonus multiplex, including myoclonus hereditary essential.

Symptoms and Signs. Onset usually in adult life. Sudden, brief, clonic jerks affecting single muscle part, entire muscle, or muscle group. With excitement contractions increase; stop during sleep.

Etiology. More a symptom than a syndrome. (1) Part of petit mal syndrome may initially be the only manifestation; (2) symptom of diffuse central nervous system degenerative diseases; (3) "sleep start," "night start," violent muscle contractions occurring in young healthy man; fatigue at time of awaking. Familial occurrence reported with autosomal dominant type of inheritance.

BIBLIOGRAPHY. Friedreich N: Paramyoclonus multiplex. Arch Pathol Anat 86:421–430, 1881
Lance JW: Myoclonic jerks and falls: An etiology, classification and treatment. Med J Aust 1:113–119, 1968
Korten JJ, Notermans SLH, Frenken CWGM, et al: Familial essential myoclonus. Brain 97:131–138, 1974

FRIEDREICH'S ATAXIA

Synonyms. Spinocerebellar ataxia; FA.

Symptoms. Onset in first year of life; only deformity of feet (pes cavus; Friedreich foot; hammer toe). Onset between 7 and 15 years of age; clumsy gait that becomes more and more ataxic and broad based, difficulty in turning arms, head, and trunk. Patients are affected later with tremor, dysmetria, asynergia, dysdiadochokinesia, slow ataxic speech, choreiform movement, and occasionally, pain and paresthesias. Blindness and deafness also reported.

Signs. Tendon reflexes decreased and then lost. Babinski sign. Nystagmus. Loss of position sense, vibratory sense, and two-point discrimination. Kyphoscoliosis in the thoracic column. Muscle wasting, more on lower extremity. High percentage of patients with signs of cardiac involvement.

Etiology. Unknown; autosomal recessive or dominant (rarely).

Pathology. Degeneration of spinocerebellar tracts, corticospinal tracts, and posterior columns of spinal cord. Optical and cochlear degeneration (possibly).

Diagnostic Procedures. *Spinal fluid.* Normal or occasionally moderate increase of protein and cells. *Electrocardiography.* Occasionally, bundle-branch block or complete heart block. *X-ray.* Marked scoliosis; pes cavus. *Blood.* Frequently, hyperglycemia.

Therapy. None.

Prognosis. Progressive; occasionally, remission; possibly incapacitating by 20 years of age. Death from intercurrent diseases or cardiac failure.

BIBLIOGRAPHY. Friedreich N: Über degenerative Atrophie der spinalen, Hinterstränge. Arch Anat Physiol 26:391–419, 1863
Spoendlin H: Optic and cochleo-vestibular degeneration in hereditary ataxia II. Temporal bone pathology in two cases of Friedreich's ataxia with vestibulocochlear disorders. Brain 97:41–48, 1974
Ackroyd RS, Finnegan JA, Green SH: Friedreich's ataxia: A clinical review with neurophysiological and

echocardiographic findings. Arch Dis Child 59:217–221, 1984

FROEHLICH'S

Synonyms. Adiposogenital; Babinski-Froehlich; hypothalamic infantilism-obesity; sexual infantilism; Leaunois-Cléret.

Symptoms. Prevalent in males. Headache; retarded growth and sexual development; mental retardation; visual troubles; polyuria; polydipsia.

Signs. Prepubertal adiposity of breast, abdomen, femoral regions, large hips. Delayed appearance of secondary sexual characteristic, hair of pubis, axillae, face. Skin remains delicate. Dysonychia.

Etiology. Hypopituitarism; hypothalamic functional alterations; tumor compressing or involving anterior pituitary gland; idiopathic. Wilkins suggests limiting the diagnosis of Froehlich syndrome to only those cases in which the pituitary disturbance is proved.

Pathology. See above; occasionally, craniopharyngioma.

Diagnostic Procedures. *Urine.* Follicle-stimulating hormone (FSH), luteinizing hormone (LH), and 17-ketosteroid determinations. Vasopressin test for polyuria if diabetes insipidus. *X-ray.* Of skull. Suprasellar calcification or destructive lesion. Skeleton shows delayed ossification.

Therapy. If tumor extirpation or x-ray, administration of pituitary extracts.

Prognosis. Depends on etiology.

BIBLIOGRAPHY. Froehlich A: Ein Fall von Tumor der Hypophysis Cerebri ohne Akromegalie. Wien Klin Rundshan 15:833–836; 906–908, 1901
Launois PE, Cléret M: Le syndrome hypophisaire adipose-génital. Gaz Hôp 83:57–64; 83–86, 1910
Bruch H: The Froehlich syndrome; Report of the original case. Am J Dis Child 58:1282–1289, 1939
Christy MP, Warren MP: Disease syndromes of the hypothalamus and anterior pituitary. In De Groot LJ, Cahill GF Jr, Odell WD, et al (eds): Endocrinology. New York, Grune & Stratton, 1979

FROIN'S

Synonyms. Lépine–Froin; Nonne's II; spinal fluid coagulation. Froin syndrome is the designation for the coagulation of spinal fluid shortly after being removed. Observed in tumor of spinal cord, in chronic arachnoiditis and other conditions where a marked increase of protein occurs.

BIBLIOGRAPHY. Froin G: Inflammation méningées avec reactions chromatiques, fibrineuse et cytologique. Gaz Hôp 76:1005–1006, 1903
Grinker RR: Chronic arachno-perineuritis with the syndrome of Froin, pseudotumor spinalis. J Nerv Ment Dis 64:616–628, 1926

FRONTONASAL DYSPLASIA

Synonym. Median cleft face.

Symptoms and Signs. Both sexes affected; present from birth. *Midline frontal bone.* Extremely variable degree of deficits: widow's peak; hypertelorism. *Nasal tip.* Variable degree of alteration from notched broad to divided nostrils; absence of prolabia with median cleft lip or without cleft palate. Mental deficiency severe in 8% of cases, mild in 12%.

Etiology. Unknown. Sporadic. Both autosomal dominant and recessive inheritance proposed.

Therapy. Cosmetic surgery.

Prognosis. Good *quoad vitam;* usually, normal mental development.

BIBLIOGRAPHY. Hoppe I: Eine angeborene Spaltung der Nase. Preuss Med 2:164–165, 1859
De Meyer W: The median cleft face syndrome. Differential diagnosis of cranium bifidum occultum, hypertelorism and median cleft nose, lip and palate. Neurology 17:961–971, 1967
Kwee ML, Lindhout D: Frontonasal dysplasia, coronal craniosynostosis, pre- and postaxial polydactyly and split nails: A new autosomal dominant mutant with reduced penetrance and variable expression? Clin Genet 24:200–205, 1983

FRUCTOSE 1, 6-DIPHOSPHATASE HEREDITARY DEFICIENCY

Synonyms. Baker-Winegrad; fructose 1, 6-Diphosphatase deficiency.

Symptoms. Both sexes affected; occur in infants, usually before 6 months of age after ingesting food containing fructose or after infections, fatigue, fasting, and stress severe hypoglycemia (fits; seizures; coma) and acidosis frequently fatal or requiring hospitalization. Nausea and vomiting do not occur after fructose ingestion. At older age no aversion to sugar and sweets.

Signs. The child is not emaciated; frequently obese and hepatomegalic.

Etiology. Autosomal recessive inheritance; deficiency of fructose 1, 6-diphosphatase.

Diagnostic Procedures. *Blood.* In normal conditions, normal values of glucose and lactic acid; in stressful situation and after ingestion of fructose: hypoglycemia, lactic acidosis; aminoacidemia; hyperglycerolemia. *Biopsy of liver.* Lack of fructose 1, 6-diphosphatase. *Caution.* Diagnostic measures such as administration of fructose, glycerol, dehydroxy-acetone are dangerous. After fasting, administration of glucagon (1 mg) is a less dangerous test. No rise of blood glucose.

Therapy. Prevention of stressful situation and of fructose administration. Glucose intravenous.

Prognosis. Severe because of difficulty in recognizing the condition.

BIBLIOGRAPHY. Baker LI, Winegard AI: Fasting hypoglycemia and metabolic acidosis associated with deficiency of hepatic fructose 1, 6-diphosphatase activity. Lancet 2:13–16, 1970.
Gitzelmann R, Steinmann B, Van den Berghe G: Essential fructosuria, hereditary fructose intolerance, and fructose-1, 6-diphosphatase deficiency. In Stanbury JB, Wyngaarden JB, Fredrickson DS, et al, The Metabolic Basis of Inherited Disease, 5th ed, p 118. New York, McGraw-Hill 1983

FRUCTOSE INTOLERANCE, HEREDITARY

Synonyms. Chambers-Pratt; fructose intolerance.

Symptoms. No symptoms as long as patients do not ingest food containing fructose. First symptoms in infancy when sucrose or fructose added to diet. Unconsciousness; convulsions; vomiting; failure to thrive; cachexia may result in death. In older children and adults, strong aversion for fruit and sweets prevent other manifestations.

Signs. In infancy, hepatomegaly, jaundice, edema, ascites.

Etiology. Congenital absence of fructose phosphate-splitting liver aldolase. Autosomal recessive trait in most, but not all families. Defect of fructose-1-phosphate aldolase B of liver, kidney cortex, and small intestine. Autosomal recessive trait in most but not all families.

Pathology. Early cirrhosis of the liver in infants. Derangement of liver and kidney; alterations possibly reversible because not found in adults.

Diagnostic Procedures. *Blood.* Hypoglycemia following ingestion of fructose 1, 6-diphosphate; aldolase, serum glutamic-oxaloacetic transaminase (SGOT), glutamic pyruvic transaminase (GPT) increase; fall of inorganic serum phosphorus. Hyperbilirubinemia; intravenous fructose tolerance test. *Urine.* Albuminuria; aminoaciduria; fructosuria (after fructose ingestion).

Therapy. Diet without fructose. In case of cirrhosis liver transplantation has been attempted with good results.

Prognosis. Good if no fructose ingested. Hypoglycemic attacks do not seem to cause serious brain damage.

BIBLIOGRAPHY. Chambers RA, Pratt RTC: Idiosyncrasy to fructose. Lancet 2:340, 1956
Froesch ER, Prader A, Labhart A, et al: Die hereditare Fructoseintoleranz, eine bisher nicht bekannte kongenitale Stoffwechsel Störung. Schweiz Med Wochenschr 86:1168–1171, 1957
Gitzelmann R, Steinmann B, Van den Berghe G: Essential fructosuria, hereditary fructose intolerance and fructose-1-6-diphosphatase deficiency. In Stanbury JB, Wyngaarden JB, Fredrickson DS, The Metabolic Basis of Inherited Disease, 5th ed, p. 118. New York, McGraw-Hill, 1983.

FRUCTOSURIA, ESSENTIAL

Symptoms and Signs. None.

Etiology. Autosomal recessive inheritance. Lack of hepatic fructokinase.

Diagnostic Procedures. After ingestion of food containing fructose: *Blood and urine.* Fructosuria; fructosemia of high level (over 25 mg/100 ml); normal glucose and galactose metabolism.

Therapy. None.

Prognosis. Harmless condition.

BIBLIOGRAPHY. Sachs B, Sternfeld L, Kraus G: Essential fructosuria: Its pathophysiology. Am J Dis Child 63:252–269, 1942
Gitzelmann R, Steinmann B, Van den Berghe G: Essential fructosuria, hereditary fructose intolerance and fructose-1,6-diphosphatase deficiency. In Stanbury JB, Wyngaarden JB, Fredrickson DS: The Metabolic Basis of Inherited Disease, 5th ed, p 118. New York, McGraw-Hill, 1983

FRYNS'

Symptoms and Signs. Broad and flat nasal bridge, receding mandible, misshapen ears, broad and short neck with additional skinfolds; brachytelephalangy with hypoplastic nails of fingers and toes; cleft palate, hypoplasia and abnormal lobation of the lungs, diaphragmatic defects, uterus bicornis/duplex, nonrotation of intestines. Less frequent are apparently heart defects, cystic dysplastic kidneys, and other abnormalities of the urinary tract, netlike form of tracheal and bronchial cartilage, and brain malformations.

Etiology. Autosomal recessive gene. The syndrome has been described in children born to consanguineous parents.

Pathology. Cystic-adenomatoid malformations; total distortion of the architecture of the various organs; multiple glioneural heterotopias.

Diagnostic Procedures. Prenatal ultrasonographic examination.

Therapy. None.

Prognosis. Lethal syndrome. After the birth of an affected child, the parents face a 25% recurrence risk for any further pregnancy.

BIBLIOGRAPHY. Fryns JP, Moerman F, Goddeeris P, Bossuyt C, Van den Berghe H: A new lethal syndrome with cloudy corneae, diaphragmatic defects and distal limb deformities. Hum Genet 50:65–70, 1979
Schwyzer U, Briner J, Schinzel A: Fryns' syndrome in a girl born to consanguineous parents. Acta Paediatr Scand 76:167–171, 1987

FUCH'S I

Synonyms. Cutaneous mucooculoepithelial; mucocutaneous ocular; ocular mucocutaneous. Eponym indicates a nonfebrile Stevens-Johnson variant.

BIBLIOGRAPHY. Fuchs E: Herpes iris congiuntival. Klin Monatsbl Augenheilkd 14:333–351, 1876

FUCHS' II

Synonym. Blepharochalasis. See Ascher's.

Symptoms and Signs. Onset at young age with transient, recurrent edemas of angioneurotic type in both eyelids (usually, only the superiors; occasionally, also the inferiors). Then with the progress of the disease, prolapse of the orbital fat and lacrimal glands and blepharoptosis.

Etiology. Unknown. Localized atrophy of the eyelids, skin, and subcutaneous tissue.

Pathology. Histologic aspect depends on stage of disease, from simple edema of subcutis, lymphocytic perivascular infiltration to atrophy of dermis and atrophy, and finally disappearance, of elastic fibers.

Therapy. Plastic surgery.

Prognosis. Progressive condition.

BIBLIOGRAPHY. Fuchs E: Ueber Blepharochalasis. (Erschlaffung der Lidhaut). Wein Klin Wochenschr 9:109, 1896
Schulze F: Beitrag zur heridetaeren Blepharocalasis. Klin Monatsbl Augenheilkd 14:863–877, 1965

FUCHS' III

Synonyms. Fuchs' heterochromia, heterochromic uveitis. Heterochromic cyclitis.

Symptoms. Onset in the third to fourth decades of life. Insidious onset; patient in most of the cases is unaware of condition until opacification of vitreous reduces vision.

Signs. Heterochromia: slight or marked difference in color between the two irides. One or both eyes may be involved (occasionally, heterochromia may be missing). Cyclitis: mild, chronic, whitish keratic precipitates, not confluent, observed in pupillary area and lower part of cornea. Cataract: develops only late in the disease. Peripheral chorioiditis may be present.

Etiology. Unknown. Possibly mild infections.

Pathology. In iris, lower number of melanocytes, diffuse fibrosis and lymphocyte and plasma cell infiltration. Ciliary body fibrosis; muscular atrophy. Focal cyclitis; peripheral chorioiditis.

Diagnostic Procedures. *Ophthalmoscopy. Tonometry.*

Therapy. None; cataract removal once developed.

Prognosis. Relatively good for its slow chronic course. Possibility of glaucoma has to be kept in mind and eventually treated.

BIBLIOGRAPHY. Fuchs E: Uber Komplikationen der Heterochromia. Klin Monatsbl Augenheilkd 15:191–212, 1906
Hart CT, Ward DM: Intraocular pressure in Fuchs' heterochromic uveitis. Br J Ophthalmol 51:739–743, 1967
Luntz MH: Clinical types of cataracts. In Duane TD (ed): Clinical Ophthalmology, vol 1, chap 73. Philadelphia, Harper & Row, 1982

FUCHS' IV

Synonyms. Endothelial corneal dystrophy; corneal erosion; endothelial-epithelial corneal dystrophy; Fuchs-Kraupa; Kraupa's.

Symptoms. Occur in elderly persons; prevalent in females. Ocular pain; photophobia; disturbed vision.

Signs. Corneal vesicles and bullae, erosions, and scarring.

Etiology. Unknown. Most cases sporadic. Suggestion of autosomal dominant inheritance with greater expression in females, possibility of X-linked dominant inheritance also formulated.

Pathology. Descemet's membrane presents hyaline deposits, endothelial erosions, edema; Bowman's membrane shows degeneration features; on posterior corneal surface evidence of pigmentation.

Diagnostic Procedures. *Ophthalmoscopy.* See Signs and Pathology.

Therapy. Hypertonic solutions; irradiation of lacrimal glands; corneal transplantation.

Prognosis. Early in disease fair response to treatment. Corneal transplantation effective in 60% of cases.

BIBLIOGRAPHY. Fuchs E: Dystrophia epithelialis corneae. Albrecht von Graefes Arch Ophthalmol 76:478–508, 1910

Rosenblum P, Stark WJ, Maumenee HI, et al: Hereditary Fuchs' dystrophy. Am J Ophthalmol 90:455–462, 1980

FUNDUS ALBIPUNCTATUS

Symptoms. Both sexes affected; increasing constriction of visual fields, night blindness, and finally blindness.

Signs. White spots scattered on the retina, more concentrated at posterior pole.

Etiology. Unknown, autosomal recessive or dominant inheritance.

BIBLIOGRAPHY. Krill AE, Falk MR: Retinis punctata albescens: A functional evaluation of an unusual case. Am J Ophthalmol 53:450–454, 1962

Krill AE: Hereditary Retinal and Choroidal Diseases: Flecked Retina Diseases, vol 2, pp 739–819. Hagerstown, Harper & Row, 1977

GAISBÖCK'S

Synonyms. Emotional polycythemia; stress erythrocytosis; benign polycythemia; polycythemia hypertonica; pseudopolycythemia; stress polycythemia.

Symptoms. Prevalent in men, usually in heavy smokers; onset at mean age 45. Tenseness; nervousness.

Signs. Moderate overweight; slight plethora; conjunctival congestion. Some patients have persistent hypertension. No splenomegaly.

Etiology. Constitutional disposition or association with emotional tension or both.

Diagnostic Procedures. *Blood.* Determination of blood volume; relative polycythemia (decreased plasma) or mild absolute polycythemia. High hematocrit. Leukocytes and platelets normal.

Therapy. None or diet; sedative; psychotherapy. Therapeutic value of phlebotomy not established.

Prognosis. Good; some develop or have associated vascular diseases.

BIBLIOGRAPHY. Gaisböck F: Die Bedeutung der Blutdruckmessung für die ärztliche Praxis. Dtsch Arch Klin Med 83:363–409, 1905
Russell RP, Conley CL: Benign polycythemia: Gaisböck's syndrome. Arch Intern Med 114:734–740, 1964
Avins LR, Krummenacher TK: Venous stasis retinopathy and Gaisböck's syndrome. Am J Ophthalmol 105:420–421, 1988

GALACTOKINASE DEFICIENCY GALACTOSEMIA

Synonyms. Galactosemia II; galactose diabetes; Giztzelmann's.

Symptoms. Both sexes affected; onset after a few weeks of life or in older age. Absence of inanition, gastrointestinal disorders, and jaundice. Irregularly progressing reduction of vision that may reach blindness. Normal intelligence. Hepatosplenomegaly only during the period of milk feeding (not consistently present). Recurrent cataract.

Etiology. Autosomal recessive inheritance. Deficiency of galactokinase activity. Cataracts caused by failure of galactose phosphorylation.

Pathology. Apparently limited to cataract formation.

Diagnostic Procedures. *Urine.* Galactosuria (especially after milk feeding). *Blood.* High galactosemia (after milk feeding); absence of galactokinase in red cells (normal galactose-1-phosphate uridyltransferase).

Therapy. Diet without milk and derivatives.

Prognosis. Variable degree of recurrence of cataracts and visual impairment.

BIBLIOGRAPHY. Fanconi G: Hochgrädige Galaktose-Intolleranz (Galaktose Diabetes) bei einem Kinde mit Neurofibromatosis Recklinghausen. Jahrb Klinderheilkd 138:1–8. 1933
Gitzelmann R: Hereditary galactokinase deficiency, a newly recognized cause of juvenile cataracts. Pediatr Res 1:14–23, 1967
Segal S: Disorders of galactose metabolism. In Stanbury JB, Wyngaarden JB, Fredrickson DS, et al: The Metabolic Basis of Inherited Diseases, 5th ed, p 167. New York, McGraw-Hill, 1983

GALEAZZI'S

Synonyms. Radius fracture–dislocation ulnar head distally. See Monteggia's.

Symptoms and Signs. Most frequent in children. Pain in the forearm. Fracture of the radius with disruption of the distal radioulnar joint.

Etiology. Blow on the forearm.

Diagnostic Procedures. *X-rays of forearm.*

Therapy. Closed reduction usually adequate.

Prognosis. Once the radius is restored to length and angulation corrected the distal radioulnar joint becomes stable.

BIBLIOGRAPHY. Galeazzi R: Di una particolare syndrome traumatica dello scheletro dell'avambraccio. Atti Mens Soc di Chir 2:12, 1934
Canale TS: Fractures and dislocation in children. In Crenshaw AH (ed): Campbell's Operative Orthopedics, 7th ed, pp 1853–1855. St. Louis, CV Mosby, 1987

GALLAVARDIN'S

Synonyms. Blockypnea; inhibited respiration.

Symptoms. Exertion of various degrees or tension cause inhibition of breathing; rest brings relief. No wheezing or dyspnea. In some cases, alternating with typical angina symptoms.

Signs. None.

Etiology. Equivalent of angina syndrome in patient with coronary arteriosclerosis and diseases central nervous system (spinothalamic tract to respiratory center in medulla stimulation). Increased susceptibility to stimulation of respiratory center.

Pathology. Coronary arteriosclerosis.

Diagnostic Procedures. All negative. *Electrocardiography.* May show anginal pattern, especially after effort.

Therapy. That of angina.

Prognosis. That of angina.

BIBLIOGRAPHY. Gallavardin L: Y a-t-il un equivalent non douloureux l'angine de poitrine d'effort? Lyon Med 134:345–358, 1924
Roesler H: Blockypnea (inhibited respiration), an equivalent of the angina syndrome. Am J Med Sci 244:85–87, 1962

GALLOWAY'S

Synonyms. Microcephaly-hiatus hernia-nephrotic syndrome.

Symptoms. Both sexes at birth. Microcephaly, large ears, vomiting from first feeding.

Etiology. Unknown. Possible autosomal recessive inheritance.

Pathology. *Kidney.* Focal glomerulosclerosis and microcystic dysplasia.

Diagnostic Procedures. *Urine.* Presence of albumin since birth or after few days.

Prognosis. All cases died within 3 years.

BIBLIOGRAPHY. Galloway WH, Mowat AP: Congenital microcephaly with hiatus hernia and nephrotic syndrome in two sibs. J Med Genet 5:319–321, 1968
Shapiro LR, Duncan PA, Farnsworth PB, et al: Congenital microcephaly, hiatus hernia, and nephrotic syndrome: An autosomal recessive syndrome. Birth Defects XII (5):275–278, 1976

GAMBLE–DARROW

Synonyms. Hypochloremic congenital alkalosis–diarrhea; chlorurrhea; chloride diarrhea, familial.

Symptoms. Usually prematurity; watery profuse diarrhea; no vomiting; failure to gain weight; good appetite except in period of dehydration.

Signs. Abdominal distention with a marked "ladder" pattern suggesting a (false) intestinal obstruction.

Etiology. Unknown. Congenital defect affecting absorption of water, chloride, sodium from intestinal tract. Possibly, autosomal recessive inheritance.

Diagnostic Procedures. *Blood.* Low plasma chloride; high bicarbonate; low sodium; normal potassium (except when diarrhea is severe); elevated *pH* (7.64); normal blood urea nitrogen (BUN), sugar, protein, and calcium. *Stool.* High chloride; low sodium; acid *pH.* *Stomach and duodenal secretion.* Normal. *Urine.* Occasionally, *pH* higher than that of plasma; no chloride; little sodium; variable amount of potassium.

Therapy. Intermittent intravenous administration of sodium chloride and potassium chloride initially and then orally (over 4 g potassium chloride daily).

Prognosis. With treatment growth almost normal; stools remain loose, causing little inconvenience; danger in period of febrile illness and warm weather.

BIBLIOGRAPHY. Gamble J: Congenital alkalosis with diarrhea. J Pediatr 26:509–518, 1945
Darrow DC: Congenital alkalosis with diarrhea. J Pediatr 26:519–532, 1945
Booth IW, Strange G, Murer H, et al: Defective jejunal brush-border Na^+/H^+ exchange: A cause of congenital diarrhea. Lancet I:1066–1069, 1985

GAMEKEEPER'S THUMB

Synonym. Ulnar collateral ligament rupture.

Symptoms. Chronic pain and weakness of thumb–index finger grip.

Signs. Swelling, tenderness of ulnar margin of metacarpophalangeal joint. While pressing thumb and index forcefully together, the thumb drifts radially.

Etiology. Traumatic rupture of ulnar collateral ligament. In gamekeepers from repeated twisting of necks of wounded hares; frequently observed in skiers after trying to break a forward fall with pole, or a backward fall, by wedging thumbs in the snow.

Diagnostic Procedures. *X-ray.*

Therapy. Surgical correction or casting.

Prognosis. In untreated cases, chronic disability.

BIBLIOGRAPHY. Campbell CS: Gamekeeper's thumb. J Bone Joint Surg [Br] 37:148–149, 1955
Schultz RJ, Fox JM: Gamekeeper's thumb. Result of skiing injuries. NY J Med 73:2329–2331, 1973

GAMMOPATHY, BENIGN MONOCLONAL

Synonym. See Kahler-Bozzolo.

Symptoms and Signs. None or associated with a variety of other conditions. Only constant feature is the presence of monoclonal protein (M-component), which remains in a constant concentration over many years.

Etiology. Many conditions may be associated with this finding and the M-component increase could represent a response to antigen stimulation (infection; neoplasia); however this has not been proved. The increase may also represent a "premyeloma" condition. Hereditary factors have also been considered.

Diagnostic Procedures. *Blood.* Presence of M-component (similar to those of malignant plasma cell conditions). Normal levels of normal globulins. *Urine.* In rare cases, presence of Bence Jones proteins. *Bone marrow.* Less than 10% of plasma cells.

Therapy. None or that of associated condition.

Prognosis. Benign, however in 5% evolution into myeloma.

BIBLIOGRAPHY. Waldenström J: Studies on condition associated with disturbed gamma globulin formation (gammopathies). Harvey Lect 56:211–231, 1961
Wintrobe MM (ed): Clinical Hematology, 8th ed. Philadelphia, Lea & Febiger, 1981

GAMSTORP'S

Synonyms. Adynamia episodica hereditaria; hyperkalemic periodic paralysis; Westphals hyperkalemic. See von Eulenberg's. Periodic paralysis hyperkalemic.

Symptoms. Both sexes affected; more severe in males; onset during first decade. Between attacks patient is free of symptoms. Precipitating factors are rest after exertion, cold and dampness, hunger. Attacks usually during the day. Attack is usually weakness of muscle, frequently localized at single muscle groups. May affect facial muscles also. Paresthesias frequent with cramping pain lasting 1 hour or longer. Mental faculties not affected.

Signs. Hyporeflexia of muscles involved. Percussion myotonia restricted to tongue in some cases, or to the eyelids or lips.

Etiology. Unknown; single autosomal dominant inheritance. Reduction of muscle membrane potential considered as cause of paralysis. Periodic paralysis represents an end of a spectrum extending to paraemimiotonia (see von Eulenberg's) since many cases present both conditions. In addition it does not appear justifiable to separate a normokalemic form from the hyperkalemic because in both syndromes serum potassium levels do not always correlate with degree of muscle weakness.

Pathology. Not well established. Some muscle fibers present areas of accumulation of sarcoplasm on cross section. No degenerative changes.

Diagnostic Procedures. *Blood.* Hyperkalemia.

Therapy. *Prophylactic.* Gentle exercise after exertion; carbohydrate intake. Acetazolamide. Avoid exposure to cold. *During attack.* Calcium gluconate.

Prognosis. Nonprogressive. Marked improvement during adult life. No muscle wasting occurs. Sudden death from bidirectional cardiac dysrhythmia reported.

BIBLIOGRAPHY. Gamstorp I: Adynamia episodica hereditaria. Acta Paediatr (Suppl) 108:1–126, 1956
Gould RJ, Steeg CN, Eastwood AB, et al: Potentially fatal cardiac dysrhythmia and hyperkalemic periodic paralysis. Neurology 35:1208–1212, 1985

GANSER'S

Synonyms. Balderdash; nonsense; prison psychosis; pseudodementia.

Symptoms. Usually appears suddenly in relation to circumstances by which it is precipitated. Approximate answers (which bear some relationship to the question but patient "passes by" the correct one and gives one near to it or says "I don't know") mixed with correct answer and absurd clouding of consciousness; apathetic indifference; lethargy; semistupor; disorientation. Somatic conversion features, manifested by motor and sensorial involvement, movements, tonus, flaccidity or rigidity, headache, backache, areas of anesthesia. Hallucination; visual or auditory.

Etiology. Unknown; hysterical dissociative reaction. To be differentiated from malingering, true dementia, and some varieties of schizophrenia.

Therapy. During acute phase, hospitalization.

Prognosis. Relatively transient condition, spontaneous complete recovery; recurrences possible. Recovery from syndrome occurs also when other depressive symptoms persist.

BIBLIOGRAPHY. Ganser SJ: Ueber einen eigenartigen hysterischen Dammerzustund. Arch Psychiatr Nervkr 30:633–640, 1898

Enoch MD, Trethwan WH, Barker JC: Some Uncommon Psychiatric Syndromes. Baltimore, Williams & Wilkins, 1967

Freedman AM, Kaplan HI, Sadock BJ: Comprehensive Textbook of Psychiatry, 2nd ed. Baltimore, Williams & Wilkins, 1975

GÄNSSLEN'S I

An obsolete eponym used in the past to indicate the bone changes occurring with any chronic hemolytic syndromes. See Thalassemic, Widal-Ravaut, and Minkowski-Chauffard.

BIBLIOGRAPHY. Gänsslen M, Zipperlen E, Schuz E: Die Hämolytische Konstitution. Nach 105 Beobachtungen von hämolytischem Ikterus, 39 Beobachtungen von leichten hämolytischen Konstitutionen und 19 Milzexstirpationen. Arch Klin Med 146:1–46, 1925

GÄNSSLEN'S II

Synonym. Neutropenia familial benign chronic.

Symptoms. Family history. From completely asymptomatic to tendency toward chronic recurrent infections (especially periodontal), and occasionally severe generalized infections.

Signs. Frequent evidence of periodontal disease and scar of previous infections; no splenomegaly. Clubbing of fingers.

Etiology. Unknown; autosomal dominant transmission.

Diagnostic Procedures. *Blood.* Leukocyte count borderline low range; absolute neutropenia; relative lymphocytosis and monocytosis; irregular increase in eosinophils occasionally seen. Hyperglobulinemia. *Bone marrow.* Erythroid and megakaryocytic series normal; myeloid series represented up to myelocytes, marked reduction of more mature elements; increase of lymphocytes and monocytes.

Therapy. Antibiotics.

Prognosis. Excellent; chronic lengthy course.

BIBLIOGRAPHY. Gänsslen M: Konstitutionelle familiäle Leukopenia (Neutropenie). Klin Wochenschr 20:922–925, 1941

Bousser J, Neyde R: La neutropénie familiale. Sang 18:521–529, 1947

Pincus SH, Boxer LA, Stossel TP: Chronic neutropenia in childhood: Analysis of 16 cases and a review of the literature. Am J Med 61:849–861, 1976

GARCIN'S

Synonyms. Half base; Schmincke's (tumor-unilateral cranial paralysis). See Foix's I.

Symptoms and Signs. Unilateral paralysis of all territories of cranial nerves. Primarily acoustic (VIII), glossopharyngeal (IX), vagus (X), spinal accessory (XI), and hypoglossal (XII). Absence of cerebral signs and symptoms, including intracranial pressure (papilledema; spinal fluid change).

Etiology and Pathology. Primary sarcoma of base of skull and meninges or primary neoplasm of nasopharynx extending into cranial cavity.

Diagnostic Procedures. *X-ray of skull. Biopsy of tumor.*

Therapy. X-rays or surgery.

Prognosis. Poor; metastasis frequent.

BIBLIOGRAPHY. Garcin R: Le syndrome paralytique unilatéral des nerves crânienes. Theses de Paris, 1927

Spiegal LA: Syndrome de Garcin—Unilateral total involvement of cranial nerves with report of one case. Ann Otol 52:706–712, 1943

Chakrabarth AK: Nasopharyngeal carcinoma with multiple cranial nerve palsies. Practitioner 212:103–106, 1974

GARDENER–DIAMOND

Synonyms. Autoerythrocyte sensitization; erythrocyte membrane sensitization; purpura-painful bruising. See David's and Purpura, psychogenic.

Symptoms. Affects only women, not infrequently at various times after operations related to reproductive organs. History of bleeding episodes of different nature before onset of manifestations. Local sensation of tingling or burning preceding by several hours (18–24), the development of purpuric lesions that persist indolent for 5 to 7 days. Usually affecting extremities, face, and scalp; seldom the back. Frequently, these patients present particular psychologic manifestations.

Signs. Purpuric lesion frequently on areas not involved in trauma.

Etiology. Autosensitization to red cells or red cell stroma component, possibly phosphatidylserine (PPD) (proved in one case). Emotional factors of importance in the development of symptoms.

Pathology. Data available from skin biopsy of lesion experimentally induced by the injection of PPD. Pattern in part resembling that of allergic vascular purpura.

Diagnostic Procedures. Injection into the skin of red cell or red cell stroma (positive reaction). For differential diagnosis, injection of deoxyribonucleic acid DNA (negative), histamine (negative), PPD (may be positive). *Blood.* Coagulation tests and platelet number. Normal.

Therapy. None (corticosteroid; antihistamine; antimalarial drugs; desensitization with erythrocyte unsuccessful).

Prognosis. Recurrent manifestation.

BIBLIOGRAPHY. Gardener RH, Diamond LK: Autoerythrocyte sensitization: A form of purpura producing painful bruising following autosensitization to red cells in certain women. Blood 10:675–690, 1955
Whitlock FA: Psychophysiological Aspects of Skin Diseases. London, WB Saunders, 1976
Rook A, Wilkinson DS, Ebling FJG, et al: Textbook of Dermatology, 4th ed, p 2265. Oxford, Blackwell Scientific Publications, 1986

GARDNER'S

Synonyms. Bone tumor–epidermoid cyst–polyposis; multiple familial colon polyposis; epidermoid cyst–osteomatosis–polyposis; intestinal polyposis III. Polyposis intestinal III; GRS.

Symptoms. Both sexes affected; average age of onset 20 years, but lesions have been found in 2-month-old children and 70-year-old person. Early mild diarrhea and small amount of mucus and blood. Some patients with intestinal polyposis are asymptomatic. In 15 to 20 years after onset of intestinal symptomatology, multifocal malignant transformation of polyps.

Signs. *Soft tissue.* Multiple epidermoid cysts; dermoid tumors; fibromas; neurofibromas. *Bone.* Self-limited benign exostosis; osteomatosis mostly localized in face and skull; multiple impactions of supernumerary teeth; (additional sign of the syndrome), long bones seldom involved. Frequently associated: retinal pigment epithelium hypertrophy (see).

Etiology. Unknown; dominant hereditary condition where soft tissue, bone tumors, and polyposis depend on same gene. Half of offspring affected.

Pathology. Benign cutaneous and subcutaneous tumors; benign bone tumor. Premalignant and eventually malignant transformation of multiple, scattered polyps most commonly in colon and rectum.

Diagnostic Procedures. *Biopsy of skin and intestine.*

Therapy. Subtotal colectomy with ileorectal anastomosis and fulguration of residual rectal adenomas. Follow-up to destroy reappearing polyps. If carcinoma develops, abdominoperineal resection and permanent ileostomy.

Prognosis. Death from cancer of colon occurs at an average age of 41 to 50 years.

BIBLIOGRAPHY. Devic, Bussy: Un cas de polypose adénomatease; généralisée a tout l'intestin. Arch Mal Appar Dig 6:278–299, 1912
Gardner EJ, Stephens FE: Cancer of the lower digestive tract in one family group. Am J Hum Genet 2:41–48, 1950
Naylor EW, Lebenthal E: Gardner's syndrome: Recent development in research and management. Dig Dis Sci 25:945–959, 1980
Bull MJ, Ellis FD, Sato S, et al: Hypertrophy of retinal pigment epithelium in Gardner syndrome. Proc Greenwood Genet Centr 4:136, 1985

GARRÉ'S

Synonyms. Sclerosing nonsuppurative osteomyelitis; osteomyelitis sicca; Osteitis Garré's.

Symptoms. Both sexes affected; onset in young adult, less frequently in late childhood. Fever. Moderate bone pain, especially during the night.

Signs. All bones may be affected, more frequently the tibia and femur; tenderness on palpation, and slow development of fusiform bone enlargement.

Etiology. Variable and frequently not clear: low grade infection (nonsuppurative acute or chronic of haversian canals); less frequently trauma; related to osteoid osteoma (see Bergstrand's) or other similar conditions.

Pathology. Scattered areas of necrosis; devascularization and fusiform thickening of cortex.

Diagnostic Procedures. *X-ray.* Subperiosteal calcification; cortex thickened with circumferential involvement and absence of nidus or rarefaction of focus.

Therapy. Guttering; drilling of multiple holes.

Prognosis. Recurrences at interval of weeks or months. Recovery with subsidence of fever and persistence of described bone changes.

BIBLIOGRAPHY. Garré C: Ueber besondere Formen und Folgezunstände der akuten intektiösen Osteomyelitis. Beitr Klin Chir 10:241–298, 1893
Carnesale PG: General principles in infection. In Crenshaw AH (ed): Campbell's Operative Orthopedics, 7th ed, pp 663–664. St. Louis, CV Mosby, 1987

GARROD'S

Synonyms. Alkaptonuria; ochronosis.

Symptoms. Both sexes affected; manifestation more severe in males; onset in first few days of life. (1) Passage of urine that becomes black on standing or if alkalinized (washed diapers become black). Black pigment excreted also with sweat. (2) Arthropathia; back pain; stiffness; onset in fourth decade; progressive involvement of several joints to complete disablement in 15 to 20 years. Severe pain over symphysis pubis. Extruded intervertebral disk frequent. (3) Renal and prostatic stones, usually during fifth decade. (4) Cardiovascular lesions; hoarseness; occasionally, deafness.

Signs. Pigmentation (blue black) of sclerae and ear cartilages (which also become stiff, a sign appearing in second decade), occasionally of tip of nose and tendons.

Etiology. Deficiency of homogentisic acid oxidase of liver and kidney. Autosomal recessive inheritance.

Pathology. Typical black pigmentation of cartilaginous structures, heart valves. Articular degenerative changes; accelerated arteriosclerotic changes. In kidney, black stones and secondary infections.

Diagnostic Procedures. *Urine.* Determination of homogentisic acid. *X-ray.* Narrowing of intervertebral space. Collapse and calcification of intervertebral disks. Degenerative changes in large joints.

Therapy. Kidney transplantation followed by recurrence of renal failure in years.

Prognosis. Arthropathy may make patient bedridden for years. Cardiovascular defects and uremia causes of death. Oldest patient reached 99 years.

BIBLIOGRAPHY. Boedeker C: Ueber das Alkapton; ein neuer Beitrug zur Frage Welche Stoff des Hanus können Kupferreduction bewirken? Ztschr Rat Med 7:130–145, 1859

Garrod AF: About alkaptonuria. Lancet 2:1484–1486, 1901

McKusick VA: Heritable Disorders of Connective Tissue, 4th ed. St. Louis, CV Mosby, 1972

La Du BN: Alcaptonuria. In Stanbury JB, Wyngaarden JB, Fredrickson DS: The Metabolic Basis of Inherited Disease, 4th ed, p 268. New York, McGraw-Hill, 1978

GASSER–KARRER

Synonyms. Acute erythroblastopenia. See pure red cell aplasia syndromes.

Symptoms and Signs. Both sexes affected; onset from first days of life. Jaundice progressing for a few days and then receding. As jaundice fades, anemia becomes evident (in second or third week). No splenomegaly.

Etiology. Exogenous toxin. Vitamin K analogues administration is frequently involved.

Pathology. Not specific.

Diagnostic Procedures. *Blood.* Anemia; reticulocytosis, hyperbilirubinemia. Presence of Heinz's bodies in 9 to 45% of red cells. (Heinz's bodies may be observed in many other conditions, such as inclusion body anemiapigmenturia, after splenectomy, red cell enzymes defect. See Widal-Ravaut.) Negative Coomb's test and absent cold-warm agglutinins.

Therapy. Transfusions.

Prognosis. Without treatment, infant deteriorates rapidly, becoming drowsy. Death may occur. If survival of hemolytic episode, the condition is self-limited.

BIBLIOGRAPHY. Gasser C, Karrer J: Delataere haemolytische Anaemie mit Spontan-innerkoerpe Bildung bei Fruehgeburt. Helv Paediatr Acta 3:387–403, 1948

Gasser C: Die hämolytische Frühgeburtenanamie mit spontaner Innenkörperbildung: Ein neues Syndrom, beobachtet an 14 Fallen. Helv Paediatr Acta 8:491–529, 1953

Sheehy TW: Inclusion body anemia with pigmenturia. Arch Intern Med 114:83–85, 1964

Wintrobe MM (ed): Clinical Hematology, 8th ed. Philadelphia, Lea & Febiger, 1981

GASSER'S II

Synonym. Hemolytic uremic.

Symptoms. Occur in seriously ill infants and children. Vomiting; diarrhea; skin, gastrointestinal or urinary bleeding; pallor. Hemolytic anemia-acute renal failure.

Signs. Mild edema; ecchymosis and petechiae; jaundice; hepatomegaly; seldom, splenomegaly; hypertension in 50% of cases.

Etiology. Unknown; may represent one manifestation of autoimmune reaction. Acute renal shutdown and hemolytic anemia. Clinical and pathologic findings demonstrate sufficient correlation to define the hemolytic uremic syndrome as an entity separate from Moschcowitz's, periarteritis nodosa, and necrotizing glomerulonephritis. In Argentina the disorder seems unusually frequent and a viral etiology has been proposed. Other endemic areas are South Africa, the West Coast of the USA, and the Netherlands. Remuzzi suggested that deficiency of a vascular prostacyclin stimulator may underlie the disorder.

Pathology. Jaundice; edema; cutaneous hemorrhages; small serous effusions; variable submucosal hemorrhages throughout gastrointestinal tract. Liver enlarged and fatty. Kidney patchy to almost total cortical necrosis; in nonnecrotic areas, glomerulitis, capillary microthrombi, and fibrinoid necrosis of efferent arterioles; casts of red cells and hemoglobin. Tubular necrosis without interstitial inflammation.

Diagnostic Procedures. *Blood.* Anemia with red cells showing morphologic alterations (fragmentation; anisopoikilocytosis; polychromasia). Reticulocytes high (10–20%). High sedimentation rate, Coomb's test negative; lupus erythematosis (LE) test negative. Thrombocytopenia; increased blood urea nitrogen (BUN). *Bone marrow.* Erythroid hyperplasia. *Urine.* Proteinuria; hematuria; casts. *Biopsy of kidney.* (During recovery) specific changes (see Pathology).

Therapy. Blood transfusion. Fresh plasma for restoring the activity of prostacyclin may be tried. Electrolyte balance; peritoneal dialysis; antihypertensive therapy; steroids. Streptokinase–streptodornase.

Prognosis. About 60% recovery; 10% residual hypertension; 30% death. Cases whose onset was within a short time of each other had a relatively good prognosis; those whose onset was more than a year apart had a poorer prognosis. This suggests an environmental agent in the first group and genetic factors in the second. Most of the first group of families came from an endemic area, whereas most of the second group came from a nonendemic area.

BIBLIOGRAPHY. Gasser C, Gantier E, Steck A, et al: Hamolytisch-urämische Syndrom: bilateral Nierenrindennenekrosen bei akuten erbworbenen hämolitisch Anämien. Schweiz Med Wochenschr 85:905–909, 1955
Remuzzi G, Mecca D, Marchesi M, et al: Familial deficiency of a plasma factor stimulating vascular prostacyclin activity. Thromb Res 16:517–525, 1979
Neild G: The haemolytic uraemic syndrome: A review. Q J Med 63:367–378, 1987

GAS SYNDROMES

AEROPHAGIA I

Synonym. Magenblase.

Symptom. Belching.

Etiology. Moderate air swallowing.

Diagnostic Procedures. *Fluoroscopy.* After swallowing air, air in the esophagous during respiratory excursion.

Therapy. Reassurance; tranquilizers; exhalation of air before swallowing.

AEROPHAGIA II

Symptoms. Belching; gastric distention; flatulence.

Etiology. Same as above; delayed eructation.

Diagnostic Procedures. Same as above.

Therapy. Same as above.

AEROPHAGIA III

Symptoms. Massive gastric distention; respiratory difficulty; abdomen tympanic.

Etiology. Marked air ingestion with stomach atony. Postoperative stage.

Therapy. Immediate intubation.

GASTRIC ACID SECRETION I

Symptoms. Abdominal distention; flatulence.

Etiology. Gastric hypoacidity.

Diagnostic Procedures. *Gastric juice analysis. Bacterial examination.* Duodenal flora.

Therapy. Acid potions, specific for bacterial flora.

GASTRIC ACID SECRETION II

Symptoms. Epigastric pain; abdominal distention, flatulence.

Etiology. Gastric hyperacidity (with or without peptic ulcer); carbon dioxide production.

Diagnostic Procedures. As above. *Stool.* Occult blood and mucus.

Therapy. Antacids; anticholinergics; surgery.

INTESTINAL MOTILITY I

Symptoms. Occur in elderly, aged patients; colonic distention; hepatic and splenic pressure complaints; delayed flatulence.

Etiology. Colonic hypomotility.

Diagnostic Procedures. *X-ray.* Motility from stomach to cecum normal; motility of cecum delayed.

Therapy. Bethanechol chloride; reduction of carbohydrate intake.

INTESTINAL MOTILITY II

Symptoms. "Frothers"; borborygmi; occasional diarrhea; abdominal distention; flatulence.

Etiology. Hypermotility of intestine; mucus increase.

Diagnostic Procedures. *X-ray.* Small bowel gas (flat plate). Increased colonic motility; decreased transit time (carmine marker or barium or both).

Therapy. Dimethicone; pancreatic enzymes; anticholinergics.

MALDIGESTION

Synonyms. Pancreatic insufficiency; small intestinal hurry.

Symptoms. Borborygmi; abdominal distention; flatulence; occasionally, diarrhea.

Etiology. Pancreatic insufficiency; disaccharidase deficiency, small intestine accelerated motility.

Diagnostic Procedures. *X-ray.* Decreased transit time. *Stool.* Presence of undigested materials (protein; fat); duodenal enzymes, lactic acid decreased or increased according to etiology. *Disaccharide tolerance test.*

Therapy. Mecholyl; bethanechol chloride.

REFLEX SMALL INTESTINE HYPOTONIA

Symptoms. Abdominal distention; delayed flatulence.

Etiology. Urologic instrumentation.

Diagnostic Procedures. *Fluoroscopy.* Increased gas in small bowel.

Therapy. Mecholyl; bethanechol chloride.

BIBLIOGRAPHY. Danhaf IE: The clinical gas syndromes, a pathophysiological approach. Ann NY Acad Sci 150:127–140, 1968

GASTRODUODENAL ULCERATION–CHRONIC PULMONARY DISEASE

Synonym. Chronic pulmonary disease–gastroduodenal ulceration. While the occurrence of gastroduodenal ulcer in the general population is in the 10% range, in patients with chronic pulmonary disease the incidence reaches 25%. This association is considered statistically significant, and the association considered as a syndrome.

BIBLIOGRAPHY. Green TP, Dundee VC: On the association of chronic peptic ulceration. Can Med Assoc J 67:438–439, 1952
West WO, Burns RO, Daniel JM, et al: The syndrome of chronic pulmonary disease and gastroduodenal ulceration. Arch Intern Med 103:897–901, 1959

GASTROINTESTINAL MILK ALLERGY (IN INFANTS)

Synonym. Cow milk allergy.

Symptoms. Onset in early infancy (2 days to 4 or 5 mo) when cow milk feeding. Vomiting; chronic diarrhea; mucus and occult blood in the stool. Various degrees of severity from minimal to fulminating diarrhea, gastrointestinal bleeding, and collapse. Colic may precede diarrhea for months. Growth retardation.

Signs. Pallor; dehydration. Hypotension and tachycardia, and in some, shock (following milk challenge). On sigmoidoscopy, mucosa of rectum and colon from slight injection to red, ulcerated surface.

Etiology. Allergy to cow milk. Frequent family history of allergy and gastrointestinal diseases.

Pathology. *Biopsy of rectum.* From slight infiltrate of lymphocyte and plasma cells to granulocyte infiltrate and destruction of surface epithelium; abscesses.

Diagnostic Procedures. *Cow milk challenge* (with caution). Lactose tolerance normal. *Stool.* Precipitating antibodies against cow milk. *Studies of sugar-splitting enzymes.* For differential diagnosis.

Therapy. Change in formula (protein hydrolysate, soybean formula, or sheep milk formula).

Prognosis. Asymptomatic after starting change of formula. Usually obtain tolerance to cow milk at 2 years of age or later.

BIBLIOGRAPHY. Scholss OM, Worthen TW: The permeability of the gastroenteric tract of infants to indigest protein. Am J Dis Child 11:342, 1916
Gryboski JD: Gastrointestinal milk allergy in infants. Pediatrics 40:354–362, 1967
Behrman RE, Vaughan RE, Nelson RE (eds): Nelson's Textbook of Pediatrics, p 926. Philadelphia, WB Saunders, 1983

GAUCHER'S

Synonyms. Familial splenic anemia; cerebroside lipidosis; Gaucher-Schlagenhaufer; glucosyl ceramide lipidosis; histiocytosis, lipid kerasin type.

TYPE I: NON-NEURONOPATHIC (ADULT) CHRONIC GAUCHER'S

Symptoms. Both sexes equally affected; high proportion of Ashkenazy Jews; onset at any age, usually as patient reaches the second part of second decade after an asymptomatic or paucisymptomatic period. Pains in extremities or trunk: episodic; severe; occasionally, accompanied by hyperthermia. In some cases, respiratory difficulties.

Signs. If symptoms appear early, stunted growth. Old patients have yellow pallor and pigmentation of face and legs. Abdominal distention. Splenomegaly; hepatomegaly (sometimes with later onset). Pathologic fractures. Pinguecula (brownish wedge-shaped thickening of subconjunctival fibrous tissue) first on nasal side, then also on temporal side.

Etiology. Autosomal recessive inheritance. Subnormal activity of glucocerebrosidase in organs and tissues, determining an accumulation of glucocerebroside.

Pathology. *Liver.* Enlarged; degree of infiltration by Gaucher's cell variable (usually not in relation to size reached by the organ). Evidence of portal hypertension. *Spleen.* As above. *Lung.* Possibly, infiltration and pneumonia. *Bone.* Rarefraction of cortex, pathologic fractures.

Diagnostic Procedures. *Blood.* Mild microcytic anemia; leukopenia; thrombocytopenia; hyposideremia. Increase of nontartrate inhibited acid phosphatase. *Bone marrow.* Infiltration by Gaucher's cells. *X-ray.* Bone cortex reduced; pathologic fractures; expansion of cortex of lower end of femur; Erlenmeyer flasklike aspect. *Assay of glucocerebroside in tissue sample.*

Therapy. Symptomatic. Splenectomy to correct hypersplenism (see). Administration of purified glucocerebrosidase.

Prognosis. Pain most severe in first 20 years; thereafter less intense. Hemorrhages, hematemesis, and pneumonia causes of death. Survival in relation to time of onset and severity of condition; poorer prognosis for early onset.

TYPE II: NEURONOPATHIC ACUTE (INFANTILE) GAUCHER'S

Symptoms. Both sexes affected; mild prevalence in male; onset between 6 months and 1 year of age; no racial prevalence. Progressive hepatosplenomegaly; strabismus; hyperextension of head; hypertonicity; rigidity of neck; dysphagia; apathy or catatonia; increased deep reflexes; laryngeal spasm; mental retardation.

Etiology. See Type I.

Pathology. *Liver, spleen, lymph nodes.* Enlargement, presence of characteristic Gaucher's cells, large cells with reticular pattern (crumpled silk) of cytoplasm. *Bone.* Infiltration and eventual replacement of other marrow elements by Gaucher's cells. Bone destruction by proliferating cells. *Central nervous system.* Focal, nonspecific, degenerative changes of neurons; active neurophagocytosis; Gaucher's cell infiltration.

Therapy. See Type I.

Prognosis. Eighty percent fatality within first year of life.

TYPE III: SUBACUTE NEURONOPATHIC (JUVENILE) GAUCHER'S

Symptoms. Both sexes affected; onset at older age than Type II, up to adulthood. Seizures; occasionally, hypertonicity; strabismus and lack of movement coordination; poor mentation.

Signs. Hepatosplenomegaly.

Etiology and Pathology. See Types I and II.

Diagnostic Procedures. See Type I. *Electroencephalography.* Abnormalities.

Therapy. As Type I.

Prognosis. Subacute course and longer survival than Type II.

BIBLIOGRAPHY. Gaucher P: De l'epithelioma primitif de la rate (thesis) p 212. Paris, 1882
Brady RO, Barranges JA: Glucosyl ceramide lipidosis: Gaucher's disease. In Stanbury JB, Wyngaarden JB, Fredrickson DS, et al: The Metabolic Basis of Inherited Disease, 5th ed, p 842. New York, McGraw-Hill, 1983
Gafe M, Thomas C, Schneider J, et al: Infantile Gaucher's disease: A case with neuronal storage. Ann Neurol 23:300–303, 1988

GAUSTAD'S

Synonyms. Postshunt encephalopathy; hepatocerebral; portal-systemic encephalopathy; Gaustad's; transient hepatargy.

Symptoms. Mental confusion; behavior disorders; apathy; drowsiness; delirium.

Signs. Precoma without loss of consciousness, as well as coma. Hyperreflexia; rigidity; flapping tremor (hands and wrists). In coma, flaccid extremities and areflexia, fetor hepaticus, jaundice.

Etiology. After portocaval shunt. Hepatic failure and toxic state (increased blood ammonia level). Precipitating causes: anoxia; intercurrent infections; exercise; pregnancy; abdominal paracentesis; gastrointestinal ammonia; blood transfusion; drugs; hypokalemia; shunts; alkalosis; cholemia.

Pathology. Liver cirrhosis. In brain, nonspecific changes in cerebral cortex, basal ganglia, thalamus, brain stem, and cerebellum. Increase of astrocytes.

Diagnostic Procedures. *Blood.* Bilirubin; prothrombin time; proteins; albumin, blood urea nitrogen (BUN), ammonia level; alkaline phosphatase.

Therapy. Recognition and treatment of precipitating causes. General supportive measures; avoidance of additional trauma to liver.

Prognosis. Reversible condition with appropriate therapy. That of severe liver cirrhosis. Mortality 60%.

BIBLIOGRAPHY. Hahn M, Massen O, Wencki M, et al: Die Eck'sche Fistel Zwischen der Unteren Holivene und der Pfortader und ihre Folgen fur den Organisms. Arch Exp Pathol 32:151, 1893
Baker AB: Interrelationship of diseases of the liver and brain. Arch Pathol 46:268–286, 1948

Gaustad V: Transient epatargia. Acta Scand 135:354–363, 1949

Langer B, Taylor BR, McKenzie DR, et al: Further report of a prospective randomized trial comparing distal splenorenal shunt with end-to-side portocaval shunt: An analysis of encephalopathy, survival, and quality of life. Gastroenterology 88:424–429, 1985

GAY BOWEL

Symptoms and Signs. In homosexual male. Enterocolitis.

Etiology. Result of oral-anal-genital sexual practices. Due to a large variety of infective agents: virus (herpes, hepatitis), chlamydiae, bacteria (shigella, salmonella, neisseria, etc), protozoa, etc.

Therapy. According to infective agents.

BIBLIOGRAPHY. Centers for Disease Control: Sexually transmitted diseases: Treatment guidelines, 1985. MMWR 34:755, 1985

G-DELETION SYNDROMES

Synonym. Monosomy G. See Antimongolism.

Symptoms and Signs. Ptosis of eyelids; epicanthal folds; flat nasal bridge; bifid uvula; cutaneous syndactyly of toes; hypotonia. Other symptoms and signs shared with antimongolism (see): growth retardation; retarded development; microcephaly; large or low set ears; normal palmar folds. Several clinical entities, including antimongolism (see); cyclopia; ring g chromosome (Weleber's), and others.

Etiology. Monosomy G (?) or mosaic monosomy G. 45, XX, G-; 46, XY/45, XY, G-; 46XX/45, XX, G-; 46, XG/ 45, XY, G-.

Diagnostic Procedures. *Chromosome study.*

BIBLIOGRAPHY. Reisman LE, Darnell A, Murphy JW, et al: A child with partial deletion of a G-group autosome. Am J Dis Child 114:336–339, 1967

Weleber RG, Hecht F, Giblett ER: Ring-G chromosome: A new G-deletion syndrome? Am J Dis Child 115:289–493, 1968

Goldberg MF: Genetic and Metabolic Eye Disease, p 563. Boston, Little Brown, 1974

GEE'S

Synonyms. Infantile celiac; Gee-Hertener-Heubener; Gee-Thoysen; Golden-Kantor; Heubener's; Herter's; gluten-enteropathy; nontropical sprue, steatorrhea idiopathic; temperature sprue. Celiac disease.

CHILDREN'S VARIETY

Symptoms and Signs. Both sexes affected; onset between 6 and 9 months of age; prodromal signs may be present from birth. Celiac triad: diarrhea; weight loss; abdominal enlargement. Watery diarrhea (seen frequently in adult group) rare; vomiting frequent. Celiac crisis: dehydration with acidosis. Growth retardation.

Etiology. Autosomal dominant inheritance with incomplete penetrance. Deficiency of peptidases in intestinal mucosa and consequent inability to hydrolyze dietary gluten. This etiology is presently disputed and direct toxicity of gluten product on intestinal mucosa emphasized.

Pathology. Intestinal villi atrophic; surface epithelium degenerative changes. Bone osteoporosis.

Diagnostic Procedures. *Blood.* Variable degree of macrocytic anemia; hypoproteinemia; hypocalcemia; hypokalemia; hypolipemia. Prothrombin time prolonged. *Stool.* Steatorrhea. *X-ray of small bowel.* Segmentation and flocculation of barium meal; coarsening of jejunal folds, Maulage sign. *Urine.* Measurement of d-xylose absorption; determination of urinary indoles. *Biopsy of jejuneum.*

Therapy. Gluten-free diet. Specific deficiencies must also be corrected (vitamin B_{12}, calcium, potassium, zinc.) Corticosteroids.

Prognosis. Dramatic improvement in a few days with gluten-free diet. Occasionally, improvement only after 2 to 6 months of dietetic treatment.

LATENT VARIETY (TEMPERATURE SPRUE)

All symptoms and signs of disease are not present, except for intermittent episodes of diarrhea (typical fatty stool) with intercurrent pulmonary infections. Presence of the condition may be demonstrated by diagnostic procedures. During adulthood the adult variety of the condition manifests itself (see).

ADULT VARIETY

Symptoms. Preponderant in females (2:1); at onset 25% of patients have history of childhood diarrhea that disappeared in later childhood, malabsorption persisting, however. Symptoms and signs between third and sixth decades, characterized by intermittent exacerbations and remissions. Stresses (psychological or physical) may trigger an acute phase with diarrhea, with foul smelling, bulky stools (during attacks may be watery), weakness, weight loss, bleeding phenomena, hypocalcemia manifestations, anorexia, skeletal disorders, hypotension.

Signs. Abdominal bloating, all degrees of malabsorption syndrome (see); muscle wasting; edema; glossitis or stomatitis; occasionally, clubbing of fingers; skin pigmentation (Addisonlike).

Etiology. See Children's variety.

Pathology. See Children's variety.

Diagnostic Procedures. See Children's variety.

Therapy. See Children's variety.

Prognosis. See Children's variety.

BIBLIOGRAPHY. Gee S: On the celiac affection. St Barth Hosp Rep 24:17–20, 1888
Golden R: The small intestine and diarrhea. Am J Roentgen 36:892–901, 1936
Kantor JL: The roentgen diagnosis of idiopathic steatorrhea and allied conditions. Practical value of the "maulage sign." Am J Roentgen 41:758–778, 1939
Weiss JB, Austin RK, Sckaufield MS: Gluten sensitive enteropathy: Immunoglobulin G heavy chain (GM) allotypes and the immune response to wheat gliadin. J Clin Invest 72:96–101, 1983
Tiwari JL, Betuel H, Gebuhrer L, et al: Genetic epidemiology of coeliac disease. Genet Epidemiol 1:37–42, 1984

GELFARD-HYMAN

Synonyms. Histiocytic dermoarthritis; Zayid-Farraj. See also Multicentrix reticulohistiocytosis.

Symptoms. Both sexes affected; onset in childhood or adolescence. Joint pain, mainly on hands and wrists, but possible also on feet and elbows. Possibly, hearing loss and visual impairment. See Signs.

Signs. Multiple intracutaneous nodules and subcutaneous plaques with skin lichenification forming on face, ears, and limbs. Arthropathic changes of above mentioned joints. Glaucoma; bilateral uveitis; cataracts. Hydronephrosis reported also.

Etiology. Unknown; autosomal dominant inheritance.

Pathology. Histology. Nodules of lipoidal histiocytoma type, characterized by the absence of multinucleated giant cells (differential element with multicentric reticulohistiocytosis).

Diagnostic Procedures. *Biopsy of skin.* See Pathology. *X-ray of skeleton.* Symmetric destructive arthritis of mentioned joints. *Kidney function evaluation.* Possible abnormalities.

Therapy. Symptomatic.

Prognosis. Progressive condition.

BIBLIOGRAPHY. Gerfarb M, Hyman AB: Multiple noduli cutanei. Arch Dermatol 85:89–94, 1962
Zayid I, Farraj S: Familial histiocytic dermatoarthritis. A new syndrome. Am J Med 54:793–800, 1973
Sauden Y: Diagnosis of peripheral arthropathies. Radiol Clin Biol 43:283–291, 1974

GELINEAU'S

Synonym. Narcolepsy.

Symptoms. Onset in adolescence or early adulthood; male to female ratio 6:1. Sudden attacks of sleep that cannot be resisted. Sleep from a few minutes to a half an hour. Intense concentration in activity may prevent attack; less concentrating activities, such as reading, facilitates attack. Driving a car does not prevent attack. Patients awake refreshed. Patients may easily be awakened by noises of different intensities depending on patient. Impossible to differentiate from normal sleep. Sleep paralysis and hypnagogic hallucinations are experienced in the early part or during REM (rapid eye movement) stage, especially when in a comfortable position. Sometimes syndrome is associated with somnambulism, and frequently (2/3) with cataplexy (attacks of weakness or paralysis) especially with strong emotions.

Signs. Patient tends to be obese. While asleep, normal deep reflexes, eyes in Bell's position; sleep induces gentle muscle relaxation; normal breathing; slowing of pulse.

Etiology. Unknown (idiopathic type). Encephalitis; head injuries; systemic infections; polycythemia vera; multiple sclerosis; tumor of third ventricle. Familial cases with autosomal dominant trait.

Pathology. None. It is assumed that disturbance of the reticular formation or of the hypothalamus may be responsible for this syndrome.

Diagnostic Procedures. *Blood.* Hematocrit; blood volume. *X-ray of skull. Angiography. Pneumoencephalography. Electroencephalography. Electrooculography. Electromyography.*

Therapy. Methylphenidate (Ritalin); amphetamine sulfate.

Prognosis. Recurrent attacks for life (idiopathic); according to etiology (secondary).

BIBLIOGRAPHY. Gélineau E: De la narcolepsie. Gaz Hôp Paris 53:626–628; 635–637, 1880

Adie W: Idiopathic narcolepsy: A disease sui generis: With remarks on the mechanism of sleep. Brain 49:275–306, 1926

Hioshikawa Y, Nan'no H, Tachibana M, et al: The nature of sleep attack and other symptoms of narcolepsy. Electroencephalogr Clin Neurophysiol 24:1–10, 1968

Langdon N, Welsh KI, Van Dam M, et al: Genetic markers in narcolepsy. Lancet II:1178–1180, 1984

GEOGRAPHIC TONGUE

Synonyms. Erythema migrans tongue; exfoliatio aerata; glossitis areata exfoliativa; migratory glossitis; fissured tongue; lingua plicata.

Symptoms. Children younger than 4 years most commonly affected. Incidence in general population around 1 to 2%. Usually, asymptomatic; occasionally, soreness or pain especially with some particular type of food.

Signs. Smooth patches on the dorsum of tongue, outlined by margin grey-yellow or whitish, constantly changing pattern, and coalescing in polycyclic maplike spots; occasionally, some lesions on lips and soft palate.

Etiology. Unknown. Benign aspecific inflammation. Association with psoriasis and seborrheic dermatosis reported. A genetic factor suspected. Autosomal dominant inheritance.

Pathology. In dermis, acute inflammatory perivascular infiltrates of neutrophils and lymphocytes invading spongious epithelium; edema of rete; thickening of filiform papillae.

Therapy. Oral hygiene. If pain, gentian violet paint or mild anesthetic in tablet form.

Prognosis. Spontaneous remission and relapses; years later may develop into "fissured tongue."

BIBLIOGRAPHY. Turpin R, Caretzali A: Contribution a l'etologie de la glossite exfoliatrice marginée. Presse Med 44:1273–1274, 1936

Rahaminoff P, Muhsauf HU: Some observations on 1246 cases of geographic tongue. Am J Dis Child 93:519–525, 1957

Seiler A: Zur Verbreitung und Vererbun der Faltenzunge (lingua plicata). Ach Klaus Stift Vererbungsforsch 11:541–569, 1963

Dowson TAJ, Pielson WD: Geographic tongue in three generations. Br J Dermatol 79:678–681, 1967

GEOMINNE'S

Synonym. Cryptorchidism–keloids–renal–torticollis.

Symptoms and Signs. Occur in males; female carriers have less severe manifestations. Facial asymmetry; congential, progressive muscular torticollis; cryptorchidism; fever; multiple pigmented nevi. At puberty appearance of spontaneous keloids, varicose veins of legs; evidence of chronic pyelonephritis.

Etiology. X-linked inheritance (?).

BIBLIOGRAPHY. Geominne L: A new probably X-linked inherited syndrome: Congenital muscular torticollis, multiple keloids, cryptorchidism and renal dysplasia. Acta Genet Med Gemellol (Rome) 17:439–467, 1968

GERBASI'S

See also Addison-Biermer; Zuelzer's syndromes.

Symptoms and Signs. Onset in neonatal period; both sexes affected. All symptoms and signs of megaloblastic anemia.

Etiology. Breast feeding from mother with marginal folate stores.

Diagnostic Procedures. See Zuelzer's.

Therapy. Integration of alimentation with folate acid.

Prognosis. Prompt remission of symptoms and signs.

BIBLIOGRAPHY. Gerbasi M: Anemia perniciosiforme osservata in bambini ad allattamento materno esclusivo e protratto. Pediatria (Napoli) 48:505–526, 1940

Wintrobe MM (ed): Clinical Hematology, 8th ed. Philadelphia, Lea & Febiger, 1981

GERHARDT'S

Synonyms. Laryngeal adductor paralysis. LABD; vocal cord dysfunction, familial.

Symptoms and Signs. Impairment of phonation or severe inspiratory dyspnea leading to suffocation.

Etiology. Hemorrhage; infections; neoplasm in medulla oblongata; pons or exit from skull, or vagus (X) nerve determining paralysis of both pharyngeal adductor muscles. Autosomal dominant inheritance reported.

BIBLIOGRAPHY. Gerhardt C: Encephalitis; Stimmbandlähmung ohne Stimmveränderung. Arch Path Anat Berl 27:309, 1863

Gerhardt C: Ueber Diagnose und Behandlung der Stimmbandlähmung. Samml Klin Vortr (Leipzig) 36: (Inn Med 13:271–282); Allg Wien Med Stg 17:410–426, 1872

Cunningham MJ, Eavey RD, Shannon DC: Familial vocal cord dysfunction. Pediatrics 76:750–753, 1985

GERLIER'S

Synonyms. Kubisagari; "Le tourniquet"; paralytic vertigo.

Symptoms. Observed in epidemic form in Switzerland and Japan. During warm summer months, affects mainly young, healthy males who are in contact with cows (in Switzerland) or horses (Japan). Symptoms disappear if contaminated stables are abandoned and in the fall and winter. Attacks of palsies precipitated by severe exertion or bright light, warmth, hunger, or looking at a moving object (optokinetic irritation). Each attack lasts about 10 minutes, and they may follow each other at very short intervals. Mild form not incapacitating, severe form prevents any activity. Ptosis; dimness of vision; vertigo; diplopia; pains in the back of neck; nodding of head during attack.

Signs. Attack of temporary palsy of muscles: levator palpebrae superior; muscles of back of neck; extensor limbs; face; pharynx; larynx. During attack, hyperemia of fundus oculi; fundus normal and eyesight normal between attacks. Hyperreflexia in intervals.

Etiology. Infective agent suspected but not definitely provided. Small gram-negative coccus from spinal fluid of patient, when injected in cats, gives multiple transient palsies. A similar syndrome may be observed in pellagra.

Pathology. Unknown; possibly brain stem lesion.

Therapy. Unknown; avoidance of contact with contaminated animals and stables.

Prognosis. Good; possible recurrence with reexposure.

BIBLIOGRAPHY. Gérlier E: Une épidémie de vertige paralysant. Rev Med Suisse Romande 7:5–29, 1887
Conchoud PL: Le Kubisagari, Maladie de Gerlier. Rev Med 34:241–296, 1914
De Raadt OLE: Paralytic vertigo (Gerlier's syndrome). Confin Neurol 8:312–320, 1947–48

GERMAN'S

Synonyms. Fetal trimethadione. Tridione.

Symptoms. Both sexes affected; prenatal onset. Growth and mental deficiencies. Speech disorders.

Signs. Mild brachycephaly; midfacial hypoplasia and synophrys. Nose short, upturned, with low and broad bridge. Eyebrows upslanted; forehead prominent. Cleft lip and palate. Micrognathia. Ear abnormalities. Signs of cardiac malformations (Fallot's tetralogy; septal defects). Genital abnormalities: hypospadias; hypertrophic clitoris. Occasionally, variable abnormalities of skin, gastrointestinal, renal, and skeletal systems.

Etiology. Trimethadione or paramethadione taken in pregnancy. The syndrome becomes manifest in two thirds of offspring of women who have received the drugs during pregnancy.

Therapy. Nonspecific. If these drugs have been used during pregnancy, therapeutic abortion is indicated.

Prognosis. Poor, because of mental deficiency and heart abnormalities.

BIBLIOGRAPHY. German J, Lowal A, Ehlers KH: Trimethadione and human teratogenesis. Teratology 3:349–361, 1970
Zackai E, Mellman MJ, Neider B, et al: The fetal trimethadione syndrome. J Paediatr 87:280–284, 1975
Dukes MN: Meyler's Side Effects of Drugs, 9th ed, p 100. Amsterdam, Elsevier, 1980

GERSTMANN-STRAUSSLER-SCHEINKER

Synonyms. GSD, encephalopathy, subacute spongiform, GSSD; cerebellar ataxia–progressive dementia, amyloid dependent; amyloidosis cerebral-spongiform encephalopathy; Straussler's.

Symptoms and Signs. Onset in the fifth decade. Initially ataxia then dementia, accompanied by spinocerebellar and corticospinal tract degeneration. Absence of leg reflexes.

Etiology. Autosomal dominant inheritance or possibly slow viruses.

Pathology. Extensive amyloid plaques throughout central nervous system, spongiform degeneration.

Prognosis. Death in 2 to 10 years.

BIBLIOGRAPHY. Gerstmann J, Straussler E, Scheinker I: Ueber eine eigenartige hereditaer-familiaere Erkrankung des Zentral Nerven Systems. Z Gensamte Neurol Psychiat 154:736–762, 1936
Hudson AJ, Fanell MA, Calnins R, et al: Gerstmann-Straussler-Scheinker disease with coincidental familial onset. Ann Neurol 14:670–678, 1983

GERSTMANN'S

Synonym. Angular gyrus. Bilateral asomatognosia. Asomatognosia bilateral.

Symptoms. Finger agnosia; right-left disorientation; dysgraphia; dyscalculia.

Etiology. Each of the symptoms component of the syndrome may be found isolated or in different combinations. The autonomous entity of this syndrome has been denied and considered an arbitrary selection of concurrent deficits. The fact that the concurrence of the four symptoms implies a localization of lesion on the angular gyrus of the dominant hemisphere has also been disproved.

Prognosis. When the four components are found, severe impairment of brain function exists, and the underlying disease compromises the patient's life.

BIBLIOGRAPHY. Gerstmann J: Fingeragnosie: Eine umschriebene Storung der orientierung am eigenen Korper. Wien Klin Wochenschr 37:1010–1012, 1924
Gerstmann J: Some notes on the Gerstmann syndrome. Neurology 7:866–869, 1957
Adams RD, Victor M: Principles of Neurology, 3rd ed, p 340. New York, McGraw-Hill, 1985
Hemiberger RF, Demeyer W, Reitan RM: Implications of Gerstmann's syndrome. J Neurol Neurosurg Psychiatr 27:52–57, 1964

GESSLER'S

Synonym. Gold polishers. See Ulnar nerve compression.

Symptoms and Signs. Muscular atrophy in hands of gold polishers.

Etiology. Ulnar neuritis (not recognized by Gessler).

BIBLIOGRAPHY. Gessler H: Eine Egenartige Form von progressive muskelatrophie bei Goldpolirinner. Med Kor Bl J Württemerg Artstl 36:281, 1929

GIANNOTTI-CROSTI

Synonyms. Papular infantile acrodermatitis; infantile lichenoid acrodermatitis; Crosti-Giannotti; eruptive papular infantile acrodermatitis. IPA; PAC.

Symptoms and Signs. Both sexes affected; onset in neonatal period or early infancy (highest frequency between 2 and 6 years of age), seldom in adults. No seasonal predilection. Incubation period 15 to 29 days; few systemic manifestations; occasionally central nervous system irritative signs. Onset abrupt; erythematous-papular-lenticular eruption; occasionally, hemorrhagic; also with isolated elements on cheeks, chin, neck, extremities, buttocks. The trunk is rarely involved. No itching. In a few cases, mild fever; eruptions last 15 to 29 days. Modest lymphadenopathy (lasting 2 months). Splenomegaly (lasting a few days). Hepatomegaly. Jaundice in 9% of cases.

Etiology. Unknown. In some cases, may follow vaccination (smallpox or poliomyelitis). Hepatitis B virus (HBV), Epstein–Barr virus and coxsackie virus have been suspected.

Pathology. *Skin.* Lymphomonocytic infiltration (histiocytic type of cells) of papillary and superficial derma; occasionally, red cell extravasation. *Lymph nodes.* Reactive intense follicular hyperplasia. *Liver.* Acute hepatitis.

Diagnostic Procedures. *Blood.* Transaminase, aldolase, phosphatase increased; sodium sulfobromophthalein (Bromsulphalein) increased retention (40%); increase of alpha-2 and beta globulins; hyperchromic anemia; monocytosis; presence of plasma cells. *Bone marrow.* Increase of reticular elements.

Therapy. None. Corticosteroids do not affect course of disease.

Prognosis. Spontaneous remission. Hepatopathy lasts 6 to 12 months; enzymatic increase may last longer.

BIBLIOGRAPHY. Crosti A: Contributo alla conoscenza della pityriasis rubra pilaris di Devergie e dei suoi rapporti con sindromi vicine. Gior It Dermatol Sif 71:305–340, 1930
Crosti A, Giannotti F: Dermatose eruptive acrosituée d'origine probablement virosique. Dermatologica 115:671–677, 1957
Giannotti F: L'acrodermatite papulosa infantile. Malattia. Gaz San 41:271–274, 1970
Rook A, Wilkinson DS, Ebling FJG, et al: Textbook of Dermatology, 4th ed, p 718. Oxford, Blackwell Scientific Publications, 1986
Draelos ZK, Hansen RC, James WD: Giannotti-Crosti syndrome associated with infections other than hepatitis B. JAMA 256:2386–2388, 1986

GIANT CELL INTERSTITIAL PNEUMONIA

Synonym. GIP. See also Pneumonia lymphoid interstitial.

Symptoms. Both sexes affected; onset at all ages. Asthenia; cough; dyspnea; fever; weight loss.

Signs. Pulmonary rales and finger clubbing.

Etiology. Unknown. In children, defective immunologic system; in adults, intact immunologic system.

Pathology. Within alveoli, numerous bizarre, giant, multinucleated cells. Interstitial tissue thickened by fibrosis and plasma lymphocyte infiltrate.

Diagnostic Procedures. *Blood.* Usually, no defective immunologic findings in adults. *X-ray.* Streaked and mottled nodular density from hilus to periphery.

Therapy. Corticosteroids.

Prognosis. Good response to treatment.

BIBLIOGRAPHY. Reddy PA, Gorelich DG, Christianson CS: Giant cell interstitial pneumonia (GIP). Chest 58:319–325, 1970
Sokolowski JW, Cordray OR, Cantow EF, et al: Giant cell interstitial pneumonia. Report of a case. Am Rev Resp Dis 105:417–420, 1972
Fraser RG, Paré JAP: Diagnoses of Diseases of the Chest, 2nd ed, p 1704. Philadelphia, WB Saunders, 1977

GIBERT'S

Synonyms. Hebra's herpes tonsurans maculosus; herpes tousurans maculosus, pityriasis rosea.

Symptoms. Both sexes affected; onset at all ages; highest frequency between 10 and 35 years of age. Malaise; mild pruritus; slight fever.

Signs. On thigh or upper arm, trunk or neck appearance of "herald patch": bright red; round or oval; covered by fine silvery gray scaling epidermis. The patch edge is slightly raised and patch rapidly reaches 2 to 5 cm in diameter or more. Usually after 5 to 15 days crops of smaller similar patches appear on the whole body with successive bursts, at 2 to 3 days' interval, for 4 to 7 weeks. Center of plaques clears and becomes wrinkled. Occasionally, lymphadenopathy.

Etiology. Unknown. Infective agent suspected.

Pathology. Not typical: edema, plus inflammatory changes.

Diagnostic Procedures. *Blood.* Negative. *Skin.* Mycelium search negative.

Therapy. In mild cases, none. In irritated cases, diluted corticosteroid ointments; ultraviolet light.

Prognosis. Self-limited condition of 1 to 2 months' duration. Recurrences 2%.

BIBLIOGRAPHY. Gilbert CM: Traité pratique des maladies de la peau, p 402. Paris, Plan, 1860

Rook A, Wilkinson DS, Ebling FJG, et al: Textbook of Dermatology, 4th ed, pp 720–723. Oxford, Blackwell Scientific Publications, 1986

GIBSON'S

Synonyms. Gibson-Scott-Griffith; hereditary methemoglobinemia with deficiency of nicotinamide adenine dinucleotide (NADH) cytochrome b₅ reductase. See also Hoerlein-Weber.

Symptoms. Both sexes affected; onset frequently from birth. Asymptomatic or fatigability and dyspnea after exercise. A minority of patients are mentally retarded or have neurologic impairment.

Signs. Slate gray cyanosis (patient more blue than sick). No evidence of pulmonary or cardiac condition; no finger clubbing.

Etiology. Autosomal recessive inheritance. Deficiency of NADH dehydrogenase in red cells and possibly in other tissues (e.g., brain).

Pathology. Apparently, none.

Diagnostic Procedures. *Oxygen administration.* Does not reverse cyanosis. *Blood.* Shaking with air does not reduce the basic dark color. Spectral absorption peaks; qualitative and quantitative determination of methemoglobinemia. Hegesh's reaction to assay NADH dehydrogenase.

Therapy. None necessary. Vitamin C and methylene blue reduce cyanosis.

Prognosis. Very good; normal life and longevity in most cases.

BIBLIOGRAPHY. Gibson QH: The reduction of hemoglobin in red blood cells and studies on the cause of idiopathic methemoglobinemia. Biochem J 42:13–23, 1948
Scott EM, Griffith IV: The enzymatic defect of hereditary methemoglobinemia. Diaphorase Biochem Biophs Acta 134:584–586, 1959
Schwartz JM, Reiss AL, Jaffé ER: Hereditary methemoglobinemia with deficiency of NADH cytochrome b₅ reductase. In Stanbury JB, Wyngaarden JB, Fredrickson DS: The Metabolic Basis of Inherited Disease, 5th ed, p 1654. New York, McGraw-Hill, 1983

GIBSON'S (A.)

Synonyms. Krabbe III; muscular hypoplasia, congenital, universal. Muscular infantilism.

Symptoms and Signs. From birth. Severe generalized muscular hypoplasia.

Etiology. Possibly heterozygous group of conditions including cases of nemaline myopathy (see) and other without specific change except small muscle fibers.

Pathology. Small muscle fibers without pathologic changes.

Prognosis. Nonprogressive nature.

BIBLIOGRAPHY. Gibson A: Muscular infantilism. Arch Intern Med 27:338, 1921
Krabbe KH: Kongenit generaliseret muskelaplasi. Nord Med 35:1756, 1947
Pelias MZ, Thurmon TF: Congenital universal muscular hypoplasia: Evidence for autosomal recessive inheritance. Am J Hum Genet 31:548–554, 1979

GILBERT-DREYFUS

See Pseudohermaphroditism male incomplete hereditary type I.

Symptoms and Signs. Male phenotype. Small phallus; hypospadias; gynecomastia; scanty body hair; absent beard; testis normal-sized.

Etiology. X-linked inheritance.

Pathology. Incompletely developed wolffian ducts.

Diagnostic Procedures. Male sex chromatin 46 XY karyotype; gonadotropin level elevated; testosterone and estradiol levels elevated.

Therapy. Resistance to the effects of testosterone.

Prognosis. Good for life; function poor.

BIBLIOGRAPHY. Gilbert-Dreyfus NI, Savoie NI, Sebaoun NI, et al: Etude d'un cas familial d'androgenoidisme avec hypospadias grave, gynécomastie et hypoestrenogénie. Ann Endocrinol (Paris) 18:93–101, 1957
Wilson JD, Harrod MJ, Goldstein JL, et al: Familial incomplete manifestations in a family with the Reifenstein syndrome. N Engl J Med 290:1097–1103, 1974

GILBERT'S (J.B.)

Synonyms. Choriogenic gynecomastia.

Symptoms. Occur in males. Tenderness and pain of nipples.

Signs. Unilateral or bilateral swelling, initially under areola, successive enlargement of breast.

Etiology. Excessive production of chorionic hormones from malignant testicular tumor.

Therapy. Orchidectomy.

Prognosis. According to time of onset and therapy.

BIBLIOGRAPHY. Gilbert JB: Studies in malignant testis tumor II. Syndrome of coriogenic gynecomastia: Report of six cases and review of one hundred and twenty nine. J Urol 44:345–357, 1940

GILBERT'S (N.A.)

Synonyms. Unconjugated benign bilirubinemia; Gilbert-Lereboullet; low-grade chronic hyperbilirubinemia; icterus intermittens juvenilis, familial nonhemolytic nonobstructive jaundice; constitutional liver dysfunction; Meulengracht's.

Symptoms and Signs. Both sexes affected; male to female ratio 4 : 1; onset usually shortly after birth, but may not be recognized for many years. Scleral jaundice only abnormal finding. Usually after diagnosis is made, fatigue, nausea, abdominal pain in right quadrant (anxiety reaction?). Symptoms and jaundice become more pronounced after exertion, alcohol, intercurrent infections.

Etiology. Unknown; possibly autosomal dominant inheritance. Benign group of metabolic abnormalities. Attempts to determine impairment of bilirubin conjugation or decrease of glucuronyl transferase activity have failed. Slight reduction of red cell survival found in 50% of patients. Reduced bilirubin uridine diphosphate (UDP) glucuronyl transferase activity could possibly explain hyperbilirubinemia and impaired clearance of pigment but it is not the only mechanism responsible for the syndrome.

Pathology. Normal hepatic histology.

Diagnostic Procedures. *Blood.* Unconjugated bilirubinemia (fasting increases hyperbilirubinemia); serum transaminases normal; serum alkaline phosphatase normal. No overt evidence of hemolysis or other conditions that may produce bilirubinemia. *Urine.* Bilirubinuria absent. *Biopsy of liver.* Normal. *Cholangiography.* Normal.

Therapy. Reassurance of the patient about benign prognosis to avoid anxiety-type symptoms. Phenobarbital administration reduces bilirubin level.

Prognosis. Excellent; jaundice with fluctuation persisting through life.

BIBLIOGRAPHY. Gilbert NA, Lereboullet P: La cholemie simple familiale. Sem Med 11:241–243, 1901
Powell LW, Hemingway E, Billing BH, Sherlock S: Idiopathic unconjugated hyperbilirubinemia (Gilbert's syndrome). N Engl J Med 277:1108–1112, 1967
Wolkoff AW, Chowdhury JR, Arias IM: Hereditary jaundice and disorders of bilirubin metabolism. In Stanbury JB, Wyngaarden JB, Fredrickson DS, et al: The Metabolic Basis of Inherited Disease, 5th ed, p 1385. New York, McGraw-Hill, 1983

GILFORD–BURNIER

Synonyms. Ateliosis; Burnier's; pituitary dwarfism; prepuberal panhypopituitarism. Ateliotic dwarfism–hypogonadism; pituitary dwarfism III, Hanhart's (see for subtypes).

Symptoms and Signs. Both sexes affected; age of onset variable. Characteristic diversity of appearance according to number of hormone deficiencies. All cases present delayed growth; symptomatic hypoglycemia is another almost constant feature; hypothyroidism features (52%); hypogonadism (88%); hypoadrenalism (56%).

Etiology. Idiopathic. Often secondary to pituitary adenoma or other destructive lesions of pituitary or other diencephalic pathology. Also possibly related to trauma at birth. Autosomal recessive inheritance also well described.

Pathology. According to etiology and type of hormone deficiencies.

Diagnostic Procedures. *Blood.* Determination of growth hormone; adrenocorticotropic hormone (ACTH); thyroid-stimulating hormone (TSH), gonadotropin, hypoglycemia. Other metabolic derangements according to hormones involved.

Therapy. Pituitary hormones, according to development of hormonal deficiencies (occasionally sequential).

Prognosis. Excellent response to hormone administration. That of primary lesion.

BIBLIOGRAPHY. Gilford H: Ateliosis: Form of dwarfism. Practitioner 70:797–819, 1903
Burnier R: A new hypophyseal syndrome; hypophyseal nanism. Ann Ophthalmol 21:263–273, 1912
Goodman GH, Grumbach MM, Kaplan SL: Growth and growth hormone. II. A comparison of isolated growth hormone deficiency and multiple pituitary-hormone deficiencies in 35 patients with idiopathic hypopituitary dwarfism. N Engl J Med 278:57–78, 1968
Frasier DS: Human pituitary growth hormone (4GH) therapy in growth hormone deficiency. Endocrinol Rev 4:155–170, 1983
McArthur RG, Morgan K, Phillips JA III, et al: The natural history of familial hypopituitarism. Am J Med Genet 22:553–566, 1985

GILLES DE LA TOURETTE'S

Synonyms. Brissaud's II; coprolalia-generalized tic; Guinon's myospasia impulsiva; Tourette's.

Symptoms. Occur generally in boys; begin at the age 7 or 8. Generalized tics limited preferably to facial muscles;

inarticulate expiratory laryngeal noises at the beginning, spreading of tics to the shoulders and arms. With progression of the form, the patient begins to exclaim in loud voice obscene words or short phrases (coprolalia). Echolalia, pallilalia, echomimesia may also develop. Tics that may be very violent stop during sleep and are intensified by emotions. It has been reported that in some cases they may be suppressed by voluntary control. Coprolalia manifests only in presence of other people; it may, by some patients, be masked by coughing. Intelligence varies from superior to subnormal.

Signs. In some cases, neurologic signs of doubtful significance.

Etiology. Unknown; not established if of organic or psychogenic origin. Emotional trauma frequently precipitating factor. Disturbed parent–child relation frequently encountered in history.

Pathology. Only two autopsies: one normal; the second showed no gross pathology, but possibly an enlargement of large neurocytes of corpus striatum.

Therapy. Chlorpromazine; haloperidol; group psychotherapy (?); prefrontal leukotomy (in extremely severe cases). The proposed differentiation of Tourette syndrome subgroups according to the presence or absence of migraine and other serotonin-related associated symptoms may aid in predicting drug response to haloperidol, clonidine, and other agents and in the development of other drugs for the treatment of this disorder.

Prognosis. Course unpredictable. Spontaneous arrest with exacerbations; lifelong symptoms. Quoad vitam good.

BIBLIOGRAPHY. Gilles de la Tourette G: Étude sur une affection nerveuse caractérisée par de l'incoordination motrice accompagnée d'écholalie et de coprolalie. Arch Neurol 9:19–42; 158–200, 1885
Hanin J, Merikangas JR, Merikangas KR: Red-cell choline and Gilles de la Tourette syndrome. N Engl J Med 301:661–662, 1979
Barabas G, Matthews WS: Homogenous clinical subgroups in children with Tourette syndrome. Pediatrics 75:73–75, 1985
Morrison JE, Lockhart CH: Tourette syndrome: anesthetic implications. Anesth Analg 65:200–202, 1986

GILLESPIE'S

Synonyms. Aniridia–cerebellar ataxia–mental deficiency.

Symptoms and Signs. Both sexes. From birth. Bilateral aniridia; physical and mental retardation; hypotonia; normal tendon reflexes, normal sensitivity; gross incoordination, attention tremor, scanning speech.

Etiology. Unknown. Autosomal recessive inheritance proposed. Normal karyotype.

Diagnostic Procedures. All laboratory exams normal.

Prognosis. With age some improvement of motor performance. Persisting mental deficiency.

BIBLIOGRAPHY. Gillespie FB: Aniridia, cerebellar ataxia and oligophrenia in siblings. Arch Ophthalmol 73:338–341, 1965
Sarsfield JK: The syndrome of congenital cerebellar ataxia, aniridia and mental retardation. Dev Med Child Neurol 13:508–511, 1971

GILLIN AND PRYSE-DAVIS

Synonyms. Pterygium, multiple, lethal type.

Symptoms and Signs. Those of pterygium in aborted fetuses. Varieties with bone fusion or spinal fusion described.

BIBLIOGRAPHY. Hall JC: The lethal multiple pterygium syndromes (editorial). Am J Med Genet 17:803–807, 1974
Gillin ME, Pryse-Davis J: Pterygium syndrome. J Med Genet 13:249–251, 1976

GILLUM-ANDERSON

Synonyms. Blepharoptosis–inherited myopia–ectopia lentis.

Symptoms and Signs. From birth bilateral ptosis. Ectopia lentis, dislocated lenses.

Etiology. Genetic defect. Responsible for weakness of orbital connective tissue.

BIBLIOGRAPHY. Gillum WM, Anderson RL: Dominantly inherited blepharoptosis, high myopia and ectopia lentis. Arch Ophthalmol 100:282–284, 1982

GIROUX-BARBEAU

Synonyms. Erythrokeratodermia–ataxia; ataxia–erythrokeratodermia.

Symptoms and Signs. Both sexes. After birth. Papulosquamous erythematous plaques more evident in winter and that disappear or are markedly reduced after 25 years of age. After a few years progressive neurologic altera-

tions: decreased tendon reflexes, nystagmus, dysarthria, and ataxia.

Etiology. Unknown. Autosomal dominant inheritance.

Pathology. Skin. Centrifugal damage with spongiosis and necrosis of malpighian layer and absence of stratum granulosum.

Therapy. None specific. Temporal effacing by stripping of the lesions.

BIBLIOGRAPHY. Giroux JM, Barbeau A: Erythrokeratoderma with ataxia. Arch Dermatol 106:183–188, 1972

GJESSING'S

Synonym. Periodic catatonia.

Symptoms. Recurring periods of catatonic stupor and psychic excitement.

Etiology. Unknown. No further report on the syndrome. It may belong in the group of thyroid psychoses.

Diagnostic Procedures. Increase of blood urea nitrogen (BUN) during episodes.

Therapy. Thyroid hormone.

Prognosis. Complete control with indicated treatment.

BIBLIOGRAPHY. Gjessing R: Disturbances of somatic function in catatonia with a period course, and their compensation. J Ment Sci 84:608–621, 1938

GLANZMANN-RINIKER

Synonyms. Swiss type agammaglobulinemia; lymphocytosis–thymic alymphoplasia; thymic dysplasia; lymphopenic agammaglobulinemia. Severe combined immunodeficiency; lymphocytophthisis. ADA deficiency, adenosine deaminase deficiency.

Symptoms and Signs. Male to female ratio 3 : 1; onset from early infancy (3–6 mo). Succession of debilitating infections (viral and bacterial); watery diarrhea; candidiasis; failure to thrive.

Etiology. Two different modes of inheritance: autosomal recessive and X-linked. In 50% of autosomal recessive cases absence of adenosine deaminase (ADA). The pathogenesis in these cases is due to ATP accumulation or S-adenosyl homocysteine toxicity on immunocompetent lymphocytes.

Pathology. *Thymus.* Small or almost absent; lack of Hassall's corpuscles. *Bone marrow, spleen, lymph nodes.* Absence or small number of lymphocytes and plasma cells; lack of germinal centers.

Diagnostic Procedures. *Blood.* Leukopenia lower than 2000; marked lymphopenia (lack of both T and B types); lymphocytes unresponsive to phytohemoagglutinin or allogenic stimulation; many lymphocytes immature (lymphoblast types); granulocytes and platelets normal; moderate eosinophilia; negative adenosine deaminase in erythrocytes. *Protein electrophoresis.* Agammaglobulinemia. *Skin tests.* Negative response to Candida antigens; absence of sensitization to dinitrochlorobenzene; acceptance of skin grafts.

Therapy. Gamma globulin injection of temporary and little effect. Bone marrow transplant failure for graft versus host reaction. Keep the patient in aseptic environment.

Prognosis. Overwhelming infections; fatal usually within first year of life.

BIBLIOGRAPHY. Glanzmann E, Riniker P: Essentielle Lymphocytophtise. Ein neues Krankheitsbild aus der Säugligspathologie. Ann Paediatr 175:1–32, 1950
Kredich NM, Hershfield MS: Immunodeficiency diseases caused by adenosine deaminase deficiency and purine nucleoside phosphorylase deficiency. In Stanbury JB, Wyngaarden JB, Fredrickson DS, et al: The Metabolic Basis of Inherited Disease, 5th ed, p 1157. New York, McGraw-Hill, 1983

GLANZMANN'S

Synonyms. Diacyclothrombopathia; Glanzmann–Naegeli; thromboasthenia.

Symptoms and Signs. Both sexes affected; onset from birth. May be asymptomatic until trauma or surgical procedures make condition evident. Recurrent petechiae; epistaxis, menorrhagia or metrorrhagia and other bleeding manifestations of different degrees of severity may spontaneously occur.

Etiology. Qualitative platelet defect. Characterized by deficient adenosine diphosphate (ADP)-induced platelet aggregation and deficient clot retraction causing lack of mechanism for viscous metamorphosis or clot retraction. Four different genotype changes apparently have been identified that lead to the phenotype of this syndrome. Several varieties of this condition have been identified to be inherited as autosomal recessive traits. Absence on platelet membrane of glycoprotein IIb-IIIa which interacts with thrombin to form the clot. Absence of glycoprotein IIb-IIIa is also accompanied by absence of PL A1 antigen.

Diagnostic Procedures. *Blood.* Bleeding time prolonged; tourniquet test positive or negative. Platelets normal number (in some varieties of this condition decreased); may present normal morphology, or be small or large and bizarre; usually appear isolated rather than clumped. Usually, inability to be aggregated by ADP in one group: low platelet adenosine triphosphate (ADT), pyruvate kinase, and phosphoglyceraldehyde; in a second variety, only ATP low; in a third variety, ATPase deficient; in a fourth variety, absence of fibrinogenlike protein from surface of platelets.

Therapy. Allogenic bone marrow transplantation gives complete correction of defect. Fresh blood transfusion may temporarily modify defect.

Prognosis. Usually benign, but death from hemorrhage may occur. Usually hemorrhagic manifestation decreases with age.

BIBLIOGRAPHY. Glanzmann WE: Hereditäre hamorrhägische Thrombasthenie. Jahrb Kinderheilkd 88:1–42, 113–141, 1918
Bellucci S, Denergic A, Gluckman E, et al: Complete correction of Glanzmann thromboasthenia by allogenic bone marrow transplantation. Br J Haematol 59:635–641, 1985

GLENARD'S

Synonyms. Enteroptosis; spleneptosis; visceroptosis.

Symptoms. Female to male ratio 4 : 1; onset at all ages. In erect position, abdominal discomfort, backache; fatigability; nausea; palpitation; occasionally, vomiting and syncope; usually, chronic constipation.

Signs. Abdominal palpation reveals muscular atony, transverse colon in lower position, sagging, occasionally, to upper edge of pelvis, and epigastric pulsation. Tachycardia.

Etiology. Weakness of abdominal muscles; congenital or acquired condition, in the latter case after severe weight loss.

Diagnostic Procedures. *X-ray of gastrointestinal tract.* In various positions to evidentiate the displacement of diaphragm, hypochondrial organs, stomach and intestinal sections. The heart too may appear elongated.

Therapy. Girdle; correction of severe weight loss; physical therapy to strengthen selected muscle groups. Surgery seldom indicated.

Prognosis. Worsening with age.

BIBLIOGRAPHY. Glénard F: Neuroasthénie et entéroptose. Sem Med 6:211–212, 1886
Freedman AM, Kaplan HI, Sadock BJ: Comprehensive Textbook of Psychiatry, 2nd ed. Baltimore, Williams & Wilkins, 1975

GLOBUS

Synonyms. Bolus hystericus. See Plummer-Vinson.

Symptoms. Sensation of lump in throat, which interferes with swallowing.

Etiology and Pathology. Carcinomas; strictures; enlarged styloid process; pharyngeal pouch; pharyngeal paralysis; hypochromic anemia (see Plummer-Vinson) and cervical spine area pathology, especially osteoarthritis, psychoneurotic disorder (bolus hystericus).

Diagnostic Procedures. *Nose and throat examination. X-ray of cervical spine.* In different projections. *Blood.* Hemoglobin determination; red cell sedimentation rate.

Therapy. According to etiology; surgical; medical; psychotherapeutic.

Prognosis. Depends on etiology. Careful examination of the spine in cases with otherwise negative findings may reveal hidden pathology and significantly decrease the psychiatric group, and provide therapeutic means to cure these patients.

BIBLIOGRAPHY. Morrison LF: The cervical spine and the globus syndrome. Ann Otol 64:753–765, 1955
Freedman AM, Kaplan HI, Sadock BJ: Comprehensive Textbook of Psychiatry, 2nd ed, p 2587. Baltimore, Williams & Wilkins, 1975
Castell DO, Johnson LF: Esophageal Function in Health and Disease. New York, Elsevier-Dutton, 1982

GLOBUS PALLIDUS NECROSIS

Symptoms. Patients who have suffered an episode of coma from carbon monoxide, nitrous oxide, carbon disulfide, or natural gas inhalation. One to 3 weeks after recovering from initial coma, either with complete recovery, or with only residual slight confusion, patient relapses into coma a second time. Relapse may onset with akinetic mute state, with generalized rigidity and flexion of arm and extension of legs, with mental confusion, with visual agnosia, or catatonic postures. In a minority of cases, only a mild parkinsonian rigidity appears within 6 weeks of recovery of first episode of coma.

Etiology. Necrosis of globus pallidus associated, with major or minor cortical damage due to coal gas toxicity (carbon monoxide) and hemorrhagic necrosis.

Pathology. When death occurs during first coma episode, usually the most anterior part of internal segments show symmetric hemorrhagic softening. When death occurs after delayed relapse, larger infarct involving external segments and even part of putamen. Patchy areas of cortical laminal necrosis may be present.

Therapy. Symptomatic.

Prognosis. Very poor; death usually follows first or second episode of coma. In some cases, longer survival with development of astasia-abasia; then rigidity, and mutism.

BIBLIOGRAPHY. Meyer A: Ueber der Wirkung der Kohlenoxydvergiftung auf das Zentralnervensystem. Z Ges Neurol Psychiatr 112:172, 1926
Denny-Brown D: Basal Ganglia. London, Oxford University Press, 1962

GLOMERULONEPHRITIS, CHRONIC

It is the clinical expression of a variety of glomerular diseases often asymptomatic which progressively obliterate renal mass. Chronic renal failure with uremia is the outcome. See specific syndromes.

BIBLIOGRAPHY. Brenner BM, Rector FC Jr: The Kidney, 3rd ed, p 946. Philadelphia, WB Saunders, 1986

GLOMUS JUGULARE TUMOR

Symptoms. Prevalent in females; onset in second to sixth decade (average 48 yr). Duration of symptoms before diagnosis 2 to 3 years. Conduction deafness; fullness or pulsation in the ear; aural discharge; facial (VII) nerve paralysis; paralysis of ninth through twelfth cranial nerves; paralysis of vocal cord.

Signs. Usually tumor behind tympanic membrane, less frequently in the external canal or cervical region.

Etiology. Unknown; tumor of glomus jugulare (including all chemodectomas arising in vicinity of ear).

Pathology. Circumscribed tumor reddish, friable, usually confined to middle ear, some extending into cochlea and eustachian tube and destroying temporal bone. No capsule submucosal involvement characteristic. Cells arranged in nest with vascular fibrous septa.

Diagnostic Procedures. *Angiography of carotid.*

Therapy. Surgical excision; total seldom possible. X-ray treatment.

Prognosis. Usually, cure with surgery; local recurrences or local invasion may develop; or metastasis in malignant type (rare).

BIBLIOGRAPHY. Rosenwasser H: Carotid body tumor of the middle ear and mastoid. Arch Otolaryngol 41:64–67, 1945

Oberman HA: Chemodectomas (nonchromaffin paraganglioma) of head and neck. Cancer 21:838–851, 1968

Horn KL, Creemley RL, Schindler RA: Facial neurolemmomas. Laryngoscope 91:1326–1331, 1981

GLOSSOPALATINE ANKYLOSIS

Symptoms and Signs. Present from birth. Tongue attached to hard palate and occasionally also to superior alveolar ridge; consequent reduced mobility. Occasionally, high-arched or cleft palate. Mandible sometimes hypoplastic; hypodontia (incisor teeth primarily); occasionally, temporomandibular joint ankylosis; occasionally, facial paralysis. Possibly associated limb anomalies (e.g., hands, feet).

Etiology. Unknown. Sporadic.

BIBLIOGRAPHY. Kettner: Kongenitaler Zungendefect. Dtsch Med Wochenschr 33:532, 1907

Kramer W: Zur Entstehung der angeborenen Gaumenspalte. Zentrabl Chir 38:385–387, 1911

Henderson JL: The congenital facial diplegia syndrome: Clinical features, pathology and aetiology. Brain 62, 381–403, 1936

Gorlin RJ, Pindborg JJ, Cohen MM, Jr: Syndromes of the Head and Neck, 2nd ed. New York McGraw-Hill, 1976

GLUCAGONOMA

Synonyms. Alpha-2 cell carcinoma; pancreas alpha-2 cell carcinoma.

Symptoms and Signs. Prevalent in females (3 : 2); onset between second and seventh decade. Weight loss in 64% of cases; pallor; necrolytic migratory erythema (individual erythematous papules that blister, ooze, crust, and spread peripherally, while clearing in the center). Superinfections common; lesions evolve in 14 days and heal, leaving bronze discoloration, without scar formation. Stomatitis and glossitis (in 33% of cases). Neuropsychiatric disturbances. Can be part of a pluriglandular syndrome.

Etiology. Alpha-2 cell tumor of the islets of Langerhans, producing excessive amount of glucagon.

Pathology. Tumor of pancreas. Metastasis in liver and other sites. Primary tumor averages 3 cm in diameter at time of surgery. *Histologically.* Alpha-2-type of islet cells.

Diagnostic Procedures. *Blood.* Normochromic anemia; plasma glucagon levels 0.3 to 96.0 ng/ml (normal less than 0.2 ng/ml); hyperglycemia or altered glucose tolerance test (or both).

Therapy. Surgery whenever feasible. Chemotherapy by streptozocin gives good response; by diaminotriazenoimidazone carboximide as an alternative. The skin manifestation responds to zinc sulfate. In case of metastatized tumor Somatostatin analogue SMS 201-995.

Prognosis. Complete removal of tumor induces full remission of all symptoms. In inoperable cases good results (symptom control) obtained with chemotherapy.

BIBLIOGRAPHY. Becker SW, Kahn D, Rothman S: Cutaneous manifestations of internal malignant tumors. Arch Dermatol Syph 45:1069–1080, 1942

McGavran MH, Unger RH, Recant L, et al: A glucagon-secreting alpha-cell carcinoma of the pancreas. N Engl J Med 274:1408–1413, 1966

Higgins GA, Recant L, Fishman AB: The glucagonoma syndrome: Surgically curable diabetes. Am J Surg 137:142–148, 1979

Bloom SR, Polak JM: Glucagonoma syndrome. Am J Med 82 (suppl 5B):25–35, 1987

GLUCOSE-GALACTOSE MALABSORPTION

Symptoms and Signs. Both sexes affected; onset with first milk feeding. Watery diarrhea following every milk intake. Failure to thrive; dehydration.

Etiology. Unknown; autosomal recessive inheritance. Basic defect in absorption of both glucose and galactose confined to mucosal cells at brush border of intestine.

Pathology. Normal jejunal mucosa; accumulation of glucose in brush border of cells.

Diagnostic Procedures. *Stool.* Acid rich in glucose, galactose, lactic acid; disaccharides absent. *Urine.* Glycosuria. *Elimination of lactose and galactose from diet.* Relieves all symptoms. *Administration of fructose.* Well tolerated and increases plasma glucose. *Glucose-galactose oral tolerance test.* No rise in blood sugar.

Therapy. Omit milk and any carbohydrate, except fructose, from diet.

Prognosis. If defect readily identified and dietetic regimen instituted, good. Permanent damage if not treated early.

BIBLIOGRAPHY. Laplane R, Polonovski C, Etienne M, et al: Intolerance to sugars of active intestinal transfer. Its relation to intolerance to lactose and the celiac syndrome. Arch Fr Pediatr 19:895–944, 1962

Milue MD: Hereditary abnormalities of intestinal absorption. Br Med Bull 23:279–284, 1968

Gray GM: Intestinal disaccharidase deficiencies and glucose–galactose malabsorption. In Stanbury JB, Wyngaarden JB, Fredrickson DS, et al: The Metabolic Basis of Inherited Disease, 5th ed, p 1740. New York, McGraw-Hill, 1983

GLUCOSE-6-PHOSPHATE DEHYDROGENASE DEFICIENCY

Synonyms. G6PD. Cluster of syndromes due to a congenital defect of normal glucose-6-phosphate dehydrogenase and presence of abnormal mutant enzymes (80 variants described), some of which may induce the different clinical manifestations.

DRUG-INDUCED HEMOLYTIC ANEMIA (G6PD)

Symptoms and Signs. Males affected; seldom seen in females, or mild symptoms onset at all ages after exposure; to drugs (antimalarials; sulfonamides; sulfones; nitrofurans; antipyretics; analgesics; others). Hemolytic crises of mild degree; abdominal and back pains; hemoglobinuria.

EPISODIC HEMOLYTIC ANEMIA (G6PD) WITHOUT DRUG EXPOSURE

Symptoms and Signs. Whites, blacks of both sexes affected; onset at any age. Moderate or severe hemolytic crises spontaneous or in association with infections; metabolic alterations (ketoacidosis). Acute renal insufficiency may result from crises.

FAVISM

Symptoms and Signs. Occurs in population from Mediterranean areas (highest incidence in Sardinians); reported also in west China; male to female ratio 6.2 : 1; onset at 2 to 5 years of age. Hemolytic crises of variable severity following ingestion of fava beans (2–3 days) or inhalation of pollen (few hours).

NEONATAL JAUNDICE (G6PD)

Symptoms and Signs. Greeks, Thais, and others affected; onset in neonatal period. Severe hemolytic crisis, with possible kidney failure, spontaneous or after vitamin K, drugs, or infections.

NONSPHEROCYTIC CONGENITAL HEMOLYTIC ANEMIA (G6PD)

Symptoms and Signs. Whites and blacks affected; onset in infancy or childhood. Symptoms and signs of chronic hemolytic anemia.

Etiology. X-linked inheritance. Glucose-6-phosphate deficiency and presence of various mutant enzymes. Different clinical syndromes precipitated by drugs, infections, other toxic factors (e.g., immunologic).

Pathology. Nonspecific.

Diagnostic Procedures. *Blood.* Anemia of various degree; hemoglobinemia. Identification of red cell deficiency and presence of various mutant enzymes. *Urine and stool.* Hemoglobin degeneration products.

Therapy. Avoidance of exposure to drugs or products that induce crises. Blood transfusions. Crisis may result in death. Usually, recovery after crisis and limited period of resistency to drug or product exposure.

BIBLIOGRAPHY. Cordes W: Experiences with plasmochin in malaria: Preliminary reports, p 66. 15th Annual Report, United Fruit Company (Med Dept), 1926

Luisada A: Favism. Medicina (B Aires) 20:229–250, 1941

Bentler E: Glucose-6-phosphate dehydrogenase deficiency. In Stanbury JB, Wyngaarden JB, Fredricksen DS, et al: The Metabolic Basis of Inherited Disease, 5th ed, p 1629. New York, McGraw-Hill, 1983

Smith CL, Snowdon SL: Anaesthesia and glucose-6-phosphate dehydrogenase deficiency: A case report and review of the literature. Anaesth 42:281–287, 1987

GLUE EAR

Synonym. Chronic exudative otitis media.

Symptoms and Signs. Affects children between the ages 5 and 8; onset also in adulthood. Incidence about 3%. Deafness occasionally discovered in 5-year-old children by teachers, and routine testing, since patients are not aware of it. The conductive deafness is usually with a threshold of 20 db or more. Detailed examination with binocular operating microscope is often required and sometimes also diagnostic myringotomy. At the onset, membrane appears normal, but at closer observation annular and radial vessels appear filled. Later, the membrane assumes yellowish color.

Etiology. Unknown. Have been considered: bacterial and viral infections, allergy; dysfunction of eustachian tubes due to muscosal swelling in the tympanic orifice or other pathologic process at pharyngeal end.

Pathology. Accumulation in middle ear of sterile, highly viscous fluid containing cellular elements (neutrophils; lymphocytes; macrophages; plasma cells; rarely eosinophils).

Diagnostic Procedures. *Myringotomy.* Different diagnosis with secretory otitis media (low-viscosity fluid).

Treatment. Aspiration of exudate by electrically driven suction through myringotomy; insertion of hourglass-shaped plastic tube to keep the middle ear at atmosphere pressure. Hearing aid needed in relapsing cases.

Prognosis. Inserted grommet is removed within 6 months and the membrane heals spontaneously. Susceptibility to this form of otitis media decreases with puberty.

BIBLIOGRAPHY. Jordan R: Chronic secretory otitis media. Laryngoscope 59:1002–1015, 1949
Glue ear. (editorial) Br Med J I:589, 1969
Eichenwald H: Development in diagnosis and treating otitis media. Am Fam Physician 31:155–164, 1985

GLUTARIC ACIDURIA I

Synonyms. Glutaricidemia I, GA I, glutaric-CoA dehydrogenase deficiency.

Symptoms and Signs. Both sexes. Onset 6 months: opisthotonos, dystonia; athetoid posture.

Etiology. Autosomal recessive inheritance.

Diagnostic Procedures. *Blood.* Increased glutaric acid. Lysed leukocytes impairment to metabolize glutaryl CoA. *Urine.* Glutariciduria (increased by L-lysine administration).

Prognosis. Progressive dystonic cerebral palsy.

BIBLIOGRAPHY. Goodman SI, Moc PG, Markey SP: Glutaric aciduria: A "new" inborn error of amino acid metabolism. Am J Hum Genet 26:36A, 1984
Stutchfield P, Edwards MA, Gray RGF, et al: Glutaric aciduria type I misdiagnosed as Leith's encephalopathy and cerebral palsy. Dev Med Child Neurol 27:514–521, 1985

GLUTARIC ACIDURIA II

Synonyms. Multiple acyl-CoA dehydrogenases deficiency (MAD); GA IIB; ethylmalonic-adipic aciduria, EMA.

Symptoms and Signs. From birth metabolic acidosis, hypoglycemia, odor sweaty feet.

Etiology. Metabolic blocks in various pathways. Dehydrogenases for different acyl-CoAs. Autosomal recessive inheritance.

Diagnostic Procedures. *Urine.* (Glutarate the principal component) various dicarboxylic acids, short chain fatty acids. *Blood.* Hypoglycemia, acidosis without ketosis.

Therapy. Bicarbonate infusion.

Prognosis. Death in early infancy.

BIBLIOGRAPHY. Przyrembel H, Wendel U, Becker K, et al: Glutamic aciduria type II: Report of a previously undescribed metabolic disorder. Clin Chim Acta 66:227–239, 1976
Jakobs C, Sweetman L, Wadman SK, et al: Prenatal diagnosis of glutaric aciduria type II by direct chemical analysis of dicarboxylic acids in amniotic fluids. Eur J Paediatr 141:153–157, 1984

GLUTARIC ACIDURIA, NEONATAL

Synonyms. GA II A; Acyl-CoA dehydrogenase multiple deficiency; ACAD

Symptoms and Signs. Males. From birth: metabolic acidosis, hypoglycemia, hyperammonemia.

Etiology. X-linked inheritance.

Prognosis. Early death.

BIBLIOGRAPHY. Mantagos S, Genel M, Tanaka K: Ethylmalonic adipic aciduria. J Clin Invest 64:1580–1589, 1979
Mitchell G, Saudubray JM, Benoit Y, et al: Antenatal diagnosis of glutaricaciduria type II. Lancet I, 1099, 1983

GLUTATHIONE DEFICIENCIES

Synonyms. Hemolytic anemia–GSH deficiency; enzymopathy–GSH hemolytic anemia. GSH deficiency anemias are classified according to the enzyme deficiency.

1. GLUTAMYL CYSTINE SYNTHETASE DEFICIENCY
Symptoms and Signs. Hemolytic anemia, spinocerebellar degeneration, peripheral neuropathy, myopathy.

Etiology. Autosomal recessive inheritance. Deficiency of glutamylsynthetase.

Diagnostic Procedures. *Blood.* Hemolytic anemia, reduced glutathione. *Urine.* Aminoaciduria.

Therapy. Avoidance of oxydizing drugs.

Prognosis. Benign.

2. GLUTAMYL TRANSPEPTIDASE DEFICIENCY
Symptoms and Signs. Two patients described, one normal, one retarded.

Etiology. Probably autosomal recessive inheritance.

Diagnostic Procedures. *Urine.* Glutathyonuria. *Blood.* Glutathyonemia.

3. 5-OXOPROLINASE DEFICIENCY

Symptoms and Signs. From birth. Enterocolitis, urolithiasis.

Etiology. Deficiency of 5-oxoproline level.

BIBLIOGRAPHY. Oort M, Loos JA, Prins HK: Hereditary absence of reduced glutathione in the erythrocytes—A new clinical and biochemical entity? Vox Sang 6:370–373, 1961

Konrad PN, Richards F, II, Valentine VN, et al: Gamma glutamyl-cysteine synthetase deficiency. A cause of hereditary hemolytic anemia. N Engl J Med 286:557, 1972

Meister A: 5-Oxoprolinuria (pyroglutamic aciduria) and other disorders of the glutamyl cycle. In Stanbury JB, Wyngaarden JB, Fredrickson DS, et al: The Metabolic Basis of Inherited Disease, 5th ed, p 348. New York, McGraw-Hill, 1983

GLUTATHIONE SYNTHETASE DEFICIENCY

Synonyms. Oxoprolinuria; pyroglutamicaciduria.

Symptoms and Signs. Two types of syndromes. (1) Congenital hemolytic anemia with slight reduction of leukocyte glutathione. Symptoms are not severe. Major predisposition to infections. (2) Hemolytic anemia accompanied by severe metabolic acidosis due to high levels of 5-oxoproline in plasma and urine. Major predisposition to infections due to impaired bactericidal activity of neutrophils.

Etiology. Autosomal recessive. Type 1 is due to unstable glutathione synthetase enzyme. Type 2 is due to absence of glutathione synthetase which leads to overproduction of 5-oxoproline by glutamyl cysteine synthetase, the first enzyme of the glutathione synthetic pathway.

Diagnostic Procedures. Study of erythrocyte and leukocyte enzymes.

Therapy. In type 2 vitamin E administration. Sodium bicarbonate for metabolic acidosis.

Prognosis. Good quoad vitam.

BIBLIOGRAPHY. Spielberg SP, Kramer LI, Goodman SI, et al: Oxoprolinuria: Biochemical observations and case report. J Pediatr 91:237–241, 1977

Spielberg SP, Corash LM, Butler JD, et al: Biochemical heterogeneity in glutathione synthetase deficiency. J Clin Invest 61:1417, 1978

GM1 GANGLIOSIDOSIS ADULT

Synonym. GM1 gangliosidosis type 3.

Symptoms and Signs. From adolescence progressive cerebellar dysarthria spasticity and ataxia. Intellectual impairment progressive with time.

Etiology. Autosomal recessive inheritance. Diminished acid-β-galactosidase. Defect on chromosome 3.

Diagnostic Procedures. See Norman Landing.

Pathology. Not known.

Therapy. None.

Prognosis. Good quoad vitam.

BIBLIOGRAPHY. Wenger DA, Sattler M, Mueller OT, et al: Adult GM1 gangliosidosis: Clinical and biochemical studies of two patients and comparison to other patients called variant or adult GM1 gangliosidosis. Clin Genet 17:323, 1980

O'Brien JS: The gangliosidoses. In Stanbury JB, Wyngaarden JB, Fredrickson DS, et al: The Metabolic Basis of Inherited Disease, 5th ed, p 945. New York, McGraw-Hill, 1983

GODFRIED-PRICK-CAROL-PRAKKEN

Eponym used to indicate an association of Von Recklinghausen's I and atrophoderma vermiculare, facies mongoloid, mental retardation, and congenital heart block.

BIBLIOGRAPHY. Carol WL, Godfried EG, Prakken MR, Prick JJ: Von Recklinghaussenische Neurofibromatosis, Atrophodermia vermiculata und kongenitale Herzanomalie als Haupkennizeichen eines familiaerhereditaere Syndromes. Dermatologica 81:345–346, 1940

GOEBEL'S

Synonyms. Spheroid body myopathy; myopathy, spheroid body.

Symptoms and Signs. Both sexes. Onset in adolescence. Slowly developing myopathy causing motor incapacitation.

Etiology. Unknown. Autosomal dominant inheritance.

Pathology. *Muscle biopsy.* Presence of spheroid bodies (mainly type 1) in fibers, devoid of organelles. *Electromyography.*

Therapy. None.

Prognosis. Progressive motor incapacitation up to degeneration. Life span normal.

BIBLIOGRAPHY. Goebel HH, Muller J, Gillen HV, et al: Autosomal dominant spheroid body myopathy. Muscle Nerve 1:14–26, 1978

GOLDBERG-MAXWELL

Synonyms. Hairless women; Morris'; testicular feminization. See Male pseudohermaphroditism, incomplete hereditary type I. Complete testicular feminization.

Signs. Individual who appears externally to be a normal, well-developed female in body contour, distribution of body hair, voice and breast development. Raised psychologically and socially as a female. Vagina well developed; external genitalia female in character, although there may be in some cases an ambiguous phallic enlargement and scant pubic hair. Often inguinal hernias.

Etiology. Unknown; possibly a sex-linked recessive gene. Inability of end organs to respond to normal circulating levels of testosterone or ectopic testes fail to secrete.

Pathology. Fallopian tubes and uterus are rudimentary or absent. Sometimes testis in the inguinal canal, intrabdominal or in the labia.

Diagnostic Procedures. *Chromosome studies.* Sexual chromatin absent; XY pattern. *Blood.* Testosterone level may be similar to those found in normal males. Elevated plasma luteinizing hormone (LH) levels.

Therapy. No attempt to change sex. If vagina inadequate, use of dilators or plastic surgery. Removal of testicles, which are undescended. Estrogen administration.

Prognosis. Good psychological adjustment and life as female possible. Removal of testicles to avoid possible neoplastic transformation.

BIBLIOGRAPHY. Goldberg MB, Maxwell AF: Male pseudohermaphroditism proved by surgical exploration and microscopic examination. A case report with speculations concerning pathogenesis. J Clin Endocrinol 8:367–379, 1948
Morris JM: The syndrome of testicular feminization in male pseudohermaphrodites. Am J Obstet Gynecol 65:1192–1211, 1953
Wilson JD, Griffin JE, Leshin M, et al: The androgen resistence syndromes: 5-α-reductase deficiency, testicular feminization and related disorders. In Stanbury JB, Wyngaarden JB, Fredrickson DS, et al: The Metabolic Basis of Inherited Disease, 5th ed, p 1001. New York, McGraw-Hill, 1983

GOLDBERG'S (M.F.)

Synonyms. Neuroaminidase–β-galactosidase deficiency, galactosialidosis.

Symptoms and Signs. From birth. Both sexes. Delayed mental and physical development, seizures, visual defects, deafness. Gargoyle facies. Dwarfism, corneal clouding; macular cherry red spot; dyastasis multiplex.

Etiology. Autosomal recessive. Defect on chromosome 10. Defects in the processing mechanism that protects the two enzymes from enzymatic digestion by other enzymes in the lysosomes.

Pathology. See sialidosis.

Diagnostic Procedures. *Enzymatic studies.* In fibroblasts lack of galactosidase and neuraminidase.

BIBLIOGRAPHY. Goldberg MF, Cottlier E, Fichenscher LG, et al: Macular cherry red spot, corneal clouding and beta-galactosidase deficiency. Clinical, biochemical, and electron microscopic study of a new autosomal recessive storage disease. Arch Intern Med 128:387–398, 1971
Andria G, Strisciuglio P, Pontarelli G, et al: Infantile neuraminidase and beta-galactosidase deficiencies (galactosialidosis) with mild clinical courses. Perspect Inherit Metab Dis 4:379–395, 1985

GOLDENHAR'S

Synonyms. Auriculovertebral; mandibulofacial dysostosis-epibulbar dermoids; oculoauriculovertebral dysplasia; facioauriculovertebral anomaly; OAV; oculovertebral dysplasia.

Symptoms. Prevalent in males (70%), present at birth. Hearing defect of various degrees from near normal to severe hearing loss (conductive type); vision defect, including diplopia of various degrees. Feeding difficulty; moderate mental retardation in only 10% of cases.

Signs. *Ocular.* Epibulbar dermoid tumor; coloboma upper eyelids and eyebrows; ptosis of eyelid; antimongoloid obliquity. *Auricular.* Microtia; auricular appendices; atresia or stenosis of external auditory meatus; blind-ended fistula. *Oral.* Micrognathia; unilateral facial hypoplasia or hypoplasia of ramus and condyle; maxillary hypoplasia; high-arched palate; macrostomia; cleft palate; malocclusion. *Musculoskeletal.* Hemivertebrae; spina bifida; scoliosis; vertebral spinal fusion; supranumerary vertebrae; hypoplastic ribs; inguinal hernia; clubfoot; congenital heart defect.

Etiology. Autosomal recessive or dominant inheritance is possible. Sporadic cases occur. Embryonic malformation due possibly to vascular abnormality involving first and second brachial arches, vertebrae, and eyes. To be differentiated from Treacher-Collins (see) and hemifacial microsomia (bilateral conditions usually without vertebral anomalies).

Pathology. See Signs.

Diagnostic Procedures. *X-rays.* Normal. *Chromosome studies.* Negative.

Therapy. Early diagnosis important; hearing aid (very efficient); plastic surgery; combined effort of pediatrician, surgeon, dentist, orthodontist.

Prognosis. Good; only minority with mental retardation. Good result from plastic surgery.

BIBLIOGRAPHY. V Arlt F von: Klinische Dortstellung der Krankheiteu des Auges. Wien, Braunmüller, 1881
Van Duyse D: Bride dermoide oculo-palpebrale et coloboma partiel de la paupiere avec remarques sur la genese de cas anomalies. Ann Ocul 88:101–132, 1882
Goldenhar M: Associations malformatives de l'oeil et de l'oreille, en particulier le syndrome dermöide epibulbaire-appendices auriculaires-fistula auris congenita et ses relations avec la dysostose mandibulo-faciale. J Genet Hum 1:243–282, 1952
Michand C, Sheridan G: Goldenhar's syndrome associated with cranial and neurological malformations. Can J Ophthalmol 3:347–350, 1974
Mansour AM, Wang F, Henkind P, et al: Ocular findings in the facioauriculovertebral sequence (Goldenhar-Gorlin syndrome). Am J Ophthalmol 100:555–559, 1985
De Filippo P, Prato M, Quarto B: La sindrome di Goldenhar. Descrizione di un caso e considerazioni genetiche. Aggiornamento Pediatrico 37:47–49, 1986

GOLDMANN-FAVRE

Synonym. Hyaloidretinal degeneration. See also Wagner's. Hyaloidoretinal degeneration; retinoschisis-early hemeralopia.

Symptoms. Only a few cases reported. Severe night blindness from early childhood.

Signs. Extensive vitreoretinal dystrophy with bone corpuscle pigmentation; pattern of foveal retinoschisis coarse; occasionally cataract.

Etiology. Autosomal recessive inheritance.

Etiology and Pathology. *Electroretinography.* Abolished b-wave (differential element to distinguish from Wagner's and X-linked retinoschisis). Liquified vitreous body with preretinal band-shaped structures, edema, macular changes, pigmentary degeneration of retina and hemeralopia.

BIBLIOGRAPHY. Favre M: A propos de deux cas de dégénérescence hyaloidéorétinienne: Two cases of hyaloid-retinal degeneration. Ophthalmologica 135:604–609, 1958
Ricci A: Clinique et transmission génétique de différentes formes de dégénérescences vitréo-rétiniennes. Ophthalmologica 139:338–343, 1960
Goldberg MF: Genetic and Metabolic Eye Disease, p 370. Boston, Little Brown, 1974
Francois J, De Rouch, A, Cambrie E. Degenerescence hyaloideo-tapeto-retinienne de Goldmann-Favre. Ophthalmologica 168:81–86, 1974

GOLDSCHEIDER'S

Synonyms. Acantholysis bullosa; epidermolysis bullosa hereditaria simplex; Koebner's. See Fox's; Hurlier's, Hallopeau-Siemens, and epidermolysis bullosa hyperplastic.

Symptoms and Signs. Present from infancy. No symptoms, except pain and discomfort when bullae rupture. Bullous elevations on the hands and feet (involvement of other areas of body: this wider extension differentiates it from the epidermolysis bullosa hyperplastic type Cockaine Touraine, see), developing after minor trauma; (e.g., walking, using tools). Associated hyperhidrosis of hand and feet. The bullae appear especially in warm weather and are frequently hemorrhagic. Scars frequently may be so severe as to affect growth of the patient.

Etiology. Autosomal recessive inheritance.

Pathology. Subepidermal bullae, containing usually clear fluid, little or no inflammatory reaction unless infection supervenes. Elastic tissue may be frayed and splintered but not destroyed.

Diagnostic Procedures. *Biopsy.* Differentiate from porphyria drug reactions and other forms of epidermolysis bullosa.

Therapy. Nonspecific. Protection from secondary infections and damage due to extensive scar retraction.

Prognosis. Chronic persistence of the condition that may result in various growth disorders up to dwarfism.

BIBLIOGRAPHY. Goldscheider A: Hereditäre Neigung zur Blasebildung. Mhefte Prakt Dermatol 1:163–174, 1882
Koebner H: Hereditaere Anlage zur Blasenbildung (Epidermolysis bullosa hereditaria). Dtsch Med Wochenschr 12:21–22, 1886
Elliot GT: Two cases of epidermolysis bullosa. J Cutan Genitourin Dis 13:10–18, 1895

Mulley JC, Nicholls CM, Propert DN, et al: Genetic linkage analysis of epidermolysis bullosa simplex Koebner type. Am J Med Genet 19:573–577, 1984

GOLDSTEIN-REICHMANN

Synonym. Acquired cerebellar.

Symptoms. Both sexes affected; onset at all ages. Tendency to fall; insecure ambulation with severe swaying. Intentional tremor; unilateral lack of normal arm movements; catalepsy.

Signs. Equilibrium disorders; posture abnormalities; adiadochokinesia; pendular knee reflex; choreiform hyperkinesia.

Etiology. Trauma; infection (ear); meningitis; encephalitis; neoplasia involving (directly or indirectly) the cerebellum.

Pathology. Cerebellar parenchymatous degeneration.

Diagnostic Procedures. *Spinal fluid. X-ray. Angiography. CT brain scan.* To show cerebellar involvement.

Therapy. According to etiology.

Prognosis. Variable.

BIBLIOGRAPHY. Goldstein K, Reichmann F: Beitraege zur Kasuistik und Symptomatologie der Kleinhiznerkrankungen (in besondersen zu den Staerungen der Bewegungen der Gewichtsraum und Zeitschaetzung). Arch Psychiatr (Nevenkr) 56:466–521, 1915–1916

GOLTZ'S

Synonyms. Focal dermal hypoplasia; FDH.

Symptoms and Signs. Cases reported in females (90%). Shortness of stature and slight build. Mental retardation frequent. Cutaneous changes; poikiloderma (linear hypoplasia with pigmentation; telangiectasia). In some areas of the thinned skin, herniation of nodules of adipose tissue. Occasionally, angiofibromas around mouth, anus, and vagina (50%); dystrophic nails (50%); syndactylism and other finger and toe abnormalities (80%); usually third and fourth fingers. Eye defects (50%); microphthalmia; colobomas; strabismus; defective dentition (60%); malocclusion, malformation, absence of teeth. Lip, vulvar, and anal papillomas.

Etiology. X-linked dominant with lethality in males.

Pathology. *Skin.* Histologic examination of fatty deposit in skin reveals normal fat separated from epidermis by fragmented fibrillary collagen, absence of collagen

bundles, decrease of normal elastic fibers. Nonaffected areas show normal skin.

Diagnostic Procedures. *Blood, urine.* Normal. *X-ray skeleton.* Striated bones.

Therapy. Surgical correction of finger abnormalities.

BIBLIOGRAPHY. Jessner M: Naerviforme, poikilodermieartige Hautveraenderungen mit Missbildungen. Zentralbl Haut Geschlkr 27:468, 1928
Goltz RW, Peterson WC, Gorlin RJ, et al: Focal dermal hypoplasia. Arch Dermatol 86:708–717, 1962
Ballesta F, Botet F, Figueras J, et al: Observation familiar de aplasia congenita de cutis. Acta Paediatr Esp 43:89–94, 1985

GOODMAN'S

Synonyms. Acrocephalopolysyndactyly IV. ACPS IV.

Symptoms and Signs. From birth. Both sexes. Clinodactyly, camptodactyly, ulnar deviation. Congenital heart malformations. No mental retardation. Difficult clinical differentiation from Carpenter's (see).

Etiology. Autosomal recessive.

Prognosis. Poor.

BIBLIOGRAPHY. Goodman RM, Steinberg M, Shem-Toy Y, et al: Acrocephalopolysyndactyly type IV: A new genetic syndrome in three sibs. Clin Genet 15:209–214, 1979
Hall JR, Reed SD, Sells CJ, et al: Autosomal recessive acrocephalosyndactyly revisited: Am J Med Genet 5:423–424, 1980

GOODPASTURE'S

Synonyms. Glomerulonephritis-pulmonary hemorrhages; lung purpura-glomerulonephritis; pneumorenal; renopneumonal. See Ceelen-Gellerstedt.

Symptoms. Prevalent in males; age of onset between 16 and 61 years of age (median 21 years). One-fifth of patients present preceding, nonspecific, viral respiratory infections. Hemoptysis, exertional dyspnea; cough; fatigue; occasionally, nausea and vomiting; weight loss; chest pains; hematuria.

Signs. Pallor; pulmonary rhonchi; seldom, hypertension, edemas, skin rash, splenomegaly. Later in the disease hypertension and edemas more frequently observed.

Etiology. Familial occurrence reported (autosomal recessive?); possibly viral agents or autoimmune condition. Postulated that kidneys play a primary role: antigen–antibody interaction at glomerular level and release of vasoactive polypeptides that enhance pulmonary capillary permeability. Antigen involved is 25,000 to 50,000 dalton non-collagen glycoprotein domain of type IV collagen on the inner aspect of lamina densa.

Pathology. *Lung.* Mottled by areas of hemorrhage, especially lower lobes. Microscopically, intraalveolar hemorrhage and siderophages, and thickening of alveolar septi with collagenization. Vasculitis absent; occasionally, infiltrate of polymorphonucleated cells. *Kidney.* Enlarged, pale, soft. Subcortical punctiform hemorrhages; capsule nonadherent. In cases of longer duration, kidney shrinks in size and capsule becomes adherent. Microscopically, diffuse involvement, capillary loops occluded by eosinophilic material PAS-negative. Immunofluorescence: linear deposits of Ig G, deposits of C3. Epithelial cell proliferation; endothelial proliferation scarce or absent. Progressive glomerular fibrosis. Interstitial inflammatory infiltration mostly lymphocytes, and then fibrillar interstitial fibrosis and dilation and atrophy of tubules.

Diagnostic Procedures. *Blood.* Normocytic, normochromic anemia; normal or increased leukocytes; later in disease, hyperazotemia; immunofluorescence of circulating (and tissue) antibasement antibodies (anti GBM). *Urine.* Proteinuria; hematuria; increased leukocytes, casts. *X-ray of chest.* Infiltrates, especially lower lobes. *Biopsy of Kidney.* Characteristic lesions (see Pathology). *Sputum.* Macrophages full of hemosiderin.

Therapy. Corticosteroids of limited value. Cytotoxic and immunosuppressant agents of potential value. Plasmapheresis and kidney transplantation: good results.

Prognosis. Invariably fatal within 6 months with few exceptions of longer survival and recovery (?).

BIBLIOGRAPHY. Goodpasture EW: The significance of certain pulmonary lesions in relation to the etiology of influenza. Am J Med Sci 158:863–870, 1919
Simonsen H, Brun C, Thomsen OF, et al: Goodpasture's syndrome in twins. Acta Med Scand 212:425–428, 1982
Brenner BM, Rector FC: The Kidney, 3rd ed, p 1032. Philadelphia, WB Saunders, 1986

GORDAN-OVERSTREET

See Turner's. Eponym to indicate the presence of mild virilization characteristics in cases of gonadal dysgenesis. It may not, in the light of present knowledge, be considered as an autonomous entity.

BIBLIOGRAPHY. Godan GS, Overstreet EW, Traut HF, et al: A syndrome of gonadal dysgenesis: variety of ovarian agenesis with androgenic manifestations. J Clin Endocrinol 15:1–12, 1955

GORDON-COOKE

Synonym. Ring 1 chromosome–dwarfism.

Symptoms and Signs. Low birth weight; delayed mental and physical development; microcephaly; disproportionately tall for weight, although dwarfed. Cheerful and pleasant behavior.

Etiology. Large monocentric autosomal ring result of terminal deletion of chromosome 1.

Diagnostic Procedures. *Chromosome study.*

BIBLIOGRAPHY. Gordon RR, Cooke P: Ring 1 chromosome and microcephalic dwarfism. Lancet 2:1212–1213, 1964
Wolf CB, Peterson JA, Logrippo GA, et al: Ring 1 chromosome and dwarfism—A possible syndrome. J Pediatr 71:719–722, 1967

GORDON'S (H.)

Synonyms. Arthrogryposis multiplex congenita (distal type II A). Camptodactyly–cleft palate–club foot.

Symptoms and Signs. Both sexes. From birth. Fixed camptodactyly (89%) sparing the thumb and affecting only the PIP joints (72%). Club feet (varus or valgus). Cleft palate (27%). Occasionally associated: short stature, nevus flammeus (see), dermatoglyphic anomalies, omphalocele.

Etiology. Autosomal dominant inheritance with variable expression.

BIBLIOGRAPHY. Gordon H, Davies D, Berman M: Camptodactyly, cleft palate and club foot. A syndrome showing the autosomal dominant pattern of inheritance. J Med Genet 6:266–274, 1969
Robinow M, Johnson GF: The Gordon syndrome: Autosomal dominant cleft palate, camptodactyly, and club feet. Am J Med Genet 9:139–146, 1981

GORDON'S (R.S.)

Synonyms. Protein-losing; lymphangiectatic enteropathy; exudative enteropathy; hypercatabolic-hypoprotein; familial hypoproteinemia–lymphangiectatic enteropathy; intestinal lymphangiectasia; lymphangiectatic enteropathy; neonatal lymphedema–exudative enteropathy.

Symptoms and Signs. Both sexes affected; onset from infancy to early adulthood. Initially, intermittent bilateral or unilateral edema, usually preceding diarrhea; then persistent edema and hydrothorax; ascites. Repeated infections, malnutrition, and wasting late stage.

Etiology. Unknown. With onset at birth, possibly congenital malformation of lymphatic system. With onset in early adulthood, acquired, secondary to several conditions, including Ormond's, infective, collagen, neoplastic, cardiovascular disorders. Familial form reported (autosomal recessive).

Pathology. Small intestine shows edema of affected areas; serosa covered with fibrinous exudate; dilatation of lymphatic vessels; yellowish nodules along their course. Mesenteric lymph nodes enlarged with yellowish foci. No mucosal atrophy; villi swollen; red brownish pigmentation in external muscular layer. Absence of inflammatory reaction.

Diagnostic Procedures. *Blood.* Moderate anemia. Hypoproteinemia; albumin and gammaglobulin decreased. Cholesterol usually normal. *Bone marrow.* Slight hyperplasia. *Absorption studies.* Steatorrhea; abnormal fat and vitamin A tolerance; normal carbohydrate and D-xylose test. Rapid degradation of radioactive iodine labelled albumin, with decreased normal half-life; increased fecal excretion of ^{131}I labelled polyvinylpyrrolidone. *Biopsy of jejunum.* (See Pathology). *X-ray.* Thickening and coarsening of jejunal fold.

Therapy. Protein administration; reduction of alimentary fat. Surgery if disease confined to limited intestinal area.

Prognosis. Immunologic deficiency (hypogammaglobulinemia) may develop. Excellent response to treatment depending, in secondary forms, on basic condition.

BIBLIOGRAPHY. Gordon RS Jr: Exudative enteropathy. Abnormal permeability of the gastrointestinal tract demonstrable with labelled polyvinylpyrrolidone. Lancet 1:325–326, 1959

Sleisinger MH, Kim YS: Protein digestion and absorption. N Engl J Med 300:659–663, 1979

Perrault J, Markowitz H: Protein-losing gastroenteropathy and the intestinal clearance of serum alpha 1-antitrypsin. Mayo Clin Proc 59:278–279, 1984

GORHAM'S

Synonyms. Disappearing bones; massive osteolysis; phantom bones. See Haferkamp's.

Symptoms and Signs. Both sexes affected; clinical onset from childhood to young adulthood. Almost constantly unilateral, focal hemangioma involving one or several contiguous bones, including adjacent vertebrae; massive osteolysis. Soft tissues near bone lesion usually involved. Diffuse muscle atrophy. Hemangiomas on overlying skin may or may not be present.

Etiology and Pathology. Angioma of bone(s) with osteolysis and replacement of bone by fibrosis. Sporadic or autosomal dominant inheritance.

Diagnostic Procedures. *X-ray of skeleton.*

Therapy. X-ray therapy.

Prognosis. Relatively benign condition, slowly progressing and self-limited. No therapy has changed significantly the course of the disease for its effects to be predictable.

BIBLIOGRAPHY. Jackson JBS: Boneless arm. Boston Med Surg J 18:368–369, 1838

Gorham LW, Wright AW, Schurtz HH, et al: Disappearing bones: A rare form of massive osteolysis. Am J Med 17:674–682, 1954

Wallis LA, Asch T, Maisel BW: Diffuse skeletal hemangiomatosis: Report of two cases and review of literature. Am J Med 37:545–563, 1964

Carnesale PG: Benign tumors of the bone. In Crenshaw AH (ed): Campbell's Operative Orthopedics, 7th ed, p 753. St Louis, CV Mosby, 1987

GORLIN-CHAUDHRY-MOSS

Symptoms and Signs. Present from birth. Craniofacial dysostosis; dental anomalies; microphthalmia; inability to close or open eyes completely; oblique palpebral fissures; horizontal nystagmus at lateral gaze; limited upper gaze. Astigmatism; hyperopia; corneal scars. Signs of patency of ductus arteriosus; hypertrichosis, hypoplastic labia majora.

Etiology. Unknown.

BIBLIOGRAPHY. Gorlin RJ, Chaudhry AP, Moss ML: Craniofacial dysostosis, patent ductus arteriosus, hypertrichosis, hypoplasia of labia majora, dental and eye anomalies, a new syndrome? J Pediatr 56:778–785, 1960

GORLIN-COHEN

Synonyms. Frontometaphyseal dysplasia; Gorlin-Holt.

Symptoms. Present from birth. Deafness (conductive type). Impaired movements from ankylosis. Feeding troubles. Recurrent respiratory tract infections.

Signs. Generalized hirsutism. Facies coarse; nose with wide bridge; eyebrows prominent; teeth partially absent; mandible small; palate high. Ankylosis of main joints; arachnodactyly. Femur and tibia metaphyseal enlargement (Erlenmeyer flask type). Cardiac murmur. Cryptorchidism. Uropathy.

Etiology. X-linked inheritance with severe manifestation in males and variable in female.

Diagnostic Procedures. *X-ray of skeleton* (see Signs). Vertebral interspaces widened; pelvis flared; carpal and tarsal bones partially fused.

Prognosis. Progressive disability.

BIBLIOGRAPHY. Gorlin RJ, Cohen MM: Frontometaphyseal dysplasia: A new syndrome. Am J Dis Child 118:487–494, 1969
Fitzsimmons JS, Fitzsimmons EM, Barrow M, et al: Frontometaphyseal dysplasia: Further delineation of the clinical syndrome. Clin Genet 22:195–205, 1982

GORLIN-GOLTZ

Synonyms. Basal cell nevus (carcinoma); Hermans-Herzberg; multiple basal cell nevi; nevus epitheliomatosis multiplex. Ward's.

Symptoms and Signs. No sex prevalence. *Skin.* Multiple nevoid basal cell carcinomas appearing in childhood or (especially) at puberty in exposed and unexposed areas. Other skin changes include palmar dyskeratosis, milia, cysts, fibromas and/or neurofibromas, especially on extremities. *Face.* Frontal and temporal bossing (pagetoid appearance); sunken appearance of eyes; broad nasal root; frequent strabismus; true hypertelorism; seldom, dystopia canthorum. Mild mandibular prognatism. *Mouth.* Multiple jaw cysts; fibrosarcoma jaws; ameloblastoma. *Skeletal system.* Rib: bifid; synostosis; partial agenesis. Vertebrae: scoliosis; cervical or thoracic fusion; deformed chest. Shortened metacarpals and distal phalanx of thumb. *Central nervous system.* Variable mental retardation; congenital hydrocephalus. *Eyes.* Congenital blindness; choroid and optic nerve coloboma. *Genitals.* Infantile genitals; female habit and hair distribution in boys; cryptorchidism. *Other.* Gastrointestinal disease also associated in some families.

Etiology. Unknown; autosomal dominant inheritance, determined by a highly penetrant gene with multiple and variable effects.

Pathology. Basal cell nevus; wide diversity of histopathologic appearance giving rise to a spectrum of skin tumor from benign to aggressive ulcerating basal cell carcinoma. Ovarian fibroma; jaw fibroma; medulloblastoma frequently found.

Diagnostic Procedures. *X-ray.* See Signs. *Biopsy.* These patients are hyporesponsive to parathyroid hormone. *Chromosome study.* Normal.

Therapy. Curettage, electrodesiccation, x-radiation, and surgical excision of nevi. For resistant lesions, topical application of dichloroacetic acid and zinc chloride followed by shaving; process repeated until all tumor removed. Systemic chemotherapy produces only incomplete results. Topical chemotherapy (colchicine and methotrexate ointment, and 5-fluorouracil ointment). For all other manifestations of the syndrome use conventional means of treatment.

Prognosis. Surgery and x-ray treatment results in a 5-year cure of nevi lesions in 90% of cases. Topical chemotherapy (colchicine and methotrexate) results in a 4-year cure in 70% of cases. 5-Fluorouracil effective in ulcerating basal cell tumor; recurrences, however, are frequent. It is not yet possible to evaluate the possible curative effect of high dose of 5-fluorouracil. Early fatality from medulloblastoma. Surviving male patients develop eunuchoid traits, while females develop ovarian fibromas and uterine calcifications.

BIBLIOGRAPHY. Jarisch A: Zur Lehre von den Hantgeschwuelsten Arch J Dematol Syph 28:163–222, 1894
Nomland R: Multiple basal cell epithelioma originating from congenital pigmented cell nevi. Arch Dermatol 25:1002–1008, 1932
Ward WH: Nevoid basal celled carcinoma associated with a dyskeratosis of the palms and soles. A new entity. Aust J Dermatol 5:204–207, 1960
Gorlin RJ, Goltz RW: Multiple nevoid basal cell epithelioma, jaw cysts and bifid rib: A syndrome. New Engl J Med 262:908–912, 1960
Totten JR: The multiple nevoid basal cell carcinoma syndrome: Report of its occurrence in four generations of a family. Cancer 46:1456–1462, 1980

GOSSELIN'S

Eponym used to indicate a V-fracture of lower end of tibia extending into ankle joint.

BIBLIOGRAPHY. Gosselin LA: Des fractures en V et de cours complications. Paris, Clayde, 1866
Sisk TD: Fractures of lower extremities. In Crenshaw AH (ed): Campbell's Operative Orthopedics, 7th ed, p 1637. St Louis, CV Mosby, 1987

GOTTRON'S (H.A.)

Synonym. Erythrokeratoderma symmetrical progressive.

Symptoms and Signs. Onset in infancy (4 mo to 4 yr) but also in adult life. On hands, feet and occasionally in other location (thighs, upper arms, neck, face), formation of strikingly symmetrical plaques of erythema with hyperkeratosis, margin frequently pigmented.

Etiology. Unknown. Autosomal dominant inheritance with variable expressivity.

Pathology. Hyperkeratosis, parakeratosis, acanthosis, and inflammatory changes.

Treatment. None or oral retinoid therapy.

Prognosis. Lesions reach greatest extent in puberty then may regress.

BIBLIOGRAPHY. Gottron HA: Congenital angelegte symmetrische progressive Erythrokeratodermie. Zentralbl HautGeschlkrank 4:493–494, 1922

Ruiz-Maldonado R, Tamayo L, del Castillo V, et al: Erythrokeratodermia progressive simmetrica. Report of 10 cases. Dermatologica 164:133–141, 1982

Rook A, Wilkinson DS, Ebling FJG, et al: Textbook of Dermatology, 4th ed, p 1433. Oxford, Blackwell Scientific Publications, 1986

GOTTRON'S (H.)

Synonyms. Familial acrogeria; familial acromicria. See Werner's. Acrogeria; acromicria. See Ehler-Danlos IV.

Symptoms and Signs. Prevalent in female. Normal hair and eyes. Senile changes affecting prevalently distal extremities. Evident subcutaneous vascular pattern over the chest.

Etiology. Autosomal recessive inheritance.

Pathology. Absence of subcutaneous fat in most severely affected zones. Atrophia of dermis, abundant clumped elastin; sparse collagen bundles.

Prognosis. General health and life expectancy normal. Short stature.

BIBLIOGRAPHY. Gottron H: Familiaere Akrogerie. Arch Dermatol Syph 181:571–583, 1940

De Groot WP, Tafelkruyer J, Woerdman MJ: Familial acrogeria (Gottron). Br J Dermatol 103:213–223, 1980

GOUGEROT-BLUM

Synonym. Pigmented purpuric lichenoid dermatitis. Prurigo pigmentosa.

Symptoms. Rare in western countries; more frequent in Japan. Both sexes affected (prevalent in females); onset in middle life. Itching at site of lesions.

Signs. Usually on lower extremities and seldom on upper extremities or trunk. Papules slightly elevated, clus-

tered in irregular areas; shape round; surface smooth; evolving toward a reddish color; showing a fine desquamation in the center.

Etiology. Unknown. Capillaritis (?).

Pathology. Hyperkeratosis and parakeratosis; decreased papillae in the corium; fragmentation of elastic tissue; perivascular infiltration by lymphocytes, plasma cells, and fibroblasts; blood vessels show edematous walls, endoartheritic process.

Diagnostic Procedures. *Biopsy.* Immunofluorescence negative. *Blood.* Occasionally eosinophils increase.

Therapy. Systemic and topical cortisone treatment; keratolytics, and antihistamine with scarce response; 30% of cases respond to dapsone.

Prognosis. Chronic condition lasting for years.

BIBLIOGRAPHY. Gougerot H, Blum P: Purpura angioscléreux prurigineux avec éléments lichénoides. Présentation de malade. Bull Soc Fr Dermatol Syph 32:161–163, 1925

Rook A, Wilkinson DS, Ebling FJG, et al: Textbook of Dermatology, 4th ed, p 416. Oxford, Blackwell Scientific Publications, 1986

GOUGEROT-CARTEAUD

Synonym. Confluent reticular papillomatosis. See Acanthosis nigricans.

Symptoms and Signs. Prevalent in females; onset after puberty. Appearance of flat warty papules, not larger than 0.5 centimeter in diameter, between the breasts and in the midline of the back; progressive extension of lesions, which become confluent to form an irregular network; extension proceeds in all directions, reaching neck, pubis.

Etiology. Unknown; usually isolated cases; however, probably, genetic condition. Autosomal dominant inheritance suggested.

Pathology. Hyperkeratosis and papillomatosis without acanthosis.

Diagnostic Procedures. *Biopsy of skin.*

Therapy. None.

Prognosis. Progression for a few years, then becomes stabilized. No symptoms or disfiguration.

BIBLIOGRAPHY. Gougerot H, Carteaud A: Papillomatose pigmentée innominée. Bull Soc Fr Dermatol Syph 34:712–719, 1927

Kesten BM, James HD: Pseudoatrophoderma colli, acanthosis nigricans, and confluent and reticular papillomatosis. Arch Dermatol 75:525–542, 1957

Henning JPH, de Wit RFE: Familial occurrence of confluent and reticulated papillomatosis. Arch Dermatol 117:809–810, 1981

GOUGEROT-HAILEY-HAILEY

Synonyms. Darier's bullous variant; dyskeratosis bullosa hereditaria; Hailey-Hailey. Pemphigus benign, familial.

Symptoms and Signs. Both sexes affected; onset usually in adolescence or early adulthood. Onset usually in hot, humid weather. Unilateral or bilateral lesions in zone of friction (neck, axillae, groin) and occasionally other areas (scalp, limbs). Cluster of small vesicles, first with clear fluid, becoming turbid; erythema of underlying skin, then breaking and crusting. Extending to periphery; center healing or moist vegetations.

Etiology. Unknown; autosomal dominant inheritance with variable penetrance.

Pathology. Similar to pemphigus vulgaris. Differences: (1) more extensive acantholysis; (2) less damage to acantholytic cells; (3) permanence of a few intercellular bridges.

Diagnostic Procedures. *Biopsy.* To differentiate with Darier's (see). *Bacteriologic examination.*

Therapy. Topical and systemic antibiotics. Topical steroids. Grenz rays.

Prognosis. Spontaneous remission in cold weather. Chronic, recurrent condition. Long remission possible, becoming less severe at later age.

BIBLIOGRAPHY. Hailey H, Hailey H: Familial benign chronic pemphigus. Report of 13 cases in four generations of a family and report of 9 additional cases in 4 generations in a family. Arch Dermatol Syph 39:679–685, 1939

Gougerot H: La priorite du pemphigus chronique familial héréditaire benin. Ann Dermatol Syph 10:361–363, 1950

Montgomery H: Dermatopathology, Vol 1. New York, Harper & Row, 1967

Michel B: Hailey-Hailey disease—Familial benign chronic pemphigus. Arch Dermatol 118:781–783, 1982

GOUGEROT-RUITER

Synonyms. Allergic vasculitis; arteriolitis allergica; leukocytoclastic angiitis; angiitis-urticarial vasculitis; pentasymptomatic Gougerot's (papules, macules, petechiae, bullae, and ulcerations); Ruiter's; tetrasymptomatic Gougerot's (papules, macules, petechiae, and bullae); trisymptomatic Gougerot's (papules, macules, and petechiae); Gougerot-Duperrat; Werther's (dermatitis nodularis necroticans—may be considered as a variant of this syndrome).

Symptoms and Signs. Prevalent in females (3:2); onset at all ages. Pruritus; local pain. Frequently, fever, malaise, arthralgia, gastrointestinal manifestations. *Acute form.* Hemorrhagic, purpuric necrotic skin eruption on legs, arms, and buttocks; seldom other locations; erythema multiformelike lesions. Seldom, involvement of viscera with relative manifestations. *Subacute form.* Papules, maculoerythematous lesions, nodules; necrotic lesions usually confluent to form plaques; urticaria common. *Chronic form.* Papules, macules, petechiae, urticaria frequent. No systemic manifestations, except mild malaise.

Etiology. *Unknown.* Possibly allergic mechanism against drug, bacteria, fungi, parasite, or tumor. Antigen-antibody reaction at vessel wall site.

Pathology. Dilatation and thrombosis of dermal capillaries and arterioles with fibrinoid and necrotic changes. Leukocytoclasis characteristic feature; erythrocyte extravasation.

Diagnostic Procedures. *Biopsy of skin. Blood.* Sedimentation rate normal or most frequently increased. Neutrophilia or eosinophilia possible. Frequently hypocomplementemia.

Therapy. Elimination of infective focus. Corticosterone, dapsone or indomethacine: variable effects.

Prognosis. Removal of foci may be followed by cure.

BIBLIOGRAPHY. Gougerot H: "Maladie trisymptomatique de H. Gougerot": Trisymptome associant petits nodules dermiques, cocardes d'erytheme polymorphe, purpura. Sem Hôp Paris 23:1311–1315, 1947

Ruiter M, Brandsman CH: Arteriolitis allergica. Dermatologica 97:265–271, 1948

Rook A, Wilkinson DS, Ebling FJG, et al: Textbook of Dermatology, 4th ed, p 1140–1143. Oxford, Blackwell Scientific Publications, 1986

GOULEY'S

Eponym is used to indicate the constriction of the pulmonary artery (partial or complete) in adhesive pericarditis. See Pick's.

BIBLIOGRAPHY. Gouley BA: Constriction of the pulmonary artery by adhesive pericarditis. Am Heart J 13:470–482, 1937

GOUT SYNDROMES

Synonyms. "Disease of kings and king of diseases"; podagra; uric acid dysmetabolism.

Etiology. The gout disorder of purine metabolism may be classified according to etiology. *Primary*. There are various subtypes of primary gout probably all with hereditary basis. There are two hypotheses as to the inheritance of gout: autosomal dominant or multifactorial. The gout syndrome appears also associated with other enzyme deficiencies: glucose-6-phosphatase deficiency (von Gierke's, see); altered kinetics of phosphoribosyl pyrophosphate synthetase. (PP-ribose-P); hypoxanthine-guanine phosphoribosyl transferase deficiency (Lesch–Nyhan, see). *Secondary*. Hematologic disorders; myeloproliferative syndromes (including polycythemia); hemolytic disease; iatrogenic (administration of hyperuricacidemic drugs); obesity; starvation; chronic renal diseases; glycogen storage disease type 1; sarcoidosis; psoriasis; idiopathic. From a clinical point of view, this condition may manifest itself with several syndromes.

ACUTE GOUTY ARTHRITIS

Symptoms. Prevalent in adult males; peak of incidence, third to fifth decade. In women, appears postmenopause. Onset frequent during night. Severe, sharp gnawing pain in the great toe; less frequently other sites (instep, ankle, heel, knee, wrist, in order of frequency). Extreme discomfort; chills and shivers; no change in posture relieves the pain.

Signs. Skin overlying affected joint inflamed.

Diagnostic Procedures. *Blood*. Uric acid determination.

Therapy. Colchicine, phenylbutazone, oxyphenbutazone, indomethacin, allopurinol, adrenocorticotropic hormone (ACTH), or corticosteroids.

Prognosis. Pain lasts a few days or weeks if untreated. Complete recovery follows. Recurrent attacks at variable intervals (weeks or years), affecting the same or different joints.

CHRONIC GOUTY ARTHRITIS

Symptoms and Signs. Average time for development of this syndrome from first acute attack 11.6 years. Onset may be insidious or sequela of a repeated attack also affecting previously uninvolved joints. Usually, after chronic form develops, acute attacks disappear. Polyarthric involvement with eventual evolution to grotesque, deforming, destructive, ulcerating changes. From ulcer of tophi, excretion of chalky material, usually painless. Tophi in ear cartilage, tendons, less frequently skin, nose cartilage, and eyes.

Pathology. Tophi are urate deposits with inflammation of foreign body reaction type of surrounding tissues. Predominately located in cartilage, epiphyses, periarticular structures, and kidney. Necrotic changes of joint cartilage with synovial proliferation, bone destruction, and sometimes ankylosis. In kidney, uric acid crystal in interstitial tissue of pyramids; necrotic changes; urolithiasis.

Diagnostic Procedures. *Blood*. Hyperuricemia. *X-ray*. Punched-out lesion of bones; deformative changes of joints. *Biopsy* (of joint) or *synovial fluid aspiration*. Presence of uric acid crystals.

Therapy. Uricosuric agents: probenecid; sulfinpyrazone; zoxazolamine; salicylates, cinchophen. Inhibitors of uric acid synthesis; allopurinol.

RENAL SYNDROME IN GOUT

Symptoms and Signs. Evidence of renal disease; albuminuria, hypertension, and urolithiasis with passage of stones.

Pathology. See Chronic gouty arthritis syndrome.

BIBLIOGRAPHY. Sydenham T: Tractatus de podagra et hydrope. London, G Kettilby, 1783.
Garrod AB: Observations on certain pathological conditions of the blood and urine in gout, rheumatism and Bright's disease. Trans Med Chir Soc Edinburgh 31:83, 1848
Wyngaarden JB, Kelley WN: Gout. In Stanbury JB, Wyngaarden JB, Fredrickson DS, et al: The Metabolic Basis of Inherited Disease, 5th ed, p 1043. New York, McGraw-Hill, 1983

GOWER-WELANDER

Synonyms. Distal muscular dystrophy; late distal hereditary myopathy; Welander's. Myopathy, late, distal, hereditary.

Symptoms. Observed in Sweden, occasionally in other areas; onset after second decade; peak at fifth decade. Initial symptom weakness of thumb and first finger, then spreading to small muscles and extensors of hands and feet. Seldom, extension of moderate weakness to proximal muscles of extremities.

Etiology. Unknown; autosomal dominant inheritance. Proposed recessive inheritance may be explained instead by an unusual mechanism: germinal mosaicism in a parent.

Pathology. Muscle fiber degeneration fibrosis.

Diagnostic Procedures. *Electromyography*. No myotonia and compatible with myopathy.

Therapy. None.

Prognosis. Extremely slow progression; remains limited to distal parts.

BIBLIOGRAPHY. Gowers WR: A lecture on myopathy and distal form. Br Med J 2:89–92, 1902

Welander L: Myopathia distalis tarda hereditaria: 249 examined cases in 72 pedigrees. Acta Med Scand (Supp) 141:1–115, 1951

Marksbery WR, Griggs RC, Herr B: Distal myopathy—Electron microscope and histochemical studies. Neurology 27:727–735, 1977

Scoppetta C, Vaccaro ML, Casali C, et al: Distal muscular dystrophy with autosomal recessive inheritance. Muscle Nerve 7:478–485, 1984

GOWERS' PANATROPHY

Symptoms and Signs. Prevalent in women; onset in second to fourth decades. On the back, buttocks, thighs or arms, occasionally forearms or lower legs, over a period of a few weeks without signs of inflammation, development of clearly defined areas of atrophy of skin with disappearance of subcutaneous tissue. Single or multiple areas (usually quadrangular or triangular in shape, from 2 to 20 cm in diameter).

Etiology. Unknown; to be differentiated from sclerotic panatrophy of scleroderma and forms of panniculitis.

Pathology. Atrophy of subcutaneous tissue and skin.

Diagnostic Procedures. *Biopsy of skin.*

Therapy. None.

Prognosis. Lesions progress for a few months, then remain unchanged indefinitely.

BIBLIOGRAPHY. Barnes S: Report on Sir William Gowers' case of local panatrophy. Trans Clin Soc London 36:164–168, 1902–1903

Barnes S: Gowers' case of local panatrophy. Br J Dermatol 51:377–380, 1939

Rook A, Wilkinson DS, Ebling FJG, et al: Textbook of Dermatology, 4th ed, p 1810. Oxford, Blackwell Scientific Publications, 1986

GOYER'S

Eponym used to indicate a form of autosomal dominant neural progressive deafness appearing in childhood, associated with glomerulosclerosis, ichthyosis of extremities, and prolinuria that falls within the spectrum of Alport's syndrome (see), and there is not actual reason to distinguish the form from it.

BIBLIOGRAPHY. Goyer RA, Reynolds J Jr, Burke J, et al: Hereditary renal disease with neurosensory hearing loss, polyuria, and ichthyosis. Am J Med Sci 256:166–179, 1968

GRADENIGO'S

Synonyms. Abducens nerve palsy–petrous osteomyelitis; Lannois-Gradenigo; temporal. See Orbital apex.

Symptoms. Frontal headache (area of ophthalmic branch of nerve); acute otitis media with persistent diplopia.

Signs. Internal strabismus due to homolateral abducens (VI) paralysis; optic (II), trochlear (IV), trigeminal (V), and facial (VII) nerves may be occasionally involved.

Etiology. Localized meningitis over the tip of petrous pyramid, and perineuritis of trigeminal (V) and abducens (VI) nerve as they contact the bone.

Pathology. Mastoiditis; purulent infection spreading from antrum to tip of petrous bone and localized pachymeningitis and perineuritis.

Diagnostic Procedures. *X-ray of mastoid.* Haziness and then sclerosis of petrous apex.

Therapy. Antibiotics and surgery frequently required.

Prognosis. Recovery with adequate treatment.

BIBLIOGRAPHY. Gradenigo G: Sulla leptomeningite circoscritta e sulla paralisi dell' abducente di origine otitica. Gior R Accad Med Torino 10:59–84, 1904

Horowitz S: Gradenigo's syndrome and report of two cases. J Laryngol 62:639–647, 1948

Adams RD, Victor M: Principles of Neurology, 3rd ed, p 503. New York, McGraw-Hill, 1985

GRAFT-VERSUS-HOST

Synonyms. Allogenic bone marrow; bone marrow transfusion; GVH; leukocyte transfusion; runt.

Symptoms. Occur in patients who, after total irradiation, have received allogenic bone marrow transfusion or leukocyte transfusion. Onset 5 to 9 days after transfusion. Fever; asthenia; anorexia; nausea; vomiting; diarrhea; severe weight loss.

Signs. Exfoliative erythroderma; occasionally, jaundice and hepatomegaly, and transitory lymphoadenopathy.

Etiology. Graft against host reaction.

Pathology. Transient hyperplasia of lymphoid tissue (proliferation of hyperbasophilic cells), then aplasia of lymphatic tissue. Skin infiltration with lymphocytes and reticulum cells; epithelial vacuolization and dyskeratosis; area of acanthosis, hyperkeratosis, and parakeratosis. (These skin manifestations are concurrent with the myeloid repopulation).

Diagnostic Procedures. *Blood.* Transient lymphocytosis, followed by intense or moderate lymphocytopenia; anemia may be present. IgA, IgM, IgG decreased. *Blood cultures:* Bacterial, viral, mycotic infections. *Studies of immunoglobulin phenotype.*

Therapy. Keep the patient in sterile environment to prevent infections. Antibiotics.

Prognosis. Complete remission of long duration of the primary leukemic condition may be obtained by the technique of total body radiation and bone marrow transplant. This secondary syndrome is one of the prices we pay for this drastic therapeutic procedure. Careful studies to establish maximum compatibility between host and graft marrow may reduce intensity of secondary reaction.

BIBLIOGRAPHY. Mathe G, Schwarzenberg L, de Vries MJ, et al: Les divers aspects du syndrome secondaire compliquant les transfusions allogéniques de moelle osseuse ou de leukocytes chez des sujets atteints d'hémopathies malignes. Eur J Cancer 1:75–113, 1965

Wintrobe MM (ed): Clinical Hematology, 7th ed, p 328, 1731. Philadelphia, Lea & Febiger, 1974

GRAHMANN'S

Synonym. Pituitary diencephalon.

Symptoms. Occur in male adolescents. Periodic psychotic episodes with or without slight temperature elevation.

Signs. Obesity; underdevelopment; hypogonadism.

Etiology. Attributed to abnormality of diencephalon; secondary to intracerebral alterations (see Engel-Aring and Transient Cushing.)

Pathology. Unknown.

Diagnostic Procedures. Not reported.

Therapy. Symptomatic.

Prognosis. Unknown.

BIBLIOGRAPHY. Grahmann H: Periodische Ausnahmezustände in der Reifezeit als diencephale Regulationstörung. Psychiatr Neurol 135:361–377, 1958

Wolff SM, Adler RC, Buskirsk ER, et al: A syndrome of periodic hypothalamic discharge. Am J Med 36:956–967, 1966

GRAM'S

Synonyms. Adiposalgia-arthritico-hypertonica; justoarticular adiposis dolorosa; postmenopausal triad. See Menopausal.

Symptoms and Signs. Occur after menopause, usually in multiparae. Rheumatoid arthritis of knee; adiposis dolorosa; blood hypertension.

Etiology. See Menopausal.

BIBLIOGRAPHY. Gram HC: A symptom-triade of the postclimateric period. (Adipositas dolorosa–arthritis genuum–hypertension arterialis). Acta Med Scand 73:139–207, 1930

GRAND MAL

Synonyms. Tonic or tonico-clonic seizures.

Symptoms. *Prodromal.*
1. Paroxysmal attacks of strangeness, short-lasting "dreamy states," giddiness, pain, isolated muscle contraction, palpitations.
2. Continuous irritability or lethargy 1 or 2 days preceding the attack; depression or euphoria; well being, bulimia; headache.
3. Auras immediately preceding the attack: epigastric, strange indefinable sensation in stomach, throat, nausea, or hunger, palpitation. Psychic terror, fright; cursive epileptic syndrome; (the patient runs in terror before unconsciousness that follows). Dreamy states, with peculiar olfactory, gustative, visual, auditory sensations. Epileptic cry, and parrot scream are respectively forced expiration or inspiration that precede the convulsion.

Attack.
1. Sudden loss of consciousness following tonic spasm of all voluntary muscles almost equally bilaterally.
2. Cyanosis; fractures or dislocation from muscle contraction or fall. Release of sphincters with emission of feces or urine. Spastic relaxation and clonic contractions.
3. Finally, cessation of spasm and bubbling saliva emission.
   Partial attack sometimes with only spastic phase or only loss of consciousness. Return of consciousness after a few minutes or hours, usually the patient falls asleep after regaining consciousness.

Signs. Typical loss of consciousness and convulsions; pupils dilated not reactive; reflexes abolished. Tachycardia; apnea during spastic phase. Increase in blood pressure.

Etiology and Pathology. Symptomatic. Cerebral injury; familial and congenital developmental defect; vascular occlusion; inflammatory disease or sequelae; tumor; paroxysmal diseases. Idiopathic.

Diagnostic Procedures. *Electroencephalography. X-ray. Spinal tap. Isotope brain scan.*

Therapy. Diphenylhydantoin; primidone; phenobarbital; methylphenylethylhydantoin. Neurosurgery (when indicated).

Prognosis. Recovery from single attacks. Possibility of status epilepticus (see). Psychic deterioration with repeated seizures.

BIBLIOGRAPHY. Temkin O: The Falling Sickness: A History of Epilepsy from the Greeks to the Beginning of Modern Neurology. Baltimore, Johns Hopkins Press, 1945

Adams RD, Victor M: Principles of Neurology, 3rd ed, pp 233–254. New York, McGraw-Hill, 1985

GRANT'S

Synonyms. Cholinergic urticaria; micropapular urticaria.

Symptoms. Both sexes affected; onset in adolescence or young adulthood. After exertion or emotional disturbances, itching irritable wheals (or both) appear on the skin. In some cases, accompanied by flushing and fainting.

Signs. Wheals 1 to 3 mm in diameter on all areas of the skin.

Etiology. Unknown. Sympathetic stimulation by heat, emotion, gustatory stimulus.

Diagnostic Procedures. Syndrome may be reproduced by intradermal administration of cholinergic drugs or intramuscular injection of nicotine or of sodium chloride solution (5 to 6%).

Therapy. No treatment required in most cases. Antihistaminic or anticholinergic drugs may prevent attacks. Exertion may relieve symptoms after induced attack for 24 hours.

Prognosis. Attacks last minutes or 1 to 2 hours. After attacks, for 24 hours, freedom from symptoms even if the patient exerts or is subject to emotional stress. Condition persists for months or years and usually regresses spontaneously.

BIBLIOGRAPHY. Grant RT, Pearson RSB, Comeau WS: Observations on urticaria provoked by emotion, by exercise and by warming the body. Clin Sci 2:253–272, 1936

Buckley RH, Mathews KP: Common "allergic" skin diseases. JAMA 248:2611–2622, 1982

Rook A, Wilkinson DS, Ebling FJG, et al: Textbook of Dermatology, 4th ed, pp 1105–1106. Oxford, Blackwell Scientific Publications, 1986

GRANULOMA ANNULARE

Symptoms. All ages. Predominant in children and young adults. Both sexes, predominant in females. Symptomless and only occasionally pruritic lesions.

Signs. Usually localized lesion. Seldom three different patterns observed: generalized, perforating, and subcutaneous. All areas of skin may be involved, most frequently dorsal aspect of hands and feet. Rings of papules smooth and firm, 1 to 5 cm of diameter; mildly erythematous. Stretching of skin makes them more evident, scaling is rare. Lesions tend to enlarge.

Etiology. Unknown. Various hypothesis (not substantiated): insect bites; trauma; gold therapy; sun exposure; immunologic reaction; diabetes (see Oppenheim-Urbach).

Pathology. Focal obstructive process of dermis with "palisading" granuloma.

Diagnostic Procedures. *Skin biopsy.*

Therapy. All useless or of scarce benefit.

Prognosis. Slow development for months or years, spontaneous regression without scar. Recurrences are common (40%) but regress faster than primary lesion.

BIBLIOGRAPHY. Rook A, Wilkinson DS, Ebling FJG, et al: Textbook of Dermatology, 4th ed. Oxford, Blackwell Scientific Publications, 1986

GRANULOSIS RUBRA NASI

Symptoms and Signs. Onset in early childhood (6 mo to 10 yr). Usually preceded by hyperhidrosis. Erythema starting on the tip of nose and progressively extending to cover nose and possibly cheeks, upper lip, and chin. Area of hyperhidrosis could be larger than that of erythema. Maculae, papules, and vesicles at sweat duct orifices. Associated symptomatology; coldness, hyperhidrosis of hands and feet.

Etiology. Unknown; possibly hereditary (undetermined mode of inheritance).

Diagnostic Procedures. Assess status of nutrition and general health.

Therapy. Usually disappointing. Improvement of nutrition and general care.

Prognosis. May recede spontaneously at puberty or after improvement of nutrition or persist complicated by cyst formation and telangiectasis.

BIBLIOGRAPHY. Maschkilleisson LN, Naeadow LA: 33 Fälle von Jodassohns Granulosis rubra nasi. Dermatol Z 71:79–84, 1935
Binazzi M: Ulteriori rilievi su una osservazione di granulosis rubra nasi ereditaria. Rass Dermat Sif 11:23–26, 1958

GRAWITZ'S

Synonyms. Kidney adenocarcinoma; hypernephroma; renal cell carcinoma; RCC.

Symptoms. Both sexes affected; onset over 50 years of age. In 40% of cases asymptomatic. Dull pain in lumbar region; occasionally, colic. Later, anorexia, asthenia, nausea, weight loss, hematuria, hyperthermia.

Signs. Palpable mass in kidney; tenderness elicited at costovertebral angle. Occasionally, varicocele; blood hypertension.

Etiology. Unknown. Considered congenital malformation, embryonic residue; trauma; infections. Familial cases with autosomal dominant pattern reported.

Pathology. In kidney, spherical, 3 to 15 cm diameter, yellow grey encapsulated masses. Histologic examination shows tubular cells arranged in various patterns invading vessels.

Diagnostic Procedures. *Blood.* Normochromic anemia; occasionally, polycythemia. *Urine.* Hematuria; pyuria; presence of malignant cells. *X-ray.* Intravenous pyelography: presence of masses displacing and invading calyces. Of skeleton, possible metastases. *Biopsy.* See Pathology.

Therapy. Surgical excision. Chemotherapy. X-ray treatment.

Prognosis. Five year survival in 30 to 50%.

BIBLIOGRAPHY. Grawitz PA: Die sogenannten Lipome der Niere. Arch Pathol 93:39–63, 1883
Goldman SM, Fishman EK, Abeshouse G, et al: Renal cell carcinoma diagnosed in three generations of a single family. South Med J 72:1457–1459, 1979

GRAY

Synonym. Neonatal chloramphenicol toxicity.

Symptoms. Occur 3 or 4 days after starting administration of chloramphenicol. Vomiting, dyspnea; failure to suckle.

Signs. Skin grayish color; cyanosis; occasionally, jaundice; muscle flaccidity; abdominal distension; tachycardia; hypotension; cardiovascular collapse.

Etiology. Failure to metabolize (liver), excrete (kidney) chloramphenicol, possibly because of immature enzymes. Probably mitochondrial lack of resistance to chloramphenicol.

Diagnostic Procedures. *Blood.* Hyperbilirubinemia. *Stool.* Green.

Therapy. Symptomatic.

Prognosis. Shock and death. Severe shock and death frequent. Bone marrow cells from patients who survive to chloramphenicol toxicity *in vitro* became more resistant.

BIBLIOGRAPHY. Burns LE, Hodgman JE, Cass AB: Fatal circulatory collapse in premature infants receiving chloramphenicol. New Engl J Med 261:1318–1321, 1959
Sutherland JM: Fatal cardiovascular collapse of infants receiving large amounts of chloramphenicol. Am J Dis Child 97:761–767, 1959
Dameshek W: Chloramphenicol aplastic anemia in identical twins—A clue to pathogenesis. N Engl J Med 281:42–43, 1968
Fine PEM: Mitochondrial inheritance and disease. Lancet II:659–662, 1978

GRAYOUT

See also Blackout.

Symptoms. In fast acceleration or deceleration of vehicles (e.g., airplane). Gradual decrease of vision; misting; reduced peripheral vision area.

Etiology. Reduction of blood pressure of retina.

Diagnostic Procedures. For pilots or exposed persons: *Testing the visual threshold.* With progressive acceleration. *Ophthalmoscopy.*

GRAY PLATELET

Synonym. Raccuglia's.

Symptoms and Signs. Both sexes. Lifelong purpura.

Etiology. Unknown. Probably autosomal recessive inheritance.

Diagnostic Procedures. *Blood.* Bleeding time prolonged; clot retraction poor; platelet number normal; lack of granules, presence of vacuolization, and peculiar gray hue in Wright's stained smears. Adenosine triphosphate

(ATP) and extractable phosphatides from platelets reduced. Platelets aggregation with adenosine diphosphate (ADP), epinephrine, and collagen normal. Absence of alpha granules. Decrease of platelet fibrinogen, factor 4, β-thromboglobulin, growth factor, and protein sensitive to thrombin, glycoprotein Ig, or thromborespondine. *Bone marrow.* Cytoplasm of megakaryocytes vacuolated and lacking vacuoles in zones. Decrease of alpha granules in megacaryocytes and platelets. Sometimes observed myelofibrosis.

Therapy. Splenectomy reduces thrombocytopenia but fails to modify purpura and other clotting abnormalities.

BIBLIOGRAPHY. Raccuglia G: Gray platelet syndrome: A variety of qualitative platelet disorder. Am J Med 51:818–828, 1971
White JG: Ultrastructural studies of the gray platelet syndrome. Am J Pathol 95:445–462, 1979
Greenberg–Sepersky SM, Simons ER, et al: Studies of platelets from patients with gray platelet syndrome. Br J Haemat 59:603–609, 1985

GRAYSON-WILBRANDT

Synonym. Anterior membrane dystrophy. See Reis-Bueckler's syndrome.

Symptoms. Onset at end of first decade. Infrequent episodes of eye redness and pain; reduction of vision; normal corneal sensation.

Signs. Corneal changes variable from a mottled scarring (as in Reis-Bueckler's syndrome, see) to small, macular, gray, raised opacities.

Etiology. Unknown; autosomal dominant trait. Considered as separated from Reis-Bueckler's, because of (1) variable effect on vision, (2) partial corneal involvement, and (3) normal corneal sensation.

Pathology. See Reis-Bueckler's.

Therapy. Corneal transplant if needed.

Prognosis. Progressive vision reduction of variable degree; in some cases vision not affected at all.

BIBLIOGRAPHY. Grayson M, Wilbrandt H: Dystrophy of the anterior limiting membrane of the cornea (Reis-Bückler type). Am J Ophthalmol 61:345–349, 1966

GREAT ARTERIES, COMPLETE TRANSPOSITION

Symptoms. Male prevalence (2 to 4 : 1); onset from birth. Feeding difficulty; dyspnea; growth retardation.

Signs. High weight at birth; squatting; syncopes; progressive cyanosis. Single accentuated first sound in second left interspace; tachypnea; digital clubbing; hepatomegaly; narrow pulse; pulmonary edema.

Etiology. Congenital malformation.

Pathology. Aorta originating from right ventricle and rotating forward to left; pulmonary artery from left ventricle and rotating backward to right. Associated various malformations (e.g., septal defects; ductus arteriosus). Arterial and venous thrombosis of gastrointestinal and cerebral, kidney, and pulmonary districts.

Diagnostic Procedures. *Electrocardiography.* Right axis deviation; right-left predominance. *X-ray.* Cardiomegaly; vascular pedicle narrow at the base; increased pulmonary vessels. *Angiography.* Evidence of vessel inversion at origin. *Blood.* Polycythemia. *Two-dimensional echocardiography, cardiac catheterization.*

Therapy. Surgery; interatrial transposition of venous returns, during cardiopulmonary bypass with hypothermia. In patients with an intact ventricular septum, the first step is to establish an adequate interatrial opening (balloon septostomy).

Prognosis. Death usually in infancy. Possible survival to adolescence and even to adulthood. Good results with surgery at the time of election (first year of age).

BIBLIOGRAPHY. Farre JR: On malformations of the heart (essay I). In Pathological Researches, p 28. London, Longman, Hurst, Rees, Orme, Brown, 1814
Van Proogh R: The story of anatomical corrected malposition of the great arteries. Chest 69:2–4, 1976
Perloff JK: The Clinical Recognition of Congenital Heart Disease, 2nd ed, p 663. Philadelphia, WB Saunders, 1978
Hurst JW: The Heart, 6th ed, pp 691–696. New York, McGraw-Hill, 1986
Williams RG, Bierman FZ, Sanders SP: Echocardiographic Diagnosis of Cardiac Malformations, pp 165–169. Boston, Little, Brown & Co, 1986

GREBE'S

Synonyms. Achondrogenesis II; brazilian achondrogenesis (limb malformation type). Nonlethal achondrogenesis: Quelce–Salgado.

Symptoms. Both sexes affected; evident from birth. Dwarfism. Obesity. Facies normal. Striking reduction of limbs, especially of distal part; legs shorter than arms; short digits (fingers similar to toes); valgus position of feet. Polydactyly (57% of cases). Mental development delayed, but mentality normal.

Etiology. Autosomal recessive inheritance.

Pathology. Missing or hypoplastic bones.

Diagnostic Procedures. *X-ray of skeleton.* Shortened forearms, greater reduction of ulnae with respect to radii. *X-ray of spine.* Clear spaces because of uncalcified vertebrae.

Therapy. Surgery to remove extra digits.

Prognosis. Stillborn; death in early infancy. Possible survival.

BIBLIOGRAPHY. Grebe H: Die Achondrogenesis ein einfach rezesives Erbmerkmal. Folia Hered Pathol (Milano) 2:23–28, 1952
Quelce-Salgado A: A new type of dwarfism with various bone aplasias and hypoplasia of the extremities. Acta Genet 14:63–66, 1964
Kumar D, Curtis D, Blank CE: Grebe chondrodysplasia and brachydactyly in a family. Clin Genet 25:68–72, 1984

GREEN NAIL

Symptoms. Prevalent in females. Occur in patient whose occupation involves prolonged exposure of hands to soap, water, and detergents. Pain of involved fingers.

Signs. Green discoloration of the nail plate, entire nail, portion (proximally, distally, or laterally), or demarcated horizontal bands (in repeated episodes).

Etiology. Paronychial infections with *Pseudomonas aeruginosa* or some species of *Aspergillus*.

Pathology. Growth of pseudomonas within nail and formation of pigment.

Diagnostic Procedures. *Culture of infected material* (beneath nail and shaving of colored portion of nail).

Therapy. Polymyxin; neomycin; amphotericin B and 5-fluorocytosine for frequently associated *Candida* infection.

Prognosis. Recovery with treatment.

BIBLIOGRAPHY. Goldman L, Fox H: Greenish pigmentation of nail plates from *Bacillus pyocyaneus* infection: Report of two cases. Arch Dermatol Syph 49:136–137, 1944

Shellow WVR, Koplon BS: Green striped nails: Chromonychia due to *Pseudomonas aeruginosa*. Arch Dermatol 97:149–153, 1968
Samman PD: Management of disorders of the nails. Clin Exp Dermatol 7:189–194, 1982

GREEN STOOL

Symptoms. None.

Signs. Passage of green bile-stained stools without diarrhea.

Etiology. Unknown. Epidemic outbreak due to unknown agent that modifies intestinal flora and consequently urobilin metabolism.

Diagnostic Procedures. *Blood.* Low prothrombin level. *Urine.* Absence of bile and urobilinogen. *Stool.* Elevated bile; absent urobilinogen. *Culture.* Negative.

Therapy. Penicillin.

Prognosis. Stool becomes normal within 24 hours after administration of penicillin; prothrombin time is normal within 48 hours, and urobilinogen appears in urine and stool within that time.

BIBLIOGRAPHY. Greenblatt IJ, Bloch H, Turin RD, et al: "Green stool syndrome" of newly born infant. Pediatrics 5:180–183, 1950

GREEN URINE

Synonym. *Pseudomonas* toxemia.

Symptoms and Signs. In patient with infection of a large surface of body with *Pseudomonas aeruginosa* (e.g., extensive burn; empyema). One or 2 days before appearance of green urine, hemolytic crisis; followed by hypothermia, oliguria, dehydration, with or without shock.

Etiology. Massive infection with *Pseudomonas aeruginosa* determining massive hemolysis and formation of verdohemoglobin.

Pathology. That of gram-negative sepsis complicating different conditions (of burn, lung, pleura, intestine).

Diagnostic Procedures. *Urine.* Presence of a dark bilious green pigment (verdohemoglobin) to be differentiated from other pigments produced by *Pseudomonas* infection. Fluorescence with ultraviolet. *Culture of pus. Blood.* Red cell volume; bilirubin; electrolytes.

Therapy. Gentamicin and other antibiotics effective against *Pseudomonas* plus general symptomatic treatment and prevention of development of other substituting flora.

Prognosis. Until now always fatal within 2 to 3 days, or if in intensive treatment, a few weeks.

BIBLIOGRAPHY. Stone HH: The green urine syndrome: An ominous manifestation of Pseudomonas toxemia. Bull Emory Univ Clin 3:81–86, 1964

GREGG'S

Synonyms. Rubella embryopathy; postrubella; congenital rubella.

Symptoms and Signs. Occur in newborns of mothers exposed to rubella virus during first trimester of pregnancy. Hepatosplenomegaly; interstitial pneumonia; congenital heart defects (patent ductus arteriosus; stenosis of pulmonary trunk); low birth weight; congenital cataracts and visual disturbance with diplopia; purpura; hearing loss; inguinal hernias; mental retardation. Ataxia. Failure to thrive.

Etiology. Rubella virus affecting tissues during development.

Pathology. See Signs.

Diagnostic Procedures. Isolation of virus from throat swab, urine, and fecal material (positivity 63%). *Blood.* Anemia; hyperbilirubinemia; reticulocytosis; thrombocytopenia. *X-ray.* Changes in long bones; cerebral calcifications.

Therapy. Symptomatic. Keep infant isolated because he remains a carrier of the virus for a long time.

Prognosis. Severe mortality (14%) within a few months.

BIBLIOGRAPHY. Gregg NM: Congenital cataract following German measles in mother. Trans Ophthalmol Soc Aust 3:35–46, 1942
Singer DB, Rudolph AJ, Harvey S, et al: Pathology of the congenital rubella syndrome. J Pediatr 71:665–675, 1967
Shoenbaum SC, Biano S, Mack T: Epidemiology of congenital rubella syndrome. The role of maternal parity. JAMA 233:151–155, 1975

GREIG'S I

Synonym. Ocular hypertelorism.

Symptoms. Mental deficiency occasionally associated. Optic atrophy (when tension of optic nerve).

Signs. Excessive distance between orbits; strabismus; paralysis of external recti. Brachycephaly; occipital flattening, prominent and separated by a groove in frontal prominence; flat, upturned nose.

Etiology. Unknown; sporadic or hereditary (autosomal dominant or sex linked). Abnormal development of sphenoid.

Diagnostic Procedures. *X-ray of skull.* No synostosis of skull sutures; no signs of intracranial pressure.

Therapy. If feasible, surgical correction of some associated features, particularly ocular muscle and palpebrae.

Prognosis. If not associated with mental deficiency, adequate mental and physical development.

BIBLIOGRAPHY. Greig DM: Hypertelorism: A hitherto undifferentiated congenital cranio-facial deformity. Edinburgh Med J 31:560–593, 1924
Meisenbach AE Jr: Bilateral paralysis of external rectus muscle in hypertelorism: Report of a case with convergent strabismus. Am J Ophthalmol 33:83–87, 1950
Gorlin RJ, Pindborg JJ, Cohen MM: Syndromes of the Head and Neck, 2nd ed. New York, McGraw-Hill, 1976

GREIG'S II

Synonyms. Craniofacial; Polysyndactyly cephalopolysyndactyly Greigs'; GCPS; Hootnick-Holmes; frontodigital; Marshall-Smith, oxycephaly.

Symptoms and Signs. Both sexes. From birth. Expanded cranial vault, high forehead, broad nose. Polysyndactyly of hands and feet. Normal intelligence. May be associated: ichthyosis, tapetoretinal degeneration, bilateral hip dislocation.

Etiology. Unknown. Autosomal dominant inheritance.

Diagnostic Procedures. *X-rays.* Markedly advanced bone age.

BIBLIOGRAPHY. Greig DM: Oxycephaly. Edinburgh Med J 33:189–218, 1928
Marshall RE, Smith DW: Frontodigital syndrome: A dominantly inherited disorder with normal intelligence. J Pediatr 77:129–133, 1970
Hootnick D, Holmes LB: Familial polysyndactyly and craniofacial anomalies. Clin Genet 3:128–134, 1972
Tommerup N, Nielsen F: A familial reciprocal translocation t (3:7) (p21.1:p13) associated with the Greig polysyndactyly-craniofacial anomalies syndrome. Am J Genet 16:313–321, 1983

GREITHER'S

Synonym. Palmoplantar progressive keratoderma. See Meleda's; Hopf's. Tylosis, keratosis Greither, Unna-Thost; including palmoplantar epidermatolytic variant; and keratosis palmoplantar striate.

Symptoms. Both sexes affected, female less severe manifestations; onset in infancy and gradual progression. Asymptomatic or painful fissure on palms or soles.

Signs. Keratosis of palms and soles extending to all hands and feet and eventually to patches of arms and legs. Epidermolysis (in the PE variant). Family has been reported with lesions consisting in streaks of hyperkeratosis running along each finger to the palm (Bologna).

Etiology. Unknown; autosomal dominant inheritance.

Pathology. Keratoderma with scaling.

Therapy. Vitamin A in high doses; topical keratolytic agents and corticosteroids.

Prognosis. Progression and extension of lesions up to 40 years of age: then frequently, spontaneous, total regression in a few years.

BIBLIOGRAPHY. Greither A: Keratosis extremitatum hereditaria progrediens mit dominantem Erbagang. Hautarzt 3:198–203, 1952
Bologna EI: Durch vier generationen dominant vererblich geshlechtsgebundene keratosis palmaris striata (linearia). Dermatol Wochenschr 152:446–457, 1966
Gamborg Nielsen P: Two different clinical and genetic forms of hereditary palmoplantar keratoderma in the northernmost county of Sweden. Clin Genet 28:361–366, 1985
Camisa C, Williams H: Epidermolytic variant of palmoplantar keratoderme. Br J Dermatol 112:221–225, 1985

GRIERSON-GOPALAN

Synonyms. Barashek's; burning feet; Chacalek's; electric feet; Gopalan's; nutritive melalgia.

Symptoms. Frequently observed in the Indian regions and in Africa. Prevalent in women; onset between 20 and 40 years of age. Burning, pain, tingling, cramplike pain on soles, occasionally in the palms; excessive sweating; tachycardia with exertion; amnesia; decreased vision; amblyopia.

Signs. Elevated skin temperature; vasomotor changes of feet; shuffling gait; reflexes decreased; sensory loss; ataxia; weight loss.

Etiology. Malnutrition; occurs in epidemic form in malnourished population of prisoner camps, jails. Observed in chronic alcoholism.

Pathology. Body wasting; trophic skin changes in affected part.

Diagnostic Procedures. *Blood.* Protein decreased; hypochromic anemia.

Therapy. Yeast extract; calcium pantothenate.

Prognosis. Rapidly fatal without treatment. Responds well to therapy.

BIBLIOGRAPHY. Grierson J: On the burning feet of natives. Trans Med Phys Soc Calcutta 2:275–280, 1826
Gopalan C: The "burning feet syndrome." Indian Med Gaz 81:22–26, 1946
Vernon S: Nutritional melalgia: A deficiency vascular disease. JAMA 143:799–802, 1950

GRIESINGER'S

Synonyms. *Ankylostoma* duodenitis; Egyptian chlorosis; Gotthard tunnel; miner's anemia; tunnel anemia.

Symptoms. Usually appear in barefoot workers operating in damp soil. Itching, usually on feet and between toes, later in perineal area. Cephalalgia; weakness; dizziness; palpitation; tinnitus, abdominal colic and diarrhea. Possibly, cough and severe dyspnea. In some cases, duodenal ulcer symptomatology.

Signs. Early erythema and edematous change at site of invasion. Later, pallor; possibly, fever.

Etiology. Infestation with *Ankylostoma duodenale* or *Necator americanus.*

Pathology. *Jejunum.* Mucosal edema and inflammation with possible ulceration. *Liver.* Fatty infiltration.

Diagnostic Procedures. *Stool.* Parasites' ova; Charcot-Leyden crystals. *Blood.* Microcytic anemia; hyposideremia; eosinophilia. *Gastric fluid.* Higher activity than in patients with duodenal ulcer. *X-ray.* Deformity of duodenal bulb; hyperperistalsis of duodenum; absence of ulcer niche.

Therapy. Tetrachlorethylene; bephenium hydroxynaphthoate; hexylresorcinol; antianemic drugs.

Prognosis. Disappearance of duodenal symptoms within 24 hours and of radiologic findings in 10 to 24 days after treatment.

BIBLIOGRAPHY. Griesinger W: Kliniche und anatomiche Beobachtungen ueber die Krankheiten von Egypten. Arch Physiol Heilk 13:528–575, 1854

Yenikombistan H, Shehadi W: Duodenal ulcer syndrome caused by ankylostomiasis. Am J Roentgen 49:39–48, 1963

Brandborg LL: Parasitic diseases. In Sleisenger MH, Fordtran JS: Gastrointestinal Disease, p 1168. Philadelphia, WB Saunders, 1978

GRISCELLI'S

Synonyms. Chediack-Higashi-like; albinism immunodeficiency.

Symptoms and Signs. Both sexes. Partial albinism; acute episodes of fever.

Etiology. Autosomal recessive inheritance.

Pathology. Large clumps of pigment in the shafts of hair; accumulation of melanosomes in the melanocytes.

Diagnostic Procedures. *Blood.* Neutropenia (with normal neutrophils) and normal leukocyte specific protease activity; thrombocytopenia; hypogammaglobulinemia. *Skin.* Absence of delayed skin reaction and skin graft rejection.

Prognosis. Adulthood may be reached.

BIBLIOGRAPHY. Griscelli C, Durandy A, Guy-Grand D, et al: A syndrome associating partial albinism and immunodeficiency. Am J Med 65:691–702, 1978

GRISEL'S

Synonyms. Nasopharyngeal torticollis; atlantoaxial torticollis.

Symptoms and Signs. Spastic contraction of sternocleidomastoid muscle, which pulls the head laterally. Condition may arise after tonsillectomy or infection of the nasal cavities.

Etiology. Synovial effusion that causes relaxation of the joint capsule of the atlas and its subluxation.

Therapy. Antibiotic, antiinflammatory, and analgesic agents. Immobilization of the head.

Prognosis. Good with treatment.

BIBLIOGRAPHY. Grisel P: Enucleation de l'atlas et torticollis nasopharyngen. Presse Med 38:50–53, 1930

GROB'S

Synonyms. Dysplasia linguofacialis II; Papillon–Léage and Psaume variant.

Symptoms. Mental deficiency. Feeding problems.

Signs. *Head.* Partial alopecia; epicanthus; cleft lip and palate; mucous membranes of mouth multiridged; fissured tongue; broad nasal bridge and small orifices. *Limbs.* Brachydactyly and clinodactyly.

Etiology. Unknown. See Papillon-Léage and Psaume.

BIBLIOGRAPHY. Grob M: Dysplasia linguo-facialis (Grob). Lehrbuch der Kinderchirurgie, Stuttgart, 1957

GROENBLAD-STRANDBERG-TOURAINE

Synonyms. Darier-Grönblad-Strandberg; elastosis dystrophica; systemic elastorrhexis; pseudoxanthoma elasticum; PXE; Touraine's.

Symptoms and Signs. The complete syndrome or subsyndromes may be observed. Symptoms and signs may appear at any age. *Cutaneous.* Bands of small yellowish papules parallel to cutaneous grooves in the neck, axillae, flexor side of elbows, groin, popliteal area. Skin inelastic; when pinched retains folds for some time (opposite of Ehlers-Danlos). *Ocular.* Wide lines; reddish or greyish around optic disk in both eyes (angioid streaks). Occasionally, retinal and choroidal degeneration. *Cardiovascular.* Alteration of peripheral pulses; angina pectoris; hypertension; occasionally, visceral hemorrhages; hematemesis and melena. Focal cerebral symptoms.

Etiology. Unknown; hereditary condition; autosomal recessive gene. Occasionally associated with Paget's, Marfan's, Herrick's, Albers-Schönberg.

Pathology. *Skin.* Degeneration and fragmentation of elastic tissue. *Eyes.* Ruptures of elastic membrane of Bruch of the choroid. *Cardiocirculatory.* Generalized. Arteritis. Rupture of vessel elastic fibers with calcification of degenerated tissue. Proliferation of intima with occlusion of vessel. Necrotic lesions and secondary hemorrhages in gastrointestinal tract, kidney, brain. Renal angioma in one case responsible for hypertension.

Therapy. Plastic surgery to improve cosmetic aspect.

Prognosis. No effect on life span. Complicating hypertension or hemorrhages. In pregnancy, high incidence of gastrointestinal bleeding.

BIBLIOGRAPHY. Rigal D: Observation pour servir à l'histoire de la cheloide diffuse xanthélasmique. Ann Dermatol Syph 2:491–501, 1881

Darier J: Pseudoxanthoma elasticum. Monatssch Prakt Dermatol 23:609–617, 1896

Grönblad E: Angoid streaks: Pseudoxanthoma elasticum. Vorläufige Mitteilung. Acta Ophthalmol 7:329, 1929

Strandberg J: Pseudoxanthoma elasticum. Zentralbl Haut Ges Krkh 31:689, 1929

Touraine A: L'elastorrhexie systématisée. Bull Soc Fr Dermatol Syph 47:225–273, 1940

Geominne L, Van Ginneken E, Bernard R: Syndrome de Grönblad-Strandberg-Touraine. Presse Med 71:2511–2514, 1963

Rook A, Wilkinson DS, Ebling FJG, et al: Textbook of Dermatology, 4th ed, pp 1841–1844. Oxford, Blackwell Scientific Publications, 1986

GROENOUW'S I

Synonyms. Buckler's; corneal granular dystrophy; macular corneal dystrophy Groenouw's I.

Symptoms. Both sexes affected; onset during first 10 years of life. Visual reduction by 50 to 60 years of age.

Signs. Grayish white opaque granules with sharp borders, mostly in central part of cornea. Cornea clear between opaque spots.

Etiology. Unknown; autosomal dominant inheritance. Sporadic cases also reported.

Pathology. Masses of hyaline substance between epithelium and Bowman's membrane. Dehiscences in Bowman's membrane. Disruption of nerve fiber.

Diagnostic Procedures. *Biopsy of cornea.*

Therapy. Corneal graft.

Prognosis. Deterioration becoming serious after fifth decade.

BIBLIOGRAPHY. Groenouw A: Knotchenformige Hornhauttrübungen. Arch Augenheilkd 21:281–289, 1890
Goldberg MF: Genetic and Metabolic Eye Disease, p 290. Boston, Little Brown, 1974

GROENOUW'S II

Synonyms. Buckler's II; corneal granular dystrophy II; macular corneal dystrophy Groenouw's II.

Symptoms. Both sexes affected; onset in early childhood. Corneal sensitivity may be reduced. Painful attacks, photophobia. Reduction of vision; significant reduction by age 30 to 40; then further progression.

Signs. Grayish opaque corneal spots; borders not sharply delimitated; scattered over entire cornea, especially dense in central zone.

Etiology. Autosomal recessive inheritance. Defect in glycoprotein processing.

Pathology. Accumulation of acid mucopolysaccharides in corneal corpuscles; mucoid degeneration of stromal lamellae; disappearance of stromal cells. Electron microscopy reveals no abnormality of skin or bulbar conjunctive.

Diagnostic Procedures. *Biopsy of cornea. Urine.* Absence of acid mucopolysaccharide.

Therapy. Corneal graft.

Prognosis. Patients may be blind by the age of 40, occasionally later.

BIBLIOGRAPHY. Groenouw A: Knötchenförmige Hornhaüttrubungen. Arch Augenheilkd 21:281–289, 1890
Hassel JR, Newsome DA, Krachmer JH, et al: Macular corneal dystrophy: Failure to synthesize a mature keratan sulfate proteoglycan. Proc Nat Acad Sci 77:3705–3709, 1980

GROLL-HIRSCHOWITZ

Synonyms. Deafness–mesenteric diverticula–neuropathy. See Refsum's.

Symptoms and Signs. In females. Onset between 3 and 24 years of age. Progressive deafness, normal vestibular function, peripheral sensory neuropathy, tachycardia; progressive impairment of digestive processes, steatorrhea (loss of gastric motility) diverticulosis.

Etiology. Autosomal recessive inheritance.

Pathology. Jejunoileal diverticula with ulceration. Peripheral nerves: demyelinization.

Diagnostic Procedures. *Feces.* Malabsorption with fat and protein loss. *Blood.* Hypocholesterolemia. *Electromyography. X-rays of intestine.* Diverticulosis of small bowel. *Electrocardiography. Biopsy.* Peripheral nerve: demyelinization.

Therapy. Symptomatic.

Prognosis. Death in the end of second or third decade.

BIBLIOGRAPHY. Groll A, Hirschowitz BI: Steatorrhea and familial deafness in two siblings. Clin Res 14:47, 1966
Potasman I, Stermer E, Levy N, et al: The Groll-Hirschowitz syndrome. Clin Genet 28:76–79, 1985

GROSS-GROH-WEIPPL

Synonyms. Thrombocytopenia radial aplasia; TAR.

Symptoms. Both sexes equally affected; present from birth.

Signs. Absence or hypoplasia of radius (usually bilateral). Frequent association of hypoplasia of ulna and hands or bones of the lower extremities Tetraphocomelia in one case. Less frequent association of cardiac or renal defects; low stature; spina bifida and other bone involvement. Hemorrhagic tendency. Pallor out of proportion to blood loss.

Etiology. Unknown; probably, autosomal recessive inheritance.

Pathology. See Signs. *Bone marrow.* Absence (66%) or hypoplasia of megakaryocytes.

Diagnostic Procedures. *Blood.* Anemia out of proportion; white blood cells; leukemoid granulocytosis (62%); eosinophilia (53%). Thrombocytopenia and disorders of blood clotting secondary to platelet deficiency. *X-ray of skeleton.* See Signs. *Electrocardiography, heart catheterization, functional studies.* Different abnormalities possible.

Therapy. Corticosteroids have symptomatic action on hemorrhages, but do not affect thrombocytopenia. Orthopedic prosthesis.

Prognosis. Improvement of hematologic condition with advancing of age.

BIBLIOGRAPHY. Gross H, Groh C, Weippl G: Kongenitale hypoplastische Thrombopenie mit Radialaplasie. Neue Osterr Zschr Kinderheilkd 1:574–582, 1956
Show S, Oliver RAM: Congenital hypoplastic thrombocytopenia with skeletal deformities in siblings. Blood 14:374–377, 1959
Gmyrek D, Otto FMG, Slym-Rapaport I: Über das familiare Auftreten von Fanconi-anamie und Thrombocytopenie mit Missbildungen (Bemerkungen zur Therapie der Fanconi-anaemie). Monatsschr Kinderheilkd 113:542–552, 1965
Adeyokunnu AA: Radial aplasia and amegakaryocytic thrombocytopenia (TAR syndrome) among Nigerian children. Am J Dis Child 138:346–348, 1984
Ayane–Yeboa K, Jaramillo S, Nagel C, et al: Tetraphocomelia in the syndrome of thrombocytopenia with absent radii (TAR syndrome). Am J Med Genet 20:571–576, 1985

GROSSHAN'S

Synonym. Cutaneous amyloid poikiloderma.

Symptoms and Signs. Two sisters affected; onset at 1 year of age. Telangiectasia; skin atrophy; pigmentary poikiloderma-like alterations; at puberty, verrucous lesions on elbows and backs of feet and hands. Absence of cataract.

Etiology. Autosomal recessive inheritance proposed.

BIBLIOGRAPHY. Grosshans VE, Bergoend H, Khochnevis A: Die erbilichen Hand-amyloidosen: Die familiaere amyloide Poikilodermie. MMW 114:1183–1190, 1972

GRUND'S

Synonyms. Gamstorp-Wahlfort; myokimia–myotonia–muscle atrophy–hyperhidrosis. See Charcot-Marie tooth.

Symptoms and Signs. Muscular stiffness with fine twitches (myokymia) followed by wasting and generalized hyperhidrosis.

Etiology. Unknown. Sporadic possibly autosomal dominant inheritance.

Therapy. Muscle stiffness reduced by anticonvulsants.

BIBLIOGRAPHY. Grund G: Ueber genetische Beziehungen zwischen Myotonie, Mustelkraempfen und Myokimie (Zugleich Beitrag zur Pathologie der neuralen Muskelatrophie). Dtsch Z Nervenheilk 146:3–14, 1938
Gamstorp I, Wahlfort G: A syndrome characterized by myokymia, myotonia, muscular wasting and increased perspiration. Acta Psychiatr Neurol Scand 34:181–194, 1959

GRUNER-BERTOLOTTI

Combination of Parinaud's (see) and von Monakow's.

GUERIN'S

Eponym used to indicate a fracture of the maxilla.

BIBLIOGRAPHY. Guérin AF: Des fractures des maxillaires supérieures. Nouveau moyen de les reconnaitre dans les cas fréquents où elles ne l'accompagnent pas de déplacement. Arch Gen Med 2:5–13, 1866

GUERRY-COGAN

Synonyms. Cogan-Guerry; microcystic corneal dystrophy. Corneal dystrophy microcystic; map-out-fingerprint pattern.

Symptoms. Prevalent in females. Initially, vision not affected, then reduced according to degree of involvement of central cornea.

Signs. Fine wavy lines (fingerprint-like) within corneal epithelium.

Etiology. Unknown. Autosomal dominant inheritance.

Pathology. Intraepithelial cysts with pyknotic nuclei and debirs. Basement membrane thickened or with multilaminar aspect (or both).

Diagnostic Procedures. *Binocular microscopy.* With retroillumination (see Signs). *Electromicroscopy.*

Therapy. None.

Prognosis. Progressive condition, eventually resulting in visual impairment.

BIBLIOGRAPHY. Guerry D: Fingerprint-like lines in the cornea. Am J Ophthalmol 33:724–726, 1950
Cogan DG, Donaldson DD, Kuwabara T, Marshall D: Microcystic dystrophy of the corneal epithelium. Trans Am Ophthalmol Soc 62:213–225, 1964
Luxenburg MN, Friedland BR, Holder JM: Superficial microcystic corneal dystrophy. Arch Ophthalmol 93:107–110, 1975

GUILLAIN-ALAJOUANINE-GARCIN

Synonyms. Half base; Garcin's; Bertotti-Garcin; Hartmann's; Schmincke's tumor; unilateral cranial palsy; hemipolyneuropathy-cranial palsy.

Symptoms and Signs. Hemilateral loss of function of all 12 cranial nerves. Seldom associated symptoms of pyramidal involvement or intracranial pressure.

Etiology and Pathology. Nasopharyngeal tumors; primary tumor of base of the skull; leukemic infiltrates (Schmincke) of basal meninges; trauma; metastases.

Diagnostic Procedures. *CT brain scan. Blood. Bone marrow biopsy. Cerebrospinal fluid.* Normal or increased protein.

Therapy. According to etiology.

BIBLIOGRAPHY. Guillain G, Alajonnaine R, Garcin R: Le syndrome paralitique unilateral global des nerfs cranieus. Bull Soc Med Hosp Paris 50:456–460, 1926
Garcin R: Le syndrome paralitique unilatèral global des nerfs cranieus. Paris (Thesis) 1927

GUILLAIN-BARRÉ

Synonyms. Guillain-Barré-Strohl; Glanzmann-Salaud; Kussmaul-Landry; Landry's; ascending paralysis; acute infective polyneuritis; postinfectious radiculoneuropathy.

Symptoms. Affects all ages and both sexes. In 50% of cases, upper respiratory infection observed a few days or weeks before start of symptoms. Paresthesia; lower leg weakness initially (may begin in other part of body); progressive diffusion to trunk, upper extremities, neck, and cranial nerves. Pain in the back; muscle tenderness; mild stiffness of neck; fever (occasionally absent).

Signs. Flaccid, atonic paralysis ascending (developing in hours or days—up to 7–10 days). Motor involvement more evident than sensory involvement. Proximal muscles more prominently affected. Tendon reflexes decreased or absent; Plantar response absent. Lassègue's sign present.

Etiology. Unknown; toxic, allergic, autoimmune mechanism. Observed following viral, bacterial, parasitic infections, leukemia and lymphoma, toxic condition, insect bite, surgery, vaccine therapy.

Pathology. Early, fragmentation of cylinder axons in peripheral nerves, spinal ganglion, nerve roots. Later, inflammatory infiltrates and degeneration of medullary nerve sheaths.

Diagnostic Procedures. *Spinal fluid.* Increased proteins; normal or slightly elevated number of cells. *Blood.* Normal. Search for etiologic agent. *Serology. Culture. Smears.*

Therapy. Supportive; respirator necessary in some cases. Steroids are of no benefit; in severe cases (i.e., those requiring ventilation) are indicated plasmapheresis and immunosuppressants. Plasmapheresis.

Prognosis. The outcome has been graded as follows:
(0) Healthy
(1) Minor symptoms or signs
(2) Able to walk 5 meters without help, walking frame or stick but unable to do manual work, including shopping or gardening
(3) Able to walk 5 meters with help, walking frame, or stick
(4) Chair or bed bound
(5) Requiring assisted ventilation (for at least part of day or night)
(6) Dead.
Children seem to have a better prognosis than adults, and the need for ventilation is not necessarily to be considered a poor prognostic factor.

BIBLIOGRAPHY. Landry JBO: Note sur la paralysie ascendante aigue. Gaz Hebd Med Chir 6:472–474; 486–488, 1859
Guillain G, Barré JA, Strohl A: Le réflexe médico-plantaire: Étude de ses caractères graphiques et de son temps perdu. Bull Soc Med Hop Paris 40:1459–1462, 1915–1916
Winer JB, Hughes RAC, Greenwood RJ, Perkin GD, Healy MJR: Prognosis in Guillain-Barré syndrome. Lancet 1:1202–1203, 1985
Cole GF, Matthew DJ: Prognosis in severe Guillain-Barré syndrome. Arch Dis Child 62:228–291, 1987
McKhann GM, Griffin JW, Cornblath DR, et al: Plasmapheresis and Guillain-Barré syndrome: Analysis of prognosis factors and the effects of plasmapheresis. Ann Neurol 23:347–353, 1988

GUILLAIN-BERTRAND-LEREBOULLET

See Choreiform syndromes.

BIBLIOGRAPHY. Guillain G, Bertrand I, Lereboullet J: Myoclonies arythmiques unilaterales des membres par lésion du noyau dentlé du cervelet. Rev Neurol (Paris) 2:73–78, 1934

GULLNER'S

Synonyms. Hypokalemia familial; hypokalemia alkalosis–renal tubulopathy.

Symptoms. Both sexes. From infancy. Weakness, muscle cramps, nausea, and intermittent vomiting. Normal blood pressure in some cases asymptomatic.

Etiology. Unknown. Possibly autosomal recessive inheritance. Suggested abnormal magnesium metabolism responsible for hypokalemia.

Pathology. *Kidney*. Changes in the proximal tubules: hypertrophy of basal membranes, intense staining of cells, pyknotic nuclei. Juxtaglomerular apparatus, glomeruli and distal tubule and Henle loops: normal.

Diagnostic Procedures. *Blood*. Inability to retain Na; elevated plasma K and renin levels or decreased plasma K levels. Plasma Mg level normal. Hypokalemia corrected by Mg administration or high Na intake and triamterene. *Urine*. Prostaglandin increased.

Therapy. See Diagnostic procedures. Hyperkalemia is corrected by Mg administration or high Na diet and triamterene.

BIBLIOGRAPHY. Potter WZ, Trygstad CW, Helmer OM, et al: Familial hypokalemia associated with renal interstitial fibrosis. Am J Med 57:971–977, 1974
Gullner HG, Gill JR Jr, Bartter FC, et al: A familial disorder with hypokalemic alkalosis hyperreninemia, aldosteronism, high urinary prostaglandins and normal pressure that is not Bartter's syndrome. Trans Assoc Am Phys 92:179–188, 1979
Gullner HG, Bartter FC, Gill JR Jr, et al: A sibship with hypokalemic alkalosis and renal proximal tubulopathy. Arch Intern Med 143:1534–1540, 1983

GULL'S

Synonyms. Adult myxedema; cachexia strumipriva. Includes myxedematous cachexia, adult myxedema.

Symptoms. Females more frequently affected than males; insidious onset in middle age. Decrease in sweating; cold hypersensitivity; decrease in activity; listlessness; lack of energy; easy fatigability. Mental dullness may follow or precede other symptoms. Progressive constipation; Decrease of menstrual flow; deafness; thick speech; dizziness; headache may be another presenting symptom or follow in various orders. Decreased libido. In cases of more rapid onset (from surgery, radioiodine therapy), acute onset with the addition of anxiety or depression and severe skeletal symptoms.

Signs. Pallor; dry skin; falling hair; weight gain; facial puffiness. Pulse rate decreased; cardiomegaly; palpitations; muscles weak and flabby; arthropathy with effusion. Later; nonpitting edema (myxedema) remaining stable for years to end (if not treated) in myxedematous cachexia (intensification of described symptoms and signs).

Etiology. Autoimmune endemic iodine deficiency, genetic, iatrogenic infiltrative diseases, hypothalamic disfunctions Seabright-Bantam mechanism (see).

Pathology. *Thyroid*. Usually, dense fibrosis; infiltration by lymphocytes and plasma cells possible; follicle and active cells may persist in scattered fashion. *Pituitary*. Increase of gamma cells; decrease of acidophilic cells. *Skin*. Hyperkeratosis; plugging of sweat glands; edema; swelling and fraying of collagen fibers; deposition of intracellular material. *Muscles*. Edematous; swollen; pale. *Serous cavities*. Free fluid. *Brain*. Possibly; atrophy gliosis; foci of degeneration.

Diagnostic Procedures. *Metabolic rate*. Decreased. *Blood*. Free T_3, T_4 and protein-bound iodide reduced; ^{131}I uptake reduced; thyroid-stimulating hormone (TSH) increased; antithyroid antibodies possibly increased; plasma creatinine phosphokinase, lactic dehydrogenase, uric acid cholesterol increased. Anemia common. *Electrocardiography*. Low voltage; QT prolonged; T wave abnormal.

Therapy. Thyroid or L-thyroxine per os.

Prognosis. Remission of all symptomatology and most of the body changes with treatment.

BIBLIOGRAPHY. Fagge CH: On sporadic cretinism occurring in England. Med Chir Trans 54:155, 1871
Gull WW: On a cretinoid state supervening in adult life in women. Trans Clin Soc 7:180–185, 1874
Tachmann MI, Guthrie GP: Hypothyroidism: Diversity of presentation. Endocrinol Rev 5:456–465, 1984

GÜNTHER'S I

Synonyms. Congenital erythropoietic porphyria; photosensitive porphyria. CEP.

Symptoms. No sex predominance; wide racial distribution; clinical onset at birth or during first year. Passage of red urine. This finding will persist showing considerable daily and seasonal variations. As exposure of the infant to sun increases, vesicular or bullous eruptions of areas exposed to sun appear (usually within first year); lesions heal slowly leaving scars. Abdominal and neurologic symptoms absent.

Signs. Acute manifestation (bullae) and scarring of different degrees of intensity from mild to severely mutilating. Hypertrichosis (fine blond lanugo); slight chronic jaundice; erythrodontia (best visible with ultraviolet light). Splenomegaly (inconstant finding; variation in size during course of disease may occur). Normal blood pressure.

Etiology. Unknown; autosomal recessive inherited metabolic defect of porphyrin, with overproduction of porphyrin type I, confined to erythroid system. Autosomal recessive inheritance. Deficiency of uroporphyrogen III cosynthase activity that causes overproduction of porphyrin type I.

Diagnostic Procedures. *Blood.* Normochromic anemia seldom severe, intermittent in type; reticulocytes high; circulating normoblasts; decreased survival of an aliquot of red cell population. *Bone marrow.* Erythroid hyperplasia; normoblasts may show central inclusion. Studies in unstained sample with fluorescent light microscope show intense fluorescence in one aliquot of nucleated red cell, maximal fluorescence in nuclear and perinuclear areas, and minor degree in some reticulocytes. *Urine.* Pale pink to deep red. Porphyrin type I dominating; small amount of porphyrin III: small amount of coproporphyrin. *Stool.* Large amount of coproporphyrin type I; only small amount of type III; increased fecal urobilinogen.

Therapy. Splenectomy (usually highly beneficial for hemolytic anemia). Avoid exposure to the sun; protect bullae from infection.

Prognosis. Following splenectomy, decrease of hemolytic process and of photosensitivity. Severe mutilation may result from scarring.

BIBLIOGRAPHY. Schultz JH: Ein fall von Pemphigus leprosus complicirt durch Lepra visceralis. (thesis). Greifswald, 1874
Günther H: Die Hämatoporphyrie. Dtsch Arch Klin Med 105:89–146, 1911
Kappas A, Sassa S, Anderson KE: The porphyrias. In Stanbury JB, Wyngaarden JB, Fredrickson DS, et al: The Metabolic Basis of Inherited Disease, 5th ed, p 1301. New York, McGraw-Hill, 1983

GUTIERREZ'S

Synonym. Horseshoe kidney.

Symptoms. Male to female ratio 2:1. Frequently asymptomatic. Chronic gastrointestinal or urinary complaints (or both).

Signs. Hyperextension of body may elicit nausea and vomiting, signs that will be relieved by opposite movement (Rovsing's signs).

Etiology. Congenital malformation: fusion of nephrogenic blastemas for mechanical reasons during fetal development.

Pathology. In great majority (90%) kidneys are fused on the inferior pole. Presence of solid mass (parenchymal fibrous) that joins the two kidneys across the midline.

Diagnostic Procedures. *Urography. Isotope scan. CT scan. Urine.* Variable changes in function. *Blood.* Features of chronic renal condition.

Therapy. Surgery according to entity of compression exerted on the ureters and technical feasibility of ureteral flow correction according to the associated malformation.

Prognosis. Variable.

BIBLIOGRAPHY. Gutierrez R: The clinical management of the horseshoe kidney. Am J Surg 15:132–165, 1932
Kissane JM: Congenital malformations. In Heptinstall RH: Pathology of the Kidney, 3rd ed. Boston, Little, Brown & Co, 1983

H

HAAB'S

Synonym. Macular retinal senile degeneration II.

Symptoms. Onset in advanced age. Moderate decrease of visual function that usually remains fairly satisfactory for long time.

Signs. Bilateral, but usually asymmetric presence of drusen or small clumps of pigment or both; thickening of inner limiting membrane gives a "beaten bruise" aspect and gliotic glistening.

Etiology. Unknown; autosomal dominant inheritance suggested.

Pathology. See Signs. With evolution, destruction of cones.

Therapy. Symptomatic.

Prognosis. Benign course with fairly satisfactory vision for a long time; strong individual variability of speed of progression.

BIBLIOGRAPHY. Kimura SJ, Wayne MC: Retinal Diseases. Philadelphia, Lea & Febiger, 1966

HAAS'

Synonym. Syndactyly type IV

Symptoms and Signs. Syndactyly complete and bilateral; six metacarpals and digits; fingers flexion. Teeth normal.

Etiology. Autosomal dominant inheritance.

Diagnostic Procedures. *X-ray.* Absence of bone fusion.

BIBLIOGRAPHY. Haas SL: Bilateral complete syndactylism of all fingers. Am J Surg 50:363–366, 1940

HABER'S

Synonym. Intraepidermal epithelioma-rosacea-like eruption.

Symptoms and Signs. Both sexes affected; onset in childhood. Rosacea-like eruption on the cheeks, nose, forehead, and chin. Erythema; telangiectasia; follicle papules; pitted areas. Later in life, appearance of warty lesions, scaly or keratotic (1 cm in diameter), not symmetric, on trunk and thighs.

Etiology. Unknown; autosomal dominant inheritance.

Pathology. Erythematous lesions: perivascular inflammation; fibrosis; acanthosis and parakeratosis; proliferation of sebaceous glands. Warty lesions: papillomatosis; acanthosis; dyskeratosis; mitotic figures.

Diagnostic Procedures. *Biopsy of skin.*

Therapy. For erythema, steroids. For warty lesions, x-ray treatment.

Prognosis. Good.

BIBLIOGRAPHY. Wilson HTH: Two cases of familial rosacea-like dermatosis with lanugo hair changes. Br J Dermatol 72:322, 1960
Sanderson KV, Wilson HTH: Haber's syndrome—familial rosacea-like eruption with intraepithelial epithelioma. Br J Dermatol 77:1–8, 1965
Rook A, Wilkinson DS, Ebling FJG, et al: Textbook of Dermatology, 4th ed, p 2393. Oxford, Blackwell Scientific Publications, 1986

HAENEL'S

Synonym. Ocular tabetic anesthesia.

Symptoms and Signs. Absence of pain on pressure applied on the eyes; associated with other symptoms of tabes dorsalis.

Etiology. Advanced stage of neurosyphilis.

BIBLIOGRAPHY. Haenel H: Eine neues Tabessymptom. Neurol Zentralbl 28: 1199, 1909

HAFERKAMP'S

Synonyms. Gorham's variant; malignant hemoangiomatosis-osteolysis.

Symptoms and Signs. Related to generalized hemoangiomatosis and bone (incomplete) osteolysis (see Gorham's).

Etiology. Unknown.

Pathology. Gorham's syndrome plus a typical fatty degeneration of the tumor tissue and fatty infiltration of liver and kidney.

Diagnostic Procedures. *Blood.* Anemia; presence of immature cells, both erythroid and myeloid, in circulation. *X-ray.* See Gorham's.

Therapy. Symptomatic.

Prognosis. Poor.

BIBLIOGRAPHY. Haferkamp O: Ueber das Syndrome generalisierte maligne Haemangiomatosis mit Osteolysis. Krebsforsch 64:418–426, 1962
Hardegger F, Simpson LA, Segmueller G: The syndrome of idiopathic osteolysis: classification, review and case report. J Bone Joint Surg 67B:89–93, 1985

HAFF*

Synonyms. Rhabdomyolysis; toxic myoglobinuria.

Myoglobinuria following the ingestion of eel or fish poisoned by waste products of cellulose factory.

BIBLIOGRAPHY. Assmann H, Bielenstein H, Hobs H, et al: Beobachtungen and Untersuchungen bei der Haffkrankeit. Dtsch Med Wochenschr 59:122–126, 1933
Adams RD, Victor M: Principles of Neurology, 3rd ed, p 1040. New York, McGraw-Hill, 1985

HAGEMAN'S FACTOR DEFICIENCY

Synonym. Factor XII deficiency.

Symptoms and Signs. Asymptomatic with few minor exceptions. Laboratory curiosity.

Etiology. Congenital deficiency of Hageman factor. Autosomal recessive inheritance. Families with autosomal dominant condition found.

Diagnostic Procedures. *Blood.* Normal bleeding time; prolonged clotting time; increased partial thromboplastin time corrected by absorbed plasma or aged serum; abnormal thromboplastin generation test when all reagents are from the patients; abnormal prothrombin consumption test; normal one-stage prothrombin time. Radioimmunoassay of factor XII: lack of factor XII.

Therapy. None.

Prognosis. Excellent.

BIBLIOGRAPHY. Ratnoff OD, Colopy JE: Familial hemorrhagic trait associated with deficiency of clot-promoting fraction of plasma. J Clin Invest 34:602–613, 1955
Saito H, Ratnoff OD, Pensky J: Radioimmunoassay of human Hageman factor (factor XII). J Lab Clin Med 88:506, 1976

HAGLUND'S

Synonym. Calcaneous fracture. Eponym used to indicate a fracture of the nucleus calcaneus at the Achilles' tendon insertion, without damage of cartilage or of the periostium. Occurs at a young age.

Etiology. Trauma, often preceding osteocondritic lesions.

BIBLIOGRAPHY. Haglund P: Ueber Fractur des Epiphysenkerns des Calcaneus, nebst allgemeinen Bemerkungen über einige aehnliche juvenile Knochenkervverletzungen. Arch Klin Chir (Berlin) 82:922–930, 1907
Haglund P: Beitzag sur Klinik der Achillessehne. Z Orthop Chir 49:49–58, 1927
Canale ST: Fracture and dislocation in children. In Crenshaw AH (ed): Campbell's Operative Orthopedics, 7th ed, pp 1988–1994. St. Louis, CV Mosby, 1987

HAIR-BRAIN

Synonyms. Amish brittle hair; brittle hair-intellectual impairment-decreased fertility-short stature; BIDS; Sabinas trichothiodystrophy. See Pollitt's; Trichorrhexis nodosa.

Symptoms. Mild intellectual impairment; decreased fertility.

Signs. Short stature, brittle hair, nails break easily.

Etiology. Autosomal recessive inheritance. Possibly identical with Pollitt's syndrome.

Pathology. Hair. Irregular grooved surface, lack of scales, reduction 50% of sulfur.

BIBLIOGRAPHY. Pollitt RJ, Jemer FA, Davis M: Sibs with mental and physical retardation and trichorrhexis nodosa with abnormal amino acid composition of hair. Arch Dis Child 43:211–216, 1968
Allen RJ: Neurocutaneous syndromes in children. Postgrad Med J 50:83–89, 1971
Jackson CE, Weiss L, Watson JHL: Brittle hair with short stature, intellectual impairment and decreased fertility: an autosomal recessive syndrome in Amish kindred. Pediatr 54:201–212, 1974

---

*From the name of a bay (Haff) in the area of Könisberg (Germany).

King MD, Gummer CL, Stephenson JBP: Trichothio-dystrophy-neurocutaneus syndrome of Pollitt: a report of two unrelated cases. J Med Genet 21:286–289, 1968

HAJDU-CHENEY

Synonyms. Acroosteolysis-osteoporosis-skull changes; arthrodentoosteo dysplasia; Cheney's; dentoarthroosteo dysplasia; Giaccai's; osteoarthrodento dysplasia.

Symptoms. Both sexes affected; onset in early teens to sixth decade. Severe backache; occasionally, headache.

Signs. Short stature. Acroosteolysis. Hypoplasia of terminal phalanges: short fingers and toes. Delayed closure of cranial sutures. Mild hypoplasia of mandibular ramus. Protuberance of occipital bone. In adult life, collapse of vertebral bodies with progressive loss of height. Bone fractures from minor traumas.

Etiology. Unknown; autosomal dominant inheritance.

Pathology. Generalized osteoporosis. Multiple wormian bones.

Diagnostic Procedures. *X-ray of skeleton.* Decalcification of bone; cranial changes; enlargement of sella turcica; basilar impression; spine; density of intervertebral disk greater than that of bones. *Blood.* Calcium, phosphorus, alkaline phosphatase normal.

Therapy. None.

Prognosis. Progressive alterations mostly osteoporosis. Progressive loss of height. Fracture prone.

BIBLIOGRAPHY. Hajdu N, Kauntze R: Cranio-skeletal dysplasia. Br J Radiol: 21:42–48, 1948
Cheney WD: Acro-osteolysis. Am J Roentgen 94:595–607, 1965
Elias AN, Pinals RS, Anderson HC, et al: Hereditary osteodysplasia with acro-osteolysis (the Hajdu-Cheney syndrome). Am J Med 65:627–636, 1978

HALBAN'S

Synonyms. Secondary amenorrhea; persistent corpus luteum; functional ovarian disturbance.

Symptoms. Appear in young women. Amenorrhea, occasionally following cycles of decreasing frequency.

Signs. Absence of objective evidence of pregnancy.

Etiology. Benign tumor of the ovary with persistence of the corpus luteum activity. One of the many functional ovary disturbances responsible for secondary amenorrhea.

Diagnostic Procedures. *Pregnancy test. Hormonal studies.*

Therapy. Excision of tumor.

Prognosis. Good.

BIBLIOGRAPHY. Ascheim S, Varangot J: Verkante schwangershaft. Arch Gynecol 183:275–280, 1953

HALF-AND-HALF NAIL

Synonym. Azotemic onychopathy.

Symptoms. Those of chronic nephropathy with hyperazotemia (25 cases of 1500 present nail findings).

Signs. Fingernail beds with red, pink brown, transverse, distal band, occupying at least 20 to 60% of nail length and with the remaining nail showing a dull, whitish aspect. Constriction of venous return does not affect the contrast between two zones. Lack of tendency of the pattern to grow out with the nail. No correlation between severity of azotemia and nail change.

Etiology. Unknown. This type of onychopathy observed in 20 to 40% of chronic hyperazotemic conditions; occasionally, in cases with cylinduria without azotemia. Association is also possible with liver cirrhosis (as an extension of the Terry's syndrome).

Pathology. Chronic nephropathies. Pathology of onychopathy unknown.

Diagnostic Procedures. *Blood.* Determination of blood urea nitrogen in all patients exhibiting this type of onychopathy. Decreased creatinine clearance.

Therapy and Prognosis. That of chronic nephropathy.

BIBLIOGRAPHY. Bean WB: A discourse on nail growth and unusual fingernails. Trans Am Clin Climatol Assoc 74:152–167, 1963
Lindsay PG: The half and half nail. Arch Intern Med 119:583–587, 1967
Rook A, Wilkinson DS, Ebling FJG, et al: Textbook of Dermatology, 4th ed, p 2069. Oxford, Blackwell Scientific Publications, 1986

HALLERMANN-STREIFF

Synonyms. Audry's I; dyscephalia oculomandibularis-hypotrichosis; mandibulo-ocular dyscephaliahypotrichosis; Ullrich-Fremerey-Dohna; Fremerey-Dohna; François' II.

Symptoms and Signs. Affects both sexes equally. Localized alopecia; beaked nose; microcornea; congenital cataracts with spontaneous rupture and absorption; occasionally, glaucoma. Proportionate nanism; atrophy of skin; retardation of psychomotor development.

Etiology. Unknown; sporadic occurrence, no chromosomal abnormalities detected. Possibly autosomal recessive inheritance.

Pathology. See Symptoms and Signs.

Diagnostic Procedures. *X-ray.* Reveals most distinctive features in the mandible: hypoplasia of rami; anterior displacement of temporomandibular joints. Condyles may be completely absent. Skull, brachycephalic, delayed closure of fontanelles. Face small; small orbits; gracile appearance of tubular bones.

Therapy. None.

Prognosis. Good *quoad vitam.*

BIBLIOGRAPHY. Audry C: Variété singulière l'alopécie congenitale. Alopécie suturale. Ann Dermatol Syph 4:899–900, 1893
Hallermann W: Vogelgesicht und Cataracta congenita. Klin Monatsbl Augenheilkd 113:315–318, 1948
Streiff EB: Dysmorphie mandibulo faciale (tete d'oiseau) et alterations oculaires. Ophthalmologica 120:79–83, 1950
Steele RW, Bass JW: Hallermann-Streiff syndrome: clinical and prognostic consideration. Am J Dis Child 120:462–465, 1970
François J: François' dyscephalic syndrome. Birth Defects Orig Art Ser 18(6):595–619, 1982

HALLERVORDEN'S

Synonyms. Poser's dysmyelinating leukodystrophy; simple orthochromatic leukodystropy; Poser's.

Symptoms and Signs. Rather heterogeneous group; age of onset varies greatly. Onset most frequently from first month to 15 years of age. Variable and aspecific. Neurologic and mental symptoms and signs of progressive loss of vision and speech, then hearing, down to decerebration.

Etiology. Unknown; possibly congenital. Autosomal recessive (?)

Pathology. Characterization of this syndrome is essentially on pathologic features. Central nervous system: no inflammation (except for simple reabsorption reaction); diffuse myelin disintegration, however, not excessively pronounced; large number of sudanophilic cells scattered throughout and not concentrated perivascularly; no metachromatic granules; nerve cells and axis well preserved.

Diagnostic Procedures. Rule out metachromatic leukodystrophy (see).

Therapy. None.

Prognosis. Slow, progressive evolution.

BIBLIOGRAPHY. Hallervorden J: Die degenerative diffuse Sklerose. In Lubarsch O, Henke F, Rossle R (ed): Handsbuch der speciellen pathologischen Anatomie und Histologie, Vol 13, pp 716–782. Berlin, Springer-Verlag, 1957
Peiffer J: Differentiation of various types of leukodystrophies. World Neurol 3:580–601, 1962

HALLERVORDEN-SPATZ

Synonyms. Globus pallidus pigmentary degeneration; progressive pallidal degeneration; neuroaxonal dystrophy, late infantile. See Seitelberger's.

Symptoms. Onset at approximately 10 years of age. Gradually increasing stiffness of all extremities; dysarthria; dysphagia; cerebellar ataxia; visual impairment to blindness, mental deterioration, occasionally hyperkinesis.

Signs. Inversion of feet. Retinitis pigmentosa occasionally observed. Pigmentary changes of the skin; muscle atrophy.

Etiology. Unknown; familial disease (some unrelated cases recorded). Considered one form of iron storage disease.

Pathology. Basal ganglia (occasionally also of the cortex) demyelinization and less demyelinization of nerve cells; deposit of iron in the globus pallidus and substantia nigra, in ganglion cells, and interstitial tissue.

Diagnostic Procedures. *X-ray of skull. Electromyography.*

Therapy. Nonspecific. Symptomatic.

Prognosis. Progressive; death 10 to 20 years after onset of symptoms.

BIBLIOGRAPHY. Hallervorden J, Spatz H: Eigenartige Erkrankung im extrapyramidalen System mit besonderer Beteiligung des Globus pallidus und der Substantia nigra; ein Beitrag zu den Beziehungen zwischen diesen beiden Zentren. Z Neurol Psychiatr 79:254–302, 1922
Jankovic J, Kirkpatrick JB, Blonquist KA, et al: Late onset Hallervorden-Spatz disease presenting as familial parkinsonism. Neurology 35:227–234, 1985

HALLOPEAU'S I

Synonyms. Csilloag's; guttate morphea; guttate sclero-derma; lichen planus sclerosis atrophicus; von Zam-busch's; white spot; Zambusch's.

Symptoms. Prevalent in females (6 to 7:1); onset at any age, usually around menopause (average age in females 50, males 43). Soreness; pruritus; dyspareunia; mouth ulceration; asymptomatic skin lesions.

Signs. Skin eruption of small whitish round papules and macules, slightly raised; seldom bullae; horny plugs. Later; atrophy, wrinkling and depression of skin involved. Lesions affect mostly trunk, neck, flexor areas. In females affect vulva, perineal areas, anus; whitish irritation; atrophy produces shrinkage of vulva and reduces vaginal introitus. In males, balanitis xerotica obliterans. Similar lesions in oral mucosa as described above.

Etiology. Unknown; hormonal factor may precipitate collagen disease; possibly, autoimmunity type of reaction.

Pathology. Hyalinization of dermal collagen; thickening hyperkeratosis; dilation of capillaries. Secondary inflammatory changes.

Diagnostic Procedures. *Biopsy.*

Therapy. No effective treatment. Bland cream and corticosteroids. Excision of areas of leukoplakia.

Prognosis. Chronic condition; possibly spontaneous remission (especially in girls after puberty). Severe atrophy of vulva usually results.

BIBLIOGRAPHY. Hallopeau H: Du lichen plan, et particuliérement de sa forme atrophique. Union Méd 43:729–733, 1887
Rook A, Wilkinson DS, Ebling FJG, et al: Textbook of Dermatology, 4th ed, pp 1368–1374. Oxford, Blackwell Scientific Publications, 1986

HALLOPEAU'S II

Synonyms. Hallopeau-Leredde; pemphigus vegetans (Hallopeau's variety); pyodermite vegetante.

Symptoms and Signs. Both sexes affected; onset in middle age. Formation of pustules (not bullae) followed by warty vegetations that spread peripherally with erosions. Flexure zones most frequently affected. Mouth erosion frequent.

Etiology. Unknown; considered as a benign variant of pemphigus.

Pathology. Nonspecific granulomas with abscess formation and pseudoepitheliomatous hyperplasia; acanthosis; little hyperkeratosis.

Diagnostic Procedures. *Biopsy.*

Therapy. Corticosteroids.

Prognosis. Chronic benign course of many years' duration. Spontaneous remissions; also complete healing.

BIBLIOGRAPHY. Hallopeau H: Nouvelle not sur la dermatose bulleuse hereditaire et traumatique. Arch Dermatol Syph 45:323–328, 1898
Rook A, Wilkinson DS, Ebling FJG, et al: Textbook of Dermatology, 4th ed, p 1639. Oxford, Blackwell Scientific Publications, 1986

HALLOPEAU-SIEMENS

Synonyms. Polydysplastic epidermolysis bullosa. Epidermolysis bullosa polydysplastic; recessive generalized dystrophic.

Symptoms and Signs. Both sexes affected, onset at birth or early infancy; exceptionally, later. Large, flaccid bullae developing spontaneously on any part of skin surface. Bullae heal leaving scar and miliary cysts. Pseudowebbing may develop between fingers and toes. Mucosae frequently involved; tongue mobility may be limited by scarring, esophagous mucosa may be involved and strictures develop. Malformation of teeth and nail frequent. Hair may be sparse and alopecia develops. Physical and mental development impaired.

Etiology. Unknown; autosomal recessive inheritance. Increased and altered synthesis of immunoreactive skin collagenase. The lethal form is now considered on histologic basis (electron microscopy) as a different entity, although clinically they overlap significantly.

Pathology. *Light microscopy.* Bullae in the upper dermal components attached to roof of blister. *Immunofluorescence study.* Antibodies pemphigoid antigen basement membrane in the roof blister. *Electron microscopy.* Dissolution of collagen fibrils (dermolysis).

Diagnostic Procedures. *Biopsy of skin. Electroencephalography.* May show abnormalities.

Therapy. Symptomatic; antibiotics; steroids.

Prognosis. Very poor; carcinoma frequently develops from scars in the skin and mucosae.

BIBLIOGRAPHY. Touraine A. L'Hérédité en Medicine. Paris, Masson, 1955
Rook A, Wilkinson DS, Ebling FJG, et al: Textbook of Dermatology, 4th ed, p 1626–1627. Oxford, Blackwell Scientific Publications, 1986

HALL-RIGGS

Synonym. Mental retardation of Hall-Riggs.

Symptoms. From birth, both sexes. Sudden episodes of vomiting during infancy; severe mental retardation; lack of development of speech; retarded growth.

Signs. Microcephaly; depressed nasal bridge, anteverted nostrils, large lips; scoliosis; short limbs.

Etiology. Autosomal recessive inheritance.

Diagnostic Procedures. *X-ray of skeleton.* Flat femoral head and neck of femorus; flat epiphyses in the fingers and at the ankle.

BIBLIOGRAPHY. Hall BD, Riggs FD: A new familial metabolic disorder with progressive osseous changes, microcephaly, coarse severe mental retardation. Birth Defects Orig Art Ser XI(5):79–90, 1975

HALL'S

Synonym. Anemic pseudohydrocephalus. Old eponym used to indicate a pseudohydrocephalic condition resulting from severe exhaustion or cachexia.

BIBLIOGRAPHY. Hall H: An Essay on a Hydrocephaloid Affection in Infants Arising from Exhaustion. London, Sherwood, 1836

HAMMAN-RICH

Synonyms. Bronchiolar emphysema; pulmonary interstitial idiopathic fibrosis; idiopathic pulmonary fibrosis; classic interstitial pneumonia; rheumatoid lung; unidentified interstitial pneumonia (UIP). See Alveolar capillary block syndrome.

Symptoms. Both sexes affected; slight male predominance; onset over broad age range (higher incidence between 40 and 70 years of age). Insidious onset. Progressive exertional dyspnea; breathing rapid and shallow; dry cough; weight loss.

Signs. Cyanosis; clubbing of fingers (common). Fine and medium rales on lower part of lungs. Signs of right heart failure late in the disease.

Etiology. Unknown. Nonspecific reaction to a variety of stimuli. Familial, autosomal dominant inheritance. In some cases; possible association with rheumatoid arthritis or scleroderma, x-ray radiation, exposure to beryllium or asbestos.

Pathology. Diffuse thickening and fibrosis of alveolar walls.

Diagnostic Procedures. *Blood.* High titer of rheumatoid factor in some cases. Pa CO_2 decreased. Hyperglobulinemia; autoantibodies, eosinophilia; Coomb's test positive. *X-ray.* Fine, diffuse mottling and reticulation from minimal in the beginning to honeycomb aspect in the end. *Pulmonary function tests.* No evidence of obstruction on expiration, diffusing capacity for carbon dioxide reduced. *Biopsy of lung.*

Therapy. Unrewarding; corticosteroid utility doubtful. If indicated, attempt lung or heart-lung transplantation.

Prognosis. Poor; death in less than a year.

BIBLIOGRAPHY. Hamman L, Rich AR: Acute diffuse interstitial fibrosis of the lungs. Bull Johns Hopkins Hosp 74:177–212, 1944
Javaheri S, Lederer DH, Pella JA, et al: Idiopathic pulmonary fibrosis in monozygotic twins: the importance of genetic predisposition. Chest 78:591–594, 1980
Beaumond F, Jansen HM, Elema JD, et al: Simultaneous occurrence of pulmonary interstitial fibrosis and alveolar cell carcinoma in a family. Thorax 36:252–258, 1981

HAMMAN'S

Synonym. Mediastinal emphysema.

Symptoms. Dyspnea; retrosternal pain accentuated on breathing; mediastinal crepitation noticed by patient.

Signs. Tachypnea; occasionally, subcutaneous emphysema of neck and upper thorax; cyanosis; hyperresonancy of chest; typical popping sounds synchronous with heart beat.

Etiology. Trauma; spontaneous from rupture of alveolus; secondary to air passage from various source (e.g., tracheostomy; trachea or esophagus perforation; retroperitoneal space); from rupture of viscus or diagnostic procedures (e.g., pneumoperitoneum; perineal air insufflation).

Diagnostic Procedures. *X-ray.* Streaks of radiolucency on lateral edges of mediastinum; outline of heart and major vessels.

Therapy. When needed, surgery.

Prognosis. Good. Spontaneous resolution in days if the air is removed.

BIBLIOGRAPHY. Hamman L: Spontaneous mediastinal emphysema. Bull Johns Hopkins Hosp 64:1–21, 1939
Hurst JW: The Heart, 4th ed, p 916. New York, McGraw-Hill, 1986

HAND-FOOT

See Herrick's.

Symptoms and Signs. Occur in infants with sickle cell disease. Painful, symmetric (usually) swelling of hands and feet, persisting for 1 to 4 weeks, accompanied by fever.

Etiology. Unusual manifestation in Herrick's syndrome (rare in the United States; more frequent in Africa). Report of hand-foot syndrome in *Salmonella* osteomyelitis and Herrick's syndrome and in streptococcal infection without sickle cell disease.

Pathology. Metacarpals, metatarsals, and phalanges are thought to be infracted by multiple small capillary red cell blocks in sickling crisis.

Diagnostic Procedures. *Blood.* Electrophoresis of hemoglobin: SS or SC pattern. Anemia; sickling phenomena; leukocytosis during attack. *X-rays.* Destruction of involved bones; subperiosteal new bone formation.

Therapy. Analgesics.

Prognosis. Spontaneous recovery within 1 to 4 weeks. Attacks may recur.

BIBLIOGRAPHY. Danford EA, Marr R, Elsey EC: Sickle cell anemia, with unusual bone changes. Am J Roentgen 45:223–226, 1941
Koren A, Garty I, Katzuni E: Bone infarction in children with sickle cell disease: early diagnosis and differential from osteomyelitis. Eur J Pediatr 142:93, 1984

HAND, FOOT, AND MOUTH

Synonyms. Exanthem-vesicularstomatitis; summer-term blains.

Symptoms. Affects especially farmers and people in contact with livestock. No distress or mild illness; fever; malaise; anorexia; diarrhea; sore throat.

Signs. Vesicular rash restricted to hands and feet. Oral enanthema on mucosa, uvula, tonsillar pillars, tongue. Occasionally, hepatosplenomegaly and cervial lymphadenopathy.

Etiology. Coxsackie virus infection (Group A type 16 or other groups).

Pathology. Gray vesicles on erythematous bases; some break. In the mouth, small ulcerative lesions.

Diagnostic Procedures. *Throat and rectal swabs, blood, fluid.* For isolation and identification of virus. Serology. During disease and convalescence. *Cytologic study.* With scrapings from lesions.

Therapy. Symptomatic.

Prognosis. Complete recovery.

BIBLIOGRAPHY. Robinson CR, Doane FW, Rhodes AJ: Report of an outbreak of febrile illness with pharyngeal lesions and exanthem: Toronto, summer 1957. Isolation of group A coxsackie virus. Can Med Assoc J 79:615–621, 1958
Cherry JD, John CL: Hand, foot, and mouth syndrome: report of six cases due to coxsackie virus, Group A type 16. Pediatrics 37:637–643, 1966
Centers for Disease Control: Enteroviral disease in the United States 1970–1979. J Infec Dis 146:103–108, 1982

HAND-FOOT-UTERUS

Synonym: HFU

Symptoms. Present from birth.

Signs. *Hands.* Normal size or moderately smaller; moderate degree of clinodactyly of fifth finger; hypoplasia of thenar eminence; thumb incompletely rotated and in some cases angulated outward. No upper limb involvement. *Feet.* Markedly small; great toe short. *Urogenital tract.* Duplication of uterus; in some cases, associated with double cervix or subseptate vagina.

Etiology. Unknown; autosomal dominant inheritance. Full penetrance and variable expression.

Diagnostic Procedures. *X-rays of hands and feet.* Short first metacarpal (75%); pointed phalanx of thumb; clinodactyly of fifth finger; unusual fusion of wrist bones; short first metatarsal; in toe same changes as thumb; short calcaneus; seldom tarsal or middle-distal phalangeal bone fusion. *Hysterosalpingography.* See pathology. *Chromosome studies.* Negative. *Dermatoglyphic studies.* Distal placed axial triradius; absence of pattern in thenar and hypothenar areas. Thumbs show low arches, no whorls or radial loops on the fingers; total ridge count reduced.

Therapy. Plastic surgery for genital malformation.

Prognosis. Good *quoad vitam.* Higher than normal incidence of stillbirth and of perinatal death.

BIBLIOGRAPHY. Stern AM, Gall JC, Perry BI, et al: The hand-foot-uterus syndrome. J Pediatr 77:109–116, 1970
Elias S, Simpson JL, Feingold M, et al: The hand-foot-uterus syndrome: a rare autosomal dominant disorder. Fertil Steril 29:239–240, 1978

HAND-SCHÜLLER-CHRISTIAN

Synonyms. Christian's; craniohypophyseal xanthoma; xanthomatous granuloma; Hand-Rowland; lipoid histiocytosis; lipoid granuloma; multifocal eosinophilic bone granuloma; nonlipoid reticuloendotheliosis; reticuloendothelial granuloma; Schüller-Christian; xanthomatosis. See Histiocytosis.

Symptoms. Both sexes affected (males slight predominance); onset mostly in children; may occur in young adults; seldom in elderly persons. Onset frequently with otitis media or externa; less frequently, with diabetes insipidus. Intermittent low-grade fever, occasionally. Seborrheic dermatitis of scalp, chest, neck, shoulders, occasionally becoming hemorrhagic. Lung involvement may be perihilar, central, or diffuse. Pulmonary fibrosis, honeycombing of the lungs, alveolocapillary block, cor pulmonale, and right heart failure are possible complications.

Signs. Lymphadenopathy; occasionally hepatomegaly; rarely, exophthalmos; rarely, splenomegaly.

Etiology. Unknown.

Pathology. Skeletal lytic lesions and visceral lesions. Proliferation of histiocytes in masses; vescicular nuclei, lobulated with phagocytic material. Rarely mitoses; large number of eosinophil aggregates, occasionally with necrotic changes. Foam cells; vacuolated histiocytes with sudanophilic material.

Diagnostic Procedures. *X-ray.* Osteolytic lesions with sharp borders (more frequently on ribs, femora, pelvic bones, skull). *Blood.* Anemia; normal cholesterol; changes due to diabetes insipidus (when present). *Biopsy of lesions.*

Therapy. Curettement or small doses of x-ray therapy to localized lesion. For widespread lesions: methotrexate, vinca alkaloids, corticotropin, adrenal steroids, cyclophosphamide, or nitrogen mustard.

Prognosis. Good response to treatment. Survival from onset variable from months to 20 years.

BIBLIOGRAPHY. Hand A Jr: Polyuria and tuberculosis. Arch Pediatr 10:673–675, 1893
Christian HA: Defects in membranous bones, exophthalmos, and diabetes insipidus: an unusual syndrome of dyspituitarism. Med Clin N Am 3:849–871, 1920
Schüller A: Dysostosis hypophysaria. Br J Radiol 31:156–158, 1926
Oberman HA: Idiopathic histiocytosis: a clinicopathologic study of 40 cases and review of the literature on eosinophilic granuloma of bone, Hand-Schüller-Christian disease and Letterer-Siwe disease. Pediatrics 28:307–327, 1961

Wintrobe MM (ed): Clinical Hematology, 8th ed, pp 1351–1353. Philadelphia, Lea & Febiger, 1981

HANEY-FALLS

Synonym. Congenital keratoconus posticus circumscriptus.

Symptoms. Mental retardation; stunted growth; visual alterations.

Signs. Sharply localized increase in curvature of posterior corneal surface; corneal nebulae; myopic astigmatism; corneal endothelial precipitate; mild hypertelorism; broad flat nose; upward displacement of lateral canthi; brachydactyly; ptergyium colli; barrel chest.

Etiology. Unknown; autosomal or (more likely) recessive inheritance reported.

Prognosis. Good *quoad vitam.*

BIBLIOGRAPHY. Butler TH: Keratoconus posticus. Trans Ophthalmol Soc U K 50:551–556, 1930
Haney WP, Falls HF: The occurrence of congenital keratoconus posticus circumscriptus in two siblings presenting a previously unrecognized syndrome. Am J Ophthalmol 52:57, 1961
Young ID, Macral WG, Hughes HE, et al: Keratoconus posticus circumscriptus, cleft lip and palate, genitourinary abnormalities, short stature and mental retardation in sibs. J Med Genet 19:332–336, 1982

HANHART'S

Synonyms. Hanhart's dwarfism; mandibular dysostosis-peromelia; Richner-Hanhart type IV. See Gilford-Burnier.

TYPE I
Symptoms. Affect closely inbred group of people in Switzerland and one Adriatic island (Veglia); both sexes equally affected. Normal infancy and early childhood. Between 1.5 and 6 years of age growth retardation becomes evident that in following years results in a slow proportionate growth. Diminished or absent libido. Occasionally, mental retardation.

Signs. Typical facies; occasionally brachycephaly. Absence of secondary sexual characteristics. Adipose tissue hyperplasia on breast and abdominal regions; late development of gonads and of secondary sexual characteristics.

TYPE II
Onset from birth. Type I signs plus micrognathia, peromelia, and missing teeth.

TYPE III

Characterized by peromelia, micrognathia. Cleft palate, mental retardation (brain microgyrus); occasionally, symptoms related to kidney, genital, and uterine defects.

TYPE IV

Hyperkeratosis of plams and soles; anhidrosis; multiple lipoma in subcutaneous tissue (Richner's). Excessive tears; photophobia; dendril lesions of cornea. Periodontia; hypotrichosis. Absence of fingers and toes. Micrognathia. Mental retardation.

Etiology. Type I autosomal recessive inheritance. Multiple pituitary hormone deficiency. Types II–IV, non-Mendelian development disturbance.

Pathology. Absence of particular features; delayed epiphyseal closure.

Diagnostic Procedures. *Hormonal studies.* Growth hormone deficiency; adrenocortotropic hormone or thyrotropic hormone deficiency or both. Protein-bound iodine level progressively falling. *X-rays.* Delayed closure of epiphyses.

Therapy. Correction of hormonal deficiency. Growth hormone, adrenocorticotropic, thyroid-stimulating hormone.

Prognosis. Good with treatment. If not treated, dwarfism with normal life expectancy.

BIBLIOGRAPHY. Hanhart E: Ueber heredodegenerativen Zwergwuchs mit Dystrophia adiposo-genitals and Hand von Untersuchungen bei drei Sippen von proportionierten Zwergen. Arch Julius Klaus 1:181–257, 1925

Richner H: Hornhaul affection bei Keratoma palmare et plantare hereditarium. Klin Monatsbl Augenheilkd 100:580–588, 1938

Hanhart E: Neuse Sonderformen von Keratosis palmoplantaris, u.a. eine regelmäss g-dominanten mit systematisierten Lipomen, ferner 2 einfach-rezessive mit Schwachsinn und Z.T. mit Hornhautveränderungen des Auges (Ektadermal syndrome). Dermatologica 94:286–308, 1947

Garner LD, Bixler D: Micrognathia, an associated defect of Hanhart's syndrome Types II and III. Oral Surg 27:601–606, 1969

Bokesoy I, Aksuyck C, Deniz E: Oromandibular limb hypogenesis, Hanhart's syndrome: possible drug influence on the malformation. Clin Genet 24:47–49, 1983

HANOT-ROESSLE

Synonyms. Intrahepatic cholangitis; cholangitis lenta. See Charcot's biliary fever.

Symptoms and Signs. Fever; jaundice; pruritus.

Etiology and Pathology. Intrahepatic suppurative cholangitis without extrahepatic duct cholangitis. (Cholangitis lenta.)

Diagnostic Procedures. *Blood.* Hyperbilirubinemia; sodium sulfobromophthalein retention; increase of enzymes; leukocytosis. *Urine.* Biliary pigments; hyperbilirubinemia. *Liver scan.*

Therapy. Antibiotics. Elimination of underlying causes of cholestasis.

Prognosis. With modern treatments this entity has almost disappeared.

BIBLIOGRAPHY. Albot G, Kopandji M: La cholangiolite obstructive ou course des cholangites diffuses non oblitérantes ou maladie de Hanot-Roessle. Semin Hôp 38:3213–3231, 1962

Wright R, Alberti KGMM, Karran S, et al: Liver and Biliary Disease, p 299. London, WB Saunders, 1979

HANOT'S

Synonyms. Cholangiolitic biliary cirrhosis; hypertrophic primary cirrhosis; hypertrophic primary liver.

Symptoms. Prevalent in middle-aged females; insidious onset. Intense itching; steatorrhea; good general condition progressing to malnutrition, melena; coma.

Signs. Jaundice; skin pigmentation; xanthomas; generalized lymphadenopathy; hepatomegaly; moderate splenomegaly.

Etiology. Unknown; infectious hepatitis, drug toxicity (chlorpromazine; methyl testosterone; arsenic preparations).

Pathology. Periportal inflammation and fibrosis; intracanalicular biliary obstruction; later, cirrhosis with granulation on periphery of lobules. Disruption of lobular pattern.

Diagnostic Procedures. *Blood.* Increased bilirubin, alkaline phosphatase level, lipid, globulins. Circulating antibodies against cells rich in mitochondria. *Urine.* Dark urobilinogen and biliary pigments increased. *Stool.* Discolored; increase in fatty acids. *X-rays.* Absence of extrahepatic obstruction; later osteomalacia. *Ultrasonography. Liver biopsy. Laparoscopy. Arteriography.*

Therapy. Correct malabsorption; fat-soluble vitamins; cholestyramine against pruritus; treatment of complication (portal hypertension; bleeding). Liver transplantation.

Prognosis. Death in approximately 5 years from onset of symptoms. Good results with transplantation.

BIBLIOGRAPHY. Hanot V: Étude sur une forme de cirrhose hypertrophique du foie (cirrhose hypertrophique avec ictère chronique) (thesis). Paris Medical Classic, 1875

Sherlock S: Primary biliary cirrhosis (chronic intrahepatic obstructive jaundice). Gastroenterology 37:574–586, 1959

Galambos J: The cirrhosis. In Bockus HL: Gastroenterology, 3rd ed, Vol 3, pp 409–416. Philadelphia, WB Saunders, 1976

HANSEN'S

Synonyms. Sclerosteosis; cortical hyperostosis-syndactyly.

Symptoms and Signs. In Afrikaners of Dutch extraction. From early infancy progressive. Headaches; deafness (childhood), blindness (adulthood); overgrowth progressing to moderate gigantism; prominent asymmetric (occasional) mandible; syndactyly, 2nd to 3rd finger; nail dysplasia.

Etiology. Autosomal recessive.

Diagnostic Procedures. *X-ray skeletal studies.*

Therapy. Skull decompression.

Prognosis. Progression of bone thickening leads to occlusion of multiple cranial foramina. Intracranial pressure if not relieved may be fatal.

BIBLIOGRAPHY. Mirsch IS: Generalized osteitis fibrosa. Radiology 13:44–84, 1929

Hansen HG: Sklerosteose. In Opitz J, Smith F (eds): Handbook der Kinderheilkunde, Berlin, Springer Vol. 6. pp 351–355, 1967

Beighton P, Durr L, Hamersma H: The clinical features of sclerosteosis. Ann Internal Med 84:393–397, 1976

Beighton P, Barnard A, Hamersma H, et al: The syndromic status of sclerosteosis and van Buchem disease. Clin Genet 25:175–181, 1984

HAPPY PUPPET

Synonyms. Puppet children. Williams and Frias suggested the use of eponym *Angelman's syndrome* because the term *happy puppet* may appear derisive and even derogatory to the patient's family.

Symptoms. Major fits and frequent infantile spasms; easily provoked and prolonged paroxysms of laughs; jerky puppetlike movements; continuous tongue protrusion; mental deficiency.

Signs. Skull alterations: brachycephaly; microcephaly; occipital depression or flattening; prognathism; incomplete development of choroid.

Etiology. Unknown; very rare form of infantile epilepsy.

Pathology. Not reported.

Diagnostic Procedures. *X-ray of skull.* Vertical inclination of base. *Electroencephalography.* Typical pattern with consistent absence of hypsarrhythmia and presence of symmetric synchronous 2/sec wave and spike activity. The persistence of such patterns represents one of the characteristic elements that differentiate it from the transitional EEG pattern of infantile spasms syndrome. *CT brain scan.* Unilateral cerebellar atrophy demonstrated in one patient.

Therapy. Prednisone; ethosuximide.

Prognosis. Temporary improvement with therapy.

BIBLIOGRAPHY. Angelman H: "Puppet" children: a report on three cases. Dev Med Child Neurol 7:681–688, 1965

Bower BD, Jeavons PM: The "happy puppet" syndrome. Arch Dis Child 42:298–302, 1967

Williams CA, Frias JL: The Angelman ("happy puppet") syndrome. Am J Med Genet 11:453–460, 1982

HARADA'S

Now considered part of the Vogt-Koyanagi-Harada syndrome (see). Initially typified by retinal separation and absent or low-grade anterior uveal involvement. The poliosis and alopecia occasionally present in the Harada's syndrome were considered as invariable features of the Vogt-Koyanagi's syndrome.

BIBLIOGRAPHY. Harada E: Clinical study of nonsuppurative choroiditis: a report of acute diffuse choroiditis. Acta Soc Ophthalmol Japn 30:356, 1926

HARBITZ'S

Synonyms. Alveolar microlithiasis; pulmonary alveolar microlithiasis.

Symptoms. Affects all races in familial form; found more often in females, but equal sex distribution in sporadic cases. Onset insidious in Western countries between 30 and 50 years of age, in Japan between 6 and 9 years of age. Paucisymptomatic; moderate exertional dyspnea; late symptoms of cor pulmonale.

Signs. Right ventricular hypertrophy.

Etiology. Several etiologic factors and idiopathic forms; among them: (1) Familial form with suggestion of autosomal and recessive types of inheritance; (2) exposure to dust rich in calcium salt. This condition may result from alteration of unknown nature of alveolar lining membrane that predisposes to local calcification.

Pathology. Intraalveolar calcific free deposits (microliths). No histologic abnormalities in alveolar membranes and capillaries.

Diagnostic Procedures. *Blood.* Moderate polycythemia may develop. Calcium metabolism studies normal. *Pulmonary function tests.* Decrease of alveolar ventilation; arterial hypoxia; lung volume reduced. *X-ray.* Typical radiologic pattern with numerous diffuse calcifications.

Therapy. Symptomatic.

Prognosis. Good; slow progressive course; cor pulmonale develops late.

BIBLIOGRAPHY. Harbitz F: Extensive calcification of the lungs as a distinct disease. Arch Intern Med 21:139, 1918
O'Neill RP, Cohn JE, Pellegrino ED: Pulmonary alveolar microlithiasis—a family study. Ann Intern Med 67:957–967, 1967
Prakash UBS, Barham SS, Rosenaw EC, III, et al: Pulmonary alveolar microlithiasis: a review including ultrastructural and pulmonary function studies. Mayo Clin Proc 58:290–300, 1983

HARD-WATER

Synonym. Extracorporeal dialysis–hypercalcemia.

Symptoms and Signs. Onset during or after hemodialysis. Nausea; vomiting; warm skin; extreme weakness; lethargy; blood pressure changes. Occasionally, clotting within the arteriovenous cannula.

Etiology. Occurs when water softening process is abruptly discontinued while hemodialysis is being performed.

Diagnostic Procedures. *Blood.* Calcium and magnesium elevation. *Analysis of water used for dialysis.*

Prognosis. Good since the simultaneous increase of calcium and magnesium in plasma reciprocally neutralizes their pharmacologic effects.

BIBLIOGRAPHY. Freeman RM, Lawton RL, Chamberlain MA: Hard water syndrome. New Engl J Med 276:113–118, 1967
Schulten HK, Sieberth HG, Deck KA, et al: Das akute Hypercalcämiesyndrom als Dialysezwischenfall. Dtsch Med Wochenschr 93:387–340, 1968

HARJOLA-MARABLE

Synonyms. Celiac axis; celiac axis compression; median arcuate ligament; Marable's. See Abdominal angina.

Symptoms. More frequent in young women. Epigastric crampy pain beginning 30 minutes to 4 hours after eating, not related to type of food. Moderate relief from knee-chest position. Occasionally, nausea, vomiting, diarrhea, eructation, flatulence.

Signs. Moderate weight loss; loud epigastric systolic bruit.

Etiology and Pathology. External compression of celiac axis during its passage through the aortic hiatus by the median arcuate ligament.

Diagnostic Procedures. *X-ray of gastrointestinal tract. Aortography.* To rule out congenital malformation.

Therapy. Incision of fibrous tissue of the anterior portion of aortic hiatus of diaphragm compressing celiac axis.

Prognosis. Disappearance of all symptoms following surgery.

BIBLIOGRAPHY. Harjola PT: A rare obstruction of the coeliac artery. Ann Chirur Gynecol Fenniae 52:547–549, 1963
Marable SA, Kaplan MF, Berman FM, et al: Celiac compression syndrome. Am J Surg 115:97–102, 1966
Jamieson CW: Coeliac axis compression syndrome. Br J Med 193:159–160, 1986

HARKAVY'S

Synonym. Kussmaul-Maier variant.

Symptoms and Signs. Asthmatic crises associated with the symptoms of Kussmaul-Maier (see).

BIBLIOGRAPHY. Harkavy J: Vascular allergy. Pathogenesis of bronchial asthma with recurrent pulmonary infiltration and eosinophilic polyserositis. Arch Intern Med 67:709–734, 1941

HARLEQUIN COLOR CHANGE

Synonyms. Particolored infant; particolored baby.

Symptoms. None.

Signs. Reddening of one side of the body and blanching of the other half. Clear demarcation between the two halves from forehead through midline to legs (one red, one blanched).

Etiology. Unknown condition of no pathologic significance, caused by gravity (reddening and blanching revert with turning the infant from one side to the other).

Pathology. Unknown.

Prognosis. Color change lasts from a few minutes to hours; disappears no later than 3 weeks from birth; if still present beyond 4th week, possibly associated to hypoxia due to cardiovascular defects.

BIBLIOGRAPHY. Neligan GA, Strang LB: "Harlequin" colour change in newborn. Lancet 2:1005–1007, 1952
Birdsong M, Edmunds JE: Harlequin color change of the newborn: report of a case. Obstet Gynecol 7:518–521, 1956

HARLEQUIN FETUS

Synonyms. Ichthyosis congenita harlequin fetus. Harlequin fetus; keratoma malignum; Riecke's type I and II ichthyosis congenita. See Collodion baby.

Symptoms and Signs. (1) *Ichthyosis fetalis.* At birth (often premature) encased in thickened skin (white armor). Difficulty in breathing and swallowing. Majority die in 3 to 4 days. (2) *Ichthyosiform erythroderma.* Present at birth or onset in first days of life, occasionally later. Generalized erythema; thickening of skin; scaling; crusting; edema; various degrees of severity from limited erythema to half of the body to encasing total body. Hair normal, hypertricosis, or alopecia. Nails normal.

Etiology. Unknown; autosomal recessive inheritance.

Pathology. Skin thickening of all layers, increased miotic rate, perivascular lymphocytic infiltrates.

Therapy. Corticosteroids; antibiotics; careful nursing.

Prognosis. Extremely variable from death in first few days, to survival with circumscribed zones of hyperkeratosis, erythema, scaling or return to normal skin after initial exfoliation.

BIBLIOGRAPHY. Seeligmann E: De Epidermis Imprimis Neonatorum Desquamatione. Inaugural Dissertation, Berlin, 1841
Thomson MS, Wakeley CPG: The harlequin fetus. J Obstet Gynecol Br Comm 28:190–203, 1921
Arnold ML, Lamprecht I: Problems in prenatal diagnosis of the ichthyosis congenita group. Hum Genet 71:301–311, 1985
Lawlor F, Peiris S: Progress of a harlequin fetus treated with etretinate. C R Soc Med 78 (suppl) 11:19–20, 1985

HARNDEN-STEWART

Synonyms. Gonadal dysgenesis (XX or XY); pure gonadal dysgenesis.

Symptoms and Signs. Female phenotype; failure of puberty and fertility. No stigma of Turner's syndrome (see). Tall stature; eunuchoid proportion.

Etiology. Failure of fetal testes to develop and thus the fetus develops on female phenotype. Claimed difference from Goldberg-Maxwell, Savage's, and Turner's.

Pathology. Streak gonads at the site where ovaries may be expected; small uterus and fallopian tubes.

Diagnostic Procedures. *Chromosome study.* XY or XX karyotype. At time of anticipated puberty, evidence of absent gonadal activity in presence of increased gonadotropins.

Therapy. As in Turner's (see). Prophylactic gonadectomy and estrogen substitution at puberty.

Prognosis. With treatment, good response and good psychological adjustment. High incidence of neoplasia (germinomas; gonadoblastomas).

BIBLIOGRAPHY. Harnden DG, Stewart JSS: The chromosomes in a case of pure gonadal dysgenesis. Br Med J 2:1285–1287, 1957
Frasier SD, Bashore RA, Mosier HD: Gonadoblastoma associated with pure gonadal dysgenesis in monozygous twins. J Pediatr 64:740–745, 1964
Sternberg WH, Barclay DL: Familial XY gonadal dysgenesis. Lancet II:946, 1967
Conte FA, Grumbach MM: Pathogenesis classification diagnosis and treatment of anomalies of sex. In De Groot L, Cahill LJ, Odell WD, et al (eds): Endocrinology, p 1329. New York, Grune & Stratton, 1979

HARRIS' (S.)

Synonyms. Hyperinsulinoma; reactive functional hypoglycemia; See McQuarrie's, Neonatal hypoglycemic, and recently described Insulin autoimmune hypoglycemia.

Symptoms and Signs. Occurs at all ages, in both sexes during the course of wide variety of diseases and is the presenting sign of many other syndromes. Increasing nervousness; tachycardia; flushing; sweating; hunger (epinephrine response); headache; visual disturbances; twitching; thick speech; transitory hemiplegia; seizures (cerebral response). Personality alterations: negativism; maniacal behavior (psychiatric response).

Etiology and Pathology. *Organic.* Alteration of organs involved in keeping normal glucose level. Pancreatic and extrapancreatic tumors; hepatic diseases; endocrine diseases, toxic and metabolic conditions. *Functional.* Organic causes for hypoglycemia cannot be established.

Diagnostic Procedures. *Blood.* Determination of glucose level in blood; usually below 40 mg/100 ml during attack. *Provocative tests.* Prolonged fasting; tolbutamide (Orinase) tolerance tests. *Insulin assay.* Also, all tests indicated in different syndromes with hypoglycemia for differential diagnosis. It must be remembered that hypoglycemic symptoms may occur in presence of normal blood glucose concentration and in some individuals without symptoms, low glucose level may be found. *Pancreas selective arteriography. CT brain scan. Ultrasonography.*

Therapy. During attack; administration of glucose by mouth or intravenously; corticosteroids. Multiple feedings to prevent attack. Specific treatment according to diagnosis.

Prognosis. Depends on etiology.

BIBLIOGRAPHY. Harris S: Hyperinsulinism and dysinsulinism. JAMA 83:729–733, 1924
Cateland S: The adult hypoglycemias. In Mazzaferri EL (ed): Textbook of Endocrinology, pp 670–676. New York, Medical Examination Publishing, 1985

HARTNUP'S

Synonyms. Aminoaciduria-pellagra-cerebellar ataxia; H disease; Hart's; tryptophan pyrrolase deficiency.

Symptoms. Intermittent and variable. From "disorders" without disease to itching rash on areas exposed to light from February to October. Headache; intermittent ataxia; pains in abdomen, chest, and extremities; emotional lability (crying spells); mental retardation, fainting attacks; psychotic reactions.

Signs. Skin thickened and scaling, hyperpigmented where exposed to light. Hair dry and hair of different color intermingled with normal hair. Nystagmus; deep tendon reflexes hyperactive; ataxic gait.

Etiology. Congenital defective tryptophan metabolism and other metabolic abnormalities (aminoaciduria). Attacks precipitated by light exposure, drugs (sulfonamides), psychological stress and inadequate or irregular diet. Autosomal recessive transmission; two forms suggested: (1) classic, with defect expressed in intestine and kidney; (2) variant, with defect expressed only in kidney.

Pathology. Skin, pellagra-like lesions.

Diagnostic Procedures. *Blood.* Normal; glucose tolerance test followed by hypoglycemia after normal curve in some cases. *Urine.* Normal at routine examination. Urinary chromatogram, aminoaciduria of renal origin with characteristic H-pattern. Tryptophan loading test and neomycin and tryptophan loading test. *Electroencephalography.* Altered in some cases.

Therapy. Nicotinamide and vitamin B complex.

Prognosis. Symptoms become milder with age, but without treatment mental deterioration may occur. Treatment effective for all symptoms except for aminoaciduria.

BIBLIOGRAPHY. Baron DN, Deut CE, Harris H, et al: Hereditary pellagra-like skin rash with temporary cerebellar ataxia, constant renal aminoaciduria and other bizarre chemical features. Lancet II:421–428, 1956
Halvorsen K, Halvorsen S: Hartnup disease. Pediatrics 31:29–38, 1963
Scriver CR, Mahon B, Levy HL, et al: The Hartnup phenotype shows epistasis and genetic heterogeneity. Am J Hum Genet 37:A16, 1985

HARTUNG'S

Synonyms. Myoclonic epilepsy Hartung's; epilepsy Hartung's. See Friedreich's.

Symptoms and Signs. From birth, those of Unverricht's (see).

Etiology. Autosomal dominant inheritance.

Pathology. Brain diffuse atrophy, absence of Lafora's bodies (see).

BIBLIOGRAPHY. Hartung E: Zwei Faelle von Paramyoclonus multiplex mit Epilesie. Z Ges Psychiatr 56:150–153, 1920
Vogel F, Hafner H, Diebald K: Zur Genetik der progressiven Myoklonusepilepsien (Unverricht-Lundberg). Humangenetik 1:437–475, 1965

HASHIMOTO-PRITZKER

Synonyms. Self-healing reticulohistiocytosis; reticulohistiocytosis self-healing. See Histiocytic syndromes.

Symptoms and Signs. Clinical and hematologic finding developing a few days after birth (instead of at birth). Pea-sized mobile nodules of dark brownish-blue color spreading over a period of two days on the face, scalp, trunk, and extremities; jaundice-hepatomegaly. No splenomegaly or lymphadenopathy.

Etiology. Unknown.

Diagnostic Procedures. *Blood.* Moderate anemia and thrombocytopenia; leukocytes normal range; lymphocytosis with atypical form. Hyperbilirubinemia, sGOT, sGPT increased. *X-ray.* Normal. *Bone marrow.* No specific pattern, few atypical cells. *Surgical biopsy of nodules.* Infiltrate of large lymphocytes and histiocytes. Histiocytes occasionally multinucleated with glassy eosinophilic cytoplasm or foamy cytoplasm and mitotic figures; PAS positive material.

Prognosis. Self-healing within one month with complete recovery.

BIBLIOGRAPHY. Hashimoto K, Pritzker MS: Electron microscopy study of reticulohistiocytoma: an unusual case of congenital self-healing reticulohistiocytosis. Arch Derm 107:263–270, 1973

Hashimoto K, Griffin D, Kohsbaki M: Self-healing reticulohistiocytosis: a clinical, histologic and ultrastructural study of a fourth case in the literature. Cancer 49:331–337, 1982

HASHIMOTO'S

Synonyms. Lymphadenoid goiter; chronic lymphadenoid; struma lymphomatosa; chronic lymphocytic thyroiditis; autoimmune thyroiditis.

Symptoms. Incidence in females 15 to 20 times higher than in males; onset at any age; highest incidence between 30 to 50 years of age. Initially, asymptomatic or vague discomfort in the neck; seldom, dysphagia or dyspnea. Periodic paralysis reported.

Signs. Gradual enlargment of thyroid, followed initially (in nearly 20% of cases) by signs of mild hypothyroidism and then by myxedema (see Gull's). In 25% of cases, musculoskeletal symptoms and rheumatoid arthritis.

Etiology. Autoimmune reaction. Possibly genetic predisposition, defect in hormonogenesis; "forbidden clone" theory; abnormal exposure to thyroid antigens. Autosomal dominant inheritance observed in some families, possibly on the same basis of other autoimmune conditions (see Polymyalgia rheumatica, Horton's, Lupus erythematosus, Addison-Biermer, etc.).

Pathology. Thyroid symmetric, rubbery consistency, pinkish to yellow color, nonadherent to perithyroid structures. Parenchymal atrophy; lymphoid infiltration and fibrosis; Colloidal space reduced; colloid absent. Typically, all gland is involved.

Diagnostic Procedures. *Basal metabolic rate.* Normal or decreased. *Blood.* Thyroxine (T$_4$) from low to high; free thyroxine iodide (FTI) normal or reduced; butanol extractable iodine increased; antithyroid globulin diagnostic elevation. *Biopsy.* See Pathology. *Fluorescent thyroid scan.* High diagnostic value.

Therapy. None if situation is stable. Thyroid hormone useful especially in early treatment of young person. Seldom, surgery may be considered. Cortisone of doubtful long-term utility.

Prognosis. Relatively benign condition; from long-term asymptomatic condition to severe, rapidly evolving hypothyroidism, associated more or less with other possible autoimmune conditions.

BIBLIOGRAPHY. Hashimoto H: Zur Kenntnis der lymphomatösen Verärderung der Schilddrüse (Strauma lymphomatosa). Arch Klin Chir 97:219–248, 1912

Leung AKC: Familial "hashitoxic" periodic paralysis. J Roy Soc Med 78:638–640, 1985

Hamburger JI: The various presentations of thyroiditis: diagnostic considerations. Ann Int Med 104:219–224, 1986

HAVERHILL FEVER

Symptoms and Signs. Both sexes affected; onset at all ages. Abrupt onset. Fever; rubellalike rash on extremities; polyarthritis.

Etiology. *Haverhillia multiformis* (*Streptobacillus*). After ratbite or drinking contaminated milk.

Diagnostic Procedures. *Blood and synovial fluid.* Culture for demonstration of *Streptobacillus*. Specific agglutinin also found.

Therapy. Penicillin; streptomycin; tetracyclines.

Prognosis. Arthritis and functional joint limitation may last months.

BIBLIOGRAPHY. Willner O, Place EH, Sutton LE: Erythema arthriticum, epidemicum: preliminary report. Med Sur J 194:285–287, 1926

Schmidt FR: Unusual features and special types of infectious arthritis. In Hollander JL, McCarty DJ: Arthritis and Allied Conditions, 8th ed, p 1268. Philadelphia, Lea & Febiger, 1972

Shanson DC, Gazzara BG, Midgley J, et al: *Streptobacillus moniliformis* isolated from blood in four cases of Haverhill fever. Lancet II:92–94, 1983

HAXTHAUSEN'S I

Synonym. Keratoderma climactericum.

Symptoms and Signs. Occur in menopausal women. Tenderness on walking; painful fissuring of feet, especially in winter. Hyperkeratosis of palms and soles appearing as discrete, sharply defined lesions, regular round or oval, lentil to pea size. Eczematous complication frequent. Obesity and hypertension and chronic arthritis frequently associated features.

Etiology. Unknown.

Pathology. Horny layer slightly frayed and sometimes with superficial fissures. Eczematous lesions with miliary vesicles developing later.

Therapy. Hormonal treatment not indicated. Weight reduction; keratolytic ointments; paring of excessive horn.

Prognosis. After months of progression, stabilization of condition or improvement. Chronic condition refractory to treatment. Eczema and itching are complicating features.

BIBLIOGRAPHY. Haxthausen H: Keratoderma climactericum. Br J Dermatol Syph 46:161–167, 1934

Rook A, Wilkinson DS, Ebling FJG, et al: Textbook of Dermatology, 4th ed, p 1461. Oxford, Blackwell Scientific Publications, 1986

HAYDEN-GROSSMAN

Synonym. Familial rectal pain. See Painful ophthalmoplegia, Thaysen's, and Frey's.

Symptoms and Signs. Both sexes affected; onset in infancy. Brief excruciating pain in submandibular, ocular, and rectal zones, with flushing of the corresponding skin areas; followed by a normal bowel movement, buttock and leg flushing, and pain cessation. The orbital pain is accompanied by tears, squinting, and blurring of vision; the submandibular is followed by salivation.

Etiology. Autosomal dominant inheritance with variable penetrance. Dysautonomic nature (?).

Pathology. Unknown.

Therapy. None.

Prognosis. Pains occur once a day or once a week 5 to 10 times, then stop for some weeks or months. Cycles eventually recur.

BIBLIOGRAPHY. Hayden R, Grossman M: Rectal, ocular, and submaxillary pain: a familial autonomic disorder related to proctalgia fugax. Report of a family. Am J Dis Child 97:479–482, 1959

Mann TP, Cree JE: Familial rectal pain. Lancet I:1016–1017, 1972

HEAD-HOLMES

Synonyms. Distorted spacial perception; visual disorientation; Verger-Déjerine; Déjerine's; cortical sensory. See Riddoch's.

Symptoms. Inability to localize stationary or moving object in the three planes of space because of lack of ability to estimate distance and improper judgment of size and length of objects. Visual acuity good; stereoscopic vision seldom lost. In some cases, associated visual inattention, difficulty in maintaining fixation when object moves; visual agnosia.

Signs. Failure to accommodate and to converge on close object; absence of blinking reflex.

Etiology and Pathology. Bilateral cerebral lesions, posterior part of parietal lobe or surface of occipital lobe. Trauma, hemorrhage.

Therapy and Prognosis. Depends on etiology.

BIBLIOGRAPHY. Head H, Holmes G: Sensory disturbances from cerebral lesions. Brain 34:102, 1911

Déjerine J, Monzon J: Un nouveau type de syndrome sensitif corticale observè dans un cas de monoplégic corticale dissociée. Rev Neurol 28:1265, 1914–1915

Holmes G: Disturbances of visual orientation. Br J Ophthalmol 2:449–468, 1918

Riddoch G: Visual disorientation in homonymous half fields. Brain 58:376–382, 1935

Adams RD, Victor M: Principles of Neurology, 3rd ed, pp 338–339. New York, McGraw-Hill, 1985

HEAD-RIDDOCH

Synonyms. Autonomic hyperreflexia; high spinal myelomalacia.

Symptoms. Occur in quadriplegic patients. Sweating; flushing; pilomotor activity; nasal stuffiness; blurred vision; headache; occasionally, generalized seizures.

Signs. Bradycardia; hypertension; dilated pupils.

Etiology. Distension of a viscus below the level of a spinal cord lesion or other type of nerve stimulation. More intense in patient with high cervical cord lesions than in the ones with low cervical or upper thoracic lesions. Lack of inhibitory impulses from high centers to control vasoconstrictor reflexes.

Pathology. High spinal myelomalacia.

Therapy.

1. Reduction of stimuli that precipitate symptoms, such as catheter obstruction, fecal impaction, bladder calculi, urinary infection, decubiti
2. Neurologic rhizotomy or pharmacologic destruction of spinal rootlets by intrathecal nerve block
3. Pharmacologic interruption of neuronal transmission by the use of ganglionic blockade with quaternary ammonium compounds or, better, by guanethidine

Prognosis. This syndrome occasionally ends in generalized seizures and death.

BIBLIOGRAPHY. Head H, Riddoch G: The automatic bladder, excessive sweating and some other reflex conditions in gross injuries of the spinal cord. Brain 40:188–263, 1917

Cole TM, Kottke FJ, Olson M, et al: Alterations of cardiovascular control of high spinal myelomalacia. Arch Phys Med Rehabil 48:359–368, 1967

Adams RD, Victor M: Principles of Neurology, 3rd ed, pp 406–407. New York, McGraw-Hill, 1985

HEART DISEASE, CONGENITAL-DEAFNESS-SKELETAL MALFORMATION

See Jervell-Lange-Nielsen.

Symptoms. Both sexes affected; onset in infancy. Deaf-mutism; dyspnea; feeding problems; growth retardation.

Signs. Hypertelorism; broad nasal root; low-set ears. Multiple variable skeletal malformations: acrocephaly; scoliosis; pectus excavatum; syndactyly; supernumerary digits. Signs of pulmonary stenosis in the heart or mitral insufficiency or both.

Etiology. Unknown; autosomal dominant inheritance with incomplete penetrance.

Pathology. Congenital heart defect (pulmonary stenosis in one family and mitral insufficiency in another family). Skeletal malformations. Malformation of stapes and other auricular bone defects (as cause of deafness).

Diagnostic Procedures. *Audiography. Electrocardiography. X-ray chest and skeleton. Biochemical studies.* Negative. *Chromosome studies.* Negative. *Cardiac catheterization.*

Therapy. Surgery for cardiac malformation when indicated.

Prognosis. Nonprogressive condition, except for heart complications.

BIBLIOGRAPHY. Koroxenidis GT, Webb NC, Jr, Moschos CB, et al: Congenital heart disease, deaf-mutism and associated somatic malformation occurring in several members of one family. Am J Med 40:149–155, 1966

Forney WR, Robinson SJ, Pascoe DJ: Congenital heart disease, deafness and skeletal malformations: a new syndrome? J Pediatr 68:14–26, 1966

HEART TAMPONADE

Synonym. Cardiac tamponade.

Symptoms. Sudden chest pain; skin pale, sweating, cold; dyspnea; asthenia; syncope.

Signs. Jugular vein distended; paradoxical pulse; apex pulse absent. Tachycardia; cardiac sound faint; pericardial friction rub; blood pressure decreased. Central venous pressure increased; low cardiac output. Oliguria.

Etiology. Chest trauma; myocardial infarction; vessel rupture; intrapericardial bleeding causing an accumulation of pericardial fluid, which causes an increase of pressure and prevents cardiac filling.

Pathology. See Etiology.

Diagnostic Procedures. *Electrocardiography.* QRS low voltage; ST elevation; T wave flattening. *X-rays.* Widening of heart shadow; obliteration of great vessels outlines. *Blood.* Anemia; elevated enzymes. *Echocardiography.* Analysis of the jugular pulsations.

Therapy. Pericardial tapping or surgery.

Prognosis. Good with prompt and appropriate treatment.

BIBLIOGRAPHY. Chevers N: Observation of diseases of the orifices and valves of aorta. Guy's Hosp Rep 7:387, 1842

Shabetai R: Diseases of pericardium. In Hurst JW: The Heart, 6th ed, pp 1259–1261. New York, McGraw-Hill, 1986

HEBERDEN'S

Synonyms. Angina pectoris; Master's; Elsner's; initial angina; Rougnon de Magny's; stable angina; stenocardia. See Preinfarction and Prinzmetal's II.

Symptoms. Sudden, mild, severe or excruciating precordial dull pain, tightness, accompanied by anxiety. Radiation to left shoulder, arm, hand. Short duration (usually less than 3 minutes), precipitated by emotion, effort, cold exposure, heavy meal. Relieved by nitroglycerin (see also Gallavardin's)

Signs. None.

Etiology. Relative myocardial hypoxia due to anatomic or functional coronary artery flow insufficiency.

Pathology. Atherosclerosis of coronary vessels.

Diagnostic Procedures. *Electrocardiography.* During attack S-T segment is depressed; in intermittent periods usually normal. Under effort (three-step test) alterations may appear. *X-ray.* Negative; cardiomegaly in advanced disease. *Catheterization with coronary angiography. Echocardiography.* Left ventriculography.

Therapy. Management of underlying disease (atherosclerosis; syphilis; aortic valvular disease). Elimination of contributing factors (anemia; arrhythmias; gastrointestinal tract pathology). Avoidance of precipitating factors (e.g., heavy meals, cold). Nitroglycerin; isosorbide dinitrate; beta-adrenergic blockers; perhexiline maleate; digitalis (in specific cases); diuretics, long-acting nitrates, sedatives. Angioplasty or bypass grafting.

Prognosis. Average survival 10 years from first attack.

BIBLIOGRAPHY. Lancisi GM: De Subitaneis Mortibus. Rome, 1707
Heberden W: Some account of a disorder of the breast. Med Tr R Coll Phys (London) 2:59–67, 1772
Anonymous: The Ebers Papyrus, XXVII, p 47 Ebbell B (trans). Copenhagen, Levin and Munksgaard, 1937
Caelius: On Swift or Acute Disease, p 261. Drabkin IE. (ed, trans). Chicago, University of Chicago Press, 1950
Hurst JW: The Heart, 6th ed, pp 882–1008. New York, McGraw-Hill, 1986

HEBERDEN'S NODES

Synonyms. Bouchard's nodes (see Symptoms and Signs); interphalangeal distal osteoarthritis; Rosenbach's.

Symptoms and Signs. More common in females; onset in middle life. Swelling at distal interphalangeal joints, which may develop unnoticed for years; or abrupt painful onset, with redness, paresthesia, and clumsiness. Followed by articular deformity and limitation of motion. When nodes are in juxtaphalangeal position, they are called Bouchard's nodes.

Etiology. Sex-linked inheritance; dominant in females; recessive in males or secondary to traumas.

Pathology. Massive areas of necrobiosis, in subcutis, with degenerated collagen and surrounding palisading of histiocytes, fibrosis, and capillary hyperplasia. Marginal osteophytes of distal phalanges of fingers not distinguishable from osteoarthritic lesions of other joints.

Diagnostic Procedures. *X-ray.* Typical osteoarthritic changes.

Therapy. Analgesic and anti-inflammatory agents.

Prognosis. Progressive condition.

BIBLIOGRAPHY. Heberden W: De Nodis Digitorum in His Commentarii de Morborum Historia et Curatione. London, Payne, 1802
Rosenback O: Die Anftreibung der Endphalangen der Finger eine bisher noch nicht beschriebene trophische Störung. Zentralbl Nerveh 13:191–205, 1890
Rook A, Wilkinson DS, Ebling FJG, et al: Textbook of Dermatology, 4th ed, pp 1386–1696. Oxford, Blackwell Scientific Publications, 1986

HEBRA'S PRURIGO

Synonyms. Prurigo ferox; prurigo mitis.

Symptoms. Both sexes affected; onset between 1 and 5 years of age. Itching of various intensities.

Signs. Prevalent on extensor side of legs and arms, less frequently on trunk; appearance of small, numerous papules that rather rapidly ulcerate and crust. Thickening of interposed skin, but absence of lichenification. Regional lymph adenopathy.

Etiology. Unknown; possible relation with atopic condition, malnutrition, poor hygiene.

Therapy. Prevention of scratching. Avoidance of exposure to possible allergens. Identify allergens and treat by desensitization. Antihistamines: chlorpheniramine or promethazine for symptomatic relief. Topical corticosteroids or systemic (only to overcome acute phases). Ultraviolet light applications.

BIBLIOGRAPHY. von Hebra F: Traité Pratique des Maladies de la Peau. Paris, 1854
Rook A, Wilkinson DS, Ebling FJG, et al: Textbook of Dermatology, 4th ed, p 417. Oxford, Blackwell Scientific Publications, 1986

HECHT-BEALS

Synonyms. Trismus-pseudocamptodactyly (TPS); camptomelic trism; Wilsons' Dutch-Kentucky. The eponym Dutch-Kentucky syndrome was proposed in 1974 by Mabry et al. after performing an extensive pedigree of a Kentucky family; the earliest affected family member that they were able to trace was a young Dutch girl who immigrated to the southern United States circa 1780.

Symptoms and Signs. Male: female 1:2. From birth, feeding problems from inability to open mouth completely; slow eaters. Hand handicaps due to campodactyly. Trismus with enlarged coronoid process of mandibula. When hands dorsiflexed, fingers partially flexed. *Feet.* Downturned toes; talipes equinovarus; metatarsus adductus; short gastrocnemius.

Etiology. Autosomal dominant inheritance.

Pathology. Short flexor tendons of hands and feet. Short muscles.

Therapy. Bilateral removal of the coronoid processes of the mandible has been performed in some cases.

BIBLIOGRAPHY. Hecht F, Beals RK: Inability to open the mouth fully: an autosomal dominant phenotype with facultative campodactyly and short stature (preliminary note). Birth Defects Orig Art Ser (3):96–98, 1969

Tsukahara M, Shimozaki F, Kajii T: Tismus-pseudocampodactyly syndrome in a Japanese family. Clin Genet 28:247–250, 1985

Wilson RV, Gaines DL, Brooks A, et al: Autosomal dominant inheritance of shortening of the flexor profundus muscle tendon unit with limitation of jaw excursion. Birth Defects Orig Art Ser 5:99–102, 1969

Mabry CC, Barnett IS, Hutcheson NW: Trismus pseudo-camptodactyly syndrome: Dutch-Kentucky syndrome. J Pediatr 85:503–508, 1974

Browder FH, Lew D, Shahbazian TS: Anesthetic management of a patient with Dutch-Kentucky syndrome. Anesthesiology 65:218–219, 1986

HEDBLOM'S*

Synonym. Acute primary diaphragmitis.

Symptoms. Sudden onset. Pain in the shoulder; upper abdominal pain.

Signs. Decreased lung expansion on inspiration. Deep inspiration prevented by pain.

Etiology. Unknown; aspecific myositis of one or both sides of diaphragm.

Pathology. Diaphragmatic leukocytic infiltration; swelling of muscle fibers; in some cases extension of inflammatory changes to pleura and peritoneum.

Diagnostic Procedures. *X-ray of chest. Fluoroscopy.*

Therapy. Antibiotic reported useful.

Prognosis. Self-limited condition; possible recurrences.

BIBLIOGRAPHY. Joannides M: Acute primary diaphragmitis (Hedblom's syndrome). Dis Chest 12:89–110, 1946

HEERFORDT'S

Synonyms. Uveoparotid fever; uveoparotic paralysis; uveoparotitis. Used also as synonym for Besnier-Boeck-Schaumann (see). See also Waldeström uveoparotitis.

Symptoms and Signs. Prevalent in females; onset in young adulthood. Bilateral uveitis; parotitis; mediastinal lymphadenopathy; splenomegaly, facial palsy; fever; skin nodules.

Etiology. Majority of cases affected by sarcoidosis. In some cases, *Mycobacterium tuberculosis* may possibly be the etiologic agent.

Pathology. Presence of tubercules that do not calcify; see Besnier-Boeck-Schaumann.

Diagnostic Procedures. See Besnier-Boeck-Schaumann.

Therapy. See Besnier-Boeck-Schaumann.

Prognosis. Swelling of parotid glands lasts from 6 weeks to 2 years. Parlaysis disappears within a few months.

BIBLIOGRAPHY. Heerfordt CF: Ueber eine Febris uveoparotidea subchronica an der Glandula parotis und der Uvea des Auges lokalisiert und haufig mit Paresen cerebrospinaler Nerven kompliziert. Graefes Arch Ophthalmol 70:254–273, 1909

Dufour R, Bourquin A: Deux cas d'uveoparotidite histologique tuberculeuse. Ophthalmologica 120:50–56, 1950

Theobald GD, Wilder HL: Heerfordt's syndrome. Trans Am Acad Ophthalmol Otol 57:332–333, 1953

Iwata K, Nanba K, Sobue K, et al: Ocular sarcoidosis: evaluation of intraocular findings. Ann NY Acad Sci 278:445–454, 1976

Adams RD, Victor M: Principles of Neurology, 3rd ed, p 1013. New York, McGraw-Hill, 1985

HEIDENHAIN'S

Synonym. Cortical blindness-presenile dementia. Myoclonic dementia, subacute; spongiform encephalopathy (to be distinguished from Creutzfeldt-Jakob [see] although this eponym is inappropriately used).

Symptoms and Signs. Occur in males; onset between 38 and 55 years of age. Progressive loss of vision; progressive mental deterioration of central type. Ataxia; dysarthria; athetoid movements and generalized rigidity.

Etiology. Unknown. Akin to kuru (see) (transmissible agent). Iatrogenic transmission (transplantation, infected electrodes, etc.) demonstrated.

Diagnostic Procedures. *Electroencephalopathy.* Distinctive pattern. *Blood and cerebrospinal fluid.* Normal.

Pathology. Cortical degeneration prevalent in the occipital cortex and more or less generalized to other cortical zones. *Histology.* Altered architecture; protoplasmic and fibrous astroycte proliferation; small nerve cell shrinkage and pigment atrophy.

Therapy. None; antiviral agents ineffective.

Prognosis. Poor; death follows quite rapidly after onset.

BIBLIOGRAPHY. Heidenhain A: Klinische und anatomische Untersuchungen uber eine eigenartige organische Enkrankung des Zentral-nervensystems im Praesenium. Z Neurol Psychiatr 118:49–114, 1929

---

*Nominated in honor.

Meyer A, Leigh D, Bagg CE: Rare presenile dementia associated with cortical blindness (Heidenhain's syndrome). J Neurol Neurosurg Psychiatr 17:129–133, 1954

Prusiner SB, Haven WJ (eds): Slow Transmissible Diseases of the Nervous System. New York, Acad Press, 1973

HEINE-MEDIN

Synonyms. Infantile paralysis; paralytic spinal poliomyelitis.

Symptoms. Both sexes affected; onset most frequently between 6 months and 15 years of age: symptoms appear from late spring to fall. In some cases, asymptomatic. Usually follows a prodromal phase characterized by fever, upper respiratory symptoms, or gastrointestinal symptoms: nausea; vomiting; diarrhea; stypsis; abdominal pain, or influenzalike symptoms (bone, muscle, and joint aches).

Signs. *Aborted type.* Initial vague signs of receding generic viral infection. *Nonparalytic type.* Prodromal signs acquiring consistency; possibly, meningeal irritation signs, then recession. *Paralytic type.* Onset of generalized or localized paralysis usually 3 to 5 days or less after onset of symptoms of nervous system involvement (onset may be later). In acute phase, irritability, tenderness and spasm of affected muscles. Loss of corresponding tendon reflexes.

Etiology. Poliovirus (strain Brunhilde, Lansing, Leon).

Pathology. Necrosis of anterior horn cells of all segments of spinal cord with more frequent involvement of cervical and lumbar enlargements: hyperemia; then edema and softening. Medulla frequently affected. Cortex of brain and cerebellum more rarely involved. Mild inflammatory changes in subarachnoid space; infiltration by mononuclear cells; edema and hemorrhages of areas affected; when inflammation subsides, parenchymatous degeneration intervenes.

Diagnostic Procedures. *Oropharynx, stool, cerebrospinal fluid.* Demonstration of virus. *Cerebrospinal fluid.* Leukocytosis (initially polymorphs; soon later lymphocytes). Protein normal or slight elevation; chloride and sugar normal; pressure increased. *Blood.* Marked leukocytosis (polymorphonucleates).

Therapy. Prophylaxis (vaccination) Symptomatic; gamma globulins. When needed, artificial ventilation.

Prognosis. Mortality 5% to 15%. Permanent paralysis rate of difficult estimation. Recovery of muscle function possible within 3 to 4 months, then poorer outlook for complete recovery and residual atrophy.

BIBLIOGRAPHY. Heine J: Beobachtungen ueber Laehmungszustaende der untern Extremitaeten und deren Behandlung. Stuttgart, Köhler, 1840

Medin O: En epidemi af infantil paralysi. Hygiea [Stockh] 52:657–668, 1890

Dalakas MC, Elder G, Hallett M, et al: A long-term follow up of patients with post-poliomyelitis neuromuscular symptoms. N Engl J Med 314:959–963, 1986

HEINER'S

Synonyms. Cow's milk precipitins pulmonary hemosiderosis; milk (bovine) precipitins pulmonary; bovine milk pulmonary sensitivity; Heiner-Sears hemosiderosis pulmonary hypersensitivity cow milk. See Allergic gastroenteritis.

Symptoms. Occur in young infants of both sexes. Failure to thrive; recurrent diarrhea; chronic respiratory distress.

Signs. Underweight; pallor; variable pulmonary findings.

Etiology. Not precisely delineated: delayed sensitivity to cow's milk products; intravascular precipitation of antigen-antibody complexes; sensitivity reactions of blood vessel.

Pathology. Suppurative bronchitis with various degrees of atelectasis. Pulmonary hemosiderosis, secondary cor pulmonale, ahypertrophied mesopharyngeal lymphoid tissue. Microhemorrhages in the intestinal mucosa.

Diagnostic Procedures. *Blood.* Hypochromic anemia; low sideremia; hypoproteinemia; high titer of circulating antibodies against cow's milk; eosinophils may be present. *Stool.* Presence of milk coproantibodies and blood. In adults, however, cow's milk sensitivity and the presence of antibodies may be associated with other diarrheal disorders (e.g., ulcerative colitis; regional enteritis; celiac disease; cystic fibrosis that have to be ruled out by specific tests). *X-ray of lung.* Variable findings: patchy infiltrates; atelectasis; peribronchial infiltrated; enlarged lymphnodes.

Therapy. Discontinuation of cow's milk feeding and substitution with carbohydrate solutions and with soybean-base or meat-base formulas. Pulmonary infections respond well to antibiotics. Iron if needed. Tonsillectomy corticosteroids useful.

Prognosis. The syndrome is limited to small infants. The symptomatology recedes in older infants. Better than pulmonary hemosiderosis.

BIBLIOGRAPHY. Heiner DC, Sears JW: Chronic respiratory disease associated with multiple circulating precipitins to cow's milk. Am J Dis Child 100:500–502, 1960

Katz J, Spiro HM, Herskovic T: Milk precipitating substance in the stool in gastrointestinal milk sensitivity. New Engl J Med 278:1191–1194, 1968

Chang CH, Whitting HJ: Heiner's syndrome. Radiology 92:507–508, 1969

Behrman RE, Vaughan VC III: Nelson's Textbook of Pediatrics, 12th ed, p 1062. Philadelphia, WB Saunders, 1983

HEINZ BODIES-CONGENITAL HEMOLYTIC ANEMIA

Synonyms. CHBA, Cathic's; hemolytic anemia (Heinz bodies).

Symptoms and Signs. From birth. Congenital nonspherocytic hemolytic anemia; jaundice; splenomegaly; pigmenturia. Symptoms vary with different types of hemoglobin variants. Hemolytic crisis may be precipitated by sulfonamides.

Etiology. Autosomal dominant inheritance. Over 90 different types of unstable hemoglobin variants that precipitate spontaneously with heat in RBC causing hemolytic anemia.

Diagnostic Procedures. Heating the blood causes copious hemoglobin precipitates.

Pathology. Heinz bodies in RBC.

Therapy. None. Prevent rise of temperature and do not administer sulfonamides or other oxidative agents. Some authors advocate splenectomy.

Prognosis. Good.

BIBLIOGRAPHY. Cathic JAB: Apparent idiopathic Heinz body anemia. Creat Ormond St J 3:43, 1952

Bunn HF, Forget BG: Hemoglobin: Molecular, Genetic, and Clinical Aspects, p 565. Philadelphia, WB Saunders, 1986

HELLER-NELSON

Synonym. Klinefelter's variant.

BIBLIOGRAPHY. Heller CG, Nelson WO: Hyalination of the seminiferous tubulus associated with normal or failing Leydig cell function. Discussion of relationship to eunuchoidism, gynecomastia, elevated gonadotropins, depressed 17-ketosteroids, and estrogens. J Clin Endocrinol 5:1–12, 1945

HELLER'S (J.)

Synonyms. Dystrophia unguis mediana canaliformis; dysonychia canaliformis; median nail dystrophy.

Symptoms and Signs. Rare. Development of a split or true canal on one nail (usually of the thumb) or several nails.

Etiology. Unknown; possibly related to trauma or to some temporary defect in the nail matrix.

Therapy. Unnecessary. Emolient cream in the nail fold.

Prognosis. After months or years nail returns to normal; relapses may occur.

BIBLIOGRAPHY. Heller J: Zur Kasuistik seltener Nagelkrankheiten. XVIII. Dystrophia unguim (*sic*) mediana canali-formis. Dermatol Z 51:416–419, 1927

Rook A, Wilkinson DS, Ebling FJG, et al: Textbook of Dermatology, 4th ed, p 2051. Oxford, Blackwell Scientific Publications, 1986

HELLER'S (T.)

Synonym. Aphonia–dementia infantilis. Term obsolete.

BIBLIOGRAPHY. Heller T: Ueber dementia infantilis. Z Kinderforsch 37:661–667, 1930

HELLERSTRÖM'S

Symptoms and Signs. Association with Afzelius'. Erythema chronicum migrans with symptoms related to meningitic involvement.

Etiology. The same as Afzelius' (see).

BIBLIOGRAPHY. Hellerström S: Erythema chronicum migrans afzelli. Acta Derm Venereol (Stockh) 11:315–321, 1930

HELMHOLTZ-HARRINGTON

Synonym. Corneal opacity-cranioskeletal dysostosis.

Symptoms and Signs. Both sexes affected; onset from birth. Zonular cataract; other ocular disorders due to oxycephaly; various apical malformations (polydactyly; syndactyly; camptodactyly; lobster-claw type of dystrophy). Mental retardation; hepatosplenomegaly.

Etiology. Unknown.

BIBLIOGRAPHY. Appenzeller GFA: Ein Beitrag zur Lehre von der Erblichkeit des grauen Staars (these). Tübingen, 1884
Helmholtz H, Harrington EFR: Syndrome characterized by congenital clouding of cornea and by other anomalies. Am J Dis Child 41:793–800, 1931
François J: Syndromes with congenital cataract. Am J Ophthalmol 52:207–238, 1961

HELWEG-LARSEN'S

Synonym. Anhidrosis-congenital neurolabyrinthitis.

Symptoms. Both sexes affected; onset from birth. Temperature disturbances due to anhidrosis or marked hypohidrosis. In 4th or 5th decade, vertigo (neurolabyrinthitis).

Signs. Normal skull configuration; no abnormalities of teeth or hair.

Etiology. Unknown; autosomal dominant inheritance.

BIBLIOGRAPHY. Helweg-Larsen HF, Ludvigsen K: Congenital familial anhidrosis and neurolabyrinthitis. Acta Dermatol Venereol (Stockh) 26:489–505, 1946
Rook A, Wilkinson DS, Ebling FJG, et al: Textbook of Dermatology, 4th ed, p 143. Oxford, Blackwell Scientific Publications, 1986

HEMATOMA, EPIDURAL

Synonym. Epidural hematoma.

Symptoms. Patient with trauma of the head, and temporary unconsciousness, who develops the following symptomatology after a more or less prolonged lucid interval (a few minutes or days). Symptoms may be subdivided in two groups: (1) Acute type with interval shorter than 7 days (82%); (2) chronic type with longer interval (18%). The patient starts to grow sleepy, then stuporous, and then comatose. Symptoms progress rapidly once started.

Signs. Bradycardia; bradypnea; hypertension; pupil side of lesion dilated and fixed; occasionally, contralateral hemianopsia or hemiplegia may be observed.

Etiology. Hemorrhage between dura and inner table of skull usually from middle meningeal artery.

Pathology. Fracture of skull and hematoma of the middle meningeal artery or laceration of dural sinuses; compression of cerebral hemisphere; occasionally, cerebral infarction.

Diagnostic Procedures. *X-ray of skull. Spinal tap. CT brain scan.*

Therapy. Immediate surgery with decompression and ligation of bleeding artery.

Prognosis. Depends on degree of consciousness, patient's age, intensity of bleeding.

BIBLIOGRAPHY. Heyser J, Weber G: Die epiduralen Hämatome. Schweiz Med Wochenschr 94:2–7; 46–52, 1964
Adams RD, Victor M: Principles of Neurology, 3rd ed, p 652. New York, McGraw-Hill, 1985

HEMATURIA, ESSENTIAL

Synonyms. Benign recurrent hematuria; essential hematuria.

Symptoms. Prevalent in male children; onset between 2 and 11 years of age. Asymptomatic.

Signs. Episodes of gross hematuria.

Etiology. Various conditions may cause the syndrome: 50% of cases, focal glomerulonephritis; some present the Berger's syndrome (see), a smaller number, chronic progressive nephropathies.

Pathology. See Etiology. Usually, nonspecific changes.

Diagnostic Procedures. *Blood.* Normal. *Urine.* Gross recurrent hematuria. In some cases, persistent microscopic hematuria between episodes. *Biopsy of kidneys.* See Etiology. *X-ray. Intravenous pyelography. Renal arteriography. Computerized axial tomography.*

Therapy. None, or according to etiology.

Prognosis. Generally good.

BIBLIOGRAPHY. Stamey T, Kindrauchuk RW: Urinary Sediment and Urinalysis: A Practical Guide for Health Professionals. Philadelphia, WB Saunders, 1985

HEMI 3

Synonym. Hemihypertrophy subtype.

Symptoms and Signs. Observed in girls. Hemihypertrophy. Hemihyperesthesia, hemiareflexia, and scoliosis. In body, larger side (usually the left), increase of muscle size and strength and bone thickness but not length.

Etiology. Neural tube defects with multifactorial inheritance.

Prognosis. Scoliosis progressive. Musculoskeletal and neurological defects stable.

BIBLIOGRAPHY. Nudleman K, Anderman E, Anderman F, et al: The hemi 3 syndrome: hemihypertrophy-hemihypoesthesia, hemiareflexia and scoliosis. Brain 107:533–546, 1984

HEMIFACIAL MICROSOMIA

Synonyms. Unilateral mandibulofacial dysostosis. See also Goldenhar's, François-Haustrate; Nager Reyner, and Weyers-Thier.

Symptoms. Both sexes equally affected. In majority of cases left side involvement. Symptoms related to presence or combination of signs (see).

Signs. *Face.* Asymmetry: maxillary and malar bone on one side reduced and flattened, with resulting lowering of eye position; palpebral fissure on affected side lowered. Occasionally; microphthalmia, congenital cystic eye, colobomas, and strabismus. Macrostomia or microstomia associated in 30% of cases with mandibular ramus agenesis; *External ear.* Malformation of variable degrees up to complete aplasia; ear canal frequently missing. *Musculoskeletal system.* Muscle hypoplasia; (masseter, temporalis, pterygoideus, and others of involved side). *Visceral system.* In some cases, pulmonary agenesis of affected side.

Etiology. Genetic defects excluded. An alteration of intrauterine environment suggested.

Pathology. See Signs.

Diagnostic Procedures. *X-rays. Blood. Urine. Biopsy.* No diagnostic value.

Therapy. If feasible, plastic surgery.

Prognosis. Stable condition.

BIBLIOGRAPHY. Ballantine JW: Manual of Antenatal Pathology and Hygiene. II The Fetus. Baltimore, William Wood, 1950

Gorlin RJ, Pindborg JJ, Cohen NM: Syndromes of the Head and Neck, 2nd ed. New York, McGraw-Hill, 1976

HEMIHYPERTROPHY

Synonyms. Asymmetric lateral; hemigigantism; hemimacrosomia. See Curtius' I and Hemi 3.

Symptoms and Signs. Prevalent in males; present at birth in 40% of cases. Prevalent on the right side; varies in extent and severity in an extremely large spectrum. (Normal asymmetry exists, although not always apparent, and may be determined only by accurate measurements). Syndrome has been divided into *total* (musculoskeletal and visceral organs of involved side), *limited,* which has been subdivided in to *segmental* and *crossed.* Possible associated features numerous and include skin, hand and foot, vertebral column, genitourinary, and neurologic abnormalities. Occasionally, association with different tumors.

Etiology. Unknown; possibly more than one cause. Nervous system, vascular and lymphatic, endocrine, chromosomal abnormalities.

Pathology. Hypertrophy of muscle, bones, and viscera.

Diagnostic Procedures. *X-rays. Chromosome studies. Endocrine studies.*

Therapy. Symptomatic and othopedic when needed.

Prognosis. Usually good; may be determined by associated conditions.

BIBLIOGRAPHY. Meckel JF: Ueber die Seitliche Asymmetrie im tierischen Körper. Anatomische physiologische Beobachtungen und Untersuchungen, p 147. Halle, Renger, 1822

Massimo L, Scarabicchi S, Tortorolo G: Le neoplasie renali primitive nell infanzia. Clin Pediatr 42:991–1026, 1960

Fraumeni JF Jr, Geiser CF, Manning MD: Wilms' tumor and congenital hemihypertrophy. Report of five new cases and review of literature. Pediatrics 40:886–899, 1967

Viljoen D, Pearn J, Beighton P: Manifestations and natural history of idiopathic hemihypertrophy: a review of eleven cases. Clin Genet 26:81–86, 1984

HEMIPLEGIA, HEMIANESTHESIA, ALTERNATING-HYPOGLOSSAL

Symptoms. Hemiplegia of arm and leg (but not the face) and loss of position and vibration sensibility on the same side (without loss of pain or temperature sensibility). Paralysis (peripheral type) of the half of the tongue on opposite side.

Signs. Tongue hemiatrophy and twitching.

Etiology. Involvement of pyramidal tract and emergent fibers of hypoglossal nerve in the medulla. Basilar meningitis or other cause determining softening of pyramidal tract (rare).

BIBLIOGRAPHY. Alpers BJ: Clinical Neurology, 6th ed. Philadelphia, FA Davis, 1971

HEMIPLEGIA, INFANTILE

See Little's (WI).

Symptoms. Both sexes affected; onset in infancy or early childhood. May develop suddenly as a complication of acute infection with high fever, or without associated illness. Generalized or focal seizures usually first symptom, followed by hemiplegia. Arms more severely affected than legs. Common, repeated uncontrollable convulsions and behavioral problems (disobedience, inattentiveness, hyperactivity, destructiveness).

Etiology. Injury to one hemisphere occurring at birth or later (e.g., encephalitis, cerebrovascular problem, developmental defects).

Diagnostic Procedures. *Scintigraphy. CT brain scan. Angiography. Electroencephalography.* Demonstration of nature and extension of lesion.

Therapy. Anticonvulsants. Removal of cerebral cortex of damaged hemisphere.

Prognosis. Little response to treatment; severe educational problems. Unilateral cerebral decortication results in striking improvement in behavior and reduction of number of seizures.

BIBLIOGRAPHY. Vick NA: Grinker's Neurology, 7th ed. Springfield, IL, CC Thomas, 1976

Adams RD, Victor M: Principles of Neurology, 3rd ed, pp 924–925. New York, McGraw-Hill, 1985

HEMOGLOBIN CONSTANT SPRING

Synonym. HbCS. See also Hemoglobin H and Thalassemia syndromes.

Symptoms and Signs. In 50% of Asian subjects with HbH disease. Mild hemolytic anemia, splenomegaly.

Etiology. Mixed inheritance of hemoglobin H disease and anomalous hemoglobin Constant Spring. Symptoms are apparent only in the homozygous state. Heterozygotes for HbCS are phenotypically similar to individuals with heterozygous alpha thalassemia 2.

Diagnostic Procedures. *Blood.* Reticulocytosis. No hypochromia and microcytosis.

Therapy. None.

Prognosis. Good.

BIBLIOGRAPHY. Milner PF, Clegg JB, Weatherall DJ: Hemoglobin H disease due to a unique hemoglobin variant with elongated chain. Lancet I:729, 1971

Clegg JB, Weatherall DJ, Milner PF: Hemoglobin Constant Spring—a chain termination mutant? Nature 234:337, 1971

Bunn HF, Forget BG: Hemoglobin Molecular Genetic and Clinical Aspects, p 331. Philadelphia, WB Saunders, 1986

HEMOGLOBIN C SYNDROMES

HEMOGLOBIN C HOMOZYGOUS (CC)

Symptoms. Mild recurrent bone and joint pains; recurrent abdominal pains of variable intensity; convulsions; hemorrhagic manifestations.

Signs. Frequently jaundice; splenomegaly; no skeletal abnormality.

Etiology. Hemoglobin abnormality; (lysine for glutamic acid in the sixth position of the beta chain); homozygous, autosomal recessive inheritance.

Diagnostic Procedures. *Blood.* Normocytic or microcytic moderate anemia; microspherocytes; target cells; reticulocytosis; moderate. Hyperbilirubinemia, osmotic fragility decreased. Thrombocytopenia frequent. *Hemoglobin electrophoresis.* Hemoglobin C represents the entire hemoglobin. *Bone marrow.* Hyperplasia.

Therapy. Symptomatic.

Prognosis. Good; normal life span.

SICKLE CELL-HEMOGLOBIN C

See Hemoglobin SC syndrome.

Symptoms. Milder than in Herrick's (see).

Prognosis. Better than in Herrick's.

HS-O ARABIA

See Hemoglobin S/Hemoglobin O.

Symptoms and Signs. Reported in Sudan, Jamaica, and the United States. See Sickle cell hemoglobin C.

Diagnostic Procedures. *Hemoglobin electrophoresis.* Migration of hemoglobin O to same position as hemoglobin C difficult to distinguish except for biochemical characteristic (hemoglobin O Arabia-beta 121 Glu→Lys).

HEMOGLOBIN C-THALASSEMIA

Synonym. Zuelzer-Kaplan.

Symptoms and Signs. Mild to severe bone pain; splenomegaly rare.

Diagnostic Procedures. *Blood.* Anemia; large, thin target cells; schistocytes; microspherocytes. Decreased osmotic fragility. *Bone marrow.* Hyperplasia.

BIBLIOGRAPHY. Itano HA: A third abnormal hemoglobin associated with hereditary hemolytic anemia. Proc Natl Acad Sci 37:775–784, 1951

Zeulzer WE, Kaplan E: Thalassemia-hemoglobin C disease: a new syndrome presumably due to the combination of the genes for thalassemia and hemoglobin C. Blood 9:1047–1054, 1954

Bunn HF, Forget BG: Hemoglobin: Molecular, Genetic, and Clinical Aspects. Philadelphia, WB Saunders, 1986

HEMOGLOBIN D SYNDROMES

(Beta 121 Glu → Gln). Hemoglobin D has subvariants in HbD-Punjab, HbD-Los Angeles, Ibadan, Iran, etc.

HEMOGLOBIN D TRAIT (AD)

Symptoms. Asymptomatic.

HEMOGLOBIN D HOMOZYGOUS (DD)

Symptoms. Mild hemolytic anemia; no splenomegaly or bone alterations.

SICKLE CELL–HEMOGLOBIN D

Symptoms. Milder than in Herrick's (see). Combination of hemoglobin D with other hemoglobinopathies also reported.

BIBLIOGRAPHY. Itano HA: A third abnormal hemoglobin associated with hereditary hemolytic anemia. Proc Nat Acad Sci 37:775–784, 1951

Chernoff AI: The hemoglobin D syndromes. Blood 8:116–127, 1958

Bunn HF, Forget BG: Hemoglobin: Molecular, Genetic, and Clinical Aspects, p 424. Philadelphia, WB Saunders, 1986

HEMOGLOBIN E SYNDROMES

(Alpha-2 beta-2 26 Glu → Lys). In orientals.

HEMOGLOBIN E TRAIT

Symptoms. Asymptomatic.

HEMOGLOBIN E HOMOZYGOUS

Symptoms. Anemia; occasionally, polycythemia; moderate or absent splenomegaly.

Diagnostic Procedures. *Blood.* Mild, microcytic normochromic anemia; target cells. Decreased osmotic fragility; mild hyperbilirubinemia.

HEMOGLOBIN E THALASSEMIA

Symptoms. Similar to Cooley's (see Thalassemia syndromes).

SICKLE CELL–HEMOGLOBIN E

Symptoms. Milder than Herrick's (see).

BIBLIOGRAPHY. Itano HA, Bergren WR, Sturgeon P: Identification of a fourth abnormal human hemoglobin. J Am Chem Soc 76:2278, 1954

Bunn HF, Forget BG: Hemoglobin: Molecular, Genetic, and Clinical Aspects, p 426. Philadelphia, WB Saunders, 1986

HEMOGLOBIN H

Synonyms. Double heterozygous alpha thalassemia 1 + alpha thalassemia 2.

Symptoms and Signs. From birth. Some patients with mongoloid facies. Splenomegaly, hepatomegaly. Hemolytic anemia of variable severity. Anemia worsens during pregnancy and oxidative drug ingestion.

Etiology. Double heterozygous condition for alpha thalassemia 1 in one parent and alpha thalassemia 2 (silent carrier state) in the other parent. Presence of HbH (beta 4).

Diagnostic Procedures. *Hemoglobin electrophoresis.* In newborn 20 to 40% Hb Bart's (gamma-4); children and adults: HbH (beta) 5 to 30%. *Peripheral blood smear.* Hypochromia, microcytosis, poikilocytosis, polychromasia, targeting. *Bone marrow.* Erythroid hyperplasia.

Therapy. None. May require transfusions.

Prognosis. Good *quoad vitam.*

BIBLIOGRAPHY. Rigas DA, Koller RD, Osgood EE: New hemoglobin possessing a higher electrophoretic mobility than normal adult hemoglobin. Science 121:372, 1955, J Lab Clin Med 47:51–64, 1956

Bunn HF, Forget BG: Hemoglobin: Molecular, Genetic, and Clinical Aspects, p 329. Philadelphia, WB Saunders, 1986

HEMOGLOBIN S-G (S-D)

Symptoms. Few individuals have symptomatic sickle cell disease.

Etiology. Double heterozygosity for HbS and HbD.

BIBLIOGRAPHY. Melurdy PR, Lorkin PA, Casey R, et al: Hemoglobin S-G (S-D) syndrome. Am J Med 57:665, 1974

HEMOGLOBIN S/HEMOGLOBIN LEPORE-BOSTON

Symptoms. Those of Herrick's with hemolytic anemia and microcytes.

Etiology. Double heterozygosity for HbS and Hb Lepore Boston.

BIBLIOGRAPHY. Stevens MCG, Lehmann H, Mason KP, et al: Sickle cell-Hb Lepore Boston syndrome. Am J Dis Child 136:19, 1982

HEMOGLOBIN S/HEMOGLOBIN O-ARAB

Symptoms. Hand-foot syndrome (see) and symptoms of Herrick's (see).

Etiology. Double heterozygosity for HbS and hemoglobin O-Arab.

BIBLIOGRAPHY. Gilman PA, Abel AS: Acute splenic sequestration in hemoglobin O-Arab disease. Bull Johns Hopkins Hosp Bull 146:285, 1980

HEMOGLOBIN SC

See Herrick's.

Symptoms. In African Blacks and Jamaicans. Milder than in Herrick's. More frequent proliferative retinopathy.

Etiology. Double heterozygosity for HbS and HbC.

Prognosis. Better than in Herrick's.

BIBLIOGRAPHY. Balls SK, Lewis CN, Noone AM, et al: Clinical, hematological and biochemical features of HbSC disease. Am J Hematol 13:37, 1984

HEMOLYTIC ANEMIA OF NEWBORN

Synonyms. Congenital newborn anemia; erythroblastosis fetalis; hemolytic disease newborn, HDN; hydrops fetalis; icterus gravis neonatorum; Pfannestiel's, Schridde's.

Symptoms and Signs. From extremely severe form (stillbirth and hydrops fetalis) to simple serologic findings. In this vast spectrum fall clinical manifestations of variable severity; infants often born anemic, jaundiced, and edematous; or normal at birth and progressively developing jaundice and anemia. Liver and spleen usually palpable. Cutaneous purpura and bleeding from mucosa occasionally observed. Kernicterus syndrome frequent sequela. In some cases the inspissated bile syndrome (see) is observed.

Etiology. Isoimmunization of the mother by her fetus of different blood group. In 93% of cases due to a Rh positive/negative infant carried by Rh positive/negative mother. Difference in ABO groups may also cause hemolytic disease and other antigens c, C, C^w, C^x, E, also, but seldom involved. If mother sensitized against fetus by previous incompatible blood transfusion, firstborn may be affected; otherwise, usually firstborn is normal and hemolytic disease appears in successive pregnancies.

Pathology. Jaundice; edema; effusions of serous cavities; occasionally, purpura; extensive extramedullary hematopoiesis and hemosiderin deposits in enlarged spleen and liver and several other organs (adrenal; genital organs). In macerated fetus, erythroblast in the lung is characteristic sign. Brain may show generalized or icteric stain localized in basal ganglia.

Diagnostic Procedures. *Blood.* Anemia; nucleated cells up to 100,000/mm³; polychromatophilia; reticulocytosis; leukocytosis (15,000 to 30,000); platelets normal or decreased. Hyperbilirubinemia increasing to a peak of 20 mg/100 ml on third day after birth. If infant survives, progressive decrease afterward. Prothrombin and fibrinogen deficiency, occasionally. If condition due to Rh or some other group antibodies, cord blood erythrocytes give a positive direct Coombs' test. If due to ABO incompatibility, the test is negative, or only slightly positive. Indirect reaction positive at birth. Prenatal testing of mother usually shows an increasing titer of anti-Rh antibodies. *Spectrophotometric examination of amniotic fluid.* Obtained transabdominally. *X-rays.* Bone within first week of life shows radiolucent metaphyseal bands.

Therapy. Prophylactic use of anti-Rh immunoglobulin for prevention of active immunization of Rh negative mother. Given intramuscularly in Rh negative mother with Rh positive baby in whom there are no antibodies detected within 48 to 72 hours. Repeated prophylaxis in successive pregnancies after each delivery. Exchange transfusions to remove antibodies and bilirubin.

Prognosis. Prior to advent of exchange transfusion, mortality up to 80% or severe sequelae. With modern treatment and prophylaxis, much improved.

BIBLIOGRAPHY. Schridde H: Die angeborene allgemeine Wassersucht. MM Wochen 57:397–398, 1910

Levine P, Stetson RE: An unusual case of intragroup agglutination. JAMA 113:126, 1939

Behrman RE, Vaughan VC: Nelson's Textbook of Pediatrics, pp 383–388. Philadelphia, WB Saunders, 1983

HEMOPHILIA, CLASSIC

Synonyms. AHG deficiency; antihemophilic globulin deficiency; bleeder's; factor VIII deficiency; hemophilia A.

Symptoms and Signs. *Incidence.* 60 to 80 per million. Occur in males (with a few exceptions in homozygous females); onset from birth (umbilical hemorrhage; circumcision); more frequently when child begins to crawl and walk; occasionally later in childhood. Spontaneous, intramuscular, mucous membrane, gastrointestinal, pulmonary, pleural, intracranial, genitourinary tract, joint (with resultant hemarthrotic changes) hemorrhages. Spontaneous hemorrhages may have cyclic (3 to 6 weeks) character. A mild form of the disease exists where manifestations are less severe.

Etiology. Congenital deficiency of Factor VIII; X-linked recessive type of inheritance. Female carrier may have a decreased amount of Factor VIII. In hemophilialike syndrome in female, circulating anticoagulant explains the hemorrhagic manifestations. Cases of females with hemophilia, without family history, are not explained. Possible mutation has been postulated; or Lyon's hypothesis, which assumes that only one of the X chromosomes is functional.

Pathology. That of bleeding in different organs and tissues; hemarthrosis.

Diagnostic Procedures. *Blood.* Normal bleeding time; normal or prolonged clotting time; usually, increased partial thromboplastin time; usually, abnormal thromboplastin generation test; abnormal absorbed plasma reagent in Factor VIII deficiency; normal or abnormal prothrombin consumption test; Factor VIII assay is diagnostic; normal one-stage prothrombin time.

Therapy. Transfusion of fresh whole blood when blood loss; for prevention, fresh, frozen plasma, plasma concentrate, or concentrate antihemophilic globulin (AHG) preparation. Local therapy with topical thrombin. Corticosteroids also useful. Initially, good results with marrow transplantation.

Prognosis. Death in first 5 years of life in 57% of cases. Surgical procedures frequent cause of death. In mild form, prognosis relatively better.

BIBLIOGRAPHY. Otto JC: An account of an hemorrhagic disposition existing in certain families. M Repository 6:1, 1803

Epstein I (ed): The Babylonian Talmud, Yebamoth Sec 64B, Vol 1, p 431. London, Soncino Press, 1936

Wright AE: On a method of determining the condition of blood coagulability for clinical and experimental purposes, and on the effect of the administration of calcium salts in haemophilia and actual or threatened hemorrhage. Br Med J 2:223–225, 1938

Aledort LM (ed): Recent advances in hemophilia. Ann NY Acad Sci 240, 1975

Wintrobe MM (ed): Clinical Hematology, 8th ed. Philadelphia, Lea & Febiger, 1981

HEMORRHAGIC, NEONATAL

Synonyms. Hemophilia neonatorum; neonatal hemorrhagic diathesis; melena neonatorum; morbus hemorrhagicus neonatorum; neonatal diathesis.

Symptoms and Signs. Both sexes affected; onset in first few days of life. Spontaneous (seldom massive; usually oozing type) external and internal hemorrhages: skin (30%), gastrointestinal tract (70%); umbilical cord (25%); brain, lungs. Signs according to site and extent of hemorrhage.

Etiology. *Maternal factors.* Dietary deficiency; poor absorption of vitamin K. *Constitutional factors.* Functional immaturity of liver. More severe physiologic hypoprothrombinemia observed in between 2nd and 6th day after birth. *Acquired factors.* Trauma or hemorrhage at delivery with depletion of coagulation factors. Not hereditary.

Pathology. According to site and extent of hemorrhage.

Diagnostic Procedures. *Blood.* Anemia; bleeding time and clotting time usually prolonged; prothrombin level low.

Therapy. Blood transfusion if needed; vitamin K parenterally immediately after delivery.

Prognosis. Cases with limited external hemorrhage not serious; internal hemorrhage, 70% mortality. Rapid course; death or complete recovery in 2 to 3 days.

BIBLIOGRAPHY. Lovegren E: Erfahrungen und Studien über Melaena neonatorum. Jahrb Kinderheilk 78:249, 1913

Wintrobe MM (ed): Clinical Hematology, 8th ed. Philadelphia, Lea & Febiger, 1981

HEMORRHAGIC SHOCK AND ENCEPHALOPATHY

Synonym. HSES.

Symptoms. Loss of consciousness; cyanosis; agonal respiration; focal and generalized convulsions.

Signs. Hypotension; extreme hypothermia; diaphoresis; hypertonicity; brisk reflexes.

Etiology. Excessive wrapping and warming of infants (hyperpyrexial) for a mild upper respiratory tract infection.

Pathology. Cell loss, swelling and pyknosis, in Purkinje cells of both cerebral as well as cerebellar cortex.

Diagnostic Procedures. Laboratory evidence of renal, hepatic, coagulation and metabolic disfunction.

Prevention. Do not keep mildly ill children excessively warm.

Therapy. Resuscitation; lowering of body temperature; anticonvulsants.

Prognosis. Significant motor and intellectual deficits.

BIBLIOGRAPHY. Levine M, Kay JDS, Gould JD, et al: Hemorrhagic shock and encephalopathy: a new syndrome with a high mortality in young children. Lancet II:64–67, 1983

Whittington LK, Roscelli JD, Parry WH: Hemorrhagic shock and encephalopathy: further description of a new syndrome. J Pediatr 106:599–602, 1985

Sofer S, Phillip M, Hershkowits J, Bennet H: Hemorrhagic shock and encephalopathy syndrome: its association with hyperthermia. Am J Dis Child 140:1252–1254, 1986

HEMORRHOIDAL-PROSTATIC-IMPOTENCE

Symptoms and Signs. Sexual impotency developing in patient with internal hemorrhoids.

Etiology. No detectable anatomic or physiologic mechanism. (Possible vascular prostatic congestion.) Psychic factors primary cause or component of etiology.

Therapy. Hemorrhoidectomy.

Prognosis. Good with therapy.

BIBLIOGRAPHY. Cantor AJ: Hemorrhoidal-prostatic-impotence syndrome. NY State J Med 46:1455–1456, 1946

HENCH-ROSENBERG

Synonyms. Hench's; palindromic rheumatism.

Symptoms. Sudden attack of pain from moderate to very severe, and swelling of joints, reaching its peak in a few hours. Attacks occur at any time of day, but most often in late afternoon. Attack lasts and completely recedes in 1 or 2 days (occasionally lasts 7 days). Finger joint, usually of dorsum or hand, knees, wrists, shoulder, ankles, elbows, temporomandibular, sternoclavicular; cervical vertebra less frequently. Absence of constitutional effects. Occasionally, periarticular attacks, painful swelling involving periarticular or soft tissues (heel bottom; finger pads; flexor or dorsal surfaces of forearms; ankle tendon).

Signs. Swelling of periarticular tissue; skin discolored, reddish, or red. Variable degree of disability of articulation. Nonarticular attacks show brown discoloration,

firm consistency, nonpitting, tenderness. Some patients show the sudden appearance of nodules that usually disappear within 1 week.

Etiology. Unknown. In some cases response to irritant or allergens.

Pathology. Acute nonspecific cellular exudates in synovial cavities, reverting to normal with cessation of attack. Nodules: nonspecific inflammation.

Diagnostic Procedures. *Blood.* Moderate lymphocytosis, moderate elevation of sedimentation rate during attack. All tests for rheumatoid arthritis or rheumatism negative. Occasionally, increase of blood lipids and fatty acids.

Therapy. None specifically indicated. Long remission reported with the use of gold salts. Corticosteroids only in severe forms. Prophylaxis of attack by indomethacin or phenylbutazone.

Prognosis. Repeated attacks 50%; complete remission 10%; evolution into rheumatoid arthritis or other collegen diseases 40%.

BIBLIOGRAPHY. Hench PS, Rosenberg EF: Palindromic rheumatism; "new" often recurring disease of joints (arthritis, periarthritis, para-arthritis) apparently producing no articular residues—report of 34 cases; its relation to "angioneural arthrosis," "allergic rheumatism" and rheumatoid arthritis. Arch Intern Med 73:293–321, 1944

Schumacher HR: Palindromic onset of rheumatoid arthritis: clinical, synovial fluid, and biopsy studies. Arthritis Rheum 25:361–369, 1982

HENNEBERT'S

Synonyms. Luetic-otitic-nystagmus; syphilitic-otitic-nystagmus; vertigo-nystagmus-luetic.

Symptoms and Signs. Occur in children. Short, spontaneous attacks of giddiness and nystagmus. Fistula symptom without fistula: compression with finger of external auditory meatus or pulling the tragus elicits spontaneous nystagmus. Tympanic membrane intact.

Etiology. Congenital syphilis.

Pathology. That of congenital syphilis.

Diagnostic Procedures. *Serology.*

Therapy. Penicillin; antisyphilitics.

Prognosis. This symptom complex is a transient phenomenon, occasionally encountered in congenital syphilis.

BIBLIOGRAPHY. Hennebert C: Réactions vestibularies dans les labyrinthites héredo-syphilitiques. Arch Int Laryngol Otol 28:93–96, 1909

Asherson N: Spontaneous nystagmus in congenital syphilis. Arch Dis Child 5:331–334, 1930

Geeraets WJ: Ocular Syndromes, 3rd ed. Philadelphia, Lea & Febiger, 1976

HENOCH'S

This eponym is sometimes used in place of the term *Schönlein-Henoch* (see) when abdominal manifestations are predominant.

HEPATIC FLEXURE

See Gas syndromes.

Symptoms. Feeling of abdominal fullness and desire to eructate. Pain in right renal zone, epigastrium, left upper abdominal hypochondrium, right shoulder.

Signs. Sometimes, increased tympansim, right hypochondrium.

Etiology. Collection of gas in hepatic flexure of colon. If gas collects in splenic flexure, called splenic flexure syndrome.

Diagnostic Procedures. *X-ray.* Flat plate of abdomen.

Therapy. Removal of anatomic or functional obstruction.

BIBLIOGRAPHY. Palmer ED, Deutsch DL, Scott NM Jr: Clinical experiences with the splenic flexure syndrome and the hepatic flexure syndrome. Am J Dig Dis 22:194–197, 1955

HEPATORENAL SYNDROMES

Synonyms. Bile nephrosis; cholemic nephrosis; Flint's; Heyd's; Urohepatic.

Vague term that means any renal disease that occurs in patient with liver pathology. Laboratory evidence of renal involvement (oliguria-azotemia), frequently found in all types of liver pathology, the pathophysiologic interrelationship between liver and kidney has not yet been clarified. Deposition of pigment and other hemodynamic alterations have been considered. Practical therapeutic considerations to be kept in mind in such conditions are to restrict salt in spite of hyponatremia and avoid administration of diuretics if at all possible.

LIVER CIRRHOSIS

1. Cirrhosis associated with prerenal uremia–functional renal failure: minimal urine sodium concentration; absence of proteinuria; normal renal histology.
2. Cirrhosis associated with acute tubular necrosis: typical biochemical changes (high urine sodium concentration; isosmolality of urine); typical histologic pattern.
3. Alpha-1 antitrypsin deficiency.

Etiology. Cause of renal dysfunction has been uncertain for a long time. In some cases compression of inferior vena cava decreases renal blood flow, glomerular filtration rate, and sodium excretion. The compression of the inferior vena cava may precede the formation of ascites when due to caudate lobe compression. Neurogenic vasoconstriction; false neurotransmitters; renin-angiotensin system role; possible role of endotoxins.

Pathology. A wide spectrum of alterations, from normal renal histology to tubular necrosis. Numerous glomerular lesions, papillary necrosis, pyelonephritis, interstitial nephritis have been described as well. Immunofluorescence: IgA in mesangium and capillary.

Diagnostic Procedures. *Hepatic function tests, kidney function tests, determination of inferior vena cava pressure.* Strong correlation observed between caval pressure and glomerular filtration rate and urinary sodium excretion.

Therapy. That of cirrhosis. Demonstration of constriction of vena cava by caudate lobe is a necessary precautionary measure prior to portacaval surgery. Conservative management of renal failure.

Prognosis. Poor.

FULMINANT HEPATIC FAILURE

The association with renal failure (functional renal failure or acute tubular necrosis) is found in 80% of patients with fulminating hepatic failure.

Etiology. Related to endotoxins.

Pathology. See Liver cirrhosis.

Therapy. That of basic condition. Results with dialysis better than in cirrhosis. Treatment (including persevering with dialysis) may result in complete recovery in some cases. *Liver transplantation.*

Prognosis. Poor.

OBSTRUCTIVE JAUNDICE

Various degrees of kidney insufficiency occurring in association with any cause of obstruction of biliary tract (e.g., neoplastic; inflammatory; surgical).

Etiology. Enhanced absorption of endotoxin from intestine due to lack of biliary salts; depression of reticuloendothelial function; sensitization of renal parenchyma to anoxia by bilirubin and bile salts.

Pathology. Fibrin deposits in kidney and tubular necrosis.

Therapy. Surgical. If needed, dialysis.

Prognosis. Fair.

SHOCK AND SEPSIS

In these conditions, frequent occurrence of jaundice and renal failure.

Etiology. Multifactorial: (e.g., large transfusion; endotoxins; reticuloendothelial system insufficiency).

Pathology. *Liver.* From simple cholestasis to centrilobular necrosis (according to length of shock period). *Kidney.* Different degrees and types of lesions from none to tubular necrosis and glomerulonephritis.

Therapy. That of shock; once stabilized, prolonged dialysis until situation is overcome.

Prognosis. Seldom, progression to hepatic failure. Good results with intensive treatment.

INFECTIVE

Some particular infections affect both liver and kidney. Hepatitis B (especially in children of certain geographic areas (Asia, Eastern Europe, Africa). See also Yellow fever.

MISCELLANEOUS

1. Polycystic disease
2. Glomerulonephritis (immune complex type) associated with chronic hepatitis B and other conditions.

BIBLIOGRAPHY. Flint A: Clinical report on hydroperitoneum based on the analysis of 46 cases. Am J Med Sci 45:306–339, 1863

Heyd CG: The liver and its relation to chronic abdominal infection. Ann Surg 79:55–77, 1924

Brenner BM, Rector FC: The Kidney, 3rd ed, p 1050. Philadelphia, WB Saunders, 1986

HERLITZ'S

Synonyms. Epidermolysis bullosa hereditaria letalis; Heinrichsbauer's; junctional, lethal epidermolysis bullosa.

Symptoms and Signs. Present at birth. Bullous skin lesions. Fever; absence of residual scarring; bullous lesions of mucosae; loss of nails from toes and fingers.

Etiology. Unknown; recessive type of inheritance.

Pathology. Skin cleavage at the dermoepidermal junction with bulla formation present but not marked. Regeneration of basal cells at the edges of areas of ulceration;

absence of inflammatory reaction and edema; characteristic vacuolization of basal part of germinal layer of epidermis. Other organs negative findings.

Diagnostic Procedures. *Biopsy of skin. Blood.* Severe progressive hypoalbuminemia.

Therapy. Symptomatic; antibiotics; steroids not effective.

Prognosis. Death within 1 year.

BIBLIOGRAPHY. Herlitz G: Kongenitaler nicht syphilitischer Pemphigus Eine Übersicht nebst Beschreibung einer neuen Krankheits-Form (Epidermolysis bullosa hereditaria letalis). Acta Paediatr 17:315–371, 1935

Roberts MH, Howell DRS, Bramhall JL, et al: Epidermolysis bullosa letalis. Pediatrics 25:283–290, 1960

Rook A, Wilkinson DS, Ebling FJG, et al: Textbook of Dermatology, 4th ed, pp 1623–1624. Oxford, Blackwell Scientific Publications, 1986

Kaplan R, Stranch D: Regional anesthesia in a child with epidermolysis bullosa. Anesthesiology 67:262–264, 1987

HERMAN'S

Not a well-defined entity, it represents the combination of possible neurologic symptomatology following a closed head injury. See Livedo reticularis.

BIBLIOGRAPHY. Herman E: Niezwyklyzespól oprazowy: livedo racemosa universalis u osobnika z objawami piramidwopozapiramidowymi i zaburzeniami psychicznymi. Warsz Czas Lek 14:107–109, 1973

Walt AJ, Wilson RF: Management of trauma. Pitfalls and Practice, p 201. Philadelphia, Lea & Febiger, 1979

HERMANSKI-PUDLAK

Synonyms. Albinism-hemorrhagic diathesis; albinism-thrombocytopathy; HPS; delta storage pool disease.

Symptoms and Signs. Prevalent in Puerto Ricans, but also in other ethnic groups. Both sexes affected; onset from birth. Pigment disorder with variable phenotypic expression of degrees of pigmentation affecting skin, hair, and eyes. Nystagmus; photophobia. Hemorrhagic episodes: usually, mild bleeding, seldom massive; easy bruisability; epistaxis; hemorrhages after tooth extraction and trauma (aspirin may intensify hemorrhages). Restrictive lung disease and ulcerative colitis may develop (see Diagnostic Procedures).

Etiology. Unknown. It is the combination of three defects (albinism, hemorrhagic diathesis, and storage of abnormal lipidlike material) attributed to a pleiotropic effect of a single autosomal recessive mutation. Suspected enzymatic defect.

Pathology. In skin, from no visible pigment to dermatization of granular melanin. Generalized infiltration by a yellow pigment (ceroid-lipofuscinlike) of spleen, liver, lungs, lymph nodes, and other organs. *Electron microscopy.* Presence of granules in circulating leukocytes and bone marrow full of pigment.

Diagnostic Procedures. *Blood.* Morphologic, chemical, and functional defects of platelets. Blood clotting abnormalities. Leukocytes with two types of cytoplasmatic inclusions: ceroidlike and fibrillar membrane-bound. *Bone marrow.* Presence of pigment-laden macrophages, which stain sea blue. *X-ray.* Changes similar to interstitial pulmonary fibrosis. *Hair incubation test.* Increased pigmentation after addition of L-tyrosine.

Therapy. None. Avoid aspirin and nonsteroidal antiinflammatory drugs.

Prognosis. Variable, from minor bleeding episodes to massive fatal hemorrhages.

BIBLIOGRAPHY. Hermanski F, Pudlak P: Albinism associated with hemorrhagic diathesis and unusual pigmentated reticular cells in bone marrow. Blood 14:162–169, 1959

Witkop CJ, Quevedo WC, Fitzpatrick TB: Albinism and other disorders of pigment metabolism. In Stanbury JB, Wyngaarden JB, Fredrickson DS, et al: The Metabolic Basis of Inherited Disease, 5th ed, p 301. New York, McGraw-Hill, 1983

HERMAPHRODITISM, TRUE

Symptoms and Signs. Present from birth. Incidence very rare. Two hundred patients have been reported. External genitalia usually ambiguous or of apparently normal male or female aspect (20%); phallus usually bound in chordee; hypospadias; labioscrotal folds incompletely fused usually present; cryptorchidism (see) frequent. At puberty, variable prevalence of one phenotypic functional features, breast development, menses, some virilization characteristics.

Etiology. Genetic disorders (70% chromatin-positive; the majority with 46 XX karyotype; a lower percentage with 46 XY). Chimerism; hidden mosaicism. Mutant gene and environmental factors have been implicated. Underlying mutation could be transmitted by the father as an autosomal dominant trait.

Pathology. Both ovarian and testicular tissue in the same gonad or opposite ones. The "ovotestis" with a fallopian tube in 65% and a vas in 45% of cases.

Diagnostic Procedures. *Hormonal studies. Karyotype. Biopsy of the gonads.*

Therapy. Planned according to the age of diagnosis. In newborn, after sex dominance assessment, removal of heterologous structures (e.g., either ovary or testis, mullerian duct) integrated with plastic surgery according to role decided upon. Eventual hormonal integration.

Prognosis. Variable according to degree of "confusion" and adequacy of treatment. Incidence of tumor higher than in people with normal gonads. In rare cases, ovulation and pregnancy described. Fertility in male not reported.

BIBLIOGRAPHY. Milner WA, Garlick WB, Fink AJ, et al: True hermaphrodite siblings. J Urol 79:1003–1009, 1958

Rosenberg HS, Clayton GW, Hsu TC: Familial true hermaphroditism. J Clin Endocrinol 23:203–206, 1963

Fraccaro M, Tiepolo L, Zuffardi O, et al: Familial XX true hermaphroditism in three siblings: plasma hormonal profile and in vitro steroid biosynthesis in gonadal structures. J Clin Endocr 42:653–660, 1976

Emery AEH, Rimoin DL: Principles and Practice of Medical Genetics, Vol. 1. Edinburgh, Churchill Livingstone, 1983

HERPES GESTATIONIS

Synonyms. Dermatitis gestationis; prurigo gestationis. Pemphigoid gestationis

Symptoms. Less than 1 case every 60,000 pregnancies; onset during second trimester. Severe form recurring after delivery, during menstrual periods. Severe burning and itching on face, arms, legs, and trunk.

Signs. Multiform erythematous, vesicular, pustular, and bullous lesions that spread over the body centripetally, beginning around the umbilicus.

Etiology. High responsiveness of patient and possibly exposure to antigens derived from sexual consort. Condition hormonally modulated (balance of estrogen/progesterone responsible).

Pathology. Epidermal and papillary edema with (nonconstant) eosinophilic spongiosis subepidermal. Bullae.

Diagnostic Procedures. *Blood.* Eosinophilia up to 30%.

Therapy. Corticosteroids; adrenocorticotropic hormone (ACTH); in most severe cases: plasmapheresis. Dapsone and pyridoxine useless.

Prognosis. Good; disappears spontaneously a few weeks after delivery. May recur (in more severe form) during successive pregnancy. Severe form recurrent at menstrual cycles. Risk to fetus is minor (neonatal death reported).

BIBLIOGRAPHY. Milton JL: The Pathology and Treatment of Disease of the Skin, p 205. London, Hardwicke, 1972
Holmes RC, Black MM: Symposium on blistering diseases. Dermatol Clin 1:195, 1983

HERPETIFORM DERMATITIS, SENILE

Synonyms. Bullous pemphigoid; old-age pemphigus; parapemphigus; pemphigoid.

Symptoms and Signs. Both sexes affected; onset usually after 60 years of age (80%). Nonspecific urticarial or eczematous rash of extremities. In urticarial type, after 2 to 3 weeks, formation of bullae; in eczematous type, after months. Sudden generalization follows (erythema multiformlike) bullae with clear serum, occasionally hemorrhagic. Reabsorption, without lesion or erosion, which heals rapidly, leaving hyperpigmentation. Mucosal lesions rare.

Etiology. Unknown; French authors consider it a variant of Stevens-Johnson syndrome.

Pathology. No acantholysis; subepidermal bullae.

Therapy. None.

Prognosis. Spontaneous remission; recurrences possible. Death from complication (pneumonia).

BIBLIOGRAPHY. Rook A, Waddington E: Pemphigus and pemphigoid. Br J Dermatol 65:425–431, 1953
Rook A, Wilkinson DS, Ebling FJG, et al: Textbook of Dermatology, 4th ed, pp 1631–1639. Oxford, Blackwell Scientific Publications, 1986

HERRICK'S

Synonyms. African hemolytic anemia; sickle cell hemolytic anemia; hemoglobinopathy S; meniscocytosis; sickle cell; Chwechweechwe, Nwiiwii, Nuiduidui, Abotutuo (African tribe names); SS disease.

Symptoms. Occur particularly in Blacks, also in Greeks, Italians (especially Sicilians), and in Turkish families; more common in females. Increased fatigability. Subject to the occurrence and spontaneous remission of several symptoms. Sudden increase in weakness; severe pain in joints (in children, see Hand and Foot) and elsewhere in extremities. Abdominal cramps, epigastrium or right abdominal quadrant (simulating acute abdomen); fever (during crisis). Spontaneous hematuria; epistaxis; neurologic manifestations: headache; drowsiness; hemiplegia; aphasia; blindness (temporary or permanent).

Signs. Skin pale; mild subicterus of skin and mucosae; underweight; short trunk and long extremities; occasionally, dorsal kyphosis and lumbar lordosis; chest anteroposterior enlargement. Facial hair scanty. Heart enlarged; tachycardia; sinus arrhythmia, systolic thrill on precordium; diastolic tap in pulmonic area; accentuation of second sound. Abdominal or extremity tenderness or both (during crisis). Mild lymphadenopathy, as a rule; moderate hepatomegaly; seldom, splenomegaly. Chronic leg ulcers.

Etiology. Congenital hemoglobinopathy; autosomal intermediate inheritance. Presence of two hemoglobin S genes produce sickle cell anemia, while only one abnormal gene produces a sickle gene trait with only partial symptomatic manifestation.

Pathology. *Bone.* Deformities with abnormal calcifications. Generalized bone marrow hyperplasia and hemosiderosis except in smaller bones where fat substitution may be observed. Infarctions, necrosis, and hemorrhages of various tissues. *Liver.* Anoxic necrosis; hemochromatosis; erythrophagocytosis; in many cases micronodular cirrhosis. *Spleen.* Congestion with sickle cells; infarctions; eventually fibrosis and shrinkage (autosplenectomy). *Kidney.* Congestion; infarctions; necrosis and fibrotic calcific changes. *Nervous system.* Infarction and small hemorrhages.

Diagnostic Procedures. *Blood.* Anemia; anisopoikilocytosis; few drepanocytes; nucleated red cells; reticulocytes increased. Sickle cell test (drepanocytes developing for lack of oxygen). Leukocytosis with shift to the left; eosinophilia; increased monocytes. Platelets increased. Increased resistance to osmotic fragility. Low sedimentation rate. Hyperbilirubinemia. *Bone marrow.* Erythroid hyperplasia. *Urine.* Hematuria, decrease of kidney concentration ability after fluid deprivation. *X-ray of skeleton.* Abnormalities of bones; ground glass appearance of skull; peculiar radial striation, which may be noticed in other bones as well (vertebrae). Osteoporosis and osteosclerosis of long bones; pathologic fractures.

Therapy. Constant medical attention. Polyvalent pneumococcal vaccine. Folic acid administration. Hypertransfusion therapy. *In crisis.* Hydration, analgesics, antibiotics. Splenectomy in case of splenomegaly with hypersplenism. Antisickling agents are still in discussion. Bone marrow transplantation.

Prognosis. Good adaptation to anemic condition; partial remission of anemia occasionally observed, crisis of 4 to 6 days' duration recurrent at variable intervals (days or years). Majority die in first 10 years of life; few survive to fourth decade. Death from shock, intercurrent infections, cardiac and renal failure.

BIBLIOGRAPHY. Herrick JB: Peculiar elongated and sickle-shaped red corpuscles in a case of severe anemia. Arch Intern Med 6:517–521, 1910

Bunn HF, Forget BG: Hemoglobin: Molecular, Genetic and Clinical Aspects, p 502. Philadelphia, WB Saunders, 1986

HERRMAN'S

Synonyms. Facio-audio symphalangism; symphalangism-brachydactyly; WL (initials of patient); synostoses-multiple brachydactyly.

Symptoms and Signs. Both sexes. Deafness conductive type; facies peculiarities; broad nose; pectus carinatum; bilateral dysplasia and synostoses of elbow, wrist, fingers, and toes. Middle phalanges and metacarpals short. Nail malformations.

Etiology. Autosomal dominant inheritance.

BIBLIOGRAPHY. Herrman S: Symphalangism-brachydactyly syndrome: report of the WL symphalangism brachydactyly syndrome: review of the literature and classification. Birth Defects Orig Art Ser 10(5):23–53, 1974

Hurvitz SA, Goodman RM, Hertz M, et al: The facio-audio-symphalangism syndrome: report of case and review of the literature. Clin Genet 28:61–68, 1985

HERS'

Synonyms. Cori's type VI glycogenosis; Glycogenosis type VI; glycogen storage defect type VI; hepatic phosphorylase deficiency.

Symptoms. Both sexes affected, onset in infancy and early childhood. Symptoms may be so mild that syndrome may pass undetected. Moderate growth retardation; mild to moderate Harris' (S.) syndrome (see).

Signs. Marked hepatomegaly.

Etiology. Unknown; possibly, autosomal dominant type of inheritance. In these patients, a reduction up to 75% of liver phosphorylase has been found. Relationship between this biochemical defect and clinical manifestation not yet clearly established.

Pathology. Marked hepatomegaly. Glycogen accumulation. Biochemical study shows deficiency of phosphorylase activity. Other enzymatic activity apparently normal. No accumulation of glycogen in heart or muscles.

Diagnostic Procedures. *Blood.* In leukocytes, deficiency of phosphorylase activity. Glycogen in erythrocytes and leukocytes normal.

Therapy. Dietary management of hypoglycemia.

Prognosis. Excellent; normal growth and development with the exception of persisting hepatomegaly.

BIBLIOGRAPHY. Hers HG: Études enzymatiques sur fragments hepatiques application à la classification des glycogenoses. Rev Intern Hepatol 9:35–55, 1959

Howell RR, Williams JC: The glycogen storage diseases. In Stanbury JB, Wyngaarden JB, Fredrickson DS, et al: The Metabolic Basis of Inherited Disease, 5th ed, p 141. New York, McGraw-Hill, 1983

HERSMAN'S

Synonyms. Progressive hand growth, Macrodactyly.

Symptoms and Signs. Progressive growth of hands without other signs of macroacromia or endocrine involvement.

BIBLIOGRAPHY. Hersman CF: A case of progressive enlargement of the hands. Intern Med Mag 3:662–665, 1894

Milford L: Congenital anomalies. In Crenshaw AH (ed): Campbell's Operative Orthopedics, 7th ed, pp 428–429. St. Louis, CV Mosby, 1987

HERTWIG–MAGENDIE

Synonyms. Vertical diplopia; Magendie-Hertwig; skew deviation.

Symptoms. Vertical diplopia. Various associated symptoms of neurologic nature. See Etiology.

Signs. One eye faces down and the other one up and out.

Etiology and Pathology. Trauma or neurosurgery; atherosclerosis or neoplasia resulting in vascular brainstem lesions; primary cerebellar tumors; metastatic posterior fossa lesions; mesencephalic lesions; demyelinizing syndromes; syringobulbia; or as an isolated neurologic sign (vertical strabismus simulating skew deviation).

Diagnostic Procedures. *Screen and cover test. Examination of old photographs. To detect previous strabismus. X-ray of skull. Angiography. Pneumoencephalography. Brain isotope scan.*

Therapy. According to etiology.

Prognosis. Depends on etiology.

BIBLIOGRAPHY. Hertwig H: Experimenta quaedam de effectibus laesionum in partibus encephali singularibus et de verosimili harum partium functione, Berolini, formis Feisterianis et Eiserdorffianis [1926]. Ind Cat Surg Gen 1st series 6:185, 1885

Pötzl O, Sittig O: Klinische Befunde wit Hertwig—Magendiescher Augeneinstellung. Z Ges Neurol Psychiatr 95:701–730, 1925

Smith JL, David NJ, Klintworth G: Skew deviation. Neurology 14:96–105, 1964

HERTWIG-WEYERS

Synonyms. Aplasia ulnae multiple bone and visceral malformations; oligodactyly-ulnar hemimelia.

Symptoms and Signs. Present from birth. Ulnar aplasia associated with variable bone (sternum; jaw) or visceral (kidney; spleen) abnormalities.

Etiology. Unknown; possibly hereditary recessive or new mutation.

BIBLIOGRAPHY. Hertwig P: Sechs neue Mutationen bei der Hausmaus in ihrer Bedeutung für allgemeine Vererbungsfragen. Z Mensch Vereb 26:1–21, 1942

Weyers H: Das Oligodactylie-syndrome des Menschen und seine Parallelmutation bei der Hausmaus. Ann Paediatr (Basel) 189:351–370, 1957

HERXHEIMER'S

Synonyms. Atrophic chronic acrodermatitis; acrodermatis chronica atrophicans; Pick-Herxheimer's; Taylor's.

Symptoms. Insidious onset in country dwellers between 30 and 90 years of age; rare in childhood; occur mostly in north central European, Italian, and Spanish peoples. Insidious onset. Itching; burning; constitutional symptoms.

Signs. Reddish nodules or plaques appear on feet or legs, less frequently on forearms and hands, rarely affecting trunk or face. Slow, progressive peripheral inflammatory extension, while the central part of lesions shows hairless skin, pigmented or poikilodermatous. The nodules concentrate around knees and elbows, the fibrous bands along ulnar margins. Possible ulcerations on the legs.

Etiology. Unknown. Incriminated infective agents transmitted by *Ixodes ricinus.*

Pathology. *Skin.* Initially, dermal edema and perivascular inflammations; later, skin atrophy with destruction of appendages. Subdermal lymphocyte and histiocyte infiltration. *Lymph nodes.* Sinus catarrh; plasma cell infiltration.

Diagnostic Procedures. *Biopsy of skin.* See Pathology. *Blood.* High red cell sedimentation rate; hypergammaglobulinemia.

Therapy. Penicillin for 1 to 2 weeks in initial stages.

Prognosis. Fair response to early treatment. Once atrophy established, no response. In some cases, involvement of joints with resulting limitation of functions of articulation (e.g., feet, hands, shoulders). Rare, squamous cell carcinoma development in atrophic cases.

BIBLIOGRAPHY. Pick PJ: Erythromelie. Festschr Kaposi Wien, p 919, 1900

Herxheimer K, Hartmann K: Ueber Acrodermatitis chronica atrophicans. Arch Dermatol Syph 61:57–76, 1902

Rook A, Wilkinson DS, Ebling FJG, et al: Textbook of Dermatology, 4th ed, pp 1807–1808. Oxford, Blackwell Scientific Publications, 1986

HIBERNOMA

Synonyms. Fetalocellulare lipoma. Granular cell lipoma.

Symptoms. Rare; occur in both sexes; onset usually in early adult life. Asymptomatic.

Signs. On the cervical, axillary, or intrascapular regions (in order of incidence), appearance of a firm, nontender nodule, with vascular dilatation of the overlying skin.

Etiology. Vestiges of brown fat.

Pathology. Encapsulated, multilobular tumor of primitive fetal fat (tan to dark brown) histologically multiloculated masses of cells with fine sudanophilic granules and solitary central nucleus.

Therapy. Excision.

Prognosis. Good.

BIBLIOGRAPHY. Jennings RC, Behr G: Hibernoma (granular cell lipoma). J Clin Pathol 8:310–312, 1955

Rook A, Wilkinson DS, Ebling FJG, et al: Textbook of Dermatology, 4th ed, p 1879. Oxford, Blackwell Scientific Publications, 1986

HIDRADENOMA ERUPTIVUM

Synonym. Syringoma.

Symptoms. More frequent in females; onset usually in adolescence. Chest, face, eyelids and neck areas mostly affected. Asymptomatic.

Signs. Small dermal papules (1–5 mm in diameter) yellowish in color, occasionally cystic; at onset, eruptive, then individual or group appearance. The lesions slowly expand to reach limited size (3–5 mm).

Etiology. Unknown; defective development of sweat ducts (?)

Pathology. Sweat ducts dilated and convoluted; lumina filled by amorphos debris. Characteristic strand of cells projecting from side of ducts like a comma.

Therapy. Diathermy for cosmetic reason.

Prognosis. Partial removal followed by relapse.

BIBLIOGRAPHY. Daicker B: Das lidsyringoma Studien über seinen geureblichen Bau und seine Histogenese. Dermatologica 128:417–463, 1964
Rook A, Wilkinson DS, Ebling FJG, et al: Textbook of Dermatology, 4th ed, pp 2407–2408. Oxford, Blackwell Scientific Publications, 1986

HIGH-ALTITUDE PULMONARY EDEMA

Synonyms. HAPE; noncardiac pulmonary edema.

Symptoms and Signs. Dyspnea; restlessness; cough. Rales heard diffusely or in an asymmetric pattern; mild fever.

Etiology. Not clear. Decrease of P_{O_2} causing marked nonuniform vasoconstriction of terminal pulmonary arterioles. Presence of preterminal arterioles emptying directly into venous side of pulmonary capillary bed and transmitting directly elevated pulmonary pressure and causing leakage of plasma or blood into parenchyma.

Pathology. See etiology. Damage of arterial walls, microthrombi obstructing pulmonary vascular bed (occasionally).

Diagnostic Procedures. *Blood.* Mild leukocytosis. P_{O_2} decreased. *Chest x-ray.* Patchy irregular infiltrates.

Therapy. Bed rest and oxygen.

Prognosis. Good.

BIBLIOGRAPHY. Kliner JP, Nelson WP: High-altitude pulmonary edema: A rare disease? JAMA 234:491–495, 1975
Overland ES, Severinghaus JW: Noncardiac pulmonary edema. Ann Rev Med 23:307–311, 1978

HIGH-OUTPUT CIRCULATORY FAILURE

Synonym. Heart failure, high output. See Hyperkinetic heart.

Symptoms. Symptoms of right, or predominantly right, heart failure.

Signs. Cardiac enlargement and venous pressure elevation; diastolic pressure usually diminished; systolic and pulse pressure increased. All signs of congestive failure.

Etiology. Cardiac failure developing as complication of diminished circulatory resistance in various conditions. Arteriovenous fistula; hyperthyroidism; anemia; beriberi; severe pulmonary emphysema with hypoxemia; pregnancy; advanced Paget's disease and Albright's.

Pathology. See Etiology. Cardiac failure features. In this type of cardiac failure, initiating pathology is in the periphery not in the heart. Diminished peripheral resistance favors speeding of circulation.

Diagnostic Procedures. *Circulation time.* Rapid or normal. *Venous pressure.* Increased. *Cardiac catheterization. Echocardiograph. Special laboratory study.* Evaluation of thyroid function, search for beriberi condition, anemia, hepatic condition. *X-ray.* Assess the possible presence of Paget's disease of the bone (see).

Therapy. Control of heart failure; digitalis, sodium restriction, diuretics to correct failure and further increase cardiac output. Treatment of basic condition will restore the cardiac output to normal.

Prognosis. Depends on etiology.

BIBLIOGRAPHY. Hurst JW: The Heart, 6th ed, pp 395–403. New York, McGraw-Hill, 1986

HILGER'S

Synonym. Carotodynia.

Symptoms. Cephalgia and homolateral pain on the neck.

Etiology. Dilatation of carotid artery (?).

BIBLIOGRAPHY. Hilger JA: Carotid pain. Laryngoscope 59:829–838, 1949

HIRANO'S

Synonyms. Dementia-parkinsonism complex; Guam parkinsonism-dementia; Parkinsonism-dementia complex.

Symptoms and Signs. Observed on the island of Guam, exclusively among members of Chamorro tribe; age of onset 32 to 64 years of age (mean 52 years); predominant in males (31%); insidious onset (no preceding history of encephalitis or other febrile illness). Akinesia; masklike expressionless face; stooped posture; slow, shuffling gait; poor coordination of alternative movements and skilled actions. Generalized slowness of movements; mental deterioration; apathetic and indifferent depression. Tremor in mild or moderate degree (never major characteristic) or absent. Moderate or no appreciable rigidity; cogwheel phenomenon only in some cases. Generalized hyperreflexia in all cases. In some patients, symptoms and signs of amyotrophic lateral sclerosis. Cerebellar dysfunction not found.

Etiology. Unknown; autosomal dominant inheritance. This syndrome may be considered a clinical entity that represents a combination of Parkinson's and presenile dementia and amyotrophic lateral sclerosis, without, however, having all the characteristic features of each one of them. Only difference from Jakob-Creutzfeldt is that this syndrome has a much faster course.

Pathology. Macroscopically, cerebral atrophy, pallidal atrophy, loss of pigmentation in the substantia nigra and locus ceruleus. Microscopically, severe neuronal alterations associated with fibroses, Alzheimer's neurofibrillary changes, intracytoplasmatic granulovascular inclusion bodies, accumulation of intracytoplasmatic lipid granules. Loss of neurons most apparent in globus pallidus and substantia nigra.

Diagnostic Procedures. *Blood, urine, stool, cerebrospinal fluid.* Normal. *Electroencephalography.* Background pattern shows generalized 8- to 9-cycle activity of moderate voltage, with superimposed occurrence of frequent, intermittent, moderate voltage slower activity present in all leads with accentuation over temporal areas.

Therapy. Symptomatic.

Prognosis. Slow evolution but steady progression to death within 4 to 5 years from onset; 7% of deaths of Chamorro due to this syndrome.

BIBLIOGRAPHY. Hirano A, Kurland LT, Krooth RS, et al: Parkinsonism-dementia complex, endemic disease on island of Guam. I. Clinical features. Brain 84:642–661, 1961

Malamud N, Hirano A, Kurland LT: Pathoanatomic changes in amyotrophic lateral sclerosis on Guam. Arch Neurol 5:401–415, 1961

Adams RD, Victor M: Principles of Neurology, 3rd ed, p 872. New York, McGraw-Hill, 1985

HIRSCHSPRUNG'S

Synonyms. Aganglionic megacolon; congenital megacolon.

Symptoms. Prevalent in males (3:1); onset from birth. Intensity of symptoms according to length of involved segment. Obstipation; vomiting; rapid dehydration; small, narrow stool eventually passed. Infrequently, diarrhea may be the main symptom. If not treated, failure to thrive and weakness.

Signs. According to length and location of segment involved. Increased peristalsis; abdominal dilatation; elevation of diaphragm. Mass of feces palpated in lower abdomen, nontender and movable. Rectal examination shows normal anus and rectum, usually empty or with small, goaty fecal pellets. Impacted feces palpated anteriorly to the rectum. Complications are impaction, perforation, bleeding, and ulceration.

Etiology. See Pathology. Familial cases reported; no definite hereditary pattern established (polygenetic).

Pathology. Colon dilatation with thickening of wall above the point of lesion. Sharp demarcation between dilated and normal part. Microscopically, all wall layer hypertrophic, absence of ganglia at end and in proximity of narrowing point.

Diagnostic Procedures. *Sigmoidoscopy.* Distal segment normal; dilated part filled with impacted feces; mucosa reddened and with small ulceration. *Biopsy of rectum.* Demonstration of aganglionosis. *X-ray.* Narrowed zone of colon with marked proximal dilatation.

Therapy. Surgical removal of aganglionic zone. In mild case, conservative medical treatment. With surgical treatment, 50% immediate recovery, 34% control within 5 years, 16% persistent mild symptoms.

Prognosis. If untreated, varies from development of megacolon in adult life to death in severe form.

BIBLIOGRAPHY. Hirschsprung H: Stuhlträgheit Neugeborener in folge von Dilatation und Hypertrophie des Colons, Jahrb Kinderheilk 27:1–7, 1888

Hirschsprung H: Erneiterung und Hypertrophie des Dickdarms. Berl Klin Wochenschr 36:977, 1899

Jayle F: La dilatation congenitale idiopathique du colon observee an XVII siecle. Presse Med 17:803, 1909

Ikeda K, Goto S: Diagnosis and treatment of Hirschsprung disease in Japan: an analysis of 1628 patients. Ann Surg 199:400–405, 1984

Garver KL, Law JC, Garver B: Hirschsprung disease: a genetic study. Clin Genet 28:503–508, 1985

HIRSUTISM, ESSENTIAL

Synonyms. Constitutional hirsutism; term *hirsutism* restricted to androgen-dependent hair patterns; term *hypertrichosis* restricted to other patterns of excessive hair growth.

Signs. Occur in females. Increased amount of body hair (on face, chest, abdomen, and extremities) without changes of secondary sexual characteristics.

Etiology. Unknown; familial, racial.

Diagnostic Procedures. *Hormone study.* Normal hormone excretion and secretion. See other hirsutism syndromes for differential diagnosis.

Therapy. Shaving.

BIBLIOGRAPHY. Lipsett MB, Migeon CJ, Kirscher MA, et al: Physiologic basis of disorders of androgen metabolism. Combined Clinical Staff Conference at the National Institutes of Health. Ann Intern Med 68:1327–1344, 1968

Fenton DA: In Dawber R, Rook A (eds): Seminars in Dermatology, Vol 4, p 43. New York: Thieme-Stratton, 1985

Rook A, Wilkinson DS, Ebling FJG, et al: Textbook of Dermatology, 4th ed, pp 1965–1966. Oxford, Blackwell Scientific Publications, 1986

HISTIDINEMIA

Synonym. Hyperhistidinemia.

Symptoms. Both sexes affected; normal at birth. General physical development normal or slight retardation in 50%. Speech retardation noticed in 50% of patients. Intelligence normal or retarded.

Etiology. Unknown; probably autosomal recessive inheritance.

Pathology. None.

Diagnostic Procedures. *Blood and urine.* Increased plasma and urinary concentration of histidine and alanine (positive ferric chloride and phenystix test).

Therapy. Trial with low histidine diet.

Prognosis. All cases described alive. Mental retardation in some cases.

BIBLIOGRAPHY. Ghadimi H, Partington MW, Hunter A: A familial disturbance of histidine metabolism. New Engl J Med 265:224, 1961

Ghadimi H: Diagnosis of inborn errors of amino acid metabolism. Am J Dis Child 114:433–439, 1967

La Du BN: Histidinemia. In Stanbury JB, Wyngaarden JB, Fredrickson DS, et al: The Metabolic Basis of Inherited Disease, 4th ed, p 317. New York, McGraw-Hill, 1978

HISTIOCYTOSIS SYNDROMES

Synonyms. Histiocytosis X (discontinuation of this term's use suggested); Lichtenstein's.

CLASS I: *Langerhans-cell histiocytosis (LCH)*
Inclusion of clinical syndromes that share the following diagnostic elements suggested:
A. For diagnostic confidence
 1. Positive stain for ATPase
 2. s-100 protein
 3. Alpha-D-mannosidase or
 4. Characteristic binding of peanut lecithin
B. For definitive confidence
 1. Birbeck granules in lesional cells by electron microscopy or
 2. Demonstration of T-6 antigenic determinants on the surface of lesional cells
Letterer-Siwe (see); Hand-Schüller-Christian (see); Lichtenstein-Jaffe's (see); Hashimoto-Pritzker (see); Pure cutaneous histiocytosis, Langerhans-cell granulomatosis; Type II histiocytosis and the old term, nonlipid reticuloendotheliosis.

CLASS II: *Histiocytoses of mononuclear phagocytes other than Langerhans cells.* Hemophagocytic lymphohistiocytosis; infection-associated hemophagocytic; sinus histiocytosis reticulohistiocytoma.

CLASS III: *Malignant histiocytic.* Acute monocytic leukemia; malignant histiocytosis; histiocytic lymphomas; histiocytic sarcomas.

BIBLIOGRAPHY. Writing group of the Histiocyte Society. Histiocytosis syndromes in children. Lancet 1:208–209, 1987

HNEVKOVSKI'S

Synonyms. Vastus intermedius contracture; progressive fibrosis vastus intermedius.

Symptoms and Signs. More common in females and in twins. Onset between 1 and 7 years of age. Monolateral (occasionally bilateral). From mild to severe limitation of flexion of knee. No effusion. Occasionally, palpable dense band, tensing during knee flexion proximal to patella in the quadriceps. Mild proximal dislocation of patella occasionally subluxated.

Etiology. Unknown.

Pathology. Fascia of thigh adherent to quadriceps muscles and fibrosis and contraction of vastus intermedius. Increase of fibrosis tissue and fat decrease in muscle fibers.

Diagnostic Procedures. *Muscle biopsy.*

Therapy. Division of fascia and vastus intermedius. Conservative treatment ineffective.

Prognosis. Excellent with surgery.

BIBLIOGRAPHY. Hnevkovsky O: Progressive fibrosis of the vastus intermedius muscle in children: a cause of limited knee flexion of the patella. J Bone Joint Surg 43B:318–324, 1961

Justis EJ Jr: Nontraumatic disorders. In Crenshaw (ed): Campbell's Operative Orthopedics, 7th ed, pp 2247–2248. St Louis, CV Mosby, 1987

HITZENBERGER'S

Synonyms. Hereditary methemoglobinemia; idiopathic methemoglobinemia. Eponym used (mostly in past literature) to indicate Gibson's (see) and Hoerlein-Weber (see).

BIBLIOGRAPHY. Hitzenberger K: Autotoxische Zyanose (Intraglobulaere Methämoglobinämia). Wien Arch Inn Med 23:85–96, 1932

HMG CoA LYASE DEFICIENCY

Synonyms. Leucine metabolism defect; hydroxymethylglutaric aciduria.

Symptoms and Signs. Normal at birth. Then vomiting, cyanosis, lypothymia, lethargy, metabolic acidosis, hypoglycemia. Recurrence of episodes.

Etiology. Autosomal recessive inheritance. Deficiency of HMG CoA lyase.

Diagnostic Procedures. *Blood.* Hypoglycemia. Metabolic acidosis. *Urine.* Excretion of HMG, and related substances.

Therapy. Correction of hypoglycemia.

Prognosis. If recovery from episodes, good, however, death occurs early.

BIBLIOGRAPHY. Faull K, Bolton P, Halpern B, et al: Patient with defect in leucine metabolism. New Engl J Med 294:1013, 1976

Wilson WG, Cass MB, Sovik O, McKusick, et al: A child with acute pancreatitis and recurrent hypoglycemia due to 3-hydroxy-3-methylglutaryl CoA lyase deficiency. Europ J Pediatr 142:289–291, 1984

HODGKIN'S

Synonyms. Bonfil's; Hodgkin's granuloma; Hodgkin-Haltauf-Stemberg; HD; multiple lymphadenoma; malignant lymphogranulomatosis; Hodgkin's paragranuloma; Sternberg's disease.

Symptoms. *Incidence Rate.* 35:1 million in white males; 26:1 million in white females. Mixed incidence: three age periods 0 to 14, 15 to 34, 50 and over. *Sex.* 63% male; 37% female. Malaise; anorexia; weight loss; nausea; fever 30 to 50% (cyclic; continuous, intermittent or Epstein type); drenching sweats; pruritus; 10 to 15% early symptoms; 85% during course of disease. Lung involvement; brassy cough; dysphagia; alcohol intolerance 17 to 20% (not specific).

Signs. Painless; progressive enlargement of lymph nodes: cervical (60–80%); axillary (6–20%); inguinal (6–12%); mediastinal (6–12% initially, 60% in course of disease). Abdominal and peritoneal involvement frequent.

Lung. Clinical involvement in 40%; simulation of various tumors or infections. *Pleura.* Effusion in 33% by clinical detection, 60% in autopsy findings. *Abdomen.* Bleeding, obstruction; infiltration of walls; extrinsic pressure from retroperitoneal mass. *Spleen.* Splenomegaly 30% initially, 80% during course of disease. Secondary hypersplenism (anemia; thrombocytopenia; leukopenia). *Liver.* Hepatomegaly 33%; jaundice. *Bone.* Clinical involvement 30%; at autopsy 60%. *Central nervous system.* 10%. *Skin.* Excoriation produced by response to pruritus, or direct involvement.

Initially, or at late stage, any organ may be involved. Association with herpes zoster frequent (13%), occasionally repeated episodes; fungus infection (*Candida albicans* 11%, *Mucor; Aspergillus; Nocardia* especially if treated with corticoid or chemotherapy). Association with active tuberculosis in only 2% of cases. Abnormalities in immune response, autoimmune hemolytic anemia, amyloidosis, collagen diseases should not be considered as complication, but, in some not yet explained way, connected with the pathogenesis of the disease.

Etiology. Unknown; malignant neoplasm or malignant inflammation. Possibly more than one disease included in this diagnosis.

In differential diagnosis "great imitator" symptomatology may be confused with that of many diseases (other lymphomas; tuberculosis; brucellosis and other infections; neoplastic diseases).

Pathology. *Gross.* Lymph node involvement initially is usually confined to a single node or cluster of nodes. Nodes enlarged, well-defined, not adherent, firm. Cut surface shows nodular aspect with areas of dense, retracted, grayish-white (fish flesh) aspect. Different organ may be involved by the lymphomatous process in the form of extensive or nodular infiltration.

Microscopic. The morphologic expression of the disease is characterized by different combinations of the following features: lymphocytic or histiocytic proliferation (with the appearance of atypical, abnormal reticular elements: Reed-Sternberg cell) or both; diffuse or nodular fibrosis and variable degree of inflammatory reaction. The different histologic patterns resulting from the combinations of the mentioned findings have been grouped into three main categories: paragranuloma; granuloma; sarcoma. More recently a finer classification, which better correlates the clinical aspects of the condition with the histologic patterns, has been proposed by Lukes (see table).

Diagnostic Procedures. *Biopsy of lymph nodes* (see Pa-

Comparison Between Pathologic Classifications

Jackson Parker (1944)	Lukes (1963)
1. Paragranuloma	1. Lymphocytic and/or
	2. Nodular
2. Granuloma	3. Mixed
	4. Diffuse fibrosis
3. Sarcoma	5. Reticular hysticytic
	a. Diffuse
	b. Nodular

thology). *Blood.* Anemia; hemolytic anemia 80% (in late disease); Coombs' test usually negative; leukocytosis with neutrophilia 50%; eosinophilia (may be seen); leukocyte alkaline phosphatase elevated during active phase, decreased in remission; sedimentation rate elevated in active disease. Hypercalcemia 30%; hypophosphatemia; high alkaline phosphatases in bone involvement. Serum albumin decreased; globulin alpha-1 increased, alpha-2 increased, beta-2 increased, gamma decreased; low zinc; high copper. *X-ray.* Lymph node enlargement or tissue infiltration. *Tomography. Pyelography. Splenoportography. Radioisotope scan.* For lymphangiography and demonstration of liver and bone marrow, bone, spleen, and lung infiltration.

Therapy. See staging and treatment.

Staging and Treatment

	Stage I	Stage II	Stage III	Stage IV
Lymph node group	Single	Multiple, all localized either above or below diaphragm	Above and below diaphragm	Decreased
Parenchymal involvement	None	None	None	Lesion in any of the following: bone; bone marrow; lung; skin; subcutaneous; gastrointestinal tract (considered secondary)
Systemic symptoms	None	A, none B, +	A, none B, +	++++
Complications	None	None	±	+++
Treatments	X-ray (3,000–4,000γ) of local and contiguous nodes	X-ray, same as Stage I Chemotherapy	X-ray (palliative, 1,000–2,000γ) Chemotherapy* Cortisone and cortisonelike drugs Transfusion Antibiotics	
Prognosis (survival based on 5 years' staging)	71%	56%	15%	0
(survival based on 10 years' staging)	58%	35%	2%	0

* Chemotherapy: MOPP (mechlorethamine, Oncovin, Procarbazine, prednisone). Resistant cases: ABVD (Adriamycin, bleomycin, vinblastine, dacarbazine).

Prognosis. Prognosis based on anatomic and pathologic features of lymph node biopsy. (1) Numerous mature, well-differentiated lymphocytes: favorable prognosis. (2) Lymphocytes depletion associated either with fibrosis or numerous Reed-Sternberg cells: poor prognosis. (3) The form designated "nodular sclerosis": good prognosis although there is lymphocyte depletion.

Complications Causing Death

Severe infections	21%
Failure of pulmonary function	20%
CNS involvement	11%
GI bleeding	10%
Liver failure	7%

BIBLIOGRAPHY. Hodgkin T: On some morbid appearances of the absorbent glands and spleen. Medico Chir Trans 17:68–114, 1832; Cancer Research 26:1045–1311, 1966
Teillet F, Bayle-Weisgerber C: Traitement de la maladie de Hodgkin. Encyclopédie Medico Chirurgicale Sang 13030 B60-6, 1981
Fuller LM, Hagemeister FB, Sullivan MP, et al: Hodgkin's disease and non-Hodgkin lymphomas in adults and children. New York, Raven, 1988

HOERLEIN-WEBER

Synonyms. Congenital methemoglobin; M hemoglobin; hereditary methemoglobinemia; Tamyra-Takahashi; Kuchikuro (black mouth); Nigremid hereditary black blood. See Gibson's.

Symptoms and Signs. Both sexes affected; onset of cyanosis at birth (alpha-substituted M hemoglobin) or at 6 to 12 months of age (beta chain mutants). In alpha-substituted, asymptomatic, no exercise intolerance. In beta-substituted, usually pallor, splenomegaly.

Etiology. Autosomal dominant inheritance.

Diagnostic Procedures. *Blood.* Color chocolate brown; color does not change with shaking in air; hemoglobin electrophoresis (better after oxidation with potassium ferrocyanide).

Therapy. None.

Prognosis. Normal longevity and health.

BIBLIOGRAPHY. Hoerlein H, Weber G: Ueber chronische familiäre Methämoglobinemia und eine neue Modifikation des Methämoglobins. Dsch Med Wochenschr 73:476–478, 1947
Bunn HF, Forget BG: Hemoglobin: Molecular Genetic, and Clinical Aspects, p 623. Philadelphia, WB Saunders, 1986

HOFFA'S

Synonyms. Infrapatellar fat pad hypertrophy; Hoffa-Kaster; patellar fat pad hypertrophy.

Symptoms. Usually, long history of pain in anterior compartment of knee related to exertion. Occasionally, sharp pain may cause the knee to "give way."

Signs. Swelling due to the presence of enlarged fat pad. Mild effusion; forced extension reproduces pain; local tenderness with deep pressure.

Etiology. Hypertrophy of infrapatellar fat pad that causes nipping of synovial fringes between the condyles on extension of joint.

Pathology. Trauma of synovial membranes; hemorrhages; hypertrophy and fibrosis; occasionally, calcification.

Diagnostic Procedures. *X-ray and arthroscopy of knee.*

Therapy. *Conservative.* Addition of 25 mm (0.5 inch) to heel of shoes; quadriceps exercises. *Surgical.* In cases that do not respond to conservative treatment, excision of tags, reduction in size of fat pad.

Prognosis. Cured by surgical correction.

BIBLIOGRAPHY. Hoffa A: The influence of adipose tissue with regard to the pathology of knee joint. JAMA 43:795–796, 1904
Kaster J: Die Verwachsung des Kniegelenkfett Koeiers als selbastaengiges Krankheitsbild. Chirurg 24:390–394, 1953

HOFFMANN'S (E.)

Synonym. Projecting ear-everted lip-woolly hair.

Symptoms and Signs. Present from birth. Projecting ears; everted lower lip; sparse woolly hair.

Etiology. Unknown. Recessive inheritance.

BIBLIOGRAPHY. Hoffmann E: Ueber einen kräuselnaevus Innerhallo sonst glatten Kopfhaares im Vergleich zum erblichen Kraushaar und zur Lockenbildung näch Röntgenepilation. Dermatologica 107:281–291, 1953

HOFFMANN'S (J.) II

Synonyms. Myopathy-myxedema; myxedema myotonic dystrophy syndromes. This eponym is used to designate the muscular manifestations described in Kocker-Debré-Semelaigne (see) associated with myxedema in children.

Most likely no fundamental difference between Hoffmann's and Kocker-Debré-Semelaigne.

BIBLIOGRAPHY. Hoffmann J: Weiterer Beitrag zur Lehre von der Tetanie. Deutsch Z Nervenkr 9:278–290, 1897
Adams RD: In Werner SC (ed): The Thyroid, 2nd ed. New York, Hoeber Harper Row, 1962

HOFFMANN-ZURHELLE

Synonym. Nevus lipomatosus cutaneous superficialis.

Symptoms. Rare. Both sexes affected; lesions present at birth or appearing later, up to adolescence. Asymptomatic.

Signs. The buttock most frequent site. Presence of soft, round papules and yellowish nodes that slowly grow to form a confluent plaque. Occasionally hairy, with comedolike plugs.

Etiology. Unknown.

Pathology. Collection of ectopic fat cells in the dermis.

Therapy. None. Excision for cosmetic reason.

Prognosis. Good.

BIBLIOGRAPHY. Hoffman E, Zurhelle E: Ueber einen Naevus lipomatodes cutaneous superficialis der linken Glutäalgegend. Arch Dermatol Syph 130:227–333, 1921
Rook A, Wilkinson DS, Ebling FJG, et al: Textbook of Dermatology, 4th ed, p 193. Oxford, Blackwell Scientific Publications, 1986

HOLLENHORST'S

Synonym. Chorioretinal infarction.

Symptoms. Observed when the patient regains consciousness after surgery, when a headrest and faulty positioning of patient causes eye trauma. Unilateral blindness or only decrease of light perception.

Signs. Proptosis; lid edema; ecchymosis; dilated and fixed pupil; hazy cornea.

Etiology. Secondary eye trauma during surgery.

Pathology. See Signs. Retinal edema; pigmentary retinopathy.

Therapy. Symptomatic. Corticosteroids.

Prognosis. From persistent unilateral blindness to partial or total recovery of vision.

BIBLIOGRAPHY. Slocum HC, O'Neal KC, Allen CR: Neurovascular complications from malposition on the operating table. Surg Gynecol Obstet 86:729–734, 1948
Hollenhorst RW, Svien HJ, Benait CF: Unilateral blindness occuring during anesthesia for neurosurgical operations. AMA Arch Ophthalmol 52:819–830, 1954
Geeraets WJ: Ocular Syndromes, 3rd ed. Philadelphia, Lea & Febiger, 1976

HOLMES' I

Synonym. Cerebellar olivary degeneration; olivocerebellar degeneration.

Symptoms and Signs. Prevalent in males; onset gradual in sixth, or seventh decade. Progressive disturbance of gait; eventual uncertainty of movements of arms; speech changes (hesitant scanning and explosive). Later, cerebellar tremor and nystagmus. Mild hyperreflexia; no ankle clonus.

Etiology. Unknown; often familial.

Pathology. Progressive atrophy of cerebellar cortex; disappearance of Purkinje's cells and preserved basket cells. Involvement of cerebellar white matter; cerebellar nuclei spared. No changes in remainder of nervous system.

Diagnostic Procedures. *Pneumoencephalography. Spinal tap. CT brain scan.*

Therapy. None.

Prognosis. Good for survival. Progressive evolution with severe neurologic impairment.

BIBLIOGRAPHY. Holmes G: A form of familial degeneration of the cerebellum. Brain 30:466–488, 1907
Dow RS, Moruzzi G: The Physiology and Pathology of the Cerebellum. Minneapolis, University of Minnesota Press, 1958
Adams RD, Victor M: Principles of Neurology, 3rd ed, p 880. New York, McGraw-Hill, 1985

HOLMES' (A.F.)

Synonyms. Holmes' heart; single ventricle–great arteries normally related. See Single ventricle. Variety of single ventricle characterized by single ventricle and aorta arising from left or primitive ventricle and pulmonary trunk from right ventricular infundibulum or rudimentary outlet chamber.

BIBLIOGRAPHY. Holmes AF: Case of malformation of the heart. Trans Med Chir Soc Edinburgh 1:252, 1824
Perloff JK: The Clinical Recognition of Congenital Heart Disease, 2nd ed, p 644. Philadelphia, WB Saunders, 1978

HOLTHOUSE-BATTEN

Synonym. Honeycombed retina degeneration. See also Retina postpole colloidal degeneration.

Symptoms. Both sexes affected. Progressive visual loss.

Signs. Characteristic honeycombed deposition of hyaline and colloidal material in and about macula and posterior pole.

Etiology. Unknown; possibly, autosomal dominant inheritance.

BIBLIOGRAPHY. Kimura SJ, Caygill WM: Retinal Diseases. Philadelphia, Lea & Febiger, 1966

HOLT-ORAM

Synonyms. Atriodigital dysplasia; cardiac-limb; hand-heart.

Symptoms. Complete syndrome: congenital heart defects and upper extremities defect. Either isolated heart or upper extremity defects observed in members of same family. May be asymptomatic or cardiac symptoms such as dyspnea, fatigue, may be observed.

Signs. Congenital heart defects and upper extremity defects, including polydactyly and syndactyly. The association of radial defects (absence of a thumb on one side; hyperphalangeal thumb on the other side; manus vara; short radii; radioulnar synostosis) with heart defect are much more frequent than are ulnar defects.

Etiology. Idiopathic autosomal dominant inheritance with high degree of penetrance or secondary to antiepileptic drugs taken during first month of pregnancy.

Pathology. Secundum atrial septal defect and radial defect.

Diagnostic Procedures. Evaluation of heart defect. *X-ray of skeleton. Chromosome studies.* Reported as normal or with suggested abnormalities of pair 16. *Dermatoglyphic studies.* Show only abnormalities secondary to the musculoskeletal defects, and do not appear to be genetically determined.

Therapy. Symptomatic; orthopedic correction if feasible.

Prognosis. Depends on heart defect.

BIBLIOGRAPHY. Holt M, Oram S: Familial heart disease with skeletal malformations. Br Heart J 22:236–242, 1960
Kaufman RL, Rimoin DL, McAlister WH, et al: Variable expression of the Holt-Oram syndrome. Am J Dis Child 127:21–25, 1974

Gladstone I Jr, Sybert VP: Holt-Oram syndrome: penetrance of the gene and lack of maternal effect. Clin Genet 21:98–103, 1982

HOLZBACH-SANDERS

Synonyms. Cholestasis, intrahepatic in pregnancy; recurrent intrahepatic cholestasis-pregnancy; pregnancy-related cholestasis.

Symptoms and Signs. During third trimester of pregnancy, pruritus, icterus (may be absent), biliary colics. Shortly after delivery, disappearance of all symptoms.

Etiology. Autosomal dominant inheritance.

Pathology. Liver normal.

Diagnostic Procedures. *Blood.* Hyperbilirubinemia. Trait can be demonstrated between pregnancies by the administration of oral contraceptive with reproduction of the symptoms.

Therapy. Symptomatic.

BIBLIOGRAPHY. Holzbach RT, Sanders JH: Recurrent intrahepatic cholestasis of pregnancy: observation on pathogenesis. JAMA 193:542–544, 1965
Holzbach RT, Sivack DA, Braun WE: Familial recurrent intrahepatic cholestasis of pregnancy: a genetic study providing evidence for transmission of a sex-limited dominant trait. Gastroenterology 85:175–179, 1983

HOLZKNECKT'S

Eponym used to indicate a roentgenologic finding: the displacement of mediastinum to the right during inspiration occurring in patients affected by bronchial stenosis.

BIBLIOGRAPHY. Holzknekt G: Ein neues radioscopisches Symptom bei Bronchialstenose und Metodisches. Wein Klin Wehsch 13:785–787, 1899

HOMEN'S

Synonyms. Repeated brain concussion; posttraumatic brain; boxer's; Friedmann's; postconcussion; posttraumatic personality; punch drunk. Dementia pugilistica.

Symptoms and Signs. Slurring of speech; rigidity of limbs and unsteady gait; poor memory; insomnia; irritability; headache; occasionally, vertigo; diminished intellectual faculties to progressive dementia.

Etiology. Lesion of lentiform nucleus, due frequently to chronic trauma (see Cerebral concussion), or as sequelae to a type of progressive subacute encephalitis due to trauma (Friedmann's).

BIBLIOGRAPHY. Homen EA: Eine eigenthümliche Familien Krankheit unter der Form progressiven Dementia, mit besanteren anatomischen Befund. Neurol Zbb 9:514–518, 1890

Friedmann AP, Brenner C, Denny Brown D: Post-traumatic vertigo and dizziness. J Neurosurg 2:36, 1945

Adams RD, Victor M: Principles of Neurology, 3rd ed, p 655–656. New York, McGraw-Hill, 1985.

HOMOCARNOSINOSIS

Synonym. Homocarnosinase deficiency.

Symptoms and Signs. In Norwegian pedigree. Both sexes. Progressive spastic paraplegia, retinal pigmentation.

Etiology. Autosomal recessive inheritance. Lack of homocarnosinase.

Pathology. *Cerebral biopsy.* Atrophy of cortex.

Diagnostic Procedures. *Liquor.* High homocarnosine content. *Blood and urine.* Normal.

Therapy. None.

Prognosis. Progressive condition.

BIBLIOGRAPHY. Gjessing LR, Sjaastad O: Homocarnosinosis: a new metabolic disorder associated with spasticity and mental retardation. Lancet II:1028, 1974

Lemey JF, Pepper SC, Kucera CM, et al: Homocarnosinosis: lack of serum carnosinase is the defect probably responsible for elevated brain and CSF homocarnosine. Clin Chim Acta 132:157–165, 1983

HOMOLOGOUS BLOOD

Synonym. Sequestration–desequestration.

Symptoms and Signs. During extracorporeal circulation, the injection of large volume of homologous blood results in decrease of effective circulating blood volume with significant hypotension, which, to be corrected, requires further blood infusion, far in excess of calculated blood balance. The hypotension is progressive and continues in the first postoperative day, during which tachypnea, cyanosis, hypoxemia, severe pulmonary congestion, vascular stasis on nail bed compression are noted. Subsequently, there is a return to normal of plasma and red cell volume. However, if large volume of blood has been used to correct the postperfusion hypotension, hypervolemia develops.

Etiology. Intensity and severity of manifestations depend on body size of patient, amount of blood injected, and duration of injection. Blood sequestration (in lungs) induced by infusion of homologous blood, resembling the changes occurring with histamine shock.

Diagnostic Procedures. *Blood.* Metabolic acidosis and postperfusion anemia.

Therapy. Use of washed red cells; reduction of extracorporeal priming volume; substitution of electrolyte solutions for a part of homologous blood; reutilization of patient's own blood collected from pleural and precordial spaces during surgery. At the completion of perfusion, maintenance of normotension, but use of only minimum amount of blood and integration with cardiotonic and vasopressor agents. Maintenance of isotopic normovolemia should not be attempted; subsequent blood loss from oozing must be only partially replaced in anticipation of expected desequestration.

Prognosis. When pulmonary complications develop, poor (about 50% survival).

BIBLIOGRAPHY. Gadboys HL, Slonim R, Litwak RS: Homologous blood syndrome. I. Preliminary observations on its relationship to clinical cardiopulmonary bypass. Ann Surg 156:793–804, 1962

Gadboys HL, Jones AR, Slonim R, et al: The homologous blood syndrome. III. Influence of plasma, buffy coat and red cells in provoking its manifestation. Am J Cardiol 12:194–202, 1963

HONEYCOMB ATROPHY

Synonyms. Atrophodermia reticulata; folliculitis ulerymatosa.

Symptoms and Signs. Both sexes. Typical skin lesion symmetrical. Limited areas of skin atrophy causing pits with sharp edges and "wormeaten" or "honeycomb" appearance. Occasionally associated: oligophrenia, neurofibromatosis (see von Recklinghausen's), cardiac defects.

Etiology. Sporadic or autosomal recessive defect.

BIBLIOGRAPHY. Carol WLL, Gotfried EG, Prakken JR, et al: Recklingausensche Neurofibromatosis, Atrophodermia vermiculata und Kongenitale Herzanomalie als Haupkennzeichen eines familiaer-hereditaeren syndroms. Dermatologica 81:345–365, 1940

Kooij R, Veuter J: Atrophodermia vermiculata with unusual localisation and associated congenital anomalies. Dermatologica 118:161–167, 1959

HONEYMOON CYSTITIS

Synonyms. Honeymoon cystitis; honeymoon pyelitis.

Symptoms. Occur in females after frequent sexual intercourse. Dysuria; pollakiuria; perineal discomfort; chills; fever; flank pain. Occasionally, nausea, vomiting, abdominal pain, ileus; or only fever and chills.

Signs. Tenderness in upper or lower abdomen, frequently on costovertebral angle palpation.

Etiology. Cystitis. Gram-positive or more frequently gram-negative bacteria.

Pathology. Inflammatory signs in bladder, ureter(s), kidney collecting system.

Diagnostic Procedures. *Blood.* Leukocytosis shift to the left. *Urine.* Proteinuria; white cells and leukocyte casts. *Intravenous urography.* To be carried out in all patients.

Therapy. Antibiotics.

Prognosis. Recovery of acute phase in 5 days (90%).

BIBLIOGRAPHY. Papper S: Clinical Nephrology, 2nd ed, p 275. Boston, Little, Brown 1978

HOOFT'S

Synonyms. Familial hypolipemia; Hypolipemia–tryptophan abnormality.

Symptoms and Signs. Present from birth. *Hair.* Thin; singed; dry. *Teeth.* Abnormal. *Skin.* Squamous, erythematous rash, and opaque leukonychia. *Eye.* Tapetoretinal degeneration. Mental retardation. Growth delay.

Etiology. Unknown; autosomal recessive inheritance. Absence of coenzymes pyridine nucleotide for transformation of tryptophan into 5-hydroxylated derivatives and indolacetic acid.

Diagnostic Procedures. *Blood.* Cholesterol 90 to 115 mg/100 ml; low phospholipids; no acanthocytosis. *Urine.* Indoluria; hyperaminoaciduria. *Fat absorption test.* Normal.

Therapy. None.

BIBLIOGRAPHY. Hooft C, De Lacy P, Herpal J, et al: Familial hypolipidemia and retarded development without steatorrhea. Another inborn error of metabolism? Helv Paediatr Acta 71:1–23, 1962
Herbert PN, Gotto AM, Fredrickson DS: Familial lipoprotein deficiency. In Stanbury JB, Wyngaarden JB, Fredrickson DS, et al: The Metabolic Basis of Inherited Disease, 4th ed, p 569. New York, McGraw-Hill, 1978

HOPF'S

Synonym. Acrokeratosis verruciformis.

Symptoms and Signs. Both sexes affected; present at birth or appearing in early childhood. On back of hands and feet, knees or elbows, and forearms, presence of verrucous papules and colored skin. Occasionally, presence of crops of similar lesions on other skin areas; in some cases, diffuse thickening of palmar skin with small areas of hyperkeratosis. Friction may produce bullae formation. Nails are thicker, whitish, in some cases stripped.

Etiology. Unknown; autosomal dominant inheritance. Apparently, linkage with Darrier's (see).

Pathology. Hyperkeratosis and acanthosis with thick granular layer. Absence of vacuolization.

Therapy. Topical application of keratolytic and emollient agents.

Prognosis. Chronic condition. Moderate response to treatment.

BIBLIOGRAPHY. Hopf G: Ueber eine bisher nicht beschriebene disseminierte Keratose (Acrodermatosis verruciformis). Dermatol Z 60:227–250, 1931
Rook A, Wilkinson DS, Ebling FJG, et al: Textbook of Dermatology, 4th ed, p 1145. Oxford, Blackwell Scientific Publications, 1986

HOPPE-THURMAN

Synonym. Congenital aneurysms of Valsalva sinuses; aortic sinus aneurysm.

Symptoms and Signs. Three clinical patterns observed:
1. *Imperforate aneurysm.* Asymptomatic in most cases; or variable symptomatology according to size and location: continuous murmur (flow to and from aneurysm); right ventricular outflow obstruction; tricuspid regurgitation; various types of heart block; anginal pains.
2. *Small perforation of the aneurysm.* Occasionally, initially, asymptomatic. Minor dyspnea and continuous murmur may precede for years the onset of congestive failure.
3. *Large perforation of the aneurysm.* Predominant in males (4:1). Onset between puberty and 30 years of age and seldom out of this range. Severe retrosternal or abdominal pain, marked dyspnea, lasting hours or days, then receding with fair subsidence of symptoms. Wide pulse pressure; vigorous pulsation in the neck. After a variable period; congestive heart failure progressing to death.

Etiology. Congenital or acquired defect.

Pathology. Blind pouch originating from one of the Valsalva sinuses (right or noncoronary 95%) and projecting fingerlike into heart cavities. Rupture usually at the tip may communicate with right atrium or ventricle, pulmonary artery, left ventricle and atrium, or pericardial cavity. Crista supraventricularis septal defect is frequently associated.

Diagnostic Procedures. *Electrocardiography, echocardiography, x-rays.* Variable findings according to pathology. *Cardiac catheterization. Aortography.*

Therapy. Surgical correction in cardiopulmonary bypass.

Prognosis. Extremely variable according to pattern. Survival into old age or sudden death in early adulthood or sooner. Interval between sudden large rupture and death from immediate to 1 year.

BIBLIOGRAPHY. Hope J: A treatise on the Diseases of the Heart and Great Vessels, 3rd ed. London, J. Churchill, 1839
Thurman J: On aneurysms, and especially spontaneous varicose aneurysms of the ascending aorta and sinuses of Valsalva; with cases. Med Chir Trans (London) 23:323–384, 1840
Hurst JW: The Heart, 6th ed, pp 620–621. New York, McGraw-Hill, 1986

HORNER'S

Synonyms. Bernard-Horner; Claude Bernard-Horner; cervical sympathetic paralysis; sympathetic ophthalmoplegia; sympathetic cervical paralysis. See Bernard's.

Symptoms and Signs. Miosis (paradoxical pupillary dilatation may occur after a few days from onset with emotional or physical stress). Ptosis; apparent or minimal exophthalmos; hypotonia oculi. Rise in temperature of homolateral side of face; lacrimation increased or decreased; hemifacial anhidrosis (lesion below bifurcation of common carotid artery). Occasionally, development of cataract. Depigmentation of iris (when syndrome occurs in children).

Etiology. Interruption of sympathetic chain in any part of its path. Trauma; surgery; neoplasm; thrombosis; aneurysm.

Pathology. See Etiology.

Diagnostic Procedures. *Ophthalmologic.* Failure of the pupil to dilate with cocaine. Supersensitivity to adrenergic amines (test for differentiation between preganglionic and postganglionic cervical lesions). *Angiography. CT brain scan. Spinal tap.*

Therapy. According to etiology.

Prognosis. Depends on etiology. Adrenergic supersensitivity may persist for many years.

BIBLIOGRAPHY. Bernard C: Des phénomènes oculopupillaires produits par la section du nerf sympathique cervical; ils son indèpendents des phénomènes vasculaires caloriques de lat tête. C R Acad Sci [D] Paris 55:381–382, 1862
Horner F: Ueber eine Form von Ptosis. Klin Monatsbl Augenheilka 7:193–198, 1869
Adams RD, Victor M: Principles of Neurology, 3rd ed, p 208. New York, McGraw-Hill, 1985
Van der Wiel HL, Van Gijn J: The diagnosis of Horner's syndrome: use and limitations of the cocaine test. J Neurol Sci 73:311–316, 1986
Woodruff G, Buncic JR, Morin JD: Horner's syndrome in children. J Pediatr Ophthalmol Strabismus 25:40–44, 1988

HORNOVÁ-DLUHOSOVÁ

Synonym. Oral conjunctival amyloidosis–mental retardation.

Symptoms. A brother and sister affected. Discovered within first year of life. Swelling of eyelids with nodular deposition of amyloid in the conjunctiva; congenital cataracts; ocular bulb atrophy; amaurosis; gingiva show amyloid deposits as well (icinglike). Mental retardation.

Etiology. Unknown.

BIBLIOGRAPHY. Hornová J, Dluhosová O: Primary amyloidosis of gingiva and conjunctiva and mental disorder, in a brother and sister. Oral Surg 25:451–466, 1968

HORTON'S

Synonyms. Cranial arteritis; temporal arteritis; Horton-Gilmour: Horton-Magath-Brown; giant cell arteritis. See Polymyalgia rheumatica.

Symptoms. Occurs in old age group (7th and 8th decade), seldom before age 55; affects both sexes equally. Unilateral or bilateral, localized, severe headache in region of temporal artery. Systemic manifestations: anorexia; insomnia; weight loss; low-grade fever. When process spreads to ophthalmic artery, blindness may result.

Signs. Swelling, tenderness over temporal artery area; arteries thickened, prominent, often pulseless.

Etiology. Unknown; included in the collagen diseases group. Autosomal dominant inheritance observed in some families, possibly on the same basis as other autoimmune conditions (see Polymyalgia rheumatica, Hashimoto's, lupus erythematoid, Addison-Biermer, etc.).

Pathology. Granulomatous arteritis and periarteritis changes. The process is often diffuse to involve arteries in several organs.

Diagnostic Procedures. *Blood.* Increase of sedimentation rate; leukocytosis; increase of alpha-2 globulin fraction. *Biopsy of artery.*

Therapy. Adrenocorticotropic hormone (ACTH) and corticosteroids; surgery in case of severe refractory pain.

Prognosis. Self-limited; course several months. Residual manifestation may be blindness.

BIBLIOGRAPHY. Hutchinson J: Diseases of arteries. Arch Surg (London) 1:323, 1890

Horton BT, Magath TB, Brown GE: An undescribed form of arteritis of temporal vessels. Proc Mayo Clin 7:700, 1932

Granato JE, Abben RP, May WS: Familial association of giant cell arteritis: a case report and brief review. Arch Intern Med 141:115–117, 1981

Adams RD, Victor M: Principles of Neurology, 3rd ed, pp 138–139. New York, McGraw-Hill, 1985

HOUSEMAID'S KNEE

Synonyms. Prepatellar bursitis; nun's knee. See "Beat Knee."

Symptoms. Pain in the knee when kneeling.

Signs. Swelling of the anterior aspect of knee; palpable granules.

Etiology. Chronic or acute trauma of prepatellar bursa; secondary infection.

Pathology. Thickening of prepatellar bursa walls; loose bodies in the cavity.

Diagnostic Procedures. *X-ray.* Acute swelling of soft tissue; chronic radiopaque bodies in the bursa.

Therapy. Protection against further irritation. Injection of corticosteroids; x-ray therapy; ultrasonic treatment; surgical removal for refractory case.

Prognosis. Good with treatment.

BIBLIOGRAPHY. Justis EJ: Nontraumatic disorders. In Crenshaw AH (ed): Campbell's Operative Orthopedics, 7th ed, pp 2253–2254. St Louis, CV Mosby, 1987

HOUSSAY'S

Synonyms. Vanishing diabetes mellitus; Houssay-Biasotti. See Pituitary apoplexy syndrome.

Symptoms and Signs. The symptoms and signs of diabetes disappear while symptoms and signs of hypopituitarism become suddenly or progressively evident. Generally there is a lack of clearly specific clinical features except in the fulminating type of hypopituitarism.

Etiology. Necrosis or infarction of pituitary in diabetic patients. (See Pituitary infarction.)

Pathology. Necrotic lesion of pituitary; according to duration of syndrome, adrenal atrophy and other features of panhypopituitarism develop.

Diagnostic Procedures. *Blood.* Hypoglycemia. Persistence of abnormal tolerance curve. Decrease in urinary gonadotropin, corticoids, and 17-ketosteroids.

Therapy. Correction of hypoglycemia, and other features of hypopituitarism with adrenocorticotropic hormone (ACTH), corticoids.

Prognosis. Poor.

BIBLIOGRAPHY. Houssay BA, Biasotti A: La diabetes pancreatica de los perros hipofisoprivos. Rev Soc Argent Biol 6:251–296, 1930

Calvert RJ, Caplin G: The Houssay syndrome. Br Med J 2:71–74, 1957

HOWSHIP-ROMBERG

Synonyms. Obturator hernia; Romberg-Howship; von Romberg-Howship.

Symptoms. More common in women; onset especially in old age. Recurrent pain along thigh, radiating to the knee; if strangulation is generalized, abdominal pain.

Signs. Moving hip exacerbates pain in leg and abdomen. Palpation of abdomen reveals rigidity; rectal examination allows palpation of mass.

Etiology. Congenital abnormality of obturator canal.

Pathology. Sac passing through obturator foramen.

Therapy. Surgery.

Prognosis. High incidence of strangulation and irreducibility.

BIBLIOGRAPHY. Howship J: Practical Remarks on the Discrimination and Appearance of Surgical Disease. London, Churchill, 1840

Romberg MH: In Dieffenbach: Operative-Chirurgie. Leipzig, 1848

Arbman G: Strangulated obturator hernia: a simple method for closure. Acta Chir Scand 150:337–339, 1984

HUGHES-STOVIN

Synonym. Pulmonary artery aneurysm–peripheral vein thrombosis.

Symptoms. Prevalent in males (all but one case reported); onset from 14 to 37 years of age. Recurrent episodes of fever that do not respond to antibiotics; hemoptysis; symptoms from recurrent pulmonary, dural sinus, and peripheral vein thrombosis; frequently at onset, intracranial hypertension and/or optic neuritis.

Signs. Murmur or thrill over aneurysm of pulmonary artery.

Etiology. Unknown.

Pathology. Aneurysm of large and small pulmonary arteries and thrombosis of veins. Association with congenital cardiac defects.

Diagnostic Procedures. *Blood.* Clotting studies. *X-rays of chest.* Variable pattern. *Electrocardiography. Angiography.* Similar findings on Behçet's.

Therapy. None effective.

Prognosis. Poor; terminal event massive hemoptysis.

BIBLIOGRAPHY. Hughes JP, Stovin PGI: Segmental pulmonary-artery aneurysm with peripheral vein thrombosis. Br J Dis Chest 53:19–34, 1959

Durieux P, Bletry O, Huchon G, et al: Multiple pulmonary aneurysms in Behçet's disease and Hughes-Stovin. Am J Med 71:736–741, 1981

HUGUIER-JERSILD

Synonyms. Genitoanorectalis elephantiasis; genitoanorectal; Jersild's; penoscrotal lymphedema. See also Lymphedema.

Symptoms. Both sexes affected, but prevalent in females; more frequent onset in adult life. Pain; dysuria; stypsis.

Signs. Presence of initial ulcer, papula, or herpetiform lesion that causes lymphedema in the pelvic region. Edema, initially pitting, then becoming harder; hyperkeratosis may develop later as well as secondary infections.

Etiology. Lymphogranuloma venereum; syphilis; seldom, gonorrhea or other infections.

Pathology. Lymphatic obstruction; edema; secondary fibrosis; infection; hyperkeratosis.

Therapy. Antibiotics.

Prognosis. Good results with early treatment. Disappointing result in advanced forms.

BIBLIOGRAPHY. Huguier PC: Mémoire sur l'esthiomène ou dartrerogeante de la région vulvo-anale. Mem Acad Med (Paris) 14:501–514, 1849

Jersild O: Elephantiasis genito-anorectalis. Dermatol Wchnscr 96:433–481, 1933

Rook A, Wilkinson DS, Ebling FJG, et al: Textbook of Dermatology, 4th ed, p 2198. Oxford, Blackwell Scientific Publications, 1986

HUIJING-FERNANDES

Synonyms. Glycogenosis type VIII; glycogenosis type VI A; phosphorylase "b" kinase defect; Hug's.

Symptoms and Signs. Occur in males. Asymptomatic except for hepatomegaly. Heterozygote females may show moderate symptoms.

Etiology. X-linked inheritance.

Diagnostic Procedures. *Blood.* In leukocytes low activity of phosphorylase "b" kinase. *Biopsy of liver.* Increased glycogen storage; 90% deficit of phosphorylase "b" kinase activity.

Therapy. None.

Prognosis. Good.

BIBLIOGRAPHY. Huijing F, Fernandes J: X-chromosomal inheritance of liver glycogenosis with phosphorylase kinase deficiency. Am J Hum Genet 21:275–284, 1964

Hug G, Schubert WK, Chuck G: Deficient activity of dephosphorylase kinase and accumulation of glycogen in the liver. J Clin Invest 48:704–715, 1969

Howell RR, Williams JC: The glycogen storage diseases. In Stanbury JB, Wyngaarden JB, Fredrickson DS, et al: The Metabolic Basis of Inherited Disease, 5th ed, p 141. New York, McGraw-Hill, 1983

HUNGRY BONES

Synonym. Postsurgical hypoparathyroidism.

Symptoms and Signs. Follows parathyroidectomy. Those of hypocalcemia (see) associated with hypomagnesemia (see) and hypophosphatemia.

Etiology. Removal of hyperfunctioning parathyroids. The condition is determined by a great excess of bone formation over bone resorption. A mild form is seen during early healing of rickets or osteomalacia and with osteoblastic metastases from breast, prostate, and lung carcinoma.

Therapy. Aggressive treatment with calcium, vitamin D, calcitonin, etidronate disodium.

Prognosis. Good with treatment.

BIBLIOGRAPHY. Sackner MA, Spivak AP, Balian LJ: Hypocalcemia with presence of osteoblastic metastases. New Engl J Med 262:173–176, 1960

Brenner BM, Rector JGJ: The Kidney, 3rd ed, p 582. Philadelphia, WB Saunders, 1986

HUNNER'S

Synonyms. Bladder submucosae ulcer; interstitial cystitis; elusive ulcer; Hunner's ulcer.

Symptoms and Signs. Occur in women; onset insidious in postmenopausal period (at 40 to 60 years of age). Pollakiuria; stranguria.

Etiology. Unknown. Apparently related to hormonal imbalance or psychological factors or both.

Pathology. Bladder contracted; wall edematous; epithelium thinned; ulcers of difficult identification. Ulcers shallow; increased vascularization with degenerative changes of vessels; submucosa infiltrated by mononucleated and polynucleated cells; fibrous tissue increased; involving all layers of bladder.

Therapy. Hormones, antibiotics, and anti-inflammatory agents.

Prognosis. Slow and progressive evolution.

BIBLIOGRAPHY. Hunner GL: Consideration of a new viewpoint on the etiology of renal tuberculosis in women. Am J Obstet 24:704–708, 1932

HUNTER'S

Synonyms. Iduronate sulfatase deficiency; mucopolysaccharidosis (MPS) II; sulfoiduronate sulfatase deficiency. (In past literature referred to as mild Hunter's gargoylism, or Hurler-Hunter.)

Symptoms. Males affected (cases in females rare but not unknown); clinical onset in infancy or childhood. A mild form and a severe form distinguished; however, the severe one is less severe than Hurler's. Symptomatology very similar in both conditions. Mental retardation (less severe than in Hurler's); deafness (constant feature); no visual impairment (or appearing late in the course of the disease). Chronic diarrhea in many cases. Hoarseness in a limited number of cases.

Signs. Dwarfism; grotesque facial features; joint stiffness; dorsal gibbus (less evident than in Hurler's); nodular lesions on posterior thorax and arms (unique to this type of mucopolysaccharidosis). Corneal clouding (evident only on slit lamp examination). In some cases, atypical retinitis pigmentosa. Hepatosplenomegaly. In adult rosy cheeks and plethoric facies.

Etiology. Autosomal; X-linked recessive inheritance; about 33% of cases represent a new mutation. Deficiency of iduronate sulfatase.

Pathology. Identical to those of Hurler's.

Diagnostic Procedures. *Serum and cells.* Test directly and indirectly for assay of iduronate sulfatase. *Urine.* Equal amount of dermatan sulfate and heparan sulfate, but high rate of the latter is frequent. *X-ray.* Dysostosis multiplex.

Therapy. None available. Experimental evaluation of normal plasma and lymphocyte infusion.

Prognosis. In severe form, death in adolescence, usually from heart failure after progressive mental deterioration; in mild forms, survival into old age with several degrees of manifestation from minimal (allowing a normal life) to relatively severe with marked impairment.

BIBLIOGRAPHY. Hunter C: A rare disease in two brothers. Proc R Soc Med 10:104–116, 1917

McKusick VA, Neufeld EF: The mucopolysaccharide storage diseases. In Stanbury JB, Wyngaarden JB, Fredrickson DS, et al: The Metabolic Basis of Inherited Disease, 5th ed, p 751. New York, McGraw-Hill, 1983

HUNTINGTON'S

Synonyms. Chronic progressive chorea; degenerative chorea; Lund-Huntington; microcellular-striatal; Mount's.

Symptoms. Insidious onset between 30 and 45 years of age or earlier. Gradual increase of choreiform movements in early stages. Patient may be mistaken for drunk. Muscle movements become very violent and finally in later stage decrease to akinesia. Mental deterioration, usually concurrent with chorea progressing to dementia. Death from coronary artery disease is frequent and may occur before 10 years of age.

Etiology. Autosomal dominant programmed, premature selective neural cell death.

Pathology. Brain small; degenerative changes in nucleus caudatus, putamen, and cerebral cortex; neuroglia proliferation; ventricles enlarged.

Diagnostic Procedures. *Pneumoencephalography. Electroencephalography. CT brain scan.*

Therapy. Haloperidol; chlorpromazine; choline chloride 150–230 mg/Kg + lecithin 350 mg/Kg. Ayres and Mihan suggested that a fault in vitamin E metabolism may be at the root of the syndrome, and recommended vitamin E therapy for its antioxidant effect.

Prognosis. Death within 10 to 15 years; suicidal tendency.

BIBLIOGRAPHY. Waters CO: Description of chorea. In Dunglison R, Practice of Medicine, Vol 2, p 312. Philadelphia, Lea & Blanchard, 1842
Huntington G: On Chorea. Med Surg Reporter Philadelphia 26:317–321, 1872
Lund JC: Chorea Sti Viti i Saetersdalen Uddrag of Distrikslaege. JC Lunds Medicinalberetuig for 1860. Norges officielle Statistikk 1882C N. 4.
Ayres SC, Mihan R: Progeria: a possible therapeutic approach. JAMA 227:1381–1382, 1974
Growdon JH, Wurtman RJ: Dietary influences on the synthesis of neurotransmitters in the brain. Nutr Rev 37:129–136, 1979
Conneally PM: Huntington disease: genetic and epidemiology. Am J Hum Genet 36:506–526, 1984

HUNT'S (A.D.)

Synonym. Pyridoxine cerebral deficiency.

Symptoms. Occur in newborn with atraumatic birth; onset a few hours after delivery. Repeated and intractable convulsions; shrill cries. Mental retardation.

Signs. Convulsions preceded by faint pallor and rolling of the eyes.

Etiology. Autosomal recessive inheritance. Possibly high intake of pyridoxine during pregnancy. Enzymatic abnormality of central nervous system in which there is a continuing high requirement for pyridoxine in excess of normal dietary intake due to glutamate decarboxylase deficiency.

Pathology. *Brain.* Edema; neural degeneration (hypoxic type). *Adrenal cortex.* Areas of degeneration. *Liver.* Fatty degeneration; local congestion.

Diagnostic Procedures. *Electroencephalography.* Marked dysrhythmia and slow wave activity (findings present when signs of incipient convulsion are present). After injection of pyridoxine, significant decrease of slow wave activity. *Tryptophan loading and xanthurenic acid excretion test.* Normal.

Therapy. Pyridoxine hydrochloride will dramatically stop the convulsions and continuous treatment prevents their recurrence.

Prognosis. Death without treatment. With treatment, control of seizures, but mental retardation persists.

BIBLIOGRAPHY. Hunt AD, Stokes J Jr, McCrory WW, et al: Pyridoxine dependency: report of a case of intractable convulsions in an infant controlled by pyridoxine. Pediatrics 13:140–145, 1954
Frimpter GW: Pyridoxine (B₆) dependency syndromes. Ann Intern Med 68:1131–1132, 1968
Goutierez F, Aicardi J: Atypical presentation of pyridoxine-dependent seizures: a treatable cause for intractable epilepsy in infants. Ann Neurol 17:117–120, 1985

HUNT'S (J.R.) I

Synonyms. Auricular herpes zoster; geniculate neuralgia; herpes zoster oticus; Ramsay Hunt.

Symptoms. Intense pain in the region of ear and mastoid process; paralysis of facial (VII) nerve; hearing loss; vertigo; tinnitus. Taste loss in two-thirds of tongue; xerostomia and xerophthalmia.

Signs. Herpetic lesions over mastoid process, and around external auditory canal and ear drum that may extend to oral mucosa, face, neck, and scalp.

Etiology. Virus infection (herpes zoster) affecting the geniculate ganglion.

Pathology. Hyperemia and lymphocytic infiltration in perivascular spaces.

Therapy. Symptomatic; calamine lotion and protective dressing. Antibiotic to protect from secondary infections. Analgesic. Specific vaccine. Surgical measures and x-ray therapy of doubtful value.

Prognosis. Prognosis for recovery, poor. Recovery of paresis occurs, but return of function is seldom complete. Intractable pain sometimes remains after recovery from herpetic lesions.

BIBLIOGRAPHY. Hunt JR: On herpetic inflammations of geniculate ganglion: a new syndrome and its aural complications. Arch Otol 36:371–381, 1907
Adams RD, Victor M: Principles of Neurology, 3rd ed, p 1013. New York, McGraw-Hill, 1985
Robillard RB, Hilsinger RL, Adour KK: Ramsay Hunt facial paralysis: clinical analyses of 185 patients. Otolaryngol Head Neck Surg 95:292–297, 1986

HUNT'S (J.R.) II

Synonyms. Hunt's ataxia; dentatorubro atrophy; dyssynergia cerebellaris myoclonica; myoclonic dysynergia cerebellaris; Ramsay Hunt II.

Symptoms and Signs. Average age of onset early adulthood. Convulsion and myoclonus; action tremor that begins locally in one of the extremities and then spreads to involve entire voluntary muscular system. Legs are disturbed less often than arms. Asthenia; dysarthria; dysmetria; hypotonia; adiadochokinesis. Mental deterioration (rare).

Etiology. Unknown; may be associated with Friedreich's ataxia. Autosomal dominant inheritance with reduced penetrance suggested.

Pathology. Almost complete loss of cells in dentate nuclei; demyelinization of the brachium conjunctivum. Atrophy of column of Gall and ventral and dorsal spinocerebellar tracts.

Diagnostic Procedure. *Electroencephalographic* brain mapping. *Cerebrospinal fluid.* Uric acid may be increased.

Therapy. Anticonvulsant therapy (see Epilepsy syndromes).

Prognosis. Slow progression of condition over 10 years or longer.

BIBLIOGRAPHY. Hunt JR: Dyssynergia cerebellaris myoclonica—primary atrophy of the dentate system, a contribution to the pathology and symptomatology of cerebellum. Brain 44:490–538, 1921
May DL, White HH: Familial myoclonus, cerebellar ataxia and deafness. Arch Neurol 19:331–338, 1968
Tanaka N, Ito K, Yoshimura J, et al: Familial chorea and myoclonus epilepsy. Neurology 28:913–919, 1978

HURIEZ'S

Synonyms. Keratoderma; scleroatrophic Huriez's.

Symptoms and Signs. Both sexes affected; onset from birth. Keratoderma of palms, and less of the soles; sclerodermalike changes of fingers; atrophy back of the hands. Not Raynaud's phenomenon.

Etiology. Unknown; autosomal dominant inheritance.

Prognosis. Squamous epitheliomas developing during adolescence.

BIBLIOGRAPHY. Huriez C, Desmons F, Bombart M: Plasmocytomes dermiques malins de la fesse. Bull Soc Fr Dermatol Syph 70:743, 1963

Rook A, Wilkinson DS, Ebling FJG, et al: Textbook of Dermatology, 4th ed, p 1813. Oxford, Blackwell Scientific Publications, 1986

HURLER'S

Synonyms. Alpha-L-iduronidase deficiency (H); dysostosis multiplex; gargoylism; Johnie MCL; Hunter-Hurler; lypochondrodystrophy (misnomer); mucopolysaccharidosis I_H; MPSH; Pfaundler-Hurler; Sheldon-Ellis; Thompson's. See Hunter's.

Symptoms. Both sexes affected; clinical onset in infancy or early childhood. After a few months of normal growth, physical and mental abilities show progressive deterioration. Troubles of vision.

Signs. Hydrocephalus; grotesque facial features; macroglossia; lumbar gibbus; stiff joints; chest deformities; dwarfism; clouding of cornea and retinal degeneration; hepatosplenomegaly. Thickened skin and nodules over scapulae; hirsutism.

Etiology. Homozygous for mucopolysaccharidosis (MPS) I_H gene. Deficiency of alpha-L-iduronidase blocking the degradation of both dermatan sulfate and heparan sulfate.

Pathology. Cellular deposition of mucopolysaccharides in cartilage, periosteum, fasciae, tendons, heart valves, meninges, cornea. Hepatic cells show diffuse discrete vacuolization. Brain may contain bodies of abnormal lipid material.

Diagnostic Procedures. *Urine.* Mucopolysacchariduria: dermatan sulfate and heparan sulfate. *Blood.* Reilly (Alder) bodies (metachromatic inclusions) in polymorphonuclear leukocytes. Direct measurement of alpha-L-iduronidase activity in leukocytes. *Bone marrow.* Reilly bodies in histiocytes and lymphocytes. *X-ray.* Enlargement of shafts of long bones; convex vertebra; backward displacement of one or two upper lumbar bodies; coxa valga. Skull thickening restricted to vault. Frontal sinuses may be absent. Pituitary fossa deformed. Jaw and teeth alteration and dental cysts.

Therapy. Some improvement reported with fresh plasma infusion.

Prognosis. Death by 10 years of age. Respiratory infections; cardiac failure.

BIBLIOGRAPHY. Hurler G: Ueber einen Typ multipler Abartungen, vorwiegend am Skelettsystem. Z Kinderheilkd 24:220–234, 1919
McKusick VA, Neufeld EF: The mucopolysaccharide storage diseases. In Stanbury JB, Wyngaarden JB,

Fredrickson DS, et al, The Metabolic Basis of Inherited Disease, 5th ed, p 751. New York, McGraw-Hill, 1983

Herrick IA, Rhine EJ: The mucopolysaccharidoses and anaesthesia: a report of clinical experience. Can J Anesth 35:67–73, 1988

HURLER-SCHEIE

Synonyms. Alpha-L-iduronidase deficiency H/S; mucopolysaccharidosis $I_{H/S}$; MPS H/S. Hurler-Scheie "compound" alpha-L-iduronidase deficiency

Symptoms and Signs. A combination of symptoms less severe than Hurler's, more severe than the Sheie's. A unique feature seems represented by the dimension and consequence of presence of arachnoid cysts, which probably have the time to grow because of longer survival of patient with this genetic combination. Distinctive micrognathism.

Etiology. Autosomal inheritance. Genetic compound of MPS I_H and I/S genes.

Pathology. See Hurler's and Scheie's.

Diagnostic Procedures. See Hurler's and Scheie's. Differential diagnosis on clinical basis only.

Therapy. None.

Prognosis. May reach adult life. All the features of the two basic conditions evolving with less severity.

BIBLIOGRAPHY. Kajii T, Matsuda K, Osawa T, et al: Hurler/Scheie genetic compound (mucopolysaccharidosis I_H/I_S) in Japanese brothers. Clin Genet 6:394–400, 1974

McKusick VA, Neufeld EF: The mucopolysaccharide storage diseases. In Stanbury JB, Wyngaarden JB, Fredrickson DS, et al: The Metabolic Basis of Inherited Disease, 5th ed, p 751. New York, McGraw-Hill, 1983

HUTCHINSON-GILFORD

Synonyms. Gilford's; premature senility; progeria; Souques-Charcot.

Symptoms and Signs. Occur in children of both sexes. Normal appearance at birth and during first year. Then, lack of weight gain, retardation of growth become evident, with height and weight below third percentile. Baldness; absence of eyelashes; loss of subcutaneous fat; appearance of dwarfism; small face; prominent eyes and beaked nose; irregular teeth; senile aspect; parchment skin with brownish pigmentation; infantile sex organs; protruding abdomen; poor muscle development.

Etiology. Unknown; possibly heterogenic phenotype, autosomal dominant or recessive type germinal mosaicism. The primary source of multiple defects unknown.

Pathology. Absence of subcutaneous fat; senile features; atherosclerosis; occlusion of coronary vessel.

Diagnostic Procedures. *Blood.* Increased lipids. Erythrocytes—heat lability of G6PD and 6-phosphogluconate dehydrogenases. *Urine.* Seldom, aminoaciduria. *X-ray.* Premature fusion of epiphyses; long thin bone with decalcification; poorly developed mandible; crowding of teeth. *Chromosome study.* Pattern normal.

Therapy. None.

Prognosis. Death by the middle of second decade.

BIBLIOGRAPHY. Hutchinson J: Congenital absence of hair and mammary glands with atrophic conditions of skin and its appendages. Med Chir Trans 69:473–477, 1886

Gilford H: Progeria: A form of senilism. Practitioner 73:188–217, 1904

De Busk FL: The Hutchinson-Gilford progeria syndrome. J Pediatr 80:697–724, 1972

Brown WT, Darlington GJ: Thermolabile enzymes in progeria and Werner syndrome: evidence contrary to the protein error hypothesis. Am J Hum Genet 32:614–619, 1980

HUTCHINSON'S (J.)

Synonyms. Choroiditis guttata senilis; Tay's choroiditis (see Retina posterior pole colloidal degeneration).

Symptoms. Both sexes affected; onset in advanced age. Gradual and progressive visual loss.

Signs. Large colloidal deposit in and about macula.

Etiology. Unknown; possibly, autosomal dominant inheritance.

BIBLIOGRAPHY. Hutchinson J: Illustration of Clinical Surgery, pp 49–52. London, J. Churchill, 1875

Kimura SJ, Caygill WM: Retinal Diseases. Philadelphia, Lea & Febiger, 1966

HUTCHINSON'S MELANOTIC WHITLOW

Synonyms. Melanotic whitlow; subungual melanotic whitlow; Hutchinson's III.

Symptoms. Rare; onset in middle to advanced age. Pain.

Signs. Three modes of presentation:
1. Pigmented band in the nail followed by granulation at the edge of nail bed
2. Chronic paronychia (single finger) with pigmentation in contiguous cutaneous area
3. Warty growth on nail bed with loss of nail

Etiology. Unknown.

Pathology. Malignant melanotic tumor.

Diagnostic Procedures. *Biopsy.* Must be performed as soon as syndrome suspected. Performed after application of a tourniquet. Frozen section analysis.

Therapy. If positive histology, immediate amputation at the metacarpophalangeal joint level.

Prognosis. Depends on the results of early surgery and prevention of metastases.

BIBLIOGRAPHY. Hutchinson J: Melanotic disease of the great toe following a whitlow of the nail. Trans Pathol Soc London 8:404–405, 1857

Rook A, Wilkinson DS, Ebling FJG, et al: Textbook of Dermatology, 4th ed, p 2336. Oxford, Blackwell Scientific Publications, 1986

HUTCHINSON'S (R.)

See Parker's.

Symptoms and Signs. Those of Parker's (see) Plus multiple bone metastases that confer on them a "moth eaten" aspect.

BIBLIOGRAPHY. Hutchinson R: On suprarenal sarcoma in children with metastases to the skull. Q J Med 1:33–38, 1907

HUTCHINSON'S TRIAD

Synonym. Deafness-interstitial keratitis-Hutchinson's teeth. Eponym indicates the association of the three signs occurring in congenital syphilis.

Symptoms and Signs. (1) Hutchinson's teeth: permanent teeth; dirty gray color; widely separated; upper incisor narrowed; small, bowed at sides; central depression of cutting edge. Lower incisors peg-shaped, center notched. First molar maldeveloped. (2) Deafness. (3) Interstitial keratitis.

Etiology. These symptoms, together with others, develop during infancy and early childhood in cases of late congenital syphilis. The Hutchinson's teeth may be observed also in rickets and traumatic lesions.

BIBLIOGRAPHY. Hutchinson J: On the different forms of inflammation of the eye consequent on inherited syphilis. Ophthalmol Hosp Rep 1:191–203; 226–244, 1858; 2:54–105, 1859

Hutchinson J: Medical Classics 5:138–146, 1940

HYALINE MEMBRANE

Synonyms. Perinatal respiratory distress; pulmonary hypoperfusion; respiratory distress; RDS.

Symptoms and Signs. Most frequently in premature infants, infants born of diabetic mothers, infants delivered by cesarean section, or infants of mothers with antepartum hemorrhages or toxemia. Less frequently in full term, normally delivered infants. Onset within a few hours from birth. Tachypnea; poor chest excursion, inspiratory retraction; expiratory grunting; weak cry; rales; frothing at lips; often, cyanosis and edema.

Etiology. Unknown; genetically determined RDS predisposing factor; high risk mothers. Possibly decreased surface activity agent in lung; damage to alveolar cells by asphyxia; toxic product or effect of reflex vasoconstriction due to hypoxemia, acidemia, hypothermia, hypovolemia.

Pathology. Lung voluminous, purplish red; poor stability of expansion; extensive atelectasis; alveolar septa vascular congestion; hemorrhages; homogeneous eosinophilic lining on bronchial epithelium and alveolar ducts (hyaline membranes). Right heart dilatation.

Diagnostic Procedures. Findings of inadequate oxygenation and carbon dioxide removal. Respiratory and metabolic acidosis. *X-ray.* Granular appearance of lung fields.

Therapy. Supportive care; oxygen, avoid oxygen toxicity to the retina (see Terry's syndrome) and the lungs with a careful monitoring of arterial P_{O_2}. Treatment in a neonatal intensive care unit by skilled personnel.

Prognosis. Mortality of low birth weight infants referred to proper intensive unit is steadily declining. About 50% of those under 1000 gm survive, and over 95% of those weighing more than 2500 gm survive.

BIBLIOGRAPHY. Swyer PR: The respiratory distress syndrome of the newly born. Chicago Med 70:12–17, 1967

Klaus MH, Fanaroff AA: Care of the High-Risk Neonate, 2nd ed. Philadelphia, WB Saunders, 1979

HYDATIDIFORM MOLE

Synonyms. Hydatid mole; vesicular mole; pregnancy molar. See Choriocarcinoma.

Symptoms. Incidence 1 : 2000 pregnancies in the Western world; more frequent in Far East. Bleeding (spotting or profuse); nausea and vomiting. Pain due to rapid uterine enlargement.

Signs. Enlargement of uterus beyond the size for the estimated period of gestation. Bilateral adnexal enlargement due to the lutein cysts of ovary. Hypertension during the second trimester.

Etiology. Unknown.

Pathology. Hydatidiform mole is placental tissue in which chorionic villi are converted to vesicles of varying sizes (a few mm to 2 to 3 cm in diameter) arranged in grapelike clusters. The contents usually distend the uterus to the size of a gestation of 6 months. Microscopically, villi show hydropic degeneration and swelling, scanty blood vessels, proliferation of chorionic epithelium, especially syncytial trophoblasts. Ovaries very often exhibit multiple lutein cysts, produced by overstimulation by chorionic gonadotropin.

Diagnostic Procedures. *Blood, urine, cerebrospinal fluid.* Chorionic gonadotropins in great amount.

Therapy. Once diagnosed, immediate evacuation of the uterus, either vaginally, by dilatation and curettage, or by abdominal hysterectomy (the latter for selected multiparas). Supportive measures: blood, antibiotics, nutrition. Because of the danger of chorionepithelioma, the patient should be followed for 1 year: look for abnormal bleeding; make serial biologic pregnancy tests. No chorionic gonadotropin should be detected 30 days after evacuation of the uterus. A persistent or rising hormone titer is an indication for exploratory laparotomy and hysterectomy. Effective contraception (birth control pills). Antitumor chemotherapy. Low risk patients: methotrexate 0.4 mg/Kg im 5 day period, or dactinomycin 10–12, μg/Kg/d iv over 5-day period. High risk patients: refer for multiple agent chemotherapy.

Prognosis. Hydatidiform mole destroys the fetus. Prognosis of mother depends chiefly on the amount of bleeding, infection, or perforation of the uterine wall. Risk of abortion and fetal anomaly not greater in patients who have had hydatiform mole. After courses of chemotherapy (even when metastases) 5-years' arrest can be expected in 85% of cases of choriocarcinoma.

BIBLIOGRAPHY. Szulman AE, Surti U: The syndromes of partial and complete molar gestation. Clin Obstet Gynecol 27:172–180, 1984

HYDE'S

Synonyms. Lailler-Brocq lichen obtusus corné; nodular lichenification; nodular prurigo.

Symptoms. Rare; prevalent in middle-aged females. Intense crisis of pruritus lasting minutes or 1 to 2 hours, daily or more frequent intervals.

Signs. On the back of forearms, but also, less frequently, on thighs and legs. Few, widespread, nodular lesions 1 to 3 cm of diameter, with hard and warty surface. Initially red in color, they become pigmented, crust, and scale. Halo of hyperpigmentation around nodules.

Etiology. Unknown. Emotional stress (?). Considered also as a variant of lichen simplex.

Pathology. Thickening of horny layer. Chronic inflammatory infiltrates; schwannomas.

Therapy. Infiltration with corticosteroids. Tranquilizers; psychiatric counseling Benaxaprofen useful in some cases.

Prognosis. New nodules may appear; old ones remain pruriginous, seldom regressing with a residual scar.

BIBLIOGRAPHY. Hyde JN: A Practical Treatise on Diseases of the Skin for the Use of Students and Practictioners, 3rd ed. Philadelphia, Lea & Febiger, 1883
Rook A, Wilkinson DS, Ebling FJG, et al: Textbook of Dermatology, 4th ed, pp 417–418. Oxford, Blackwell Scientific Publications, 1986

HYDROARTHROSIS INTERMITTENS

Synonyms. Intermittent hydroarthrosis; periodic arthritis; Perrin's.

Symptoms. Prevalent in females; onset after puberty or in old age. Usually, single joint pain (knee most frequently affected, less frequently ankle). Functional limitation lasting 7 to 20 days. In some cases, symptoms parallel menses.

Signs. Swelling and distension of affected joint. Absence of systemic manifestation and local signs of inflammation.

Etiology. Unknown; familial (?). In many cases, history of allergy.

Pathology. No specific changes.

Diagnostic Procedures. *Blood, urine, synovial fluid.* Negative. *X-ray.* Soft tissue swelling.

Therapy. None satisfactory.

Prognosis. Length of recurrences unpredictable (months, lifetime).

BIBLIOGRAPHY. Perrin ER: J Med 3:82, 1845
Ehrlich GE: Intermittent and periodic arthritic syndromes. In Hollander JL, McCarty DJ: Arthritis and Allied Condition, 8th ed, p 822. Philadelphia, Lea & Febiger, 1972

HYDROA VACCINIFORME

Synonym. Hydroa aestivale (term is best reserved for a variant of polymorphic light eruption).

Symptoms. Male to female ratio 2 : 1; onset in infancy or early childhood; onset after exposure to sun. Malaise; light hyperthermia; restlessness; pruritus absent; after 12 hours, skin eruption.

Signs. On the face, arms, and any other area exposed to light, red papules that evolve into bullae and then into crusted lesions and, finally, into scars. Various developmental anomalies may be associated.

Etiology. Unknown; type of inheritance not established; possibly, autosomal recessive.

Diagnostic Procedures. *Blood and urine.* To exclude porphyria.

Therapy. Sunscreen of little effect. Chloroquine possibly useful; estrogen (in a girl) and gonadotropin (in a boy) claimed useful.

Prognosis. Attacks last about 2 weeks; become milder and less frequent with early adult life (at 20 to 30 years of age), but may persist.

BIBLIOGRAPHY. McGrae JD, Perry HO: Hydroa vacciniforme. Arch Dermatol 87:618–625, 1963
Rook A, Wilkinson DS, Ebling FJG, et al: Textbook of Dermatology, 4th ed, p 647. Oxford, Blackwell Scientific Publications, 1986

HYDROLETHALUS

Symptoms and Signs. The syndrome is lethal and is characterized by polydactyly and central nervous system malformation, as observed in the Meckel-Gruber syndrome (see), but unlike the latter disorder does not show cystic kidney and liver and the central nervous system derangement is hydrocephalus not encephalocele. Other possible malformations in this syndrome are heart defects, stenosis of the airway, and abnormal lobation of the lungs.

Etiology. Recessive inheritance.

Diagnostic Procedures. Prenatal diagnosis by ultrasonography. *CT brain scan.*

Therapy. None. Cerebrospinal fluid shunt for hydrocephalus as palliative treatment.

Prognosis. Poor.

BIBLIOGRAPHY. Salonen R, Herva R, Norio R: The hydrolethalus syndrome: delineation of a "new" lethal malformation syndrome, based on 28 patients. Clin Genet 19:321–330, 1981
Toriello HV, Bauserman SC: Bilateral pulmonary agenesis: association with the hydrolethalus syndrome and review of the literature from a developmental field prospective. Am J Med Genet 21:93–103, 1985

HYDROPS FETALIS-Hb BART'S

Synonym. Homozygous alpha thalassemia 1.

Symptoms and Signs. Individuals from Southeast Asia, Greece, and Cyprus. Premature delivery with stillborn fetus or death few hours after birth. Hydrops fetalis.

Etiology. Autosomic recessive. Absence of alpha chain synthesis.

Diagnostic Procedure. *Peripheral blood smear.* Large hypochromic RBC, reticulocytosis. Hb electrophoresis: Hb Bart's (gamma 4) prevalent; absence of alpha chains.

Pathology. Hydrops fetalis. Hepatosplenomegaly.

Therapy. Cesarean section. Exchange transfusions.

Prognosis. Poor.

BIBLIOGRAPHY. Lie-Injo LE, Jo BH: A fast-moving hemoglobin in hydrops fetalis. Nature 185:698, 1960
Bunn HF, Forget BG: Hemoglobin Molecular Genetic and Clinical Aspects, p 332. Philadelphia, WB Saunders, 1986

HYPERALGESIC PSEUDOTHROMBOPHLEBITIS

Symptoms and Signs. In male homosexuals. Frequent association with Kaposi's sarcoma (see). Painful swelling in the legs, with overlying skin showing erythematous and intensely tender reactions. Hyperthermia.

Etiology. Unknown. Unusual manifestation of AIDS (see).

Diagnostic Procedures. *Venography.* No evidence of venous occlusion.

Therapy. Diagnosis needed to prevent unnecessary anticoagulation. Nonsteroidal anti-inflammatory agents.

Prognosis. Erythema and pain persisting for one month.

BIBLIOGRAPHY. Abramson SB, Odajnyk CM, Grieco AJ, et al: Hyperalgesic pseudothrombophlebitis: new syndrome in male homosexuals. Am J Med 78:317–320, 1985

HYPERBILIRUBINEMIA, BREAST-FEEDING

Synonyms. Transient nonhemolytic unconjugated hyperbilirubinemia associated with breast-feeding; maternal milk hyperbilirubinemia; breast milk jaundice.

Symptoms and Signs. Both sexes. From birth, only in breast-fed children. Progressive jaundice. Ameliorated only by discontinuation of breast-feeding. No kernicterus.

Etiology. Presence of inhibitor of UDP-glucuronyl transferase in maternal milk: 3 alpha, 20 beta-pregnanediol.

Diagnostic Procedures. *Blood.* Unconjugated hyperbilirubinemia. *Maternal milk.* 3 alpha-20 betapregnanediol.

Prognosis. Recession of jaundice with artificial feeding.

BIBLIOGRAPHY. Arthur LJH, Bevan BR, Holton JB: Neonatal hyperbilirubinemia and breast feeding. Dev Med Child Neurol 8:279, 1966

HYPERCALCEMIA

Symptoms. Malaise; muscular weakness; polyuria; polydipsia; constipation; dehydration; nausea; vomiting; anorexia. Mental derangement from depression to delirium.

Signs. Cardiac arrhythmias; muscle hypotonia, areflexia; band keratopathy.

Etiology and Pathology. Increase of calcium in circulation observed in many different conditions: malignancy of bones; myeloma; sarcoidosis; hypervitaminosis D; primary and secondary hyperparathyroidism; Burnett's; hypophosphatasia. In patients subject to prolonged immobilization, and patients treated with estrogen or testosterone.

Diagnostic Procedures. *Blood.* Elevation of calcium level; associated with other findings typical of various pathologic entities. *Electrocardiography.* Short Q-T interval.

Therapy. *In crisis.* Electrocardiographic monitoring; sodium chloride 0.9% infusion and potassium as needed; vasopressor agents; furosemide or etiodronate intravenously. If inadequate response, phosphate infusion, then per os; mithramycin. If no response (renal failure), corticosteroids and calcitonin. Treatment of underlying condition by specific measures.

Prognosis. Depends on etiology.

BIBLIOGRAPHY. Goldsmith RS, Ingbar SH: Inorganic phosphate treatment of hypercalcemia of diverse etiologies. New Engl J Med 274:1–7, 1966
Mundy GR: The hypercalcemia of cancer. Clinical implication and pathogenesis mechanisms. N Engl J Med 310:1718–1727, 1984
Ryzen E, Martodam RR, Troxeu M, et al: Intravenous etiodronate in the management of malignant hypercalcemia. Arch Intern Med 145:449–452, 1985

HYPERCALCEMIA, INFANTILE IDIOPATHIC

Comprehensive designation to indicate a constant complication of the SAS syndrome (Williams-Beuren) and to designate a variant of this syndrome that presents all symptoms and signs *except* the presence of supravalvular aortic stenosis and peripheral pulmonary stenosis.

Etiology. Possibly defect concerning vitamin D inactivation. A later onset of the process (hypercalcemia) has been considered responsible for the absence of these particular vascular injuries.

BIBLIOGRAPHY. Smith DW, Blizzard RM, Harrison HE: Idiopathic hypercalcemia: a case report with assay of vitamin D in the serum. Pediatrics 24:258–269, 1959
Wiltse HE, Goldbloom RB, Antia AU, et al: Infantile hypercalcemia syndrome in twins. New Engl J Med 275:1157–1160, 1966
Marx SJ: Familial hypocalciuric hypercalcemia. New Engl J Med 303:810–811, 1980

HYPERCALCIURIA, FAMILIAL IDIOPATHIC

Symptoms and Signs. Urolithiasis; hematuria; urinary tract infections; abnormal urinary concentrating ability; enuresis. Hypercalciuria is defined as a 24 hours urine excretion of calcium greater than 0.094 mmol/kg/day (4 mg/kg/day) and/or a calcium/creatinine ratio greater than 0.56 mmol/mmol (0.2 mg/mg).

The condition has been classified into three different pathogenic types based on response to changes in dietary calcium and sodium.

Group I. Absorptive hypercalciuria. Low calcium excretion on low-calcium diet (400–600 mg/day) with sodium excretion >2.5 mmol/kg/day.

Group II. Renal hypercalciuria. Low calcium excretion only when hydrochlorothiazide (HCT) is administered.

Group III. Sodium-dependent hypercalciuria. Low calcium excretion only if sodium excretion (<2.5 mmol/kg/day).

Etiology. Autosomal dominant inheritance.

Therapy. Varies according to the response to dietary manipulation described above. A high fluid intake is recommended to all patients. Patients belonging to group II should receive HCT 1 to 2 mg/kg/day. Excessive sodium intake can block HCT effect. Patients belonging to groups I and III should follow a low-calcium, low-sodium diet.

Warning. A severely calcium-restricted diet can produce a negative calcium balance, which may be harmful in childhood.

Prognosis. Good if early institution of treatment.

BIBLIOGRAPHY. Berlin LJ, Clayton BE: Idiopathic hypercalciuria in a child. Arch Dis Child 39:409–414, 1964

Moore ES: Hypercalciuria in children. Contr Nephrol 27:20–32, 1981

Cervera A, Corral MJ, Gomez JM, et al: Idiopathic hypercalciuria in children: classification, clinical manifestations, and outcome. Acta Pediatr Scand 76:271–278, 1987

HYPERCHOLESTEROLEMIA, FAMILIAL

Synonyms. Harbiz-Mueller; familial hyperbetalipoproteinemia; hyperlipoproteinemia II: xanthomatosis-hypercholesterolemia; xanthoma tuberosum simplex.

Symptoms. Both sexes affected; age of detection from infancy to third or fourth decade. Anginal pain; symptoms of arterial obstruction in different organs. Possibly, recurrent attacks of polyarthritis and tenosynovitis without temperature elevation.

Signs. Xanthoma tendinosum or tuberosum, especially elbows, knees, hands, feet; arcus senilis; no hepatosplenomegaly.

Etiology. Autosomal dominant inheritance. Autosomal dominant inheritance with gene dosage effect. Mutant alleles for LDL receptors (Rb^0, Rb^-, Rb^{+10}), (all inactive), do not allow LDL uptake from plasma and as a consequence low density proteins accumulate in arteries and macrophages.

Pathology. Diffuse atheromatosis.

Diagnostic Procedures. *Blood.* Subtype a: plasma aspect clear increased LDL; normal very low-density lipoproteins (VLDL); increased cholesterol and normal triglycerides. Subtype b: aspect clear or slightly turbid; increased LDL and VLDL; increased cholesterol and triglycerides. Sedimentation rate frequently increased; fibrinogen marked increase. Normal glucose tolerance test. *Electrocardiography. X-ray.* Calcification of vascular atheromas. Prenatal diagnosis possible on amniotic cells.

Therapy. Diet: cholesterol intake below 300 mg/day for adult; reduction of saturated fats and increase of polyunsaturated fats. Cholestyramine, preferably in combination with nicotinic acid. Three new experimental approaches: (1) Intravenous hyperalimentation; (2) end-to-side portocaval anastomosis; (3) use of continuous-flow blood-cell separator for repeated plasma exchange. Lovastatin-Simvastatin.

Prognosis. Vast spectrum of possibilities, from simple increase of beta-lipoprotein without limitation of life span to fatality from atheromatosis during first year of life.

BIBLIOGRAPHY. Fagge CH: General xanthelasma or vitiligoidea. Trans Pathol Soc London 24:242–250, 1872

Rayer PFO: Traite theorique et pratiques des maladies de la peau. Paris 1836

Harbitz F: Svulster indeholdente xanthomaev I. Sarkomer utgaaende fra sense-skeder og ledkapler. II. Multiple symmetriske xanthomer III Xantosarkomer. Norsch Mag Laegevid 86:321–348, 1925

Mueller C: Xanthomate hypercholesterolemia, angina pectoris. Acta Med Scand [Suppl] 89:75–84, 1938

Goldstein JL, Brown MS: Familial hypercholesterolemia. In Stanbury JB, Wyngaarden JB, Fredrickson DS, et al: The Metabolic Basis of Inherited Disease, 5th ed, p 672. New York, McGraw-Hill, 1983

Grundy SM, Bearn AG (eds): The Role of Cholesterol in Atherosclerosis. Philadelphia, Hanley & Belfus, 1987

HYPERCYANOTIC ANGINA

Synonym. Angina hypercyanotic.

Symptoms and Signs. Chest pain in patient with congenital heart diseases and pulmonary hypertension.

HYPEREMESIS GRAVIDARUM

Synonyms. Emesis gravidarum; pregnancy vomiting; pernicious vomiting pregnancy.

Symptoms. Begins as simple vomiting around sixth week, gradually increasing in spite of treatment, so that no food or water can be retained. Nervousness and insomnia; polyneuritis, coma.

Signs. Dehydration; starvation; emaciation.

Etiology. Not known; some metabolic change is the fundamental factor, but psychoneurosis plays a role also.

Pathology. Most marked morbid changes occur in liver: fatty degeneration of central portion of lobule extending to acute yellow atrophy; liver glycogen is depleted. Kidney lesions.

Diagnostic Procedures. *Urine.* High concentration; albuminuria; casts. *Blood.* Electrolyte imbalance; hyperbilirubinemia; increased blood urea nitrogen.

Therapy. *Prophylaxis.* Good antenatal care; differentiation between neurotic and toxic type. *Curative.* Complete rest in bed; intravenous fluid medication with maintenance of electrolyte balance. Sedation (sodium phenobarbital; thorazine as central nervous system depressant). If intractable, therapeutic abortion.

Prognosis. Can be prevented by proper antenatal care. Death if inadequate therapeutic measures.

BIBLIOGRAPHY. Pritchard-McDonald-Gant: Williams Obstetrics, 17th ed, pp 260–261. Norwalk, (Conn), Appleton-Century-Croft, 1985

HYPEREOSINOPHILIC

Synonyms. Loeffler's fibroblastic endocarditis; eosinophilic leukemia; eosinophilic disseminated collagen disease. See Eosinophilic lung, secondary.

Symptoms and Signs. The term *idiopathic* hypereosinophilic syndrome is applied when the following criteria are fulfilled: (1) eosinophilia 1.5 × 10/1; (2) persists for at least 6 months or fatal in a shorter time; (3) results in organ system disfunction; (4) absence of a recognized cause for the eosinophilia. Three different forms have been recognized: (a) hypereosinophilia with lung involvement and angioedema; (b) severe cardiac and central nervous system complications; (c) eosinophilic cytogenic abnormalities and other features of a leukemic disease.

Etiology. Unknown. Various theories have been put forward: autoimmune disease; neoplastic disease; exaggerated response to a parasite or allergic disease.

Pathology. *Lung.* Eosinophilic infiltration; signs of pulmonary hypertension. *Myocardium.* Increase of collagen connective tissue and eosinophilic infiltration. *Other organs.* Mature eosinophil infiltration and proliferation of collagen tissue.

Therapy. Corticosteroids. Hydroxyurea is used in patients who do not respond to steroids and also to allow the steroid dosages to be reduced. Vincristine has been used in patients with aggressive disease. Anticoagulants are required in most patients. Leucophoresis and plasma exchange are useful in cases with increased blood viscosity and widespread vessel occlusions.

Prognosis. Favorable prognostic factors are high IgE concentrations, the presence of angioneurotic edema, and eosinopenia within a few hours after the first dose of prednisone. Unfavorable signs are leucocytosis and myeloblasts in peripheral blood and congestive heart failure.

BIBLIOGRAPHY. Chusoil MJ, Dale DC, West BC, et al: The hypereosinophilic syndrome: analysis of fourteen cases with review of literature. Medicine 54:1–27, 1975
Weller PF: Eosinophilia. J Allergy Clin Immunol 73:1–10, 1984
Alfaham MA, Ferguson SD, Sihna B, Davies J: The idiopathic hypereosinophilic syndrome. Arch Dis Child 62:601–613, 1987
Lovisetto P, Manachino D, Olivetto L, et al: Le grandi eosinofilie del sangue. Aspetti clinico-nosografici. Rec Progr Med 79:525–532, 1988

HYPERHIDROSIS

Synonyms. Asymmetric hyperhidrosis; gustatory hyperhidrosis; mental sweating; thermoregulatory hyperhidrosis. Four clinical variants of this condition recognized.

ASYMMETRIC HYPERHIDROSIS

Symptoms and Signs. Both sexes affected; onset at all ages. Localized excessive sweating occurring in any area of the body. Usually associated with various neurologic or visceral symptoms and signs.

Etiology. Neurologic or visceral lesion producing an abnormal stimulation of selected sympathetic pathway.

Therapy. Topical atropinelike drugs; aluminum salts; ethanol glycerine of little effect. Atropinelike drugs have limited effect. Sympathectomy of temporary utility; removal of area with affected sweat gland could be beneficial.

Prognosis. That of main neurologic condition.

GUSTATORY HYPERHIDROSIS

See also Bogorad's and Von Frey's.

Symptoms and Signs. Both sexes affected; onset in childhood. It also appears frequently (50–80%) 4 to 7 months after surgery on the parotid glands. Localized sweating on lips, nose, and forehead or, seldom, on other areas of the body (e.g., knee) after eating especially hot or spicy foods.

Etiology. In most cases, unknown reflex mechanism; in others, lesion within central nervous system or damage to sympathetic and parasympathetic systems of face or neck.

Therapy. See Asymmetric hyperhidrosis.

Prognosis. Form of no clinical significance and lifelong persistence, or symptomatic, where the syndrome may wane after 3 to 5 years.

MENTAL SWEATING

Symptoms and Signs. Both sex affected; onset in childhood or early puberty. Following emotions or mental activity sweating (usually very profuse) on palms, soles, axillae, groin, and face. Hands usually cold and show tendency to acrocyanosis (see). Sweating could be also continuous. Pompholyix (see) and contact dermatitis possible complications.

Etiology. Unknown; overactivity of eccrine glands.

Therapy. See Asymmetric hyperhidrosis.

Prognosis. Persistent condition; tendency to improvement after the 25th year of life.

THERMOREGULATING HYPERHIDROSIS

Synonym. Sweating sickness.

Symptoms. Bonus of persistent sweating, not related to exogenous heating and without fever. More frequent during sleep.

Etiology. Extremely variable. Following infective processes or as presenting manifestation; intoxications (e.g., alcohol) or metabolic disorders (e.g., diabetes; endocrinopathies; obesity) or malignancies.

Therapy. See Asymmetric hyperhidrosis.

Prognosis. Variable.

BIBLIOGRAPHY. Guttmann L, List CF: Zur Topik und Pathophysiologie der Schweiss-Secretion. Ztschr Neurol Psychiatr 116:504–536, 1928
Sulzberger MB, Hermann F: The clinical significance of disturbances in the delivery of sweat. Springfield, IL, CC Thomas, 1954
Rook A, Wilkinson DS, Ebling FJG, et al: Textbook of Dermatology, 4th ed, pp 1887–1889. Oxford, Blackwell Scientific Publications, 1986

HYPERHYDROXYPROLINEMIA

Synonym. Hydroxyprolinemia.

Symptoms and Signs. Only a trait. Some cases with association of mental retardation reported.

Etiology. Autosomal recessive. Probably absence of 4 hydroxy-L-proline oxidase.

Diagnostic Procedures. *Urine.* Hyperhydroxyprolinuria.

Prognosis. Good.

BIBLIOGRAPHY. Efron ML, Bixby EM, Palattao LG, et al: Hydroxyprolinemia associated with mental deficiency. New Engl J Med 267:1193, 1962
Scriver CH, Smith RJ, Phang JM: Disorders of proline and hydroxyproline metabolism. In Stanbury JB, Wyngaarden JB, Fredrickson DS, et al: The Metabolic Basis of Inherited Disease, 5th ed. p 360. New York, McGraw-Hill, 1983

HYPERKALEMIC

Synonym. Potassium intoxication.

Symptoms. None in mild form. In severe attack (potassium 6 mEq/liter), nausea, vomiting, abdominal pain, weakness, flaccid paralysis, dysarthria, oliguria, respiratory arrest, syncope.

Signs. Earliest sign is provided by the electrocardiographic changes: tall tent-shaped T waves; decreased P wave amplitude; and finally atrial systole. Hypotension; arrhythmias; ileus; cardiac arrest.

Etiology. Renal damage: acute tubular necrosis; chronic renal failure; diabetic coma; postsurgical electrolyte imbalance. As component of Addison's syndromes, Conn's. Iatrogenic: spironolactone; triamterene; blood transfusion; excessive potassium administration.

Diagnostic Procedures. *Blood.* Total serum. Determination of serum potassium. *Urine.* Urinary potassium excretion; pH; base excess; osmolarity. *Electrocardiography.* See Signs.

Therapy. Interdiction of all intake of potassium. If there is trauma and necrosis, removal of necrotic tissue. Infusion of glucose and insulin. Administration of sodium bicarbonate, calcium gluconate to counteract potassium effect on myocardium. Cation exchange resin in sodium cycle (per os or per rectum) to remove potassium from body. Hemodialysis (if other therapeutic approach unsuccessful). Pacemaker if there are severe arrhythmias.

Prognosis. According to etiology. Good response to treatment.

BIBLIOGRAPHY. Schwartz WB: Fluid, electrolyte, and acid-base balance. In Beeson PB, McDermott W (eds): Cecil-Loeb Textbook of Medicine, 12th ed. Philadelphia, WB Saunders, 1967

Tanner RL (ed): Symposium on potassium homeostasis Kidney Int 11:389 (whole issue), 1977

Brenner BM, Rector FC: The Kidney, 3rd ed, p 533. Philadelphia, WB Saunders, 1986

HYPERKINETIC HEART

Synonyms. Athletic heart; circulatory hyperkinetic; hyperdynamic heart.

Symptoms. Occur in patients of all ages. Less than 50% have cardiorespiratory symptoms (dyspnea; orthopnea; chest discomfort); about 20% are participating in athletic activities. Occur in young or early middle age.

Signs. Overactivity of heart and great vessels; thrusting ventricles; pulse full and quick; basal or left parasternal ejectionlike systolic murmur, up to grade 4 in intensity. Systolic ejection click and split second pulmonic sound (50%). Over femoral vein, in the inguinal trigone, venous murmur increasing with lifting of leg or on exertion. Labile blood pressure (50%).

Etiology. Unknown; possibly, psychic pressure; anxiety, prehypertensive condition, superficial similarities to the effects of catecholamine stimulation. Time used for ejection shorter than normal; volume per beat not necessarily increased. Unknown. Related to hyperstimulation of beta-adrenergic system.

Diagnostic Procedures. *Electrocardiography.* Left ventricular hypertrophy; in some patients completely normal tracing. *X-ray.* Usually normal. Pulmonary plethora only in minority of patients. *Echocardiography.* Normal thickness of walls.

Therapy. Beta-adrenergic reception blockade.

Prognosis. This syndrome, usually observed in hypertensive or prehypertensive patients, may lead to circulatory failure.

BIBLIOGRAPHY. Starr I, Jonas L: Supernormal circulation in resting subjects (hyperkinemia) with a study of the relation of the kinetic abnormalities to the basal metabolic rate. Arch Intern Med 71:1–22, 1943

Gorlin R: The hyperkinetic heart syndrome. JAMA 182:823–829, 1962

Stano A, Di Renzi L, Pennelti V: On the peripheral venous murmur of the circulatory hyperkinetic syndrome. Angiology 17:213–222, 1966

Gillium RF, Teichholz LE, Herman MV, et al: The idiopathic hyperkinetic heart syndrome: clinical course and long term prognosis. Am Heart J 102:728, 1981

HYPERLEUCINE-ISOLEUCINEMIA

Synonym. Branched-chain amino transaminase.

Symptoms and Signs. Rare. Both sexes. From birth seizures failure to thrive, mental retardation. Retinal degeneration, hearing loss.

Etiology. Unknown. Defective metabolism of leucine, isoleucine, and proline.

Diagnostic Procedures. *Blood.* High leucine, isoleucine, and proline. *Urine.* Leucine, isoleucine normal; increased glycine and delta-pyrolidine-5-carboxylic acid.

Therapy. Low-protein diet.

Prognosis. Death in early age.

BIBLIOGRAPHY. Jeune M, Collombel E, Michel M, et al: Hyperleucine isoleucinemie par defaut partial de transamination associée a une hyperprolinemie de type 2: observation familiale d'une double aminoacidopathie. Ann Pediatr 17:85–99, 1970

Tanaka K, Rosenberg LE: Disorders of branched chain acid metabolism. In Stanbury JB, Wyngaarden JB, Fredrickson DS, et al: The Metabolic Basis of Inherited Disease, 5th ed, pp 450–451. New York, McGraw-Hill, 1983

HYPERLIPEMIC RETINITIS

Adult form of Coat's (see). Same findings as in children's form, with the exception of constant history of some preceding uveal inflammation and constant findings of hypercholesterolemia.

Therapy. This form does not respond to diathermy or photocoagulation; dietary treatment and anticholesterolemic agents are indicated.

HYPERLIPOPROTEINEMIA TYPE III

Synonyms. Broad beta; carbohydrate-induced hyperlipemia; dysbetalipoproteinemia; familial type III hyperlipoproteinemia; floating beta; xanthoma tuberosum.

Symptoms. Both sexes affected; age of detection 3rd to 4th decade. Anginal pain and symptoms of arterial obstruction in different organs. Attacks of abdominal pain may occur.

Signs. Appearance, during 3rd or 4th decade, of nodules in tendons in various locations, and other xanthomas, both planar (xanthoma striata palmaris) and tuberous types. Hepatosplenomegaly.

Etiology. Autosomal dominant inheritance (?); pathogenesis unknown. Possibly, aberrant synthesis and direct release of the unusual lipoproteins into the blood. Uncertain relationship with hyperlipoproteinemia type II since, to the feature of this form is added the increase of prebetalipoprotein that is carbohydrate-dependent. Homozygosity for the E^d allele, which determines synthesis of an inactive type of apoprotein (E-3) combined with other factors elevating blood cholesterol (i.e., other inherited hyperlipidemias or thyroid deficiency, obesity, glucose intolerance). The necessary presence of two cofactors causes a pseudodominant inheritance. It is hypothesized that deficiency of normal E-3 causes altered degradation of chylomicrons and VLDL determining the appearance of B-VLDL. The B-VLDL alone among lipoproteins rich in cholesterol have the capacity of accumulating in macrophages determining foam cells and xanthomas.

Pathology. Diffuse atheromatosis; gallstones, and cholecystitis frequent. Foam cells in various organs.

Diagnostic Procedures. *Blood.* Plasma aspect usually turbid, often faint cream layer; presence of beta very low-density lipoproteins (VLDL) (floating beta; low-density lipoproteins [LDL] of abnormal composition). Abnormal glucose tolerance test; frank diabetes in some cases. Hyperuricemia in 50% of cases. *Electrocardiography. X-ray.* To demonstrate calcification of atheromas.

Therapy. Diet: low calory intake; 40% carbohydrates; 40% fats; cholesterol below 300 mg/day; alcohol restriction. Clofibrate; nicotinic acid; d-thyroxine; cholestyramine not indicated.

Prognosis. Wide variation, from death in early infancy or in 5th or 6th decade. Good with therapy.

BIBLIOGRAPHY. Gofman JW, De Lalla O, Glazier F, et al: The serum lipoprotein transport system in health metabolic disorders, atherosclerosis and coronary artery disease. Plasma 2:413–484, 1954
Fredrickson DS, Levi RI, Lees RS: Fat transport in lipoproteins: an integrated approach to mechanisms and disorders. New Engl J Med 276:32, 94, 148, 251, 273, 1967
Brown MS, Goldstein JL, Fredrickson DS: Familial type 3 hyperlipoproteinemia (dysbetalipoproteinemia). In Stanbury JB, Wyngaarden JB, Fredrickson DS, et al: The Metabolic Basis of Inherited Disease, 5th ed, p 655. New York, McGraw-Hill, 1983
Grundy SM, Bearn AG (eds): The Role of Cholesterol in Atherosclerosis. Philadelphia, Hanley & Belfus, 1987

HYPERLIPOPROTEINEMIA TYPE IV

Synonym. Carbohydrate-inducible hyperlipemia.

Symptoms and Signs. Early atherosclerotic changes, eruptive xanthoma may be present.

Etiology. It represents a phenotype including many conditions: hypertriglyceridemia (see); combination of III and V hyperlipoproteinemias (see); uremia; hypopituitarism, anticonceptional steroids, von Gierke's (see). Carbohydrate and ethanol consumption strongly influence the degree of biochemical alterations.

Diagnostic Procedures. *Plasma.* High VLDL and triglycerides, normal cholesterol, and phospholipids.

Therapy. *Diet.* Antilipid agents.

Prognosis. Variable. Early atherosclerosis and increased incidence of myocardial infarction.

BIBLIOGRAPHY. Sprinz N: Carbohydrate-induced lipemia: report of a familial occurrence. New Engl J Med 271:291–293, 1964
Fredrickson DS, Goldstein JL, Brown MS: The familial hyperlipoproteinemia. In Stanbury JB, Wyngaarden JB, Fredrickson DS, et al: The Metabolic Basis of Inherited Disease, 4th ed, p 641. New York, McGraw-Hill, 1978
Grundy SM, Bearn AG (eds): The Role of Cholesterol in Atherosclerosis. Philadelphia, Hanley & Belfus, 1987

HYPERLIPOPROTEINEMIA TYPE V

Synonyms. Essential hyperlipemia; familial hyperlipoproteinemia type V; fat-carbohydrate-induced hyperlipemia; mixed hyperlipemia.

Symptoms and Signs. Occur in both sexes; onset in adulthood. Recurrent abdominal pain related to high fat intake; symptoms and mild diabetes (occasionally). Seldom, eruptive xanthomas; no tuberous or tendinous lesions. No striking history of heart ischemia. Hepatosplenomegaly. Mild paresthesias of extremities. Gout in 10 to 20% of cases.

Etiology. Dominant inheritance (?); familial inheritance of undetermined type, probably carrying mutations different from those of other reported hyperlipoproteinemias (see); can also be secondary to diabetes, alcoholism, nephrotic syndrome, hypothyroidism.

Pathology. Nonspecific changes.

Diagnostic Procedures. *Blood.* Plasma, cream layer on top, turbid below; presence of chylomicrons; increased very low-density lipoproteins VLDL cholesterol and triglycerides. Removal of fat from diet causes temporary fall in triglyceride concentration. Abnormal glucose tolerance tests (80%). Hyperuricemia almost constant. Postheparin lipoprotein lipase; and hepatic triglyceride lipase activities in plasma are normal.

Therapy. Restriction of dietary fat to 50 g/day to prevent abnormal attacks. Reduction of carbohydrates. Nicotinic acid 1.0 to 1.5 g/day and clofibrate induce only a moderate reduction of blood hyperlipemia. Steroid hormones more effective in women.

Prognosis. Myocardial ischemia not abnormally prevalent in this condition.

BIBLIOGRAPHY. Malmros H, Swahn B, Truedsson E: Essential hyperlipaemia. Acta Med Scand 149:91–108, 1954
Fredrickson DS, Lees RS: Familial hyperlipoproteinemia. In Stanbury JB, Wyngaarden JB, Fredrickson DS, et al: The Metabolic Basis of Inherited Disease, 2nd ed, p 429. New York, McGraw-Hill, 1966
Nikkilä EA: Familial lipoprotein lipase deficiency and related disorders of chylomicron metabolism. In Stanbury JB, Wyngaarden JB, Fredrickson DS, et al: The Metabolic Basis of Inherited Disease, 5th ed, p 622. New York, McGraw-Hill, 1983
Grundy SM, Bearn AG (eds): The Role of Cholesterol in Atherosclerosis. Philadelphia, Hanley & Belfus, 1987

HYPERLYSINEMIA, PERIODIC

Synonyms. Colombo's; hyperlysinemia-hyperammonemia; lysine intolerance; hyperlysinuria-hyperammonemia. See Hyperlysinemia, persistent.

Symptoms and Signs. Present from birth. Episodes of vomiting; abdominal pain; diarrhea; dehydration; spasticity; episodes of convulsions and comas. Severe motor retardation; hepatosplenomegaly; protein aversion; intelligence retarded or normal.

Etiology. Partial defect in L-lysine nicotinamide adenine dinucleotide (NAD) oxidoreductase activity; incapacity of degrading lysine. Since this amino acid inhibits arginase, it most likely interferes with urea synthesis and leads to ammonia intoxication.

Diagnostic Procedures. *Blood.* Increased plasma lysine and arginine level. Extremely high blood ammonia during attacks. Protein intake (3 g/kg/day) precipitates crisis lasting weeks. Dietary protein restriction and fluid therapy correct and prevent crisis.

Therapy. Diet with reduced amount of lysine. Attacks always follow an excessive protein ingestion.

Prognosis. Poor; treatment prevents acute attacks. If treatment started early enough, may also prevent brain damage.

BIBLIOGRAPHY. Colombo JP, Richterich R, Spahr DA, et al: Congenital lysine intolerance with periodic ammonia intoxication. Lancet I:1014–1015, 1964
Colombo JP, Bürgi W, Richterich R, et al: Congenital lysine intolerance with periodic ammonia intoxication: a defect in L-lysine degradation. Metabolism 16:910–925, 1967
Dancis J, Hutzler J, Cox RP: Familial hyperlysinemia: enzyme studies, diagnostic methods, comments on terminology. Am J Hum Genet 31:290–299, 1979

HYPERLYSINEMIA, PERSISTENT

Synonyms. Ghadimi-Woody; Woody-Ghadimi; lysine-ketoglutarate reductase deficiency. See Hyperlysinemia, periodic.

Symptoms and Signs. Both sexes; age of detection from infancy to early adulthood. Severe mental retardation; occasionally, convulsions. Physical development variable from retardation to normality. Occasionally, laxity of joints and synophrys. Absence of secondary sex characteristics; strabismus, hepatosplenomegaly; altered facial features.

Etiology. Inherited condition; autosomal recessive.

Diagnostic Procedures. *Blood.* Mild anemia; persistent hyperlysinemia with absence of hyperammonemia, even under lysine loading. Lysine loading abnormal response. *Urine.* Hyperlysinuria; usually absence of other basic amino acids. *Electroencephalography.* From normal to petit mal pattern.

Therapy. Symptomatic. Diet.

Prognosis. Poor.

BIBLIOGRAPHY. Woody NC: Hyperlysinemia (abstr). Proc Am Pediatr Soc VII Ann Meeting (Seattle): p 33, 1964
Ghadimi H, Bimington VL, Pecora F: Hyperlysinemia associated with retardation. New Engl J Med 273:723–729, 1965
Dancis J, Hutzler J, Ampola MG, et al: The prognosis of hyperlysinemia: an interim report. Am J Hum Genet 35:438–442, 1983

HYPERMAGNESEMIA

Symptoms. Nausea; vomiting; malaise; micturition; central nervous system depression (drowsiness; lethargy; slight slurring of speech); ataxic gait. Coma (with very high concentration). Cardiac arrest.

Signs. Blood hypotension (if high magnesium plasma concentration); absent tendon reflexes; bradypnea.

Etiology. In newborn (if mother received large doses of magnesium intravenously prior to delivery); in patients who ingest high doses of magnesium, antacids, or receive parenteral administration of magnesium salts, and in patients with renal disease where ability to excrete magnesium is seriously impaired.

Pathology. Unknown.

Diagnostic Procedures. *Blood.* Serum magnesium determination. *Electrocardiography.* P-R prolongation; slight reduction of P waves and QRS duration; nodal rhythm with branch block; Q-T interval increased.

Therapy. Calcium administration; avoidance of magnesium administration in patients with reduced renal function. In severe intoxication, hemodialysis or peritoneal dialysis.

BIBLIOGRAPHY. Randall RE, Cohen MD, Spray CC, et al: Hypermagnesemia in renal failure: etiology and toxic manifestations. Ann Intern Med 61:73–88, 1964

Beck LH (ed): Symposium on body fluid and electrolyte disorders. Med Clin North Am 65:249 (whole issue): 1981

Brenner BM, Rector FC: The Kidney, 3rd ed, pp 588–593. Philadelphia, WB Saunders, 1986

HYPERMOBILE CECUM

Synonym. Mobile cecum.

Symptoms and Signs. Lower right quadrant pain; symptoms mimicking partial bowel obstruction and acute appendicitis.

Etiology. Large range of mobility of cecum and lower half of ascending colon.

Diagnostic Procedures. *X-ray.* Cecum located in midline with dilatation and stasis.

BIBLIOGRAPHY. Rogers RL, Hartford FJ: Mobile cecum syndrome. Dis Colon Rectum 27:399–402, 1984

HYPERMOBILITY

Symptoms. Pain localized to the knees, hands, and fingers.

Signs. The diagnosis of the syndrome is made if the patient is able to perform at least three of the following maneuvers: (1) extension of the wrists and metacarpal phalanges so that the fingers are parallel to the dorsum of the forearm; (2) passive apposition of thumbs to the flexor aspect of the forearm; (3) hyperextension of knees (> 10 degrees); (4) hyperextension of elbows (> 10 degrees); (5) flexion of trunk with knees extended so palms rest on the floor. The absence of easy bruising, lens dislocation, and characteristic skin changes makes posssible the differential diagnosis with Ehlers-Danlos syndrome (see). The hypermobility syndrome may be seen also in association with rheumatic diseases and does not seem to affect the course of these conditions.

Diagnostic Procedures. Serum and x-ray examinations for ruling out rheumatic diseases.

Therapy. Reassurance, physical therapy, and symptomatic therapy (aspirin).

BIBLIOGRAPHY. Biro F, Gewanter HL, Baum J: The hypermobility syndrome. Pediatrics 72:701–706, 1983

HYPERORNITHINEMIA-HYPERAMMONIEMIA-HOMOCITRULLINURIA

Synonyms. HHH; Shih.

Symptoms and Signs. After breast-feeding is stopped, vomiting, lethargy, delayed milestones. After infancy, spontaneous selection of low-protein diet. From moderate to severe mental retardation.

Etiology. Autosomal recessive. Suggested defect of ornithine entry in mitochondria, which decreases urea cycle and impairs ammonia detoxification.

Diagnostic Procedures. *Blood.* Post prandial hyperammonemia, hyperornithinemia. *Urine.* Homocitrullinuria.

Therapy. Protein restriction.

Prognosis. Good *quoad vitam.*

BIBLIOGRAPHY. Shih VE, Efron ML, Moser HW: Hyperornithinemia, hyperammonemia and homocitrullinuria: a new disorder of aminoacid metabolism associated with myoclonic seizures and mental retardation. Ann J Dis Child 117:83–92, 1969

Valle D, Simeel O: The hyperornithinemias. In Stanbury JB, Wyngaarden JB, Fredrickson DS, et al: The Metabolic Basis of Inherited Disease, 5th ed, p 382. New York, McGraw-Hill, 1983

HYPEROSMOLALITY SYNDROMES

1. Part of classic diabetes insipidus (traumatic, see) syndrome (with sodium increase)
2. Intracranial lesions with hypernatremia
3. Essential hypernatremia
4. Asymptomatic hypovolemic hypernatremic (Goldberg's variant)
5. Pure water depletion (with sodium increase)
6. Part of renal failure and urea retention (without sodium increase)
7. As part of uncontrolled diabetes (without sodium increase).

BIBLIOGRAPHY. Bartter FC: Hyper- and hypoosmolality syndromes. Am J Cardiol 12:650–655, 1963

Goldberg M, Weinstein G, Adesman J, et al: Asymptomatic hypovolemic hypernatremia: a variant of essential hypernatremia. Am J Med 43:804–810, 1967

Christie SBM, Ross EJ: Ectopic pinealoma with adipsia and hypernatremia. Br Med J 2:669–679, 1968

DeGroot L, Cahill GF Jr, Odell WD, et al (eds): Endocrinology, p 1025. New York, Grune & Stratton, 1979

HYPERPARATHYROIDISM FAMILIAL

Symptoms. Variable manifestation of hyperparathyroidism in members of same family. Frequent association with glandular pathology. Most frequent association with peptic ulceration, pancreatitis, and renal calculi. See multiple endocrine neoplasia.

Etiology. Unknown; autosomal dominant inheritance.

Pathology. Primary chief-cell hyperplasia most common finding.

Diagnostic Procedures. *Blood.* Calcium; phosphorus; alkaline phosphatase. *X-ray of gastrointestinal tract. Intravenous pyelogram.*

Therapy. Excision of enlarged parathyroid gland. Abdominal operation for gastrointestinal hemorrhage and for calculi of kidney.

Prognosis. Depends upon complications.

BIBLIOGRAPHY. Goldmann L, Smith FS: Hyperparathyroidism in siblings. Ann Surg 104:971–981, 1936

Cutler RE, Reiss E, Ackerman LV: Familial hyperparathyroidism: A kindred involving eleven cases with a discussion of primary chief cell hyperplasia. N Engl J Med 270:859–865, 1964

Sandler LM, Moncrieff MF: Familial hyperparathyroidism. Arch Dis Child 55:146–147, 1980

HYPERPARATHYROIDISM SYNDROMES

Synonyms. Primary hyperparathyroidism; parathyroid hyperfunction. Prevalent in female; onset usually in adulthood. The full blown, complete syndrome is seldom seen initially. A cluster of different syndromes with various degrees of overlapping is the rule.

MYOPATHY

Symptoms. Rare condition (3:76 cases of hyperparathyroidism). Fatigue; muscle weakness (subjective weakness frequent symptom of primary hyperparathyroidism, but presence of objective weakness and atrophy characterize this syndrome).

Signs. Objective muscle weakness; atrophy suggesting diagnosis of primary muscle disease.

Etiology. Unknown; adenoma of parathyroid.

Pathology. Scattered areas of muscle fiber degeneration and neutrophilic infiltration. Presence of functioning adenoma in parathyroid.

Diagnostic Procedures. *Blood.* Typical finding of hyperparathyroidism (see). *Urine.* Increased creatine excretion. *Biopsy of muscle. Electromyography.* High percentage of polyphasic potentials.

Therapy. Surgery to excise adenoma.

Prognosis. Removal of adenoma results in complete recovery of muscle function.

BIBLIOGRAPHY. Vicale CT: The diagnostic features of a muscular syndrome resulting from hyperparathyroidism, osteomalacia, owing to renal tubular acidosis and perhaps to related disorders of calcium metabolism. Trans Am Neurol Assoc 74th Meeting, p 143, 1949

Frame B, Heinze EG, Block MA, et al: Myopathy in primary hyperparathyroidism. Ann Intern Med 68:1022–1027, 1968

SKELETAL SYNDROME OF HYPERPARATHYROIDISM

See von Recklinghausen's.

Symptoms. Seldom seen in pure form (without urologic syndrome). Fifteen percent of cases of hyperparathyroidism. Bone or articular discomfort; fractures and vertebral collapse.

Signs. Cystic formation in various bones (frequent site: mandible or maxilla).

Etiology. Unknown; sporadic adenoma hyperplasia or cancer of parathyroid; familial form of hyperparathyroidism. Adenomas also found in association with multiple different endocrine adenomas (see Wermer's).

Pathology. *Parathyroid.* Edema usually limited to one gland (in 90–95% of cases); size of gland, from pea to large egg. The gland may be ectopically found in mediastinum or embedded in thymus; orange brown mass; necrosis and hemorrhage into the gland frequent; water-clear cells. Carcinoma rare. *Bones.* Increased osteoclastic and osteoblastic activity; generalized reabsorption and rarefaction; cyst formation and fibrous tissue replacement of marrow space.

Diagnostic Procedures. *Blood.* Increased calcium and decreased phosphorus; increased alkaline phosphatase activity. *Urine.* Hypercalcuria. *X-ray of skeleton.* Evidence of generalized osteoporosis; coarse trabeculation; increased size; partial fractures; cyst formation.

Therapy. Exploration and excision of parathyroid tumor.

Prognosis. Good; recovery of bone defects of calcification once tumor is removed.

UROLOGIC SYNDROME OF HYPERPARATHYROIDISM

Symptoms and Signs. Most common manifestation in 75% of hyperparathyroid patients. It is almost constantly associated with major or minor degree of skeletal changes. Symptoms of renal calculosis. Pain in lumbar region with radiation along the ureters to testes or groin.

Etiology. See skeletal syndrome section.

Pathology. Parathyroid, see Skeletal syndrome. Kidneys more frequently present definite concretions; seldom, generalized nephrocalcinosis. Associated inflammatory changes. Tubular damage from calcium deposition.

Diagnostic Procedures. *Blood.* See Skeletal syndrome, plus increase of blood urea nitrogen. *Urine.* Abnormality of urine-concentrating ability. *X-ray.* Demonstration of kidney lesions.

Therapy. See Skeletal syndrome.

Prognosis. Depending on time of surgical excision of tumor. If process too advanced, irreversible kidney changes and death from uremia. If early treatment, good recovery.

HYPERCALCEMIC SYNDROME IN HYPERPARATHYROIDISM

See Hypercalcemic; occurs usually in mild form with other manifestation of hyperparathyroidism.

PEPTIC ULCER SYNDROME IN HYPERPARATHYROIDISM

See Wermer's.

Symptoms and Signs. The association of peptic ulcer symptoms and hyperparathyroidism is higher than incidence of peptic ulcer in general population. Symptoms and signs are those of peptic ulcer. Distinctive features are (1) preponderance of duodenal ulcer in females; (2) relative high frequency of gastric ulcer in males; (3) absence of gastric hypersecretion; (4) more refractoriness to direct medical and surgical treatment; (5) prompt healing after removal of parathyroid tumor (but not in Wermer's, see).

ACUTE PANCREATITIS IN HYPERPARATHYROIDISM

Symptoms and Signs. Those of acute pancreatitis.

Etiology. Calcium precipitate in alkaline pancreatic ducts.

CENTRAL NERVOUS SYSTEM

Symptoms and Signs. Apathy, depression, malaise, fatigue. Mental depression or other psychiatric manifestations (occasionally, anxiety or psychiatric behavior). Mental obtundation up to coma when severe hypocalcemia.

Diagnostic Procedures. *Electroencephalography.* No specific abnormalities.

BIBLIOGRAPHY. von Recklinghausen FD: Die Fibröse oder Deformirende Ostitis, die Osteomalacie und die Osteoplastische Carcinose in Ihren Gegenseitigen Beziehungen. Festschrift Rudolf Virchow (Berlin), 1891
Ellis C, Nicoloff DM: Hyperparathyroidism and peptic ulcer disease. Arch Surg 96:114–118, 1968
Hahn TJ: Parathyroid hormone, calcitonin, vitamin D. Mineral and bone: metabolism and disorders. In Mazzaferri EL (ed): Endocrinology, 3rd ed, pp 199–502. New York, Medical Examination Publishing, 1985

HYPERPATHIA

Synonym. Thalamic hyperpathia. See Dejerine-Roussy.

Symptoms. Hemilateral disagreeable sensations caused by different stimuli (heat; cold; touch; vibration) but usually with a raised threshold to stimulation. Seldom, sensations may give a pleasurable effect that may be isolated or associated with other symptoms of Dejerine-Roussy (see).

Etiology. Release of thalamic activity from cortical control (?); observed also with peripheral nerve diseases.

Therapy. Painful sensations unresponsive to analgesics.

BIBLIOGRAPHY. Head H, Holmes G: Sensory disturbances from cerebral lesions. Brain 34:102–254, 1911

Vick NA: Grinker's Neurology, 7th ed. Springfield, CC Thomas, 1976

HYPERPHENYLALANINEMIA SYNDROMES

TYPE 1

See Foelling's.

TYPE 2 PERSISTENT HYPERPHENYLALANINEMIA

Asymptomatic.

TYPE 3 TRANSIENT MILD HYPERPHENYLALANINEMIA

Asymptomatic.

TYPE 4 DIHYDROPTERIDINE REDUCTASE DEFICIENCY

Symptoms and Signs. Normal at birth. Within 1 year of life; seizures, abnormal mental development; at 18 months, voluntary movements and social awareness have stopped.

Etiology. Dihydropteridine reductase deficiency. Autosomal recessive inheritance.

Diagnostic Procedures. *Electroencephalography.* Gross abnormalities.

Therapy. Dopa, 5-OH-tryptophan, carbidopa.

Prognosis. Physical growth fair in spite of severe cerebral damage.

TYPE 5

Symptoms. Myoclonus, tetraplegia, recurrent hyperthermia, greasy skin.

Etiology. Dihydrobiopterin synthesis defect.

Diagnostic Procedures. *Urinalysis.* Abnormal biopterin metabolites.

Therapy. DOPA, 5-OH-tryptophan, carbidopa.

TYPE 6 PERSISTENT HYPERPHENYLALANINEMIA AND TYROSINEMIA

Symptoms and Signs. Progressive ataxia and seizures appearing between 12 and 18 months.

Etiology. Perhaps defect of catabolism of tyrosine.

Diagnostic Procedures. *Urinalysis.* Phenylethylamine, mandelic acid, p-OH mandelic acid.

Therapy. Diet.

TYPE 7 TRANSIENT NEONATAL TYROSINEMIA

Asymptomatic.

Therapy. Vitamin C

TYPE 8 HEREDITARY TYROSINEMIA (SEE)

BIBLIOGRAPHY. Smith J: Atypical phenylketonuria accompanied by a severe progressive neurological illness unresponsive to dietary treatment. Arch Dis Child 49:245–250, 1974

Kaufman S, Helzman NA, Milstein S, et al: Phenylketonuria due to a deficiency of dehydropteridine reductase. New Engl J Med 293:785, 1979

Tourian A, Sidbury JB: Phenylketonuria and hyperphenylalaninemia. In Stanbury JB, Wyngaarden JB, Fredrickson DS, et al: The Metabolic Basis of Inherited Disease, 5th ed, p 270. New York, McGraw-Hill, 1983

HYPERPROLINEMIA

Synonyms. Familial renal iminoglycinuria; Joseph's.

Two types described. Both are autosomal recessive traits not associated with symptoms and signs of disease. The association of hyperprolinemia with renal disease is today considered obsolete.

Type I is due to proline oxidase deficiency. Type II is due to delta-pyrrolidine 5-carboxylate dehydrogenase deficiency.

BIBLIOGRAPHY. Joseph R, et al: Maladie familiale associant des convulsions à début très précoce, une hyperaminoacidurie. Arch Fr Pediatr 15:374–387, 1958

Berlow S, Efron ME: A new cause of hyperprolinemia associated with the excretion of Δ pyrrolidine-5-carboxylic acid. Proc Soc Pediatr Res 34th Ann Meet, Seattle, WA 1974, p 43

Scriver CR, Smith RJ, Phang JM: Disorders of proline and hydroxyproline metabolism. In Stanbury JB, Wyngaarden JB, Fredrickson DS, et al: The Metabolic Basis of Inherited Disease, 5th ed, p 360. New York, McGraw-Hill 1983

HYPERSARCOSINEMIA

Synonym. Sarcosinemia.

Symptoms and Signs. Mild mental retardation and few morphological abnormalities.

Etiology. Autosomal recessive.

Diagnostic Procedures. *Liver biopsy.* Deficiency of sarcosine dehydrogenase.

BIBLIOGRAPHY. Gerritsen T, Waisman HA: Hypersarcosinemia: an inborn error of metabolism. New Engl J Med 275:66–69, 1966

Kang ES, Seyer J, Tood TA, et al: Variability in the phenotypic expression of the abnormal sarcosine metabolism in a family. J Hum Genet 64:80–85, 1983

HYPERSOMNIA

Synonyms. Von Economo. See Gélineau's, Kleine-Levin, Pickwickian, and Elpenor's.

Symptoms. Gradual onset of irresistible desire to sleep, which allows the patient enough time to withdraw and go to bed; prolonged sleep (not associated with cataplexy, sleep paralysis, or hypnagogic hallucination, as in narcolepsy). Sleep is prolonged for hours, days, or weeks. Difficult to arouse; irritable; drowsy; slow mentation after awaking. Introverted; slightly anxious; mildly depressed.

Etiology and Pathology. Multiple conditions are responsible for this syndrome: trauma; brain tumors; destructive lesions or inflammation of brainstem; menarche or menstrual cycle; psychogenic basis; diencephalic dysfunction. The syndrome of Kleine-Levin may be considered a particular form of hypersomnia, as well as pickwickian and Elpenor's.

Diagnostic Procedures. *Electroencephalography.* Normal sleep stage pattern. Cyclic regularity of (no rapid eye movement) NREM-REM (rapid eye movement) stages for all periods of sleep. *X-ray of skull. CT brain scan. Angiography of skull. Basal metabolism.*

Therapy. Stimulant drugs useful.

Prognosis. According to etiology.

BIBLIOGRAPHY. Bonkalo A: Hypersomnia: a discussion of psychiatric implication based on three cases. Br J Psychiatr 114:69–75, 1968

Hartmann E: Sleep requirements: long sleepers, short sleepers, variable sleepers and insomniacs. Psychosomatics 14:95–103, 1973

HYPERSPLENISM SYNDROMES

Symptoms and Signs. All clinical manifestations associated with any combination of anemia, thrombocytopenia, and leukopenia. In patient with enlarged spleen, bone marrow not primarily involved. According to some authors, all cases in which there is a return to normal values of blood elements after splenectomy. See Doan-Wright, Doan-Wiseman, Felty's, Hodgkin's syndromes, Banti's, Besnier-Boek-Schaumann.

Etiology. Sequestration and increased rate of destruction of blood cells due to idiopathic or secondary splenomegaly. Splenic suppression of bone marrow cell production postulated but not confirmed.

BIBLIOGRAPHY. Doan CA: Hypersplenism. Bull NY Acad Med 25:625–650, 1949

Cooney DP, Smith BA: The pathophysiology of hypersplenic thrombocytopenia. Arch Intern Med 121:332–337, 1968

Wintrobe MM (ed): Clinical Hematology, 8th ed. Philadelphia, Lea & Febiger, 1981

HYPERSTIMULATION

Synonym. Secondary Meigs'.

Symptoms. Occur in patients receiving human menopausal gonadotropins for treatment of amenorrhea and infertility. Abdominal pain and distension; acute abdominal crisis; tachycardia; oliguria; hematuria; chest pain; dyspnea.

Signs. Ascites; ovarian enlargement; hydrothorax.

Etiology. Administration of human menopausal gonadotropins, clomiphene.

Pathology. Ovarian enlargement, necrosis. Ascites; hydrothorax; in some cases; intraabdominal hemorrhages.

Diagnostic Procedures. *Blood and urine.* Electrolytes. Nonprotein nitrogen. *Electrocardiography.*

Therapy. Discontinuation of administration of drug; rest; fluid therapy. If surgery necessary, wedge resection indicated rather than castration, except in uncontrollable hemorrhage.

Prognosis. Generally good. Cases of death reported.

BIBLIOGRAPHY. Vandiest L, DeBast A: Syndrome adbominal aigü par dégénérescence kystique massive et totale des ovaires due a l'administration des gonadotrophines. Brux Med 38:1636–1642, 1958

Neuwirth RS, Turksoy RN, Vande Wiele RL: Acute Meig's syndrome secondary to ovarian stimulation with human menopausal gonadotropins. Am J Obstet Gynecol 91:977–981, 1965

HYPERTELORISM-HYPOSPADIAS

Synonyms. BBB; telecanthus-associated abnormalities; Opitz-Christian; Christian-Opitz.

Symptoms and Signs. Female carriers only telecanthus. In males, telecanthus (more marked than in females) and hypospadias; sometimes cryptorchidism, cleft lip and palate, urinary malformation, and mental retardation.

Etiology. Unknown. Possible X-linked inheritance.

BIBLIOGRAPHY. Opitz JM, Summit RL, Smith DW: The BBB syndrome: familial telecanthus with associated congenital anomalies. Birth Defects Orig Art Ser V (2):86–94, 1969

Christian JC, Bixler D, Blythe S, et al: Familial telecanthus with associated congenital anomalies. Birth Defects Orig Art Ser V (2):82–85, 1969

Silva EO: The hypertelorism-hypospadias syndrome. Clin Genet 23:30–34, 1983

HYPERTRICHOSIS LANUGINOSA CONGENITAL

Symptoms and Signs. Present at birth. Overgrowth of lanugo hair and precocious teeth.

Etiology. Autosomal dominant with varying expressivity.

Therapy. Dental care; counseling; shaving; bleaching the hair; chemical and electrical epilation.

Prognosis. Good. In some cases, hypertrichosis diminishes later in childhood. Shaving does not increase the profusion or rate of regrowth of hair.

BIBLIOGRAPHY. Beighton P: Congenital hypertrichosis lanuginosa. Arch Dermatol 101:669–672, 1970

Partridge JW: Congenital hypertrichosis lanuginosa: neonatal shaving. Arch Dis Child: 62:623–625, 1987

HYPERTRIGLYCERIDEMIA

Synonym. Combined hyperlipidemia.

Symptoms and Signs. Both sexes affected; age of detection second to sixth decades. Uncertain clinical features. Moderate obesity; increased risk of coronary heart disease. Absence of pancreatic involvement and eructive xanthomas.

Etiology. Autosomal dominant inheritance. The syndrome encompasses a wide variety of several biochemical defects. The phenotype is that of hyperlipoproteinemia IV (see).

Pathology. Nonspecific.

Diagnostic Procedures. *Blood.* Type IV hyperlipoproteinemia; plasma turbid, no cream layer; very low-density lipoproteins (VLDL) increased; chylomicrons "absent"; low-density lipoproteins (LDL) not increased; cholesterol normal; triglycerides increased. Fasting hyperglycemia; insulin resistance; glucose intolerance, hyperuricemia.

Therapy. No specific treatment. Carbohydrate and caloric restriction. Clorofibrate. Trial with human plasma if associated with apolipoprotein II deficiency (drop of triglycerides lasting 6 days). New antilipemic agents under investigation: Lovastatin.

Prognosis. Association with myocardial ischemia and early death.

BIBLIOGRAPHY. Fredrickson DS, Goldstein JL, Brown MS: The familial hyperlipoproteinemias. In Stanbury JB, Wyngaarden JB, Fredrickson DS: The Metabolic Basis of Inherited Disease, 4th ed, p 641. New York, McGraw-Hill, 1978

Breckenridge WC, Little, Steiner G, et al: Hypertriglyceridemia associated with deficiency of apolipoprotein C-II. New Engl J Med 298:1265–1273, 1978

Karathanasis SK, McPherson J, Zannis VI, et al: Linkage of human apolipoproteins A-1 and C-III genes. Nature 304:371–373, 1983

HYPERVALINEMIA

Synonym. Valinemia.

Symptoms and Signs. Present from early infancy. Vomiting; diarrhea; failure to thrive; mental retardation; hyperkinesia. Muscular hypotonia; nystagmus.

Etiology. Deficiency of enzyme converting valine to corresponding keto-acid.

Diagnostic Procedures. *Plasma and urine.* Increased valine concentration. *Electroencephalography. Electromyography.*

Therapy. Low-protein diet. Plasmapheresis of questionable benefit: Penicillamine, corticosteroids and azathioprine.

Prognosis. Poor.

BIBLIOGRAPHY. Tanaka K, Rosenberg LE: Disorders of branched chain amino acid and organic acid metabolism. In Stanbury JB, Wyngaarden JB, Fredrickson DS: The Metabolic Basis of Inherited Disease, 5th ed, p 440. New York, McGraw-Hill, 1983

Chen LB, Amlinder EP, Wolke AM, et al: Role of plasmapheresis in primary biliary cirrhosis. Gut 26:291–294, 1985

HYPERVENTILATION

Synonyms. Carbonic acid deficit; psychophysiologic hyperventilation; respiratory alkalosis.

Symptoms. Rare; most often females between 20 and 40 years of age. Precipitating factor nervous tension accompanied by headache, apprehension, indigestion, irritable colon. Presyncopal symptoms: palpitation; weakness; dizziness; trembling; sweating; paresthesias in extremities and perioral region; flushed face; chest pain; shortness of breath; sighing respiration. Attack occurs with patient standing or sitting, not lying down. Syncope (there may be short loss of consciousness or just brief dimming of consciousness as only manifestation). Dimming of consciousness may sometimes last hours because, after losing and regaining consciousness, the patient hyperventilates again for a few seconds. Tetany is rarely associated. Postsyncopal: weakness; apprehension for hours.

Symptoms and Signs. Tetany (rare); sweating; tachycardia.

Etiology. (1) Fast breathing and susceptibility to syncope. Combination of factors: emotion, tenseness; drop of P_{CO_2}; reduced cerebral flow and decreased oxygen release by oxihemoglobin. (2) Central nervous lesions. (3) Salicylate, sulfonamides administration. (4) Compensatory reaction in respiratory acidosis (tracheotomy or sudden increase in ventilation).

Pathology. According to etiology.

Diagnostic Procedures. Rule out other causes of syncope (see Syncope syndromes). Many patients may reproduce voluntary syncope by overbreathing. *Blood.* P_{CO_2} low; pH high; carbon dioxide content, actual bicarbonate low, carbon dioxide capacity and standard bicarbonate normal. Chloride high; serum sodium low or normal.

Therapy. Correct the tension and advise the patient about the mechanism precipitating the syncope; correct other causes when different etiology.

Prognosis. Good.

BIBLIOGRAPHY. Maytum CK: Tetany caused by functional dyspnea with hyperventilation: Report of case. Proc Staff Meet Mayo Clin 8:282–284, 1933
Magarian GJ: Hyperventilation syndromes: infrequently recognized common expression of anxiety and stress. Medicine 61:219–236, 1982
Weissler AM, Warren JV: Syncope: pathophysiology and differential diagnosis. In Hurst JW: The Heart, 6th ed, p 518. New York, McGraw-Hill, 1986

HYPOBETALIPOPROTEINEMIA

Synonym. Beta-lipoprotein deficiency.

Symptoms and Signs. Similar to Bassen-Kornzweig (see) in the homozygous state. In the heterozygotes only, blood lipid abnormalities. In homozygous neurological symptoms are less severe than in the classical form.

Etiology. Autosomal dominant inheritance. Represents a mutation different from Bassen-Kornzweig syndrome.

Diagnostic Procedures. *Blood.* LDL low but present; HDL normal.

Therapy. Vitamin E.

Prognosis. Good for heterozygotes. For homozygotes, see Bassen-Kornzweig.

BIBLIOGRAPHY. Van Buchem FSP, Pol G, De Grier J, et al: Congenital beta-lipoprotein deficiency. Am J Med 40:794, 1966
Herbert PN, Assman G, Gatto AM Jr, Fredrickson DS: Familial deficiency: abetalipoproteinemia, hypobetalipoproteinemia, and Tangier disease. In Stanbury JB, Wyngaarden JB, Fredrickson DS, et al; The Metabolic Basis of Inherited Disease, 5th ed, p 589. New York, McGraw-Hill, 1983

HYPOCALCEMIA

Symptoms. Tetany. In infants, laryngospasm, facial muscle spasm, paresthesia, change of mood, asthmatic attacks, convulsions.

Signs. Trousseau's, Chvostek's signs. Skin dry, coarse; absent or patchy scalp hair; scant body hair. Other signs associated with basic condition (see Etiology).

Etiology. As part of (1) rickets and osteomalacia; (2) malabsorption syndromes; (3) Balser's; (4) hypoparathyroidism; (5) pseudohypoparathyroidism; (6) renal insufficiency, (7) Epstein's. As result of use of chelating agent in administration of large amount of citrated blood.

Pathology. According to etiology.

Diagnostic Procedures. *Blood.* Hypocalcemia; potassium normal, low, or high. *Urine.* Absence of calcium; Ellsworth-Howard test. *Electrocardiography.* Q-T interval prolonged; normal RS-T segment and T wave. *X-ray.* According to etiology. *Stool.*

Therapy. If tetany, calcium gluconate or calcium lactate intravenously. High calcium, low phosphorus, vitamin D in diet. Specific treatment of basic condition (see etiology).

Prognosis. Depends on etiology.

BIBLIOGRAPHY. Rabin D, McKenna TJ: Calcium and phosphate homeostasis. In Clinical Endocrinology and Metabolism, Vol 9, pp 324–371 of Science and Practice of Medicine. Philadelphia, Grune & Stratton, 1982

Brenner BM, Rector FC: The Kidney, 3rd ed, p 577. Philadelphia, WB Saunders, 1986

HYPOFIBRINOGENEMIA, HEREDITARY

Synonyms. Factor I deficiency; fibrinogen synthesis partial deficiency. See Dysfibrinogenemias and Rabe-Salomon.

Symptoms. Both sexes affected; onset not as early as above. Same hemorrhagic manifestations as above; both less severe and infrequent.

Etiology. Deficient synthesis of fibrinogen. Possibly autosomal recessive or dominant with incomplete penetration.

Diagnostic Procedures. Fibrinogen markedly reduced; poor clot formation.

Therapy. Fibrinogen during bleeding episodes.

Prognosis. All patients reached adulthood.

BIBLIOGRAPHY. Revol L: Les grandes hypofibrinémies cos-titutionalles hémorrhagiques. Étude clinique, hémato-logique, génetique et thérapeutique. Hemostase 2:243–254, 1962

Gilabert J, Regañon E, Vila V, et al: Congenital hypofi-brinogenemia and pregnancy: obstetric and hematologi-cal management. Gynecol Obstet Invest 24:171–176, 1987

Vila V, Regañon E, Aznar J, et al: Congenital dysfibrino-genemia characterized by defective release of fibrino-peptide A and fibrinogen degradation products. Thrombs Res 45:437–449, 1987

HYPOGLOBULINEMIA, TRANSIENT INFANTILE

Symptoms and Signs. Both sexes affected. After a few months of normal life, severe irritability, mild gastrointestinal disturbance. Edema in periorbital region; pallor. Moderate liver enlargement. Lineal growth continues at normal rate.

Etiology. Transitory deficiency that develops because of delayed onset of production of immunoglobulin, after catabolism of placental transferred maternal IgG.

Diagnostic Procedures. *Blood.* Anemia; hypoglobuline-mia; absence of gamma globulin. *Liver function.* Minor alterations. *Urine.* Normal.

Therapy. Injection of gamma globulin.

Prognosis. Cases with early onset more severe manifestation. Recovery with normalization of protein; disappearance of hepatomegaly in 3 to 5 months.

BIBLIOGRAPHY. Ulstrom RA, Smith NJ, Heimlich EM: Transient dysproteinemia in infants: a new syndrome. Am J Dis Child 92:219–253, 1956

Sell S: Immunological deficiency diseases. Arch Pathol 86:95–107, 1968

Tiller TL, Buckley RH: Transient hypoglobulinemia of infancy: review of the literature, clinical and immuno-logical features of 11 new cases, a long-term follow-up. J Pediatr 92:347–353, 1978

HYPOGLYCEMIA, TRANSIENT NEONATAL

Synonym. Neonatal hypoglycemia.

Symptoms. Predominant in males born of mothers reported to have had preeclampsia (50% of cases); in normal newborn infants who breathed and cried spontaneously, symptoms beginning from 2 hours to 7 days after birth. Tremor; cyanosis; convulsion; apnea or respiratory distress; eye rolling; limpness; apathy; weak or high-pitched cry; difficulty in feeding.

Signs. Usually underweight; below the 10th percentile. When twin birth, the syndrome usually is present in the lower weight twin. Prompt response to intravenous administration of glucose.

Etiology. Unknown; possibly malnutrition in intrauterine environment, primary brain defect, of faulty glyco-genolytic mechanism.

Pathology. Unknown.

Diagnostic Procedures. *Blood.* Blood sugar level lower than 20 mg/100 ml; calcium usually low; polycythemia. *Spinal fluid.* Normal except for hypoglycorrhachia. *Glu-cagon, tolbutamide, leucine tolerance tests. Glucose toler-ance test. Epinephrine and glucagon combined tolerance test.*

Therapy. Glucose intravenously. Adrenocorticotropic hormone (ACTH) or corticosteroids.

Prognosis. Self-limited course. Dramatic improvement after glucose administration.

BIBLIOGRAPHY. Cornblath M, Odell GB, Levin EY: Symptomatic neonatal hypoglycemia associated with toxemia of pregnancy. J Pediatr 55:545–562, 1959

Cornblath M, Reisner SH: Blood glucose in neonate and its clinical significance. New Engl J Med 273:378–381, 1965

Koivisto M, Benco-Sequiros M, Krause V: Neonatal symptomatic and asymptomatic hypoglycemia: a follow-up of 151 children. Dev Med Chil Neurol 14:603–614, 1972

HYPOGLYCEMIC, TRANSIENT HEMIPLEGIA

Symptoms. No sex preference; all age groups affected. Usually, attacks precipitated by fasting or exercise. Transient flaccid or spastic paralysis, with various degrees of muscle weakness, involving the right side more frequently. Attack may last a few hours or a few days, recurring frequently about three times within a period of a few days.

Signs. Babinski's sign, often bilateral; sensory change inconstant. Tachycardia; profuse sweating usually precedes the paralysis and convulsions (often coma). Occasionally, however, hemiplegia may be an isolated manifestation.

Etiology. Hypoglycemia of endogenous or exogenous origin. Insulin administration; adrenal tumor; pancreatic adenomas; idiopathic hypoglycemia.

Pathology. Damage from hypoglycemia is usually transient, and no data are available.

Diagnostic Procedures. *Blood.* Hypoglycemia. *Functional studies* (see Hypoglycemic) *and x-ray.* To determine cause of hypoglycemia.

Therapy. Glucose intravenous infusion.

Prognosis. Easily reversible if treated promptly.

BIBLIOGRAPHY. Miller WL, Trescher JH: Amnesia, epileptiform convulsive seizures and hemiparesis as manifestations of insulin shock. Am J Med Sci 174:453, 1927

Montgomery BM, Pinner CA: Transient hypoglycemic hemiplegia. Arch Intern Med 114:680–684, 1964

Koivisto M, Blenco-Sequiros M, Krause V: Neonatal symptomatic hypoglycemia: a follow-up of 151 children. Dev Med Chil Neurol 14 :603, 1972

HYPOKALEMIA

Synonyms. Hypopotassemia; potassium deficiency. See also Siegal-Cattan-Manou.

Symptoms. Anorexia; nausea; vomiting; abdominal distention; paralytic ileus; generalized weakness; mental depression. Thirst and polyuria (occasional). Tetany may also occur.

Signs. Abdominal tympanism; tendon hyporeflexia.

Etiology. (1) Excessive fluid administration. (2) As part of the metabolic alkalosis syndrome. (3) Loss of potassium from gastrointestinal tract or through urine. (4) Chronic malnutrition. (5) Potassium redistribution in the body (i.e., into liver, muscles).

Pathology. *Kidney* (in chronic deficiency). Degenerative changes of tubules; no glomerular vascular changes. *Heart.* Degeneration of myocardium; loss of muscle cell striation; karyorrhexis; karyolysis; infiltration with neutrophils and monocytes, progressing to fibrosis.

Diagnostic Procedures. *Blood.* Potassium low; calcium normal, low, or high; features of metabolic alkalosis (see). *Urine.* Potassium may be increased, normal, or low. *Electrocardiography.* Best diagnostic tool for this condition. Lowering and broadening of T wave; prolongation of Q-T interval; with more severe hypokalemia, progression of those findings up to downward shifting of T wave, appearance of a prominent U wave, depression of RS-T segment.

Therapy. Potassium through a peripheral IV line can be given at rates up to 40 mEq/hour. It is better not to exceed 100–200 mEq/daily. Correct the underlying cause (alkalosis, gastrointestinal pathology, etc.).

Prognosis. Severe condition that may result in death if not efficiently corrected.

BIBLIOGRAPHY. Brenner BM, Rector FC: The Kidney, 3rd ed, p 525. Philadelphia, WB Saunders, 1986

HYPOKALEMIC PERIODIC PARALYSIS

Synonyms. Shakhonovich's; paroxysmal myoplegia. See Albright-Hadorn and Hypokalemia.

Symptoms. Prevalent in males in most affected families and in the sporadic cases; age of onset from first year to 5th decade (between 7 and 21 years in 90% of cases). Between attacks, patients are free of symptoms; occasionally, slight decrease of muscle strength. Attacks of migraine may precede for years the onset of the muscular syndrome. Precipitating factors: stresses (infection; surgery; emotions; menstruation; cold); large meal rich in carbohydrates; rest after intense exercise; various drugs (epinephrine; adenocoticotropic hormone [ACTH]; desoxycorticosterone; thyroid; licorice). Prodromal symptoms: most of the time attacks occur in early hours of the morning at awaking. During the day stiffness, cramps, paresthesia, irritability, severe thirst may warn of attack. Exercise may "work out" the attack. Attack: onset in the legs, spreading to the rest of the body of a flaccid type of paralysis. Limited paralysis also reported. Eye movement, speech, swallowing, respiration, mental faculties, and sensory acuity unaffected during attack. Occasionally, nausea, vomiting, or constipation. Recovery in 1 hour or 1 day, or later, following diuresis and sweating; strength returns first in neck and arms.

Signs. Between attacks, increased muscular size (in some cases suggesting pseudohypertrophic muscular dystrophy). During attacks muscles may have firmer consistency and increased circumference. Tendon reflexes are diminished or absent. In some cases, bradycardia, cardiomegaly during attack. In these cases, tachycardia precedes attack.

Etiology. Unknown. Adrenal hypersecretion; alteration of carbohydrate metabolism. Primary defect of muscle. Autosomal dominant in most families; sporadic cases reported.

Pathology. Mainly normal muscle fiber; some fiber degenerative changes (especially after years of attacks). Typical lesion observable with light and electron microscope, consisting in small subsarcolemmic vacuolization.

Diagnostic Procedures. *Blood.* During attack, neutrophilia, leukocytosis, and eosinopenia; followed, after recovery, by lymphocytosis and eosinophilia. Between attacks, potassium normal or low; during attack, low. Sodium retention preceding the attacks; slight serum elevation preceding and during attack. Phosphorus (inorganic) falls during attack. Cholesterol rises during attack. *Urine.* Potassium excretion falls simultaneously with serum value fall; after end of attack, potassium diuresis for 1 to 2 days. Sodium increases at termination of attack. During attack mild proteinuria, glycosuria, acetonuria, and cylindruria. *Electromyography.* Normal between attacks; during attack, progressive increase in latent period, action potential more prolonged in duration and reduced in amplitude. *Electrocardiography.* Changes typical of hypokalemia. *Biopsy muscle.* See Pathology.

Therapy. Potassium chloride 5–10 g daily; if unsuccessful, low-sodium, low-carbohydrate diet and slowly releasing potassium preparation. During attack 10g of KCl (or other salt). Exceptionally intravenous K^+ administration (40 mEq/h).

Prognosis. Severity and frequency of attacks increasing up to 20 years, stable up to 30 years, and declining or disappearing afterward, especially in females. In some patients, especially male, severe attacks may continue in middle and later life. Progressive muscular atrophy may supervene in elderly patients.

BIBLIOGRAPHY. Shakhnovitch: On a case of intermittent paraplegia. Russk Vratch 32:537, 1882; London M Rec 12:130, 1884 (abstr by Idelson V)

Adams RD, Victor M: Principles of Neurology, 3rd ed, pp 1085–1086. New York, McGraw-Hill, 1985

HYPOMAGNESEMIA

Synonym. Magnesium deficiency.

Symptoms. Tremor and twitching; liability to severe potentially fatal epileptiform seizures. Occasionally, mental disturbance, confusion, agitation, hallucination.

Signs. Chvostek's sign; no Trousseau's sign.

Etiology. Magnesium deficiency in severe gastroenteritis, malnutrition, and diarrhea. Increased calcium intake after prolonged severe diarrhea. Primary forms with autosomal (with later onset) dominant, recessive, and X-linked (early onset) inheritance.

Diagnostic Procedures. *Blood.* Determination of magnesium, calcium, protein levels.

Therapy. Administration of magnesium.

Prognosis. Symptoms respond rapidly to treatment with magnesium deficient diet, children deteriorate rapidly, developing neurologic complications; recovery is rapid with treatment.

BIBLIOGRAPHY. Flink EB, McCollister R, Prasad AS, et al: Evidences for clinical magnesium deficiency. Ann Int Med 47:956–968, 1957

Albertson PD, Krauss M (eds): The pathogenesis and clinical significance of magnesium deficiency. Ann NY Acad Sci 162:705–984, 1969

Teeby AS: Primary hypomagnesemie, an X-borne allele? Lancet I:701, 1983

Dudin KI, Teebi AS: Primary hypomagnesemia. Eur J Pediatr 146:303–305, 1987

HYPONATREMIA SYNDROMES

Synonyms. Dehydration; (also used as synonym of "pure water depletion syndrome"); desalting water loss; hypoosmolality; low sodium; pure salt depletion; sodium loss.

Symptoms. In acute loss, shock. In chronic loss; weakness, apathy, faintness, no thirst, anorexia, nausea, muscle cramps, orthostatic hypotension, cold extremities. Progression to confused state, brain syndrome, acute (see).

Signs. Eyeballs sunken and soft; glassy stare, tongue shrunken, longitudinal wrinkling; skin lacks elasticity and when pinched, remains folded. Tachycardia; low blood pressure; small pulse; absent peripheral pulse; vein collapse. In severe form; clammy, sweating skin.

Etiology. Sodium loss: from vomiting, diarrhea, gastrointestinal or biliary fistula, intestinal tubing and lavage, intense sweating (and drinking). Burns; as part of mucoviscidosis. Small bowel obstruction: salt loss into and from serous cavities. In immediate postoperative period, as component of Addisonian syndromes (see), Thorn's (see), Schwartz-Bartter (see). Iatrogenic: administration of diuretics or forced fluid, in syndromes of secondary hyperaldosteronism, and sodium retention (see Schroeder's), and after hypodermoclysis of dextrose in water.

Diagnostic Procedures. *Blood.* Hemoconcentration, with high mean corpuscular volume of red cells. Blood volume low; sodium low; chloride and bicarbonate low; potassium usually high; blood urea nitrogen high; serum osmolality low.* *Urine.* Volume low; specific gravity normal; sodium and chloride very low.

Therapy. Treatment of shock. Arrest of further sodium loss and replacement of sodium to compensate for loss; addition of other electrolytes as necessary. Plasma transfusion indicated. Treatment of basic pathology.

Prognosis. Severe outcome according to severity of form and etiology.

BIBLIOGRAPHY. Schroeder HA: Renal failure associated with low extracellular sodium chloride; the low salt syndrome. JAMA 141:117–124, 1949

Bartter FC: Hyper and Hypo-osmolality syndromes. Am J Cardiol 12:650–655, 1963

Goldberger E: A Primer of Water, Electrolyte, and Acid-Base Syndromes, 3rd ed. Philadelphia, Lea & Febiger, 1965

Flear CT, Gill GU: Burn J: Hyponatremia mechanisms and management. Lancet II:26–31, 1981

Barton IK: Fluid and electrolyte disorders: sodium. Br J Hosp Med 32(1):15–18, 1984

Anderson RJ, Chung HM, Kluge R, et al. Hyponatremia: A prospective analysis of its epidemiology and the

pathogenetic role of vasopressin. Ann Intern Med 102:164–168, 1985

HYPOPARATHYROIDISM ISOLATED SYNDROMES

Synonyms. Hypoparathyroidism acquired; hypoparathyroidism isolated (autosomal dominant); hypoparathyroidism isolated (autosomal recessive); hypoparathyroidism isolated (X-linked).

Symptoms. *Acquired.* Onset at all ages, both sexes. *Congenital.* Onset in first year of life in X-linked, only in males. Muscle spasm and tetany; nervousness; weakness; paresthesia of hands; blurred vision; headache; memory loss. In congenital forms, edema in neonatal period.

Signs. Chvostek's, Trousseau's signs. Papilledema; teeth and nail disorders; dry, coarse skin; patchy hair; alopecia; cataracts. Absence of candida infection and other endocrine gland deficiencies. Differentiate these syndromes from Multiple endocrine neoplasia (see).

Etiology. *Acquired.* Surgery; miscellaneous pathologic processes. *Congenital.* Autosomal dominant, recessive, or X-linked inheritance.

Pathology. Absence or hypoplasia of parathyroid.

Diagnostic Procedures. *Blood.* Hypocalcemia; hyperphosphatemia; no circulating antibodies antiparathyroid; subnormal level of immunoreactive PTH. *X-ray.* Absence of rickets, osteomalacia or kidney calcification. *Electrocardiography. Urine.* Absence of signs of renal insufficiency. After parathyroid hormone administration, acute phosphate diuresis.

Therapy. Parathyroid hormone; vitamin D; dihydrotachysterol (DHT); calcium; low-phosphorous diet; dihydroxycholecalciferol (1–25 (OH2)); acetazolamide (to increase phosphate excretion).

Prognosis. Good with treatment.

BIBLIOGRAPHY. Buchs S: Familiarer hypoparathyroidism. Ann Paediatr 188:124–127, 1957

Ahn TG, Autonarakis SE, Kronenberg HM, et al: Familial isolated hypoparathyroidism: a molecular genetic analysis of 8 families with 23 affected persons. Medicine 81, 65:73–84, 1986

Han TJ: Parathyroid hormone, calcitonin vitamin D, mineral and bone: metabolism and disorders. In Mazzaferri EL (ed): Endocrinology, 3rd ed, pp 458–573. New York, Medical Examination Publishing, 1985

---

* Hyponatremia without hypoosmolality may be seen in hyperlipemia (where serum lipid displaces serum water, and produces low sodium concentration) and hyperglycemia, and when mannitol is given for therapeutic use in patient with defective mannitol excretion. In those cases, asymptomatic and no treatment is necessary if primary sodium loss has been ruled out.

HYPOPHYSEAL, SENILE, SYNDROMES

According to Herman, based upon Kretschmer types of physical constitution, analysis of senile signs occurring in Cushing's syndrome makes it possible to establish two types of physiologic senescence: (1) Asthenic (leptosome) corresponding to the Simmonds' syndrome; and (2) pyknic type corresponding to Cushing's.

BIBLIOGRAPHY. Kretschmer E: Körperbau und Charakter Untersuchungen zun Konstitutionsproblem und zur Lehre von den Temperamenten. Berlin, Springer, 1921
Herman E: Senile hypophyseal syndromes. J Neurol Sci 4:101–110, 1966

HYPOPLASTIC LEFT HEART

Synonyms. HLHS; Aortic arch atresia or interruption; aortic arch hypoplasia; aortic valve atresia; mitral valve atresia. See Mitral valve atresia.

This definition has been used interchangeably with hypoplasia of aortic tract complex including coexistent aortic and mitral atresia or stenosis, preductal coarctation, hypoplasia of ascending aorta, hypoplasia of transverse aortic arch. Considering the functional and anatomic adequacy of the left ventricle as the basic factor in these lesions, Sinha prefers the term *hypoplastic left ventricle syndrome* and excludes from the entity the conditions where a functionally adequate left ventricular chamber exists.

Symptoms and Signs. Sudden onset of severe respiratory distress and slate-gray cyanosis; moist rales; severe hepatomegaly.

Etiology. Multifactorial inheritance. Subtype with autosomal recessive type possible.

Diagnostic Procedure. *X-ray.* Cardiac enlargement, pulmonary arterial and venous engorgement. *Electrocardiography.* Right axis deviation and marked right ventricular hypertrophy. M-mode and two-dimensional echocardiography. Cardiac catheterization.

Therapy. Palliative operations cause only temporary benefit. Heart replacement by allotransplantation is a potential definitive form of treatment.

Prognosis. Inexorably progressive and fatal without transplant.

BIBLIOGRAPHY. Lev M: Pathology, anatomy and interrelationship of hypoplasia of the aortic tract complex. Lab Invest 1:61–70, 1952

Brownell LG, Shokeir MHK: Inheritance of hypoplastic left heart syndrome (HLHS): further observations. Clin Genet 9:245–249, 1976
Baily LL, Nehlsen-Cannarella SL, Doroshow RW, et al: Cardiac allotransplantation in newborns as therapy for hypoplastic left heart syndrome. New Engl J Med 315:949–951, 1986

HYPOPLASTIC RIGHT HEART

This definition is used to designate a group of congenital cardiac anomalies that share anatomic atresia or stenosis on right hemicardium, with hypoplasia of right ventricle and hypertrophy of left ventricle and functionally a right-to-left shunt (usually) at atrial level. In this group are included tricuspid atresia, pulmonary atresia, severe pulmonary stenosis with intact ventricular septum, and congenital isolated hypoplasia of right ventricle (rare).

BIBLIOGRAPHY. Peacock TB: On Malformation of the Human Heart, 2nd ed. London, J. Churchill, 1866
Morgan AD, McLoughlin TG, Bartley TD, et al: Endocardial fibroelastosis of the right ventricle in the newborn: presenting the clinical picture of the hypoplastic right heart syndrome. Am J Cardiol 18:933–937, 1966
Perloff JK: The Clinical Recognition of Congenital Heart Disease, 2nd ed, p 605. Philadelphia, WB Saunders, 1978
Williams RG, Bierman FZ, Sanders SP: Echocardiographic Diagnosis of Cardiac Malformations, pp 103–107. Boston, Little, Brown 1986

HYPOTENSION, ORTHOSTATIC

Synonyms. Postural hypotension; orthostatic hypotension. See Bradbury-Eggleston and Sly-Dragger.

Symptoms. Prevalent in men (4:1); slow progression of symptoms; sometimes years before patient seeks medical attention. Impotence (usually first symptom). Episodic feelings of exhaustion, lightheadedness, blurring of vision, slow mentation, and faintness in upright position. Syncope common, preceded by the described premonitory symptoms. Convulsive seizures may occur (especially if bystander helps the patient up after he falls). Chronic diarrhea; nocturnal polyuria; intolerance to heat.

Signs. Usually, youthful appearance. Pallor precedes the attack. Decrease in systolic and diastolic pressure in erect position. Valsalva maneuver results in marked fall of arterial blood pressure and the characteristic "overshoot" and bradycardia (that are present in normal individual) are absent. Various degrees of anhidrosis can be demonstrated by sweating tests.

Etiology. Unknown; autonomic dysfunction: impaired arteriolar constriction; anhidrosis; xerostomia; heat intolerance; impotence. It is distinguished from a primary form (see Bradbury-Eggleston and Sly-Dragger) and secondary form due to impairment of autonomic function from peripheral neuropathy due to infections, toxins, malnutrition, amyloidosis, age.

Pathology. Unknown.

Diagnostic Procedures. *Blood pressure.* Vasopressin increases systolic and diastolic pressure in patients (and not in normal individuals). *Sweat tests. Basal metabolism rate.* Low. *Blood.* Moderate increase in blood urea nitrogen; mild anemia.

Therapy. Various therapeutic measures usually fail or present several disadvantages like vasopressin (water intoxication and myocardial ischemia). Best treatment appears to be wearing a special custom-fitted counterpressure suit, made of elastic mesh, which allows adequate ventilation (Jobst garment).

Prognosis. In early stage of disease, patients are able to work. With progression of disease, wearing the described special suit becomes necessary. Fluctuation of intensity of symptoms. Progression of neurologic symptoms. General debility and sudden death reported.

BIBLIOGRAPHY. Bradbury S, Eggleston C: Postural hypotension: a report of three cases. Am Heart J 1:73–86, 1925
Lanbry C, Doumer E: L'hypotension orthostatique. Presse Med 1:17–20, 1932
Adams RD, Victor M: Principles of Neurology, 3rd ed, pp 404–405. New York, McGraw-Hill, 1985

HYPOTHALAMIC CARREFOUR

Symptoms. Occur in middle-aged females with blood hypertension; sudden onset. Hemiplegia; hemianesthesia; astereognosis; apraxia; asynergy.

Etiology. Unknown.

Therapy. Symptomatic.

Prognosis. Tendency to regression.

BIBLIOGRAPHY. Ramirez F, Iniguez A: Sindrome de la encrucijada hipotalamica. An Fac Med Montevideo 37:109–116, 1952

HYPOTHALAMIC POSTINFECTIVE

Synonym. Hyperphagia-hyperthermia-hypothyroidism.

Symptoms and Signs. Occur following infections, trauma, or without preceding causes. Development of hyperthermia with good appetite and weight gain, with or without secondary hypothyroidism symptoms and signs.

Etiology and Pathology. Lesion of hypothalamus due to infection (viral), trauma, or leukemia.

Diagnostic Procedures. *Blood.* Cultures; complete blood count. *Basal metabolic rate. Thyroid function tests. Adrenal function tests. X-ray of skull.*

Therapy. Symptomatic.

Prognosis. Poor; sudden death.

BIBLIOGRAPHY. Grossman M: Late results of epidemic encephalitis. Arch Neurol Psychiatr 5:580, 1921
Lipsett MB, Dreifuss FE, Thomas LB: Hypothalamic syndrome following varicella. Am J Med 32:471–475, 1962

HYSTERICAL SYNCOPE

Symptoms. In young adult with severe emotional illness. Attacks always in presence of public. Slumping is gentle and graceful, may last long time (1 hour or longer)

Signs. Unresponsive to verbal stimulation. Skin calor, pulse, blood pressure normal. Changing position (recumbency) does not modify symptoms.

Etiology. Emotional imbalance.

Treatment. Psychotherapy.

Prognosis. Good. Possible conversion to other hysterical symptoms.

BIBLIOGRAPHY. Weissler AM, Warren JV: Syncope: pathophysiological and differential diagnosis. In Hurst JW (ed): The Heart, 6th ed, p 519. New York, McGraw-Hill, 1986

I

IATROGENIC HYPOTHYROIDISM

Synonym. Iodide-induced hypothyroidism.

Symptoms and Signs. Onset following prolonged iodine administration for treatment of thyroid disorders or for any other therapeutic reason (e.g., for chronic bronchitis or for radioiodine therapy and other drugs such as lithium carbonate).

Etiology. Probably depending on preexistent defect in thyroid metabolism.

Pathology. Varies; cases studied histologically: showed colloid storage goiter; thyroid hyperplasia with tendency to colloid depletion.

Diagnostic Procedures. *Basal metabolic rate. Blood.* Serum cholesterol; butanol extractable iodine determination. *Radioiodine uptake.* Rapid thyroidal uptake in first few hours; followed by decline to low value within 24 hours; enlarged thyroidal iodide space; discharge of ^{131}I with thiocyanate. Rebound phenomena following discontinuation of iodide.

Therapy. Discontinuation of treatment and then thyroid administration.

Prognosis. Good with therapy.

BIBLIOGRAPHY. Thompson WO, Thompson PK, Brailey AG, et al: Myxedema during the administration of iodide in exophthalmic goiter. Am J Med Sci 179:733–749, 1930
Oppenheimer JH, McPherson HT: The syndrome of iodide-induced goiter and myxedema. Am J Med 30:281–288, 1961
Jefferson JM: Lithium carbonate-induced hypothyroidism: its many faces. JAMA 242:271–272, 1979

ICHTHYOSIFORM ERYTHRODERMA

Synonym. Brocq congenital nonbullous form. See also Harlequin fetus.

Symptoms and Signs. Onset at birth. Lesions localized on flexor areas. Growth retardation. Spastic paralysis; oligophrenia; hypotrichia, genital hypoplasia.

Etiology. Autosomal recessive inheritance.

Prognosis. Shortened life expectancy.

BIBLIOGRAPHY. See Bullous ichthyosiform hyperkeratosis.

ICHTHYOSIFORM ERYTHRODERMA, UNILATERAL

Synonym. Congenital hemidysplasia-ichthyosiform erythroderma-limb deformity (CHILD).

Symptoms and Signs. Prevalent in females (19:1). From birth. Unilateral ichthyosis and limb malformation accompanied by hypoplasia of several organs on the same side (lung, thyroid), as well as psoas muscle, central nervous system, and cranial nerves.

Etiology. X-linked inheritance.

Prognosis. Males stillbirth or early death.

BIBLIOGRAPHY. Falek A, Heath CW Jr, Ebbin AJ, et al: Unilateral limb and skin deformities with congenital heart disease in two siblings: a lethal syndrome. J Pediatr 73:910–913, 1968

Wettke-Schafer R, Cantiner G: X-linked dominant inherited disease with lethality in homozygous males. Hum Genet 64:1–23, 1983

ICHTHYOSIS HEPATO-SPLENOMEGALY-ATAXIA

Synonym. Dykes'.

Symptoms and Signs. See ichthyosis vulgaris dominant. Hepatosplenomegaly and dysarthria and ataxia begin after age 50.

Etiology. Suggested storage disease, nature not yet evident. Autosomal recessive inheritance. X-linked inheritance not excluded.

BIBLIOGRAPHY. Dykes PJ, Markes R, Harper PS: A syndrome of ichthyosis, hepatosplenomegaly and cerebellar degeneration. Br J Derm 100:585–590, 1979

ICHTHYOSIS HYSTRIX

Etiology.
1. Spriegler-Fendt (see)
2. Lambert's (see)
3. Ichthyosis hystrix Curth-Macklin type (see)
4. Ichthyosiform erythroderma (BIE) (see) and localized form warty linear nevus.
5. Ichthyosis hystrix gravior of Rheydt.

Pathology. The different forms mentioned in the etiology are difficult to distinguish by light microscopy. Only electron microscopy provides the differential characteristics.

Therapy. Specific. Emolients and keratolytic topical retinoic or etretinate per os or isotretinoid are also helpful in some cases.

BIBLIOGRAPHY. Anton-Lamprecht I: Hereditaire ichthyosen. In Herzberg JJ (ed): Paediatrische Dermatologie, p 161. Stuttgart, Schattauer, 1978
Kanerva L, Kardonen J, Oikarinen A, et al: Light and electronic microscopic studies performed before and after etretinate treatment. Arch Dermatol 120:1218–1223, 1984

ICHTHYOSIS HYSTRIX, CURTH-MACKLIN TYPE

Symptoms and Signs. See Ichthyosis hystrix.

Pathology. Continuous perinuclear tonofibril shell in spinous and granular cell layers and absence of tonofilament clumps (typical of ichthyosiform erythroderma).

BIBLIOGRAPHY. Curth HO, Macklin MT: The genetic basis of the various types of ichthyosis in a family group. Am J Hum Genet 6:377–381, 1954
Curth HO, Allen FH Jr, Schneider VW, et al: Follow-up of a family group suffering of ichthyosis hystrix, type Curth-Macklin. Hum Genet 17:37–48, 1972
Kanerva L, Kardonen J, Oikarinen A, et al: Light and electron microscopic studies performed before and after etretinate treatment. Arch Dermatol 120:1218–1223, 1984

ICHTHYOSIS HYSTRIX, GRAVIOR OF RHEYDT

Synonyms. Nevus linear; nevus verrucosus; porcupine man; Rheydt's.

Symptoms and Signs. Both sexes affected; present from infancy. Marked hyperkeratosis with quill-like projection involving entire body with the exception of face, palms, soles, and genitalia.

Etiology. Unknown; autosomal dominant inheritance. Variant of harlequin fetus (see).

Pathology. Extreme hyperkeratinization of skin.

Therapy. None.

Prognosis. No change with age.

BIBLIOGRAPHY. Penrose LS, Stern C: Reconsideration of the Lambert Pedigree (ichthyosis hystrix gravior). Ann Hum Genet 22:258–283, 1957
Anton-Lamprecht I: Electron microscopy in the early diagnosis of genetic disorders of the skin. Dermatologica 157:65–85, 1978

ICHTHYOSIS-MALE HYPOGONADISM

Synonym. Lynch's.

Symptoms and Signs. Males. Two families described. Those related to congenital ichthyosis-secondary hypogonadism.

Etiology. Possibly X-linked inheritance.

Diagnostic Procedures. Low titer of pituitary gonadotrophic hormones.

Prognosis. Males do not reproduce.

BIBLIOGRAPHY. Lynch HT, Ozer FL, Mevutt CW, et al: Secondary male hypogonadism and congenital ichthyosis: an association of two rare genetic diseases. Am J Hum Genet 12:440–447, 1960
Dodinval PA, Husquinet HA, Legros JS: Ichthyosis, hypogonadotrophic hypogonadism and mild epilepsy in

two young male sibs, p 260. Sixth Int Cong Hum Genet, Jerusalem 1981

ICHTHYOSIS VULGARIS, DOMINANT

Synonyms. Ichthyosis nitidus; ichthyosis simplex; xeroderma.

Symptoms. Both sexes affected; onset between 1 and 4 years of age. No symptoms except irritation of skin in cold weather.

Signs. From dryness and roughness of skin in cold weather (milder form: xeroderma) to dryness with small, white, shiny scales, progressively becoming more severe over a few years. Affected are extensor areas of limbs and sometimes the trunk, the back more severely than abdomen or anterior chest; axillae and groin always unaffected. Face affected in childhood, usually clears at later age. Seasonal variations with enhancing of manifestation during winter and remission during summer. High percentage of patients manifest asthma and eczema.

Etiology. Unknown; autosomal dominant inheritance.

Pathology. Horny layer slightly thickened, reduced or absent granular layer, low mitotic count, dermal and perivascular lymphocytic infiltrates.

Therapy. Moving to warm climate regions. Salicylic acid (3%) in emulsifying ointment. Bath oil in bath water. Ultraviolet light application; vitamin A.

Prognosis. Chronic condition never too severe; tendency to improve with age.

BIBLIOGRAPHY. Felsher Z, Rothman S: Insensible perspiration of skin in hyperkeratotic conditions. J Invest Dermatol 6:271–278, 1945
Wells RS: Ichthyosis. Br Med J 2:1504–1506, 1966
Sybert VP, Dale BA, Holbrook KA: Ichthyosis vulgaris: evidentiation of a defect in synthesis of filaggrin correlated with an absence of keratohyaline granules. J Invest Dermatol 84:191–194, 1985

ICHTHYOSIS VULGARIS, SEX-LINKED

Synonyms. Ichthyosis negricans; ichthyosis nigricans; steroid sulfatase deficiency.

Symptoms. Only males (1 in 6000 male births); onset in very early infancy. Lesions may be troublesome and disfiguring.

Signs. Scattered, large, brownish scales, affecting all areas of skin, including axilla, groin, antecubital and popliteal fossas; front of trunk more markedly affected than back. Tendency to shed in autumn and spring. Alopecia may develop. Corneal opacities. Palms and soles are spared; nails are normal. Possible association with mental retardation, skeletal abnormalities, hypogonadism. Mothers of affected males may have trouble in parturition.

Etiology. X-linked recessive inheritance. Deficiency of steroid sulfatase with probable accumulation of cholesterol esters in skin.

Pathology. Horny and granular layer thickened with acanthosis; constant dermal lymphocytic infiltrates.

Diagnostic Procedures. *Maternal urine.* Low estrogens. *Fibroblast culture.* Absence of steroid sulfatase.

Therapy. None.

Prognosis. Chronic condition; no improvement with age.

BIBLIOGRAPHY. Kerr CB, Wells RS: Sex-linked ichthyosis. Ann Hum Genet 29:33–50, 1965
Shapiro LJ: Steroid sulphatase deficiency and X-linked ichthyosis. In Stanbury JB, Wyngaarden JB, Fredrickson DS, et al: The Metabolic Basis of Inherited Disease, 5th ed, p 1027. New York, McGraw-Hill, 1983

IDIOPATHIC DIFFUSE CRESCENTIC GLOMERULONEPHRITIS, TYPE I

Synonyms. Antiglomerular basement membrane antibody mediated; crescentic glomerulonephritis without pulmonary hemorrhage.

Symptoms and Signs. Usually young or middle-aged males. Sometimes preceded by exposure to hydrocarbon fumes or respiratory illness. Onset like acute glomerulonephritis (see Bright's) but more insidious, with fever, myalgia, or abdominal pain.

Etiology. Unknown. Antiglomerular basement membrane antibodies (IgG) are probably the pathogenetic mechanism. This may be a partial type of Goodpasture's syndrome (see).

Pathology. Light microscopy. Accumulation of cells (crescents) in Bowman's space in 50% of glomeruli; in time, glomerular sclerosis. *Electromicroscopy.* Widened zones in subendothelial space with detachment gaps in basement membrane. *Immunofluorescence.* Glomeruli with linear deposits of IgG (rarely IgA); C3 deposits are rare. Pattern similar to Goodpasture's syndrome

Diagnostic Procedures. *Urine.* Dysmorphic RBC, casts. Decreased glomerular filtration rate. *Blood.* Circulating antiglomerular basement membrane antibodies; signs of uremia. HLA-DR2 in 85% of patients. Fibrin degradation products high in urine and serum.

Therapy. Plasmapheresis; steroids; cyclophosphamide; azathioprine.

Prognosis. Without therapy, progression to renal insufficiency in 6 months. With therapy, better prognosis. Renal transplantation is followed by a 10 to 30% recurrence of disease.

BIBLIOGRAPHY. Brenner BM, Rector FC Jr: The Kidney, 3rd ed, p 940. Philadelphia, WB Saunders, 1986

IDIOPATHIC DIFFUSE CRESCENTIC GLOMERULONEPHRITIS, TYPE II

Synonym. Immune complex mediated crescentic glomerulonephritis.

Symptoms and Signs. Middle-aged patients, no sex predominance. Fever; malaise; hypertension. Occult visceral sepsis or necrotizing vasculitis may be present.

Etiology. Unknown. Basement membrane lesion is due to immune complex deposition. The antigen is occult but infection is usually the cause (virus).

Pathology. *Light microscopy.* Lesions similar to type I. *Electron microscopy.* Electron-dense deposits in mesangium and subendothelial space. *Immunofluorescence.* Scattered deposits (mesangial and capillary) of IgG and IgM often with C3.

Diagnostic Procedures. *Urine.* Hematuria; proteinuria. *Serum.* C3 decreased; cryoimmunoglobulins and circulating immune complex.

Therapy. Plasma exchange; cortisone (pulses of corticosteroid). Quadruple therapy (anticoagulant, antithrombotic, glucorticoid, immunosuppressive).

Prognosis. Better than in type I. Spontaneous resolution is possible; response to therapy is good.

BIBLIOGRAPHY. Brenner BM, Rector FC Jr: The Kidney, 3rd ed, p 944. Philadelphia, WB Saunders, 1986

IDIOPATHIC DIFFUSE CRESCENTIC GLOMERULONEPHRITIS, TYPE III

This syndrome is disputed.

Symptoms and Signs. Older patients, predominantly males. Fever, arthralgias, abdominal pain.

Etiology. Unknown.

Pathology. *Light microscopy.* Absence of proteinaceous deposits. *Electromicroscopy.* Absence of electron-dense deposits. *Immunofluorescence.* Absence of IgG deposits.

Diagnostic Procedures. See types I and II. No antiglomerular basement membrane antibodies, immune complexes, or rheumatoid factors.

Therapy. Pulses of corticosteroids.

Prognosis. Better than in type I. In case of chronic renal failure, kidney transplantation gives good results.

BIBLIOGRAPHY. Brenner BM, Rector FC Jr: The Kidney, 3rd ed, p 945. Philadelphia, WB Saunders, 1986

IDIOPATHIC HYPERTROPHIC SUBAORTIC STENOSIS

Synonyms. IHSS; subvalvular aortic stenosis; Bernheim Schmincke; familial cardiomyopathy; obstructive cardiomyopathy; noncoronary cardiopathy; Schmincke-Bernheim; hypertrophic obstructive cardiomyopathy; hypertrophic cardiomyopathy, HC.

Symptoms. Both sexes affected; familial form: 1:1; male to female ratio: 1:1; sporadic: 4:1. Onset from birth to late age, most common in 3rd or 4th decade. Exertional dyspnea; angina pectoris; dizziness especially in assuming upright position.

Signs. Patients are physically well-developed; many may have practiced athletic activities before onset of symptomatology. Heart enlarged; left ventricular lift. Findings suggesting ventricular defect or mitral regurgitation. Protodiastolic gallop in 50% of cases; systolic murmur (100%); second sound single. Friedreich's ataxia (see) frequently associated.

Etiology. Variable sporadic cases and autosomal dominant inheritance. Several etiologic causes under this heading. "Aberration of catecholamine function" in the embryo heart proposed.

Pathology. Hypertrophy of left ventricle, with marked hypertrophy in the septal region, centimeters below the aortic valve, septum bulges into right ventricle. Muscle bundles arranged into whorls, separated; bizarre nuclei of fibers.

Diagnostic Procedures. *Electrocardiography.* Left ventricular hypertrophy; Wolf-Parkinson (see) in 25% of cases; abnormal Q waves. *X-ray.* In 50% of cases, abnormally large cardiothoracic ratio. *Angiocardiography.* Thickening of left ventricle walls. *Hemodynamic studies.* Variable results. *Echocardiography. Radionuclide imaging. Phonocardiogram. Systolic time intervals. Apex cardiogram.*

Therapy. In case of syncope, antishock position and phenylephedrine or methoxamine. Basic treatment: propranolol and other beta-blocking agents (symptoms of failure may be enhanced). Calcium blocking agents; Amiodarone. Surgical treatment. Laser myoplasty.

Prognosis. Sudden death frequent occurrence.

BIBLIOGRAPHY. Frank S, Brunewald E: Idiopathic hypertrophic subaortic stenosis: clinical analysis of 126 patients with emphasis on natural history. Circulation 37:759–788, 1968
Wenger NK, Goodwin JF, Roberts WC: Cardiomyopathy and myocardial involvement in systemic disease. In Hurst JW: The Heart, 6th ed, pp 1193–1208. New York, McGraw-Hill, 1986

IgA SELECTIVE DEFICIENCY

Synonym. Primary IgA immunodeficiency.

Symptoms and Signs. Incidence 1/700 individuals. Asymptomatic. Infections of upper respiratory and/or intestinal tract. Associated allergic manifestations.

Etiology. Unknown. Sporadic and familial cases reported. In some cases deletion of chromosome 14.

Diagnostic Procedures. *Blood.* Selective decrease of IgA1 and A2. In some cases increased IgE.

Therapy. No treatment. Immunoglobulin administration not advised.

Prognosis. Good.

BIBLIOGRAPHY. Ugazio AG, Out TA, Plebani A, et al: Record infections in children with "selective IgA deficiency": association with IgG2 and IgG4 deficiency. Birth Defect 19:169–171, 1983

ILIOCAVAL COMPRESSION SYNDROME

Symptoms and Signs. More frequent in females. Classic form on the left side; rarely on the right. Characteristic lower extremity pains, moderate to severe swelling, varicosities.

Etiology. Left common iliac vein compressed between right common iliac artery and lumbar spine. Occasionally, other sources of compression that may cause the manifestation on the right side (e.g., metastatic nodes, bone spur).

Diagnostic Procedures. *Doppler venous survey. Exercise strain gauge venous plethysmography. Ambulatory venous pressure. Descending and ascending venography.*

Therapy. *Surgical.* Direct operative repair of the iliocaval junction, rerouting of the iliac artery, and excision of ileocaval webs with vein patch angioplasty.

Prognosis. Long-term sequelae of venous insufficiency.

BIBLIOGRAPHY. McMurrich JP: The occurrence of congenital adhesion in the common iliac veins and their relation to thrombosis of the femoral and iliac veins. Am J Med Sci 135:342, 1908
Cockett B, Thomas ML: The iliac compression syndrome. Br J Surg 51:816–821, 1965
Toheri SA, Williams J, Powell S, et al: Iliocaval compression syndrome. Am J Surg 154:169–172, 1987

ILLIG'S

Synonym. See Isolated growth hormone deficiency.

Symptoms and Signs. Features more severe than in the isolated growth hormone deficiency (see): shorter at birth; more marked dwarfism; puppet facies.

Etiology. Unknown. Autosomal recessive inheritance.

Diagnostic Procedures. *Blood.* Hypoglycemia; total absence of growth hormone; presence of growth hormone antibodies after treatment characterizing feature of the syndrome.

Therapy. Growth hormone. Presence of antibodies makes treatment more difficult. Recent availability of synthetic preparations reduces antibody formation.

BIBLIOGRAPHY. Zilig R: Growth hormone antibodies in patients treated with different preparations of human growth hormone (HGH). J Clin Endocr Metab 31:679–688, 1970
Zachmann M, Fernandez F, Tassinari D, et al: Anthropometric measurements in patients with growth hormone deficiency before treatment with human growth hormone. Eur J Pediatr 133:277–282, 1980

ILLUSION OF FREGOLI

Symptoms. Patient identifies persecutors in several persons (e.g., doctor; nurse; aide; postman) accusing them of being the same person and changing faces to persecute him.

Etiology. Considered an extension of Capgras' syndrome (see). Form of illusion of positive doubles as contrasted with the Capgras' syndrome illusion of negative doubles. To be differentiated also from Illusion of Intermetamorphosis (see).

BIBLIOGRAPHY. Courbon P, Fail G. Syndrome d' "illusion de Frégoli" et schizophénie. Bull Soc Clin Med Ment 15:121–125, 1927

Enoch MD, Trethowan WH, Barker SC: Some Uncommon Psychiatric Syndromes. Baltimore, Williams & Wilkins, 1967

ILLUSION OF INTERMETAMORPHOSIS

Symptoms. Patient has the illusion that the persons with whom he is in contact change one with another: A becomes B; B becomes C; C becomes A.

Etiology. Considered an extension of Capgras' (see). Differs from illusion of Fregoli. In the intermetamorphosis, physical resemblance is claimed in addition to false identification.

BIBLIOGRAPHY. Courbon P, Tusques J: Illusions d'intermétamorphose et de charme. Ann Med Psychol 90:401–406, 1932

Enoch MD, Trethowan WH, Barker SC: Some Uncommon Psychiatric Syndromes. Baltimore, Williams & Wilkins, 1967

IMERSLUND-GRAESBECK

Synonyms. Megaloblastic hereditary anemia; familial selective B$_{12}$ vitamin malabsorption.

Symptoms. Both sexes affected; clinical onset in second year of life. Fatigue; weakness.

Signs. Pallor.

Etiology. Unknown. Autosomal recessive inheritance. Defect in the process of vitamin B$_{12}$ transport in the ileum.

Pathology. Gastric, jejunal mucosa normal. Kidney, glomerular changes suggestive of mild subacute glomerulonephritis.

Diagnostic Procedures. *Blood.* Megaloblastic anemia. *Bone marrow.* Typical megaloblastic changes. *Gastric fluid.* Normal free acid and intrinsic factor. *Urine.* Proteinuria; in some cases aminoaciduria. *Biopsy of kidney.* See Pathology.

Therapy. Vitamin B$_{12}$.

Prognosis. Administration of vitamin B$_{12}$ corrects anemia but does not affect albuminuria or aminoaciduria.

BIBLIOGRAPHY. Graesbeck R, Gordin R, Kantero I, et al: Selective vitamin B$_{12}$ malabsorption and proteinuria in young people: a syndrome. Acta Med Scand 167:289–296, 1960

Imerslund O: Idiopathic chronic myeloblastic anemia in children. Acta Paediat (suppl 119) 49:1–115, 1960

Broch H, Imerslund O, Monn E, et al: Imerslund-Graesbeck anemia: a long-term follow-up study. Acta Paediatr Scand 73:248–253, 1984

IMINOGLYCINURIA

Synonym. Iminoglycinuria familial.

Symptoms and Signs. Benign condition associated with other pathologies and syndromes but not pathological per se.

Etiology. Deficiency of tubular carriers for amino acids. Autosomal recessive inheritance.

Diagnostic Procedures. *Urine.* Excessive amounts of proline, hydroxyproline, and glycine.

Therapy. None.

Prognosis. Good.

BIBLIOGRAPHY. Joseph R, Ribierre M, Job J, et al: Maladie familiale associante des convulsions a debut tres precoce, une hyperalbuminorachie et une hyperamminoacidurie. Arch Fr Pediatric 15:374, 1948

Scriver CR: Familial iminoglycinuria. In Stanbury JB, Wyngaarden JB, Fredrickson DS, et al: The Metabolic Basis of Inherited Disease, 5th ed, p 1792. New York, McGraw-Hill, 1983

IMMERSION FOOT

Synonyms. Paddy foot; swamp foot; trench foot; tropical immersion foot. See Pernio.

Symptoms and Signs. Occur in individuals (e.g., soldiers; hunters) subjected to prolonged exposure of lower extremities to cold and moisture as well as dependency and immobility.

1. *Initial vasospastic, ischemic phase.* Edema; pallor; cyanosis of feet; followed by petechiae, shallow ulcerations. Anesthesia of patchy type.
2. *Postimmersion, hyperemic phase.* After removal from cold exposure, feet red and hot; peripheral pulsation full (changes similar to erythromelalgia syndrome). Bullae filled by hemorrhagic fluid. Ecchymosis; ulcerations; gangrene. Burning paresthesia starts at the 10th day. Condition lasts about 2 weeks if gangrene complication does not supervene.
3. *Late vasospastic, ischemic phase.* (In mild case properly treated, this stage is absent.) Coldness, pain, stiffness,

and paresthesia of lower extremities. Exposure to cold results in Raynaud's phenomenon, hyperhidrosis.

Etiology. Changes of peripheral circulation due to prolonged exposure to cold and dampness.

Pathology. In early stage similar to Pernio (see). In later stages fibrosis, intimal thickening of small arteries, mild periarterial fibrosis. Secondary damage to veins, perivenous fibrosis thrombosis, muscle fiber degeneration.

Therapy. Prevent by minimizing exposure to moisture (silicone grease most effective) and heat dispersion; avoid constriction. Practice movement and avoid prolonged dependency of legs (standing or sitting, especially with feet immersed in the water). During hyperemic phase: avoid trauma and infections; elevate feet to reduce edema; warm body, cool feet. During vasospastic phase: avoid cold exposure; passive exercises; mild heat application; fever treatment (may be tried); stop smoking. Sympathectomy in selected cases.

Prognosis. According to stage reached. In full course, patient cannot work in cold climate; also reduced ability in warmer climate.

BIBLIOGRAPHY. Wright IS, Allen EV: Frostbite, immersion foot, and allied conditions. Army Med Bull 65:136–150, 1943
Taplin D, Zaias N, Blank H: The role of temperature in tropical immersion foot syndrome. JAMA 202:546–549, 1967
Killian H: Cold and frost injuries. Berlin, Springer 1981

IMMOTILE CILIA

Synonyms. See also Kartagener's; incomplete Kartagener's; Polynesian bronchiectasis; Dyskinetic cilia; Afzelius'.

Symptoms and Signs. Prevalence 1:20,000. Symptoms and signs the same as in Kartagener's. Half the affected patients have situs viscerum inversus. Males are sterile.

Syndrome is diagnosed in: (1) patients with complete Kartagener's; (2) men without situs inversus but typical history (chronic bronchitis and rhinitis) with living but immobile spermatozoa; (3) patients without situs inversus but with typical clinical signs and sibs with complete Kartagener's; (4) patients without situs inversus but with clinical signs if biopsy shows classical signs of ciliary immotility.

From birth. Neonatal asphyxia; chronic bronchial disease; chronic rhinitis; nasal polyps; chronic sinusitis; otitis. *In childhood.* Bronchiectases; moderate hearing loss; recurrent headaches. Dextrocardia. Rare associated polydactyly anomalies.

Etiology. Recessive autosomal inheritance. Due to abnormal structure and function of body cilia because of defective protein formation.

Pathology. *Electron microscopy.* Variable alterations of cilia structure.

Diagnostic Procedures. Examination of cilia is easier in ejaculate when spermatozoa are poorly motile or immotile. Biopsy or brushing of nasal canti, bronchi, middle ear, nasal polyps, or endometrium show same alterations. *Radioactive aerosol.* Mucociliary transport absent or reduced.

Therapy. Symptomatic. Surgery for complications. Abstinence from smoking.

Prognosis. Good *quoad vitam.* Decrease of pulmonary function with age. Sterility in males.

BIBLIOGRAPHY. Afzelius BA: A human syndrome caused by immotile cilia. Science 193:317, 1976
Afzelius AB, Mosberg B: The immotile-cilia syndrome including Kartagener's syndrome. In Stanbury JB, Wyngaarden JB, Fredrickson DS, et al: The Metabolic Basis of Inherited Disease, 5th ed, p 1986. New York McGraw-Hill, 1983

IMMUNOGLOBULIN DEFICIENCY–ADDISON-BIERMER

Synonyms. Anemia pernicious–Addison-Biermer; Pernicious anemia-immunoglobulin deficiency; transcobalamine II deficiency, hereditary.
See also Addison-Biermer.

Symptoms and Signs. Prevalent in males (70%); onset at mean age of 34 years. Recurrent bacterial infection (predominantly pneumococcal) preceding other symptoms. Episodic diarrhea. All symptoms of Addison-Biermer (see). In some cases, rheumatoid arthritis, idiopathic ulcerative colitis, allergic manifestations.

Etiology. Unknown. The pernicious anemia and the immunoglobulin deficiency are independent consequences of single defect, based (or not based) on genetic abnormality. Gastric atrophy (responsible for pernicious anemia) resulting from delayed-type cellular immune hyperactivity, host hypersensitivity, or both, role of giardiasis to be considered. Autosomal recessive inheritance deficiency of transcobalamine 2.

Pathology. Gastric mucosal atrophy, with infiltrates of lymphocytes and lack of plasma cells. Typical pattern of pernicious anemia, deficiency in plasma cells of bone marrow. Biopsy of small intestine mucosa normal. Findings typical of recurrent infections and of pernicious anemia.

Diagnostic Procedures. *Blood.* Hyperchromic anemia and other findings of pernicious anemia; Coombs' test negative; absence of serum antibodies against parietal cell, thyroid antigens, or against binding of B_{12} to intrinsic factor. *Gastric fluid.* Achlorhydria, absence of intrinsic factor in gastric juice; vitamin B_{12} malabsorption, not corrected by exogenous intrinsic factor. Presence of *Giardia* infestation in majority of cases. *Immunologic studies.* IgG, IgA, IgM strongly decreased or absent. Positive delayed cutaneous response; positive mitotic response to phytohemoagglutinin (PHA).

Therapy. That of Addison-Biermer; antibiotics; gamma globulins.

Prognosis. Not reported. According to chronic nature of disease: poor. Possibility of development of gastric adenocarcinoma, and of different immunologically based (?) disorders (e.g., rheumatic arthritis; ulcerative colitis).

BIBLIOGRAPHY. Twomey JJ, Jordan PH, Jarrold T, et al: The syndrome of immunoglobulin deficiency and pernicious anemia. Am J Med 47:340–350, 1969

Hitzig WH, Dohmann H, Pluss HJ, et al: Hereditary transcobalamine II deficiency: clinical findings in new family. J Pediatr 85:622–628, 1984

IMMUNOHEMOLYTIC ANEMIAS

Synonyms. Acquired hemolytic anemia; acute hemolytic anemia; antiglobulin positive hemolytic anemia; autoimmune hemolytic anemia, AIHA; Druyfus-Dausset-Vidal; Dyke-Young (chronic macrocytic type); Hayem-Widal-Loutit; Lederer-Brill; Lederer's anemia (acute transient type). See Dressler's; Hemolytic anemia, newborn; and Marchiafava-Micheli.

WARM ANTIBODY TYPE

Symptoms. Slightly more prevalent in females; onset at all ages. Extremely variable clinical features. Onset acute or insidious; occasionally, history of previous infection. From acute hemolytic crisis with pyrexia, shocklike prostration up to coma, to chronic mild anemia with moderate tiredness and exertional dyspnea. Hemoglobinuria frequent feature. Dark stool. Occasional features: superficial thrombophlebitis; gallstones (usually asymptomatic); precordial pain headache; complex neurologic syndrome (Dreyfus-Dausset-Vidal) accompanying hemolytic crisis. Bleeding features (see Evans').

Signs. Pallor; jaundice; splenomegaly; occasionally, liver enlargement.

Etiology. Primary and idiopathic; usually sporadic cases; familial occurrence reported. Occurrence in member of family with other types of autoimmune syndromes (e.g., lupus erythematosus; rheumatoid arthritis; perni-

cious anemia) suggests the possibility of an hereditary fundamental aberration of immune apparatus. Other associations: virus infections; drug-dependent antibodies; lymphomas; lymphatic leukemia; other nonlymphoreticular tumors.

Pathology. Spleen enlarged; congestion of pulp; histiocytic proliferation; giant cell formation; erythrophagocytosis; myeloid metaplasia. Areas of thrombosis and infarction. Hemosiderosis of spleen and liver. Liver enlarged, congested; occasionally, areas of focal necrosis. Renal lesion may be (seldom) observed. Normoblastic hyperplasia of bone marrow.

Diagnostic Procedures. *Blood.* Variable degree of anemia; usually, macrocytosis; considerable anisopoikilocytosis; spherocytosis; autohemoagglutination; reticulocytosis; small number of siderocytes; normoblastemia; erythrophagocytosis. In acute episode, leukocytosis; in chronic, usually neutropenia. Platelets normal or low (see Evans'). Hyperbilirubinemia; haptoglobulin absent in acute stage. Osmotic fragility moderately or markedly increased; autohemolysis markedly increased. Positive Coombs' test, direct and indirect. Special techniques to demonstrate special antibodies. Red cell survival time shortened. Normal complement concentration.

Therapy. Corticosteroids; splenectomy. In chronic cases, immunosuppressant agents.

Prognosis. Unpredictable; potentially dangerous. Quick recovery; several relapses; may become chronic. Overall mortality for this condition 50%.

COLD AGGLUTINATION SYNDROME

Synonym. Cryoglobulinemia.

Symptoms. Slightly more prevalent in females; onset usually in older age than warm antibody type; 30 to 80 years of age. Variable features: anemia and associated symptoms, usually severe and usually more severe in winter, occasionally, main sensory neuropathy may develop; Raynaud's phenomenon (see); hemoglobinuria with cold exposure.

Signs. Pallor; jaundice; spleen and liver only occasionally enlarged. Purpuric eruptions followed by hyperpigmentation. Ulceration about ankles.

Etiology. Primary disease or in many cases, secondary to infections such as primary atypical pneumonia (*Mycoplasma pneumoniae*) virus, collagen disorders, lymphoma.

Pathology. See warm antibody type. The possibility, although rare, of acute renal failure reported. Occasionally, tissue gangrene of finger or toes.

Diagnostic Procedures. *Blood.* Anemia; erythrocytes show minor abnormalities when compared with warm agglutination type; seldom erythrophagocytosis; moderate reticulocytosis; autohemoagglutination markedly increased. Osmotic fragility normal or slightly increased. Leukocytes and platelets decreased, normal, or increased. Hyperbilirubinemia variable. Coombs' direct positive, cold agglutination test with temperature ranging between 2°C and 28°C. Patient serum may lyse normal erythrocytes in vitro at low temperature (20°C; pH 6.5 to 7.5). Decreased serum complement. Wasserman and Kahn negative. *Urine.* Increased urobilin all the time; hemoglobinuria associated with cold exposure. *Stool.* Increased stercobilin.

Therapy. Corticosteroid. Avoid exposure to cold.

Prognosis. Relatively benign; usually no recovery (except in the secondary cases), but patients may live many years with the condition.

BIBLIOGRAPHY. Hayem G: Sur une variété particuliére d'ictére chronique; ictére infectieux chronique splénomégalique. Presse Méd 1:121–125, 1898

Widal F, Abrami P: Types divers d'ictéres hémolytiques non congénitaux, avec anémie; la recherche de la résistance globulaire par le procédé des hématies déplasmatisées. Bull Mem Soc Méd Hôp Paris 24:1127–1169, 1907

Dreyfus B, Dausset J, Vidal G: Étude clinique et hématologique de douze cas d'anémie hémolytique acquise avec anti corps. Rev Hématol 6:349, 1951

Dacie JV: The Haemolytic Anaemias. New York, Grune & Stratton, 1963

Lawson DH, Lindsay RM, Sawers JD, et al: Acute renal failure in the cold-agglutination syndrome. Lancet II:704–705, 1968

Pirofsky B: Hereditary aspects of autoimmune hemolytic anemia: a retrospective analysis. Vox Sang 14:334–347, 1968

Logothetis J, Kennedy WR, Ellington A, et al: Cryoglobulinemic neuropathy: incidence and clinical characteristics. Arch Neurol 19:389–397, 1968

Wintrobe MM (ed): Clinical Hematology, 8th ed, pp 734–752. Philadelphia, Lea & Febiger, 1981

INDIAN CHILDHOOD CIRRHOSIS

Synonyms. Liver cirrhosis of Indian children; Sen's.

Symptoms and Signs. Occur in Indian subcontinent; both sexes equally affected; onset usually from 1 to 3 years of age. In some cases asymptomatic. *First stage.* Gastrointestinal symptoms; abdominal distension; hepatosplenomegaly; fever. *Second stage.* Marked hepatosplenomegaly; ascites; jaundice (75%). *Third stage.* Liver size reduction; gastrointestinal bleeding; other signs of liver failure up to hepatic coma and death.

Etiology. Unknown. No consistent association with foods, viruses; possibly multifactors including genetic predisposition.

Pathology. Liver swelling and vacuolization of hepatocytes followed by necrosis; lymphocytes and polymorphonuclear infiltration; later fibrotic changes; in advanced stages cholestasis. Characteristic lack of regeneration and presence of deposits of hepatocellular hyaline material.

Diagnostic Procedures. *Blood and urine.* Standard liver function test abnormal. Hypoalbuminemia; presence of alphafetoprotein in the serum. Serum complement fractions low.

Therapy. Symptomatic.

Prognosis. Very severe. Cases with milder course have been reported.

BIBLIOGRAPHY. Chaudhuri A, Chaudhuri KC: The karyotype in Sen's syndrome (infantile cirrhosis of liver). Indian J Pediatr 31:309–311, 1964

Nelson Textbook of Pediatrics, p 979. Philadelphia, WB Saunders, 1983

INFANTILE

Synonym. Coronary artery origin from pulmonary artery.

Symptoms and Signs. Rare. Onset within 4 months of life in 80% of patients with defect; angina pectoris or congestive heart failure, with mitral regurgitation. In the remaining 20%, onset during childhood or adult life; asymptomatic murmur, mitral insufficiency, angina pectoris, and sudden death.

Etiology. Unknown.

Pathology. Origin of coronary artery from pulmonary artery. Origin of left coronary artery from left posterior pulmonary sinus, 90%; origin of right coronary artery or both, rare. Patients surviving develop large intercoronary collateral flow with vessel dilatation.

Therapy. Early surgical correction to eliminate left to right shunt and establish good flow to anomalous vessel or to reimplant anomalous vessel into aortic root.

Prognosis. See symptoms. High morbidity and mortality.

BIBLIOGRAPHY. Levin DC, Fellows KE, Abrams HC: Hemodynamically significant primary anomalies of the coronary arteries. Angiograph Aspects Circ 58:25–32, 1978

Hurst JW: The Heart, 6th ed, p 1018. New York, McGraw-Hill, 1986

INFECTIOUS MONONUCLEOSIS

Synonyms. Filatov's; kissing disease; mononucleosis infectiva; Pfeiffer's (misnomer, see); Sprunt's; Türck's.

Symptoms. Both sexes equally affected; onset at all ages, but higher frequency in 20 to 25 year bracket. Epidemics in young communities. Symptoms variable: malaise and fatigue (100%); increased sweating (80–95%); dysphagia and throat angina (80–85%); anorexia (50–80%); cephalalgia (50–70%); chills (50%); cough (40%); myalgia (35%); ocular muscle pain (15%); photophobia (10%); diarrhea (10%); epistaxis (5%). Seldom at 3rd to 4th week, spleen rupture.

Signs. Adenopathy (100%); hyperthermia (90%); splenomegaly (50%); bradycardia (40%); periorbital edema (35%); palatal enanthema (30%); hepatosplenic tenderness (20%); hepatomegaly (20%); rhinitis (20%); jaundice (5–10%); skin rash (5%).

Etiology. Due to the Epstein-Barr (EB) virus, herpesvirus (human herpesvirus 4)

Pathology. Generalized and marked perivascular infiltration with normal and abnormal lymphocytes. *Lymph nodes.* Lymphocytic and reticular hyperplasia with moderate simple distortion of normal architecture; diminished follicular prominence; focal proliferation of macrophages and presence of atypical lymphocytes (Downey's cells-virocytes). *Spleen.* Hyperplastic and markedly infiltrated by equal type of cells. *Liver.* Minimal cellular damage, infiltration with lymphocytes and virocytes. *Other organs* (including brain, spine, and meninges). May show moderate, scanty, similar cell infiltrations.

Diagnostic Procedures. *Blood.* Increase of white blood cells (10,000 to 20,000, seldom up to 60,000 to 80,000). Presence (60–90%) of abnormal lymphocytes (Downey's cells), which vary in size and shape and show peculiar characteristics. Decrease of red cells and platelets seldom observed; coagulation abnormalities frequently observed (suggesting thrombocytopathia). Hyperbilirubinemia 5 to 10%. Heterophil antibodies present, anti-EBV antibodies (see Etiology) almost always observed.

Therapy. No therapy is indicated in majority of cases. Salicylates and/or other symptomatic drugs for treatment of fever, headache, and sore throat. Antibiotics are employed only if throat cultures are positive for group A B-hemolytic streptococci. Corticosteroids are indicated in severe tonsillitis with pharyngeal edema and impending respiratory obstruction; acute hemolytic anemia and thrombocytopenia; neurological complications; myocarditis and pericarditis. Specific antiviral chemotherapy is under evaluation: adenine arabinoside, acyclovir, human interferon.

Prognosis. Condition usually benign, hepatitis, myocarditis and encephalitis possible complications. Recovery within 15 to 20 days, followed by a period of variable length of asthenia and easy fatigability. Observed cases with lengthy course and persistent thrombocytopenia; seldom, fulminating cases (fatal complication 1 : 3000 cases).

BIBLIOGRAPHY. Filatov N: Leksii ob ostrykh infeksionnykh bolezniakh u detei. Moska, 1887
Türck W: Vorlesungen ueber klinische Haematologie, Vol 2. Wien, 1904
Sprunt TPV, Evans FA: Mononuclear leukocytosis in reaction to acute infection (infectious mononucleosis). Bull Johns Hopkins Hosp 31:410–417, 1920
Betts RF: The infectious mononucleosis syndromes in hematology and oncology. In Lichtman MA (ed): The Science and Practice of Clinical Medicine. New York, Grune & Stratton, 1980
Audiman WA: Epstein-Barr virus associated syndromes. Pediatr Infec Dis 3:198–203, 1984
Reese RE, Gordon Douglas R (ed): A practical approach to infectious diseases. Boston, Little, Brown, 1986

INSPISSATED BILE

Synonym. Jaundice obstructive infantilis.

Symptoms and Signs. Occur in newborns. Jaundice developing within first 2 days of life and lasting about 3 weeks. Anemia; splenomegaly; hepatomegaly.

Etiology. Bile inspissation due to excessive hemolysis. See Hemolytic anemia of newborn.

Pathology. Distortion of bile canalculi due to massive hepatic hematopoiesis, bile thrombosis, and liver necrotic changes.

Diagnostic Procedures. See Hemolytic anemia of newborn. *Blood.* Direct and indirect bilirubin in blood and urine markedly increased, negative flocculation tests.

Therapy. See Hemolytic anemia of newborn syndrome.

Prognosis. That of hemolytic anemia of newborn, progression to liver cirrhosis as sequela considered.

BIBLIOGRAPHY. Hsia DY, Patterson P, Allen FH Jr, et al: Prolonged obstructive jaundice in infancy. I. General survey of 156 cases. Pediatrics 10:243–252, 1952
Dacie JV: The Haemolytic Anaemias, 2nd ed. New York, Grune & Stratton, 1967

INSTITUTIONALISM

Symptoms. Psychological changes developing in people kept in segregated communities. Apathy; resignation; dependence; depersonalization, and reliance on fantasy.

BIBLIOGRAPHY. Bettelheim B, Sylvester E: A therapeutic milieu. Am J Orthopsychiatry 18:191–206, 1948
Wing JK: Institutionalism in mental hospitals. Br J Soc Clin Psychol 1:38–51, 1963
Freedman AM, Kaplan HI, Sadock BJ: Comprehensive Textbook of Psychiatry, 2nd ed. Baltimore, Williams & Wilkins, 1975

INTENSIVE CARE

Synonym. ICU.

PATIENTS

Symptoms. Acute disorganization of behavior occurring in many patients when exposed to a variety of intense diagnostic and therapeutic procedures (monitoring; infusion; contact with other acutely ill patients). Observed in particular in coronary care units and intensive care units.

Etiology. Incapacity to handle stress plus basic pathologic conditions.

Diagnostic Procedures. Monitoring of signs and symptoms of organic brain syndromes.

Therapy. Prevention by establishing personal relationship with attendant involved in care, active participation, physical presence, visits, and explanations of procedures by personal physician. Avoid or minimize delirifacient drugs. Make environment look as familiar as possible.

STAFF

Symptoms. Complex psychological reactions that may go through phases from enthusiasm to discouragement; in some cases, with acquired tendency to become less attentive to hygienic prophylactic measures. From intense, disturbing participation in patient fate, to indifference and resentment. Conflict and tension between nurses and physicians.

Etiology. Life under stressful physical and psychological situation.

Therapy. Rotation through different departments and avoid excessively lengthy period in intensive care unit. Psychological evaluation before assignment of personnel to the unit. Recognize the inevitability of conflict and tension. Maximize communication between and within professional groups in the unit and with other groups in the hospital.

BIBLIOGRAPHY. Nahum LH: Madness in the recovery room from open heart surgery or "They kept waking me up." Conn Med 29:771–772, 1965
McKegney FP: The intensive care syndrome. Conn Med 30:633–939, 1966
Kachoris PJ: Psychodynamic considerations in the neonatal ICU. Crit Care Med 5:62–65, 1977
Youngner S, Jackson DH, Allen M: Staff attitude towards the care of the critically ill in the medical intensive care unit. Crit Care Med 7:35–40, 1979
Harrell RC, Othmer E: Postcardiotomy confusion and sleep loss. J Clin Psychiatry 48:445–446, 1987

INTERMITTENT VERTEBRAL COMPRESSION

Synonyms. Bärtschi Rochain's; cervical-vertigo; vertebral artery compression. See Barré-Lieou.

Symptoms. Onset unpredictable. Precipitating factors include emotional tension, rotation or extension of head. Vertigo; dizziness; decreased hearing; tinnitus (which may persist when vertigo is over and in some patients is continuous); headache. Gastrointestinal symptoms: nausea; vomiting; explosive diarrhea. Visual disturbances; paresthesia; numbness; coldness of ipsilateral arm.

Signs. Diminution or obliteration of radial pulse with Adson maneuver; supraclavicular bruit may be heard (30% of cases) or appear with change of position of head.

Etiology and Pathology. Anomaly of vertebral artery system, which results in intermittent compression at the origin or at site of cervical course of the artery. Defect of cervical spine that intermittently compresses the artery. Vertebrobasilar aneurysm.

Diagnostic Procedures. *X-ray. Arteriography.*

Therapy. According to etiology, different surgical procedures: surgical mobilization of the artery with stripping of vertebral plexus; fusion of vertebrae; correction of aneurysm.

Prognosis. Good response to surgery.

BIBLIOGRAPHY. Pratt-Thomas HR, Berger KE: Cerebellar and spinal injuries after chiropractic manipulation. JAMA 133:600–603, 1947
Bärtschi-Rochain W: Migrain cervicale (Das encephale Syndrome nach halswirbel Trauma). Berne, Huber, 1949
Morley JB: Unruptured vertebro-basilar aneurysms. Med J Austr 2:1024–1027, 1967

Adams RD, Victor M: Principles of Neurology, 3rd ed, p 600. New York, McGraw-Hill, 1985

INTESTINAL CARBOHYDRATE DYSPEPSIA

Synonym. Carbohydrate dyspepsia. See Irritable bowel.

Symptoms. Prevalent in middle-aged females with depressive tendency, anxiety, nervousness. Characteristic intermittent attacks following emotional stress. Attacks are extremely variable in length (days or many years). Abdominal pains, usually after meals; nocturnal distress; abdominal fullness; distension; flatus; belching; intolerance to certain foods (starches, vegetables, milk). Constipation or diarrhea; asthenia; fatigability.

Signs. In some patients, weight loss, chronic choroidoretinitis (in 25% of patients), hypotension (30%), tachycardia.

Etiology. Alteration of intestinal flora; deficiency of diastatic enzymes; intestinal hypermotility; dietary disorders; sensitivity to carbohydrates, aerophagia.

Pathology. No constant pathologic changes; chronic state of congestion and increased mucosal desquamation reported.

Diagnostic Procedures. *Blood.* Moderate anemia. *Stool.* Rich in undigested carbohydrates; increased mucus and gas bubbles. *Sigmoidoscopy.* Normal. *X-ray.* Colon dilatation, spasm, accelerated transit (in some cases).

Therapy. Difficult. Psychotherapy to correct emotional factors; correction of aerophagia; dietary measures; vitamin supplementation; pancreatic enzymes; atropine in diarrhea; modification of flora with short course of antibiotic also useful.

Prognosis. Periodic recurrence with period of freedom from symptoms.

BIBLIOGRAPHY. Althausen TL, Gunnisin JB, Marshall MD, et al: Carbohydrate intolerance and intestinal flora: A clinical study based on sixty cases. Tr Am Gastro-enterol A 36:143–174, 1935
Bargen JA: Irritable bowel syndrome. Writings & Reports Scott and White Clinic 4:57–62, 1965–66
Sleisenger MH, Fordtran JS: Gastrointestinal Disease, p 1181. Philadelphia, WB Saunders, 1978
Gray GM: Intestinal disaccharidase deficiencies and glucose-galactose malabsorption. In Stanbury JB, Wyngaarden JB, Fredrickson DS, et al: The Metabolic Basis of Inherited Disease, 5th ed, pp 1733–1734. New York, McGraw-Hill, 1983

INTESTINAL IDIOPATHIC PSEUDOOBSTRUCTION

Synonym. IIP. See Diffuse esophageal spasm.

Symptoms and Signs. Both sexes affected; onset at all ages. Recurrent signs of esophageal obstruction and, later, recurrent signs of small and large bowel dysfunction.

Etiology. Unknown.

Diagnostic Procedures. *Manometry.* Lower esophageal sphincter pressure in the normal range with incomplete relaxation. *X-rays.* Barium swallow.

Therapy. Medical management. Nifedipine and isosorbide dinitrate (modest results). If unsuccessful, surgical myotomy; pneumatic dilatation.

Prognosis. Good.

BIBLIOGRAPHY. Schuffer MD, Pope CH II: Esophageal motor dysfunction in idiopathic intestinal pseudoobstruction. Gastroenterology 70:677–682, 1976
Castell DO, Johnson LF: Esophageal Function in Health and Disease. New York, Elsevier, 1982

INTESTINAL KNOT

Synonyms. Compound volvulus; double volvulus.

Symptoms and Signs. Prevalent in males (85%); maximal incidence in 5th and 6th decades. Relatively rare. Sudden, severe, abdominal pain and nausea. Abdomen boardlike with generalized tenderness. Chest examination normal.

Etiology and Pathology. Knotting strangulation of both cecal and sigmoid segments. Variations reported such as appendiceal knot and subsequent closed loop, ileal obstruction, and others. No precipitating factor identified. Possibly, underlying mesenteric inflammatory change with shortening of proximal and distal sigmoid segments. Intestinal parasites a predisposing factor in some cases.

Diagnostic Procedures. *Blood.* White blood cells increased. *Abdominal paracentesis.* Cloudy fluid with low amylase content. *X-ray of abdomen.* Oval loop of dilated bowel in right lower quadrant. With patient erect, no free air, several gas-filled and dilated loops of small bowel. Classical "breaking" of barium column at site of sigmoid volvulus.

Treatment. Immediate surgical intervention. When possible, separation and unwinding of loops; resection with end-to-end anastomoses of both ileum and colon, with decompressing cecostomy.

Prognosis. Determined by promptness of surgical intervention.

BIBLIOGRAPHY. Parker E: Case of intestinal obstruction: sigmoid flexure strangulated by the ileum. Edinburgh Med Surg J 64:306, 1845

Boyden FM, Tappan WM: The intestinal knot syndrome. JAMA 211:662–663, 1970

Gumbs MA, Kashan F, Shumofsky E, et al: Volvulus of the transverse colon: report of cases and review of literature. Dis Colon Rectum 26:825–828, 1983

Northeast ADR, Dennison AR, Lee EG: Sigmoid volvulus: new thoughts on the epidemiology. Dis Colon Rectum 27:260–264, 1984

INTESTINAL POLYPOSIS, FAMILIAL

Symptoms. Onset before the age of 40, usually in late childhood or young adulthood. Symptoms not specific; occasionally, diarrhea and weakness, with development of malignant changes. Change in bowel habits. Pain; obstruction; malnutritional findings.

Signs. Pallor; pain over colon.

Etiology. Familial autosomal dominant trait (about half of offspring of person with disease affected).

Pathology. Benign adenomas, small usually sessile, densely packing the entire colon mucosal surface; frequent malignant transformation at early age; adenocarcinomas enlarge and spread rather rapidly.

Diagnostic Procedures. *Barium enema. Sigmoidoscopy.* Appearance pathognomonic.

Therapy. Subtotal colectomy with ileoproctostomy and careful follow-up for possible development of carcinoma on remaining stump. Fulguration of remaining polyps also recommended.

Prognosis. Guarded; occasionally, remission of remaining polyps.

BIBLIOGRAPHY. Cripps H: Two cases of disseminated polyps of rectum. Trans Med Soc Lon 33:165, 1882

Lynch HT, Krush AF: Heredity and adenocarcinoma of the colon. Gastroenterology 53:517–527, 1967

Hrabovsky EE, Watne AL, Carrier JM: Changing management in familial polyposis: role of ileoanal endorectal pull-through. Am J Surg 147:130, 1984

INTRAMURAL CORONARY ARTERY ANEURYSM

See Coronary artery steal syndrome.

Symptoms. Angina pectoris, dyspnea, and fatigue on exertion.

Signs. Harsh systolic and diastolic murmur along left sternal border and on apex.

Etiology and Pathology. Intramural coronary artery aneurysm.

Diagnostic Procedures. *Electrocardiography.* Suggests posterior myocardial infarction. *X-ray.* Heart normal size. *Heart catheterization.* Normal output; normal pressure; no shunt. *Left ventricular angiography and aortography.* Left ventricle normal size and normal contraction. Right coronary normal. Left descending coronary dilated to 1 cm in diameter; tortuous emptying into an aneurysmal sac at the apex of heart; aneurysm large in diastole, contracted in systole.

Therapy. Closure of aneurysmal neck and approximation of walls. Anticoagulant or antiplatelet therapy.

Prognosis. Variable; good result with surgery.

BIBLIOGRAPHY. Björk VO, Björk L: Intramural coronary artery aneurysm: a coronary artery steal syndrome. J Thorac Cardiovasc Surg 54:50–52, 1967

Baue AE, Baum S, Blakemore WS, et al: A large stage of anomalous coronary circulation with origin of the left coronary artery from pulmonary artery-coronary artery steal. Circulation 36:878–885, 1967

Perloff JK: The Clinical Recognition of Congenital Heart Disease, 2nd ed. Philadelphia, WB Saunders, 1978

Hurst JW: The Heart, 6th ed, p 1020. New York, McGraw-Hill, 1986

INTRINSIC FACTOR I, CONGENITAL DEFICIENCY

Synonyms. Addison-Biermer, infantile; pernicious infantile anemia.

Symptoms and Signs. Both sexes, affected; onset in early childhood. Pallor; absence of malabsorption signs.

Etiology. Unknown; autosomal recessive inheritance.

Diagnostic Procedures. *Blood and bone marrow.* Evidence of megaloblastic anemia. *Gastric fluid.* Normal, free acid. *Biopsy.* Absence of gastric atrophy. *Urine.* Shilling's test positive.

Therapy. Vitamin B_{12}.

Prognosis. Anemia responds to treatment with vitamin B_{12}.

BIBLIOGRAPHY. Herbert V, Streiff RR, Sullivan LW: Notes on vitamin B_{12} absorption: autoimmunity and pernicious anemia: relation of intrinsic factor to blood group substance. Medicine (Baltimore) 43:679–687, 1964

McIntyre OR, Sullivan LW, Jeffries GH, et al: Pernicious anemia in childhood. New Engl J Med 272:981–986, 1965

Yang Y, Ducos R, Rosenberg AJ, et al: Cobalamin malabsorption in three siblings due to an abnormal intrinsic factor that is markedly susceptible to acid and proteolysis. J Clin Invest 76:2657–2665, 1985

IRRITABLE BOWEL

Synonyms. IBS; adaptive colitis; mucous colitis; colonic neurosis; spastic colitis; dyssynergia colon; irritable colon; unstable colon; neurogenic mucous colitis.

Symptoms. More frequent in women. From adult age. *Precipitating factors.* Psychogenic: cancer phobia; emotional tension; fatigue; weakness; menstrual periods; tobacco; diet; bowel irritants. Constipation alternated with normal bowel movement and diarrhea (in about 25% of cases); epigastric pains. *Associated symptoms.* Aerophagy; anxiety; insomnia; nervousness; fatigue. *Vasomotor symptoms.* Flushing, faintness; sweating, cardiac arrhythmias, headache; urinary frequency; dysuria; dysmenorrhea; pruritus ani and vulvae.

Signs. Symptoms during attack: palpation of spastic colon (lower descending portion), tenderness over ascending and transverse parts; absence of muscle guarding (except for excessive reaction of patient). Rectal examination negative.

Etiology. Emotional tension, as manifestation of numerous endocrinopathies. Unknown. Probably due to alteration of vagus nerve function. May be part of autonomic failure syndrome.

Diagnostic Procedures. *Stool.* Abnormal, small, hard, narrow cylindrical or fragmented; mucus. *Sigmoidoscopy.* Colon irritability and spasm; absence of organic lesion or dilatation. *X-ray.* *Barium enema and barium meal* reveal increased speed of transit; smooth narrowing of lumen of colon; other spastic features. Gastric secretory response to insulin hypoglycemia impaired.

Therapy. Psychotherapy; sedatives; diet; bulking agent and mild laxative when needed.

Prognosis. Recurrence in most patients. Gratifying result may be obtained with adequate treatment.

BIBLIOGRAPHY. Ryle JA: Chronic spasmodic affections of the colon. Lancet II:1115–1119, 1928

Bockus HL, Bank J, Wilkinson SA: Neurogenic mucous colitis. Am J Med Sci 176:813–829, 1928

Dotevall G, Svendlund J, Sjodin I: Symptoms in irritable bowel syndrome. Scand J Gastroenterol 17 (suppl 79):16–19, 1982

Smart HL, Atkinson M: Abnormal vagal function in irritable bowel syndrome. Lancet II:475–478, 1987

IRVINE-GASS

Synonyms. Cataract extraction; vitreous cataract extraction; vitreous tug; vitreous wick.

Symptoms. Posttraumatic or onset 2 to 3 weeks after intraocular surgery. Sensation of light flashes. Decreasing vision.

Signs. Irregular pupils. Vitreous strand passing through pupil attached to corneal scar. Possibly, vitreous detachment.

Etiology. Trauma that causes attachment or entrapment of a vitreous strand in the corneal wound, and where pupillary constriction causes forward pull on vitreous and then on retina.

Diagnostic Procedures. *Ophthalmoscopy.* Loss of foveal reflex; localized edema retinae; occasionally, posterior retinal detachment.

Therapy. Surgical repair.

Prognosis. Good with surgery.

BIBLIOGRAPHY. Irvine SR: Newly defined vitreous syndrome following cataract surgery: Interpreted according to recent concepts of structure of vitreous (Seventh Francis P Proctor Lecture). Am J Ophthalmol 36:599–619, 1953

Stainer GA, Binder PS: Vitreous wick syndrome following a corneal relaxing incision. Ophthal Surg 12:567–570, 1981

ISAACS-MERTENS

Synonym. Continuous muscle fiber activity. See Moersch-Waltmann.

Symptoms and Signs. Both sexes. Persistent myokymia from first months, then diminishing motor activity with flexion, contractures of lower limbs. Increased muscular tone persists during sleep. Cyanotic episodes. At later age persistence of myokymia and transient stiffness after initiation of movements.

Etiology. Autosomal dominant inheritance.

Diagnostic Procedures. *Electromyography.* Continuous motor activity that persists in spite of peripheral nerve blockade or anesthesia. *X-rays, thoraco-abdominal, CT scan, sonography.* Eventration of diaphragm with poor motion.

Therapy. Phenytoin sodium.

Prognosis. Considerable improvement with therapy.

BIBLIOGRAPHY. Isaac HA: A syndrome of continuous muscle fiber activity. J Neurol Neurosurg Psychiatr 24:319–325, 1961

Martens HG, Zschocke S: Neuromyokymia. Klin Wchnsch 43:917–925, 1965

McGuire SA; Tomasovic JJ, Ackermann N Jr: Hereditary continuous muscle fiber activity. Arch Neurol 41:395–396, 1984

ISCHEMIC COLON

Synonym. Transient intestinal ischemic attack. See Abdominal angina.

Symptoms. In patient over 50. Acute onset. Cramping lower or left side abdominal pain; urge to defecate, nausea, vomiting. Occasionally fever, bloody diarrhea.

Signs. Abdominal tenderness and/or rigidity of abdominal wall.

Etiology. Occlusion spontaneous or following surgery of branches of interior mesenteric artery with transient ischemia of portion of colon. In younger patients association with diabetes mellitus, lupus erythematosus, sickle cell crisis. Usually without intestinal infarction.

Pathology. See etiology. Minor atherosclerotic changes of vessels, intestinal lesions, edema, and then necrotic changes leading to strictures.

Diagnostic Procedures. *X-ray. Barium enema.* Mass lesion or edema of mucosa (pseudotumor). In advanced cases lesions similar to ulcerative colitis and strictures splenic flexure-descending colon most frequent location. Mesenteric arteriography. *Blood.* Leukocytosis. *Stool.* Blood.

Therapy. Symptomatic. Immediate surgery not required and reserved only for severe form.

Prognosis. Usually self-limited condition; may heal without permanent lesion. Fair for severe form.

BIBLIOGRAPHY. Williams LF, Nittenberg J: Ischemic colitis: a useful clinical diagnosis. But is it ischemic! Ann Surg 182:439–448, 1975

Abel ME, Russel TR: Ischemic colitis: a comparison of surgical and non operative management 26:113–118, 1983

ISOLATED GROWTH-HORMONE DEFICIENCY

Synonyms. Ateliosis; pituitary dwarfism I. See Gilford-Burnier and Illig's.

Symptoms and Signs. Both sexes affected; birth weight and gestational age usually normal. Usually, normal growth during first year, then continuing at markedly diminished rate. Occasionally, later onset (up to 10 years) of slowed growth. Normal or delayed pubertal development; height more retarded than weight. Symptomatic Harris' syndrome (see).

Etiology. Isolated deficiency of secretion of growth hormone. Usually sporadic cases. Familial cases reported with autosomal dominant inheritance.

Diagnostic Procedures. *Plasma.* Low or absent growth hormone; lack of increase after insulin stimulation. Normal level of thyroid-stimulating hormone (TSH), adrenocorticotropic hormone (ACTH), gonadotropins. Hypoglycemia. *X-ray.* Markedly retarded bone age. No lesions of sella turcica.

Therapy. Growth hormone.

Prognosis. Striking growth with administration of hormone. Pubertal development may also be accelerated by treatment.

BIBLIOGRAPHY. Gilford H: Ateliosis: form of dwarfism. Practitioner 70:797–819, 1903

Antonin JMF: Hypothalamo-hypophysarer Zwergwuchs mit spontaner Pubertat. Helv Paediat Acta 16:267–276, 1961

Goodman HG, Grumbach MM, Kaplan SL: Growth and growth hormone. II. A comparison of isolated growth-hormone deficiency and multiple pituitary-hormone deficiencies in 35 patients with idiopathic hypopituitary dwarfism. New Engl J Med 278:57–68, 1968

Van Gelderen HH, Van der Hoog CE: Familial isolated growth hormone deficiency. Clin Genet 20:173–175, 1981

Grossman A, Savage MO, Wass JAH, et al: Growth hormone-releasing factor in growth hormone deficiency: demonstration of a hypothalamic defect in growth hormone release. Lancet II:137–138, 1983

ISOVALERIC ACIDEMIA

Symptoms and Signs. Both sexes affected. At birth normal; after a few days, attacks of vomiting, acidosis, coma, strong objectionable body odor that increases with recurrence of symptoms. During attacks, ataxia and tendon hyperreflexia. Mild psychomotor retardation; aversion to protein-rich foods. Two clinical cases described: acute severe type and chronic intermittent type (sweaty feet)

Etiology. Inborn error of leucine metabolism with accumulation of isovaleric acid in serum; defect of isovaleric coenzyme A (CoA) dehydrogenase. Autosomal recessive inheritance.

Diagnostic Procedures. *Blood.* High accumulation of isovaleric acid and inability of leukocytes to degrade $2^{14}C$ leucine normally. Leukopenia. Ketonemia during crisis. *Urine.* Excretion of isovaleric acid (typical odor). Leucine tolerance test.

Therapy. Low-protein diet.

Prognosis. Neonatal death may be associated with this condition. Patients have survived to childhood since syndrome identified.

BIBLIOGRAPHY. Holmes LB, Tanaka K, Budd MA, Isselbacher KJ, et al: Isovaleric acidemia (abstr). Soc Pediat Res 69:961, 1966
Tanaka K, Rosenberg LE: Disorders of branched chain aminoacid and organic acid metabolism. In Stanbury JB, Wyngaarden JB, Fredrickson DS, et al: The Metabolic Basis of Inherited Disease, 5th ed, p 440. New York, McGraw-Hill, 1983

ISRAEL'S

Synonym. Hyperbilirubinemia shunt.

Symptoms and Signs. Prevalent in males; onset between 16 and 40 years of age. Modest signs of anemia and jaundice; 50% with splenomegaly, without hepatomegaly.

Etiology. Autosomic recessive inheritance. Primitive increase of early labeled bilirubin diphasic or multiphasic. The first (diphasic) deriving from nonerythropoietic source; the second (multiphasic) from premature destruction of newly formed erythrocytes.

Pathology. *Spleen.* Enlarged, no remarkable changes; little deposit of iron pigment. *Liver.* Heavy infiltration of brown pigment in granules of irregular size and shape into parenchymal cells. Kupffer's cells increased and pigment loaded. *Bone marrow.* Erythroblastic hyperplasia.

Diagnostic Procedures. *Blood.* Anemia; reticulocytosis (2–5%). Occasionally, spherocytosis. Autohemolysis and mechanical fragility of red cells normal. Red cell survival normal or reduced. Moderate hyperbilirubinemia (2 to 7 mg/100 ml); prevalent nonconjugated form. Liver func-

tion test normal. *Urine.* Urobilinogen increased. *Stool.* Stercobilinogen increased.

Therapy. Hemolysis when present, corrected by splenectomy.

Prognosis. Persistent benign condition, hyperbilirubinemia persists after splenectomy and consequent correction of hemolysis and bone marrow hyperplasia.

BIBLIOGRAPHY. Kalk H, Wildhirt E: Die posthepatitische Hyperbilirubinaemie. Z Klink Med 153:354–387, 1955
Israel LG, Suderman HJ, Ritzmann SE: Hyperbilirubinemia due to an alternate path of bilirubin production. Am J Med 27:693–702, 1959
Berk PD, Wolkoff AW, Berlin NI: Inborn errors of bilirubin metabolism. (Symposium on Diseases of Liver.) Med Clin North Am 59:803–816, 1979

ITCHING PURPURA

Synonyms. Pruritic angiodermatitis; angiodermatitis pruriginosa, disseminata; eczematidelike purpura. See Schamberg's.

Symptoms. Prevalent in males; onset in adulthood. Pruritus around ankles, extending to entire legs and also, occasionally, elsewhere.

Signs. Purpuric lesions appearing on lower part of body. Typical orange color.

Etiology. Unknown.

Pathology. Perivascular inflammatory reaction in upper corium; endothelial swelling and lymphohistiocytic-red cell infiltration.

Therapy. None specific. Topical steroids.

Prognosis. Spontaneous improvement in months. Frequent recurrences.

BIBLIOGRAPHY. Davis E: Schoenlein-Henoch syndrome of vascular purpura. Blood 3:129–136, 1948
Rook A, Wilkinson DS, Ebling FJG, et al: Textbook of Dermatology, 4th ed, p 1117. Oxford, Blackwell Scientific Publications, 1986

ITO'S

Synonym. Nevus depigmentosus systematicus bilateralis; incontinentia pigmenti achromians; hypomelanosis Ito's, confused with Naegeli's syndrome.

Symptoms and Signs. Reported only in females; onset early in life and persisting for years. Progressive pigment loss without preceding inflammation. Sharply demarcated, linear or bandlike, depigmented, bizarre macules. (Negative picture of pigmentation observed in patient with Bloch-Sulzburger.) Frequently associated: mental retardation; strabismus; alopecia; congenital dislocation of the hip.

Etiology. Unknown. Developmental defect. Autosomal dominant inheritance suggested in some cases.

Pathology. Biopsy of lesion shows absence of inflammatory changes, decreased amount of granules of melanin in basal layer, epidermal melanocytes weaker in dopa reaction.

Prognosis. Lesions may disappear or remain for undetermined time.

BIBLIOGRAPHY. Ito M: Studies on melanin. XI. Incontinentia pigmenti achromians: a singular case of nevus depigmentosus systematicus bilateralis. Tohoku J Exp Med (suppl) 55:57–59, 1952

Rosemberg S, Arita FM, Campos C, et al: Hypomelanosis of Ito: case report with involvement of the central nervous system and review of the literature. Neuropediatrics 15:52–55, 1984

IVE'S

Synonym. Actinic reticuloid.

Symptoms and Signs. Only males, elderly subjects. History of contact dermatitis and mild photosensivity. Progressively increasing photosensitivity: erythema, edema, "leonine" aspect of areas exposed to light.

Etiology. Enhanced sensitivity to light entire spectrum. Relationship among allergy to plants (particularly compositae), light sensitivity and reticulosis not yet clarified.

Pathology. *Skin.* Intense superficial and deep infiltration of lymphocytes (some atypical). Collagen damaged.

Therapy. Light avoidance; sun screens; systemic mild steroid or azathioprine.

Prognosis. Recovery difficult (lifelong condition). Few cases evolve into frank Alibert-Bazin (see).

BIBLIOGRAPHY. Ive FA, Magnus IA, Warin RP, et al: "Actinoid reticuloid": a chronic dermatosis associated with severe photosensitivity and the histological resemblance to lymphoma. Br J Dermat 81:469–485, 1969

Rook A, Wilkinson DS, Ebling FJG, et al: Textbook of Dermatology, 4th ed. Oxford, Blackwell Scientific Publications, 1986

IVEMARK'S

Synonyms. Asplenia; congenital spleen absence; splenic agenesis.

Symptoms. Prevalent in males. Maternal pregnancy history and familial history occasionally significant. Dyspnea; retardation of growth.

Signs. Cyanosis from neonatal period; clubbing of fingers and toes in oldest patients. Systolic cardiac murmur diffuse along left sternal border in about 50% of patients. Symptoms and signs are of no value in differentiating this form from other types of cyanotic heart diseases.

Etiology. Unknown. Most cases sporadic. Maternal virus infection during pregnancy and familial form reported with autosomal recessive inheritance.

Pathology. Asplenia or hypoplasia of spleen; pulmonary stenosis or atresia (100%); ostium primum atrial septal defect (100%); transposition of great vessels (95%); persistent complete atrioventricular canal (95%); bilateral superior venae cavae (85%); infundibular inversion (85%); common atrium (80%); anomalous pulmonary venous connection (75%). Cases may be subdivided as follows: those with two ventricles and large ventricular septal defect; those with common ventricle.

Diagnostic Procedures. *Spleen scan.* Absence of spleen. *Blood.* Signs of asplenia; normoblast and presence of Howell-Jolly and normoblast and presence of Howell-Jolly and Heinz bodies. *Electrocardiography.* Features of persistent common atrioventricular canal. *X-ray.* Hepatic symmetry; diminished pulmonary blood flow; transposed blood vessels. *CT brain scan. Ultrasonography.*

Prognosis. For patient with these lesions, no indication for surgery. Death at young age from heart failure, overwhelming bacterial infections; in oldest patient (19 years) multiple systemic thrombosis was cause of death.

BIBLIOGRAPHY. Martin MG: Observation d'une deviation organique de l'estomac, d'une anomalie dans la situation, dans la configuration du coeur et des vaisseaux qui en partent on qui s'y rendent. Bull Soc Anat Paris 1:39, 1826

Ivemark BI: Implications of agenesis of the spleen on the pathogenesis of conotruncus anomalies in childhood: an analysis of the heart malformations in the splenic agenesis syndrome with fourteen new cases. Acta Paediatr 44 (suppl 104): 1–110, 1955

Ruttenberg HD, Neufeld HN, Lucas RV Jr, et al: Syndrome of congenital cardiac disease with asplenia: distinction from other forms of congenital cyanotic cardiac disease. Am J Cardiol 13:387–406, 1964

Hurvitz RC, Caskey CT: Ivemark syndrome. In Siblings Clin Genet 22:7–11, 1982

IVEMARK'S II

Synonyms. Asplenia-kidney, liver, pancreas dysplasia. See Polycystic, prevalent renal cystic syndrome, infantile type.

Symptoms and Signs. See Ivemark I and Polycystic, prevalent renal cystic syndrome, infantile type.

Etiology. Autosomal recessive lethal disorders.

BIBLIOGRAPHY. Ivemark BI, Oldfeld V, Zetterstrom R: Familial dysplasia of kidneys, liver, and pancreas: a probably genetic determined syndrome. Acta Paediatr 48:1–11, 1959

Crawford MDA: Renal dysplasia and aplasia in two sibs. Clin Genet 14:338–344, 1978

IVIC

(Acronym for Istituto Venezolano Investigationes Cientificas).

Synonyms. Radial ray defects-deafness-internal ophthalmoplegia-thrombocytopenia.

Symptoms and Signs. From birth. In most cases strabismus, deafness, and occasional upper limb radial ray defect (from almost normal thumbs to thumbs with longer metacarpal and shorter phalanx). Radial bone always affected. In a few cases imperforated anus.

Etiology. Autosomal dominant inheritance.

Diagnostic Procedures. *Blood:* Thrombocytopenia (mild); leukocytosis (mild).

Prognosis. Fair.

BIBLIOGRAPHY. Arias S, Penchaszadeh VB, Pinto-Cisternas J, et al: The IVIC syndrome: a new autosomal dominant complex pleiotropic syndrome with radial ray hypoplasia, hearing impairment, internal ophthalmoplegia, thrombocytopenia. Am J Med Genet 6:25–29, 1980

J

JABS'-BLAUS

Synonym. Granulomatous synovitis-uveitis-cranial neuropathies, familial. See Rotenstein's.

Symptoms and Signs. Onset; childhood. Granulomatous synovitis; symmetric, boggy polysynovitis of the hands and wrists, resulting in boutonniere deformities. Recurrent nongranulomatous acute iridocyclitis. Cranial neuropathies: bilateral neurosensory hearing loss; 6th cranial nerve palsy.

Etiology. Hereditary syndrome with an autosomal dominant inheritance pattern.

Diagnostic Procedures. Synovectomy specimens. Granulomatous inflammation with giant cells. *X-rays of hand.* No erosions or joint destruction.

Therapy. Corticosteroids (both local and systemic administration). Mydriatics.

Prognosis. The major long-term problems are iritis and joint contractures.

BIBLIOGRAPHY. Jabs DA, Honk JL, Bias WB, et al: Familial granulomatous synovitis, uveitis and cranial neuropathies. Am J Med 78:801–804, 1985
Blaus EB: Familial granulomatous arthritis, iritis and rash. J Pediatr 107:689–693, 1985

JACCOUD'S (S.)

Synonym. Jaccoud's arthritis.

Symptoms and Signs. After severe repeated attacks of rheumatic fever, development of articular changes, especially of metacarpophalangeal joints: ulnar deviation, followed by subluxation with little pain and minor mobility loss.

Etiology. Unknown; possibly, consequence of rheumatic fever or rheumatoid arthritis (see Diagnostic Procedures).

Pathology. Progressive periarticular fibrosis of selected joints.

Diagnostic Procedures. *Blood.* Rheumatoid factor seldom present. All features of acute rheumatic fever.

Therapy. Antibiotics; anti-inflammatory agents.

Prognosis. Long course. Characteristically, joint deformities may be voluntarily corrected by the patient.

BIBLIOGRAPHY. Jaccoud S: Leçons de Clinique Médicale Faites à l'Hôpital de la Charité, 2nd ed. Paris, Delahaye, 1869
Beausang E, Barnett E, Goldstein S: Jaccoud's arthritis. Ann Rheum Dis 26:239–245, 1967

JACKSONIAN

Synonyms. Focal epilepsy; Jackson's I; Bravais-Jackson.

Symptoms. Contraction starts from a focus such as tip of toe, finger, corner of mouth, and then gradually spreads to other muscles. If it remains hemilateral, consciousness is preserved.

Etiology and Pathology. Organic brain diseases are usually recognized as responsible for this type of epilepsy (e.g., neoplastic, vascular lesion).

Therapy. Surgical removal of lesion; diphenylhydantoin; phenobarbital.

Prognosis. Depends on etiology.

BIBLIOGRAPHY. Bravais LF: Recherches sur les symptomes et le Traitement de l'Épilepsie Hémiplégique, Paris (thesis), 1827
Jackson JH: Epileptiform convulsions from cerebral disease. Trans Int Med Congr 2:6–15, 1881
Adams RD, Victor M: Principles of Neurology, 3rd ed, pp 238–239. New York, McGraw-Hill, 1985

JACKSON-LAWLER

Synonyms. Murray's; pachyonychia congenita. See Jadassohn-Lewandowsky.

Symptoms and Signs. Both sexes affected; present from birth. Hoarse voice; natal teeth (poor calcification; occasionally, erupted at birth). Pachyonychia; palmoplantar hyperkeratosis and hyperhydrosis; follicular keratosis; large epidermoid cysts on the head, neck, upper chest (onset at puberty); corneal dystrophy; absence of oral leukokeratosis.

Etiology. Unknown; autosomal dominant inheritance.

Diagnostic Procedures. None specific.

BIBLIOGRAPHY. Murray FA: Four cases of hereditary hypertrophy of the nail bed associated with a history of erupted teeth at birth. Br J Dermatol 33:409–411, 1921

Jackson ADM, Lawler SD: Pachyonychia congenita: a report of six cases in one family. Ann Eugen 16:142–146, 1951

Gorlin RJ, Pindborg JJ, Cohen MM Jr: Syndromes of the Head and Neck, 2nd ed. New York, McGraw-Hill, 1976

JACKSON'S II

Synonyms. Hughlings Jackson's; McKenzie's; Jackson's paralysis; vagoaccessory-hypoglossal.

Symptoms and Signs. Paralysis of half of soft palate and larynx, sternocleidomastoid and trapezius muscles; hemiatrophy of tongue. Tachycardia.

Etiology and Pathology. Paralysis of vagus (X), spinal accessory (XI), and hypoglossal (XII) nerves usually due to vascular lesion, seldom neoplasia, trauma, or infections; affecting one lateral half of medulla oblongata at the level of the hypoglossus, ambiguous and spinal nuclei or pathways of the above mentioned cranial nerves.

BIBLIOGRAPHY. Jackson JH: Paralysis of tongue, palate, and vocal cord. Lancet I:689–690, 1886

Adams RD, Victor M: Principles of Neurology, 3rd ed, p 1010. New York, McGraw-Hill, 1985

JACKSON'S CEREBELLAR

Synonyms. Cerebellar seizures; cerebellar epilepsy; Wurffbain's.

Symptoms and Signs. Both sexes affected; onset at all ages. Seizure occasionally preceded by a loud cry. Head drawn back and back curved; no twitching of face nor deviation of eyeballs. Hands clenched; forearms flexed; upper arm (usually) kept to the sides; legs extended; feet arched backward. Urine and fecal loss (occasional). Between attacks, persistent hyperextended posture remains (cerebellar attitude).

Etiology. Midline cerebellar tumor. Brainstem lesions are also considered necessary for occurrence of these seizures.

Pathology. Neoplastic, inflammatory, vascular lesions with cerebellar involvement and brain stem lesions.

Diagnostic Procedures. *Angiography. Electroencephalography. CT brain scan.*

Therapy. According to etiology.

Prognosis. Depends on etiology.

BIBLIOGRAPHY. Jackson JH: Case of tumor of the middle lobe of the cerebellum: cerebellar paralysis with rigidity (cerebellar attitude), occasional tetanus-like seizures. Brain 29:425–440, 1906

Fulton JF: A case of cerebellar tumor with seizures of head retraction described by Wurffbain in 1691. J Nerv Ment Dis 70:577–583, 1929

Dow RS, Moruzzi G: The Physiology and Pathology of the Cerebellum. Minneapolis, University of Minnesota Press, 1958

JACOB-DOWNEY

Synonyms. Arthropathy-camptodactyly; hypertrophic synovitis congenita familial.

Symptoms and Signs. Both sexes. At birth, flexor contracture of fingers, camptodactyly; polyarticular large joint arthritis in early infancy.

Etiology. Autosomal recessive inheritance.

Pathology. Synovial membrane: hyperplasia, necrotic villi deposits of eosinophilic and periodic acid-Schiff positive material, presence of multinucleated giant cells.

Therapy. Synovectomy when needed.

Prognosis. Spontaneous tendency to regression in older age.

BIBLIOGRAPHY. Jacob JC, Downey JA: Juvenile rheumatoid arthritis. In Downey JA, Low NL: The Child with Disabling Illness, p 524. Philadelphia, WB Saunders, 1974

Di Liberti JM, McKean R, Hecht F: Progressive tenosynovitis with contractures and possible systemic involvement: a new heritable disorder of connective tissue? Birth Defects Orig Art Ser 11(6):81–82, 1975

Martin JR, Huang SN, Lacson A, et al: Congenital contractural deformities of the fingers and arthropathy. Ann Rheum Dis 44:826–830, 1985

JACOBS' (E.C.)

Synonyms. Genital oculo oral; oculogenital; oro-oculo-genital.

Symptoms. Intense burning and itching of the scrotum; conjunctivitis; stomatitis; fissuring of alae nasi.

Signs. Scrotal dermatitis and pigmentation with scaling and superficial ulceration.

Etiology. Riboflavin deficiency and other vitamin B complex components and zinc. Local inflammation may play a role. (In prisoners of war other causes of malnutrition.) Prolonged antibiotic treatment.

Diagnostic Procedures. *Blood.* Anemia; other signs of malnutrition.

Therapy. Diet and vitamin B complex.

Prognosis. Complete recovery with treatment.

BIBLIOGRAPHY. Jacobs EC: Oculo-oro-genital syndrome: a deficiency disease. Ann Intern Med 35:1049–1054, 1951
Rook A, Wilkinson DS, Ebling FJG, et al: Textbook of Dermatology, 4th ed, p 2325. Oxford, Blackwell Scientific Publications, 1986

JACOB'S (J.C.)

Synonym. Brachial plexus neuritis-cleft palate.

Symptoms and Signs. Both sexes affected; present from birth. Facial asymmetry; mongoloid slant of palpebrae; hypotelorism; cleft palate. At 3 years of age, sudden pain in the shoulder, radiating to arm and hand and gradually subsiding; leaving paresthesia and weakness; after repeated attacks, sensory loss, limitation of elbow extension.

Etiology. Autosomal dominant inheritance. Palsy precipitated by exogenous factors because of abnormalities of Schwann cells.

Pathology. Nerve biopsy; tomaculous neuropathy.

Diagnostic Procedures. *Electromyography.* Partial denervation of some arm and hand muscles.

BIBLIOGRAPHY. Jacob JC, Andermann F, Robb, JP: Heredofamilial neuritis and brachial predilection. Neurology (Minneapolis) 11:1025–1033, 1961
Erickson A: Hereditary syndrome consisting in recurrent attacks resembling brachial plexus neuritis, special facial features and cleft palate. Acta Paediatr Scand 63:855–888, 1974
Araksinen EM, Iivanainen M, Karli P, et al: Hereditary recurrent brachial plexus neuropathy with dysmorphic features. Acta Neurol Scand 71:309–316, 1985

JACOBSEN-BRODWALL

Synonyms. Oculo-oto-reno anemia; reno-oculo-oto-oro anemia; oculo-oto-oro-reno anemia; oro-oculo-oto-reno anemia; oto-oculo-oro-reno anemia.

Symptoms. One case in female reported; present from birth. Dizziness; weakness; hearing loss (neurogenic); progressive visual loss up to blindness. Abdominal colic.

Signs. Pallor. Atypical development of periodontium and caries; high arched palate. Glaucoma; iridocyclitis; cataract. Genu valgum and pes excavatus.

Etiology. Has not been classified. Possibly, genetic defect.

Pathology. Renal biopsy shows dysplasia with smooth muscle in parenchyma and absent Henle's loops.

Diagnostic Procedures. *Blood.* Hypochromic anemia; anisocytosis and few target cells. *Urine.* Lack of concentration. *Bone marrow.* Increased erythropoiesis. *X-ray of skull.* Enlargement of lateral and 3rd ventricles. *Electroencephalography.* Possible changes in medial structures; generalized dysrhythmia. *Kidney function test.* Altered. *Ophthalmoscopy.* Mild macular changes, hemorrhages, and exudates.

Therapy. Symptomatic; blood transfusion.

Prognosis. Slowly progressive to blindness and severe kidney insufficiency (patient age 28 at time of report).

BIBLIOGRAPHY. Jacobsen CD, Brodwall EK: A clinical syndrome with inborn defect in erythropoiesis, dysplastic kidneys, eye lesions, malformation of the teeth and impaired hearing: a new syndrome in a 28 year old woman. Acta Med Scand 195:231–235, 1974
Geeraets AJ: Ocular Syndromes, 3rd ed. Philadelphia, Lea & Febiger, 1976

JACOBSEN'S

Synonyms. SED tarda; X-linked; spondyloepiphyseal dysplasia tarda; X-linked spondyloepiphyseal dysplasia.

Symptoms and Signs. Occur only in males. Dwarfish short trunk variety. Limbs relatively long. Female may present arthritic complaints.

Etiology. Unknown; sex-linked inheritance.

Pathology. Degenerative changes of cartilages.

Diagnostic Procedures. *X-ray of spine.* Posterior portion of superior plate of vertebrae is "humped" (distinctive feature). Osteoarthrosis of other joints (hips, knees, shoulders) is precocious.

Therapy. None.

Prognosis. Progressive condition.

BIBLIOGRAPHY. Nilsonne H: Eigentuemliche Wirbelkorper-veraenderungen mit familiaerem Auftreten. Acta Chir Scand 62:550–554, 1927
Jacobsen AW: Hereditary osteochondrodystrophia deformans: a family with 20 members affected in 5 generations. JAMA 113:121–124, 1939

Maroteaux P, Lamy M: Les formes pseudo-achondroplas-tiques des dysplasies spondylo-epiphysaires. Presse Med 67:383–386, 1959

Monteiro de Pina Neto J, Bonfim MD, et al: Classic X-linked spondyloepiphyseal dysplasia tarda in a woman with normal karyotype. In Papadatos CJ, Bartsocas CS (eds): Skeletal Dysplasias, pp 127–132. New York, Alan R Liss, 1982

JACOD'S

Synonyms. Jacod-Rollett, petrosphenoidal carrefour; Negri-Jacod; petrosphenoidal paralysis; retrosphenoidal space; Silvio Negri's. See orbital apex.

Symptoms and Signs. Unilateral trigeminal neuralgia (first 2nd branch area, then 3rd branch) and optic tract lesion (unilateral amaurosis); total unilateral ophthalmo-plegia, sometimes optic (II), oculomotor (III), and troch-lear (VI) nerves may escape. Then deafness (middle ear type) and palatal muscle paralysis. Unilateral or bilateral cervical nodes involved in 30% of cases.

Etiology and Pathology. Neoplastic lesion, primary or metastatic beginning at medial part of medial cranial fossa, near cavernous sinus; expanding to foramen rotun-dum, foramen ovale, superior orbital fissure (optic fora-men) to the base of skull, involving eustachian tubes and palatal muscles; total loss of function of optic (II), oculo-motor (III), trochlear (IV), trigeminal (V), and abducens (VI) nerves.

Diagnostic Procedures. *X-ray. CT brain scan.*

Therapy. Deep x-rays.

Prognosis. Extremely poor.

BIBLIOGRAPHY. Jacob M: Sur la propagation intracra-nienne de sarcomes de la trompe d'Eustache, syndrome du carrefour pétrosphenoidal paralysie des 2e, 3e, 5e, and 6e pairs craniennes. Rev Neurol 28:33–38, 1921

Adams RD, Victor M: Principles of Neurology, 3rd ed, p 503. New York, McGraw-Hill, 1985

JACQUET'S

Synonyms. Alopecia reflex; circumscribed congenital alopecia.

Signs. Circumscribed alopecia occurring in association with other ectodermal dysplasias (e.g., nail; dental, see Hallermann-Streiff, Pseudopelade, Bloch-Sulzberger, and others), or associated with epidermal nevi (most common form). Alopecia may be present at birth, or develop in first month of life.

Etiology. Autosomal dominant inheritance reported; autoimmune mechanism suggested.

BIBLIOGRAPHY. Jacquet L: Des érythémes papuleux fes-siers post-érosifs. Rev Mal Enf 4:208–218, 1886

Valsecchi R, Vicari O, Frigeni A, et al: Familial alopecia areata—genetic susceptibility or coincidence? Acta Derm Venereol 65:175–177, 1985

JADASSOHN-LEWANDOWSKY

Synonyms. Pachyonychia congenita. Jackson-Lewan-dowsky.

Symptoms and Signs. Both sexes affected; evident at birth or developing in early infancy. Nails of fingers and toes: a yellow wedgelike thickening and prominent trans-verse curve, inflammatory changes, and nail shedding oc-cur frequently. Teeth may be already erupted at birth; occasionally corneal dyskeratosis. In 2nd or 3rd year, ker-atoderma of palms and soles appear. Hyperhidrosis with bullae occasionally developing on toes, edges of foot, and ankles. Horny papules in the extremities, face. Leukopla-kia of oral and anal mucosa develops frequently in second decade. Hair normal or abundant, or hypotrichosis.

Etiology. Unknown; autosomal dominant inheritance with variable penetrance.

Pathology. Subungual keratosis; various dyskeratosis features.

Therapy. None. Watch for possible malignant changes of leukoplakias.

Prognosis. If nails are removed, they regrow abnor-mally. Slowly progressing condition.

BIBLIOGRAPHY. Jadassohn J, Lewandowsky F, Neisser A, Jacobi E: Ikonographia Dermatologica, pp 29–31. Berlin, Urban & Schwarzenburg, 1906

Young LL, Lenox JA: Pachyonychia congenita: a long term evaluation. Oral Surg 36:663–666, 1973

Stieglitz JB, Centerwall WR: Pachyonychia congenita (Jadassohn-Lewandowsky syndrome): a seventeen member, four generation pedigree with unusual respi-ratory and dental involvement. Am J Med Genet 14:21–28, 1983

JADASSOHN-PELLIZZARI

Synonyms. Anetoderma; Pellizzari-Jadassohn; macular atrophy; dermatitis atrophicans maculosa. See Schwen-inger-Buzzi.

Symptoms and Signs. Predominant in women; onset usually in 2nd to 4th decade. Crops of round-oval, pink, small maculae usually on trunk and extremities, seldom on face or neck. Larger erythema plaques may be present.

Etiology. Focal elastolysis due to release of elastase from inflammatory cells. Inflammatory onset that distinguishes this syndrome from Schweninger-Buzzi, in which there is no such sequence. Distinction between the two forms today seems of historical interest.

Pathology. Early edema and perivascular lymphocytic infiltrates of dermis. Later, flattening of epidermis, fragmentation, and disappearance of elastic fibers leaving cone-shaped areas.

Diagnostic Procedures. *Biopsy.*

Therapy. Some cases respond to penicillin during the inflammatory stage, later no treatment effective.

Prognosis. Slow fading with residual maculae of atrophic skin, yielding to pressure, admitting finger in a sort of ring; defect remaining for life.

BIBLIOGRAPHY. Pellizzari C: Eritema orticato atrofizzante; atrofia parziale idiopatica della pelle. Gior Ital Mal Ven 19:230–243, 1884

Jadassohn J: Ueber eine eigenartige Form von Atrophia maculosa cutis. Verh Dtsch Dermatol Ges 342–358, 1891

Rook A, Wilkinson DS, Ebling FJG, et al: Textbook of Dermatology, 4th ed, pp 1805–1807. Oxford, Blackwell Scientific Publications, 1986

JAFFE-GOTTFRIED-BRADLEY

Synonym. Hemolytic nonspherocytic anemia-lipid membrane abnormality; high red cell phosphatidylcholine hemolytic anemia, HPCHA.

Symptoms and Signs. Both sexes affected; onset in infancy. Chronic moderate hemolysis.

Etiology. Altered phospholipid composition of erythrocyte; autosomal dominant inheritance.

Pathology. Not specific.

Diagnostic Procedures. *Blood.* Moderate anemia; reticulocytosis (6–15%); mild hyperbilirubinemia; osmotic fragility decreased, and less increase in fragility after 24 hours' incubation than normal cells. Autohemolysis slightly increased. Correction with addition of glucose. Normal red cell enzymes.

Therapy. None.

Prognosis. Relatively benign condition.

BIBLIOGRAPHY. Jaffe ER, Gottfried EL, Bradley TB Jr: Hereditary nonspherocytic hemolytic disease associ- ated with altered phospholipid composition of erythrocytes. J Clin Invest 45:1027, 1966

Jaffe ER, Gottfried EL: Hereditary nonspherocytic hemolytic disease associated with an altered phospholipid composition of the erythrocytes. J Clin Invest 47:1375–1388, 1968

Yawata Y, Sugihara T, Mori M, et al: Lipid analysis and fluidity studies by electron spin resonance of red cell membranes in hereditary high red cell membrane phosphatidylcholine hemolytic anemia. Blood 64:1129–1134, 1984

JAFFE-LICHTENSTEIN

Synonyms. Monostotic fibrous dysplasia; Jaffe's II; Jaffe-Lichtenstein-Uehlinger.

Symptoms and Signs. Occur in healthy children. Swelling, tenderness, pain in one long bone or ribs, facial bone, or skull. Absence of systemic endocrine or other skeletal manifestations.

Etiology. Unknown; congenital anomaly or possibly disturbance of normal reparative process after trauma.

Pathology. Solitary bone cyst usually affecting metaphyseal end of long bones; however, each single bone may be involved. Lacunar absorption of bone and fibrous replacement. Giant cells.

Diagnostic Procedures. *X-ray.* Cystic area in the bone cortex. *Blood.* Slight elevation of calcium and alkaline phosphatase occasionally observed.

Therapy. Osteotomy indicated to prevent fracture. Bone grafting is indicated.

Prognosis. Excellent with treatment.

BIBLIOGRAPHY. Jaffe HL, Lichtenstein L: Non-osteogenic fibroma of bone. Am J Pathol 18:205–215, 1942

Ross DW, Vitale CC: Monostotic fibrous dysplasia of the metacarpal. J Bone Joint Surg [Am] 37:196–200, 1955

JAFFE-LICHTENSTEIN-SUTRO

Synonyms. Jaffe's I; pigmented villonodular synovitis; tendon sheath xanthogranuloma.

Symptoms. Pain in one or several of the large joints with functional limitation of articulation (knee most frequently affected). Absence of systemic symptoms.

Signs. Mild to moderate limitation of movement in joint affected by pain.

Etiology. Unknown; aspecific inflammation, neoplasm, trauma have been suggested as causes.

Pathology. Formation of brownish mosslike villi or nodular proliferation of synovial membrane, localized or diffuse, in one joint or several articulations. Hyperplasia and proliferation of synovial lining cells. Large spindle-shaped stromal cells and multinuclear giant cells. Dark serohemorrhagic synovial fluid.

Diagnostic Procedures. *X-ray. Biopsy synovial membrane. Blood.* Rheumatoid arthritis (RA) test; sedimentation rate.

Therapy. Debridement of joint and arthroplasty.

Prognosis. Very benign process; good response to treatment.

BIBLIOGRAPHY. Jaffe HL, Lichtenstein L, Sutro CJ: Pigmented villonodular synovitis, and bursitis, tenosynovitis. A discussion of the synovial and bursal equivalents of the tenosynovial lesion commonly denoted as xanthoma, xanthogranuloma, giant-cell tumor, or myeloplaxoma of the tendon sheath, with some consideration of this tendon sheath lesion itself. Arch Pathol 31:731–765, 1941

Chung SMK, Jones JM: Diffuse pigmented villonodular synovitis of hip joint. J Bone Joint Surg [Am] 47:293–303, 1965

Cohen AS: Tumor of synovial joints, bursae and tendon sheaths. In Hollander JL, McCarty DJ: Arthritis and Allied Conditions, 8th ed, p 1374. Philadelphia, Lea & Febiger, 1972

Richardson EG: Miscellaneous non traumatic disorders. In Crenshaw AH (ed): Campbell's Operative Orthopedics, 7th ed, pp 1006–1007. St Louis, CV Mosby, 1987

JAKE PARALYSIS

Symptoms and Signs. Headache; myosis; vomiting; sweating; abdominal cramps; salivation; whizzing; muscular weakness; areflexia.

Etiology. Drinking of extract of Jamaican ginger contaminated with triorthocresylphosphate (TOCP). Other epidemics have been reported in Morocco (contaminated olive oil) and other regions of the world (grain, cooking oil, etc.).

Pathology. "Dying back" from terminal ends of largest medullated motor nerve fibers.

Diagnostic Procedures. *Blood:* acetylcholinesterase level.

Therapy. Atropine; pralidoxime mesylate.

Prognosis. Variable according to amount of TOCP ingested.

BIBLIOGRAPHY. Nambe IT, Nalte CT, Jackerel J, et al: Poisoning due to organophosphate insecticides: acute and chronic manifestations. Am J Med 50:475, 1971

Gosselin RE, Smith RP, Hodge HC: Clinical Toxicology of Commercial Products, 5th ed. Baltimore, Williams & Wilkins, 1984

JAKSCH'S

Synonyms. Pseudoleukemic anemia infantilis; Jaksch-Hayem-Luzet; pseudoleukemia anemia; von Jaksch's.

Symptoms. Occur in young children (under 3 years of age). Listlessness; weakness; gastrointestinal troubles; irregular fever.

Signs. Pallor; hepatosplenomegaly; lymphadenopathy.

Etiology and Pathology. Represents a symptom complex with a large variety of etiologic factors from malnutrition to infections, thalassemia, hemolytic diseases of newborn. This eponym, in view of better understanding of pathology of anemia in childhood, has become obsolete.

Diagnostic Procedures. Anemia; anisopoikilocytosis; leukocytosis with relative lymphocytosis.

Therapy and Prognosis. Depends on etiology.

BIBLIOGRAPHY. von Jaksch R: Ueber Leukämie und Leukocytose im Kindesalter. Wien Klin Wochenschr 2:435–437; 456–458, 1889

JAMAICAN VOMITING SICKNESS

Synonyms. Ackee fruit intoxication; intoxication ackee fruit.

Symptoms and Signs. Predominant in children, but also in adults. After ingestion of unripe ackee fruit, vomiting, convulsions, coma, and death.

Etiology. Intoxication by toxins (hypoglycins A and B) from unripe ackee fruit.

Diagnostic Procedures. *Blood, urine.* Findings, like those of glutaric aciduria type II (see).

Pathology. *Liver.* Fatty infiltration.

Therapy. Supportive.

Prognosis. Death.

BIBLIOGRAPHY. Hill KR: The vomiting sickness of Jamaica: a review. West Indian Med J 1:243, 1952

Billington D, Osmundsen H, Sherratt HSA: The biochemical basis of Jamaican ackee poisoning. New Engl J Med 295:1482, 1976

Sherratt HSA, Al-Bassan SS: Glycine in ackee poisoning. Lancet II:1243, 1976

JANSEN'S

Synonyms. Dysostosis enchondralis metaphysaria (type C-I); Jansen's metaphyseal dysostosis; spondylometaphyseal dysostosis (type C-I).

Symptoms and Signs. Both sexes affected. Dwarfism evident from childhood; variable deafness. Mental deficiency. Mild supraorbital frontonasal hyperplasia; micrognathia. Metaphysis of all bones affected with marked widening. Hands and feet not spared; short diaphysis. Squatting stance from flexion deformities of knee.

Etiology. Unknown; autosomal dominant inheritance. Most cases sporadic.

Pathology. Metaphysis enlarged, spongelike and granite in appearance; epiphysis normal.

Diagnostic Procedures. *X-ray* Abnormalities described; condyles and glenoid appear irregular. Vertebrae irregular, some cuneiform or with irregular contours. Hyperostosis of calvaria; thick dense skull base. *Blood.* Hypercalcemia.

Therapy. Orthopedic.

Prognosis. Severe articular dysfunction.

BIBLIOGRAPHY. Jansen M: Ueber atypische Condrodystrophie (Achondroplasie) und Über eine noch nicht beschriebene angeborene Wachstumsstöring des Knochensystems: Metaphysare Dysostosis. Orthop Chir 61:253–286, 1934

Bailey JA: Disproportionate Short Stature: Diagnosis and Management, p 296. Philadelphia, WB Saunders, 1973

JARCHO'S

Synonyms. Carcinoma disseminated-thrombocytopenic purpura; paraneoplastic thrombocytopenic purpura-disseminated carcinoma.

Symptoms. Purpura and hemorrhagic manifestation in patient with carcinoma, and hematologic malignancies.

Etiology. Autoimmune destruction of platelets.

Diagnostic Procedures. Platelet-bound IgG has been demonstrated in some patients.

Prognosis. The time of onset of the purpura bears little relation to the duration, severity, or state of activity of the neoplasm, and, except for the hazard posed by thrombocytopenia itself, has no adverse prognostic implications.

Therapy. Prednisone, splenectomy, platelet transfusion.

BIBLIOGRAPHY. Jarcho S: Diffusely infiltrative carcinoma. A hitherto undescribed correlation of several varieties of tumor metastasis. Arch Pathol 22:674–696, 1936

Wintrobe MM (ed): Clinical Hematology, 8th ed. Philadelphia, Lea & Febiger, 1981

JAUNDICE, BREAST-MILK

Synonyms. Breast-feeding hyperbilirubinemia, transient nonhemolytic unconjugated hyperbilirubinemia associated breast-feeding; maternal milk hyperbilirubinemia; breast milk jaundice.

Symptoms. Jaundice associated with breast-feeding, becoming maximal during first 10 to 20 days of life and disappearing after 30 to 60 days, in spite of continuation of breast-feeding.

Etiology. Presence of inhibitor of UDP-glucuronyl transferase in maternal milk: 3(alpha), 20(beta) pregnanediol.

Diagnostic Procedures. *Blood.* Unconjugated hyperbilirubinemia. *Maternal milk.* 3(Alpha), 20(beta) pregnanediol.

Therapy. Discontinuation of breast feeding.

Prognosis. Recession of jaundice with artificial feeding. No kernicterus usually develops.

BIBLIOGRAPHY. Arias IM, Gardner LM, Seifter S, et al: Prolonged neonatal unconjugated hyperbilirubinemia associated with breast feeding and a steroid pregnane-3(alpha),20(beta)-diol in maternal milk, that inhibits glucoronide formation in vitro. J Clin Invest 43:2037–2047, 1964

Schmid R, McDonath AF: Hyperbilirubinemia. In Stanbury JB, Wyngaarden JB, Fredrickson DS, et al: The Metabolic Basis of Inherited Disease, 4th ed, p 1234. New York, McGraw-Hill, 1978

JAYLE-OURGAUD

Synonym. Internuclear ophthalmoplegia.

Symptoms and Signs. Paresis of internal rectus muscles, becoming apparent in attempted lateral gaze, while convergence is usually preserved; nystagmus of abducted eye (?).

Etiology. Lesion in the median longitudinal fasciculus. Usually observed in multiple sclerosis (see).

BIBLIOGRAPHY. Hugonnier R, Magnard P: Paralysie internucléaire antérieure. Bull Soc Ophthalmol Fr 71:265–268, 1958
Vick NA: Grinker's Neurology, 7th ed. Springfield, Il, CC Thomas, 1976

JEJUNITIS, CHRONIC ULCERATIVE

Synonym. Regional nongranulomatous enteritis. See Crohn's and ulcerative colitis.

Symptoms and Signs. All symptoms and signs of malabsorption syndromes of differing degrees.

Etiology. Unknown; distinct from (1) nontropical sprue, (2) lymphoma, and (3) dysgammaglobulinemia because of lack of response to gluten-free diet and type of pathologic lesions, and return to normal of protein after treatment.

Pathology. Ulceration of jejunum with adjacent atrophic and normal mucosa.

Diagnostic Procedures. See Gee's. *Biopsy of jejunum.*

Therapy. Corticosteroids.

Prognosis. Temporary remission or unremitting course with no response to treatment.

BIBLIOGRAPHY. Jeffries GH, Steinberg H, Sleisenger MH: Chronic ulcerative (nongranulomatous) jejunitis. Am J Med 44:47–59, 1968
Sleisenger MH, Fordtran JS: Gastrointestinal Disease, p 1090. Philadelphia, WB Saunders, 1978

JENSEN'S

Synonym. Opticoacoustic nerve atrophy-dementia.

Symptoms and Signs. In males. Onset in infancy; sensineural deafness; in adolescence, optic nerve atrophy; in adulthood, progressive dementia.

Etiology. Unknown. X-linked recessive inheritance.

BIBLIOGRAPHY. Jensen PKA: Nerve deafness, optic nerve atrophy and dementia: a new X linked recessive syndrome. Am J Med Genet 9:55–60, 1981

JERVELL–LANGE-NIELSON

Synonym. Cardioauditory.

Symptoms and Signs. Occur in child of either sex with bilateral conduction type deafness; onset in infancy or early childhood. Repeated attacks of syncope. Seizures may begin with a piercing scream followed by pallor and then cyanosis and loss of consciousness of short duration, followed by deep sleep. Attack may result in sudden death. Seizures precipitated by exertion or emotional strain.

Etiology. Unknown; congenital recessive condition.

Pathology. No gross or pathologic cardiac abnormality. In two cases infarction of sinoatrial node, abnormality of Purkinje fibers.

Diagnostic Procedures. *Electrocardiography.* Prolongation of Q-T interval. *Audiography.* Bilateral perceptive hearing loss. *Blood.* Moderate hypochromic anemia. Other changes (electrocardiographic, electroencephalographic, and biochemical) not constant features of condition.

Therapy. Beta-blocking drugs, left sympathetic atelectomy with or without beta-blockade therapy.

Prognosis. Most cases terminate fatally during childhood. Sudden death follows a syncopal attack. In surviving cases, it seems that attacks become less frequent as patients grow older.

BIBLIOGRAPHY. Meissner F: Taubstummheit and Taubstummenbildung. Leipzig und Heidelberg, Wenter 120, 1856
Jervell A, Lange-Nielson F: Congenital deaf mutism, functional heart disease with prolongation of Q-T interval and sudden death. Am Heart J 54:59–68, 1957
Locati E, Moss AJ, Schwartz PJ, et al: The long Q-T syndrome. J Am Cardiol 3:516, 1948

JERVIS'

Synonym. Early familial cerebellar degeneration. See Marinesco-Sjögren.

Symptoms and Signs. Both sexes affected; present from birth. Inconspicuous and nonprogressive cerebellar signs; mental deficiency.

Etiology. Unknown; familial and sporadic cases reported.

Pathology. Shrinking of all divisions of cerebellum, cerebellar cortex site of primary involvement, granular cells rather than Purkinje cells affected. Some Purkinje cells show "torpedoes" in the axon and "cactuslike" formation on their dendrites. Several "basket cells."

Diagnostic Procedures. *CT brain scan.*

Therapy. None.

Prognosis. Death in first year of life, or in less severe form, some improvement in walking and talking.

BIBLIOGRAPHY. Jervis GA: Early familial cerebellar degeneration (report of three cases in one family). J Nerv Ment Dis 111:398–407, 1950
Dow RS, Moruzzi G: The Physiology and Pathology of the Cerebellum. Minneapolis, University of Minnesota Press, 1958

JESSNER-KANOF

Synonym. Lymphocytic benign skin infiltration.

Symptoms and Signs. Occur predominantly (almost exclusively) in men; onset between 2nd and 8th decades. Single or multiple flat, reddish papules, occasionally circinate, becoming firm. Face (molar region) usually affected; any other body region may be involved. Sun exposure may irritate or aggravate lesion. No systemic symptoms or visceral involvement.

Etiology. Lymphocyte infiltration of skin, without follicular pattern (see Spiegler-Fendt).

Pathology. Normal epidermis; diffuse lymphocytic infiltration of dermis, perivascular and periadnexal. Basophilic degeneration of dermis; no germinal center.

Diagnostic Procedures. *Biopsy. Blood.* Occasionally, lymphocytosis.

Therapy. Trials with antimalarial agents; topical steroids; gold; x-rays; carbon dioxide.

Prognosis. Improvement with treatment. Condition persists for years, spontaneous remission, and relapses. No systemic effect; no progression of lesion to skin atrophy (lupus erythematosus).

BIBLIOGRAPHY. Jessner M, Kanof NB: Lymphocytic infiltration of the skin. Arch Dermatol Syph 68:447–449, 1953
Willemze R, Dijkstra A, Meijer CJ: Lymphocytic infiltration of the skin (Jessner): a T cell lymphoproliferative disease. Br J Dermatol 110:523–529, 1984

Rook A, Wilkinson DS, Ebling FJG, et al: Textbook of Dermatology, 4th ed, pp 1716–1717. Oxford, Blackwell Scientific Publications, 1986

JEUNE'S

Synonyms. Asphyxiating thoracic dystrophy; infantile thoracic dystrophy; suffocating thoracicdystrophy; thoracic-pelvic-phalangeal dystrophy.

Symptoms. The syndrome is thought to be genetically heterogeneous because it occurs in both a neonatal form, with life-threatening thoracic deformity, and a form that develops in later childhood, manifested as renal dysfunction.

Signs. Hypoplastic horizontal ribs; elevated clavicles; reduced growth and motility of thorax. Long bones wide and short; fraying of epiphyses; distal bones more severely affected. Pelvic changes: "squaring" of iliac wings; "sawtoothing" of acetabular roofs. Occasionally, lacunar skull.

Etiology. Unknown; autosomal recessive condition. Variant of Ellis-van Creveld (see) characterized by lower incidence of ectodermal dysplasia, and by more severe thoracic deformity. Suggested also autosomal dominant inheritance with incomplete penetrance.

Pathology. See Ellis-van Creveld.

Diagnostic Procedures. *X-ray of chest and skeleton.* Multiple ossification centers in body of sternum; shortened ulnae and fibulae; notches at the ends of metacarpal and metatarsal bones; lacking typical knee alterations (distinctive characteristic from Ellis-van Creveld).

Therapy. Antibiotics and prevention of pulmonary infections. Corrective thoracoplasty; long-term ventilatory support; renal transplantation.

Prognosis. Some patients die from asphyxia when pulmonary infection occurs. Pulmonary complication tends to decrease with age.

BIBLIOGRAPHY. Jeune M, Carron R, Beraud C, et al: Polychondrodystrophie avec blocage thoracique d'evolution fatale. Pediatrie 9:380–392, 1954
Langer LO: Thoracic-pelvic-phalangeal dystrophy, asphyxiating thoracic dystrophy of the newborn, infantile thoracic dystrophy. Radiology 91:447–456, 1968
Tahernia AC, Stamps P: Jeune syndrome. Clin Pediatr 16:903–908, 1977
Borland L: Anesthesia for children with Jeune's syndrome (asphyxiating thoracic dystrophy). Anesthesiology 66:86–88, 1987

JEUNE-TOMMASI

Synonym. Ataxia-Deafness-Cardiomyopathy.

Symptoms and Signs. In Gypsies. Onset 6 years of age circa. Cerebellar ataxia; sensineural deafness; mental deficiency. Diffuse lentigines. Cardiomegaly.

Etiology. Autosomal recessive inheritance.

Diagnostic Procedures. Heart block frequently develops.

BIBLIOGRAPHY. Jeune M, Tommasi M, Freycon F, et al: Syndrome familial associant ataxia, surdité et oligophrenie: sclerose myocardique d'evolution fatale chez l'un des enfants. Pediatrie 18:984–987, 1963
Koenigsmark BW, Gorlin RJ: Genetic and Metabolic Deafness, pp 306–307. Philadelphia, WB Saunders, 1976

JOB'S

Synonyms. Granulomatous disease variant; hyper IgE; hyperimmunoglobulin E–recurrent infection; HIE.

Symptoms and Signs. Occur in fair-skinned, red-haired females; onset from birth. Recurrent suppurative infections of the skin. Pulmonary infections, lymphadenitis and conjunctivitis may be features. As part of the syndrome (to justify its name) a feeling of depression, guilt, and rejection from relatives and friends may also be considered.

Etiology. Unknown. It appears that this syndrome is not an isolated entity, but part of the spectrum of chronic granulomatous disease. Agent responsible for infections is usually *Staphylococcus*.

Pathology. Not reported for original cases. Biopsy material from other cases does not show granuloma formation.

Diagnostic Procedures. *Blood.* Normal leukocytes activities or insignificant changes possibly unrelated to infection proneness. *Immunoglobulin studies.* High IgE level. Culture for determination of bacteria.

Therapy. Antibiotics.

Prognosis. Various degrees of disability according to extent and type of infections.

BIBLIOGRAPHY. Job 2:7–8, 19:1–29
Davis SD, Schaller J, Wedgewood RJ: Job's syndrome recurrent "cold" staphylococcal abscesses. Lancet I:1013–1015, 1966
Dreskin SC, Goldsmith PK, Gallin JI: Immunoglobulin in the hyperimmunoglobulin E and recurrent infection

(Job's) syndrome: deficiency of anti-*Staphylococcus aureus* immunoglobulin A. J Clin Invest 75:26–34, 1985

JOHANSON-BLIZZARD

Synonyms. Deafness-hypothyroidism-hypoplasia alae nasi; oligodontia–hypoplasia alae nasi-mental retardation.

Symptoms and Signs. Prenatal onset. Both sexes. From normal to severe mental and growth deficiencies. Microcephaly. Sparse hair. Hypoplasia alae nasi. Hypoplastic deciduous; absent permanent teeth. Imperforate anus; septate or double vagina; hypotonia; joint hyperextensibility.

Etiology. Unknown. Sporadic and autosomal recessive inheritance.

Pathology. Small thyroid filled with colloid, replacement with fat of the pancreas, abnormalities in central nervous system (cortex).

Diagnostic Procedures. *Blood.* Cholesterol normal; macrocytic anemia. *Thyroid studies.* Malabsorption mainly due to pancreatic insufficiency. *X-ray of kidney.* From dilatation of calix of ureters to hydronephrosis.

Therapy. Thyroid and pancreatic extracts.

Prognosis. Poor because of scarce response to treatment of growth and mental deficiencies. Need for institutionalization in some cases. Death from pancreatic exocrine insufficiency reported.

BIBLIOGRAPHY. Grand RJ, Rosen SN, di Sant'Agnese PA, et al: Unusual case of XXY Klinefelter's syndrome with pancreatic insufficiency, hypothyroidism, deafness, chronic lung disease, dwarfism and microcephaly. Am J Med 41:478–485, 1966
Johanson A, Blizzard RA: A syndrome of congenital aplasia of alae nasi, deafness, hypothyroidism, dwarfism, absent permanent teeth, and malabsorption. J Pediatr 79:982–987, 1971
Baraitser M, Hodgson SV: The Johanson-Blizzard syndrome. J Med Genet 19:302–303, 1982

JOHNSON'S

Synonyms. Adherence; ocular rectus muscles pseudoparalysis.

Symptoms and Signs. Observed in children under 3 years of age, occasionally between 3 and 5 years, and seldom later. Strabismus simulating bilateral lateral rectus paralysis. Four possible variants of this syndrome depending on anomalous adhesions simulating paralysis of (1) lateral rectus (usually bilateral); (2) inferior oblique (theoretical); (3) superior rectus; (4) superior oblique (manifest when tilting head.)

Etiology. Congenital anomalous development.

Diagnostic Procedures. *"Fixed muscle" deduction test.*

Therapy. Adherent area separated by closed lysis or open lysis.

Prognosis. Normal rotation reestablished by surgery. Spontaneous recovery also observed.

BIBLIOGRAPHY. Johnson LV: Adherence syndrome: Pseudoparalysis of lateral or superior rectus muscles. Arch Ophthalmol 44:870–878, 1950
Geeraets WJ: Ocular Syndromes, 3rd ed. Philadelphia, Lea & Febiger, 1976

JOHNSON'S NEUROECTODERMAL

Synonyms. Anosmia-alopecia-deafness-hypogonadism; AADH.

Symptoms and Signs. From birth, deafness; anosmia; occasionally, mental retardation; microtia; protruding ears or aural atresia (external ear canal); alopecia; occasionally undeveloped secondary sexual characteristics; dental caries; congenital heart defect; cleft palate.

Etiology. Autosomal dominant inheritance. Involvement of ectoderm and neuroectoderm of the first two brachial arches, Rathke's pouch and diencephalon.

BIBLIOGRAPHY. Johnson VP, McMillin JM, Aceto T Jr, et al: A newly recognized neuroectodermal syndrome of familial alopecia, anosmia, deafness, hypogonadism. Am J Med Genet 15:497–506, 1983

JOLLIFFE'S

Synonyms. Nicotinic acid deficiency encephalopathy. See Jacob's.

Symptoms and Signs. Clouding of consciousness; cogwheel rigidities; grasping and sucking reflexes. Association with polyneuritis features and oculomotor signs of central neuritis.

Etiology. Complete nicotinic acid deficiency as part of the pellagra syndrome, where a partial nicotinic acid deficiency is present.

Pathology. Focal demyelination and ganglion cell degeneration in the cerebrum.

Therapy. Nicotinic acid and other vitamins of the B group as indicated by associate symptomatology.

Prognosis. If treatment of nicotinic acid given before irreversible stage is established, mortality of 14% in contrast to a mortality of nearly 100% without treatment or with treatment with hydration and thiamine only.

BIBLIOGRAPHY. Jolliffe N, Bowman KM, Rosenblum LA, et al: Nicotinic acid deficiency encephalopathy. JAMA 114:307–312, 1940
Adams RD, Victor M: Principles of Neurology, 3rd ed, pp 772–773. New York, McGraw-Hill, 1985

JONES'

Synonyms. Cherubism; fibrous jaw dysplasia (misnomer); mandibular cystic dysplasia.

Symptoms and Signs. Both sexes affected; present from birth. Rounded cheeks and jaw fullness; submandibular region swelling and narrow V-shaped palate. On sclera, beneath the iris, presence of a white line.

Etiology. Unknown. Autosomal dominant inheritance, with variable penetrance ranging from 80–100% in male patients to 50–70% in female patients.

Pathology. In affected bones, presence of multinucleated giant cells of osteoclastic type, small hemorrhages and fibroblasts. In the bone cortex lacunar absorption and replacement by connective tissue.

Diagnostic Procedures. *X-ray. Biopsy of bone.*

Therapy. None.

Prognosis. Permanent condition. The syndrome generally regresses during puberty and on into adult life. Maxillary regression generally precedes mandibular regression.

BIBLIOGRAPHY. Jones WA: Familial multilocular cystic disease of the jaw. Am J Cancer 17:946–950, 1933
Salinas CF, Bradford BL, Laden SA, et al: Cherubism associated with rib anomalies. Proc Greenwood Center 2:129–130, 1983
Maydew RP, Berry FA: Cherubism with difficult laryngoscopy and tracheal intubation. Anesthesiology 62:810–812, 1985

JOUBERT'S

Synonyms. Familial cerebellar vermis agenesis.

Symptoms and Signs. Both sexes affected; onset in early infancy. Episodic hyperpnea, alternating with periods of apnea, with occasional single deep inspiration; episodes initiated or intensified by stimulation (e.g., emotional upsets; crying). Abnormalities of eye movements (e.g., conjugate; irregular jerky movements; rotatory nystagmus). Ataxia; psychomotor retardation. Associated nonspecific malformations.

Etiology. Unknown. Frequently related to other midline malformations (See Dandy-Walker and Bailey-Cushing). Autosomal recessive with pleotropic manifestations or variable expressivity. Sporadic cases also reported.

Pathology. Agenesis of vermis (partial or complete); more widespread cerebral involvement suggested by clinical findings has not as yet been confirmed histologically.

Diagnostic Procedures. *CT brain scan.* Findings suggesting agenesis of vermis. *Ultrasonography. Blood.* Negative. Rule out metabolic causes for altered respiration. *Electroretinogram.*

Therapy. Symptomatic.

Prognosis. The respiratory abnormality tends to improve with age. Prognosis *quoad vitam* fair; *quoad functionem* poor.

BIBLIOGRAPHY. Joubert M, Eisenring JJ, Robb JP, et al: Familial agenesis of the cerebellar vermis. Neurology 19:813–825, 1969
King MD, Dudgeon J, Stephenson JBP: Joubert's syndrome with retinal dysplasia: neonatal tachypnoea as the clue to a genetic brain-eye malformation. Arch Dis Child 59:709–718, 1984

JOUSSEF'S

Synonyms. Vesicovaginal postcesarean fistula; menstrual hematuria.

Symptoms. Occur after cesarean section or after prolonged labor. Urinary incontinence; vaginal irritation. Odor of decomposing urine.

Signs. Urinary incontinence. Hematuria at period of menses.

Etiology. Vesicovaginal fistula due to surgical lesion or possibly infection, irradiation, neoplasia.

Diagnostic Procedures. Methylene blue injected into vagina passes into urine. *Cytoscopy.* Evidence of fistula. *Urine.* Features of cystitis.

Therapy. Surgical.

Prognosis. Good.

BIBLIOGRAPHY. Joussef AF: "Hemouria" following lower segment cesarean section: a syndrome. Am J Obstet Gynecol 73:759–767, 1957

Pritchard-McDonald-Gant: Williams Obstetrics, 17th ed, pp 678–679. Norwalk, Conn, Appleton-Century-Crofts, 1985

JUBERG-HAYWARD

Synonyms. Orocraniodigital; cleft lip-palate–abnormal thumbs–microcephaly.

Symptoms and Signs. Both sexes. From birth. Cleft lip and palate; microcephaly; hypoplasia or absence of thumbs; elbow deformity; occasionally, toe anomalies; short stature.

Etiology. Unknown. Autosomal recessive inheritance.

Diagnostic Procedures. *X-ray.* Sella turcica normal or absent. No endocrine dysfunction; in one case deficiency of growth hormone.

BIBLIOGRAPHY. Juberg RC, Hayward JR: A new familial syndrome of oral, cranial and digital anomalies. J Pediatr 74:755–762, 1969
Kingston HM, Hughes IA, Harper PS: Orocraniodigital (Juberg-Hayward) syndrome with growth hormone deficiency. Arch Dis Child 57:790–792, 1982

JUBERG-HOLT

Synonyms. Multiple epiphyseal dysplasia tarda; MEDT type I e.

Symptoms and Signs. Present from birth. Dwarfism. Waddling gait; limited motion of hips and elbows; short fingers; abnormal position of thumbs.

Etiology. Autosomal recessive inheritance.

Diagnostic Procedures. *X-ray.* Flattening of epiphyses of all bones; clefting of patellae.

BIBLIOGRAPHY. Juberg RC, Holt JF: Inheritance of multiple epiphyseal dysplasia tarda. Am J Hum Genet 20:549–563, 1968
Maroteaux P, Stanescu R, Cohen-Solal D: Dysplasie poly-epiphysaire probablement recessive autosomique. Apport de l'etude ultrastructurale dans l'isolement de cette forme autonome. Nouv Presse Med 4:2169–2172

JUHLIN-MICHÄLSSON

Synonym. Basophils-eosinophils absence.

Symptoms. Repeated infections; asthma; vasomotor rhinitis; hemolytic anemia; alopecia totalis; scabies; extensive warts.

Signs. Those of repeated infections; burrows of scabies on several areas of the body; warts on hands, resistant to treatment.

Etiology. Unknown; possibly, immunologic destruction of eosinophils and basophils.

Pathology. *Bone marrow.* Normal erythropoiesis. Scarce plasma cells. Absence of eosinophils and basophils.

Diagnostic Procedures. *Blood.* Absence of eosinophils and basophils, differential counts otherwise normal. Immunoglobulin levels low, but within normal limits. Demonstration of an eosinophil-basophil destruction factor in plasma. *Sputum.* Absence of eosinophils and basophils. *Biopsy of bone marrow.* See Pathology.

Therapy. Antibiotic or surgical treatment (or both) of infections and infestations.

Prognosis. Fair.

BIBLIOGRAPHY. Juhlin L, Michälsson G: A new syndrome characterized by absence of eosinophils and basophils. Lancet I:1233–1235, 1977

JUNG'S

Symptoms and Signs. Recurrent and persistent pyoderma, folliculitis, and atopic folliculitis.

Etiology. Unknown. Hypotheses include (1) defects of histamine metabolism resulting in raised histamine levels; (2) increase in histamine receptor expression on cell surfaces, leading to increased sensitivity to histamine.

Diagnostic Procedures. *Immunological studies.* Abnormalities of lymphocyte function, including defective proliferative responses to phytomitogens, and subnormal response in immunoglobulin production after stimulation of the lymphocytes by pokeweed mitogen; defective leucocyte chemiluminescence responses, associated with defective ability for intracellular killing of microbial organisms.

Therapy. Chlorpheniramine (histamine-1 antagonist).

Prognosis. Good with lifelong treatment.

BIBLIOGRAPHY. Joung LKL, Engelhard D, Kapoon N: Pyoderma eczema and folliculitis with defective leucocyte and lymphocyte function: a new familial immunodeficiency disease responsive to a histamine-1-antagonist. The Lancet II:185–187, 1983

JUNIUS-KUHNT

Synonyms. Kuhnt-Junius; macula senile disciform degeneration; macula lutea juvenile degeneration.

Symptoms. *Macula senile disciform degeneration.* Onset in advanced age. Impairment of central vision; central scotoma. Atrophic macular degeneration surrounded by retinal hemorrhages resulting in moundlike lesion.
Macula lutea juvenile degeneration. Onset in juvenile period. Same symptoms. Exudative and atrophic reaction with deposit in and about macula.

Etiology. Unknown; possibly autosomal dominant or recessive inheritance.

Treatment. None effective. Trial with vasodilator and lipid-clearing agent and general psychological support.

Prognosis. Usually, improvement of visual acuity of temporary nature and then relapse, up to ultimate degeneration; however, usually, the patient remains able to manage his daily activities.

BIBLIOGRAPHY. Kimura SJ, Caygill WM: Retinal Diseases. Philadelphia, Lea & Febiger, 1966

KABURI MAKEUP

Symptoms and Signs. Mental retardation. Recurrent otitis. Reduced physical development leading to dwarfism. *Facies.* Long palpebral fissures; eversion of lateral third of lower eyelids (Kaburi mask); broad, depressed nose; large ears; high arched or cleft palate. *Limbs.* Short 5th finger. *Spine.* Scoliosis.

Etiology. Unknown.

Diagnostic Procedures. *X-ray.* Abnormalities of vertebrae, joints, hands.

BIBLIOGRAPHY. Kuroki Y, Suzuki K, Chyo H, et al: A new malformation syndrome of long palpebral fissures, large ears, depressed nasal tip and skeletal anomalies associated with post natal dwarfism and mental retardation. J Pediatr 99:570–573, 1981
Nukawa N, Kuroki Y, Kajii T: The dermatographic pattern of the Kaburi make-up syndrome. Clin Genet 21:315–320, 1982

KAESER'S

Synonym. Scapuloperoneal amyotrophy.

Symptoms and Signs. Both sexes. At onset, bilateral foot drop and talipes equinovarus; then in a second phase, the shoulder girdle and finally bulbar involvement may occur.

Etiology. Unknown. Autosomal dominant inheritance. Clinically indistinguishable from Kugelberg-Welander (see) (which is recessive); similarity with Landouzy-Dejerine and perhaps also with Charcot-Marie-Tooth.

Pathology. Muscular atrophy. Involvement of caudal cranial nerves.

Diagnostic Procedures. *Electromyography.* Suggestion of anterior horn cell pathology.

Therapy. None.

Prognosis. Progressive condition.

BIBLIOGRAPHY. Kaeser HE: Die familiaere scapuloperoneale Muskelatrophie. Dtsch Z Nervenheilk 186:379–394, 1964

Kazakov VM, Bogorodiusky DK, Skorometz AA: The myogenic scapuloperoneal syndrome. Muscular dystrophy in the K kindred: clinical study and genetics. Clin Genet 10:41–50, 1976

KAHLER-BOZZOLO

Synonyms. Myelopathic albuminuria; Bence Jones; Huppert's; McIntyre's; multiple myeloma; plasma cell myeloma; multiple plasmacytoma; sarcomatous osteitis; von Rustitski's; myeloma multiple.

Symptoms and Signs. Prevalent in males; onset at all ages, usually after age 50. Asthenia; anorexia; weight loss; weakness; bone pains (at onset wandering and intermittent; usually at the back, less frequently chest and extremities; then at site of bone tumefactions and spontaneous fractures). Usually, later hepatomegaly, seldom splenomegaly. Neurologic complications frequent.

Etiology. Unknown. Genetic factors, chronic stimulation of the reticuloendothelial system, viruses considered.

Pathology. *Bones.* Thinning of shell; cortex may be reabsorbed; in marrow presence of gelatinous reddish substance. Microscopically, plasma cells, hemorrhages. *Kidney.* Atypical nephritis. *Liver, spleen,* and *various organs.* Para-amyloid deposition (10%).

Diagnostic Procedures. *Blood.* Moderate normocyte anemia. Leukocytes usually normal; occasionally, presence of plasma cells in peripheral blood. Platelets usually normal; coagulation test usually abnormal. Hyperproteinemia; typical electrophoretic pattern; cryoglobulinemia; hypercalcemia; hyperuricemia; frequently high blood urea nitrogen; usually normal phosphorus; alkaline phosphatase normal or slightly elevated. *Urine.* Albumin; casts; Bence Jones protein; abnormal kidney function test. *Bone marrow.* Characteristic infiltration with myeloma cells. Hemogenic series usually normal. *X-ray of skeleton.* Rounded punched-out lesions; diffuse osteoporosis may also be observed.

Therapy. Encourage an increase of physical activity with the use of analgesics, corsets, and walkers. Radiation therapy for bone pain from pathological fractures, and for areas of spinal cord compression. Adequate hydration to prevent and control renal complications from the precipitation of Bence Jones protein. Hemodialysis.

Antibiotics against bacterial infections. Chemotherapy with a combination of melphalan, cyclophosphamide, doxorubicin, vincristine, carmustine, intermittent course at 3 to 4 week intervals. Other agents: androgens, interferon, vindesine.

Prognosis. Wide variation.

BIBLIOGRAPHY. Dalrymple J: On the microscopical character of mollities ossium. Dublin Q J Med Sci 2:85–95, 1846

Jones HB: On a new substance occurring in the urine of a patient with mollities ossium. Philosoph Trans R Soc Lond 138:55–62, 1848

Kahler O: Zur Symptomatologie des multiplen Myeloms; Beobachtung von Albumosurie. Prag Med Wochenschr 14:33–45, 1889

Bozzolo: Sulla malattia di Kahler. Archochen Internat Med Chir (Napoli) 409, 1897

Nadeau LA, Magalini SI, Stefanini M: Familial multiple myeloma. Arch Path 61:101–106, 1956

Alexanian R: Plasma cell neoplasms and related disorders. In Thorn GW, Adams RD, Braunwold E et al: Harrison's Principles of Internal Medicine. New York, McGraw-Hill, 1983

Horwitz LJ, Levy RN, Rosner F: Multiple myeloma in three siblings. Arch Intern Med 145:1449–1450, 1985

KALLMANN'S

Synonyms. Anosmia eunuchoidism; olfactogenital dysplasia; hypogonadism anosmia; De Morsier's III.

Symptoms and Signs. Both sexes affected; prevalent in males (3 : 1); possibility of female carrier. Body proportions and lack of development of secondary sexual characteristics consistent with gonadotropic hypogonadism. Anosmia. Hypertension. Mental retardation. Occasionally, color blindness.

A patient with this syndrome was found to have an atrial septal defect, mitral valve prolapse, and a large intracranial cyst.

Other clinical abnormalities observed include obesity, cryptorchidism, osteopenia, mild neurosensory hearing loss, gynecomastia, diabetes mellitus, cleft lip or palate.

Etiology. Unknown. Condition appears to be X-linked or of autosomal recessive or dominant inheritance. Dysfunction of hypothalamus and pituitary.

Pathology. *Male.* In testis, absence of spermatogenesis and Leydig's cells; abiotrophy of tubules. *Female.* Hypoplastic ovary and uterus. *Nasal mucosa.* Agenesis of olfactory nerve cells. Slight atrophy of part of telencephalon.

Diagnostic Procedures. *Blood.* Hyposecretion of gonadotropin. Evaluation of loss of sense of smell. *Biopsy of the testis.*

Therapy. Gonadotropin. Testosterone or estrogen.

Prognosis. Treatment affects eunuchoidism but not anosmia.

BIBLIOGRAPHY. Maester de San Juan A: Falta total de los nervios olfatorios con anosmia en un individus en quien existia una atrofia congenita de los por el Dr. M. de San Juan, p 211. Madrid, El Siglo Medico, 1856

Kallmann FJ: The genetic aspects of primary eunuchoidism. Am J Ment Defic 48:203–236, 1943–44

De Morsier G: Median cranioencephalic dysraphias and olfactogenital dysplasia. World Neurol 3:485–506, 1962

Lieblich JM, Rogol AD, White BJ, et al: Syndrome of anosmia with hypogonadotropic hypogonadism (Kallmann syndrome). Am J Med 73:506–519, 1982

Moorman JR, Crain B, Osborne D: Kallman's syndrome with associated cardiovascular and intracranial anomalies. Am J Med 77:369–372, 1984

KANDINSKII-CLÉRAMBAULT

Synonym. Clérambault's II.

Symptoms and Signs. Confusing clinical entity characterized by automatism of mental apparatus: automatic obedience to any command or suggestion as well as echolalia, echopraxia, and waxy muscle flexibility; feeling of being possessed by dissociated forces, internal (e.g., fluid; humors; spirits) or external (e.g., metereologic; magnetic).

Etiology. Part of schizophrenia or expression of organic cerebral (i.e., hypophysiodiencephalic) disturbance. The frequency of the occurrence of these symptoms and their indistinct nature suggest the discontinuation of the use of this eponym.

BIBLIOGRAPHY. Kandinskii VK: Opsevdogalliutsinatsiiakh. Kritiko-klini-cheskii étud. St. Petersburg, 1890

de Clérambault CG: Syndrome mécanique et conception mécaniciste des psychoses hallucinatoire. Ann Med Psychol 85:398–413, 1927

Freedman AM, Kaplan HI, Sadock RJ: Comprehensive Textbook of Psychiatry, 2nd ed, p 1729. Baltimore, Williams & Wilkins, 1975

KANDORI'S

Synonym. Flecked retina–night blindness.

Symptoms. Both sexes affected; onset at young age. Mild anomaly of dark adaptation; no changes in visual acuity or field.

Signs. Large, irregular, yellowish, well-outlined flecks under retinal vessels, especially in midperipheral area.

Etiology. Unknown; possibly hereditary autosomal recessive (?). Toxic causes also considered.

Pathology. Unknown.

Diagnostic Procedures. *Ophthalmologic examination.* To differentiate from fundus flavimaculatus and Drusen. *Functional studies* and *angiography.* Focal alteration of retinal pigment epithelium. *Electro-oculography.* Normal.

Therapy. None.

Prognosis. Nonprogressive condition.

BIBLIOGRAPHY. Kandori F: Very rare cases of congenital non-progressive night blindness with flecked retina. Jpn J Ophthalmol 13:394, 1956
Bullock JD, Albert DM: Flecked retina. Arch Ophthalmol 93:26–31, 1975

KANNER'S

Synonyms. Autistic child; infantile autism; Asperger's; "wild boy of Aveyron."

Symptoms. Frequency 4.5 : 10,000; more frequent in males; no special birth order. In mother, increased incidence of pregnancy complications or perinatal complications. Parents in above average occupation-intelligence bracket. Siblings normal. Onset in first years of life (usually before second birthday). Lack of responsiveness to other human beings. Insistence on preservation of sameness in environment. The child appears alert and attractive in spite of odd behavior. Usually not intellectually subnormal; 50% show marked delay in motor milestones. Speech development abnormality very frequent.

Etiology. Unknown; organic causes suspected, possibly derangement in tryptophan metabolism. Genetic predisposition proposed: Fragile X (see) has been found in autistic boys (16%) but not in girls.

Therapy. Early psychiatric treatment. These children are highly vulnerable to understimulating environment.

Prognosis. With early treatment, good results possible. If inadequately treated in institution, development of institutionalism syndrome.

BIBLIOGRAPHY. Stard JMG: The Wild Boy of Aveyron. Humphrey G, Humphrey M (trans). New York, 1932
Kanner L: Autistic disturbances of affective contact. Nerve Child 2:217–250, 1943
Blomquist HK, Bohman M, Edvinsson SO, et al: Frequency of the fragile X syndrome in infantile autism: a Swedish multicentric study. Clin Genet 27:113–117, 1985
Rutter M: The treatment of autistic children. J Child Psychol Psychiatr 26:193–214, 1985
Spence MA, Ritvo ER, Marazite, et al: Gene mapping studies with the syndrome of autism. Behav Genet 15:1–13, 1985
Bryson SE, Smith IM, Eastwood D: Obstetrical suboptimality in autistic children. J Am Acad Child Adolesc Psychiatr 27:418–422, 1988
Strayhorm JM, Rapp N, Donina W, Strain PS: Randomized trial of methylphenidate for an autistic child. J Am Acad Child Adolesc Psychiatr 27:244–247, 1988
Van Lancker D, Cornelius C, Kreiman J, et al: Recognition of environmental sounds in autistic children. J Am Acad Child Adolesc Psychiatr 27:423–427, 1988

KARPATI'S

Synonym. Systemic carnitine deficiency, SCD.

Symptoms and Signs. In children. Encephalopathy; vomiting; stupor; coma; weakness of proximal muscles, also of head and neck; cardiomyopathy.

Etiology. Autosomal dominant inheritance. Deficit of carnitine synthesis or metabolism.

Pathology. *Muscle.* Biopsy, liver biopsy: neutral lipid droplets.

Diagnostic Procedures. *Urine.* Carnitine above normal levels. *Blood.* Hyperglycemia, hypoprothrombinemia, hyperammoniemia, elevation of transaminases.

Therapy. Administration of L-carnitine not always beneficial. During attacks, glucose administration.

Prognosis. Half of affected patients die before 20 years of age.

BIBLIOGRAPHY. Karpati G, Carpenter S, Engel AG, et al: The syndrome of systemic carnitine deficiency: clinical, morphologic, biochemical, and pathophysiologic features. Neurology 25:16–24, 1975
Rebouche CJ, Engel AG: Carnitine metabolism and deficiency syndromes. Mayo Clin Proc 58:533–540, 1983

KAPOSI-IRGANG

Synonyms. Lupus erythematosus profundus; lupus panniculitis.

Symptoms. Male to female ratio 1 : 2. Onset in females usually in the 4th decade; in males, the 5th decade. Good general health.

Signs. Under normal skin, appearance of firm nodules (1–10 cm in diameter) most frequent on the cheeks, less frequent in other areas of face, arms, hands, trunk, or legs. In 20% of patients, telangiectasis of face.

Etiology. Unknown. Genetic factors (?); somatic mutation (?). Environmental factors (coagent?). Autoimmune etiology suggested. Considered an unusual clinical variant of lupus erythematosus, systemic (see).

Pathology. Epidermal atropy; basal layer hydropic degenerative changes; dermal collagen degenerated; foci of lymphocytes; occasionally, vasculitis and panniculitis.

Diagnostic Procedures. *Blood.* Anemia; leukopenia; thrombocythemia (33%); hypergammaglobulinemia (30%); erythrocyte sedimentation rate increased in 20% of cases. Rheumatoid arthritis (RA) test positive (17%); lupus test positive (2%). *Biopsy.* See Pathology.

Treatment. Antimalarial drugs. Intralesional injection of corticosteroids.

Prognosis. Chronic and relapsing. Healing results in depressed scarring and pigmentation. Risk of systemic lupus development less than 5%.

BIBLIOGRAPHY. Kaposi M: Pathologie und therapie der Hautkrankheiten, 2nd ed, p 642. Urban & Schwarzenberg, 1883
Irgang S: Lupus erythematosus profundus: report of example with clinical resemblance to Darrier-Roussy sarcoid. Arch Dermatol Syph 42:97–108, 1940
Rook A, Wilkinson DS, Ebling FJG, et al: Textbook of Dermatology, 4th ed, p 1865. Oxford, Blackwell Scientific Publications, 1986

KAPOSI'S I

Synonyms. Endotheliosarcoma; multiple idiopathic hemorrhagic sarcoma; hemoangiosarcoma, multiple pigmented.

Symptoms and Signs. Predominant in males (10:1); occurs with major frequency in European Jews, Italians, and blacks. Onset in Europeans at late age; in blacks at all ages, or in subjects with AIDS (see). Dark, bluish macular skin lesions, usually on extremities, enlarging to 1 to 3 cm in diameter. Adjacent maculae may fuse and form a plaque. Edema may develop. Lesions may involute, leaving scar, or ulcerate and fungate. Progressive invasion, along course of superficial vein to involve both limbs symmetrically. Lymph node enlargement; occasionally, visceral involvement (e.g., liver; spleen). Association with diabetes, lymphomas.

Etiology. Unknown. Possible correlation with acquired cellular immunodeficiency (HTLV III) and opportunistic infections (*Pneumocystis carinii*).

Pathology. At onset, invasion of middermis by bands of spindle cells in a network of reticulin and vascular spaces; around spindle bands, macrophages and inflammatory changes are found. Invasion proceeds along course of vein. Proliferative endarteritis of vessel surrounding tumor. Similar features in lymph node and visceral organs when involved.

Diagnostic Procedures. *Blood.* Humoral and cellular immune response may be impaired. *Biopsy.* See Pathology.

Therapy. If localized, excision and radiotherapy. If diffuse, intra-arterial injection of nitrogen mustard.

Prognosis. Course of progression extremely variable. When initial lesion excised, recurrences in other sites.

BIBLIOGRAPHY. Kaposi M, Kohn M: Idiopathisches, multiples Pigmentsarkom der Haut. Arch Dermatol Syph 4:265–273, 1872
Durak DT: Opportunistic infections and Kaposi's sarcoma in homosexual men. New Engl J Med 305:1465–1467, 1981
Finzi A: Mediterranean Kaposi's sarcoma. It Gen Rev Dermatol 23:11–27, 1986
Warner LC, Fisher BK: Cutaneous manifestations of the acquired immunodeficiency syndrome. Int J Dermatol 25:337–350, 1986
Bouquety JC, Siopathis MR, Ravisse PR, et al: Lymphocutaneous Kaposi's sarcoma in an African pediatric AIDS case. Am J Trop Med Hyg 40:323–325, 1989

KAPOSI'S II

Synonyms. Atrophoderma pigmentosum; progressive melanosis lenticularis; xeroderma pigmentosum (XP); xeroderma pigmentosum types C, E, F, and "variant"; xeroderma pigmentosum, nonneurologic form. See De Sanctis-Cacchione.

Symptoms. Occur in many races; both sexes affected; onset in first year, in early life (75%), or later. Increased sensitivity to sunlight; photophobia.

Signs. Freckling and dryness of skin areas exposed to light, followed by sunburn and persistent erythema. Freckles tend to enlarge and become confluent to form patches. Initially they fade in winter; later, remain unchanged year round. Successive formation of telangiectasis, small angiomas, white atrophic spots, and warty keratosis. Sunburned areas are followed by ulcerations, crustings, scarrings, and contractions. From 3rd and 4th year or later malignant transformation (basal cells; squamous cell; melanoma). Teeth are occasionally defective.

Type C. Classical XP: only skin disorders

Type D. Skin disorders plus late-developing neurologic signs of group A (see De Sanctis-Cacchione)

Type E. Slight skin lesions

Type F. Mild skin involvement; in Japanese

Variant (pigmented xerodermoid). Mild to severe symptoms starting in old age

Etiology. Increased sensitivity to sunlight. Autosomal recessive inheritance. Defective capacity for excision repair of damaged DNA at pyrimidine dimers because of enzyme deficiency. All the various forms have different enzymatic alterations in the fibroblasts. Fibroblasts from one group of patients may correct defects of another group when hybridized.

Pathology. Skin of senile type; lack of special characteristics. Malignant transformation (see Signs).

Diagnostic Procedures. *Biopsy.* Identification of malignancies. *Blood.* In some cases increased serum glutamic-oxaloacetic transaminase (SGOT), serum glutamic-pyruvic transaminase (SGPT), and alpha-2-globulin. *Urine.* In some cases, aminoaciduria. *Cell culture studies.*

Therapy. Protection from sunlight (physical and cosmetic). Early excision of tumors. Genetic counseling.

Prognosis. Frequently, fatal before 10 years of age; 66% die before age 20 from metastases. With adequate protection and treatment, prognosis improved. High variability of course and possibility of longer survival even in the same family.

BIBLIOGRAPHY. Kaposi M: Xeroderma pigmentosum. Med Jahrb:619–633, 1882
Cleaver JE: Xeroderma pigmentosum. In Stanbury JB, Wyngaarden JB, Fredrickson DS, et al: The Metabolic Basis of Inherited Disease, 5th ed, p 1227. New York, McGraw-Hill, 1983

KAPOSI'S III

Synonyms. Dermatitis, Kaposi-Juliusberg; eczema herpeticum; varicelliform eruption.

Symptoms. Unexplained prevalence in males; highest incidence in infancy. Usually affects patients with active or recently suppurated atopic manifestation of other type of dermatitis. Incubation period from time of exposure to virus (herpes simplex or vaccinia). Severe itching. Severe constitutional symptoms in many cases.

Signs. Sudden appearance of crops of vesicles-pustules (varicelliform) in areas already affected by dermatitis, or generalized. After 1 week new crop eruption may follow. Pustules crust in 4 to 5 days, then heal with moderate scarring. Lymphadenopathy.

Etiology. Infection usually primary to virus (herpes simplex or vaccinia) and other viruses (Coxsackie A16 etc.) in patients with skin affected by atopic condition.

Pathology. Necrosis of epidermis; presence of intranuclear (herpes) or intracytoplasmic (vaccinia) bodies in corium cells. In addition, in the herpes condition multinucleated giant cells.

Diagnostic Procedures. *Cytologic examination of lesion smears.*

Therapy. Isolation. Acyclovir. Antibiotics for secondary infections. Corticosteroids contraindicated. Hyperimmune gammaglobulins: vaccinal or herpetic Lupidion; inosine p-acetaminobenzoate 1-dimethylamino-2-propanole (1 : 3).

Prognosis. Fever subsides in 4 to 5 days. Majority of patients recover completely. Possibly, encephalitis, transverse myelitis. Mortality for vaccine form 6%; for herpetic form not known.

BIBLIOGRAPHY. Kaposi M: Pathologie und Therapie der Hautkrankheiten, p 483, Berlin, 1887
Juliusberg F: Ueber Pustulosis acuta varioliformis. Arch Dermatol Syph 46:21–28, 1898
Rook A, Wilkinson DS, Ebling FJG, et al: Textbook of Dermatology, 4th ed, pp 691–693. Oxford, Blackwell Scientific Publications, 1986

KARSCH-NEUGENBAUER

Synonyms. Split hand–congenital nystagmus–fundal changes–cataracts; nystagmus–split hand.

Symptoms and Signs. From birth. Both sexes. Split hand and foot deformity. Nystagmus (modulatory); fundal changes; cataracts (possibly at latter age).

Etiology. Autosomal dominant inheritance.

BIBLIOGRAPHY. Karsch J: Erbliche Augenmissbildung in Verbindung mit Spalthand und-fuss. Z Augenheilk 89:274–279, 1936
Neugenbauer H: Spalthand und-fuss mit familiaerer Besonderheit. Z Orthop 95:500–506, 1962
Piparski RT, Pauli RM, Bresnick GH, et al: Karsch-Neugenbaur syndrome: split foot, split hand, and congenital nystagmus. Clin Genet 27:97–101, 1985

KARTAGENER'S

Synonyms. Bronchiectasis-dextrocardia-sinusitis; situs inversus-sinusitis-bronchiectasis; Kartagener's triad; dextrocardia-bronchiectasis-sinusitis–immotile cilia; Siewert's.

Symptoms. Onset in early infancy (90% before 15 years of age). Dyspnea; productive cough; recurrent respiratory infections; palpitation; otitis media; nasal speech; conductive hearing loss. Anosmia.

Signs. Clubbing of fingers. In chest, diffuse crepitant rales, dextrocardia (right-sided apical beat and sounds). Features of sinusitis. Hepatic dullness on left side.

Etiology. Unknown; autosomal recessive inheritance with incomplete penetrance. See Immotile cilia.

Pathology. Dextrocardia alone or situs inversus totalis; bronchiectasis; maldevelopment of frontal paranasal sinuses; edema; hyperemia of nasal mucosa; nasal polyposis (frequent). See Immotile cilia.

Diagnostic Procedures. *X-ray of skull and chest. Electrocardiography. Sputum.* Culture and bacterial sensitivity. *Blood.* In infancy transient immunoglobulin deficiency.

Therapy. Antibiotics for recurrent pulmonary infections. Lobectomy or lung resection when indicated.

Prognosis. Relatively good. Recurrent pulmonary infections. Congestive heart failure and infection causes of death.

BIBLIOGRAPHY. Siewert AK: Ueber einen Fall vor bronchiectasie bei einem Patieten mit situs inversus viscerum. Berl Klin Wochr 41:139–141, 1904

Kartagener M: Zur Pathogenese der Bronchiektasien: Bronchiektasien bei Situs viscerum inversus. Beitr Klin Tuberk 83:489–501, 1933

Rott HD: Genetics of Kartagener's syndrome. Eur J Respir Dis 64(suppl 127):1–4, 1983

Eavey RD, Madol JB, Holmes LB, et al: Kartagener's syndrome: a blind, controlled study of cilia ultrastructure. Arch Otolaryngol Head Neck Surg 112:646–650, 1986

KASABACH-MERRITT

Synonyms. Capillary angioma-thrombocytopenia; hemangioma-thrombocytopenia; thrombocytopenia-purpura-hemangioma.

Symptoms. Occur in infants. Purpura and bleeding.

Signs. Large capillary angioma; pallor; petechiae and ecchymosis.

Etiology. Angioma causes sequestration of platelets and platelet deficiency.

Pathology. Capillary angioma containing platelet thrombi.

Diagnostic Procedures. *Blood.* Thrombocytopenia; injected ^{51}Cr tagged platelets collect in the tumor. Anemia; increased fibrinolytic activity (release of plasmin from clotting into the tumor).

Therapy. X-ray or radium treatment of the tumor. Surgical excision.

Prognosis. Recovery (platelet number returns to normal) following destruction of tumor.

BIBLIOGRAPHY. Kasabach HH, Merritt KK: Capillary hemangioma with extensive purpura: Report of a case. Am J Dis Child 59:1063–1070, 1940

David TJ, Evans DIK, Stevens RF: Haemangioma with thrombocytopenia (Kasabach-Merritt syndrome). Arch Dis Child 58:1022–1023, 1983

El-Dessouky M, Raine PAM, Young DG: Kasabach-Merritt syndrome. J Pediatr Surg 23:109–111, 1988

El-Dessouky M, Azmy AF, Raine PAM, Young DG: Kasabach-Merritt syndrome. J Pediatr Surg 23:109–111, 1988

Loh W, Miller JH, Gomperts ED: Imaging with technetium 99m–labeled erythrocytes in evaluation of the Kasabach-Merrit syndrome. J Pediatr 113:856–859, 1988

KASHIN-BECK

Synonyms. Aso's; Lin Kuatang-tz'w; osteochondroarthrosis deformans endemica; Tokut-ze; Urov's.

Symptoms. Example of regional disease occurring principally in childhood; endemic in Korea, northern China, and Siberia. Onset asymptomatic or ache, muscular weakness, cramps, paresthesias, fatigability. After 6 months to 1 year, joint stiffness. Clinical classification of 3 degrees according to degree of joint involvement and clinical findings: *1st degree.* Mild form; initial stage moderate involvement and few symptoms. *2nd degree.* Increased involvement of joints; pain and systemic symptoms. *3rd degree.* Chronic deforming arthritis and general manifestations. Reduction of height; involvement of vertebral column; chronic gastritis.

Signs. Most often wrist and interphalangeal joint deformities; crepitation; no inflammation or effusion. Symmetric involvement; slow progression of osteoarthosis to other joints. Atrophy of muscles adjacent to joints involved.

Etiology. Toxic origin following ingestion of a cereal grain infected with the fungus *Fusarium sporotrichiella.*

Pathology. Necrobiotic degenerative changes of the aseptic focal necrosis type, involving those parts of the growing skeleton associated with hyaline cartilage. Abnormalities most marked in epiphyses and metaphyses. Muscle atrophy; no pathology of viscera except chronic gastritis during the 3rd stage.

Diagnostic Procedures. *X-ray.* Narrowness and rarefaction of zone of preliminary calcification; dystrophic process of growth of tubular bones and shortening of extremities; vertebral bodies flatten with beak osteophytes. *Blood.* Normal; in 3rd degree, anemia with lymphocytosis. Calcium and phosphorus always normal.

Therapy. Avoidance of use of contaminated bread, and importation of "healthy" food in regions where disease occurs.

Prognosis. Slow progression. Emigration or change of diet prevents further development of the disease.

BIBLIOGRAPHY. Kashin NI: The description of the endemic and other disease, prevailing in the Urov-river area. The records of physico-medical scientific society attached to the Moscow University, 1859
Beck EB: To the problem of deforming endemic osteoarthritis in the Baikal area. Russian Physician 5:74–75, 1906
Nesterov AI: The clinical course of Kashin-Beck disease. Arthritis Rheum 7:29–40, 1964
Sokoloff L: The pathology and pathogenesis of osteoarthritis. In Hollander JL, McCarty DJ: Arthritis and Allied Conditions, 8th ed, p 1020. Philadelphia, Lea & Febiger, 1972

KATAYAMA

Synonyms. Bilharziasis (invasive phase); cardiopulmonary schistosomiasis; schistosomiasis japonica. See Marchand's and Manson's schistosomiasis–pulmonary artery obstruction.

Symptoms. Fever; headache; angioneurotic edema; urticaria; abdominal pain; diarrhea; melena (later massive hematemesis). Pulmonary migration: dyspnea. Cerebral migration: disorientation; coma; aphasia; paraplegia; jacksonian epilepsy and other neurologic manifestations.

Signs. *Early.* Hepatomegaly; pain on palpation of liver edge; splenomegaly. *Later.* Smaller liver; ascites; caput medusae; progressive weight loss.

Etiology. Infestation with *Schistosoma japonicum;* katayama snails intermediate host. Infestation with *S. mansoni* and *S. haematobium* gives a similar clinical pattern and the term *Katayama syndrome* may be applied to all three conditions.

Pathology. Eggs of parasite in different tissues surrounded by eosinophils. *Colon.* Rigid, mucosa edematous and congested; hemorrhages; ulcerated polyps. *Liver.* Early, enlarged and congested; later, cirrhosis; periportal fibrosis. *Spleen.* Enlarged.

Diagnostic Procedures. *Blood.* Marked eosinophilia; anemia; leukopenia; thrombocytopenia; hypoproteinemia. *Stool.* Ova.

Therapy. Nutritional; correction of anemia; improvement of general condition prior to chemotherapy. Praziquantel metrifonate; oxamniquine; niridazole; antimonial trivalent compounds. Surgery (filtering worms from the portal system).

Prognosis. Good in early moderate infestation if adequate treatment. Severe in chronic infestation and complication.

BIBLIOGRAPHY. Walt F: The Katayama syndrome. South Afr Med J 28:89–93, 1954
Schistosomiasis: a review of recent abstracts. Tropical Dis Bull 82:R1–R3, 1985

KAUFMAN-McKUSICK

Synonyms. Hydrometrocolpos–postaxial polydactyly-congenital heart malformations; McKusick-Kaufman.

Symptoms. Onset in newborn. Respiratory embarassment; urinary, intestinal, circulatory obstruction.

Signs. Abdominal mass; transvaginal membrane (vaginal atresia) or imperforate hymen; accumulation of fluid in upper vagina and uterus. Occasionally, swelling of breast and "witches milk" production. Postaxial polydactyly (may be limited to one limb) and/or congenital heart malformation.

Etiology. Lack of patency of vaginal canal; excessive secretion from uterus and cervical glands in response to maternal hormone. Presence of transvaginal membrane transmitted as female-limited autosomal recessive inheritance in members of the Amish community; occasionally, associated with other somatic malformations.

Pathology. Accumulation of fluid proximal to vaginal obstruction. See Signs.

Diagnostic Procedures. *Hydrometrocolpos fluid.* Presence of glycogen-containing vaginal cells.

Therapy. Surgical removal of obstruction.

Prognosis. Marked variation of intensity of manifestation from minimal to very severe; it may even be lethal if treatment is not instituted. Cases with minimal symptomatology that escape diagnosis will manifest hematocolpos at age of menarche. Possibly infection (pyocolpos).

BIBLIOGRAPHY. McKusick VA, Bauer RL, Koop, CE, et al: Hydrometrocolpos as a simply inherited malformation. JAMA 189:813–816, 1964
Kaufman RL, Hartman AF, McAlister WH: Family studies in congenital heart disease II: a syndrome of hydrometrocolpos, postaxial polydactyly and congenital heart disease. Birth Defects Orig Art Ser VIII(5):85–87, 1972
Jabs EW, Leonard CO, Phillips JA: New features of the McKusick-Kaufman syndrome. Birth Defects Orig Art Ser XVIII(3B):161–166, 1982
Chitayat D, Hahn SYE, Marion RW, et al: Further delineation of the McKusick-Kaufman hydrometrocolpos-polydactyly syndrome. Am J Dis Child 141:1133–1136, 1987

KAUFMAN'S

Synonym. Mental retardation–microcorneamicrocephaly.

Symptoms. Present from birth. Mental and physical retardation; myopia; congenital hypotonia; respiratory distress; constipation.

Signs. Microcephaly; hypertelorism; epicanthus, eyelid ptosis; mongoloid slant of palpebral fissures; microcornea; eyebrows sparse and brooding laterally; flat filtrum; high and narrow palate; lordosis; flat feet.

Etiology. Autosomal recessive or dominant inheritance or sporadic.

BIBLIOGRAPHY. Kaufman RL, Rimoin DL, Prensky AL et al: An oculocerebrofacial syndrome. Birth Defects 7:135–138, 1971
Jureka SB, Evans J: Kaufman oculocerebrofacial syndrome: case reported. Am J Med Genet 3:15–19, 1979

KAWASAKI'S

Synonym. Mucocutaneous lymph node, MLN.

Symptoms. Observed in Japan. Higher incidence in summer. Male to female ratio 1 : 5.1; occur in infants and children 2 months to 9 years. Hyperthermia (1–2 weeks duration). Dry lips; pharyngeal angina; stomatitis; arthralgia; dyspnea; diarrhea. In some cases, symptoms related to meningitis.

Signs. "Strawberry tongue" and oral and pharyngeal hyperemia; polymorphic exanthema; indurative edema; red palms and soles; and (during convalescence) desquamation of fingertips. Cervical adenopathy. Signs of myocardial involvement. Occasionally, icterus and signs of meningitis. Coronary aneurysms.

Etiology. Unknown. Considered an allergic reaction or unusual reaction to various types of infections. Possible connection with Stevens-Johnson (see).

Diagnostic Procedures. *Blood.* Leukocytosis; erythrocyte sedimentation rate increased; alpha-2-globulin and C-reactive protein increased, moderate anemia. Bilirubin increased (occasionally). *Electrocardiography.* Myocarditis (70%). *Spinal fluid.* Aseptic meningitis (occasionally). *Urine.* Proteinuria.

Therapy. Clinical evolution affected by antibiotics. Symptomatic. To prevent coronary aneurysms, some children have been treated with salicylate and high-dose intravenous gamma globulin, by analogy with the treatment of idiopathic thrombocytopenic purpura. The clinical, electrical, radiological, echographic cardiac surveillance did not show any sign of aneurysms more than 6 months after the onset of the disease.

Prognosis. Self-limited; sudden death from coronary thrombosis (1–2%).

BIBLIOGRAPHY. Kawasaki T: Acute febrile mucocutaneous syndrome with lymphoid involvement with specific desquamation of fingers and toes in children. Jpn J Allergol 16:178–222, 1967
Furusho K, Nakano H, Shinomiya K, et al: High dose intravenous gammaglobulin for Kawasaki disease. Lancet II:1055–1058, 1984
Rowley AH, Duffy E, Shulman ST: Prevention of giant coronary artery aneurysms in Kawasaki disease by intravenous gamma globulin therapy. J Pediatr 113:290–294, 1988

KEARNS-SAYRE

Synonyms. Heart block–retinitis pigmentosa–ophthalmoplegia; Kearns-Shy. See Barnard-Scholz.

Symptoms and Signs. Prevalent in females. Onset before 20 years of age. Progressive external ophthalmoplegia (see Barnard-Scholz); pigmentary degeneration of retina; symptoms and signs related to heart block. Limb weakness.

Etiology. Unknown. Sporadic (nonhereditary). Sporadic and familial forms known.

Pathology. See Barnard-Scholz. Abnormal mitochondria with paracrystalline inclusion in muscle cells.

Diagnostic Procedures. *Electrocardiography.* Heart block. *Spinal fluid.* Elevated proteins. *Study of intact mitochondria from skeletal muscle.* Deficiency of mitochondrial protein synthesis, and absence of a translation product with the mobility of a 5 KDa protein. *Evaluation of intracellular respiration.* Shows that the absent protein is not a functional subunit of a respiratory chain complex.

Therapy. Pacemaker frequently required.

Prognosis. Heart involvement may cause sudden death.

BIBLIOGRAPHY. Kearns TP, Sayre GP: Retinitis pigmentosa, external ophthalmoplegia and complete heart block. Arch Ophthalmol 60:280–289, 1958
Jean R, Bonnet H, Dumas R: Kearns' syndrome with metabolic disorders. Arch Fr Pediatr 29:436, 1972
Eagle RC, et al: The atypical pigmentary retinopathy of Kearns-Sayre syndrome. Ophthalmology 89:1433–1440, 1982
Byrne E, Marzukis S, Sattayasai N, et al: Mitochondrial studies in Kearns-Sayre syndrome: normal respiratory chain function with absence of a mitochondrial translation product. Neurology 37:1530–1534, 1987

KEIPERT'S

Symptoms. Male siblings affected. Sensorineural deafness.

Signs. *Facies.* Large nose; high bridge; prominent alae. *Mouth.* Upper lip protruding; cupid bow laterally overlapping the lower lip. *Extremities.* Broad terminal phalanges of all toes and of thumbs and first, second, and third fingers; 5th fingers shortness and clinodactyly.

Etiology. Autosomal recessive (?) or X-linked inheritance.

Diagnostic Procedures. *X-ray.* Bifid terminal phalanges (one case) of both indexes.

BIBLIOGRAPHY. Keipert JA, Fitzgerald MG, Damks DM: A new syndrome of broad terminal phalanges and facial abnormalities. Austr Paediatr J 9:10–13, 1973

KENNEDY'S

Synonyms. Bulbospinal muscular atrophy, X-linked; spinal-bulbar muscular atrophy; muscular atrophy, spinal bulbar. See Kugelberg-Welander.

Symptoms and Signs. In males. Onset in 3rd to 4th decade. Muscle weakness, fasciculation, and atrophic changes. *Bulbar signs.* Dysphagia. Absent pyramidal (negative Babinsky) sensory and cerebellar signs. Occasionally, gynecomastia.

Etiology. Unknown. X-linked recessive inheritance.

Prognosis. Slow progression.

BIBLIOGRAPHY. Kennedy WR, Alter M, Sung JH: Progressive proximal spinal and bulbar muscular atrophy of late onset: a sex-linked recessive trait. Neurology 18:671–680, 1980
Paulson GW, Liss L, Sweeney PJ: Late onset spinal muscle atrophy: a sex-linked variant of Kugelberg-Welander. Acta Neurol Scand 61:49–55, 1980

KEMP-ELLIOT-GORLIN

Synonym. Angina pectoris-normal coronary arteriography. See Heberden's.

Symptoms. Represents 9% of patients with angina pectoris. Prevalent in females (66% of cases). Typical angina pectoris symptoms.

Etiology. Unknown. Possibly, disease of small heart arteries beyond resolution of coronary arteriography; regional functional small artery constriction.

Pathology. Unknown.

Diagnostic Procedures. *Electrocardiography.* Normal or abnormal after effort. *Cineangiocardiography.* Normal. *Blood.* Normal. Lactate myocardial production during isoproterenol infusion or tachycardia induced by right atrial pacing (in 30% of cases).

Therapy. That of classic angina (see Heberden's).

Prognosis. Much better than that for other patients with other forms of angina.

BIBLIOGRAPHY. Kemp HG, Elliott WC, Gorlin R: The anginal syndrome with normal coronary arteriography. Trans Assoc Am Physicians 80:59–70, 1967
Hurst JW: The Heart, 6th ed, pp 894–895, 1011. New York, McGraw-Hill, 1986

KENNY-CAFFEY

Synonym. Dwarfism–tubular bone stenosis.

Symptoms. Both sexes with equal severity. Onset a few days after birth. Tetanic convulsions; delayed physical development; activity and intelligence normal. Myopia; nanophthalmos with hyperopia. Papilledema; vascular tortuosity; macular crowding.

Signs. Proportionate dwarfism; large anterior fontanelle.

Etiology. Unknown. Autosomal dominant inheritance suggested, but X-linked inheritance not excluded.

Pathology. Narrow long-bone shafts with stenosed medullary cavities; lack of differentiation of calvaria into a diploic space; relative craniofacial disproportion.

Diagnostic Procedures. *Blood.* Transient hypocalcemia; hyperphosphatemia; microcytic anemia. *X-ray of skeleton.* See Pathology.

Therapy. Convulsions and hypocalcemia and hyperphosphatemia fully corrected by vitamin D and calcium. Anemia corrected by iron administration.

Prognosis. Skeletal configuration persists unchanged. Proportionate dwarfism results.

BIBLIOGRAPHY. Kenny FM, Linarelli L: Dwarfism and cortical thickening of the tubular bones: Transient hypocalcemia in mother and son. Am J Dis Child 111:201–207, 1966
Caffey J: Congenital stenosis of medullary spaces in tubular bones and calvaria in two proportionate dwarfs—mother and son; coupled with transitory hypocalcemic tetany. Am J Roentgen 100:1–11, 1967
Lee WK, Vargas A, Barnes J, et al: The Kenny-Caffey syndrome—a rare type of growth deficiency with tubular stenosis, transient hypoparathyroidism and anomalies of refraction. Eur J Pediatr 136:21–30, 1981

KENTEL'S

Symptoms. Both sexes. Neural hearing loss.

Signs. Short terminal phalanges; calcification and ossification of cartilage in the ears, nose, larynx, trachea, ribs; respiratory difficulty.

Etiology. Autosomal recessive inheritance.

Pathology. See Signs. Same as in multiple peripheral pulmonary stenosis.

BIBLIOGRAPHY. Kentel J, Jorgensen G, Gabriel P: A new autosomal recessive syndrome: peripheral pulmonary stenosis, brachytelephalangism, neural hearing loss, and abnormal cartilage calcification-ossification. Birth Defects Orig Art Ser 8(5):60–68, 1972
Fryus JP, Van Fleteren A, Mattalaer P, et al: Calcification of cartilages, brachytelephalangy, and peripheral pulmonary stenosis: confirmation of the Kentel syndrome. Eur J Pediatr 142:201–203, 1984

KERATITIS FUGAX HEREDITARIA

Synonym. Valle's. See Francescetti-Kauffman.

Symptoms. Both sexes affected; onset between 2 and 12 years of age. Pain; photophobia; impairment of vision; recurrent attacks 2 to 8 times a year.

Signs. Corneal bullae and vescicles; edema; erosions.

Etiology. Unknown; hereditary dominant inheritance.

Pathology. Acute, subacute and then chronic keratitis.

Diagnostic Procedures. *Ophthalmoscopy.* See Pathology.

Therapy. Hypertonic fluids; irradiation of lacrimal glands.

Prognosis. Recurrent, becoming milder after 50 years of age.

BIBLIOGRAPHY. Valle D: Keratitis fugax hereditaire. Duodecim 80:659–664, 1964
Pouliquen Y: Précis d'optalmologie. Masson, Paris, 1984

KERATOSIS, FOCAL PALMOPLANTAR–GINGIVAL

Synonym. Fred's.

Symptoms and Signs. Prevalent in males. Onset in early childhood. Marked hyperkeratosis in weight-bearing area of feet and palms, marginal gingival hyperkerato-

sis; plaques of hyperkeratosis on other areas of buccal mucosa.

Etiology. Autosomal dominant inheritance.

Pathology. Condensation of tonofilaments appearing as paranuclear bodies in keratocytes.

Therapy. See Papillon-Lefevre.

Prognosis. Progressive condition.

BIBLIOGRAPHY. Fred HL, Gieser RG, Berry WR, et al: Keratosis palmaris et plantaris. Arch Int Med 113:866–871, 1964
Young WG, Newcomb GM, Daley TJ: Focal palmoplantar and gingival hyperkeratosis syndrome: report of a family, with cytology syndrome ultrastructural and histochemical findings. Oral Surg 53:473–482, 1982

KERATOSIS, PALMOPLANTAR–CLINODACTYLY

Synonym. See Greither's.

Symptoms and Signs. Keratosis, palmoplantar; clinodactyly.

Etiology. Autosomal dominant inheritance.

BIBLIOGRAPHY. Anderson IF, Klinworth GK: Hypovitaminosis A in a family with tylosis and clinodactyly. Br Med 1:1293–1297, 1961
Hernandez A, Aguirre-Negrete MG, Gonzales-Mendoza A, et al: Autosomal dominant keratosis palmaris et plantaris with clinodactyly. Birth Defects Orig Art Ser 18(3B):207–210, 1982

KERATOSIS, PALMOPLANTAR–ESOPHAGEAL CANCER

Symptoms and Signs. Those of Greither's (see) with late onset plus oral leukoplakia and development of esophageal cancer around 60 years of age.

Etiology. Autosomal dominant inheritance; unknown if allelic with Greither's.

Pathology. See Greither's. Lower esophagus lined by gastric mucosa; sliding hiatal hernia.

BIBLIOGRAPHY. Howel-Evans W, McConnell RB, Clarke CA, et al: Carcinoma of the esophagus with keratosis palmaris et plantaris (tylosis) a study of two families. Q J Med 27:413–429, 1958
Yesudian P, Premalatha S, Thambiah AS: Genetic tylosis with malignancy: a study of a South Indian pedigree. Br J Derm 102:597–600, 1980

KERNICTERUS

Synonyms. Bilirubin encephalopathy; nuclear jaundice; neonatal hyperbilirubinemia.

Symptoms and Signs. Occur in icteric infant during first 2 or 3 weeks of life. Hypotonia; lethargy and diminution of sucking reflex; spasticity; opisthotonos; convulsions; fever; high-pitched cry. If surviving, neurologic signs develop: seizures; mental deficiency; ataxia; bilateral choreoathetosis.

Etiology. Hyperbilirubinemia with deposition of pigment in the brain and damage of cells. Hemolytic diseases of newborn: Rh, ABO incompatibility; administration of vitamin K water-soluble analogue; congenital hyperbilirubinemic conditions (see Crigler-Najjar).

Pathology. Edema and enlargement of brain; yellowish, orange stain of nuclear masses, especially basal ganglia; degenerative changes of ganglion cells. In patients who survive the acute phase, the brain loses the brilliant stain and shows only loss of ganglion cells and gliosis.

Diagnostic Procedures. *Blood.* Hyperbilirubinemia (indirect); anemia; nucleated red cells.

Therapy. Exchange transfusion with Rh-negative blood. Keep the bilirubin below 20 mg/100 ml. Phototherapy.

Prognosis. Usually fatal in first days when patient survives development of clinical manifestations from neurologic damage.

BIBLIOGRAPHY. Van Praagh R: Diagnosis of kernicterus in the neonatal period. Pediatrics 28:870–876, 1961
Adam RD, Victor M: Principles of Neurology, 3rd ed, p 926. New York, McGraw-Hill, 1985

KERSHNER-ADAMS

Synonym. Obsolete. Eponym used to indicate a nonspecific suppurative pneumonitis.

BIBLIOGRAPHY. Kershner RD, Adams WE: Chronic nonspecific suppurative pneumonitis. J Thorac Surg 17:495–511, 1948

KERSTING-HELLWIG'S

Synonyms. Spiradenoma; eccrine spiradenoma, Werther's syringoadenomatosus papilliferus; Stokes' spiroadenoma.

Symptoms. Male to female ratio 2 : 1; onset between 15 and 35 years of age. Pain at location of lesion.

Signs. On any area of skin, appearance of a usually solitary, well-defined nodule, diameter 0.5 to 3.0 cm, overlying skin of normal color or various colors (e.g., blue; yellow).

Etiology. Unknown.

Pathology. Diagnosis is made by histologic examination. Cells of two kinds: around lumina, larger, paler cells; in the periphery, smaller and darker (mioepithelial) cells forming the edges of the lobulated mass. Possibly, cystic spaces in the centers of masses.

Diagnostic Procedure. *Biopsy.*

Therapy. Excision.

Prognosis. Slow growth for years; removal curative. Recurrence if excision incomplete.

BIBLIOGRAPHY. Kersting DW, Helwig B: Eccrine spiradenoma. Arch Derm 73:199–227, 1956
Rook A, Wilkinson DS, Ebling FJG, et al: Textbook of Dermatology. 4th ed, pp 2412–2413. Oxford, Blackwell Scientific Publications, 1986

KESAREE-WOOLEY

Synonyms. Penta-X; 49 (XXXXX); XXXXX.

Symptoms and Signs. Present from birth. Postnatal growth deficiency; failure to thrive; mental deficiency of variable degrees. *Head.* Moderate mongoloid slant; low nasal bridge. *Neck.* Short. *Extremities.* Clinodactyly of 5th fingers. Patency of ductus arteriosus. Occasionally, colobomas; hypertelorism, low ears, and arms and feet malformations.

Etiology. XXXXX.

Prognosis. Variable. Failure to thrive.

Diagnostic Procedures. *Chromosome studies.* Presence of five X chromosomes.

BIBLIOGRAPHY. Kesaree N, Wooley PV Jr: A phenotypic female with 49 chromosomes presumably: a case reported. J Pediatr 63:1099–1103, 1963
Jones KL: Smith's recognizable patterns of human malformations. Philadelphia, WB Saunders, 1988

KETOTIC HYPERGLYCINEMIA

This syndrome is becoming obsolete because the condition can be attributed to different errors of metabolism:
1. Beta-ketothiolase deficiency
2. Propionic acidemia (types I and II)
3. Methylmalonic acidema

Synonyms. Glycinemia infantilis; secondary hypergly-cinemia; hyperglycinuria-hyperglycinemia.

Symptoms. Both sexes affected; onset in first months of life. Episodic vomiting; lethargy; dehydration. Repeated episodes of infection and purpura. Mental retardation.

Signs. Small babies, pale; all muscles poorly developed.

Etiology. Syndrome may be seen in a number of differ-ent disorders (e.g., propionic acidemia; methylmalonic ac-idemia; isovaleric acidemia) crisis precipitated by infec-tions or protein intake in majority of cases. Defect of oxidation of propionate and deficiency of propionyl-coenzyme A (CoA) carboxylase, and defect of glycine oxidation.

Pathology. Nonspecific changes.

Diagnostic Procedures. *Blood.* Anemia; recurrent neu-tropenia and thrombocytopenia; hypogammaglobuline-mia; ketonemia; hyperglycinemia. *Urine.* Ketonuria, gly-cinuria. Other amino acid levels normal. *X-ray.* Osteoporosis.

Therapy. Restricted protein intake.

Prognosis. Diet improves all symptoms including neu-tropenia. The outcome is, however, fatal.

BIBLIOGRAPHY. Rosenberg LE: Disorders of propionate and methylmalonate metabolism. In Stanbury JB, Wyngaarden JB, Fredrickson DS, et al: The Metabolic Basis of Inherited Disease, 5th ed, p 474. New York, McGraw-Hill, 1983

KIDNEY ARTERIOVENOUS FISTULA

Symptoms. Headache and other common symptoms of blood hypertension, and early symptoms of cardiac failure.

Signs. Blood hypertension; bruit heard best over upper part of abdomen, anteriorly or posteriorly; palpable thrill. Cardiac enlargement, edema, and other signs of cardiac failure.

Etiology. Arteriovenous fistula of the kidney.

Pathology. See Etiology.

Diagnostic Procedures. *Excretory urography. Aortogra-phy. CT scan. Blood.* Polycythemia.

Therapy. Surgery.

Prognosis. Early cardiac failure; good response to sur-gery with remission of all signs.

BIBLIOGRAPHY. Kirby CK, et al: Arteriovenous fistula of renal vessels: case report. Surgery 37:267–271, 1955

Scheifley CH: A new clinical syndrome producing hyper-tension—arteriovenous fistula of the kidney. JAMA 174:1625–1627, 1960

KIENBÖCK'S

Synonyms. Lunatomalacia; lunate bone osteochondro-sis. See Epiphyseal ischemic necrosis.

Symptoms and Signs. More common in males. Onset at young age (15–40 years), usually after severe trauma with wrist in dorsiflexion (75% of cases). Symptoms be-came manifest 18 months prior to X-ray showed lesions. Recurrent pain, stiffness, and limitation of extension of wrist. Swelling over lunate bone area, with thickening of skin and tenderness on palpation.

Etiology. See Epiphyseal ischemic necrosis.

Treatment. Not standardized. Surgical based on ulnar lengthening. Conservative; early casting (4 months, with uncertain results).

Prognosis. According to success of treatment.

BIBLIOGRAPHY. Kienböck R: Ueber traumatische Malazie des Mondbeins und ihre Folgezustaende: Entartungs-formen und Kompressions-frakturen. Forschr Roentgen 16:77–103, 1910
Milford L: Fractures. In Crenshaw AH (ed): Campbell's Operative Orthopedics, 7th ed, pp 219–222. St Louis, CV Mosby, 1987

KIENBÖCK'S SYRINGOMYELIA

Eponym used to indicate the traumatic form of Morvan's I (see).

BIBLIOGRAPHY. Kienböck R: Kritik der sogennanten "Traumatischen Syringomyelie." Jahrbuch Psychiatr 21:50–110, 1910

KILOH-NEVIN II

Synonyms. Anterior interosseous nerve; interosseus neuritis. See Parsonage-Turner.

Symptoms and Signs. Spontaneous onset or following injury of bones. Isolated paralysis of flexor pollicis longus and flexor digitorum profundus; absence of sensory in-volvement (may be combined with partial medium nerve paresis). *Square pinch sign.* Contact between pulps of thumb and index.

Etiology. Idiopathic or associated with fracture or in-jury of forearm bones. Fingers more proximal than nor-mal.

Pathology. Lesion of anterior interosseous nerve.

Therapy. Surgery when indicated.

Prognosis. Within 2 years, almost complete recovery in idiopathic cases.

BIBLIOGRAPHY. Parsonage MJ, Turner JWA: Neurologic amyotrophy: the shoulder-girdle syndrome. Lancet I:973–978, 1948
Kiloh LG, Nevin S: Isolated neuritis of anterior interosseous nerve. Br Med J 1:850–851, 1952
Chan KM, Lamb DW: The anterior interosseous nerve syndrome. J Roy Coll Surgeons Edinburgh 29:350–353, 1984

KIMMELSTIEL-WILSON

Synonym. Diabetic glomerulosclerosis; intercapillary glomerulosclerosis.

Eponym used in the past to indicate the various forms of diabetic glomerulopathies. It is better to restrict its use to the anatomic-pathologic finding of nodular glomerular sclerosis. This lesion is characterized by tubular atrophy and dilatation, balllike hyaline acidophilic masses situated at the periphery of glomerular tuft containing nuclei, and thickening of basal membrane. Kimmelstiel himself writes: "We have learned that this correlation is much closer to nonspecific glomerular changes which were carefully excluded in the original presentation. The term Kimmelstiel-Wilson syndrome is, therefore, not justified."

BIBLIOGRAPHY. Kimmelstiel P, Wilson C: Benign and malignant hypertension and nephrosclerosis: a clinical and pathological study. Am J Pathol 12:45–48, 1936
Brenner BM, Rector FC: The Kidney, 3rd ed, p 1054. Philadelphia, WB Saunders, 1986

KINDLER'S

Synonyms. Poikiloderma, acrokeratoic, hereditary; bullous acrokeratotic poikiloderma; Weary's.

Symptoms and Signs. Both sexes. Pigmentary anomalies in majority of cases; tendency to blistering following mild trauma. Four clinical expressions identified.
1. *Onset 1–3 months.* Vescico-pustule on hands and feet resolving in late childhood.
2. *Onset 3–6 months.* Eczematoid diffuse dermatitis resolving at age 5 years.
3. *Onset in 1st month.* Gradual diffuse poikiloderma striate and reticulate atrophy (sparing face and ears) persisting into adulthood.
4. *Onset before age 5.* Keratotic papules on hands, feet, elbows, knees. Persisting into adulthood.

Etiology. Unknown. Autosomal dominant inheritance; recessive also suggested (with photosensitivity in addition to other symptoms). The nosologic status of this syndrome is under revision.

BIBLIOGRAPHY. Kindler T: Congenital poikiloderma with traumatic bulla formation and progressive cutaneous atrophy. Br J Derm 66:104–111, 1954
Weary PE, Manley WF Jr, Graham GF: Hereditary acrokeratotic poikiloderma. Arch Derm 103:409–422, 1971
Hacham-Zadeh S, Garfunkel AA: Kindler syndrome in two related Kurdish families. Ann Med Genet 20:43–48, 1985

KING'S

Synonym. Malignant hyperthermia–myopathy–multiple anomalie.

Symptoms and Signs. All males and 1 female. From childhood. Short stature; delayed motor development; malar hypoplasia; micrognathia; ptosis or blepharophimosis; downslanting of palpebral fissures; malignant hyperthermia; pectus carenatum; cryptorchidism.

Etiology. Unknown. Apparently nonfamilial. Increase of creatinine phosphokinase in some cases in healthy members of family may suggest an autosomal dominant trait.

Pathology. *Fresh muscle biopsy.* Increased contracture on exposure to halotane. *Muscle histologic examination.* Predominance of type 2 fibers.

Diagnostic Procedures. *Muscle biopsy. Electromyography. Blood.* Creatine phosphokinase level occasionally increased.

Therapy. Physical therapy with some improvement of muscle strength. Surgery for the correction of kyphoscoliosis, pectus carinatum, and cryptorchidism. Prior to surgical operation, pretreatment with dantrolene for the prevention of malignant hyperthermia (MH). Avoid drugs like halothane and succinylcholine that can trigger an MH episode.

Prognosis. Relatively mild, slowly progressing course. High risk for malignant hyperthermia (usual cause of death in reported cases).

BIBLIOGRAPHY. King JO, Denborough MA: Anesthetic-induced malignant hyperpyrexia in children. J Pediatr 83:37–40, 1973
McPherson EW, Taylor CA, Jr: The King syndrome: malignant hyperthermia, myopathy, and multiple anomalies. Am J Med Genet 8:159–165, 1981
Steenson AJ, Torkelson RD: King's syndrome with malignant hyperthermia: potential outpatient risks. Am J Dis Child 141:271–273, 1987

KINSBOURINE'S

Synonyms. Dancing eye; oculogyric crisis. See also West's.

Symptoms and Signs. Occur in infants 1 to 3 years old. Irregular jerky eye movements; twitching of eyelids and eyebrows, enhanced or promoted by activity. Occasionally, lateral nystagmus. Lack of coordination; ataxia; irritability; generalized myoclonic attacks; mental retardation.

Etiology. Unknown.

Diagnostic Procedures. *Electromyography.* Myoclonic action potentials.

Therapy. See West's.

BIBLIOGRAPHY. Kinsbourine M: Myoclonic encephalopathy of infants. J Neurol Neurosurg Psychiatr 27:271–276, 1962

Adams RD, Victor M: Principles of Neurology, 3rd ed, pp 198–922. New York, McGraw-Hill, 1985

KIRNER'S

Synonym. Dystelephalangy.

Symptoms. Male to female ratio 1:2. *Females.* More frequently bilateral. *Male.* Monolateral. Becomes evident from 5th year of life. Asymptomatic.

Signs. The tip of the 5th finger points toward the thenar eminence.

Etiology. Unknown; autosomal dominant inheritance.

Diagnostic Procedures. *X-ray of hand.* Metaphyses of distal phalanx of 5th finger angulated.

Therapy. Orthopedic surgery.

BIBLIOGRAPHY. Brailsford JF: Radiology of Bones and Joints, 5th ed, p 64. Baltimore, Williams & Wilkins, 1953

Blank E, Girdany BR: Symmetric bowing of the terminal phalanges of the fifth fingers in a family (Kirner's deformity). Am J Roentgen 93:367–373, 1965

KITAMURA'S

Synonym. Periodic thyrotoxic paralysis.

Symptoms. Occur more often in males; onset in 3rd or 4th decade. Occur mostly in people of Japanese extraction (2% to 8% of hyperthyroid Japanese patients suffer from this syndrome). Usually occur in the early morning; episodes during day occur when resting after either heavy exertion or large meals. Painless episodes of paroxysmal symmetric muscle weakness that makes the patient unable to rise or move. Eye movements, speech, swallowing, respiration unimpaired. Attacks last from 1 to several hours. Between attacks, completely normal. When attack occurs during the day, initial weakness announces attack. This may be prevented by activity. All symptoms of hyperthyroidism (see Flajani's). Clinical manifestation of hyperthyroidism may appear after months of muscle syndrome. In some cases, thyroid may be enlarged without other signs of hyperthyroidism.

Signs. During attack; reflexes of group of muscles involved reduced or absent; in unaffected muscles, normal reflexes. No myotonia. Signs of hyperthyroidism.

Etiology. Shift of extracellular potassium into cells causing paralysis in patients in whom a latent defect has been unmasked by the hyperthyroid condition.

Pathology. *Muscle biopsy.* Shows mainly normal, rare fibers undergoing degenerative changes. *Light and electron microscopy.* Disclose in affected muscles small, central subsarcolemmal vacuolization.

Diagnostic Procedures. Paralytic attack induced by 10 U of insulin. *Electromyography.* During attack, myopathic type paresis. *Blood.* Glucose tolerance test altered. Lymphocytosis during attack. Hypokalemia accompanies every induced attack. *All tests for hyperthyroidism.*

Therapy. Treatment of hyperthyroidism. Episodes aborted by potassium administration or propranolol. Prophylaxis by avoiding precipitating causes or heavy meals.

Prognosis. Correction of thyroid function induces complete remission of periodic paralysis and associated findings.

BIBLIOGRAPHY. Shinosaki T: Klinische Studien ueber die periodischen paralyse der extremitaten. Zt Ges Neurol Psychiatr 100:564–611, 1926

Norris FH, Panner BJ, Stormont JM: Thyrotoxic periodic paralysis; metabolic and ultrastructural studies. Arch Neurol 19:88–98, 1968

McKenzie JM, Zakarija M: Hyperthyroidism. In De Groot LJ, Cahill FG Jr, Odell WD, et al (eds): Endocrinology. New York, Grune & Stratton, 1979

Adams RD, Victor M: Principles of Neurology, 3rd ed, p 1060. New York, McGraw-Hill, 1985

KJELLIN'S

Symptoms and Signs. All symptoms and signs of Barnard-Scholz except ophthalmoplegia.

BIBLIOGRAPHY. Kjellin KG: Hereditary spastic paraplegia and retinal degeneration (Kjellin syndrome and Barnard-Scholz syndrome). In Vinken PJ, Bruyn GW (eds): Handbook of Clinical Neurology, vol 22, pp 467–473. Amsterdam, North Holland, 1975

KLEINE-LEVIN

Synonyms. Bulimia-hypersomnia; morbid hunger; periodic somnolence; hibernation. See Gelineau's syndrome.

Symptoms. Usually affects adolescent males. Attacks of somnolence lasting several days or weeks; ravenous appetite when awake. Sometimes attacks accompanied by motor unrest, irritability, incoherent speech, hallucination, absence of nocturnal disturbance of sleep.

Etiology. Unknown; occasionally, appearing after acute illness (suggesting postencephalitic condition) or following trauma. A family with autosomal inheritance reported.

Pathology. Unknown; possibly, lesion of prefrontal zone or hypothalamus or both.

Diagnostic Procedures. *Electroencephalography.* Occasional spiking as in epilepsy.

Therapy. Amphetamine; lithium.

Prognosis. Interval of months or years between attacks. Patient normal in the interval. Attacks tend to disappear as full adulthood is reached.

BIBLIOGRAPHY. Kleine W: Periodische Schlafsucht. Mschr Psychiatr Neurol 57:285–320, 1925
Levin M: Periodic somnolence and morbid hunger: a new syndrome. Brain 59:494–504, 1936
Popper JS, Hsia YE, Rogers T, et al: Familial hibernation (Kleine-Levin) syndrome. Am J Hum Genet 32:123A 1980
Goldberg M: The treatment of Kleine-Levin syndrome with lithium. Can J Psychiatr 28:491–493, 1983

KLEINSCHMIDT'S

Obsolete eponym used to indicate the respiratory distress secondary to laryngeal stenosis, dyspnea, tachycardia, hyperthermia, associated with nucal rigidity, observed as complications of influenza.

BIBLIOGRAPHY. Kleinschmidt H: Ein charakteristisches Syndrom durch Influenzabazilleninfektion. Kinderaerztl Prax 10:52–58, 1939

KLEINST'S

Synonyms. Apraxia; constructive apraxia; Mayer-Gross.

Symptoms. Inability to assemble elements to form a significant or correct whole (arranging; building; drawing). Is the 4th form of apraxia (see Liepmann's).

Etiology. Resulting from lesions of right hemisphere in left-handed persons.

BIBLIOGRAPHY. Kleinst K: Gehirnpathologie. Vornehmlich Aufgrund der Kriegerfahrungen. Aus: Handboch der Artzlichen Weltkriege, Band IV, TL 9. Leipzig, Clothbarth, 1934. Leipzig, 1934.
Mayer-Gross W: Some observations on apraxia. Proc R Soc Med 28:1203–1212, 1935
Adams RD, Victor M: Principles of Neurology, 3rd ed, pp 46–47. New York, McGraw-Hill, 1985

KLEIN-WAANDERBURG

Synonym. Waanderburg III, WS III.

Symptoms and Signs. Those of Waanderburg's (see) with associated limb anomalies: hypoplasia of musculoskeletal system; flexion contractures, fusion of carpal bones; syndactyly.

Etiology. Autosomal dominant inheritance.

BIBLIOGRAPHY. Klein D: Albinism partial (leucisme) avec surdi-mutism, blepharophimosis et dysplasie myo-osteo-articulaire. Helv Paediatr Acta 5:38–58, 1950
Klein D: Historical background and evidence for dominant inheritance of the Klein-Waanderburg syndrome (type III). Am J Med Genet 14:231–239, 1983

KLINEFELTER'S

Synonyms. Aspermatogenesis-gynecomastia; seminiferous tubule dysgenesis; Reifenstein-Albright XXY; XXXY; XXYY.

Symptoms. Manifestations become evident at adolescence. Infertility; usually asymptomatic except for a decrease of libido in about 30% of cases and many psychopathologic manifestations: immaturity; shyness; lack of judgment; assertive unrealistic activity.

Signs. Testes small and firm. Gynecomastia (usually minimal); tendency toward obesity; secondary sex characteristics well developed except in some patients, who may present sparsity of facial hair and other eunuchoid characteristics (arm span that exceeds body length by more than 4 inches). Frequently associated with this syndrome are asthma, chronic pulmonary diseases, hypothyroidism, diabetes mellitus (8%).

Etiology. Syndrome due to chromosomal polysomy. Presence of 47 chromosomes including two X's and one

Y's. Other patterns of chromosomal aberration such as XXXY, XXYY, and some mosaic patterns may result in the same syndrome.

Pathology. Testes: variable degree of hyalinization of tubules; absence of elastic fibers around tunica propria; Leydig cells adequate number, frequently clumped.

Diagnostic Procedures. *Urine.* Follicle-stimulating hormone (FSH) levels usually elevated; 17-ketosteroids and 17-hydroxycorticoids low, normal, or diminished. *Buccal smears.* Sex chromatin positive. *Blood.* Drumsticks in smears. *Chromosome studies.* Forty-seven chromosomes or other abnormal patterns. *Biopsy of testes.* See Pathology.

Therapy. When secondary sex characteristics do not develop properly, androgen. For gynecomastia, plastic surgery.

Prognosis. Good; infertility; normal life span.

BIBLIOGRAPHY. Klinefelter HR Jr, Reifenstein EC Jr, Albright F: Syndrome characterized by gynecomastia, aspermatogenesis without A-leydigism, and increased excretion of follicle-stimulating hormone. J Clin Endocrinol 2:615–627, 1942
Ratcliffe SG, Bancroft J, Axworthy D, et al: Klinefelter's syndrome in adolescence. Arch Dis Child 57:6–12, 1982

KLIPPEL-FEIL

Synonyms. Brevicollis, congenital cervicothoracic vertebrae synostosis; congenital osseous–torticollis.

Symptoms. Females prevalently affected (65%). Difficulty in breathing and swallowing. Occasionally, associated neurologic disturbance due to congenital myeloid dysplasia. Convergent strabismus; horizontal nystagmus; deafness. "Mirror movements" syndrome may be said to be present in the condition where voluntary movements of one arm are involuntarily mimicked by the other one.

Signs. Shortening of neck; lowering of hairline on back of neck; platybasia; limited neck motion; occasionally associated, torticollis; facial asymmetry; scoliosis and kyphosis; Sprengel's (see) deformity of scapula (congenital displacement upward) sometimes also associated. This syndrome may be subdivided into 3 types:

Type 1. Extensive anomalies with elements of several vertebrae incorporated into a single block.

Type 2. Failure of complete segmentation of one or two cervical interspaces.

Type 3. Includes type 1 or type 2 with coexisting abnormalities of lower dorsolumbar spine.

Etiology. Unknown; autosomal dominant or recessive disorder with various degrees of penetrance. Congenital fusion of two or more cervical vertebrae.

Pathology. See Signs. Webbed trapezius muscle.

Diagnostic Procedures. *X-ray.* Cervical spine shortened and vertebrae fused; associated malformation. Complete radiological evaluation, including a metrizamide-enhanced computerized tomography scan with sagittal reconstruction. Magnetic resonance imaging can be useful, particularly if an associated syringomyelia is suspected.

Therapy. *Various surgical approaches.* Posterior cervical fusion with autogenous bone graft is indicated in presence of unstable fusion pattern. Anterior or posterior decompression if there is cranio-cervical anomaly and radiological evidence of a compression area. Decompressive laminectomy in presence of cervical spine stenosis symptomatic.

Prognosis. Malformation static during life. Progressive paraplegia possible later in life.

BIBLIOGRAPHY. Klippel M, Feil A: Un cas d'absence des vertebres cervicales avec cage thoracique remontant jusqua à la base du crane (cage thoracique cervicale). Nouv Icon Salpetrière 25:223–250, 1912
Naguib MG, Maxwell RE, Chou SN: Klippel-Feil syndrome in children: clinical features and management. Child's Nerv Syst 1:255–263, 1985
Naguib M, Farag H, Ibrahim AEW: Anesthetic considerations in Klippel-Feil syndrome. Can Anesth Soc J 33:66–70, 1986

KLIPPEL'S

Eponym used to indicate motion incapacitation due to severe osteoarthritic ankylosing changes in elderly people suffering also from arteriosclerotic changes. A generalized arthritic pseudoparalysis results.

BIBLIOGRAPHY. Klippel M: De la pseudoparalysie génerale arthritique. Rev Med 12:280–285, 1892

KLIPPEL-TRENAUNAY-WEBER

Synonyms. Angio-osteohypertrophy; hemangiectasia hypertrophicans; osteohypertrophic nevus flammeus; nevus verucosus hypertrophicans; Ollier-Klippel; Parkes-Weber; Trenaunay's; Weber's (P.F.).

Symptoms and Signs. Nevi unilaterally located; varicose veins; hypertrophy of soft tissue and bones of affected extremity (usually upper), which makes it longer and warmer than the unaffected one. (If hypertrophy secondary to arteriovenous aneurysm is present the syndrome is called Parkes-Weber). Varicose veins and osteohypertrophy not always present at birth but develop during first few months or years of life. Syndactyly and polydactyly frequently associated. Other internal anomalies also associated.

Etiology. Unknown; possibly, hereditary weakness of mesenchymal tissue of vascular walls. Autosomal dominant inheritance.

Pathology. Nevi with dilated capillaries, lined with single layer of endothelial cells; in some cases arteriovenous fistula. Hypertrophy of muscles and bones of affected limb (see Signs).

Diagnostic Procedures. *X-ray.* (Not diagnostic.) Thickening of bone cortex.

Therapy. None. If arteriovenous fistula, surgery.

Prognosis. Very rapid period of enlargement, then sudden cessation of growth; residual deformity.

BIBLIOGRAPHY. Klippel M, Trenaunay P: Naevus variqueux osteohypertrophique. Arch Gen Med (Paris) 3:641–642, 1900

Weber PF: Angioformation in connection with hypertrophy of limbs and hemihypertrophy. Br J Derm 19:231–235, 1907

Servelle M: Klippel and Trenaunay's syndrome: 768 operated cases. Ann Surg 201:369–373, 1985

Chomette G, Auriol M: Classification des angiodysplasies et tumeurs vasculaires. Rev Stom Clin Maxillo 87:1–5, 1986

Viljoen DL: Klippel-Trenaunay-Weber syndrome (angio-osteohypertrophy syndrome). J Med Genet 25:250–252, 1988

KLÜVER-BUCY

Synonym. Temporal lobectomy behavior.

Symptoms. Symptoms appear soon after bilateral removal of temporal lobes. Loss of recognition of people, including close relatives; loss of fear and rage reaction; hypersexuality, also hypersexuality in the form of masturbation; homosexual tendency; bulimia; hypermetamorphosis (response by motor action to every object or event); marked memory deficiency.

Etiology. Surgery attempting removal of bilateral epileptogenic foci. In humans this operation in some cases reproduces the syndrome experimentally induced by Klüver and Bucy in rhesus monkeys. The syndrome has been observed also after treated herpes encephalitis.

Pathology. Bilateral removal of anterior portion of temporal lobes, uncus, anterior part of the hippocampus, and amygdaloid nucleus.

Diagnostic Procedures. *X-ray of skull.* Atrophy of temporal lobe. *Angiography. CT brain scan.*

Therapy. Carbamazepine.

Prognosis. Result of the operation for treatment of the epileptic attacks arising from temporal lobes is poor. In the postencephalitic syndrome, improvement can occur over an extended period, and chronic residual sequelae may be relatively mild.

BIBLIOGRAPHY. Klüver H, Bucy PC: An analysis of certain effects of bilateral temporal lobectomy in the rhesus monkey, with special reference to "psychic blindness." J Psychol 5:33–54 1938

Bucy PC, Klüver H: Anatomic changes secondary to temporal lobectomy. Arch Neurol Psychiatr 44:1142–1146, 1940

Hart RP, Kwentus JA, Frazier RB, et al: Natural history of Klüver-Bucy syndrome after treated herpes encephalitis. South Med J (Birmingham) 79:1376–1378, 1986

KNEE JOINT, INTERNAL DERANGEMENT

Synonyms. IDK; internal knee derangement; knee locking; weak knee.

Symptoms. Pain on movement of knee; locking, buckling; snapping.

Signs. Local tenderness; thigh atrophy; joint swelling; special maneuvers to reproduce symptoms.

Etiology and Pathology. IDK is a loose term that includes many etiologic causes: tears of menisci; cyst of menisci; discoid meniscus; calcified meniscus; ligament tears; incomplete tears; fractures of tibial plateaus; tears of patellar tendons; fracture of patella; chondromalacia of patella; traumatic synovial effusions; plica articularis syndrome; Pellegrini-Stieda, osteochondritis dissecans; Osgood-Schlatter; Baker's cyst; osteoarthritis; pigmented villonodular synovitis rheumatoid arthritis. (Many of these syndromes have been described under these headings.)

Diagnostic Procedures. *X-ray. Aspiration of fluid. Biopsy of synovial membrane.*

Therapy. Rest; immobilization or surgical correction or repair according to etiology or systemic medication.

Prognosis. Depends on etiology.

BIBLIOGRAPHY. Hey W: Practical Observations in Surgery. London, Cadell and Davis, 1803

Sisk TD: Knee injuries. In Crenshaw AH (ed): Campbell's Operative Orthopedics, 7th ed, pp 2299. St Louis, CV Mosby, 1987

KNIEST-LIKE, LETHAL

Symptoms and Signs. Those of Kniest's (see). Neonates severely hydropic, death in first few days.

Etiology. Autosomal recessive inheritance.

Pathology. Bone and cartilage lesion similar to those of Kniest's (Swiss cheese appearance) with other distinctive changes in cartilage and growth plate. Electron microscopy shows stronger differences from Kniest's lesions.

Diagnostic Procedures. *X-ray.* Dumbbell-shaped long bones (as in Kniest's), but with noticeably shortened diaphyseal and metaphyseal changes.

BIBLIOGRAPHY. Stevenson RE: Micromelic chondrodysplasia: further evidence for autosomal recessive inheritance. Proc Greenwood Genet Center 1:52–57, 1982
Scouyers SM, Rimoin DL, Lachman RS, et al: A distinct chondrodysplasia resembling Kniest dysplasia: clinical, roentgenographic, histologic, and ultrastructural findings. J Pediatr 103:898–904, 1983

KNIEST'S

Synonyms. Kniest's dwarfism; metatrophic dwarfism II.

Symptoms and Signs. Present from birth. Moon facies with prominent eyes; saddle nose; short arms and legs. Incapacity to make a fist; violaceous hue of the palms. Swelling of joints; lack of full elbow extension. Reduced length; variable weight. Delay of motor milestones. Poor vision; decreased hearing; muscle weakness. Frequently, cleft palate. Intelligence normal. First and 2nd cervical nerve irritability with secondary myelopathy signs.

Etiology. Autosomal dominant inheritance. Abnormal proteoglycan synthesis suggested.

Pathology. Only one report of soft bones; hiatal hernia.

Diagnostic Procedures. *Urine.* High excretion of keratan sulfate. *X-rays.* General skeletal hypoplasia (that of odontoid process of greatest clinical significance). See Atlantoaxial-spinal dislocation. Characteristic pelvic changes (wineglass deformity).

Therapy. Stabilization of unstable atlantoaxial joint. Prevention of joint contractures.

Prognosis. Poor. Bony fusion between anterior arch of atlas and odontoid and posterior arch of atlas and cranial base.

BIBLIOGRAPHY. Kniest W: Zur Abrenzung der Dysostosis enchondralis von der Chondrodystrophie. Z Kinderheilkd 70:633–640, 1952

Friede H, Matalon R, Harris V, et al: Craniofacial and mucopolysaccharide abnormalities in Kniest dysplasie. J Craniofac Genet Devel Biol 5:267–276, 1985

KNOBLOCH'S

Synonym. Retinal detachment-occipital encephalocele.

Symptoms and Signs. Myopia; vitreoretinal detachment; and occipital encephalocele (meningocele?). Normal mental development.

Etiology. Autosomal recessive inheritance

BIBLIOGRAPHY. Knobloch WA, Layer JM: Retinal detachment and encephalocele. J Ped Ophthalmol 8:181–184, 1971
Cohen MM Jr, Lemire RJ: Syndromes with cephaloceles. Teratology 25:161–172, 1972

KNUCKLE PADS–
DEAFNESS–LEUKONYCHIA

Synonyms. Bart-Pumphrey; deafness-knuckle-leukonychia; Schwann's.

Symptoms. Sensorineural and conductive hearing loss.

Signs. Knuckle pads; total leukonychia. Keratoderma of palms and soles may also be a feature.

Etiology. Unknown; congenitally transmitted as an autosomal dominant trait. The knuckle pad feature is variably expressed.

Diagnostic Procedures. *Audiometry.* Indicates cochlear neural defect. *Blood, urine, chromosome studies.* Unrevealing.

BIBLIOGRAPHY. Schwann J: Keratosis palmaris et plantaris cum surditate congenita et leuconychia totali unguium. Dermatologica 126:335–353, 1963
Bart RS, Pumphrey RE: Knuckle pads, leukonychia, and deafness. New Engl J Med 276:202–207, 1967
Crosby EF, Vidurrizaga RH: Knuckle pads, leukonychia, deafness and keratosis palmoplantaris of a family. John Hopkins Med J 139:90–92, 1976

KOBY'S

Synonym. Floriform cataract.

Symptoms. Both sexes affected. Asymptomatic or visual impairment.

Signs. Multiple opacities of different shapes: (anular, floriform, and of different colors) found especially around structures of embryonic nucleus.

Etiology. Unknown; possibly, autosomal dominant inheritance.

Therapy. None.

Prognosis. Usually static.

BIBLIOGRAPHY. Koby FE: Cataracte familiale d'un type particulier, se transmettant apparent suivant le mode dominant. Arch Ophthalmol 40:492–503, 1923
Tosch C: Beitrag zur Stammbaumforschung der Cataracta floriformis. Klin Monatstbl Augenheilkd 133:60–66, 1958

KOCKER-DEBRÉ-SÉMÉLAIGNE

Synonyms. KDS; cretinism–muscular hypertrophy; Debré-Sémélaigne; myxedema–muscular hypertrophy. See Hoffmann's syndrome.

Symptoms. Occur in children and adults. Typical clinical manifestations of cretinism, associated with a sense of stiffness and discomfort in large muscles; some movements painful. Slow muscle contractions and slow clumsy gait; cold weather enhances slowness of movements (paramyotonia); dysarthria (due to big tongue).

Signs. Firm, large, well-developed muscles (true hypertrophy). Prolongation of tendon reflexes.

Etiology. Unknown; association of clinical manifestations of cretinism and muscular disorder constitute KDS; the combination of myxedema and myotonoid muscular disorder constitute Hoffmann's; most likely no fundamental difference between the two conditions. Familial occurrence reported.

Pathology. No consistent pathologic changes have been found in skeletal muscles, except a volumetric increase of muscle fibers.

Diagnostic Procedures. *Electromyography.* "Wormlike" contraction persisting for nearly a second after stimulation. *Urine.* Lack of creatinuria; high creatine tolerance. *Blood.* Elevated serum cholesterol, lowered iodine uptake and other thyroid functional studies.

Therapy. Thyroxine.

Prognosis. Complete recovery may follow the administration of thyroxine.

BIBLIOGRAPHY. Kocker T: Zur Verhütung des Cretinismus und cretinoider Zustände nach neuen Forschungen. Dtsch Z Chir 34:556–626, 1892
Hoffmann J: Weiterer Beitrag zur Lehre von der Tetanie. Dtsch Z Nervenkr 9:278–290, 1896
Debré R, Sémélaigne G: Syndrome of diffuse muscular hypertrophy in infants causing athletic appearance: its connection with congenital myxedema. Am J Dis Child 50:1351–1361, 1935

Adams RD, Victor M: Principles of Neurology, 3rd ed, p 1060. New York, McGraw-Hill, 1985

KOEBBERLING-DUNINGAN

Synonyms. Lipoatrophic diabetes; lipodystrophy, reverse partial. See Lawrence-Seip and Symmetric adenolipomatosis.

Symptoms and Signs. Full syndrome only in females. Fat accumulation on the neck, shoulder, buffalo hump area, and genitalia. *Limbs.* Lean muscles. Phlebectasia. Symptoms of diabetes mellitus and gout.

Etiology. Unknown. Sporadic and familial cases. Possibly autosomal dominant trait or X-linked (lethality in hemizygous males?).

Diagnostic Procedures. *Blood.* Hyperglycemia (insulin-resistant), hyperlipoproteinemia (type IV) (see). Hyperuricemia.

BIBLIOGRAPHY. Greene ML, Gheck CJ, Fujimoto WY, et al: Benign symmetric lipomatosis (Lannosis-Bensaude adenolipomatosis) with gout and hyperlipoproteinemia. Am J Med 48:239–246, 1970
Dunningan MG, Cochrane M, Kelly A, et al: Familial lipodystrophic diabetes with dominant transmission: a new syndrome. Q J Med 43:33–48, 1974
Koebberling J, Willms B, Kattermann R, et al: Lipodystrophy of extremities: a dominantly inherited syndrome associated with lipoatrophic diabetes. Hum Genet 29: 111–120, 1975
Wettke-Schafer R, Kantner G: X-linked dominant diseases with lethality in hemizygous males. Hum Genet 64:1–23, 1985

KOENIG'S I

Synonyms. Arthrolithiasis; joint loose body; joint mice; osteochondrolysis; Paget's (quiet bone necrosis); osteochondritis dissecans.

Symptoms. Both sexes affected; onset at all ages. Asymptomatic for a long time; occasional or persistent sharp pain in joint caused or exacerbated by pressure. Occasionally, locking of joint (transitory).

Signs. Usually the knee involved. Crepitus; swelling; inflammatory signs. Occasionally loose bodies may be palpated.

Etiology. Various conditions may be responsible: osteochondritis dissecans; osteoarthritis; synovial chondromatosis; osteocartilage fracture.

Pathology. In cartilage cavity, round, smooth, cartilagineous or fibrous loose bodies; secondary synovial inflammatory changes.

Diagnostic Procedures. *X-ray.* Visibility of bodies according to their degree of calcification.

Therapy. Removal when interfering with motion; debridement of cartilagineous tabs, spurs.

Prognosis. Good with removal; frequent consequence: chronic persistent synovitis.

BIBLIOGRAPHY. Koenig F: Lehrbuch der allgemeinen Chirurgie fuer Ärtze und Studierende, p 751. Berlin, 1889
Sisk TD: Knee injuries. In Crenshaw AH (ed): Campbell's Operative Orthopedics, 7th ed, pp 2471–2476. St Louis, CV Mosby, 1987

KOENIG'S II

Synonym. Ileocecal valve.

Symptoms and Signs. Alternating diarrhea and constipation. Recurrent abdominal pain; meteorism; borborygmi in right iliac fossa. A mass may or may not be palpated in right lower abdominal quadrant.

Etiology. Tuberculous lesion at the level of ileocecal valve or other conditions interfering with ileocecal valve function. See Ischemic colon.

Diagnostic Procedures. *X-ray of intestinal tract, chest. Sputum. Stool.* Microscopic examination and culture. *Mantoux test.*

Therapy. Antitubercular chemotherapy.

Prognosis. Good with treatment.

BIBLIOGRAPHY. Koenig F: Die strieturirende Tuberculose des Darmes und ihre Behandlung. Dstch Z Chir 34:65–81, 1892

KOFFERATH'S

Synonym. Diaphragmatic obstetric paralysis.

Symptoms and Signs. Occur in newborn, especially when forceps has been used in delivery. Dyspnea; cyanosis, unilateral edema of the neck; asymmetric thoracic movements on breathing. Frequently associated, Duchenne-Erb paralysis (see).

Etiology. Lesion of one phrenic nerve associated, in some cases, also with lesions of cervical nerves.

Therapy. Symptomatic. Protection from respiratory infections.

Prognosis. Good *quoad vitam.* Nerve function may return according to extent of lesion.

BIBLIOGRAPHY. Kofferath W: Ueber eine Fall von rechtsseitigen erbscher Lähmung und Phrenikuslaehmung nach Zangenextraktion. Mschr Geburtshecol 55:33–38, 1921
Robotham JL: A physiological approach to hemidiaphragm paralysis. Crit Care Med 7:563–566, 1979

KÖHLER'S I

Synonyms. Köhler-Mouchette; Panner's I. See Epiphyseal ischemic necrosis.

Symptoms and Signs. More common in males; onset at 3 to 10 years of age. Asymptomatic or pain on medial side of foot. Tenderness on palpation and swelling over area of navicular bone. Slight, usually unilateral, limp.

Etiology. See Epiphyseal ischemic necrosis.

BIBLIOGRAPHY. Köhler A: Ueber eine häufige, bisher anscheinen unbekannte Erkrankung inzelner kindlicher knochen. MMW 55:1923–1925, 1908
Canale ST: Osteochondrosis or epiphysitis? In Crenshaw AH (ed): Campbell's Operative Orthopedics, 7th ed, p 989. St Louis, CV Mosby, 1987

KOK'S

Synonyms. Startle; hyperexplexia; hyperekplexia, Stiff baby.

Symptoms and Signs. Both sexes. At birth. Hypertonia in flexion; exaggerated startle response to minor stimuli (e.g., light touch of the nose, light hand clapping), which may cause generalized hypertonia and falling "like a log" to the ground; exaggerated brainstem reflexes; and, occasionally, seizures. Symptoms disappear during sleep (in one family reported nocturnal myoclonic jerks); occasionally congenital hip dislocation and inguinal hernia.

Etiology. Hyperactive long-loop reflexes proposed as mechanism for exaggerated startle. Autosomal dominant inheritance.

Diagnostic Procedures. *Electrophysiological studies.* Prominent C response after nerve stimulation.

Therapy. Barbiturates, clonazepam usually effective in reducing symptoms. Some resistant cases reported.

Prognosis. After 1 year usually reduction of intensity of symptoms, which may, however, persist for life.

BIBLIOGRAPHY. Kok O, Bruyn GW: An unidentified hereditary disease (letter). Lancet I:1359, 1962

Mazkand ON, Garg BP, Weaver DD: Familial startle disease (hyperexplexia): electrophysiologic studies. Arch Neurol 41:71–74, 1984

Cook W, Kaplan RF: Neuromuscular blockade in a patient with stiff baby syndrome. Anesthesiology 55:525–528, 1986

KÖHLMEIER-DEGÓS

Synonyms. Cutaneo intestinal; Degós'; Degós-Delort-Tricot; atrophic dermatitis papulo squamosa; malignant atrophic papulosis; arteriolar cutaneogastrointestinal thrombosis.

Symptoms and Signs. Predominate in males; onset in third decade of life. *Stage 1. Skin.* Of varying duration from weeks to years; affecting trunk, proximal extremities, neck, occasionally face. Palms and soles spared. Appears as circular erythematous papules that enlarge and assume irregular form, umbilicate, and ulcerate leaving depressed atropic scar. At any time, different degrees of evolution. *Ocular manifestations.* White avascular plaque on bulbar conjunctiva; chorioretinal lesions. *Stage 2.* Abdominal symptoms and signs of peritonitis.

Etiology. Unknown; possibly clinical variation of polyarteritis; immune or autoimmune process.

Pathology. *Skin.* Vascular changes affecting both arteries and veins; inflammatory changes mostly in intima. Elastica and media rarely involved. Endothelial proliferation; fibrinoid degeneration; thrombosis. Epithelial changes appear as secondary. *Small bowel.* White subserous plaque; shallow ulcers; perforation followed by peritonitis. *Stomach and colon.* May be similarly affected.

Diagnostic Procedures. *Biopsy.*

Therapy. None; exploratory laparotomy. Does not respond to corticosteroids. Trials with phenylbutazone, aspirin, dipyridamole, and fibrinolytics.

Prognosis. Fatal. Few cases with only skin lesions reported to have survived.

BIBLIOGRAPHY. Köhlmeier W: Multiple Hautnekrosen bie Thromboangiitis obliterans. Arch Dermatol Syph 181:783–792, 1941

Degós R, Delort J, Tricot R: Dermatitie papulo-squamense atrophiante. Bull Soc Fr Dermatol Syph 49:148–150, 1942

May RE: Degós' syndrome. Br Med J 1:161–162, 1968

KOHLSCHUTTER'S

Synonyms. Amelogenesis imperfecta–epilepsy–mental deterioration; epilepsy–yellow teeth.

Symptoms. Occur in males; normal at birth; onset between 1 and 4 years of age. Epileptic attacks sudden and generalized, followed by progressive mental deterioration.

Signs. Amelogenesis imperfecta; associated with hypohidrosis and myopia.

Etiology. Unknown. Autosomal recessive (?) or X-linked (?) inheritance.

Diagnostic Procedures. *Sweat test. Blood.* Mild hypernatremia and chloremia; marked hyperkalemia. *Electroencephalography.*

BIBLIOGRAPHY. Kohlschutter A, Chappuis D, Meier C, et al: Familial epilepsy and yellow teeth: a disease of the central nervous system associated with enamel hypoplasia. Helv Paediatr Acta 29:283–294, 1974

Witkop CJ Jr, Sank JJ Jr: Heritable defects of enamel. In Stewart RE, Prescott GH (eds): Oral Facial Genetics, pp 200–202. St Louis, CV Mosby, 1976

KOREAN HEMORRHAGIC FEVER

Synonyms. Hemorrhagic epidemic fever; hemorrhagic nephroso nephritis fever.

Symptoms. Reported in Manchuria, Siberia, Korea, eastern Russia, Czechoslovakia, and Hungary. Two seasonal peaks of incidence, but endemic cases during the entire year. Onset at all ages; both sexes affected. Abrupt onset. Headache; fever; chills; anorexia; nausea; vomiting, backache. In Scandinavia and the rest of Europe less severe form, epidemic nephropathy, without hemorrhagic phenomena.

Signs. *Day 1.* Conjunctival congestion; skin flushed; especially face and neck. *Day 2.* Petechiae on the face, oral mucosa, conjunctiva, axillar areas. *Day 4.* Periorbital edema. *Day 5.* Fever stops; hypotension, oliguria. *Day 10.* Diuretic phase lasting days or weeks with fluctuation between shock and hypertension and with pulmonary edema according to fluid balance. Convalescence 3 to 12 weeks, with gradual recovery.

Etiology. The disease is caused by Hantaan virus, first recovered from the striped field mouse, *Apodemus agrarius* excreta in Korea. Sometimes arthropod vector.

Pathology. *Kidney.* Pallor of cortex; congested pyramids. *Heart.* Hemorrhagic lesions of right atrial wall. *Anterior pituitary.* Intense congestion; various degrees of necrosis. *Capillaries.* Generalized dilatation. *Small vessels.* Lack of inflammatory changes.

Diagnostic Procedures. *Blood.* High hematocrit; leukocytosis up to 50,000 with immature elements. Thrombocytopenia. Electrolyte imbalance. In oliguric phase, high blood urea nitrogen and creatinine. *Urine*. Proteinuria. Specific diagnosis is made by immunofluorescent techniques, using lung sections from *Apodemus* rodents as source of antigen.

Therapy. Limit fluid intake; human serum albumin; treatment of the acute renal failure, with careful control of the electrolytes; if necessary, hemodialysis. Trials with antiviral agents.

Prognosis. Oriental, including Russia form, overall mortality with proper treatment seldom surpasses 5%. In Europe and the United States mild symptoms and rapid recovery.

BIBLIOGRAPHY. Symposium on epidemic hemorrhagic fever. Am J Med 16:617, 1954
Myhrman G: Nephropathia epidemica: a new infectious disease in Northern Scandinavia. Acta Med Scand 140:52–56, 1951
PHLS Report. Febbre emorragica con interessamento renale: infezione da Hantaan virus. Br Med J (Italian ed) 5:177–179, 1986

KORO

Synonyms. Depersonalization; depersonalization psychosis.

Symptoms. Occur mostly in people of Malayan archipelagos. Prevalent in males, who are possessed by fear of penis shrinking and disappearing inside the abdomen, with death to follow. Usually patients try to secure penis by putting a ribbon around it or clamping in a wooden box. In females, fear of shrinkage of vagina and breast.

Etiology. Unknown. Type of depersonalization syndrome resulting from cultural-social and psychologic factors. Sexual excess or physical injuries, including cold exposure of penis, may be precipitating factors.

Therapy. Psychotherapy; tranquillizer.

Prognosis. Only 30% recover completely.

BIBLIOGRAPHY. Yap PM: Koro—a culture-bound depersonalization syndrome. Br J Psychiatr 111:43–50, 1965
Freedman AM, Kaplan HI, Sadock BJ: Comprehensive Textbook of Psychiatry, 2nd ed, p 1731. Baltimore, Williams & Wilkins, 1975

KORSAKOFF'S

Synonyms. Anamnestic; anamnestic confabulatory. See Wernicke-Korsakoff.

Symptoms. *Retrograde anamnesia.* Impaired capacity to recall events and information that were known before onset. *Anterograde anamnesia.* Impaired capacity to acquire new information; concentration, spatial organization, visual and verbal abstraction partially affected. *Confabulation.* Fabrication of stories of recent events occasionally present. Remote memory and immediate memory (digit repetition) intact.

Etiology. Not well defined. Medial temporal lobe and median thalamic regions lesion. Can be observed in several clinical conditions, atherosclerosis, trauma, hemorrhages, CO_2 poisoning, concussion, Wernicke-Korsakoff's (see), virus encephalitis, tuberculous meningitis, tumor and brain degenerative disorders (e.g., Alzheimer's).

Pathology. Critical structures damaged seem to be the hippocampus and mostly the underlying temporal stem.

Diagnostic Procedures. *CT brain scan. Electroencephalography. Cerebrospinal fluid. Examination of mental status.*

Therapy. General care. Symptomatic to reduce restlessness, anxiety, and aggressive symptoms or to stimulate.

Prognosis. Poor.

BIBLIOGRAPHY. Korsakoff SS: Ob alkogol'nom paraliche Vest. Psychiatr (Moskva) 4, 1887
Adam RD, Victor M: Principles of Neurology, 3rd ed, New York, McGraw-Hill, 1985, p 318.

KOSTMANN'S

Synonyms. Infantile genetic agranulocytosis; agranulocytosis, infantile genetic. Hereditary neutropenia.

Symptoms. Onset usually in early infancy. Recurrent infections.

Signs. According to localization of infections; no splenomegaly.

Etiology. Unknown; an autosomal recessive mode of inheritance has been suggested.

Pathology. Necrotic ulceration of oral and genital mucosae. Diffuse inflammatory reactions with lymphocytes, plasma cells, and histiocytes, and without neutrophils, in various tissue. Liver and spleen moderately congested. Extramedullary hematopoiesis in various tissues.

Diagnostic Procedures. *Blood.* Leukocytes in normal number with absolute or very marked neutropenia. Absolute and relative eosinophilia and monocytosis. No anemia or only secondary at later stage of the disease. *Bone marrow.* Erythropoiesis and megakaryocytes normal; myeloid series—absence of myeloid precursors beyond early myelocyte stage. *Epinephrine stimulation test.* Window test (Rebuck). Reveals absence of neutrophils. Addition of sulfur-containing aminoacids to tissue cultures leads to maturation of neutrophils.

Therapy. Antibiotics. All types of treatment, medical and surgical (splenectomy), fail.

Prognosis. Poor, death a few months after discovery of condition (usually before age 3 years) because of severe infections. Meningitis frequent.

BIBLIOGRAPHY. Kostmann R: Infantile genetic agranulocytosis (agranulocytosis infantilis hereditaria): new recessive lethal disease in man. Acta Paediatr (suppl 105) 45:1–78, 1956

Iselius L, Gustavson KH: Spatial distribution of the gene for infantile genetic agranulocytosis. Hum Hered 34:358–363, 1984

KOZHEVNIKOV'S

Synonyms. Epilepsia partialis continua; Kojewnikoff's; Koshewnikow's.

Symptoms. *Onset.* High fever, delirium, localized muscular spasms, and generalized convulsion then clonic twitching of one group of muscles (face, upper (more frequently) or lower limbs) at regular intervals (a few seconds) lasting for hours or months, remaining always localized. May be reduced but not abolished during sleep and enhanced by passive or active movements.

Etiology. Focal motor status epilepticus. (Kozhevnikov reported it on the occasion of an encephalitis epidemic in Russia in spring.) May be caused by acute or chronic brain lesions. Cortical origin favored.

Pathology. Lesion of opposite side of brain cortex and involvement of deeper structures.

Diagnostic Procedures. *Electroencephalography.*

Therapy. Same as for epilepsy.

Prognosis. Difficult treatment. Partial recovery from acute stage; paralysis recedes, but after some time, continuous muscular contractions persisting for years only in limbs affected. Major seizures may occur.

BIBLIOGRAPHY. Kozhevnikov A: Ia Osobyi vid Kortical noĭ épilepsii. Moskva, 1952

Thomas JE, Regan TJ, Klass DW: Epilepsie partialis continua: a review of 32 cases. Arch Neurol 34:266, 272, 1977

KOZLOWSKI'S

Synonym. Spondylometaphyseal dysplasia (type GII).

Symptoms. Both sexes affected; onset at 1 year of age.

Reduction of growth (especially of trunk) between 1 and 4 years of age. Waddling gait; limitation of joint mobility.

Signs. Dwarfism (adult height 130 to 165 cm). Short neck and trunk. Kyphosis; dorsal kyphoscoliosis; platyspondylisis; pectus carinatum; bowed legs; irregular metaphyses.

Etiology. Autosomal recessive (?) inheritance.

Pathology. Cellular reduction in proliferation cartilage zone; vacuolization of cells and reduction of calcification of bony precursors.

Diagnostic Procedures. *X-ray of spine and pelvis.* Evident at age 2. Platyspondylisis in "tongue" form; anterior deformity in spine. In infancy, horizontal and trident acetabular roof.

Therapy. Control of evolution of hypoplastic odontoid process (see Atlantoaxial spine dislocation).

Prognosis. Limited growth; joint degeneration producing pain and limiting motion.

BIBLIOGRAPHY. Kozlowski K, Maroteaux P, Spranger G: Le dysotose spondylo-metaphysaire. Presse Med 75:2769–2774, 1967

Le Quesne GW, Koslowski K: Spondylometaphyseal dysplasia. Br J Radiol 46:685–691, 1973

Kozlowski K, Beemer FA, Bens G, et al: Spondylometaphyseal dysplasia: report of 7 cases and assay of classification. In Papadatos CJ, Bartsocas CS (eds): Skeletal Dysplasias. New York, Alan R Liss, 1982

KRABBE'S I

Synonyms. Globoid cell brain sclerosis; galactocerebroside beta-galactosidase deficiency; galactosylceramide lipoidosis; globoid cell leukodystrophy; galactosyl ceramide lipoidosis.

Symptoms and Signs. Both sexes affected; onset usually in childhood (1st year of life); described also in adults. Ambiguous onset: irritability or hypersensitivity to stimuli, followed rapidly by mental and motor deterioration and visual and hearing disorders. Hypertonicity in early phase, then hypotonicity. Variable clinical pattern according to areas of cerebral lesions, prevalent involvement of internal capsula (abnormal reflexes, paralysis, contractures), optic nerve, optic tract. Systemic manifestations are rare.

Etiology. Autosomal recessive inheritance. Deficiency of galactocerebroside beta-galactosidase and accumulation of galactocerebroside and psychosine in macrophages, which causes degeneration of oligodendroglia (the cells that produce myelin).

Pathology. Demyelinization of central nervous system

areas. In demyelinized areas, appearance of globoid cells, giant cells with peripherally displaced nucleus and homogeneous cytoplasm, clustering around small blood vessels or diffuse in border areas of demyelinization areas. Similar cells may be found also in lung, spleen, and lymph nodes. Absence of metachromatic leukodystrophy nodes. Absence of metachromatic breakdown product (see Metachromatic leukodystrophy).

Diagnostic Procedures. *Blood.* Galactocerebroside beta-galactoside assay in white cells (and fibroblasts) decreased. *Spinal tap. Electroencephalography. Electromyography. X-ray of skull. Pneumoencephalography. Angiography. CT brain scan.* Progressive brain atrophy.

Therapy. None specific; symptomatic.

Prognosis. In infantile form death within 2nd year. In later onset (from 2 to 6 years) possible survival up to 5 years. Most surviving infants show early slowing and then arrest of growth, leading progressively to microcephaly and severe failure to thrive. In adult type, 2 to 10 years survival from onset.

BIBLIOGRAPHY. Krabbe KH: A new familial; infantile form of brain sclerosis. Brain 39:74–114, 1916
Suzuki K, Suzuki Y: Galactosylceramide lipidosis: globoid cell leukodystrophy (Krabbe's disease) In Stanbury JB, Wyngaarden JB, Fredrickson DS, et al: The Metabolic Basis of Inherited Disease, 5th ed, p 857. New York, McGraw-Hill, 1983
Zlotogora J, Regev R, Hadar S, et al: Growth pattern in Krabbe's disease. Acta Paediatr Scand 75:251–254, 1986

KRABBE'S II

Synonyms. Facial-meningeal angiomas; Sturge-Weber-Krabbe. See also Sturge-Weber.

Symptoms and Signs. Both sexes affected; present from birth, developing more or less rapidly. Mental deterioration; hemiplegia; epileptic attacks; facial hemiatrophy and flat angioma in the distribution area of the trigeminal V nerve.

Etiology. Unknown; congenital malformation with irregular dominant inheritance.

Pathology. *Skin.* Nevus flammeus (see). *Brain.* Atrophy; cerebral angiomas.

Diagnostic Procedures. *X-rays of skull.* Presence of calcium deposits that follow cerebral gyri. *Angiography. CT brain scan.*

Therapy. Surgery and x-rays.

Prognosis. Variable, but generally poor.

BIBLIOGRAPHY. Krabbe KH: Facial and meningeal angiomas associated with calcification of the brain cortex. A clinical and anatomopathologic contribution. Arch Neurol Psychiatr 32:737–755, 1934
Chomette G, Auriol M: Classification des angiodysplasics et tumeurs vasculaires. Rev Stom Clin Maxillo Fac 87:1–5, 1986

KRAEMER'S

Synonyms. Metastatic furunculiformi episcleritis; suppurative scleritis.

Symptoms. Severe ocular pain; lacrimation; photophobia.

Signs. Abscess in scleral vessels.

Etiology. Septic embolus, especially staphylococcal.

Therapy. Systemic and topical antibiotics.

Prognosis. Good.

BIBLIOGRAPHY. Kraemer R: Episkleritis metastatic furunculiformis. Klin Monatstbl Augenheilkd 66:441–450, 1921

KRAMER-POLLNOW

Eponym indicating an entity of doubtful individuality consisting in a sudden onset, between 1 and 4 years of age, of progressive hyperkinesia, followed by retardation of mental development, anxiety, and regression of expressive capacities. See Little's.

BIBLIOGRAPHY. Kramer F, Pollnow H: Ueber eine hyperkinetische Erkrankung in Kindersalter. Mschr Psychiatr Neur 82–83: 1–40, 1932

KRAMER'S

Synonyms. Ankyloglossia superior; glossopalatine ankylosis–microglossia hypodontia–limb anomalies; Kettner's. It may be included in the Oromandibular-limb hypogenesis spectrum (hypoglossia-hypodactyly; aglossia-adactyly; Moebius'; Charlie M; facial limb disruptive spectrum).

Symptoms. Rare. Both sexes affected. Congenital symptoms related to signs and their association.

Signs. *Mouth.* Tongue small, with anterior part attached to hard palate or upper alveolar ridge or both; tip could be cleft. Upper lip and mandible hypoplastic. Palatal vault high; occasionally, hypodontia and ankylosing of temporomandibular joint. *Limbs.* Various anomalies both in the hands and feet, unilateral or bilateral syndactyly, clinodactyly, hypoplasia of digits, nail absence, lobster claw deformity. Occasionally, associated paralysis of abducens (VI) or facial (VII) nerve.

Etiology. Unknown. Possible alteration of environment between the eighth and twelfth week in utero.

BIBLIOGRAPHY. Kettner H: Kongenitaler Zungendefekt Dtsch Med Wochenschr 38:352, 1907

Kramer W: Zur Entstehung der angeborenen Gaumenspalte. Zentralbl Chir 38:385–387, 1911

Gorlin RJ, Pindborg JJ, Cohen MM: Syndromes of the Head and Neck, 2nd ed. New York, McGraw-Hill, 1976

Jones KL: Smith's recognizable patterns of human malformations, p 588. Philadelphia, WB Saunders, 1988

KRAUSE'S

Synonyms. Encephalo-ophthalmic dysplasia; ophthalmo-encephalic dysplasia; Yudkin's; Krause-Reese. See Reese-Blodi and Patau's.

Symptoms. Usually discovered months after birth in premature infants. Ocular symptoms of variable degrees from minimal vision trouble in only one eye to total vision loss. Cerebral symptoms also of variable degrees from mild symptoms of mental deficiency to cerebral agenesis.

Signs. Ocular signs range from small areas of retinal atrophy and slight structural eye anomaly to ptosis, enophthalmos, strabismus, glaucoma, microphthalmia, retinal and choroid optic nerve malformation. Microcephaly; hydrocephalus. Visceral malformations possibly associated.

Etiology. Unknown; neuroectodermal congenital defect. Autosomal recessive inheritance (?); chromosomal basis.

Pathology. Microphthalmia; retinal dysplasia of hyaloid artery, intraocular hemorrhages. Brain hyperplasia; hypoplasia and aplasia of cerebrum and cerebellum.

Therapy. Symptomatic.

Prognosis. Poor; death in early infancy or mental retardation.

BIBLIOGRAPHY. Yudkin AM: Congenital bilateral microphthalmos accompanied by other malformations of the body. Am J Ophthalmol 11:128–131, 1928

Krause AC: Congenital encephalo-ophthalmic dysplasia. Arch Ophthalmol 36:387–444, 1946

Reese AB, Blodi FC: Retinal dysplasia. Am J Ophthalmol 33:23–32, 1950

Matthes A, Stenzel K: Familiaere, encephalo-retinale Dysplasie (Krause-Reese Syndrome) mit myoklonischastatischem petit mal. Z Kinderheilk 103:81–89, 1968

KREIBIG'S

Synonym. Opticomalacia atherosclerotica.

Symptoms. Usually occur in people past middle age; onset acute. Unilateral vision disturbance, which progresses up to unilateral blindness.

Signs. Irregular narrow arteries, with wide light reflex and nicking of crossing veins. Hemorrhages (if associated with hypertension).

Etiology. Atherosclerosis.

Pathology. Degeneration of optic nerve.

Diagnostic Procedures. *Ophthalmoscopy.*

Therapy. None.

Prognosis. Progressive condition.

BIBLIOGRAPHY. Hruby K: Ueber einige neue Krankheitsbilder in der Angenheilkunde. Wien Klin Wochenschr 61:693–695, 1949

KRETSCHMER'S

Synonyms. Coma vigile; apallic syndrome; persistent vegetative state.

Symptoms. Patient is mute and immobile; eyes may follow people's movements or may be diverted by sound. Pain reflexes are present, but no emotional change accompanies them. If fed, patient swallows but does not always chew. Sleep is prolonged; arousal by normal stimuli. Catatonia may be present during recovery period.

Etiology. Diffuse bilateral degeneration of cerebral cortex, sometimes following anoxia, head injury, or encephalitis.

Diagnostic Procedure. *CT brain scan. Nuclear magnetic resonance. Angiography. Cerebral blood flow measurements. Electroencephalography. Evoked potentials.*

Therapy. According to etiology. General assistance. Levodopa and cytidine diphosphate choline seem to shorten the recovery period.

Prognosis. Poor. Variable according to etiology and entity of lesions.

BIBLIOGRAPHY. Kretschmer E: Das apallishce Syndrom. Z Ges Neurol 169:576–579, 1940

Dalle Ore G, Gerstenbrand F, Lucking CH (eds): The Apallic Syndrome. New York, Springer-Verlag, 1977

Inguar DH, Brun A, Johansson L: Survival after severe cerebral anoxia with destruction of the cerebral cortex: the apallic syndrome. In Koscin J (ed): Brain death: interrelated medical and social issues. Ann New York Acad Sci 315:184–214, 1978

Kaufman HH, Lynn J: Brain Death. Int Crit Care Digest 8:18–22, 1989

KRISHABER'S

Synonym. Cerebrocardiac.

Symptoms. Both sexes affected; predominant in females; onset at all ages. Patient complains of "empty head," vertigo, or dizziness, and insomnia.

Signs. Tachycardia. No other objective signs.

Etiology. Form of psychoneurosis. Diagnosis of exclusion after ruling out all other possibilities, especially Barré-Liéou (see).

Therapy. Psychotherapy and mild tranquilizers.

Prognosis. Difficult to cure. Possibly, conversion into other symptoms.

BIBLIOGRAPHY. Krishaber M: De la Néuropathie Cérébro-cardiaque. Paris, Masson, 1873

KRUKENBERG'S

Synonym. Ovary carcinoma mucocellulare.

Symptoms. Occur in elderly women. In early stage asymptomatic. Weight in lower abdomen; fatigue.

Signs. Ascites. Palpation in adnexal zones of abdominal masses.

Etiology. Unknown. Metastatic tumor from gastrointestinal tract or breast, occasionally of primary ovarian origin.

Pathology. Metastatic tumor of the ovary, usually bilateral. Histologically, signet ring cells (mucin pushing and flattening nucleus at periphery). Stroma areas of hypercellularity and edema.

Diagnostic Procedures. *Vaginal smear.* Presence of malignant cells. *X-ray of gastrointestinal tract.* For identification of primary tumor.

Therapy. Surgery; chemotherapy; x-rays.

Prognosis. Poor.

BIBLIOGRAPHY. Krukenberg F: Ueber das Fibrosarcom Ovarii mucocellulare (carcinomatodes). Arch Gynecol (Berlin) 50:287–321, 1896

Scully RE: Tumors of the ovary and maldeveloped gonads. Armed Forces Inst Path Fasc 16, 1979

KUESS'

Symptoms. Complaints of small-caliber stools, difficult and unsatisfactory evacuation frequently accompanied by pain or bleeding.

Etiology. Stenosis of rectum and sigmoid due to inflammatory process (e.g., fissure) or secondary to habitual use of laxatives.

Diagnostic Procedures. *Proctoscopy.*

Therapy. Cortisone and antibiotic suppository or ointment. Surgical division of fibrotic strictures usually needed; mobilization of normal epithelium to cover defect.

Prognosis. Good with treatment.

BIBLIOGRAPHY. Kuess G: Les retrécissements pseudocancéreux péricoliques pelviens. Bull Acad Natl Med 134:377–380, 1950

Sleisenger MH, Fordtran JS: Gastrointestinal Disease, p 1884. Philadelphia, WB Saunders, 1978

KUFS'

Synonyms. Adult chronic GM_2 gangliosidosis; gangliosidosis, GM_2, adult type.

Symptoms. Onset in adolescence. Progressive gait and postural deterioration; mild ataxia and dysarthria. Normal vision and intelligence. Clinical picture may be confused with Batten-Spielmeyer-Vogt.

Signs. Ascending muscular atrophy; pes cavus. Normal fundus oculi.

Etiology. Deficiency of hexosaminidase A. Autosomal recessive inheritance.

Diagnostic Procedures. *Blood, urine, spinal fluid, tissue, and cell cultures.* Assay of hexosaminidase levels.

Therapy. None.

Prognosis. Slow progression. Death within 19 or 20 years of onset.

BIBLIOGRAPHY. Kufs H: Ueber eine Spätform der amaurotishchen Idiotie und ihre heredofamiliaren Grundlagen. Z Neurol Psychiatr 95:169–188, 1925

Rapin I, Suzuki K, et al: Adult (chronic) GM_2 gangliosidosis: atypical spinocerebellar degeneration in a Jewish sibship. Arch Neurol 33:120–130, 1976

O'Brien JS: The gangliosidoses. In Stanbury JB, Wyngaarden JB, Fredrickson DS, et al: The Metabolic Basis of Inherited Disease, 5th ed, p 945. New York, McGraw-Hill, 1983

KUGELBERG-WELANDER

Synonyms. KWS; juvenile spinal muscular atrophy; Wohlfart-Kugelberg-Welander. Spinal muscular atrophy-juvenile; SM III; muscular atrophy.

Symptoms and Signs. Both sexes affected; onset in late childhood or adolescence. Weakness and atrophy of proximal muscles (muscular dystrophylike); frequently, fasciculation. Normal reflexes; sphincters seldom affected. Slow progression. Later onset and milder course distinguish it from Strümpell-Lorrain.

Etiology. Unknown; autosomal recessive (more severe in males than females), or dominant (equal severity in both sexes) inheritance.

Pathology. In muscle; neurogenic type of atrophy and hypertrophic hyalinized fibers with central nuclei. Degeneration of anterior horn cells of spinal cord and motor nuclei of brain stem and Betz cells in the cortex. Degeneration of anterior spinal roots and peripheral nerves.

Diagnostic Procedures. *Electromyography. Biopsy of muscle. Blood. Serum enzymes.* Creatine phosphokinase (CPK) normal or slight elevation.

Therapy. None.

Prognosis. Slow progression; subject can still walk 20 years after onset.

BIBLIOGRAPHY. Strümpell A: Ueber spinale, progressive, muskelatrophic und amyotrophische Seitenstrangsklerose. Dtsch Arch Klin Med 42:230–260, 1888

Wohlfart G, Fex J, Eliasson S: Hereditary proximal spinal muscular atrophy—clinical entity simulating progressive muscular dystrophy. Acta Psychiatr Neurol Scand 30:395–406, 1955

Kugelberg E, Welander L: Heredofamilial juvenile muscular atrophy simulating muscular dystrophy. Arch Neurol Psychiatr 75:500–509, 1956

Hausmanowa-Petrusewicz I, Zaremba J, et al: Chronic proximal spinal muscular atrophy of childhood and adolescence: problems of classification and genetic counseling. J Med Genet 22:350–353, 1985

KUGEL-STOLOFF

See Cardiomegaly, idiopathic. Obsolete eponym denoting onset in children in first year of life. Dyspnea; progressive cardiomegaly; cyanosis, and sudden death; no temperature elevation.

BIBLIOGRAPHY. Kugel MA, Stoloff EG: Dilatation and hypertrophy of the heart in infants and young children, with myocardial degeneration and fibrosis (so-called congenital idiopathic hypertrophy). Am J Dis Child 45:828–864, 1933

KULENKAMPFF-TORNOW

Synonyms. Cervico-linguo-masticatory; chlorpromazine toxicity; neck-face.

Symptoms and Signs. Occur in patients during first days of chlorpromazine therapy. Spasmodic contraction of neck, mouth floor, pharynx, and tongue muscles that causes speech alterations; respiratory disorders. Tachycardia and hypotension.

BIBLIOGRAPHY. Kulenkampff C, Tornow G: Ein eigentümliches Syndrom in oralen Bereich bei Magaphenapplikation. Nervenarzt 27:178–180, 1956

Antonelli F: Therapy in Psychosomatic Medicine. Rome, Pozzi, 1979

KÜMMELL'S

Synonyms. Kümmell-Verneuil; osteoporotic vertebra collapse.

Symptoms and Signs. Occur months after trauma, direct or indirect, of major or minor entity of vertebrae. Formation of gibbus and kyphosis associated or not associated with neurologic symptoms: pain; paralysis of legs; sphincter disturbances.

Etiology. Degenerative change of vertebrae following trauma.

Pathology. Rarefaction of vertebral structure without inflammatory signs and with deformation and collapse of body.

Diagnostic Procedures. *X-ray of spine. Biopsy. Myelogram. Electromyography.*

Therapy. Orthopedic correction.

Prognosis. Good.

BIBLIOGRAPHY. Kümmell H: Ueber traumatische Erkrankungen der Wirbelsäuld. Dtsch Med Wochenschr 21:180–181, 1895

Alpers BJ: Clinical Neurology, 6th ed. Philadelphia, FA Davis, 1973

Wright PE: Peripheral nerve injuries. In Crenshaw AH (ed): Campbell's Operative Orthopedics, 7th ed, pp 2791–3170. St. Louis, CV Mosby, 1987

KURTZ-SPRAGUE-WHITE

Synonym. Fallot's tetralogy—pulmonary valve absence.

Symptoms and Signs. Both sexes affected; onset in first weeks of life. Neonatal cyanosis that tends to disappear in a few weeks. Early development of right ventricular failure. Frequent respiratory distress. Emphysema, frequently marked. Right ventricular impulse conspicuous; systolic thrills common; pulmonic ejection sound; absent pulmonic component of pulmonic sound. Gap between aortic component of second sound and onset of diastolic murmur is maximal in second-third intercostal space. Loud midsystolic murmur.

Etiology. Congenital malformation.

Pathology. Absence of pulmonary valve associated with large ventricular septal defect and dilatation of pulmonary trunk and stenotic pulmonary valve ring.

Therapy. Medical or, according to severity, surgical (high risk).

Diagnostic Procedures. *Electrocardiography.* Right axis deviation greater than in classic Fallot's. *X-rays.* Marked dilatation of pulmonary trunk and its branches; right ventricle enlarged. Lungs show variable (reduced, normal, or increased) blood flow.

Prognosis. Modified by surgical correction.

BIBLIOGRAPHY. Kurtz CM, Sprague HB, White PD: Congenital heart disease: interventricular septal defects with associated anomalies in series of three cases examined post-mortem and living patient 58 years old with cyanosis and clubbing of fingers. Am Heart J 3:77–90, 1927

Hurst JW: The Heart, 6th ed, p 667. New York, McGraw-Hill, 1986

KURU

Synonym. Laughing death.

Symptoms. Restricted to the Fore tribe of eastern New Guinea; prevalent in children and adult women. Ataxia, trembling of leg muscles; incoordination spreading to the arms; exaggeration of voluntary movements; jerks; slurred speech; fecal incontinence. Finally, aphonia and dysphagia.

Signs. Ataxia; hyperreflexia. Sensory abnormalities; nystagmus and strabismus rarely associated.

Etiology. Unknown; possibly, virus affecting only members of tribe (transmitted experimentally to chimpanzees with inoculation from brain of patients); or toxic, nutri-

tional factors. It is probably common in this tribe because cannibalism is practiced.

Pathology. Changes widespread through brain; demyelinization; loss of neuron; microglia proliferation; perivascular infiltration.

Diagnostic Procedures. *Blood.* High level of globulins; all other tests normal.

Therapy. None.

Prognosis. In seventy percent of females in the tribe, death due to this condition.

BIBLIOGRAPHY. Gajdusek DC, Zigas V: Degenerative disease of the central nervous system in New Guinea. The endemic occurrence of "Kuru" in the native population. New Engl J Med 257:974–978, 1957

Gajdusek DC, Gibbs CJ, Alpes M: Experimental transmission of a Kuru-like syndrome to chimpanzees. Nature 209:794–796, 1966

Johnson RT, Meulen V: Slow infections of the nervous system. Adv Intern Med 23:353–383, 1978

KURZ'S

Eponym used to indicate a confusing condition of congenital blindness, high grade of axial hyperopia; enophthalmos; wandering eye movements. In 2nd stage, a delay of mental development becomes noticeable.

BIBLIOGRAPHY. Kurz J: Syndrom Vrozené slepoty. Cesk Oftalmol 7:377–387, 1951

KUSKOKWIM

Named for the river delta where original cases were found.

Synonym. Arthrogryposis variant. See also Guerin's.

Symptoms. Found in Alaskan Eskimos; more males than females affected. From birth, impaired movements, especially of the limbs because of joint contractures. Propensity to walk on knees or develop ducklike waddle. Normal mental development.

Signs. Multiple joint contractures affecting especially the knee and ankles; muscle atrophy or hypertrophy (compensatory). Deep tendon reflexes normal. Absent or diminished corneal reflex, may be associated pigmented nevi.

Etiology. Unknown; autosomal recessive inheritance suggested.

Pathology. Abnormal muscle attachment, involving primarily the extensor muscles.

Diagnostic Procedures. *Blood.* Normal. *Urine.* Normal. *X-ray.* Cyst formation in proximal part of long bone (occasional). *Electromyography.* Normal. *Biopsy of muscle.* Normal. *Enzyme study.* Normal.

Therapy. Standard orthopedic procedure and physiotherapy manipulation as soon as possible, at 15 to 18 months fitting with long leg braces and surgical shoes.

Prognosis. Good *quoad vitam.* Function, according to degree of lesions and treatment.

BIBLIOGRAPHY. Patjan JH, Momberg GL, Aasc J, et al: Arthrogryposis syndrome (Kuskokwim disease) in the Eskimo. JAMA 209:1481–1486, 1969

KUSSMAUL-MAIER

Synonyms. Necrotizing arteritis; nodosa panarteritis; periarteritis nodosa; polyarteritis nodosa.

Symptoms. Male to female ratio 2.4 : 1; onset at all ages. Respiratory infection (21%) or drug reaction (24%). During preceding years protean features: fever (50%); malaise; weight loss; myalgia and arthralgia; abdominal pain; anginal pain; polyneuritis (motor and sensory changes); hemiplegia; convulsion; acute brain syndrome; visual troubles.

Signs. Skin lesion (25%), polymorphic manifestation: diffuse erythema; purpura; urticaria; various types of rash; ulcers; painful, tender, occasionally pulsating, cutaneous or subcutaneous nodules; Raynaud's phenomenon (frequent); gangrene in acute cases. Blood hypertension (67%); tachycardia (out of proportion with temperature elevation), edema (50%); pericarditis; aoritis. Fundus oculi exudates; uneven caliber of vessels; retinal detachment.

Etiology. Idiopathic. Belongs to collagen disease (autoimmune) group. See also Zeek's and Strauss-Churg-Zak.

Pathology. Widespread inflammatory necrotizing panangiotis in small elastic arteries, arterioles, and veins; aneurysm formation. Ischemia and infarction of organs involved. Limited to selected organs or widespread. Renal involvement (87%). Usually, absence of vasculitis in pulmonary circulation and splenic follicular arteries (see Zeek's).

Diagnostic Procedures. *Blood.* Anemia; neutrophil leukocytosis; leukopenia in some cases; eosinophilia up to 75%; high sedimentation rate; protein increase of gamma globulin, lupus erythematosis (LE) test negative; high blood urea nitrogen. *Urine.* Albumin; red cell; casts. *Biopsy of nodules and muscles.*

Therapy. Adrenocorticotropic hormone (ACTH) or corticosteroids in high doses, then maintenance doses. Elimination of septic foci. Antibiotics (rule out sensitivity first).

Prognosis. Severe; survival variable: from fulminating cases dying in a few days, to complete recovery. Before steroid 50% spontaneous remission. If renal involvement, poor prognosis. Cutaneous variety (Lindberg's) better prognosis.

BIBLIOGRAPHY. Kussmaul A, Maier R: Ueber eine bisher nicht beschriebene eigenthumliche Arterienerkrankung (Périarteritis nodosa), die mit Morbus Brightii und rapid fortschreitender allgemeiner, Muskellähmung einhergeht. Dtsch Arch Klin Med 1:484–518, 1866
Moskowitz RW, Baggenstoss AH, Slocumb CH: Histopathologic classification of perirarteritis nodosa: a study of 56 cases confirmed at necropsy. Proc Staff Meet Mayo Clinic 38:345–357, 1963
Rook A, Wilkinson DS, Ebling FJG, et al: Textbook of Dermatology, 4th ed, pp 1171–1176. Oxford, Blackwell Scientific Publications, 1986

KWASHIORKOR–DISPLACED CHILD

Synonyms. Nutritional dystrophy; malignant malnutrition; mehlährschaden; nutritional edema; plurideficiency; polycarential.

Symptoms. Prevalent in infants and young children (rarely observed in full-blown form in adults, except as complication of alcoholism); onset after child has been weaned and kept for some time on any diet very poor in protein. Failure to grow; apathy; irritability; weak cry; diarrhea.

Signs. The child appears well nourished (because fat is still present, more or less in normal amount). Edema (that further contributes to hide muscle wasting). Skin pigmentation, desquamation, oozing areas, dryness that may give a particular aspect called "crazy pavement skin." Hair changes colors from black to brown, and then to red. If hair curly before onset, it becomes straight. Marked hepatomegaly; no tenderness of liver.

Etiology. Protein deficiency.

Pathology. Fatty liver; atrophy of pancreas; muscle wasting.

Diagnostic Procedures. *Blood.* Anemia; hypoproteinemia; all fractions, including albumin, markedly decreased.

Therapy. Milk or protein-rich preparation providing 1

to 1.5 mg/kg body weight daily. Multivitamin preparation; potassium, if depleted and good excretion observed.

Prognosis. If treated, reversal of symptoms. Fatty liver, infiltration recedes without sequelae. Lack of treatment results in death.

BIBLIOGRAPHY. Williams CD: Kwashiorkor. JAMA 153:1280–1285, 1953

Adams EB, Scragg JN, Naidoo BT, et al: Observation on the aetiology and treatment of anaemia in Kwashiorkor. Br Med J 3:451–454, 1967

Rook A, Wilkinson DS, Ebling FJG et al: Textbook of Dermatology, 4th ed, pp. 2328–2329. Oxford, Blackwell Scientific Publications, 1986

KYRLE'S

Synonym. Hyperkeratosis follicularis penetrans.

Symptoms and Signs. Age of onset 20 to 63 years; no sex difference. Bilateral, asymptomatic, chronic, scattered, generalized papular eruptions having hyperkeratotic cone-shaped plugs. Lesions may coalesce into hyperkeratotic verrucous plaques. Mucous membranes, palmar and plantar surfaces are consistently respected. Symptoms and signs of hepatic insufficiency or diabetes mellitus frequently associated.

Etiology. Unknown; association in siblings suggests heredofamilial condition. Frequent association with diabetes mellitus suggests that this syndrome belongs in the diabetic syndromes.

Pathology. Histologic criteria for diagnosis: keratotic plug filling epithelial invagination; parakeratosis in part of plug, basophilic cellular debris not staining with elastic tissue stains in the plug; epidermal disruption with keratinized cells in dermis and surrounding granuloma reaction.

Diagnostic Procedures. *Biopsy of skin.* (See Pathology.) *Blood: Glucose tolerance test, Liver function test. Urine.* Albuminuria (frequent); glycosuria.

Therapy. High doses of vitamin A. Topical keratolytics improve appearance. Topical isotretinoin. *Large lesions.* Cautery or CO_2 snow.

Prognosis. Good response to vitamin A administration after 1 month of treatment. No patients reported cured. Correction of systemic disease when associated, accompanied by clearing of Kyrle's lesions.

BIBLIOGRAPHY. Kyrle J: Hyperkeratosis follicularis et parafollicularis in cutem penetrans. Arch Dermatol Syph 123:466–493, 1916

Carter VH, Costantine VS: Kyrle's disease I. Arch Dermatol 97:624–632, 1968

Costantine VS, Carter VH: Kyrle's disease II. Arch Derm 97:633–639, 1968

Rook A, Wilkinson DS, Ebling FJG, et al: Textbook of Dermatology, 4th ed, pp 1449–1451. Oxford, Blackwell Scientific Publications, 1986

LABAND'S

Synonyms. Acrodefects–gingival fibromatosis–hepatosplenomegaly; fibromatosis gingival–abnormal fingers, nose, ears–splenomegaly.

Symptoms and Signs. Both sexes affected; present from birth. Nose and ears poorly structured; gingival fibromatosis (present at birth or appearing in first months of life); generalized hirsutism. Hypoplasia of thumb and other digits; hypoplasia or absence of nails; occasionally absence of terminal phalanges; joint hypermobility; hepatosplenomegaly (Zimmermann denies this feature). Occasionally, mental retardation.

Etiology. Possibly, autosomal dominant inheritance.

Diagnostic Procedures. *X-ray.* See Symptoms and Signs. Spina bifida occulta; 3rd thoracic vertebra may be sagittally divided and the 4th flattened.

BIBLIOGRAPHY. Zimmermann KW: Ueber Anomalien des Ektoderms (Cases 1 und 2). Vjschr Zahnh 44:419–434, 1928
Laband PF, Habib G, Humphreys OS: Hereditary gingival fibromatosis: report of an affected family with associated splenomegaly and skeletal and soft tissue abnormalities. Oral Surg 17:339–351, 1964
Gorlin JK, Pindborg JJ, Cohen MM Jr: Syndromes of the Head and Neck, 2nd ed, p 331. New York, McGraw-Hill, 1976

LABBÉ'S

Eponym used to indicate the hypertensive paroxysmal crisis in pheochromocytoma (see).

BIBLIOGRAPHY. Labbé M, et al: Crises solaires et hypertension paroxystique en rapport avec une tumeur surrénale. Bull Soc Med Hôp 46:982–990, 1922

LACTIC ACIDOSIS, IDIOPATHIC

Synonym. Idiopathic acidosis of infancy.

Includes several errors of metabolism:
1. Glycogen storage disease (type 1)
2. Pyruvate carboxylate or pyruvate dehydrogenase deficiency
3. Branched chain ketonuria (maple syrup disease)
4. Isovaleric acidemia
5. Beta-ketathiolase deficiency
6. Propionic acidemia
7. Methylmalonic acidemia

BIBLIOGRAPHY. Intensive Care World 4, no. 4 (whole issue), 1987

LACUNAR

Synonyms. Cerebral atherosclerosis; état lacunaire; lacunar state; arteriopathic dementia; multi-infarct dementia. See Pseudobulbar palsy and Binswanger's.

Symptoms. Onset usually past middle age. Mental symptoms always present. Impairment of memory for recent events; usually, vivid recall of past events; repetition of facts or repeated requests for some information in a more or less monotonous tone. Lack of grasp and storage of recent facts. Altered mental processing of facts and manifestations of paranoid tendencies that may lead to foolish acts. Headache; vertiginous attacks, or, more commonly, giddiness; occasionally, convulsions.

Signs. Several clinical syndromes may be recognized in this condition, which derives its name from anatomic-pathologic findings: homolateral cerebellar ataxia, with pyramidal tract signs; isolated hemiplegia; pure sectorial sensory stroke; the dysarthria–clumsy hand syndrome.

Etiology. Cerebral atherosclerosis or systemic hypertension or both.

Pathology. Brain microinfarctions that produce a number of lacunae (irregular cavities 0.9 to 15.0 mm in diameter) irregularly distributed in all cerebral nervous system structures. In these areas, ganglion cells are degenerated or necrotic, little increase of fibrous glial elements and microglial stimulation. Lacunae are located in the periphery of sclerosed and occluded arterioles.

Diagnostic Procedures. *Angiography.* Not necessary because clinical symptoms are so evident. *CT brain scan.* Useless, because of size of lesions.

Therapy. None; antihypertensive agents; mild sedatives; some success reported with the use of vincamine and phosphacoline.

Prognosis. Progressive mental deterioration, although in many cases with abrupt onset the situation may become stabilized and remain at the same level for years.

BIBLIOGRAPHY. Fisher CM: The arterial lesions underlying lacunes. Acta Neuropathol (Berlin) 12:1–15, 1969

LADD-GROSS

Synonym. Bile duct atresia.

Symptoms and Signs. Both sexes affected; present from birth or onset at 2 to 3 weeks of life. Jaundice of progressive intensity. Hepatosplenomegaly. Fetor hepaticus.

Etiology. Arrest of canalization of biliary ducts in fetal life.

Pathology. Lack of canalization at extrahepatic or intrahepatic level or both.

Diagnostic Procedures. *Urine.* Bilirubin increased. *Stool.* Acholic. *Blood.* Hyperbilirubinemia over 6 mg/100 ml; prothrombin time increased; alkaline phosphatases increased.

Therapy. Surgical correction (possible in 16%). Chemotherapy. Vitamin K. In patients with end-stage liver disease: liver transplantation.

Prognosis. Good with surgery. If surgery not feasible, fatal within 1 year. Longer survival with defect limited to intrahepatic region. Many patients after correction develop recurrent cholangitis. Reexploration and surgical revision may be needed.

BIBLIOGRAPHY. Ladd WE, Gross RE: Abdominal Surgery in Infancy and Childhood, pp 260–275. Philadelphia, WB Saunders, 1971
Howard ER: Extrahepatic biliary atresia: a review of current management. Br J Surg 70:193–197, 1983
Lilly JR: Biliary atresia and liver transplantation: the National Institutes of Health point of view. Pediatrics 74:159–160, 1984

LADD'S

Synonyms. Duodenal stenosis; includes Weyer's I.

Symptoms and Signs. Occur in newborn within a few hours of birth or after first feeding. Usually bilious, continuous vomiting indicates complete obstruction; distension of epigastrium; meconium may be excreted; jaundice in 30% of cases. Intermittent vomiting at variable times after birth (days, weeks, months, or years) indicates partial obstruction.

Etiology. Not well defined. In atresia, possibly autosomal recessive inheritance. In atresia or stenosis, vascular defects in embryo, lack of relief of normal temporary obstruction occurring during fetal life (6th or 7th week of embryonic development). If multiple zones of intestinal atresia, called also Weyer's I.

Diagnostic Procedures. *X-ray, plain film.* Evidence of gastric and duodenal gas distension proximal to the "double bubble" sign. Presence or absence of gas in intestinal lumen indicates partial or total obstruction; rule out extrinsic compression (annular pancreas).

Therapy. Duodenojejunostomy or gastrojejunostomy (if atresia of first part of duodenum).

Prognosis. Related to the time of intervention and, eventually, to complications.

BIBLIOGRAPHY. Ladd WE: Congenital obstruction of the duodenum in children. New Engl J Med 206:277–283, 1932
Andrass RJ, Weizman JJ, Brennan LP: Operative technique for the correction of congenital obstruction of the duodenum in the neonate. Surg Gynecol Obstet 150:247–248, 1980

LAENNEC'S

Synonyms. Alcoholic cirrhosis; fatty nutritional cirrhosis; portal liver cirrhosis; Morgagni-Laennec; portal cirrhosis; septal cirrhosis. See also Zieve's.

Symptoms. Prevalent in males. Onset insidious; becomes symptomatic usually at 50 years of age. Anorexia; fatigability; later nausea; emesis; diarrhea; abdominal pain.

Signs. Initially, progressive hepatomegaly with smooth surface; then reduction of size and firm edge becoming sharp, then nodular. Initially, liver tender on palpation; weight loss; jaundice (in two-thirds of patients) of variable degree and progression; ascites, leg edema; spider nevi; caput medusae; gynecomastia and loss of axillary and pubic hair; splenomegaly. Frequently, low-grade and continuous fever. Encephalopathy with asterixis; bleeding tendency and interstitial hemorrhages from esophageal or gastric varices.

Etiology. Direct action of ethanol on the liver plus (more important) dietary insufficiency. Increased peripheral fat mobilization; enhanced hepatic lipogenesis; decreased lipid oxidation; alterated hepatic protein production and release.

Pathology. Early, presence on the surface of gold yellow micronodules (Laennec's cirrhosis). Size variable, from 4 kg to a small hard mass. Later, increase in nodule size and appearance of scars. Early nodules are regular in size and shape, then they become irregular and "relobulized"; scar tissue distorts architecture of parenchyma. Bands of connective tissue between portal and central zones; changes in hepatic circulation, limited by neovascularization of connective tissue septae. Fat deposits; inflammatory changes; cholestasis; iron deposits.

Diagnostic Procedures. *Blood.* Sodium sulfobromophthalein retention; hyperbilirubinemia; hypoalbuminemia; hyperglobulinemia (beta and gamma); IgA and to lesser degree IgG and IgM elevated; esterified fraction of cholesterol decreased, serum glutamic-oxaloacetic transaminase (SGOT) and serum glutamic pyruvic transaminase (SGPT) and alkaline phosphatase moderately elevated. Impaired glucose tolerance. Anemia; leukocytosis. *Biopsy of liver.* See Pathology. *Liver scan.*

Therapy. Alcohol abstension; correction of diet. Silimarin: corticosteroids of little benefit. Portosystemic shunting. Vegetable protein diet; branched-chain amino acids; removal of fecal material from the colon, using oral or rectal lactulose; oral or rectal neomycin; treatment of infections; correction of electrolyte abnormalities; salt restriction; bed rest; diuretics and/or dopamine if needed. In patients with ascites refractory to medical therapy, peritoneovenous shunt (Le Veen or Denver shunt).

Prognosis. Five years survival for patients without jaundice, ascites, and hematemesis 88.9% in abstainers and in 62.8% drinkers. If mentioned signs present, 50% in abstainers and 33% in drinkers.

BIBLIOGRAPHY. Laennec RT: Traité de l'auscultation médical et des maladies du poumon et du coeur. Paris, 1819
Wright R, Alberti KGMM, Karan S, et al: Liver and biliary disease, p 735. London, WB Saunders, 1979
Orland MJ, Saltman RJ (ed): Manual of Medical Therapeutics, 25th ed, p 264. Boston, Little, Brown, 1986

LAFORA'S BODIES

Synonyms. Myoclonus epilepsy–Lafora's body; Lafora's body form–myoclonus epilepsy. See Unverricht's.

Symptoms and Signs. Onset in the 2nd decade. Progressive seizures; myoclonus; dementia; ataxia; dysarthria; visual troubles. Symptoms and signs of extrapyramidal and bulbar musculature involvement.

Etiology. Unknown; autosomal recessive inheritance. On the basis of presence of bodies considered different from Unverricht's; although it presents similar clinical features and evolution.

Pathology. Presence of Lafora bodies (bodies resembling plant starch formed by insoluble polyglucosan) in ganglion cells (substantia nigra and dentate nuclei predilected), retina, and axons of spinal nerves. Little demyelinization. Lafora's bodies presence may be demonstrated also in heart, liver, and striated muscles.

Diagnostic Procedures. *Blood.* Decreased mucoprotein content. *Electroencephalography. Muscle and liver biopsy.*

Therapy. That of Unverricht's myoclonus epilepsy.

Prognosis. Death 2 to 10 years from onset of symptoms.

BIBLIOGRAPHY. Lafora GR, Gluck G: Beitrag zur Histologie der myoklonischen Epilepsie. Z Neurol Psychiatr 6:1–14, 1911
Yokoi S, Austin J, Witmer F, et al: Studies in myoclonus epilepsy (Lafora body form). Arch Neurol 19:15–32, 1968
Noris R, Koskiniemi M: Progressive myoclonus epilepsy: genetic and nosological aspects with special reference to 107 Finnish patients. Clin Genet 15:382–398, 1979

LAGER

Synonyms. Concentration camp I; persecution victim; postdetention; survived. See also Todeserwartung.

Symptoms and Signs. Observed in victims who have survived prolonged detention in concentration camps, or mental and psychological stresses caused by persecution (hiding and fighting for survival). Chronic state of tension; alertness; irritability; depression; restlessness and timor; sleep disturbed; nightmares; cephalalgia; prostration; excessive sweating. Patients usually avoid company and in most severe cases seek complete isolation. They have a feeling of guilt because of their survival, especially when they are the only survivers of a family or a group. Frequent also are memory defects and parapraxia.

Etiology. Aftereffect of severe psychological traumas.

Prognosis. Difficult treatment and generally poor results.

BIBLIOGRAPHY. Niederland WG: Psychiatric disorder among persecution victims; a contribution to the understanding of concentration camp. Pathology and its after-effects. J Nerv Ment Dis 139:458–474, 1964

LAHEY'S

Eponym used to indicate the thyroid crisis in its two main forms: "agitating" Lahey's I (see also Waldenström's II) and "apathetic" Lahey's II (see Apathetic thyrotoxin storm).

BIBLIOGRAPHY. Lahey FH: The crisis of exophthalmic goiter. New Eng J Med 199:235–257, 1928

LAIGNEL-LAVASTINE-VIARD

Mitchell's II (see) with hypertrophy of subcutaneous fat of the lower part of the body.

BIBLIOGRAPHY. Laignel-Lavastine M, Viard M: Adipose

segmentaire des membres inférieurs. Nouv Icon Salt-pétrière 25:473–482, 1912

Rook A, Wilkinson DS, Ebling FJG: Textbook of Derma-tology, 2nd ed. Philadelphia, FA Davis, 1972

LAMBERT'S

Lambert is the name of a family affected by ichthyosis hystrix and exhibited at fairs in Suffolk, at the end of the 19th century.

Synonyms. Porcupine man. See Ichthyosis hystrix.

LAMBLING'S

Synonym. Postgastrectomy malabsorption. See also Postgastrectomy dumping syndromes.

Eponym used to indicate the symptom complex due to malabsorption appearing in variable combinations in a percentage of patients after gastrectomy: diarrhea (post-prandial); weight loss; specific nutritional deficiencies; mild anemia; bone disease; metabolic neuropathy.

BIBLIOGRAPHY. Lambling A: Syndrome carential com-plexe chez des gastrectomisés. Étude biologique. Bull Soc Med Hôp 65:161–164, 1949

Meyer JH: Chronic morbidity after ulcer surgery. In Sleisenger HM, Fortran JS (eds): Gastrointestinal dis-eases. pp 757–779. Philadelphia, WB Saunders, 1983

LANDOUZY-DEJERINE

Synonyms. Facioscapulohumeral muscular dystrophy, FSH, FSHD; muscular dystrophy, facioscapulohumeral.

Symptoms. Onset between 12 and 14 years of age, to as late as 30 to 40 years of age; males and females equally affected. First symptoms, weakness in the use of shoulder muscles (in female, noticed while combing hair). Facial weakness results in difficulty in closing the eyes, sucking through straw, blowing cheeks, whistling. Later, involve-ment of pelvic muscles and legs.

Signs. Typical pouting of lips; "ironing out" of facial expression. Scapulae winging; muscular hypertrophy very rare in this form.

Etiology. Unknown; usually autosomal dominant inher-itance, but hereditary autosomal recessive and X-linked transmission also observed. Decreased adult form of myoglobin and increased fetal form.

Pathology. Atrophic muscles; loss of striation in swol-len fibers; increased number of sarcolemma nuclei; in-crease of endomysial collagen and fat.

Diagnostic Procedures. *Electromyography.* Interference to mixed pattern. *Urine.* Slight creatinuria. *Blood.* Ele-vated serum glutamic oxaloacetic transaminase (SGOT), aldolase; decreased creatinine.

Therapy. None specific; keep the patient ambulatory; passive and active physical therapy. Treatment of cardiac condition, digitalis.

Prognosis. Normal life span, with incapacitation at late age.

BIBLIOGRAPHY. Landouzy L, Déjérine J: De la Myopathie Atrophique Progressive; Myopathie Héréditaire, sans Neuropathie, de-Butant d'Ordinaire dans l'Enfance par la Face. Paris, F Alcan, 1885

Gieron MA, Korthals JK, Kousseff BG: Facioscapulohu-meral dystrophy with cochlear hearing loss and tortu-osity of retinal vessels. Am J Med Genet 22:143–147, 1985

LANDOUZY'S I

Eponym used to indicate the secondary muscular atrophy caused by sciatica. See Cotugno's.

BIBLIOGRAPHY. Landouzy JT: De la sciatique et de l'atrophie musculair qui peut la compliquer. Arch Gen Med 25:303–325, 1875

LANE'S (J.E.)

Synonyms. Acroerythema symmetricum naeviforme; er-ythema palmare hereditarium; palmoplantar erythema; red palms.

Symptoms and Signs. Evident at birth or onset in early infancy or during adult life. Symmetric, stable, perma-nent erythema of the palms (localized especially on thenar, hypothenar eminences, and pads of fingers) and soles (talon, lateral margin of foot, and plantar surface). No signs of sympathetic excitability (changes with tem-perature or emotion). Pregnancy may cause appearance of hereditary erythema.

Etiology. Unknown; hereditary autosomal dominant condition, isolated form also observed. Mildest form of keratoderma may be considered in the group of palm and sole dyskeratosis syndromes. One family with autosomal recessive inheritance reported with associated clubfoot and dental anomalies.

Pathology. Uniform thickening of all layers of epider-mis; hyperkeratosis; but epidermis normal appearance (except for the change in color). No parakeratosis, no evidence of spongiosis or inflammation. Normal architec-ture respected; increased number of capillaries.

Therapy. None.

Prognosis. Stable, permanent; no evolving lesions; no functional troubles.

BIBLIOGRAPHY. Lane JE: Erythema palmare hereditarium (red palms). Arch Dermatol Syph 20:445–448, 1929
Poinso R, Calas E, Stahl A, et al: Le "syndrome" des paumes rouges. Presse Med 61:275–278, 1953
Montgomery, H: Dermatopathology, p. 66. New York, Hoeber, 1967
Bryan HG, Coskey RJ: Familial erythema of acral regions. Arch Dermatol 95:283–286, 1967
Rook A, Wilkinson DS, Ebling FJG, et al: Textbook of Dermatology, 4th ed, p 1431. Oxford, Blackwell Scientific Publications, 1986

LANE'S (W.A.)

Synonyms. Chronic ileal obstruction; intestinal stasis. Eponym obsolete; used to indicate the intestinal stasis resulting from congenital or acquired obstructive ileum.

BIBLIOGRAPHY. Lane WA: The kink of the ileum in chronic intestinal stasis. Nisbet, 1910

LANGE-AKEROYD

Synonyms. Hemolytic anemia–congenital Heinz body; CIBHA infuscuria; unstable hemoglobin.

Symptoms. Both sexes affected; onset from birth. Variable jaundice, cholelithiasis, and splenomegaly. Symptoms are of variable degrees of severity. Classified according to intensity of hemolysis in four groups from I (very severe hemolysis) to IV (not associated with signs of hemolysis).

Etiology. Autosomal dominant inheritance; sporadic. Presence of one type of unstable hemoglobin (Hb); (numerous variants have been identified and named according to towns where discovery has occurred, e.g., Hb Zurich, Hb Torino, Hb Saint Louis, Hb Sidney); variable clinical manifestations occur according to type of hemoglobin (see groups in Symptoms and Signs).

Pathology. Nonspecific. According to severity of form.

Diagnostic Procedures. *Hemoglobin electrophoresis.* To identify type. Presence of Heinz body in red cells of all groups; increased after splenectomy. *Blood.* Group I: Hemoglobin from below 4 g/100 ml to 8 g/100 ml; reticulocytes, hyperbilirubinemia very high. Group II: episodic hyperbilirubinemia; hemoglobin from 6 to 9 g/100 ml; reticulocytes 4% to 20%. Group III: normal hemoglobin level; reticulocytes 4% to 10%. Group IV: normal findings. Heat denaturation test; isopropanol precipitation

test. *Urine.* Groups I, II, III: dark urine. Presence of pigmenturia in almost all patients; pigment appears to be a dipyrrole related to mesobilifuscin. *Bone marrow.* Erythroid hyperplasia.

Therapy. Mildly affected patients require little therapy. Avoid sulfonamides and other oxidant drugs. Prompt treatment of infections (infections can precipitate hemolytic crisis). Blood transfusions in cases of severe anemia. Splenectomy is of little, if any, therapeutic value.

Prognosis. Unknown; only recent definition of syndrome.

BIBLIOGRAPHY. Lange RD, Akeroyd JH: CIBHA infuscuria: a new clinical syndrome. Clin Res Proc 4:234, 1946
Lange RD, Akeroyd JH: Congenital hemolytic anemia with abnormal pigment metabolism and red cell inclusion bodies: A new clinical syndrome. Blood 13:950–958, 1958
Sheehy TW: Inclusion body anemia with pigmenturia. Arch Intern Med 114:83–88, 1964
Wintrobe MM (ed): Clinical Hematology, 8th ed., p 828. Philadelphia, Lea & Febiger, 1981

LANGER-GIEDION

Synonyms. Acrodysplasia V; Klingmüller's; trichorhinophalangeal II; LG. See also Trichorhinophalangeal I.

Symptoms. Both sexes affected; present from birth. Moderate mental deficiency; recurrent respiratory infections (in first 5 years of life); growth deficiency; hypotonia; delayed speech, hyperextensible joints. Redundant skin.

Signs. Redundance of skin, nevi; scalp and body hair scarce. *Head.* Mild microcephaly; full, bushy eyebrows; large nose, less bulbous than in trichorhinophalangeal syndrome; elongated philtrum; thin upper lips; recessed mandible, protruding large ears. *Skeleton.* Multiple exostoses (for onset and distribution see Ehrenfried's); tendency to fractures.

Etiology. Unknown. Sporadic.

Diagnostic Procedures. *X-ray of skeleton.* Multiple exostoses.

Prognosis. After 5th year, good health except for tendency to fractures.

BIBLIOGRAPHY. Langer LO Jr: The thoracic-pelvic-phalangeal dystrophy. Radiology 91:447–456, 1968
Giedion A: Autosomal dominant transmissions of the tricorhino-phalangeal syndrome. Helv Pediatr Acta 28:249–259, 1973
Buhler EM, Malik NJ: The tricho-rhinophalangeal syn-

drome(s): chromosome 8 long arm deletion: is there a shortest region of overlap between reported cases? TRP I and TRP II syndromes: are they separate entities? Am J Med Genet 19:113–119, 1984

LANGER'S

Synonyms. Langer's mesomelic dwarfism; Leri-Weill homozygous dyschondrosteosis; ulna-fibula-mandible hypoplasia; mesomelic dwarfism, Langer's.

Symptoms and Signs. Present at birth. Short upper and lower limbs, especially of the middle segments. Hands and feet rarely involved. Lack of Madelung's deformity. Mandible with mesomelic micromelia. Trunk normal.

Etiology. Autosomal recessive (?) inheritance.

Pathology. Hypoplasia of ulna (minor hypoplasia of radius), fibula, and mandible.

Diagnostic Procedures. X-ray. Lack of ossification in distal half of ulna and proximal half of fibula.

BIBLIOGRAPHY. Braisford JF: Dystrophies of the skeleton. Br J Radiol 8:533–569, 1935
Langer LO Jr: Mesomelic dwarfism of the hypoplastic ulna, fibula, mandible type. Radiology 89:654–660, 1967
Goldblatt J, Wallis C, Viljoen D, et al: Heterozygous manifestations of Langer's mesomelic dysplasia. Clin Genet 31:19–24, 1987

LANGER-SALDINO

Synonyms. Achondrogenesis type Ib; Spranger's type II; pseudochondrogenesis with fractures.

Symptoms and Signs. Fewer stillbirths, longer survival and less marked features than Parenti-Fraccaro (see). *Characteristic craniofacial signs.* Prominent forehead; flat face; micrognathia. Short trunk; prominent abdomen; hydropic aspect; marked micromelia.

Etiology. Autosomal recessive inheritance.

Diagnostic Procedures. *X-ray of skeleton.* Thin ribs with multiple fractures.

BIBLIOGRAPHY. Saldino RM: Lethal short limb dwarfism: achondrogenesis and thanotophoric dwarfism. Am J Roentgen 112:185–197, 1971
Chen H, Liu CT, Yang SS: Achondrogenesis: a review with special consideration of achondrogenesis type II: Langer-Saldino. Am J Med Genet 10:379–394, 1981

LANGE-SHADE

Synonyms. Myogelosis; occupational myalgia; painful myosis.

Symptoms. Pain in one or several muscles.

Signs. Nodular change in texture of affected muscles. The nodules persist during sleep and anesthesia.

Etiology. Unknown; possibly, localized cramps due to exertion or posture. According to most authors, it cannot be distinguished from muscle cramps.

Pathology. Biopsy of nodules does not show microscopic abnormalities or shows only minor changes of doubtful significance.

Diagnostic Procedures. *Electromyography.*

Therapy. Rest and massage.

Prognosis. Good.

BIBLIOGRAPHY. Lange M: Die Muskelhaerten (Myogelosen). Munich, Lehmann, 1931
Jordon HH: Myogeloses: the significance of pathologic conditions of musculature in disorders of posture and locomotion. Arch Phys Ther 23:36–41, 1942
Adams RD, Victor M: Principles of Neurology, 3rd ed, p 1097. New York, McGraw-Hill, 1985

LANZIERI'S

Synonym. Craniofacial malformation–dwarfism–fibula absence.

Symptoms and Signs. Present from birth. Dwarfism. *Head.* Dyscephalia; microphthalmia; anophthalmia; congenital cataracts; coloboma (iris and optic nerve); dental anomalies. *Skin.* Atrophic changes; hypertrichosis. *Skeleton.* Absence of fibula and some tarsal and metatarsal bones.

Etiology. Unknown. Developmental anomaly.

BIBLIOGRAPHY. Lanzieri M: Su una rara associazione di una sindrome malformativa cranio facciale e assenza congenita della fibula. Ann Ital Clin Ocul 87:667–673, 1961

LARON'S

Synonyms. Dwarfism Laron; GH-resistance. See Seabright-Bantam.

Symptoms and Signs. Children from Middle East born of consanguineous unions. Dwarfism.

Etiology. Autosomal recessive. Anomalies of growth hormone (GH) receptor or postreceptor defect.

Diagnostic Procedures. Elevated GH concentration; exaggerated GH response to stimuli; no response to exogenous human (pituitary) growth hormone (h-GH); serum somatomedin low.

BIBLIOGRAPHY. Laron Z, Pertzelan A, Mannheimer S: Genetic pituitary dwarfism with high serum concentration of growth hormone: a new inborn error of metabolism? Isr J Med Sci 2:152–155, 1966
Eshet R, Laron Z, Pertzelan A, et al: Defect of human growth hormone receptors in the liver of two patients with Laron-type dwarfism. Isr J Med Sci 20:8–11, 1984

LARSEN-JOHANSSON

Synonyms. Patellar chondropathy; osteochondritis patellae; chondromalacia patellae; Sinding-Larsen.

Symptoms and Signs. Prevalent in boys in early teenage years. Pain and tenderness over inferior pole of patella. Limping; pain on flexion and slight swelling at area of tenderness.

Etiology. Inflammation of a secondary or accessory center of calcification of patella (accessory center present in 3% of cases, in most cases remaining asymptomatic). Trauma or vascular disturbance considered important factor in initiating the osteochondritic process. Occasionally, autosomal dominant inheritance (male-to-male transmission).

Pathology. Synovial thickening; effusion; cartilage gray or yellow, fissured and flaking; loose bodies.

Diagnostic Procedure. X-ray.

Therapy. Rest; reassurance; immobilization seldom required. Testosterone to accelerate ossification.

Prognosis. Mild course. Recovery.

BIBLIOGRAPHY. Sinding-Larsen CMF: A hitherto unknown affection of the patella in children. Acta Radiol 1:171–173, 1921
Johansson S: En foerut icke beskriven sjnkdom i patella. Hygiea 84:161–166, 1922
Lopez R, Lewis H: Larsen-Johansson disease: osteochondritis of the accessory ossification center of the patella. Clin Pediatr 7:697–700, 1968

LARSEN'S

Synonyms. Flat facies–short fingernails–multiple joint dislocation; dish face; McFarland's.

Symptoms. Prevalent in females. Mentally normal; occasionally, respiratory difficulty at young age.

Signs. *Facies.* Flat; depressed nasal bridge; bossed forehead; hypertelorism. *Joints.* Bilateral dislocation of tibia and femur, elbows, and hip; feet equinovalgus or equinovarus. *Fingers.* Long and cylindrical; spatulate thumbs. Short metacarpals. Occasionally associated, palatoschisis (50%); teeth abnormalities, abnormal vertebral segmentation, congenital cardiac defects, hydrocephalus, laryngotracheomalacia.

Etiology. Unknown; autosomal recessive (probably); in some families possibly dominant.

BIBLIOGRAPHY. McFarland BL: Congenital dislocation of the knee. J Bone Joint Surg II:281–285, 1929
Larsen LJ, Schottstaedt ER, Bost FC: Multiple congenital dislocations associated with characteristic facial abnormality. J Pediatr 37:574–581, 1950
Houston CS, Reed MH, Desansch JEL: Separating Larsen's syndrome from the "arthrogryposis basket." J Can Assoc Radiol 32:206–214, 1981

LARVA VISCERAL MIGRANS

Synonyms. Eosinophilia-hepatomegaly.   See   Eosinophilic lung, secondary; toxocariasis.

Symptoms. Occur in children, predominantly in boys. Pica; cough; wheezing; fever; convulsions; vision impairment (in order of frequency).

Signs. Hepatomegaly; pulmonary rales or wheezes; malnutrition; skin lesions; lymphadenopathy; eye ground lesion (in order of frequency).

Etiology. Visceral infiltration with larvae of *Toxocara canis* or *T. cati*. *Capillaria hepatica, Ascaris suis, A. hominis,* and *Strongyloides* may also produce this syndrome.

Pathology. Hepatic and cerebral infestation with parasites. Eosinophilic granulomas with necrotic centers containing larvae; lymphoplasmocytic and giant cell halo.

Diagnostic Procedures. *Blood.* Hypochromic anemia; leukocytosis; chronic peripheral blood and bone marrow eosinophilia (over 30%); hypoalbuminemia; increase gamma globulins and IgM globulin. Precipitating antibodies to A and B blood group substances or helminth antigens or both. Isohemoagglutinin titers elevated; sheep cell agglutination titers slightly elevated; presence of heat-stable antiglobulins. *Biopsy of liver.* Presence of larvae. *X-ray of chest.* Bilateral peribronchial infiltration. *Stool.* Presence of intestinal parasites.

Therapy. No specific treatment. Trials with thiabendazole, levamisole, mebendazole. *Symptomatic.* Cortisone antibiotics, analgesics, antihistamines.

Prognosis. Depends on spread of infestation and specific organ involvement (e.g., brain, eyes). Usually clears in 1 to 2 years.

BIBLIOGRAPHY. Beaver PC, Snyder CH, Carrera GM, et al: Chronic eosinophilia due to visceral larva migrans, report of 3 cases. Pediatrics 9:7–19, 1952

Danis P, Parmentier N, Maurus R, et al: Syndrome de "visceral larva migrans" et atteinte oculaire. Bull Soc Belge Ophthalmol 144:899–908, 1966

Fraser RG, Paré JAP: Diagnosis of Diseases of the Chest, 2nd ed, p 876. Philadelphia, WB Saunders, 1977

Molk R: Ocular toxocariasis: a review of literature. Ann Ophthal 15:216–219, 1983

Bekhti A: Mebendazole in toxocariasis. Ann Int Med 100:463, 1984

LARYNGEAL NEURALGIA, SUPERIOR

Symptoms. Severe, lancinating paroxysmal pain of larynx, usually localized to small area over hypothyroid membrane.

Etiology. Unknown.

BIBLIOGRAPHY. Smith LA, Moersch HJ, Love JG: Superior laryngeal neuralgia. Proc Staff Meet Mayo Clin 16:164–167, 1941

LASEGUE-FALRET

Synonyms. Association psychosis; double insanity; folie a deux; folie communiquée.

Symptoms and Signs. Prevalent among women living more or less confined. (1) Coincidental appearance of psychotic symptoms in members of a family while living together; (2) appearance of psychotic symptoms in two closely associated persons and retention of symptoms once initiated, in spite of separation; (3) transmission of psychotic symptoms from a sick person to one person or several healthy individuals who elaborate on the induced delusions.

Etiology. Unknown; hereditary factors frequently involved.

Therapy. Separation frequently results in recovery of the secondary (usually less affected) person. Psychiatric treatment for primarily affected one.

BIBLIOGRAPHY. Lasègue C, Falret J: La Folie à deux ou folie communiquée. Ann Med Psychol 18:321–355, 1877

Freedman AM, Kaplan HI, Sadock BJ: Comprehensive Textbook of Psychiatry, 2nd ed, p 1725. Baltimore, Williams & Wilkins, 1975

LASEGUE'S I

Synonym. Persecution mania.

Symptoms and Signs. Delusion of being persecuted by a particular person, by groups of people (e.g., police; army; organized groups), or by everybody. Manifestation may vary from a feeling of unexpressed discomfort to complaints limited to relatives, friends, doctors, or public authorities with minor or major emphasis or violence. Reaction may vary from aggression to suicide.

Etiology. Unknown.

Therapy. Psychotherapy and pharmacotherapy.

Prognosis. Variable. Tendency to chronicity or conversion to other psychotic delusions.

BIBLIOGRAPHY. Lasègue CE: Du Délire des Persécutions. Arch Gen Med (Paris) 28:129–159, 1852

Freedman AM, Kaplan HI, Sadock BJ: Comprehensive Textbook of Psychiatry, 2nd ed, p 793. Baltimore, Williams & Wilkins, 1975

LASEGUE'S II

Synonyms. Amblyopic hysteric paralysis. See Briquet's.

Symptoms. Prevalent in females. Anesthesia and paralysis of an extremity appearing when the patient closes eyes. Accompanied by other hysterical symptoms.

Signs. Reflexes normal; the patient can move and feel as long as the part involved can be seen.

Etiology. Unknown.

Therapy. Psychotherapy.

Prognosis. Good recovery; relapse possible or substitution of other hysteric manifestation.

BIBLIOGRAPHY. Lasègue C: Anesthésie et ataxie hystériques. Arch Gen Med (Paris) 3:385–402, 1864

Lasègue C: Des hysteriques périphériques. Arch Gen Med (Paris) 1:641–656, 1878

Freedman AM, Kaplan HI, Sadock BJ: Comprehensive Textbook of Psychiatry, 2nd ed. Baltimore, Williams & Wilkins, 1975

LASSUER–GRAHAM-LITTLE

Synonyms. Brocq's pseudopelade; Graham-Little's; folliculitis decalvans et atrophicans; lichen planopilaris; Piccardi's.

Symptoms and Signs. Cicatricial alopecia of scalp, trunk, and limbs; follicular plugging and keratosis pilaris.

Occasionally, alopecia of axillae, pubes, and trunk. Prevalent in females, age range 30 to 70.

Etiology. Unknown. Distinctive syndrome, suggestion of relationship with lichen planopilaris.

Pathology. Destruction of follicles. No scarring.

Diagnostic Procedures. *Skin biopsy. Immunofluorescence studies.*

Therapy. None. Keratolytics.

BIBLIOGRAPHY. Brocq L: Alopecia. J Cutan Venereol Dis 3:49–51, 1885

Piccardi G: Cheratosi spinulosa del capillizio e suoi rapporti con la pseudo-pelada di Brocq. Gior Ital Malad Vener Pelle 35:416–422, 1914

Graham-Little EG: Folliculitis decalvans et Atrophicans. Brit J Dermatol 27:183–185, 1915

Horn RT Jr, Goette DK, Odom RB, et al: Immunofluorescent finding and clinical overlap in two cases of follicular lichen planus. J Am Acad Dermatol 7:203–207, 1982

LATAH

Symptoms. Mostly observed in Malaysian people, predominantly in women. Patterns of manifestation: (1) Following a sudden stimulus, all normal activities stop and inappropriate uncontrollable motor and verbal manifestations occur. (2) Following a sudden stimulus, person exhibits a complete echolalia, echopraxia, and automatic obedience. The person remains aware of situation, but in spite of his protestation against unacceptable actions, performs them as commanded.

Etiology. Disorganization of ego and ego boundaries following sudden fright.

Therapy. Psychotherapy; tranquilizers. If associated with chronic mental disorders, pharmacotherapy and electroconvulsive therapy may be indicated.

Prognosis. If it becomes chronic, leads to automatic obedience and echo reaction with severe personality deterioration.

BIBLIOGRAPHY. Yap PM: The latah reaction: its pathodynamics and nosological position. J Ment Sic 98:515–564, 1952

Freedman AM, Kaplan HI, Sadock BJ: Comprehensive Textbook of Psychiatry, 2nd ed. Baltimore, Williams & Wilkins, 1975

LATERAL SINUS THROMBOSIS

Synonym. Sigmoid sinus thrombosis.

Symptoms. Children more frequently affected than adults; onset acute or secondary to chronic otitic infections. Fever; pain behind the eye; temporal headache; nausea; vomiting; muscle palsies; possible lesions of glossopharyngeal (IX), vagus (X), spinal accessory (XI) nerves (involvement of jugular bulb). Occasionally, swelling over mastoid region; tenderness of homolateral jugular vein; symptoms and signs of intracranial hypertension. Papilledema (50%). Seldom, seizures and hemiplegia.

Etiology. Any microorganism may be responsible for infection and secondary thrombosis.

Pathology. Thrombosis of lateral sinus and venous congestion of perimastoid area.

Diagnostic Procedures. *Cerebrospinal fluid.* Cloudy; leucocytes, proteins, and pressure increased. Tobey-Ayer test negative on affected side. Queckenstedt sign on affected side. *Blood.* Leukocytosis; culture positive in 50% of cases. *X-ray. Angiography. CT brain scan.*

Therapy. Antibiotics. Thrombolytics. Surgery if indicated.

Prognosis. High mortality without treatment.

BIBLIOGRAPHY. Goldberg RA: Lateral sinus thrombosis: medical or surgical treatment? Arch Otolaryngol 3:56–58, 1985

LATHYRISM

Synonym. Neurolathyrism.

Symptoms. Prevalent in males, in persons who consume large amounts of *Lathyrus* peas; onset sudden, preceded by exposure to cold or dampness. On awakening, pain in lumbar region, weakness of legs, slight fever (occasionally), paresthesias, weakness progressing slowly to spastic paralysis; then loss of control of bladder and rectum and impotence. Arms may successively become involved. Later, loss of sensation to pain and thermal changes.

Signs. Tendon hyperreflexia; Babinski's sign.

Etiology. Toxic effect of *Lathyrus* peas. In some cases, nutritional deficiences may result in this syndrome (lathyrismlike syndrome).

Pathology. Sclerosis of anteroposterior part of spinal cord.

Diagnostic Procedures. *Spinal tap. Electromyography. Biopsy of muscle. Chemical analysis.* Identification of the gamma L-glutamyl-L-beta-cyanoalanine and of the beta-cyanoalanine that may be responsible for the toxicity.

Therapy. Stop ingestion of peas.

Prognosis. Neural lesions permanent.

BIBLIOGRAPHY. Minchin R: Primary lateral sclerosis of South India. Lathyrism without lathyrus. Br Med J 1:253–255, 1940

Gopalan C: Lathyrism syndrome. Trans Roy Soc Trop Med Hyg 44:333–338, 1950

Jouglard J: Intoxications d'origine vegetale. In Encyclopédie médico-chirurgicale, Vol 2. Paris, Laffont et Durieux, 1977

Arya LS, Qurescima, Jabor A, Singh M: Lathyrism in Afghanistan. Indian J Pediatr 55:440–442, 1988

LATISSIMUS DORSI

Symptoms. Pain in lower back and lower extremities (sclerotomes of second lumbar and first sacral nerves) with occasionally associated pain of upper back, shoulder, upper extremities, neck, and chest.

Signs. Diagnostic injection of local anesthetic on the lumbodorsal fascia produces remission of pain within minutes.

Etiology. Irritation of sensory fibers in aponeurosis of latissimus dorsi muscle due to fibrosis of subfascial fat, adhesion of tissue to fascia, and defect of the fascia.

Diagnostic Procedures. See Signs. *X-ray of spine.*

Therapy. Resection portion of aponeurosis of latissimus dorsi (narrow strip that arises from lumbodorsal fascia).

Prognosis. Good with treatment.

BIBLIOGRAPHY. Copeman WSC, Ackerman WL: Edema or herniations of fat lobules as a cause of lumbar and gluteal "fibrositis." Arch Intern Med 79:22–35, 1947

Dittrich RJ: The latissimus dorsi syndrome. Ohio Med J 51:973–975, 1955

LAUBER'S

Synonyms. Stationary retinitis punctata albescens; fundus albipunctatus hemeralopia. See also Punctata albescens, progressive.

Symptoms. Both sexes affected. Static or slowly progressing hemeralopia.

Signs. Minute white spots scattered on all retinal area, with some concentration at the posterior pole.

Etiology. Unknown; both autosomal recessive and dominant inheritance have been proposed.

BIBLIOGRAPHY. Lauber H: Die sogenannte Retinitis punctata albescens. Klin Monatsbl Augenheilkd 48:133–148, 1910

Krill AE: Hereditary Retinal and Choroidal Disease: Flecked Retina Diseases, vol. 2, pp 739–819. Hagerstown, MD, Harper & Row, 1977

LAUBRY-PEZZI

Synonym. Aortic valve regurgitation–ventricular septal defect.

Symptoms. Male-to-female ratio 2 : 1; onset of symptoms in childhood, between 2 and 10 years of age. Pulsation in the neck; precordial movements especially when lying on left side. Eventually, chest pain, diaphoresis, sudden death.

Signs. Good general development and normal health during first years of life. Bounding water-hammer pulse; capillary pulsation (nails); head shocks; left ventricular pulsation; holosystolic and early diastolic murmurs. Cardiomegaly.

Etiology. Congenital heart defect.

Pathology. Supracristal ventricular defect and fault in aortic valve leaflet support, or infracristal ventricular defect and above mentioned aortic valve lesion. Infundibular pulmonic stenosis occasionally coexisting.

Diagnostic Procedures. *Electrocardiography.* Left ventricular hypertrophy of marked degree. *X-ray.* Disproportion between large left ventricle and aspect of pulmonary trunk and vasculature. Aorta prominent. *Echocardiography, cardiac catheterization. Angiography.*

Therapy. Prevention of bacterial endocarditis. Surgical correction.

Prognosis. Slowly developing clinical pattern. Survival into adulthood possible; cardiac failure develops and is cause of death. Accelerated course in case of complicating subacute bacterial endocarditis.

BIBLIOGRAPHY. Laubry C, Pezzi C: Traite de Maladies Congenitales de Coeur. Paris, JB Baillière et Fils, 1921

Perloff JK: The Clinical Recognition of Congenital Heart Disease, 2nd ed, p 421. Philadelphia, WB Saunders, 1978

Hurst JW: The Heart, 6th ed, pp 591, 595, 741. New York, McGraw-Hill, 1986

LAUNOIS

Synonyms. Acromegaloid gigantism; pituitary gigantism; fractional hypopituitarism-gigantism; Neurath-Cushing.

Symptoms. Onset in adolescents who show retarded skeletal growth, delayed puberty, muscle weakness.

Headache; perspiration; joint pain. At approximately 18 to 20 years of age abnormal growth starts and continues until 27 to 30 years of age. Possibly, mental retardation.

Signs. Pallor; smooth skin; youthful appearance; broad face; scanty facial and body hair; small penis and testes; eunuchoid aspect; high-pitched voice; large limbs, hands, and feet; slipped epiphysis. In one case, hypothyroidism and hypoadrenalism.

Etiology. Idiopathic or due to chromophobe adenoma; craniopharyngioma with diminished production of gonadotropic hormones and occasionally thyroid-stimulating hormone (TSH) and adrenocorticotropic hormone (ACTH). Increase of secretion of growth hormone.

Diagnostic Procedures. *Blood.* Determination of gonadotropins, 17-ketosteroids, 11-desoxicortisol metabolites, protein-bound iodine. Thyroidal ^{131}I uptake. *X-ray.* Sella turcica normal or signs of tumor; bone age determination.

Therapy. Correction of hormonal deficiency. If tumor, surgery, X-ray radiation, or radium implantation.

Prognosis. Determined by etiology and time of diagnosis.

BIBLIOGRAPHY. Launois PE, Roy P: Études biologiques sur les Géants, p 50. Paris, Masson, 1904
Goldman JK, Cahill GF Jr, Thorn GW: Gigantism with hypopituitarism. Am J Med 34:407–416, 1963
Sarver ME, Sabeh G, Fetterman GH et al: Fractional hypopituitarism with gigantism and normal sella turcica. New Engl J Med 271:1286–1289, 1964
Williams RH: Textbook of Endocrinology, 5th ed. Philadelphia, WB Saunders, 1974
Malarkey WB: The pituitary and hypothalamus. In Mazzaferri EL: Textbook of Endocrinology, pp 55–58. New York, Medical Examination Publishing, 1985

LAURENCE-MOON

Synonym. Incorrectly called Laurence-Moon-Bardet-Biedl. See Bardet-Biedl.

Symptoms. Twice as frequent in males; onset in childhood. Mental deficiency. Initially, problem of night vision; then central vision and then peripheral vision loss progressing to blindness. Spastic paraplegia.

Signs. All or only some of the characteristic features may be present: hypogenitalism; pigmentary degeneration of retina; cataract; strabismus; microphthalmia; body hair scanty or absent. In male, pseudogynecomastia, azoospermia. In female, amenorrhea, lack of breast development.

Etiology. Unknown; single recessive autosomal gene, or two genes in same chromosome, acting early in embryo-

logic life producing secondary manifestations according to variable degrees of penetrance.

Pathology. Most remarkable lesions observed in kidney (chronic glomerulonephritis or hydronephrosis), pituitary, testicles, eyes (retinitis pigmentosa); features of secondary hypogenitalism.

Diagnostic Procedures. *Electroretinography. Hormonal studies. Chromosome studies.*

Therapy. None.

Prognosis. Usually fatal at early age with infection. If adulthood reached, eye lesions progress to blindness at 20 years of age (73%); other signs stay stationary. A great proportion of the patients with this syndrome have significant renal abnormalities with risk of progression to renal insufficiency.

BIBLIOGRAPHY. Laurence JZ, Moon RC: Four cases of "retinitis pigmentosa," occurring in the same family, and accompanied by general imperfections of development. Ophthalmol Rev 2:32–41, 1866
Biedl A: Retinitis pigmentosa: Ein Geschwisterpaar mit adiposogenitaler Dystrophie. Dtsch Med Wochenschr 48:1630, 1922
Linné T, Wikstad I, Zetterström R: Renal involvement in the Laurence-Moon-Biedl syndrome. Acta Paediatr Scand 75:240–244, 1986
Cheng IKP, Chan KW, Chan MK, et al: Glomerulopathy of Laurence-Moon-Biedl syndrome. Postgrad Med J 64:621–625, 1988
Williams B, Jenkins D, Walls J: Chronic renal failure: an important feature of the Laurence-Moon-Biedl syndrome. Postgrad Med J 64:462–464, 1988

LAWRENCE-SEIP

Synonyms. Berardinelli-Seip; generalized lipodystrophy; lipoatrophic diabetes; lipodystrophy-gigantism; lipohistiodieresis; Seip's. See Sotos'.

Symptoms. Onset in both sexes; prevalent in females (2 : 1); apparent at birth or developing later. Mental retardation. Diabetic symptoms eventually appear.

Signs. *In children.* Increased stature; generalized fat loss; patients appear wasted and prematurely aged; pigmentation; hirsutism; prominence of muscles; hepatomegaly; genital enlargement (male: penis; female: clitoris without other sign of virilization); umbilical hernia; cardiac enlargement (not constant). *In adults.* Normal or slightly elevated stature; muscle and abdominal prominence not too evident; hepatomegaly; cardiac enlargement (not constant); hypertension. Acanthosis nigricans.

Etiology. Autosomal recessive inheritance. Secretion of

abnormal pituitary hormone with melanotrophic and growth hormone properties.

Pathology. Lack of subcutaneous fat; retained normal skin elasticity; hirsutism; scalp hair abundant and often curly; pigmentation. Hepatomegaly; periportal foci of round cell infiltration; nuclear syncytial formation; fatty infiltration; glycogen deposition; fibrosis. Kidney frequently enlarged; features of glomerulonephritis.

Diagnostic Procedures. *Blood.* Hyperglycemia (without ketosis, and insulin-resistant). Insulinlike activity of blood increased. Hyperlipemia (mostly, elevation of triglycerides). Basal metabolic rate increased. Serum colloidal lability affected. *Urine.* Albumin; casts. *X-ray.* Children show advanced bone age in relation to chronologic age. Cardiac enlargement. *Pneumoencephalography.* In some cases, ventricular dilatation (these cases may represent cerebral gigantism in childhood). *Bone marrow.* Absence of fat. *Biopsy of liver.* Fatty vacuolization (see Pathology).

Therapy. Treatment of diabetes. Hypophysectomy.

Prognosis. Renal disease or hepatic failure frequent causes of death. Improvement with hypophysectomy.

BIBLIOGRAPHY. Lawrence RD: Lipodystrophy and hepatomegaly with diabetes, lipaemia, and other metabolic disturbances; a case throwing new light on the action of insulin. Lancet I:724; 773–775, 1946
Berardinelli W: An undiagnosed endocrinometabolic syndrome: report of two cases. J Clin Endocrinol Metab 14:193–204, 1954
Seip M: Lipodystrophy and gigantism with associated endocrine manifestations; a new diencephalic syndrome? Acta Paediatr 48:555–574, 1959
Dorasamy DS: Congenital lipodystrophy: a case report. South Afr Med 58:417–420, 1980

LAZZARONI-FOSSATI

Synonym. Fibrochondrogenesis.

Symptoms and Signs. Rare. Both sexes. From birth. Chondrodysplasia rhizomelic (dwarfism).

Etiology. Sporadic and autosomal recessive inheritance.

Pathology. Cartilage: Characteristic interwoven fibrous septa and fibroblastic dysplasia.

Diagnostic Procedure. *X-ray of skeleton.* Broad long-bone metaphyses; pear-shaped vertebral bodies.

Prognosis. Neonatal death.

BIBLIOGRAPHY. Lazzaroni-Fossati F, Stanescu V, Stanescu R, et al: La fibrochondrogenese. Arch Fr Pediatr 35:1016–1104, 1978

Eteson DJ, Adomian GE, Ornoy A, et al: Fibrochondrogenesis: radiologic and histologic studies. Am J Med Genet 19:277–290, 1984

LAZY LEUKOCYTE

Symptoms and Signs. Both sexes affected; onset in early childhood. Recurrent stomatitis, gingivitis, and various infections.

Etiology. Deficiency of response of granulocytes to chemotactic stimuli, believed to be related to a structural/functional abnormality of actomycinlike microfilaments of cytoplasma.

Diagnostic Procedures. *Blood.* Neutropenia; few granulocytes released into blood after endotoxin injection. Random mobility, phagocytic activity, opsonin activity, complement-mediated chemotaxis: normal. *Bone marrow.* Normal number of mature neutrophils.

BIBLIOGRAPHY. Miller ME, Oski FA, Harris MB: Lazy leukocyte syndrome: a new disorder of neutrophil function. Lancet I:665–669, 1971
Goldman JM, Foroozanfar N, Gazzard BG, et al: Lazy leukocyte syndrome. J Roy Soc Med 77:140–141, 1984

LEAKING DUODENAL STUMP

Symptoms. Onset 3 to 6 days after gastric resection. Severe, constant pain in the right upper abdomen, initially remaining localized. If condition not recognized, peritonitis spreading slowly. Eventually, abscess or fistula develops.

Signs. Tenderness and moderate muscle spasm; progressive rise of pulse and temperature.

Etiology. Leaking duodenal stump.

Therapy. Prompt surgical treatment.

Prognosis. If not recognized, mortality 85%.

BIBLIOGRAPHY. Larsen BB, Foreman RC: Syndrome of leaking duodenal stump. Arch Surg 63:480–485, 1951
Woodward ER: The blown duodenal stump: an avoidable complication. Arch Surg 115:693, 1980

LEBER'S I

Synonyms. Hereditary optic neuritis; optic atrophy, Leber's; neuroretinopathy.

Symptoms. Occurs usually in males; acute onset usually between 15 and 25 years of age (in Europe). Unilateral or bilateral visual loss; affecting primarily central vision. Association with hereditary-familial ataxia frequent.

Signs. At onset, optic disk normal or swelling of optic (II) nerve head; later, atrophy of disks. Signs of widespread central nervous system damage may be associated (protean clinical manifestations).

Etiology. Unknown; possibly, sex-linked recessive. Possibly a toxic metabolic disorder, or an abnormality of cyanide metabolism, or related to smoking. Cytoplasmic inheritance and vertical transmission of an infectious agent (a slow virus) have also been considered.

Pathology. Neuronal degeneration of the retina and optic (II) nerve with secondary degenerative changes of optic system, except for calcarine cortex.

Diagnostic Procedures. *Neurologic examination. Spinal fluid. Urine. Culture.*

Therapy. Avoiding exposure to cyanide is theoretically advisable: no smoking; prevention and treatment of infection, particularly urinary (formation of cyanide by *Escherichia coli, Pseudomonas pyocyanea*). Hydroxocobalamin in massive doses; sodium thiosulfate (both yet untried).

Prognosis. Marked visual loss.

BIBLIOGRAPHY. Leber T: Beitrage zur Kenntniss der Atrophischen Veranderungen des Sehnerven nebst Bemerkungen uber die normale Structur des Nerven. Arch Ophthalmol 14:164–176, 1868
Adams JH, Blackwood W, Wilson J: Further clinical and pathological observation on Leber's optic atrophy. Brain 89:15–26, 1966
Nikoskelainen E, Hassinen IE, Palijarvi L, et al: New aspects of the genetic, etiologic, and clinical puzzle of Leber's disease. Neurology 34:1482–1484, 1984

LEBER'S II

Synonyms. Congenital amaurosis; neuroepithelial dysgenesis of retina; congenital amaurosis I and II; congenital retinal blindness (CRB). See Alstroem's-Olsen.

Symptoms. Both sexes affected; may be present at birth, but usually onset between 15 and 30 (most frequent in younger years). Decreased visual acuity; mental retardation.

Signs. Microcephaly; mongoloidlike face; oculodigital reflex. Nystagmus of various types, keratoconus (20–40%). Initially, normal appearing retina, then narrowing of retinal arteries (67%). Macular lesions, "salt and pepper"; retinal pigment changes or "bone corpuscle."

Etiology. Autosomal recessive inheritance. Two types of amaurosis congenita have been described. Type I limited to the eye, and type II with possible associated mental disorders. Both have autosomal recessive inheritance.

Diagnostic Procedure. *Electroretinography.* Extinguished or decreased response.

Therapy. None.

Prognosis. Progressive visual loss.

BIBLIOGRAPHY. Leber T: Ueber Retinitis pigmentosa und angeborene Amaurose. Arch Ophthalmol 15:1–25, 1869
Leber T: Ueber hereditare und kongenitalangelegte Sehennervenleiden. Arch Ophthalmol 17:249–291, 1871
Godel V: Congenital Leber's amaurosis, keratoconus and mental retardation in familial juvenile nephrophthisis. J Ped Ophthalmol Strabismus 15:89–91, 1978
Nickel B, Houyt CS: Leber's congenital amaurosis: is mental retardation a frequent associated defect? Arch Ophthalmol 100:1089–1092, 1982

LEDDERHOSE'S

Synonym. Plantar fibromatosis.

Symptoms. Both sexes affected; onset usually in young age. Asymptomatic; then pain on walking.

Signs. Multiple fibrous nodules, adherent to the plantar aponeurosis, localized in the medial region of the plantar arch. In some cases, nodules cause retraction of the tendons of last four toes (hammer toes).

Etiology. Unknown. Frequent association with other varieties of fibromatosis suggests a common etiology. Familial occurrence (hereditary pattern not yet established).

Pathology. In different areas formation of bands of connective tissue with variable cellular density and discrete hyaline component. In some areas, polymorphic nuclei with hyperchromic scarce mitotic figures.

BIBLIOGRAPHY. Ledderhose G: Ueber Zerreisungen der Plantarfascie (Langenbeeks). Arch Klin Chir 48:853–856, 1894
Terragni R, Zuccoli E: Su un caso di malattia di Ledderhose bilaterale associata a noduli interfalangei alle mani. Gazz San 44:298–304, 1974

LEFT CORONARY ARTERY ARISING FROM PULMONARY ARTERY

Symptoms and Signs. *Phase 1.* Neonatal. Infant appears normal at birth and for a short time afterward. *Phase 2.* Transitory. Death or survival according to development of adequate intercoronary anastomosis. Distress; myocardial ischemia symptoms and signs. *Phase 3.* Progressive improvement of symptoms and signs of ischemia. Frequently, dilatation of left side of heart and secondary mitral insufficiency. In later period arrhythmias. *Phase 4.* Coronary artery steal syndrome (see).

Etiology. Congenital malformation where the left coronary artery arises from pulmonary artery.

Pathology. Myocardial ischemic changes. If patient survives second phase, abundant collateral circulation.

Diagnostic Procedures. *Electrocardiography. Cardiac catheterization. Cinecardioangiography. X-ray of chest.*

Therapy. If adequate collateral circulation is demonstrated, ligation of anomalous artery at its origin. If collateral circulation inadequate, vascular graft from aorta to the left coronary artery.

Prognosis. Second phase is most dangerous period; death from acute myocardial ischemia. In third phase, death from fatal arrhythmia.

BIBLIOGRAPHY. Brooks H St J: Two cases of an abnormal coronary artery of the heart arising from the pulmonary artery: with some remarks upon the effects of this anomaly in producing cirsoid dilatation of vessels. Trans Acad Med Ireland (Dubl) 3:447–449, 1885

Bane AE, Baum S, Blakemore WS, et al: A later stage of anomalous coronary circulation with origin of the left coronary artery from the pulmonary artery; coronary artery steal. Circulation 36:878–885, 1967

Perloff JK: The Clinical Recognition of Congenital Heart Disease, 2nd ed, p 561. Philadelphia, WB Saunders, 1978

LEGAL'S

Synonyms. Cephalalgia pharyngotympanica; pharyngotympanic neuralgia. Eponym obsolete. See Hunt's syndrome.

BIBLIOGRAPHY. Legal E: Ueber eine öftere Ursache des Schlaefen und hinterhapts Kopfschmerzes (Cephalagia pharyngotympanica). Dtsch Klin Med 40:201–216, 1886–1887

LEGG-CALVÉ-PERTHES

Synonyms. Calvé-Perthes; capital femoral epiphysis coxa plana; femoral osteochondrosis; Perthes'.

Symptoms. Sudden or gradual onset between 6 and 12 years of age. Moderate pain in the hip; limitation of motion and limp of involved leg that become progressively more intense.

Signs. Tenderness and muscular spasm in the hip. Eventually atrophy of muscles and shortening of leg.

Etiology. Idiopathic ischemia of ossification centers. Trauma. Occasionally associated with Herrick's (see). Polygenic inheritance suggested (risk in affected parent 3%).

Pathology. Osteocyte disappearance; reactive hyperemia; osteoclast and osteoblast invasion; replacement with normal bone.

Diagnostic Procedures. *Blood.* Sedimentation rate slightly elevated. *X-ray.* Initially, bone resorption; then sclerosis; indentation of subchondral tissue; fragmentation of epiphysis; joint irregularity.

Therapy. Bed rest; relative immobility for 2 or 3 years.

Prognosis. Self-limiting; may persist for years; heals with residual deformity (30% good recovery; 30% fairly normal; 25% continuous pain, limited movements).

BIBLIOGRAPHY. Legg AT: The cause of atrophy in joint disease. Am J Orthop Surg 6:84–90, 1908–1909

Calvé F: Sur une forme particulière de pseudocoxalgie greffée sur des deformations caractéristiques de l'extrémite supérieure du fémur. Rev Chir (Paris) 42:54–84, 1910

Perthes G: Ueber arthritis deformans juvenilis. Dtsch Z Chir 107:111–159, 1910

Harper PS, Brotherton J, Cochlin D: Genetic risks in Perthes' disease. Clin Genet 10:178–182, 1976

LEIGH'S

Synonyms. Subacute necrotizing encephalopathy, Wernicke's infantilis (misnomer). SNE; necrotizing encephalopathy, infantile; See Pyruvate carboxylase deficiency.

Symptoms and Signs. Both sexes affected; onset in early infancy. Lack of evidence of primary dietary deficiency or hepatic-gastroenteric diseases. Slow development, "mild hypotonia," brief "spasms," moderate tendon hyporeflexia, evolving through progressive deterioration to terminal stupor, hypertonia, myoclonic spasms, or severe hypotonia and areflexia.

Etiology. Apparently, autosomal recessive inheritance; X-linked inheritance also reported. A common expression of several genetic defects involving pyruvate metabolism.

Pathology. In brain, rarefaction of interstitial neuroglia or "ground substance" proceeding to vacuolization and parenchymal cavitation, associated with mesoglial proliferative reaction. Tendency to preserve nerve cell bodies. Changes affecting primarily pons, globus pallidus, optic nerve, chiasm tract, and spinal cord. Mammillary bodies are spared.

Diagnostic Procedures. *Blood.* Leukocytosis; mild

metabolic acidosis; increased lactate, pyruvate, and alanine. *Cerebrospinal fluid.* Increase in protein. *CT brain scan.* Ventricles dilatated.

Therapy. None.

Prognosis. Death within few years; a few patients have survived to midteens.

BIBLIOGRAPHY. Leigh D: Subacute necrotizing encephalomyelopathy in an infant. J Neurol Neurosurg Psychiatr 14:216–221, 1951.

Richter RB: Infantile subacute necrotizing encephalopathy (Leigh's disease): its relationship to Wernicke's encephalopathy. Neurology 18:1125–1132, 1968

Benke PJ, Parker JC Jr, Lubs M, et al: X-linked Leigh's syndrome. Hum Genet 62:52–59, 1982

LEINER'S

Synonym. Erythroderma desquamativum.

Symptoms and Signs. Prevalent in infant females; onset in 2nd to 4th month of life. Rapid onset. Severe seborrheic dermatitis of scalp and flexures associated with maculae or plaques of erythema with scaling on trunk and limbs. Gastrointestinal crusting troubles frequent; fever; lymphadenopathy (mild).

Etiology. Unknown.

Pathology. Seborrheic dermititis, plus superimposed infection (*Staphylococcus* and *Candida* 66%).

Diagnostic Procedures. *Blood.* Anemia; hypoproteinemia. *Culture and biopsy of skin.*

Therapy. Incubator control of heat loss; control of fluid and food intake; antibiotics; vitamins, transfusion if needed. Corticosteroids if other measures insufficient.

Prognosis. Without careful management, 50% mortality (from pneumonia, meningitis, nephritis). With good management, 10% mortality.

BIBLIOGRAPHY. Leiner C: Erythrodermia desquamativa (universal dermatitis of children at the breast). Br J Dis Child 5:244–251, 1908

Rook A, Wilkinson DS, Ebling FJG, et al: Textbook of Dermatology, 4th ed, pp. 249–251. Oxford, Blackwell Scientific Publications, 1986

LEIRI'S

See Choreiform syndromes.

BIBLIOGRAPHY. Leiri F: Ueber Tremor bei Kleinhirnaffektionen. J Psychol Neurol 29:429–433, 1923

LEISHMANIOSIS, NEW WORLD

Synonyms. American Leishmaniosis; bush yaws; Chichero's ulcer (Guatemala, Honduras, Mexico); Espundia (Peru); Pian bois (Guiana); Picatura de Pinto; Uta (Peru).

Symptoms and Signs. Distinct clinical patterns according to different species of *Leishmanias*. *Primary lesion.* In exposed parts; small papula, then red nodule, and finally ulceration. In Central America frequently affecting the ear. *Secondary infection.* Regional adenitis and lymphangitis. *Secondary lesions.* Mucosae of nose, mouth, nasopharynx eroding the cartilage and forming necrotic ulcers.

Etiology. *Phlebotomus* bite transmitting various species of *Leishmanias.*

Pathology. Central necrotic infected areas surrounded by edema and epithelial hyperplasia. *Secondary mucosal lesions.* Macrophages with leishmanias; inflammatory signs; capillary blockage, necrosis.

Therapy. Sodium antimony gluconate; pentamidine isothionate; stilbamidine isothionate (in antimony-resistant cases); allopurinol (under clinical trial in antimony-resistant cases); amphotericin B; antibiotics for secondary infection. Cauterization in some cases.

Prognosis. Good with early treatment. If untreated or late treatment, death from secondary infection.

BIBLIOGRAPHY. Pessoa SB, Barretto MP: Leishmaniose Tegumentar Americana. Rio de Janeiro Imprensa National, 1948.

Rook A, Wilkinson DS, Ebling FJG, et al: Textbook of Dermatology, 4th ed, pp 1024–1026. Oxford, Blackwell Scientific Publications, 1986

LEITNER'S

Synonyms. Eosinophilia–pulmonary tubercolosis. Loeffler's syndrome associated with tubercular infection. Used occasionally as synonym for Loeffler's.

BIBLIOGRAPHY. Leitner J: Ueber flüchtige hyperergische Lungeninfiltrate mit Eosinophilie bei Tuberkulose. Beitr Klin Tuberk 88:388–420, 1936

LENEGRE'S

See Lev's.

Symptoms and Signs. Both sexes affected; onset over 50 years of age. Those of progressive heart block.

Etiology. Obscure degenerative process limited to the heart conductive system.

Pathology. Sclerodegenerative process limited to the conduction system.

Diagnostic Procedures. *Electrocardiography.* Right bundle heart block; or left anterior hemiblock or other varieties or combinations of conductive defects.

Therapy. After pharmacologic trials; pacemaker as last resort.

Prognosis. Slow progression (in years) toward complete heart block.

BIBLIOGRAPHY. Lenègre J: Etiology and pathology of bilateral bundle branch block in relation to complete heart block. Prog Cardiovasc Dis 6:409–444, 1964
Rosenbaum MB: Interventricular trifascicular block. Heart Lung 1:216, 1972

LENNIEUX-NEEMEH

Synonym. Charcot-Marie-Tooth–deafness. See Rosenberg-Chutorian.

Symptoms and Signs. Both sexes. *In childhood.* Progressive weakness of peroneal muscles; poor balance; steppage gait; legs—hypoesthesia and absent reflexes, then muscle atrophy, clubfoot, and muscle involvement. *In 2nd decade.* Deafness (severe to deep) becomes apparent. The nephropathy of the original cases of Lennieux-Neemeh has not been reported in other families.

Etiology. Autosomal dominant trait; a family with possible recessive trait also reported (Cornell).

Diagnostic Procedures. *Electromyography. Audiography. Blood.* To exclude amyloidosis and uremic polyneuropathy.

BIBLIOGRAPHY. Lennieux G, Neemeh JA: Charcot-Marie-Tooth disease and nephritis. Can Med Assoc J 97:1193–1198, 1967
Lennieux G, Neemeh JA: Charcot-Maire-Tooth disease with sensorineural hearing loss: An autosomal dominant trait, p 241. Sixth Cong Hum Genet Jerusalem, 1981
Cornell J, Sellar S, Beighton P: Autosomal recessive inheritance of Charcot-Marie-Tooth disease associated with sensorineural deafness. Clin Genet 25:163–165, 1984

LENNOX-GASTAUT

Synonyms. Astatic petit mal; Doose's (when strong genetic basis); Gastaut's; hemiconvulsion-hemiplegia-epilepsy, HHE; Lennox's variant; petit mal variant.

Symptoms. It is a form of epilepsy that usually appears in the preschool age. Several seizure types, with atypical absences, head nodding, and drop attacks particularly prominent, in association with mental retardation and brain damage due to a diverse group of conditions.

Etiology. Diverse conditions. Doose described a group of patients with a similar syndrome, but a strong familial disposition to convulsive diseases, normal development, and good response to treatment with sodium valproate.

Diagnostic Procedures. *Electroencephalography.* In the awake patient slow spike and wave pattern; tonic seizures associated with low-amplitude fast activity are common during sleep.

Therapy. Nitrazepam; clorazepam.

Prognosis. Poor.

BIBLIOGRAPHY. Gastaut H, Vigoroux M, Trevisan C, et al: Le syndrome hemiconvulsion-hémiplégie-épilepsie (syndrome HHE). Rev Neurol (Paris) 97:37–52, 1957
Lennox WG: Epilepsy and Related Disorders. Boston, Little Brown, 1960
Hopkins IJ: The Lennox Gastaut syndrome. Aust Paediatr J 22:269–270, 1986

LENOBLE-AUBINEAU

Synonym. Myoclonia-nystagmus.

Symptoms and Signs. Prevalent in males; manifested in first years of life. Lateral nystagmus; myoclonic movements of extremities and trunk. Cold or tapping muscles enhances the symptoms. Patient partially controls them. Tendon hyperreflexia. Frequently associated, abnormalities of teeth, hypospadias, facial asymmetry, local hyperhidrosis, and localized edema.

Etiology. Unknown; possibly congenital and familial.

Pathology. Nonspecific meningovascular and glial changes in brain.

Therapy. Symptomatic. Ethosuximide; phenobarbital may be associated; ACTH or corticosteroid are also effective.

Prognosis. Incurable, but not progressive.

BIBLIOGRAPHY. Lenoble E, Aubineau E: Une variété nouvelle de myoclonie congénitale pouvant être héréditaire et familiale á nystagmus constant. Rev Med 26:471–515, 1906
Alpers BJ: Clinical Neurology, 6th ed. Philadelphia, FA Davis, 1971

LENZ-MAJEWSKI

Synonym. Osteosclerosis-syndactyly; Braham-Lenz; hyperostotic dwarfism.

Symptoms and Signs. Rare; Two cases reported. Present from birth. Progeroid skin; vein dilatation; large anterior fontanelle; large ears (Choanal atresia); hands and feet syndactyly; joint hyperextension; enamel hypoplasia.

Etiology. Unknown.

Diagnostic Procedures. *X-ray.* Increased density of skull base, mandible, clavicles, ribs, and long bones diaphyses.

BIBLIOGRAPHY. Braham RL: Multiple congenital abnormalities with diaphyseal dysplasia (Camurati-Engelmann syndrome). Oral Surg 27:20–26, 1969

Lenz WD, Majewski FA: A generalized disorder of the connective tissues with progeria, choanal atresia, symphalangism, hypoplasia of dentine and craniodiaphyseal hyperostosis. Birth Defects 10:133–136, 1974

Robinow M, Johanson AJ, Smith TH: The Lenz-Majewski hyperostotic dwarfism a syndrome of multiple congenital anomalies, mental retardation and progressive skeletal sclerosis. J Pediatr 91:417–421, 1977

LEOPARD

Synonyms. Cardiocutaneous; lentigo-electrocardiographic changes; multiple lentigines.

Symptoms and Signs. Both sexes affected; present from birth. Generalized freckling (not related to sunlight exposure), especially on neck and trunk, increasing with time. Systolic murmur that diffuses, more intense at heart base. Mild sensorineural deafness; mild growth deficiency; hypertelorism; prominent ears; scapula alata; pectus carinatum or excavatum. Delayed sexual development. Occasionally, mental deficiency, hypospadias, hypogonadism.

Etiology. Autosomal dominant inheritance with variable expression (incomplete syndrome a possibility).

Pathology. Pulmonary stenosis. Occasionally, unilateral kidney agenesis, subaortic stenosis, unilateral gonadal agenesis.

Diagnostic Procedures. *Electrocardiography.* Prolonged PR and QRS; abnormal P waves. *Hormonal studies.* Hypopituitarism and primary or secondary hypogonadal hormones. *X-ray of lung.* Vascular engorgement.

Therapy. Hormone replacement, if indicated.

Prognosis. Fair.

BIBLIOGRAPHY. Walther RJ, Polansky BJ, Crotis IA: Electrocardiographic abnormalities in family with generalized lentigo. New Engl J Med 275:1220–1225, 1966

Senn M, Hess OM, Krayenbuhl HP: Hypertrophe Kardiomyopathic und Lentiginose. Schweiz Med Wochenschr 114:838–841, 1984

LEPOUTRE'S

Synonyms. Primary hyperoxaluria; oxalosis.

Symptoms and Signs. Clinical onset in early adulthood. Those of nephrolithiasis and nephrocalcinosis progressing to chronic renal insufficiency. Some cases of congenital type: onset in early childhood. Nausea; vomiting; dry burning mouth; abdominal pain; renal colic; passage of calculi in urine; occasionally, tetany.

Etiology. Congenital form: autosomal recessive inheritance. Acquired forms: metabolic disorders with accumulation in tissues of oxalic acid. *Type I.* Glycolic aciduria; defect of 2-oxoglutarate/glyoxylate carboligase. *Type II.* L-glyceric aciduria; defect of D-glyceric dehydrogenase. Numerous other acquired conditions exist where calcium oxalate accumulates in tissues: oxalate poisoning; ethylene glycol poisoning; glyoxylate administration; pyridoxine deficiency; liver cirrhosis; renal tubular acidosis syndrome.

Pathology. In kidneys, deposits of crystal of calcium oxalate, calculi formation. Fibrosis; necrotic changes of tubules and glomeruli. Deposits of crystals observed in other tissues as well.

Diagnostic Procedures. *Blood.* Increase of oxalates; hypocalcemia. *Bone marrow.* Crystal of calcium oxalate may be observed. *Urine.* Oxalate excretion 3 to 5 times normal; albuminuria; hematuria; casts and stones of calcium oxalate. *X-ray of kidney.* Bilateral kidney calculosis. Osteoporosis.

Therapy. Magnesium oxide; sodium bicarbonate, mandelic acid. Alkalinization of urine, especially during night, and keeping volume abundant; diet low in calcium, high in phosphate. If specific cause such as pyridoxine deficiency, correction of deficiency. Renal transplantation is followed by recurrence of the disease.

Prognosis. Progressive course. Death in early adulthood (in congenital form), from various causes according to etiology, from renal failure in acquired forms.

BIBLIOGRAPHY. Lepoutre C: Calculs multiples chez un enfant: Infiltration du parenchyme renal par des depots cristallins. J Urol (Paris) 20:424, 1925

Williams HE, Smith LH Jr: L-Glyceric aciduria: a new genetic variant of primary hyperoxaluria. New Engl J Med 278:233–239, 1968

Williams HE, Smith LH Jr: Primary hyperoxaluria. In Stanbury JB, Wyngaarden JB, Fredrickson DS, et al: The Metabolic Basis of Inherited Disease, 5th ed, p 204. New York, McGraw-Hill, 1983

LEPTOMENINGEAL ADHESIVE THICKENING

Synonyms. Chronic adhesive arachnoiditis; circumscribed serum meningitis. See also Spinal chronic arachnoiditis.

Symptoms and Signs. Onset insidious. According to localization of process: headache; diplopia; nausea; vomiting; vertigo; epileptic seizures.

Etiology. Follows a chronic leptomeningeal infection, trauma, or after spontaneous subarachnoid hemorrhages. Occasionally, unknown.

Pathology. Fibrous tissue proliferation in limited areas of leptomeninge with chronic inflammatory cellular reaction.

Diagnostic Procedures. *Blood.* Leukocytosis. *Cerebrospinal fluid.* Increased proteins; xanthochromia. *X-ray. Angiography of brain. Scintigraphy. CT brain scan.*

Therapy. If infections demonstrated, antibiotics; corticosteroid of relative benefit. Surgery when indicated.

Prognosis. Progressive condition.

BIBLIOGRAPHY. Adams RD, Victor M: Principles of Neurology, 3rd ed, p 512. New York, McGraw-Hill, 1985

LERICHE'S

Synonyms. Abdominal thrombosis of aorta; aortic bifurcation. Aortoiliac obstruction (chronic).

Symptoms. Occur in males. Intermittent claudication; pain and discomfort at high level (thighs, hips, buttocks); impotence.

Signs. Arterial pulses in the legs decreased or absent; bruits occasionally heard over abdominal aorta and iliac and femoral arteries. Muscle atrophy; in skin, usually good perfusion (high obstruction and fair collateral circulation) or coldness, pallor, cyanosis, trophic changes, and gangrene. Hypertension.

Etiology. Atheromatous plaques at bifurcation of aorta; segmental arteritis; gradual thrombosis at terminal portion of aorta.

Pathology. Thrombus (red, white, or mixed), eventually organized.

Diagnostic Procedures. *Oscillography.* Absence of pulsation *X-ray.* Basketlike calcification at bifurcation of aorta. *Aortography.* To determine site and extent of obstruction.

Therapy. Conservative therapy or surgery.

Prognosis. Cerebral and coronary arteriosclerosis cause of death.

BIBLIOGRAPHY. Leriche R: De la résection du carrefour aortico-iliaque avec double sympathectomie lombaire pour thrombose artéritique de l'aorte. Le syndrome de l'oblitération terminoaortique par arterite. Presse Méd 48:33–604, 1940
Lindsay J, De Backey ME, Beals AC: Diseases of the aorta. In Hurst JW: The Heart, 6th ed, pp 1335–1336. New York, McGraw-Hill, 1986

LERI-JOHANNY

Synonyms. Flowing hyperostosis; monomelic hyperostosis; melorheostosis; osteosis eburnisans; monomelic periostitis.

Symptoms and Signs. Both sexes affected; onset in infancy. Severe pain of difficult localization, involving one bone or several. In 75% of cases, only the bones of a single extremity (monomelic) affected; side of pelvis or shoulder contiguous to affected limbs also involved. If condition has an early onset, premature closure of epiphysis and dwarfism may result. Limb motion may be reduced, because of ankylosis or muscle involvement or both.

Etiology. Unknown; congenital.

Pathology. Along shaft of long bones growth of bone that protrudes externally, beneath periosteum (melorheostosis: like melted candle wax) and internally into medulla. Microscopically, normal bone structure.

Diagnostic Procedure. *X-ray.* Peculiar bone malformation with long irregular streaks.

Therapy. None.

Prognosis. Severe incapacitation and dwarfism may result according to area affected and time of onset.

BIBLIOGRAPHY. Leri A, Johanny: Une affection non décrite des os: hyperostose "en coulée" sur toute la longuer d'un membre ou "melorhéostose." Bull Soc Med Hôp 46:1141–1145, 1922
Aagerter E, Kirkpatrick JA Jr: Orthopedic diseases, 3rd ed, p 178. Philadelphia, WB Saunders, 1968
Maroteaux P: Les désordres de la transparence osseuse. Encycl Méd Chir, p 3. Appareil Locomoteur 14023 B10, 1982

LERI'S

Synonyms. Premature bone ossification; pleonosteosis.

Symptoms. Both sexes affected; onset in early infancy. Usually, normal mental development. Some cases of impaired intelligence reported. Physical disabilities; limited motion of joints, including spine. Carpal tunnel syndrome, Morton's metatarsalgia may result.

Signs. Mongoloid facies (inconstant). Broadening and deformity of thumbs and great toes; hands short, thick. Flexion contractures of interphalangeal articulations; semiflexed internal rotation of upper limbs. Semiflexed external rotation of lower limbs.

Etiology. Unknown; autosomal dominant inheritance.

Pathology. Thickening of bones; joint deformities; capsular contraction; capsule formed by dense fibrous fibrocartilaginous tissue without elastic fibers.

Diagnostic Procedure. *X-ray.*

Therapy. Orthopedic treatment of complications.

Prognosis. Life expectancy not affected. Progressive articular impairment.

BIBLIOGRAPHY. Leri A: Une dystrophie osseuse géneralisée et hereditaire la pleonosteose familiale. Presse Med 30:13–16, 1922
Friedman M, Lawrence BM, Shaw DG: Leri's pleonosteosis. Br J Radiol 54:517–518, 1981

LERI-WEILL

Synonyms. Leri-Weill mesomelic dwarfism; Leri-Weill dyschondrosteosis; Lamy-Bienefeld.

Symptoms and Signs. Both sexes affected but prevalent in females; detection at birth to end of growing period. Bilaterality of lesions characterizing element (unilateral lesions, see Madelung's). Wrist pain when lifting objects. Forearms shorter with respect to hands and upper arm; distal ulna dorsal dislocation; dislocation easily reduced but unstable. Limited motion of elbows and wrists; legs shorter with respect to thighs.

Etiology. Autosomal dominant inheritance (sex influenced?).

Diagnostic Procedures. *X-ray of limbs.* Shortening of radius; triangularity of the distal radius epiphyses; wedging of carpal bones between radius and ulna.

Therapy. Splinting; orthopedic intervention for cosmetic reasons.

Prognosis. Pain stops with growth cessation. Mild dwarfism results.

BIBLIOGRAPHY. Leri A, Weill J: Une affection congénitale et symétrique du développement osseaux. La dyschondrostéose. Bull Soc Med Hôp 53:1491–1494, 1929
Lamy M, Bienefeld C: La Dyschondrosteose. In Gedda (ed): Analecta Genetica, pp 153–164. Rome, Mendel Institute, 1954
Jackson LG: Dyschondrosteosis: clinical study of a sixth generation family. Proc Greenwood Genet Center 4:147–148, 1985

LERMOYEZ'S

Synonyms. Deafness-tinnitus-vertigo; allergic vestibulitis; labyrinthitis, nonsuppurative.

Symptoms and Signs. Onset in the 30s and 40s (as opposed to Ménière's syndrome's onset in the 50s and 60s). The sequence of tinnitus and deafness, which diminishes or disappears after vertigo becomes established, (as opposed to the sequence of vertigo followed by tinnitus and deafness, characteristic of Ménière's). Allergic manifestations, especially urticaria, sometimes preceding the syndrome.

Etiology. Vasospasm of internal auditory artery. Allergic origin, especially urticaria.

Pathology. Unknown.

Diagnostic Procedures. *Otologic examination. Audiography. Skin tests.*

Therapy. See Ménière's.

Prognosis. Excellent; recovery of normal health and disappearance of tinnitus and deafness (as opposed to Ménière's, which causes a more or less permanent disability).

BIBLIOGRAPHY. Lermoyez M: La Vertige qui fait entendre (angiospasme labyrinthique). Presse Med 27:1–3, 1919
Eagle WW: Lermoyez's syndrome—an allergic disease. Ann Otol 57:453–464, 1948
Eckhardt J, Claussen CF: Ein Beitrag zum Lermoyez-Syndrom. Arch Klin Exp Ohr Nas Kehlk Heilk 201:159–171, 1972
Maragos NE, Neel HB III, McConald RJ: Dissection of dizziness: with emphasis on labyrinthine vertigo. Postgrad Med 69:113–115, 1981
Sweetlow R: Counseling the patient with tinnitus. Arch Otolaryngol 111:283–287, 1985

LEROY'S I-CELL

Synonyms. Mucolipidosis II, ML II; I-cell.

Symptoms and Signs. High frequency in Arab community. Both sexes affected; present at birth or onset in early postnatal period. Lack of striking corneal clouding. Minimal hepatomegaly. Dislocation of hips. Thoracic deformities. Hyperplastic gums. Hernia. Restricted joint mobility. Retarded psychomotor development. Recurrent respiratory infections.

Etiology. Autosomal recessive inheritance. Defect of phosphorylation of hydrolases that prevents them from entering lysozomes and thus becoming active. Many mucopolysaccharides are not metabolized.

Pathology. Subepithelial connective tissue hypercellular with numerous vacuolated histiocytes and fibroblasts. Containing numerous inclusion cells (I-cells). Also affected: chondrocytes, Schwann's cells, glomerular epithelial, vascular parietal cells, and peripheral neurons. Lipid content of I-cell three times above normal.

Diagnostic Procedures. *Fibroblast culture.* See Pathology. High levels of lysosomal enzymes in medium of culture. *Urine.* Moderate mucopolysacchariduria or normal level. *X-ray.* Radiologic features suggesting Hurler's syndrome. *Blood.* No metachromatic granules in leukocytes; increased lysosomal enzyme values. Ten- or twentyfold increase of beta-hexosaminidase; presence of iduronate sulfatase and aryl sulfatase A in serum is diagnostic.

Therapy. None.

Prognosis. Most patients die by age 5 or 6.

BIBLIOGRAPHY. Leroy JG, De Mars RI: Mutant enzymatic and cytological phenotypes in cultured human fibroblasts. Science 158:1097–1103, 1968
Leroy JG, O'Brien JS: Mucolipidosis II and III: differential residual activity of beta-galactosidase in cultured fibroblasts. Clin Genet 9:533–539, 1976
Neufeld EF, McKusick VA: Disorders of lysosomal enzyme synthesis and localization: I-cell disease and pseudo-Hurler polydystrophy. In Stanbury JB, Wyngaarden JB, Fredrickson DS, et al: The Metabolic Basis of Inherited Diseases, 5th ed, p 778. New York, McGraw-Hill, 1983

LESCH-NYHAN

Synonyms. Choreoathetosis—self mutilation; juvenile gout; hyperuricemia-oligophrenia; Nyhan's; uric acid disorder–oligophrenia; hypoxanthine guanine phosphoribosyltransferase deficiency; HGPRT deficiency.

Symptoms and Signs. Major manifestation in affected males; onset at 3 to 4 months of age. Extensor spasm of the trunk; generalized muscular weakness; athetoid or clonic movements; hypotonia when at rest; occasionally seizures; increased deep tendon reflexes; Babinski's sign. No sensory disturbances. Self-destructive behavior usually starts at 2 years of age. Lip, thumb, and foot biting; dislocation of eyes; face scratching; head banging. Mental

retardation usually severe. If speech develops, it remains extremely limited; dysarthria. Growth severely impaired.

Etiology. Unknown; sex-linked recessive type of inheritance. Deficient activity of hypoxanthine guanine phosphoribosyltransferase (HGPRT) demonstrated in some patients. X-linked inheritance. Complete deficiency of hypoxanthine guanine phosphoribosyltransferase. Patients with partial deficiency of HGPRT have severe gout (see).

Pathology. Lesions from biting and trauma. In brain, no characteristic pathologic changes. Urate-staining granules may be associated with lesions.

Diagnostic Procedures. *Blood.* Hyperuricemia. Anemia (usually megaloblastic type). Erythrocytes: HGPRT absent, and increased adenine phosphoribosyl transferase. *Urine.* Yellow staining of diaper from uric acid from first days of life. High uric acid excretion. *X-ray.* Negative. Tophaceus deposits in some older patients. *Pneumoencephalography, CT brain scan.* Ventricular dilatation and cortical atrophy.

Therapy. Allopurinol; alkalinization of urine (sodium citrate/citric acid) prevents complication from uric acid stones and renal damage. Restraints to prevent biting and self-inflicted damage.

Prognosis. Poor; treatment does not affect neurologic defect, which appears not to be progressive. Death in 2nd or 3rd decade from infections or renal failure.

BIBLIOGRAPHY. Catel W, Schmidt J: Ueber familiare gichtische Diathese in Verbindung mit zerebralen und renalen Symptomen bei einem Kleinkind. Dtsch Med Wochenschr 84:2145–2147, 1959
Lesch M, Nyhan WL: A familial disorder of uric acid metabolism and central nervous system function. Am J Med 36:561–570, 1964
Kelley WN, Wyngaarden JB: Clinical syndromes associated with hypoxanthine guanine phosphoribosyltransferase deficiency. In Stanbury JB, Wyngaarden JB, Fredrickson DS, et al: The Metabolic Basis of Inherited Disease, 5th ed, p 1115. New York, McGraw-Hill, 1983

LETHAL MIDLINE GRANULOMA

Synonym. Stewart's type of malignant granuloma.

Symptoms and Signs. Affects all ages, most common between 30 and 50 years of age; prevalent in men and whites. *Prodromal.* For 1 year or longer nasal stuffiness with serous or serous-hemorrhagic discharge. *Disease.* Increased discharge, which becomes purulent; areas of necrotic tissue in the nasal cavity that spread to involve entire nose and pharynx; production of fistula through skin. Tongue not involved. Eye involved directly by granulomatous process or because of involvement of adnexae. Pain minimal; episodes of high spiking fever only late in the course.

Etiology. Unknown; possibly, autoimmune condition. Possible relation with Wegener's granuloma discussed.

Pathology. Nonspecific lesions; chronic inflammation; granulation tissue; necrosis.

Diagnostic Procedures. *Serology, biopsy, cultures.* Rule out tuberculosis, syphilis, Hodgkin's, mycosis fungoides, fungus infections, leishmaniasis, leprosy, granuloma venereum and neoplasms of the upper airways, particularly midline malignant reticulosis and certain lymphomas.

Therapy. The treatment of choice is local radiation therapy. Surgery is not useful and can actually worsen the clinical course. Corticosteroids and cytotoxic agents are ineffective.

Prognosis. High dose radiotherapy to the involved areas results in a high percentage of remissions. The disease should no longer be referred to as lethal.

BIBLIOGRAPHY. McBride P: Case of rapid destruction of the nose and face. J Laryngol 12:64, 1897

Stewart JP: Progressive lethal granulomatous ulceration of nose. J Laryngol Otol 48:657–701, 1933

Eisenlohr JE: Lethal midline granuloma: clinical aspects. Tex J Med 61:188–192, 1965

Douglas AC, Anderson TJ, McDonald M, et al: Midline and Wegener's granulomatosis. Ann New York Acad Sci 278:618–655, 1976

Rook A, Wilkinson DS, Ebling FJG: Textbook of Dermatology, 4th ed, p 1180. Blackwell, Oxford, 1986

LETTERER-SIWE

Synonyms. Abt-Letterer-Siwe; aleukemic reticulosis; aleukemic reticuloendotheliosis; Siwe's. See Histiocytosis syndromes.

Symptoms. Occur in infants and growing children (under 3 years of age); onset occasionally later, up to young adulthood. Fatigue; anorexia; irritability; wasting; chronic otitis media. Low-grade, persistent fever.

Signs. On the scalp (primarily), face, and trunk, cutaneous maculopapular lesions, yellowish brown papules with red edge and yellow center. Weeping erosion on skin folds, ecchymoses, and petechiae. Edema; generalized lymphadenopathy and hepatosplenomegaly.

Etiology. Unknown; Autosomal recessive trait reported. Disseminated condition of histiocytosis syndromes (see).

Pathology. Histiocytic proliferation resembling generalized reticular cell sarcoma or monocytic leukemia. Gener-

alized eosinophilia, hepatomegaly, and splenomegaly. Histiocytic infiltration of lungs.

Diagnostic Procedures. *Blood.* Leukocytosis, anemia, thrombocytopenia. *X-ray.* Destructive lesions of bones, especially skull.

Therapy. Corticosteroids; vinblastine; vincristine; cyclophosphamide; antibiotics; and other chemotherapeutic agents.

Prognosis. Acute form: rapidly fatal; possibility of chronicity or remission; variable duration from weeks to years.

BIBLIOGRAPHY. Letterer E: Aleukämische Retikulose. Frank Z Pathol 30:377–394, 1924

Siwe S: Die Reticuloendotheliose-ein neues Krankheitsbild unter den Hepatosplenomegalien. Z Kinderheilkd 55:212–247, 1933.

Schoeck VW, Peterson RDA, Good RA: Familial occurrence of Letterer-Siwe disease. Pediatrics 32:1055–1063, 1963

LEUKOCYTE GLUCOSE-6-PHOSPHATE DEHYDROGENASE DEFICIENCY

Synonym. Leukocyte G6PDH deficiency.

Symptoms and Signs. Very rare. From birth, severe infections. Congenital nonspherocytic hemolytic anemia (due to G6PDH deficiency also in erythrocytes).

Etiology. X-linked. Associated to erythrocyte G6PDH deficiency.

Diagnostic Procedures. *Neutrophil function tests.* Normal particle ingestion and degranulation. Defective killing of catalase positive bacteria.

Therapy. Prevention and treatment of infections.

Prognosis. Patients described have reached adulthood.

BIBLIOGRAPHY. Cooper MR, De Chatelet LR, McCall CE, et al: Complete deficiency of leukocyte glucose-6-phosphate dehydrogenase with defective bactericidal activity. J Clin Invest 51:769–772, 1972

LEVINE-CRITCHLEY

Synonyms. Acanthocytosis–neurologic disease; choreoacanthocytosis; neuroacanthocytosis.

Symptoms and Signs. Both sexes. From infancy. Various patterns of neurologic conditions recalling Gilles de la Tourette's (see); Huntington's (see); Friedreich's (see); chorea syndromes (see); self-mutilation of tongue, lips, and cheeks; parkinsonism.

Etiology. Unknown. Heterogenous inheritance (autosomal dominant and recessive).

Pathology. *Brain.* Neural loss, gliosis, and degeneration of basal ganglia.

Diagnostic Procedures. *Blood.* Acanthocytosis. Normal serum lipoproteins. *CT brain scan. Electroencephalography.*

Therapy. Symptomatic.

Prognosis. Survival into adulthood.

BIBLIOGRAPHY. Critchley EMR, Clark DB, Wikler A: An adult form of acanthocytosis. Trans Am Neurol Assoc 92:132–137, 1967

Levine IM, Estes JW, Looney JM: Hereditary neurological disease with acanthocytosis: a new syndrome. Arch Neurol 19:403–409, 1968

Spitz MC, Jankovic J, Killian JM: Familial tic disorder, parkinsonism motor neuron disease, and acanthocytosis: a new syndrome. Neurology 35:366–370, 1985

LEVIN'S I

Synonym. Cranioectodermal dysplasia.

Symptoms and Signs. Dolicocephaly; slow-growing fine hair; epicanthal folds; hypomicrodontia; brachydactyly; thin thorax. Normal intellectual development.

Etiology. Autosomal recessive inheritance.

BIBLIOGRAPHY. Levin LS, Perrin JCS, Ose L, et al: A hereditable syndrome of craniostenosis, short thin hair, dental abnormalities and short limbs: cranioectodermal dysplasia. J Pediatr 90:55–61, 1977

LEVIN'S II

Synonym. Osteogenesis imperfecta–skeletal lesion (unusual).

Symptoms and Signs. Those of osteogenesis imperfecta. Normal teeth; frequent infection of jaws.

Etiology. Autosomal dominant inheritance.

Diagnostic Procedures. *X-ray of maxilla and mandible.* Multiocular radiolucent-radiopaque lesions. Coarseness of trabecular and osteopenia of skeleton.

Prognosis. Good.

BIBLIOGRAPHY. Levin LS, Wright JM, Byrd DL, et al: Osteogenesis imperfecta with unusual skeletal lesions: report of three families. Ann J Med Genet 21:257–259, 1985

LEV'S

Symptoms and Signs. See Lenègre's. Usually occur in elderly persons. Those of atrioventricular (AV) block of various degrees up to complete.

Etiology. Exogenous invasion of heart conduction system. See Pathology.

Pathology. Fibrosis or calcification spreading into conducting system from adjacent fibrous structures: e.g., calcification of aortic valve; fibrosis of summit of muscular septum; fibrosis or calcification of mitral ring.

Diagnostic Procedure. *Electrocardiography.* Heart block.

Therapy. Permanent pacemaker.

Prognosis. Variable according to basic condition. Optimal results with pacemaker implantation.

BIBLIOGRAPHY. Lev M: The pathology of complete atrioventricular block. Am J Med 37:742–748, 1964

Hurst JW: The heart, 5th ed., p 464. New York, McGraw-Hill, 1986

LEVY-HOLLISTER

Synonyms. Lacrimo-auriculo-dento-digital, LADD; lacrimo-auriculo-radio-digital, LARD.

Symptoms and Signs. Both sexes. From birth. Lack of lacrimation; conjunctivitis; cupped pinnas; mixed hearing defects. Small peg-shaped teeth and enamel dysplasia. *Hands.* Variable malformations; clinodactyly, syndactyly, duplication of phalanx; radial aplasia.

Etiology. Sporadic cases and autosomal dominant inheritance.

Pathology. Aplasia or hypoplasia of puncta of lacrimal ducts. See Signs.

BIBLIOGRAPHY. Levy WJ: Mesoectodermal dysplasia: a new combination of anomalies. Am J Ophthalmol 63:978–982, 1967

Hollister DW, Klein SH, Dejager HL, et al: The lacrimo-auriculo-dento-digital syndrome. J Pediatr 83:438–444, 1973

Thompson E, Pembray M, Graham JM: Phenotypic variation in LADD syndrome. J Med Genet 22:382–385, 1985

LEWANDOWSKY-LUTZ

Synonyms. Epidermodysplasia verruciformis; generalized verrucosis; Lutz's.

Symptoms. Both sexes affected; onset at any age; develops more rapidly in infancy.

Signs. On the face, neck, back of hands, and feet; more rarely on trunk. Development of flat, verrucous warts (2 cm in diameter). The warts on the face (most frequent site) are the flat type, while those on the trunk and extremities are larger and firmer. In some cases, they present a pink or violet color. The confluence of neighboring lesions forms lines or large plaques.

Etiology. Wart virus (papova). To develop this syndrome, a special hereditary predisposition is needed. Autosomal recessive or dominant and X-linked inheritance.

Pathology. Typical histologic changes observed in common warts.

Diagnostic Procedures. *Biopsy.* Electron and fluorescent microscopic examination to show presence of virus.

Therapy. Unsatisfactory. Frequent recurrence, even after large excision.

Prognosis. The lesion may remain static for decades. In nearly 20% development of squamous epithelioma in one or more lesions. Malignancy only in cases affected with HPV4.

BIBLIOGRAPHY. Lewandowsky F, Lutz W: Ein Fall einer bisher nicht beschriebenen Hauterkrankung (Epidermodysplasia verruciformis). Arch Dermatol Syph 41:193–202, 1922
Jablonka S, Orth G, Jarzabel-Chorzelske M, et al: Twenty-one years of follow-up studies of familial epidermodysplasia verruciforms. Dermatologica 158:309–327, 1979
Androphy EJ, Dvoretzky I, Lowy DR: X-linked inheritance of epidermodysplasia verruciforms: genetic and virologic studies of a kindred. Arch Derm 121:864–868, 1985

LEWANDOWSKY'S

Synonym. Periporitis staphylogenes.

Symptoms and Signs. Occur in infants of both sexes. Inflammation of sweat glands evolving into small abscesses.

Etiology. Pyogenic microorganisms associated with variable systemic conditions depressing immune response and defenses. Secondary infection by *Staphylococcus aureus;* miliaria progresses to abscesses of the sweat glands.

Pathology. Abscesses and pustules associated with sweat glands.

Diagnostic Procedures. Screening for identification of possible systemic condition.

Therapy. Antibiotics and correction of basic disorder.

Prognosis. Good with adequate treatment.

BIBLIOGRAPHY. Lewandowsky F: Zur Pathogenese der multiplen Abszesse im Säuglingsalter. Arch Dermatol Syph 80:179–191, 1906
Rook A, Wilkinson DS, Ebling FJG, et al: Textbook of Dermatology, 4th ed, p 260. Oxford, Blackwell Scientific Publications, 1986

LEWIS' (C.S.)

Synonym. Symphalangism, Lewis type; stiff thumbs.

Symptoms and Signs. Presumed synostosis involving the first metacarpophalangeal joint. Lewis described his own condition.

Etiology. Autosomal dominant inheritance.

Prognosis. Manual clumsiness (which the eponymous author says drove him to become a writer).

BIBLIOGRAPHY. Lewis CS: Surprised by Joy: The Shape of My Early Life, p 12. New York, Harcourt, Brace and World, 1955

LEWIS' (F.)

Synonyms. Heart-hand II; cardiovascular-arm; ventriculo-radial dysplasia. See Holt-Oram.

Symptoms. Present from birth. Association of multiple heart and upper limb defects:
1. Atrial septal defect; ventricular septal defect; great vessel transposition; single coronary artery; retroesophageal right subclavian artery
2. Absence or deformity of thumbs; phocomelia; deformed long bones (humerus, radius, and ulna) and metacarpal bones

Etiology. Autosomal dominant inheritance very likely does not differ from that of Holt-Oram.

BIBLIOGRAPHY. Lewis F: High defects of atrial septum. J Thorac Cardiovasc Surg 36:1–11, 1958
Harris LC, Osborne WP: Congenital absence or hypoplasia of the radius with ventricular septal defect: ventriculo-radial dysplasia. J Pediatr 68:265–272, 1966

LEWIS' (R.A.)

Synonym. Ocular   albinism–lentigines–sensorineural deafness.

Symptoms and Signs. Both sexes. From birth. Reduced visual acuity; pathophobia nystagmus; translucent irises; refractive errors. Sensorineural deafness.

Etiology. Autosomal dominant inheritance.

Diagnostic Procedures. *Fundus.* Albinotic with hypoplasia of fovea.

Therapy. None.

Prognosis. Good.

BIBLIOGRAPHY. Lewis RA: Ocular albinism and deafness. Twenty-ninth Annual Meeting, American Society of Human Genetics, Vancouver. Am J Hum Genet 30:57 (abstr), 1978

LEWKOJEWA'S

Synonym. Amyloid hereditary corneal deposits.

Symptoms. Three siblings affected. Photophobia; excessive lacrimation.

Signs. Raised gelatinous mulberrylike masses over central cornea.

Etiology. Unknown. Possibly autosomal recessive inheritance.

Therapy. Corneal graft.

BIBLIOGRAPHY. Lewkojewa EF: Ueber einen fall primaerer degeneration amyloidose der kornea. Klin Monatsbl Augenheilkd 83:117–137, 1930
Kirk HQ, Rabb M, Hattenhauer J, et al: Primary familial amyloidosis of the cornea. Trans Am Acad Ophthalmol Otoryngol 77:411–417, 1973
Mondino BJ, Rabb HF, Sugar J, et al: Primary familial amyloidosis of the cornea. Am J Ophthalmol 92:732–736, 1981

LEYDEN-MÖBIUS

Synonyms. Femoral dsytrophy; limb-girdle inferior dystrophy; pelvifemoral muscular dystrophy.

Symptoms and Signs. Muscular dystrophy of lumbosacral muscles. See Erb's III.

BIBLIOGRAPHY. Leyden E: Klinik der Rueckenmarks-Krankheiten, vol 2. Berlin, Hirschwald, 1876

LEYDEN'S II

Symptoms and Signs. Tetraparesis with fatal evolution following an epileptic attack.

Etiology. Hemorrhage in the pons or bulb.

BIBLIOGRAPHY. Leyden E: Klinik der Rueckenmarks-Krankheiten, vol. 2, p 64. Berlin, Hirschwald, 1875.

LHERMITTE-CORNIL-QUESNEL

Synonym. Extrapyramidal–pyramidal degeneration (obsolete).

Symptoms and Signs. Appear in middle age or later. Periods of excitation and depression. Gradual onset and slow progression; absence of sudden vascular accidents that are usually at the onset of pseudobulbar palsy. Pain and paresthesia and rigidity of lower limbs. Dysarthria; aphonia; dysphagia; involuntary laughing and crying. Further retrograde mental changes; apathy and negativism. Muscular hypertonia, more marked in proximal muscles. Hand posture similar to that observed in paralysis agitans: extended wrist; finger flexed at metacarpophalangeal joints and extended at other joints. Lower limb posture not particularly characteristic. Good muscular power (slowness of movement associated with extrapyramidal hypertonia). Tendon hyperreflexia; presence of ankle clonus; Babinski's sign. Normal fundus oculi.

Etiology. Unknown; observed in cases of epidemic encephalitis. Considered by the authors a distinct entity from very similar conditions: Parkinson's; pseudobulbar palsy; Creutzfeld-Jakob; amyotrophic lateral sclerosis; paralysis agitans.

Pathology. In putamen reduction of cells, neuroglial overgrowth, degeneration of fibers originating in the putamen. Globus pallidus shows similar pattern, but less severe. Pyramidal tract degeneration below level of medulla. In the cord, degeneration of crossed pyramidal tracts.

Diagnostic Procedures. *Blood* and *cerebrospinal fluid.* Normal.

Therapy. None.

Prognosis. Rapid evolution; death within 1 year.

BIBLIOGRAPHY. Lhermitte J, Cornil L, Quesnel: Le syndrome de la dégénération pyramidopallidale progressive. Rev Neurol 27:262–269, 1920
Lhermitte J, McAlpine D: A clinical and pathological résumé of combined disease of the pyramidal and extrapyramidal systems, with especial reference to a new syndrome. Brain 49:157–181, 1926

LHERMITTE-LEVY

Synonyms. Hallucinosis–red nucleus; peduncular hallucinosis; Lhermitte-Delthil-Garnier.

Symptoms. Occurs in elderly people. Slowly progressing paralysis after a stroke. Incessant choreiform movement of arms and legs (rhythmic trembling). Visual and auditory hallucinations.

Etiology. The combination of movements and hallucination attributed by the authors to a lesion of unknown nature in the upper portion of peduncle and subthalamic region.

BIBLIOGRAPHY. Lhermitte MJ, Levy G: Phenomenes d'allucinose chez une malade presentant une torsion et une contracture athetoides intentionnelles du bras. Soc Neurol May 7, 1931

Lhermitte MJ, Delthil, Garnier: Syndrome controlateral du noyau rouge avec hallucinations visuelles et auditives. Rev Neurol 70:623–628, 1938

Adams RD, Victor M: Principles of Neurology, 3rd ed, p 307. New York, McGraw-Hill, 1985

LIAN-SIGUIER-WELTI

Eponym used to indicate a venous thrombosis complicating eventration or diaphragmatic hernia.

BIBLIOGRAPHY. Lian G, Siguier F, Welti JJ: Le syndrome "hernia diaphragmatique ou éventration diaphragmatique et thrombose veineuses." Presse Med 61:145–146, 1953

LIBAN-KOZENITZKY

Synonyms. Renal hamartomas–nephroblastomatosis–fetal gigantism; Perlman's.

Symptoms and Signs. Both sexes. At birth. Large body size; unusual facies; ascites; polyhydramnios.

Etiology. Unknown. Possibly autosomal recessive inheritance.

Pathology. Bilateral renal hamartomas with or without nephroblastomatosis. Pancreas; hypertrophy of Langerhans islets.

Diagnostic Procedures. *Blood.* Hyperinsulinism. *X-rays. Echography.*

Therapy. None attempted. Correction of hyperinsulinism could improve survival chances.

Prognosis. All patients died as infants.

BIBLIOGRAPHY. Liban E, Kozenitzky IL: Metanephric hamartomas and nephroblastomatosis in siblings. Cancer 25:885–888, 1970

Perlman M, Goldberg GM, Bar-Ziv J, et al: Renal hamartomas and nephroblastomatosis with fetal gigantism: a familial syndrome. J Pediatr 83:414–418, 1973

Greenberg F, Stein F, Gresik MV, et al: Perlman's syndrome: familial nephroblastomatosis, fetal ascites, polyhydramnios, macrosomia, and Wilms' tumor—follow-up. Proc Greenwood Genet Center 4:150, 1985

LIBMAN-SACKS

Synonyms. Atypical verrucous endocarditis. Nonbacterial verrucous endocarditis; nonrheumatic endocarditis; Kaposi-Besnier-Libman-Sacks; Osler-Libman-Sacks. See Lupus erythematosus, systemic.

Symptoms. Those of lupus erythematosus.

Signs. Systolic and diastolic apical murmurs.

Etiology. Associated with lupus erythematosus, systemic (see).

Pathology. Mucoid degeneration of cardiac valves; fibrinoid necrosis; necrotic fibrinoid vegetation without bacteria.

Diagnostic Procedures. Those of lupus erythematosus, systemic.

Therapy. Same as for lupus erythematosus, systemic.

Prognosis. Same as for lupus erythematosus, systemic.

BIBLIOGRAPHY. Libman E, Sacks B: A hitherto undescribed form of valvular and mural endocarditis. Arch Intern Med 33:701–737, 1924

Hurst JW: The Heart, 6th ed, p 1436. New York, McGraw-Hill, 1986

LICHEN PLANUS

Synonyms. Wilson's (E.) including lichen planus familial; Hebra.

Symptoms. More common in men; onset in young adulthood (recorded in infancy and old age as well). Pruritus; malaise. Familial form earlier onset, tendency to chronicity, more severe and atypical manifestations.

Signs. Usually, insidious onset (chronic type) or less frequently (5%) sudden (acute). On inner side of thighs, knees, back, less frequently on genitalia and mucosae, appearance of papules varying in shape (polygonal), size (pinpoint to over 1 cm), and distribution (widely scattered or aggregated). Papular surface is shining, flat; the color is violet with dots and striae.

Etiology. Unknown. Toxic, viral, psychogenic factors blamed without proof or confirmation. Families with autosomal dominant inheritance reported.

Pathology. Moderate increase of horny layer; increase of granular layer; irregular acanthosis; liquefaction necrosis of basal layer. Dermis is infiltrated by lymphocytes and histiocytes. Presence of colloid bodies.

Therapy. Corticosteroids; adrenocorticotropic hormone (ACTH) in severe cases. Antipruritic drugs also useful. Symptomatic; topical fluorinated steroid creams or ointments; in hypertrophic form, occlusive dressing with tar, ichthammol, or cream with salicyclic acid added. Retinoic acid. Photochemotherapy (warning: danger of carcinogenesis).

Prognosis. Acute form: average duration 8 months (from weeks to years). Chronic form: average duration 3 years (up to 20). May leave areas or atrophy or hyperpigmentation.

BIBLIOGRAPHY. Wilson E: On lichen planus: The lichen ruber of Hebra. Br Med J 2:399–402, 1866
Rook A, Wilkinson DS, Ebling FJG, et al: Textbook of Dermatology. 4th ed, pp 1665–1678. Oxford, Blackwell Scientific Publications, 1986
Mahood JM: Familial lichen planus: a report of nine cases from four families with a brief review of the literature. Arch Derm 119:292–294, 1983

LICHTENSTEIN-JAFFE

Synonyms. Unifocal eosinophilic bone granuloma; eosinophilic granuloma. See Histiocytosis syndromes.

Symptoms and Signs. Males more frequently affected (3 : 2); onset all ages. At onset, asymptomatic or low-grade fever (intermittent), pain, tenderness, and, occasionally, tumor on affected bone site. Most frequently affected are the head and femur in children and the ribs in adults. Moderate shotty cervical lymphadenopathy; no otitis media; cutaneous manifestation or exophthalmos at onset (see Hand-Schüller-Christian). Seldom (after years), diabetes insipidus may develop.

Etiology. Unknown.

Pathology. Single or multiple lytic lesions in bone. Histiocytic proliferation with eosinophilia.

Diagnostic Procedures. *X-ray. Biopsy.*

Therapy. Curettement of the lesion, simultaneously with the biopsy. Modest doses of x-ray therapy (500–1500 rads).

Prognosis. Relatively benign condition; long survival; spontaneous remission observed.

BIBLIOGRAPHY. Lichtenstein L, Jaffe HL: Eosinophilic granuloma of bone, with report of case. Am J Path 16:595–604, 1940
Oberman HA: Idiopathic histiocytosis: a clinico-pathologic study of 40 cases and review of the literature on eosinophilic granuloma of bone, Hand-Schüller-Christian disease and Letterer-Siwe disease. Pediatrics 28:307–327, 1961
Wintrobe MM (ed): Clinical Hematology, 8th ed, p 382. Philadelphia, Lea & Febiger, 1981

LICHTENSTERN'S

Eponym used to indicate an association of pernicious anemia (see Biermer-Addison) and tabes dorsalis.

BIBLIOGRAPHY. Lichtenstern O: Ueber progressive perniziöse Anaemie bei Tabeskranken. Dtsch Med Wochenschr 10:849–850, 1884

LICHTHEIM'S I

Synonyms. Lichtheim's aphasia. See Broca's Aphasia. Eponym used to indicate a form of anamnestic aphasia (nominal) where the patient is unable to say words but may indicate (indirectly) the number of syllables or letters of the word in question.

BIBLIOGRAPHY. Lichtheim L: On aphasia. Brain 7:433–484, 1885

LICHTHEIM'S II

Synonyms. Ataxic paraplegia; combined system; Dana's; spinal funicular; neuroanemic; posterolateral sclerosis; Putnam-Dana; subacute combined; spinal cord degeneration; subacute combined degeneration (SCD). See Addison-Biermer.

Symptoms. Condition widely disseminated, but more common in blond Nordic races; male and female same incidence. Onset most commonly in 4th decade. Great variability of symptoms, onset subacute or chronic. Slowly progressing: paresthesias that cannot be rubbed away; aggravated by cold; relieved by heat. Ataxia of various degrees. Motor symptoms may be present (weakness and easy fatigability). Spasticity or flaccid paralysis of various degrees; sphincter disturbances. Sensory symptoms rare; visual disturbances; mental changes (not specific).

Signs. Position and vibration senses lost. Babinski's sign; hyperreflexia initially, then areflexia. Eyes may present retinal hemorrhage, changes in visual field. If pernicious anemia, pallor and typical tongue. This syndrome may precede the blood changes for a long time.

Etiology. Pernicious anemia most frequent cause; chronic alcoholism, sprue, and other conditions may be responsible; lack of intrinsic factor in gastric secretion.

Pathology. If limited to spinal cord, thoracic and lumbar tracts most frequently affected. Degeneration of posterior columns, pyramidal tract, spinocerebellar tract, and anterior portion. Loss of myelin and axis cylinders; glyosis in old lesion. Spongy appearance. Cerebral cortex may show evidence of damage and infarcts.

Diagnostic Procedures. *Blood.* If associated with pernicious anemia, macrocytic anemia. *Bone marrow.* Megaloblastosis. *Gastric fluid.* Achlorhydria.

Therapy. Vitamin B$_{12}$ and thiamine. Curare and intensive care for spasms.

Prognosis. Poor; improvement with treatment. Complete regression with early treatment.

BIBLIOGRAPHY. Lichtheim: Zur Kenntniss der perniciösen Anämia. Verh Cong Innere Med 6:84–96, 1889
Adams RD, Victor M: Principles of Neurology, 3rd ed, pp 773–776. New York, McGraw-Hill, 1985

LIDDLE'S

Synonyms. Inappropriate excessive renal sodium conservation; pseudohyperaldosteronism.

Symptoms and Signs. See Conn's.

Etiology. Unknown; Autosomal dominant inheritance. Primary defect in membrane transport.

Diagnostic Procedures. As in primary hyperaldosteronism except low level of aldosterone and the patients do not respond to spironolactone administration. Excessive renal reabsorption of sodium; potassium depletion; plasma renin activity suppression and inhibition of aldosterone secretion.

Therapy. Potassium loss corrected by triamterene.

BIBLIOGRAPHY. Liddle GW, Bledsoe T, Coppage WS Jr: A familial renal disorder simulating primary aldosteronism, but with negligible aldosterone secretion. Trans Assoc Am Physicians 76:199, 1963
Rodriguez JA, Biglieri EG, Schambelan M: Pseudohyperaldosteronism (PHA) with tubular resistance to mineralocorticoid hormone (MCH). Clin Res 29:567 A, 1981

LIEBENBERG'S

Synonym. Brachydactyly–joint dysplasia.

Symptoms and Signs. Flexion deformity simulating anterior dislocation of elbow. Wrist slight flexion and radial deviation. Fingers short, club form of distal phalanges. Groved nails. Absence of other bone fusions.

Etiology. Autosomal dominant inheritance.

Diagnostic Procedures. *X-rays of hand.* Multiple anomalies. Of *wrist.* Triquetrous-pisiform fusion; small capitate; trapezium; and trapezoid; enlarged tetriquetum and hammate. Aplasia of bones at elbow.

BIBLIOGRAPHY. Liebenberg F: A pedigree with unusual anomalies of elbow, wrists and hands in five generations. S Afr Med J 47:745–747, 1973

LIEBOW-CARRINGTON

Synonym. Wegener's lymphomatoid variant. See Carrington-Liebow and Angioimmunoblastic lymphoadenopathy.

Symptoms and Signs. Those of Wegener's (see); without renal complication.

Etiology. Unknown.

Pathology. Histologic features difficult to differentiate from reticuloendothelial neoplasia except for the intense and prominent vasculitis and the fact that lymph nodes are not involved.

Therapy. Corticosteroids of uncertain benefit. Cyclophosphamide: benefits in few cases.

Prognosis. Some cases have subsequently developed malignant lymphoma. Seventy percent: death within 5 years from onset.

BIBLIOGRAPHY. Liebow AA, Carrington CB: The lymphomatoid variant of limited Wegener's granulomatosis (abstr). Am J Pathol 55:78–83, 1969
Friedman PJ: Idiopathic and autoimmune type III-like reactions: interstitial vasculitis and granulomatosis. Semin Roentgenol 10:43–51, 1975

LIEPMANN'S

Synonym. Apraxia.

Symptoms and Signs. Inability to carry out purposeful or skilled actions, while general mental capacity and motor power are present. Varieties of the condition are recognized:
1. *Kinetic or motor.* Usually one hand or arm affected
2. *Ideational.* Inability to program a plan of action
3. *Ideokinetic.* Lack of coordination between ideation and motor pattern
4. *Constructional.* Inability to assemble objects (see Kleinst's)

Etiology. Organic brain lesions.
1. Focal lesion of precentral contralateral cortex
2. Bilateral diffuse lesions or toxic state

3. Supramarginal gyrus unilateral or bilateral lesion
4. Right hemisphere (usually) lesion

BIBLIOGRAPHY. Liepmann H: Das Krankheitsbild der Apraxie ("motorischen Asymbolye") auf Grund eines Falles von einseitiger Apraxie. Mschr Psychiatr Neurol 8:15–44; 10–32, 182–197, 1900

Adams RD, Victor M: Principles of Neurology, 3rd ed, pp 46–47. New York, McGraw-Hill 1985

LIGHT ERUPTION POLYMORPHOUS

Synonyms. Solar dermatitis; solar eczema; polymorphic light eruption. See Magnus' and Solar elastosis.

Symptoms. All races, both sexes affected; onset at any age; it becomes manifest in spring and early summer and diminishes later in the year. After exposure to the sun, the latent period ranges from hours to a week. Itching.

Signs. In areas exposed to the sun, usually on the face, triangle of neck, and arms, formation of small papules or vesicular papules (hydroa aestivalis) or large diskoid plaque resembling those observed in erythema multiforme or lupus erythematosus.

Etiology. Phototoxicity (most active wavelength 290 to 320 μ).

Pathology. Dermal inflammatory response.

Diagnostic Procedures. *Skin test.* With light to assess active wavelength.

Treatment. Avoidance of sun exposure during season. Antimalarial drugs intermittently; protection with topical cream and lotions.

Prognosis. Tendency to yearly recurrence without improvement or increase in severity.

BIBLIOGRAPHY. McGrae JDV, Perry HO: Chronic polymorphic light eruption: a review. Arch Dermatol 43:364–379, 1963

Norris PG, Murphy GM, Hawk JL, et al: A histological study of the evolution of solar urticaria. Arch Dermatol 124:80–83, 1988

LIGHTWOOD-ALBRIGHT

Synonyms. Renal tubular acidosis (I, II, & IV); Albright's III; Butler-Albright. Old eponym for renal tubular acidosis (see individual syndromes).

BIBLIOGRAPHY. Lightwood R: Calcific infarction of the kidneys in infants. Communication, Proc Br Paediatr Soc Arch Dis Child 10:205–206, 1935

Albright F, et al: Metabolic studies and therapy in a case of nephrocalcinosis with rickets and dwarfism. Bull Johns Hopkins Hosp 66:7–33, 1940

LIJO PAVIA'S

Synonym. Retinohypophyseal (obsolete).

Symptoms. Onset at all ages, more frequent in women. Headache; psychic disturbances; vertigo and diminution of vision. Atypical alteration of visual field.

Signs. Narrowing of retinal vessel; optic neuritis; optic atrophy.

Etiology and Pathology. Unknown.

Diagnostic Procedures. *Urine.* Glycosuria. *X-ray of skull.* Alteration of bone structure of sella turcica with decalcification and osteolysis of posterior clinoid processes.

Therapy. Gonadotrophic hormone injection.

Prognosis. With treatment, vision only slightly improved, but increase of well-being remarkable.

BIBLIOGRAPHY. Lijo Pavia J: Sindrome retinohipofisario tratado por la gonadotropina suérica: Cuatro neuvas observaciones. Rev Oto Neuro Oftal 22:5–9, 1947

Lijo Pavia J, Lis M: Sindrome retinohipofisario binigno. Sobre 30 observaciones. Rev Oto Neuro Oftal 24:41–45, 1949; 73–76, 1949

LILLIPUTIAN

Synonym. Micropsia.

Symptoms and Signs. Occur in patients suffering from acute infection, toxic delirium (from drugs or alcohol), dementia, or traumatic brain injuries. Visual aura, where little people appear, usually with offensive attitude. Left-sided hemianopia; transient deviation of head and eyes to the left.

Etiology. Psychovisual phenomenon correlated to brain alteration.

BIBLIOGRAPHY. Kauders O: Drehbewegungen um die Körperlangsachse, Hallucination im hemianopischen Gesichtsfeld als Folge eines Schädeltraumas. Z Ges Neurol Psychiatr 98:602–614, 1925

Bender MB, Savitzky N: Micropsia and teleopsia limited to the temporal fields of vision. Arch Ophthmol 29:904–908, 1943

LINEAR NEVUS SEBACEOUS

Synonym. Choristoma-convulsions–mental retardation.

Symptoms. Onset at birth. Nevus sebaceous on scalp or face (midline); convulsion and mental retardation developing during early childhood; failure to thrive.

Signs. Nevus sebaceous: smooth, yellowish papules and nodules in well-delimited patches. In one case hydrocephalus, various deformities, and coarctation of aorta.

Etiology. Unknown; congenital abnormality (only 3 cases reported). Normal chromosomal studies.

Pathology. Microscopic examination of skin lesion: thickening and hyperkeratosis of epidermis and hyperplasia of sebaceous glands (normal in appearance) increased in vascularity of dermis.

Diagnostic Procedures. *Biopsy of skin. Electroencephalography.* Focal abnormalities. *X-ray of skull.* Normal. *Pneumoencephalography.* Lateral ventricular enlargement.

Therapy. Treatment of epilepsy.

Prognosis. Repeated infections; occasionally, seizures, failure to thrive.

BIBLIOGRAPHY. Feuerstein RC, Mims LC: Linear naevous sebaceous with convulsions and mental retardation. Am J Dis Child 104:675–679, 1962
Marden PM, Venters HD: A new neurocutaneous syndrome. Am J Dis Child 112:79–81, 1966
Monahan RH, Hill CW, Venters HD: Multiple choristomas, convulsions and mental retardation as a new neurocutaneous syndrome. Am J Ophthalmol 64:529–532, 1967
Monk BE, Vollum DI: Familial naevus sebaceous. J Roy Soc Med 75:660–661, 1982

LINGUA NIGRA

Synonym. Black hairy tongue.

Symptoms. Occur only in adults. Usually, asymptomatic; in some cases tickling of mouth and retching.

Signs. Proliferation of papillae on the dorsum of tongue, assuming colors that vary from yellow brown to black.

Etiology. Unknown. In some cases, related to antibiotics; in others, to poor oral hygiene or smoking.

Pathology. Hyperplasia of filiform papillae (up to 2 cm) with increased pigmentation.

Therapy. Oral hygiene; gentle brushing with soft toothbrush, after application of strong (long-steeped) tea or 40% solution of urea.

Prognosis. Condition that may persist for months or years.

BIBLIOGRAPHY. Tomaszewski W: Incidence of black tongue in antibiotic treatment. Br Med J I:1249–1251, 1953
Rook A, Wilkinson DS, Ebling FJG, et al: Textbook of Dermatology, 4th ed, p 2118. Oxford, Blackwell Scientific Publications, 1986

LIPOMATOSIS, MULTIPLE

Synonyms. Systemic multicentric lipoblastosis; metastasizing lipoma, Tedeschi's.

Symptoms and Signs. Onset from puberty to 40 years of age. Lipoma localized in the limbs.

Etiology. Unknown. Sporadic or autosomal dominant or polygenic inheritance.

Pathology. Nonencapsulated fat growth affecting (in scattered and disordered pattern) subcutaneous tissue, internal cavity, organs, and bones. Predominance of mature fat cells with transitional forms; lack of cellular anarchy and mitotic figures suggesting neoplastic process.

Diagnostic Procedures. *Biopsy.* Lipid biochemical studies.

Therapy. Excision of masses, affecting function or for esthetic reasons.

Prognosis. Long duration; years of the process. Tendency of fat tissue to regrow after excision.

BIBLIOGRAPHY. Tedeschi CG: Systemic multicentric lipoblastosis. Arch Pathol 42:320–337, 1946
Humphrey AA, Kingsley PC: Familial multiple lipomas: Report of a family. Arch Dermatol Syph 37:30–34, 1938
Rabbiosi G, Borroni G, Scuderi N: Familial multiple lipomatosis. Acta Dermatol Venerol 57:265–267, 1977

LISKER'S

Synonym. Peripheral motor neuropathy/autonomic dysfunction.

Symptoms and Signs. Distal, slowly progressive muscle weakness and hypotrophy beginning in childhood; evidence of autonomic dysfunction starting a few years later and consisting of profuse sweating, distal cyanosis related to cold weather, orthostatic hypotension, and achalasia appearing in the 3rd decade of life.

Etiology. Autosomal recessive/dominant inheritance with reduced penetrance. The disease results from an abnormality of cholinergic innervation.

Pathology. Light and electron microscopic studies of a nerve specimen show nonspecific demyelinization.

Diagnostic Procedures. *Electromyography. Muscle biopsy. Upper gastrointestinal X-ray.*

Therapy. Surgical correction of achalasia; symptomatic medical therapy.

Prognosis. Good *quoad vitam;* variable for the various disturbances.

BIBLIOGRAPHY. Lisker R, Garcia G, de la Rosa-Laris C, et al: Peripheral motor neuropathy associated with autonomic dysfunction in two sisters: new hereditary syndrome? Am J Med Genet 9:255–259, 1981

LISSAUER'S

Synonym. Lissauer's paralysis. See Dementia paralytica.

Symptoms. Occur in patients affected by dementia paralytica (see). Mild or severe strokes, usually following convulsive attacks and leaving hemiplegia, monoplegia, cranial nerve palsy, which after a short period partially or totally recede and leave only mild permanent defects.

Etiology. See Dementia paralytica.

BIBLIOGRAPHY. Storch E: Ueber einige Fälle atypischer progressiver. Paralyse. Nach einem hinterlassenen Manuscript Dr. H. Lissauer. Mschr Psychiatr 9:401–434, 1901

LIST'S

Synonyms. Foraminal impaction; tonsillar herniation. See Arnold-Chiari and Klippel-Feil.

Symptoms. Recurrent headache; dizziness, tinnitus; nausea; stiffness of neck on exertion and after coughing, sneezing.

Signs. Absent or few neurologic signs.

Etiology and Pathology. Congenital malformation. Transitory tonsillar herniation because of minor foraminal malformation.

Diagnostic Procedures. *Spinal tap. X-ray of skull.*

Therapy. Surgical.

Prognosis. Good.

BIBLIOGRAPHY. List CF: Neurologic syndromes accompanying developmental anomalies of occipital bone, atlas, and axis. Arch Neurol Psychiatr 45:577–616, 1941
Michie I, Clark M: Neurological syndromes associated with cervical and craniocervical anomalies. Arch Neurol 18:241–247, 1968

Adams RD, Victor M: Principles of Neurology, 3rd ed, p 688. New York, McGraw-Hill, 1985

LITTLE'S (W.J.)

Synonyms. Cerebral palsy; cerebral diplegia; infantile cerebral diplegia; cerebral paralysis infantilis. See Hemiplegia, infantile.

Symptoms. Both sexes affected; firstborn more frequently affected. Prematurity frequent. Onset at 6 months of age or later. Slow and delayed first motor milestones and speech development; paucity of voluntary movements; scissorlike gait.

Signs. Spasticity, sometimes limited to the legs. Tendon reflexes exaggerated; Babinski's, Oppenheim's, Gordon's signs; clonus; spared abdominal reflexes. In double hemiplegia, bilateral paresis and spasticity more severe in upper extremities. Focal damage signs possibly present. Athetosis and chorea may be present; frequently generalized seizures; frequently mental deficiency (however, remarkable intelligence possible).

Etiology. Widely differing. Prenatal, natal, and postnatal factors (see Pathology). Encephalitis; toxic defect in development.

Pathology. *Brain.* Small defects in individual gyri. Diffuse degenerative process or atrophic lobar sclerosis; gross malformations or developmental defects; grossly normal but pathologic alteration in neurons and cellular architecture.

Diagnostic Procedures. *X-ray; angiography; scintigraphy; CT brain scan.* Variable patterns of degenerative processes and primitive or secondary malformations.

Therapy. Pharmacologic control of convulsion. Antispastics (little effect). Orthopedic measures. Special schooling.

Prognosis. Poor.

BIBLIOGRAPHY. Little WJ: On the influence of abnormal parturition, difficult labour, premature birth, and asphyxia neonatorum on the mental and physical condition of the child, especially in relation to deformities. Trans Obstet Soc 3:293–344, 1862
Adams RD, Victor M: Principles of Neurology, 3rd ed, pp 923–924. New York, McGraw-Hill, 1985

LITTRE'S

Synonyms. Hernia, Littre's.

Symptoms and Signs. More common in men and on the right side. Hernia (50% inguinal, 20% femoral, 20%

umbilical, 10% miscellaneous). When strangulation occurs: pain, fever while small bowel obstruction symptoms and signs are delayed.

Etiology. Hernia sac containing a Meckel's diverticulum.

Treatment. Repair of hernia and excision of diverticulum.

Prognosis. Good with appropriate treatment.

BIBLIOGRAPHY. Littre A: Observation sur la nouvelle espace de hernia. Hist Acad Roy d Sc 1700, Paris 1719, no 300–310

Zuniga D, Zupanec R: Littre's hernia. JAMA 237:1599, 1977

Perlman JA, Hoover HC, Safer PK: Femoral hernia with strangulated Meckel's diverticulum. Am J Surg 139:286–289, 1980

LIVEDO RETICULARIS

Synonyms. Asphyxia reticularis multiplex; dermatopathia pigmentosa reticularis; inflammatio cutis racemosa; livedo annularis; livedo racemosa. See also Cutis marmorata.

Symptoms. Manifestation different according to etiology. *Congenital.* Present from birth. *Idiopathic.* Occur in young adults and middle-aged females. *Secondary.* Onset at all ages. In all forms usually no symptoms except tingling or numbness on cold exposure.

Signs. Dilatation of small vessels; reticular, blotchy red bluish discoloration of the skin of extremities (legs in particular); ulcerations; scaling.

Etiology. Variable: congenital; idiopathic; secondary to collagen and infective process; from chronic close exposure to heating sources, charcoal containers, or hot-water bottles (*ab igne*); cold intensifies manifestations.

Pathology. Pigmentary changes; scaling; ulcers.

Therapy. None satisfactory. Severe cases with ulceration are helped by anticoagulants.

Prognosis. Changes initially reversible when cause may be abolished, but subsequently vessel dilatation and skin changes become permanent. Congenital form may improve with growth.

BIBLIOGRAPHY. Unna PG: The Histopathology of the Diseases of the Skin. Walker N (trans). Edinburgh, Clay, 1896

Champion RH: Livedo reticularis: a review. Br J Dermatol 77:167–179, 1965

Rook A, Wilkinson DS, Ebling FJG, et al: Textbook of Dermatology, 4th ed, pp 627–631. Oxford, Blackwell Scientific Publications, 1986

LIVER, MASSIVE NECROSIS

Synonyms. Acute fatty metamorphosis of the liver; acute parenchymatous hepatitis; icterus gravis; pregnancy, fatty metamorphosis of the liver; yellow liver atrophy. See Reye's (R.K.D.) II.

Symptoms. Occur in young women in 3rd trimester of pregnancy. Epigastric and right upper quadrant pain. Excessive fatigue; fainting episodes; nausea and vomiting. Later, confusion, disorientation, stupor, coma, and death.

Signs. Jaundice.

Etiology. Unknown, but among possible etiologic agents: (1) Medications given to pregnant woman during 3rd trimester of pregnancy, e.g., tetracyclines, especially intravenously; chlorothiazides; (2) overwhelming viral hepatitis during pregnancy; (3) lipotropic deficiency; (4) hepatotoxins.

Pathology. At autopsy, the main findings are in liver: centrolobular fatty metamorphosis; occasionally, hepatocellular necrosis.

Diagnostic Procedures. *Blood.* Total serum bilirubin increased. *Liver profile.* Liver function deterioration.

Therapy. Liver transplant.

Prognosis. Fatal outcome.

BIBLIOGRAPHY. Peters RL, Edmondson HA, Kunelis CT: Acute fatty metamorphosis of the liver in pregnancy. JAMA 180:767, 1962

Czernobilsky B, Bergnes MA: Acute fatty metamorphosis of the liver in pregnancy with associated liver cell necrosis. Obstet Gynecol 26:792–798, 1965

Kaplan MM: Recent concepts: acute fatty liver of pregnancy. New Engl J Med 313:367–370, 1985

LIVER PELIOSIS

Synonyms. Liver angiomatosis; hepatic peliosis; peliosis hepatis; purpura hepatis; sinusoidal ectasia (closely related condition).

Symptoms and Signs. Markedly variable. Hepatomegaly and jaundice main features.

Etiology. In the past associated mainly with neoplastic marasmus or tuberculosis; today associated with contraceptive pill and prolonged androgenic steroid treatment; attributed also to azathioprine treatment in a patient with kidney transplant. Possibly, direct toxic mechanism acting on lining cells of sinusoids.

Pathology. In liver; cavernous cysts filled with blood in continuity with the sinusoids. Minor changes of the hepatocytes contiguous to the cysts.

Diagnostic Procedures. *Biopsy of liver.* Caution: danger of hemorrhagic complication. *Liver scan.* Isotopes; ultrasound.

Therapy. Symptomatic. Discontinuation of previous therapy.

Prognosis. Related mainly to basic condition, possibility, however of progression to hepatic failure.

BIBLIOGRAPHY. Zak FG: Peliosis hepatis. Am J Pathol 26:1–15, 1950
Zafrani ES, Pinaudeau Y, Dhumeaux D: Drug induced vascular lesions of the liver. Arch Int Med 143:495–503, 1983

LIVER, RADIATION

Synonym. Radiation hepatitis.

Symptoms and Signs. Onset usually 4 weeks after radiation of liver area. Mimics Budd-Chiari (see): jaundice; ascites; painful hepatomegaly.

Etiology. Radiation.

Pathology. Intrahepatic venules damaged with resulting congestion of liver. Minimal histologic changes in the parenchyma.

Diagnostic Procedures. Demonstration of patency of hepatic vein. *Biopsy of liver. Angiography. Liver scan. Blood: Liver function tests.* Alkaline phosphatase high.

Prognosis. Variable according to amount of radiation. Acute venous congestion may result in death.

BIBLIOGRAPHY. Ingold JA, Reed GB, Kaplan HS, et al: Radiation hepatitis. Am J Roentgenol 93:200–208, 1965
Lansing AM, Davis WM, Brizel HE: Radiation hepatitis. Arch Surg 96:878–882, 1968

LLOYD'S

Eponym used to indicate the association of pituitary, parathyroid, and pancreatic adenomas. See Wermer's.

BIBLIOGRAPHY. Lloyd PC: A case of hypophyseal tumor with associated tumorlike enlargement of the parathyroides and islands of Langerhans. Bull John Hopkins Hosp 45:1–14, 1929

LOBAR EMPHYSEMA

Synonyms. Congenital lobar emphysema, including Hislop-Reid syndrome.

Symptoms and Signs. Male predominance (3 : 1); onset at birth in 30% of cases, in the remainder, onset after some weeks, occasionally months, of life. Respiratory distress; cyanosis in severe forms; thoracic asymmetry (unilateral overinflation); breath sounds reduced; rales and local wheeze; tachypnea.

Etiology. Lobar emphysema caused by congenital malformations; vascular type; idiopathic (e.g., unrecognized infection); absence or hypoplasia or bronchial cartilage; gigantism of pulmonary acini (Hislop-Reid syndrome). Familial cases autosomal dominant inheritance.

Pathology. Severe overinflation of pulmonary lobe with predilection for left upper lobe and, slightly less, for right middle lobe.

Diagnostic Procedures. *X-ray.* Overinflation of a particular lobe; depression of corresponding hemidiaphragm and mediastinum displacement; vascular markings in the lobe are separated. Usually hyperlucency of affected lobe; occasionally, increased density (impaired fluid drainage). *Cardiac catheterization. Angiography.*

Therapy. Surgery according to evolution, or supportive therapy.

Prognosis. Usually, course rapid and progressive; in many cases, spontaneous regression.

BIBLIOGRAPHY. Sloan H: Lobar obstructive emphysema in infancy treated by lobectomy. J Thorac Cardiovasc Surg 26:1–20, 1953
Hislop A, Reid L: New pathologic findings in emphysema of childhood. I. Polyalveolar lobe with emphysema. Thorax 25:682–690, 1970
Wall MA, Eisenberg JD, Campbell JR: Congenital lobar emphysema in a mother and daughter. Pediatrics 70:131–133, 1982

LOCKED-IN SYNDROME

Synonym. De-efferentation.

Symptoms. Paralysis of all four extremities and the lower cranial nerves without interference with consciousness. Possibility of maintaining the capacity to use vertical eye movements and blinking to communicate awareness of internal and external stimuli.

Etiology. Midbrain infection, pontine tumor, or hemorrhage; myelinolysis; head injury; polyneuritis; myasthenia gravis.

Pathology. Lesions of ventral and paramedian pontine tegmentum.

Diagnostic Procedures. *CT brain scan. Angiography. Transcranial Doppler. Nuclear magnetic resonance.*

Prognosis. Poor.

Therapy. Same as for apallic coma (see).

BIBLIOGRAPHY. Hawkes CH: Locked-in syndrome: report of seven cases. Br Med J 4:379–382, 1976
Feldam MH: Physiological observation in a chronic case of locked-in syndrome. Neurology 21:459–478, 1978

LOCKED LUNG

Synonym. Paradoxical bronchospasm.

Symptoms and Signs. Status asthmaticus unresponsive to adrenalin, steroids, aminophylline, and intermittent positive pressure treatment occurring in patients who use an excess of nebulized isoproterenol.

Etiology. Excessive exposure to nebulized isoproterenol determining a cumulative irritating effect on respiratory tract mucous membranes. No allergic factor seems involved, but a direct effect of the drug is responsible for the syndrome.

Therapy. Discontinuation of use of isoproterenol. Asthmatic patient should be advised to use only isoproterenol spray, as little as possible, preferably less than seven times a day. Other bronchodilator drugs have become available with beta-2-adrenergic selectivity, to be used alone or in combination, with prolonged action compared to isoproterenol.

Prognosis. Death may result from abuse of isoproterenol. Discontinuation of drug cures the condition. Reexposure to the drug in usual therapeutic doses after recovery does not induce discomfort.

BIBLIOGRAPHY. Keighley JF: Iatrogenic asthma associated with adrenergic aerosols. Ann Intern Med 65:985–995, 1966
Death from asthma (Annotation). Lancet I:1412–1413, 1968
Whitsett TL, Manion CV: Cardiac and pulmonary effects of therapy with albuterol and isoproterenol. Chest 74:251–255, 1978
Dukes MNG: Side Effects of Drugs, vol. 2, p 121. Amsterdam, Excerpta Medica, 1978

LOEFFLER'S

Synonyms. Idiopathic eosinophilic lung disease; transient eosinophilic pneumonia. See Eosinophilic lung, secondary.

Symptoms. Malaise; anorexia; fever; cough; pain in the chest and dyspnea. Occasionally asymptomatic.

Signs. Pleural rales; pericardial effusion; prolonged expiration and wheezing.

Etiology. Unknown. History of atopy.

Pathology. Lung infiltration with eosinophils, giant cells, interstitial proliferation, serous exudation, and vascular alterations.

Diagnostic Procedures. *Blood.* Leukocytosis: 20,000 white blood cells, in great part eosinophils. *Sputum.* Rich in eosinophilis. *X-ray of lung.* Migratory patchy infiltration.

Therapy. Corticosteroids.

Prognosis. Acute, self-limited form with benign outcome.

BIBLIOGRAPHY. Loeffler W: Zur Differential-diagnose der Lungeninfiltrierungen: ueber flüchtige Succedaninfiltrate (mit Eosinophilie). Beitraege Klin Tubercolose 79:338–367, 1932
Hall JW, Kozak M, Spink WW: Pulmonary infiltrates, pericarditis and eosinophilia. Am J Med 36:135–143, 1964
Lynch JP, Flint A: Sorting out the pulmonary eosinophilic syndromes. J Respir 5:61, 1984

LÖFGREN'S

Synonym. Hilar bilateral lymphadenopathy. See Besnier-Boeck-Schaumann and erythema nodosum.

Symptoms and Signs. Prevalent in females, especially during pregnancy or puerperium. Fever; erythema nodosum; signs of bilateral enlargement of mediastinal lymph nodes.

Etiology. Unknown; sarcoidosis leading cause. In Hodgkin's syndrome, viral, bacterial, or atypical tuberculosis infections.

Diagnostic Procedures. *X-ray of chest.* Bilateral enlargement of mediastinal lymph nodes, sometimes, also right paramediastinal glands. *Kveim's test.* Frequently positive. *Tuberculin test.* Negative or weak. *Biopsy of lymph node and liver.*

Therapy. According to etiology.

Prognosis. Benign course, that subside in 3 weeks (mild) or 6 weeks (severe). Exceptionally, recurrences after these periods. Fatigue and general depression may continue for months.

BIBLIOGRAPHY. Löfgren S: Erythema nodosum: Studies on etiology and pathogenesis in 185 adult cases. Acta Med Scand (suppl) 174:1–197, 1946
Rook A, Wilkinson DS, Ebling FJG, et al: Textbook of Dermatology, 4th ed, pp 1162–1164. Oxford, Blackwell Scientific Publications, 1986

LOEHR-KINDBERG

Synonyms. Subacute allergic pneumonia; chronic eosinophilic pneumonia; subacute eosinophilic pneumonitis; Loeffler's variant; pulmonary eosinophilia.

Symptoms. Predominantly in women. High fever; malaise; dyspnea; occasionally, hemoptysis.

Signs. All features of pneumonia with slow resolution. Weight loss.

Etiology. Unknown; atopic background common, but not always demonstrated.

Pathology. Massive infiltration of alveolar walls by polymorphonuclear leukocytes, especially eosinophils and macrophages, histiocytes, lymphocytes. In some cases, mild angiitis and granulomas.

Diagnostic Procedures. *Blood.* Eosinophilia (frequently, but not always). *Pulmonary function test.* Nonconstant reduced diffusing capacity. *X-ray.* See Loeffler's.

Therapy. Corticosteroids.

Prognosis. Prompt and dramatic response to treatment. Clinical resolution in 3 to 10 days of onset of therapy. Chronic evolution without specific treatment.

BIBLIOGRAPHY. Loehr H: Ueber flöchtige Lungeninfiltrierungen mit und ohne Eosinophilie des Blutes. Z Klin Med 137:297, 1940
Kindberg LM: Pneumopathie à eosinophiles. Presse Med 48:277–278, 1940
Christoforidis AJ, Molnar W: Eosinophilic pneumonia. Report of two cases with pulmonary biopsy. JAMA 173:157–161, 1960
Lynch JP, Flint A: Sorting out of pulmonary eosinophilic syndromes. J Respir Dis 5:61, 1984

LOEWENTHAL'S

Symptoms and Signs. Present from birth. Hyperhidrosis; atony of limbs; flaccidity or poorly developed muscles; joint hyperextension; rhizomelic contractures; reduced movements; blepharoptosis.

Etiology. Unknown. Congenital hereditary condition.

Diagnostic Procedures. *Biopsy of muscle.* Sclerosis of connective tissue and of subcutaneous fat as well. *X-ray.* Kyphoscoliosis; spurs on calcaneus.

Therapy. Orthopedic.

Prognosis. Gradual spontaneous improvement from birth.

BIBLIOGRAPHY. Loewenthal A: Étude sur les myosites. IV. Sur une forme congénitalisée avec blépharoptose (contribution à l'étude des maladies congénitales des muscles et du tissue conjonctif). Acta Neurol Belg 52:141–145, 1952

LOEWENTHAL'S II

Synonym. Congenital myosclerosis of Loewenthal.

Symptoms and Signs. From birth. Sclerosis of skin and muscles.

Etiology. Unknown. Occurrence in 4 sibs from normal parents.

BIBLIOGRAPHY. Loewenthal A. Une groupe heredodegenerative nouveau: le myoscleroses heredofamiliales. Acta Neurol Belg 54:155–165, 1954

LOIN PAIN–HEMATURIA

Symptoms. Occur in young women (19 to 34 years of age). Repeated attacks of unilateral or bilateral (nonradiating) intense, and usually incapacitating, loin pain of variable duration, from 2 days to 2 weeks, followed by hematuria. Low-grade fever.

Signs. Loin tenderness.

Etiology. Unknown. Relationship to treatment with estrogen compounds, and to consistent renal angiographic abnormalities (intravascular coagulation within the kidneys).

Pathology. *Kidney biopsy.* Normal glomeruli. Thickening of interlobular arteries with deposit of C3 but not Ig. *Arteriography.* Narrowing of intrarenal vessels.

Diagnostic Procedures. *Urine.* Mild proteinuria. *Blood.* Platelet factor 3 availability increased and platelet lifespan diminished; heparin-thrombin clotting time reduced. *X-ray.* Renal arteriography shows abnormalities of smaller vessels and local variations in the rate and flow of contrast.

Therapy. Suspension of estrogens or warfarin or both.

Prognosis. Good with treatment.

BIBLIOGRAPHY. Little PJ, Sloper JS, de Wardener HE: A syndrome of loin-pain and hematuria associated with disease of peripheral renal arteries. Q J Med 36:253–259, 1967
Burden RP, Dathan JR, Etherington MD, et al: The loin pain syndrome. Lancet I:897–900, 1974
Brenner BM, Rector FC: The Kidney, 3rd ed, p 953. Philadelphia, WB Saunders, 1986

LONGER LEG

Synonyms. Leg discrepancy; lower limb length discrepancy. See hemihypertrophy.

Symptoms. Fifteen percent of population have a leg length disparity of 1 cm or more. Patients with 0.5 cm to 1 cm usually present no symptoms or may have the same symptoms as patients with larger disparity. Pain in buttock, thigh, sometimes low back, knee, occasionally calf.

Signs. Leg length disparity. Five types of discrepancies have been classified according to slope pattern versus age, from continuous increase to various patterns of deceleration.

Etiology. Various causes. Idiopathic congenital short femur; coxa vara; proximal femoral focal deficiency; epiphyseal destruction; Ollier's (see) anisomelia; hemihypertrophy (see); hemoangiomatosis; poliomyelitis; juvenile rheumatoid arthritis; neurofibromatosis syndromes (see); Legg-Calvé-Perthes (see); septic arthritis of hip; fractures.

Diagnostic Procedures. Serial observation at 6-month intervals initially and later at 12-month intervals. *Teleoroentgenograms* (before 5 years of age) and *orthoroentgenograms* at older age.

Therapy. According to diagnosis of basic disorder and age of patients.

Prognosis. Variable according to basic disorder and stage of evolution.

BIBLIOGRAPHY. Codivilla A: On the means of lengthening in the lower limbs, the muscle and tissues which are shortened through deformity. Am J Orthop Surg 2:353–370, 1905
Beaty JH: Congenital anomalies of lower extremities. In Crenshaw AH (ed): Campbell's Operative Orthopedics, 7th ed, pp 2683–2703. St Louis, CV Mosby, 1987

LONG Q-T SYNDROMES

Congenital. See Jervell–Lange-Nielsen (1) and Romano-Ward (2).
Acquired (1) due to class 1 antiarrhythmic drugs, tricyclic antidepressants, and phenothiazines. (2) Electrolyte abnormalities; myocarditis; acute ischemia; cardiomyopathies; mitral valve prolapse syndrome (rarely).

BIBLIOGRAPHY. Locati E, Moss AJ, Schwartz PJ, et al: The long Q-T syndrome. J Am Coll Cardiol 3:516, 1984

LONG THUMB-BRACHYDACTYLY

Synonym. Brachydactyly–long thumb.

Symptoms and Signs. Both sexes. From birth. Limitation of hand motion (inability to form fist). Symmetric brachydactyly; long thumbs; 5th finger clinodactyly. Shoulders (limitation of rotation), pectus excavatum. Rhizomelic shortness of limbs. Murmur of pulmonic stenosis; apparent cardiomegaly, possible cardiac conduction defects.

Etiology. Consistent with autosomal dominant inheritance.

Therapy. Symptomatic.

Prognosis. Rhizomelic shortness does not produce shortness of stature, but only reduced length of arms.

BIBLIOGRAPHY. Hollister DW, Hollister WG: The "long thumb" brachydactyly syndrome. Am J Med Genet 8:5–16, 1981

LORAIN-LEVI

Synonyms. Brissaud's III; Brissaud-Meigs; snubnosed dwarfism; Levi's; essential microsomia; Nebecourt's. See also Gilford-Burnier.

Symptoms. History of normal growth with successive periods of impaired growth; delayed puberty; precocious senility; hypoglycemic attacks.

Signs. Relatively normal proportions; face childish; skin dry, loose, wrinkled; sparse subcutaneous fat; dwarfism.

Etiology. Lack or deficient secretion of growth hormone; lesions involving pituitary (cyst; craniopharyngioma; idiopathic fibrosis). The distinction between sexual ateleiosis and primordial short stature is not clear. Possibly autosomal recessive inheritance.

Pathology. Craniopharyngioma (most common lesion); suprasellar cysts; fibrosis of pituitary gland.

Diagnostic Procedures. *Urine.* Absence of gonadotrophin. *Blood.* Reduced protein-bound iodine; hypoglycemia; subnormal elevation of plasma corticoid level after intravenous adrenocorticotropic hormone (ACTH) injection. *X-ray.* Delayed fusion of epiphyses; destruction of sella turcica by tumor or cyst.

Therapy. Growth hormone, thyroid hormone, and gonadal steroid.

Prognosis. Spectacular results with growth hormone treatment. Some results with thyroid and gonadal steroids alone. Depends on etiology.

BIBLIOGRAPHY. Lorain PJ quoted in Faneau de la Cour, Ferdinand-Valére: Du féminisme et de l'infantilisme chez les tuberculeux, No 1 Paris, 1871
Levi E: Contribution à l'étude de l'infantilisme du type Lorain. Nouv Icon Saltpetriére 21:297–324; 421–471, 1908
Soyka LF, Ziskind A, Crawford JD: Treatment of short stature in children and adolescents with human pituitary growth hormone. New Engl J Med 271:754, 1964
Bailey JA: Disproportionate Short Stature: Diagnosis and Management. Philadelphia, WB Saunders, 1973

LORTAT-JACOB–DEGÓS

Synonyms. Mucosynechial dermatitis; Duhring-Brocq variant; mucosynechial atrophic bullous dermatitis; ocular pemphigus; cicatricial pemphigoid; benign pemphigoid mucosal.

Symptoms and Signs. Prevalent in women (2 : 1); onset (on average) over 65 years of age. Recurrent bullae of mucosal and skin zones adjacent to body orifices. Conjunctivae affected in 75% of patients. Bullae eventually break and leave erosions slow to heal. No severe discomfort.

Etiology. Unknown.

Pathology. Subepidermal bullae; no acantholysis. Infiltration of derma by lymphocytes, plasma cells, and eosinophils leading to fibrosis.

Therapy. None; corticosteroids of little use; skin grafting for persistent erosions.

Prognosis. Scar formation after healing; adhesions may develop.

BIBLIOGRAPHY. Lortat-Jacob E: Benign mucosal pemphigoid: dermatite bulleuse muco-synéchante et atrophiante. Br J Dermatol 70:361–367, 1958
Mitchell RD, Smith NH: Cicatricial pemphigoid: a review of 11 cases. Austr Dent J 24:260–265, 1979

LOUIS-BAR'S

Synonyms. Ataxia-telangiectasia syndrome I; Boder-Sedgwick; cephalo-oculocutaneous–telangiectasis; cerebello-cutaneous–telangiectasia; teleangiectasia-ataxia I. See Paine-Efron.

Symptoms. Affects both sexes equally. Choreoathetosis beginning at early age; progressive ataxia; apraxia of ocular movement; seldom, mental retardation (50%); respiratory infections.

Signs. Telangiectasia of bulbar conjunctivae, zygomatic areas, palate, ears, and neck; antecubital and popliteal fossas showing at 4 to 6 years of age; growth deficiency.

Etiology. Unknown; autosomal recessive inheritance. Suggested defect of interaction necessary for differentiation of organs: liver, thymus.

Pathology. Loss of Purkinje cells; degenerative lesions in cortex of cerebellum; venules dilated in cerebellar leptomeninges and white matter. Association of bronchiectasis. Thymus atrophic or absent. Lymphoid tissues devoid of lymphocytes.

Diagnostic Procedures. *CT brain scan.* Atrophy of cerebellum. *Blood.* Hypogammaglobulinemia; IgA low (50%); rarely, IgG low (5%); IgM normal; IgE low; 80–85% decrease in insulin receptor activity of circulating monocytes. Lymphopenia. *Urine.* Presence of unusual substance reported by Pelc and Vis.

Therapy. Symptomatic. X-ray treatment of malignancies may be fatal.

Prognosis. Slowly progressing; treatment of recurrent respiratory infection. High incidence of malignancy (reticuloendothelial system) with this condition.

BIBLIOGRAPHY. Louis-Bar D: Sur an syndrome progressif comprenant des télangiectasies capillaires cutanées et conjonctivales symétriques a disposition naevoïde et des troubles cérébelleux. Confin Neurol, 4:32–42, 1941
Pelc S, Vis H: Ataxia familiale avec Telangiectasies oculaires. Acta Neurol Belg 60:905–922, 1960
Waldmann TA, Misiti J, Nelson DL, et al: Ataxia-telangiectasia: a multisystem hereditary disease with immunodeficiency, impaired organ maturation, X-ray hypersensitivity, and high incidence of neoplasia. Ann Int Med 99:367–379, 1983

LOWENBERG-HILL

Synonym. Pelizaeus-Merzbacher (adult type).

Symptoms. Both sexes affected; onset in adulthood (4th–5th decades). Progressive, increasing tremor of head, jaw, extremities. Transitory attacks (not well definable) during which the patient becomes helpless. Mild depression.

Signs. Absence of abdominal reflexes; tendon hyperreflexia.

Etiology. Unknown; autosomal dominant or recessive.

Pathology. Incomplete patchy demyelinization (similar to carbon monoxide poisoning); dense fiber gliosis; perivascular sudanophilic microglia cells.

Diagnostic Procedures. *Electroencephalography. Spinal tap. CT brain scan.* Symmetric decrease of white matter density. *Magnetic resonance imaging.*

Therapy. None.

Prognosis. Slow progression to complete incapacitation. Usually 20 years' survival.

BIBLIOGRAPHY. Lowenberg K, Hill TS: Diffuse sclerosis with preserved myelin islands. Arch Neurol Psychiatr 29:1232–1245, 1933

Norman RM, Tingey AH, Harvey PW, et al: Pelizaeus-Merzbacher disease: a form of sudanophil leukodystrophy. J Neurol Neurosurg Psychiatr 29:521–529, 1966

Eldridge R, Anayotos CP, Schlesinger S, et al: Hereditary adult-onset leukodystrophy simulating chronic progressive multiple sclerosis. New Engl J Med 311:948–953, 1984

LOWER LEG STASIS

Synonym. Gravitational leg.

Symptoms. Four times more frequent in women than in men. Burning; itching; pain; muscle cramps in the legs.

Signs. Dilatation and tortuosity of leg veins. Chronic edema; induration; ulceration; pigmentation; stasis; dermatitis.

Etiology. Venous antigravitational failure resulting from incompetence of venous valves, a familial trait; postphlebitic lesions; increase in venous pressure.

Pathology. Elongation, tortuosity of veins; medial fibrosis; fragmentation of tunica elastica; disappearance or atrophy of valves.

Therapy. Bed rest; elastic stockings; sponge rubber dressing; injection of sclerosing solutions; high ligation or excision; skin grafting.

Prognosis. Good response to treatment.

BIBLIOGRAPHY. Bauer G: Pathophysiology and treatment of the lower leg stasis syndrome. Angiology 1:1–8, 1950

Rook A, Wilkinson DS, Ebling FJG, et al: Textbook of Dermatology, 4th ed, pp 1196–1201. Oxford, Blackwell Scientific Publications, 1986

LOWER NEPHRON NEPHROSIS

Of historical interest only. See acute tubular insufficiency.

BIBLIOGRAPHY. Strauss MB: Acute renal insufficiency due to lower nephron nephrosis. New Engl J Med 239:693–700, 1948

LOWE'S

Synonyms. Organic aciduria; ammonia, reduced renal production; cerebro-oculorenal dystrophy; Lowe-Bickel; Lowe-Terrey-MacLachlan; oculocerebrorenal dystrophy; renal-oculocerebrodystrophy.

Symptoms. Males affected (a few cases reported in females); symptoms apparent in very early infancy. Mental retardation; generalized hypotonia; hyperactivity with bizarre choreoathetoid movements and screaming. Blindness; no deafness; difficulty in feeding and thriving.

Signs. Striking resemblance of all affected children. Blond (except one Mexican patient). At younger age, chubby, then emaciation. Hypotonic; flabby musculature; areflexia or severe hyporeflexia. Cataracts, and in some congenital glaucoma. Joint hypermobility; cryptorchidism.

Etiology. Unknown; inherited metabolic error affecting only males and transmitted by heterozygous female (X-linked trait). Renal lesions appear as secondary manifestation.

Pathology. No common features from general observation at autopsy. Histologically, kidney tubule dilatation, protein casts, interstitial fibrosis, glomeruli hyalinized, no inflammatory components. *Testes.* Increased interstitial fibrous tissue; diminution of size of tubules. *Eye.* Suprachoroidal layer; prominence of vessels (dilatation); retinal abnormalities of ganglion cells. *Brain.* Diffuse alteration of cortex; tendency for vacuolization of subpial parenchyma; perivascular rarefaction. Proliferation of endothelial elements of arterioles with formation of granulation.

Diagnostic Procedures. *Blood.* Normal or slightly elevated nonprotein nitrogen; variable metabolic acidosis; serum chloride elevated, sodium and potassium normal or low. *Urine.* Usually dilute, but good concentration with fluid restriction. Intolerance to acid stress; organic aciduria; hyperaminoaciduria; proteinuria.

Therapy. Symptomatic.

Prognosis. Poor; mental retardation and metabolic defects. The result of cataract surgery poor.

BIBLIOGRAPHY. Lowe CU, Terrey M, MacLachlan EA: Organic aciduria, decreased renal ammonia production, hydrophthalmos and mental retardation. Am J Dis Child 83:164–184, 1952

Witzleben CL, Schoen EJ, Tu WH, et al: Progressive morphologic renal changes in the oculo-cerebro-renal syndrome of Lowe. Am J Med 44:319–324, 1968

Matsuda I, Takeda T, Sugai M, et al: Oculocerebrorenal syndrome, in a child with a normal urinary acidification and a defect in bicarbonate reabsorption. Am J Dis Child 117:205–212, 1969

Tripathi R, Cibis GW, Harris DJ, et al: Lowe's syndrome. Birth Defects Orig Art Ser 18(6):629–644, 1982

LOWN-GANONG-LEVINE

Synonyms. LGL; Clerc-Levy-Cristeco, CLP; coronary nodal rhythm; short P-R interval; short P-Q interval. Eponym used to indicate an electrocardiographic pattern: right P waves in leads II, III and a VF with short P-Q interval, and normal QRS complex. Clinically, this pattern may be observed in paroxysmal tachycardia. Experimentally, this pattern can be obtained by a stimulating electrode in the right atrium, in front of coronary sinus, close to the AV node.

Symptoms and Signs. Young patients. Both sexes. Paroxysmal supraventricular tachycardia or atrial fibrillation flutter. Sometimes ventricular tachycardia.

Etiology. Anomalous atrioventricular conduction pathways. Either reentry using the AV node or reentry using slow AV nodal pathways anterograde and a fast AV nodal pathway retrograde.

Diagnostic Procedures. *ECG.* Short P-R interal, narrow QRS complexes various and/or arrhythmias.

Therapy. Antiarrhythmic drugs. Surgery.

Prognosis. In a small percentage sudden cardiac death.

BIBLIOGRAPHY. Clerc A, Levy R, Cristesco C: A propos du raccourcissement permanent de l'espace P-R de l'electrocardiogramme sans déformation du complexe ventriculaire. Arch Mal Coeur 31:569–582, 1938

Lown B, Ganong W, Levine S: The syndrome of short PR interval, normal QRS complex and paroxysmal rapid heart action. Circulation 8:693–706, 1952

Castellanos A, Zaman L, Moleio F, et al: The Lown-Ganong-Levine syndrome. PACE 5:715, 1982

Weiner I: Syndromes of Lown-Ganong-Levine and enhanced atrioventricular nodal conduction. Am J Cardiol 52:637–639, 1983

LOW OUTPUT

Synonyms. Heart forward failure; heart power failure.

Symptoms and Signs. Recognition from clinical data alone impossible. Diagnosis reached with the aid of monitoring equipment. Usually observed following cardiac surgery. Oliguria.

Etiology and Pathology. Inadequate cardiac output to meet the needs of tissues for oxygen and other nutrients. Increase of the vascular systemic resistences. Reductions of the cardiac pumping ability.

Diagnostic Procedures. *Hemodynamic measurements; oxygen consumption. Blood: Lactic acid production; plasma catecholamine; pH.* Cardiac index (CI): < 2.2 L/min/m^2. Systemic vascular resistance (SVR): > 1500 dyne sec/cm^3. Mixed venous O$_2$ saturation (SVO$_2$): $< 55\%$. O$_2$ consumption index (VO$_2$J): < 100 ml/mn/m^2. Lactic acid > 20 mg%.

Therapy. Digitalis; vasopressors; inotropes, vasodilators. Correction metabolic acidosis. Mechanical circulatory support.

Prognosis. Usually poor. If not given early after onset, vasopressors are frequently ineffective in preventing death.

BIBLIOGRAPHY. Lillehei RC, Dietzman RH, Block JH: Hypotension and low output syndrome following cardiopulmonary bypass. In Norman JC (ed): Cardiac Surgery, pp 437–456. New York, Appleton-Century-Crofts, 1967

Dietzman RH, Ersek A, Lillehei CW, et al: Low output syndrome, recognition and treatment. J Thorac Cardiovasc Surg 57:138–150, 1969

Gray R, Shah PK, Singh B, et al: Low cardiac output states after open heart surgery: comparative hemodynamic effects of dobutamine, dopamine and norepinephrine plus phentolamine. Chest 80:16–25, 1981

Pharmacologic therapy of low output syndromes after cardiac surgery. Arch Int Physiol Biochem 92:S21–S31, 1984

LOW SALT

Synonyms. Cellular hypo-osmolality; essential hyponatremia.

Symptoms and Signs. Occur in patient with advanced congestive heart failure (treated as well as untreated), protracted wasting diseases, malnutrition, or severe chronic infection. No specific symptoms; laboratory diagnosis of hyponatremia; or same symptoms and signs as

Schroeder's. Lethargy; anorexia; disorientation; edema; ascites; pleural cavity fluid accumulation.

Etiology and Pathology. Not well understood. Continuous potassium release from the cells with replacement by sodium ions. Two sodium ions replace three potassium ions with fall of osmotic pressure of cells, consequent antidiuretic hormone (ADH) secretion and water retention with lowering of extracellular sodium concentration. Not to be confused with Schroeder's (see), which occurs in intensively treated congestive heart failure and presents the same feature of hyponatremia.

Diagnostic Procedures. *Blood.* Low serum sodium and potassium; blood urea nitrogen normal; anemia, with decreased mean corpuscular red cell volume. Hypoproteinemia. Estimation of total body water and electrolytes reveals normal sodium values. *Urine.* May show increase in potassium.

Therapy. Treatment of underlying disease and complication. Administration of sodium contraindicated; continuation of salt restriction; limitation of fluid intake. Ammonium chloride and potassium chloride; mercurial diuretics at long intervals, and with caution.

Prognosis. That of associated condition; persisting indefinitely in chronically ill patients.

BIBLIOGRAPHY. Vogl A: The low-salt syndrome in congestive heart failure. Am J Cardiol 3:192–198, 1959
LaRotonda ML, Grace WJ: The low salt syndrome: an extreme example in heart failure. Am J Cardiol 6:676–677, 1960
Packer M, Medina N, Yushak M: Correction of dilutional hyponatremia in severe chronic heart failure by converting enzyme inhibition. Ann Int Med 100:782–789, 1984
Schrier RW: Treatment of hyponatremia: editorial retrospective. New Engl J Med 312:1121–1122, 1985

LUBARSCH-PICK

Eponym used to indicate the association of macroglossia with primary amyloidosis, or amyloidosis syndromes (see).

BIBLIOGRAPHY. Königstein H: Ueber Amyloidose der Haut. Arch Dermatol Syph 148:330–383, 1925
Lubarsch O: Zur Kenntnis ungewöhnlicher Amyloidablagerungen. Virchows Arch [Pathol Anat] 271:867–889, 1929

LUBS'

Synonyms. Male pseudohermaphroditism familial; male familial pseudohermaphroditism; androgen insensitivity;

testicular feminization; dihydrotestosterone receptor deficiency. See pseudohermaphroditism, male, incomplete hereditary (type I).

Symptoms and Signs. Male pseudohermaphrodites. Signs variable with age. Enlarged clitoris; labia with scrotal characteristics containing testes; pseudohernia; urogenital sinus containing urethra. Female breast development and hair distribution. Phenotype voluptuously feminine.

Etiology. X-linked inheritance. Represents the variant toward the feminine end of the spectrum of the male pseudohermaphroditism, hereditary (Type I). End-organ unresponsiveness to androgen (see Seabright-Bantam).

Pathology. Presence of testicular tissue bilaterally with marked degree of Leydig-cell hyperplasia. Tubules appearance variable, usually with almost normal spermatogenesis. Epididymis; rete testis; vas deferens normal.

Diagnostic Procedures. *Biopsy of testis. Endocrine studies.* Lack of significant abnormalities. *Sex chromatin studies.* No chromatin positive cells. *Chromosome studies.*

Therapy. Removal of testes.

Prognosis. Good *quoad vitam.*

BIBLIOGRAPHY. Pallaillon NI: Observation d'hermaphroditisme. Bull Neur Soc Obstet Gynec (Paris) 123–130, 1891
Dieffenbach H: Familiarer Hermaphroditism. Inaugural Dissertation Stuttgart, 1912
Lubs HA, Vilar, O, Bergenstal DM: Familial male pseudohermaphroditism with labial testes and partial feminization: endocrine studies and genetic aspects. J Clin Endocrinol Metab 19:1110–1120, 1959
Wilson JD, Carlson BR, Weaver DD, et al: Endocrine and genetic characterization of cousins with male pseudohermaphroditism: evidence that the Lubs phenotype can result from a mutation that alters the structure of the androgen reception. Clin Genet 26:363–370, 1984

LUCEY-DRISCOL

Synonyms. Lucey-Arias; transient familial neonatal hyperbilirubinemia.

Symptoms and Signs. Both sexes; from birth. Rapidly progressive jaundice; kernicterus. Sudden death.

Etiology. Unidentified inhibitor of uridine diphosphate (UDP) glucuronosyltransferase. Possible autosomal recessive inheritance.

Pathology. At autopsy, kernicterus.

Diagnostic Procedures. *Blood.* Unconjugated hyperbilirubinemia up to 60–65 mg/dl. *Maternal serum.* Inhibitor of UDP glucuronosyltransferase.

Therapy. Phototherapy; exchange transfusion.

Prognosis. Death in some cases; in others, neurological sequelae.

BIBLIOGRAPHY. Lucey JF, Arias IM, McKay RJ Jr: Transient familial neonatal hyperbilirubinemia. Am J Dis Child 100:787–789, 1960

Lucey JF, Driscol JJ: Physiological jaundice re-examined. In Saal-Korttsak A (ed): Kernicterus, p 29. Toronto, University of Toronto Press, 1961

Arias IM, Wolfson S, Lucey JF, et al: Transient familial neonatal hyperbilirubinemia. J Clin Invest 44:1442–1450, 1965

LUDWIG'S

Synonym. Parapharyngeal abscess.

Symptoms and Signs. Most frequent in males; onset in childhood. Dysphagia; dyspnea; trismus; fever; malaise. Pharyngeal and laryngeal edema; cellulitis of the submaxillary region and oral cavity floor and tongue, and possibly extending to anterior part of neck. Tachycardia; occasionally, cyanosis.

Etiology. Severe pharyngitis caused, usually, by streptococci, less frequently by other infective agents; usually, secondary to tooth extraction, trauma of interior of mouth, dental caries, or paradental infections.

Pathology. Cellulitis with possible pus formation involving submaxillary ducts, sublingual space, fascial neck spaces.

Diagnostic Procedures. *Blood.* Polymorphonuclear leukocytosis. *Swab culture. Streptococcus pyogenes* frequently identified. *Ultrasonography.*

Therapy. Antibiotics. Surgery if needed.

Prognosis. Good with treatment. Possible complications: jugular thrombosis; mediastinitis; pneumonia; metastatic infection of myocardium; cavernous sinus; meninges.

BIBLIOGRAPHY. Ludwig D, et al: Ueber eine in neuere Zeit wiederholt beier vorgkommene Form von Halsentzündung. Med Corresp Wuertt Aerztl Vereims 6:21–25, 1836

Fliacher I, Peleg H, Joackims HZ: Mediastinitis and bilateral pneumothorax complicating a parapharyngeal abscess. Head Neck Surg 3:438, 1981

LUETSCHER'S I

Synonyms. Fever dehydration; pure dehydration; dehydration-hypertonicity; dessication; transitory fever newborn; water depletion.

Symptoms. Thirst (this symptom may be missing in patient with cerebral lesions); inability to swallow dry food; weakness; weight loss; fever; change in personality (forced vivacity); hallucination; delirium.

Signs. Skin flushed; sweating decreased; xerostomia; lack of tears; tongue dry and fissured; skin doughy-feeling. Tachycardia, hyperpnea, and then coma (terminal signs).

Etiology and Pathology. (1) Lack of water; (2) difficulty in swallowing; (3) adipsia in debilitated infants because of cerebral lesions; (4) diabetes insipidus neurohypophyseal (see); (5) water-losing nephritis; (6) diarrhea (mild, especially in infants and young children); (7) hyperventilation or tracheostomy; (8) burns; (9) sudden water loading; (10) diabetes insipidus syndromes, antidiuretic hormone (ADH)-resistant (see).

Diagnostic Procedures. *Blood.* Early stage normal, then hemoconcentration (high hematocrit, serum electrolytes, and protein); high blood urea nitrogen. *Urine.* Small volume; high specific gravity (except if previous inability to concentrate); hematuria; proteinuria; casts.

Therapy. Water alone (if ion deficiency has been ruled out), orally or rectally, or intravenous isotonic solution, or intravenous 10% dextrose in water. One half replacement water and daily requirement given on first day; the remainder the second day. If diabetes insipidus, vasopressin; if vasopressin-resistant diabetes, drug of chlorothiazide group.

Prognosis. According to amount of water loss and pathogenetic mechanism; cases of 12% water loss, inability to swallow: 12% to 25% mortality.

BIBLIOGRAPHY. Luetscher JA Jr, Blackman SS, Jr: Severe injury to kidneys and brain following sulfathiazole administration: high serum sodium and chloride levels and persistent cerebral damage. Ann Int Med 18:741–756, 1943

Schoolman HM, Dubin A, Hoffman WS: Clinical syndromes associated with hypernatremia. Arch Int Med 95:15–23, 1955

Gennari FJ: Serum osmolality: uses and limitation. New Engl J Med 310:102–105, 1984

LUPUS ERYTHEMATOSUS, DISCOID

Synonyms. Discoid lupus erythematosus; cutaneous lupus erythematosus.

Symptoms. Female to male ratio 2 : 1; onset at any age; however, usually, it begins in the 4th decade in females and slightly later in males. Onset may occur coincidentally with trauma of different types: mechanical; sun; cold; psychological (e.g., worry). Frequently, history of

Raynaud's phenomenon (see) and pernio (see). Itching or tenderness of affected areas may be present.

Signs. Facial areas more frequently involved; extremities and trunk less frequently. Unilateral or bilateral lesions represented by erythematous plaques, sharply circumscribed, covered by adherent grayish scales of variable diameter (a few millimeters to 10 to 19 cm). Under the scales, in the pilosebaceous canals, horny plugs are present. Regional lymph node enlargement.

Etiology. Unknown. Genetic factor plus somatic mutations may be implicated, plus environmental factors that precipitate the onset by interfering with defense mechanisms.

Pathology. Degeneration of basal cell layer; degenerative changes of connective tissue (hyalinization; edema; fibrinoid changes); lymphocyte infiltration; keratotic plugs in follicular openings.

Diagnostic Procedures. *Biopsy.* See Pathology. *Blood.* Erythrocyte sedimentation rate increased in 20% of cases; antinuclear factor in 35%; leukopenia in 13%.

Therapy. Screening from sun. Protective topical creams and corticosteroid creams (or intralesional injection of corticosteroid). Oral antimalarial agents (e.g., chloroquine sulfate; hydroxychloroquine).

Prognosis. Tendency toward persistence of lesions. Good response to treatment, determined however, by type and duration of lesion. Scarring and pigmentation frequent. Relapses with trauma, sun, cold. General good health is maintained.

BIBLIOGRAPHY. Kaposi M: Pathologie und Therapie der Hautkrankheiten, 2nd ed, p 642. Vienna, Urban & Schwarzenberg, 1883
Rook A, Wilkinson DS, Ebling FJG, et al: Textbook of Dermatology, 4th ed, pp 1285–1302. Oxford, Blackwell Scientific Publications, 1986

LUPUS ERYTHEMATOSUS, SYSTEMIC

Synonyms. SLE; disseminated lupus erythematous.

Symptoms. Predominantly in women in childbearing age. Malaise; weakness; anorexia; migratory joint pains; intermittent abdominal pleuritic pains; "anaphylactoid" pneumonitis (tachypnea, dyspnea, and cyanosis); mental reaction; anxiety; hallucination; convulsions; recurrent fever. Exposure to sunlight may induce manifestations.

Signs. Butterfly face eruption (in 50%), and maculopapular erythematous eruptions on neck, extremities; telangiectasis; chronic leg ulcers; scarring of nail bed and fingertips; frequently cotton-wool retinal exudates. Enlargement of lymph nodes; splenomegaly; hepatomegaly. Signs of involvement of cardiovascular system (pericarditis, endomyocarditis in 50% of cases) and of kidney (in 75%).

Etiology. Unknown; alteration of immune mechanism. Congenital susceptibility. Primary lesion appears to be cellular breakdown releasing cellular antigens. Antigens combine with anti-DNA and are phagocytized, resulting in release of lysosomal products. These cause further tissue breakdown and a continuous cycle.

Pathology. *Kidney biopsy.* Various histological patterns are seen: mesangial glomerulonephritis chronic (see), focal and segmental proliferative glomerulonephritis, diffuse proliferative glomerulonephritis, membranous GNF, glomerular sclerosis.

Diagnostic Procedures. *Blood.* Leukopenia; eosinophils reduced; anemia; thrombocytopenia; lupus erythmatosus cell; hypergammaglobulinemia; presence of anticoagulant in plasma. A chronic false-positive serology test for syphilis may antedate the onset of clinical manifestations of SLE by many years. Antinuclear antibodies (IgG, but also IgM, IgA, and IgE), antibodies to double stranded DNA (ds DNA), antibodies to ribonuclear antigens, serum complement depression, circulating immune complexes. Association with HLA B7 and B8. Rheumatoid factor, cryoglobulins, abnormalities of T4/T8 ratio. *Urine.* Albuminuria.

Therapy. Corticosteroids; adrenocorticotropic hormone; immunosuppressant agents (azanthioprine; mercaptopurine). Transplantation.

Prognosis. Periods of activity of different durations. Hypertension, cardiac and renal failure, hemorrhages causes of death. Recurrence in transplanted kidney is rare.

BIBLIOGRAPHY. Kaposi MK: Neue Beiträqe zur Kenntniss des Lupus Erythematosus. Arch Dermatol Syph 4:36–78, 1872
Tan EM, Cohen AS, Fries JF, et al: The 1982 revised criteria for the classification of systemic lupus erythematosus. Arch Rheum 25:1271, 1982
Rook A, Wilkinson DS, Ebling FJG, et al: Textbook of Dermatology, 4th ed, pp 1303–1334. Oxford, Blackwell Scientific Publications, 1986
Mandell BF: Cardiovascular involvement in systemic lupus erythematosus. Semin Arthr Rheum 17:126–141, 1987
Wallace DJ, Dubois EL: Dubois's Lupus Erythematosus, 3rd ed, p 71. Philadelphia, Lea & Febiger, 1987
McHugh NJ, Maymo J, Skinner RP, et al: Anticardiolipin antibodies livedo reticulosis and major cerebrovascular and renal disease in systemic lupus erythematosus. Ann Rheum Dis 47:110–115, 1988
Lehman TJA, McCurdy DK, Bernstein BH, et al: Sys-

temic lupus erythematosus in the first decade of life. Pediatrics 83:235–239, 1989

LUTEMBACHER'S

Synonyms. Atrial septal defect–mitral stenosis.

Symptoms. Predominantly in women; onset in young adulthood. History of rheumatic fever; cardiac disease; slow growth; congestive heart failure. Varying hemodynamic patterns depending on the size of the atrial septal defect and the severity of the mitral stenosis.

Signs. Left atrial enlargement; systolic murmur on the apex; atrial fibrillation at older age.

Etiology. Congenital atrial septal defect with mitral stenosis.

Pathology. Interatrial septal defect; mitral stenosis; dilated pulmonary artery. This syndrome makes up 6% of all general atrial defects.

Diagnostic Procedures. *Electrocardiography.* P waves broadened, notched; right ventricular hypertrophy; right bundle branch block; possibly, atrial fibrillation or flutter. *X-ray.* Small aorta; dilated pulmonary artery; large pulmonary trunk; hypertrophy, right side. *Angiocardiography. Cardiac catheterization. Echocardiography.*

Therapy. Surgical treatment when symptoms and systemic manifestation indicate.

Prognosis. Average life span 35 years; longevity possible.

BIBLIOGRAPHY. Lutembacher R: De la stenose mitrale avec communication interauriculaire. Arch Mal Coeur 9:237–250, 1916
Perloff JK: The Clinical Recognition of Congenital Heart Disease, 2nd ed, p 318. Philadelphia, WB Saunders, 1978
Hurst JW: The Heart, 6th ed, pp 597–603. New York, McGraw-Hill, 1986

LUTZ-JEANSELME

Synonyms. Jeanselme's; periarticular nodosities; Steiner's.

Symptoms and Signs. Mobile, periarticular, nodular formations appearing during treponemic infections.

Etiology. Syphilis and pinta.

Therapy. Antibiotics.

Prognosis. Regression with therapy.

BIBLIOGRAPHY. Lutz A: Mhefte Prakt Derm 14:30, 1892
Jeanselme E: Nodosités juxtarticulaires. Cong, p 15. Colonial, Paris, Sect Med Hyg Colon, 1904

LUTZ-MIESCHER

Synonyms. Elastosis perforans serpiginosa; keratosis follicularis serpiginosa; Miescher's; elastoma intrapapillare perforans serpiginosa.

Symptoms and Signs. Prevalent in males; onset before 30 years of age in 90% of cases (youngest patient 5 years old; oldest patient, 84); all races. Usually, localized to the neck; less frequently to upper extremities, face, lower extremities, trunk (in this order). Asymptomatic or slight pruritus. Slight erythematous keratotic papules (2 to 5 mm in diameter), with small central scaling arranged in diffuse, serpiginous, or circular pattern; satellite lesions usually appear. Frequently, symmetric distribution on both sides of neck, both forearms. Also, frequently associated with various disorders of Van Der Hoeve's, Grönblad-Strandberg-Touraine, Marfan's, and Rothmund's, Ehlers-Danlos, Down's.

Etiology. Unknown; familial incidence has been reported; autosomal dominant (?).

Pathology. Areas of skin perforation in the form of narrow canals, whose openings are plugged with keratinous corium, which shows foreign body granulomas. Peripheral canal part: loose parakeratinous flakes; central part: mixture of degenerated epithelial cells, inflammatory cells, and eosinophilic fibers. Staining for elastic fibers reveals increase of these fibers in the corium, thicker than those seen in normal skin.

Therapy. Dry ice; electrosurgery (may induce formation of keloid scar). Best treatment: cellophane tape and stripping of keratinous material.

Prognosis. Difficult to predict. From spontaneous regression without scar, to persistence and recurrences up to 5 years with or without scar. Very good results with cellophane tape technique; recurrences are possible, however.

BIBLIOGRAPHY. Jones PE, Smith DC: Porokeratosis, review and report of cases. Arch Dermatol 56:425–436, 1947
Lutz W: Keratosis follicularis serpiginosa. Dermatologica 106:318, 1953
Miescher G: Elastoma intrapapillare perforans verruciforme. Dermatologica 110:254–266, 1955
Ayala F, Donofrio P: Elastosis perforans serpiginosa: report of a family. Dermatologica 166:32–37, 1983

LUTZ-RICHNER

Synonyms. Biliary malformation, renal tubular insufficiency, cholestatic jaundice.

Symptoms and Signs. Neonatal jaundice. Failure to thrive. Repeated infections. Occasionally micrognathia, low-set ears, highly arched palate, barrel chest, club feet, hypotonia.

Etiology. Autosomal recessive inheritance.

Pathology. *Liver.* Intrahepatic biliary hyperplasia. *Kidney.* Normal structure with calcification of some distal tubules.

Diagnostic Procedures. *Blood.* Hyperbilirubinemia; defect of polymorphonucleates cell migration and intracellular killing. *Blood gas.* Metabolic acidosis. *Urine.* Aminoaciduria, proteinuria, glycosuria.

Therapy. Symptomatic.

Prognosis. Death within few months.

BIBLIOGRAPHY. Lutz-Richner AR, Landolt RF: Familiaere Gallengangmissbildungen mit tubolaerer Niereninsuffizienz. Helv Paediatr Acta 28:1–12, 1973
Mikati MA, Barakat AY, Suhl HB, et al: Renal tubular insufficiency, cholestatic jaundice, and multiple congenital anomalies: a new multisystem syndrome. Helv Paediatr Acta 39:463–471, 1984

LUXURY-PERFUSION

Synonyms. Cerebral hypoxia–relative hyperemia; Lassen's I.

This designation is used to indicate the dissociation between overabundant cerebral blood flow and cerebral oxygen uptake and arterial carbon dioxide tension. It is observed in many acute brain diseases, such as apoplexy, acute neurosurgical conditions, tumor, head injury, encephalitis; and in patients with severe diabetic acidosis, sickle cell anemia, other chronic anemias, severe ethanol intoxication, and prolonged hypoglycemia. The diminution of cerebral oxygen uptake is the main feature; arterial-jugular venous oxygen difference is small.

Etiology. Acute metabolic acidosis (probably due to increased cerebral lactic acid concentration) of the whole (or part) of brain is the most likely mechanism responsible for this syndrome.

Pathology. Cerebral hyperemia; edema; plus specific lesions according to the etiology.

Diagnostic Procedures. *X-ray. Serial angiography* (with special attention to capillary phase and early filling of vein). *Regional cerebral blood flow measurements: Arteriovenous oxygen difference; arterial pH, cerebrovascular resistance, cerebral oxygen uptake. Blood-brain barrier, using radioisotope scanning. Cerebrospinal fluid: Bicarbonate content.*

Therapy. Hyperventilation that may normalize local pH at expense of alkalosis in other parts of the body.

Prognosis. Extremely poor, depends on etiology.

BIBLIOGRAPHY. Lassen NA: The luxury-perfusion syndrome and its possible relation to acute metabolic acidosis localized within the brain. Lancet II:1113–1115, 1966
Shapiro W, Eisenberg S: Cerebral blood flow and metabolism in the coma of St Louis encephalitis. JAMA 202:145–147, 1967
Davis S, Ackerman R: Cerebral blood flow and cerebrovascular CO_2 reactivity in stroke age normal controls. Neurology 33:391–399, 1983

LYME*

Symptoms and Signs. Oligoarticular arthritis with the unique skin lesion erythema chronicum migrans. May be accompanied by headache, stiff neck, fever, arthralgias and meningoencephalitis.

Etiology. A tick believed to transmit the disease has been identified, and recently spirochetal etiology has been proposed (*Borrelia burgdorferi*).

Pathology. A round papule, which expands peripherally to form an erythematous ring with central clearing.

Diagnostic Procedures. Circulating immune complexes; specific test for *Borrelia burgdorferi;* high titers of complement.

Therapy. Penicillin.

Prognosis. Good.

BIBLIOGRAPHY. Steere AC, Malawista SE, Hardin JA, et al: Erythema chronicum migrans and Lyme arthritis: the enlarging clinical spectrum. Ann Intern Med 86:685–698, 1977
Steere AC, Malawista SE, Snydman DR, et al: Lyme arthritis: an epidemic of oligoarticular arthritis in children and adults in three Connecticut communities. Arthritis Rheum 20:7–17, 1977
Sturfelt G, Cavell B: Lyme disease in a 12-year-old girl. Acta Pediatr Scand 74:133–136, 1985
Seligmann J, Hager M, Drew L, et al: Tiny tick, big worry. Newsweek, May 22, 1989

LYMPHADENOSIS BENIGNA ORBITAE

Symptoms and Signs. Onset reported at 18 to 66 years of age; possibly, higher incidence in women. Exoph-

---

* First recognized in Lyme, Connecticut, in 1975 in an epidemic.

thalmos (may be absent); tumorlike swelling in the orbita, growing slowly, well circumscribed, painless. Affecting one eye or both eyes; if both, developing symmetrically and simultaneously. Not adherent to the skin; eye movements slightly restricted; no palsy; no papilledema. In one case development of glaucoma (lymphadenoglaucomatous syndrome). Absence of lymphadenopathy.

Etiology. Localized inflammatory process of undetermined origin. (Individual reaction to different stimulation: trauma; insect bite; malignant tumor in another part of organism.) Localized manifestation of Spiegler-Fendt (see).

Pathology. In lymphoreticular tissue, mature lymphocytes, plasma cells, eosinophils, leukocytes; absence of Langhans' or Sternberg cells.

Diagnostic Procedures. *Biopsy; blood; bone marrow.* Normal.

Therapy. X-ray therapy.

Prognosis. Duration of disease from 2 to 12 months, occasionally years. Prompt response to x-ray treatment; recurrence seldom.

BIBLIOGRAPHY. Bäfverstedt B, Lundmark C, Mossberg H, et al: Lymphadenosis benigna orbitae. Acta Ophthalmol 34:367–376, 1956

Orlowski WJ, Korobowicz J: The lymphadenoglaucomatous syndrome. Am J Ophthalmol 52:101–106, 1961

LYMPHOHISTIOCYTOSIS, FAMILIAL

Synonyms. Erythrophagocytic familial lymphohistiocytosis; hemophagocytic reticulosis; familial reticulendotheliosis; Omenn's (could be a distinct entity); Farquhar's reticulosis, familial histiocytic.

Symptoms and Signs. Onset in infancy or early childhood. Two phases: (1) *Chronic.* Eczema, failure to thrive, multiple abscesses, chronic otitis media, frequent respiratory tract infections, fever. (2) *Fulminating.* Progressing lymphadenopathy, hepatosplenomegaly, jaundice, pulmonitis.

Etiology. Unknown; possibly autosomal recessive inheritance or virus or both. Nosologically confused group.

Pathology. Generalized reticular cell infiltration of all body tissue, including central nervous system, disruption of lymphoid architecture, and increased presence of plasma cells and eosinophils. Absence of granulomatous formation, necrosis, erythrophagocytosis, and storage-laden histiocytes.

Diagnostic Procedures. *Blood.* Anemia; moderate reticulocytosis; leukopenia. Platelets increased in number in a family report. Hypergammaglobulinemia terminally; hyperbilirubinemia. *Bone marrow.* Reticular cell infiltration; erythroid hyperplasia.

Therapy. Temporary improvement with splenic irradiation or splenectomy and corticosteroids.

Prognosis. Death 2 to 6 weeks after onset; pneumonia; bacteriemia; candidiasis. Longest survival 2 years.

BIBLIOGRAPHY. Farquhar JW: Familial haemophagic reticulosis. Br Med J 2:1561, 1958

Nelson P, Santamaria A, Olson RL, et al: Generalized lymphohistiocytic infiltration: a familial disease not previously described and different from Letterer-Siwe disease and Chediak-Higashi syndrome. Pediatrics 27:931–950, 1961

Omenn GS: Familial reticuloendotheliosis with eosinophilia. New Engl J Med 273:427–432, 1965

Miller DR: Familial reticuloendotheliosis: concurrence of disease in five siblings. Pediatrics 38:986–995, 1966

Petersen RA, Kuwabara T: Ocular manifestations of familial lymphohistiocytosis. Arch Ophthalmol 79:413–416, 1968

Martin VJ, Cras P: Familial erythrophagocytic lymphohistiocytosis: a neuropathologic study. Acta Neuropath 66:140–144, 1985

McARDLE'S

Synonyms. Cori's type V glycogenosis; glycogenosis, type V; McArdle-Schmid-Pearson; myophosphorylase deficiency; muscle phosphorylase deficiency.

Symptoms. Onset usually in childhood, although diagnosis may be made later. First pain; then stiffness following exercise of any muscle, including masseter. Rest makes symptoms disappear. Transient myoglobinuria may appear in some cases.

Signs. Size and initial power tone of muscle normal at outset of exercise. No fasciculation or fibrillation; no myoclonia; reflexes normal. After 3 decades, some muscle atrophy and permanent weakness may be noted.

Etiology. Myophosphorylase deficiency. Autosomal recessive inheritance. Dominant form also reported.

Pathology. Increased glycogen deposits in muscle; no detectable phosphorylase with diphosphopyridine nucleotide (DPNH) stain.

Diagnostic Procedures. *Routine laboratory analyses.* All normal. *Venous return.* From exercised muscle, poor in concentration of lactate and pyruvate (opposite of that in normal). *Epinephrine test.* Smaller lactate response than normal. *Biopsy of muscle.* Usually no immunologic cross reacting material to normal phosphorylase. *Biochemical study. Electromyography.* Normal prior to exercise; no activity after. *Urine.* Myoglobinuria (90%).

Therapy. Avoidance of extreme exercise. Oral fructose and glucose. Isoproterenol.

Prognosis. Usually, stable condition, progression to atrophy according to amount of exercise.

BIBLIOGRAPHY. McArdle B: Myopathy due to a defect in muscle glycogen breakdown. Clin Sci 10:13–35, 1951
Porte D, Crawford DW, Jennings DB, et al: Cardiovascular and metabolic responses to exercise in a patient with McArdle's syndrome. New Engl J Med 275:406–412, 1966
Howell RR, Williams JC: The glycogen storage diseases. In Stanbury JB, Wyngaarden JB, Fredrickson DS, et al: The Metabolic Basis of Inherited Disease, 5th ed, p 141. New York, McGraw-Hill, 1983
Schmidt B, Servidei S, Gabbai AA, et al: McArdle's disease in two generations: autosomal recessive transmission with manifesting heterozygote. Neurology 37:1558–1561, 1987

McCUNE-ALBRIGHT

Synonyms. Albright's I; Albright-McCune-Stenberg; fibrous dysplasia; Fuller-Albright's; osteitis fibrosa disseminata; osteodystrophia fibrosa; polyostotic fibrous dysplasia.

Symptoms. Occur in children or young adults; predominantly in females (3:2). Difficulty in walking; pain in the legs; pathologic fractures; sexual precocity with early development.

Signs. Bone deformities and pathologic fractures especially of lower extremities and pelvic ring; cutaneous brownish pigmentations (absent in some cases) of various sizes, more frequently observed on head, neck, sacrum, thighs. In monostotic variety, unilateral exophthalmos, unilateral optic atrophy, loss of hearing, convulsions, mental retardation. Signs of precocious development (genitals; breasts; early menarche). In some cases, associated with hyperthyroidism (19%). Differential diagnosis with hyperparathyroidism and adrenocortical and ovarian tumors.

Etiology. Unknown; sporadic conditions. Families with autosomal dominant trait reported.

Pathology. Bone cysts; avascular fibrous tissue replacing normal medullary structure. Pigmented spots on the skin with melanin in the inner layer of epidermis.

Diagnostic Procedures. *X-ray.* Reveals fusiform enlargement of bone with thin cortex; translucent foci. *Blood.* Serum phosphatase elevated; calcium, phosphorus normal. *Urine.* 17-ketosteroids and follicle-stimulating hormone (FSH) excretion normal.

Therapy. Treatment of fractures and orthopedic correction of deformities.

Prognosis. Disease progressive until growth stops.

BIBLIOGRAPHY. McCune DJ: Osteitis fibro-cystica: the case of a nine year old girl who also exhibits precocious puberty, multiple pigmentation of the skin and hyperthyroidism. Am J Dis Child 52:743–747, 1936
Albright F, Butler AM, Hampton AO, et al: Syndrome characterized by osteitis fibrosa disseminata, areas of pigmentation and endocrine dysfunction with precocious puberty in females. New Engl J Med 216:727–746, 1937
McCune DJ, Bruch H: Osteodystrophia fibrosa. Am J Dis Child 54:806–848, 1937

Gorlin RJ, Sedano H: Albright's syndrome, polyostotic fibrous dysplasia, cutaneous pigmentation, and endocrine disorders. Mod Med 36:160–161, 1968

Alvarez-Arretia MC, Rivas F, Avila-Abundis A, et al: A probable monogenic form of polyostotic fibrous dysplasia. Clin Genet 24:132–139, 1983

McKITTRICK-WHEELOCK

Symptoms and Signs. Eponym used to indicate severe electrolyte imbalance, caused by the presence of a large villous adenoma in the colon or rectum.

Therapy. Correction of electrolyte imbalance and surgery.

Prognosis. Good with treatment.

BIBLIOGRAPHY. McKittrick LS, Wheelock FC Jr: Carcinoma of the Colon, 3rd ed. Springfield, Ill, CC Thomas, 1954

McKUSICK-CROSS

Synonyms. Lymphopenic agammaglobulinemia–dwarfism; ataxia telangiectasia III.

Symptoms. Present from birth. Failure to thrive. Repeated infections. Diarrhea.

Signs. Growth deficiency; short limbs; small thorax. Redundant skin; erythema; dyskeratosis; hair loss.

Etiology. Unknown; possibly, autosomal recessive inheritance. In the two original sibs described: one presented Louis-Bar's syndrome (see) and the other Swiss-type agammaglobulinemia (see), thus suggesting possible relationship between these two disorders.

Diagnostic Procedures. *Blood.* Anemia; lymphopenia; agammaglobulinemia; *X-ray.* Radial and ulnar metaphyseal cusping. Hypoplastic thymus. *Bone marrow.* Occasionally, aplasia of all erythropoietic elements.

Prognosis. Death in early infancy.

BIBLIOGRAPHY. McKusick VA, Cross HE: Ataxia-telangiectasia and Swiss-type agammaglobulinemia: two genetic disorders of the immune mechanism in related Amish. JAMA 195:739–745, 1966

Gatti RA, Platt N, Pomerance HH, et al: Hereditary lymphopenic agammaglobulinemia associated with a destructive form of short-limbed dwarfism and ectodermal dysplasia. J Pediatr 75:679–684, 1969

MACLENNAN'S

Synonyms. Proctalgia fugax; Thaysen's.

Symptoms. Attacks of sharp, severe, brief pain in the area of rectal sphincter. Frequently associated with pallor, sweating, precordial oppression, and fainting.

Etiology. Unknown.

BIBLIOGRAPHY. MacLennan A: A short note on rectal crises of nontabetic origin. Glasgow Med J 88:129–131, 1917

Thaysen TE: Proctalgia fugax. Lancet II:243–246, 1935

Mann TP, Cree JE: Familial rectal pain. Lancet I:1016–1017, 1972

McQUARRIE'S

Synonym. Infantile familial hypoglycemia. See Cochrane's.

Symptoms. Onset in early infancy (84% under 2 years); prevalent in males. Vague clinical signs of hypoglycemia usually attributed to hunger, teething, fatigue, or environmental changes. Generalized convulsions recurring at specific times, without fever or evidence of other illness.

Signs. None.

Etiology. Unknown; possibly, familial or hereditary character.

Pathology. Unknown. In two cases, biopsy of pancreas showed absence of alpha cells; in other two cases, normal pancreas.

Diagnostic Procedures. *Blood.* Fasting sugar; glucose tolerance curve; epinephrine test; glucagon test; adrenocorticotropic hormone (ACTH) and cortisone administration test. *Biopsy of pancreas.*

Therapy. Glucose stops convulsion. ACTH and corticosteroids.

Prognosis. Normal physical and mental growth if treated. Permanent improvement possible following prolonged ACTH treatment. Possible brain damage if condition goes unrecognized and maltreated (i.e., with antiepileptic drugs).

BIBLIOGRAPHY. McQuarrie I: Idiopathic spontaneously occurring hypoglycemia in infants. Am J Dis Child 87:399–428, 1954

Cornblath M, Reisner SH: Blood glucose in the neonate and its clinical significance. New Engl J Med 273:378–381, 1965

Koh THH, Eyre JA, Anysley-Green A: Neonatal hypoglycaemia—the controversy regarding definition. Arch Dis Child 63:1386–1398, 1988

MACROAMYLASEMIA MALABSORPTION

Symptoms and Signs. Apparently restricted to elderly females (four cases reported). Chronic diarrhea; malabsorption symptoms and signs.

Etiology. Unknown; the nature of correlation of malabsorption with presence of 11S amylase is unknown. Patients with persistent macroamylasemia of 7S type have no malabsorption.

Pathology. Subtotal villous atrophy of small intestine with mononuclear cell infiltration.

Diagnostic Procedures. *Blood.* Persistent amylasemia, 11S type (normal type, increased in pancreatitis to 4.5S). Low xylose absorption. *Stool.* Significantly increased fat.

Therapy. Trial with pancreatic supplement, tetracycline, gluten-free diet.

Prognosis. Poor response to treatment. Progressive deterioration due to malabsorption.

BIBLIOGRAPHY. Wilding P, Cooke WT, Nicholson GI: Globulin-bound amylase: a cause of persistently elevated levels in serum. Ann Intern Med 60:1053–1059, 1964
Levitt MD, Goetzl EJ, Cooperband SR: Two forms of macroamylasaemia. Lancet I:957–958, 1968

MACULA VITELLIFORM DEGENERATION

Synonyms. Best's; macula lutea congenital degeneration; vitelliform macula degeneration (including Ferrell's atypical vitelliform); vitelliruptive macular dystrophy; polymorphic macular degeneration; Bradley's.

Symptoms. Both sexes affected; onset very early; observed at 1 week of age, more frequently between 5 and 15 years of age. Visual function affected slightly or not at all. Sometimes absolute or relative central scotoma; chromatic discrimination frequently normal; adaptation to dark usually normal.

Signs. Usually bilateral, subretinal, sharply defined discoid formation at the macula; yellow, orange yellow, or pink yellow (resembling yolk of poached egg); no vessels; size one-half to two disk diameters. Later in life, the initial homogeneous content of vitelliform disk forms a sediment (resembling pseudohypopyon) or fragment. (At this stage, serious visual loss may occur.)

Etiology. Unknown; many observations suggest autosomal recessive inheritance, with reduced penetrance and variable expressivity, or autosomal dominant.

Pathology. Extensive defect in receptor layers with absence of pigmented epithelium; pigment and neuroepithelium replaced by glial membrane; calcification and fragmentation of Bruch's membrane. Choriocapillaris absent.

Diagnostic Procedures. *Electro-oculography.*

Therapy. None.

Prognosis. Degeneration is progressive, very slow course; around age 50 the lesion becomes atrophic.

BIBLIOGRAPHY. Adams JE: Case showing peculiar changes of the macula. Ophthalmol Soc UK 3:113–114, 1883
Best F: Ueber eine hereditare Macule affection Beitrage zur Vererbungleschre. Z Augenheilkd 13:199–212, 1905
Nordstrom S, Thornburn W: Dominantly inherited macular degeneration (Best's disease) in a homozygous father with 11 children. Clin Genet 18:211–216, 1980
Mohler CW, Fine SL: Long-term evaluation of patients with Best's vitelliform dystrophy. Ophthalmology 88:688–692, 1981
Ferrell RE, Hittner HM, Autoszyk JH: Linkage of atypical vitelliform macular dystrophy (UMD-1) to the soluble glutamate pyruvate transaminase (GPT1) locus. Am J Hum Genet 35:78–84, 1983

MADELUNG'S I

Synonyms. Carpus curvus; manus valga. See Leri-Weill (different type of the same condition?).

Symptoms. Females more frequently affected (4 : 1); diagnosed usually in adolescence. Moderate stature shortness (failure of growth of tibia and resulting genu varum); typical wrist pain and deformity: fork deformity because of backward subluxation of distal end of ulna, due to failure of growth in distal radial growth plate.

Etiology. Autosomal dominant inheritance.

Diagnostic Procedures. *X-ray.*

Therapy. Orthopedic measures. Ulnar subluxation may be reduced, but only temporarily.

Prognosis. Short stature; limitation of wrist and elbow motion.

BIBLIOGRAPHY. Madelung OW: Die spontane Subluxation der Hand nach Vorne. Verh Dent Ges Chir 7:259–276, 1878
Anton JI, Reitz GB, Spiegel MB: Madelung's deformity. Am J Surg 108:411–439, 1938

Lichtenstein JR, Sundaram M, Burdge R: Sex-influenced expression of Madelung's deformity in a family with dyschondrosteosis. J Med Genet 17:41–43, 1980

MAD HATTER

Synonym. Chronic mercury intoxication. See Minamata.

BIBLIOGRAPHY. Freedman AM, Kaplan HI, Sadock BJ: Comprehensive Textbook of Psychiatry, 2nd ed, p 1119. Baltimore, Williams & Wilkins, 1975

MADIDA

Symptoms and Signs. Hypersecretion of hypotonic tears (as contrasted to the sicca syndrome).

Etiology. Supposed response to central nervous system lesion due to toxic irritation of hypothalamus.

Pathology. Unknown.

BIBLIOGRAPHY. Prinz CW: Das Madida-Syndrom bei Akrodinie als gegensatz sum Sicca syndrom. Klin Monatsbl Augenheilkd 141:749–463, 1932

MAFFUCCI'S

Synonyms. Chondrodystrophy-hemangiomas; dyschondroplasia-hemangiomas; multiple enchondromatosis; Kast's; vascular hamartoma–dyschondroplasia. See Ollier's.

Symptoms. Both sexes affected. Normal at birth; bone and cartilage deformities appear during childhood. Usually, no history of pain; orthostatic hypotension in sitting or standing position (pooling of blood in dependent hemangiomas). Normal intelligence. Fracture of bones (26%) following minimal trauma; slow union.

Signs. Before puberty a hard nodule appears on finger or toe, followed by other tumors with asymmetric distribution in the cylindrical bones. In the subcutaneous and soft tissue, bluish hemangiomas appear. Deformities and inequality of bones due to tumors and fractures. Tumor of flat bones less common. No visceral involvement.

Etiology. Unknown; combination of enchondromatosis and hemangiomatosis. Does not appear to be hereditary. Chromosomal abnormalities have not been found.

Pathology. *Bone.* Areas of dyschondroplasia. Sarcomatous degeneration of bone lesion frequent (19%). *Skin.* Vascular malformation; hemangioma. No relation between the two types of lesions.

Diagnostic Procedures. *X-ray of skeleton. Arteriography. Venography. Biopsy of skin and bones.*

Therapy. Surgical removal of sarcomatous transformation; orthopedic measures and corrective surgery when indicated.

Prognosis. Progression of lesions to the end of second decade, then stabilization. Malignant transformation may be cause of death.

BIBLIOGRAPHY. Maffucci A: Di un caso di encondroma ed angioma multiplo. Contribuzione alla genesi embrionale dei tumori. Movimento Medico-Chirurgico 3:399–412, 1881
Sun TC, Swee RG, Schives TC, et al: Chondrosarcoma in Maffucci's syndrome. J Bone Joint Surg 67A:1214–1219, 1985
Ben-Itzhak I, Denolf F, Versfeld GA, et al: The Maffucci syndrome. J Pediatr Orthoped 8:345–348, 1988

MAGNUS'

Synonyms. Erythropoietic protoporphyria, EPP; hydroa aestivale; PP.

Symptoms. Both sexes affected; onset in childhood or adolescence. Various intensities of manifestations, from minimal to relatively severe, with fluctuation of intensity also in the same individual. After exposure to sun, from a few minutes to a prolonged time (according to individuals), intense pruritus, erythema, edema of areas exposed. Usually, receding completely in 12 to 24 hours without sequelae. Exceptionally, formation of chronic eczema persisting for days and leaving scars. Frequently associated, cholelithiasis symptoms at early age.

Signs. Erythrodontia; abnormal mechanical fragility of skin; hirsutism; pigmentation absent. Occasionally, splenomegaly.

Etiology. Unknown; autosomal dominant inheritance. Excessive production of protoporphyrin in bone marrow and possibly in other organs. Generalized deficiency of ferrochelatase activity.

Pathology. Fluorescence of skin. No particular pathologic findings in liver.

Diagnostic Procedures. *Blood.* Mild hypochromic anemia; seldom, hemolysis; frequently, evidence of liver insufficiency. *Urine.* Normal. Only positive findings are increased concentration of protoporphyrin in circulating erythrocytes (isomer type III [9a] protoporphyrin) and increase of same pigment in the feces. *Stool.* Large excretion of protoporphyrin. *Bone marrow.* Increased fluorescence limited to cytoplasm of erythroid cells.

Therapy. Avoidance of exposure to sun; prolonged treatment with cholestyramine; beta-carotene ameliorates skin symptoms.

Prognosis. Relatively mild condition with possible severe hepatic damage leading to cirrhosis and liver failure.

BIBLIOGRAPHY. Magnus IA, Jarrett A, Prankerd TAJ, et al: Erythropoietic protoporphyria: a new porphyria syndrome with solar urticaria due to protoporphyrinaemia. Lancet II:448–451, 1961
Kappas A, Sassa S, Anderson KE: The porphyrias. In Stanbury JB, Wyngaarden JB, Fredrickson DS, et al: The Metabolic Basis of Inherited Disease, 5th ed, p 1301. New York, McGraw-Hill, 1983

MAJOCCHI'S

Synonyms. Purpura annularis telangiectoides; telangiectasia follicularis annulata.

Symptoms and Signs. Both sexes affected; onset usually in adolescence or early adulthood. Any site of body skin may be affected. Small annular plaques (1 to 3 cm in diameter), purple, yellow-brownish, with or without "cayenne spots." Centrifugal extension; slight atrophy in the center of lesion.

Etiology. Unknown.

Pathology. Hemosiderin deposit; telangiectases.

Therapy. None.

Prognosis. Persistence for months or years.

BIBLIOGRAPHY. Majocchi D: Sopra una dermatosi telangettode non ancora descritta "purpura annularis" "telangiectasia follicularis annulata." Studio clinico Giorn Ital Mal Venereol 37:242–250, 1896
Rook A, Wilkinson DS, Ebling FJG, et al: Textbook of Dermatology, 4th ed, p 1118. Oxford, Blackwell Scientific Publications, 1986

MALABSORPTION SYNDROMES

Symptoms. Both sexes affected; onset at all ages. One or more, frequently severe, attacks of diarrhea with passage of gray or yellowish, soft, greasy stools. Anorexia; weight loss; borborygmi; muscle tenderness; bone pain; weakness; fatigue; dyspnea; paresthesias. Primary mucosal disease.

Signs. Abdominal bloating; muscle wasting; dehydration; hyperkeratosis; folliculitis; bleeding manifestations; glossitis; cheilosis.

Etiology and Pathology. Numerous hereditary and acquired conditions may be responsible for this syndrome.

On the basis of clinical features and diagnostic procedures it may be subdivided under different headings.

Group 1. Inadequate digestion. Postgastrectomy syndromes; pancreatic exocrine insufficiency; biliary insufficiency.

Group 2. Metabolic defects. Sprue; sugar-splitting enzyme deficiency.

Group 3. Inadequate absorptive area. Fistulas; resection; gastroileostomy; jejuneal exclusion.

Group 4. Intestinal wall pathology or lymphatic obstruction. Radiation syndromes; amyloidosis; enteritis (bacterial; viral; parasitic); scleroderma; carcinoid syndrome; pneumatosis cystoides intestinalis; lymphomas; Whipple's; tuberculosis; Crohn's; chronic ulcerative jejunitis (nongranulomatous).

Group 5. Altered bacterial flora. Blind loop syndrome; multiple jejunal diverticula; antibiotic enterocolitis.

Group 6. Endocrinopathies. Diabetes mellitus; hypoparathyroidism; hyperparathyroidism; islet cell tumor of pancreas (Zollinger-Ellison; watery diarrhea–hypokalemia associated with pancreatic islet cell adenoma).

Group 7. Protein abnormalities. Dysgammaglobulinemia; Bassen-Kornzweig; intestinal lymphangiectasia; intestinal lymphangiectasia-hypobetalypoproteinemia.

Group 8. Vascular. Superior mesenteric artery syndrome; congestive heart failure; Pick's I; tricuspid regurgitation–protein-losing enteropathy.

Diagnostic Procedures. See specific condition.

Therapy. According to etiology.

Prognosis. Depends on etiology.

BIBLIOGRAPHY. Sleisenger MH, Fordtran JS: Gastrointestinal Disease. Philadelphia, WB Saunders, 1983
Sleisenger MH: Malabsorption and nutritional support. Clin Gastroenterol 12:323-A, 1983

MALE CLIMACTERIC

Synonym. Male climacterium.

Symptoms and Signs. Diminished libido; impotence; fatigue; hot flushes; nervousness. Depression; memory and concentration decreased; sleep disturbed; loss of interest.

Etiology. Rare disorder, usually due to emotional disturbances.

Pathology. Variable degrees of decreased spermatogenesis and of parenchymal atrophy.

Diagnostic Procedures. *Blood: Plasma level of testoster-*

one, follicle-stimulating hormone (FSH), luteinizing hormone (LH). *Semen analysis.* Normal or variable degree of decreased number and mobility of spermatozoa. *Urine.* 17-ketosteroids usually normal; gonadotropins usually normal. In rare cases, positive findings make a legitimate climacteric condition.

Therapy. Psychotherapy; androgen may be beneficial.

Prognosis. Good in many cases if psychological block is removed.

BIBLIOGRAPHY. Heller CG, Myers GB: The male climacteric, its symptomatology, diagnosis and treatment. Use of urinary gonadotropins, therapeutic tests with testosterone proprionate and testicular biopsies in delineating the climacteric from psychoneurosis and psychogenic impotence. JAMA 126:472–477, 1944
Landau R: The concept of the male climacteric. Med Clin N Am 35:279–288, 1951
Ryan RJ: Uncertain and hypothetic disorders; unclassifiable syndromes. Dis Mon 27–36, 1961
Smith, KD: Testicular function in the aging male. In De Groot LJ, Cahill FG Jr, Odell WD, et al (eds): Endocrinology, p 1577. New York, Grune & Stratton, 1979

MALHERBE'S

Synonyms. Calcified epithelioma; benign calcifying epithelioma; Malherbe-Chenantais; pilomatrixoma.

Symptoms. Females more frequently affected; onset at any age (majority of cases under 30 years). Frequently associated with myotonic dystrophy.

Signs. On the head, neck, or upper extremities, solitary dermal tumor, which on palpation feels smooth or lobulated and of stone-hard consistency; overlying skin normal. Frequent and repeated associated infections.

Etiology. Hamartoma of hair matrix. Familial autosomal dominant cases reported.

Pathology. Encapsulated tumor, well defined, surrounded by inflammatory cells; tumoral peripheral cells small and dark; rarely, mitotic figures; scanty cytoplasm; intracellular connections; internal zone calcified and surrounded by cells with larger eosinophilic cytoplasm.

Diagnostic Procedures. *Biopsy.*

Therapy. Excision.

Prognosis. No recurrence if completely excised.

BIBLIOGRAPHY. Malherbe A, Chenantais J: Note sur l'épithéliome calcifié des glandes sébacées. Prog Med 8:826–828, 1880
Geiser JO: Malherbe's calcified epithelioma. Ann Dermatol Syph 86:383–403, 1959

Rook A, Wilkinson DS, Ebling FJG, et al: Textbook of Dermatology, 4th ed. Oxford, Blackwell Scientific Publications, 1986

MALIGNANT HYPERTHERMIA*

Synonym. Pharmacogenic myopathy.

Symptoms. Both sexes affected; onset at any age. Inducted by general anesthesia or triggered by various pharmacologic agents or environmental stresses (temperature; infection; emotion; injuries; exercise).

Signs. *Early manifestations.* Rapid multifocal ventricular arrhythmias; unstable blood pressure; rapid and deep respiration; excessive heat; mottled cyanosis. In 80% of cases, skeletal muscle rigidity (especially after injection of succinylcholine). *Later manifestations.* High fever, rapidly rising to 44°C to 46°C and not controllable by physical or pharmacologic means. Oliguria; anuria; pupils fixed and dilated; deep tendon reflexes absent; convulsions. Milder reaction (fever without muscle rigidity) may also occur, because of minor defect (see Etiology) or weaker agents.

Etiology. Autosomal dominant inheritance or weaker recessive gene. Crisis caused by sudden rise in concentration of myoplasmic calcium induced by the administration of several drugs.

Pathology. Muscle contraction: rigor that may precede death.

Diagnostic Procedures. *Blood.* Metabolic acidosis; hypoxia; electrolytes, enzymes, and myoglobin alterations. *Urine.* Myoglobinuria. *Muscle biopsy.* Vigorous in vitro contracture of the specimen in presence of halothane, and reduced contracture threshold to caffeine.

Therapy.
1. Stop anesthesia and surgery immediately.
2. Hyperventilate patient with 100% oxygen.
3. Administer dantrolene (Dantrium) 2.5 mg/kg IV and procainamide (up 15 mg/kg IV slowly if required for arrhythmias) as soon as possible.
4. Initiate cooling.
5. Correct acidosis.
6. Secure monitoring lines: electrocardiograph, temperature, Foley catheter, arterial pressure, central venous pressure.
7. Maintain urine output.
8. Monitor patient until danger of subsequent episodes is past (48–72 hr).
9. Administer oral or IV dantrolene for 48 to 72 hr.

---

* The Malignant Hyperthemia Association of the United States has a hotline number (209-634-4917) which is available 24 hours a day for any information.

Prognosis. With constant vigilance and proper, aggressive treatment, the syndrome can be treated adequately for a successful outcome.

BIBLIOGRAPHY. Denborough MA, Forster JFA, Lovell RRH, et al: Anaesthetic deaths in a family. Br J Anaesth 34:395–396, 1962
Britt BA: Etiology and pathophysiology of malignant hyperthermia. Fed Proc 38:44–48, 1979
Britt BA: Malignant hyperthermia. Boston, Martinus Nijhoff, 1987
Williams CH (ed): Experimental malignant hyperthermia. New York, Springer-Verlag, 1988

MALLORY-WEISS

Synonym. Gastroesophageal laceration.

Symptoms. Prevalent in males, usually onset after 30 years of age. Vomiting; severe retching, and then hematemesis and melena.

Signs. Pallor; tachycardia; in some patients shock.

Etiology. Longitudinal laceration of mucosa and submucosa of gastroesophageal junction following severe retching. Usually following large ingestion of alcohol.

Pathology. See Etiology. Acute and chronic gastritis; pancreatitis; liver cirrhosis may or may not be associated.

Diagnostic Procedures. *Blood: Blood cell count; liver function test; serum amylase; blood urea nitrogen; glucose; clotting studies. Esophagogastroscopy.* As soon as condition of patient allows it, followed by *X-ray* of upper gastrointestinal tract.

Therapy. Stomach emptied and washed with iced saline. Blood replaced. Coagulants, atropine, and sedative. If bleeding does not stop, surgery: high gastrotomy; laceration identified and repaired. Sengstaken-Blakemore tube and blind gastric resection in these cases not useful.

Prognosis. Fair with adequate treatment; affected by preexisting general conditions (e.g., liver cirrhosis).

BIBLIOGRAPHY. Mallory GK, Weiss S: Hemorrhages from lacerations of the cardiac orifice of the stomach due to vomiting. Am J Med Sci 178:506–515, 1929
Sugawa C, Benishek D, Walt AJ: Mallory-Weiss syndrome: a study of 224 patients. Am J Surg 145:30–33, 1983
Watts DM, et al: Lesions brought on by vomiting: the effect of hiatus hernia on the site of injury. Gastroenterology 71:683–688, 1986
Rimer U, et al: Mallory-Weiss syndrome. An analysis of

haemostatic function in a bleeding free period. Acta Chir Scand 152:39–41, 1986

MANSON'S SCHISTOSOMIASIS-PULMONARY ARTERY OBSTRUCTION

Synonyms. Cardiopulmonary bilharziasis; pulmonary schistosomiasis; protopulmonary bilharziasis; cardiopulmonary schistosomiasis. See Katayama.

Symptoms. Occur in young adults living (or who have lived) in areas with endemic schistosomiasis. Progressive dyspnea; pain in upper abdomen.

Signs. Cyanosis; engorgement of neck vessels; edema of legs; scanty pulmonary findings (contrasted with severe dyspnea); hepatosplenomegaly. In heart, loud P2, systolic and diastolic murmurs.

Etiology. Manson's *Schistosoma* infestation.

Pathology. Widespread pulmonary obliterative arteriolitis due to repeated emboli; ova of *Schistosoma*; granulomas; para-arterial angiomatosis arteritis with fibrinoid necrosis; hyaline thrombi. Right ventricular hypertrophy.

Diagnostic Procedures. *Stool.* Demonstration of *Schistosoma. Biopsy of rectum. Blood.* Moderate anemia; normal white blood cells. *Electrocardiography.* Cor pulmonale pattern. *X-ray of chest.* Right ventricular hypertrophy; dilated pulmonary arteries.

Therapy. Digitalis; oxygen and salt restriction; diuretics. To avoid myocardial damage, no intense antimony treatment.

Prognosis. Poor; death usually within 1 year. These patients do not tolerate surgical procedures well.

BIBLIOGRAPHY. Belelli V: Les oeufs de Bilharzia haematobia dans les poumons. Unione med Egiz Alessandria 1: No. 22–23, 1884–1885
Marchang EJ, Marcial-Rojas RA, Rodriguez R, et al: The pulmonary obstruction syndrome in schistosoma pulmonary endarteritis. Arch Intern Med 100:965–980, 1957
Macieira-Coelho E, Duarte CS: The syndrome of portopulmonary schistosomiasis. Am J Med 43:944–950, 1967
Bores DL: Schistosomiasis Manson: a granulomatous disease of cell-mediated immune etiology. Ann New York Acad Sci 278:36–46, 1976
Schistosomiasis: a review of recent abstracts. Tropical Disease Bull 82:R1, R3, 1985
Bennet JL, Depenbusch JW: The chemotherapy of schistosomiasis. In Mansfield JM (ed): Parasitic Disease, vol 2, pp 73–117. New York, Marcel Dekker, 1984

MANUBRIOSTERNAL

Synonyms. Pseudoangina; thoracic pain.

Symptoms. Occur in patients with rheumatoid arthritis or without any joint changes. Sharp pain over or on either side of manubrium; pain induced or aggravated by exercise (walking, climbing stairs, bending or straightening), coughing and sneezing.

Signs. Tenderness; occasionally, slight swelling of manubriosternal joint. Relief by procaine infiltration.

Etiology. Unknown; part of rheumatoid arthritis syndrome or isolated inflammatory condition.

Diagnostic Procedures. *X-ray.* Occasionally, slight changes of manubriosternal joint; usually no changes. *Electrocardiography.* Normal.

Therapy. Relief by procaine or corticoid infiltration.

Prognosis. Symptoms may persist and recur for years.

BIBLIOGRAPHY. Söderstrom N: Manubrial pain and angina pectoris. Svensk Lakartidn 48:1845–1847, 1951
Fisher CM, Light W: Manubriosternal arthralgia. New Engl J Med 256:799–801, 1957

MAPLE SYRUP

Synonyms. Branched chain ketonuria I; ketoaciduria; Menkes' I; maple syrup urine disease (MSUD); thiamine-responsive MSUD; ketoacid decarboxylase deficiency.

Symptoms and Signs. Both sexes affected; onset in first week of life. Vomiting; difficulty in feeding; failure to thrive; absence of grasping reflex; irregular gaspy breathing. Later, generalized rigidity and opisthotonos. Hypoglycemic crisis may occur. Severe mental retardation. Maple syrup odor in the urine. Five different phenotypes recognized: (1) classic; (2) intermittent; (3) intermediate; (4) thiamine-responsive; (5) E_3 deficiency.

Etiology. Deficient activity in various components of branched-chain 2-ketoacid dehydrogenase (BCKADH). Classic type is autosomal recessive; other types, genetic heterogeneity.

Pathology. In central nervous system, marked deficiency in myelin, and astrocytosis.

Diagnostic Procedures. *Blood: Investigation of enzymatic activity of leukocytes.* Shows block of branched chain ketoacid metabolism. Elevation of plasma level of leucine, isoleucine, valine, and presence of alloisoleucine. *Urine, cerebrospinal fluid.* Alloisoleucine found in increased amounts.

Therapy. Trial with diet in which branched amino acids are omitted. After level of these amino acids falls to normal, resumption of administration without exceeding minimum requirement.

Prognosis. Death occurs early; if not in first week, then usually within first year. If patient survives long enough, mental damage becomes evident. Therapeutic approach, if instituted before brain damage occurs, may result in prevention of serious complications. The difficulty of this treatment has to be pointed out.

BIBLIOGRAPHY. Menkes JH, Hurst PL, Craig JM: A new syndrome: progressive familial infantile cerebral dysfunction associated with an unusual urinary substance. Pediatrics 14:462–466, 1954
Tanaka K, Rosenberg LE: Disorders of the branched-chain amino acid and organic acid metabolism. In Stanbury JB, Wyngaarden JB, Fredrickson DS, et al: The Metabolic Basis of Inherited Disease, 5th ed, p 440. New York, McGraw-Hill, 1983

MARAÑON'S I

Symptoms and Signs. Flatfoot, scoliosis, and various spinal disorders associated with ovary insufficiency.

BIBLIOGRAPHY. Marañon G: Syndrome ostéomusculaire douloureux de l'insuffisance ovarique juvénile. Paris Med 1:414–419, 1930

MARAÑON'S II

Eponym used to indicate the particular aspect of a wrestler that may be conferred by generalized symmetric muscle lipomas.

BIBLIOGRAPHY. Jablonski S: Illustrated Dictionary of Eponymic Syndromes and Diseases and Their Synonyms. Philadelphia, WB Saunders, 1969

MARAÑON'S III

Association of a thyrotoxic status (see Flajani's), fever, and adiposity.

BIBLIOGRAPHY. Marañon G: Vei Sindrome adiposidad-Basedow-distermia (ABD). Med Espan 30:509–516, 1953

MARAÑON'S IV

Eponym used to indicate a clinical association of hypertrophy of testicle (?) and gynecomastia.

BIBLIOGRAPHY. Marañon G: Contribution casuistica al sindrome ambihipergenital hipertesticulismo con ginecomastia. Bull Inst Pat Med 12:237–240, 1957

MARBLE BRAIN

Synonyms. Carbonic anhydrase II deficiency syndrome; recessive osteopetrosis–renal tubular acidosis and cerebral calcification; carbonic anhydrase B deficiency; Guibaud-Vainsel.

Symptoms and Signs. Osteopetrosis; renal tubular acidosis with both proximal and distal components; cerebral calcification; mental retardation; growth failure; typical facial features; abnormal teeth. Sometimes, restrictive lung disease.

Etiology. Inborn error of metabolism consisting of carbonic anhydrase II deficiency. Autosomal recessive inheritance.

Pathology. Osteopetrosis; cerebral calcification; stiff and deformed rib cage.

Diagnostic Procedures. *Blood.* Deficiency of carbonic anhydrase II; metabolic acidosis; hyperchloremia; normal anion gap. Analysis of carbonic anhydrase II in fetal blood or amniotic cells might prove to be of value in this syndrome for antenatal diagnosis. *X-rays of skull.* Intracranial calcifications. *Electroencephalography.* Abnormal for age. *Urine.* Alkaline, pH 6.0.

Therapy. Symptomatic; sodium bicarbonate; whether bone marrow transplantation could alleviate some of the manifestations of this syndrome is not known.

Prognosis. Variable.

BIBLIOGRAPHY. Guibaud P, Larbre F, Freycon MT: Osteopetrose et acidose renale tubulaire deux cas de cette association dans une fraterie. Arch Fr Pediatr 29:269–286, 1972
Vainsel M, Fondu P, Cadranel S, et al: Osteopetrosis associated with proximal and distal tubular acidosis. Acta Paediatr Scand 61:429–434, 1972
Ohlsson A, Stark G, Sakati N: Marble brain disease: recessive osteopetrosis, renal tubular acidosis, and cerebral calcification in three Saudi Arabian families. Dev Med Child Neurol 22:72–96, 1980
Sly WS, Whyte MP, Sundaram V, et al: Carbonic anhydrase II deficiency in 12 families with autosomal recessive syndrome of osteopetrosis with renal tubular acidosis and cerebral calcification. New Engl J Med 313:139–145, 1985
Ohlsson A, Cumming WA, Paul A, et al: Carbonic anhydrase II deficiency syndrome: recessive osteopetrosis with renal tubular acidosis and cerebral calcification. Pediatrics 77:371–381, 1986

MARCHAND'S

Synonyms. Postnecrotic liver; cirrhosis; toxic cirrhosis; posthepatitic cirrhosis. See Posthepatitis. Includes Cryptogenic cirrhosis.

Symptoms and Signs. Those of liver cirrhosis (see Laennec's). Pathologic pattern (see) distinguishes it and seems to represent a common end-stage cirrhosis evolving from other less advanced stages.

Etiology. Difficult to assess, except when clear anamnesis or specific microscopic features are present: e.g., hepatitis B; alpha-antitrypsin deficiency (see); iron storage.

Pathology. In liver, nodules separated by large bands of dense collagen; bile ductal proliferation and lymphocyte infiltration into the band may be observed. In some areas the hepatic parenchyma is missing and the fibrotic area includes different portal tracts. Nodules appear encapsulated by concentric collagen fiber; bile retention in hepatocytes and canaliculi may be observed; all forms of hepatocyte degeneration may be present, up to uniform coagulation necrosis of entire nodules.

Diagnostic Procedures. *Blood.* See Laennec's. *Biopsy of liver* (see Pathology).

Therapy. See Laennec's.

Prognosis. Variable according to different authors; may be better or worse than for Laennec's.

BIBLIOGRAPHY. Gordon BL, Barclay WR, Rogers HC (eds): Current medical Information and Terminology, 4th ed. Chicago, American Medical Association, 1971
Wright R, Alberti KGMM, Karan S, et al: Liver and Biliary Disease, p 688. London, WB Saunders, 1979

MARCHAND'S (E.J.)

Synonyms. Hepatosplenic bilharziasis; cyanosis in schistosomiasis; hepatosplenic schistosomiasis; portal hypertension–cyanosis in schistosomiasis. See Katayama.

Symptoms and Signs. Chronic severe cyanosis. Clubbing of fingers; hepatosplenomegaly. No significant signs of pulmonary and cardiac abnormalities.

Etiology. Hepatosplenic schistosomiasis with portal hypertension (see Manson's schistosomiasis–pulmonary artery obstruction).

Pathology. Hepatosplenic schistosomiasis with or without complicating portal cirrhosis. Evidence of portal hypertension and abnormal ramification of both pulmonary arteries and veins; increase of vascular bed of lung parenchyma; presence of arteriovenous fistula.

Diagnostic Procedures. *Stool.* Ova of schistosoma. *Electrocardiography.* No evidence of cardiac disease. *Blood: Liver function test.* Moderate liver impairment or cirrhosis. *Right heart catheterization.* Normal pressure of right side of heart and associated vessels. *Pulmonary function test.* Demonstration of lack of arterial oxygen saturation even after administration of 100% oxygen.

Therapy. Treatment of infestation. In some cases, portal shunt and splenectomy.

BIBLIOGRAPHY. Marchand EJ, De Jesus M, Biascoechea ZA: Cyanotic syndrome of portal hypertension in hepatosplenic schistosomiasis and portal cirrhosis. Am J Cardiol 10:496–506, 1962

Boros DL: Schistosomiasis mansoni: a granulomatous disease of cell-mediated immune etiology. Ann New York Acad Sci 278:36–46, 1976

Bennet JT, Depenbusch JW: The Chemotherapy of Schistosomiasis. In Mansfield JM (ed): Parasitic Disease, vol 2, pp 73–117. New York, Marcel Dekker, 1984

MARCHIAFAVA-BIGNAMI

Synonyms. Corpus callosum degeneration; demyelinating callosal encephalopathy.

Symptoms. Observed in middle-aged or old people who have consumed large quantities of wine. Gradual mental changes from excitement to apathy. Convulsions; tremors; dysarthria; ataxia; sphincter alteration; remission and exacerbations.

Etiology. Alcohol abuse and/or nutritional disorder.

Pathology. Symmetric demyelinization of central part of corpus callosum; involvement of white matter and anterior commissure.

Diagnostic Procedures. *Electroencephalography. Spinal fluid. Liver function tests. CT brain scan. Magnetic resonance imaging of brain.*

Therapy. Vitamins, correct diet.

Prognosis. Death 4 to 6 years after onset.

BIBLIOGRAPHY. Marchiafava E, Bignami A: Sopra un alterazione del corpo calloso osservata in soggetti alcoolisti. Riv Patol Nerv Ment 8:544–549, 1903

Poser CM: Central pontine myelinolysis and Marchiafava-Bignami disease. Ann New York Acad Sci 215:373–381, 1973

Adams RD, Victor M: Principles of Neurology, 3rd ed, pp 780–781. New York, McGraw-Hill, 1985

MARCHIAFAVA-MICHELI

Synonyms. Hemolytic anemia–paroxysmal nocturnal hemoglobinuria; paroxysmal nocturnal hemoglobinuria; Strübing-Marchiafava.

Symptoms. Onset usually between 3rd and 4th decade in both sexes; rarely in childhood or old age. Frequently asymptomatic. Abdominal, lumbar, substernal pain; malaise and fever. Urine passed during night or in the morning is dark; day urine has normal appearance. Atypical forms common (chronic hemolysis; pancytopenia; thrombotic episodes).

Signs. Pallor with yellowish discoloration of skin and mucosae; sometimes, bronzing discoloration. Functional cardiac murmur; splenomegaly; occasionally, hepatomegaly.

Etiology. Intracorpuscular defect makes red cells abnormally susceptible to lytic action of complement. Nature of abnormality unknown; not a familial condition.

Pathology. Venous thrombosis in systemic or portal circulation. Splenomegaly; hepatomegaly (central zone necrosis). In bone marrow, erythroid hyperplasia.

Diagnostic Procedures. *Blood.* Anemia; reticulocytosis. Icterus index high, free hemoglobin in plasma; leukopenia; low neutrophil alkaline phosphatase; moderate thrombocytopenia; iron deficiency; *Ham's test or acidified serum test. Sucrose hemolysis test; sugar-water test. Urine.* Urobilinuria; hemosiderinuria; free hemoglobin.

Therapy. There is no specific therapeutic agent for the erythrocyte membrane abnormality. In cases with severe anemia, frequent hemolytic crisis, thromboses, and infection: bone marrow grafts; adrenal steroids; blood transfusions; iron; anticoagulants; dextran.

Prognosis. Chronic condition; great variability of survival time (median survival 10 years). The severity of the disease is reflected in the degree of anemia. In some patients the severity lessens with time. In 50% of cases venous thrombosis cause of death.

BIBLIOGRAPHY. Strübing P: Paroxysmale Haemoglobinurie. Dtsch Med Wochenschr 8:17–21, 1882

Marchiafava E, Nazari A: Nuovo contributo allo studio degli itteri cronici emolitici. Policlinico (Sez Prat) 18:241–254, 1911

Micheli F: Uno caso di anemia emolitica con emosideriuria perpetua. Accad Med Torino 7:148, 1928

Mengel CE, Kann HE, Meriwether WD: Studies of paroxysmal nocturnal hemoglobinuria erythrocytes: increased lysis and lipid peroxide formation by hydrogen peroxide. J Clin Invest 46:1715–1723, 1967

Bell WR, Zerhouni E, Spitz R: Proxysmal nocturnal hemoglobinuria. Johns Hopkins Med J 142:218–223, 1978

Wintrobe MM (ed): Clinical Hematology, 8th ed, p. 869. Philadelphia, Lea & Febiger, 1981

Pittiglio DH, Sacher RA: Clinical Hematology and Fundamentals of Hemostasis. Philadelphia, FA Davis, 1987

MARCUS GUNN'S

Synonyms. Gunn's; jaw-winking. See Marin Amat.

Symptoms and Signs. Present from birth. Moderate ptosis of one eyelid when opening mouth. Jaw has lateral deviation toward the opposite side of the ptosis and results in elevation of upper lid and widening of palpebral fissure. When acquired, condition may appear at any age.

Etiology. Unknown; inherited (irregular dominant), congenital, or acquired condition.

Therapy. Surgery.

Prognosis. Usually remains constant for life; may also be transient, may progress, or may disappear while only the ptosis remains.

BIBLIOGRAPHY. Gunn RM: Congenital ptosis with peculiar associated movements of the affected lid. Trans Ophthalmol Soc UK 3:283–286, 1883

Reo MV, Syeda A: Jaw-winking movement (Marcus Gunn phenomenon). Indian J Med Sci 27:925–929, 1973

Doucet TW, Crawford JS: The quantification, natural course and surgical results in 57 eyes with Marcus Gunn (jaw-winking) syndrome. Am J Ophthalmol 92:702–707, 1981

MARDEN-WALKER

Synonyms. Blepharophimosis–joint contractures–muscular hypotonia; generalized connective tissue.

Symptoms and Signs. Present at birth. Fixed facial expression; micrognathia; cleft soft palate and uvula; blepharophimosis; pectus carinatum; kyphoscoliosis; arachnodactyly. Myotonia and contractures limiting adduction of hips and extension of elbows and knees that disappear during first year of life. Failure to thrive. Decreased deep tendon reflexes.

Etiology. Unknown; very similar to Schwartz-Jampel. Claimed to be different by Marden and Walker on the basis of the presence of cardiac and renal abnormalities, lack of respiratory system abnormalities, and presence of lesions at birth. Autosomal recessive (?) inheritance.

Pathology. *Heart.* Inferior vena cava common opening with superior vena cava. *Kidney.* Microscopically revealed diffuse dilation of large collecting tubules and hydropic degeneration of proximal and distal tubules (microcystic disease). *Skeletal muscles.* Atrophic without infiltrates. *Liver.* Mild fatty degeneration. *Other organs.* Normal.

Diagnostic Procedures. Laboratory tests, including chromosome studies, normal. *X-rays of skull.* Small frontal region. *Of skeleton.* Metacarpal phalanges metatarsal longer than normal. Bilateral talipes equinovarus. *Dermatoglyphic study.* Simian creases. *Pneumoencephalography.* Partial or complete agenesis of cerebellum and brainstem. *Electromyography.* No myotonia or myotonic discharge on percussion.

Prognosis. Death by 3 months.

BIBLIOGRAPHY. Marden PM, Walker WA: A new generalized connective tissue syndrome. Am J Dis Child 112:225–228, 1966

Jaatoul NY, Haddad NE, Khoury LF, et al.: The Marden-Walker syndrome. Am J Med Genet 11:259–271, 1982

MARFANOID HYPERMOBILITY

Symptoms and Signs. Patients present some features of Marfan's: increased height and slenderness; arachnodactyly; fibrous tendon contractures in hand; sparse subcutaneous fat; pectus excavatum; genu recurvatum; scoliosis; abnormalities of external ear; skin striae; and features of Ehlers-Danlos (skin hyperextensibility and joint laxity far exceeding the degree occasionally observed in Marfan's) Valvular heart disease reported in some cases.

Etiology. Considered by some authors a separate clinical entity, within the heterogeneous Marfan's group of conditions.

Pathology. *Biopsy of skin.* No abnormalities.

Diagnostic Procedures. *X-ray.* Bone alteration reported above; mild generalized osteoporosis; absence of calcified subcutaneous spheroids. *Urine.* Absence of abnormal excretion of amino acids.

Therapy. None.

Prognosis. Not reported.

BIBLIOGRAPHY. Roederer C: Syndrome d'Ehlers-Danlos atypique coincidant avec une dolichostenomélie. Arch Fr Pediatr 8:192–195, 1951

Walker BA, Beighton PH, Hurdoch JL: The Marfanoid hypermobility syndrome. Ann Intern Med 71:349–352, 1969

Daneshwar A, Tavakoli D, Nazarian J: Marfanoid hypermobility syndrome associated with coarctation of the aorta. Br Health J 41:621–623, 1979

MARFAN'S I

Synonyms. Arachnodactyly-dolichostenomelia; congenital mesodermal dystrophy.

Symptoms. Both sexes affected. Variable symptoms according to type and extent of organs involved (see Signs).

Signs. Slender elongated body; dolichocephalic skull; prominent ears; arched palate; long arms and legs; hands with long slender fingers (arachnodactyly); kyphoscoliosis; pectus excavatum; flat feet; hammer toes. Subcutaneous fat scanty; hyperextensibility and dislocation of articulations; muscles hypotonic. Eyes involved in 50% of cases: myopia; strabismus; myosis; nystagmus; subluxation of lens; tremulous irides; cataract; coloboma. Heart and vascular system involved in 40% to 60% of cases: valvular deformities; septal defects; aneurysm of aorta and pulmonary arteries. Pulmonary and kidney defects. A rare case of Marfan's syndrome presenting as intrapartum death has been described. Recognizable mitral valve lesions were present.

Etiology. Unknown; congenital disorder of connective tissue; autosomal dominant inheritance.

Pathology. Mesodermal dystrophy; loss of elastic fibers; hyperplasia and dilatation of vessel; valvular defects of heart; fusion of vertebrae.

Diagnostic Procedures. *Blood.* Decreased mucoprotein in serum. *X-ray.* Aorta dilatation or other cardiovascular defects. *Metacarpal index.* Greater length-to-width ratio than normal. *Echocardiography.*

Therapy. Early repair of cardiovascular defects when indicated (surgery difficult because of poor consistency of tissues).

Prognosis. Long life possible according to degree of heart involvement.

BIBLIOGRAPHY. Marfan AB: Un cas de déformation congénitale des quatre membres, plus prononcée aux extrémités, caracterisée par l'allongement des os avec un certain degre d'amincissement. Bull Soc Med Hôp Paris 13:220–226, 1896

Prockop DJ, Kivirikko KI: Heritable diseases of collagen, New Engl J Med 311:376–386, 1984

Buchanan R, Wyatt GP: Marfan's syndrome presenting as an intrapartum death. Arch Dis Child 60:1074, 1985

Scherer LR, Arn PH, Dressel DA, et al: Surgical management of children and young adults with Marfan syndrome and pectus excavatum. J Pediatr Surg 23:1169–1172, 1988

MARIE-BAMBERG

Synonyms. Bamberg's III; Hagner's; hypertrophic osteoarthropathy; Mankowsky's; hypertropic pulmonary osteoarthropathy; secondary pachydermoperiostosis; Von Bamberger's.

Symptoms. Warm sensation at fingertips; sweating of hands and feet; arthralgia.

Signs. Clubbing of fingers; swelling of joints; followed by enlargement of epiphyses of long bones. Deformity of cyanotic nails.

Etiology. Unknown. See Dysacromelias. This particular syndrome may be hereditary (autosomal dominant), idiopathic, or secondary to chronic pulmonary, cardiac, gastrointestinal, hepatic, endocrine, infective, or neoplastic conditions.

Pathology. Chronic inflammatory changes of synovial membranes; articular capsules; and adjacent tissues; infiltration of periosteum with round cells.

Diagnostic Procedures. *X-ray.* Osteoporosis; thickening of periosteum along shaft of long bones; thinned cortex; enlargement of terminal phalanges.

Therapy. With treatment of primary condition, pain ceases and periostitis is decreased.

Prognosis. That of primary condition. The appearance of this syndrome may serve as the only clue to a silent lesion.

BIBLIOGRAPHY. Marie P: De l'osteo-arthropathie hypertrophiante pneumique. Rev Med 10:1–36, 1890

Kuhlewein H: Hyppocratis opera quae feruntur omnia. Leipzig, 1894–1902

von Bamberger E: Ueber Knochenveranderungen bei chronischen Lungenund Herzkrankheiten. Zschr Klin Med 18:193–217, 1891

Fischer DS, Singer DH, Feldman SM: Clubbing: a review with emphasis on hereditary acropachy. Medicine 43:459–479, 1964

Bhate DV, Pizarro AJ, Greenfield GB: Idiopathic hyperthrophic osteoarthropathy without pachyderma. Radiology 129:378–381, 1978

Rook A, Wilkinson DS, Ebling FJG, et al: Textbook of Dermatology, 4th ed, pp 156–157. Oxford, Blackwell Scientific Publications, 1986

MARIE-LERI

Synonyms. Acro-osteolysis, rheumatoid; trophopathy myelodysplastica. See Hajdu-Cheney.

Symptoms. Peculiar hand alteration; the fingers may be extended and shortened like a telescope. Syndrome seen in congenital indifference to pain; in congenital sensory neuropathy, in Thevenard's syndrome.

Etiology. The authors attributed the syndrome to a peculiar form of rheumatoid arthritis causing acro-osteolysis. Likely related to Ehlers-Danlos. A toxic acro-osteolysis has been reported due to exposure to vinylchloride.

BIBLIOGRAPHY. Marie P, Leri A: Une varieté de rheumatisme chronique: la main en largnette (présentation de pièces et de coupes). Bull Soc Ed Hôp 36:104–107, 1913

Dodson VN, Dinman BD, Whitehous WN, et al: Occupational arteriosclerosis: a clinical study. Arch Environ Health 22:83–91, 1971

Largauer-Lewowicka H: Nailford capillari abnormalities in polyvinyl chloride production workers. Int Arch Occup Environ Health 51:337–340, 1983

MARIE'S II

Synonyms. Acromegalic; anterior pituitary adenoma; growth hormone hypersecretion; pituitary eosinophilic adenoma; somatotropic growth hormone hypersecretion. From a clinical point of view, it is useful to distinguish two syndromes: (1) The *endocrine* syndrome due to the hormonal secretion and (2) the *neurologic* syndrome due to the mechanical compression of the growing tumor.

ENDOCRINE SYNDROME

Symptoms. Slow gradual onset, usually between 30 and 50 years of age. Headache; backache; pain in limbs; sweating; hypomenorrhea or anemorrhea in women or loss of libido and potency in men (early symptoms). Sometimes temporary increase of libido at the onset of disease; polyuria; polydipsia; later muscular weakness.

Signs. Facial changes; prognathism and separation of teeth; coarsening of nose; prominence of supraorbital ridges; enlargement of lips and tongue. *Skin changes.* Fibroma; pigmentation; hirsutism, increased sebaceous secretion. *Trunk and limb changes.* Enlargement of hands and feet (changing size of shoes impresses the patient). *Thoracic cage changes.* Kyphosis, muscle and joint hypertrophy. *Genitalia changes.* Testes become small and flabby. *Other changes.* Enlargement of heart size; tachycardia; hypertension.

Etiology. Excessive secretion of growth hormone (GH) after puberty. Can be secreted by (1) hypothalamus (growth hormone releasing hormone [GH-RH]-producing gangliocytoma; hyperfunctioning neuronal hamartoma/adenohypophyseal choristoma with pituitary GH cell hyperplasia, with pituitary GH cell hyperplasia adenoma); (2) anterior pituitary (GH adenomas; GH cell adenomas; mixed GH-prolactin adenoma; plurihormonal

adenoma; mammosomatotropic adenoma; acidophilic stem cell adenoma; ectopic adenomas (GH cell)); (3) ectopic neoplasms (GH-producing; GHRH-producing).

Pathology. Hyperplasia or adenoma of pituitary, splanchnomegaly (liver; spleen; heart; kidney; intestine); enlargement of terminal parts of bones. Metachromatic material in muscles, which are atrophic. Frequently, goiter; adrenal enlarged; thymus usually large.

Diagnostic Procedures. *Blood.* Glucose tolerance curve; increased alkaline phosphatase and phosphorus level; increased follicle-stimulating hormone (FSH). *Urine.* Decreased FSH; increased 17-ketosteroids; glycosuria; increased creatine; occasionally, elevated basal metabolic rate. *X-ray.* Skull thickened; enlargement of sella turcica; paranasal sinus. Osteolytic process together with cortical periosteal thickening; conspicuous excrescences of muscle insertion. Osteoarthritis; tufted distal phalanges.

Therapy. *Surgery.* Total or partial hypophysectomy; radiation therapy; ^{90}yttrium implantation. *Medical treatment.* Pergolide, bromocriptine, somatostatin analogs after surgery or radiation therapy to compensate for deficient secretion.

Prognosis. Progressive evolution usually in several years, but variable. Stabilization at later stage.

NEUROLOGIC SYNDROMES
Different syndromes may develop according to direction of adenoma expansion. See Chiasma and cavernous sinus.

BIBLIOGRAPHY. Marie P: In Major RH: Classic Descriptions of Diseases, 2nd ed. Springfield, Ill, CC Thomas, 1939

Kendall-Taylor P, Upstill-Goddard G, Cook D: Long-term pergolide treatment of acromegaly. Clin Endocrinol 19:711–719, 1983

Brennan MD, Jackson IT, Keller EE, et al: Multidisciplinary management of acromegaly and its deformities. JAMA 253:682–683, 1985

Scheithauer BW, Kovacs K, Randall RV, et al: Pathology of excessive production of growth hormone. Endocrin Metab 15:3:655–677, 1986

Bauman G: Acromegaly. Endocrin Metab 16:685–705, 1987

MARIE-SAINTON

Synonyms. Cleidocranial dysplasia; cleidocranial dysostosis; Hulkcrantz's anosteoplasia; Scheuthaurer's; "Arnold head".

Symptoms and Signs. Widespread racial, ethnic, and regional occurrence; family history; also cases of spontaneous occurrence. Varying degrees of aplasia of clavicles that allow unusual mobility of shoulders. Neurologic and vascular symptoms from compression of clavicular stumps. Excessive development of head (brachycephaly). Metopic suture remains open in childhood and adulthood. Incomplete closure of fontanelles. Facial bones small, poorly developed; mastoid air cells absent or small. Hyptertelorism may be present; frequently, dwarfism; kyphosis; scoliosis; lordosis; spina bifida. Also, frequently, pathologic fractures. Epilepsy, schizophrenia, and mental retardation also reported in association.

Etiology. Disorder of ossification primarily affecting bones that ossify earliest in life. Autosomal dominant inheritance; also cases of spontaneous occurrence.

Pathology. Tendency for ossification to proceed slowly in skull, hands, pelvis; concurrent osteosclerosis also noticed.

Diagnostic Procedures. *X-ray of skeleton.* See Signs.

Therapy. Surgical correction of defect when feasible.

Prognosis. Disability rarely severe; normal activities and life span.

BIBLIOGRAPHY. Marie P, Sainton P: Sur la dysostose cléido-crânienne héréditaire. Bull Mém Soc Méd Hôp Paris 15:436, 1898
Scheuthauer G: Kombiantion rudimentärer. Schlüssel beine mit Anomalien des Schädels beim erwachsen Menschen. All Weir Med Ztg 16:293–295, 1871
Jackson WPU: Osteo-dental dysplasia (cleidocranial dysostosis): the "Arnold Head." Acta Med Scand 139:292–307, 1951
Arvystas MG: Familial generalized delayed eruption of dentition with short stature. Oral Surg 41:235–243, 1976

MARIE-SEE

Synonyms. Julien Marie-See; hydrocephalus-hypervitaminosis.

Symptoms. Occur in infants within 24 hours of receiving a massive doses of vitamin A and D. Vomiting; somnolence.

Signs. Brusque and intense fontanelles bulging. All other findings negative.

Etiology. Acute vitamin A toxicity. Equivalent of cephalalgia reported in adult receiving massive doses of vitamin A.

Pathology. Hydrocephalus.

Diagnostic Procedures. *CT scan of fundus oculi.*

Therapy. Spinal tap (with caution).

Prognosis. Within 24 hours all signs and symptoms disappear spontaneously.

BIBLIOGRAPHY. Marie J, See G: Hydrocéphalie aiguë bénigne du nourrisson apres ingestion d'une dose massive et unique de vitamines A et D. Arch Fr Pediatr 8:563–565, 1951
Dukes MN: Meyler's side effects of drugs, 10th ed, p 716. Amsterdam, Elsevier, 1984

MARIE UNNA'S

Synonyms. Hereditary hypotrichosis; Unna's (M.).

Symptoms and Signs. Very rare. Both sexes affected; onset in childhood. Eyebrows and eyelashes could be missing from birth or fall out shortly later; usually, however, they eventually grow back to normal. Later in childhood, loss of hair; hair loss progressively extends from the vertex to produce a partial or complete bald vertico-occipital patch by adulthood. Scanty growth of nails and of axillary and pubic hair; limited growth of teeth and nails. Mental development and health are normal. In women, hair is thick and abundant but seldom exceeds 20 cm in length.

Etiology. Autosomal dominant inheritance.

Pathology. Hairs show several irregularities of calibre, pigmentation, and are rotated 180 degrees on their axis.

Therapy. None.

Prognosis. See Signs.

BIBLIOGRAPHY. Unna M: Ueber hypotricosis congenita hereditaria. Derm Wochenschr 81:1167–1178, 1925
Bentley-Phillips B, Grace HJ: Hereditary hypotrichosis: a previously undescribed syndrome. Br J Derm 101:331–339, 1979

MARIN AMAT'S

Synonyms. Corneo-mandibular reflex; inverted Marcus Gunn's; Mueller-Kannberg; pterygo corneal reflex; winking-jaw.

Symptoms. Automatic, involuntary, or reflex closure of the eye.

Signs. With pressure on the cornea (with eye open) to produce winking, and quick movement of the mandible of contralateral side, sometimes mandible moves slightly forward. Movement very rapid and minimal; easily overlooked.

Etiology. Unknown; not found in normal subject. It can be demonstrated best a few weeks after hemiplegic attacks, and in cases of amyotrophic lateral sclerosis. Considered an associated movement between orbicularis oculi and external pterygoid muscles; release phenomenon due to supranuclear lesion.

BIBLIOGRAPHY. Mueller-Kannberg: Eigentumliche Mitbewegung eines ptotischen Lides bei Unterkiefer–Bewegungen. Der Artz Prack, 7:1177–1180, 1894

Marin Amat M: Sur le syndrome ou phenomene de Marcus Gunn. Ann Ocul 156:513–528, 1919

Wartenberg R: Winking-jaw phenomenon. Arch Neurol Psychiatr 59:734–753, 1948

Adams RD, Victor M: Principles of Neurology, 3rd ed, p 208. New York, McGraw-Hill, 1985

MARINESCO-SJÖGREN

Synonyms. Ataxia-cataract-dwarfism; hereditary oligophrenic cerebellolental degeneration; oligophrenic cerebellolenticular degeneration; Garland-Moorhause; Sjögren's II; Torsten's; MMS.

Symptoms and Signs. Both sexes affected; clinical onset when child learns to walk. Ataxia; rotary and horizontal nystagmus; dysarthria; physical and mental development retarded, weakness with or without muscle hypotonia; association with variable skeletal defects (short stature; kyphoscoliosis; genu valgum; reduced extensibility of the knee; digital defects). Hair sparse, short, fine, usually poor in pigment. Congenital cataract. Hypersalivation.

Etiology. Autosomal recessive inheritance. Possibly a lysosomal storage disorder.

Pathology. Degenerative process in the cortical areas of the cerebellum. Biopsy suggests chronic atrophy of nerve cells rather than inflammation. Electron microscopy shows enlarged lysosomes containing whorled lamellar or amorphous inclusion bodies.

Diagnostic Procedures. *X-ray. Electroencephalography. Biopsy of muscle. Electromyography. Ophthalmoscopy.*

Therapy. None.

Prognosis. Normal life expectancy.

BIBLIOGRAPHY. Marinesco G, Draganesco S, Vasiliu D: Nouvelle maladie familiale, caractérisée par une cataracte congenitale et un arrét du dévelopement somatoneuro-psychique. Encéphale 26:97–109, 1931

Sjögren T: Hereditary congenital spinocerebellar ataxia accompanied by congenital cataract and oligophrenia. Confinia Neurol 10:293–308, 1950

Walker PD, Blitzer MG, Shapira E, et al: Sjögren syndrome: evidence for a lysosomal storage disorder. Neurology 35:415–419, 1985

MARION'S

Synonyms. Female prostatic obstruction. See bladder neck.

Symptoms. Dysuria, from simple difficulty in voiding to complete retention.

Signs. Urinary bladder distension.

Etiology. Inflammation or hypertrophy (or both) of the group of glands surrounding the posterior part of the female urethra.

Diagnostic Procedures. *Urine.* No pathologic findings or varying degree of albuminuria, and variable number of granulocytes in different stages of degeneration (pus). *Cystography.* Filing defect in the region of the internal orifice similar to the defects seen in men in prostatic hypertrophy; in bladder wall, various degree of trabeculation.

Therapy. Transurethral resection.

Prognosis. Good with treatment.

Comment. Not all authors accept hypertrophy of adenomatous tissue equivalent to the male prostate as the pathogenesis of this syndrome. The following have been considered as etiologic factors for the rare obstruction of the neck of bladder observed in women: granulomatous inflammation; neurologic causes; cystocele. Folsom and O'Brien, however, presented a good pathologic demonstration of the nature of the tissue in their patients.

BIBLIOGRAPHY. Caulk J: Contracture of the vesical neck in the female. J Urol 6:341–343, 1921

Marion G: De l'hypertrophie congenitale du col vésical. J Urol Méd Chil 23:97–101, 1927

Grasset D: Maladie du col vescical. Encicl Med Chir Techniques Chirurgicales. Edition Techniques, Paris, Urologic 41225, 1978

MARJOLIN'S

Synonym. Marjolin's ulcer.

Symptoms and Signs. Occur in both sexes, usually in elderly persons; onset a few months after burn. Cicatricial scar; then 30 to 40 years later, pruritus, hyperesthesia, pain, malodorous discharge.

Etiology. Carcinomatous degeneration of burn scar, or of lesions due to lupus vulgaris or erythematosus.

Pathology. On margin of ulcer or scar, epidermoid carcinoma, dense fibrosis, reduced vascularization; seldom, basal cell carcinoma type.

Diagnostic Procedures. *Biopsy.*

Therapy. Surgery; radiotherapy; local destruction.

Prognosis. Poor.

BIBLIOGRAPHY. Marjolin Ulcère. Dictionnaire de Méde-cine 2nd ed, vol 30, pp 10–31. Paris, 1846

Ghosh J: A case report of extensive bilateral Marjolin's ulcer. Br J Plast Surg 19:97–100, 1966.

Way LW (ed): Current Surgical Diagnosis and Treat-ment, p 731. Los Altos, Calif, Lange Medical Publica-tions, 1982

MARKOVITS'

Synonym. Ophthalmodynia hypertonica copulationis.

Symptoms. Ocular pain during copulation in prone po-sition.

Etiology. Prone position enhancing the closure of a nar-row-angle glaucoma.

BIBLIOGRAPHY. Markovits AS: Ophthalmodynia hyper-tonica copulationis. Can J Ophthalmol 9:484–485, 1974

MAROTEAUX-LAMY I

Synonyms. Polydystrophic dwarfism; mucopolysac-charidosis VI; MPS VI; N-acetylgalactosamine-4-sulfa-tase deficiency; arylsulfatase B deficiency.

Symptoms. Both sexes affected; clinical onset at 2 to 3 years of age (severe form) or later. Visual impairment; restriction of articular movements; dyspnea; neurologic manifestations. Normal intelligence.

Signs. Short stature; hydrocephalus (in some cases); coarse facies; clouding of cornea. Progressive sternal pro-trusion. Murmurs indicating valvulopathies. Lumbar kyphosis. Genu valgum. Atlantoaxial subluxation (see) (in some cases). Hips severely involved.

Etiology. Autosomal recessive inheritance. Two or more alleles producing, respectively, more or less severe clinical patterns. Inability to hydrolyze the sulfate group from N-acetylgalactosamine-4-sulphate (arylsulfatase B).

Pathology. Abnormal metachromatic inclusion in many tissues and leukocytes.

Diagnostic Procedures. *Urine.* Excretion of dermatan sulfate only. Measurement of arylsulfatase activity. *X-ray.* See Hurler's.

Therapy. None.

Prognosis. Variable according to severity of the condi-

tion. In severe cases, maximal survival to the late 20s. In mild cases, longer survival reported.

BIBLIOGRAPHY. Maroteaux P, Levéque B, Marie J, et al: Une nouvelle dysostose avec élimination urinaire de chondroitine-sulfate. B Presse Med 71:1849–1852, 1963

Williams HE: Heritable disorders of mucopolysaccharide metabolism. Calif Med 106:306–311, 1967

McKusick VA, Neufeld EF: The mucopolysacharide stor-age diseases. In Stanbury JB, Wyngaarden JB, Fred-rickson DS, et al: The Metabolic Basis of Inherited Disease, 5th ed, p 751. New York, McGraw-Hill, 1983

MAROTEAUX-LAMY II

Synonyms. Pycnodysostosis; pyknodysostosis.

Symptoms and Signs. Both sexes affected; evident from early infancy. Dwarfism; easy fractures of bones; partial agenesis of terminal digits of hands and feet; per-sistent opening of cranial fontanelles; occipital bossing; parrotlike nose; micrognathism; scoliosis (Toulouse-Lau-trec seems to have suffered from this syndrome). Occa-sionally, mental retardation. Two-thirds of patients had fractures, especially of lower extremities; poor dentition and frequent caries.

Etiology. Unknown; autosomal recessive inheritance.

Pathology. Osteopetrosis.

Diagnostic Procedures. *Blood.* Normal; no anemia. *X-ray.* Skull dolichocephaly; opening of fontanelles. Bone dense; absence of diploë; absence of frontal sinuses. In other bones, diffuse osteopetrosis.

Therapy. Special dental care; orthopedic provision for fractures.

Prognosis. Good; no anemia, blindness, or other compli-cation as observed in similar syndromes (e.g., Albers-Schönberg's). There may be, however, progressive loss of distal phalanges; persistence of open fontanelles.

BIBLIOGRAPHY. Montanari U: Acondroplasia e disostosi cleidocranica digitale. Chir Organi Mov 7:379–391, 1923

Collado–Otero F: Una forma mas de distrofia osea. Acta Pediatr Esp 14:1–27, 1956

Maroteaux P, Lamy M: La pycnodysostose. Presse Med 70:999–1002, 1962

Maroteaux P, Lamy M; The malady of Toulouse-Lautrec. JAMA 191:715–717, 1965

Sedano HD, Gorlin RJ, Anderson VE: Pycnodysostosis: clinical and genetic considerations. Am J Dis Child 116:70–77, 1968

Meneses de Almeida L: A genetic study of pycnodysostosis. In Papadatos CJ, Barsocas CS (eds): Skeletal Dysplasias, pp 195–198. New York, Alan R Liss, 1982

MAROTEAUX'S

Synonyms. Metaphyseal dysplasia (type A-III); metaphyseal dysostosis (type A-III). See Schmid's.

Symptoms and Signs. Present from birth. Metaphyseal dysostosis limited to knees.

Etiology. Autosomal recessive inheritance.

Diagnostic Procedures. X-ray. Limited metaphyseal abnormalities.

BIBLIOGRAPHY. Maroteaux P, Savart P, Lefebvre J, et al: Les formes partielles de la dysostoses metaphysaire. Presse Med 71:1523–1526, 1963

Sutcliffe J: Metaphyseal dysostosis (dysostosis methaphysaire). Ann Radiol 9:215–223, 1966

MAROTEAUX'S MEDT

Synonyms. Multiple epiphyseal dysplasia tarda (type Id), MEDT (type Id).

Symptoms and Signs. Both sexes affected. Moderate dwarfism (mainly trunk shortness). Normal length of extremities. Frequently, arthrosis of hips.

Etiology. Autosomal dominant or recessive inheritance.

Diagnostic Procedures. X-ray of spine. Vertebral irregularity and decreased height; corpus spongiosum hernial changes. *Extremities.* In hips, alteration of femoral epiphyses; minor alteration of proximal epiphyses of humeri.

BIBLIOGRAPHY. Maroteaux P: Spondiloepiphyseal dysplasias and metatropic dwarfism. Birth Defects 5:35–41, 1969

MAROTEAUX-SPRANGER-WIEDEMANN

Synonyms. Hyperchondrogenesis; metatrophic dwarfism I.

Symptoms. Both sexes affected; evident at birth and progressing during infancy. Motor milestones delayed. Birth length normal or slightly decreased (long trunk—especially thorax—and short limbs). Linear fold that overlies the coccyx and may extend as a taillike process. Waddling gait. Knobby and lax joints. Elbow may not fully extend. Occasionally, inguinal hernia and cleft palate. In infancy and childhood, retarded growth, severe kyphoscoliosis, short neck, upward displacement of sternum, generalized weakness. In adolescence, progressive disability. Dyspnea.

Etiology. Unknown; both autosomal dominant and recessive (lethal) types of inheritance.

Pathology. Lack of endochondral ossificatn in growth areas and irregular arrangement of trabeculae.

Diagnostic Procedures. X-rays. Delayed ossification; kyphoscoliosis; pelvic supraacetabular notch; squared iliac wings; bell-shaped ends of long bones. *Blood.* Phosphorus elevated.

Therapy. Mainly orthopedic.

Prognosis. Few survive beyond adulthood because of cardiopulmonary complications and atlantoaxial instability.

BIBLIOGRAPHY. Kaufmann E: Untersuchungen ueber die sogenanute foetale Rachitis Chondrodystrophia foetalis. Berlin, G Reimer, 1892

Maroteaux P, Spranger J, Wiedemann HR: Der metatropische Zwergwuchs. Arch Kinderheilkd 173:211–226, 1966

Beck M, Roubicek M, Roger JG et al: Heterogeneity of metatropic dysplasia. Eur J Pediatr 140:231–237, 1983

MARSHALL'S

Synonym. Atypical ectodermal dysplasia. See Wagner's and Stichler's.

Symptoms. Both sexes affected; present from birth. Partial (usually) deafness; myopia; hypohidrosis.

Signs. Facial malformation with saddle nose. Cataract; fluid vitreous.

Etiology. Autosomal dominant inheritance.

Therapy. None.

Prognosis. Frequently, spontaneous absorption of cataract; in some cases; luxation. Permanent condition.

BIBLIOGRAPHY. Marshall D: Ectodermal dysplasia: report of kindred and ocular abnormalities and hearing defect. Am J Ophthalmol 45:143–156, 1958

Zellweger H, Smith JK, Grutzner P: The Marshall syndrome: report of a new family. J Pediatr 84:868–871, 1974

Gorlin RJ, Pindborg JJ, Cohen MM Jr: Syndromes of the Head and Neck, 2nd ed, p. 757–758. New York, McGraw-Hill, 1976.

MARSHALL'S (J.)

Synonyms. Acquired cutis laxa; postinflammatory elastolysis.

Symptoms and Signs. Reported in Afroeuropean children in South Africa; onset before the age of 3 years. Eruption of red edematous papules, slowly progressing up to 2 to 10 cm, followed by successive sporadic new eruptions for 1 year. During eruptive phase, some patients develop pneumonia.

Etiology. Unusual reaction to arthropod bite (?).

Pathology. Reduction and degenerative changes of elastic fibers in affected areas.

Therapy. None.

Prognosis. Papules disappear to leave areas of cutis laxa.

BIBLIOGRAPHY. Marshall J: Alopecia after tick bite. S Afr Med J 40:1555–1556, 1966
Rook A, Wilkinson DS, Ebling FJG, et al: Textbook of Dermatology, 4th ed, p 1835. Oxford, Blackwell Scientific Publications, 1986

MARSHALL'S (R.E.)

Synonyms. Accelerated growth-failure to thrive, Marshall-Smith. See Weaver's.

Symptoms. Present from birth. Noisy breathing; repeated respiratory infections; failure to thrive; mental retardation; accelerated skeletal growth.

Signs. Underweight for length. Long cranium; prominent forehead; head hyperextension. Bulging eyes; blue sclerae; megalocornea; thick eyebrows; small upturned nose, small mandible. Broad middle and maximal phalanges.

Etiology. Unknown; sporadic.

Diagnostic Procedures. *X-ray.* Bone age markedly advanced; mandibular rami hypoplastic; absence of normal angle. Of chest. Frequently, pneumonia.

Therapy. Prevention of respiratory infections. Feeding.

Prognosis. All patients died with pneumonia before the 20th month of age.

BIBLIOGRAPHY. Marshall RE, Graham CB, Scott CR, et al: Syndrome of accelerated skeletal maturation and relative failure to thrive: a newly recognized clinical growth disorder. J Pediatr 78:95–101, 1971
Fitch N: Update on the Marshall-Smith-Weaver controversy. Am J Med Genet 20:559–562, 1985

MARSHALL-WHITE

Synonym. Bier's.

Symptoms. Sporadic periods of insomnia and tachycardia, with the appearance of spots in the palms that are colder and paler than surrounding skin.

Etiology. Unknown; vasospastic phenomenon.

BIBLIOGRAPHY. Bier A: Die Entstehung des Collateralkreisedlaufs. II Der Rueckfluss des Bluts aus ischaemichen Koerperteilen. Virchows Arch [Pathol Anat] 153:306–334, 1898
Marshall W, White C: Localized area of ischemia of the hands. J Lab Clin Med 18:386–388, 1932–33

MARTIN-ALBRIGHT

Synonyms. Albright's IV; Albright's hereditary osteodystrophy; pseudohypoparathyroidism. See also Pseudopseudohypoparathyroidism.

Symptoms. Female to male ratio 2 : 1; onset of symptoms at about 8 years of age. Headache; weakness; lethargy; numbness; paresthesia; dyspnea; laryngeal stridor; photophobia and blurred vision. Muscular cramps; abdominal pain; convulsion. Some degree of mental deficiency.

Signs. Short stature; round face; thick neck; shortness of limbs in relation to trunk. Hands fat; stubby short fingers; short metacarpal and metatarsal bones. Chvostek's and Trousseau's signs.

Etiology. Hereditary condition with diminished end-organ responsiveness (Seabright-Bantam syndrome) to parathyroid hormone, which is secreted in normal amount. No longer accepted X-dominant inheritance. Genetics are under discussion. Two forms are described according to the pathogenesis. Pseudohypoparathyroidism type 1: renal (end-organ) resistance to parathyroid hormone due to defect of N protein (receptor for PTH and stimulating cAMP production) (type IA) or defect in adenylate cyclase enzyme complex (type 1B), bone resistance of the same nature.

Pseudohypoparathyroidism type 2: normal receptor mechanism but inability of intracellular cAMP to initiate cascade of events in bone and kidney.

Pathology. Normal or hyperplastic parathyroid glands. Subcutaneous calcification; calcification of basal ganglia of brain.

Diagnostic Procedures. *Blood.* Normal serum phosphatase activity; low calcium; increased serum phosphate. *Urine.* Decreased urinary excretion of calcium and phosphate. Ellsworth-Howard test: No response of kidneys to parathyroid hormone. Patients with pseudohypothyroidism show no change of urinary excretion of adenosine 3':5'-cycle phosphate (cyclic AMP) while normal and patients with true hypoparathyroidism show a 10-fold to 20-fold increase. *X-ray.* Early epiphyseal closure; subcutaneous and basal ganglia of brain calcifications.

Therapy. Large dose of parathyroid hormone has little or no effect on serum calcium and phosphorus and urinary phosphate excretion. Fair response to large dose of vitamin D and calcium salts.

Prognosis. Satisfactory response to treatment indicated.

BIBLIOGRAPHY. Martin D, Bourdillon J: Un cas de tétanie idiopathique chronique. Échec thérapeutique de la graffe d' un adénome parathyroïdien. Rev Med Suisse Rom 60:1166–1177, 1940

Albright F, Burnett CH, Smith PH, et al: Pseudo-hypoparathyroidism-example of "Seabright-Bantam syndrome"; report of three cases. Endocrinology 30:922–932, 1942

Drezner MK, Neelon FA, Lebovitz HE: Pseudohypoparathyroidism type II: a possible defect in the reception of the cyclic AMP signal. New Engl J Med 289:1056, 1973

Drezner MK, Neelon FA: Pseudohypoparathyroidism. In Stanbury JB, Wyngaarden JB, Fredrickson DS, et al, The Metabolic Basis of Inherited Diseases, 5th ed, p. 1508. New York, McGraw-Hill, 1983.

MARTIN DU PAN-RUTISHAUSER

Synonym. Laminar osteochondritis. See Epiphyseal ischemic necrosis.

Symptoms and Signs. Prevalent in males; onset in adolescence. Pain; progressive motion reduction, due to ankylosis of a single joint.

Etiology. Unknown.

Pathology. Destruction of cartilage from infiltration of connective tissue between cartilage and spongious tissue.

BIBLIOGRAPHY. Martin du Pan C, Rutishauser E: Un type d'hartrose infantile nouvelle: ostéochondrite laminaire. Schweiz Med Wochenschr 75:955–956, 1945

MARTIN'S

Synonyms. Apoplexia uvulae; Bosviel-Martin; staphylohematoma.

Symptoms and Signs. Hemoptysis.

Etiology. Hemorrhage from hematoma of uvula.

BIBLIOGRAPHY. Martin A: Ueber das Staphylohaematoma. Neue Med Chir Ztg 225–227, 1846

MARTORELL'S I

Synonym. Hypertensive ischemic ulcer.

Symptoms and Signs. Predominant in women, onset in middle or old age. Painful ulceration of the leg (frequently bilateral) above the ankle. Other symptoms and signs of blood hypertension.

Etiology. Blood hypertension.

Pathology. Arteries present accumulation of hyalin material between elastica and endothelium.

Therapy. Excision; control of pressure and sympathectomy. Grafting valid quick method.

Prognosis. Control of pressure cures the condition.

BIBLIOGRAPHY. Martorell R: Ulcera hypertensiva. Barcellona Ediciones BTP, 1953

Rook A, Wilkinson DS, Ebling FJG, et al: Textbook of Dermatology, 4th ed, pp. 1218–1219. Oxford, Blackwell Scientific Publications, 1986

MASSETERIC HYPERTROPHY

Synonym. Benign masseteric hypertrophy.

Symptoms and Signs. Unilateral or bilateral masseter muscle hypertrophy manifesting itself as a painless swelling below and anterior to the ear, with or without ear ache or temporomandibular arthralgia. Habitual grinding of teeth during sleep. Usually, tense personality.

Etiology. Acquired condition due to different mechanisms: primary or secondary malocclusion; displacement of the mandible by "cracking" jaw while reading; tension and teeth grinding.

Pathology. Masseter hypertrophy; wearing of teeth surfaces; temporomandibular joint changes.

Diagnostic Procedures. *X-ray.* When unilateral condition, severe distortion of mandible. *Dental consultation.* Malocclusion.

Therapy. Restoration of normal bite; frequently, simple explanation of nature of condition reassures the patient and cures associated complaints arising from fear of cancer or incurable infections. Sedative may be useful in particularly tense patients to break the habit.

Prognosis. Good with proper treatment.

BIBLIOGRAPHY. Gurney GE: Chronic bilateral benign hypertrophy of masseter muscles. Am J Surg 73:137–139, 1947

Barton RT: Benign masseteric hypertrophy: a syndrome of importance in the differential diagnosis of parotid tumors. JAMA 164:1646–1647, 1957

MASSHOFF'S

Eponym used to designate the mesenteric lymphadenitis (see Brennemann's) associated with *Pasturella pseudotuberculosis* (*Yersinia pseudotuberculosis*) infection.

BIBLIOGRAPHY. Masshoff W: Eine neuartige Form der Mesenterialen Lymphadenitis. Dtsch Med Wochenschr 78:532–535, 1953

MASSIVE ASPIRATION

Synonyms. Massive fetal aspiration; atelectasia neonatorum; fetal aspiration. See Meconium aspiration.

Symptoms. Occur in newborn: they may be stillborn, die in a few hours after birth, or survive. Tachypnea; wheezing; apnea; flaccidity; rigidity and convulsions in more severe cases. In milder form, dyspnea soon after birth, lasting 2 or 3 days followed by rapid recovery.

Signs. Intercostal retraction; asphyxia pallida; brain damage in severe cases; chest percussion diminished resonance; generalized or localized area of hyperresonance possible. Rales may or may not be present; temperature normal (except when infection develops); no cough.

Etiology. Fetal asphyxia causes the fetus to gasp in the uterus or birth canal (postmaturity may also play an important role) and to inhale amniotic, vaginal, or oropharyngeal fluids.

Pathology. Lung firm, poorly aerated; bronchi full of mucus or fluid; alveoli collapsed; some expanded; squamae and amniotic debris elements recognized. Edema and hemorrhages present. Brain hemorrhages and edema may coexist. Right heart dilatation in many cases.

Diagnostic Procedures. *X-ray of chest.* Coarsely granular pattern with irregular aeration.

Therapy. Bronchoscopic suction; oxygen; humidity control; antibiotic prophylaxis.

Prognosis. Brief course unless complications develop (hours or days later). Severe form lethal.

BIBLIOGRAPHY. Farber S, Wilson JL: Atelectasis of the newborn: a study and critical review. Am J Dis Child 4b:572–589, 1933

Schaffer AJ: Diseases of Newborn, 2nd ed. Philadelphia, WB Saunders, 1965

MATERNAL-FETAL TRANSFUSION

See Neonatal polycythemia.

Symptoms and Signs. Neonatal polychythemia (see).

Etiology. Maternal-fetal transfusion.

Pathology. Polycythemia.

Diagnostic Procedures. *Blood.* High hemoglobin and hematocrit values. Demonstration of maternal erythrocytes in newborn (Ashby's differential agglutination method). Presence in the newborn blood of beta-2-M-globulin.

Therapy. See Neonatal polycythemia.

Prognosis. See Neonatal polycythemia.

BIBLIOGRAPHY. Hedenstedt S, Naeslund J: Investigations of the permeability of the placenta with the help of elliptocytes. Acta Med Scand 170 (suppl):126–134, 1946

Michael AF, Mauer AM: Maternal-fetal transfusion as a cause of plethora in neonatal period. Pediatrics 28:458–461, 1961

Fouron JC: Polycythemie neo-natale. Union Med Can 96:1388–1393, 1968

Van der Zee DC, Poelmann RE, Vermeij-Keers C, et al: Materno-embryonic transfusion and congenital malformations: an experimental study using rat embryos. J Pediatr Surg 23:266–269, 1988

Rosenkrantz TS, Oh W.: Neonatal polycythemia and hyperviscosity. In Milunsky A, Friedman EA, Gluck L, et al: Advances in Perinatal Medicine, Vol 5, p 93. New York, Plenum Medical Book Co, 1986

MATHES'

Synonym. Puerperal mastitis.

Symptoms. Occur 10 days after delivery, or later (parenchymatous type). Fever; chills; malaise; breast pain, initially slight, then progressive, accentuated by nursing.

Signs. Two types distinguished: *Interstitial.* Inflammatory area tense and hard, from nipple to breast margin. *Parenchymatous.* Localized, tender masses in breast lobe, evolving into abscesses.

Etiology. Infections, most common agent responsible is *Micrococcus aureus.*

Pathology. Interstitial inflammatory features, extending among septa between lobes; parenchymatous infection, involving lactiferous ducts and glands.

Diagnostic Procedures. *Blood.* Leukocytosis.

Therapy. Antibiotics; breast support; nursing interruption; oral stilbestrol. If abscess formation, surgery.

Prognosis. Good with adequate therapy.

BIBLIOGRAPHY. Mathes P: Eine typische Form der Brustentzündung im Wochenbett. Munch Med Wochenschr 68:15, 1921

Nelson Textbook of Pediatrics, 12th ed. Philadelphia, WB Saunders, 1983

MATSOUKAS'

Synonym. Articulo-oculo-cerebro-skeletal dysplasia.

Symptoms. Both sexes affected; present from birth. Mental retardation; myopia.

Signs. Small stature; multiple joint dislocation. Small mouth; high palate; microphthalmia; reduced palpebral fissures. Senile cataract; corneal sclerosis. In-curved little finger.

Etiology. Autosomal dominant inheritance. Not well differentiated from Larsen's, Schwartz's, Hallermann-Streiff, Mieter's and Stickler's.

BIBLIOGRAPHY. Matsoukas J, Liarikos S, Giannikas A: A newly recognized dominantly inherited syndrome: short stature, ocular and articular anomalies, mental retardation. Helv Pediatr Acta 28:383–386, 1973

MATZENAUER-POLLAND

Synonym. Dermatitis symmetrica dysmenorrhoica.

Symptoms and Signs. Include the periodic activation or exacerbation of many existing dermatoses during premenstrual and menstrual periods. Associated with the dermatologic manifestation are emotional tension, headache, and abdominal, articular and urinary symptoms (see Premenstrual).

Etiology. Part of premenstrual syndrome (see); no reason to separate this dermatologic syndrome from premenstrual. Some of the dermatologic manifestations have been attributed to autoimmune mechanism or hypersensitivity to progesterone.

BIBLIOGRAPHY. Matzenauer R, Polland R: Dermatitis symmetrica dysmenorrhoica Beitrag zur Angioneurosefrage. Arch Dermatol Syph 111:385–394, 1912

Shelley WB: Autoimmune progesterone dermatitis: cure by oophorectomy. JAMA 190:35–38, 1964

Rook A, Wilkinson DS, Ebling FJG, et al: Textbook of Dermatology, 4th ed, pp 1001, 1917. Oxford, Blackwell Scientific Publications, 1986

MAUGERI'S

Synonym. Silicotic mediastinitis.

Symptoms. Onset after chronic (10 to 30 years) exposure to silicates. Frequently asymptomatic. Dyspnea; congestive heart failure symptoms; cough.

Signs. Evidence of thoracic deformity; pleural effusion; basal crepitations; finger clubbing. Broadbent's sign; systolic retraction of apex during inspiration; pulsus paradox; frequently, hepatosplenomegaly.

Etiology. Chronic exposure to silicate products.

Pathology. Silicates, usually in fibrous forms (asbestos; talc), in bronchioles and alveoli of lungs with typical formation of reacting bodies and secondary fibrosis; distortion; microcysts and honeycombing formations. Striking pleural thickening, in this case fibrous attachment with pericardium and other mediastinal structures. Congestive heart failure features.

Diagnostic Procedures. *X-ray.* Pleural changes: plaques; calcifications; effusion. Pulmonary changes: small or large opacities. *Electrocardiography.* Low voltage especially of QRS complex; T waves flattened or inverted. Right axis deviation. *Blood.* Polycythemia; hypercapnia.

Therapy. Symptomatic.

Prognosis. Progressive evolution. Possibly, development of mesothelial neoplasm of pleura.

BIBLIOGRAPHY. Maugeri S: La mediastinite silicotica. Folia Med 36:136–143, 1953

Fraser RG, Paré JAP: Diagnosis of Diseases of the Chest, p 1510. Philadelphia, WB Saunders, 1977

MAUMENEE'S

Synonyms. Congenital hereditary corneal dystrophy, CHCD; congenital hereditary endothelial dystrophy. Including Dystrophy-deafness syndrome.

Symptoms and Signs. Both sexes affected; corneal edema present at birth. Corneas show diffuse milky or ground-glass opacity and thickening. Opacity may be central or peripheral. Vision variously impaired, sometimes worse at wakening. Occasionally, nystagmus or sensorineural deafness.

Etiology. Autosomal dominant or recessive inheritance.

Pathology. Corneal endothelial cells reduced or atrophic, pigmented or absent pigment; increased thickness in Descemet's membrane, replacement by a mixture of long-spacing and regular collagen.

Diagnostic Procedures. *Biopsy.*

Prognosis. Some cases static; in others slow progression of visual impairment.

BIBLIOGRAPHY. Maumenee AE: Congenital hereditary corneal dystrophy. Am J Ophthalmol 50:1114–1124, 1960

Kenyon KR, Maumenee AE: The histological and ultrastructural pathology of congenital hereditary corneal dystrophy: a case report. Invest Ophthalmol 7:475–500, 1968

Goldberg MF: Genetic and Metabolic Eye Disease, p 305. Boston, Little, Brown, 1974

MAURIAC'S (C.)

Synonym. Syphilitic erythema nodosum.

Symptoms and Signs. Those of erythema nodosum (see), among other manifestations of tertiary syphilis.

BIBLIOGRAPHY. Mauriac C: Pathologie générale de la syphilis terziarie. Paris, Capiomont et Renault, 1886

MAURIAC'S (P.)

Synonym. Diabetes-dwarfism-obesity. See Wolcott-Rallison.

Symptoms. Slowly developing in diabetic children of the "brittle" type. Hard-to-manage diabetes; slow growth; abdominal colic.

Signs. Dwarfism; obesity with moon facies; hepatomegaly, splenomegaly, hypersensitivity to quick-acting insulin; favorable response to slow acting types.

Etiology. Nutritional deficiencies; lack of insulin. Possibly, metabolic derangement due to diabetes or associated conditions.

Pathology. Liver fat infiltration; lesion typical of diabetes (see).

Diagnostic Procedures. Evaluation of diabetes, adrenal cortex and pituitary functions. Rule out storage diseases. *X-ray.* Retarded ossification; osteoporosis.

Therapy. Slow-acting insulin; adequate diet.

Prognosis. That of juvenile diabetes.

BIBLIOGRAPHY. Mauriac P: Gros ventre, Hépatomégalie. Troubles de la croissance cher les enfants diabétiques, traités depuis plusieurs années par l'insuline. Gaz Hebd Sci Med Bordeaux 51:402–404, 1930

Guest GM: The Mauriac syndrome. Diabetes 2:415–417, 1953

Wolcott CD, Rallison ML: Infancy-onset diabetes mellitus and multiple epiphyseal dysplasia. J Pediatr 80:191–197, 1972

Sims EAH: Syndromes of obesity. In De Groot LJ, Cahill FG Jr, Odell WD, et al (eds): Endocrinology, p 1941. New York, Grune & Stratton, 1979

MAYER-ROKITANSKY-KÜSTER-HAUSER

Synonyms. Vaginal congenital absence; Rokitansky-Küster-Hauser, RKH; nonRokitansky-Küster-Hauser; uterus bipartitus solidus rudimentarius cum vagina solida.

Symptoms and Signs. Incidence statistics differ from 1 : 4000 (at birth) to 1 : 20,000 at female hospital admissions. Recognized usually at time of expected menarche. Primary amenorrhea; congenital absence of vagina; uterus normal or rudimentary; bicornate cords or complete absence; normal ovulation; normal breast development; normal body and hair. Frequent association with urinary tract anomalies (34%); skeletal abnormalities (12%); congenital heart conditions (4%); inguinal hernia (7%).

Etiology. Usually sporadic. Possibly, karyotype abnormalities. Normal initial phases of Müller's duct development and impairment of subsequent development; defect in organization of mesoderm. Familial form consistent with autosomal recessive trait.

Pathology. See Symptoms and Signs.

Diagnostic Procedures. *Chromosome studies.* Karyotype 46XX; *Basal body temperature.* Biphasic. *Hormone studies.* Normal ovulation pattern. *X-rays.* Evaluation of urinary tract anatomy. *Pneumography. Ultrasonography.*

Therapy. *Surgical.* Vagina construction. *Nonsurgical.* Repeated application of pressure against vaginal dimple with a dilator.

Prognosis. High success rate with both surgical and nonsurgical correction of defect.

BIBLIOGRAPHY. Mayer CAJ: Ueber Verdoppelungen des Uterus und ihre Arten, nebst Bemerkungen über Hasenscharte und Wolfsrachen. J Chir Augenheilked 13:525–564, 1829

Rokitansky KF: Ueber die sogenannten Verdoppelungen des Uterus. Med Jahrb Ostet Staat 26:39–77, 1838

Las Casas dos Santos NI: Missbildungen des Uterus, 2 Geburtsh Gynaeck 14:140–184, 1888

Küster H: Uterus bipartitus solidus rudimentarius cum vagina solida. Z Gebur Gynaekol 67:692–718, 1910

Hauser GA, Keller M, Koller T, et al: Das Rokitansky-Küster-Syndrom. Uterus bipartitus solidus rudimentarius cum vagina solida. Gynaecologia 151:111–112, 1961

Griffin JE, Edwards C, Madden JD, et al: Congenital absence of the vagina. Ann Intern Med 85:224–236, 1976

MAY-HEGGLIN

Synonyms. Döhle's bodies—myelopathy; Hegglin's.

Symptoms and Signs. Both sexes affected; detection possible from birth. Usually asymptomatic; seldom, minor hemorrhagic manifestation.

Etiology. Autosomal dominant inheritance.

Pathology. Inclusion bodies may be paracrystalline arrays of depolymerized ribosomes.

Diagnostic Procedures. *Blood.* Mild leukopenia; increased percentage of polymorphonuclear leukocytes, these cells show in the cytoplasma fusiform or semilunar basophilic inclusion bodies (same features as Döhle's or Amato's bodies). Mild thrombocytopenia; platelets giant and poorly granulated. *Clotting tests.* Tourniquet: frequently positive; increased time of clot retraction. *Bone marrow.* Megakaryocytes clamping (impaired fragmentation?).

Therapy. None.

Prognosis. Good.

BIBLIOGRAPHY. May R: Leukocytenanschlüfsse. Kausistiche Mitteilung. Dtsch Arch Klin Med 96:1–6, 1909
Hegglin R: Gleichzeitige konstitutionelle Veränderungen an Neutrophilen und Thrombozyten. Helv Med Acta 12:439–440, 1945
Davis JW, Wilson SJ: Platelet survival in the May-Hegglin anomaly. Br J Haematol 12:61–65, 1966
Cabrera JR, Fontan G, Lorente, F, et al: Defective neutrophyl mobility in the May-Hegglin anomaly. Br J Haemat 47:337–343, 1981

MAY-WHITE

Synonyms. Cerebellar ataxia-deafness-myoclonus; myoclonus-cerebellar ataxia-deafness (including Latham-Munro).

Symptoms and Signs. Both sexes affected; onset at various ages, usually in adolescence. Progressive cerebellar ataxia; myoclonic seizures and neural hearing loss. In some members of the affected family, *forme fruste* may be present.

Etiology. Unknown; autosomal dominant inheritance. One family with autosomal recessive inheritance re-

ported (Latham) in which manifestation occurred at 10–12 years of age.

Diagnostic Procedures. *Electroencephalography.*

Therapy. Attacks controlled by phenytoin and valproic acid.

Prognosis. Chronic progressive condition. Life expectancy may be within normal limits.

BIBLIOGRAPHY. Latham AD, Munro TA: Familial myoclonus epilepsy associated with deaf-mutism in a family showing other psychobiological abnormalities. Ann Eugen 8:166–175, 1937
May DL, White HH: Familial myoclonus, cerebellar ataxia and deafness. Arch Neurol 19:331–338, 1968
Chayasirisobhon S, Walters B: Familial syndrome of deafness, myoclonus and cerebellar ataxia. Neurology 34:78–79, 1984.

MEADOW'S

Synonyms. Dilantin fetal; fetal hydantoin.

Symptoms and Signs. Variable; combinations of the following: mild mental deficiency; mild growth deficiency; craniofacial abnormalities (hypertelorism; broad and depressed nasal sella; abnormal ears; gingival hypertrophy; cleft lip and palate); limb abnormalities (hypoplasia of distal phalanges, hypo-onychon) and various others (hirsutism; coarse hair; hernias). Occasionally other malformations may be present; microcephaly; strabismus; congenital heart; pulmonary; gastrointestinal and genital defects.

Etiology. Teratogenic effect of hydantoin (or combination of hydantoin plus barbiturates) on the fetus. Risk of the complete syndrome 10%; of only some isolated sign 33%.

Therapy. Symptomatic.

Prognosis. Some manifestations regress with growth gingival hyperplasia, dysonychia. Mild degrees of mental deficiency (average IQ of 71).

BIBLIOGRAPHY. Meadow SR: Anticonvulsant drugs and congenital abnormalities. Lancet II:1296, 1968
Smith DW: Recognizable patterns of human malformation. Philadelphia, WB Saunders, 1982

MEADOWS'

Synonyms. Postpartum myocardiopathy; puerperium myocardiopathy. See Cardiomegaly, idiopathic.

Symptoms. Occur in mothers between 2nd week and the 2nd month after delivery. Cough; nocturnal paroxysmal dyspnea; hemoptysis; chest pain. Gastrointestinal symptoms: nausea; vomiting. Symptoms of cerebral embolism with hemiplegia or pulmonary embolism.

Signs. The physical findings are those of congestive heart failure: left-sided first; then right-sided. Diastolic hypertension; pulsus alternans; gallop rhythm; cyanosis; liver enlargement; fundus oculi abnormal.

Etiology. Unknown; myocarditis or myocardiopathy possibly of viral origin or autoimmune disease; familial occurrence has been reported.

Pathology. Heart dilated, soft and flabby, average weight 500 g. Left and right ventricular mural thrombi. Microscopically, focal and diffuse areas of degeneration of myocardial fibers with occasional hemorrhages; lymphocytic and fat droplets infiltration.

Diagnostic Procedures. *X-ray.* Enlargement of the transverse diameter of heart. *Electrocardiography.* T-wave inversion; significant Q-wave and conduction defects.

Differential Diagnosis. Clinical or subclinical toxemia of pregnancy; specific infections; unrecognized preexisting renal or cardiac disease; autoimmune condition.

Therapy. Bed rest until diameter of heart returns to normal. Control of symptoms of congestive heart failure with digitalis, diuretics. Anticoagulation if embolization occurs.

Prognosis. About two-thirds of cases make complete recovery; syndrome tends to recur.

BIBLIOGRAPHY. Hull E, Hafkesbring E: Toxic post-partal heart disease. New Orleans Med Surg J 39:550–557, 1937

Woolford RM: Post-partum myocardosis. Ohio Med J 48:924–930, 1952

Meadows WR: Idiopathic myocardial failure in the last trimester of pregnancy and the puerperium. Circulation 15:903–914, 1957

Hurst JW: The Heart, 6th ed, pp. 1383–1394. New York, McGraw-Hill, 1986

MECKEL-GRUBER

Synonyms. Splanchnocystic dyscephalia; Gruber's; von Hippel-Lindau, lethal form; Simopoulos'.

Symptoms. Prevalent in females; present from birth. Symptoms related to signs.

Signs. *Head.* Microcephaly; posterior encephalocele; sloping forehead; micrognathia; cleft lip and palate; olfactory hypoplasia; cryptophthalmos; mongoloid slant of lids; sclerocornea; cataract; retinal dysplasia. *Neck.* Short. *Limbs.* Polysyndactyly; clubfeet. *Heart.* Congenital de-

fects. *Urogenital tract.* Cryptorchidism. *Other.* Spina bifida.

Etiology. Unknown; autosomal recessive inheritance.

Pathology. See Signs. Polycystic kidney; occasionally, absence of adrenal glands; intestinal malrotation; accessory spleen; imperforate anus; hydrocephalus; absent olfactory lobes and pituitary; incompletely developed forebrain, basal and hypothalamic areas. Septal heart defect; patent ductus; coarctation of aorta; pulmonary stenosis. Lung hypoplasia. Liver cysts; fibrosis.

Diagnostic Procedures. See Signs. *Chromosome studies.* Normal.

Prognosis. Early death (in days or weeks).

BIBLIOGRAPHY. Meckel JF: Beschreibung zweier durch sehr ähnliche Bildungsabweichungen entstellter Geschwister. Dtsch Arch Physiol 7:99–172, 1822

Gruber GB: Beiträge zur Frage "gekoppelter" Missbildung (Akrocephalo-Syndactylie und Dysencephalia splanchnocystica). Beitr Pathol Anat 93:459–476, 1934

Simopoulos AP, Breunan GC, Alwan A, et al: Polycystic kidneys, internal hydrocephalus, and polydactylism in newborn siblings. Pediatrics 39:931–934, 1967

Valenzuela A, Muñor A, Bayes R, et al: Sindrome de Meckel-Gruber: tres casos en una misma fratria. Acta Pediatr 43:44–47, 1985

MECONIUM ASPIRATION

See Massive aspiration.

Symptoms and Signs. Occur in newborns, usually with weight over 2500 g, shortly after birth. Tachypnea and mild cyanosis, resolving in 24 to 72 hours, or worsening, respiration becoming irregular and gasping, cyanosis deeper, and appearance of gross, diffuse rales.

Etiology. Aspiration of meconium-stained amniotic fluid at moment of delivery.

Diagnostic Procedures. *Apgar score.* Below 6 at 1 and 5 minutes (predisposing factor). *X-rays.* Nonuniform, coarse, patchy infiltrates of the lungs; areas of atelectasis and of emphysema; chest hyperexpansion; diaphragm flattening.

Therapy. Aspiration of all traces of meconium fluid first from airways as soon as possible, and, then from pharynx and trachea under laryngoscopic vision. Gastrolysis. Intubation and repeated aspiration and, if needed, ventilatory assistance (expiratory pressure) and general intensive care assistance. Hydrocortisone therapy is not of benefit. For severe cases, extracorporeal membrane oxygenation (ECMO) has been tried with success.

Prognosis. Mortality 4.6%.

BIBLIOGRAPHY. Bacsik RD: Meconium aspiration syndrome. Pediatr Clin N Am 24:463–477, 1977

Davis RO, Philips JB III, Harris BA, et al: Fatal meconium aspiration syndrome occurring despite airway management considered appropriate. Am J Obstet Gynecol 151:731–736, 1985

Byrne DL, Gan G: In utero meconium aspiration: an unpreventable cause of neonatal death. Br J Obstet Gynaecol 94:813–814, 1987

Ortitz RM, Cilley RE, Bartlett RH: Exracorporeal membrane oxygenation in pediatric respiratory failure. Pediatr Clin N Am 34:39–46, 1987

MacFarlane PI, Heaf DP: Pulmonary function in children after neonatal meconium aspiration syndrome. Arch Dis Child 63:368–372, 1988

MECONIUM PLUG

Synonyms. Meconium ileus; meconium peritonitis.

Symptoms. Occur in newborns. Inability to defecate with 48 hours from birth. Nausea; vomiting; abdominal distention.

Signs. Rectal examination reveals meconium plug.

Etiology. Impaction of the meconium plug into the sigmoid flexure of colon, lower ileum, or ileocecal valve. Causes of impaction; deficiency of biliary secretion; deficiency of pancreatic secretion; diminution of amniotic fluid swallowed during intrauterine life. Associated with aganglionosis (see Hirschsprung's) or mucoviscidosis (10%).

Pathology. Meconium plug formed by solidly packed material. Aganglionosis of segment of rectum demonstrated in some cases.

Diagnostic Procedures. *Insertion of rectal catheter. X-ray.* Flat plate of abdomen. Intraluminal or extraluminal calcification in 10 to 25% of cases. *Sweat test.* Later.

Therapy. Enema and meconium plug removal and concurrent intravenous fluid therapy to counteract the hyperosmolar effect of enema. If aganglionosis demonstrated, colostomy and Swenson pull-through procedure and later, colostomy closure.

Prognosis. Survival in both complicated and uncomplicated cases about 50%. Patient with this syndrome must be followed, and aganglionosis and cystic fibrosis ruled out.

BIBLIOGRAPHY. Van Leeuwen G, Riley WC, Glenn L, et al: Meconium plug syndrome with aganglionosis. Pediatr 40:665–666, 1967

Meconium ileus (editorial) Lancet I:1000, 1982

Shwachman H: Meconium ileus: ten patients over 28 years of age. J Pediatr Surg 18:570–575, 1983

MEESMANN'S

Synonyms. Dystrophia epithelialis cornea; juvenile epithelial dystrophy; Meesmann-Wilke; corneal dystrophy juvenile, epithelial.

Symptoms and Signs. Both sexes affected; onset in first 2 years of life. Slight corneal irritation; slight, but progressive visual impairment. Multiple punctiform opacities on the cornea, extending in some cases to Bowman's membrane.

Etiology. Unknown; autosomal dominant inheritance.

Pathology. Corneal dystrophy, characterized by vacuoli full of glycogen and cysts containing degenerated cells.

Therapy. Corneal transplant.

BIBLIOGRAPHY. Meesmann A: Ueber eine bisher nicht beschriebene, dominant vererbte Dystrophyie epithelialis cornae. Ber Dtsch Ophthalmol Ges 52:154–158, 1938.

Meesmann A, Wilke F: Klinische und anatomische Untersuchungen ueber eine bisher unbekannte, dominant vererbte Epitheldystrophie der Hornhaut. Klin Monatsbl Augenheilkd 103:361–391, 1939

Fine BS, Yanoff M, Pitts E, et al: Meesmann's epithelial dystrophy of the cornea. Am J Ophthalmol 83:633–642, 1977

MEGACONIAL MYOPATHY

Synonym. Mitochondrial (megaconial) myopathy.

Symptoms. Onset in infancy. Hypotonia and weakness (floppy infant); proximal muscle weakness (Werdnig-Hoffmann-like); difficulty in walking, climbing stairs.

Signs. Tendon reflexes decreased or absent; no myotonia; no fasciculation; no sensory loss; no incoordination.

Etiology. Unknown; other similar cases reported as lipoid myopathy.

Pathology. Muscle biopsy shows presence of giant mitochondria up to 100 times normal size; fat infiltration.

Diagnostic Procedures. *Biopsy of muscle.* See Pathology. *Electromyography.* Myopathic pattern. *Blood enzymes.* Normal. *Basal metabolic rate.* Normal.

Therapy. None.

Prognosis. Slowly progressing weakness; temporary improvements noticed.

BIBLIOGRAPHY. Shy GM, Gonatas NK, Perez M: Two childhood myopathies with abnormal mitochondria. I Megaconial myopathy. II Pleoconial myopathy. Brain 89:133–158, 1966

D'Agostino AN, Ziter TA, Rollison ML, et al: Familial myopathy with abnormal mitochondria. Arch Neurol 18:388–401, 1968

Adams RD, Denny-Brown D, Pearson CM: Diseases of the Muscles, 3rd ed, p 248. New York, Harper & Row, 1976

MEGADUODENUM-MEGACYSTIS

Synonyms. Intestinal pseudoobstruction; megacystis-microcolon-intestinal hyperperistalsis.

Symptoms and Signs. Both sexes affected; onset from infancy, or later. Symptoms related to dilated duodenum or urinary bladder or both. Subjects with marfanoid habitus (see Marfan's syndrome). Within families, high variability of severity.

Etiology. Unknown; autosomal dominant inheritance.

Pathology. *Biopsies.* Duodenum, jejunum, ileum, colon, urinary bladder. Thinning and collagen replacement of muscle layer—normal ganglion cells.

Diagnostic Procedures. *Sonography. X-rays. Biopsy.*

Therapy. Avoid unnecessary laparatomy for presumed obstruction.

Prognosis. Variable from asymptomatic cases to severe impairment.

BIBLIOGRAPHY. Weiss W: Zur Actiologie des Mega-duodenums. Dtsch Z Chir 251:317–330, 1938

Newton WT: Radical enterectomy for hereditary mega-duodenum. Arch Surg 96:533–549, 1968

Schuffler MD, Rohrmann CA, Chaffee RG, et al: Chronic intestinal pseudoobstruction: a report of 27 cases and review of literature. Medicine 60:173–196, 1981

MEGASIGMOID

Symptoms. Observed in elderly patients, and also in young patients, when neurologic damage is present. Psychotic reaction preceding or following manifestation of this syndrome. Mental deterioration (that may mask symptoms of megasigmoid even in progressed stage). Long-standing constipation, masked by fluid fecal incontinence; loss of tone of sphincter. Abdominal pain; fever, nausea; vomiting.

Signs. Abdominal distension; sudden peritonitis or intermittent or recurring volvulus. Occasionally; liver dislodged medially.

Etiology. It is always acquired (as contrasted with megacolon, which may be acquired or congenital). Neurogenic disorder of sigmoid in association with mental deterioration, cerebral concussion or arteriosclerosis, Parkinson's syndrome, multiple sclerosis, tabes.

Pathology. Only sigmoid enlarged; it may fill entire peritoneal cavity and also push diaphragm into chest cavity. Feces from semiliquid to very compact; deep ulcers with embedded fecaliths. Histologic features of acute and chronic inflammation. Mucosal atrophy; necrosis; hemorrhages of sigmoid walls; hypertrophic ganglion cells preserved.

Diagnostic Procedures. *X-ray of abdomen.* According to amount of gas and location of fecal material three well-defined radiodiagnostic patterns may be obtained. *Barium enema.* Very informative, but difficult to perform.

Therapy. Difficult because of anal sphincter relaxation. Digital removal of feces; tube inserted to remove gas. Cholinergic drug to stimulate peristalsis. Surgical intervention difficult; emergency operation for stercoraceous ulcer. Sigmoidoscopic management for removal of impaction.

Prognosis. Permanent localized and irreversible condition (as opposed to megacolon, which is reversible or changed into total megacolon).

BIBLIOGRAPHY. Kraft E, Finby N: Megacolon and mega-sigmoid syndrome. GP 36:104–114, 1967

MEIGS'

Synonyms. Ascites-pleural effusion-ovarian; Demons-Meigs; Meigs-Cass.

Symptoms. Abdominal distension; pain in the chest; dyspnea; edema of legs not uncommon; weight loss; urinary incontinence.

Signs. Ascites; hydrothorax (62% left side; 11% right side; 24% both sides); adnexal mass; uterine prolapse.

Etiology and Pathology. Solid ovarian tumor, usually benign fibroma, thecoma, granulosa cell tumor, or Brenner tumor. Mechanism of formation of ascites and hydrothorax is unknown. Removal of tumors eliminates fluid effusions.

Diagnostic Procedures. *Ascitic and pleuric fluid.* Transudates (SG 1015 clear, amber, or yellowish). Nonprotein nitrogen (NPN) normal; total serum proteins normal. Carbon particles injected into ascitic fluid pass rapidly and irreversibly into thoracic cavity.

Therapy. Removal of tumor.

Prognosis. Good. If malignant, disease according to histologic grade and extent.

BIBLIOGRAPHY. Meigs JV, Cass JW: Fibroma of the ovary with ascites and hydrothorax, with a report of 7 cases. Am J Obstet Gynecol 33:249–267, 1937
Novak ER: Textbook of Gynecology, 7th ed. Baltimore, Williams & Wilkins, 1965

MELEDA

Synonyms. Keratosis palmoplantaris transgradiens Siemens'; mal de Meleda; Mljet; Siemens'.

Symptoms. Both sexes affected; onset in first month of life. Redness of palms and soles, followed by scaling and thickening, localized or diffuse, extending progressively to dorsal surface. Erythema remains. Hyperhidrosis is frequently associated; frequently, eczematization; continuous patchiform progression of new lesions on extremities. Poor physical development and mental retardation.

Etiology. Autosomal recessive inheritance.

Pathology. Different from tylosis: marked acanthosis; irregular hyperkeratosis and parakeratosis and perivascular lymphohistiocyte infiltration.

Diagnostic Procedures. *Biopsy. Electroencephalography.* Frequently, abnormalities.

Therapy. None.

Prognosis. Progresses through life.

BIBLIOGRAPHY. Neuman NI: Ueber das keratoma hereditarism. Arch Derm Syph 42:163–174, 1898
Kogoj F: Die Krankheit von Mljet ("Mal de Meleda") Acta Dermatovener (Stockh) 15:264–299, 1934
Franceschetti A, Peinhart V, Schnyder UN: La maladie de Meleda. J Genet Hum 20:267–296, 1972

MELENA NEONATORUM

Synonyms. Hemorrhagic newborn; morbus hemorrhagicus neonatorum; newborn hemorrhagic disease; swallowed blood.

Clinically important in the newborn. Differentiate (1) maternal blood swallowed by the newborn; (2) intrinsic bleeding in the gastrointestinal tract of the newborn. Differentiation between the two conditions is of utmost importance. If the blood in the stools is proved to be of maternal origin, the newborn must be spared all the elaborate laboratory tests, x-rays, and even surgical exploration that should be done instead if blood is suspected to be of fetal origin.

Diagnostic Procedures. *Blood.* Fetal hemoglobin is resistant to denaturation by alkalis. Adult hemoglobin is readily denaturalized by alkaline solution. Comparison between clinical findings in both conditions:

EXTRINSIC BLEEDING

Onset. Bloody stools are passed within the first 12 hours. *Anemia.* No anemia found in the newborn. No change in bleeding time, clotting time, or prothrombin time. Usually associated with complications of labor: e.g., placenta previa or premature separation of placenta. The general clinical condition of newborn is good.

INTRINSIC BLEEDING

Onset. Bloody stools are passed usually after first 24 hours. *Anemia.* Gradual and proportionate decrease in the hemoglobin level of the newborn. Change may be found. No associated complications of labor. The clinical condition of the newborn is poor.

Pathology. If the bleeding is intrinsic: (1) evidence of severe infection in the newborn; (2) evidence of bowel pathology (e.g., volvulus); (3) evidence of hepatitis; (4) evidence of upper gastrointestinal tract pathology (e.g., esophageal ulcer). For extrinsic causes of bleeding, no pathology is found.

Therapy. Therapy is needed if bleeding is of fetal origin. Depending on the etiology, from medical management to surgical exploration.

Prognosis. If detected early, the prognosis is good for those patients with intrinsic bleeding.

BIBLIOGRAPHY. Singer K, Chernoff AI, Singer L: Studies on abnormal hemoglobins; I. their demonstration in sickle cell anemia and other hematologic disorders by means of alkali denaturation. Blood 6:413–428, 1951
Apt L, Downey WS: "Melena" neonatorum: the swallowed blood syndrome. A simple test for the differentiation of adult and fetal hemoglobin in bloody stools. J Pediatr 47:6–12, 1955
Wintrobe MM (ed): Clinical Hematology, 8th ed, p 1206. Philadelphia, Lea & Febiger, 1981

MELKERSSON'S

Synonyms. Cheilitis granulomatosis; Melkersson-Rosenthal; Rossolino's. See Miescher's II.

Symptoms and Signs. No sex or racial preference; onset in childhood or youth. Facial paralysis (unilateral or bilateral); facial edema (nonpitting, involving one or both lips, chin, cheeks, or tongue) appearing in association with the paralysis or spaced by as long as 25 years. Lingua plicata (scrotal tongue). Episodes of facial paralysis and edema associated or independently recurrent (*formes* *fruste*). Migraine, corneal ulcers, parotitis may occasionally be associated.

Etiology. Autosomal dominant inheritance with variable expressivity.

Pathology. Intracellular edema; nonspecific round cell infiltration, of lymphohistiocytic, sarcoidal, or tuberculoid type. Thickening of epithelium; dilated lymph vessels in corium.

Therapy. During the stage of acute facial paralysis, moisture chamber eye shields, artificial tears, and analgesics. Facial massage, electrical stimulation, and warm compresses may be helpful. Possible benefit from corticosteroid therapy. If the bouts of facial palsy are frequent, consider surgical decompression of the facial nerve. If the lip swelling becomes unsightly, a cheiloplastic reduction is indicated. Cheiloplasty plus continuously repeated injection of triamcinolone into the lips. Dapsone reported beneficial.

Prognosis. Recurrent episodes with complete remission initially; then tendency to become chronic.

BIBLIOGRAPHY. Rossolimo GJ: Recidivirende Facialislähmung bei Migräne. Neurol Zenbl 20:744–749, 1901

Melkersson E: Ett fall av recidiverande facialispares i samband med angioneurotiskt ödem. Hygiea 90:737–741, 1928

Rosenthal C: Klinisch-erbbiologischer Beitrag zur Konstitutions-Pathologie: Gemeinsames Auftreten von (rezidivierender familiairer) Facialislähmung, angioneurotischem Gesichtsödem und Lingua plicata in Arthritismus-Familien. Z Neurol Psychol 131:475–501, 1931

Wadlington WB, Riley HD, Lowbeer L: The Melkersson-Rosenthal syndrome. Pediatrics 73:502–506, 1984

MELZER'S

Synonym. Cryoglobulinemia, familial mixed.

Symptoms and Signs. Both sexes. In adolescence, evidence of progressive deterioration of renal function: hematuria, edema, anasarca, blood hypertension.

Etiology. Unknown. Autosomal dominant inheritance.

Diagnostic Procedures. *Blood.* Mixed IgG and IgM cryoglobulins and blood urea nitrogen and creatinine increase. Other signs of kidney functions altered.

BIBLIOGRAPHY. Meltzer M, Franklin EC: Cryoglobulinemia: a clinical and laboratory study. Ann J Med 40:837–856, 1966

Nightingale SD, Pelley RP: A shared cryoglobulin antigen in familial cryoglobulinemia. Ann J Hum Genet 33:722–734, 1981

MELNICK-NEEDLES

Synonym. Osteodysplasty.

Symptoms and Signs. Both sexes affected male-to-female 1:7 present from birth. Facial abnormalities; micrognathia; malocclusion. Recurrent respiratory and ear infections. Generalized bone dysplasia (see Diagnostic Procedures).

Etiology. Autosomal dominant inheritance; strong possibility for X-linked inheritance, reported, however.

Diagnostic Procedures. *X-rays.* Of head. Delayed closure of anterior fontanelle; sclerosis of skull base and mastoids; underdevelopment of paranasal sinuses. Of spinal column. Vertebral bodies tall (more so axis, atlas, and occipital condyles); thoracic vertebrae show anterior concavity and beaking. Of sternum. Delayed ossification. Of ribs. Ribbonlike. Of pelvis. Flaring of the crest of iliac bones and constriction in superacetabular area; tapering of ischial bones. Of long bones. Bowing of tibia and radius; flaring of ends of humerus, fibia, and tibia; coxa valga.

BIBLIOGRAPHY. Melnick JC, Needles CF: An undiagnosed bone dysplasia: a 2 family study of 4 generations and 3 generations. Am J Roentgenol 97:39–48, 1966

Wettke-Schaeffer R, Kantner G: X-linked dominant inherited diseases with lethality in homozygous males. Hum Genet 64:1–23, 1983

MENDELSON'S

Synonyms. Acid-pulmonary-aspiration; aspiration pneumonitis; chemical pneumonitis; acid aspiration pneumonitis.

Symptoms and Signs. The syndrome has been described in association with obstetric anesthesia. Can occur also in states of altered consciousness, neuromuscular disease, gastrointestinal disease, and with the use of medical devices such as nasogastric tubes or uncuffed tracheostomy tubes. Aspiration may be liquid or solid. Two distinct clinical pictures are present depending upon the nature of the aspiration. *If liquid.* Cyanosis; tachycardia; tachypnea; hypotension; acute asthmalike syndrome in form of wheeze, rales, and bilateral rhonchi. *If solid.* Laryngeal or bronchial obstruction with atelectasis; mediastinal shift; signs of consolidation; decreased breath sounds; cyanosis; tachycardia.

Etiology. Aspiration of acid gastric content during general anesthesia. It has been demonstrated experimentally that the acidity of the gastric contents is responsible for the whole clinical and pathologic picture. The critical pH is 2.5 or below. Experimentally, in cats and rabbits, injection into trachea of distilled water, normal saline, 11.3% sodium bicarbonate solution; did not give rise to the above pathologic changes, while the injection of an acid solution reproduced the typical syndrome.

Pathology. At autopsy the pathologic findings are limited to the lung. The heart may show cardiac enlargement if cardiac failure supervenes. Trachea and bronchi are infarcted with areas of necrosis. Pleural cavities contain serum and hemorrhagic fluid. Peribronchiolar hemorrhage and exudate; bronchiolar epithelium is necrotic and sloughed into lumen. Alveolar walls are hyaline, and edema around the blood vessels is noticed.

Diagnostic Procedures. *Blood.* Signs of hypoxia and sometimes acidosis. *X-ray.* Homogeneous density with mediastinal shift. In liquid aspiration, usually irregular soft, mottled densities in both lungs.

Therapy. Prompt establishment of an adequate airway; suction of the airway; single lavage with 10 ml of saline; avoid lavage with larger volumes and intratracheal instillation of sodium bicarbonate and steroid. Fluid replacement with crystalloid or colloid solutions; oxygen and positive-pressure ventilation with PEEP; aminophylline; avoid diuretics (the pulmonary edema in this syndrome is not cardiogenic and is usually associated with intravascular volume depletion); avoid systemic corticosteroids. Intensive care.

Prognosis. High mortality (28–62%).

BIBLIOGRAPHY. Mendelson CL: Aspiration of stomach contents into the lungs during obstetric anesthesia. Am J Obstet Gynecol 52:191–205, 1946
Berkman YM: Aspiration and inhalation pneumonias. Semin Roentgenol 15:73–84, 1980
Mimmo WS: Aspiration of gastric contents. Br J Hosp Med 34:76–179, 1985
James FM: Anesthetic complications in obstetric anesthesia. American Society of Anesthesiologists. 37th annual refresher course lectures and clinical update program, Las Vegas, Nevada, 1986

MENDES DA COSTA'S

Synonyms. Da Costa's (M.); erythrokeratodermia variabilis, EKV; keratitis rubra figurata.

Symptoms and Signs. Both sexes affected; onset usually at early infancy up to 3 years; occasionally, much later. Trunk and buttocks most common sites; may occur, however, in any other site: (1) plaques of erythema and hyperkeratosis, polycyclic, occasionally darker edges (2) plaques of erythema that vary in intensity and location.

Etiology. Unknown; autosomal dominant inheritance.

Pathology. Edema; cellular infiltration; hyperkeratosis; acanthosis of variable degree.

Diagnostic Procedures. *Biopsy of skin.*

Therapy. Vitamin A (of temporary benefit); oral retinoic acid; etretinate: good results.

Prognosis. Condition persisting for life; general health not affected.

BIBLIOGRAPHY. Mendes da Costa S: Erythrodermia and keratodermia variabilis in mother and daughter. Acta Dermvenereol 6:255–261, 1925
Brown J, Kierland RR: Erythrokeratodermia variabilis. Arch Dermatol 93:194–201, 1966
Van der Schroeff JG, Nijenhuis LE, et al.: Genetic linkage between erythrokeratodermic variabilis and Rh locus. Hum Genet 68:165–168, 1984

MENETRIER'S

Synonyms. Giant hypertrophic gastritis; protein-losing gastroenteropathy.

Symptoms. Onset at all ages; prevalent in males. Epigastric distress; ulcerlike pain relieved by alkali. Anorexia; nausea and vomiting; weight loss. Food may relieve or enhance symptoms. Occasionally, diarrhea, melena, hematemesis, and steatorrhea.

Signs. Usually none; occasionally, epigastric tenderness, edema, ascites.

Etiology. Unknown.

Pathology. Stomach with large swollen folds, separated by deep sulci; mucosal erosions; hemorrhagic effusions; covered by abundant mucus; hyperplasia of epithelium; mucous cysts. Eosinophils abundant; edema of muscularis; lack of inflammatory or neoplastic changes.

Diagnostic Procedures. *Blood.* Hypoproteinemia. *X-ray of stomach. Gastroscopy. Biopsy of stomach.*

Therapy. High-protein diet if hypoproteinemia; alkai for relief of pain. Partial or total gastrectomy as last resort. Postoperative course difficult, especially if hypoproteinemia not previously corrected.

Prognosis. Severe; occasionally, uncontrollable ulcer. Malignant transformation possible. Reported duration from 2 months to 22 years.

BIBLIOGRAPHY. Menétrier P: Des polyadénomes gastriques et des leurs rapports avec le cancer de l'estomac. Arch Physiol. Norm Pathol 1:32–55, 1888
Jeffries GH, Holman HR, Sleisenger MH: Plasma proteins of the gastrointestinal tract. New Engl J Med 266:652–660, 1962

Searcy RM, Malagelada JR: Menétrier's disease and idiopathic hypertrophic gastropathy. Ann Intern Med
100:565–570, 1984

MENIERE'S

Synonyms. Labyrinthine; recurrent aural vertigo; labyrinthine hydrops; cochlear Ménière (Episodic deafness
without vertigo).

Symptoms. Onset usually between 3rd and 5th decade.
Initial stage. Unilateral (90%) hearing loss, fluctuating
inner ear type, affecting first only low tones, then both
low and high. Tinnitus, first low-pitched, then high-
pitched tone. Sudden appearance of vertigo: violent;
totally incapacitating, lying still in bed to minimize
symptoms is all patient can do. Nausea and vomiting
frequently accompany vertigo. Repeated attacks.

Signs. Nystagmus (may be present); psychological maladjustment.

Etiology. Not clear; labyrinthine hydrops best explanation.

Pathology. Dilatation of endolymph spaces of cochlea
and saccule; degenerative changes of vestibular sense organs.

Diagnostic Procedures. *Audiometry.* Hearing severely
reduced in affected ear; caloric response not much affected. *X-ray of skull.*

Therapy. Low-salt diet; nicotinic acid; dimenhydrinate;
fair results with betahistine hydrochloride. If medical
management fails, surgical destruction of labyrinth.

Prognosis. Recurrent progressive condition. Complete
hearing loss is frequently followed by cessation of vertigo
spells.

BIBLIOGRAPHY. Ménière P: Maladie de l'oreille interne of-
frant les symptômes de congestion cérébrale apoplectiforme. Gaz Med Paris 3 s 16:88, 1861
Ménière P: Mémoire sur des lésions de l'oreille interne
donnant lieu è des symptômes de congestion cérébrale apoplectiforme. Gaz Med J Paris 16:597–601,
1861
Wladislavosky-Waserman P, Facer GW, Mokri B,
Kurland LT: Ménière's disease: a 30-year epidemiological and clinical study in Rochester, Minnesota, 1951–
1980. Laryngoscope 94:1098–1102, 1984
Paparella MM: Pathogenesis of Ménière's disease and
Ménière's syndrome. Acta Otolaryngol (Stockh),
(Suppl 106):10–25, 1984
Eggermont JJ, Schmidt PH: Ménière's disease: a long-
term follow-up study of hearing loss. Ann Otol Rhinol
Laryngol 94:1–9, 1985

MENINGOCOCCEMIA

Symptoms and Signs. Occur in relatively healthy appearing individual. Fever; malaise; joint pain. A few days
after onset of fever; rash, ill-defined erythematous macules in dependent parts of the body (frequently sparing
palms and soles) developing in irregular hemorrhagic areas. Most characteristic element: pink lesions with central petechial element. Splenic enlargement.

Etiology. Chronic meningococcemia; allergic basis for
the skin rash suggested; individual with partial immunity
to meningococcus.

Pathology. Biopsy of the skin lesion at 36 to 48 hours
after appearance shows perivascular infiltrate of lymphocytes and macrophages, few granulocytes, no fibrin or
thrombus occlusion, vascular wall intact, no endothelial
swelling, edema in upper dermis, normal epithelium. Absence of bacteria (pattern strikingly differing from that of
acute meningococcemia).

Diagnostic Procedures. *Blood culture.* Meningococcus.
Inability to agglutinate meningococci isolated from blood.
White blood cells increased. *Spinal fluid.* Normal.

Therapy. Penicillin; streptomycin; sulfonamides.

Prognosis. Afebrile within 24 to 48 hours of onset of
treatment; skin lesion and splenomegaly disappear in a
few days.

BIBLIOGRAPHY. Salomon H: Ueber Meningokokkensepti-
kämie. Klin Wochenschr 39:1045–1048, 1902
Ognibene AJ, Dito WR: Chronic meningococcemia.
Arch Intern Med 114:29–32, 1964
Foltzer MA, Reese RE: Bacteremias and Sepsis. In Reese
RE, Gordon DR Jr (eds): A Practical approach to infec-
tious diseases, p 47. Boston, Little, Brown, 1986

MENKES' II

Synonyms. Kinky hair; steely hair; trichopolydys-
trophy; X-linked copper deficiency; pili torti; copper
transport; MK; MNK.

Symptoms. Only males affected; present from early infancy. Spasticity; refractory motor seizures; dementia; retarded growth; decreased visual function.

Signs. Small at birth; lack of facial expression; skin thick
and dry. Transient jaundice. Hair normal at birth; at 6
weeks begins to lose pigmentation and assumes the typical aspect: twisting and breaking.

Etiology. X-linked recessive inheritance. Malabsorption
of copper and sequestration of the metal in tissues where
it cannot be accessible for copper enzyme synthesis. Defi-

ciency of lysyl oxidase activity which creates disulfide bond in hair (pili torti).

Pathology. *Brain.* Small, diffuse degenerative changes of both gray and white matter in cerebrum and cerebellum. *Hair.* Monilethrix. *Bones.* Wormian bones of the skull; ribs and femur, metaphyseal widening with spur formation. Arterial elongation and tortuosity with fragmentation and reduplication of the internal elastic lamina.

Diagnostic Procedures. *X-ray.* Arteriopathic and skeletal changes. *Blood.* Decreased copper and ceruloplasmin levels.

Therapy. Parenteral administration of copper salts.

Prognosis. Death in infancy. Treatment reverses clinical features. One case survived (decerebrated) for 12 years.

BIBLIOGRAPHY. Menkes JH, Alter M, Steigeeder GK, et al: A sex-linked recessive disorder with retardation of growth, peculiar hair, and focal cerebral and cerebellar degeneration. Paediatrics 29:764–769, 1962

Bray PF: Sex-linked neurodegenerative disease associated with monilethrix. Paediatrics 36:417–420, 1965

McKusick VA: Heritable Disorders of Connective Tissue, 4th ed. St Louis, CV Mosby, 1972

Danks DM: Hereditary disorders of copper metabolism in Wilson's disease and Menkes' disease. In Stanbury JB, Wyngaarden JB, Fredrickson DS, et al: The Metabolic Basis of Inherited Disease, 5th ed, p 1251. New York, McGraw-Hill, 1983

Leone A, Pavlakis GN, Hamer DH: Menkes' disease: abnormal metallothionein gene regulation in response to copper. Cell 40:301–309, 1985

Gupta A, Arora NK, Desai N, et al: Menkes disease. Indian J Pediatr 55:445–447, 1988

MENOPAUSAL

Synonym. Female climacteric.

Symptoms. Experienced by some women during climacteric. Hot facial flashes; chills; sweats, tachycardia; palpitations; nervousness; irritability; depression; headaches; lost or increased libido; abnormal uterine bleeding; pruritus valvae; atrophic vaginitis; breast pain; hypertrophy of breasts; bursitis and bone pains; hypertension.

Etiology. Waning ovarian function and deficiency of estrogen secretion.

Pathology. Changes associated with decreased estrogen secretion: climacteric changes of ovary, genital tract, uterus, cervix, vagina, external genitalia, breasts.

Diagnostic Procedures. *Blood.* Increased follicle-stimu-

lating hormone (FSH), increased cholesterol. *X-ray.* Osteoporosis; arthritic changes.

Therapy. Sedation, barbiturate and benzodiazepines. If depression, amphetamine or bromazepam. Hormonal therapy: cyclic estrogen administration (3 weeks therapy and 1 week rest) for several months.

Prognosis. Condition tends to disappear spontaneously, lasting months, sometimes years. With treatment, symptoms may be well controlled.

BIBLIOGRAPHY. Greenblatt RB, Emperaire JC: Changing concepts in the management of the menopause. Med Times 98:153, 1970

Odell WD: The menopause. In De Groot LJ, Cahill FG Jr, Odell WD, et al (eds): Endocrinology, p 1489. New York, Grune & Stratton, 1979

Margolis AJ, Greenwood S: Gynecology and obstetrics. In Krupp MA, Schroeder SA, Tierney LM (eds): Current medical diagnosis and treatment, pp 471–472. Norwalk, Conn, 1987

MENOPAUSAL MUSCULAR DYSTROPHY

Synonyms. "Late life" muscular dystrophy; necrotizing myopathy. See Polymyositis, Group I.

MENSTRUAL PERIOD, UNEXPLAINED DELAY

Synonym. Psychosexual menstrual period.

Symptoms. Usually associated with beginning of sexual life or a change in its pattern. Menstrual delay of 10 to 60 days followed by abnormal uterine bleeding.

Signs. Normal anatomic and functional capacities.

Etiology. Psychogenic origin: beginning of sexual relations; change in its patterns; fear of or desire for pregnancy. To be differentiated from (1) incomplete abortion, (2) incipient abortion, (3) extrauterine pregnancy.

Pathology. Endometrial curettage: proliferative endometrium or early secretory endometrium or both. Puncture of Douglas pouch: 5 to 20 ml of serohematic fluid.

Diagnostic Procedures. *Pregnancy tests.* Negative (see Pathology).

Therapy. Psychotherapy.

Prognosis. Good; condition will spontaneously correct itself.

BIBLIOGRAPHY. Soferman N, Haimov M: The syndrome

of unexplained delayed menstrual period. Am J Obstet Gynecol 91:137–141, 1965

Yen SSC: Chronic anovulation. In Yen SSC, Jaffe RB (eds): Reproductive endocrinology. Philadelphia, WB Saunders, 1986

MENZEL'S

Synonyms. Marie's I; Nonne-Marie; Sanger-Brown; hereditary spastic ataxia. See Déjerine-Thomas, Friedreich's, and Olivopontocerebellar atrophy (OPCAI).

Symptoms and Signs. Both sexes affected; onset after 20 years of age. Cerebellar ataxia with moderate or severe coordinative disturbances. Deep reflexes normal or exaggerated. Hyperreflexia (as contrasted with hyporeflexia observed in Friedreich's ataxia) is one of the main differentiating features. Spasticity.

Etiology. Possibly, heterogeneous group; autosomal dominant recessive forms (?). This syndrome is subject of intense discussion and disagreement. Considered similar or identical to Déjerine's and Friedreich's ataxia.

Pathology. Lack of agreement on typical features, so that no specific anatomic findings may be assigned. Importance of pontoolivocerebellar atrophy emphasized by certain authors. Less involvement of Purkinje cells of cerebellar cortex. Involvement of spinal cord relatively frequent.

Diagnostic Procedures. *Pneumoencephalography. Brain scan. Electromyography. Biopsy of muscle. Spinal tap.*

Therapy. Symptomatic.

Prognosis. A milder course than Friedreich's ataxia.

BIBLIOGRAPHY. Menzel P: Beitrage zur Kenntnis der hereditaren Ataxie und Kleinhirnatrophie. Arch Psychiatr Nervenkr 22:160–190, 1891

Brown S: On hereditary ataxia, with a series of twenty-one cases. Brain 15:250–282, 1892

Marie P: Sur l'hérédo-atasie cerebelleuse. Semin Med 13:444–447, 1893

Pedersen L, Platz P, Ryder LP, et al: A linkage study of hereditary ataxias and related disorders: evidence of heterogeneity of dominant cerebellar ataxia. Hum Genet 54:371–383, 1980

MERETOJA'S

Synonym. Amyloidosis V, Finland type. See also Biber-Haab-Dimmer.

Symptoms and Signs. Both sexes equally affected; onset in 3rd decade. First symptom: lattice corneal dystrophy (see Biber-Haab-Dimmer). Visual acuity preserved up to late age. Repeated temporary corneal erosion; occasionally, secondary iritis or iridocyclitis. Simple glaucoma (25% of cases); frequently corneal anesthesia. In older age, upper facial paresis (smoothing of forehead skin); sporadic abnormalities of other cranial nerves (decreased auditory activity). Late: mild peripheral nerve involvement (rarely). In 5th decade, skin changes, blepharochalasis, lichenification of skin of extremities. From 7th decade, skin atrophic and pendulous. Arthropathy and gastrointestinal symptoms are inconstant features.

Etiology. Unknown; autosomal dominant inheritance.

Pathology. *Eyes.* Small, round, yellow masses in the epithelium or under Bowman's membrane; leukomatous lesions. Lattice lines possibly represent degenerated corneal nerves with amyloid deposits. *Skin.* Amyloid deposits, especially around eccrine glands, diffuse into the dermis. *Kidney.* Amyloid interstitial accumulation; concentrated in the glomeruli. *Arteries.* Amyloid deposits in the media and intima. *Heart.* Variable myocardial deposits. *Central nervous system.* Deposits restricted to the leptomeninges.

Diagnostic Procedures. *Ophthalmoscopy.* Lattice trunks running from limbus to corneal centrum. Nodular opacities. *Urine.* Proteinuria. *Electrocardiography. X-rays.* Evidence of cardiac involvement (after 40 years of age). *Biopsy of skin, kidney.*

Therapy. Symptomatic.

Prognosis. Relatively benign condition.

BIBLIOGRAPHY. Meretoja J: Familial systemic paramyloidosis with lattice dystrophy of the cornea, progressive cranial neuropathy, skin changes, and various internal symptoms: a previously unrecognized heritable syndrome. Ann Clin Res 1:314–324, 1969

Sack GH Jr, Dumars KW, Gummerso KS, et al: Three forms of dominant amyloid neuropathy. Johns Hopkins Med J 149:239–247, 1981

MERMAID

Synonyms. Caudal dysplasia; caudal regression; sirenomelia. See Townes-Brocks.

Symptoms and Signs. Variable anomalies:
1. Lower limbs. Symmelia; flexion and turning of independent leg into external rotation; atrophy; clubfoot; defective motion of joints
2. Rectum. Imperforate anus
3. Kidney and urinary tract. Bilateral or unilateral agenesis
4. Genital organ. Agenesis with exception of gonads

5. Lumbosacral spine. Agenesis or increase in number of vertebrae epistasis
6. Other visceral or somatic anomalies may also be associated. Some anomalies incompatible with life.

Etiology. Genetic (autosomal and X-linked inheritance) and nongenetic teratogenic mechanisms. Of great interest is the presence of the syndrome in infants born from diabetic mothers.

BIBLIOGRAPHY. Feller A, Sternberg H: Zur Kenntnis der Fehlbildungen der Wirbelsäule. III. Mitteilung. Ueber den vollständigen Mangel der unteren Wirbelsäulenabschinitte und seine Bedeutung für die formale Genese der Defektbildungen des hinteren Körperendes. Virchows Arch Pathol Anat 280:649–692, 1931

Duhamel B: From the mermaid to anal imperforation: the syndrome of caudal regression. Arch Dis Child 36:152–155, 1961

Passarge E, Lenz W: Syndrome of caudal regression in infants of diabetic mothers; observations of further cases. Pediatrics 37:672–675, 1966

Gellis SS: Denouncement and discussion: caudal dysplasis syndrome. Am J Dis Child 116:407–408, 1968

Aylsworth AS: The Townes-Brocks syndrome: a member of the anus-hand-ear family of syndromes (abstr). Am J Hum Genet 37:A43, 1985

MERWARTH'S

Synonym. Rolandic vein occlusion.

Symptoms. Progressively developing hemiplegia, starting and affecting particularly the foot and leg. Sensory and motor disturbances. Arm weakened; hand usually not affected.

Signs. Leg tendon hyperreflexia; mucle tone varies from spasticity (usually) to hypotonia.

Etiology. Idiopathic thrombosis of cortical veins.

Pathology. Cerebral venous thrombosis. Areas of hemorrhage and softening of variable degrees.

Diagnostic Procedures. *Clotting studies. Spinal tap. Venography. Electroencephalography.*

Therapy. Anticoagulants.

Prognosis. Complete recovery seems to be the rule. Function returns progressively in the arm first, then eventually to leg, and last in the foot.

BIBLIOGRAPHY. Merwarth HR: Hemiplegia of cortical or venous origin (occlusion of rolandic veins). Brooklyn Hosp J 2:193–212, 1940

Vick NA: Grinker's Neurology, 7th ed. Springfield, Ill, CC Thomas, 1976

MESENTERIC ARTERY, SUPERIOR

Synonym. SMA; including cast chronic forms (Wilkie's syndrome). See Dorph's.

Symptoms. Usually begin in early childhood. The syndrome may also appear in patients with chronic illness or after surgery when remaining for prolonged period in supine position. Postprandial fullnss; abdominal cramps and pains; nausea; vomiting; failure to gain weight.

Signs. Height to weight ratio with tendency toward slender habitus seems to be of significance. Prone or knee chest position may relieve pain.

Etiology and Pathology. Many structural abnormalities that reduce the angle formed by the aorta and vertebrae posteriorly, and the root of superior mesenteric artery and vein anteriorly. Reduction of this angle compresses the duodenum. Kyphoscoliosis; lordosis; weight loss with decrease of fat; lymphadenopathy; tumors in the retroperitoneum; rotation of intestine with abnormal fibrous bands; wearing constrictive girdles or body cast.

Diagnostic Procedures. *Fluoroscopy.* Permanence of barium in obstructed areas.

Therapy. Medical: small feedings with bland, low-residue, high-calorie food. Removal of extrinsic obstruction (e.g., girdle; cast). If failure, surgery: division of ligament of Treitz and freeing the duodenum, or, if needed, bypass of obstruction by gastrojejunostomy or duodenojejunostomy.

Prognosis. In many cases, good response to conservative treatment, and child may grow out of the situation (gain weight). In incapacitating cases (vomiting; dehydration; failure to grow), surgery indicated and good results obtained.

BIBLIOGRAPHY. Von Rokitansky C: Lehrbuch der pathologischen Anatomie, p 187. Vienna, Braumüller, 1861

Wilkie DPD: Chronic duodenal ileus. Br J Surg 9:204, 1921

Hyde JS, Swarts CL, Nicholas EE, et al: Superior mesenteric artery syndrome. Am J Dis Child 106:25–34, 1963

Edmond AS: Scoliosis. In Crenshaw AH (ed): Campbell's Operative Orthopedics, pp 3212–3215, 7th ed, St Louis, CV Mosby, 1987

METACHROMATIC LEUKODYSTROPHY

Synonyms. MLD; Greenfield's; Scholz's; Scholz-Bielschowsky-Henneberg; sulfatide lipoidosis; Van Bogaert-

Nyssen-Peiffer; cerebroside sulfatase deficiency, arylsulfatase A.

LATE INFANTILE FORM

Symptoms. Both sexes affected; onset before 30 months of age. Early development normal (locomotion and speech at normal age); then progressive weakness and hypotonia of legs; ataxia or spastic paralysis; seizures (in 50% of cases); optic atrophy (30%); dementia.

Signs. *Early stages.* Muscle tone decreased; reflexes absent, decreased, or increased. *Later stages.* Muscle tone increased; Babinski's sign; reflexes absent or increased. *Final stage.* Decerebrated posture; unreactive to visual and auditory stimuli.

Etiology. Autosomal recessive inheritance. Deficiency of arylsulfatase A (cerebroside sulfatase). Sulfatides accumulate in nervous tissue and in other organs.

Pathology. In brain; white matter symmetric diffuse involvement, increased consistency, grayish or brown discoloration, sometimes cavitation. Loss of normal myeline sheaths; accumulation of lipoid granular masses that are typically stained (metachromatic). Certain group of neurons and peripheral nerves also involved. Kidney, gallbladder (mucosa contains macrophages with some granules), liver, pancreas, pituitary, adrenal cortex, and testes are also involved.

Diagnostic Procedures. *Urine.* Direct examination of urine sediment with the addition of toluidine blue reveals metachromatic bodies; application of lipid extracted from urine to filter paper and staining with toluidine blue; arylsulfatase test, absence of the enzyme. *Biopsy.* Of sural nerve.

Therapy. Trials with low vitamin A diet and thiosulfate are under study.

Prognosis. Death occurs 5 months to 10 years after onset.

CONGENITAL FORM

Symptoms and Signs. Apnea, cyanosis, tonic-clonic movements. Death after few weeks.

Pathology. See late infantile form.

ADOLESCENT FORM

Symptoms. Onset (between 4 and 14 years) of age. First symptoms: failure in schoolwork; emotional disturbances; visual trouble.

Prognosis. Progression slower than above.

ADULT FORM

MLD WITHOUT ARYLSULFATASE A
DEFICIENCY

Synonyms. Cerebroside sulfatase activator deficiency, sphingolipid activator protein 1, SPA 1.

Symptoms and Signs. Clinical course of juvenile form but without arysulfatase A deficiency. What is probably lacking is an activator protein for arylsulfatase activity.

ARYLSULFATASE A DEFICIENCY
WITHOUT MLD

Synonyms. Pseudoarylsulfatase A deficiency. This defect without clinical manifestations is sometimes present in relatives of people with MLD or in patients with neurological disabilities different from MLD.

Etiology. It has been suggested that autosomal dominant inheritance, sex-linked factors, and mutation are genetic possibilities to be considered in different families.

Pathology. While in the infantile form, metachromatic material may be demonstrated only in frozen section; in adult form, it may also be demonstrated in paraffin-or celloidin-treated material.

Prognosis. Long course.

BIBLIOGRAPHY. Scholz W: Klinische, patologischanatomische und erbbiologische Untersuchungen bei familiarer, diffuser Hirnsklerose im Kindersalter. Z Neurol Psychiat 99:651–717, 1925

Kolodny EH, Moser HW: Sulfatide lipidosis: metachromatic leukodystrophy. In Stanbury JB, Wyngaarden JB, Fredrickson DS, et al: The Metabolic Basis of Inherited Disease. 5th ed, p 881. New York, McGraw-Hill, 1983

Dewji N, Wenger D, Fujibayashi S, et al: Molecular cloning of sphingolipid activator protein 1 (SAP1): the sulfatide sulfatase activator. Am J Hum Genet 37:A 150, 1985

METHYLMALONIC ACIDEMIA

Synonym. Ketosic hyperglycinemia (see).

Symptoms and Signs. Includes at least five biochemical derangments (see Etiology) with similar but not identical clinical features. The four etiologic groups (1, 2, 3, and 4) show a common clinical pattern: Both sexes affected; onset within first months (50%) or within first year of life (50%). Failure to thrive; vomiting; lethargy; developmental retardation; recurrent infections (50%). A fifth group (5) shows instead variable manifestation from asymptomatic to critical illness from birth. Manifestations include seizures; failure to thrive, psychosis, and abnormal cerebellar and spinal cord function.

Etiology.
1. Methylmalonyl coenzyme A (CoA) racemase deficiency
2. Methylmalonyl CoA mutase apoenzyme deficiency
3. AdoCbl synthesis defect I

4. AdoCbl synthesis defect II
5. Combined synthesis defect of AdoCbl and MeCbl.

Pathology. *Groups 1, 2, 3, 4.* Osteoporosis; absence of megaloblastic changes. Features secondary to overwhelming infection. *Group 5.* Brain and spinal cord abnormalities similar to that of Lichtheim's (see).

Diagnostic Procedures. *Blood (1, 2, 3, 4).* Neutropenia and thrombocytopenia (in 50% of cases) absence of megaloblastic changes; hyperglycinemia; severe ketoacidosis (pH 6.9 to 7.1). *Urine.* (1) Hyperglycinemia. *Bone marrow.* Absence of megaloblastic change. *Blood.* (5) Absence of ketoacidosis; occasionally, megaloblastic anemia.

Therapy. *Groups 1, 2, 3, 4.* Fifty percent of cases respond to cobalamine administration.

Prognosis. Extremely severe. Death between 40 days and 3 years (40%); survival 2 to 8 years 60%.

BIBLIOGRAPHY. Oberholzer VG, Levin B, Burgess EA, et al: Methylmalonic aciduria: an inborn error of metabolism leading to chronic metabolic acidosis. Arch Dis Child 42:492–504, 1967
Rosenberg LE: Disorders of propionate and methylmalonate metabolism. In Stanbury JB, Wyngaarden JB, Fredrickson DS, et al: The Metabolic Basis of Inherited Disease, 5th ed, p. 474. New York, McGraw-Hill, 1983

MEYER-BETZ'S

Synonyms. Guenther's II; myoglobinuria type II; paroxysmal idiopathic myoglobinuria.

Symptoms and Signs. Predominant in males (4:1). Clinically divided into two types. (1) Onset at puberty to early adulthood, few hours after exertion. (2) Onset in childhood, associated with an infection. Sudden severe pain and cramping in the muscle; usually followed by temporary weakness or paralysis. Chills; vomiting; pallor; abdominal pain; fever and shock may also occur at time of attack.

Signs. After a few hours, urine becomes first pink, then deep red brown. Oliguria and anuria in some cases. Urine coloration persists for 72 hours. Affected muscles, swollen "woody" consistency, tender. After repeated attacks, muscles may become atrophic.

Etiology. Unknown; usually sporadic appearances; some familial cases reported.

Pathology. Muscle biopsy obtained after attack shows coagulative muscle necrosis and necrotic discolored fibers dispersed among normal fibers. In kidney, myoglobin casts.

Diagnostic Procedures. *Urine.* After attack, color red to chocolate brown; presence of myoglobin. *Blood.* Serum, normal color; leukocytosis; *Biopsy of muscle.*

Therapy. Force fluid to prevent anuria.

Prognosis. Attack usually recurs with major and minor episodes, with differing frequency, sometimes at intervals of years. Muscular atrophy may result from repeated attacks.

BIBLIOGRAPHY. Meyer-Betz F: Beobachtungen an einem eigenartigen mit Muskellahmungen verbundenen Fall von Hämoglobinurie. Dtsch Arch Klin Med 101:85–127, 1911
Guenther H: Myositis myoglobinuria. 70:517, 1913
Rainey RL, Estes PW, Neely CL, et al: Myoglobinuria following diabetic acidosis. Arch Intern Med 111:564–571, 1963
Knochel JP: Rhabdomyolysis and myoglobinuria. Ann Rev Med 33:435–443, 1982
Adams RD, Victor M: Principles of Neurology, 3rd ed, p 1040. New York, McGraw-Hill, 1985

MIBELLI'S

Synonyms. Hyperkeratosis eccentrica; keratoderma eccentrica; Mantoux's; porokeratosis, including Guss's (porokeratosis palmo-plantaris et disseminate) and actinic porokeratosis.

Symptoms and Signs. Both sexes affected; male-to-female ratio 3:1; onset usually in young adulthood. On palms, soles, and fingers, eruption in crops of miliary translucent papules, slowly enlarging and forming a dark center. Shedding after weeks, leaving small pits that eventually fade away.

Etiology. Autosomal dominant type of inheritance with lower penetrability in females. (Guss claims a separated entity for prevalent localization on palm and soles and with possible autosomal or X-linked dominant inheritance. A photosensitive variety has also been recognized, affecting areas exposed to the sun, with particular histologic pattern: Chernosky-Freeman.)

Pathology. Cavernous capillary dilatations.

Therapy. None.

Prognosis. Recurrences for years; occasionally, short duration. Seven percent of patients develop skin cancer.

BIBLIOGRAPHY. Mibelli V: Di una nuova forma di cheratosi "angiocheratoma." Giorn Ital Mal Vener 30:285–301, 1889
Mantoux C: Porokératose pokillomateuse palmaire et plantaire. Ann Dermatol Syph 4:15–31, 1903
Chernosky ME, Anderson DE: Disseminated superficial actinic porokeratosis: clinical studies and experimental production of lesions. Arch Derm 99:401–407, 1969
Guss SB, Osbourn RA, Lutzner MA: Porokeratosis plantaris, palmaris et disseminate. A third type of porokeratosis. Arch Derm 104:366–373, 1971

Machino H, Miki Y, Teramoto T, et al: Cytogenetic studies in a patient with porokeratosis of Mibelli, multiple cancers and a *forme fruste* of Werner's syndrome. Br J Derm 111:579–586, 1984

MICROMYOMAS UTERI

Synonym. Uterine adenomyoma uterus.

Symptoms. Menorrhagia, unresponsive to hormone therapy, curettage, or oxytocics, with normal timing of menstrual periods.

Signs. Rectovaginal examination: uterus slightly enlarged and firm without irregular nodules on the surface.

Etiology. Unknown; micromyomas interfere with contractile power of myometrium so that bleeding results.

Pathology. Myometrium of uterus with muscular hypertrophy resembling diffuse miliary fibroid process; increased tortuosity of vessels with hyalinized walls.

Diagnostic Procedures. *Curettage. Biopsy. Blood clotting studies. Doppler.*

Therapy. Total hysterectomy.

Prognosis. Benign condition.

BIBLIOGRAPHY. Hiller RI: Micromyomas of the uterus with severe menorrhagia: a syndrome. Am J Obstet Gynecol 87:163–165, 1963
Vardi JR, Tovell HMM: Leiomyosarcoma of the uterus. Clinopathological study. Obstet Gynecol 56:428–434, 1980

MICTURITION SYNCOPE

Symptoms. Syncope occurring during or after termination of voiding urine. Usually, attacks occur at night, when arising after some hours of sleep. Pallor; lightheadedness may precede the syncope or occasionally not progress to it. Attacks may be aborted by sitting down promptly.

Signs. Bradycardia; hypotension.

Etiology. Unknown; represents one form of the vasovagal syndrome (see).

Diagnostic Procedures. *Electroencephalography.* To differentiate from epilepsy. *Valsalva maneuver.* Occasionally, may reproduce the syndrome.

BIBLIOGRAPHY. Gastaut H, Gastaut Y: Etude électroencéphalographique des syncopes. III. Formes cliniques des syncopes vasovagales: differentiation d'avec l'épilepsie. Rev Neurol (Paris) 95:547–549, 1956
Godec CJ, Cass AS: Micturition syncope. J Urol 126:551, 1981

Weissler AM, Warren JV: Syncope: pathophysiology and differential diagnosis. In Hurst JW: The Heart, 6th ed. New York, McGraw-Hill, 1986

MIEHLKE-PARTSCH

Synonym. Wiedemann's variant.

Symptoms and Signs. Observed in neonates. Deformities limited to face and ears; abduction palsy.

Etiology. Thalamidone-induced embryopathy. See Wiedemann's.

BIBLIOGRAPHY. Miehlke A, Partsch CH: Ohrmissbildung, Facialis und Abducenslähmung als Syndrom der Thalamidomidschädigung. Arch Ohr Heilk 181:154–164, 1963

MIESCHER-LEDER

Synonyms. Granuloma disciformis; Miescher's III; necrobiosis maculosa.

Symptoms and Signs. Prevalent in women; onset at 50 to 75 years of age; reported also in adolescents. Plaques, reddish, margined, usually polycyclic shape, center atrophic, edges indurated, present on shins, thighs; abdominal and chest walls may be involved.

Etiology. Today is not considered as an autonomous syndrome but part of the necrobiosis (not diabetic forms). See Granuloma annulare and Oppenheim-Urbach.

BIBLIOGRAPHY. Miescher G, Leder M: Granulomatosis disciformis chronica et progressiva (atypiche tubercolosi) Dermatologica 97:25–34, 1948
Miescher G: Nekrobiosis maculosa. Dermatologica 98:199–204, 1949
Rook A, Wilkinson DS, Ebling FJG, et al: Textbook of Dermatology, 4th ed, p 1693. Oxford, Blackwell Scientific Publications, 1986

MIESCHER'S I

Synonyms. Acanthosis nigricans-diabetes mellitus (insulin resistant); insulin receptor defect-acanthosis nigricans.

Symptoms and Signs.
Type A. Young females, signs of virilization; accelerated growth.

Type B. Older females, immunologic disease with circulating antibodies, insulin receptors.

Lesions may be present at birth, but usually develop in childhood, seldom after puberty. Pigmentation, dryness, roughness of skin, which assumes a gray, brown, or black color; increased thickness and formation of small papillomatous elevations from velvety to rugose and mammillary. Most frequently involved, unilateral or bilateral axilla, back and sides of neck, groins; less frequently, other flexures, submammary, and umbilical areas. Palms and soles may be thickened. Mucoses rarely show a velvety pattern. Diabetes. Other anomalies have been described in these patients.

Etiology. Autosomal recessive inheritance. Insulin receptor defect.

Pathology. Hyperkeratosis; papillomatosis; acanthosis and pigmentation of variable degree even within single section. Occasionally, horny inclusion cysts.

Diagnostic Procedures. *Blood.* Glycemia (frequent association with lipodystrophic diabetes); insulin in plasma 100 times normal; marked increase in C-peptide. *Biopsy of skin.*

Therapy. Symptomatic.

Prognosis. Slow progression of lesions, which become more severe at puberty and, afterward, may regress, or remain static.

BIBLIOGRAPHY. Miescher G: Zwei Faelle von congenitaler familiaerer Akanthosis nigricans, kombiniert mit Diabetes mellitus. Dermatol 32:276–305, 1921
Leme CE, Waichenberg BL, Lerario AC, et al: Acanthosis nigrans, hirsutism, insulin resistance and insulin receptor defect. Clin Endocrinol 17:43–49, 1982
Tasjian D, Jarratt M: Familial acanthosis nigricans. Arch Derm 120:1351–1354, 1984

MIESCHER'S II

Synonym. Granulomatous cheilitis. Used to designate the granulomatous cheilitis as a monosymptomatic form of the Melkersson's (see).

BIBLIOGRAPHY. Miescher G: Ueber essentielle granulomatöse Makrocheilie (cheilitis granulomatosa). Dermatologica 91:57–85, 1945
Hornstein O: Problems in granulomatous cheilitis (Miescher from an expert testimony viewpoint). Hautarzt 13:302–309, 1962

MIETENS-WEBER

Synonyms. Corneal opacity-nystagmus-elbow contracture-mental retardation-dwarfism; mental retardation Mietens-Weber.

Symptoms and Signs. *Facies.* Bushy eyebrows; low hairline; ptosis; external ear defects. *Musculoskeletal sys-*

tem. Muscular defects; digital defects (primarily of hands). Hypertrichosis.

Etiology. Unknown. Autosomal recessive (?) inheritance.

Therapy. Keratoplasty.

BIBLIOGRAPHY. Mietens C, Weber H: Syndrome characterized by corneal opacity, nystagmus, flexion contractures of elbows, growth failure and mental retardation. J Pediatr 69:624–629, 1966
Waring GO, Rodiguez MM: Ultrastructural and successful keratoplasty of sclerocornea in Mietens syndrome. Am J Ophthalmol 90:469–475, 1980

MIGRAINE, CLASSIC

Synonyms. Common migraine; sick headache; hemicrania vera; familial migraine; hemiplegic migraine; abdominal migraine. See Möbius' I.

Symptoms. Prevalent in women (variable female-to-male ratio according to different authors); occasionally, onset in childhood (10% of patients with migraine have this form); may begin in puberty and cease in menopause; or onset at 40 years of age and termination at 60 years of age. Peak onset between 2nd and 3rd decades. Attacks of unilateral throbbing pain (hemicrania), periodic and recurrent. Nervous tension (usually in these patients starting when relaxed). Prodromes include contralateral visual manifestations, occasionally motor and sensory phenomena. Attacks last from 4 to 6 hours, partially relieved by darkness and quiet. Anorexia; Abdominal colic of variable intensity lasting minutes or days. Vomiting (may relieve pain), diarrhea. Followed occasionally by polyuria.

Signs. Hyperidrosis; pallor or flushing of skin.

Etiology. Personality factors of significant importance in precipitating and establishing condition. Autosomal dominant (70% penetrance) or recessive.

Diagnostic Procedures. *Electroencephalography.* May show minimal changes. *Ergotamin test.* Prevention of attack in aureal stage.

Therapy. Once attack is begun, no medication completely relieves the pain, Ergotamin in association with caffeine and other compounds taken in prodromal state may abort the attacks. Methysergide for prophylaxis (with care because of risk of retroperitoneal fibrosis, see Ormond's); good results also with propranolol.

Prognosis. Lifelong condition. See symptoms. Attacks may be followed by permanent deficit of visual field.

BIBLIOGRAPHY. Allan W: Inheritance of migraine. Arch Intern Med 42:590–599, 1928

Alvarez WC: Was there sick headache in 3,000 B.C.? Gastroenterology 5:524, 1945

Friedman AP: The migraine syndrome. Bull New York Acad Med 44:45–62, 1968

Adams RD, Victor M: Principles of Neurology, 3rd ed, pp. 133–138. New York, McGraw-Hill, 1985

Elmaleh C, Dubuisson C, Fouret C, Thibaut J: A propos d' un cas de migraine ophtalmique ayant entraîne une hémianopsie latérale homonyme définitive chez une jeune fille de 19 ans. Bull Soc Opht France, 11:1223–1224, 1987

MIGRATORY OSTEOLYSIS

Synonyms. Transient osteoporosis of hip; regional migratory osteoporosis. See Observation hip.

Symptoms. Prevalent in males; onset in youth and middle age. Intensely painful regional swelling in one of the lower extremities, seldom preceded by trauma. Pain aggravated by weight-bearing and motion. Similar segmental episodes may occur in other areas of opposite leg without an initiating cause.

Signs. Swelling of hip, knee, or foot. Overlying skin is dry; superficial veins are dilated.

Etiology. Unknown. Condition similar to Sudeck's (see).

Pathology. Periosteal reaction under edematous areas; increase of synovial fluid; membrane injected and thickened. Microscopically, minimal or absent signs of inflammation.

Diagnostic Procedures. *X-ray.* Normal during first 2 to 3 weeks, then severe localized osteoporosis.

Therapy. Analgesics.

Prognosis. Self-limited condition. Spontaneous resolution in months with return to normal density of the bone. Possibly recurrence in other areas.

BIBLIOGRAPHY. Curtiss PH, Kincaid WE: Transitory demineralization of the hip in pregnancy: a report of three cases. J Bone Joint Surg [Am] 41:1327–1333, 1959

De Marchi E, Santacroce A, Salarino GB: Su di una peculiare artropatia rarefacente dell'anca. Arch Putti 21:62–75, 1966

Hunder GG, Kelly PJ: Roentgenologic transient osteoporosis of the hip: a clinical syndrome? Ann Intern Med 68:538–552, 1968

Pinals RS: Traumatic arthritis and allied conditions. In Hollander JL, McCarty DJ: Arthritis and Allied Conditions, 8th ed, p 1397. Philadelphia, Lea & Febiger, 1978

MILIAN'S I

Synonym. Ninth day erythema.

Symptoms. Onset after the injection of arsphenamine, neoarsphenanine, oxophenarine hydrochloride (Mapharsen) or acetylglycarsenobenzene. Abrupt onset of prodromal symptoms between the 5th and 19th days. Malaise; chills; fever; anorexia; vomiting; headache; sore throat; followed after 1 day (average 9 days) by generalized rash, lasting between 1 and 12 days, and followed by desquamation.

Signs. Rash described as macular erythematous, rarely urticarial; generalized lymphadenopathy; conjunctival suffusion. Occasionally, hepatomegaly, jaundice, and splenomegaly.

Etiology. Unknown; not observed since penicillin has been substituted for arsenical compounds in the treatment of syphilis. Reaction to arsenophenamine compounds not related to presence of syphilis.

Pathology. In addition to the skin manifestation, visceral manifestations have been observed; hepatomegaly; splenomegaly; nephritis. Pathology reports are not available, however.

Therapy. Palliative.

Prognosis. Self-limited condition; spontaneous recovery; never fatal. Recurrence not constant when the drugs are administered again.

BIBLIOGRAPHY. Milian G: Arsénobenzol, érythème et rubéole. Paris Med 23:131–135, 1917

Peters EE: The syndrome of Milian's erythema of the ninth day: Report of 54 cases. Am J Syph 25:527–556, 1941

De Francisci G, Magalini S: Reazioni Immunologiche a farmaci. Il Pensiero Scientifico editore. Roma, 1983

MILIAN'S II

Synonyms. Atrophia alba; progressive fibrosis telangiectasis; progressive telangiectasis; white atrophy; livedoid vasculitis.

Symptoms and Signs. Prevalent in women. On the foot or ankle, formation of a white plaque with stippled telangiectasia and pigmented edges. Tender petechiae, blistering, and crusting may precede the lesion. Associated usually with venous incompetence (see Lower leg stasis). Ulceration follows in 30% of cases.

Etiology. Unknown; defect of circulation (possibly, primary capillaritis).

Pathology. Atrophy of epidermis; sclerodermalike changes; no inflammatory changes. Thrombosis of small vessels; fibrinoid changes. Ulcer necrosis bordered by acanthosis and hyperkeratosis.

Therapy. Rest; compression (with poor results). Steroids accelerate ulcer healing. Low molecular weight dextran, phenformin, ethyl estradiol, stanazol, heparin among the many agents tried.

Prognosis. Ulcer slow to heal. Chronic condition.

BIBLIOGRAPHY. Milian G: Les atrophies cutanées syphilitiques. Bull Soc Fr Dermatol 36:865–871, 1929

Rook A, Wilkinson DS, Ebling FJG, et al: Textbook of Dermatology, 4th ed, pp 1203–1205. Oxford, Blackwell Scientific Publications, 1986

MILIARY HEMANGIOMAS, CONGENITAL

Synonyms. Hematoangiomatosis eruptive neonatal; diffuse neonatal hemoangiomatosis.

Symptoms and Signs. Both sexes affected; evident at birth. Two clinical forms: I, benign, and II, malignant. The malignant form is associated with visceral lesion. In the malignant form, large number of hemangiomas scattered over skin, mucosae. Dyspnea; tachycardia; jaundice.

Etiology. Unknown; no evidence of hereditary transmission. Possible relation with Rendu-Osler-Weber syndrome.

Pathology. Hemangiomas on skin, mucosae, and practically all organs (liver; spleen; mesentery; pancreas; trachea; central nervous system). Some invasion and destruction of normal tissue, but no evidence of malignancy.

Diagnostic Procedures. *Biopsy. Angiography.* (If feasible.) *Echography of liver.*

Therapy. Systemic corticosteroids. Hepatic artery ligation, partial lobectomy, transarterial embolization when indicated.

Prognosis. *Benign form.* Favorable outlook. *Malignant form.* Death in early infancy generally from high output failure.

BIBLIOGRAPHY. von Falkowski A: Ueber eigenartige mesenchymale Hämartome in Leber and Milz neben multiplen eruptiven. Angiomen der Haut bei einem Säugling. Beitz Pathol Anat 57:385–414, 1914

Burman D, Mansell PWA, Warin RP: Miliary hemangiomata in the newborn. Arch Dis Child 42:193–197, 1967

Rook A, Wilkinson DS, Ebling FJG, et al: Textbook of Dermatology, 4th ed, pp 207–208. Oxford, Blackwell Scientific Publications, 1986

MILKMAN'S

Synonyms. Looser-Milkman; Looser's zones; osteoporosis-osteomalacia; pseudofractures.

Symptoms. Prevalent in females; onset in middle age. Fatigue; pain in back, legs.

Signs. Tenderness on pressure of affected bones; possibly, limping.

Etiology. Disorder of phosphorus, calcium metabolism; osteomalacia (adult counterpart of rickets). The eponym *Milkman's syndrome* has been used to indicate the radiologic feature of pseudofractures.

Pathology. Ribbonlike zone of calcification. Decalcification along paths of vessels; incomplete fractures; defect filled by active osteoblasts; lack of calcification of matrix.

Diagnostic Procedures. *Blood.* Low serum calcium and phosphorus; high alkaline phosphatase level. *X-ray.* Pseudofractures zone of Looser or Milkman, small fissures in cortex of long bones in symmetric locations; generalized demineralization.

Therapy. Vitamin D.

Prognosis. Chronic condition; occasionally, spontaneous disappearance of manifestations during pregnancy or menopause.

BIBLIOGRAPHY. Looser E: Ueber pathologische Foramen von Infraktionen und Callusbildungen bei Rachitis und Osteomalackie und anderen Knochenerkrankungen. Zentralbl Chir 47:1470–1474, 1920

Milkman LA: Pseudofractures (hunger osteopathy late rickets, osteomalacia). Am J Roentgenol 24:29–37, 1930

Steinback HL, Noetzli M: Roentgen appearance of the skeleton in osteomalacia and rickets. Am J Roentgenol 91:955–972, 1964

Wahner HW: Assessment of metabolic bone disease: review of new nuclear medicine procedures. Mayo Clin Proc 60:827–835, 1985

MILLARD-GUBLER

Synonyms. Abducens-facial hemiplegia alternans; Gubler's; alternating inferior hemiplegia. See Foville's.

Symptoms and Signs. Hemiplegia and contralateral internal strabismus, diplopia, and loss of power to rotate eye outward.

Etiology. Vascular lesions; encephalitis; tumors at the base of pons, affecting abducens (VI) and facial (VII) nerves and pyramidal tract.

BIBLIOGRAPHY. Gubler A: De l'hémiplégie alterne envisagée comme signe de lesion de la protubérance annulaire

et comme preuve de la décussation des nerfs faciaux, Gaz Hebd Med Paris 3:749–789; 811, 1856
Adams RD, Victor M: Principles of Neurology, 3rd ed, p 1010. New York, McGraw-Hill, 1985

MILLES'

Sturge-Weber (see) associated with choroid angioma without glaucoma.

BIBLIOGRAPHY. Milles (1884)
Jablonski S: Illustrated Dictionary of Eponymic Syndromes and Diseases. Philadelphia, WB Saunders, 1969

MILLIKAN-SIEKERT

Synonyms. Basilar artery insufficiency; brachial-basilar insufficiency; subclavian steal; vertebral basilary artery.

Symptoms. Numbness; coldness; pain; claudication of arm and hand (left arm more frequently involved; bilateral involvement also possible). Exercise of involved arm precipitates neurologic symptoms: syncopal attacks; facial paresthesia; blindness; headache. Neurologic symptoms, however may be absent.

Signs. Bruit over supraclavicular area; pulse reduction and reduction of blood pressure in ipsilateral arm.

Etiology. Stenosis of proximal part of subclavian artery (congenital atherosclerosis) draining the blood from the vertebral artery to upper extremity resulting in basilar insufficiency.

Pathology. Congenital or acquired (atherosclerosis; thrombosis; extrinsic compression) stenosis of subclavian artery proximal to vertebral artery branch.

Diagnostic Procedures. *Angiography.* Reversed blood flow in vertebral artery.

Therapy. Ligation of vertebral artery close to its origin or (better) end-to-side bypass graft, between common carotid artery and subclavian artery distal to vertebral origin. Antiaggregant and/or anticoagulant therapy.

Prognosis. Symptoms disappear with surgical correction.

BIBLIOGRAPHY. Millikan CH, Siekert RG: Studies in cerebrovascular disease: the syndrome of intermittent insufficiency of the basilar arterial system. Proc Staff Meetings Mayo Clin 30:61–68, 1955
Berger RL, Sidd JJ, Ramaswamy K: Retrograde vertebral-artery flow produced by correction of subclavian-steal syndrome. New Engl J Med 277:64–69, 1967
Hurst JW: The Heart, 6th ed, p 514. New York, McGraw-Hill, 1986

MILLS'

Synonym. Ascending progressive spinal paralysis.

Symptoms. Paralysis affecting one leg and gradually ascending to involve the arm. The other side is affected later in the same fashion.

Signs. Slowly developing muscular atrophy without fibrillations. Extrapyramidal signs may develop during course of disease.

Etiology. Unknown; considered by Mills and Spiller a spinal paralysis and by Cossa and colleagues of cerebral origin, due to an abiotrophic process (form of senile paraplegia). The characterization of this very doubtful clinical entity is given by the exclusive involvement of the motor neurons. Many different agents show this selective action clinically.

Pathology. Cortical atrophy; ventricular dilatation.

Diagnostic Procedures. *Cerebrospinal fluid.* Pleocytosis. *Electroencephalography. CT scan of brain and spine.*

Therapy. None.

Prognosis. Very slow progressive evolution lasting decades.

BIBLIOGRAPHY. Mills CK, Spiller WG: On Landry's paralysis, with the report of a case. J Nerv Ment Dis 25:365–391, 1898
Spiller WG, Llongcope WT: Multiple motor neuritis including Landry's paralysis and lead palsy with reports of cases. Med Record 70:81–88, 1906
Cossa P, et al: Revision du syndrome de Mills. Presse Med 60:419–420, 1952

MINAMATA

Named for the bay in Japan near where the condition was first observed.

Synonym. Alkyl-mercury poisoning.

Symptoms. Both sexes affected; onset several weeks or months after ingestion of fish from water contaminated by methyl mercury (industrial wastage) or ingestion of animals (hogs) fed with grain treated with methyl mercury fungicide. From very severe to extremely mild. Mouth, tongue, and extremity paresthesia; constriction of visual fields up to blindness; hearing decreases up to complete loss; asthenia; fatigue; inability to concentrate; disarthria; tremors; apallic syndrome (see Kretshmer's) or persistent vegetative state.

Etiology. Chronic alkyl-mercury poisoning. Paresthesias are associated with an estimated total body burden of 40 mg, whereas death occurred at an estimated 200 mg.

Pathology. Degenerative changes in cerebral cortex and cerebellum.

Diagnostic Procedures. *Blood, hair, and tissues.* Presence of mercury. *Electroencephalography.* Severe abnormalities.

Therapy. Withdrawal from exposure. No specific treatment. BAL not useful. Trial with DMPS (2,3-dimercapto-1-propanosulfonic acid).

Prognosis. Poor. Severe residual effects after remission of acute phase. More than 100 fatal cases and 17 babies with cerebral palsy.

BIBLIOGRAPHY. Kurland LT, Faro SN, Siedler HL: Minamata disease. World Neurology 1:370–395, 1960
Takeuchi T, Eto N, Eto K: Neuropathology of childhood cases of methylmercury poisoning (Minamata disease) with prolonged symptoms, with particular reference to the decortication syndrome. Neurotoxicology 1:1–20, 1979
De Francisci G, Magalini SI: L'avvelenamento da mercurio. Rec Progr Med 74:438–450, 1983
Gosselin RE, Smith RP, Hodge HC: Clinical Toxicology of Commercial Products, 5th ed, pp 267–270. Baltimore, Willkins & Williams Co, 1984

MINKOWSKI-CHAUFFARD

Synonyms. Gaensslen-Erb alcoholic jaundice; congenital hemolytic icterus; congenital hemolytic anemia; HS; familial spherocytosis.

Symptoms. Recognized at all ages; both sexes equally affected. Positive family history. At least one of the parents affected (mother-gallbladder disease) and about 50% of siblings. Rarely, sporadic cases. Usually first noticed in childhood or early adolescence, with various degrees of intensity; occasionally so mild as to pass unnoticed. Anorexia; lassitude; delayed puberty. Recurrent acute episodes characterized by fever, tachycardia, abdominal pain, dyspnea, vomiting.

Signs. Persistent slight jaundice; not infrequently, chronic leg ulcer, splenomegaly; occasionally, moderate hepatomegaly and various developmental anomalies may be present.

Etiology. Autosomal dominant inheritance. Primary defect of red cell membrane: abnormal spectrin that binds protein 4.1 poorly and interacts weakly with actin. When red blood cells pass through the spleen they are conditioned by the inhospital environment and become spherocytes which in circulation are more susceptible to destruction by the reticuloendothelial system or during successive passages through the spleen.

Pathology. *Spleen.* Splenomegaly, absence of adhesions, pulp dry, dark, homogeneous, malpighian bodies undistinguished. Sinus apparently empty (containing red cell stromas); macrophages increased; active erythrophagocytosis. *Liver.* Increased iron content. *Gallbladder.* Bilirubin stones. *Bone marrow.* Hyperplastic erythroid hyperplasia; myeloid metaplasia in bones.

Diagnostic Procedures. *Blood.* Hemoglobin 9 to 12 g/100 ml; during crisis 3 to 4 g/100 ml; mean corpuscular volume (MCV) variable (83 ± 85); mean corpuscular hemoglobin (MCH) variable; mean corpuscular hemoglobin concentration (MCHC) 37 to 39 g/100 ml. Mean diameter of red cells reduced; absence of central pallor. Reticulocytes increased. Polychromatophilia; red cell fragility increased. Coombs' negative. Leukocytes normal. Serum bilirubin (indirect) increased. Serum iron normal or increased. *Urine.* Urobilin increased. *Stool.* Urobilin increased.

Therapy. Splenectomy.

Prognosis. Death possible during crisis. Repeated crises may cause several complications (e.g., cerebral, cardiac, biliary tract). Possibly, spontaneous improvement without recurrence of jaundice.

BIBLIOGRAPHY. Minkowski O: Ueber eine hereditäre, unter dem Bilde eines chronischen Ikterus mit Urobilinurie, Splenomegalie und Nierensiderosis verlaufende Affection. Verh Dtsch Kongr Inn. Med 18:316–319, 1900
Chauffard MA: Pathogenie de l'ictére congenital de l'adulte. Sem Med (Paris) 27:25–29, 1907
Lux SE: Disorders in red cell membrane skeleton: hereditary spherocytosis and hereditary elliptocytosis. In Stanbury JB, Wyngaarden JB, Fredrickson DS: The Metabolic Basis of Inherited Disease, 5th ed, p 1573. New York, McGraw-Hill, 1983

MINOR'S

Synonyms. Central hematomyelia; hematorrhachis; Minor-Oppenheim.

Symptoms and Signs. Onset usually after trauma (e.g., bending, falling); onset sudden, occasionally, delayed. Complete or almost complete paralysis; below lesion vasomotor changes, absence of sphincter control, absence of deep reflexes (according to spinal shock), extensor plantar reflex usually elicited. Sensory changes variable according to extension and location of primitive injury.

Etiology. Direct and indirect injury to spine. Blood dyscrasias, syphilis, tumor, myelitis, angioma, aneurysm, administration of anticoagulants are other possible causes.

Pathology. Bleeding in spinal cavity, without direct spinal cord involvement.

Diagnostic Procedures. *Spinal fluid.* Hemorrhagic. *Myelography.* Not indicated. *Selective spinal angiography.*

Therapy. Microsurgery if needed.

Prognosis. After progression of symptoms for 2 to 3 days, static period; then improvement up to complete disappearance of symptoms if spinal cord is not involved.

BIBLIOGRAPHY. Minor L: Central haematomyelia. Arch Psychiatr (Berlin) 24:693–729, 1892
Vick NA: Grinker's Neurology, 7th ed. Springfield, Ill, CC Thomas, 1976
Adams RD, Victor M: Principles of Neurology, 3rd ed, p 681. New York, McGraw-Hill, 1985

MIRIZZI'S

Synonym. Ductus hepaticus obstruction.

Symptoms and Signs. Those of hepatocholangitis.

Etiology. Local organic (possibly spastic) stenosis of hepatic duct.

Pathology. Segmental hepatocholangitis.

Diagnostic Procedures. *Cholangiography. Timed biliary drainage. Combined cholecystokinin-pancreozymin-secretin test. Echography.* ^{99m}Tc *IDA cholescintigraphy.*

Therapy. Surgery or antispastic agent according to etiology.

Prognosis. Good if stenosis treated.

BIBLIOGRAPHY. Mirizzi PL: Sindrome del conducto hepatico. G Int Chir 8:731–777, 1948
Albot G, Corteville M: De pathologie van de ductus hepaticus. Belg Geneesk 10:452–465, 1954
Blumgart LH (ed): The Biliary Tract. New York, Churchill & Livingstone, 1982

MIRROR PSEUDOTOXEMIA

Synonyms. Toxemic maternal; pseudotoxemic.

Symptoms. Occur in Rh-negative isoimmunized pregnant patients around 28th or 30th week of pregnancy.

Signs. Increased weight gain; edema refractory to the usual diuretics; mild elevation of blood pressure. These signs and symptoms in an Rh-negative isoimmunized pregnant woman represents an ominous complex and universally predicts a rather immediate intrauterine fetal death or delivery of a baby who cannot survive.

Etiology. Unknown; possibly disturbance in aldosterone secretion leading to fluid accumulation in the fetus and mother. This increased size of uterine content could conceivably produce anoxia of the decidua and perhaps result in the increased production of the oxytocin and hence symptoms of toxemia.

Pathology. Hydrops fetalis; large placenta.

Diagnostic Procedures. *Urine.* Mild proteinuria.

Therapy. Nothing can be done at that stage to save the baby, except to induce labor. The management is that of Rh-isoimmunized pregnant women, namely repeated amniocentesis if necessary, induction of labor around 34th to 36th week if deemed necessary. If earlier, intrauterine blood transfusion and then induction of labor at 34th to 36th week. Finally, intramuscular injection in all Rh-negative primigravidas after delivery, of Rh_0 (D antigen) immune globulin (RhoGAM) to immunize against further isoimmunization in susequent pregnancies.

Prognosis. Poor for the baby; good for the mother after termination of pregnancy.

BIBLIOGRAPHY. Jeffcoate TNA, Scott JS: Some observations on the placental factor in pregnancy toxemia. Am J Obstet Gynecol 77:475–489, 1959
Speck G: Eclampsia at the sixteenth week of gestation, with Rh isoimmunization and cystic degeneration of the placenta. Obstet Gynecol 15:70–72, 1960
Nicolay KS, Gainey HL: Pseudotoxemic state associated with severe Rh isoimmunization. Am J Obstet Gynecol 89:41–45, 1964
Morison DH: Anaesthesia and preeclampsia. Can J Anesth 34:415–422, 1987

MITCHELL'S I

Synonyms. Erythermalgia; primary erythromelalgia; Gerhardt's II; Weir Mitchell's I.

Symptoms and Signs. Burning distress of extremities; redness; increased skin temperature; often induced by increased environmental temperature, during summer months, and at night in bed. Relieved by cooling. Trophic changes rare. Both sexes; onset usually over middle age.

Etiology. Unknown; often preceding for years the onset of a myeloproliferative syndrome. Autosomal dominant inheritance reported in some families.

Pathology. Little known.

Diagnostic Procedures. *Blood.* Studies for typical blood changes of myeloproliferative syndromes. Thrombocythemia reported in several cases. Induction of attack by application of heat.

Therapy. Treatment of underlying condition if present. Aspirin may produce relief for days. Avoidance of causes of vasodilation in extremities.

Prognosis. As mentioned, often an early clue, preceding for years, the development of severe, often fatal conditions.

BIBLIOGRAPHY. Mitchell SW: Clinical lecture on certain painful affections of the feet. Philadelphia, Med Times 3:81–82, 113; 115, 1872

Rook A, Wilkinson DS, Ebling FJG, et al: Textbook of Dermatology. 4th ed, pp 1190–1191. Oxford, Blackwell Scientific Publications, 1986

MITCHELL'S II

Synonyms. Barraquer-Simons; Holländer's; Partial lipodystrophy; Simond's; Smith's; Weir Mitchell's II.

Symptoms and Signs. Most frequently, onset between 5 and 15 years of age; prevalent in females (4:1). Symmetric loss of facial fat occurring over some months, with or without disappearance of fat from arms, chest, abdomen, and hips, but with retention of distal fat deposits. Mental retardation in some cases.

Etiology. Unknown; congenital derangement of mesenchyma. May follow damage of midbrain or diencephalon.

Pathology. Absence of fat in indicated locations; kidney frequently affected: enlarged; nephritis; pyelonephritis; nephrotic changes. Liver occasionally enlarged; mild fibrosis; fat vacuolization.

Diagnostic Procedures. *Blood.* Absence of diabetes (see Total lipodystrophy). In some cases, however, disturbed glucose metabolism and hyperlipemia. Blood urea nitrogen and creatinine elevated. *Urine.* Albuminuria; hematuria. *X-ray.* Pyelograms normal or caliceal dilatation with or without ureter dilatations. *Pneumoencephalography.* In some cases, abnormal.

Therapy. Symptomatic treatment of kidney condition.

Prognosis. The presence of pathologic kidney findings makes the prognosis guarded.

BIBLIOGRAPHY. Mitchell SW: Singular case of absence of adipose matter in upper half of the body. Am J Med Sci 90:105, 1885

Senior B, Gellis SS: The syndromes of total lipodystrophy and of partial lipodystrophy. Pediatrics 33:593–612, 1964

Rook A, Wilkinson DS, Ebling FJG, et al: Textbook of Dermatology, 4th ed, pp 1876–1877. Oxford, Blackwell Scientific Publications, 1986

MITRAL VALVE ATRESIA

Synonyms. Hypoplastic heart ventricle; hypoplastic left ventricle. (Hypoplasia of aortic tract complex associated with functionally adequate left ventricular chamber not to be considered within this entity).

Symptoms and Signs. Predominant in male infants. Mild cyanosis; pallor; tachypnea; congestive heart failure; frequently, peripheral pulses absent or weak. Systolic murmur (grade 2-3/6) at left sternal border. Second sound loud and single. Failure to thrive. Syncope.

Etiology. Unknown; congenital heart malformation.

Pathology. Hypoplasia of left ventricle associated with a small aortic arch and small ascending and transverse aorta, large pulmonary artery and orifice, and normally related arterial trunks.*

Diagnostic Procedures. *X-ray.* Cardiomegaly; passive congestion increases vascularity of the lungs. *Electrocardiography.* Right axis deviation and right ventricular hypertrophy; vectorcardiography: P Wave broad, tall, notched. *Cardiac catheterization.* Elevated left atrial pressure. *M mode; two-dimensional echocardiography.*

Therapy. Surgery only palliative to reinforce the interatrial communication left to right and patency of ductus arteriosus right to left. Medical treatment of intercurrent infection and congestive failure.

Prognosis. Very poor; death in early infancy.

BIBLIOGRAPHY. Noonan JA, Nadas AS: The hypoplastic left heart syndrome, an analysis of 101 cases. Pediatr Clin N Am 5:1029–1056, 1958

Gittenberger-de Groot AC, Weuick ACG: Mitral atresia: morphological details. Br Heart J 51:252, 1984

MITRAL VALVE REGURGITATION

Symptoms. Both sexes affected but prevalent in males; onset at all ages. Initially asymptomatic; then cough, asthenia. Occasionally, dyspnea, palpitation, hemoptysis, angina.

Signs. Strong left-downward displaced apical beat. Holosystolic murmur replacing first apical sound and radiating toward axilla; systolic thrill; second pulmonic sound accentuated; frequently, third sound.

---

* Blind dimple in floor of left atrium; frequently association with aortic atresia; patent foramen ovale; transposition of great vessels; hypoplasia of left ventricle (see) ventricular septal defects.

Etiology. Rheumatic infection; subacute bacterial endocarditis; ischemia; trauma; hereditary (see Leopard). Undue restraint upon leaflets or chordae (bacterial endocarditis, myxomatous mitral valve, Loeffler's endomyocardiac fibrosis, lupus erythematosus). Calcification mitral ring.

Pathology. Mitral valve insufficiency; left ventricle hypertrophy.

Diagnostic Procedures. *Electrocardiography.* Left ventricular predominance. *X-rays. Fluoroscopy. Angiography. Cineangiography. Echocardiography. Cardiac catheterization. Radionuclide studies.*

Therapy. Surgical treatment. Valve prothesis and prevention of bacterial endocarditis. If indicated, medical management of cardiac failure.

Prognosis. From asymptomatic to various degrees of cardiac failure.

BIBLIOGRAPHY. Hope J: Signs of disease of the mitral valve. In A Treatise on the Diseases of the Heart, p 387. London, Churchill, 1939
Hurst JW: The Heart, 6th ed, pp 764–780. New York, McGraw-Hill, 1986

MITRAL VALVE STENOSIS

Symptoms. *Congenital form.* Equal distribution in both sexes (possibly, female prevalence); onset before 6 months of age. From asymptomatic to severe acute illness (see below); seldom syncope; no hemoptysis. *Acquired form.* Onset in childhood, adolescence, seldom later. Palpitation; distress in cardiac area; dyspnea; orthopnea; cough; frequent respiratory infections; hoarseness or aphonia; weakness; abdominal discomfort; hemoptysis; angina; syncope.

Signs. Left displaced apical beat and thrust; presystolic or early diastolic crescendo rumble (with onset of atrial fibrillation the rumble disappears). First sound loud and high pitched; second sound reinforced. Congestion of neck veins; later, edema and pulmonary congestion.

Etiology. Congenital defect (rare); rheumatic infection. Thrombus formation; atrial myxoma; bacterial vegetation and calcification.

Pathology. Narrowing of mitral valve from various morphologic defects.

Diagnostic Procedures. *Electrocardiography.* QRS vertical axis; seldom, right deviation; large, broad P waves. *X-rays.* Left atrium and right ventricle enlarged; displacement of esophagus. *Heart catheterization. Echocardiography.* Most reliable noninvasive technique. Decrease of the E-F slope of the anterior leaflet of mitral valve, abnor-

mal posterior leaflet movement, decreased valve motion, thick echoes around valve (calcification). *Radionuclide studies.*

Therapy. Surgical treatment if indicated. Medical management of cardiac failure and prevention of bacterial endocarditis.

Prognosis. According to degree of lesions. Common complications and causes of death are atrial fibrillation, pulmonary edema, bacterial endocarditis, peripheral and pulmonary embolism, cardiac failure.

BIBLIOGRAPHY. Vienssen SR: Traite nouveau de la structure et des causes du mouvement naturel du coeur, p 101. Toulouse, Guillemette 1715
Hurst JW: The Heart, 6th ed, pp 754–764. New York, McGraw-Hill, 1986

MITRAL VALVE STENOSIS–BALL VALVE THROMBUS

Synonyms. Massive atrial thrombosis; massive mitral thrombosis.

Symptoms. Occur in 9% to 20% of mitral stenosis patients (percentage increasing with age); insidious onset. Dyspnea; disorientation; mental confusion; rarely, syncope.

Signs. Severe pulmonary congestion with intervals of temporary improvement. Occasionally, episodes of acrocyanosis; absence or weakness of pulse; engorgement of neck veins, relieved by sitting up or leaning forward.

Etiology. Rheumatic disease. Large thrombus of left atrium occluding mitral valve. Myxoma or pedunculated sarcoma may produce the same syndrome.

Pathology. See Etiology.

Diagnostic Procedures. *Electrocardiography. Angiocardiography.* Interatrial filling defect. *Echocardiography. Radionuclide studies.*

Therapy. Anticoagulants; digitalis ineffective.

Prognosis. Poor.

BIBLIOGRAPHY. Surawicz B, Nierenberg MA: Association of silent mitral stenosis with massive thrombi in the left atrium. New Engl J Med 263:423–431, 1960
Hurst JW: The Heart, 6th ed, p 761. New York, McGraw-Hill, 1986

MITTELSCHMERZ

Synonym. Graafian follicle cyst.

Symptoms. Sharp abdominal pain, recurrent at periodic intervals. Menstrual irregularity and pelvic discomfort.

Etiology. Follicular ovary cyst; atresia of ovarian follicle.

BIBLIOGRAPHY. Pritchard JA, McDonald P, Gant NF: Williams Obstetrics 7th ed, p 43. Norwalk, Conn, Appleton-Century-Crofts, 1985

MÖBIUS' I

Synonyms. Hemicrania hemiplegic; hemiplegic-ophthalmoplegic migraine; hemiplegic familial migraine; neurologic migraine.

Symptoms. Occur in young adults. Moderate hemicrania accompanied by extraocular palsy (oculomotor [III] and other oculomotor nerves); frequently followed (after 3 to 5 days of onset and when pain subsides) by hemiparesis. Recovery usually follows after a few days.

Etiology and Pathology. Unknown; indirect indications of unilateral cerebral edema due to vasomotor phenomena; in some cases aneurysm of internal carotid or neoplasia.

Diagnostic Procedures. *X-ray of skull. Angiography. CT Brain scan.*

Therapy. Same as for migraine, classic (see). Corticosteroids; diuretics; if aneurysm identified, surgery.

Prognosis. Permanent damage of oculomotor (III) nerve may occur.

BIBLIOGRAPHY. Möbius PJ: Ueber periodische wiederkehrende Oculomotoriuslachennung. Klin Wochenschr 21:604–608, 1884
Ad hoc Committee: Classification of headache. JAMA, 179:717–718, 1962
Frideman AP: The migraine syndrome. Bull New York Acad Med 44:45–62, 1968

MÖBIUS' II

Synonyms. Akinesia algera; arthrogryposis; congenital facial diplegia; Graefe's II; nuclear agenesis; oculofacial paralysis; paralysis congenita 6th to 12th cranial nerves; von Graefes'.

Symptoms. Facial paralysis; inability to abduct the eyes beyond midpoint; nutritional difficulty because of tongue and palate atrophy or deformities. Mental deficiency often associated.

Signs. Masklike expression; open mouth; paralysis of soft palate and muscles of mastication; atrophy of tongue.

Also observed, absence of pectoralis muscles, talipes, syndactyly.

Etiology. Possibly, failure of development of facial nerve cells or primary defect of muscles deriving from first two branchial arches or both. Chromosomal abnormalities (short arm of chromosome 1 or long arm of chromosome 13). Congenital myopathies may also cause this syndrome.

Pathology. Studies are few, incomplete, and inadequate to draw any conclusions about real pathology of the condition. Extensive asymmetric changes in brain stem, medulla, and pons. Aplasia, hypoplasia of facial and extraocular muscles. Facial nerves small or absent.

Diagnostic Procedures. *Electromyography. Biopsy of muscle. X-ray of skull. Electroencephalography. Pneumoencephalography. Brainstem auditory evoked potentials (BAEP). Abnormal.*

Therapy. Surgery to protect cornea. Surgical correction of associated defects.

Prognosis. Recovery in a few weeks or nonprogressive permanent paralysis of face, always bilateral, often asymmetric, and when incomplete, usually sparing lower face and platysma.

BIBLIOGRAPHY. von Graefe A: Graefe-Saemisch Handbuch, Vol 6, p 60. Leipzig, Engelmann, 1880
Möbius PJ: Ueber angeborene doppelseitige Abduces-Facialis-Lahmung. Munch Med Wochenschr 35:91–94; 108–111, 1888
Thomas HM: Congenital facial paralysis. J Nerv Ment Dis 25:571–593, 1898
Von Allen MW, Blodi FC: Neurologic aspect of Möbius syndrome. Neurology 10:249–259, 1960
Stabile M, Cavaliere ML, Scarano G, et al: Abnormal BAEP in family with Möbius syndrome: evidence for supranuclear lesion. Clin Genet 25:459–463, 1984
Krajcirik WJ, Azar I, Opperman S, Lear E: Anesthetic management of a patient with Moebius syndrome. Anesth Analg 64:371–372, 1985

MOELLER-HUNTER

Synonyms. Hunter's (W.); atrophic glossitis; Hunter's glossitis; glossitis Moeller's.

Symptoms. Pain on the tip and side of tongue.

Signs. Vivid red patches on edges of tongue.

Etiology. Pernicious anemia (see Addison-Biermer).

Prognosis. With treatment, rapid regression of symptoms and signs; papillae may be regenerated in a week.

BIBLIOGRAPHY. Moeller JOL: Klinische Bemerkungen

über einige weniger bekannte Krankheiten der Zunge. Dtsch Klin 3:273–275, 1851

Hunter W: Further observation on pernicious anaemia (severe cases). A chronic infective disease: its relation to infection from the mouth and stomach; suggested serum treatment. Lancet I:221–224, 1900

MOENCKEBERG'S

Synonyms. Medial arteriosclerosis; medial calcified sclerosis.

Symptoms. Prevalent in males; onset after 50 years of age. Intermittent claudication with pain in foot, calf, thigh, or buttock.

Signs. Palpation of leg vessels reveals nodularity.

Etiology. Unknown. Various factors correlated with arteriosclerotic changes: stress; diet; toxic; nicotine.

Pathology. Larger arteries involved: rings or plaques of calcification of media; tortuosity and elongation. Adventitia respected; endothelium intact, but deformed.

Diagnostic Procedures. Evaluation of arterial flow. *X-ray.* Calcium deposits along arterial tracts.

Therapy. None. Or surgical bypass.

Prognosis. That of associated atherosclerotic changes.

BIBLIOGRAPHY. Moenckeberg JG: Ueber die reine Mediaverkalkung der Extremitätenarterien und ihr Verhalten zur Arteriosklerose. Virchows Arch Pathol 171:141–167, 1903

MOERSCH-WOLTMANN

Synonyms. Muscular rigidity–progressive spasm; stiff-man.

Symptoms. Predominant in men (70%). Prodromal intermittent aching and tightness of body and limb muscles, evolving into a permanent stiffness that affects voluntary mobility. In addition, paroxysmal, painful spasms that are precipitated by physical and emotional stimuli and that may result in bone fractures. Profuse sweating, tachycardia associated with spasms. Sleep suppresses contractions. Sensory system and intellect are not affected.

Signs. Boardlike stiffness of muscles. Reflexes normal.

Etiology. Unknown. Postulated: abnormal activity of small gamma motor neurons that induce contraction of muscle spindles, which in turn, maintain excitability of lower motoneuron system correlation with hyperthyroidism or hypothalamic dysfunction or both. Familial occur-

rence reported (autosomal dominant (?) X-linked (?). Autoimmunity.

Pathology. *Biopsy.* Of muscle. Normal or various abnormalities; increase in fibers and collagen; degeneration phenomena; sarcolemmal hyperplasia.

Diagnostic Procedures. *Urine.* In 30% of cases, abnormal reducing substance. *Blood.* Increased serum phosphorus during glycogen deposition (insulin administration). *Basal metabolic rate.* Increased. *Electromyography.* Tonic contraction continuing at rest.

Therapy. Dramatic improvement with diazepam; cortisol or correction of other hormone specific derangements may produce good remission.

Prognosis. Long range unknown. Progressive condition; weight loss and fractures.

BIBLIOGRAPHY. Moersch FP, Woltmann HW: Progressive fluctuating muscular rigidity and spasm ("stiff-man" syndrome): report of case and some observations in 13 other cases. Proc Staff Meet Mayo Clinic 31:421–427, 1956

Gordon EE, Januszku DM, Kaufman L: A critical survey of stiff-man syndrome. Am J Med 42:582–599, 1967

George TM, Burke JM, Sobotka PA, et al: Resolution of stiff-man syndrome with cortisol replacement in a patient with deficiency of ACTH, growth hormone and prolactin. New Engl J Med 310:1511–1513, 1984

Layzer RB: Stiff-man syndrome: an autoimmune disease? New Engl J Med 318:1060–1061, 1988

MOHR'S

Synonyms. Acrocephalosyndactyly IV; Mohr-Claussen; orofacial-digital II; OFD II. See Papillon-Leage-Pseume.

Symptoms. Both sexes affected equally; present from birth. Feeding difficulties; mental and physical development retardation; deafness (conductive type).

Signs. *Facies.* Broad nasal bridge; hypoplasia alae nasi, pleudocleft (median) of upper lip; irregular teeth; multiple hypertrophic frenula of labia; cleft tongue; narrow arched palate; molar and maxillar hypoplasia. *Limbs.* Short humerus, femur, and tibia; in some cases, partial duplication of toes. *Muscle.* Hypotonia. *Hair and skin.* No changes.

Etiology. Unknown; autosomal recessive inheritance.

BIBLIOGRAPHY. Mohr OL: A hereditary sublethal syndrome in man. Avhandl Norske Videnskaps-Akademi Oslo. J Mat Naturwiss Klasse 14:1–3, 1941

Claussen O: Et arvelig syndrom omfattende tugemisdannelse of polydactyly. Nord Med 30:1147–1151, 1946

Rimoin DL, Edgenton MT: Genetic and clinical heterogeneity in the oral-facial-digital syndromes. J Pediatr 71:94–102, 1967

Anneren G, Arvidson B, Gustavson K-H, et al: Oro-facio-digital syndromes I and II: radiological methods for diagnosis and the clinical variations. Clin Genet 26:178–186, 1984

MOLLARET'S

Synonym. Benign recurrent meningitis.

Symptoms and Signs. Observed particularly in infants. Recurrent hyperthermia; cephalalgia; nausea; vomiting; nuchal rigidity; myalgia; Kernig's and Brudzinski's signs. Occasionally, convulsions.

Etiology. Suspected, viral infection.

Diagnostic Procedures. *Cerebrospinal fluid.* Pleocytosis of mixed type; lymphocytes, neutrophils and endothelial cells.

Therapy. Symptomatic.

Prognosis. Good. Symptoms recede in 2 to 3 days but may recur for weeks or months. Apparently, however, a self-limited condition.

BIBLIOGRAPHY. Mollaret P: Méningite endothélio-leucocytaire multirécurrente benigne. Syndrome nouveau ou maladie nouvelle? (Documents cliniques). Rev Neurol (Paris) 76:57–76, 1944

Adams RD, Victor M: Principles of Neurology, 3rd ed, p 556. New York, McGraw-Hill, 1985

MONBRUN-BENISTY

Synonym. Ocular stump causalgia.

Symptoms. Occur a month after rupture of the eyeball. Severe refractory pain starting from orbital cavity and extending on the face and the corresponding hemicranium. Congestion and hyperhidrosis of region involved.

Etiology. Sympathetic irritation of resected sympathetic fiber to the eye.

Pathology. Neuroma of resected sympathetic fibers.

Therapy. Cervical ganglion or Gasser's ganglion resection; alcoholization of superior branch of trigeminal (V) nerve brings temporary relief.

Prognosis. Ablation of stump ineffectual. Good result with cervical or Gasser's ganglion resection.

BIBLIOGRAPHY. Monbrun M, Mme Benisty: C R Soc Neurol Paris, 1916

Barre JA, Klein M: Un cas de syndrome de Monbrun-Benisty (causalgie du moignon oculaire) gueri par Gasserectomie. Rev Otoneuro-ophthalmol 11:755–758, 1934

Barraco P, Morax S: Chirurgie mutilante du globe. Encycl Méd Chir (Paris, France) Ophtalmologie 213000 A10, 10, 1987

MONDAY FEVER

Synonyms. Byssinosis; cotton mill fever; cotton miller fever. See Allergic alveolitis syndromes.

Symptoms. Occupational disease. Wheezing; dyspnea; cough with mucoid expectoration. Onset on Monday morning when returning to work at place with high concentration of industrial cotton dust.

Signs. Rales; hyperresonance on chest percussion.

Etiology. Hypersensitivity to cotton dust.

Pathology. Emphysema; chronic bronchitis; interstitial fibrosis; small granuloma contains bodies similar to asbestos.

Diagnostic Procedures. *X-ray of chest. Skin test.* Reaction to cotton dust.

Therapy. Avoidance of exposure to cotton dust.

Prognosis. Good if exposure discontinued; otherwise, chronic bronchitis, respiratory failure, or cor pulmonale.

BIBLIOGRAPHY. Chan-Yeung M, Lam S: Occupational asthma. Am Rev Respir Dis 133:686–703, 1986

MONDOR'S

Synonyms. Superficial breast phlebitis; superficial chest wall phlebitis; sclerosing breast periphlebitis; sclerosing breast phlebitis.

Symptoms. Predominant in females; onset in 3rd to 6th decade. None or slight discomfort.

Signs. Usually, unilateral red linear cord from lateral margin of breast, crossing costal margin to abdominal wall, attached to skin, not to deep fascia.

Etiology. Obliterative phlebitis of thoracoepigastric vein. Frequently, history of trauma.

Pathology. Periphlebitis of lateral thoracic or thoracoepigastric vein. Thrombosis; adventitia and media destruction.

Therapy. Topical application of heparinoid compounds.

Prognosis. Usually, all manifestations disappear in a few weeks.

BIBLIOGRAPHY. Mondor H: Tronculite souscutanée sub-aiguë de la paroi thoracique antérolatérale. Mem Acad Chir (Paris) 65:1271–1278, 1939

Hogan GF: Mondor's disease. Arch Intern Med 113:881–885, 1964

Hurst JW: The Heart, 6th ed, p 910. New York, McGraw-Hill, 1986

MONGE'S

Synonyms. Chronic mountain sickness; chronic secondary mountain polycythemia; Seroche.

EMPHYSEMATOUS TYPE
Symptoms. Dyspnea; frequently, bronchitis; laryngitis.

Signs. Cyanosis; globular chest.

ERYTHREMIC TYPE
Symptoms. Fatigue; exertional dyspnea; decrease in mental fitness; headache; epistaxis; gum bleeding; hemoptysis; anorexia; nausea; vomiting; decreased visual acuity; tinnitus; cough. Loss of libido; paresthesia and pain in the extremities. Aphonia, lethargy up to coma.

Signs. Severe cyanosis (increasing with exertion); frequently purpura. Eyelids edematous; bluish scleral injection; thickening of tongue; turgor of hands; clubbing of fingers; hepatosplenomegaly (in 10% of cases).

Etiology. Unknown; possibly, minimal intrinsic pulmonary disease too mild to give manifestation at low altitude. Similar to Ayerza's, differentiated by the fact that the latter condition does not respond to transfer to low altitude.

Pathology. Polycythemia.

Diagnostic Procedures. *Blood.* Erythrocytosis; reticulocytes normal or increased. Leukocytes normal; platelets normal; indirect bilirubin high; increase of blood volume; increased excretion of urobilinogen.

Therapy. Transference to sea level.

Prognosis. Remission and relapses frequently observed. Complete remission if patient transferred to sea level. Death from hemorrhages, bronchopneumonia; or cardiac disorders late and frequently cause of death.

BIBLIOGRAPHY. Monge C: High altitude disease. Arch Intern Med 59:32–40, 1937

Monge C, Lozano R, Carcelen A: Renal excretion of bicarbonate in high altitude natives and in natives with chronic mountain sickness. J Clin Invest, 43:2303–2309, 1964

Houston CS: Altitude illness. Emerg Med Clin N Am, 2:503–512, 1984

Pittiglio DH, Sacher RA: Clinical Hematology and Fundamentals of Hemostasis, p 185. Philadelphia, FA Davis, 1987

MONGOLIAN BLUE SPOTS

Synonym. Dermal melanocytosis.

Symptoms and Signs. Present in 90% of Oriental neonates and in 1% of white infants (maximal frequency in those of Mediterreanean areas). Incidence in other nationalities range between these two. Faint, blue-grayish, macular pigmentation, usually a single patch in lumbosacral area that, occasionally, may extend to loins and shoulders.

Etiology. Unknown.

Pathology. Dermal collagen fibers and neurovascular bundles mixed with melanocytes, disposed parallel to skin. Absence of macrophages and no alteration of collagen and elastic fibers.

Prognosis. For some time after birth, pigmentation tends to increase in depth; then, usually, it fades completely in 7th and occasionally, 13th year. Rarely discoloration remains for life.

BIBLIOGRAPHY. El Bahrawy AA: Arch Dermatol Syph 141:171, 1922

Rook A, Wilkinson DS, Ebling FJG, et al: Textbook of Dermatology, 4th ed, pp 49, 1580, 2443. Oxford, Blackwell Scientific Publications, 1986

MONTEGGIA'S

Synonym. Ulnar fracture-radial head dislocation. See Galeazzi's.

Symptoms. More common in children. Pain in forearm.

Signs. Fracture dislocation of forearm with dislocation of radial head proximally. Elbow partially flexed and rotated inward.

Etiology. Blow on forearm.

Diagnostic Procedures. *X-ray of elbow.* Fracture of ulna radial head points through the middle of the capitellum. Four types of this fracture have been described.

Therapy. Most fractures treated by closed methods. If unsuccessful, open reduction is needed.

Prognosis. If not recognized and treated, poor function may result.

BIBLIOGRAPHY. Monteggia GB: Istituzioni Chirurgiche, Vol 5. Milan, Pirotta Maspero, 1814

Canale TS: Fractures and dislocation in children. In Crenshaw AH (ed): Campbell's Operative Orthopedics, 7th ed, pp 1849–1853. St Louis, CV Mosby, 1987

MOORE-FEDERMAN

Synonym. Familial dwarfism-stiff joints. See also Leri's.

Symptoms and Signs. Both sexes affected; apparently normal at birth; noticed between 3 and 5 years of age. Joint stiffness. Symptoms slowly progress to produce inability to completely clench hand. Delayed growth: adult reaches 130 cm to 150 cm. Hyperopia; asthma; hoarseness; hepatomegaly.

Etiology. Autosomal dominant inheritance.

Diagnostic Procedures. *X-rays.* Diminished height of vertebrae; slightly widened phalangeal metaphyses. *Urine.* No mucopolysaccharides and amino acid excretion.

Prognosis. Good *quoad vitam*. Dwarfism. Frequent respiratory infections.

BIBLIOGRAPHY. Moore WT, Federman DD: Familial dwarfism and "stiff joints." Report of a kindred. Arch Intern Med 115:398–404, 1969
McKusick VA: Heritable Disorders of Connective Tissue, 4th ed. St Louis, CV Mosby, 1972

MOOREN'S

Synonyms. Ulcus rodens corneal; serpiginous cornea ulcer.

Symptoms. No significant race or sex incidence. Primarily affects adults. Ocular pain (in one eye or both eyes) and photophobia that appear simultaneously or at different times in the absence of any known systemic disease.

Signs. Superficial corneal erosion starting as a corneal infiltrate, just inside the limbus and spreading in serpiginous manner. Central margin presents an overhanging lip; the anterior corneal layers are involved. Lesion is progressive and chronic; the cicatricial reaction is minimal. Signs of iritis are frequently present. The perforation of cornea and hypopyon are rarely seen. Conjunctiva and sclera are never affected by the ulcer.

Etiology. Unknown; allergy and hypersensitivity have been considered. Other postulated etiologic mechanisms: metabolic disorders; malnutrition; hereditary familial primary changes in trigeminal (V) nerve or sympathetic fibers; trophic disturbances secondary to local disease.

Pathology. Ulceration of cornea undermined at its central edge. Microscopically, scanty inflammatory reaction in the region of the cleft and central lip of ulcer, absence of neovascularization of the cornea. Intracellular edema of basal layer of corneal epithelium. Lip of ulcer covered by thinned epithelium, curled into thick squamous fragments. Bowman's membrane absent beneath ulcer. Inflammatory pannus of limbus formed by plasma cells in anterior chamber; eosinophilic material bordering the endothelium and polymorphonuclear cells, filling angle and trabecular meshwork behind ulcer. Iris may be normal or show signs of inflammation.

Diagnostic Procedures. Search for bacteria, viruses, fungi.

Therapy. Analgesic and topical agents for secondary infections; trial with antiallergic or corticosteroid compounds.

Prognosis. Chronic progressive disease; usual duration 2 to 12 months.

BIBLIOGRAPHY. Nettleship E: Chronic serpiginous ulcer of the cornea (Mooren's ulcer). Trans Ophthalmol Soc UK 22:103–115, 1902
Edwards WC, Reed RE: Mooren's ulcer. Arch Ophthalmol 80:361–364, 1968

MOORE'S (E.M.)

Eponym used to indicate a fracture of distal end of radius, dislocation of the ulna, and trapping of styloid process under the annular ligaments.

BIBLIOGRAPHY. Moore EM: A luxation of the ulna not hitherto described, with a plan of reduction and mode of after-treatment; including the management of Colles' fracture. Albany, NY, Weed, 1872

MOORE'S (M.T.)

Synonyms. Abdominal epilepsy; paroxysmal pain; visceral epilepsy.

Symptoms. Cramps, pain; nausea; strange feeling in the abdomen and chest, followed or not followed by seizures. General pattern of attack remains the same in each patient, although initiating symptoms may vary. Percentages of incidence of paroxysmal symptoms: gastrointestinal (Moore's) (65%); cardiorespiratory (50%); genitourinary (5%); rising visceral sensation (17%); generalized convulsions (50%); psychiatric disturbances (46%).

Etiology. Usually, lesions of frontal parasagittal regions, or idiopathic.

Diagnostic Procedures. *Electroencephalography. X-ray of skull and organ involved.* For differential diagnosis.

Therapy. Anticonvulsant drugs.

Prognosis. Good response to treatment. Recovery with possible development of recurrent convulsions in later years.

BIBLIOGRAPHY. Morgagni GB: The Seats and Causes of Diseases Investigated by Anatomy; in Five Books, Containing a Great Variety of Dissection with Remarks, Vol I, pp 192–195. Alexander B (trans) London, Millar Cadell, 1769

Moore MT: Paroxysmal abdominal pain. A form of focal symptomatic epilepsy. JAMA 124:561–563, 1944

Mulder DW, Daly D, Bailey AA: Visceral epilepsy. Arch Intern Med 91:481–493, 1954

Adams RD, Victor M: Principles of Neurology, 3rd ed, p 237. New York, McGraw-Hill, 1985

MOREL-WILDI

Eponym used to indicate nodular formations (of probably dysgenetic origin) of the frontal cortex. Asymptomatic.

BIBLIOGRAPHY. Morel F, Wildi F: Dysgénésie nodulaire disséminée de l'écorce frontale. Rev Neurol (Paris) 87:251–270, 1952

MORGAGNI-ADAMS-STOKES

Synonyms. MAS; Adams-Stokes; Stokes-Adams; cardiac syncope (arrhythmic); atrioventricular heart block; Spen's.

Symptoms. Onset usually after 40 years of age. Episodes of sudden weakness, fainting, convulsions regardless of body position or particular time. Syncope, however, occurs more readily when patient is standing or sitting.

Signs. Paleness becoming cyanosis; unconsciousness; clonic jerks; during attacks pulse very slow (usually under 20), or absent (asystole of 4 to 15 seconds duration); fall of blood pressure; difficult breathing; fixed pupils; incontinence; bilateral Babinski's with resumption of heart beats; flushing of the face.

Etiology. Intensity and progression of symptoms and signs depend on degree of bradycardia. Cerebral hypoxia due to atrioventricular block; asystolic fibrillation.

Pathology. Atherosclerotic heart disease findings; congenital or rheumatic heart disease; myocarditis (infections, particularly diphtheria).

Diagnostic Procedures. *Electrocardiography.* Atrioventricular block, transient or permanent.

Therapy. During attacks and if no pulse, strike a blow over precordium. If ineffective, institute resuscitation procedures (massage; artificial respiration; defibrillation). If ventricular fibrillation etiologic cause, start intravenous injection of isoproterenol in dextrose; epinephrine (intramuscular, or intravenous, or intracardiac if needed). Type and severity of attacks or failure of medical management (long-term oral isoproterenol, atropine, epinephrine, corticosteroid therapy, chlorothiazide) indicate the need for implantation of an artificial cardiac pacemaker.

Prognosis. Guarded, depending upon pathogenetic factors.

BIBLIOGRAPHY. Morgagni JB: De Sedibus et Causis Morborum. Letter the Ninth—which Treats of the Epilepsy [description of heart block], 1761

Adams R: Cases of diseases of the heart accompanied with pathological observations. Dublin Hosp Reports 4:353–453, 1827

Stokes W: Memoir on slow pulse. Dublin Q J Med Sc 2:73–85, 1846

Bondoulas H, Lewis RP: Cardiac syncope: diagnosis, mechanism and management. In Hurst JW: The Heart, 6th ed. New York, McGraw-Hill, 1986

MORNING GLORY

Synonym. Optic disk central glial anomaly.

Symptoms. Present from birth. Severe decrease in visual acuity.

Signs. Strabismus. Unilateral enlarged pink optic disk, flowerlike with fluffy dot in the center nerve head, inscribed in a ring of alterated chorioretinal pigment. At the edge of disk, narrow branches of retinal arteries, presence of exudates, subretinal hemorrhages, and neovascularization. Periphery of retina normal. Possibly abnormality of anterior chamber.

Etiology. Unknown; no hereditary factor proved.

BIBLIOGRAPHY. Handmann M: Erbliche, vermütlich angeborene zentrale Gliöse; Entartung des Sehenerven mit besonderer Beteiligung der Zentralgefaesse. Klin Monatsbl Augenheilkd 83:145–152, 1929

Kindler P: Morning glory syndrome: unusual congenital optic disk anomaly. Am J Ophthalmol 69:376–384, 1970

MORPHEA

Synonyms. Addison keloid; Alibert keloid; circumscribed scleroderma. See Scleroderma and Romberg-Wood.

Symptoms. Prevalent in females (3 : 1); onset usually in 2nd to 4th decades. Migraine; arthralgia; abdominal pain in only 15% of cases; generalized joint pain in 40% of cases.

Signs. Five varieties recognized: (1) Plaques, usually multiple, asymmetric (2 to 15 cm in diameter), zones of skin induration that in months become smooth, shiny, hairless, nonsweating, and ivory color with purplish edges. Bullae, vesicles, hemorrhages, and telangiectases may develop. Hypoesthesia of zone involved. Trunk, limbs, face, and genital areas may be involved. (2) Guttate lesions, bigger and less numerous lesions, similar to white-spot (see). (3) Linear lesions, usually single (occasionally bilateral) lesions of linear shape similar to plaque lesion described. (4) Frontoparietal scleroderma *en coupe de sabre*. Linear scleroderma affecting frontal or frontoparietal region of face and scalp, associated more or less with minor subcutaneous atrophic changes. (5) Generalized, larger plaques usually appearing first on the trunk, sometimes involving the entire body. Face becomes expressionless; contractures appear.

Etiology. Unknown; occasionally, onset associated with trauma, pregnancy, menopause. Nature of relationship not established.

Pathology. Epidermis normal or atrophic. Dermis edematous, swelling, and degeneration of collagen; moderate perivascular lymphocytic infiltrates. Reduction of elastic tissue. Atrophy of hair, follicle, and sweat glands.

Diagnostic Procedures. *Biopsy of skin. Blood.* Normal; occasionally eosinophilia, hypocomplementaemia; increased sedimentation rate; rarely, anti DNA and ENA antibodies. *X-ray.* Spine abnormality in 47% of patients (especially linear lesions).

Therapy. Penicillamine and pyridoxine per os in early stage; sapazopyrin (enteric coated) to slow down rapidly developing forms; antimalarials useful for inflammation aspects. Infiltration with corticosteroids if indicated. Surgery occasionally used if sclerosis interferes with different functions.

Prognosis. Plaque: spontaneous improvement; 3 to 5 years duration. Linear: spontaneous improvement; lasts longer. Occasionally, development of systemic sclerosis syndrome. Generalized form: improvement after 3 to 5 years; severe disability in some cases. Death from other causes.

BIBLIOGRAPHY. Fagge CH: On keloid, sclerosis, morphoea and some allied affections. Guy's Hosp Rep 13:255–328, 1868
Wartenberg R: Progressive facial hemiatrophy. Arch Neurol Psychiatr 54:75–96, 1945
Rook A, Wilkinson DS, Ebling FJG, et al: Textbook of Dermatology, 4th ed, pp 1341–1343. Oxford, Blackwell Scientific Publications, 1986

MORQUIO'S

Synonyms. Brailsford-Morquio; chondrosteodystrophy; eccentro-osteochondrodysplasia; keratan sulfaturia; hereditary osteochondrodystrophy deformans; mucopolysaccharidosis IV; MPS IV A and B; Dale's (Morquio type B).

Symptoms. Both sexes affected; become clinically evident at end of first year of life. Deafness; weak extremities; waddling gait. Absence of mental retardation; subtle or evident symptoms of myelopathy up to quadriplegia.

Signs. Dwarfism (growth stops at 6 years of age); short trunk and neck. *Facies.* Coarse broad mouth; spaced teeth. *Thorax.* Pectus carinatum. Aortic regurgitation in some cases. *Extremities.* Knock-knees; joints very loose and unstable. Absence of hypoplasia of odontoid process, possibly resulting in atlantoaxial subluxation (see).

Etiology. Autosomal recessive inheritance. Two forms are now recognized. Type A due to absence of N-acetylgalactosamine-6-sulfatase and type B (milder Dale's syndrome due to B-galactosidase deficiency). Both give defective degradation of keratan sulfate.

Pathology. Irregular growth of cartilage and epiphysis and focal aseptic necrosis. Chondrocytes packed with vacuoles.

Diagnostic Procedures. *Urine.* Excretion of keratan sulfate. *X-rays.* Skeletal survey. Platyspondyly; epiphyseal changes; spotty calcification. *Blood.* Reilly's bodies in lymphocytes.

Therapy. Orthopedic surgery.

Prognosis. After 6 to 7 years of age situation becomes stabilized without further growth, however, death usually occurs before 20 to 30 years of age. Longer survival reported. Myelopathy and pulmonary complications are the leading causes of death.

BIBLIOGRAPHY. Morquio L: Sur une forme de dystrophie osseuse familiale. Bull Soc Pediatr Paris 27:145–152, 1929
Dale T: Unusual forms of familial osteochondrodystrophy. Acta Radiol 12:337–358, 1931
McKusick VA, Neufeld EF: The mucopolysaccharide storage disease. In Stanbury JB, Wyngaarden JB, Fredrickson DS, et al: The Metabolic Basis of Inherited Disease, 5th ed, p 751. New York. McGraw-Hill, 1983

MORQUIO-ULLRICH

Terminology proposed by Wiedemann to distinguish these patients from those with classic Morquio's.

Symptoms and Signs. Typical symptoms and signs of Morquio's, plus one or more features usually associated with Hurler's: hepatosplenomegaly; corneal opacity; deafness; granulation in leukocytes. This eponym is unnecessary since it appears that in all patients with Morquio's syndrome, if they survive to adolescence, these extraskeletal manifestations develop.

BIBLIOGRAPHY. Wiedemann HR: Ausgedehnte und allgemeine erblich bedingte Bildungs-und Wachstumsfehler des Knockengerüstes. Mschr Kinderheilkd 102:136–140, 1954

Kaplan D, McKusick V, Trebach S, et al: Keratosulfate-chondroitin sulfate peptide from normal urine and from urine of patients with Morquio syndrome (mucopolysaccharidosis IV). J Lab Clin Med 71:48–55, 1968

MORROW-BROOKE

Synonyms. Brooke's epidemic acne; epidemic acne; keratosis follicularis contagiosa.

Symptoms. Outbreak in different world regions; in each episode, it may be prevalent in one sex or age group. Pruritus; general discomfort.

Signs. On the face and ears, but possibly also on limbs and trunk. At onset, erythematous follicular papules, which rapidly change into comedo and follicular cysts that later form large keratinized brown plaques, tending to become confluent.

Etiology. Not clearly established. Strongly suspected toxic nature, especially chlorinated compounds, Acne venenata; DDT, neat cutting oils, crude petroleum, distilled, heavy coal-tar cosmetics, asbestos, topical corticosteroids.

Therapy. Avoid contact with suspected agents. Exfoliative pastes; retinoic acid.

Prognosis. Regression. Little or no scarring. Chloracne may persist for years.

BIBLIOGRAPHY. Morrow PA: Keratosis follicularis associated with fissuring of the tongue and leukoplakia buccalis. J Cutan Dis NY 4:27–65, 1886

Brooke HA: Keratosis follicularis contagiosa. In International Atlas of Rare Skin Diseases, No 7, plate 22. 1892

Rook A, Wilkinson DS, Ebling FJG, et al: Textbook of Dermatology, 4th ed, pp 573–575. Oxford, Blackwell Scientific Publications, 1986

MORT D'AMOUR

Symptom and Sign. Sudden death during sexual intercourse.

Etiology. Increase in blood pressure; arrhythmia; heart ischemia; rupture of cerebral aneurysm.

Therapy. Prophylaxis: a skillful, cooperative partner.

Prognosis. Pleasant death.

BIBLIOGRAPHY. Heggveit HA: La mort d'amour. Am Heart J 69:287–294, 1965

MORTENSEN'S

Synonyms. Di Guglielmo's II; hemorrhagic thrombocythemia; hyperthrombocytic myelosis Revol; Revol's. See Myeloproliferative.

Symptoms. Both sexes equally affected; onset in 3rd decade or later. Spontaneous bleeding manifestations of variable severity (e.g., hemoptysis, melena, menorrhagia). Excessive bleeding after minor trauma and at surgery. Thrombotic manifestations may be present in splenic vein and superficial and deep veins of legs.

Signs. Splenomegaly of variable size.

Etiology. Possible autosomal dominant trait. Suggested but not confirmed relationship to 21 chromosome deletion.

Pathology. No characteristic changes in spleen. Seldom, myeloid metaplasia in liver, spleen, or lymph nodes.

Diagnostic Procedures. *Blood.* Usually, anemia; occasionally, moderate erythrocytosis. Leukocytes increased (10,000 to 30,000, occasionally, over 60,000). Platelets extremely increased (millions); bizarre morphologic changes; various functional abnormalities. In some cases, mild deficiency of clotting factors II, V, and VI. *Bone marrow.* Panhyperplasia with marked increase of megakaryocytes, some showing morphologic abnormalities.

Therapy. Busulfan; radioactive phosphorus. Splenectomy usually disastrous. Controversial results with anticoagulants. Encouraging results with aspirin and other platelet antiaggregating agents.

Prognosis. Survival at 5 years with 75%. May progress to myeloproliferative disease, Vaquez's.

BIBLIOGRAPHY. Di Guglielmo G: Megacariociti e piastrine negli organi emopoietici e nel sangue circolante. Atti R Acad Chir Napoli 83:19, 1919

Epstein E, Goedel A: Hämorrhagische Thrombocythamie bei vascularer Schrumpfmilz. Virchows Arch 292:233–248, 1934

Mortensen O: Thrombocythemia hemorrhagica. Acta Med Scand 129:547–549, 1948

Révol L: La myélose hyperthrombocytaire (thrombocytemie hémorragique). Sang 21:409–423, 1950

Emilia G, Torelli G, Sacchi S, et al: Chromosomal abnormalities in essential thrombocytemia. Cancer Genet 18:91–93, 1985

Brière J, Brière JF: Thrombocythèmies, Encicl Med Chir (Paris) Sang Fasc. 13006, R-10(7-1987)

MORTON'S (D.)

Synonyms. Short first metatarsal syndrome; metatarsus primus brevis varus; Morton's triad.

Symptoms. Usually bilateral condition. Excessive foot fatigue; burning pain under metatarsal heads and meta-tarsophalangeal articulations of 2nd and 3rd metatarsal bones; longitudinal arch pain; radiation of pain to the calf, hamstring, and back muscles; pain typically beginning while walking or after long standing and is relieved by rest.

Signs. Feet appear nearly normal. Careful inspection may reveal that first metatarsal may be slightly displaced upward and medially, abnormally movable, and covered with soft smooth skin, while the heads of 2nd and 3rd metatarsal are prominent and a hard callus is localized under their heads.

Etiology. Congenital malformation of 1st metatarsal bone. Autosomal dominant trait. Acute symptoms due to synovitis of 2nd or 3rd metatarsal joints and middle cuneiform; chronic symptoms due to secondary hypertrophic osteoarthritis.

Diagnostic Procedures. X-ray. Short 1st metatarsal bone and secondary changes.

Therapy. Compensating insoles; metatarsal pad or transverse bar.

Prognosis. In 75% of cases, fast recovery (1 week) with treatment; in 15% minor functional residual impairment; in 10% require further treatment.

BIBLIOGRAPHY. Morton DJ: Metatarsus atavicus: the identification of a distinct type of foot disorder. J Bone Joint Surg 9:531–544, 1927
Morton DJ: Foot disorders in general practice. JAMA 109:1112–1119, 1937
Jahss MR: Disorders of the foot. Philadelphia, WB Saunders, 1982
Beaty JH: Congenital anomalies of the lower extremity. In Crenshaw AH (ed): Campbell's Operative Orthopedics, 7th ed, pp 2629–2630. St Louis, CV Mosby, 1987

MORTON'S (T.)

Synonyms. Digital neuroma; metatarsalgia; Morton's.

Symptoms. Predominant in women. Unilateral or, occasionally, bilateral. Recurrent burning pain between 3rd and 4th metatarsal space, radiating to adjacent part of foot. Soreness may persist also when at rest and prevent sleep.

Signs. Foot appears normal. Pain may be elicited by pressure applied between 3rd and 4th metatarsal heads.

Etiology. Compression of digital nerve between metatarsal head and ground; syndrome may also occur with neurofibromas and angioneurofibromas of medial plantar nerve.

Pathology. Swelling not true neuroma of digital nerve affected; initially, simple perineural edema, then fibrosis.

Diagnostic Procedures. X-ray of foot.

Therapy. Felt pad proximal to head of 4th metatarsal. Injection of procaine and steroid relieves the pain. In very severe cases, excision of tumor.

Prognosis. Responds well to conservative or surgical treatment.

BIBLIOGRAPHY. Durlacher L: A treatise on corns, bunions and diseases of nails and the general management of the feet. London, Simpkin Marshall, 1845
Morton TG: Peculiar and painful affection of the fourth metatarso-phalangeal articulation. Am J Med Sci 71:37–45. 1876
Bichel WH, Docherty MB: Plantar neuromas. Morton toe. Surg Gynec Obstetr 84:111, 1947
Guilloff RJ, Scadding JW, Kelnerman L: Morton's metatarsalgia (clinical, electrophysiological and histological observations). J Bone Joint Surg 66B:586, 1984
Regnault B: Le pied. Springer-Verlag, Berlin, 1986

MORVAN'S I

Synonym. Syringomyelia.

Symptoms. Insidious onset in 2nd to 3rd decade. (1) Cervical lesions (most frequent); unilateral numbness of finger; localized analgesia (loss of pain and temperature; preservation of touch and deep sensibilities). At onset, in one arm and upper part of chest; then involving both sides. Later, weakness and atrophy of hands (claw deformity) and loss of deep reflexes. Stiffness of neck; deep boring spontaneous pain. (2) Lumbar lesion, unilateral and then bilateral. Same symptoms as above in lower extremities and pelvic girdle. (3) Medulla oblongata lesions (syringobulbia); same symptoms as above in the face.

Signs. Insensitivity to pain and temperature in areas affected. Burns, scars, and injuries. Trophic changes, ulcerations, Charcot's joints may be seen. Muscular atrophy and fasciculation. Spasticity; ataxia; neurogenic bladder. Horner's syndrome frequently seen.

Etiology. Unknown; possibly, neoplasm. Disorderly proliferation of ependyma; anomalies of blood supply. Probably congenital in origin. Both autosomal dominant and recessive traits have been reported.

Pathology. At onset, proliferation of glial cells in the region of central canal; then cavity formation spreading longitudinally. Gliosis is not limited to central gray matter, but tends to send projection ventrally and dorsally. Cervical cord most frequent site of origin.

Diagnostic Procedures. *Cerebrospinal fluid.* Increase of total protein (50% of cases) does not differentiate from tumors.

Therapy. Deep roentgen radiation may be effective in stopping progression. Surgery provides temporary improvement.

Prognosis. Slowly progressing for years.

BIBLIOGRAPHY. Morvan AM: De la parésie analgésique a panaris des extrémitiés supérieures ou paréso-analgésie des extrémités supérieures. Gaz Hebd Med Paris 20:580–583; 624–626, 1883

Adams RD, Victor M: Principles of Neurology, 3rd ed, pp 692–696. New York, McGraw-Hill, 1985

Brown LK, Stacy C, Schick A, Miller A: Obstructive sleep apnea in syringo–myelia–syringobulbia. New York State J Med 88:152–154, 1988

MORVAN'S II

Synonyms. Chorea fibrillaris; myoclonus multiplex fibrillaris. See also Chorea.

Symptoms and Signs. Attacks of chorea limited to calves and thighs, seldom involving the trunk.

Etiology. See Chorea.

BIBLIOGRAPHY. Morvan AM: De la chorée fibrillaire. Gaz Hebd Med 27:173–176, 1890

MOSCHCOWITZ'S

Synonyms. Baehr-Schiffrin; hemolytic thrombocytopenic purpura; thrombohemolytic purpura; TTP; Upshaw factor deficiency; Schulman-Upshaw; microangiopathic hemolytic anemia.

Symptoms. Prevalent in females; onset from infancy to old age; majority of cases between 10 and 40 years of age. Constant fluctuation of neurologic symptoms: headache; mental changes; paresis; syncope; aphasia; dysarthria; visual changes; coma. Almost constant hemorrhagic manifestations: purpura; retinal hemorrhages; melena; hematemesis; hematuria. Less frequently observed: weakness; myalgia; arthralgia; nausea; vomiting.

Signs. Pallor; petechiae; ecchymosis; jaundice (not constant); moderate adenopathy; hepatomegaly (25%); splenomegaly (20%).

Etiology. Deficiency of a plasma factor (thrombopoietin-like substance). Defect in processing of a very large VIII: vWF multimers after synthesis and secretion by endothelial cells. Autosomal recessive inheritance postulated.

Pathology. Widespread hyaline occlusion (platelets and fibrin) of arterioles and capillaries; absence of inflammatory signs; rarely infarctions.

Diagnostic Procedures. *Blood.* Various degrees of thrombocytopenia; anemia occasionally very severe; reticulocytosis; presence of fragmented and altered cells (burr cells; helmet cells); accelerated red cell breakdown; hyperbilirubinemia. Coombs' test negative; marked increase of leukocyte number (leukemoid reaction); azotemia. Biopsy revealing typical pattern (see Pathology). *Bone marrow.* Increased number of immature megakaryocytes and myeloid-erythroid hyperplasia. *Urine.* Proteinuria; hematuria; casts.

Therapy. Steroids and splenectomy of little or no benefit; conflicting reports with heparin. Dextran, aspirin, and dipyridamole reported as useful. Good results reported with plasma transfusions and plasmapheresis, also in terminal cases.

Prognosis. Progressive course; death in 3 months. Cases of recovery and apparent cure reported.

BIBLIOGRAPHY. Moschcowitz E: Acute febrile pleiochromic anemia with hyaline thrombosis of terminal arterioles and capillaries; an undescribed disease. Arch Intern Med 36:89–93, 1925

Schulman I, Pierce M, Lukens A, et al: Studies on thrombopoiesis I. A factor in normal human plasma required for platelets production; chronic thrombocytopenia due to its deficiency. Blood 16:943–957, 1960

Upshaw JD: Congenital deficiency of a factor of normal plasma that reverses microangiopathic hemolysis and thrombocytopenia. New Engl J Med 298:1350–1352, 1978

Marcus AJ: Moschcowitz revisited. New Engl J Med 37:1447–1448, 1982

MOSSE'S

Synonym. Liver cirrhosis-polycythemia.

Symptoms and Signs. According to Mosse, polycythemic symptoms and signs appearing first, followed by clinical features of liver cirrhosis.

Etiology. Not established if this may be considered a pathologic entity or rather a simple coincidence.

Pathology. That of polycythemia vera and liver cirrhosis. Occlusion of hepatic vein in polycythemia (Budd-Chiari syndrome) frequently observed.

Diagnostic Procedures. *Blood.* Polycythemia; liver functions altered; low fibrinogen. *Bone marrow.* Hyperplasia. *Biopsy of liver.* Cirrhosis.

Therapy. That of polycythemia and cirrhosis.

Prognosis. Poorer than for simple polycythemia.

BIBLIOGRAPHY. Mosse, M: Ueber Polycythemie mit Uro-blinikterus und Milztumor. Dtsch Med Wochenschr 33:2175–2176, 1907

Wintrobe MM (ed): Clinical Hematology, 8th ed, p 1599. Philadelphia, Lea & Febiger, 1981

MOTION SENSITIVITY

Synonyms. Air sickness; kinetosis; motion sickness; naupathia.

Symptoms and Signs. Occur in persons traveling in automobiles, trains, ships, or airplanes. Pallor; sweating; sialorrhea; nausea; vomiting. Prostration may follow when condition persists.

Etiology. Not clear. Familial aggregation reported. Labyrinth stimulation by motion, plus psychic factors. Visual and olfactory stimuli may play important part.

Therapy. Prophylaxis with many drugs; Scopolamine, meclizine (Bonine), dimenhydrinate (Dramamine) given 30 minutes before starting trip. Avoiding the intake of fluid and eating only solid foods. Pure lemon juice taken immediately before trip often prevents vomiting. Nausea may be repelled by lying down with a firm support for the head, closing the eyes, and breathing fresh air. Exhaustion due to prolonged vomiting cured by fluid replacement.

Prognosis. Symptoms disappear following termination of journey.

BIBLIOGRAPHY. Treisman M: Motion sickness: an evolutionary hypothesis. Science 197:493–495, 1977

MOTOR-SCOOTER HANDLEBAR

Symptoms and Signs. Occur usually in young subjects after falling from motor scooter. Evidence of trauma in the groin may or may not be present. Typical history of claudication of one leg developing soon after trauma.

Etiology and Pathology. Compression of external iliac with damage of the intima and reactive proliferation and occlusion of the vessel.

Diagnostic Procedures. Femoral and distal arteries of involved leg not palpable. *Oscillometry.* Confirms absence of pulsation. *Lumbar aortography.* Obstruction of vessel.

Therapy. If recognized early, simple arteriotomy; if recognized later, complicated bypass procedures necessary.

Prognosis. If unrecognized, spontaneous rupture may occur. Good with treatment.

BIBLIOGRAPHY. Deutsch V, Sinkover A, Bank H: The motor-scooter handlebar syndrome. Lancet II:1051–1053, 1968

MOUCHET'S

Eponym used to indicate the paralysis of the cubital nerve following fracture of external humeral condyle.

BIBLIOGRAPHY. Mouchet A: Paralyses tardives du nerfe cubital à suite de fractures du condyle externe de l'humerus. J Chir (Paris): 437–456, 1914

MOUNIER-KUHN'S

Synonyms. Bronchiectasis-ethmoid sinusitis; sinusitis-bronchiectasis; tracheobronchomegaly.

Symptoms. Predominant in males; onset in 3rd to 4th decade. Symptoms indistinguishable from those of chronic bronchitis and ethmoiditis: cough; inability to expectorate.

Signs. On chest auscultation, harsh, rasping sounds.

Etiology. Unknown. Familial incidence of congenital malformation of the trachea, that leads to increased compliance of its own and of the bronchial walls.

Pathology. Cartilagineous and membranous parts of trachea and bronchi show thin atrophic muscular and elastic tissue; tracheobronchial collapse and signs of chronic infections.

Diagnostic Procedures. *X-ray of chest.* Increased caliber of trachea and bronchi; in lateral projection (especially) the air columns present corrugated aspect. Diagnosis is made when coronal diameter of trachea (measured 2 cm from projection of aortic arch) exceeds 30 mm. *Bronchoscopy.* Aspect may simulate multiple diverticula.

Therapy. Antibiotics. Fluidification. In some cases, surgery.

Prognosis. Variable. Repeated infections lead to respiratory insufficiency and pulmonary heart.

BIBLIOGRAPHY. Mounier-Kuhn P: Dilatation de la trachée, constatations radiographiques et broncoscopiques. Lyon Med 150:106–109, 1932

Mounier-Kuhn P: Le syndrome "ethmoidoantrie et bronchiectasis." Clinique. Etiologie, Hypothèse. Pathogéniques. Ann d'OtoLaryngol 12:387–404, 1945

Davis PB, Hubbard VS, McCoy K: Familial bronchiectasis. J Pediatr 102:177–185, 1983

MOYA-MOYA

Synonyms. Progressive arterial intracranial occlusions; intracranial arteries progressive occlusions; Kawakita's; Leed's; Maki's; multiple progressive intracranial arterial occlusions; Taveras.

Symptoms and Signs. Most cases in Japanese; a few Black and Caucasian patients. Both sexes affected with slight female prevalence; onset from infancy to young adulthood, usually following some nonspecific infectious process or cold.

Paralysis and focal epileptic attacks, alternating between both sides, usually evidence onset of the condition, together with twitching, speech disturbances, unsteady gait, hemianopia, and headache. In some cases (especially in adults), psychiatric manifestations are prominent. These manifestations may be followed by signs of intracranial hemorrhage.

Etiology. Unknown; considered a nonspecific inflammation due to autoimmune reaction.

Pathology. Occlusion of distal internal carotid artery, proximal anterior and middle cerebral arteries, and sometimes basilar and proximal posterior cerebral arteries. Absence of atherosclerotic changes.

Diagnostic Procedures. *X-ray of Skull.* Usually normal. *Angiography.* Occlusion usually situated in internal carotid artery at its bifurcation; development of a large network of vessels in basal ganglia and upper brainstem areas from basilar artery and trunk of anterior and middle cerebral arteries. Marked degree of vascularization and visualization of rete mirabile. *CT brain scan.* Cerebral atrophy. *Spinal tap.* Occasionally, hemorrhagic.

Therapy. The first attempts at treatment were medical, seeking to increase blood flow pharmacologically, either by vasodilatation or reduction of blood viscosity. Today, surgical intervention is increasingly popular, and a variety of operations have been described, including cervical carotid sympathectomy and superior cervical ganglionectomy, intracranial transplantation of omentum or temporalis muscle with an intact vascular supply, direct superficial temporal artery-middle cerebral anastomosis and more recently, encephalo-duro-arterio synangiosis.

Prognosis. Serious progress to complete obstruction of most of major arterial network along base of brain that eventually stops spontaneously. Majority of patients survive with moderate or no disability. Mental retardation in one-third of children.

BIBLIOGRAPHY. Kawakita Y, Abe K, Miyata Y, et al: Spontaneous thrombosis of internal carotid artery in children. Folia Psychiatr Neurol Japn 19:245–255, 1965
Leed NE, Abbott KH: Collateral circulation in cerebro-vascular disease in childhood via rete mirabile and perforating branches of anterior choroidal and posterior cerebral arteries. Radiology 85:628–634, 1965
Maki Y, Nakata Y: Autopsy case of hemangiomatous malformation of bilateral internal carotid artery at the base of brain. Brain Nerve (Tokyo) 17:764–766, 1965
Taveras JM: Multiple progressive intracranial arterial occlusion: A syndrome of children and young adults. Am J Roentgenol Rad Ther Nucl Med 106:235–268, 1969
Yamada H: Moya-moya disease in monocular twins: case report. J Neurosurgery 53:109–112, 1980
Bingham RM, Wilkinson DJ: Anaesthetic management in moya-moya disease. Anaesthesia 40:1198–1202, 1985

MOYNAHAN'S

Synonym. XTE. See Rapp-Hodgkin.

Symptoms and Signs. Cleft palate; hypohidrosis; defective enamel; nail anomalies; hair coarse and dry; absence of eyelashes of lower lid; short-lasting skin bullae.

Etiology. Unknown; autosomal dominant inheritance.

BIBLIOGRAPHY. Moynahan E: X.T.E. (Xeroderma, talipes and enamel defect). A new heredo-familial syndrome. Two cases. Homozygous inheritance of a dominant gene. Proc Roy Soc Med 63:447–448, 1970

MUCHA-HABERMANN

Synonyms. Parapsoriasis guttata; parapsoriasis varioliformis; pityriasis lichenoides-varioliformis; varicelliform parapsoriasis; Wise's; lymphomatoid papulosis.

Symptoms and Signs. Prevalent in men; onset in adolescence and adulthood; seldom in childhood. (In childhood, acute form prevalent; in other ages chronic form more usual). *Acute.* Mild systemic manifestations occasionally may precede by 2 or 3 days; eruptions; fever; malaise; headache; joint swelling, arthralgia. Crops of edematous pinkish papules with central vesiculation and hemorrhagic necrosis evolving to superficial crusting or to scarring ulcerations. Moderate burning, or no symptoms with eruptions. Trunk, thighs, flexor sides of upper arms preferred zones; generalized form involving occasionally also palms and soles. Face and scalp usually spared. *Chronic.* Small lichenoid papules, brownish color, scaling, leaving shining brown surface. Scarring seldom. Leukoderma transitory or (seldom) permanent may follow both acute and chronic forms.

Etiology. Unknown; possibly virus or allergic vasculitis.

Pathology. Variable according to form and stage. Early

lymphocyte infiltration; dilated capillaries with endothelial proliferation. Necrotic changes. Chronic similar to resolving eczema or psoriasis.

Diagnostic Procedures. *Blood.* Exclude syphilis. *Biopsy of skin.*

Therapy. No specific treatment. *Acute.* Systemic steroids. *Chronic.* Ultraviolet light, tar preparations; or no treatment.

Prognosis. *Acute.* New crops stop appearing after a few weeks. Most cases clear in 6 months; others recur for years. *Chronic.* Scaling for 3 to 4 weeks; then clearing. Recurrence of new manifestations for years.

BIBLIOGRAPHY. Mucha V: Ueber einen der Parakeratosis variegata (Unna) bzw. Pityriasis lichenoides chronica (Neisser-Juliusberg) nahestehenden eigentüflmlichen Fall. Arch Derm Syph 123:586–592, 1916
Habermann R: Ueber die akut verlaufende, nekrotisierende Unterart der Pityriasis lichenoides (Pityriasis lichenoides et varioliformis acuta). Dermatol Z 45:42–48, 1925
Rook A, Wilkinson DS, Ebling FJG, et al: Textbook of Dermatology, 4th ed, pp 1181–1185. Oxford, Blackwell Scientific Publications, 1986

MUCKLE-WELLS

Synonym. Amyloidosis-deafness-urticaria-limb pain.

Symptoms and Signs. Both sexes affected; onset in adolescence. Recurrent attacks of urticarialike rash, with systemic manifestations; paresthesia; limb pain (aguelike bouts); pain; progressive perceptive deafness; premature loss of libido with relative infertility. Associated physical malformation: pes cavus; skin thickening; glaucoma. Nephrotic syndrome appears in middle age: *forme fruste* with one or more features missing.

Etiology. Unknown; autosomal dominant inheritance.

Pathology. Kidney small, shrivelled; adherent capsules; narrowed cortex; poor corticomedullary demarcation. Temporal bone section shows complete absence of Corti's organ and vestibular sensory epithelium; atrophy of cochlear nerve; amyloidosis.

Diagnostic Procedures. *Blood.* High sedmentation rate; polycythemia. *Urine.* Trace of reducing substances; hyperglycinuria.

Therapy. Symptomatic.

Prognosis. Progressive, ending in uremia.

BIBLIOGRAPHY. Muckle TJ, Wells M: Urticaria, deafness and amyloidosis: a new heredo-familial syndrome. Q J Med 31:235–248, 1962

Glenner GG, Ignaczak TF, Page DL: The inherited systemic amyloidoses and localized amyloid deposit. In Stanbury JB, Wyngaarden JB, Fredrickson DS: The Metabolic Basis of Inherited Disease, 4th ed, p 1331. New York, McGraw-Hill, 1978

MUCOLIPIDOSIS I

Synonyms. Lipomucopolysaccharidosis (old term); ML I; pseudo-Hurler; GAL plus disease; neuramidase deficiency.

Symptoms and Signs. Both sexes affected; present from birth. Moderate, progressive mental retardation. Skeletal abnormalities typical of dysostosis multiplex (see Hurler's).

Etiology. Unknown; familial or sporadic. Storage of both adenylosuccinic acids (AMPS) and glycolipids in lysosomes. Neuramidase deficiency.

Diagnostic Procedures. *Urine.* Moderate mucopolysacchariduria. *Fibroblast culture.* Inclusion bodies periodic acid-Schiff and sudan black positive, which stain metachromatically with toluidine blue after chloroform methanol treatment.

Therapy. Orthopedic.

Prognosis. Poor. Degenerative neuropathy, muscle wasting, hypotonic choroathetoid movements.

BIBLIOGRAPHY. Terry K, Linker A: Distinction among four forms of Hurler's syndrome. Proc Soc Exp Biol Med 115:394–402, 1964
Kelly TE, Bartoshesky L, Harris DJ, et al: Mucolipidosis I (acid neuramidase deficiency): three cases and delineation of the variability of the phenotype. Am J Dis Child 135:703–708, 1981

MUCOLIPIDOSIS IV

Synonym. ML IV.

Symptoms and Signs. Fifty percent of cases reported (17) had Ashkenazy ancestry. Corneal clouding from birth. Progressive psychomotor retardation. Skeletal dysplasia; facial anomalies; absence of hepatosplenomegaly.

Etiology. Unknown. Possibly autosomal recessive inheritance, "Inborn metabolic error still to be elucidated." Possibly ganglioside sialidase deficiency: neuramidase deficiency.

Diagnostic Procedures. *Fibroblast culture.* Lysosomal inclusions, with accumulation of 1-hyaluronic acid. Partial deficiency of ganglioside sialidase. *Electroretinogram.* In older children retinal degeneration.

Therapy. Conjunctival transplantation.

Prognosis. All cases still alive (into the 20s).

BIBLIOGRAPHY. Berman ER, Livni N, Shapiro E, et al: Congenital corneal clouding with abnormal systemic storage bodies: a new variant of mucolipidosis. J Pediatr 84:519–526, 1974
Zeigler M, Bach G: The nature of the sialidase deficiency in mucolipidosis type IV, p 78. Jerusalem, Sixth Int Congr Hum Genet, 1981
Crandall BF, Phillipart M, Brawn WJ, et al: Mucolipidosis IV. Am J Med Genet 12:301–308, 1982
Dangel ME, Bremer DL, Rogers GL: Treatment of corneal opacification in mucolipidosis IV with conjunctival transplantation. Am J Ophthalmol 99:137–141, 1985

MUELLER-KUGELBERG

Synonyms. Myopathy-Cushing's; steroid myopathy; corticosteroid myopathy. See Perkoff's.

Symptoms and Signs. Insidious onset years after the first manifestations of the endocrine disorder, Cushing's syndrome. Weakness of the pelvic girdle and thighs, minor in legs and shoulders.

Etiology. Excessive corticosteroids causing atrophy of muscle fibers.

Pathology. Muscle fiber degeneration and hyalinization. Increased fat content of muscles.

Diagnostic Procedures. *Biopsy of muscle.* See Pathology. *Electromyography.* Decreased duration and voltage; no fibrillation or pronounced irritability.

Therapy. Removal of adrenocortical tumor.

Prognosis. Complete recession of symptoms after tumor excision.

BIBLIOGRAPHY. Mueller R, Kugelberg E: Myopathy in Cushing's syndrome. J Neurol Neurosurg Psychiatry 32:314–320, 1959
Adams RD, Victor M: Principles of Neurology, 3rd ed, pp 1060–1061. New York, McGraw-Hill, 1985

MUELLER-WEISS

Synonym. Os naviculare pedis malacia. See Epiphyseal ischemic necrosis.

Symptoms. Pain in the feet enhanced by ambulation, or asymptomatic.

Etiology. Unknown.

Pathology. Symmetric malacia of os naviculare pedis.

BIBLIOGRAPHY. Mueller W: Ueber eine eigenartige doppelseitige Veraenderung des Os naviculare pedis beim Erwachsenen. Dtsch Z Chir 201:84–87, 1927
Weiss K: Ueber die "Malazie" des Os naviculare pedis. Fortschr Roentgenol 45:63–67, 1927

MUENZER-ROSENTHAL

Eponym used to indicate the triad of hallucination anxiety, catalepsy that may be found in several psychotic disorders.

BIBLIOGRAPHY. Muenzer ET: Zur Frage der symptomatischen Narkolepsie nach Enzephalitis lethargica. Mschr Psychiatr Neurol 63:97–111, 1927
Rosenthal C: Ueber das Auftreten von halluzinatorisch-kataleptischem Angstsydrom, Wachanaefallen und ählichen Storerungen bei Schizophrenen. Mschr Psychiatr Neurol 102:11–38, 1939

MULTICENTRIC RETICULOHISTIOCYTOSIS

Synonyms. Lipoid dermatoarthritis; reticulocytoma cutis.

Symptoms and Signs. Prevalent in females (3 : 1); all races affected; age of onset from 2nd to 10th decade. Gradual development of nodules in skin, mucosae, subcutaneous tissues, synovia, periostium, and bone, resulting in deforming polyarthritis. In about 25%, nodules and arthritis appear simultaneously; in 60% arthritis precedes the nodules by months or years; seldom, nodules precede arthritis. Other symptoms: weight loss; pruritus; weakness; fever; paresthesias; xanthelasma (40%): hypertension (27%); lymphadenopathy (16%).

Etiology. Unknown; granulomatous histiocytic reaction to unidentified stimulus; association with malignancies (25%) unknown if genetic or casual.

Pathology. Nodular lesions: finely vacuolated histiocytes close to small blood vessels; lymphocytes and plasma cells dispersed in the nodules; multinucleated giant cells with small vacuoles and excentric nuclei with one or two large nucleoli. Vacuoli stained by oil red (partially). Destructive arthritis.

Diagnostic Procedures. *Blood.* Hyperlipemia; all fractions increased; high beta lipoprotein. *Biopsy. X-ray.*

Therapy. Trial with adrenocorticotropic hormone (ACTH) nitrogen mustard, chlorambucil, hydroxychloroquine. Cyclophosphamide seems to bring better results.

Prognosis. In majority of cases, disease becomes spontaneously inactive after 10 years and nodules become stable or decrease. Patients are left crippled by arthritis and with leonine facies.

BIBLIOGRAPHY. Targett JH: Giant cell tumours of the integuments. Trans Pathol Soc (London) 48:230–255, 1897

Parkes-Weber F, Freudenthal W: Nodular non-diabetic cutaneous xanthomatosis with hypercholesterolemia and typical histologic features. Proc Roy Soc Med 30:522–526, 1937

Rook A, Wilkinson DS, Ebling FJG, et al: Textbook of Dermatology, 4th ed, pp 1709–1711. Oxford Blackwell Scientific Publications, 1986

MULTIFIDUS TRIANGLE

Symptoms. Single or, more frequently, recurrent attacks of sharp, localized pain followed by persistent discomfort below posterior superior iliac spine, often initiated by physical exercise (bending and twisting of lumbar spine).

Signs. Point of localized tenderness; pressure on trigger point increases pain and causes typical radiation.

Etiology and Pathology. Deep liagmentous or myofascial injury, exacerbated by trauma, inflammations. Referred to the area involved as the multifidus triangle (inferior portion of multifidus muscle).

Diagnostic Procedures. *X-ray of spine.*

Therapy. Injection of procaine or corticosteriods at trigger point.

Prognosis. Majority of attacks cured by a single injection at trigger point.

BIBLIOGRAPHY. Livingston WK: Back disabilities due to strain of multifidus muscle; cases treated by novocain injection. West J Surg 49:259–265, 1941

Bauwens P, Coyer AB: The "multifidus triangle" syndrome as a cause of recurrent low-back pain. Br Med J 2:1306–1307, 1955

MULTIPLE ENDOCRINE DEFICIENCY

Synonyms. Familial endocrinopathy-candidiasis. See Beck-Ibrahim. Candidiasis endocrinopathy, Medac multiple endocrine deficiency–autoimmune candidiasis; PGA1.

Symptoms and Signs. Both sexes affected; onset after first year of life. Chronic mucocutaneous candidiasis associated with symptoms of one (or more) endocrinopathies

(*e.g.,* hypoparathyroidism; hypothyroidism; hypoadrenalism; Hashimoto's; diabetes mellitus; ovarian failure; adrenocorticotropic hormone [ACTH] deficiency), as well as conditions such as pernicious anemia, vitiligo, premature canities, myasthenia gravis, active chronic hepatitis, pulmonary fibrosis, enamel hypoplasia, and keratoconjunctivitis.

Etiology. Autosomal recessive inheritance. Defective immunoregulation binding together the chronic mucocutaneous candidiasis, the selective IgA deficiencies, and the thyrogastric cluster of autoimmune conditions.

Pathology. Extremely variable according to the manifestations of the syndrome.

Diagnostic Procedures. *Blood.* Hypocalcemia; IgA absent; IgE elevated; polyclonal hypergammaglobulinemia. *Humoral immunity studies.* With search of antibodies to endocrine glands. *Histocompatibility profile. Other.* Enumeration of T and B lymphocytes; lymphocyte stimulation and suppressor T-cell activity. Search for biochemical changes due to various endocrine gland deficiencies and tests of hormone deficiency corrections. *X-ray.* Absence of rickets; osteomalacia (in hypoparathyroidism form). Nonspecific findings.

Therapy. Symptomatic correction of specific hormone deficiencies or of various condition clusters, and antimycotic agents.

Prognosis. Only temporary benefit from various therapeutic interventions.

BIBLIOGRAPHY. Thorpe ES, Jr, Handley HE: Chronic tetany and chronic mycelial stomatitis in a child aged four and one half years. Am J Dis Child 38:328–338, 1929

Sutphin A, Albright F, McCune DJ: Five cases (three in siblings) of idiopathic hypoparathyroidism associated with moniliasis. J Clin Endocrinol 3:625–634, 1943

Appel GB, Holub DA: The syndrome of multiple endocrine gland insufficiency. Am J Med 61:129–138, 1976

Arulananthan K, Dwyer JM, Genel M: Evidence for defective immunoregulation in the syndrome of familial candidiasis endocrinopathy. New Engl J Med 300:164–168, 1979

Ahonen P: Autoimmune polyendocrinopathycandidosis ectodermal dystrophy (APECED): Autosomal recessive inheritance. Clin Genet 27:535–542, 1985

MULTIPLE ENDOCRINE NEOPLASIA III

Synonyms. MEN III; MEN IIb, neuromata-mucosal endocrine tumors; mucosal neuroma. See also Wermer's and Sipple's.

Symptoms and Signs. Both sexes equal incidence;

may be present at birth or develop later. Fifty percent show complete syndrome of multiple neuromas (lips; tongue; eyelids), bumpy lips, pheochromocytoma, and medullary carcinoma; 7% show neuromas, pheochromocytoma, and medullary carcinoma; the others exhibit variable combinations of the above, without the pheochromocytoma. Some patients have diarrhea. Marfanoid habitus in about 50% of patients.

Etiology. Unknown; autosomal dominant inheritance. MEN III has been separated from the MEN II because of low incidence of associated parathyroid disease in these cases.

Pathology. Neuromas: masses of convoluted nerves, enveloped by thick perineurium; absence of capsule; less connective tissue than in von Recklinghausen's (see). For features of other neoplasias, see Wermer's and Sipple's.

Therapy. Surgical excision when indicated and feasible.

Prognosis. Poor.

BIBLIOGRAPHY. Braley AE: Medullated corneal nerves and plexiform neuroma associated with pheocromocytomata. Trans Am Ophthal Soc 52:189–197, 1954
Carney JA, Hayles AB, Pearse AGE, et al: Abnormal cutaneous innervation in multiple endocrine neoplasia type 2 b. Ann Intern Med 94:362–363, 1981

MULTIPLE EPIPHYSEAL DYSPLASIA TARDA

Synonyms. Multiple epiphyseal dysplasia tarda (type IV), MEDT (type IV); Orkel's.

Symptoms and Signs. Both sexes affected; normal at birth. At age of 4 or 5 ambulation problems; ankle and foot deformities; hip joint abnormally wide; bowlegs. At age 15, evidence of paraparesis; hyperactive leg reflexes; dorsal Babinski's sign; ankle clonus; visual trouble (retinitis pigmentosa).

Etiology. Autosomal recessive inheritance (?); of uncertain classification.

Diagnostic Procedures. *X-ray.* See Symptoms and Signs. *Blood and Urine.* Normal. *Ophthalmoscopy.* Retinal (retinitis pigmentosa) and vascular abnormalities.

Therapy. Orthopedic and surgical.

Prognosis. Difficulty in walking in spite of therapy. Progression of vision impairment.

BIBLIOGRAPHY. Bailey JA: Disproportionate Short Stature: Diagnosis and Management, p 429. Philadelphia, WB Saunders, 1973

MULTIPLE SCLEROSIS

Synonyms. MS; disseminated sclerosis; insular sclerosis; sclerosis, multiple; sclerose en plaques.

Symptoms. Prevalent in females; onset difficult to identify, usually between 20 and 40 years of age. Variable; multiple combinations of symptoms may represent the initial episode; because of their occasional mildness and spontaneous remission they may be forgotten or not associated with the disease. Unilateral blurring of vision; pain of the eye at rest; remission and recurrences typical, eventually resulting in central and paracentral scotoma. Attacks of double vision; trigeminal neuralgia; attacks of vertigo; intentional tremor (usually later manifestation); speech changes (usually later): slurring; long pause; monotony. Spastic paresis (80% of cases) starting with weakness, usually in legs, and "jumping of legs" at night or before falling asleep. Hemiplegia attacks; mild sensory changes; bladder disorders. Mental symptoms: deterioration; depression; hypomania; euphoria (most common symptom).

Signs. In eyes; optic disk normal or moderately hyperhemic or abnormal temporal pallor (occasional); pupillary reaction normal; nystagmus. Pathologic reflexes; abdominal reflexes absent. Atrophy of muscles (rare).

Etiology. Unknown; possibly, toxic viral, allergic or metabolic. Familial cases reported without definite genetic pattern.

Pathology. Large gray yellowish areas, consistency soft or firm, scattered throughout neuraxis from optic (II) nerve to conus medullaris, particularly in white matter. Microscopically, plaques of demyelination scattered with no perivascular distribution, and edema. In old lesion, fragmentation and destruction of axons. In recent lesion, axons are intact, microglial reaction, phagocytic cells laden with fat, perivascular round cell infiltration.

Diagnostic Procedures. *Blood, urine,* and *cerebrospinal fluid.* Normal. Occasionally, moderate pleocytosis and increase in protein of cerebrospinal fluid. *Electroencephalography.* Nonspecific changes in acute stage (90%), in subacute (68%), in remission (33%).

Therapy. No specific treatment. Symptomatic, physical therapy, good nutrition, and vitamins. Hyperbaric oxygen of some benefit, especially in early stage.

Prognosis. Remission and relapses usually with downhill course characterize the disease. Years of well-being may follow any episode. Benign form with early arrest and clinically silent forms reported. Average survival 10 to 20 years from initial episode (except in benign form). In late onset (over 40), faster evolution and shorter length of survival.

BIBLIOGRAPHY. Cruveilhier J: Anatomie pathologique du corps humain, ou descriptions avec figures lithographiées et coloriées, des diverses alterations morbides dont le corps humain est susceptible, Vol 2. Paris, Baillière, 1829–1852

Mackay RP, Hirano A: Forms of benign multiple sclerosis: Report of two "clinically silent" cases discovered at autopsy. Arch Neurol 17:588–600, 1967

Adams RD, Victor M: Principles of Neurology, 3rd ed, pp 700–711. New York, McGraw-Hill, 1985

Poser CM: MRI and CT scan in multiple sclerosis. JAMA 253:3250, 1985

Mussini JM: Sclérose en plaques. Encyclop Méd Chir Paris Neurology Fasc 17074 B–10 (3–1978)

MÜNCHAUSEN'S

Synonyms. Baron Münchausen's; factitious chronic; hospital addiction; hospital hoboes; hysterical malingering; peregrinating problem patient.

Symptoms. Male-to-female ratio 3 : 1; age range from 19 to 62 (mean 39). Subject feigns severe illness of dramatic or emergency nature; pathologic lying; aggressive, truculent, and at the same time evasive behavior; departure from hospital against medical advice; history of many hospital admissions and extensive traveling; police record and borderline drug addiction.

Signs. Evidence of many previous surgical procedures; laparotomies; cranial burr holes; evidence of interference with diagnostic procedures and self-mutilation.

Etiology. Psychopathologic entity distinct from vagrancy, self-mutilation, and malingering, but including all features of these conditions; stemming from antisocial personality, neurosis, brain damage, or unknown causes.

Pathology. Resulting from iatrogenic procedures or self-inflicted.

Diagnostic Procedures. Hypnosis may be useful to elucidate repressed affect or memories.

Therapy. No cure reported. Sympathetic attitude toward patient; long term supervision, psychotherapy, and institutionalization.

Prognosis. Patient may die of iatrogenic procedures, suicide, intercurrent real diseases; or, losing vitality, abandon hospital addiction.

BIBLIOGRAPHY. Asher R: Münchausen's syndrome. Lancet I:339–341, 1951

De Francisci G, Parisi N, Magalini SI: La sindrome di Münchausen. Il Policlinico, sezione medica 88:292–303, 1981

MURCHISON-PEL-EBSTEIN FEVER

Synonyms. Murchison-Saunderson; Pel-Ebstein fever.

Symptoms. Observed more frequently in children than in adults. Relapsing fever; intermittent periods of normal or subnormal temperature. Cycles of various length, usually 15 to 28 days, varying from patient to patient, but constant in the same patient. Sweats usually associated with pyrexia. Weakness and fatigue often out of proportion to extent of disease or anemia; weight loss.

Signs. Pulse rate usually slightly higher than expected from temperature. If lymph nodes are present, increase in size during febrile episode observed.

Etiology and Pathology. This syndrome is observed in the majority of cases associated with Hodgkin's syndrome (see); occasionally observed also with reticular cell sarcoma, some cases of malignant nephroma, other necrotic tumors, or tuberculosis.

Diagnostic Procedures. *X-ray of chest, abdomen. Skin test.* For tuberculosis. *Biopsy of lymph node.*

Therapy. Good remission with chemotherapy (nitrogen mustard or similar agent) or radiation therapy when associated with Hodgkin's disease. Cortisone and adrenocorticotropic hormone (ACTH) also control the temperature.

Prognosis. That of the disease responsible.

BIBLIOGRAPHY. Murchison C: Case of "lymphoadenoma" of the lymphatic system, etc. Trans Pathol Soc (London) 21:372–389, 1870

Pel PK: Zur Symptomatologie der sogenannten Pseudo-Leukamie. Berl Klin Wochenschr 22:3–7, 1885

Ebstein W: Das chronische Rückfallsfieber, eine neue Infektionskrankheit. Berl Klin Wochenschr 24:565; 837, 1887

MURRI'S

Synonyms. Presenile ataxia cerebellaris; parenchymatous cortical cerebellum degeneration; presenile cerebellar ataxia; toxic cerebellar degeneration. See Holmes I.

Symptoms. Prevalent in males; gradual onset in 4th to 7th decade. Difficulty in walking. Manifestation usually remains localized to legs; occasionally spreads to trunk and arms.

Signs. Hyperreflexia (occasionally); usually, absence of nystagmus.

Etiology. Uncertain; toxic factor (primarily alcohol); heart; stroke; malignancy; chronic gastrointestinal diseases; hereditary familial trait; subacute form reported with Hodgkin's. Question of nutritional cause considered.

Pathology. Cerebellar atrophy: loss of Purkinje cells and preservation of basket cells; granular and molecular layer of cerebellum sparse.

Diagnostic Procedures. *Electroencephalography. Angiography. Echoencephalography. Brain isotope scan. Spinal fluid.* Increase in protein; lymphocytic pleocytosis. *CT brain scan.*

Therapy. Symptomatic.

Prognosis. Progressive course from 1 to 15 years. Spontaneous arrest occasionally observed, especially if patient abstains from alcohol. In idiopathic form, subacute or chronic course.

BIBLIOGRAPHY. Murri A: Degeneratione cerebellare da intossicazione endogena. Riv Crit Clin Med 1:593; 609, 1900

Vick NA: Grinker's Neurology, 7th ed. Springfield, Ill, CC Thomas, 1976

Adams Rook A, Wilkinson DS, Ebling FJG, et al: Textbook of Dermatology, 4th ed, pp 1823, 2461. Oxford, Blackwell Scientific Publications, 1986

MUSCULOAPONEUROTIC FIBROMATOSIS

Synonym. Desmoid tumor.

Symptoms and Signs. Prevalent in women (70%); onset in 3rd to 5th decade, frequently after pregnancy. Tender, firm, subcutaneous mass arising usually from muscular aponeurosis of lower abdominal wall, and progressively spreading.

Etiology. Unknown; possibly, trauma, endocrine factors. Reported in association with Gardner's (see).

Pathology. Gray white, not encapsulated, consistent mass that invades the muscle. Histologically, fibroblast proliferation and infiltration, areas of mucoid degeneration.

Diagnostic Procedures. *Biopsy. Bioassay.* Could reveal elevated levels of estrogenic and gonadotropic hormones.

Therapy. Wide surgical excision.

Prognosis. Cured by surgery. No metastasis.

BIBLIOGRAPHY. Thorbjarnarson B, Pack GT, et al (eds): Treatment of Cancer and Allied Diseases, Vol 8. New York, Hoeber, 1964

Rook A, Wilkinson DS, Ebling FJG, et al: Textbook of Dermatology, 4th ed, pp 1823, 2461. Oxford, Blackwell Scientific Publications, 1986

MYCOBACTERIA-ATYPICA

Synonym. Aplastic anemia-mycobacteria.

Symptoms. Prolonged disease with remissions and relapses. Fever; weight loss; sweating; anorexia; pulmonary infections.

Signs. Pallor; hepatomegaly or splenomegaly or both; adenopathy.

Etiology. Congenital defect (autosomal recessive type) of monocytes function activity, that are unable to protect against mycobacterial agents.

Pathology. Miliary pulmonary infiltrates (30% of cases); other pulmonary infections common. Osteolytic infections; noncaseating granulomas in lymph nodes, pancreas, spleen, liver, and kidney.

Diagnostic Procedures. *Blood.* Severe anemia; thrombocytopenia; leukopenia with neutropenia (occasionally, leukocytosis). *Bone marrow.* Generally hypoplastic or increased erythropoiesis (in cases with leukocytosis-hyperplastic). Bone marrow culture for mycobacteria. *Skin test* (PPD). Negative or mildly positive.

Therapy. Patients respond poorly or not at all to antitubercular therapy, corticosteroids, splenectomy, or radiation.

Prognosis. Poor; death within 2 to 3 years.

BIBLIOGRAPHY. Engback HC: Three cases in the same family of fatal infection of M. avium. Acta Tuber Scand 45:105–117, 1964

Kilbridge TM, Gonnella JS, Bolan JT: Pancytopenia and death. Arch Intern Med 120:38–46, 1967

Uchiyama N, Greene GR, Warren BJ, et al: Possible monocyte killing defect in familial atypical mycobacteriosis. J Pediatr 98:785–788, 1981

MYELOFIBROSIS

Synonyms. Osteopathia condensans disseminata-myeloid-megakaryocytic hepatosplenomegaly; chronic nonleukemic myelosis (see Myeloproliferative syndromes); agnogenic myeloid metaplasia; Vaughan's; Harrison-Vaughan.

Symptoms. Both sexes affected; onset usually after 5th decade; very rare in childhood. Insidious onset. Weakness; fatigue; weight loss; anorexia; left quadrant or generalized abdominal discomfort. Mild hemorrhagic manifestations.

Signs. Pallor; splenomegaly; frequently hepatomegaly; seldom, moderate lymphadenopathy.

Etiology. Unknown.

Pathology. Spleen huge; liver usually enlarged; myeloid metaplasia is found in spleen, liver, renal capsules, and lymph nodes. Increased bony trabeculae and replacement of marrow space by connective tissue, with few scattered areas of hematopoiesis.

Diagnostic Procedures. *Blood.* Normocytic (seldom macrocytic) anemia of variable degree; seldom, polycythemia, reticulocytosis, polychromatophilia. Occasionally, nucleated red cells. Leukocytes initially normal (40%), elevated (40%, seldom 50,000), decreased (20%); immature cells occasionally found; increased basophils. Leukocyte alkaline phosphatase elevated. Uric acid high; hyperbilirubinemia moderate. Platelet normal or decreased; occasionally, giant platelets or megakaryocyte fragment. *Bone marrow.* Increased bone consistency, usually dry tap. *Biopsy of bone.* Typical feature (see Pathology). *Splenic puncture.* Myeloid hyperplasia. *X-ray of bone.* Typical findings.

Therapy. Symptomatic. Androgens. Busulfan, splenic radiation, or splenectomy only when splenic symptoms including hemolysis are overwhelming.

Prognosis. Usually, slow progressive course leading to death after 1 to 33 years. A "malignant" form with rapid evolution described.

BIBLIOGRAPHY. Heuck, G: Zwei Faelle von Leukämie mit eigent-hünlichen Blut-Resp Knochenmarksbefunde. Virchows Arch Pathol Anat 78:475–496, 1879
Meyer E, Heineke A: Ueber Blutbildung bei schweren Anaemien und Leukaemie. Dtsch Arch Klin Med 88:435–492, 1907
Stephens DJ, Bredek JF: A leukemic myelosis with osteosclerosis. Ann Intern Med 6:1087–1096, 1933
Vaughan JM: Leuco-erythroblastic anaemic. J Pathol Bacteriol 42:541–564, 1936
Vaughan JM, Harrison CV: Leukoerythroblastic anaemia and myelosclerosis. J Pathol Bacteriol 48:339–352, 1939
Oberling F: Myélosclérose primitive. In Encyclopedie Medico Chirurgicale. Paris, Sang 130 II D 10 (4-1986).

MYELOPROLIFERATIVE, FAMILIAL

Symptoms. Familial occurrence; onset before 4th birthday. Weakness; respiratory infections; bleeding; distended abdomen; poor growth; vomiting.

Signs. Pallor; purpura, marked splenomegaly; hepatomegaly; retarded growth.

Etiology. Unknown; only one family reported with this very rare disease. Nine children, 1st or 2nd cousins, are affected by it. This condition does not fit with any other known myeloproliferative disorder. Appears to be transmitted by an autosomal dominant inheritance with variable penetrance.

Pathology. Bone marrow: see Diagnostic procedures. Liver and spleen do not reveal typical leukemic infiltration, but only extramedullary hematopoiesis.

Diagnostic Procedures. *Blood.* Anemia; leukocytosis (25,000 to 100,000) with immature granulocytes. Leukocytes and alkaline phosphatase low; Philadelphia chromosome not found; thrombocytopenia. *Bone marrow.* Simulating myelogenous leukemia without characteristic predominance of one-cell stage. Erythroid hyperplasia. Reverting to normal as patient grows older.

Therapy. No response to antileukemic agents. Secondary hypersplenism corrected by splenectomy.

Prognosis. Variable course; acute with death, or chronic with complete recovery.

BIBLIOGRAPHY. Randall DL, Reignam CW, Githens JH, et al: Familial myeloproliferative disease (a new syndrome closely simulating myelogenous leukemia in childhood). Am J Dis Child 110:479–500, 1965

MYELOPROLIFERATIVE SYNDROMES

Included in this category are all the idiopathic persistent proliferations in the bone marrow of erythroid, myeloid, megakaryocytic, or fibroblastic types, singly or in various combinations with corresponding changes in peripheral blood. This group includes Vaquez-Osler (see), myelofibrosis (see), chronic myelocytic leukemia, primary thrombocythemia and intermediate forms (see DiGuglielmo's) including combinations with multiple myeloma.

BIBLIOGRAPHY. Dameshek W: Some speculations on the myeloproliferative syndromes. Blood 6:372–375, 1951
Lopas H, Josephson AM: Myeloproliferative syndrome: evaluation of myelosclerosis and chronic myelogenous leukemia to polycythemia vera. Arch Intern Med 114:754–759, 1964
Wintrobe MM (ed): Clinical Hematology, 8th ed. Philadelphia, Lea & Febiger, 1981

MYOSITIS, LOCALIZED

Symptoms and Signs. Muscle tenderness; enlargement and induration of all or part of a muscle.

Etiology. Inflammatory reaction secondary to injury to muscle fibers and connective sheaths.

Pathology. Inflammatory cells infiltrating regenerated muscle fibers and connective tissue.

Diagnostic Procedures. *Biopsy of muscle.*

Therapy. None specific.

Prognosis. Subsidence of the condition with residual permanent pseudocontraction of the affected muscle.

BIBLIOGRAPHY. Adams RD, Denny-Brown D, Pearson CM: Diseases of the Muscles, 3rd ed, p 367. New York, Harper & Row, 1975

Adams RK, Kakulas BA: Diseases of Muscle: Pathological Foundations of Clinical Myology, 4th ed. Philadelphia, Harper & Row, 1985

MYOTUBULAR MYOPATHY

Synonym. Centronuclear myopathy.

Symptoms and Signs. Both sexes affected; onset at birth or in early childhood. Ptosis; symmetric weakness of limbs (in one case, facial diplegia).

Etiology. Unknown; familial incidence; both autosomal recessive and dominant inheritance.

Pathology. In muscle, variation in size of fiber, increase of internal nuclei. Abnormal cell resembling myotube seen in muscle specimen from fetus (between 12 and 20 weeks' gestation).

Diagnostic Procedures. *Biopsy of muscle* (see Pathology). *Electromyography.* Myopathy pattern. *Blood, urine.* Not contributory.

Therapy. Symptomatic.

Prognosis. Usually progressive. Improvement reported.

BIBLIOGRAPHY. Spiro AJ, Shy GM, Gonatas NK: Myotubular myopathy. Arch Neurol 14:1–14, 1966

Kinoshita M, Cadman TE: Myotubular myopathy. Arch Neurol 18:265–271, 1968

Pavone L, Mollica F, Grasso A, et al: Familial centronuclear myopathy. Acta Neurol Scand 62:33–40, 1980

MYXEDEMA-COMA

Symptoms and Signs. Prevalent in females. In hypothyroid patients, infections are usually precipitating cause; other causes; anesthesia; drugs. Hypothermia, hypotension, cardiac failure progressing to shock, coma.

Etiology. Inability to cope with stress; adrenal insufficiency.

Pathology. That of hypothyroidism.

Diagnostic Procedures. *Blood.* Sodium and chloride low. *Urine.* 17-ketosteroids low. Usually no time to do studies because emergency treatment required.

Therapy. Triiodothyronine (10 to 25 mcg or more) by gastric tube or parenterally every 8 hours, or sodium levothyroxine (Synthroid, 200 to 400 mcg intravenously and 100 to 200 mcg/24 hr). Hydrocortisone (100 mg) every 8 hours. Do not warm the patient. Provide ventilation.

Prognosis. Very poor; high mortality.

BIBLIOGRAPHY. LeMarquand HS, Hausmann W, Hemsted EH: Myxoedema as a cause of death: report of two cases. Br Med J 1:704–706, 1953

Catz B, Russell S: Myxedema, shock and coma. Arch Intern Med 108:407–417, 1961

Murkin JM: Anesthesia and hypothyroidism: a review of thyroxine physiology, pharmacology, and anesthetic implications. Anesth Analg 61:371–383, 1982

Mazzaferri EL: The thyroid. In Mazzaferri EL (ed), Textbook of Endocrinology. pp 236–238. Med Exam Pub Co, New York, 1985

MYXEDEMA, JUVENILE

Synonyms. Juvenile hypothyroidism. See also Gul's and Cryptothyroidism.

Symptoms and Signs. Both sexes affected, onset in adolescence. After a period of normal growth and mental development, variable slowing of growth, from complete to mild delay. Dentition delayed; constipation; placid behavior (often considered normal and pleasant by parents). Puberty delayed or, occasionally, isosexual maturation may be precocious.

Etiology. Associated with defects in thyroid hormone synthesis (presence of goiter) or exhaustion atrophy of small amounts of aberrant thyroid tissue (see Cryptothyroidism) or examples of Hashimoto's (see).

Pathology. See Etiology.

Diagnostic Procedures. *Blood.* T_4; T_3; thyroid antibodies; thyroid-stimulating hormone (TSH) and, eventually, measurements of other pituitary hormones (e.g., gonadotropins, prolactin).[131] *I uptake X-ray.* Sella turcica normal; bone age and growth delayed.

Therapy. Thyroid hormone by slow, gradual increases up to needed dose.

Prognosis. Optimal response to a well-conducted treatment. Growth resumes; obesity and myxedematous changes revert. Precocious puberty, including galactorrhea, also reverts.

BIBLIOGRAPHY. Mazzaferri EL: The thyroid. In Mazzaferri EL (ed), Textbook of Endocrinology. pp. 238–241. Med Exam Pub Co, New York, 1985

MYXEDEMA, NODULAR-THYROTOXICOSIS

Symptoms and Signs. Occur in patients with thyrotoxicosis. Appearance of nonpitting, elevated plaques on the skin of lower extremities (seldom upper extremities) after onset of thyrotoxicosis or more frequently after thyroidectomy. Hypertrophic osteoarthropathy may also be associated.

Etiology. Unknown.

Pathology. Thyroid; see Flajani's. Typical skin changes for myxedema.

Therapy. None.

Prognosis. Lesion persists despite thyroidectomy or thyroid administration after surgery.

BIBLIOGRAPHY. Sollier P: Maladie de Basedow avec Myxoédeme. Rev Med 11:1000–1013, 1891

Cohen BC, Benua RS, Rawson RW: Localized myxedema involving upper extremity. Arch Intern Med 111:641–645, 1963

MYXEDEMATOUS, CEREBELLAR

Synonyms. Hypothyroidism-cerebellar ataxia; ataxia cerebellaris-myxedema; cerebellar ataxia-myxedema.

Symptoms and Signs. Occur in patients with hypothyroidism. Signs of myxedema and cerebellar symptoms (ataxia; incoordination) appearing at the same time or years after onset of myxedema.

Etiology. Thyroid hormone deficiency.

Pathology. That of myxedema.

Diagnostic Procedures. *Thyroid function.*

Therapy. Thyroid hormone.

Prognosis. Cerebellar symptoms and signs disappear after 2 to 3 weeks of treatment.

BIBLIOGRAPHY. White EW: Myxoedema associated with insanity. Lancet I:974–976, 1884

Jellinek EH, Kelly RE: Cerebellar syndrome in myxoedema. Lancet II:225–227, 1960

Cremer GM, Goldstein NP, Paris J: Myxedema and ataxia. Neurology 19:37–46, 1969

NAEGELI'S

Synonyms. Chromatophore nevus; Franceschetti-Jadassohn; hyperhidrosis-skin pigmentation-keratosis pilaris-enamel dysplasia; Jadassohn Franceschetti; melanophoric nevus.

Symptoms. Both sexes affected with equal frequency, onset in 2nd or 3rd year of life. Development of reticular pigmentation (in fine network) that becomes generalized, without preliminary inflammatory changes. Usually, keratoderma and hypohidrosis of palms and soles. Temperature regulation may be disturbed by reduction of number of sweat glands. Hair, nails normal. Teeth normal or defective with yellow spotting. Nystagmus, strabismus, and optic atrophy.

Etiology. Unknown; autosomal dominant inheritance (rare).

Diagnostic Procedure. *Biopsy of skin.*

Therapy. None.

Prognosis. Progressive condition. Mental and physical development normal.

BIBLIOGRAPHY. Naegeli O: Familiärer Chromatophore-naevus. Schweiz Med Wochenschr 57:48, 1927

Franceschetti A, Jadassohn W: "A propos de l'incontinentia pigmenti" delimitation de deux syndromes différents figurants sous le même terme. Dermatologica 108:1–28, 1954

Sparrow GP, Samman PD, Wells RS: Hyperpigmentation and hypohidrosis. (The Naegeli-Franceschetti-Jadassohn syndrome): report of a family and review of literature. Clin Exp Derm 1:127–140, 1976

NAGER-REYNIER

Synonyms. Mandibulofacial dysostosis: acrofacial dysostosis. See Treacher-Collins and Franceschetti-Klein.

Symptoms and Signs. Bilateral hypoplasia of mandibular ascending ramus; aplasia of temporomandibular joint; atresia of external auditory canal, frequently, with cleft palate and without lid anomalies or macrostomia. Thumbs hypoplastic or absent; radius and ulna may be fused or one of the two may be absent.

Etiology. Unknown. Autosomal inheritance suggested.

Therapy. Avulsion of abnormally implanted teeth and protheses.

BIBLIOGRAPHY. Nager FR, de Reynier JP: Das Gehoerorgan bei den angeborenen Kopfmissbildung. Pract Otorhinolaryngol (Basel) (suppl 2) 10:1–128, 1948

Halal F, Herrmann J, Pallister P, et al: Differential diagnosis of Nager acrofacial dysostosis syndrome: report of four patients with Nager syndrome and discussion of other related syndromes. Am J Med Genet 14:209–224, 1983

Thompson E, Cadbury R, Baraitser M: The Nager acrofacial dysostosis syndrome with tetralogy of Fallot. J Med Genet 22:408–410, 1985

Chemke J, Mogilner BM, Ben-Itzhak I, et al: Autosomal recessive inheritance of Nager acrofacial dysostosis. J Med Genet 25:230–232, 1988

NANCE-HORAN

Synonyms. Brachymetacarpia-cataract-mesiodens; cataract-dental; mesiodens-cataract.

Symptoms and Signs. Both sexes affected; present from birth. *Male.* Supernumerary central incisor (mesiodens); incisors screwdriverlike; cataract posterior suture microcornea; short 4th metacarpals. *Female heterozygous.* Punctate cataracts; diastemata; incisor teeth with edges narrower than normal (Hutchinsonlike).

Etiology. X-linked inheritance.

Diagnostic Procedure. *Blood.* Serum alkaline phosphatase elevated.

BIBLIOGRAPHY. Nance WE, Warburg M, Bixler D, et al: Congenital sex-linked cataract, dental anomalies, and brachymetacarpalia. Birth Defects 10:285–291, 1974

Horan MB, Billson FH: X-linked cataract and Hutchinsonian teeth. Aust Paediatr J 10:98–102, 1974

Bixler D, Higgins M, Hartfield J Jr. The Nance-Horan syndrome: a rare X-linked ocular-dental trait with expression in heterozygous females. Clin Genet 26:30–35, 1984

NANCE-SWEENEY

Synonyms. Nance's dwarfism; chondrodystrophy-sensineural deafness; Nance-Insley; otospondylomegaepiphyseal dysplasia, OSMED.

Symptoms and Signs. Both sexes. Deafness. Rhizomelic micromelia; ear deformities; saddle nose; thin hair; thick leathery skin; soft tissue calcification. Cleft palate, occasionally.

Etiology. Autosomal recessive inheritance.

Diagnostic Procedure. *X-ray.* Scoliosis; flattened base of skull; cartilage calcifications; achondroplasia-type deformity of pelvis.

Prognosis. Deafness severe and progressing. Adult height 120 cm.

BIBLIOGRAPHY. Nance WE, Sweeney A: A recessively inherited chondrodystrophy. Birth Defects 6:25–27; 1970
Insley J, Astley R: A bone dysplasia with deafness. Br J Radiol 47:244–251, 1974
Miny P, Lenz W: Autosomal recessive deafness with skeletal dysplasia and facial appearance of Marshall syndrome. Am J Med Genet 21:317–324, 1985

NARCOLEPSY AND DIABETOGENIC HYPERINSULINISM

Synonyms. Chronic refractory fatigue; euthyroid hypometabolism; hyperinsulinism-narcolepsy; hypothyroid hypometabolism; metabolic obesity; psychosomatic obesity. See Pickwickian.

Symptoms. Family history of narcolepsy (48%). Irresistible drowsiness with pathologic and inappropriate sleep (100%); cataplexy (50%); usually following sudden emotion; hypnagogic hallucination (56%); sleep paralysis (49%); inability to move on awaking or predormitum. Frequently associated, vascular headache (65%) (see cluster headache syndrome), peripheral neuropathy, especially of lower limbs (34%), spontaneous leg cramps (37%) (see Wittmaak-Ekbon). Angina pectoris and arrhythmias (32%). Psychiatric features; anxiety and depression.

Signs. Obesity (75%); therapeutic response to trial of analeptic agent (100%). Frequently associated; recurrent edema (50%), *cafe au lait* spots (29%); occipital nevus and white forelock.

Etiology. Hypoglycemia related to feeding habit; narcoleptic hypokinesia; accelerated lipogenesis related to chronic hyperinsulinism; deranged nervous system function.

Pathology. Obesity.

Diagnostic Procedures. *Blood.* Glucose determination with fasting; morning glucose tolerance test; afternoon glucose tolerance test. Insulin and insulinlike activity determination. Electrolytes; cholesterol; uric acid; protein bound iodine. *Urine.* Volume (diurnal and nocturnal collection). *Pulmonary function tests. Electrocardiography. Electroencephalography metabolic rate. Pharmacologic studies.* (1) Methylphenidate hydrochloride; (2) insulin; (3) tolbutamide; (4) liothyronine.

Therapy. Diet (gradual decrease); moderate exercise; analeptics (ritalin). If diabetes, treat; if prediabetic state, institute preventive measures. Avoid needless administration of thyroid; decrease fluid intake; avoid therapeutic fasting.

Prognosis. Good response to treatment; realistic weight reduction and analeptics.

BIBLIOGRAPHY. Roberts HJ: Obesity due to the syndrome of narcolepsy and diabetogenic hyperinsulinism: clinical and therapeutic observations on 252 patients. J Am Geriatr Soc 15:721–743, 1967

NARCOLEPTIC TETRAD

Includes narcolepsy, cataplexy, sleep paralysis, and hypnagogic hallucinosis. See Gelineau's.

NÉKAM'S

Synonyms. Keratosis lichenoides chronica; porokeratosis striata lichenoides; lichen ruber moniliformis; lichen verucosus et reticularis. Morbus Moniliformis Lichenoides.

Symptoms and Signs. *Face.* Seborrheic dermatitis-like eruption. *Limbs.* Violaceus papular and nodular lesions in linear and reticulate pattern most marked on hands and feet.

Etiology. Unknown.

Pathology. Nonspecific. Unusual variant of lichen planus.

Therapy. Favorable response to photochemotherapy.

BIBLIOGRAPHY. Kaposi M, Lichen Ruber Planus. p 571 Vierteljahr, 1886
Nékam L. Lichen moniliformis. Presse Med. 46:1000, 1938
Rook A, Wilkinson DS, Ebling FJG, et al: Textbook of Dermatology, 4th ed, p 1682. Oxford, Blackwell Scientific Publications, 1986

NELATON'S

Synonyms. Acro-osteolysis; mutilating ulcer; acropathy Denny-Brown's; neuropathy, hereditary sensory-radicular; hereditary, sensory, autonomic neuropathy, HSAN I; Hicks'; Thevenard's.

Symptoms and Signs. Onset at puberty. Ulceration of the soles of feet. Occasionally development of "elephant foot." In some cases later extension to upper extremities. Sensory disturbance of lower extremities; hypoesthesia or total anesthesia, or thermoanalgesia. Vasomotor troubles; hyperhidrosis; decreased oscillometry and Döppler determination; occasionally, progressive deafness.

Etiology. Autosomal dominant or X-linked recessive inheritance.

Pathology. Trophic ulceration of foot; osteoporosis and compression of metatarsals and phalanges.

Diagnostic Procedure. *X-ray of feet.*

Therapy. Symptomatic; amputation sometimes required.

Prognosis. Successive attacks with intermittent periods of various length. Danger of infections.

BIBLIOGRAPHY. Hicks EP: Hereditary perforating ulcer of the foot. Lancet I:319–321, 1922

Nélaton A: Affection singulière des os du pied. Gaz Hop 4:13, 1852

Thevenard A: L'acropathie ulcero-mutilante familiale. Rev Neurol (Paris) 74:193–212, 1942

Denny-Brown D: Hereditary sensory neuropathy. J Neurol 14:237–252, 1951

Danon MJ, Carpenter S: Hereditary sensory neuropathy: biopsy study of an autosomal dominant variety. Neurology 35:1226–1229, 1985

NELSON'S

See Addisonian syndromes.

Symptoms and Signs. Occur in patients with adrenal hyperplasia; onset 6 months to 12 years after adrenalectomy. Deep pigmentation of the skin and mucosae, restricted visual fields, and other neurologic signs of pituitary tumor.

Etiology. Chromophobe tumor of the hypophysis developing after removal of hypertrophic adrenal. Excessive secretion of adreno corticotropic hormone (ACTH) and beta-lipotropin.

Pathology. Chromophobe tumor of the hypophysis.

Diagnostic Procedures. *X-ray of skull. Blood.* Plasma ACTH level.

Therapy. Radiation of hypophysis or hypophysectomy Nivazol.

Prognosis. Fair; pigmentation and other neurologic and metabolic signs may respond to treatment.

BIBLIOGRAPHY. Nelson DH, Meakin JW, Thorn GW: ACTH-producing pituitary tumors following adrenalectomy for Cushing's syndrome. Ann Intern Med 52:560–569, 1960

Nelson DH: Cushing's syndrome. In De Groot LJ, Cahill FG Jr, Odell WD, et al (ed), Endocrinology, p 1187. New York, Grune & Stratton, 1979

Kasperlik-Zaluska AA, Nielubowicz J, Wislawski J, et al: Nelson's syndrome: incidence and prognosis. Clin Endocrinol (OxG) 19:693–698, 1983

Ball JA, Williams G, Yeo TH, Joplin GF: Effect of nivazol in Nelson's syndrome. Postgraduate Med J 64:220–221, 1988

NEMALINE MYOPATHIES

Synonym. Rod body myopathy. See Floppy infant syndromes.

EARLY ONSET TYPE

Symptoms. Onset at birth. Delayed motor development; proximal limb weakness.

Signs. Reduced muscle bulk; muscle hypotonia. Reflexes usually absent, normal in some cases. Associated malformations; high palate; pigeon breast; pes cavus; kyphosis or scoliosis.

Etiology. Unknown; autosomal dominant and possibly recessive inheritance.

Pathology. In muscles, 20 to 40% of fibers affected. Fibers containing variable amount of rods or filamentous formation. Nuclei of affected cell vesicular with prominent nucleoli.

Diagnostic Procedures. *Biopsy of muscle* (see Pathology). *Blood.* Creatine index increased, serum glutamicoxaloacetic transaminase (SGOT) normal. *Urine.* Aminoacid excretion normal. *Electromyography.* Decreased duration of potentials.

Therapy. Symptomatic.

Prognosis. Static weakness; unexplained death reported in some cases.

LATE ONSET TYPE

Symptoms. Both sexes affected; onset in 4th to 6th decade in reported cases. Occur in subjects previously well and without developmental abnormalities. Gradual onset of distal leg or pelvic girdle weakness, progressing to affect proximal part and then distal part of all limbs and neck flexors.

Signs. Muscle hypotonia, some wasting. Reflexes usually normal or decreased.

Etiology. Unknown; nonfamilial (or clinical variant of the above). Nonspecific reaction of Z band to various insults.

Pathology. See Early onset type.

Diagnostic Procedures. See Early onset type.

Therapy. Symptomatic.

Prognosis. Progressive course.

BIBLIOGRAPHY. Shy GM, Engel WK, Somers JE, et al: Nemaline myopathy: A new congenital myopathy. Brain 86:793–810, 1963
Heffernan LP, Rewcastle NB, Humphrey JG: The spectrum of rod myopathies. Arch Neurol 18:529–542, 1968
McMemamin JB, Curry B, Taylor GP, et al: Fatal nemaline myopathy in infancy. J Neurol Sci 11:305–309, 1984
Roig M, Hernandez Ma, Salcedo S: Survival from symptomatic nemaline myopathy in the newborn period. Pediatr Neurosci 13:95–97, 1987

NEOCEREBELLAR

Synonym. Posterior cerebellar lobe.

Symptoms and Signs. Both sexes affected; onset at all ages. Generalized or homolateral hypotonia; pendular reflexes; static tremor; during voluntary movements, disturbance in station, past-pointing, and spontaneous deviation of limbs; gait disturbances (deviation and tendency to fall toward side of lesion); asthenia; delay in starting and stopping muscular contractions; dysmetria; adiadochokinesia; speech disturbances: slow, monotonous, scanning; later, utterance, jerkiness, explosiveness; disturbances in writing.

Etiology and Pathology. Neoplastic vascular, inflammatory, or traumatic lesion of posterior lobe or of lateral part of cerebellum.

Diagnostic Procedures. *Angiography. CT brain scan. Spinal tap.*

Therapy. Surgery if indicated.

Prognosis. Depends on etiology.

BIBLIOGRAPHY. Holmes G: The symptoms of acute cerebellar injuries due to gunshot injuries. Brain 40:461–535, 1917
Bremer F: Le cervelet. In Roger GH, Benet L: Traite de Physiologie Normale et Pathologique, Vol 10, Pt 1–2. Paris, Masson, 1935

Dow RS, Moruzzi G: The Physiology and Pathology of the Cerebellum. Minneapolis, University of Minnesota Press, 1958

NEONATAL HEPATITIS

Synonyms. Giant cell hepatitis; thick bile.

Symptoms and Signs. Both sexes affected; at birth infant appears normal. In first weeks of life becomes icteric. Hepatomegaly develops. Slow weight gain and thriving. Hemorrhagic tendency may develop. Frequently, splenomegaly.

Etiology. Unknown in 70% of cases. In other cases: infective; genetic-metabolic defects; chromosomal abnormalities; toxins; various cholestatic conditions. *Familial form.* Probably autosomal recessive inheritance, with manifestation extremely variable from very severe to very mild.

Pathology. In liver; multinuclear giant cells, cholestasis, and occasionally fibrosis.

Diagnostic Procedures. *Blood and urine.* Standard tests of liver function abnormal, but do not distinguish various forms of the syndrome; general evidence of cholestasis. *Biopsy of liver.* Pathologic findings are diagnostic.

Therapy. Symptomatic.

Prognosis. Long-term studies still lacking; 6 to 12 months after recovery, two-thirds in good health; in the rest, signs of cirrhosis or dead.

BIBLIOGRAPHY. Craig JM, Landing BH: Form of hepatitis in neonatal period simulating biliary atresia. Arch Pathol 54:321–333, 1952
Aagenaes O, Van Der Hagen CB, Refsum S: Hereditary recurrent intrahepatic cholestasis from birth. Arch Dis Child 43:646–657, 1968
Sandor T, Surinya M, Monus Z: Familial occurrence of giant cell hepatitis in infancy. Acta Hepato-Gastroent 23:101–104, 1976
Steinhoff MC: Neonatal sepsis and infections. In Reese RE, Gordon D R Jr, A Practical Approach to Infectious Diseases. p 75. Boston, Little, Brown, 1986

NEONATAL LUPUS ERYTHEMATOSUS

Synonym. Congenital heart block.

Symptoms and Signs. In newborns of mothers with lupus erythematosus, more frequent in females. Petechiae, hemorrhages, pneumonitis, splenomegaly, cutaneus lupus lesions from 2nd to 6th month of life: macules, papules, plaques; congenital heart block, with associated malformation (transposition of great vessels). Hemolytic anemia.

Etiology. Due to antibodies present in mother that pass to fetus and determine inflammatory myocarditis (causing endocardial fibroelastosis and atrioventricular block). Possibly antibodies involved are SS-A (Ro) and SS-B (La) (RNA protein complexes).

Pathology. *Heart.* Replacement of atrial septal musculature by elastic, fibrous, and adipose tissue

Diagnostic Procedures. *Blood.* Thrombocytopenia, anemia; presence of lupus markers (see SLE), leukopenia.

Therapy. Permanent pacemaker. Plasmapheresis during pregnancy. Surgery.

Prognosis. In some cases progression to adult SLE, in others resolution.

BIBLIOGRAPHY. McCuistion CH, Schoch EP Jr: Possible discoid lupus erythematosus in newborn infants. Arch Derm Syph 70:782–785, 1954
Watson RM, Lane AT, Barnett NK, et al: Neonatal lupus erythematosus: a chemical serological and immunogenetic study with review of the literature. Medicine 63:362–378, 1984
Neonatal lupus syndrome. Editorial. Lancet II:489–490, 1987

NEONATAL POLYCYTHEMIA

Synonyms. Neonatal erythrocytosis; neonatal plethora.

Symptoms and Signs. By 3rd day after birth, cyanosis, little or no cardiorespiratory distress, occasionally, cardiomegaly (50%). Myoclonic jerks may be present. Moderate hepatosplenomegaly occasionally. Systolic murmur (+), second heart sound normal or slightly increased in intensity, splitting, variable or fixed, narrow or wide. All cardiovascular changes are transient.

Etiology. Different conditions may be responsible for the neonatal polycythemia. (1) *Polycythemia with hypervolemia.* (a) Twin-to-twin transfusion (see); (b) transfusion maternal-fetal in utero (see); (c) placental transfusion (delay in clamping cord); (d) diabetes in mother; (e) congenital cardiopulmonary defects. (2) *Polycythemia without hypervolemia.* (a) Placental insufficiency; (b) erythrocytosis, benign familial (see); (c) congenital adrenal hyperplasia with polycythemia; (d) chronic fetal hypoxia.

Pathology. Transitory polycythemia.

Diagnostic Procedures. *Blood.* High hematocrit and hemoglobin level; nucleated erythrocytes; fetal hemoglobin level, beta-alpha-globulin determination; differential red-cell agglutination. *Serial electrocardiography.* Transient and not constant abnormalities. *X-ray of chest.*

Therapy. Continuous oxygen treatment (decreases red cell volume and depresses bone marrow activity); digitalis; phlebotomy when respiratory distress requires.

Prognosis. Excellent: spontaneous or therapeutic remission. Cardiovascular abnormalities disappear after decrease of polycythemia. In some cases, brain damage may result with neurologic sequelae.

BIBLIOGRAPHY. Chaptal J, Jean R, Izarn P, et al: La polyglobulie pathologique néonatale: a propos de cinq observations. Pédiatrie 13:515–525, 1958
Tchernia G, Dreyfus M: Hématologie neo-natale. Encycl Méd Chir (Paris) Sang 13050 a 10 (11, 1979)
Rosenkrantz TS, Oh W: Neonatal polycythemia and hyperviscosity. In Milunsky A, Friedman EA, Gluck L, et al: Advances in Perinatal Medicine. Vol 5, p 93. Plenum Medical Book Co, New York, 1986

NEOPLASTIC PORPHYRIA TARDA

Synonym. Porphyria cutanea tarda-hepatic tumor.

Symptoms and Signs. Those of porphyria cutanea tarda (see).

Etiology. Hepatic tumor exhibiting defect of porphyrin metabolism.

Pathology. Benign or malignant primary tumor of the liver, not associated with cirrhosis. Fluorescence limited to tumoral tissue.

Diagnostic Procedures. See Porphyria cutanea tarda.

Therapy. Surgical excision of tumor.

Prognosis. Disappearance of all symptoms of porphyria tarda after removal of neoplastic tissue.

BIBLIOGRAPHY. Kordac V: Frequency of occurrence of hepatocellular carcinoma in patients with porphyria cutanea tarda in long-term follow-up. Neoplasia 19:135–139, 1972
Kappas A, Sassa S, Anderson KE: The porphyrias. In Stanbury JB, Wyngaarden JB, Fredrickson DS, et al: The Metabolic Basis of Inherited Disease. 5th ed, p 1301. New York, McGraw-Hill, 1983

NEPHRITIS, RADIATION

Symptoms. Onset 6 to 12 months after exposure to radiation (proteinuria, elevation of blood pressure may be evident sooner). Anorexia; cephalalgia; nausea; vomiting, dyspnea.

Signs. Generalized edema; pallor; high blood pressure; heart failure.

Etiology. Exposure to 2,500 or more rads in a period of 5 weeks.

Pathology. Kidney normal size; occasionally, surrounded by fibrous tissue; glomeruli show thick basement membrane, hyalinization, and swollen cells; tubular atrophy.

Diagnostic Procedures. *Blood.* Anemia; high blood urea nitrogen and creatinine. *Urine.* Proteinuria; reduced glomerular filtration rate.

Therapy. Symptomatic. Kidney transplantation.

Prognosis. Poor; death within months or years, or evolution into chronic renal disease.

BIBLIOGRAPHY. Luxton RW: Radiation nephritis. Q J Med 22:215, 1953

Maher JF: Toxic and irradiation nephropathies. In Earley LE, Gottschalk CW (ed), Strauss and Welt's Diseases of the Kidney, 3rd ed. Boston, Little, Brown, 1979

NEPHROPHTHISIS, FAMILIAL JUVENILE

Synonyms. Fanconi's III; medullary cystic kidney.

Symptoms. Reported in children and young adults. Polydipsia and polyuria; night blindness followed by progressive constriction of peripheral fields and, finally, blurred vision.

Signs. In eyes, retinal arterioles narrowed, disk pale, yellow pigment deposit present throughout retina, macular degeneration, no lens opacity. Blood pressure usually normal until late stage of disease.

Etiology. Unknown; autosomal dominant inheritance.

Pathology. *Kidney.* Contracted; cortex thin. Thickening of Bowman's capsule to hyalinization of glomeruli; nephrons coiled; tubular basal membrane thickened; tubules atrophic (areas of hypertrophy may be observed); interstitial fibrosis. *Eyes.* See Signs. In older subject, medullary cysts may be found in the kidney.

Diagnostic Procedures. *Urine.* Normal, low specific gravity, or moderate proteinuria and minimal hematuria; high excretion of K. Cultures negative. *Pyelography.* Reduction in size of kidney. Creatine tolerance and phenolsulfonphthalein excretion abnormal. *Blood.* Hyperazotemia. *Electroretinography.* Pattern consistent with retinitis pigmentosa. *Audiography.* Normal.

Therapy. Symptomatic. Hemodialysis.

Prognosis. Usually, death from renal failure before reaching adulthood. Some longer survivals reported.

BIBLIOGRAPHY. Fanconi G, Hanhart E, von Albertini A, et al: Die familiare juvenile Nephronophthise. Helv Pediat Acta 6:1–49, 1951

Steele BT, Lirenman DS, Beattie GW: Nephrophthisis. Am J Med 68:531–538, 1980

NETHERTON'S

Synonym. Ichthyosiform erythroderma variant.

Symptoms and Signs. Occur almost exclusively in females; present from infancy. Ichthyosiform erythroderma; sparse, brittle hair; trichorrhexis invaginata. Atopic manifestations.

Etiology. Autosomal recessive inborn error of metabolism (?).

Diagnostic Procedures. *Biopsy of skin. Urine.* In one case reported, aminoaciduria. *Blood.* Hypoglobulinemia.

BIBLIOGRAPHY. Netherton EW: A unique case of trichorrhexis nodosa: bamboo hairs. Arch Dermatol 78:483–487, 1958

Julius CE, Heeran M: Netherton's syndrome in a male. Arch Derm 104:422–424, 1971

NETTLESHIP'S (E.) I

Synonyms. Infantile; Urticaria perstans hemorrhagica; urticaria pigmentosa; xanthelasmoidea; mastocytosis.

Symptoms and Signs. No sex prevalence; onset in infancy and childhood, or later. Solitary lesion or multiple lesions. Tan macules on the skin, which when stroked, produce urticariation (Darier's sign), itching. Vesiculation not constantly present (absent in patient with later onset). When present, gradual decline and disappearance in 2 years. Frequently associated with history of hay fever and asthma. Dermatographia in more than half of cases. Generalized flushing; tachycardia; headache; gastrointestinal complaints. Various bone abnormalities may also be associated. Occasionally, hepatosplenomegaly.

Etiology. Unknown; sporadic cases and congenital inheritance with simple autosomal dominance, with reduced penetrance described or recessive inheritance. In family affected, frequent occurrence in twins.

Pathology. On skin biopsy, dense mast cell infiltrates.

Diagnostic Procedures. *Biopsy of skin. Urine.* Elevated level of histamine in some cases.

Therapy. Excision of lesion only if symptoms acute, attacks of excessive vesiculation and flushing, or occasionally for cosmetic reasons. Calcium lactate gives some symptomatic benefit.

Prognosis. Usually, spontaneous regression of cutaneous lesions in a few years; lightly pigmented asymptomatic macular lesions may persist. In patients with onset after childhood, symptomatic activity persists indefinitely and systemic mast cell involvement may occur. About 30% develop malignant variety.

BIBLIOGRAPHY. Nettleship E: Rare forms of urticaria. B Med J 2:323–324, 1869
Shaw JM: Genetic aspects of urticaria pigmentosa. Arch Dermatol 97:137–138, 1968
Fowler JF, Parseley WM, Cotter PG: Familial urticaria pigmentosa. Arch Derm 122:80–81, 1986

NETTLESHIP'S (E.) II

Synonyms. X-linked ocular albinism; sex-linked nystagmus; Nettleship-Falls, ocular albinism sex-linked; OA1.

Symptoms and Signs. Onset from birth. *Males.* Severely affected. Skin normal or mottled with presence of pigmented nevi and freckles. Hair normal to light colored. Eyes normal color range. Nystagmus and photophobia present; moderate to severe vision reduction. Head nodding and tilting (50%). Strabismus (60%). Reproductive system anomalies common. *Females.* Carriers with absent signs or, occasionally, as severely affected as males.

Etiology. X-linked inheritance.

Diagnostic Procedures. *Ophthalmoscopy.* Transillumination of iris: males show cartwheel; females diaphanous aspect. In males red reflex present; fundal pigment absent; in females mosaic retina ("splashes of mud") present. *Incubation of hair bulb.* With tyrosine. Pigmentation.

Therapy. None.

Prognosis. With age, possibly, darkening of iris and decreased nystagmus.

BIBLIOGRAPHY. Nettleship E: On some hereditary diseases of the eye. Trans Ophthalmol Soc UK 29:57–198, 1908–1909
Witkop CJ, Quevedo WC Jr, Fitzpatrick TB: Albinism and other disorders of pigment metabolism. In Stanbury JB, Wyngaarden JB, Fredrickson DS, et al: The Metabolic Basis of Inherited Disease, 5th ed, p 301. New York, McGraw-Hill, 1983

NEUHAUSER-BERENBERG

Synonyms. Chalasia cardiac sphincter; cardioesophageal relaxation; esophagus chalasia.

Symptoms and Signs. Affects both sexes, usually in infancy; onset a few days after birth. Vomiting occurs following feeding of child and when he is positioned horizontally. Excessive regurgitation, failure to thrive, and danger of aspiration.

Etiology. Unknown. Transitory motor disorder of esophagus with lack of closure of gastroesophageal junction after passage of food.

Diagnostic Procedure. *Fluoroscopy.* Retrograde filling of esophagus in inspiration and with increase of intraabdominal pressure.

Therapy. Keep infant in orthostatic position during and after feeding.

Prognosis. Spontaneous cure after 2 months.

BIBLIOGRAPHY. Neuhauser EB, Berenberg W: Cardioesophageal relaxation as a cause of vomiting in infants. Radiology 48: 480–483, 1947
Castell DO, Johnson LF: Esophageal Function in Health and Disease. New York, Elsevier, 1982

NEU-LAXOVA

Synonym. Microcephaly-growth retardation-flexion deformities.

Symptoms and Signs. Both sexes affected. Intrauterine growth retardation; flexion deformities; overlapping fingers; rocker-bottom feet; protruding heels; toes syndactyly. Marked microcephaly; ocular hypertelorism; absent eyelids; short neck. Occasionally, tiny nose.

Etiology. Unknown; possibly autosomal recessive inheritance.

Pathology. Brain atrophy; absence corpus callosum.

Prognosis. Early death.

BIBLIOGRAPHY. Neu RL, Kajii T, Gardener LI, et al: A lethal syndrome of microcephaly with multiple congenital anomalies in three siblings. Pediatrico 47:611–612, 1971
Laxova R, Ohdra PT, Timothy JAD: A further example of a lethal autosomal recessive condition in sibs. J Ment Defic Res 16:139–143, 1972
Mueller RE, Winter RM, Naylor CPE: Neu-Laxova syndrome: two further case reports and comments on proposed sub-classification. Am J Med Genet 16:645–649, 1983

NEUMANN'S (E.)

Synonyms. Congenital epulis; neonatal myoblastoma. See Abrikossov's myoblastoma.

Symptoms. Both sexes affected; observed in newborns. Pedunculated tumor in the oral mucosa, usually on the margin of tongue, but may be found also anywhere. Smooth nodule 1 to 3 cm in diameter.

Etiology. Unknown.

Pathology. See Abrikossov's.

Therapy. Surgical excision.

Prognosis. No tendency to recur after excision.

BIBLIOGRAPHY. Neumann E: Eine Fall von congenitaler Epulis. Arch Heilk 12:189, 1871
Rook A, Wilkinson DS, Ebling FJG, et al: Textbook of Dermatology, 4th ed, p 2107. Oxford, Blackwell Scientific Publications, 1986

NEUMANN'S (I.)

Synonym. Pemphigus vegetans (Neumann's variety).

Symptoms and Signs. Both sexes affected; onset in young and middle-aged adults. Localized lesions in the mouth and other mucosae (e.g., vaginal) may or may not precede skin lesions; usually present in some stage of the disease. *Skin.* Bullae that break and develop into exudative vegetative lesions with small pustules; when drying, hyperkeratosis and fissures occur. Skin in flexure zones most frequently involved.

Etiology. Unknown; it may develop in the recuperation phase of pemphigus vulgaris.

Pathology. Bullae as in pemphigus vulgaris; acantholysis associated with acanthosis; microabscesses with eosinophils.

Therapy. Corticosteroids.

Prognosis. Spontaneous remission reported, but usually fatal without treatment.

BIBLIOGRAPHY. Neumann I: Ueber Pemphigus vegetans (frambosioides). Vrtljschr Dermatol 13:157–178, 1886
Rook A, Wilkinson DS, Ebling FJG, et al: Textbook of Dermatology, 4th ed, pp 1634–1635. Oxford, Blackwell Scientific Publications, 1986

NEUMANN'S (M.A.)

Synonyms. Dementia familial (Neumann type). Subcortical glyosis.

Symptoms and Signs. See Senile dementia.

Etiology. Autosomal recessive inheritance.

Pathology and Diagnostic Procedures. *Brain biopsy.* Normal level of neurotransmitters; subcortical glyosis. *Cerebrospinal fluid.* Normal level of neurotransmitters.

BIBLIOGRAPHY. Neumann MA: Pick's disease. J Neuropath Exp Neurol 8:255–282, 1949
Kronbesserian P, Davons P, Bianco C, et al: Demence familiale de type Neumann (glyose sous corticale) Rev Neurol (Paris) 141:706–712, 1985

NEURITIS MULTIPLEX CUTANEA

Synonym. Multiple sensory neuritis acquired.

Symptoms. Minimal and unnoticed for a long time. Changes of skin sensitivity from hypoesthesia to anesthesia. Spontaneous pain rare, elicited by slight trauma of the skin; distribution of affected areas is disseminated but never symmetric. Most frequently involved nerves are digital, upper and lower extremity, saphenous, femoral cutaneous, lateralis calcanei.

Signs. Subjecting an involved sensory nerve to brisk "stretching," a brief sharp pain is elicited in the area innervated. Motor nerves never involved. No vasomotor or trophic manifestations; no general or systemic disturbances.

Etiology. Unknown; the syndrome may be an expression of diabetes, carcinoma, malnutrition, or abuse of alcohol or drugs.

Pathology. Unknown.

Prognosis. Chronic course with remission and intermission, affecting one sensory nerve or another one remotely located.

BIBLIOGRAPHY. Schlesinger H: Ueber Neuritis multiplex cutanea. Neurol Centralbl 30:1218–1221, 1911
Wartenberg R: Multiple sensory neuritis: A clinical entity. Trans Am Neurol Assoc 71:101–104, 1946
Rook A, Wilkinson DS, Ebling FJG, et al: Textbook of Dermatology, 4th ed, p 2235. Oxford, Blackwell Scientific Publications, 1986

NEURITIS, PATELLAR PLEXUS

Synonyms. Gonalgia paresthetica (similar condition); neuralgia traumatic prepatellar (similar condition).

Symptoms. Complaint of "electric shock" when well-defined unilateral or bilateral trigger areas of prepatellar or adjacent zones are even lightly touched. Sensation appears, disappears, and recurs without apparent reason.

Etiology. Unknown; previous minor and forgotten injury. Anatomic accident in misplacement of infrapatellar branch of saphenous or other nerve of prepatellar plexus, vulnerable to mechanical trauma or ischemia produced by movement.

BIBLIOGRAPHY. Wartenberg R: Digitalgia paresthetica and gonyalgia paresthetica. Neurology 4:106–115, 1954

Smillie IS: Injuries of the Knee Joint. Edinburgh, Livingston, 1962

NEUROBLASTOMA

Synonyms. Congenital neuroblastoma; sympathicoblastoma, sympathicogonioma. See Hutchinson's and Pepper's.

Symptoms and Signs. Both sexes affected. Seldom symptomatic until tumor reaches a massive size or metastasis occurs.

Etiology. Unknown; autosomal dominant or recessive inheritance with variable penetrance or expression suggested.

Pathology. Primary site not always easily identified. Most common areas involved are adrenal, retroperitoneal (other organs), mediastinal. In the least differentiated type, grade III, cell structure small, no evident cytoplasm, presence of rosettes. In grade II, cell separated by fibrillar eosinophilic stroma. In grade I, ganglion cell present.

Diagnostic Procedures. *X-ray. Bone marrow.* Presence of cancer cells (50%). *Urine.* Increased excretion of dopamine, norepinephrine, vanillylmandelic acid.

Therapy. Extended radical surgery within reason (see prognosis). X-ray treatment; systemic chemotherapy.

Prognosis. *Surgery.* Sixty-one percent cure in patients with known gross residual tumor. *X-rays.* No recurrence at site of irradiation, but possible metastasis. Spontaneous involution and regression well documented.

BIBLIOGRAPHY. Dodge HJ, Benner MC: Neuroblastoma of adrenal medullar in siblings. Rocky Mt Med J 42:35–38, 1945

Hecht F, Hecht BK, Northrup JC, et al: Genetics of familial neuroblastoma: long-range studies. Cancer Genet Cytogenet 7:227–230, 1982

Hayes FA, Smith EI: Neuroblastoma. In Pizzo PA, Poplack DG, Pediatric Oncology, p 607. Philadelphia, JB Lippincott, 1989

NEUROCUTANEOUS MELANOSIS

Synonyms. Hamartomatous meningeal melanosis; melanoblastic hyperplasia; melanosis neurocutaneous.

Symptoms. Both sexes affected; onset in fetal life. Variable neurologic symptoms from normality to severe mental deficiency and other neurologic deficits.

Signs. Numerous pigmented skin nevi; frequent typical feature is "bathing trunk" nevus, involving skin of lower abdomen, buttocks, and upper parts of legs.

Etiology. Congenital dysplasia of neural crest. Autosomal recessive inheritance.

Pathology. *Skin.* Typical appearance of pigmented dermal nevi. *Central nervous system.* Dura-pia-arachnoid or brain, cerebellum (almost entirely confined to gray matter) pigmented cells; pigment-laden macrophages; melanophoric cells.

Therapy. None.

Prognosis. Variable; stillbirth or death, in early childhood. Survival up to adulthood possible. Possibility of malignant transformation of lesions to be considered.

BIBLIOGRAPHY. Rokitansky J: Ein ausgezeichneter Fall von Pigmentmal mit ausgebreiteter Pigmentierung der inneren Hirn- und Rückemarks-häute. Allg Wien Met Ztg 6:113, 1861

Van Bogaert L: La melanose neurocutanée diffuse heredofamiliale. Bull Acad R Med Belg (6th series) 13:397, 1948

Kaplan AM, Itabashi HH, Hanelin LG, et al: Neurocutaneous melanosis with malignant leptomeningeal melanoma. Arch Neurol 32:669–671, 1975

NEUROFIBROMATOSIS SYNDROMES

1. NF I: Von Recklinghausen's (see)
2. NF II: Familial acoustical neurinoma
3. NF III: Riccardi's (NF III)
4. NF IV: Riccardi's (NF IV)

BIBLIOGRAPHY. Riccardi's VM, Eichner JE: Neurofibromatosis: Phenotype, Natural History, and Pathogenesis. Baltimore, Johns Hopkins University Press, 1986

NEUROGENIC BLADDER

SPASTIC BLADDER SYNDROME, REFLEX BLADDER SYNDROME

Symptoms. Precipitous micturition; nicturia; leakage around catheters; intolerance of catheter. Throbbing headache; profuse sweating; nasal obstruction; "goose bumps" accompany the spastic contractions.

Signs. Blood hypertension, bradycardia accompany spastic contraction.

Etiology. Spinal cord lesions above the conus medullaris.

Pathology. Tumor; trauma; infections; degenerative changes of spine at level immediately above the conus medullaris. Hydronephrosis may develop.

Diagnostic Procedures. *X-ray of spine. Myelography. Cystometrography.*

Therapy. Propantheline and oxybutine in cases refractory to pharmacological treatment. Convert spastic to flaccid bladder. (1) Subarachnoid injection of alcohol to abolish hyperreflexia. (2) Cordectomy. (3) Selective rhizotomy of 3rd and 4th sacral roots bilaterally is best procedure since it is not accompanied by extensive damage to nervous structure and by the resulting conus medullaris syndrome.

Prognosis. That of etiology, plus renal complication. Good result with last procedure indicated.

FLACCID BLADDER SYNDROME

Symptoms and Signs. Desire, initiation, and inhibition of micturition are absent. Usually, part of the conus medullaris syndrome.

Etiology and Pathology. Trauma, tumor, vascular lesion, or infection at level of conus medullaris.

Diagnostic Procedures. *X-ray. Spinal tap. Myelogram. Urologic evaluation. Cystometry. Cystoscopy.*

Therapy. Bethanecol or, if feasible, surgery to remove compression of cord. Symptomatic.

Prognosis. Infection of bladder a common complication.

BIBLIOGRAPHY. Bors E: Neurogenic bladder, Urol Surv 7:177–250, 1957
Manfredi RA, Leal JF: Selective sacral rhizotomy for the spastic bladder syndrome in patients with spinal cord injuries. J Urol 100:17–20, 1968
Krane RJ, Siroky MD (eds): Clinical Neurology. Boston, Little, Brown, 1979

NEUROPATHY, HEREDITARY, SENSORY, RADICULAR

Synonyms. Hicks-Camp; Denny-Brown; HSAN I.

Symptoms. Both sexes. Onset between 15 and 35 years of age. Deafness and shooting pains from the feet to the legs. No loss of sensation of touch, heat, and cold on the feet initially.

Signs. Starting with a corn on big toe, development of painless ulcer deepening to the bone and extending to other toes. Reduction then disappearance of tendon reflexes. Arms and cranial reflexes normal (except auditory).

Etiology. Unknown. Autosomal dominant trait. Relationship with other foot ulceration syndromes (see

Nelaton's; Morvan's; Biemond's III) not yet completely elucidated; restless legs and lancinating pain could be minor presentation of the same condition (?).

Pathology. Marked loss of ganglion cells in sacral and lumbar dorsal root ganglia with, in some cases, clear hyaline bodies (amyloid?).

Diagnostic Procedures. *X-ray. Electrophysiologic studies of nerve. Biopsy of nerve and ganglia.*

Prognosis. Progressive condition leading to severe ulceration and complete deafness.

BIBLIOGRAPHY. Hicks EP, Camp MB: Hereditary perforating ulcer of the foot. Lancet I:319–321, 1922
Denny-Brown D: Hereditary sensory radicular neuropathy. J Neurol Neurosurg Psychiatr 14:237–252, 1951
Danon MJ, Carpenter S: Hereditary sensory neuropathy biopsy study of an autosomal dominant variety. Br Med J 2:737–740, 1985

NEUROPATHY, SERUM

Symptoms and Signs. Predominant in males; onset 7 to 10 days after injection of serum (preventive or curative) for conditions such as tetanus, diphtheria. Local pain; swelling of tissues and joints; edema of mucous membranes; hyperthermia. After 2 or 3 days paralysis of one or more spinal nerve territories, usually of shoulder-girdle, but occasionally more extensive involvement. Possibly convulsions, meningeal reaction. Absence of sensory alterations (usually).

Etiology. Complication of injection of foreign proteins.

Pathology. Polyneuritis changes; edema of involved areas.

Diagnostic Procedure. *Electromyography.*

Therapy. During acute stage, antihistaminic drugs. Physical therapy after onset of paralysis.

Prognosis. Variable recovery in 1 to several months.

BIBLIOGRAPHY. Garvey JL: Serum neuritis: 20 cases following use of antitetanic serum. Postgrad Med 13:210–213, 1953
Vick NA: Grinker's Neurology, 7th ed. Springfield, Ill, CC Thomas, 1976

NEUTROPENIA, NEONATAL

Symptoms and Signs. Occur in newborns. Mild recurrent infections or fulminating infections. Skin infection is the most frequent clinical finding.

Etiology. Passage to the fetus of leukocyte antibodies

produced by the mother. The phenomenon of passage of these antibodies is rather frequent, while the effect on neutrophil number and clinical manifestations is very rare.

Diagnostic Procedures. *Blood.* Leukopenia with severe neutropenia, accompanied by monocytosis. No anemia or thrombocytopenia. Maternal blood contains agglutinins against neutrophils. *Bone marrow.* Rich myeloid series, but few or absent mature neutrophils. Severe neutropenia, with a normal total leukocyte count. Monocytosis is frequent, and eosinophilia is sometimes observed.

Therapy. Antibiotics (if infections); corticosteroid or adrenocorticotropic hormone.

Prognosis. Usually excellent; complete spontaneous recovery, except in fulminating cases. (The duration of the neutropenia varies from 2 to 17 weeks.)

BIBLIOGRAPHY. Hitzig WH, Gitzelmann R: Transplacental transfer of leukocyte agglutinins. Vox Sang (NS) 4:445–456, 1959
Lalezari P, Nussbaum M, Gelman S, et al: Neonatal neutropenia due to maternal isoimmunization. In Miale JB: Laboratory Medicine, Hematology, 3rd ed. St Louis, CV Mosby, 1967
Wintrobe MM (ed): Clinical Hematology, 8th ed, p 1326. Philadelphia, Lea & Febiger, 1981

NEVUS FLAMMEUS

Synonyms. Capillary nevus; plane nevus; telangiectatic nevus; Unna's nevus; salmon patches; port-wine nevus.

Symptoms and Signs. May present three distinct groups of features: (1) *Salmon patches.* Both sexes affected; present at birth. On the nape, forehead, and eyelids; pinkish patches, with fine telangiectasis. They may disappear within 1 year, or later; 5% to 7% of those of the nape persist throughout life (Unna's nevus) (2) *Port-wine nevus.* Both sexes affected; present at birth. In any part of the body, more frequent on face and upper trunk (membranes may be involved) patches, pink to bright red of various dimensions (a few millimeters to several centimeters in diameter) (3) *Nevus increasing in size.* Same characteristics as above, but appearing after a traumatic injury of the part.

Etiology. Unknown; neurogenic factor related to birth postulated. Autosomal dominant inheritance. Part of many hereditary syndromes.

Pathology. Variable. Ectasia of superficial or deeper vessels associated more or less with connective hypertrophic changes.

Therapy. Several approaches, but all unsatisfactory. Excision and grafting; ionizing radiation; dermabrasion.

Cosmetic masking remains the safest and most efficient procedure.

Prognosis. From spontaneous disappearance to permanence.

BIBLIOGRAPHY. Shelly WB, Livingood CS: Familial multiple nevi flammei. Arch Derm Syph 59:343–345, 1949
Merlob P, Reisner SH: Familial nevus flammeus of the forehead and Unna's nevus. Clin Genet 27:165–166, 1985

NEZELOF'S

Synonyms. Lymphopenia-normoglobulinemia. See Beck-Ibrahim.

Symptoms and Signs. Both sexes affected; onset in infancy. Virus and fungus infections.

Etiology. It represents the other end of the spectrum of the combined immunodeficiency, which originates from the De Vaal's syndrome (see). (See also intermediate form of Glanzmann-Rinikier). Autosomal recessive inheritance.

Pathology. Thymic dysplasia; lymphocyte depletion. In the spleen and other organs, numerous plasma cells.

Diagnostic Procedures. *Blood.* Coombs' test positive. Hemolytic anemia; leukopenia; lymphopenia. Normal immunoglobulins; however, antigen stimulation does not produce increase in antibodies. Cases reported with selective deficit of immunoglobulins IgG, IgM, and IgA.

Prognosis. Death by 3rd to 4th year of life.

BIBLIOGRAPHY. Nezelof C, Jammet ML, Lortholary P, et al: L'hypoplasie héréditaire du thymus sa place et sa responsabilité dans une observation d'aplasie lymphocytare normoplasmacytaire et normoglobulininémique du nourissau. Arch Fr Pediatr 21:897–920, 1964
Rosen FS: Genetic defects in gammaglobulin synthesis. In Stanbury JB, Wyngaarden JB, Fredrickson DS, et al: The Metabolic Basis of Inherited Disease, 5th ed, p 1921. New York, McGraw-Hill, 1983

NICOLAU'S I

Synonyms. Nicolau-Hoigné; accidental therapeutic embolization; accidental embolization.

Symptoms. Occur following an intramuscular injection of bismuth (original report), penicillin, tetracyclines. Somnolence; acoustic sensation; occasionally, visual loss; sudden pain in extremities or abdomen; paresis or paralysis; shock.

Signs. Pallor; cyanosis; peripheral edema; tachycardia; motor irritability; arterial hypotension.

Etiology. Accidental injection of drug into artery. Reaction of nonallergic type, but of embolic nature.

Pathology. According to arterial district involved.

Therapy. Symptomatic.

Prognosis. Variable. Death in severe cases.

BIBLIOGRAPHY. Nicolau S: Dermite livédoïde et gangrëneuse de la fesse, consécutive aux injections intramusculaires, dans la syphilis. A propos d'un cas de'embolie artérielle bismuthique. Ann Mal Vénéreol (Paris) 20:321, 1925
Hoigné R: Akute Nebenreaktionen auf Penicillin-präparate. Acta Med Scand 171:201–208, 1962
Domula M, Weissbac G, Lenk H: Das Nicolau-Syndrom nach Benzathinpenizillin. Ein Überblick an Hand von 5 eigenen Beobachtungen. Kinderärztl Praxis 40:437–448, 1972

NIEDEN'S

Synonym. Cataract-telangiectasia.

Symptoms and Signs. Both sexes affected; onset from birth. Telangiectasia of face and upper limbs; sparse eyebrows; skin thickened; increased pigmentation of neck; signs of heart enlargement and congenital valvular defects. Bilateral cataract. Glaucoma.

Etiology. Unknown; familial cases reported.

Pathology. Telangiectasia. Heart enlargement; valvular defects; hypoplasia of aorta. Defect of iris mesenchyma.

Therapy. Heart surgery where indicated.

Prognosis. Variable. Reported cases still alive in their 3rd and 4th decades.

BIBLIOGRAPHY. Nieden A: Cataractbildung bei teleangiectätischer Ausdehnung der Capillaren der ganzen Gesichtshaut. Centbl Prarkt Augenheilkd 11:353–357, 1887
Waardenburg PJ, Franceschetti A, Klein D: Genetics and Ophthalmology, Vol 1, p 906. Springfield, Ill, CC Thomas, 1961

NIELSEN'S (H.)

Synonym. Congenital dystrophia brevicollis.
Eponym (obsolete) used to indicate a combination of Klippel-Feil (see) and Bonnevie-Ulrich.

BIBLIOGRAPHY. Nielsen H: Dystrophia brevicollis congenita. Hospitalstidende 77:409–431, 1934

NIELSEN'S (J.M.) I

Synonyms. Exhaustive psychosis; neuromuscular exhaustion; disaster syndromes.

Symptoms. Develops subacutely after severe overexertion during a period of euphoria. Degree of overwork is variable and depends on age and other factors. Feeling of deep exhaustion of entire body, more severe in abused muscles. Pain, tenderness, twitching, and then atrophy of muscles involved. Generalized restlessness that prevents sleeping and rest; weight loss.

Signs. In acute stage, muscle flaccidity, absence of deep reflexes. Later, reflexes return to normal.

Etiology. Unknown; metabolic disturbance due to overwork.

Pathology. Unknown.

Diagnostic Procedures. *Cerebrospinal fluid.* Normal. *Electromyography. Thyroid function tests.*

Therapy. Symptomatic; rest; diet.

Prognosis. Very slow; partial recovery of moderate activity. Lack of recovery of previous tone and strength.

BIBLIOGRAPHY. Nielsen JM: Subacute generalized neuromuscular exhaustion syndrome. Bull Los Angeles Neurol Soc 5:128–130, 1940
Nielson JM: Subacute generalized neuromuscular exhaustion syndrome. Report of 3 cases. Calif Med 66:338–340, 1947
Stutman RK, Bliss EL: Postraumatic stress disorder: hypnotizability and imagery. Am J Psychiatr 142:741–743, 1985

NIELSEN'S (J.M.) II

Synonyms. Agnosia-apraxia-aphasia; anterior cingulate gyri; cingulate gyri.

Symptoms. Apathy; akinesia; mutism; incontinence.

Signs. Open eyes; normal muscle tone; indifference to pain. Babinski's sign bilaterally. Increased respiration rate.

Etiology. Bilateral damage to the cingulate gyri.

Prognosis. Coma; death in 3 to 5 weeks.

BIBLIOGRAPHY. Nielsen JM: Agnosia, Apraxia and Aphasia. New York, Hoeber, 1946
Ford FR: Diseases of Nervous System, 4th ed. Springfield, Ill, CC Thomas, 1960
Grinker RR, Sahs AL: Neurology, p 734–772, 6th ed. Springfield, Ill, CC Thomas, 1966

NIEMANN-PICK

Synonyms. Lipid histiocytosis; sphingomyelin lipidosis; sphingomyelin reticuloendotheliosis.

TYPE A (ACUTE NEURONOPATHIC)

Symptoms. Affects both sexes equally; about 40% of patients are Jewish, but all races may be affected. Usually normal at birth; onset at 1 to 2 months. Failure to thrive; mental retardation; progressing to apathy and dullness.

Signs. Debility and wasting of extremity; abdominal enlargement; hepatosplenomegaly. Cherry red spot in macular region (50%). Skin may show plaques of brown pigmented areas; blue brown discoloration; xanthomas are rare.

Etiology. Unknown; altered metabolism of sphingomyelin; lack of sphingomyelinase. Autosomal recessive inheritance with different phenotype manifestations; types A, B and C are allelic forms of altered sphingomyelinase.

Pathology. All organs show infiltration with typical foamy vacuolated cells, containing sphingomyelin-sterol. Organs primarily involved are liver, spleen, lungs, lymph nodes, bone marrow. Brain shows marked degenerative changes.

Diagnostic Procedures. *Blood.* Anemia; vacuolated leukocytes. High cholesterol level. Kampine-Brady-Kanfer test on washed white blood cells shows low level of enzymatic activity for hydrolysis of sphingomyelin and glucocerebrosides. *Bone marrow.* Presence of typical cells. *Biopsy and biochemical studies.* Of tissues.

Therapy. None; however, in some cases, splenectomy, although it does not change the final prognosis.

Prognosis. Death within 3 years.

TYPE B (CHRONIC NON-NEURONOPATHIC)

Symptoms and Signs. Onset at the same age as above or, more typical, slightly later. Splenomegaly first sign; hepatomegaly later. Respiratory infection. Absence of signs of central nervous system involvement; possibly, high intellectual capacity.

Etiology. See above.

Pathology. In spleen, liver, lungs, bone marrow, presence of birefringent foam cells.

Diagnostic Procedures. *Blood.* Anemia; evidence of minor liver function impairment. *Bone marrow.* See Pathology. *X-ray of chest.* Diffuse infiltration.

Therapy. Symptomatic.

Prognosis. Poor.

TYPE C (CHRONIC NEURONOPATHIC)

Symptoms. Normal at birth and for first 2 years (occasionally, longer). Loss of speech; ataxia; grand mal seizures. Hypertonia; hyperreflexia.

Signs. Moderate hepatosplenomegaly.

Etiology. See above.

Pathology. Presence of foamy cells in bone marrow and other organs.

Diagnostic Procedures. See above.

Prognosis. Progressive failure of mental and motor skills. Death between 5 and 15 years of age.

TYPE D (NOVA SCOTIA)

Synonym. Crocker-Farber.

Symptoms. Limited to population from Nova Scotia; onset in 2nd to 4th year of life. Unsteady gait; lack of coordination; epilepsy (grand and petit mal); mental deterioration.

Signs. Hepatosplenomegaly. Jaundice.

Etiology. See above. Sphingomyelinase normal or slightly reduced.

Pathology. Foamy cells in bone marrow and different organs.

Prognosis. Poor.

TYPE E (ADULT NON-NEURONOPATHIC)

Symptoms and Signs. Few cases reach adult life without neurologic manifestation.

Signs. Moderate hepatosplenomegaly.

Etiology. See above.

Diagnostic Procedures. *Bone marrow.* Foam cells. *Liver and spleen biopsy.* Increase of sphingomyelin.

Prognosis. Good.

BIBLIOGRAPHY. Niemann A: Ein unbekanntes Krankheitbild. Jahrb Kinderh N F 29:1–10, 1914

Pick L: Ueber die lipoidzellige Splenohepatomegalie Typus Niemann-Pick als Stoffwecheslerkrankung. Med Klin 23:1483–1488, 1927

Pick L, Bielschowsky M: Ueber lipoidzellige Splenomegalie (Typus Niemann-Pick) und amaurotische Idiotie. Klin Wochenschr 5:1631, 1927

Brady RO: Sphingomyelin lipidosis: Niemann-Pick disease. In Stanbury JB, Wyngaarden JB, Fredrickson DS: The Metabolic Basis of Inherited Disease, 5th ed, p 831. New York, McGraw-Hill, 1983

NIERHOFF-HUEBNER

Synonym. Endochondral dysostosis.

Symptoms. Onset during first days of life. Convulsion; somnolence; muscular flaccidity.

Signs. From birth, normal body length, micromelia; short neck; microcephaly (occasional); mild cyanosis; jaundice.

Etiology. Considered a variant of Morquio's (osteochondrodystrophy). Autosomal recessive inheritance or dominant with incomplete penetrance.

Pathology. Cranial sutures dehiscent. *Rib junctures.* Rachitic rosary. *Heart.* Ventricle dilatation and myocardial swelling. *Kidney.* Swelling. *Leptomeninges.* Hemorrhages. Microscopically, bone structure changes especially of proximal end of femur and distal end of ulna.

Diagnostic Procedures. *Blood.* Hyperazotemia. *X-ray of skeleton.* Abnormal calcification of epiphyseal and metaphyseal part of bones and cranial vault. *Cerebrospinal fluid.* Normal. *Electroencephalography.* Altered patterns.

Therapy. None.

Prognosis. Fatal within a few weeks.

BIBLIOGRAPHY. Nierhoff H, Heubner O: Familiaere systemisierte enchondrale Dysostose bei 3 Geschwistern. Z Kinderh 78:497–521, 1956

NIEVERGELT'S

Synonyms. Nievergelt-Erb; radioulnar synostosis.

Symptoms. Both sexes affected, prevalent in males; onset from birth. Symmetric dysplasia of elbows; luxation of ulna or radial heads; radioulnar synostosis; brachydactyly; flexion of fingers; symmetric dysplasia of lower legs; genu valgum; clubfoot; deformed great toes.

Etiology. Unknown; autosomal dominant inheritance.

Diagnostic Procedures. *X-ray of skeleton.* Superior radioulnar synostosis; fibula relatively longer; tarsal bone synostosis; epiphyseal line obliquity. *Chromosome studies.* Negative.

Therapy. Orthopedic procedures.

Prognosis. Poor *quoad functionem.*

BIBLIOGRAPHY. Nievergelt K: Positiver Vaterschafs nachweis auf Grund erblicher Missbildungen der Extremitäten. Arch Klaus Stift Vererbungforsch 19:157–160, 1944.
Hess OM, Goebel NH, Strenh R: Familiärerer mesomeler

Kleinwuchs (Nievergelt syndrome) Schweiz Med Wochenschr 108:1202–1206, 1978

NIGHT EATING

Synonym. Morning anorexia–hyperphagia–insomnia.

Symptoms. Apparently prevalent in women; occur in obese patients or patients with weight disorders. Nocturnal hyperphagia, insomnia, and anorexia in the morning. Difficulty in losing weight.

Etiology. Unknown; response to stress in emotionally disturbed individual.

Therapy. Psychotherapy; environmental manipulation; diet; amphetamine and similar medications.

Prognosis. This syndrome influences the result of weight reduction programs.

BIBLIOGRAPHY. Stunkard AJ, Grace WJ, Wolff HG: The nighteating syndrome: a pattern of food intake among certain obese patients. Am J Med 19:78–86, 1955
Adams RD, Victor M: Principles of Neurology, 3rd ed, p 293. New York, McGraw-Hill, 1985
Field HL, Domanque BB: Eating disorders throughout the life span. London, Greenwood Press, 1988

NOACK'S

Synonyms. Acrocephalopolysyndactyly I; progressive synostosis. Now considered included in Pfeiffer's syndrome (see).

BIBLIOGRAPHY. Noack M: Ein Betrag zum Krankheitsbild der Akrozephalosyndaktylie (Apert). Arch Kinderh 160:168–171, 1959
Vanek J, Losan F: Pfeiffer's type of acrocephalosyndactyly in two families. J Med Genet 19:289–292, 1982

NOCTURNAL FREQUENCY IN WOMEN

Synonym. Nocturnal stranguria.

Symptoms. Nocturnal frequency in women with or without disturbance of micturition during the day, with or without menstrual irregularity in the premenopausal group, and vasomotor disturbances or atrophic vaginitis in the menopausal group.

Signs. Majority have fibromyomas.

Etiology. Cardiovascular renal diseases; anatomic defects of urinary tract; genitourinary infections, psychogenic factors. Possibly, hormonal factors.

Diagnostic Procedures. *Urine and culture.* Frequently negative.

Therapy. Recommended by Greenblatt: implantation of testosterone pellets.

Prognosis. According to Greenblatt, total or partial relief of symptoms with testosterone. Surgery for fibromyomatas not necessary in many cases to eliminate nocturia.

BIBLIOGRAPHY. Greenblatt RB: Syndrome of nocturnal frequency alleviated by testosterone propionate. J Clin Endocrinol 2:321–324, 1942.

NOMA

Synonyms. Cancrum oris; gangrenous stomatitis.

Symptoms and Signs. Usually occur in children. On oral mucosae, ulcer rapidly extending into a gangrenous greenish black lesion. Possible complications: alveolar bone destruction and sepsis.

Etiology. Fusospirochetal infection in debilitated patient; frequently associated with severe basic conditions (e.g., leukemia; virus infection; lymphomas).

Pathology. Cellulitis and necrosis of affected zone.

Diagnostic Procedures. *Blood.* Leukocytosis. *Culture.* *Bacillus fusiformis* and many secondary infectious agents.

Therapy. Antibiotics; treatment of the basic condition. Topical clorhexidine. Metronidazole per os (7 days treatment).

Prognosis. Severe; fundamental control of basic condition for a positive outcome.

BIBLIOGRAPHY. Trible GB, Dick A: Noma. Arch Otolaryngol 16:1–8, 1932
Rook A, Wilkinson DS, Ebling FJG, et al: Textbook of Dermatology, 4th ed, p 2089. Oxford, Blackwell Scientific Publications, 1986

NONKETOTIC HYPERGLYCINEMIA

Symptoms and Signs. Onset in first days of life. Listlessness; lack of spontaneous movements; spasticity; seizures; myoclonus; opisthotonos; hiccups; failure to thrive; severe mental retardation.

Etiology. Autosomal recessive inheritance. Metabolic inborn error, causing impairment of glycine utilization and its accumulation in body fluids; probably a block in glycine decarboxylase reaction.

Diagnostic Procedures. *Blood and urine.* Glycine mark-edly elevated. *Glycine metabolism studies. Electroencephalography.* Abnormal.

Therapy. None effective. Exchange transfusion lifesaving, but with temporary effect. Glycine restriction. Sodium benzoate.

Prognosis. Overwhelming illness in early life.

BIBLIOGRAPHY. Gerritsen T, Kaveggia E, Waisman HA: A new type of hyperglycinemia with hypoxaluria. Pediatrics 36:882–891, 1965
Nyham WL: Nonketotic hyperglycinemia. In Stanbury JB, Wyngaarden JB, Fredrickson DS, et al: The Metabolic Basis of Inherited Disease, 5th ed, p 561. New York, McGraw-Hill, 1983

NONNE-MILROY-MEIGE

Synonyms. Congenital elephantiasis; hereditary tropholymphedema; lymphedema hereditary I (Nonne-Milroy); Lymphedema hereditary II (Meige).

Symptoms. Prevalent in females (70% to 80%); onset gradual and asymptomatic; two varieties: *precox* (Nonne-Milroy), at birth to 35 years of age; *tarda* (Meige), after 35 years.

Signs. Unilateral or bilateral edema of ankle ascending to the knee and eventually above; initially easily pitting; disappearing with elevation of the leg; seldom on the arms, genitalia, face, and other areas. Skin smooth, firm, and natural color. Later, harder edema, not relieved by elevation with rough, pigmented skin over swollen parts. Persistent pleural effusion; in the variety tarda, possible association with deafness, primary pulmonary hypertension, cerebrovascular malformations, peculiar facial features (puffiness, deep creases, excessive wrinkling, cleft palate).

Etiology. Autosomal dominant inheritance. Cases of secondary lymphedema (malignancy; surgery; roentgen; pressure; filariasis; inflammation) were described by authors together with the hereditary ones. Today the use of eponym is restricted to the hereditary variety.

Pathology. Layer of spongy subcutaneous tissue; replacement of part of adipose tissue by lymphatic spaces. Fibrosis; thickening of blood vessel walls.

Diagnostic Procedures. *Blood.* Hypoproteinemia. *Pleural tap.* Hyperproteinemia.

Therapy. *Early stage.* Frequent elevation and elastic stockings. *Later stage.* Kondoleon operation is palliative.

Prognosis. Chronic course; permanent condition; normal life span. Rarely, lymphosarcoma may arise.

BIBLIOGRAPHY. Nonne M: Vier Fälle von Elephantiasis

congenita hereditaria. Arch Pathol Anat (Paris) 125:189–196, 1891

Milroy WF: Undescribed variety of hereditary oedema. New York Med J 56:505–508, 1892

Meige H: Dystrophie oedematose hereditaire. Presse Med 6:341–343, 1898

Schirger A, Harrison EG Jr, Janes JM: Idiopathic lymphedema: review of 131 cases. JAMA 182:14–22, 1962

Herbert FA, Bowen PA: Hereditary late onset lymphedema with pleural effusion and laryngeal edema. Arch Intern Med 143:913–915, 1983

NONNENBRUCH'S

Synonym. Extrarenal oliguria (see Hepatorenal).
Eponym (obsolete) used to indicate all forms of oliguria due to extrarenal factors: e.g., dehydration, shock.

BIBLIOGRAPHY. Nonnenbruch W: Ueber das entzüdliche dem der Niere und das hepatorenale Syndrom. Dtsch Med Wochenschr 63:7–10, 1937

NONNE'S

Synonyms. Benign intracranial hypertension; meningeal hydrops; hydrops; otitic hydrocephalus; pseudotumor cerebri; Quincke's; serous meningitis; Symond's.

Two types are recognized: Borries' and benign hydrocephalus.

BORRIES' SYNDROME

Symptoms. Occur in both sexes; onset at all ages. Headache; nausea; vomiting; listlessness; mild fever; diplopia; blurred vision; occasionally tinnitus. Mental state unchanged; no seizures.

Signs. Bilateral papilledema; all other neurologic signs usually negative; (benign abducens (VI) nerve palsy syndrome, possible in children). In some cases, otologic examination reveals perforated tympanic membrane with purulent discharge or discolored, distorted drum (prevalence in right ear); mastoid tenderness. In other cases, no otologic findings.

Etiology. Multiple etiologies; infection of middle ear or head injury.

Pathology. Mastoiditis with obstruction of lateral sinus, most frequently observed on the right side. A localized associated edema of cerebrum adjacent to the focal infection has been postulated.

Diagnostic Procedures. *Blood.* Mild leukocytosis; moderate increase of erythrocyte sedimentation rate. Serology for syphilis negative. *Cerebrospinal fluid.* Increased pres-

sure. Lack or minimal increase with compression of jugular vein ipsilateral to infected mastoid; normal response contralaterally. Sugar and cells normal. *Electroencephalography.* Minimal alterations or normal. *X-ray of mastoid.* Clouding air cells and disruption of normal trabecular pattern. Widening of skull sutures observed in some children. *Carotid angiography. Pneumoencephalography.*

Therapy. Antibiotic therapy and serial spinal punctures. If this fails, simple mastoidectomy.

Prognosis. Two weeks after mastoidectomy majority of cases cured; if intracranial pressure persists after mastoidectomy, recovery takes up to 6 months. Eventually, 100% recovery with adequate treatment.

BENIGN HYDROCEPHALUS SYNDROME

Symptoms and Signs. Prevalent in women; onset in middle age. Symptoms and signs as above with exception of absence of otologic pathology. If in pregnancy, evidence of progressive ocular signs due to atrophy of retina.

Etiology. Unknown; frequently associated with pregnancy, obesity, Addison's syndrome, steroid or other hormone and vitamins A and D imbalances (see Marie-See).

Pathology. None, except increased amount and tension of cerebral fluid.

Diagnostic Procedures. As above.

Therapy. Repeated spinal tap may relieve all symptoms.

Prognosis. Generally good; disappearance of symptoms in 2 to 6 months. In pregnancy, good prognosis for mother and child.

BIBLIOGRAPHY. Quincke, 1897

Nonne M: Ueber Falle vom Symptomenkomplex "tumor cerebri" mit Ausgang in Heilung (pseudotumor cerebri). Ueber lethal verlaufene Falle von "pseudotumor cerebri" mit Sektionsbefund. Dtsch Z Nervenheilk 27:169–216, 1904

Mestrezat W: Le liquide cephalo-rachidien normal and pathologique: Valeur clinique de l'examen clinique: Le syndromes humoraux dans le diverses affections. Paris, A Maloin, 1912

Borries GVT: Otogene encephalitis. Soc Danoise d'Oto-laryngology, 2 Feb., 1921; Zschz Ges Neurol Psychiatr 70:93–101, 1921

Symonds CP: Otitic hydrocephalus. Brain 54:55, 1931

Gneer M: Benign intracranial hypertension I. Mastoiditis and lateral sinus obstruction. Neurology 12:472–476, 1962

Nickerson CW, Krik RF: Recurrent pseudotumor cerebri in pregnancy. Report of 2 cases. Obstet Gynecol 26:811–813, 1965

Adams RD, Victor M: Principles of Neurology, 3rd ed, pp 468–469. New York, McGraw-Hill, 1985

NOONAN'S

Synonyms. Pseudo-Turner's; Turner-like.

Symptoms. Both sexes affected. Mental retardation (rare in gonadal dysgenesis); stunted growth. Functional fetal gonads: in male, differentiation of male genitalia or complete absence or disappearance; in female, from normal sexual development, to absent development and primary amenorrhea.

Signs. Many different types of congenital anomalies (in most cases minor) none characteristic or obligatory for diagnosis. Generally, shortness of stature (not as severe as in gonadal dysgenesis). Pulmonary valvular or arterial stenosis or other congenital heart malformation (as a general rule, lesions prevalent in right heart as contrasted with gonadal dysgenesis, in which the left lesions predominate). Facial anomalies: ptosis; hypertelorism; antimongoloid slanting of palpebrae; ear abnormalities; micrognathia; dental anomalies; uvula and, less frequently, palate anomalies. Chest anomalies: pectus carinatum; vertebral anomalies; digital anomalies; dysonychia; hirsutism; occasionally webbing of neck. Some cases have been reported in which the syndrome was associated with multiple *cafe au lait* spots, compatible in size and number with Von Recklinghausen's neurofibromatosis. These features may represent a distinct genetic entity rather than the coincidence of two diseases.

Etiology. Unknown; multifactor inheritance. Male-to-male transmission has been reported, suggesting an autosomal dominant gene with variable expressivity.

Pathology. See Symptoms and Signs. Gonads normal or rudimentary.

Diagnostic Procedures. *Chromosome studies.* Normal karyotypes. *X-rays. Cardiologic studies. Hormone secretion studies.* One family reported with high alkaline phosphatase in all members of family with or without major or minor manifestation of syndrome.

Therapy. If hormonal deficiency, replacement either in continuous or cyclic fashion. Treatment has to be started early and continued as long as needed. Surgery for heart malformation when feasible.

Prognosis. According to degree, number, and type of anomalies. Relatives of proband are as a general rule affected much less severely.

BIBLIOGRAPHY. Kobilinski O: Ueber eine flughautähnliche Ausbreitung am Halse. Arch Anthropol 14:342–348, 1883

Noonan JA, Ehmke DA: Associated noncardiac malformations in children with congenital heart disease. J Pediatr 63:468–470, 1963

Caralis DG, Char F, Graber JD, et al: Delineation of multiple cardiac anomalies associated with the Noonan syndrome in an adult and review of the literature. Johns Hopkins Med J 134:346–355, 1974

Mendez HM, Opitz JM: Noonan syndrome: a review. Am J Med Genet 21:493–506, 1985

Shuper A, Mukamel M., Mimouni M, Steinherz R: Noonan's syndrome and neurofibromatosis. Arch Dis Child 62:196–198, 1987

NORMAN-LANDING

Synonyms. Beta-galactosidase deficiency; Caffey's pseudo-Hurler; familial neurovisceral lipoidosis; generalized gangliosidosis (type I); GM1; infantile GM1; neurovisceral pseudo-Hurler lipoidosis.

Symptoms. Both sexes affected; onset from birth. Mental and motor retardation; startle response to sound; seizures; blindness; deafness; spastic quadriplegia. Poor appetite, feeding difficulties. Recurrent bronchopneumonia.

Signs. Facial and peripheral edema; macrocephaly. Facial abnormalities: coarse features; broad nose; frontal bossing; long philtrum; prominent maxilla; mild macroglossia. Cherry-red macular spot (50%); retinitis pigmentosa. Joint movement limitation; kyphoscoliosis. Hepatosplenomegaly.

Etiology. Autosomal recessive inheritance. Severe deficit of lysosomal enzyme beta-galactosidase. Defect on chromosome 3.

Pathology. Neural lipidosis. Visceral histiocytosis: foamy cells in bone marrow, lymph nodes, liver, spleen, and various visceral organs. Ballooning renal glomeruloepithelial cytoplasm.

Diagnostic Procedures. *Blood.* Vacuolated lymphocytes. Beta-galactosidase assay of leukocytes. *Bone marrow.* Foamy histiocytes. *Urine.* Mucopolysacchariduria. Beta-galactosidase assay. *Biopsy of skin.* Presence of foamy cells. *Fibroblast culture.* Beta-galactosidase assay.

Therapy. Symptomatic.

Prognosis. Death at 6 months to 2 years.

BIBLIOGRAPHY. Caffey J: Gargoylism (Hunter-Hurler disease), dystomatosis multiplex, lipochondrodystrophy; prenatal and neonatal bone lesions and their early postnatal evolution. Bull Hosp Joint Dis 12:38–66, 1951

Norman RM, Tingey AH, Newman CGH, et al: Tay Sachs disease with visceral involvement and its relation to gargoylism. Arch Dis Child 39:634–640, 1964

Landing BH, Silverman FN, Craig JM, et al: Familial neurovisceral lipidosis. Am J Dis Child 108:503–582, 1964

Suzuki K, Chen GC: Morphological, histochemical and biochemical studies on a case of systemic late infantile lipidosis (generalized gangliosidosis). J Neuropathol Esp Neurol 27:15–38, 1968

O'Brien JS: The gangliosidoses. In Stanbury JB, Wyngaarden JB, Fredrickson DS, et al: The Metabolic Basis of Inherited Disease, 5th ed, p 945. New York, McGraw-Hill, 1983

NORMAN-ROBERTS

Synonym. Lissencephaly II.

Symptoms and Signs. From birth. Similar to Miller-Dieker. Low, sloped forehead, prominent nasal bridge are the distinguishing features.

Etiology. Autosomal recessive inheritance. Chromosomal normality.

BIBLIOGRAPHY. Norman MG, Roberts M, Sirois J, et al: Lissencephaly. Can J Neurol Sci 3:39–46, 1976

Dobyns WB, Stratton RF, Greenberg F. Syndromes with lissencephaly I: Miller-Dieker and Norman-Roberts syndromes and isolated lissencephaly. Ann J Med Genet 18:509–526, 1984

NORRBOTTEN*

Symptoms and Signs. Those of Greither's. Extremely severe symptoms that may reach mutilating degree.

Etiology. Autosomal recessive inheritance.

BIBLIOGRAPHY. Gamborg Nielsen P: Two different clinical and genetic forms of hereditary palmoplantar keratoderma in the northernmost county of Sweden. Clin Genet 28:361–366, 1985

NORRIE'S

Synonyms. Andersen-Warburg; atrophia bulborum hereditaria; fetal iritis; oligophrenia microphthalmus; bilateral retinal pseudotumor; Whitnall-Norman; Episkopi blindness; oculoacoustic dysplasia, congenital.

Symptoms. Only males affected; present from birth. Blindness; in some cases, mental retardation that begins at any age; deafness of different severity developing between ages of 9 and 45.

Signs. Presence of a mass behind clear lens; cataract (developing later); corneal opacification; phthisis bulbi, and, occasionally, iris atrophy and synechiae.

Etiology. Unknown; sex-linked inheritance; complete penetrance but different expressivity. Blindness a constant feature.

Pathology. Malformation of retinal layers of sensory cells, optic nerves, and tracts. Persistent hyperplastic primary vitreous intraocular hemorrhages. Other organs not studied.

Therapy. None.

Prognosis. Blindness; possibly, development of mental retardation (two-thirds of cases) and deafness (one-third of cases).

BIBLIOGRAPHY. Clarke E: Pseudo-glioma, in both eyes. Trans Ophthalmol Soc UK 18:136–138, 1898

Norrie G: Causes of blindness in children: twenty-five years' experience of Danish Institutes for the blind. Acta Ophthalmol (Kopenh) 5:357–386, 1927

Warburg M: Norrie's disease: a congenital progressive oculo-acoustic-cerebral degeneration. Acta Ophthalmol 89 (suppl):1–147, 1966

Dela Chapelle A, Sankila E-M, Lindlof M, et al: Norrie disease caused by a gene deletion allowing carrier detection and prenatal diagnosis. Clin Genet 28:317–320, 1985

Donnai D, Mountford RC, Read AP: Norrie disease resulting from a gene deletion: clinical features and DNA studies. J Med Genet 25:73–78, 1988

NORUM'S

Synonyms. Lecithin cholesterol acyltransferase deficiency familial; LCAT deficiency; serum cholesterol ester familial deficiency.

Symptoms and Signs. Prevalent in Scandinavia. From childhood, corneal opacities which form an arcus lipoides, impairment of vision. Normochromic anemia; progressive renal failure; early atherosclerotic manifestations.

Etiology. Autosomal recessive inheritance. Absence of LCAT (chromosome 16), which impairs metabolism of HDL and consequently alters lipoprotein pattern.

Pathology and Diagnostic Procedures. *Cornea.* Grayish dots that cause "misty" appearance. *Blood.* Erythrocytes, altered lipid composition. *Plasma.* High unesterified cholesterol and lecithin and low cholesterol ester and lysolecithin. No pre-beta-lipoprotein band; hypertriglyceridemia. Alteration of composition of VLDL and HDL; LDL2 are abnormally large. *Bone marrow and spleen.* Foam cells (sea blue histiocytes). *Urine.* Proteinuria, hematuria, hyaline casts. *Renal biopsy.* Foam cells.

Therapy. Plasma transfusion, restriction of dietary fat intake. Kidney transplantation (good results).

Prognosis. Increased incidence of myocardial infarction.

BIBLIOGRAPHY. Norum KR, Gjone E: Familial serum cho-

---

* Town in Sweden.

lesterol esterification failure: a new inborn error of metabolism. Biochim Biophys Acta 144:698–700, 1967

Glomset JA, Norum KR, Gjone E: Familial lecithin: cholesterol acyltransferase deficiency. In Stanbury JB, Wyngaarden JB, Fredrickson DS, et al: The Metabolic Basis of Inherited Disease, 5th ed, p 643. New York, McGraw-Hill, 1983

Vergani C, Catapano AL, Roma P, et al: A new case of familial LCAT deficiency. Acta Med Scand 214:173–176, 1983

NOTHNAGEL'S II

Synonym. Ophthalmoplegia-cerebellar ataxia. See Brun's.

Symptoms. Unilateral oculomotor palsy (ipsilateral to lesion); ataxia of gait. Poorly coordinated upper extremity movements.

Etiology and Pathology. Unilateral midbrain lesion; infarction; neoplasia.

Diagnostic Procedures. *Angiography. Spinal tap. CT brain scan.*

Therapy. According to etiology.

Prognosis. Depends on etiology.

BIBLIOGRAPHY. Nothnagel H: Topische Diagnostik der Gehirnkrankheiten: Eine klinische Studie, p 220. Berlin, Hirschwald, 1879
Dow RS, Moruzzi G: The Physiology and Pathology of the Cerebellum. Minneapolis, University of Minnesota Press, 1958
Adams RD, Victor M: Principles of Neurology, 3rd ed, p 1010. New York, McGraw-Hill, 1985

NOWAKOWSKI-LENZ

Synonyms. Androgen-resistant (type II); incomplete hereditary male pseudohermaphroditism (type II); pseudovaginal-perineoscrotal-hypospadias; 5-alpha-reductase deficiency.

Symptoms and Signs. At birth, external female phenotype; bilateral testes and normal virilized wolffian structures terminating in vagina. At puberty, variable degrees of virilization of external genitalia and partial development of secondary sexual characteristics; prostatic tissue not palpable; no gynecomastia; no acne.

Etiology. Deficiency of 5-alpha-reductase; autosomal recessive inheritance.

Pathology. See Symptoms and Signs.

Diagnostic Procedures. *Chromosome study.* 46XY. *Hormonal study.* Testosterone normal or elevated; dihy-

drotestosterone low in adulthood; ratio of urinary 5-beta-reduced to 5-alpha-reduced steroids decreased; reduction in vitro of testosterone to dihydrotestosterone; decreased 5-alpha-reductase activity in tissues.

Therapy. If decision is to raise as female, castration is needed before puberty to prevent virilization. If decision is to raise as male, repair of hypospadias and cryptorchidism.

Prognosis. As female (with early castration), usually successful adjustment; as male, at puberty usually a change in gender role.

BIBLIOGRAPHY. Nowakowski H, Lenz W: Genetic aspects on male hypogonadism. Rec Proc Horm Res 17:53–95, 1961
Griffin JE, Wilson JD: The syndromes of androgen resistance. New Engl J Med 302:198–209, 1980
Wilson JD, Griffin JE, Leshin M, et al: The androgen resistance syndrome: 5-α-reductase deficiency, testicular feminization, and related disorders. In Stanbury JB, Wyngaarden JB, Fredrickson DS, et al: The Metabolic Basis of Inherited Disease, 5th ed, p 1001. New York, McGraw-Hill, 1983

NUMB CHIN

Symptoms and Signs. Numbness of chin and lower lip, possibly associated with pain and swelling.

Etiology. Considered a potentially ominous symptom indicating the presence of metastasis or primary tumor of the lower jaw. Trauma, inflammatory disorders, cyst, or benign tumor seldom responsible for such a clinical manifestation.

Diagnostic Procedures. *X-ray.* Frequently, symptoms may precede the x-ray evidence by a month.

Therapy. Surgical, roentgen, ray or chemical treatment of primary or metastatic lesions.

Prognosis. If neoplasia, ominous.

BIBLIOGRAPHY. Seldin HM, Seldin SD, Rakower W: Metastatic carcinoma of the mandible: Report of cases. J Oral Surg 11:336–340, 1953
Coverley JR, Mohnec AM: Syndrome of numb chin. Arch Intern Med 112:819–821, 1963

NUTRITIONAL AMBLYOPIA

Synonyms. Alcohol amblyopia; deficiency amblyopia; Obal's; retrobulbar neuropathy; tobacco-alcohol amblyopia.

Symptoms. Occur in chronic undernourished individuals; onset slow, insidious. Progressive visual loss; dimness for close and far objects; difficulty in reading; photophobia; retrobulbar discomfort.

Signs. Initially, slight redness of temporal margins of optic disks; later pallor; symmetric bilateral central or paracentral scotoma; intact peripheral fields.

Etiology. Chronic malnutrition in vitamin B_{12} deficiency; diabetes mellitus, after isonicotinic acid–hydrazide treatment. The notion that tobacco or cyanide could be responsible has been discarded by logic and by experimental data.

Pathology. Bilateral symmetric loss of myelinated fibers in central part of optic (II) nerve. In severe forms, loss of ganglion cell in the macula.

Diagnostic Procedures. *Blood.* Hypoproteinemia; hypochromic microcytic or macrocytic anemia. Low level of B_{12} (occasional); low transketolase activity. *Urine.* Abnormal excretion of methylmalonic acid.

Therapy. Improved nutrition; vitamin B complex.

Prognosis. Degree of recovery according to degree of damage and time of onset of treatment.

BIBLIOGRAPHY. Obal A: Nutritional amblyopia. Am J Ophthalmol 34:857–865, 1951

Dreyfus PM: Nutritional disorders of obscure etiology. Med Sci 17:44–48, 1966

Adams RD, Victor M: Principles of Neurology, 3rd ed, pp 770–771. New York, McGraw-Hill, 1985

NUTRITIONAL RECOVERY

Symptoms and Signs. Occur in undernourished children when they begin to recover, following the administration of adequate food. The symptoms and signs appear in the following order, increase for 2 weeks, and then slowly decrease and disappear within about 3 months: transient weight loss followed by progressive increase; edema that disappears in approximately 20 days; progressively increasing hepatomegaly, normal consistency, sharp edge, no tenderness, appearing at the 20th day; abdominal distension; moderate congestion of thoracoabdominal venous network; ascites (in 50% of cases) of short duration (1 to 2 weeks); persistent hypertrichosis of shoulders, thighs, and face (in 50% of cases).

Etiology. Unknown; complex metabolic disorder. It is supposed that following the removal of fat infiltration, binding of water at the liver level determines intrahepatic-portal hypertension.

Pathology. Liver biopsies show the progressively decreasing fatty infiltrations.

Diagnostic Procedures. *Blood.* Before syndrome; total proteins, albumin, alpha and beta globulins low; gamma globulins high. Two weeks after beginning of syndrome, total protein normal, albumin still low; gamma-globulin rising. After disappearance of edema, same pattern plus correction of alpha-globulin level, hepatic function tests abnormal, with the exception of cephalincholesterol. Increase of eosinophils in blood 60 to 75 days after onset. *Biopsy of liver* (see Pathology).

Prognosis. Disappearance of the syndrome in about 3 months.

BIBLIOGRAPHY. Gomez F, Galvan RR, Munoz JC: Nutritional recovery syndrome. Pediatrics 10:513–526, 1952

Symposium on Nutrition. The pediatric clinics of North America. vol 32, n 2. Philadelphia, WB Saunders, 1985

NYGAARD-BROWN

Synonyms. Essential thrombophilia. See also Trousseau's syndrome.

Symptoms and Signs. Variable manifestations related to venous obstruction involving localized districts.

Etiology. Unknown; possibly, a paraneoplastic syndrome.

Diagnostic Procedure. *Blood.* Enhanced coagulation.

Therapy. Heparin.

Prognosis. According to basic pathology and district(s) affected. Gangrene a frequent complication.

BIBLIOGRAPHY. Nygaard KK, Brown GE: Essential thrombophilia. Report of five cases. Arch Intern Med 59:82:106–107, 1937

Wintrobe MM (ed): Clinical Hematology, 8th ed, p 1251. Philadelphia, Lea & Febiger, 1981

NYSTAGMUS COMPENSATION

Symptoms. Onset preceded by nystagmus. Infantile esotropia; abnormal head posture toward the adducted fixing eye, amblyopia. Nystagmus is reduced with fixing eye adduced.

BIBLIOGRAPHY. Von Noorden GK: The nystagmus compensation (blockage) syndrome. Am J Ophthalmol 82:287, 1976

Frank JW: Diagnostic signs in the nystagmus compensation syndrome. J Pediatr Ophthalmol Strabism 16:317–320, 1979

OAST-HOUSE

Synonyms. Beery baby; Smith-Strang; methionine malabsorption.

Symptoms and Signs. Onset in infancy. White hair; severe mental defect; unresponsiveness to stimuli; flaccidity. Recurrent episodes of generalized edema. Distinctive odor of dried malt or hops.

Etiology. Unknown; congenital enzymatic block. This condition resembles phenylketonuria but is considered a separate entity because of a different enzymatic block. Autosomal recessive inheritance, defect of utilization of alphaketoacids of essential aminoacids.

Pathology. No specific changes. Unduly soft consistency of all parts of brain; widespread defect of myelinization in cerebrum, brainstem, and cord.

Diagnostic Procedures. *Urine.* Large amounts of alpha-hydroxybutyric and phenylpyruvic acids; ferric chloride test positive.

Therapy. None specific; symptomatic.

Prognosis. Poor; condition persists until death, which may occur within first year of life.

BIBLIOGRAPHY. Smith AJ, Strang LB: An inborn error of metabolism with the urinary excretion of a hydroxybutyric acid and phenyl-pyruvic acid. Arch Dis Child 33:109–113, 1958
Cone TE: Diagnosis and treatment: some diseases, syndromes, and conditions associated with an unusual odor. Pediatrics 41:993–995, 1968
Hooft C, Carton D, Snoeck J, et al: Further investigation in the methionine malabsorption syndrome. Helv Paediatr Acta 23:334–349, 1968

OBSERVATION HIP

Synonyms. Transitory coxitis; coxitis serosa seu simplex; acute transient epiphysitis; toxic synovitis; transient synovitis. See Migratory osteolysis of the hip.

Symptoms. Occur in children. Limp with or without referred pain to the knee, thigh, or groin.

Signs. Slight limitation of passive hip movements.

Etiology. Varied: minor injury; focal infections; allergy; most frequently, idiopathic.

Pathology. Mild osteoarthritis or synovitis.

Diagnostic Procedures. *X-ray.* Normal. *Blood.* Sedimentation rate normal. *Mantoux test.* Positive only in some subjects. *Biopsy of lymph node.* Slight hyperplasia; no evidence of tuberculosis.

Therapy. Preventon of weight bearing and observation (hence the name of the syndrome).

Prognosis. Symptoms disappear spontaneously in weeks or months, seldom recur. Sequelae long after the episodes are sometimes observed with radiologic changes in hip joint.

BIBLIOGRAPHY. Lovett RW, Morse JL: A transient or ephemeral form of hip disease with report of cases. Boston Med Surg J 127:161–163, 1892
Hunder GG, Kelly PJ: Roentgenologic transient osteoporosis of the hip: a clinical syndrome? Ann Intern Med 68:539–552, 1968

OCCUPATIONAL NOSEBLEEDS

Synonyms. Apple packer; rosaniline nosebleeds.

Symptoms. Mild rhinorrhea and conjunctival irritation. Nosebleeds occurring in people working with tray manufacturing for apple and apple-packing or other industries that use rosaniline dyes.

Signs. Seldom (1%), septal ulcer ringed with blue dust.

Etiology. Mucosal irritation by rosaniline dyes (gentian violet; crystal violet; methyl violet).

Pathology. Hyperemia and hemorrhage of nasal mucosa.

Therapy. Corticosteriods may prevent bleeding and minimize irritation. Ulcer requires cautery or other prolonged treatment.

Prognosis. Nosebleeds stop with cessation of exposure, except when ulcer is present.

BIBLIOGRAPHY. Quinby GE: Epidemic nosebleeds in apple packers. JAMA 197:165–168, 1966
Quinby GE: Gentian violet as a cause of epidemic occupational nosebleeds. Arch Environ Health 16:485–489, 1968

OCKULY-MONTGOMERY

Synonyms. Lichenoid tuberculid; papulonecrotic tuberculid.

Symptoms. On the limbs, sudden, symmetric eruption of pealike, brownish lesions, possibly, annular shape and in groups.

Etiology. Unknown. Considered by the authors a tuberculid rash, which, however, is similar to sarcoidosis (see Besnier-Boeck-Schaumann).

Pathology. In upper dermis; well-defined, usually perivascular, tubercle; inconstant caseation. Coexistent (occasionally) glandular or systemic tuberculosis.

Therapy. *Biopsy. Tuberculosis tests. X-ray,* Sputum cultures. Mantoux test generally negative.

Prognosis. Lesion fades with residual brown discoloration, without scarring.

BIBLIOGRAPHY. Ockuly OE, Montgomery H: Lichenoid tuberculid: clinical and histopathologic studies. J Invest Dermatol 14:415–426, 1950
Rook A, Wilkinson DS, Ebling FJG, et al: Textbook of Dermatology, 4th ed, pp 815–816. Oxford, Blackwell Scientific Publications, 1986

OCULO-CEREBELLO-TEGMENTAL

Symptoms and Signs. Both sexes affected; onset at older ages. Transitory hemiplegia of sudden onset associated with bilateral cerebellar manifestations and paralysis of associated ocular movements.

Etiology and Pathology. Vascular lesion of mesencephalon. Softening of peduncular tegmentum.

BIBLIOGRAPHY. Rodriquez B, Rodriquez BR, Oreggia A: Un nuevo tipo de sindrome peducolar; oftalmoplejia internuclear anterior y sindrome cerebelosobilateral par lesion tegmental. Arch Urug Med 10:353–370, 1945
Fournier A, Ducoulombier H, Coussin J, et al: Oculocerebellar-myoclonic syndrome and neuroblastoma. J Sci Med Lille 90:189–197, 1972

OCULODENTAL DYSPLASIA

Synonyms. Dysplasia oculodentodigitalis; dyscraniopygophalangia; Gillespie's; Lohman's; Weyers III; microphthalmos; oculodentodigital, ODD, Mohr's; acrocephalopoly syndactyly IV, Mohr-Clausen; orofacial-digital II, OFDII; Meyer's; Schwickerath-Weyers. See also Hallermann-Streiff, Rieger's, Peter's, Rutherford's, Gorlin-Chandhry-Moss

Symptoms and Signs. Both sexes affected; present from birth. Two types. *Dysplasia oculodentodigitalis.* Symptoms and signs less severe than in type II. *II Dyscraniopygophalangial.* Hypertelorism. Microphthalmia; microcornea; eccentric pupil; changes in iris structure; remnant of pupillary membrane. Myopia; hyperopia. Thin small nose; anteverted nostrils; hypoplastic teeth; mandible wide, alveolar ridge. Syndactyly (4th and 5th fingers; 3rd and 4th toes.) Camptodactyly (5th finger) Hypoplasia of one or more digits. Sparse hair growth. Visceral malformations. Mentally normal.

Etiology. Autosomal dominant with variable expressivity.

Diagnostic Procedures. *X-ray.* Broad tubular bones.

Prognosis. *Type I.* Fair. *Type II.* Fatal because of associated visceral malformations.

BIBLIOGRAPHY. Lohmann W: Beitrug zur Kenntnis des reinen Mikrophthalmus. Arch Augenheilkd 86:136–141, 1920
Mohr, OL: A hereditary sublethal syndrome in man. Avhandl Norske Videnskaps-Akademi Oslo. J Mat Naturwiss Klasse 14:1–3, 1941
Claussen O: Et arvelig syndrom omfattende tugemis-dannelse of polydactyly. Nord Med 30:1147–1151, 1946
Meyer-Schwickerath G, Gruterich E, Weyers H: Mikrophthalmus-Syndrome. Klin Monatsbl Augenheilkd 131:18–30, 1957
Pfeiffer RA, Majewski F, Mannskopf H: Das syndrom von Mohr und Claussen. Klin Paediatr 184:224–226, 1972
Patton MA, Lawrence KM: Three cases of oculodentodigital (ODD) syndrome: development of the facial phenotype. J Med Genet 22:386–389, 1985

OCULOPHARYNGEAL MUSCULAR DYSTROPHY

Synonyms. Dysphagia-ptosis-muscular dystrophy; Von Graefe; Graefe's.

Symptoms and Signs. Equal sex distribution onset from infancy to 5th decade; insidious onset and slow progression. Progressive ptosis and dysphagia (cardinal symptoms); occasionally associated, weakness of facial, extraocular, and limb-girdle muscles. Dysphagia precedes the ptosis by an interval of a month or years. All patients share common ethnic background (six pedigrees of hereditary oculopharyngeal syndrome families have been reported). A few sporadic cases also reported.

Etiology. Unknown; inherited condition of dominant type. A variety with predominant distal myopathy has also been reported (Satoyoshy). A family with recessive form has been reported as well (Serimgeour).

Pathology. *Muscle biopsy.* Isolated or clustered fibers with accumulation of sarcoplasmic matter. *Electronmi-*

croscopy. Degenerative fiber changes and abnormalities in muscle cell mitochondria.

Diagnostic Procedures. *Deglutition studies.* Abnormality confined to pharynx, hypopharynx, and upper third of esophagus. *Electromyography.* Consistent with myopathic process.

Therapy. None.

Prognosis. Slow progression (years of ptosis and dysphagia), and wasting of affected muscles.

BIBLIOGRAPHY. Von Graefe AF: Demonstration in der Berlin medizinschen Gesellschaft. Berlin Klin Wochenschr 5:127, 1868

Taylor EW: Progressive vagus glossopharyngeal paralysis and ptosis: contribution to a group of family diseases. J Nerv Ment Dis 42:129–139, 1915

Kiloh LG, Nevin S: Progressive dystrophy of external ocular muscles (ocular myopathy). Brain 74:115–143, 1951

Satoyoshy E, Kinoshita M: Oculopharyngo distal myopathy: report of four families. Arch Neurol 34:89–92, 1977

Ozobor A: Data on the oculopharyngeal syndrome: a clinicopathological study. Eur Neurol 9:242–259, 1973

Knoblanch A, Koppel M: Die okulopharyngeale Muskeldystrophie. Schweiz Med Wochenschr 114:557–561, 1984

O'DONNELL-PAPPAS

Synonyms. See Karsch's-Neugenbauer's.

Symptoms and Signs. Nystagmus and presenile cataract; nystagmus and mild foveal hypoplasia; peripheral corneal pannus.

Etiology. Unknown autosomal dominant.

BIBLIOGRAPHY. O'Donnell FE Jr, Pappas HR: Autosomal dominant foveal hypoplasia and presenile cataracts. Arch Ophthalmol 100:279–281, 1982

OECKERMAN'S

Synonyms. Acid-alpha-mannosidase deficiency; alpha-mannosidase deficiency; mannosidosis; See Mucopolysaccharidosis syndromes (Hurler's, Scheie's, etc.). Syndrome is today divided into type I with infantile onset and type II with juvenile onset and less severe course.

Symptoms and Signs. Both sexes affected. In first year of life, normal, except for recurrent respiratory infections; then, in succeeding years the following progressive changes and manifestations: delayed early motor and speech development; clumsy movements; coarse facies (more minor than in MPS I and later than in ML II); low nasal bridge; prominent forehead and mandible; occasionally, macroglossia and wide teeth; lens opacities and vision reduction; frequently, neural deafness. Generalized muscle hypotonia; brisk tendon reflexes; protuberant abdomen.

Etiology. Autosomal recessive inheritance. Lysosomal condition with deficiency of acid-alpha mannosidase. Enzyme defect on chromosome 19.

Pathology. Lymphocytes: vacuolated; liver biopsy: vacuolated cells with reticulogranular pattern.

Diagnostic Procedures. *Blood.* Vacuolization of peripheral lymphocytes; presence of dark granules in neutrophils; presence of reduced alpha-mannosidase in serum, leukocytes, tissues, and urine. *X-ray.* Dysostosis multiplex.

Therapy. None.

Prognosis. Adult cases reported.

BIBLIOGRAPHY. Oeckerman PA: A generalized storage disorder resembling Hurler's syndrome. Lancet II:239–241, 1967

Beaudet AL: Disorders of glycoprotein degradation: mannosidosis, fucosidosis, sialidosis and aspartyl-glycosaminuria. In Stanbury JB, Wyngaarden JB, Fredrickson DS et al: The Metabolic Basis of Inherited Disease. 5th ed, p 788. New York, McGraw-Hill, 1983

OGILVIE'S

Synonyms. Acute colonic pseudoobstruction; pseudoobstruction of colon; false colonic obstruction; intestinal pseudoobstruction; colonic ileus.

Symptoms and Signs. In old age, both sexes. In patients presenting various pathological conditions (systemic or metabolic disorders, postoperative or posttraumatic states).

Etiology. Unknown. Imbalance between sympathetic and parasympathetic innervation hypothesized.

Pathology. Distended colon, with possible cecal perforation.

Diagnostic Procedures. *X-ray, plain film of abdomen.* Signs of intestinal obstruction without fluid level. *Barium enema.* No signs of mechanical obstruction. *Blood.* Mild imbalance of electrolytes.

Therapy. *Conservative.* Nasogastric aspiration, colonic decompression. Correction of electrolyte imbalance. *Surgery.* To correct perforation.

Prognosis. Mortality rate 25% to 30%.

BIBLIOGRAPHY. Ogilvie H: Large intestine colic due to sympathetic deprivation: new clinical syndrome. Br Med J 2:671–673, 1948

MacFarlane JA, Kay SK: Ogilvie's syndrome of false colonic obstruction: is it a new clinical entity? Br Med J 2:1267–1269, 1949

Nanni G, Garbini A, Luchetti P, et al: Olgivie's syndrome (acute colonic pseudoobstruction): review of literature and report of 4 additional cases. Dis Colon Rectum 25:157–177, 1982

OGUCHI'S

Synonyms. Night blindness; stationary night blindness; nyctalopia. See also Uyemura's.

Symptoms. Majority of cases observed in Japan; reported also in Caucasians and Blacks; both sexes affected; manifest at early age. Stable nyctalopia in dimmed illumination; reduced dark adaption fields and visual acuity.

Signs. Unusual color of fundus, from grayish white to yellow, extending throughout entire fundus or in small section(s); Mizno's phenomenon (in the dark the fundus assumes a normal reddish appearance).

Etiology. Unknown; autosomal recessive inheritance.

Pathology. Indirect evidence of thinning or defect in the pigmented epithelium of fundus. Cones longer and anatomically modified.

Diagnostic Procedures. *Ophthalmoscopy.* Evidence of Mizno's phenomenon using eye patches. *Electroretinography.* Absence of B waves. *Fluorescent angiography.*

Therapy. None; vitamin A may be tried.

Prognosis. Static nyctalopia.

BIBLIOGRAPHY. Oguchi C: Ueber du eigenartige Hemeralopic mit diffuser weissgränlicher Verfarhung des Augenhintergrundes. Graefe Arch Ophthalmol 81:109–117, 1912

Winn S, Tasman W, Spaerh G, et al: Oguchi's disease in Negroes. Arch Ophthalmol 81:501–507, 1969

Pau H: Differential Diagnosis of Eye Diseases. Philadelphia, WB Saunders, 1980

OLD SERGEANT

Synonym. Neurotic battle behavior.

Symptoms. Occur in well-motivated, previously efficient soldiers without neurotic factors in previous history, who are able to handle responsibility (60% noncommissioned officers) have leadership quality, strong self-esteem; onset after a long period of combat, without rest. Abnormal tremulousness; first into foxhole, last to leave shelter; decreased effectiveness in battle to complete incapacitation; inability to make quick decision and assume responsibility. No complaining and seldom on sick call. Symptoms disappear once patient is removed from environment, but quickly return if reexposed, despite willingness to perform. Strong sense of discipline and devotion to unit (squad, company) in which he is serving. Frequently, dyspepsia.

BIBLIOGRAPHY. Sobel R: "Old sergeant" syndrome. Psychiatry 10:315–321, 1947

Belenky G: Contemporary studies in combat psychiatry. London, Greenwood Press, 1987

OLIVER-MCFARLANE

Synonyms. Gray's; trichomegaly; mental retardation-dwarfism-retina pigmentary degeneration.

Symptoms and Signs. Normal development in first few months of life. Bilateral destruction of tear canals. Slow dentition; poor vision (pigmentary degeneration of retina); heterochromia; hypertrichosis of eyebrows and eyelashes; alopecia (developing at 4 to 5 years of age), dwarfism; normal mentality, or retardation.

Etiology. Unknown; form of ectodermal dysplasia. Usually sporadic. Partial trisomy of chromosome 13 suggested.

Pathology. See Signs. Biopsy of scalp skin shows degenerated hair follicles with patchy lymphocytic infiltration.

Diagnostic Procedures. *Blood.* Normal. *Spinal fluid.* Normal. *Chromosome study.* Normal.

Therapy. None.

Prognosis. Normal mental development; partially sighted.

BIBLIOGRAPHY. Gray H: Trichomegaly or movie lashes. Stanford Med Bull 2:157–158, 1944

Oliver GL, McFarlane DC: Congenital trichomegaly with associated pigmentary degeneration of the retina, dwarfism, and mental retardation. Arch Ophthalmol 74:169–171, 1965

Cant JS: Ectodermal dysplasia. J Pediatr Ophthalmol 4:13–17, 1967

Delleman JW, Van Walbeek K: The syndrome of trichomegaly, tapetoretinal degeneration and growth disturbances. Ophthalmologica 171:313–315, 1975

OLIVER'S

Synonym. Postaxial polydactyly-mental retardation.

Symptoms and Signs. Two girls and one boy with said combination reported.

Etiology. Autosomal recessive inheritance.

BIBLIOGRAPHY. Oliver CP: Recessive polydactylism associated with mental deficiency. J Hered 31:365–367, 1940

OLIVOPONTOCEREBELLAR ATROPHY III

Synonyms. OPCA III; OPCA-retinal degeneration; Froment's.

Symptoms and Signs. Both sexes. Onset in middle age, occasionally in adolescence or in severe cases in infancy. Progressive loss of vision and ataxia.

Etiology. Autosomal dominant inheritance.

Pathology. Retinal degeneration (various patterns mainly macular). Cerebellar degenerative changes.

Prognosis. Variable period of survival according to severity. Variable in different families.

BIBLIOGRAPHY. Froment J, Bonnet P, Colrat A: Heredo-degenerations retinienne et spino-cerebeleuse; variantes ophthalmoscopiques et neurologique presentees par trois generations successive. J Med Lyon, 153–163, 1937
Konigsmark BW, Weiner LP: The olivopontocerebellar atrophy: a review. Medicine 49:227–241, 1970

OLIVOPONTOCEREBELLAR ATROPHY V

Symptoms and Signs. Prevalent in male. Cerebellar signs followed at later age by rigidity and progressive mental deterioration up to dementia.

Etiology. Autosomal dominant inheritance.

Pathology. Cerebellolivary and substantia nigra degeneration up to atrophy. Cortical evidence of degenerative process.

BIBLIOGRAPHY. Chandler JH, Bebin J: Hereditary cerebellar ataxia: olivopontocerebellar type. Neurology 6:187–195, 1956
Carter HR, Sukavajane C: Familial cerebello-olivary degeneration with late development of rigidity and dementia. Neurology 6:876–884, 1956
Konigsmark BW, Lipton HL: Dominant olivopontocerebellar atrophy with dementia and extrapyramidal signs: report of a family through three generations. Birth Defects Orig Art Ser VII (1):178–191, 1971

OLLIER'S

Synonyms. Unilateral chondromatosis; multiple endochondromatosis; Ollier's osteochondromatosis. See Maffucci's.

Symptoms. Various functional disturbances of hands, feet, femora, fibulas, and pelvis (in that order), usually unilateral. Occasionally, pathologic fractures and vision impairment.

Signs. Deformity of mentioned bones; occasionally, abnormally short distal end of ulna. Ophthalmoplegia.

Etiology. Unknown; nonhereditary condition.

Pathology. Epiphyseal plates fail to undergo normal bone replacement and become incorporated in mature bone. Expansion of enchondromas with resulting deformities of bones.

Diagnostic Procedures. *X-ray of skeleton.* Radiolucent patches or fragmented, explosionlike pattern in metaphysis. *Biopsy of bone.*

Therapy. Orthopedic correction of deformities and pathologic fractures.

Prognosis. Severe disease may result in crippling and invalidism. Enchondroma sometimes develops into chondrosarcoma (10%). Growth of enchondroma may stop after puberty and calcification take place; sometimes it continues to grow throughout life. Tendency in some cases to become malignant.

BIBLIOGRAPHY. Ollier M: Sur une nouvelle affection: La dyschondroplasie. Rev Chir Paris, 21:396–398, 1900
Carnesale PG: Benign tumors of the bone. In Crenshaw AH (ed), Campbell's Operative Orthopedics, 7th ed, p 762. St Louis, CV Mosby, 1987

OMOHYOID

Symptoms. May occur when patient is in state of well-being; more frequent in subjects suffering from cramps in other areas. Onset usually following the act of yawning and swallowing at the same time as turning the head. Immediate excruciating pain in side of neck extending from the hyoid region to the omolateral scapula. Pain eases after a few minutes, but does not disappear. Inability to swallow saliva. Voice alteration and slurring of speech.

Signs. Pain on pressure over omohyoid muscle. Throat and larynx normal.

Etiology. Acute spasm or cramps of omohyoid muscle.

Therapy. Parenteral analgesic if pain lasts more than 1

hour. In cases of refractory pain or repeated attacks, division of central tendon of affected muscle.

Prognosis. Usually a little residual discomfort for 1 or 2 days.

BIBLIOGRAPHY. Zuchary RB, Young A, Hammond JDS: The omohyoid syndrome. Lancet II:104–105, 1969

ONDINE'S CURSE

Synonyms. Primary alveolar hypoventilation; idiopathic hypoventilation-nonobese; congenital central hypoventilation syndrome, CCHS. See Pickwickian.

Symptoms and Signs. Most cases reported have presented the syndrome within a few hours of birth. In 50% of patients prior history of central nervous system disease. Patient breathes relatively normally during the day but presents long periods of apnea during the night. Even death may occur during sleep. Possibly, various symptoms of hypothalamic dysfunction present.

Etiology. Diagnosis by exclusion. Rule out central nervous system disease, upper airway obstruction, neuromuscular disorders. It appears to result from a defect in the brainstem control and possibly a deficient transmission chemoreceptor.

Diagnostic Procedures. *Pulmonary function tests.* With patient awake, gas exchange normal or almost normal; during sleep, respiratory failure. *X-ray.* Normal lung findings and diaphragm movement. Of skull. Normal. *Electrocardiography.* Absence of right cardiac hypertrophy. *Blood.* Absence of polycythemia.

Therapy. Various drugs have been tried, with variable results. The most beneficial include doxapram and almitrine. The mainstay of treatment is tracheostomy with mechanical ventilation during the night. Phrenic nerve pacing (bilateral) has been used both in adults and children.

Prognosis. Children can grow up with mechanical ventilation; there is a definite risk of death due to respiratory infection, cor pulmonale or autonomic disturbances with cardiorespiratory failure or cardiac arrest.

BIBLIOGRAPHY. Giraudoux J: 'Ondine.' In Four Plays, Vol 1, p 253. New York, Hill & Wang, 1958
Severinghaus JW, Michell RA: Ondine's curse: failure of respiratory center automaticity while awake. Clin Res 10:122, 1962
Fishman LS, Samson JH, Sperling DR: Primary alveolar hypoventilation syndrome (Ondine's curse). Am J Dis Child 110:155–161, 1965
Coleman M, Boros SJ, Huseby TL, et al: Congenital central hypoventilation syndrome: a report of successful experience with bilateral diaphragmatic pacing. Arch Dis Child 55:901–903, 1980
Mather SJ: Ondine's curse and the anesthetist. Anaesthesia, 42:394–404, 1987

ONYALAI

Synonym. Werlhof's variant.

Symptoms and Signs. Occur in Bantu tribes in Africa. Only males affected; onset at any age, mostly in adulthood. Hemorrhagic bullae in mouth and other mucosal cavities.

Etiology. Unknown; variant of idiopathic thrombocytopenic purpura.

Diagnostic Procedures. *Blood.* Thrombocytopenia.

BIBLIOGRAPHY. Strongway WE, Strongway AK: Ascorbic acid deficiency in the African disease onyalay. Arch Intern Med 83:372–376, 1949
Lewis SM, Lurie A: Onyalai: a clinical and laboratory survey. J Trop Hyg 96:281–285, 1958
Wintrobe MM (ed): Clinical Hematology, 8th ed, pp 1098–1105. Philadelphia, Lea & Febiger, 1981

OPHTHALMIA, SYMPATHETIC

Synonym. Sympathetic uveitis.

Symptoms. Occur 3 to 8 weeks after injury to one eye. Development in contralateral eye, photophobia, pain, lacrimation, and vision impairment.

Signs. Tenderness; uveitis.

Etiology. Penetrating injury to one eye that causes sympathetic reaction in the other eye through reflex mechanism.

Pathology. Changes in uninjured eye: granulomatosis; inflammation; nodular accumulation of lymphocytes in uveal tract, followed by epithelioid cell infiltration.

Diagnostic Procedures. *Ophthalmoscopy.* Uveitis; retineal edema up to detachment.

Therapy. Rapid intervention up to removal of injured eye before changes in the contralateral one became established.

Prognosis. Without treatment, progressive condition leading to blindness.

OPITZ-FRIAS

Synonyms. Dysphagia-hypospadias; G; hypertelorism-esophageal abnormality.

Symptoms. Males affected (in female carriers, partial expression); present from birth. Swallowing problems with recurrent aspiration. Stridulous breathing; nonconstant wheezing; hoarse cry.

Signs. Hypertelorism. Palpebral fissures slanted; nasal bridge flat; mild to severe micrognathia. Occasionally, short frenulum of tongue, bifid scrotum, imperforate anus, prominent parietal-occipital areas. Females have normal genitalia.

Etiology. Unknown; considered autosomal dominant, sex limited or sex-linked.

Diagnostic Procedures. *Cinefluorography of swallowing.*

Therapy. If repeated aspirations, gastrostomy or jejunostomy considered.

Prognosis. Persistence of respiratory problems; bronchiectasis. Intelligence development normal; mild mental retardation in one family.

BIBLIOGRAPHY. Opitz JM, Frias JL, Gutenberger JE, et al: The G syndrome of multiple congenital anomalies. Birth Defects 5:95–103, 1969
Chemke J, Shor E, Ankori-Cohen H, et al: Male to male transmission of the G syndrome. Clin Genet 26:164–167, 1984
Bolsin SN, Gillbe C: Opitz-Frias syndrome. Anaesthesia 40:1189–1193, 1985

OPITZ-KAVEGGIA

Synonyms. FG (initial patient's surname); Keller's.

Symptoms and Signs. In males. Congenital macrocephaly; striking facies; imperforate or displaced anus; hypotonia; joint contractures; heart defects. Mental retardation; seizures, occasionally sensineuronal deafness, short stature. Striking personalities.

Etiology. X-linked inheritance.

Pathology. Partial agenesis of corpus callosum; variable gastrointestinal and heart malformations.

Prognosis. From death in first days of life to adulthood with short stature, muscle hypotonia, constipation, and variable degrees of mental retardation.

BIBLIOGRAPHY. Opitz JM, Kaveggia EF: The FG syndrome: an X-linked recessive syndrome of multiple congenital anomalies and mental retardation. Z Kinderheilk 117:1–18, 1974
Keller MA, Jones KL, Nyhan WL, et al: A new syndrome of mental deficiency with craniofacial, limb and anal abnormalities. J Pediatr 88:589–591, 1976

Thompson EM, Baraitser M, Lindenbaum RH, et al: The FG syndrome: 7 new cases. Clin Genet 27:582–594, 1985

OPITZ'S (Z.)

Synonyms. Cauchois-Eppinger-Frugoni; congestive fibrosplenomegaly; Frugoni's; thrombophlebitic splenomegaly. See Banti's and Hypersplenism.

Symptoms and Signs. Both sexes affected; onset at all ages. Low-grade or high temperature; abdominal discomfort; "dragging" feeling on left abdominal quadrant. Splenomegaly.

Etiology. Thrombophlebitis of splenic vein.

Diagnostic Procedures. See Banti's and Hypersplenism.

Therapy. Antibiotics; anticoagulants; surgery.

Prognosis. Guarded.

BIBLIOGRAPHY. Opitz Z: Zur kenntnis der thrombophlebitischen Splenomegalie. Jahr Zinderh 107:211–222, 1925
Frugoni C: La splénomegalie thrombophlébitique. Rev Belg Sci Med 10:227–236, 1938
Coon WW: Splenectomy for spenomegaly and secondary hypersplenism. World J Surg 9:437–443, 1985

OPPENHEIMER'S (A.)

Synonyms. Spondylitis ossificans ligamentosa I; physiologic vertebral ligamentous calcification. See Forestier-Rotes Querol.

Symptoms. Occur in patients over 50 years of age. Mild or no symptoms in the back, but decreased mobility of spinal column. No symptoms or evidence suggestive of rheumatoid arthritis.

Etiology. Limitation of spinal motion; degenerative changes followed by calcification of longitudinal vertebral ligaments.

Diagnostic Procedures. *X-ray.* One or multiple interspaces involved; thoracic region most frequently affected with calcification of ligament and a tortuous appearance. Vertebrae normal density; apophyseal and costovertebral joints normal. *Blood.* Normal; normal sedimentation rate.

Therapy. Physical therapy. Patients should be instructed to sleep supine on a firm bed without a pillow and to practice postural and deep-breathing exercises regularly. Indomethacin can be used for the control of pain. Surgical treatment to correct some spine and hip deformities can be of value in selected cases.

Prognosis. Good.

BIBLIOGRAPHY. Oppenheimer A: Calcification and ossification of vertebral ligaments (spondylitis ossificans ligamentosa) roentgen study of pathogenesis and clinical significance. Radiology 38:160–173, 1942

Smith CF, Pugh DG, Polley HE: Physiologic vertebral ligamentous calcification: an aging process. Am J Roentgenol 74:1049–1058, 1955

Kaine JL: Arthritis and rheumatologic disease. In Orland MJ, Saltman RJ (eds): In Manual of Medical Therapeutics, 25th ed, p 381. Boston, Little, Brown, 1986

OPPENHEIM'S

Synonyms. Amyotonia congenita; myotonia congenita; benign congenital hypotonia; congenital benign muscle hypoplasia.

Obsolete term. Hypotonia represents a symptom of various conditions. The old syndrome, representing a too-heterogeneous group, has been subdivided into Nording-Hoffman; infantile muscular atrophy; myopathies (Shy-Magee; nemaline mitochondrial; myotubular); and undifferentiated forms of hypotonia and muscle underdevelopment (see Walton's, Krabbe's and Floppy infant). Tendency to use the eponym to indicate generically primary nonprogressive myopathies and differentiate them from forms secondary to central nervous system pathology.

BIBLIOGRAPHY. Oppenheim H: Textbook of Nervous Disease. New York, GE Steckert, 1911

Adams RD, Denny-Brown D, Pearson CM: Diseases of the Muscle, 3rd ed, p 256. New York, Harper & Row, 1975

OPPENHEIM-URBACH'S

Synonyms. Extracellular cholesterosis; dermatitis atrophicans maculosa lipoides diabetica, necrobiosis diabeticorum; necrobiosis lipoidica, Urbach's.

Symptoms and Signs. Rare. Prevalent in females; 75% in patients have diabetes. Onset at all ages. *Variety I.* Purple red plaque with yellow brown center and nodules developing rapidly on extremities and dorsa of hands and feet. Ears, tongue, and chest may also be involved. *Variety II.* Purplish macular lesions interspersed with yellowish nodules and papules. Liver and spleen may be enlarged in both forms.

Etiology. Two-thirds to three-fourths of patients have diabetes mellitus; association not clear (only 0.3% of diabetic patients present the syndrome). Deposition of glycoprotein in small vessel walls may underlie the development of the condition as well as other forms of microangiopathies.

Pathology. Granulomatous reaction and fat deposit to necrobiotic and inflammatory localized changes with minimal evidence of vascular changes (except for lesion of the legs).

Diagnostic Procedures. *Biopsy of skin. Blood. Glucose* (in etiology); in many cases increase of alpha-2-macroglobulin.

Therapy. Proposed (in uncontrolled studies): aspirin and dipyridamole and perilesion infiltration with heparin.

Prognosis. Chronic, possibly incapacitating, but relatively benign course. Possibly, spontaneous remission after years.

BIBLIOGRAPHY. Oppenheim M: Eine noch nicht beschrieben Hauterkrankung bei Diabetes mellitus (Dermatitis atrophicans lipoides diabetica). Wien Klin Wochenschr 45:314–315, 1932

Urbach E: Beiträge zu einer physiologischen und pathologischen chemie der Haut; eine neue diabetische Stoffwechseldermatose: Nekrobiosis lipoidica diabeticorum. Arch Derm Syph 166:273–285, 1932

Rook A, Wilkinson DS, Ebling FJG, et al: Textbook of Dermatology, 4th ed, pp 1691–1694. Oxford, Blackwell Scientific Publications, 1986

ORBITAL APEX

Synonyms. Déjean; orbital apex-sphenoidal; orbital superior fissure; Rollet's; Rochon-Duvigneaud; sensorimotor ophthalmoplegia; sphenocavernous; sphenoid fissure; SO. A group of syndromes with extremely similar clinical characteristics. Four groups of Déjean recognized: In complete form, 2nd through 6th cranial nerves and sympathetic fibers involved; in sphenoidal, exclusion of second nerve; in partial, 3rd, 4th, and 6th cranial nerves involved; isolated nerve lesions.

Symptoms. Sudden onset, sometimes following recent respiratory infection. Impairment or loss of vision; diplopia. Severe pain in retroorbital and temporoparietal areas (area of ophthalmic branch of trigeminal (V) nerve).

Signs. Little or no displacement of bulb, from limited movement in various directions, to complete ophthalmoplegia. Bulb fixed in straight ahead position due to the paralysis of 3rd, 4th, and 6th cranial nerves. Tenderness slight or absent.

Etiology and Pathology. Infection, cysts, aneurysm, neoplasm, or trauma of sinuses (primarily frontal and ethmoidal) affecting the sphenoid fissure. Low-grade, nonspecific inflammation of cavernous sinuses.

Diagnostic Procedures. *X-ray, angiography.* Patterns according to etiology. *Blood.* In some cases, elevation of leukocytes and sedimentation rate. *Cerebrospinal fluid.* Highly variable; sugar normal or depressed; protein and cell normal or slightly elevated.

Therapy. Antibiotics or surgery. Heparin in cases with thrombosis.

Prognosis. Depends on etiology. Much improved by use of antibiotics; some cases of nonspecific infection respond to corticosteroids.

BIBLIOGRAPHY. Hirschfeld L: Epanchemant de sang dans de sinus caverneux du cote gauche diagnostique pendant la vie. C R Soc Biol 138, 1858
Rochon-Duvigneaud A: Quelques cas de paralysie de tous les nerfs orbitaires (ophtalmoplegie totale avec amaurose et anesthésie dans le domaine de l'ophtalmique d'origine syphilitique). Arch Ophthalmol 16:746–760, 1896
Déjean C: Les syndromes paralytiques du sommet de l'orbite. Arch Ophthalmol 44:657–690, 1927
Hedstrom J, Parson J, Maloney PL, et al: Superior orbital fissure syndrome: report of a case. J Oral Surg 32:198–202, 1974
Adams RD, Victor M: Principles of Neurology, 3rd ed, p 503. New York, McGraw-Hill, 1985

ORGANIC HYPERINSULINISM

Synonym. Endogenous hyperinsulinism. See Harris's and hypoglycemic, neonatal.

Symptoms and Signs. Those of acute and chronic hypoglycemia, sometimes with irreversible brain damage. Whipple's triad: (1) history of attack of hunger, weakness, sweating, and paresthesias coming during the fasting state; (2) blood glucose level of 40 mg/100 ml during the attacks; (3) immediate recovery with administration of glucose. Sudden hunger; weakness; headache; faintness; vertigo; sweating; paresthesias (on the face); tremors; palpitation. Central nervous system changes: diplopia; ataxia; aphasia; paralysis; convulsion; coma.

Etiology and Pathology. Adenoma of islets of Langerhans (beta cells), multiple, small, a few malignant with functional metastasis. Familial (usually), associated often with adenoma of parathyroids and pituitary. Hypertrophy or hyperplasia of pancreas in children.

Differential Diagnosis. Other causes of hypoglycemia: *Organic.* (1) Hypopituitarism; (2) hypoadrenocorticism; (3) chronic passive congestion of the liver; (4) tumors of different types (e.g., mesodermal; hepatomas; adrenal); (5) central nervous system lesions. *Functional.* (1) Functional hypoglycemia; (2) alimentary hypoglycemia; (3) early diabetes; (4) alcohol abuse; (5) lactation; intense

muscular exertion; (6) renal glycosuria. *Factitious hepatic enzyme defects.* (1) Glycogen storage diseases; (2) hereditary fructose imbalance; (3) hereditary galactosemia. *Therapeutic.* Overdosage in treatment of diabetes. *Idiopathic in infancy.* (1) Newborn of diabetic mother; (2) leucine sensitivity; (3) leucine insensitivity (a) absence of alpha cells, (b) poor epinephrine secretion.

Diagnostic Procedures. (1) Prolonged fasting; no food for 72 hours; only water. Only mild exercises. If patient has islet cell adenoma there is a reduction of blood glucose of 30%. (2) Five-hour glucose tolerance test: 1 g injected intravenously. If adenoma, in 30 minutes the glucose falls 50 to 80% and remains low for several hours. If functional, glucose falls but then rises to normal level in 1 to 2 hours. (3) Tolbutamide tolerance test. (4) Assay of insulin (excessive rise after tolbutamide) may be of great value. More important the longer hypoglycemia persists. (5) Leucine tolerance test. (6) Liver function test: fructose-galactose tolerance test, glucagon and epinephrine tolerance test. (7) *Angiography.* Selective celiac and superior mesenteric arteries studies.

Therapy. Surgery; blood glucose monitoring and glucose infusion with the aid of closed loop artificial pancreas; glucagon; diazoxide (300–600 mg daily orally) with concomitant thiazide diuretic. (Verapamil can be used in patients unable to tolerate diazoxide.) For islet cell carcinomas, streptozocin has been tried with success, without kidney toxicity.

Prognosis. Complete remission with adequate therapy. *Complications.* Retinal cerebrovascular hemorrhage; coronary insufficiency; central nervous system irreversible damage (fast drop; muscle atrophy; pyramidal signs); after surgery, transient or permanent diabetes; pancreatic insufficiency; gastric ulcerations.

BIBLIOGRAPHY. Arki RA: Hypoglycemia. In De Groot LJ, Cahill FG Jr, Odell WD, et al (eds): Endocrinology, p 1112. New York, Grune & Stratton, 1979
Service FJ (ed): Hypoglycemia Disorders: Pathogenesis, Diagnosis and Treatment. Hall, 1983
Schroeder SA, Krupp MA, Tierny LM (eds): Current Medical Diagnosis and Treatment. Lange, 1988

ORMOND'S

Synonyms. Gerota's fascitis; periureteral fibrosis; periureteritis plastica; retroperitoneal fibrosis; retroperitoneal idiopathic fibrosis.

Symptoms. More frequent in males; average age at onset 46 years for males, 32 years for females. Pain in the back, of variable intensity, usually progressing and radiating in pattern of ureteral colic, or abdominal pain without specific localization. Pain usually persisting for a month.

Frequently associated: vomiting; nausea; anorexia; malaise; fatigue; weight loss, constipation or diarrhea. Seldom associated: ADH-resistant diabetes insipidus syndromes (see) with nocturia; oliguria; backache; edema; headache; dysuria; thirst.

Signs. Not contributory. Moderate blood pressure elevation; seldom, fever. A mass may be palpated and tenderness elicited in the costal vertebral angle.

Etiology. Unknown; possibly a fasciculitis of collagen disease; multiple etiologies possible. See Sclerosing lipogranulomatosis syndromes. Methysergide and ergotamine can occasionally cause this syndrome.

Pathology. Periureteral fibrosis; fibrous band that locally constricts ureter, sometimes iliac vessel or aorta as well. Microscopically, chronic inflammatory reaction with prevalent lymphocytes and fibroblastic proliferation. Pyelonephritis frequently observed. Fibrous band occluding bile duct also occasionally present (suggesting systemic disease).

Diagnostic Procedures. *Blood.* Anemia (constant); high blood urea nitrogen, high sedimentation rate. *Retrograde pyelography. CT scan. Ultrasonography. Biopsy.* Multiple deep biopsies to rule out neoplastic disease.

Therapy. Surgery, nephrectomy, or nephrostomy with ureterolysis, and subsequent operation of other side to free the ureter. Antibiotics.

Prognosis. Good with therapy; diabetes insipidus-like syndrome disappears as a result of treatment of local condition. Pyelonephritis may persist. In patients with unilateral involvement, involvement of other side occurs in about 25% of cases. Surgical treatment for relief of ureteral obstruction from the fibrous encasement. Steroid therapy of questionable value.

BIBLIOGRAPHY. Oberling C: Retroperitoneal xanthogranuloma. Am J Cancer 23:477–489, 1935

Ormond JK: Bilateral ureteral obstruction due to envelopment and compression by an inflammatory retroperitoneal process. J Urol 59:1072–1079, 1948

Srinivas V, Dow D: Retroperitoneal fibrosis. Can J Surg 27:111–113, 1984

Mitchison MJ: Retroperitoneal fibrosis revisited. Arch Pathol Lab Med 110:784–786, 1986

Morad N, Strongwater SL, Eypper S, Woda BA: Idiopathic Retroperitoneal and Mediastinal Fibrosis Mimicking connective tissue disease. AM J Med 82:363–366, 1987

ORO-FACIAL-DIGITAL III

Synonyms. OFD III; Sugarman's.

Symptoms. From birth, both sexes. Mental retardation.

Signs. Eye abnormalities (in some cases "see-saw winking"); hypertelorism; hamartomatous tongue; teeth abnormalities; uvula bifida; hexadactyly of hands and feet; pectus excavatum; kyphosis; spasticity.

Etiology. Possibly autosomal recessive inheritance.

BIBLIOGRAPHY. Sugarman GI, Katakia M, Menkes JH: See-saw winking in a familial oro-facial-digital syndrome. Clin Genet 248–254, 1971

OROTIC ACIDURIA

Synonyms. Hereditary orotic aciduria; megaloblastic orotic anemia.

Symptoms. Nine cases (seven males, two females) reported. No abnormalities at birth. During first year, failure to thrive. Apathy; some degree of mental retardation, lassitude; repeated infections.

Signs. Pallor; muscle hypotonia; no neurologic defects.

Etiology. In seven cases, reduced activity in both orotate phosphoribose-transferase (OPRT) and orotidine 5' phosphate decarboxylase (ODC); in two cases, atypical different condition. Autosomal recessive inheritance.

Diagnostic Procedures. *Blood.* Hypochromic anemia with marked anisopoikilocytosis; leukogenic normal platelets. *Urine.* Excessive excretion of orotic acid. *Bone marrow.* Atypical megaloblastic changes.

Therapy. Yeast nucleotides (poorly tolerated: gastrointestinal symptoms) uridine; glucocorticoids.

Prognosis. Good remission with yeast nucleotides. Good remission with uridine. Partial hematologic remission with glucocorticoids.

BIBLIOGRAPHY. Huguley CM Jr, Bain JA, Rivers SL, et al: Refractory megaloblastic anemia associated with excretion of orotic acid. Blood 1:615–634, 1959

Kelly WN: Hereditary orotic aciduria. In Stanbury JB, Wyngaarden JB, Fredrickson DS, et al, The Metabolic Basis of Inherited Disease, 5th ed, p 1202. New York, McGraw-Hill, 1983

ORTHOSTATIC SYNCOPE

Synonyms. Hypotension orthostatic; hyperadrenergic orthostatic hypotension.

Symptoms. More frequent in tall, asthenic subjects with poor muscle structure. In the morning hours, enhanced by heat, humidity, heavy meals and exercise and when assuming upright posture. Lightheadedness, blurred vision, weakness, and unsteadiness may reach loss of consciousness.

Signs. Progressive hypotension over seconds or minutes, tachycardia, pallor, cold extremities, and sweating.

Etiology. May be classified into three categories: (1) venous pooling and/or blood volume depletion (anemia, hemorrhage, gastrointestinal fluid loss, prolonged fever, dialysis, intense sweating, diabetes insipidus); (2) pharmacological agents (antihypertensive, diuretics, nitrates, vasodilatotors, antidepressants, tranquilizers, and other central nervous system agents); 3) neurogenic (neuropathies, spinal cord diseases, intracranial tumors, Parkinson's, CNS atherosclerosis, etc.). Deficiency of autonomic functions.

Pathology. According to etiology.

Diagnostic Procedures. Evaluation of possible general causes (see Etiology) for autonomic imbalances differential diagnosis (see Bradbury-Eggleston and Shy-Drager syndromes)

Therapy. See Bradbury-Eggleston.

Prognosis. Variable according to basic condition. Single episodes tend to be overcome spontaneously.

BIBLIOGRAPHY. Schatz IJ: Orthostatic hypotension. Arch Intern Med 144, 773–777; 1037–1041, 1984

ORTNER'S

Synonym. Cardiovocal.

Symptoms. Hoarseness plus symptoms of cardiovascular conditions: aortic arch lesions; mitral stenosis; congenital cardiac defects; hypertensive heart disease; coronary artery disease.

Signs. Faulty movements or palsy of left vocal cord.

Etiology and Pathology. Left laryngeal nerve injury by compression between aorta and dilated pulmonary artery.

Diagnostic Procedures. Those for cardiac disease.

Differential Diagnosis. In infancy, vocal cord paralysis has usually been associated with central nervous system lesions, especially meningocele with Arnold-Chiari malformation. Increased intracranial pressure can compress the vagus nerves at the foramen magnum, causing bilateral vocal cord paralysis. Birth trauma could cause either bilateral or unilateral paralysis. If the traction on the left recurrent laryngeal nerve is relieved in infancy, full recovery of vocal cord function is to be expected.

Therapy. That of cardiac disease.

Prognosis. Depends on etiology.

BIBLIOGRAPHY. Ortner N: Recurrenslähmung bei Mitralstenose. Wien Klin Wochenschr 10:753–755, 1897
Stocker HH, Enterline HT: "Cardiovocal syndrome": laryngeal paralysis in intrinsic heart disease. Am Heart J 56:51–59, 1958
Condon LM, Katkov H, Singh A et al: Cardiovocal syndrome in infancy. Pediatrics 76:22–25, 1985

OSEBOLD-REMONDINI

Synonyms. Brachydactyly type A6; brachymesophalangy mesomelic short limbs–carpal and tarsal abnormalities.

Symptoms and Signs. Middle phalanges of all digits hypoplastic or absent. Mesomelic shortening of limbs. Clinodactyly of index fingers. Normal intelligence.

Etiology. Autosomal dominant inheritance.

Diagnostic Procedures. *Rx wrist*. Ammate and capitate bones fused; delayed coalescence of bipartite calcanei.

BIBLIOGRAPHY. Osebold WR, Remondini DS, Lester EL, et al: An autosomal dominant syndrome of short stature with mesomelic shortness of limbs, abnormal carpal and tarsal bones, hypoplastic middle phalanges and bipartite calcanei. Am J Med Genet 22:791–809, 1985

ORZECHOWSKI'S

Synonyms. Truncular ataxia-opsoclonia; encephalitis-opsoclonia-tremulousness.

Symptoms. Follows a benign upper respiratory infection. (1) Opsoclonia: involuntary oscillations of eyes in horizontal and vertical directions, persisting with closed eyes. Sometimes associated with blinking, lacking the rhythmicity, and regularity of nystagmus. (2) Incapacitating postural tremulousness of the body. (3) Fever and various symptoms and signs of encephalitis.

Etiology. Unknown; very likely viral. No virus, however, has yet been demonstrated.

Pathology. Unknown.

Diagnostic Procedures. *Spinal tap*. Pleocytosis, or normal. Viral isolation studies should be performed on cerebrospinal fluid, stool, and pharyngeal secretion.

Therapy. Tetracycline (?). Supportive and symptomatic.

Prognosis. Alarming and incapacitating for a few weeks. Spontaneous resolution without sequelae.

BIBLIOGRAPHY. Orzechowski K: De l'ataxie dysmetrique des yeux: Remarques sur l'ataxie des yeux dite myoclonique (opsoclonie, opsochorie). J Psychol Neurol 35:1–18, 1927

Winkler GF, Baringer JR, Sweeney VP: An acute syndrome of ocular oscillations and truncal ataxia. Trans Am Neurol Assoc 91:96–99, 1966

Cogan DG: Opsoclonus, body tremulousness and benign encephalitis. Arch Ophthalmol 79:545–551, 1968

Van Voris LP, Roberts NJ: Central nervous system infections. In Reese RE, Gordon DR (eds): A Practical Approach to Infectious Diseases, p 123. Boston, Little, Brown, 1986

OSGOOD-SCHLATTER

Synonyms. Tibial tubercle osteochondrosis; Schlatter's. See Epiphyseal ischemic necrosis.

Symptoms. More common in males; onset in early adolescence. Pain in the medial area of knee, aggravated by active extension.

Signs. Swelling over tibial tubercle; tenderness on palpation.

Etiology. Epiphyseal ischemic necrosis trauma (see).

Therapy. Conservative treatment: restriction of activities, cast immobilization for 3 to 6 weeks. Surgery seldom indicated; if symptoms persist, bone pegs may be inserted into tibial tuberosity.

Prognosis. Conservative treatment frequently successful.

BIBLIOGRAPHY. Osgood RB: Lesions of the tibial tubercle occurring during adolescence. Boston Med Surg J 148:114–117, 1903

Schlatter C: Verletzungen des schnabelförmigen Forsatzes der oberen Tibiaepiphyse. Beitr Klin Chir 38:874–887, 1903

Kujala UM, Kvist M, Heinonen O: Osgood-Schlatter's disease in adolescent athletes: retrospective study of incidence and duration. Am J Sports Med 13:236–241, 1985

Canale T: Osteochondrosis or epiphysitis. In Crenshaw AH (ed): Campbell's Operative Orthopedics, 7th ed, pp 989–991. St Louis, CV Mosby, 1987

OSLER'S (W.) II

Synonym. Ball-valve gallstone.

Symptoms. Recurrent episodes of colic pain, with typical radiation to back; possibly jaundice.

Etiology. Presence of mobile gallstone in Vater's diverticulum periodically obstructing the bile outflow.

Diagnostic Procedures. *Cholecystography.*

Therapy. *Surgery.* Antispastic medication.

Prognosis. Fair.

BIBLIOGRAPHY. Osler W: The ball-valve gallstone in the common duct. Lancet I:1319–1323, 1897

Rajagopalan AE, Pickleman J: Biliary colic and functional gallbladder disease. Arch Surg 117:1005–1008, 1983

OSTEOARTHRITIS HYPERTROPHIC GENERALIZED

Synonyms. Generalized hypertrophic osteoarthritis; Kellgren-Moore.

Symptoms. Prevalent in women; onset in middle age. Acute inflammatory phase usually precedes articular symptoms; pain and functional limitation, usually milder than anatomic changes suggest.

Signs. Predilected sites are interphalangeal and carpometacarpal joints of hands; other articulations are usually successively involved.

Etiology. Unknown; hereditary. Two groups recognized: one has more severe symptoms (associated with Heberden's nodes, see); the second is occasionally associated with inflammatory polyarthritis (negative rheumatoid arthritis [RA] test).

Pathology. Narrowing of joint spaces; osteophytes.

Diagnostic Procedures. *X-ray.* Facets, arches, and spinous processes of column enlarged ("kissing spines"); molten-wax osteophytes. *Blood.* Sedimentation rate.

Therapy. Physical therapy. Calcium; vitamin D; testosterone derivates; antiinflammatory agents.

Prognosis. Variable rate of progression toward incapacitation.

BIBLIOGRAPHY. Kellgren JH, Moore R: Some concepts of rheumatic disease. Br Med J 1:1152–1157, 1952

Richardson EG: Miscellaneous nontraumatic disorders. In Crenshaw AH (ed): Campbell's Operative Orthopedics, 7th ed. St Louis, CV Mosby, 1987

OSTEOGENESIS IMPERFECTA

Synonyms. Adair-Dighton; blue sclerae-brittle bones-deafness; Dighton-Adair; Ekman-Lobstein; Eddowes'; fragilitas ossium; Hoeve-Dekleyn; Lobstein's; osteopsathyrosis; OIC; OIT; Porak-Durante; Spurway's; van der Hoeve's; Vrolick's. Four clinical varieties are distinguished.

OI TYPE I

Synonyms. OI tarda; OI with blue sclerae.

Symptoms and Signs. All races affected; time of onset variable. Blue sclerae may be only manifestation. Fractures may or may not occur at a later age, usually from minor traumas. Decrease in fracture incidence after puberty; incidence may increase again after menopause. Short legs (bowing or sequela of fractures); round back; conical thorax; joint hypermobility.

Etiology. Autosomal dominant inheritance. Metabolic defect of collagen causing extreme fragility of bones.

Pathology. Thin cortical layer and trabeculae; normal periosteum and epiphyseal cartilage; metaphysis shows calcified cartilage, which tends to fracture. Normal osteoblasts. Bone fragmentation; fractures and healing, usually with hypertrophic callus.

Diagnostic Procedures. *X-ray.* Thin cortices; long bones have slender shaft widening at epiphyses. *Blood.* Normal calcium; phosphorus alkaline phosphatase may be increased. Coagulation studies: occasionally abnormalities.

Therapy. Calcitonin. Surgical correction of deformities.

OI TYPE I A AND B

Synonyms. OI imperfecta-opalescent teeth; dentino genesis imperfecta-osteogenesis imperfecta.

Symptoms and Signs. Same as above. Some patients may lack blue sclerae. Opalescent teeth (type IA) or normal teeth (type IB).

Etiology. Autosomal dominant inheritance.

Prognosis. Type IA more severe growth impairment due to greater occurrence of fractures. Type IB milder.

OI TYPE II

Synonym. OI congenita-neonatal lethal form.

Symptoms and Signs. All races, both sexes affected; present from birth (stillborn or short survival). Caput membranaceum (cranium soft and membraneous); extremities short and clumsy; pelvic, spinal, scapular abnormalities; cleft palate; micrognathia; flat face; flail chest; severe respiratory troubles. Fracture liability. Blue sclerae (ocular hallmark of the condition). Embryotoxon and hyperopia are frequent. Cornea may be thinned, leading to keratoconus and megalocornea. Skin thin and translucent; subcutaneous hemorrhages. Deafness. Teeth abnormal color: amber or bluish.

Etiology. Autosomal dominant. Metabolic defect of collagen: point mutation of aminoacids involved in sulfide bonds. Forms with autosomal recessive inheritance have been called *Vrolik's syndrome.*

Prognosis. Death at birth or early age.

OI TYPE III

Synonyms. OI progressively deforming-normal sclerae.

Symptoms and Signs. Sclerae bluish color at birth that normalizes with growth: Progressive deformity of limbs in childhood and of spine in adolescence. Dentinogenesis imperfecta.

Etiology. Autosomal recessive inheritance. Metabolic defect of collagen: altered collagen glycosylation.

Prognosis. Progressive deformity.

OI TYPE IV

See Beighton's.

BIBLIOGRAPHY. Ekman OJ: Dissertation Medica. Descriptionem et Casus Aliquot osteomalaciae Sistens. Upsala, 1788.

Lobstein J: De la Fragilité des Os ou l'Osteopsathy Rose, Traite de l'anatomie pathologique, Vol 2, pp 204–212. Paris, 1883

Vrolick W: Tabulae ad Illustrandan Embryogenesis Hominis et Mammalium. Tam Naturalem quam Abnormen. Lipsiae, Weigel, 1854

Spurway J: Hereditary tendency to fracture. Br Med J 2:844, 1896

van Der Hoeve J, Kleyn A: Blaue Sclera, Knochenbruchigkeit und Schwerhorigkeit. Arch Ophthalmol 95:81–93, 1918

Patterson CR, McAllion S, Miller R: Heterogeneity of osteogenesis imperfecta type I. J Med Genet 20:203–205, 1983

Horowitz AL, Lazda V, Byers PH: Recurrent type II (lethal) osteogenesis imperfecta: apparent dominant inheritance. Am J Hum Genet (abst) 37:A59, 1985

Cetta G, Ramirez F, Tsipouras P: Third Intern Conference on Osteogenesis Imperfecta, New York. Ann NY Acad Sci, 543, 1988

OSTEOGENESIS IMPERFECTA-MICROCEPHALY, CATARACTS

Synonym. Buyse-Bull. See Osteogenesis imperfecta.

Symptoms and Signs. Both sexes (3 sibs). Stillborn or afterbirth. Microcephaly, bilateral cataract, prenatal bone fractures. Blue sclerae.

Etiology. Autosomal dominant inheritance.

Pathology. Short and bowed long bones. Soft calvaria, small and smooth cortex.

BIBLIOGRAPHY. Buyse M, Bull MJ: A syndrome of osteogenesis imperfecta microcephaly and cataracts. Birth Defects Orig Ser 14:6 B:95–98, 1978

OSTEOGLOPHONIC DWARFISM

Symptoms and Signs. Both sexes. Facies distorted; depression of nasal bridge; frontal bossing; prognathism; craniostenosis; rhizomelic dwarfism.

Etiology. Autosomal dominant inheritance.

Pathology. *Biopsy of lytic lesion.* Benign, whorled, fibrous tissue.

Diagnostic Procedures. *X-ray of skeleton.* Typical Rx appearance of unusual spondyloepimetaphyseal dysplasia; symmetrical lucent metaphysis defects. *Blood.* In some cases reported hypophosphatasia (see).

BIBLIOGRAPHY. Fairbank T: An atlas of general affections of the skeleton, pp 181–183. Baltimore, Williams & Wilkins, 1951

Kelley RI, Borns PF, Nichlas D, et al: Osteoglophonic dwarfism in two generations. J Med Genet 20:436–440, 1983

OSTEOMESOPYKNOSIS

Symptoms and Signs. Pelvic pain; low back pain; thigh pain; sterility.

Etiology. Autosomal dominant trait.

Pathology. Localized increased density of bones. The lesions are localized to the spine, the pelvis, and the heads of femora. "Ovarian sclerosis" and infertility in one proband.

Diagnostic Procedures. *X-rays of the pelvis, the spine, and the femora.* Increased radiodensity.

Therapy. Symptomatic.

Prognosis. Unknown.

BIBLIOGRAPHY. Simon D, Cazalis P, Dryll A, et al: Une osteosclerose axiale de transmission dominante autosomatique: nouvelle entite? Rev Rheum 46:375–382, 1979

Maroteaux P: L'osteomesopycnose. Une nouvelle affection condensante de transmission dominante autosomique. Arch Fr Pediatr 37:153–157, 1980

Stoll C, Collin D, Dreyfus J: Brief clinical report: osteomesopyknosis: an autosomal dominant osteosclerosis. Am J Med Genet 8:349–353, 1981

OSTEOPATHIA STRIATA-CRANIAL STENOSIS

Synonyms. See Voorhoeve's.

Symptoms and Signs. Both sexes. Possible prenatal diagnosis. From mild cranial enlargement to abnormalities (with Pierre Robin syndrome). Possibly associated: hearing defects; scoliosis; spondylolisthesis.

Etiology. Unknown. Autosomal dominant trait.

Diagnostic Procedures. *X-rays.* Typical bone striation (see Voorhoeve's) and craniostenosis. Ultrasound examination: for prenatal diagnosis.

BIBLIOGRAPHY. Fairbank T: An Atlas of General Affections of the Skeleton, Baltimore, Williams & Wilkins, 1951

Ruker TN, Afidi RJ: A rare familial systemic affection of the skeleton: Fainbank's disease. Radiology 82:63–66, 1964

Paling MR, Hyde I, Denis NR: Osteopathia striata with sclerosis and thickening of the skull. Br J Radiol 54:344–348, 1981

OSTEOPATHIA STRIATA-PIGMENTARY DERMOPATHY

Synonyms. See Voorhoeve's.

Symptoms and Signs. In females. From birth. Macular, hyperpigmented dermopathy including white forelock.

Etiology. Unknown. Consistent with X-linked inheritance.

Diagnostic Procedures. *X-rays.* Typical osteopathia striata (see Voorhoeve's).

BIBLIOGRAPHY. Whyte MP, Murphy WA: Osteopathia striata associated with familial dermopathy and white forelock: evidence for postnatal development of osteopathia striata. Ann J Genet 5:227–234, 1980

OSTEOPOROSIS PSEUDOGLIOMA

Symptoms and Signs. Appear to be more frequent in Mediterranean area. Those of osteogenesis imperfecta (see) plus bilateral retinoblastoma manifesting after a few weeks of life. Muscular hypotonia; ligaments laxity. Occasionally mental retardation.

Etiology. Autosomal recessive inheritance.

Pathology. Retinal pseudoglioma.

Therapy. Eye enucleation after irrigation. Calcitonin.

BIBLIOGRAPHY. Bianchine JW, Murdoch JL: Juvenile osteoporosis in a boy with bilateral enucleation of the eyes for pseudoglioma. Birth Defects Orig Art Ser V (4):225–226, 1969

Frontali M, Stomeo C, Dalla Piccola B: Osteoporosis-pseudoglioma syndrome: report of three affected sibs and an overview. Am J Med Genet 22:35–47, 1985

OSTERTAG'S

Synonyms. Hereditary amyloid nephropathy; Amyloidosis familial visceral; amyloidosis VIII; German amyloidosis; amyloidosis familial renal.

Symptoms and Signs. Both sexes affected; age of onset variable. Arterial hypertension; marked hepatosplenomegaly; hematuria; pitting edema (clinical impression of nephritis or nephrosis).

Etiology. Unknown; possibly, autosomal dominant inheritance.

Pathology. Widespread amyloidosis, most striking in the kidneys.

Diagnostic Procedures. *Blood and urine.* Evidence of nephropathy. *Biopsy. Congo Red test.*

Therapy. Hemodialysis.

Prognosis. That of chronic renal failure.

BIBLIOGRAPHY. Ostertag B: Demonstration einer eigenartigen familiaren paramyloidose. Zbl Path 56:253–254, 1932
Ostertag B: Familiäre Amyloid-Erkrankung. Z Menschl Vererb Konstit-Lehre 30:105–115, 1950
Mornaghi R, Rubinstein P, Franklin EC: Familial renal amyloidosis case reports and genetic studies. Am J Med 73:609–614, 1982

OSUNTOKUN'S

Synonyms. Pain indifference-deafness; deafness-analgesia congenita.

Symptoms and Signs. Brother and half sister with different father. Analgesia congenital (see Biemond's I) and deafness.

Etiology. Unknown.

BIBLIOGRAPHY. Osuntokun's BO, Odeku EL, Luzzatto L: Congenital pain asymbolia and auditory imperception. J Neurosurg Psychiatr 31:291–296, 1968

OTA'S

Synonyms. Nevus fuscoceruleus-ophthalmomaxillaris; oculodermal melanocytosis.

Symptoms. Frequent in Japanese, rarer in Caucasians and Blacks; onset in childhood. Asymptomatic.

Signs. Bluish pigmented spots in the periorbital area and of sclera; may extend to include cheeks, forehead, scalp, nose, and ears (seldom, the trunk). Not always unilateral.

Etiology. Unknown.

Pathology. See Mongolian spot. Area affected usually that of first and second division of trigeminal (V) nerve.

Diagnostic Procedures. *Biopsy.*

Therapy. Cosmetics. Carbon dioxide snow may lighten the pigmentation.

Prognosis. Lesions may become confluent in some areas; they usually become darker with time and persist in adult life.

BIBLIOGRAPHY. Ota M: Nevus, fusco-coeruleus ophthalmomaxillaris. Tokyo Med J 63:143–145, 1939
Fraunfelder FT, Roy FH: Current ocular therapy. Philadelphia, WB Saunders, 1984

OTHELLO

Synonyms. Erotic jealousy; psychotic jealousy; sexual jealousy.

Symptoms. Both sexes may be affected; apparently prevalent in men; sudden onset. Minor symptoms of a few months of suspicion. Onset usually in 4th decade. Delusion of infidelity of sexual partner; accusation on the basis of a particular episode that allegedly proves the fact, misinterpretation, and distortion of past episodes. Meticulous and obsessive search for proof. Continuous repeated interrogations to obtain confession. Increased sexual activity; if rejection interpreted as proof of infidelity, avoids partner to seek certain proof. Irritability, tension, and depression distracting from proper performance of job. Frequently explosion of violence particularly against spouse.

Etiology. Unknown; pure form is a special variety of paranoia. It may be a feature of maniac depressive psychosis, epilepsy, alcoholism.

Therapy and Prognosis. If part of psychosis, follows evolution of basic condition. If pure form, long lasting, often persisting, and resistant to therapy.

BIBLIOGRAPHY. Todd J, Dewhurst K: Othello syndrome: a study in psychopathology of sexual jealousy. J Nerv Ment Dis 122:367–374, 1955
Enoch MD, Trethowan WH, Barker JC: Some Uncommon Psychiatric Syndromes. Baltimore, Williams & Wilkins, 1967
Adams RD, Victor M: Principles of Neurology, 3rd ed, p 821. New York, McGraw-Hill, 1985

OTTO-CHROBAK

Synonyms. Sunken acetabulum; acetabular protrusion; arthrokatadysis; Otto's pelvis.

Symptoms. Onset in puberal period or later. Progressive and frequently bilateral loss of hip joint movement without pain.

Signs. Deformity on hip flexion and abduction.

Etiology. Unknown. Degenerative condition. Usually, congenital defect and familial occurrence.

Diagnostic Procedures. *X-ray.* Acetabulum assumes a spherical form, completely surounding the femoral head; thinning of acetabulum floor, which appears displaced medially and bulges into pelvis.

Therapy. None for basic defect. Othopedic treatment of secondary osteoarthropathy.

Prognosis. Osteoarthropathic changes during adult life.

BIBLIOGRAPHY. Sokoowsky A, Kopera Z: Przypadek pierwotnego wgobiemia panewki stawn biodrowego (protrusio acetabuli primaria Otto-Chrobak) viekn modocianym. Post Reum Warszava 3:140–145, 1957
Richardson EG. Miscellaneous non traumatic disorders. In Crenshaw AH (ed): Campbell's Operative Orthopedics, 7th ed, pp 1060, 1361, 1363. St Louis, CV Mosby, 1987

OVARIAN HYPERTHECOSIS

Symptoms and Signs. Amenorrhea; infertility; hirsutism; virilism occasionally noted.

Etiology. Unknown. Regarded as one form of Stein-Leventhal (see) (severe form).

Pathology. Endometrial hyperplasia. Ovaries are enlarged and firm with nests of theca-lutein cells in stroma and hyperthecosis. Differential diagnosis: Stein-Leventhal syndrome; differentiation possible only on the basis of the microscopic findings. Adrenal tumor and masculinizing ovarian tumor.

Diagnostic Procedures. *Blood.* Levels of androgen higher in Stein-Leventhal.

Therapy. Wedge resection of ovaries; clomiphene citrate.

Prognosis. Good.

BIBLIOGRAPHY. Givens JR, Niser WL, Coleman SA, et al: Familial ovarian hyperthecosis, a study of two families. Am J Obstet Gynec 110:959–972, 1971

Gompel C, Silverberg SG: Pathology in Gynecology and Obstetrics, 3rd ed, p 544. Philadelphia, JB Lippincott, 1985

OVARIAN VEIN

Symptoms and Signs. Onset in 2nd or 3rd decade. Rarely observed in nulliparous women; primarily occurring or beginning during pregnancy. Periodic pain in the flank on the right side and right lower quadrant, which appears several days before onset of menstruation and disappears after 1 or 2 days of menstruation. Infection of urinary tract and administration of progesterone aggravate the symptoms.

Etiology. Related to hydronephrosis and pyelonephritis of pregnancy; extension of this condition. May result from repeated frequent pregnancies, use of oral contraceptives, and increased vascularity from gynecologic disorders, causing incompetence of ovarian vein valves.

Pathology. Right ovarian vein is larger than the left one, and dilatation and incompetence of valves occur during pregnancy and may persist in multiparas. Connective tissue sheath is thickened with adherence of vein and ureter, where the iliac vessels are crossed. The wall of the vein is thick, its muscle hypertrophic.

Diagnostic Procedures. *Excretory urography.* Right side abnormalities; mild to moderate coliectasis; pyelectasis; ureterectasis; upper portion of ureter dilated; tortuous middle portion lateral deviation; junction of middle pelvic portion medial deviation. *Cystoscopy.* Negative. *Right retrograde urography.* Normal pelvic ureter; poor filling at iliac vessels crossing; in the middle portion, minor deformities; in the proximal portion, irregular extrinsic deformities. *Pelvic phlebography.* Evidence of closeness of right ovarian vein and ureter.

Treatment. Prolonged medical treatment for urinary tract infection. In case of failure with persistence of infection and signs of progressive obstructive changes, excision of ovarian vein and arterolysis (excision of vein does not prevent pregnancy).

Prognosis. Good. If medical treatment fails, surgery succeeds in 75% of cases.

BIBLIOGRAPHY. Clark JC: The right ovarian vein syndrome. In Emmitt JL: Clinical Urography, 2nd ed, pp 1227–1236. Philadelphia, WB Saunders, 1964
Dykhuizen RF, Roberts JA: The ovarian vein syndrome. Surg Gynecol Obstet 130:443–452, 1970
Gompel C, Silverberg SG: Pathology in Gynecology and Obstetrics, 3rd ed, pp 580–581. Philadelphia, JB Lippincott, 1985

OVERLAP

Synonym. Mixed connective tissue disease, MCTD.

Symptoms and Signs. Prevalent in females; onset in adolescence or early adulthood. Symptoms and signs of scleroderma (see Morvan's) combined with those of lupus erythematosus systemic (SLE, see). Observed in about 10% of patients with scleroderma. Other overlapping conditions are SLE and rheumatoid arthritis; scleroderma and Sjogren's (see); scleroderma and Hashimoto's (see); and scleroderma and hypoglobulinemic syndromes.

Etiology. Autoimmune conditions.

Diagnostic Procedures. *Blood.* Extractable nuclear antigen (ENA) that contains ribonucleoproteins and is associated with a speckled pattern of antinuclear antibodies (ANA).

Therapy. Corticosteroid and Nonsteroidal antiinflammatory agents.

Prognosis. Six years after onset, mortality 6%. Patient finally develops scleroderma.

BIBLIOGRAPHY. Bianchi FA, Bistue AR, Wendt VE, et al: Analysis of 27 cases of progressive systemic sclerosis and a review of literature. J Chron Dis 19:953–977, 1966
Sullivan WD: A prospective evaluation emphasizing pulmonary involvement in mixed connective tissue disease. Medicine 63:92, 1984

OVERSUPPRESSION

Synonyms. Contraceptive amenorrhea; anovulation following oral contraceptive; postcontraceptive anovulation. Postpill amenorrhea.

Symptoms and Signs. Amenorrhea of 3 months or longer, or marked irregularity of menstrual cycles, and infertility following discontinuation of oral contraceptive therapy, sometimes with galactorrhea.

Etiology. Suspected dysfunction of hypothalamic centers concerned with gonadotropin release.

Diagnostic Procedures. Determination of follicle-stimulating hormone (FSH), luteinizing hormone (LH), and estrogen levels, and prolactin level (if elevated, a pituitary prolactinoma may be present).

Therapy. Usually, recover without treatment. Bromo-criptine (Parlodel) if elevated level of prolactin; otherwise clomiphene (Clomid).

Prognosis. Good response to treatment.

BIBLIOGRAPHY. Whitelow MJ, Nola VF, Kalman CF: Irregular menses, amenorrhea, and infertility following synthetic progestational agents. JAMA 195:780–782, 1966
Horowitz BJ, Solomkin M, Edelstein SW: The oversuppression syndrome. Obstet Gynecol 31:387–389, 1968
Rosenfield A (ed): Update on oral contraceptive. J Reprod Med 29(Suppl 1):501–502, 1984

OWREN'S

Synonyms. Factor V deficiency; labile factor deficiency; parahemophilia; proaccelerin deficiency. See Prothrombin deficiency syndromes.

Symptoms and Signs. Both sexes; great variability in time of onset and severity. Symptoms similar to those of hemophilia with the exception of the lack of hemarthrosis. Menorrhagia usually serious problem. Postpartum bleeding a few days after delivery. In heterozygous relatives, only epistaxis or minor manifestations.

Etiology. Absence of proaccelerin in the plasma. Autosomal recessive inheritance; autosomal dominant inheritance also suggested.

Diagnostic Procedures. *Prothrombin time.* Prolonged; corrected by fresh plasma deprived of vitamin K–dependent clotting factors; not corrected by proaccelerin-poor plasma (stored or oxalated). Thromboplastin generation usually abnormal. *Other coagulation tests.* May be abnormal.

Therapy. Fresh plasma or fresh frozen plasma. Vitamin K ineffective.

Prognosis. Good, but death from bleeding may occur.

BIBLIOGRAPHY. Owren PA: The coagulation of blood: Investigations of a new clotting factor. Acta Med Scand (Suppl 194) 128:1–327, 1947
Friedman IA, Quick AJ, Higgins F et al: Hereditary labile factor (factor V) deficiency. JAMA 175:370–374, 1961
McKee PA: Hemostasis and disorders of blood coagulation. In Stanbury JB, Wyngaarden JB, Fredrickson DS, et al: The Metabolic Basis of Inherited Disease, 5th ed, p 1531. New York, McGraw-Hill, 1983

PACEMAKER

Symptoms and Signs. In one fifth of patients with well-functioning pacemakers. Dizzy spells, syncope, breathlessness, impaired exercise capacity, postural hypotension. Palpable liver pulsations and common waves in jugular venous pulse.

Etiology. Atrial contraction stimulated by pacemaker occurring during ventricular systole. Atria contract against closed valves producing raised pressure and reduced cardiac output and blood pressure. Occurs when retrograde AV conduction is intact.

Diagnostic Procedure. *Ventricular pacing.* Observation of symptoms and signs.

Therapy. Dual chamber pacing or reprogramming ventricular pacemaker. Antiarrhythmics: flecainide and dysopyramide.

Prognosis. Good with therapy.

BIBLIOGRAPHY. Alicardi C, Fonad FM, Tarazi RC et al: Three cases of hypotension and syncope with ventricular pacing: Possible role of atrial reflexes. Am J Cardiol 42:136–142, 1978

Morley CA, Perrins EJ, Grant P et al: Carotid sinus syncope treated by pacing. Analysis of persistent symptoms and role of atrioventricular sequential pacing. Br Heart J 47:411–418, 1982

Torresani J, Ebogosti A, Allard–Latour G: Pacemaker syndrome with DDD pacing. PACE 7:1148–1151, 1984

Kenny RA, Sutton R: Pacemaker syndrome. Br J Med 293:902–903, 1986

PACEMAKER–TWIDDLER'S

Caused by repeated turning of implanted pulse generator under the skin in case of lead retraction from endocardium.

BIBLIOGRAPHY. Mond HG: The Cardiac Pacemaker: Function and Malfunction. New York, Grune–Stratton, 1983

PACHYDERMOPERIOSTOSIS

Synonyms. Acropachyderma hypopituitaric; hypopituitaric acropachyderma, pachydermoperiostosis. Simond's (A); Brugsch's; Leva's. Variant; see Touraine-Solente-Golé (same condition but associated with acromegaly).

Symptoms. Reported in many races; prevalent in males; onset after puberty. Low working capacity.

Signs. Face and scalp skin thickens and folds (expression of despair); increased sebaceous secretion. Hand and foot skin thickens but does not fold and presents hyperhidrosis. Bones of limbs, fingers, and toes thicken, determing cylindrical deformation of fingers and clubbing of toes. Hands and feet remain small (main differential sign). Joint effusions. Occasionally; decrease of facial and pubic hair, gynecomastia.

Etiology. Autosomal dominant inheritance of variable expressivity (sex influenced) and/or recessive.

Pathology. *Skin.* Hypertrophy of connective tissue of epidermis and appendages. *Bones.* Proliferative periostitis with irregular periosteal ossification. Ligaments, tendons, and membranes may ossify.

Diagnostic Procedures. *Blood.* hyponatremia. *X-rays of skeleton.* (See Pathology.) *Endocrine studies.* Normal.

Therapy. None.

Prognosis. Normal life expectancy. Irreversible condition, which, once started, progresses for 5 to 10 years and then stabilizes.

BIBLIOGRAPHY. Leva J: Ueber familiare Ackromegalia. Med Klin 11:1266–1268, 1915.

Simond's A: Familiare Trommelschlaegelbildung und Knochenhypertrophy. Dtsch Z Nezvenheilk 59:301–321, 1918

Brugsch T: Akromikrie oder Dystrophia osteogenitalis. Med Klin 23:81–82, 1927

Hedayati H, Barmada R, Skosey JL: Acrolysis in pachydermoperiostosis (primary or idiopatic hypertrophic osteoarthropathy). Arch Int Med 140:1087–1088, 1980

PACKARD–WECHSEL

Rare eponym used to designate chronic adrenal insufficiency of adult type. See Addisonian syndromes.

PADDED DASH

Synonyms. Larynx–trachea trauma; tracheolaryngeal trauma.

Symptoms. Occur in passengers involved in car accidents. Seat belt may increase chance of occurrence of this type of lesion. Respiratory distress due to obstruction of airway; aspiration of saliva, fluid, or solid into airway; hoarseness; pain on swallowing. Neck may appear normal. Presence of subcutaneous emphysema; free cartilage in severe injury. Multiple lacerations of forehead and midface frequently encountered.

Etiology. During crash, forehead strikes windshield, causing hyperextension of neck and exposing anterior neck to trauma from collision with dashboard and injuring laryngotracheal structures.

Pathology. In female (because of longer neck) lesion more frequently supraglottic; in men subglottic. Hematomas; fracture of cartilage; mucosal lacerations.

Diagnostic Procedures. *Laryngoscopy. X-ray.*

Therapy. Maintainance of respiratory exchange (positive-pressure breathing equipment) until tracheostomy may be performed. Conservative treatment in some cases. Surgical exploration, however, frequently indicated.

Prognosis. Asphyxia is cause of death if early treatment not instituted.

BIBLIOGRAPHY. Butler RM, Moser FH: The padded dash syndrome: Blunt trauma to the larynx and trachea. Laryngoscope 78:1172–1182, 1968
Delany HN, Berlin AW: Multiple injuries. In Tinker J, Rapin M (eds): Care of the Critically Ill Patient, p 611. Berlin, Springer–Verlag, 1983

PAGE'S

Synonyms. Hypertensive diencephalic. Mental sweating.

Symptoms. Prevalent in young or middle-aged women, occasionally in men: onset without any cause or brought on by embarrassment and excitement. Periodic appearance of blotchy flushes covered by small beads of perspiration in the face, upper chest, and seldom, abdomen. Extremities during attack are cold, pale, and show a dusky mottled hue. Watery lacrimation without emotional causes or changes. Headache, tachycardia, and abdominal hyperperistalsis. Emotional polyuria; deep sighing respiration.

Signs. Lability of blood pressure; elevation during attacks. Occasionally presence of low-grade fever.

Etiology. Unknown; hypothalamic disturbance. A similar syndrome is observed in some patients with tumor compressing hypothalamus (see Penfield's).

Pathology. Vascular disease secondary to hypertension minimal in these cases.

Diagnostic Procedure. Injection of 0.25 mg of histamine base intradermally, precipitates the attack.

Therapy. Sedatives: reserpine. Topical: ionophoresis. Medical: atropinelike drugs, probanthine, poldine, sedatives, tranquilizers, psychiatric treatment. Sympathectomy (in refractory cases).

Prognosis. Relatively benign course with usual minimal complications of essential hypertension (vascular, renal). After sympathectomy the manifestation of syndrome disappears, and may not further be induced by the injection of histamine, but may relapse after few years.

BIBLIOGRAPHY. Page IH: A syndrome simulating diencephalic stimulation occurring in patients with essential hypertension. Am J Med Sci 190:9–14, 1935
Schroeder HA, Goldman ML: Test for the presence of the "hypertensive diencephalic syndrome" using histamine. Am J Med 6:162–167, 1949
Adams RD, Victor M: Principles of Neurology, 3rd ed, pp 1887–1889. New York, McGraw-Hill, 1985

PAGET'S I

Symptoms. Occur in women between 50 and 60 years of age (breast), in elderly men and women (extramammary), or in men (scrotum). Burning sensation, itching, soreness of the affected area (nipple or apocrine gland areas of genital, perigenital, and axillary areas); scratching lesions.

Signs. In nipple, fissured areola, ulceration, oozing, hyperemia; retraction. Other areas: in acute stage moist erythema; then eczemalike lesion; then denudation and crusting.

Etiology. Unknown. Relationship to or, possibly, extension of carcinoma of mammary duct or ducts of apocrine sweat gland.

Pathology. *Breast.* Intraductal proliferation; pastelike plugs of material; invasion by typical Paget's cells. *Other areas.* Invasion by Paget's cells of skin and apocrine glands.

Diagnostic Procedure. *Biopsy.*

Therapy. Surgery advised in all conditions.

Prognosis. Slow progression. Treatment helpful.

BIBLIOGRAPHY. Paget J: On diseases of the mammary areola preceding cancer of the mammary gland. St Bartholomew Hosp Rep 10:87–89, 1874
Lagios MD, Westdahl PR, Rose MR, et al: Paget's disease of the nipple: Alternative management in cases without or with minimal extent of underlying breast carcinoma. Cancer 54:545–551, 1984

PAGET'S II

Synonyms. Congenital hyperphosphatasemia; hyperostosis corticalis deformans; osteitis deformans; Pozzi's.

Symptoms. More frequent in men, but more severe in women; insidious onset after 40 years of age. Frequently asymptomatic. Headache; deep, dull, constant pain in one knee; deafness; waddling gait.

Signs. Enlarged cranial vault; bowing deformities of bones subjected to greater stress (arms, legs); flattening of vertebrae; broadening of pelvis; shortening of stature; kyphosis.

Etiology. Unknown; possibly, hereditary condition of autosomal dominant type; slow virus infection has also been proposed.

Pathology. Increased circulation in bones affected, with reabsorption of bone and replacement with osteoid matrix, and fibrotic changes, disorganization of trabeculae. Frequently development of osteogenic sarcoma.

Diagnostic Procedures. *Blood.* Hyperphosphatemia and marked increase of alkaline phosphatase; hypercalcemia; hypercalciuria. *X-ray.* See pathology. Typical mosaic pattern. *Urine.* Elevated excretion of hydroxyproline peptides. *Calcium exchange.* Marked increase.

Therapy. High calcium phosphate intake. Anabolic steroids; corticosteroids (if cardiac failure or hypercalcemia). With immobilized patients, low calcium and phosphate diet, increased fluids, edetate (EDTA), corticosteroids, or sodium phytate for hypercalcemia, sodium etidronate (5 mg/kg/day), calcitonin.

Prognosis. Progressive condition. Complications: cardiac failure, renal calculi, fractures, osteogenic sarcoma.

BIBLIOGRAPHY. Paget J: On a form of chronic inflammation of bones (osteitis deformans). Med Chir Trans (London) 60:37–63, 1877
Singer FR: Paget's Disease of Bone. New York, Plenum, 1977
Harvey L, Gray T, Beneton MNC et al: Ultrastructural features of the osteoclasts from Paget's disease of the bone in relation to a viral etiology. J Clin Pathol 35:771–779, 1982

PAGET'S ABSCESS

Eponym used to indicate an abscess recurrence at the same site after apparent cure.

BIBLIOGRAPHY. Paget J: On residual abscesses. St Bartholomew Hosp Rep 5:73–79, 1869

PAGET–SCHRÖTTER

Synonyms. Axillary vein traumatic thrombosis, intermittent venous claudication; Schrötter's.

Symptoms. Occur in active healthy males; onset usually between 18 and 40 years of age. Symptoms occur after vigorous work, or occasionally after minimal effort or no exercise. Onset gradual or very rapid. Right arm most often affected. Swelling of all arm from fingers to shoulder girdle and lower part of neck, with dull pain in the joints (particularly intense in the axilla); pain sometimes absent. Absence of systemic manifestations.

Signs. Arm swelling; cyanosis diffuse or mottled; superficial veins prominent; occasionally, hard cordlike mass palpated in the axilla.

Etiology. Idiopathic obstruction of axillary or subclavian vein (not secondary to aneurysm of aorta, cardiac failure, or breast neoplasia). Probably, compressions of vein between muscles and first rib or clavicle. A recent cause of subclavian and axillary vein thrombosis is represented by the introduction of total parenteral nutrition and subclavian cannulas for hemodialysis.

Pathology. In most cases, no signs of thrombus formation. Compression of vein by muscle of phrenic nerve demonstrated.

Diagnostic Procedures. *Blood gas.* Venous pressure; oxygen saturation, and circulation time show stasis. *X-ray.* Normal. *Blood.* Normal.

Therapy. In most cases, conservative. Various surgical procedures to remove obstruction. Anticoagulant helpful. Paravertebral cervical sympathetic block also valuable.

Prognosis. Usually, spontaneous, partial or total recovery in a few days or weeks. Symptoms usually recur.

BIBLIOGRAPHY. Paget J: Clinical Lectures and Essays, p 292. London, 1875
von Schrötter L: Erkrankunger der Gefasse. In Nothnagels Handbuch der Pathologie und Therapie. Wein, 1884; Holder (Nothnagel), 1884.
Kieny R, Fontaine R, Suhler A et al: Thirty-four cases of so-called "exertion" thrombophlebitis of upper extremity (Paget–Schrötter syndrome). J Cardiovasc Surg 13:181–185, 1964
Fabri PJ, Mirtallo JM, Roberg RL, Kudsk KA et al: Incidence and prevention of thrombosis of the subclavian vein during total parenteral nutrition. Surg Gynecol Obstet 155:238–240, 1982

PAGET'S JUVENILE

Synonyms. Osteoectasia-hyperphosphatasia; hyperphosphatasemia-osteoectasia; hyperostosis corticalis deformans juvenilis; familial, osteoectasia.

Symptoms and Signs. Both sexes affected. Bluish sclerae, becoming evident during first year of life. Occasionally, deafness (nerve compression); growth deficiency. Enlarging of head; broadening and then bowing of diaphyses. Pectus carinatum; kyphoscoliosis; teeth caries. Occasionally, fractures. Usually, normal intelligence.

Etiology. Unknown; possibly autosomal recessive inheritance.

Diagnostic Procedures. *X-ray.* Severe osteoporosis of flat and long bones (see Symptoms and Signs). *Blood.* Serum alkaline and acid phosphatase leucine aminopeptidase, hydroxyproline, uric acid elevated. *Urine.* Leucine-amino acid peptidase and uric acid elevation.

Therapy. Orthopedic measures of some value; calcitonin.

Prognosis. Fair.

BIBLIOGRAPHY. Bakin H, Eiger MS: Fragile bones and macrocranium. J Pediatr 49:558–564, 1956
Iancu TC, Almagor G, Friedman E et al: Chronic familial hyperphosphatasemia. Radiology 129:669–676, 1978
Whalen JP, Horwith N, Krook L et al: Calcitonin treatment in heriditary bone dysplasia with hyperphosphatasemia: a radiographic and histologic study of bone. Am J Roentgen 129:29–35, 1987

PAGON'S

Synonym. Anemia sideroblastic–ataxia spinocerebellar.

Symptoms and Signs. In males. Anemia from birth; ataxia becomes evident by age 1 year, accompanied by clonus, positive Babinski sign.

Etiology. X-linked recessive inheritance.

Pathology. Moderate parenchymal iron storage in tissue.

Diagnostic Procedures. *Blood and bone marrow.* Hyperchromic microcytic anemia; ring sideroblasts; raised free erythrocyte protoporphyrin levels.

Therapy. None specific.

Prognosis. Nonprogressive neurologic findings.

BIBLIOGRAPHY. Pagon RA, Bird TD, Detter JC et al: Hereditary sideroblastic anemia and ataxia an X-linked recessive disorder. J Med Genet 22:267–273, 1985

PAINE–EFRON

Synonym. Ataxia telangiectasia II.

Symptoms. Onset in late childhood or adulthood. Pain in back and thigh; then slowly progressing ataxia. No sinopulmonary symptoms (see Louis–Bar). Greater sensory deficit than in Louis–Bar.

Signs. Diffuse telangiectasia (late onset); darkly pigmented nevi.

Etiology. Unknown; dominant pattern of inheritance. Possibly, spinocerebellar degeneration of a type not classifiable because of lack of histologic reports.

Pathology. Unknown.

Diagnostic Procedures. *Urine.* Absence of urinary substance reported in Louis–Bar (see). *Blood and cerebrospinal fluid.* Normal.

Prognosis. Much slower evolution in adult life and slight incapacitation.

BIBLIOGRAPHY. Paine RS, Efron ML: Atypical variants of "ataxia-telangiectasia syndrome." Dev Med Child Neurol 5:14–23, 1963
Tadjoedin MK, Fraser FC: Heredity of ataxiatelangiectasia (Louis–Bar syndrome). Am J Dis Child 110:64–68, 1965

PAINE'S

Synonym. Microcephaly–spastic diplegia. See Seemanova's.

Symptoms. Occur only in males; onset from birth. Poor swallowing, requiring gavage feeding. Retarded physical and mental development; seizures (like myoclonic jerks progressing into opisthotonic fits); lack of interest in environment.

Signs. Microcephaly; below third percentile in weight and height; limbs spastic and hyperreflexic. In eye, normal light reflex; early optic atrophy.

Etiology. Unknown; sex-linked inheritance.

Pathology. Microcephaly; cerebellar hypoplasia. Decreased number of cells in the cerebrum, no gliosis; small interior pontine. Olives only rudimentary. Marked underdevelopment of cerebellar nuclei. Spinal cord normal.

Diagnostic Procedures. *Blood. Cerebrospinal fluid.* Amino acid ratio reverted (marked increase of cerebrospinal fluid amino acid). *Urine.* Mild aminoaciduria. *X-ray of skull. Electroencephalography.*

Therapy. Orthopedic surgery. Dextroamphetamine; anticonvulsants.

Prognosis. Poor; death usually within first year. Frequently pulmonary complications.

BIBLIOGRAPHY. Paine RS: Evaluation of familial biochemically determined mental retardation in children, with special reference to amino aciduria. N Engl J Med 262:658–665, 1960

Oka E, Mandarini M: Paine's syndrome in two siblings. Dev Med Child Neurol 10:259, 1968

Opitz JM, Sutherland GR: International workshop on the fragile X and X-linked mental retardation. Am J Med Genet 17:5–94, 1984

PAINFUL HEEL

Synonym. Idiopathic heel pain.

Symptoms. In patients 40 to 70 years of age, male, active. Pain beneath the anteriolateral prominence of calcaneal tuberosity usually unilateral; pain worse in the morning and after resting, decreases after walking, when tired in the evening, pain may reappear.

Signs. Normally arched foot. Localized tenderness at the inferomedial aspect of calcaneal tuberosity. Swelling and edema may be present.

Etiology. Still unknown. Differential diagnosis includes rheumatoid arthritis, ankylosing spondylitis, Reiter's, osteoarthritis, etc. Possibly related to degenerative process in the calcaneal heel pad of elastic adipose tissue.

Diagnostic Procedure. *X-ray.* Calcaneal spur in 50% of cases (of uncertain significance).

Therapy. Surgery useless. Shoe insert, non-steroidal anti-inflammatory agents and local corticosteroid injection.

Prognosis. Symptoms last weeks, months, or years. Good response to conservative treatment.

BIBLIOGRAPHY. Still WF: Painful heel. Practitioner 108:345, 1922

Richardson EG: The foot in adolescents and adults. In Crenshaw AH (ed): Campbell's Operative Orthopedics, 7th ed, pp 933–936. St Louis, CV Mosby, 1987

PALANT–FEINGOLD–BERKMAN

Synonym. Cleft palate–face unusual–mental retardation-limb abnormality.

Symptoms. Occur in females; clinical features present from birth. Normal birth weight. Feeding difficulties; mental, motor, and developmental milestone retardation.

Signs. Short stature; midline cleft palate. *Facies.* Almond-shaped; deep-set eyes; narrow palpebral fissure; mongoloid slant; epicanthal folds; bulbous nose; low hair line. *Limbs.* Bilateral camptodactyly of fourth and fifth fingers; broad distal phalanges of toes; syndactyly of second and third toes; valgus deformity of feet.

Etiology. Unknown; possibly, autosomal recessive inheritance.

Diagnostic Procedures. *X-ray of skeleton. Dermatolglyphic pattern.* Normal.

Therapy. Institutionalization.

Prognosis. Good *quoad vitam.* Severly retarded mental and motor development.

BIBLIOGRAPHY. Palant DI, Feingold M, Berkman MD: Unusual faces, cleft palate, mental retardation, and limb abnormalities in siblings—A new syndrome. J Pediatr 78:686–689, 1971

PALATAL MYOCLONUS

Symptoms and Signs. Continuous rhythmic contraction of the palate, frequently associated and synchronous with contraction of pharynx, larynx, tongue, floor of the mouth, neck, and diaphragm. Nodding of the head. Seldom, tremor of the hand associated. Ocular movements may also be associated. Frequency of contraction 100 to 180/min. Persists during sleep and anesthesia.

Etiology and Pathology. Vascular disorders of brain stem that involve inferior olive and olivodenate connection.

Diagnostic Procedures. *Spinal tap. Electroencephalography. Angiography. Electrooculogram. CT brain scan.*

Therapy. Symptomatic. Barbital decreases frequency, but does not suppress myoclonus.

Prognosis. Depends on nature and extension of lesion.

BIBLIOGRAPHY. Gallet J: Le nystagmus du voile le syndrome myoclonique de la calotte protubërantielle (thesis). Paris, 1927

Yap CB, Mayo C, Barron K: "Ocular bobbing" in palatal myoclonus. Arch Neurol 18:304–310, 1968

Adams RD, Victor M: Principles of Neurology, 3rd ed, pp 73–81. New York, McGraw-Hill, 1985

PALEOCEREBELLAR

Synonym. Anterior lobe cerebellar.

Symptoms. Disturbed postural reflexes; increased extensor tone; tremor; incoordinate, awkward, ataxic movements. Stiff-legged gait.

Signs. Hypotonia or flaccidity of affected muscles.

Etiology. Neoplastic or degenerative lesions of anterior lobe of cerebellum.

Pathology. According to etiology.

Diagnostic Procedures. According to etiology.

Therapy. According to etiology.

Prognosis. Depends on etiology.

BIBLIOGRAPHY. Bailey P: Reflections aroused by an unusual tumor of the cerebellum. J Mt Sinai Hosp 9:299–310, 1942

Dow RS, Moruzzi G: The Physiology and Pathology of the Cerebellum. Minneapolis, University of Minnesota Press, 1958

Adams RD, Victor H: Principles of Neurology, 3rd ed, pp 70–73. New York, McGraw-Hill, 1985

PALLISTER'S

Synonym. Ulnar–mammary.

Symptoms and Signs. Both sexes. Absence of body odor and axillary sweating; absence of breast tissue and hypoplasia of nipples and areolas. Postaxial polydactyly or unilateral oligodactyly and abdominal development of ulnar rays. Abnormal development of teeth, palate, vertebral column.

Etiology. Unknown. Autosomal dominant inheritance.

Pathology. See Symptoms and Signs, plus occasionally absence of kidney.

BIBLIOGRAPHY. Pallister PD, Herrmann J, Opitz JM: A pleiotropic dominant mutation affecting skeletal, sexual and apocrine-mammary development. Birth Defects XII (5):247–254, 1976

Gonzales CH, Herrmann J, Opitz JM: Mother and son affected with ulnar-mammary syndrome of Pallister. Eur J Pediatr 123:225–235, 1976

PALSY, SIXTH NERVE, BENIGN

Synonyms. Benign abducens (VI) nerve paralysis; benign VI nerve palsy.

Symptoms. Occur in children of any age. Painless paralysis of the abducens (VI) nerve developing 7 to 21 days after upper respiratory disease. Alertness; no ataxia.

Signs. No papilledema, enlarged head, or other neurologic signs except the paralysis of abducens (VI) nerve.

Etiology. Two mechanisms possible: otitis media and complication or neuritis as part of systemic viral infection. Syndrome to be differentiated from other forms of paralysis expressing presence of tumor, hydrocephalus, meningitis.

Pathology. Not known except in a case in which otitis present.

Diagnostic Precedures. *Blood.* Frequently present, relative lymphocytosis. *Cerebrospinal fluid.* Normal (seldom, transient lymphocytosis). Defer complicated diagnostic studies (arteriogram, pneumoencephalogram,) until lack of regression of the palsy is established.

Therapy. None.

Prognosis. Usually, palsy begins to improve within 3 to 6 weeks, and clears completely within 10 weeks.

BIBLIOGRAPHY. Symond CP: Comment on a paper by Purdom Martin J et al: Venous thrombosis in central nervous system. Proc R Soc Med 37:383–392, 1944

Knox DL, Clark DB, Schuster FF: Benign VI nerve palsies in children. Pediatrics 40:560–564, 1967

Dick PJ, Thomas PK, Lambert EH et al (eds): Peripheral Neuropathy, 2nd ed. Philadelphia, WB Saunders, 1984

PANCOAST'S

Synonyms. Apicocostovertebral; Ciuffini's; Hare's; Pancoast–Tobias–Ciuffini; superior pulmonary sulcus.

Symptoms. Severe shoulder pain; paresthesias, paresis, or weakness of one arm.

Signs. Muscle atrophy of shoulder, arm, and hand involved. Signs of apical mass. Mild enophthalmos, ptosis, miosis (Horner's).

Etiology. Tumor of pulmonary apex (in less than 5% of cases).

Pathology. Bronchogenic carcinoma or any other tumor in this location. Erosion first of ribs and eventually vertebral involvement.

Diagnostic Procedures. *X-ray of chest. Bronchoscopy. Cytology.* Of expectorate. *CT scan of chest.*

Therapy. Surgery if feasible; chemotherapy; roentgen therapy.

Prognosis. Poor; death usually within 1 year.

BIBLIOGRAPHY. Hare ES: Tumor involving certain nerves. London Med Gaz 23:16–18, 1838

Pancoast HK: Importance of careful roentgen-ray investigations of apical chest tumors. JAMA 83:1407–1411, 1924

Pancoast HK: Superior pulmonary sulcus tumor; tumor characterized by pain, Horner's syndrome, destruction of bone, and atrophy of hand muscles. JAMA 99:1391–1396, 1932

Fraser RG, Paré JAP: Diagnosis of Diseases of the Chest, 2nd ed. Philadelphia, WB Saunders, 1977

Stanford W, Barnes PP, Tucker AR: Influence of staging in superior sulcus (Pancoast) tumor of lung. Ann Thorac Surg 29:406–409, 1980

Ginsberg RT, Feld RJ (eds): Fourth World Conf on Lung Cancer. Chest 89:(Suppl) 199 (all issue), 1986

PANCREATIC PSEUDOCYSTS

Symptoms. Occur following (sometimes) severe abdominal trauma. One or more attacks of acute pancreatitis, or history of gallbladder disease. Pain mild to severe, usually at epigastrium, right to left quadrant. Nausea and vomiting suggesting paralytic ileus or pyloric obstruction. Loss of weight.

Signs. Abdominal mass smooth, 10 to 15 cm in diameter in the epigastrium or either lateral upper quadrant. Moderate tenderness; fever; occasionally, paralytic ileus and, less frequently, left side hydrothorax or jaundice or both.

Etiology. Abdominal trauma, or following one or more attacks of acute pancreatitis.

Pathology. Fluid-containing, abnormal sac not lined with epithelium; in the pancreas, usually in the lesser peritoneal sac.

Diagnostic Procedures. *X-ray.* Plain film; contrast medium in stomach, duodenum. *Abdominal CT scan. Ultrasound. Chest.* Intravenous cholangiography. *Blood.* Serum amylase usually increased (twice normal value). Leukocytosis in about half of cases.

Therapy. Surgery: drainage by cystogastrostomy when feasible.

Prognosis. If untreated, eventually becomes infected, hemorrhagic; develops fistula or produces duodenal or common biliary tract obstruction. Very seldom resolves spontaneously. Cured by cystogastrostomy. Optimal results also obtained by tube drainage; however, recurrences are possible. Once treated, symptoms disappear; patient regains his weight.

BIBLIOGRAPHY. Gussenbayer C: Zur operativen Behandlung der Pankreas-Cysten. Arch Klin Cir 29:358–364, 1883

Goulet RJ, Goodhan J, Schaffer R et al: Multiple pancreatic pseudocyst disease. Ann Surg 199:6–13, 1984

PANCREATOMETAPHYSEAL

Synonym. Metaphyseal pancreatic dysplasia.

Symptoms. Onset shortly after birth. Steatorrhea. Diabetes mellitus develops in childhood or early adolescence. Sometimes associated with Shwachman's (see).

Signs. Coxa vara.

Etiology. Unknown; autosomal recessive inheritance (?).

Diagnostic Procedures. *X-ray of skeleton.* Metaphyseal dysostosis. *Pancreatic fluid.* Reduction of pancreatic enzymes. *Blood.* Hyperglycemia and diabetic features. *Biopsy of intestinal mucosa normal.*

Therapy. Symptomatic. Administration of pancreatic enzymes, insulin.

BIBLIOGRAPHY. Theodorou SD, Adams J: An unusual case of metaphysial dysplasia. J Bone Joint Surg [Br] 45:364–369, 1963

Giedion A, Prader A, Hadorn B et al: Metaphysäre Dysostose und angeborene Pankreasinsuffizienz. Fortschr Roentgenstr 108:51–57, 1968

PANIC ATTACK

Symptoms and Signs. Many peripheral manifestations of sudden, massive autonomic nervous system discharge, with fear of dying, of going crazy, or of "doing something uncontrolled during an attack." The attacks occur suddenly, without warning, and for little apparent reason.

Etiology. Predisposition to this disorder may be transmitted as an autosomal dominant trait. The syndrome is not a true psychologic problem, but an organic illness.

Pathology. In patients with disorder the incidence of mitral valve prolapse has been estimated to be as high as 30% to 50%. Recent studies oppose any direct relation, however, between panic attacks and mitral valve prolapse.

Diagnostic Procedures. High catecholamine concentrations and elevated lactate levels have been found in affected subjects.

Therapy. One of these drugs can be prescribed: imipramine hydrochloride (the drug usually chosen); phenelzine sulfate; alprazolam.

BIBLIOGRAPHY. Sheehan DV: Current perspectives in the treatment of panic and phobic disorders. Drugs Therapy 179–190, 1982
Sheehan DV: Panic attacks and phobias. N Engl J Med, 307:156–159, 1982
Coryell W, Noyes R, Clancy J: Panic disorder and primary unipolar depression. J Aff Dis 5, 311–317, 1983
Van Winter J, Stickler GB: Panic attack syndrome. J Pediatr 105:661–665, 1984

PANNER'S II

Synonyms. Capitellum humeri epiphyseal necrosis; Haas'; capitellum humeri osteochondrosis; "little league elbow." See Epiphyseal ischemic necrosis.

Symptoms and Signs. Pain in the shoulder aggravated by active movement; swelling and redness over capitellum humeri.

Etiology. See Epiphyseal ischemic necrosis.

BIBLIOGRAPHY. Panner HJ: An affection of the capitellum humeri resembling Calve-Perthes disease of the hip. Acta Radiol (Stockh) 8:617, 1927
Canale ST: Osteochondrosis or epiphysitis? In Crenshaw AH (ed): Campbell's Operative Orthopedics, 7th ed, p 991. St Louis, CV Mosby, 1987

PAPILLARY MUSCLE

Synonym. Papillary muscle dysfunction.

Symptoms. Occur usually in patients over 40. No specific symptoms. Possibly, symptoms of disease responsible for papillary muscle dysfunction (*e.g.*, angina; congestive failure).

Signs. Apical systolic murmur: delayed in onset; "diamond shaped" with midsystolic accentuation, to moderately loud; "blowing" in quality; best heard at apex radiating at axilla, seldom associated with thrill. If papillary muscle dysfunction associated with left ventricular dilatation and congestive failure, murmur of decrescent quality. Murmur may be a fixed feature (in healing of fibrotic

lesions) or transient (in evolving lesions). Absence of late systolic clicks.

Etiology and Pathology. 1. Circulatory insufficiency: angina; infarction of papillary muscle; systemic circulatory disturbances. 2. Left ventricular dilatation: generalized; localized. 3. Nonischemic atrophy of papillary muscle. 4. Defective development. 5. Endocardial diseases. 6. Heart muscle diseases. 7. Functional disturbances of papillary muscle. 8. Rupture.

Diagnostic Procedures. *Electrocardiography.* Type 1: moderate depression of junction J; concavity-upward or slight convexity-downward deformity of ST-T interval. Type II: slight to moderate depression of junction J; prominent convexity-upward deformity of ST interval and terminal inversion of T. Type III: marked depression of junction J; slight convexity-upward deformity of the initial ST interval. *Phonocardiography.* See Signs. *Two-dimensional echocardiography.*

Therapy. That of determining condition and associated manifestations (*e.g.*, congestive failure, angina). Mitral valve replacement if severe mitral regurgitation is present and if left ventricular contractility is preserved.

Prognosis. Depends on etiology.

BIBLIOGRAPHY. Burch GE, DePasquale NP, Phillips JH: Clinical manifestations of papillary muscle dysfunction. Arch Intern Med 112:112–117, 1963
Burch GE, DePasquale NP, Phillips JH: The syndrome of papillary muscle dysfunction. Am Heart J 75:399–415, 1968
Hurst JW: The Heart, 6th ed, p. 984. New York, McGraw-Hill, 1985

PAPILLON-LEAGE-PSAUME

Synonyms. Orofacial digital dysostosis I; facial orodigital I; Gorlin's; linguofacial dysplasia I, OFD, OFD II; Psaume's; orofacial digital I.

Symptoms. Limited to females; lethal in males (reported in males; one of the males who had chromosomal study done showed a 47 XXY pattern. See Klinefelter's). Mental retardation and trembling (not constant).

Signs. Constant features: cleft or defect of hard palate; hypertrophic frenulum; cleft of tongue with two or more lobules. Inconstant features: soft palate or uvular cleft; syndactyly; clinodactyly; bradydactyly; hypoplastic nasal cartilages; seborrheic changes; dystopia canthum; pseudocleft of upper lip; alopecia; missing mandibular lateral incisors. A variety of central nervous system malformations.

Etiology. Unknown; possibly, X-linked dominant mutant condition with variable penetrance.

Diagnostic Procedures. *Blood and urine.* Normal. *Chromosome study.* No consistent chromosomal abnormality detectable. *X-ray.* Typical findings.

Therapy. None.

Prognosis. Poor.

BIBLIOGRAPHY. Duplouy MS: Communication. Bull Mem Soc Nat Chir Paris 9:456, 1883

Papillon-Léage M, Psaume J; Une malformation héréditaire de la muqueuse buccale, brides et freins anormaux: Generalities. Rev Stomatol 55:209–227, 1954

Gorlin RJ, Psaume J: Orodigitofacial dysostosis: A new syndrome. A study of 22 cases. J Pediatr 61:520–530, 1962

Majewski F, Lenz W, Pfeiffer RA et al: Das oro-faciodigitale Syndrom. Symptome und Prognose. Z Kinderheilkd 112:89–112, 1972

Towfighi J, Berlin CM Jr, Ladda RL et al: Neuropathology of oral-facial-digital syndromes. Arch Pathol Lab Med 109:642–646, 1985

PAPILLON–LEFÈVRE

Synonyms. Palmoplantar hyperkeratosis–periodontitis. Keratosis palmoplantaris–periodontopathia; see Schoepf's.

Symptoms and Signs. Appear within first 4 years of life. Hyperkeratosis of palms and soles, usually diffuse type, seldom punctate type, generally not severe, similar to those of Meleda syndrome (see). In some cases, lesion more severe in winter and receding or disappearing during summer. Fetid hyperhidrosis, especially of feet. At the same time of appearance of hyperkeratosis, gingivae become red and swollen and bleed. Bad breath and destruction of periodontal ligament begins and periodontal pockets with pus form. Teeth become mobile and are lost. Period in which the patient is edentulous follows, then the process is repeated with the permanent teeth. In more severe type, complete edentia by 6 to 10 years of age.

Etiology. Unknown; autosomal recessive pattern of inheritance suspected.

Pathology. Hyperkeratosis of palms and soles; acanthosis without parakeratosis; gingival pattern similar to ordinary periodontoclasia. Teeth grossly normal with some resorption of cementum and dentin. Calcification of dura mater (third component of syndrome).

Diagnostic Procedures. *X-ray.* Occasionally, ectopic calcification in the tentorium and choroid (third feature of syndrome). Destruction of periodontal structures.

Blood. In some cases, polycythemia and glucose curve elevated.

Therapy. Vitamin A; antibiotics; oral hygiene. Acitretin.

Prognosis. Loss of teeth; dentures well tolerated.

BIBLIOGRAPHY. Papillon MM, Lefèvre P: Deux cas de kératodermie palmaire et plantaire symétrique familiale (maladie de Meleda) chez le frère et la soeur; coexistence dans les deux cas d'alterations dentaires graves. Bull Soc Fr Dermatol Syph 31:82–87, 1924

Cheung HS, Landow RK, Bauer M: Increased collagen synthesis by gingival fibroblasts derived from a Papillon–Lefèvre patient. J Dent Res 61:378–381, 1982

Nazzaro V, Blanchet-Bardon C, Mimoz C et al: Papillon–Lefèvre syndrome. Ultrastructural study and successful treatment with Acitretin. Arch Dermatol 12:533–539, 1988

PARANA HARD-SKIN

Synonym. See Stiff skin.

Symptoms and Signs. Onset 2 to 3 months of age. The same as that of stiff skin plus growth retardation.

Etiology. Probably autosomal recessive inheritance.

Prognosis. Malignant course (if compared with stiff skin).

BIBLIOGRAPHY. Cat I, Rodriguez-Magdalena NI, Parolin-Marinoni L et al: Parana hard-skin syndrome: Study of seven families. Lancet I:215–216, 1974

PARAPLEGIA PAINFUL

See Putti–Chavany.

Symptoms. Extremely severe pain due to vertebral root compression (typical specific irradiation) followed by paraplegia, cachexia.

Signs. Pain on compression of specific point of vertebral column. Signs of paraplegia.

Etiology and Pathology. Osteogenic or osteolytic lesions of vertebrae. Multiple myeloma; metastasis of prostate, lung, breast, kidney, or colon malignancy.

Diagnostic Procedures. *X-ray of spine, skeleton. Blood.* Search for primary anemia, hyperproteinemia (myeloma). *Biopsy of bone marrow.*

Therapy. Myeloma: Cyclophosphamide; melphalan, testosterone. Prostate: castration; estrogens. Breast: radiation; oophorectomy.

Prognosis. Sometimes dramatic improvement with treatment.

BIBLIOGRAPHY. Vick NA: Grinker's Neurology, 7th ed. Springfield, CC Thomas, 1976

PARAPLEGIC PHANTOM

See Phantom limb.

Symptoms. Occur in patients with paraplegia and complete cord injury. Phantom phenomena or painful phantom limb of the paraplegic extremity. Phenomena of shortening, telescoping, and decreasing size of phantom, observed in phantom limb syndrome in amputee, are not noted in paraplegic patient with analogous syndrome. In many paraplegic patients, dissociation between position of phantom and actual position of paralyzed limb is eventually noticed within a few days or weeks.

Signs. Paraplegia.

Etiology and Pathology. Different type of cord lesion.

Diagnostic Procedures. See Phantom limb.

Therapy. See Phantom limb.

Prognosis. See Phantom limb.

BIBLIOGRAPHY. Bors E: Phantom limbs of patients with spinal cord injury. Arch Neurol Psychiatry 66:610–631, 1951
Weiss AA: The phantom limb. Ann Intern Med 44:668–677, 1956

PARASPASM, BILATERAL

See Ziehen–Oppenheim.

Symptoms. Gradually increasing intermittent attacks of contractions of all facial muscles and muscles of tongue and neck. Contractions enhanced by emotions, until attacks become almost continuous.

Signs. The patient may sometimes stop the attack temporarily with special maneuvers.

Etiology. Unknown; extrapyramidal lesions; possibly, part of dystonia lenticularis syndrome (localized form). May occasionally be of psychogenic origin.

Therapy. Phenytoin or carbamazepine (inconstant effect). Quinine sulphate (better result). Diazepam.

BIBLIOGRAPHY. Zeman W, Kaelbling R, Pasamanick B: Idiopathic dystonia musculorum deformans. II. The formes frustes. Neurology 10:1068–1075, 1960
Adams RD, Victor M: Principles of Neurology, 3rd ed, pp 1090–1092. New York, McGraw-Hill, 1985

PARENTI–FRACCARO

Synonyms. Achondrogenesis I; lethal achondrogenesis; achondrogenesis Ia.

Symptoms and Signs. Stillbirth or neonatal death. Short limbs; dwarfism. Trunk as wide as it is long; wide pelvis.

Etiology. Autosomal recessive inheritance.

Pathology. Endochondral ossification severely disorganized. Lack of matrix between resting cartilage cells.

Diagnostic Procedures. *X-ray.* Normal or enlarged skull; normal base; short horizontal ribs; absent sternum ossification; vertebral, sacral, iliac, and pubic anomalies; marked metaphyseal widening and spurs; micromelia.

BIBLIOGRAPHY. Donath J, Vogl A: Untersuchungen ueber den chondrodysteophischen Zwergunchs das Verholten der Wirbelsaule beim chondrodystrophischen Zwerg. Wein Arch Inn Med 10:1–44, 1925
Parenti GC: La anosteogenesi (una varietà della osteogenesi imperfetta). Pathologica 28:447–462, 1936
Fraccaro M: Contributo allo studio delle malattie del mesenchima osteopoietico; l'acondrogenesi. Folia Hered Pathol 1:190–208, 1952
Bokesoy I, Aydm E, Gazilerli S: A case of achondrogenesis type I. Hum Genet 67:349–350, 1984

PARINAUD'S I

Synonyms. Sylvian aqueduct; nystagmus retractorius; sylvian; Koerber-Salus-Elschnig; superior colliculus; divergence paralysis; subthalamus; supranuclear. See Benedikt's and Weber-Gubler.

Symptoms. Headaches; dizziness; vertigo; impaired vertical gaze; ataxia; hemitremor; possible, hemiparesis.

Signs. Retraction nystagmus; convergence nystagmus, vertical nystagmus (best demonstrated by asking patient to attempt upward gaze or by using target moving downward). Pupils usually normal in size, but poor reaction to light and near vision. Extraocular palsies. Babinski's sign; systemic hypertension.

Etiology and Pathology. Neoplastic, vascular, or inflammatory lesions adjacent to periductal gray matter of aqueduct of Sylvius.

Diagnostic Procedures. *X-ray. Isotope brain scan. Angiography. CT scan.*

Therapy. According to etiology.

Prognosis. Poor because this syndrome is observed most frequently with neoplastic lesion.

BIBLIOGRAPHY. Parinaud H: Paralisie des mouvements associés des yeux. Arch Neurol 5:145–172, 1883

Koerber HL: Ueber drei Fälle von Retraktionsbewegung des Bulbus. Ophthalmol Klin 7:65–67, 1903

Salus R: Ueber erworbene Retractionsbewegungen der Augen. Arch Kinderheilkd 47:61–76, 1910

Elschnig A: Nystagmus Retractorius, ein cerebrales Herd-Symptom. Med Klin 1:8–11, 1913

Bielschowsky A: Lectures on motor anomalies of the eyes. Arch Ophthalmol 13:569–583, 1935

Hatcher MA, Klintworth GK: Sylvian aqueduct syndrome. Arch Neurol 15:215–222, 1966

Adams RD, Victor M: Principles of Neurology, 3rd ed, p 198. New York, McGraw-Hill, 1985

PARINAUD'S OCULOGLANDULAR

Synonyms. Cat-scratch–oculoglandular; Parinaud's conjunctiva adenitis.

Symptoms. Both sexes affected; more frequent in children. Tenderness at site of scratch. Irregular fever.

Signs. Granular or ulcerative conjunctivitis; anterior cervical lymphadenopathy; parotid gland swelling.

Etiology. Cat-scratch fever; tularemia; leptotrichosis; tuberculosis; lymphogranuloma venereum; coccidioidomycosis; sporotrichosis; syphilis, sarcoidosis; listeriosis.

Pathology. Conjunctivitis with granulomatous reaction; aspecific lymphadenopathy.

Diagnostic Procedures. *Cultures.* For viruses, mycobacteria, bacteria, and fungi. *Skin test.* For tuberculosis, cat-scratch fever, Kveim's test, and fungi. *Complement fixation. Biopsy of conjunctiva.*

Therapy. According to etiology.

Prognosis. Spontaneous recovery (in a week or month). Specific treatment speeds recovery.

BIBLIOGRAPHY. Parinaud H, Galezowski X: Conjonctivite infectieuse transmise par les animaux. Ann Ocul 101:252–253, 1889

Müller F: Die differential diagnose des konjunktivoglandulären Syndrome von Parinaud. Dtsch Med Wochenschr 80:152–154, 1955

Wood TR: Ocular coccidioidomycosis. Report of a case presenting as Parinaud's oculoglandular syndrome. Am J Ophthalmol 64:587–590, 1967

Margeleth AM: Cat-scratch disease update. Am J Dis Child 138:711–713, 1984

Rook A, Wilkinson DS, Ebling FJG et al: Textbook of Dermatology, 4th ed, p 708. Oxford, Blackwell Scientific Publications, 1986

PARKER'S

Synonyms. Abercrombie's; adrenal medullary neuroblastoma; gangliosympathicoblastoma; malignant hypernephroma; neuroblastoma; Smith's; sympathicoblastoma. See also Hutchinson's (R.) and Pepper's.

Symptoms. Both sexes affected; present from birth or early infancy or onset in childhood (under age 10 yr). Abdominal and back pain. Anorexia; debilitation; diarrhea or constipation.

Signs. Jaundice (occasionally). Abdominal mass that crosses the midline. Possible association with various congenital malformations: spina bifida; hydrocephalus; polydactyly; aorta coarctation; visceral malformations.

Etiology. Autosomal recessive inheritance. Chromosomal aberration reported.

Pathology. Typically, retroperitoneal neoplasm, usually of adrenal medulla or adjacent sympathetic chain or, less frequently, on ganglia of other areas. Gray or purplish tumor. Microscopically, dense uniform cells, occasionally producing rosettes. *Liver.* Frequently, metastases that may replace the normal tissue almost completely (*Pepper's*). *Long bones.* Typial "onion skin" layering. *Flat bones.* Vertical periosteal spines (*Hutchinson's [R.]*).

Diagnostic Procedures. *Bone marrow.* Frequently, presence of typical cells and rosettes. *X-ray.* Typical bone changes. *Biopsy.* See Pathology. *Urine.* Nonconstant increase of catecholamines and vanillylmandelic acid.

Therapy. Roentgen treatment; chemotherapy.

Prognosis. Rapid evolution: death in weeks or months. Spontaneous regression in 3% of cases.

BIBLIOGRAPHY. Parker RW: Diffuse (?) sarcoma of the liver, probably congenital. Trans Pathol Soc London 31:290–293, 1880

Abercrombie J: Multiple sarcomata of the cranial bones. Trans Pathol Soc London 31:216–223, 1880

Smith J: Case of adrenal neuroblastoma. Lancet 2:1214–1215, 1932

Hecht F, Hecht BK, Northrup JC et al: Genetics of familial neuroblastoma: Long-range studies. Cancer Genet Cytogenet 7:227–230, 1982

PARKINSON'S

Synonyms. Amyostatic; paralysis agitans; nonencephalitic parkinsonism.

Symptoms and Signs. Both sexes affected; gradual and insidious onset between 50 to 65 years of age. Tremors at rest, mostly in upper limbs, particularly in the hands (pill-rolling movements); disappear when initiating movements and during sleep. Usually monolateral at onset, then generalized. Muscle rigidity; slowing of voluntary movements initially, then generalized stiffness, fatigue, mild muscle pain, progressing to generalized stiffness. Face masklike; no wrinkling (youthful aspect); no expression; infrequent winking; pupil reaction prompt; drooling; slow swallowing. Semiflexed posture of head, hand, arm, and trunk; difficulty in straightening. Movements (active or passive) interrupted by cogwheel jerks. Handwriting: small letters; akathisia. Gait: steps short and shuffling; because of postural defect (stooping) the patient has to take a short run to keep his balance while moving; no arm swinging. Voice: monotonous; low pitched.

Etiology. Unknown; degenerative lesion of central nervous system, in particular of basal ganglia. Some familial cases reported.

Pathology. Degenerative changes mostly in globus pallidus and substantia nigra.

Diagnostic Procedures. *Electroencephalography. Serology.*

Therapy. Medical: belladonna; trihexyphenidyl, orphenadrine; levodopa; association of levodopa and decarboxylase inhibitor; benzatropine; ethopropazine; amantadine; bromocriptine; experimental deprenil (B monoamino-oxidase inhibitor); domperidone (to reduce collateral effects of bromocriptine); pergolide mesylate; lisuride; terguride; ciladopa; L-leucyl-glycinamide. Surgical: transplantation of adrenal medullary tissue to striatum or caudate nucleus.

Prognosis. Progressive course; symptomatic relief of some manifestations by medical or surgical treatment.

BIBLIOGRAPHY. Parkinson J: An Essay on the Shaking Palsy. London, Sherwood Neeley-Jones, 1817

Current concepts and controversies in Parkinson's disease. Can J Neurol Sci 11 (Suppl) 1984

Backlund ED, Granberg P, Hamberger B et al: Transplantation of adrenal medullary tissue to striatum in parkinsonism. First clinical trials. J Neurosurg 62:169–173, 1985

Madrazo I, Drucker–Colin R, Diaz V et al: Open microsurgical autograft of adrenal medulla to the right caudate nucleus in two patients with intractable Parkinson's disease. N Engl J Med 316:831–834, 1987

Various Authors: Pharmacotherapeutic Trends in Parkinson's Disease. In Parkinson's Disease—Advances in Neurology, Vol 45, pp 511–605. New York, Raven Press, 1987

PARROT'S I

Synonyms. Bednar–Parrot; Parrot's pseudoparalysis; Parrot's syphilitic osteochondritis, Wegner's.

Symptoms. Onset most commonly in first 3 weeks of life, seldom after 3 months. Upper extremities affected more frequently than lower. Pseudoparalysis; periarticular swelling.

Etiology. Congenital syphilis.

Pathology. Complete epiphyseal separation of long bones or fractures. Gelatiniform changes in bone and cartilage forming yellowish fluid.

Diagnostic Procedures. *X-ray.* Widening of joint space; irregular epiphyseal lines; periosteal thickening; bone decalcification.

Prognosis. Adequate, prompt antibiotic treatment brings complete recovery. Deformity if growing line severely affected.

BIBLIOGRAPHY. Wegner G: Ueber hederitäre knochensyphilis bei jungen kindern. Arch Pathol Anat (Berlin) 50:305–322, 1870

Parrot JM: Sur une pseudo-paralysie causée par une altération du système osseux chez les nouveau-nés atteints de syphilis héréditaire. Arch Physiol Norm Pathol Paris 4:319–333; 470–490; 612–623, 1871–72

McCord JR: Osteochondritis in the stillborn. Am J Obstet Gynecol 42:667–676, 1941

Mascola L, Pelosi R, Blount JH et al: Congenital syphilis revisited. Am J Dis Child 139:579–580, 1985

PARROT'S II

Synonyms. Athrepsia; inanition; infantile atrophy; marasmus.

Symptoms and Signs. Occur in infants. Failure to thrive; weight loss; emaciation; edema; skin dry and subcutaneous fat loss. Abdomen flat or distended; muscles hypotonic and atrophic; hypothermia; pulse slow; basal metabolic rate decreased. Fretfulness and then listlessness; constipation or diarrhea.

Etiology. Inadequate calorie intake due to insufficient supply, improper feeding habits, metabolic abnormalities, or congenital malformations. Disturbed parent–child relations.

Diagnostic Procedures. *Blood.* Hypochromic anemia; hypoproteinemia T_3, T_4 and thyroid-stimulating hormone (TSH). *X-ray.*

Therapy. Dietary correction and correction of specific anatomic or functional defects. Usually there is a slow response to dietary therapy during the first 4 weeks.

Prognosis. Usually poor.

BIBLIOGRAPHY. Parrot JM: L'Athrepsie. Paris, Masson, 1877
Nelson's Textbook of Pediatrics, 12th ed, p 166. Philadelphia, WB Saunders, 1983

PARRY–ROMBERG

Synonyms. Hemifacial atrophy; progressive facial hemiatrophy; progressive laminar aplasia trophoneurosis facialis progressiva. Romberg's. See Scleroderma ("en coupe de sabre").

Symptoms and Signs. Both sexes affected; onset in first two decades, but possible also later. At early stage on paramedian area of face, hair of skull and of face affected by alopecia, blanching, often preceding other symptoms. Atrophy of fat and subcutaneous tissue. The process may be bilateral in 5% to 10% of cases. Extension of the process homolaterally; occasionally occurs involving trunk, extremities, and visceral organs. Cerebral manifestation homolateral to lesion frequently occurs, especially jacksonian type elipsy and migraine. Sympathetic manifestations may also be present.

Etiology. Unknown; distinguishing between hemiatrophy and secondary localized scleroderm impossible.

Pathology. Atrophic and secondary inflammatory changes of fat and subcutaneous tissue; skin usually spared except occasionally at later stages. Various degenerative brain lesions; calcification may be found.

Diagnostic Procedures. *Biopsy. Electroencephalography.*

Therapy. Plastic surgery. Symptomatic for neurologic manifestations.

Prognosis. The process usually progresses for number of years, but may become arrested at any stage and then become stable for the rest of life.

BIBLIOGRAPHY. Parry CH: Collections from Unpublished Papers, p 178. London, Unterwood, 1825
Romberg MH: Trophoneurosen. In his Klinische Ergebnise, pp 75–81. Berlin, Förstner, 1846
Dilley JJ, Perry HO: Bilateral linear scleroderma en coupe de sabre. Arch Dermatol 97:688–689, 1968
Miller MT, Sloane H, Goldberg MF: Progressive hemifacial atrophy (Parry–Romberg disease). J Pediatr Ophthalmol Strabismus 24:27–36, 1987

PARSONAGE–TURNER

Eponym obsolete. Once used to indicate many forms of cryptogenic neurologic amyotrophy of the shoulder and cervical plexus. Today different mononeuropathies are described as syndromes and cervical plexus neuropathies are indicated by their etiology.

Synonyms. Neurologic amyotrophy; shoulder girdle, Feinberg's, Tinel's, Kiloh–Nevin II (see), brachial neuritis, acute brachial neuritis, cryptogenic neuropathy of brachial plexus.

Symptoms and Signs. Sharp pain across the shoulder and proximal part of arm, followed by atrophic paralysis of some muscles of shoulder girdle.

Etiology. Infection or minor surgery with involvement of branches of cervical plexus.

BIBLIOGRAPHY. Parsonage MJ, Turner JWA; Neuralgic amyotrophy, the shoulder-girdle syndrome. Lancet 1:973–978, 1948

PASINI–PIERINI

Synonyms. Atrophoderma progressivum; atrophic morphea variant.

Symptoms. Affects more females than males; may begin in infancy or old age, but usually appears in adolescence and early adult life.

Signs. Slight depression below level of normal skin. Lesions are distributed primarily on back of trunk and shoulders, less on the abdomen, seldom on the limbs; they have different shapes (round or oval) colors (violet, brown), and dimensions (2 cm in diameter or larger). They may become confluent and form patches.

Etiology. Unknown; no genetic basis. See Morphea (may represent one of its variants). Some authors maintain that there may exist two forms of such condition: (1) variant of morphea, (2) stable lesion, possibly congenital.

Pathology. Moderate changes at the lesion sites. At onset edema in lower dermis, and clamping of elastic tissue. Later, reduction of dermal thickness.

Therapy. None.

Prognosis. Lesions extend very slowly for 10 years, then stabilize. Eventually, sclerodermatous and other changes are possible.

BIBLIOGRAPHY. Pasini A: Atrofodermia idiopatica progressiva (studio clinico ed istologico). G Ital Mal Venereol 64:785–809, 1923

Pierini LE, Vivoli D: Atrofodermia idiopatica progressiva (Pasini). G Ital Dermatol 77:403–409, 1936

Rook A, Wilkinson DS, Ebling FJG et al: Textbook of Dermatology, 4th ed, pp 1809–1810. Oxford, Blackwell Scientific Publications, 1986

PASINI'S

Synonyms. Albopapuloid epidermolysis bullosa. Epidermolysis bullosa Pasini's.

Symptoms and Signs. Both sexes affected; onset seldom in infancy, usually in late childhood or adulthood. Small, firm, white perifollicular papules appearing on the trunk, especially lumbosacral region, slowly enlarging to 15 mm. Features of hyperplastic epidermolysis bullosa.

Etiology. Unknown; autosomal dominant inheritance. Deranged glycosaminoglycan metabolism.

Pathology. Connective tissue hyperplasia.

Diagnostic Procedures. *Biopsy of skin.*

Therapy. Treatment symptomatic.

Prognosis. Healing with scar, frequently of keloid type, or leaving atrophic macula.

BIBLIOGRAPHY. Pasini A: Distrofia cutanea bollosa—atrofizzante ed albo-papuloide. G Ital Dermatol Sifil 69:558–564, 1928

Rook A, Wilkinson DS, Ebling FJG et al: Textbook of Dermatology, 4th ed, p 1628. Oxford, Blackwell Scientific Publications, 1986

PASQUALINI

Synonyms. "Fertile eunuch"; pseudoeunuchoidism.

Symptoms. No libido or potency; erection rarely occurs.

Signs. Obesity; skin dry; axillary and pubic hair scanty; no beard; penis small, scrotum well formed; testes normal size; prostate small.

Etiology. Not entirely clear; isolated deficiency of luteinizing hormone (LH).

Pathology. Testes normal size; Leydig cells very scarce or absent. Tubules contain normal or reduced number of spermatozoa.

Diagnostic Procedures. *Semen analysis.* Low spermatozoa count. *Blood and urine.* Follicle-stimulating hormone (FSH) normal; LH decreased or undetected; testosterone decreased; 17-ketosteroids markedly decreased. *Biopsy of testes.* See Pathology. *Chromosome studies. X-ray of skull.*

Therapy. Testosterone and human chorionic gonadotropins effective in stimulating spermatogenesis and virilization.

Prognosis. Good response to treatment. More frequent erections and increased spermatozoa count.

BIBLIOGRAPHY. Nathanson I, Towne LE, Aub JC: Normal excretion of sex hormones in childhood. Endocrinology 28:851–865, 1941

Pasqualini RQ, Bur G: Syndrome hipoandrogénica con gametogénesis conservada. Classification de la insuficiencia testicular. Rev Assoc Méd Argent 64:6–10, 1950

McCullagh EP, Beck JC, Schaffenburg CA: A syndrome of eunuchoidism with spermatogenesis, normal urinary FSH and low or normal ICSH (fertile eunuchs). J Clin Endocrinol 13:489–509, 1953

Behrman RE, Vaughan VC: Nelson's Textbook of Pediatrics, 12th ed, p 1499. Philadelphia, WB Saunders, 1983

Faiman C, Hoffman DL, Ryan RJ et al: The "fertile eunuch" syndrome: Demonstration of isolated luteinizing hormone deficiency by radioimmunoassay technique. Mayo Clin Proc 43:661–667, 1968

PASSOW'S

Synonyms. Bremer's status dysraphicus; status dysraphicus.

Symptoms and Signs. Variable; muscular weakness; trophic changes; facial hemiatrophy; abducens (VI) and facial (VII) nerve paralysis; anesthesia first branch of trigeminal (V) nerve; myosis; heterochromia iridis; cervical rib symptoms; kyphoscoliosis; spina bifida; extremities malformations.

Etiology. Congenital lack of neural tube closure.

BIBLIOGRAPHY. Passow A: Analogie und Koordination von Symptomen der Arachnodactylie und des Status dysraphicus (zur Frage der Wesensgleichheit beider Komplexe). Klin Monatsbl Augenheilkd 94:102–103, 1935

Bremer FW: Status dysraphicus und Syringomyelie. Fortschr Neurol Psychiatr 14:109–122, 1942

PASSWELL'S

Synonym. Ichthyosis—mental retardation—dwarfism—renal changes.

Symptoms and Signs. Both sexes. From birth. Ichthyosis, mental and physical growth retardation; altered renal functions.

Etiology. Unknown. Autosomal recessive inheritance.

BIBLIOGRAPHY. Passwell JH, Goodman RM, Zprkowski M et al: Congenital ichthyosis, mental retardation, dwarfism, and renal impairment: A new syndrome. Clin Genet 8:59–65, 1975

PATAU'S

Synonyms. Bartholin–Patau; D_1 trisomy; trisomy 13–15.

Symptoms. Present from birth. Recurrent respiratory infections with episodes of cyanosis and apnea. Severe mental retardation. A few cases with motor seizures.

Signs. Arhinencephalia; microphthalmia; coloboma of iris; cleft palate and lip; polydactyly; digit fixed in flexion; cardiac and renal defects. All patients are virtually totally deaf. Diffuse capillary hemangiomas.

Etiology. Congenital condition resulting from the presence of an extra chromosome of the 13–15 group (D). Translocation chromosome or isochromosome for long arm of a group D chromosome; mosaicism for trisomy D has been described.

Pathology. Arhinencephalia with absent olfactory bulbs; fusion of frontal poles; occasionally, agenesis of corpus callosum and defect of cerebellum; double alveolar ridges of upper jaw; cleft palate and lips. *Heart.* Cardiomegaly; ventricular septal defect; patent ductus arteriosus and foramen ovale; other congenital defects. *Kidney.* Bilateral hydronephrosis. *Other organs.* Various abnormalities.

Diagnostic Procedures. *Chromosome study. Dermatoglyphic pattern.* Transverse palmar crease on one or both hands. Bilateral arch fibular S patterns on the feet (typical findings for this condition). *Blood.* Increased amount of hemoglobin F, Bart's and Gower's, peduncular projections of leukocytes.

Therapy. None; symptomatic.

Prognosis. Frequently, stillbirth. Death in infancy from cardiac or other malformations; 70% die within first 3 months of life; survival to childhood extremely rare. Because of the high infant mortality, surgical or orthopedic corrective procedures should be withheld in early infancy to await the outcome of the first few months. Furthermore, because of the severe brain defect, some authorities believe that no medical means should be used to prolong the life of infants with this syndrome.

BIBLIOGRAPHY. Patau K, Smith DW, Therman E et al: Multiple congenital anomalies caused by an extra autosome. Lancet 1:790–793, 1960

Valentine GH: The Chromosome Disorders. Philadelphia, JB Lippincott, 1966
Marden PM, Yunis JJ: Trisomy D_1 in a 10-year-old girl. Normal neutrophils and fetal hemoglobin. Am J Dis Child 114:662–664, 1967
Shinzel A: Autosomal chromosomenaberationen. Arch Genet 52:180, 1979
Smith DW: Recognizable Patterns of Human Malformation. Philadelphia, WB Saunders, 1982

PATIN'S

Synonyms. Fibrodysplasia ossificans progressiva; fibrosis ossificans progressiva; FOP; Guy–Patin's; interstitial ossifying myositis; Muenchmeyer's; myositis ossificans progressiva (misnomer, see Calcinosis universalis) stone man.

Symptoms. Both sexes affected; prevalent in males (according to various authors 4 : 1, 3 : 1, 3 : 2, or 2 : 1); onset usually before 10 years of age. Pain and tenderness during contraction of some muscles (which in time become generalized).

Signs. Localized swelling first in neck region, then in the back and, finally, in the limbs; initially, lumps may appear and disappear several times; stiffness of muscles; synostoses of various joints. Frequently associated with microdactyly of little fingers, valgus deviation of great toes, development of exostoses. Progressive rigidity of thorax with respiratory and cardiac insufficiency. Tendency to ecchymosis. Tongue, heart, larynx, diaphragm, and sphincters not affected.

Etiology. Autosomal dominant inheritance; 90% of cases represent fresh mutation.

Pathology. Biopsy of initial lesions shows extensive proliferation of interstitial cellular connective tissue with very moderate inflammatory changes; formation of reticular fibers and collagen, which retracts and compresses muscle fibers; finally, the muscle fibers fragment and degenerate. The whole process is followed by osteoid formation, which extends peripherally like normal bone (muscle fibers may remain within bone tissue).

Therapy. None; symptomatic.

Prognosis. Progressive disability and incapacitation. Possibly, arrest of ossifying process. Long survival possible. Death from intercurrent conditions.

BIBLIOGRAPHY. Muenchmeyer E: Ueber Myositis ossificans progressive. Z Ration Med 34:1, 1869
Helferich H: Ein Fall von sogenamter Myositis ossificans progressiva. Aerztl Intelligenz-Blatl 26:485, 1874
Connor JM, Evans DAP: Fibrodysplasia ossificans progressiva: The clinical features and natural history of 34 patients. J Bone Joint Surg 64:76–83, 1982

PAUTRIER–WORINGER

Synonyms. Dermatopathic lymphadenopathy; hypomelanotic reticulosis exfoliative.

Symptom. Severe pruritus (not constant).

Signs. Various generalized dermatoses: exfoliative dermatitis of different etiologies; different types of neurodermatitis; prurigo; seborrheic dermatitis; lichen planus; pemphigus; psoriasis. Lymphadenopathy.

Etiology. That of the dermatosis responsible. To be differentiated from similar malignant processes, *e.g.*, Hodgkin's disease, Brill–Simmers disease.

Pathology. *Skin.* That of various dermatoses. *Lymph nodes.* Histopathologic pattern of granulomatous hyperplasia with respect to normal architecture (exceptionally, may be altered); marked degree of hyperplasia of reticular cells, especially cortical areas. Varying deposits of melanin and lipid. Eosinophilic, polymorphonuclear, and plasma cell infiltration.

Diagnostic Procedures. *Biopsy of lymph node and skin.*

Therapy. That of specific dermatosis. Infiltration with half-strength triamcinolone.

Prognosis. Lymph node hyperplasia regresses with cure of dermatosis.

BIBLIOGRAPHY. Pautrier LM, Woringer F: Note preliminaire sur un tableau histologique particulier de lésions ganglionnaires accompagnant des eruptions dermatologiques généralisées, prurigineuses, des types cliniques différents. Bull Soc Fr Dermatol Syph 39:947–955, 1932
Pautrier LM, Woringer F: Contribution á l'étude de l'histo-physiologie cutanée; á propos d'un aspect histopathologique nouveau du ganglion lymphatique; la réticulose lipo-mélanique accompagnant certaines dermatoses généralisées; les échanges entre la peau et le ganglion. Ann Dermatol Syph 8:257–273, 1937
Schnyder UW, Schirrer CG: So-called "lipomelanotic reticulosis" of Pautrier–Woringer. Arch Dermatol Syph 70:155–165, 1954
Rook A, Wilkinson DS, Ebling FJG et al: Textbook of Dermatology. 4th ed, p 413. Oxford, Blackwell Scientific Publications, 1986

PAVOR NOCTURNUS

Synonym. Nightmare.

Symptoms. Observed especially in children. Sleep disturbance resulting in moaning, agitation, and difficulty in waking rapidly, or the child awakens abruptly in a state of intense fright, screaming. Possible association with sleep-walking. Usually in the morning no memory of the dream.

Signs. Tachycardia, tachypnea.

Etiology. Unknown; in association with frightening dreams.

Diagnostic Procedures. *Electroencephalography.* For differential diagnosis with epilepsy. EEG during the episode shows a waking type of mixed frequency of alpha pattern.

Therapy. None, or psychiatric consultation. Diazepam prevents episode (do not use for protracted periods).

Prognosis. When not expressing major psychotic disturbances, excellent.

BIBLIOGRAPHY. Adams RD, Victor M: Principles of Neurology, 3rd ed, pp 291–292. New York, McGraw-Hill, 1985

PAVY'S

Synonyms. Cyclic albuminuria; functional proteinuria; asymptomatic proteinuria; transient proteinuria, postural proteinuria; orthostatic proteinuria.

Symptoms and Signs. Asymptomatic. Finding usually discovered accidentally on routine analysis.

Etiology. Unknown. Diagnosis by exclusion after ruling out all possible systemic and local disorders. May represent an aftereffect of subclinical glomerulonephritis.

Diagnostic Procedures. *Urine.* Proteinuria usually less than 2 g/day. Careful analysis to search for other possible findings. *Blood.* Electrophoresis; creatinine clearance.

Therapy. None. Follow-up for possible identification of basic pathologic process.

Prognosis. Good. Sometime subsides spontaneously after months or years.

BIBLIOGRAPHY. Pavy FW: Cyclic albuminuria (albuminuria in the apparently healthy). Lancet 2:707–708, 1885
Brenner BM, Rector FC Jr (eds): The Kidney, 3rd ed, p 954. Philadelphia, WB Saunders, 1986

PAYR'S

Synonyms. Splenic flexure. See Irritable bowel.

Symptoms. Occur in about 20% of patients with irritable colon, usually postprandially. The abdominal pain is present in the left upper quadrant, radiation pain may be manifested in precordial area, left thoracic or shoulder areas, neck and arm, or pain and pressure in the rectum. Systemic manifestations may also occur; tachycardia; dyspnea.

Signs. Abdominal distention (occasional) on palpation of spastic colon.

Etiology. See Irritable colon. Spasm or intrinsic or extrinsic compression of colon resulting in gas accumulation in splenic flexure.

Diagnostic Procedures. *X-ray.* Gas accumulation and distention localized in the splenic flexure.

Therapy. See Irritable bowel or treat organic obstruction if present.

Prognosis. Depends on etiology.

BIBLIOGRAPHY. Payr E: Ueber eine eigentümliche, durch abnorm starke Klickunge und Adhäsionen bedinge gucartige Stenose der Flexura lienalis und hepatice coli. Verh Dtsch Keng Inn Med 27:276–305, 1910
Lasser RB, Bond JH, Levitt MD: The role of intestinal gas in functional abdominal pain. N Engl J Med 293:524–526, 1975
Eastwood MH, Eastwood J, Ford MJ: The irritable bowel syndrome: a disease or a response? (Discussion paper). J Roy Soc Med 80:219–221, 1987

PEARSON'S

Synonym. Marrow–pancreas.

Symptoms and Signs. Both sexes. In infancy. Severe refractory anemia (transfusion dependency); malabsorption or other signs of pancreatic exocrine insufficiency.

Etiology. Unknown. Possibility of autosomal inheritance.

Pathology. *Pancreas.* Fibrosis. *Spleen.* Aplasia.

Diagnostic Procedures. *Blood.* Sideroblastic anemia. *Bone marrow.* Normal cellularity, sideroblastic anemia with vacuolization of marrow precursors. *Hepatosplenic-pancreatic echography.*

Therapy. Blood transfusions.

Prognosis. Death in early infancy; if survival, hematologic improvement.

BIBLIOGRAPHY. Pearson HA, Lobel JS, Kocoshis SA et al: A new syndrome of refractory sideroblastic anemia with vacuolization of marrow precursors and exocrine pancreatic dysfunction. J Pediatr 95:976–984, 1979

PECTUS EXCAVATUM

Synonyms. Hollow chest; cobbler's chest; funnel chest.

Symptoms and Signs. Usually asymptomatic. Deformity of sternum.

Etiology. Autosomal inheritance reported. Observed in Marfan's and other congenital syndromes. Occupational deformity (cobbler's).

Therapy. Surgery to correct defect.

BIBLIOGRAPHY. Peiper A: Ueber die Erblichkeit der Trichterburst. Klin Wschz 1:1647, 1922
Sugiura Y: A family with funnel chest in three generations. Jap J Hum Genet 22:287–289, 1977

PEDERSEN'S

Synonyms. Dix–Hallpike; neurolabyrinthitis; epidemic vertigo; vestibular neuronitis.

Symptoms. Occur in young adulthood or from third to fifth decades, onset abrupt, associated with upper respiratory infections. Vertigo; nausea and vomiting. Head movements enhance the symptoms. Tinnitus rare.

Signs. Fever, gait, and stance disturbed. Absent response to caloric stimulation on one side, nystagmus with quick component to the opposite side. Normal hearing; occasionally response positive on both sides.

Etiology. Unknown; evidence of viral origin lacking.

Diagnostic Procedures. *Cochlear function.* Normal. *Hearing.* Normal. *Caloric response.* Reduced bilaterally.

Therapy. Nonspecific. Dimenhydinate and similar agents.

Prognosis. Transient and benign condition.

BIBLIOGRAPHY. Pedersen E: Epidemic vertigo: Clinical picture, epidemiology and relation to encephalitis. Brain 82:566–580, 1959
Dix MR, Hallpike CS: The pathology, symptomatology and diagnosis of certain common disorders of vestibular system. Proc R Soc Med 45:341–347, 1962
Adams RD, Victor M: Principles of Neurology, 3rd ed, p 227. New York, McGraw-Hill, 1985

PELGER'S

Synonyms. Pelger's granulocyte anomaly; Pelger–Huet.

Symptoms and Signs. Found chiefly in Germany and Holland (1 : 1000); in United States (1 : 10,000). No symptoms. In spite of abnormal leukocytes, resistance to infections is not lowered. Occasionally, other congenital or familial anomalies are associated.

Etiology. Unknown; autosomal dominant transmission with partial carrier of the trait reported. Some type of leukocyte anomaly may be observed in different conditions: pelgeroid anomalies reported in cases of leukemia, Fanconi's anemia syndrome, and following treatment with myelotoxic agents.

Pathology. None.

Diagnostic Procedures. *Blood.* Neutrophils with eccentric and frequently fragmented nuclei with coarse chromatin. Normal cytoplasmic maturation. Condensation of chromatin in lymphocytes, monocytes, and even in megakaryocytes and erythroblasts. *Bone marrow.* Some anomaly demonstrable.

Therapy. None.

Prognosis. Benign condition.

BIBLIOGRAPHY. Pelger K: Demonstratie van een paar zeldzaam voorkomende typen van bloedlichaampjes en bespreking der patiënten. Ned Tijdschr Geneeskd 72:1178, 1928

Huët GJ: Over een familiare anomalie der leucocyten. Mschr Kindergeneesk 1:173–181, 1932; (abstr) Ned Tijdschr Geneeskd 75:5965–5969, 1931

Miale JB: Laboratory Medicine, Hematology. St Louis, CV Mosby, 1967

Aznar J, Vaya A: Homozygous form of Pelger–Huet leukocyte anomaly in men. Acta Haematol 66:59–62, 1981

PELIZAEUS–MERZBACHER (INFANTILE TYPE)

Synonyms. Congenital aplasia axialis extracorticalis; diffuse familial brain sclerosis; sudanophilic leukodystrophy; Spielmeyer type PMD. See Schilder's.

Symptoms. Almost exclusively in males (a few cases reported in females, see Etiology); onset in infancy. Aimless, wandering eye movements, usually not rhythmic, "eye waggers." Failure to develop normal head control, "head nodders" head and eye movements may later disappear. General lag of development; slow growth and weight gain. Further evolution: spasticity of all extremities, subnormal mental development, and frequently, optic atrophy.

Signs. Head size low-normal or microcephaly; height below third percentile. Sensory sytem usually well preserved.

Etiology. Unknown; a certain amount of confusion exists in classification of this syndrome since different criteria are used. If clinical and genetic criteria are used: only male patients (exceptionally, female in Lyon's theory) in whom the disease develops in infancy and who have a history of sex-recessive type of genetic inheritance will be included. If pathologic criteria are used, a vast heterogenous group of different clinical syndromes will be included.

Pathology. Widespread demyelinization in centrum semiovale, cerebellum, and part of brain stem; axis cylinder preserved; throughout white matter, diffuse gliosis and small amounts of perivascular sudanophilic lipid (perinuclear or in fat granules cell). The presence of "myelin islands" in demyelinated areas ("tiger" or "leopard" skin) is considered by many authors the characteristic pathologic finding, and on the basis of its presence the diagnosis of Pelizaeus–Merzbacher made; this diagnosis includes Lowenberg–Hill (dominant inheritance occurring in adult) and other syndromes with this pathologic finding (see Norman–Landing). On the basis of presence or absence of myelin islands, the clinical Pelizaeus–Merzbacher syndrome has also been subdivided in Pelizaeus–Merzbacher type (present) and Seitelberg type (absent).

Diagnostic Procedures. *Cerebrospinal fluid.* Normal. *X-ray.* Osteoporosis; kyphoscoliosis (to be interpreted as secondary and not as genetic associated defects). *Electroencephalography.*

Therapy. None.

Prognosis. In many cases, death in early childhood. Course chronic. Some patients may live to be 60 years old.

BIBLIOGRAPHY. Pelizaeus F: Über eine eigenthumliche Form spastischer Lähmung mit Cerebraler Scheinungen auf hereditärer Grundlage (Multiple Sklerose). Arch Psychiatr Nervenkr 16:698–710, 1885

Merzbacher L: Eine eigenartige familiärhereditare Erkrankungsform (Alpasia axialis extracorticalis congenita). Z Ges Neurol Psychiatr 3:1–138, 1910

Spielmeyer W: Der anatomische Befund bei einem zweiten Fall von Pelizaeus–Merzbacherscher Krankheit. Zentralbl Ges Neurol Psychiatr 32:203, 1923

Zeman W, Demyer W, Falls HF: Pelizaeus–Merzbacher disease. A study in nosology. J Neuropath Exp Neurol 23:334–354, 1964

Norman RM, Tingey AH, Harvey PW et al: Pelizaeus–Merzbacher disease: A form of sudanophil leukodystrophy. J Neurol Neurosurg Psychiatry 29:521–529, 1966

Renier WO, Gabreels FJM, Hustinx TWJ et al: Connatal Pelizaeus–Merzbacher disease with congenital stridor in two maternal cousins. Acta Neuropathol 54:11–17, 1981

PELLEGRINI–STIEDA

Synonyms. Koehler–Stieda; knee, medial collateral ligament calcification; perarticular knee calcification; Stieda–Pellegrini.

Symptom. Stiffness and pain in and above knee.

Signs. Swelling (not constant).

Etiology. Controversial.

Pathology. Periosteal proliferation or osseous metaplasia of ligament; detached fractured bone fragments from medial femoral condyle; calcified epiperiosteal or soft tissue hematoma; bursa or tendon calcification.

Diagnostic Procedure. *X-ray.*

Therapy. Conservative: physical therapy; roentgen therapy. Surgery: last resort.

Prognosis. Good; many patients recover spontaneously.

BIBLIOGRAPHY. Pellegrini A: Ossificazione traumatica del legamento collaterale tibiale dell' articolazione del ginocchio sinistro. Clin Mod Firenze 11:433–439, 1905
Justis EJ: Nontraumatic disorders. In Crenshaw AH (ed): Campbell's Operative Orthopedics. 7th ed, pp 2250–2252. St Louis, CV Mosby, 1987

PELLIZZI'S

Synonyms. Macrogenitosomia precox; pineal; pubertas precox; quadrigeminal plate. See 21 and 11β-Hydroxylase deficiency.

Symptoms and Signs. Onset in childhood. Accelerated increase in height, weight, musculature, and development of sexual characteristics; frequently associated with pineal tumor neurologic syndrome (see).

Etiology. Unknown; usually associated with destructive tumors of pineal gland. Suppression of an hypothetical pineal hormone that inhibits gonadal development or indirect stimulation of gonadotropin secretion by pressure on the hypothalamus and pituitary.

Pathology. Gliomas, teratomas, or necrotic and anaplastic pinealoma.

Diagnostic Procedures. *X-ray of skull.* Occasionally, calcification of pineal gland. *Pneumoencephalography. Hormone study.* Gonadotropin determination.

Therapy. Surgery. Radiation therapy.

Prognosis. Depends on etiology and result of surgery.

BIBLIOGRAPHY. Heubner O: Fall von Tumor der Glandula pinealis mit ergenthümlichen Washsthumanomalien. Ver Ges Dtsch Naturf Aerzte, 1898; Leipzig, 1899
Pellizzi GB: La sindrome epifisaria "macrogenitosomia precoce," Riv Ital Neuropatol (Catania) 3:193–207; 250, 1910–11
Cohen RA, Wurtman RJ, Axelrod D et al: Some clinical, biochemical, and physiological actions of the pineal gland. Ann Intern Med 61:1144–1161, 1964
Rao YTR, Medini E, Haselow RE et al: Pineal and ectopic pineal tumors: The role of radiation therapy. Cancer 48:708–713, 1981

PEL'S

Synonyms. Ciliary tabetic neuralgia; neuralgic ciliary tabetic; ophthalmic crisis. See Duchenne's.

Symptoms and Signs. One of the many possible crises occurring in tabes dorsalis: neuralgic paroxysmal pains affecting the eyes and the ophthalmic area(s).

Etiology. Syphilis (See Duchenne's).

Therapy. Specific therapy of little value.

Prognosis. That of tabes.

BIBLIOGRAPHY. Pel PK: Augenkrisen bei Tabes dorsalis (Crisen ophthalmiques). Berl Klin Wochenschr 25:25–27, 1898

PEMPHIGOID, JUVENILE

Synonym. Juvenile dermatosis herpetiformis.

Symptoms and Signs. Prevalent in males; onset usually before 5 years of age. Acute onset. Minor systemic symptoms; extensive formation of clear, tense bullae (1–2 cm) on previously normal skin of face, lower abdomen, buttocks, less frequently, extremities. Seldom, pruritus. Bullae persist for a long time. After breaking, fast healing. Hyperpigmentation and no scars result. Mucous membrane seldom involved.

Etiology. Unknown.

Pathology. Bullae of dermoepithelial junction. Epidermis intact.

Diagnostic Procedures. *Blood.* Normal, except for eosinophilia (5–10%).

Therapy. None. If disease is persistent and severe, corticosteriods and sulfapyridine.

Prognosis. Spontaneous remission usually in 3 to 4 years, occasionally only after a few weeks.

BIBLIOGRAPHY. Kim R, Winkelmann RK: Dermatitis herpetiformis in children. Relationship to bullous pemphigoid. Arch Dermatol 83:895–902, 1961

Rook A, Wilkinson DS, Ebling FJG et al: Textbook of Dermatology, 4th ed, p 1655. Oxford, Blackwell Scientific Publications, 1986

PEMPHIGUS VULGARIS

Symptoms. Both sexes affected, common in Jews; onset in middle age (between 40 and 60 years of age.). At first localized lesion in the mouth, bullae, and painful erosion of mouth; other mucosae may also be involved. Eventual appearance of skin lesion: bullae; crusting; erosion; easy bleeding; no tendency to heal; no itching. Any part of skin involved, zones of friction and face more often involved. Eventual healing; no scar; hyperpigmentation.

Etiology. Unknown; possibly familial condition, virus or autoimmune reaction(?).

Pathology. Suprabasal acantholysis, with intraepithelial splitting and bullae.

Therapy. Corticosteroids. Immunosuppressive agents: azathioprine; cyclophosphamide; methotrexate. Gold sodium thiomalate. Plasma exchange.

Prognosis. Death within 2 years if not treated; 40% mortality with treatment.

BIBLIOGRAPHY. Rook A, Wilkinson DS, Ebling FJG et al: Textbook of Dermatology. 4th ed, p 1631–1635. Oxford, Blackwell Scientific Publications, 1986

PENA-SHOKEIR II

Synonyms. Cerebro-oculo-facio-skeletal; COFS. See also Cockayne's, Hallermann-Streiff, Seckel's, and Bowen's (P.).

Symptoms. Onset from birth. Vomiting; regurgitation. Failure to thrive.

Signs. *Head.* Microcephaly; micrognathia; prominent nasal root; large ears, microphthalmia; blepharophimosis; cataract. *Extremities.* Contractures of elbow and knee; camptodactyly; single palmar crease; clenched fists; longitudinal groove on feet; rocker-bottom feet; coxa valga. *Trunk.* Kyphosis; scoliosis; widely spaced nipples. Muscle hypotonia.

Etiology. Autosomal recessive inheritance. Considered as a different degree of clinical value of the Bowen's (P.) (or Pena-Shokeir I).

Pathology. See signs. Generalized cerebral subcortical gliosis.

Diagnostic Procedures. *X-ray.* Osteoporosis; intracranial calcifications; vertical tali and displacement of second metatarsal bone. *Blood and urine.* Normal.

Therapy. Orthopedic.

Prognosis. Repeated respiratory infections cause of death, usually, within first 3 years.

BIBLIOGRAPHY. Pena SDJ, Shokeir MKH: Autosomal recessive cerebro-oculo-facio skeletal (COFS) syndrome. Clin Genet 5:285–293, 1974

Silengo MC, Davi G, Bianco R, et al: The NEU-COFS (cerebro-oculo-facio-skeletal) syndrome: Report of case: Clin Genet 25:201–204, 1984

PENDRED'S

Synonym. Familial goiter–deaf mutism.

Symptoms. Affects both sexes equally. Various degrees of bilateral deafness from birth (perceptive in type; in some cases associated with defective vestibular function); more complete loss in high, than in low tones. Goiters dating from middle childhood that may be of any degree of severity from just detectable to goitrous cretinism. Usually, normal physical and mental development.

Signs. Size of thyroid from just detectable to 200 g. In children, diffuse enlargement; in adults, more clearly nodular.

Etiology. Unknown; recessive inherited defect. The deafness and goiter are independent expressions of same gene defect.

Pathology. Not well known.

Diagnostic Procedures. *Audiography.* Sensorineural loss. *Blood and urine.* Normal except mild glucose intolerance protein-bound iodine (PBI) butanol-extractable iodine (BEI), total and free thyroxine low or normal; antithyroid antibodies absent. Low to absent T_4; accumulation and turnover of radioiodine. Perchlorate test (method described to recognize the type of thyroid defect found in this syndrome); rapid discharge of radioiodine from thyroid after administration of perchlorate or sulphocyanide (SCN). *Biopsy.* Hyperplasia; low iodine content; absent or abnormal peroxidase activity.

Therapy. No specific treatment. After partial thyroidectomy, thyroxine or thyroid extract may prevent regrowth of thyroid.

Prognosis. No treatment may correct deafness. Goiter usually recurs after partial thyroidectomy.

BIBLIOGRAPHY. Pendred V: Deaf-mutism and goiter. Lancet 2:532, 1896

Thould AK, Scowen EF: Genetic studies of the syndrome of congenital deafness and simple goiter. Ann Hum Genet 27:283–293, 1964

Milutinoy PS, Stanbury JB, Wicken JV et al: Thyroid function in a family with the Pendred syndrome. J Clin Endocrinol 28:961–969, 1969

Stanbury JB, Dumont JE: Familial goiter and related disorders. In Stanbury JB, Wyngaarden JB, Fredrickson DS: The Metabolic Basis of Inherited Disease, 5th ed, p 231. New York, McGraw-Hill, 1983

PENFIELD'S

Synonym. Autonomic diencephalic epilepsy.

Symptoms and Signs. Prevalent in males; onset at 6 or 7 years of age. Seizures accompanied by vegetative manifestations: congestion of face; sialorrhea; perspiration; tears; exophthalmos; tachycardia; polypnea; restlessness; logorrhea. The attacks are of different duration and terminate with a short period of obnubilation.

Signs. Proptosis; excessive lacrimation; pupillary abnormalities; tachycardia; blood pressure elevated.

Etiology. Hypothalamic dysfunction and epileptic stimulus from lesions located on the floor of third ventricle. Possibility of intermittent hydrocephalus.

Pathology. One case reported of third ventricle tumor.

Diagnostic Procedures. *Electroencephalography. CT scan.*

Therapy. Phenobarbital; carbamazepine; primidone. Surgery.

Prognosis. Depends on etiology.

BIBLIOGRAPHY. Penfield W: Diencephalic autonomic epilepsy. Arch Neurol Psychiatr 22:358–374, 1929

Kohler MC: L'association "comitialité, croissance excessive et puberte précoce, arriération mentale", une forme particulière de séquelles d'encéphalopathies ou d'encéphalite infantile. J Med (Lyon) 48:1437–1503, 1967

Adams RD, Victor M: Principles of Neurology, 3rd ed, pp 390–391. New York, McGraw-Hill, 1985

PEPPER'S

See Parker's.

Symptoms and Signs. Those of Parker's (see) plus those consequent to liver metastasis.

BIBLIOGRAPHY. Pepper W: A study of congenital sarcoma of the liver and suprarenal with report of a case. Am J Med Sci 121:287–299, 1901

PERHEENTUPA'S

Synonyms. Mulibrey dwarfism; pericardial constriction–growth failure; growth failure–pericardial constriction.

Symptoms. In Finns. Low birth weight. Progressive growth failure and delayed puberal development with oligomenorrhea; quiet voice. Amblyopia.

Signs. At birth, asphyxia or cyanosis. Dwarfism with thin limbs; fibrous dysplasia of tibia. *Skin.* Nevus flammeus (see). *Muscle.* Hypotonia. *Facies.* Triangular, bulging forehead; low nasal bridge; alternating esotropic-exotropic strabismus. *Fundus oculi.* Yellowish retinal spots; hypoplasia of chorion capillaries. *Neck.* Prominent veins. *Chest.* Pulmonary congestion; cardiac enlargement; evidence of pericarditis and health failure. *Abdomen.* Ascites; hepatomegaly.

Etiology. Unknown; autosomal recessive inheritance.

Pathology. See Signs. Myocardial fibrosis.

Diagnostic Procedures. *Electrocardiography.* Evidence of myocardial hypertrophy and failure. *X-ray of chest.* Pericardial calcium deposit. *Of head.* Shallow sella turcica; large cerebral ventricles and cisterns. *Electroretinography.* Normal.

Therapy. Surgery for pericardial constriction.

Prognosis. According to cardiac involvement.

BIBLIOGRAPHY. Perheentupa J, Autio S, Leirti S et al: Mulibrey nanism: dwarfism with muscle, liver, brain and eye involvement. Acta Paediatr Scand 59:74, 1970

Raitta C, Perheentupa J: Mulibrey nanism: An inherited dysmorphic syndrome with characteristic ocular findings. Acta Ophthalmol (Suppl 123) 52:162–171, 1974

Perheentupa J: Mulibrey nanism. In Erikson AW, Forsius HR, Nevanlinna HR et al: Population Structure and Genetic Disorders, pp 641–646. New York, Academic Press, 1980

PERHEENTUPA–VISAKORPI

Synonyms. Protein intolerance defective transport of basic amino acids. Dibasic aminoaciduria II.

Symptoms and Signs. Prevalent in Finns. From birth feeding difficulties, vomiting, diarrhea, lethargy, convulsions, hyperammonemic coma. Mental retardation, hepatosplenomegaly, short stature, osteoporosis, lens opacities. Skin hyperelastic, joint hyperextensible, hair brittle.

Etiology. Autosomal recessive. Defect of intestinal and renal transport of dibasic amino acids.

Pathology. Liver biopsy: minimal fatty degeneration.

Diagnostic Procedures. *Blood.* Hyperammonemia, transaminase elevation; low dibasic amino acid levels, glutamine and alanine increased. *Urine.* Excretion of dibasic amino acids increased. Diagnosis is based on dibasic aminoaciduria without cystinuria.

Therapy. Low protein diet.

Prognosis. Reduced life expectancy.

BIBLIOGRAPHY. Perheentupa J, Visakorpi JK: Protein intolerance with deficient transport of basic amino acids. Lancet 2:813–816, 1965
Carpenter TO, Levy HL, Holtrop ME et al: Lysinuric protein intolerance presenting as childhood osteoporosis: Clinical and skeletal response to citrulline therapy. N Engl J Med 312:290–294, 1985

PERICENTRIC

Symptoms and Signs. Microcephaly; hypertelorism; broad nasal bridge; epicanthic folds; divergent squint; arched palate; hyperextensibility of elbows. Dermatoglyphics normal, but left hand shows single transverse crease and right hand three palmar creases radiating from radial border.

Etiology. Unknown.

Pathology. See Signs.

Diagnostic Procedures. *Chromosome study.* Leukocyte chromosomes show a pericentric inversion of a chromosome of C group (absence of such feature in parents of probands).

BIBLIOGRAPHY. Pitt DB, Wiener S, Sutherland G, et al: The pericentric syndrome. Lancet 2:568, 1967
Pergament E: The pericentric syndrome. Lancet 2:777, 1967

PERINEAL

Symptoms and Signs. Periodic intense perineal itching localized on raphe, accompanied by local sweating; usually worse after prolonged driving, sitting, or fatigue.

Etiology. Unknown; no clear organic basis.

Therapy. Sedatives. Topical corticosteroids.

Prognosis. Period of remission or relapse not always correlated with treatment or alleged pathogenetic factors.

BIBLIOGRAPHY. Rook A, Wilkinson DS, Ebling FJG et al: Textbook of Dermatology. 4th ed, p 2178. Oxford, Blackwell Scientific Publications, 1986

PERIODIC ARTHRALGIA

Synonym. Bone pain, periodic.

Symptoms and Signs. Episodic pain located in the shafts of the long bones. It is reminiscent of the pain of sickle cell anemia.

Etiology. Unknown. No instance of male-to-male transmission has been noted; 33 persons in 7 generations were considered affected.

Diagnostic Procedures. *X-ray.* For ruling out other diseases.

Therapy. Symptomatic.

Prognosis. Good.

BIBLIOGRAPHY. Reimann HA, Angelides AP: Periodic arthralgia in 23 members of five generations of a family. JAMA 146:713–716, 1951
McKusick V: Mendelian Inheritance in Man. Baltimore, Johns Hopkins University Press, 1986

PERIODIC PARALYSIS, NORMOKALEMIC (TYPE A)

Synonym. Pleoconial myopathy.

Symptoms. Onset in early infancy. Stable symmetric proximal weakness (floppy babies); episodes of quadriparesis lasting 2 to 3 weeks. Trunk ataxia and tremor may be present. Characteristic craving for salt, intense thirst, and stomach pains at onset of attacks, which begin usually in the morning after awaking.

Signs. Muscle hypotonia; no fasciculation or fibrillation; no sensory disturbances; tendon reflexes hypoactive; good coordination taking into consideration degree of hypotonia.

Etiology. Unknown; inherited as heterozygous trait; autonomy of the condition challenged.

Pathology. Muscle biopsy shows two types of fibers: one staining lighter with hematoxylin and eosin (normal); one staining darker, containing small vacuoles that do not stain and are diffuse in the intermyofibrillar areas. Granular material is also contained in the same areas in a lesser number of dark fibers. Cytochemistry shows increased and enlarged mitochondria in 20% to 40% of muscle cells. Fatty infiltrates in muscle cells.

Diagnostic Procedures. *Blood and urine.* Normal. *Electromyography.* Myopathic pattern. *Biopsy of muscle.* See Pathology.

Therapy. Sodium chloride, potassium salts do not improve or precipitate attacks.

Prognosis. Improvement between attacks as years pass.

BIBLIOGRAPHY. Poskanzer DC, Kerr DNS: A third type of periodic paralysis with normokalemia and favorable response to sodium chloride. Am J Med 31:328–342, 1961

Shy GM, Gonatas NK, Perez MC: Two childhood myopathies with abnormal mitochondria. I. Megaconial myopathy. II. Pleoconial myopathy. Brain 89:133–158, 1966

Spiro AJ, Prineas JW, Moore CL: A new mitochondrial myopathy in a patient with salt craving. Arch Neurol 22:259–269, 1970

PERIODIC SIALADENOSIS

Synonyms. Recurring salivary adenitis; periodic sialorrhea. Sialoadenitis chronica.

Symptoms. Sudden, recurrent episodes of discomfort on parotid, submaxillary, or submandibular glands; saliva formation increased or decreased. Cephalalgia; vomiting; diarrhea; occassionally, pain in the abdomen, thorax or extremities.

Signs. Swelling of involved glands. In some cases, dermographia, urticaria.

Etiology. Unknown; neurovascular (?); allergic (?); infective (?).

Pathology. Salivary gland edema; after repeated episodes, possibly, signs of chronic inflammation and aspecific eosinophil and monocyte infiltration.

Diagnostic Procedures. *Blood.* Leukocytes normal. Sedimentation rate normal. *Sialography.* Normal.

Therapy. None.

Prognosis. Episode may last hours or days. Recurrence typical.

BIBLIOGRAPHY. Isacsson G, Ahlner B, Lundquist PG: Chronic sialoadenitis of the submandibular gland. A retrospective study of 108 cases. Arch Otorhinolaryngol 232:91–100, 1981

Schultz PW, Woods JE: Subtotal parotidectomy in the treatment of chronic sialadenitis. Ann Plast Surg 11:459–461, 1983

Rice DH: Advances in diagnosis and management of salivary gland disease. West J Med 140:238–249, 1984

PERKOFF'S

Synonyms. Poststeroid myopathy; Cushing's–therapeutic myopathy; Slocumb's; steroid myopathy; steroid pseudorheumatism. See Mueller–Kugelberg.

Symptoms and Signs. Both sexes affected; onset at all ages. Following prolonged administration of corticosteroids, muscle weakness, mostly of the thighs; moderate muscle atrophy; mild tendon hyporeflexia. Association with other feature of Cushing's syndrome (see). Weakness is relieved by short periods of sleep.

Etiology. Corticosteroid administration.

Pathology. Moderate muscle fiber vacuolization.

Diagnostic Procedures. *Urine.* Excretion of large amount of creatine (200–1000 mg/day), reduced creatinine (1 g/day). *Blood.* See Cushing's.

Therapy. Cessation of corticosteroid administration.

Prognosis. Prompt restoration of muscle power after discontinuation of steroids.

BIBLIOGRAPHY. Perkoff GT, Silber R, Tyler FH et al: Myopathy due to the administration of therapeutic amounts of 17-hydroxycorticosteroids. Am J Med 26:981–988, 1959

Slocumb CH: Rheumatoid arthritis. In Brown J, Pearson GM (eds): Clinical Use of Adrenal Steroids, pp 30–43. New York, McGraw-Hill, 1962

Adams RD, Victor M: Principles of Neurology, 3rd ed, pp 1060–1061. New York, McGraw-Hill, 1985

PERNIO

Synonyms. Acute chilblain; dermatitis hiemalis; erythema pernis; erythrocyanosis; lupus pernio. See Immersion foot.

Symptoms and Signs. *Acute chilblain.* More frequent in children and women. Usually bilateral and symmetric lesions. Dermatitis, bluish red; slight edema. Itching and burning worsened by warm temperature, affecting fingers, toes, and legs (parts exposed to cold). Acute stage lasting usually 1 week; brownish pigmentation may appear and persist for months after lesion heals. Occasionally, hemorrhagic reaction, ulceration, and infection may appear as complications. *Chronic childblain.* Repeated acute episodes result in chronic lesions with residual fibrosis and atrophy of skin and subcutaneous tissues. During warm season, lesions may disappear completely.

Etiology. Reaction of peripheral blood vessels to cold (slow-freeze variety).

Pathology. Angiitis; necrosis of panniculus adiposus; chronic inflammatory reaction of subcutaneous tissues. In long-standing lesions, hyperpigmentation and iron deposits.

Therapy. Avoidance of exposure to cold. In chronic severe form, production of fever may clear the lesions quickly. Priscoline hydrochloride (intramuscularly or intravenously) may help. Ultraviolet radiation weekly (three doses) at onset of winter. Antipruritic local application. In severe form not responding to conservative treatment, sympathectomy.

Pathology. *Acute.* Benign, self-limited. *Chronic.* Avoiding exposure to cold prevents recurrences.

BIBLIOGRAPHY. Miller W: De Pernionibus. Jence, 1680
Rook A, Wilkinson DS, Ebling FJG et al: Textbook of Dermatology, 4th ed, p 625. Oxford, Blackwell Scientific Publications, 1986

PERONEAL COMPARTMENT

Synonyms. Peroneal muscles ischemic necrosis; March gangrene. Shin Splint.

Symptoms. Follows continuous and prolonged exertion; rapid onset. Leg tired and aching; then swelling and severe pain. Elevation and heat treatment do not relieve the pain.

Signs. Loss of dorsiflexion and inversion; any motion produces pain. Firm consistency of anterolateral portion of leg. Pulses of dorsalis pedis and posterior tibial arteries not palpable.

Etiology. Severe exertion determining diminished blood flow to muscles.

Pathology. Muscle ischemic necrosis of various degrees from massive necrosis to spotty muscle necrosis; no evidence of thrombosis of vessels.

Diagnostic Procedures. *X-ray of leg* (to rule out bone trauma).

Therapy. Extensive fasciotomy.

Prognosis. Fasciotomy helpful up to 6 to 9 days after onset. If condition allowed to progress, both anterior tibial (because of secondary compression) and peroneal compartments become impaired, and inversion and clubfoot result.

BIBLIOGRAPHY. Blandy JP, Fuller R: March gangrene: Ischemic myositis of the leg muscles from exercise. J Bone Joint Surg 39 B:679, 1957
Reszel PA, Janes JM, Spittell JA Jr: Ischemic necrosis of the peroneal musculature: A lateral compartment syndrome; report of a case. Proc Staff Meet Mayo Clinic 38:130–136, 1963
Lunceford EM Jr: The peroneal compartment syndrome. South Med J 58:621–623, 1965
Slocum DB: The shin splint syndrome. Am J Surg 114:875–881, 1967
Justis EJ Jr: Traumatic disorders. In Crenshaw AH (ed): Campbell's Operative Orthopedics. 7th ed, p 2224. St Louis, CV Mosby, 1987

PERRAULT'S

Synonym. Ovarian dysgenesis–deafness.

Symptoms and Signs. In females. Bilateral neural-sensory deafness and symptoms of Turner's (see). In males (of same family) facultative deafness and normal sexual development.

Etiology. XX dysgenesis; demonstrated a 46 XX karyotype.

BIBLIOGRAPHY. Perrault M, Klotz B, Houset E: Deux cas de syndrome de Turner avec surdi-mutism dans une meme fratrie. Bull Neur Soc Med Hosp (Paris) 16:79–84, 1951
McCarthy DJ, Opitz JM: Perrault's syndrome in sisters. Am J Med Genet 22:629–631, 1985

PETER'S

See also Ruthenfurd's, Gorlin–Chaudhry–Mass, Rieger's, and Fraser's.

Symptoms and Signs. Visual impairment due to incomplete separation of lens vesicle, central corneal opacity, synechiae residues of pupillary membrane.

Etiology. Possibly, autosomal recessive inheritance. Defect of corneogenic mesoderm.

Therapy. Corneal transplant.

BIBLIOGRAPHY. Peters A: Ueber angeborene Defekbildung der descemetschen Membran. Klin Monatsbl Augenhkeilkd 44:27–40, 1906

PETGES–CLÉJAT

Synonyms. Poikiloderma atrophicans vasculare; poikilodermatomyositis; Petges–Jacobi; Jacobi's. Poikiloderma–mycosis fungoides stage I A (see Etiology). To be considered obsolete.

Symptoms. Usually occur in young adults. Muscular weakness.

Signs. Areas of skin with pigmented poikiloderma; telangiectasis, atrophy, and calcinosis may also be observed. Muscular wasting.

Etiology. Once excluded lupus erythematodes, dermatomyositis, and drug eruption this condition is better termed poikilodermatous mycosis fungoides (MF T_1, or stage I A). Practically the poikiloderma atrophicans vasculare includes MF-associated poikiloderma and forms of poikiloderma non-MF associated.

BIBLIOGRAPHY. Petges G, Cléjat C: Sclérose atrophique de la peau et myosite généralisée. Arch Dermatol Syph 7:550–568, 1906

Guy W, Grauer RC, Jacob FM: Poikilodermatomyositis. Arch Dermatol Syph 40:867–878, 1939

Rook A, Wilkinson DS, Ebling FJG et al: Textbook of Dermatology, 4th ed, p 1747. Oxford, Blackwell Scientific Publications, 1986

PETIT MAL

Synonyms. Lennox's triad; minor epilepsy; pyknoepilepsy.

Symptoms. Condition starts in childhood; often so mild that no attention is paid to it. Loss of consciousness with or without minimal muscle spasms; loss of contact with environment; usually after a few seconds the patient resumes his activity. No sequelae.

Signs. Eyes look ahead without seeing; small spastic contractions of eyelids, face, or arm occasionally present. Lennox's triad: *petit mal;* akinetic seizures; myoclonic jerks.

Etiology. Unknown; it is felt that this syndrome may represent an hereditary and probably a metabolically determined form of epilepsy.

Diagnostic Procedure. *Electroencephalography.*

Therapy. Trimethadione; paramethadione; phensuximide; ethosuximide.

Prognosis. This type of attack tends to decrease or disappear with age; it may be followed in older age by the development of the *grand mal* syndrome.

BIBLIOGRAPHY. See Epileptic syndromes.

Matthes A, Weber H: Klinische und electroenzephalographische Familienunter-suchungen bei Pyknolepsien. Dsch Med Wochenschr 93:429–435, 1968

Adams RD, Victor M: Principles of Neurology, 3rd ed, p 235. New York, McGraw-Hill, 1985

PETIT'S

Eponym used to indicate mydriasis, increased intraocular pressure, and alterations of retina vessels due to an irritation of sympathetic nervous system. See Bernard's and Horner's.

BIBLIOGRAPHY. Petit F: Mémoire dans laquel il est Démontré que les Nerfs Intercosteaux Fournissent des Rameaux qui Portens des esprits dans les Yeux, Hist Acad Sci Paris: 1–18, 1727

PETZETAKIS'

Synonyms. Cat scratch; Debré's; Foshay–Mollaret cat-scratch fever; regional nonbacterial lymphadenitis; benign inoculation lymphoreticulosis.

Symptoms. In temperate climate most cases occur in fall and winter. More frequent in children and young adults, in patients who have been scratched or bitten by cats or exposed to penetrating wounds (thorn, splinters, hooks) 7 to 14 days, or as long as 2 months, before symptoms appear. Slight fever; headache; chills; backache; anorexia; abdominal pain. Alteration of mental status and convulsions, with favorable final prognosis.

Signs. Small area of ulceration surrounded by erythema; vesicles; pustules; regional lymph nodes greatly enlarged, tender with red, hot skin, later (25%) becoming fluctuant; absence of lymphangitis. Spleen occasionally palpable.

Etiology. Unknown; possibly a virus of Chlamydial group or mycobacteria transmitted by carrier cat or wounding objects. The most common offender is *Pasteurella multocida.*

Pathology. Lymph node, reticuloendothelial hyperplasia, necrotic centers; irregular microabscesses surrounded by reticular endothelial cells, fibroblasts, macrophages; evolving colliquation.

Diagnostic Procedures. *Hanger–Rose skin test.* Positive. *Rice–Hyde test* (incubation of white blood cells with cat-scratch disease skin test antigen). Positive. *Blood.* Slight elevation of sedimentation rate. Slight elevation of eosinophils. Complement fixation test with antigen of psittacosis; lymphogranuloma venereum-trachoma group positive in 26% adult patients; lower positivity in children. Low complement fixation antibody titer against lygranum (50%).

Therapy. Aspiration of pus; no incision if liquefaction of lymph node. Penicillin. Tetramicin or cefuroxime in the penicillin-allergic patient.

Prognosis. Fever lasts 2 to 3 weeks, lymphadenopathy sometimes several months. If sinus complication, encephalitis of variable severity that passes without sequelae.

BIBLIOGRAPHY. Petzetakis M: Monoadénite subaigüe multiple de nature inconnue. Soc Med Athens 16:229, 1935

Debré R et al: La maladie des griffes de chat. Bull Med Soc Hôp Paris 66:760–769, 1950

Carithers HA: Cat-scratch disease: An overview based on a study of 1200 patients. Am J Dis Child 139:1124–1133, 1985

Gerber MA, McSlister TJ, Ballow M: The aetiological agent of cat-scratch disease. Lancet 1:1236–1239, 1985

Magnussen CR: Animal bites. In Reese RE, Gordon DR (eds): A Practical Approach to Infectious Disease. Boston, Little, Brown & Co, 1986

Lewis DW, Tucker SH: Central nervous system involvement in cat-scratch disease. Pediatrics 77:714–721, 1986

PETZETAKIS–TAKOS

Synonyms. Phlyctenular keratoconjunctivitis; trophopenic keratitis.

Symptoms and Signs. Superficial keratitis (presence of multiple phlyctenules on cornea); palpebral edema; cornea hyperesthesia; photophobia; blepharospasm; decreased iridic reflexes; xerophthalmia; impaired vision; lymph node hypertrophy.

Etiology. Malnutrition; lack of hygiene.

Pathology. Break in corneal epithelium; scars; hypertrophy of preauricular lymph nodes.

Therapy. Diet; antibiotics. Hygienic measures.

Prognosis. Fair with adequate treatment.

BIBLIOGRAPHY. Petzetakis M: Le troubles oculaires pendant la trophopénie (maladie aedémateuse) et l'épidémie de la pellagre. (1941–1944). La keratopathie superficielle trophopenique (Kératopathie épithéliale). Presse Med 58:1082–1084, 1950

PEUTZ–JEGHERS

Synonyms. Cutaneous pigmentation–intestinal polyposis; Hutchinson–Weber–Peutz; Jeghers'; lentigiopolypose–digestive; melanoplakia–intestinal polyposis; Peutz–Touraine; intestinal polyposis II.

Symptoms. Both sexes, all ethnic groups affected; symptoms begin in adolescence. Recurrent severe abdominal pain, relieved by vigorous abdominal manipulation; unusual borborygmus; later, occasionally, massive intestinal hemorrhage.

Signs. From birth "black freckles": melanotic pigmentation 2 to 5 mm in diameter sometimes coalescing on the lips, oral mucosa, cheek, nose, fingers, palms, toes, forearm, or abdominal area. Mucosa pigmentation permanent; cutaneous lesion may appear and fade at puberty or afterward.

Etiology. Congenital autosomal dominant condition.

Pathology. Multiple adenomatous polyps growing in crops in ileum, jejunum, and less frequently, stomach and colon.

Diagnostic Procedures. *X-ray of intestine.* Multiple polyps. *Blood.* Anemia. *Stool.* Occult blood.

Therapy. Gastrointestinal tract roentgenograms every 2 years from puberty to full maturity. Uncomplicated polyps removed by excision; if intussusception with necrosis, extensive resection.

Prognosis. If all polyps removed when full adult life reached, no additional polyps develop. If not removed, they may grow and complications arise (hemorrhage; intussusception). Possibly, malignant transformation of gastric and duodenal polyps at early age.

BIBLIOGRAPHY. Hutchinson J: Pigmentation of the lips and mouth. Arch Surg London 7:290, 1896
Peutz JLA: Over een zeer merkwaardige, gecombineerde familiairie polyposis van de slimjmvliezen van den tractus intestinalis met die van de neuskeelholte en gepaard met eigenaardige pigemntaties van huiden slijmvliezen. Ned Maandschr Geneesk 10:134–146, 1921
Jeghers H, McKusick VA, Katz KH: Generalized intestinal polyposis and melanin spots of the oral mucosa, lips and digits: Syndrome of clinical significance. New Engl J Med 241:993–1005; 1031–1036, 1949
Bundick D, Prior JT: Peutz–Jeghers syndrome: A clinicopathologic study of a large family with 27-year follow-up. Cancer 50:2139–2146, 1982
Tweedic JH, Mc Cann BJ: Peutz–Jeghers syndrome and metastasizing colonic adenocarcinoma. Gut 25:1118–1123, 1984

PEYRONIE'S

Synonyms. Buren's; corpora cavernosa plastic induration; penile fibrosis; induratio penis plastica; penis plastic induration; van Buren's.

Symptoms. Onset in middle-aged or elderly males. Pain and curvature of penis; ability to achieve erection distal to process; interference with coitus.

Signs. Palpation of irregular lump along dorsum of penis.

Etiology. Unknown; frequent association with Dupuytren's contracture (see). Induced by adrenergic blockers (propanolol, practolol). Possibility of familial transmission (autosomal dominant male limited).

Pathology. Pearly gray fibrous area in cavernous sheaths extending linearly or in separate bodies; flat plaques. Microscopically, keloidlike lesion, absence of inflammatory changes, occasionally calcified lesions.

Diagnostic Procedures. *Serology.* Rule out syphilis. *Biopsy.* Rule out malignancy.

Therapy. Reassurance about benign nature of process. Alpha-tocopherol has been used with some benefit. X-rays, diathermy, massage, electrolysis occasionally helpful.

Prognosis. Chronic condition; poor response to all types of therapeutic approach. Surgical removal of lesion followed by recurrences.

BIBLIOGRAPHY. de la Peyronie F: Sur quelques obstacles qui s'opposent à l'éjaculation naturelle de la semence. Mem Acad Chir Paris 1:425, 1743

Kristensen BO: Labetalol-induced Peyronie disease? A case report. Acta Med Scand 206:510–512, 1979

Bias WB, Nybery LM Jr, Hochberg MC et al: Peyronie disease: A newly recognized autosomal dominant trait. Am J Genet 12:227–235, 1982

PFEIFFER'S (E.)

Synonyms. Acute epidemic infective adenitis; glandular fever; Drüsenfieber. See Infectious mononucleosis. Infectious mononucleosislike syndrome.

Symptoms. Both sexes affected; onset usually in childhood. Slightly contagious.

Signs. Mild throat inflammation; adenopathy limited to cervical nodes; absence of splenomegaly (except in prolonged cases).

Etiology. Unknown. Several viruses and toxoplasma have been reported. Condition separated from infectious monocytosis (mononucleosis) on clinical and epidemiologic grounds by Hoagland, particularly cytomegalovirus.

Therapy. General supportive measures; for serious infections caused by *Toxoplasma,* sulfadiazine with pyrimethamine.

Prognosis. Much shorter duration than infectious monocytosis.

BIBLIOGRAPHY. Pfeiffer E: Drüsenfieber. Jahrb Kinderheilkd 29:257–264, 1889

Hoagland RJ: Infectious mononucleosis. NY, Grune & Stratton, 1967

Magnussen CR, Chessin LN: Infectious mononucleosis and mononucleosislike syndromes. In Reese RE, Gordon DR (eds): A Practical Approach to Infectious Diseases, p 463. Boston, Little, Brown & Co, 1986

PFEIFFER–PALM–TELLER

Synonym. PPT.

Symptoms and Signs. Brother and sister. Unique amimic facies, ears cup shaped, narrow palpebral fissure with epicanthal folds, enamel hypoplasia, short stature, progressive joint stiffness; congenital aortic stenosis.

Etiology. Unknown. Possibly autosomal recessive inheritance.

BIBLIOGRAPHY. Pfeiffer RA, Palm D, Teller W: A syndrome of short stature, amimic facies, enamel hypoplasia, slowly progressing stiffness of joint and high-pitched voice in two siblings. J Pediatr 91:955–957, 1977

PFEIFFER'S (R.A.)

Synonyms. Acrocephalosyndactyly V; ACS V; See Noack's.

Symptoms and Signs. Present from birth. *Head.* Brachycephaly; high forehead; hypertelorism; antimongoloid palpebrae; small nose; narow maxilla; gothic palate. *Hands and feet.* Syndactyly (second and third digits); broach thumbs (pointing outward); broad short great toes. Normal intelligence. Occasionally, elbow synostosis; choanal atresia.

Etiology. Autosomal dominant inheritance.

Pathology. Craniosynostosis; phalangeal malformations and fusion with adjacent bones.

Therapy. None usually required or according to degree of craniosynostosis.

Prognosis. With age facies tends to improve. Normal mental development.

BIBLIOGRAPHY. Pfeiffer RA: Dominante erbliche Akrocephalosyndactylie. Z Kinderheilkd 90:301–320, 1964

Martsolf JT, Cracco JB, Carpenter GG et al: Pfeiffer syndrome. An unusual type of acrocephalosyndactyly with broad thumbs and great toes. Am J Dis Child 121:257–262, 1971

Naveh Y, Freidman A: Pfeiffer's syndrome. Report of a family and review of literature. J Med Genet 13:272–280, 1976

PHANTOM LIMB

Signs. Amputee. Occur following amputations: 20% of patients no phantom; 67% phantom phenomena; 13% painful phantom. Eighty-five percent of the last groups combined present the syndrome immediately, 7% in less than a month, and remainder within 1 year. "Natural" phantom or phantom phenomena: sensation that amputated part is still present, aligned with the stump and moving with it. Painful phantom limb: phantom pains felt in missing limb from vague unpleasant feeling to crushing pain. Patient may feel missing finger and toes curled up and that they cannot be unclenched.

Etiology. Organic: neuroma of cut nerve or other irritative mechanism in the stump. Psychogenic.

Pathology. Scar of stump; neuroma.

Diagnostic Procedures. *X-ray of stump and spine and joints involved indirectly by amputations.*

Therapy. Intrathecal fentanyl. Excision (not satisfactory because neuroma reforms). Infiltration of the area of stump (under light anesthesia) with hydrocortisone; elastic stump sock to be worn day and night; postural correction for muscular imbalance. Reamputation to improve vascularity and mobility. Psychotherapy with sedatives or tranquilizers; electroconvulsive therapy. Cordotomy; tractotomy; ablation of postcentral cortex.

Prognosis. "Natural" phantom tingling sensation becomes weaker and usually disappears within 2 or 3 years, sometimes persisting longer. Best results in painful phantom limb when treatment started early and when local causes of irritation promptly found and removed. Central pain much more difficult to treat.

BIBLIOGRAPHY. Paré A: La manière de traicter les playes faictes tat par hacquebutes que par flèche: et les accidentz d'icelles, côme fractures et caries d'os, gangrene et mortification; avec les pourtraictz des instrumentz necessaires pour leur curation. Et la méthode de curer les combustions principalement faictes par la pouldre à canon, 2nd ed. Paris, Ieau de Brie, on Arnoul l'Angelier, 1552
Mitchell SW: Phantom limbs. Lippincott's Mag 8:563–569, 1871
Gillis L: The management of the painful amputation stump, and a new theory for the phantom phenomena. Br J Surg 51:87–95, 1964
Jacobson L, Chabal C, Brody MC: Relief of persistent postamputation stump and phantom limb pain with intrathecal fentanyl. Pain 37:317–322, 1989

PHEOCHROMOCYTOMA

Synonyms. Chromaffinoma; paroxysmal hypertension; medullary paraganglioma. See also Multiple endocrine neoplasia III, Wermer's, and Sipple's.

Symptoms. Equal incidence in both sexes; onset from childhood to old age (highest incidence between third and fourth decades). Headache, frequently paroxysmal and associated with palpitations and sweating. Postural hypotension or tachycardia. Psychic changes.

Signs. Paroxysmal hypertension; weight loss; possibly, neurocutaneous lesions.

Etiology. Autosomal dominant inheritance.

Pathology. Tumor arising from chromaffin cells of paraganglia from the neck through posterior mediastinum, along the aorta to the pelvis. In 19% of cases, multiple; adrenal most frequent site; in 10% of cases, malignant.

Diagnostic Procedures. *Urine and plasma.* Catecholamines and metabolites increased. *Provocative tests.* Tyramine, glucagon, histamine, or phentolamine (depressor test). *Intravenous pyelography, angiography, iodoscan, venography, vena cava catheterization, and venous sampling. CT scan.* Localization of tumor.

Therapy. Surgery preceded by and integrated with medical control. Medical therapy: (for inoperable cases only) alpha- and beta-adrenergic blocking agents. Alpha-methylparatyrosine.

Prognosis. Good with surgery. Fair with medical treatment.

BIBLIOGRAPHY. Masson P, Martin J: Paraganglioma surrenal, étude d'un cas humain de tumeurs malignes de la medullo-surrenale. Bull Assoc Fr Cancer 12:135–141, 1923
Mayo C: Paroxysmal hypertension with tumour of retroperitoneal nerve: Report of a case. JAMA 89:1047–1050, 1927
Bravo EL, Gifford RW Jr: Pheochromocytoma: Diagnosis, localization and management. N Engl J Med 311:1298–1303, 1984

PHLEBECTASIA OF JEJUNUM, ORAL CAVITY, AND SCROTUM

Symptoms. Peptic ulcer symptoms and occasionally symptoms of gastrointestinal bleeding.

Signs. Caviar spot of the tongue; angiokeratoma (spot) of Fordyce of the scrotum; melena.

Etiology. Unknown.

Pathology. *Stomach.* Chronic gastritis; pyloric hypertrophy; duodenal ulcer. *Jejunum.* Thin-walled vessels within submucosa and in the serosa. In some cases, cecum also mildly involved. Phlebectasis of tongue and scrotum.

Diagnostic Procedures. *X-ray of gastrointestinal tract. Stool, gastric analysis.* Search for occult blood.

Therapy. Treatment of ulcer; if blood loss; exploratory laparotomy and measures to correct bleeding.

Prognosis. Depends on extent of intestinal tract lesions and bleeding.

BIBLIOGRAPHY. Rappaport I, Schiffman MA: Multiple phlebectasia involving jejunum, oral cavity, and scrotum. JAMA 185:437–440, 1963
Miller DA, Akers WA: Multiple phlebectasia of the jejunum, oral cavity, and scrotum. Arch Intern Med 121:180–182, 1968

PHLEBODYNIA

Synonym. Vein pain.

Symptoms. Prevalent in adult females; occurs in epidemic form in community. Severe pain along superficial and deep veins and legs. Mild constitutional symptoms: malaise, headache, and minimal fever.

Signs. Tenderness over affected extremities; no redness or that over course of vein; sensation of turgor of the vein along its course (thickened wall or thrombus?). Homans' sign; moderate swelling on one leg or both.

Etiology. Unknown; the possibility of mass hysteria considered.

Pathology. Biopsy of vein shows no gross abnormality. Absence of thrombus; possibly, moderate edema of wall.

Diagnostic Procedures. All negative.

Therapy. No response to conventional method of phlebitis treatment.

Prognosis. Prolonged course; tendency to recur.

BIBLIOGRAPHY. Pearson JS: "Phlebodynia" a new epidemic (?) disease. Circulation 7:370–372, 1953
Brosius GR, Calvert MD, Chin TDY: Epidemic phlebodynia. Arch Intern Med 108:442–447, 1961

PHLEGMASIA ALBA DOLENS

Synonyms. Femoral thrombophlebitis; milk leg; postpartum thrombophlebitis.

Symptoms. Postpartum, postsurgical complication. Legs painful.

Signs. Pale, edematous, cool extremity.

Etiology. Thrombosis of deep veins of legs; extension of thrombosis into uterine veins accompanied by arterial spasm and diminished pulse.

Diagnostic Procedures. *Phlebography; Ultrasound; Plethysmography; Fluximetry; Radioactive fibrinogen; Venous pressure measurement. Blood.* Coagulation studies. Fibrin products identification.

Pathology. New and preexisting thrombosis of veins, inflammation of vein walls.

Therapy. Antibiotic; heparin intravenous injection.

Prognosis. Fair with treatment. Possibly, not frequently, pulmonary embolism.

BIBLIOGRAPHY. Barnes RW: Current status of noninvasive tests in the diagnosis of venous disease. Surg Clin North Am 62:489–500, June, 1982

Schaub RG, Simmonds CA, Koets MM et al: Early events in the formation of the venous thrombus following local trauma and stasis. Lab Invest 51:218–221, 1984

PHLEGMASIA CERULEA DOLENS

Synonyms. Blue of Gregoire; Gregoire's blue; ileofemoral thrombophlebitis; venous phlebitis–gangrene; thrombophlebitis cerulea dolens.

Symptoms. Usually, sudden pain in all toes; occasionally, gradual following recurrent episodes of vein thrombosis; always severe. In some cases progression from phlegmasia alba dolens to cerulea form.

Signs. Clear line of demarcation between involved area and viable tissue; swelling and cyanosis; increase in temperature of discolored parts. Peripheral pulses always palpable, stronger and fuller than unaffected side in early stage till obliterated by progressive edema. In some cases sheathlike appearance involving all sole of foot.

Etiology. Syndrome observed frequently in association with malignancy, or it may be idiopathic. Cessation of blood flow through capillary bed determined by venous thrombosis and edema.

Pathology. Venous thrombosis; edema; gangrene; patency of arterial system.

Diagnostic Procedures. *Blood.* Anemia, high blood urea nitrogen (BUN). Arteriovenous pressure gradient decreased. *Phlebography; Ultrasound; Plethysmography; Fluximetry; Radioactive fibrinogen venous pressure measurements. Blood.* Coagulation studies. Fibrin products identification.

Therapy. Antibiotics. Continuous intravenous heparin. After demarcation of gangrenous tissue, amputation.

Prognosis. Final loss of tissue less than anticipated. High mortality and morbidity associated with this syndrome.

BIBLIOGRAPHY. Hueter C: Fall von Gangrän in Folge von Venenobliteration. Virchows Arch [Pathol Anat] 17:482–488, 1859
Loewenthal J, May J: Phelgmasia caerulea dolens. Br J Surg 52:584–587, 1965
Bertelsen S, Anker W: Phelgmasia caerulea dolens: Pathophysiology, clinical features, treatment and prognosis. Acta Chir Scand 134:107–112, 1968
Hurst JW: The Heart, Arteries and Veins, 3rd ed, p 1626. New York, McGraw-Hill, 1976
Sandler DA, Martin JF, Duncan SS et al: Diagnosis of deep-vein thrombosis: Comparison of clinical evaluation, ultrasound, plethysmography and venoscan with X-ray venogram. Lancet 2:716–719, 1984

PHOBIC

Symptoms and Signs. Onset at all ages; both sexes affected (women more than men). Exaggerated and pathologic dread of some precise situation, object, or stimulus, promoting complex maneuvers to avoid it. For example:

Acrophobia. Dread of high places.

Agoraphobia. Dread of open places.

Hydrophobia. Dread of water.

Xenophobia. Dread of strangers.

Etiology. Usually, resulting from negative experiences during learning stage, or inculcated by parents or teachers. Psychoanalytic role in emphasizing some phobic forms (of higher symbolic value).

Therapy. Psychotherapy.

Prognosis. For phobic reaction in children, good prognosis; in adults, it is more resistant to treatment and seldom spontaneously regresses.

BIBLIOGRAPHY. Westphal (1871).
Freedman AM, Kaplan HI, Sadock BJ: Comprehensive Textbook of Psychiatry, 2nd ed, p 790. Baltimore, Williams & Wilkins, 1975

PHOSPHORUS DEPLETION

Symptoms and Signs. Occur in patients receiving prolonged treatment with nonabsorbable antacids, such as magnesium-aluminum hydroxides, in peptic ulcer therapy, prophylaxis of kidney stones, and others. Weakness, anorexia, and malaise. In severe form, bone pain and joint stiffness; occasionally, intentional tremor.

Etiology. Depletion of phosphorus following the prolonged administration of antacids.

Pathology. Osteomalacia.

Diagnostic Procedures. *Urine.* Hypophosphaturia; hypercalciuria. *Blood.* Hypophosphatemia. Increased calcium gastrointestinal absorption. *X-ray.* Osteomalacia.

Therapy. Adequate dietary phosphorus.

Prognosis. Excellent once adequate amount of phosphorus is given. Severe phosphorus depletion, induced in animals, brings debilitation followed by death.

BIBLIOGRAPHY. Bloom WB, Flinchum D: Osteomalacia with pseudofractures caused by ingestion of aluminum hydroxide. JAMA 174:1327–1330, 1960
Lotz M, Zisman E, Bartter FC: Evidence for a phosphorus-depletion syndrome in man. N Engl J Med 278:409–415, 1968
Knochel JP: The clinical status of hypophosphatemia: An update. N Engl J Med 313:447–449, 1985

PHOTOPHTHALMIA

Synonyms. Desert blindness; electric ophthalmia; snow blindness; ultraviolet keratitis; actinic keratitis.

Symptoms. Onset 4 to 5 hours after exposure. Severe ocular burning pain; itching; smarting of lids; photophobia; lacrimation; blepharospasm; seeing halos around lights.

Signs. Myosis; congestion and swelling of conjunctiva; edema; ulceration of cornea; mucopurulent secretion.

Etiology. Lesion from ultraviolet rays, snow reflection, welding arc, or strong lights.

Pathology. Inflammatory change; eosinophils in secretion.

Therapy. Prevention through use of colored lenses and general anesthetic.

Prognosis. Decrease in vision may result. Usually self-limited. Healing occurs in 12 hours.

BIBLIOGRAPHY. Newell FW: Ophthalmology, Principles and Concepts. St Louis, CV Mosby, 1965
Vaughan D, Asbury T: General Ophthalmology, 11th ed. Norwalk, Appleton–Lange, 1986

PIBLOKTO

Synonym. Arctic hysteria.

Symptoms. Occur in eskimos, predominantly in women. Sudden attack of screaming, tearing away clothing, and running wildly. Attacks lasts 1 to 2 hours. Afterward, complete recovery and amnesia.

Etiology. Hysterical state of dissociation.

BIBLIOGRAPHY. Brill AA: Piblokto or hysteria among Peary's Eskimos. J Nerv Ment Dis 40:514–520, 1913
Willis JS, Martins M: Mental Health in North. Ottawa, Canada, Dept Nat Health Welfare, 1962
Freedman AM, Kaplan HI, Sadock BJ: Comprehensive Textbook of Psychiatry, 2nd ed, p 1732. Baltimore, Williams & Wilkins, 1975

PICK'S (A.)

Synonyms. Aphasia–agnosia–apraxia; Arnold Pick's; circumscribed brain atrophy; presenile dementia (see Alzheimer's); lobar sclerosis.

Symptoms and Signs. Both sexes affected; onset usually in fifth or sixth decade. Progressive dementia; focal symptoms and signs according to anatomic sites of involvement; temporal and frontal lobes most frequently involved. Anamnestic aphasia. Overall symptomatology very similar to Alzheimer's.

Etiology. Unknown; autosomal dominant inheritance reported.

Pathology. Localized atrophy of temporal lobes; frontal and parietal lobes less involved; basal ganglia normal or shrunken. Cell loss in areas involved; abundant glial proliferation; argentophilic bodies in cell cytoplasm. Absence of senile plaques and intracellular fibrillary degeneration. Blood vessel not involved.

Diagnostic Procedures. *Electroencephalography.* Diffuse changes. *CT brain scan. Electroencephalographic brain mapping.* Cerebral atrophy. *Cerebrospinal fluid.* Normal; occasionally, increase in protein.

Therapy. Symptomatic. Institutional care.

Prognosis. Death in a few years.

BIBLIOGRAPHY. Pick A: Apperzeptive Blindheit der Senilen. Arb Dtsch Psychiatr Klin In Prag: 43, 1908
Pick A, Thiele R: Aphasia. Handbuch der normalen und pathologischen Physiologie. Berlin, Springer, 1931
Morris JC, Cole M, Banker BQ et al: Hereditary dyphasic dementia and Pick–Alzheimer spectrum. Ann Neurol 16:455–466, 1984

PICK'S (F.)

Synonyms. Constrictive pericarditis; Friedel Pick; Hutinel–Pick; liver pseudocirrhosis; mediastinopericarditis; pericarditis–liver pseudocirrhosis.

Symptoms. Occur in patients with previous history of chest infection. Dyspnea; weakness; precordial discomfort; anorexia.

Signs. Cervical venous distention: ankle edema; heart normal or slightly enlarged; paradoxic pulse; protodiastolic gallop rhythm, or no significant murmur; hepatomegaly; ascites. Blood pressure usually low.

Etiology. Tuberculosis, various bacterial or viral, radiotherapy, neoplastic infections, or idiopathic, causing obliteration of pericardial cavity. Modern classification distinguishes the following forms: chronic calcific constrictive pericarditis; subacute constrictive pericarditis (rheumatoid arthritis, *Hemophilus influenzae* infections); postoperative constricting pericarditis, occult constrictive pericarditis; effusive constricting pericarditis (combined tamponade (and constrictive lesion).

Pathology. Obliteration, fibrosis, and calcification of pericardial space; chronic inflammatory reaction.

Diagnostic Procedures. *Blood and urine.* Normal; low serum albumin; sodium sulfobromophthalein retention

usually elevated. Increase of peripheral venous pressure. Circulation time elevated. *X-ray.* Occasionally, calcification of pericardium; diminished cardiac pulsation on fluoroscopy; pulmonary and pleural pathology frequent. *Electrocardiography.* Flattening or inversion of T waves, elevated RT segment, and possibly elevated ST segment in leads I and II; later, inverted T wave and diminution of QRS. *Cardiac catheterization.* Signs of constrictive pericarditis.

Therapy. Surgical. Decortication of heart; antitubercular treatment (when indicated).

Prognosis. From complete recovery after surgery to no improvement and death from cardiopulmonary insufficiency according to degree of pulmonary, cardiac, and hepatic involvement.

BIBLIOGRAPHY. Lower R: Tractatus de Corde, pp 104–107. Amstelodami, Apud Danielem Elzevirium, 1669
Pick F: Ueber chronische, unter den Bilde der Lebercirrhose verlaufende Pericarditis (pericarditische Pseudolebercirrhose) nebst Bemerkungen über die Zuckergussleber (Curschmann). Klin Med 29:385–410, 1896
Shabetai R: Diseases of Pericardium. In Hurst JW: The Heart, 6th ed, pp 1263–1266. New York, McGraw-Hill, 1986

PICK'S (L.)

Synonym. Cachectic retinitis.

Symptoms. Decreased visual acuity; reduced field of vision; distortion of shapes of objects.

Signs. Diffuse clouding of retina; peripapillary whitish gray macula; small hemorrhagic areas; distention of vessels.

Etiology. Cachexia; secondary anemia to carcinoma or severe, chronic, intestinal hemorrhages, or chronic infection conditions.

Pathology. Retinal elements showing fatty degeneration, edema, leukocyte exudates; swelling of nervous fibers; thickening and, occasionally obliteration of vessel walls.

Therapy. Treatment of basic condition.

Prognosis. Poor.

BIBLIOGRAPHY. Pick L: Netzhautveraenderungen bei chronischen Anaemien. Klin Monatsbl Augenheilkd 39:177–192, 1901

PICKWICKIAN

Synonyms. Cardiopulmonary obesity. Obesity–hypoventilation. See Narcolepsy–diabetogenic ("functional") hyperinsulinism.

Symptoms. Occur in about 10% of obese adults; rare in obese children. Somnolence; bulimia. Headache; dyspnea; drowsiness. In children, mental retardation may develop.

Signs. Obesity; limited respiratory chest excursion; cyanosis; nocturnal Cheyne–Stokes respiration; right ventricular failure. Retinal hemorrhages and papilledema.

Etiology. Obesity imposing excessive work load on respiration. Chronic hypoxemia; relative hyperinsulinism may be present. It may be considered as part of the narcolepsy or diabetogenic hyperinsulinism syndromes, where the cardiorespiratory symptoms are present as prominent feature. Role of genetic factors debated.

Pathology. Generalized obesity; excessive fat under diaphragm. Ascites and edema when right ventricular failure develops. Signs of pulmonary hypertension and right heart hypertrophy.

Diagnostic Procedures. *Blood.* Polycythemia; hypoxiemia. *Pulmonary function tests.* Alveolar hypoventilation; carbon dioxide retention; total and vital capacity decreased; reduction of expiratory reserve volume. *Electrocardiography.* Right axis deviation; changes suggesting ischemia of anterior wall.

Therapy. Diet; analeptic agent; treatment of right ventricular failure. Physical activity.

Prognosis. Fatal if unrecognized; reversible if treated.

BIBLIOGRAPHY. Burwell CS, Robin ED, Whaley RD et al: Extreme obesity associated with alveolar hypoventilation—a Pickwickian syndrome. Am J Med 21:811–818, 1956

Stunkard AJ, Sorensen TIA, Hanis C et al: An adoption study of human obesity. N Engl J Med 314:193–198, 1986

Sugarman HY, Baron PL, Fairman RP et al: Hemodynamic dysfunction in obesity hypoventilation syndrome and the effects of treatment with surgically induced weight loss. Ann Surg 207:609–613, 1988

PIE

Synonym. Pulmonary infiltrate–eosinophilia. The acronym PIE is used to indicate all eosinophilic lung diseases which has led to confusion because eosinophilia may not be a constant feature of these conditions.

PIERRE ROBIN

Synonyms. Cleft palate–glossoptosis–micrognathia; Robin's. See First arch syndromes.

Symptoms. Difficulty in breathing; difficulty in feeding.

Signs. Micrognathia; cleft palate; glossoptosis; ocular abnormalities; cyanosis; sternum retraction evidence of malnutrition.

Etiology. See First arch syndrome. Autosomal recessive inheritance.

Pathology. See Signs.

Diagnostic Procedures. *X-ray. Chromosome studies.* Normal pattern.

Therapy. Orthostatic nursing (feeding while neonate lying on the abdomen with chest elevated by small pillow). Prevent tongue from slipping backward. False palate of acrylic material.

Prognosis. Usually, infant outgrows feeding and breathing difficulties in weeks or months. There is a significant risk of major airway embarrassment in this disorder, even if the infant seems initially well. Early management of infants with this anomaly should, therefore, be undertaken at centers where skilled airway support is available.

BIBLIOGRAPHY. Sahukowsky WP: Zur Aetologie des Stridor inspiratorisu congenitalis. Jahrb Kinderheilkd NF 73:459–474, 1911.

Robin P: La glossoptose: Son diagnostic, ses consequences, son traitement. J Med Paris 43:235–237, 1923

Davies PA: Management of the Pierre Robin syndrome. Dev Med Child Neurol 15:359–362, 1973

Ogborn MR, Peruberton PJ: Late development of airway obstruction in the Robin anomalad (Pierre Robin syndrome) in the newborn. Aust Paediatr J 21:199–200, 1985

PIETRANTONI'S

Eponym used to indicate areas of neuralgia or anesthesia on the face or oral cavity, reported by patients affected by still undetected paranasal tumors.

BIBLIOGRAPHY. Pietrantoni L: Zone nevralgiche e zone di anestesia della regione facciale e della cavità orale come sintomi precoci di alcune forme di tumori maligni delle cavità paranasali. Arch Ital Otol 59:105–108, 1948

PIGEON BREEDER'S I

Synonyms. Bird breeder's lung; bird fancier's; pneumonitis of pigeon breeder. See Allergic alveolitis syndromes.

Symptoms. Occur in individuals who take care of pigeons; onset 4 to 6 hours after exposure. Malaise; fever; chills; dyspnea; cough; arthralgia.

Signs. Diffuse crepitant rales in both sides of chest.

Etiology. Hypersensitivity reaction to pigeons.

Pathology. Interstitial pneumonitis.

Diagnostic Procedures. *Blood.* Eosinophilia (not a prominent, constant feature). Presence of specific precipitating antibodies. *X-ray of chest.* Diffuse coarsening of bronchovascular markings; fine nodulation and reticulation.

Therapy. Corticosteroids.

Prognosis. If contact with birds avoided, symptoms disappear spontaneously in 12 to 24 hours, pulmonary signs in several days. Repeated, prolonged exposure results in chronic lung disease.

BIBLIOGRAPHY. Reed CE, Sosman A, Barbee RA: Pigeon breeder's lung: A newly observed interstitial pulmonary disease. JAMA 193:261–265, 1965
Unger JD, Fink JN, Unger GF: Pigeon breeder's disease. Radiology 90:683–687, 1968
Reed CE, de Shazo R: Immunologic aspects of granulomatous and interstitial lung disease. JAMA 248:2683–2691, 1982

PIGMENTARY GLAUCOMA

Synonym. Pigmentary ocular dispersion.

Symptoms and Signs. Males affected more frequently than females (4:1); onset in fourth and fifth decades. Myopia (70%); glaucomatous field changes (39%). Iris translucency (65%); insert anteriorly into the scleral spur (75%); pigment in the posterior trabecular mesh; pigment on equatorial edge of lens capsule.

Etiology. Unknown; polygenic inheritance. Pigment not cause of glaucoma, but possibly secondary to atrophy of iris epithelium.

Diagnostic Procedures. *Tonometry and tonography.* Ocular hypertension.

Therapy. That of glaucoma.

Prognosis. Progressive condition.

BIBLIOGRAPHY. Sugar HS: Pigmentary glaucoma—A 25-year review. Am J Ophthalmol 62:499–507, 1966

Lichter RP: Pigmentary glaucoma—Current concepts. Trans Am Acad Ophthalmol Otolaryngol 78:309, 1974
Maida JW, Spaeth GL: Pigmentary ocular dispersion syndrome. Presented at the 27th Wills Annual Conference, Philadelphia, Jan 30, 1975
Vaughan D, Asbury T: General Ophthalmology, 11th ed. Norwalk, Appleton–Lange, 1986

PILI ANNULATI

Synonyms. Hair ringed: thrix annulata.

Symptoms. Present at birth or developing in first 2 years of life. Asymptomatic.

Signs. Alternate light and dark bands of scalp hair (occasionally also axillary). Normal or increased hair fragility; hairs breaking at 15 to 20 cm lengths. Possible association with other congenital defects.

Etiology. Unknown; 50% sporadic cases; 50% hereditary usually autosomal dominant (recessive type possible in some cases).

Pathology. On microscopic examination affected hairs show alternating normally pigmented bands and lighter ones.

Diagnostic Procedures. On transmitted light, light hairs appear black (see Pathology).

Therapy. None.

Prognosis. Permanent condition.

BIBLIOGRAPHY. Ashley LM, Jacques RS: Four generations of ringed hair. J Hered 41:82–84, 1950
Degos R: Dermatologie. Paris, Flammarion, 1953
Rook A, Wilkinson DS, Ebling FJG et al: Textbook of Dermatology, 4th ed. Oxford, Blackwell Scientific Publications, 1986

PILLAY'S

Synonym. Ophthalmomandibulomelic dysplasia.

Symptoms and Signs. Both sexes affected. Corneal opacities; temporomandibular fusion; obtuse mandibular angle, short forearms.

Etiology. Autosomal dominant inheritance.

Diagnostic Procedures. *X-ray.* Aplasia of lateral condyle head of radius and lower third of ulna; dislocation of radiohumeral and proximal radioulnar joints.

BIBLIOGRAPHY. Pillay VK: Ophthalmo-mandibulomelic dysplasia. An hereditary syndrome. J Bone Joint Surg [Am] 46:858–862, 1964

PINCER NAIL

Symptoms. Severe pain in involved fingers.

Signs. Excessive transverse curvature of nail plate; loss of soft tissue of involved fingers.

Etiology. Unknown.

Diagnostic Procedures. *X-ray of finger.* Resorption of phalanx of involved fingers.

Therapy. Surgical avulsion of dystrophic nails.

BIBLIOGRAPHY. Samman PD: The Nails in Disease, p 79. London, Heinemann, 1965
Cornelius CE, Shelley WB: Pincer nail syndrome. Arch Surg 96:321–322, 1968

PINEAL-GONADAL

See Pellizzi's and Pineal tumor.

Symptoms and Signs. Occur in young males (hypogonadism and pineal tumor never reported in female). Delayed or absent development of primary and secondary sexual characteristics, associated with pineal tumor neurologic syndrome (see).

Etiology. Unknown; increased secretion of a hypothetical pineal hormone that inhibits gonadal development.

Pathogenesis. Adenoma or functioning pinealoma.

Diagnostic Procedures. *X-ray of skull. Pneumoencephalography. Gonadotropins secretion evaluation.*

Therapy. Surgery; substitutional therapy.

Prognosis. Depends on benign or malignant etiology.

BIBLIOGRAPHY. Kitay JI: Pineal lesions and precocious puberty: A review. J Clin Endocrinol 14:622–625, 1954
Cohen RA, Wurtman RJ, Axelrod J et al: Some chemical, biochemical, and physiological actions of the pineal gland. Ann Intern Med 61:1144–1161, 1964

PINEAL TUMOR NEUROLOGIC

Symptoms. Occur most often in young males. Weakness; headache; vomiting; diplopia; deafness; incoordination; polydipsia; polyphagia; convulsions; mental changes.

Signs. Lack of pupillary reaction; paresis of oculomotor muscle, nystagmus; papilledema; facial paralysis; tremor; ataxia; Romberg's sign; hypertonia; tendon hyperreflexia; Babinski's sign. Parinaud's I syndrome (see) most characteristic localizing sign.

Etiology. Unknown; neoplasia of pineal gland.

Pathology. Gliomas and teratomas (invasion mass, necrosis, and hemorrhage). Cystic hydrops of pineal (lined by glial cells). Pinealoma (composed of pineal parenchymal cells reproducing the mosaic pattern seen in the developing organ). Adenomas and metastasis very rare.

Diagnostic Procedures. *X-ray of skull.* Sometimes gland calcified. *CT brain scan.*

Therapy. Surgery.

Prognosis. Depends on etiology and result of surgery.

BIBLIOGRAPHY. Anderson WAD: Pathology, 5th ed. St Louis, CV Mosby, 1966
Adams RD, Victor M: Principles of Neurology. 3rd ed, pp 493–494. New York, McGraw-Hill, 1985

PINGELAPESE BLINDNESS

Synonyms. Color blindness–myopia; achromatopsia–myopia.

Symptoms and Signs. Affects 4% to 10% of Pingelapese people. Both sexes. Horizontal pendular nystagmus, photophobia, amaurosis, color blindness, gradually developing cataracts.

Etiology. Autosomal recessive.

Prognosis. Nonprogressive disorder.

BIBLIOGRAPHY. Brodie JA, Hussels I, Brink E et al: Hereditary blindness among Pingelapese people of Eastern Caroline Island. Lancet I:1253–1257, 1970

PINKUS' (F.)

Synonym. Lichen nitidus.

Symptoms. Both sexes affected; onset usually in childhood and young adulthood. Usually, asymptomatic.

Signs. Eruption of discrete (occasionally grouped) pinhead size, pink or red papules on abdomen, genitalia, forearms, chest, buttocks, seldom on palms and soles. Mucosae rarely affected. Coincidence with lichen planus frequent.

Etiology. Unknown; possibly related to lichen planus.

Pathology. Papules are formed by a dense circumscribed, infiltrated margin located under the epidermis and formed by lymphocytes, histiocytes, and rarely Langhans' cells.

Diagnostic Procedures. *Biopsy of skin.* Differential diagnosis with lichen planus, lichen scrofulosum, keratosis pilaris.

Therapy. No treatment required for majority of cases, or topical steroids.

Prognosis. Course unpredictable. Finally, recovery without scars.

BIBLIOGRAPHY. Pinkus F: Uber eine neue knoechnfoernige Hauteruption: Lichen nitidus. Arch Dermatol Syph (Berlin) 85:11–36, 1907
Rook A, Wilkinson DS, Ebling FJG et al: Textbook of Dermatology, 4th ed, pp 1682–1685. Oxford, Blackwell Scientific Publications, 1986

PINKUS (H.)

Synonym. Fibroepithelial tumor. Obsolete since represents a confusing condition including benign and malignant conditions of the fibromatosis group.

Symptoms and Signs. Appearance and slow growth of a sessile, firm, pink tumor with domed surface, on the abdomen or loins. Associated frequently with seborrheic keratosis or basal cell carcinoma or both.

Etiology. Unknown; possibly, correlation with x-ray exposure, or arsenic treatment.

Pathology. Tumor formed by fibrotic, cellular, enlarged dermal papillae, enclosed in a nest of small dark cells.

Therapy. Local excision.

Prognosis. Treatment curative.

BIBLIOGRAPHY. Pinkus H: Premalignant fibroepithelial tumors of skin. Arch Dermatol Syph 67:598–615, 1953
Rook A, Wilkinson DS, Ebling FJG et al: Textbook of Dermatology, 4th ed, p. 1823. Oxford, Blackwell Scientific Publications, 1986

PINKUS' (H.) II

Synonym. Eccrine poroma.

Symptoms. Both sexes equally affected. Onset in middle age or later. Asymptomatic.

Signs. Usually on the sole, less frequently on palm, and elsewhere on the body, solitary tumor, flat (sole), sessile, or pedunculated, with smooth surface or slightly kera-

totic; occasionally vascular or ulcerated. Diameter varying from several millimeters to several centimeters.

Etiology. Benign and seldom malignant tumor from eccrine sweat duct epithelium, juxta epidermal localization. Clinically same manifestation of hidroacanthoma simplex (intraepidermal) and dermal duct tumor (intradermal).

Pathology. Cells are small malpighian cells and rich in glycogen. Histochemical reaction of tumor cells similar to those of sudoriparous glands.

Therapy. Surgical excision. Curettage and diathermy sometimes adequate.

Prognosis. Cured by removal.

BIBLIOGRAPHY. Pinkus H et al: Eccrine poroma. Tumours exhibiting features of the epidermal sweat duct unit. Arch Dermatol 74:511–521, 1956
Rook A, Wilkinson DS, Ebling FJG et al: Textbook of Dermatology, 4th ed, pp 2408–2410. Oxford, Blackwell Scientific Publications, 1986

PINKUS' (H.) III

Synonyms. Alopecia mucinosa; follicular mucinosis.

Symptoms. Both sexes affected; onset in two age groups: (1) children over 5 and adults under 30; (2) older subjects.
Group 1. Asymptomatic or paucisymptomatic.
Group 2. Irritative skin changes and pruritus.

Signs. *Group 1.* On the face, scalp, neck or shoulders, eruption of single or multiple papules or erythematous plaques, with fine scaling, raised follicles, and hair loss.
Group 2. More numerous lesions with variable aspects: papules, plaques, and nodules; some ulcerated and some developing jelly consistency. Various signs of skin or systemic reticulosis may appear at various times after onset.

Etiology. Unknown; virus infection(?); nonspecific reaction(?).

Pathology. Edema and mucinous degeneration of sebaceous glands and hair root sheaths. Variable degree of inflammatory changes.

Diagnostic Procedures. *Biopsy.* In group 2 search for evidence of local or systemic reticulosis.

Therapy. None effective.

Prognosis. *Group 1.* Few, self-limiting lesions, and eventual recovery.
Group 2. Extensive, polymorphic, persistent lesions with frequent association with malignant reticulosis (20%).

BIBLIOGRAPHY. Pinkus H: Alopecia mucinosa. Inflammatory plaques with alopecia characterized by roots-sheath mucinosis. Arch Dermatol 76:419–426, 1957

Tappeiner J: Zuer Problem der Symtomatischen Mucinosis follicularis. Arch Klin Exp Dermatol 227:937–948, 1966

Rook A, Wilkinson DS, Ebling FJG et al: Textbook of Dermatology, 4th ed, pp 2004–2005. Oxford, Blackwell Scientific Publications, 1986

PIRINGER–KUCHINKA'S

Synonyms. Lymphadenitis subacuta; lymphadenitis nuchalis and cervicalis.

Obsolete eponym used to indicate lymphadenopathy of cervical and nuchal stations (lymphadenitis nuchalis and cervicalis) due to chronic and subacute infection (*e.g.*, toxoplasmosis).

BIBLIOGRAPHY. Piringer–Kuchinka A: Eigerartiger mikroskopischer Befund an exzidierten Lymphknoten. Verh Dtsch Ges Pathol 36:352–362, 1952

PITT–WILLIAMS

Synonym. Brachydactyly (B+E types).

Symptoms and Signs. Hypoplasia of distal phalanges of ulnar side of hand and shortening of one or several metacarpals. Absence of dwarfism.

Etiology. Autosomal dominant inheritance.

BIBLIOGRAPHY. Pitt P, Williams I: A new brachydactyly syndrome with similarities to Julia Bell type B and E. J Med Genet 22:202–204, 1985

PITUITARY APOPLEXY

Symptoms and Signs. Acute onset. Headache, ophthalmoplegia, amaurosis bilateral, drowsiness or coma.

Etiology. Infarction of a pituitary adenoma.

Diagnostic Procedures. *Cerebrospinal fluid.* Protein, leukocytes increased; possible presence of red cells. *CT brain scan.* Infarction of the tumor, enlarged sella.

Therapy. Dexamethazone (6–12 mg every 6 hr) and if no improvement transnasal decompression.

Prognosis. Life-threatening situation. Good result with immediate diagnosis and treatment.

BIBLIOGRAPHY. Brougham M, Henser AP, Adams RD: Acute degenerative changes in adenomas of the pitui-

tary body with special reference to pituitary apoplexy. J Neurosurg 7:421–439, 1950

Cooperman D, Maeazkey WB: Pituitary apoplexy. Heart Lung 7:450–454, 1978

PITUITARY DWARFISM TYPE IV

Synonym. Biodefective growth hormone.

Symptoms and Signs. Growth retardation and delayed bone age.

Etiology. Presumably mutation in the growth hormone (GH) on chromosome 17, causing a biologically ineffective GH molecule, unable to stimulate somatomedin.

Diagnostic Procedures. Normal immunoreactive GH after stimulation and low level of somatomedin.

Therapy. Exogenous GH administration induces normal level of somatomedin and increase in growth rate.

BIBLIOGRAPHY. Kowarski AA, Schneider JJ, Ben Galim E et al: Growth failure with normal serum RIA–GH and low somatomedin activity: Somatomedin restoration and growth acceleration after exogenous GH. J Clin Endocrinol 47:461–464, 1978

Valenta LJ, Sigel MB, Lesnik MA et al: Pituitary dwarfism in a patient with circulating abnormal growth hormone polymers. N Engl J Med 312:214–217, 1985

PITUITARY INSUFFICIENCY–HYPOTHYROIDISM

This group of syndromes includes six syndromes to date, which are schematically reported.

Isolated TSH deficiency. Manifested as congenital hypothyroidism. Autosomal recessive.

Panhypopituitarism. With congenital hypothyroidism and associated defects of FSH, HGH, LH and ACTH—two forms are known—*autosomal recessive and X-linked.*

Pituitary agenesis. Only congenital hypothyroidism. Autosomal recessive.

Panhypopituitarism with absent sella turcica. Congenital hypothyroidism with associated defects of HGH, FSH, LH, ACTH. Autosomal recessive.

Panhypopituitarism with enlarged sella turcica. Congenital hypothyroidism. Associated deficiency of GH.

BIBLIOGRAPHY. Stanbury JB, Dumont JE: Familial goiter and related disorders. In Stanbury JB, Wyngaarden JB, Fredrickson DS: The Metabolic Basis of Inherited Disease, 5th ed, p 231. New York, McGraw-Hill, 1983

PIULACHS–HEDERICH

Eponym used to indicate a sudden abdominal colic caused by a sudden idiopathic colic gas distention.

BIBLIOGRAPHY. Piulachs P, Hederich H: La "dilatation aguda del colon" complication del dolicomegacolon. Acta Med Hisp 5:131–135, 1947

PLACENTAL HEMANGIOMAS

Synonyms. Chorioangiofibromal; fibroangioma; hemangioblastoma; reticulohemangioendothelioma.

Symptoms and Signs. Hemangiomas of the placenta; associated hydramnios in 33% of cases, without fetal anomalies or maternal abnormalities. Often associated with premature labor, premature rupture of membranes, an increased incidence of antepartum and postpartum hemorrhage, and, rarely, dystocia.

Etiology. Not known.

Pathology. Placental hemangiomas vary in size from 2 mm to 22 cm; produce an elevation of the fetal surface. They vary in color from yellow gray to deep blue red color and are firm in consistency. Microscopically, hemangioma consists of embryonic cellular tissue with numerous small blood vessels supported by a loose network of chorionic stromal cells. These tumors are well demarcated from the surrounding placental tissue.

Therapy. No special treatment is necessary. The treatment is governed by obstetric conditions.

Prognosis. Good for the newborn, unless causing prematurity.

BIBLIOGRAPHY. Clarke J: Account of a tumor found in the substance of the human placenta. Philos Trans 88:361–368, 1798
Asadourian LA, Taylor HB: Clinical significance of placental hemangiomas. Obstet Gynecol 31:551–555, 1968

PLACENTAL INSUFFICIENCY

Synonyms. Prolonged gestation II; placental dysfunctional II; postmaturity small baby.

Symptoms and Signs. Retardation of uterine growth at about the 30th week of pregnancy; decrease in fetal movements; delivery of an "immature" baby despite the fact that the baby is full-term. Very often intrauterine fetal death.

Etiology. Unknown; possibly, inability of placenta to transfer, synthesize, transport nutritional and chemical elements necessary for growth of the fetus.

Pathology. A decreased vascular supply and increased fibrosis of the placental tissue; small placenta (200 g).

Diagnostic Procedures. *Urine.* Decrease in urinary estriol excretion; increase of atropine transfer time.

Therapy. Increased vigilance and active intervention for termination of pregnancy, either vaginally or by cesarean section if and when fetal distress becomes apparent.

Prognosis. Guarded because etiology is unknown. Recurrence of condition is high (40%).

BIBLIOGRAPHY. Rumbolz WL, Edwards MC, McCoogan LS: The small full term infant, placental insufficiency. West J Surg 69:53–60, 1961
Pritchard JA, McDonald PC, Gant NF: Williams Obstetrics, 17th ed, p 756. Norwalk, Appleton–Lange, 1985

PLACENTA PREVIA

Symptoms and Signs. Occur in 1:100 to 1:200 deliveries; more frequent in multiparas and in Caucasian patients. Painless hemorrhage during the third trimester of pregnancy. Hemorrhage may come at any time, without warning and even when the patient is asleep. Usually this bleeding is not accompanied by symptoms and signs of preeclampsia. Vaginal examination under sterile conditions and double set-up reveals the presence of placenta in lower segment of the uterus, partially or totally covering the internal os of the cervix.

Etiology. Little is known about the etiology. It has been suggested that defective vascularization of the decidua, as the result of inflammatory or atrophic processes, may be a contributing factor.

Pathology. According to the degree with which placenta covers the internal os: (1) total or central placenta previa; (2) partial placenta previa; (3) marginal placenta previa.

Diagnostic Procedures. *Ultrasound. Magnetic resonance imaging.*

Therapy. The uterus should be emptied by the most conservative method as soon as the placenta previa is diagnosed. Such patients should always be hospitalized and be kept under constant observation. *Before labor.* When the fetus is viable and the pregnancy more than 36th week, rupture of the membranes may permit the presenting part to compress the placenta and stop bleeding. If the bleeding does not stop and in case of total placenta previa, cesarean section. If the fetus is not viable, a policy of conservation is taken: complete bed rest; hospitalization; observation. If the fetus is dead, Willett forceps attached to fetal scalp used to obtain additional pressure against the placenta. *During labor.* Depends on variety of previa, dilatation and effacement of cervix, general condition of patient. If dilatation is almost complete, with marginal placenta previa and condition of the patient is good, rupture of membranes and forceps delivery. Under all other circumstances, cesarean section. *Management of third stage.* Beware of alarming postpartum hemorrhage. If bleeding is profuse, Crede's method of expression of placenta. If not successful, manual removal of placenta.

Prognosis. Threatened maternal morbidity and mortality. Increased perinatal mortality.

BIBLIOGRAPHY. Hibbard LT: Placenta praevia. Am J Obstet Gynecol 104:172–176, 1969

Gorodeski IG, Neri A, Haimovich L, Bahari CM: Placenta praevia: The ultrasonographic localization and its influence on the mode of delivery. J Reprod Med 27:655–657, 1982

Powell MC, Buckley J, Price H, Worthington BS, Symonds EM: Magnetic resonance imaging and placenta praevia. Am J Obstet Gynecol 154:565–569, 1986

PLAGIOCEPHALY–FACIAL ASYMMETRY–DENTAL ARTICULATION DERANGEMENT

Synonym. Facial malformation–skull base asymmetry. See Bencze's.

Symptoms and Signs. Malformations of vault and base of skull and disturbances of dental articulation. Mandibular compensation may sometimes reduce disturbances of articulation or various degrees of malocclusion may result, associated with various degree of plagiocephaly. Severity of one feature not always correlated with the others.

Etiology. Congenital malformation; hereditary transmission considered.

Pathology. Not specific.

Diagnostic Procedure. X-ray.

Therapy. Adequate data not yet available for an evaluation.

Prognosis. Tendency toward self-correction of the dental articulation disturbances.

BIBLIOGRAPHY. Korkhaus G: L'influence de l'hérédité et du milieu sur l'architecture du crane facial. Rev Belge Sci Dent 385–403, 1952

Delaire J, Billet J, Ferré JC et al: Malformations faciales et asymétrie de la base du crane. Rev Stomatol 66:379–396, 1965

PLOTT'S

Synonyms. Laryngeal abductor paralysis; vocal cord dysfunction familial (see Gerhardt's).

Symptoms and Signs. From birth. Impairment of phonation or severe inspiratory dyspnea. Psychomotor retardation.

Etiology. X-linked inheritance.

Pathology. Brain damage secondary to respiratory difficulties. Dysgenesis of nucleus ambiguus considered.

BIBLIOGRAPHY. Plott D: Congenital laryngeal abductor paralysis due to nucleus ambiguus dysgenesis in three brothers. N Engl J Med 271:593–597, 1964

Opitz JM, Kaveggia EG, Durkin-Stamm MV et al: Diagnostic-genetic studies in severe mental retardation. Birth Defects XIV (6B):1–38, 1978

PLUMMER'S

Synonyms. Toxic nodular goiter; toxic adenoma.

Symptoms. Prevalent in females; onset after 40 years of age. The same symptoms as Flajani's, but, typically, slower rate of appearance, sometimes asymptomatic. Usually, predominance of cardiac symptoms and absence of ophthalmopathy, pretibial myxedema, and acropathy.

Signs. Adenomatous thyromegaly precedes the symptoms. Single node usually hot, palpable; multinodular. Other findings similar to those of the Flajani's syndrome.

Etiology. Unknown. Benign neoplasm.

Pathology. Minimal to gross asymmetry of thyroid. Section: variegated surface showing normal tissue with areas of gelatinous aspect. Hyperplastic nodules not encapsulated, occasionally cystic with interposed fibrous scars.

Diagnostic Procedures. Thyroidal ^{123}I normal in 50% of cases; T_4 slightly elevated (frequently is the only laboratory finding).

Therapy. Radioiodine: treatment of choice. If surgery necessary, make the patient euthyroid first with antithyroid drugs.

Prognosis. Unrelenting course. Frequently destructive therapy required.

BIBLIOGRAPHY. Plummer HS: The clinical and pathological relationship of simple and exophthalmic goiter. Am J Med Sci 146:790–795, 1913

Mazzaferri EL: The thyroid. In Mazzaferri EL (ed): Textbook of Endocrinology, 3rd ed, pp 182–185. New York, Med Exam Publ Co, 1985

PLUMMER–VINSON

Synonyms. Plummer–Vinson anemia; sideropenic dysphagia; Kelly–Paterson; Paterson's; Paterson–Brown–Kelly; postcricoid web. Waldenström–Kjellberg.

Symptoms. Occur most often in middle-aged women, rarely in men. Pain and burning sensation behind larynx when swallowing solid food, or sensation of food stuck into the larynx. Fatigue.

Signs. Pallor of skin and mucosae (not constant). Other signs of sideropenic anemia (in hair; nails).

Etiology. An association between sideropenia and one or more webs of mucosa at the juncture between the hypopharynx and the esophagus.

Pathology. Webs of mucosa in the lumen of the esophagus that can narrow the lumen itself. Biopsy of these lesions shows chronic inflammation.

Diagnostic Procedures. *Blood.* Hypochromic anemia (not consistently present); sideropenia (constant). *Stool.* Occult blood. *X-ray.* Thick barium and very short exposures in upper part of esophagus, below cricoid cartilage, shows thin defect of opacity.

Therapy. Repletion of iron stores; rupture the webs or dilate the stenosis by means of bouginage.

Prognosis. Good with therapy. In untreated patients, the dysphagia can interfere with nutrition. Carcinoma *in situ* is a rare complication.

BIBLIOGRAPHY. Plummer HS: Diffuse dilation of the esophagus without anatomic stenosis (cardiospasm). A report of ninety-one cases. JAMA 58:2013–2015, 1912
Vinson PP: A case of cardiospasm with dilation and angulation of the esophagus. Med Clin North Am 3:623–627, 1919
Wintrobe MM: Idiopathic hypochromic anemia. Medicine 12:187–243, 1933
Wintrobe MM (ed): Clinical Hematology, 8th ed, p 630. Philadelphia, Lea & Febiger, 1981

PNEUMATIC HAMMER

Synonym. Vibration.

Symptoms. Occur in individuals exposed to the percussion of vibrating tools. Exposure to cold induces a typical Raynaud's phenomenon (see). First affecting only the hand that has been nearer to the end of tool, then all fingers. When attack is severe, complete sensory loss over the fingers may be experienced.

Signs. During attacks, color changes in the fingers; between attacks, normal fingers. No trophic changes.

Etiology. Unknown; possibly, alteration of the digital vessels, so that spasm follows exposure to cold.

Pathology. Unknown; some degree of thickening of intima of digital arteries and arterioles.

Diagnostic Procedures. Rule out other causes of Raynaud's phenomenon (see).

Therapy. Relief from attack by rubbing hands and then immersing them in warm water. Alcohol injection. If intolerable pain, change of activity; if change impossible, sympathectomy may be considered.

Prognosis. Relatively benign course; change of occupation may cure the condition.

BIBLIOGRAPHY. President's Monthly Report. The Stonecutter's J 32:5, 1917
Allen EV, Barker NW, Hines EA: Peripheral Vascular Diseases, 4th ed. Philadelphia, WB Saunders, 1972
Hurst JW: The Heart, 6th ed, p 1578. New York, McGraw-Hill, 1986

PNEUMONIA, LYMPHOID INTERSTITIAL

Synonyms. LIP; plasma cell interstitial pneumonia; PIP.

Symptoms. Both sexes affected; onset at all ages. Cough; dyspnea.

Signs. Cyanosis and clubbing in 50% of cases.

Etiology. Unknown.

Pathology. Lung infiltrate formed by a mixture of small lymphocytes, plasma cells, and a few large mononuclear elements; in some cases, prevalence of plasma cells (it could represent a variant of this condition). Relative absence of pleural infiltration, involvement of lymph nodes and extrapulmonary tissues.

Diagnostic Procedures. *Blood.* Occasionally, monoclonal gammopathy (IgM and less frequently, IgG). *X-ray.* No specific findings.

Therapy. Trial with corticosteroids.

Prognosis. Progressive condition leading to pulmonary fibrosis.

BIBLIOGRAPHY. Carrington CB, Liebow AA: Lymphocytic interstitial pneumonia. Am J Pathol 48:36A, 1966

Fraser RG, Paré JAP: Diagnosis of Diseases of the Chest, 2nd ed, p 1699. Philadelphia, WB Saunders, 1977

POLAND–MOEBIUS

Combination of the two syndromes (see Poland's and Mobius') that is considered to represent a specific genetic malformation with autosomal dominant inheritance.

BIBLIOGRAPHY. Gadot N, Biedner B, Torok G: Moebius syndrome and Poland anomaly case report and review of the literature. J Paediatr Ophthalmol 16:374–376, 1979

Stevenson RE: The Poland–Moebius syndrome. Proc Greenwood Genet Center 1:26–28, 1982

POLAND'S

Synonym. Pectoralis muscle deficiency–syndactyly.

Symptoms. Incidence 10% of patients with syndactyly. No history. Patient cannot draw arm of affected side across the chest.

Signs. Syndactyly associated with ipsilateral absence of sternal head of pectoralis major. If in a female, asymmetry of breasts; patchy absence of axillary hair; absence of the nipple on affected side.

Etiology. Unknown; sporadic or occasionally in successive generations autosomal dominant inheritance.

Pathology. Absence of pectoralis major; syndactyly.

Diagnostic Procedures. *X-ray of hand and chest. CT scan.* To identify possible associated anomalies.

Therapy. Surgical correction of syndactyly in late childhood.

Prognosis. Surgical correction of syndactyly usually brings good results.

BIBLIOGRAPHY. Poland A: Deficiency of the pectoral muscles. Guy Hosp Rep 6:191–193, 1841

David TJ, Winter RM: Familial absence of the pectoralis major, serratus anterior and latissimus dorsi muscles. J Med Genet 22:390–392, 1985

POLLITT'S

Synonyms. Trichothiodystrophy–neurocutaneous; trichorrhexis nodosa. See Sabouraud's.

Symptoms. Both sexes. From birth. Delayed mental and physical retardation. Spastic diplegia.

Signs. Microcephaly; head titubation, jerky eye movements; length and weight below normal. Facies unusual (receding chin, large ears, stubby eyebrows). Trichorrhexis nodosa (hair progressively thinning, brittle, beaded, easily breakable and falling), ichthyosis and eczema, hypoplastic nails. Absent deep tendon reflexes.

Etiology. Possibly autosomal recessive inheritance.

Pathology. Brain: abnormal cortical cell layering.

Diagnostic Procedures. *Hair.* Cystine content 50% normal. *Electroencephalography.*

BIBLIOGRAPHY. Pollitt RJ, Jenner FA, Davies M: Sibs with mental and physical retardation and trichorrhexis nodosa with abnormal amino acid composition of the hair. Arch Dis Child 43:211–216, 1968

POLYARTERITIS NODOSA CUTANEA

Synonyms. Livedo nodules. Sneddon–Champion.

Symptoms and Signs. Prevalent (*i.e.*, described) in male; onset at all ages (2 mo to 69 yr). Monosymptomatic: chronic eruption of numerous small (0.5–2 cm), firm, hard, pink, painful nodules on (but not exclusively) the legs; or polysymptomatic: associated with livedo reticularis myalgia (50%), ulcerations, gangrenous complications, polyneuritis, or arthralgia (50%).

Etiology. Unknown. Cutaneous vasculitis. Allergy(?); autoimmune disorder(?); toxic(?).

Pathology. Necrotizing arteritis at junction of dermis and subcutis; infiltration of vascular walls and fibrinoid necrosis. No inflammatory reaction (in synthesis presence of changes similar to Kussmaul's (see), but less intense).

Diagnostic Procedures. *Blood.* Normal; increase of sedimentation rate; moderate leukocytosis. *Biopsy of skin.* (See Pathology).

Therapy. Corticosteroids.

Prognosis. Benign. Attacks last a month and may relapse for years; however, no visceral complications have been observed.

BIBLIOGRAPHY. Lyell A, Church R: Cutaneous manifestations of polyarteritis nodosa. Br J Dermatol 66:335–363, 1954

Isolement d'une forme cutanée, pure benigne de periarterite nodeuse (PAN). Instantanés médicaux N.5. Encyclopédie Médico-Chirurgicale, 1979

Rook A, Wilkinson DS, Ebling FJG et al: Textbook of Dermatology, 4th ed, pp 1170–1171. Oxford, Blackwell Scientific Publications, 1986

POLYARTHRITIS, EPIDEMIC TROPICAL ACUTE

Symptoms and Signs. Epidemic, seasonal (fall) occurrence of mild fever, cutaneous rash (rubellalike), polyarthritis, lymphadenopathy.

Etiology Unknown. Mosquito bite(?).

Diagnostic Procedures. *Blood.* Agglutination and culture tests negative.

Therapy. Symptomatic.

Prognosis. Self-limited condition lasting 10 to 20 days; recovery without sequelae.

BIBLIOGRAPHY. Halliday JH, Horan JP: Epidemic of polyarthritis in northern territory. Med J Aust 2:293–295, 1943
Schmidt FR: Unusual features and special types of infectious arthritis. In Hollander JL, McCarty DJ: Arthritis and Allied Conditions, 8th ed, p 1269. Philadelphia, Lea & Febiger, 1972

POLYCYSTIC

Synonyms. Hepatic cystic; renal cystic. See Caroli's. Clinically two varieties are recognized: (1) prevalent renal cystic syndrome, (a) infantile type and (b) adult type; (2) hepatic cystic syndrome, (a) infantile, adolescent type and (b) adult type.

PREVALENT RENAL CYSTIC SYNDROME
INFANTILE TYPE
Symptoms. Nausea; vomiting; dehydration.

Signs. Abdominal distention; palpation of bilateral renal masses (except in small cyst variety). Symptoms and signs may also be observed due to the presence of cysts in other organs (brain, lung, liver, pancreas) but are usually clinically subordinate to kidney pathology.

Etiology. Unknown; may be autosomal recessive. The pathogenetic hypothesis: (1) failure of union of the ureteric bud with convoluted tubules (metanephric; metanephroblastemic); (2) tubules canalization failure; (3) persistence of various generations of "nephrons."

Pathology. Kidney size may be normal or increased and asymmetric. Cysts of various sizes; cystic fluid watery, yellow, bloody, always totally isolated. Degenerative changes of parenchyma, due to compression, calculi, secondary infections.

Diagnostic Procedures. *Urine.* Albumin; hematuria; epithelial cells. *Blood.* Hyperchloremic acidosis. *X-ray.*

Intravenous pyelography. Renal scan with radioactive isotopes.

Therapy. Medical treatment of infection, renal insufficiency, hypertension. Kidney transplantation.

Prognosis. Excellent results with kidney transplantation.

ADULT TYPE
Symptoms. May be asymptomatic for several decades. Lumbar pains; palpable mass; hypertension; bladder symptoms of dysuria; hematuria; painful or painless. Weakness; abdominal enlargement.

Signs. Hypertension; palpable kidneys.

Etiology. Unknown; hereditary dominant (in large family, affects 50% of membranes).

Pathology. See Infantile type. Adult cyst may communicate and sometimes contain urinous fluid.

Diagnostic Procedures. See Infantile type.

Treatment. See Infantile type.

Prognosis. Seldom, does not interfere with normal life; usually, progressive symptomatology (*e.g.*, hypertension, uremia infections). Death usually in the middle of sixth decade. Kidney transplantation gives normal life expectancy.

HEPATIC CYSTIC SYNDROME
See Caroli's.

INFANTILE, ADOLESCENT TYPE
Symptoms. Both sexes equally affected. Bleeding from esophageal varices is presenting manifestation.

Signs. Splenomegaly.

Etiology. Unknown; variant of polycystic disease. Other cysts usually present (including kidney) are clinically subordinate. Autosomal dominant.

Pathology. *Liver.* Connective tissue proliferation in periportal spaces; ductules more or less ectasic; lobular architecture preserved; hepatic cell normal. *Kidney.* From minimal microcystic dilatation of tubules in the cortex to macroscopic cysts in cortex and medulla.

Diagnostic Procedures. *Blood.* Normal or slight elevation of bilirubin; elevation of phosphatase; serum glutamic-oxalacetic transaminase (SGOT); serum glutamic-pyruvic transaminase (SGPT); moderate decrease of prothrombin. Normal sodium sulfobromophthalein (Bromsulphalein) excretion. *Biopsy of liver.* See Pathology. *Urography.* From normal to polycystic pattern. Increase of portal pressure.

Therapy. Portacaval shunt well supported. Liver transplantation attempted.

Prognosis. Fair with treatment.

ADULT TYPE

Symptoms. Dyspepsia; abdominal pain; hemorrhages from esophageal varices.

Signs. Massive hepatomegaly; splenomegaly.

Etiology. See Infantile, adolescent type.

Pathology. See Infantile, adolescent type.

Diagnostic Procedures. See Infantile, adolescent type.

Therapy. See Infantile, adolescent type.

Prognosis. See Infantile, adolescent type.

BIBLIOGRAPHY. Poinso R, Mouges H, Payan H: La maladie kystique du foi. Expansion Scientifique Francaise, 1954

Wilcox RG, Isselbacker KJ: Chronic liver disease in young people. Am J Med 30:185–195, 1961

Clermont RJ, Maillard JN, Benhamon JP et al: Fibrose hepatique congenitale. Can Med Assoc J 97:1272–1278, 1967

Bear JC, McManamon P, Morgan J et al: Age at clinical onset and at ultrasonographic detection of adult polycystic kidney disease: Data for genetic counseling. Am J Med Genet 18:45–53, 1984

POLYFIBROMATOSIS

See Dupuytren's contracture. Association of Dupuytren's contracture (see) with other fibromatoses: knuckle pads; keloid scarring; Duplay's (see), Peyronie's (see).

Etiology. Genetically determined syndrome.

POLYMER FUME FEVER

Symptoms. Occur several hours after exposure to fumes of heated polymer. Severe cold symptoms; rigor; shaking of limbs; headache; sore throat.

Signs. None or mild reddening of throat.

Etiology. Inhalation of fumes of pyrolysis of polytetrafluoroethylene (Teflon–fluon). Particles contaminating cigarettes of people smoking when handling these chemicals may be responsible.

Therapy. None; avoidance of exposure to fumes and smoking when handling these chemicals.

Prognosis. Symptoms disappear spontaneously within a few hours.

BIBLIOGRAPHY. Harris DK: Polymer-fume fever. Lancet 2:1008–1011, 1951

Barnes R, Jones AT: Polymer-fume fever. Med J Aust 2:60–61, 1967

Hamilton A, Hardy HL: Industrial Toxicology, 3rd ed, p 331. Acton (Mass.) Publishing Group, 1974

Sax NI: Dangerous Properties of Industrial Materials, 6th ed, p 2500. New York, Van Nostrand Reinhold, 1984

POLYMYALGIA RHEUMATICA

Synonyms. Anarthritic rheumatoid; anarthritic; Barber's (HS); Bargantum's; Bruce's; Forestier–Certonciny; myalgic syndrome of aged; *pseudopolyarthrite rhizomelique;* senile arthritis.

Symptoms. Affects mostly elderly persons; onset acute or insidious. Pain and stiffness of the shoulder and hip girdle; occasionally, severe and incapacitating. Fatigue, anorexia, weight loss, and fever. Horton's syndrome frequently associated.

Signs. Muscular stiffness and tenderness; absence of joint deformity.

Etiology. Unknown; the diagnosis is based mostly on negative criteria (absence of a definitive alternative diagnosis and exclusion of definitive and probable rheumatoid arthritis, see Diagnostic procedures). Is strongly contested by many rheumatologists who considered the association of pain, fatigue, elevated sedimentation rate, and good response to steroid inadequate criteria to define a clinically separate entity from the fibrositis syndrome. Recent interpretations tend to identify this syndrome with that of Horton's.

Pathology. No specific changes in muscle biopsy. Possible association of arteritis (see Horton's syndrome).

Diagnostic Procedures. *Blood.* High sedimentation rate; absence of rheumatoid factor and LE cells. *Biopsy of skin, muscle, mucosa.* Normal.

Therapy. Good response to corticosteroids and to phenylbutazone.

Prognosis. Duration of symptoms 6 months to 6 years. Complete recovery; possibility of recurrences.

BIBLIOGRAPHY. Bruce W: College of GP Research Newsletter (9:157); Brit Med J 2:811, 1888

Forestier J, Certonciny A: Pseudopolyarthrite rhizomelique. Rev Rheum (Paris) 20:854–862, 1953

Barber HS: Myalgic syndrome with constitutional effects. Polymyalgia rheumatica. Ann Rheum Dis 16:230–237, 1957

How J, Hirst PJ, Bewsher PD et al: Familial polymyalgia rheumatica. Scot Med J 26:59–61, 1981

Healey LA, Polymyalgia rheumatica and the America Rheumatism Association criteria for rheumatoid arthritis. Arthritis Rheum 26:1417–18, 1983

POLYMYOSITIS SYNDROMES

Synonym. Idiopathic polymyositis. See Wagner–Unverricht.

Symptoms. Common to all groups: symmetric muscle weakness (more frequently affecting proximal muscle), shoulder girdle first group to be affected; tenderness; occasionally, increased consistency; occasionally, progression to fibrotic contractures. Frequently, associated are the Raynaud's phenomenon and dysphagia.

Signs. Tendon reflex may be lost when severely affected.
Group 1. A. Acute. More frequent in young people (1–20 yr). B. Subacute. I: in childhood; chronic; II: early adult life; chronic; III: "late life" muscular dystrophy.
Group 2. Polymyositis dominant feature; associated connective tissue diseases minor clinical role.
Group 3. Polymyositis minor feature, associated connective tissues diseases major role.
Group 4. Polymyositis associated with carcinoma.

Etiology. Unknown.

Pathology. Common feature of the polymyositis is acute or subacute degeneration of muscle fibers with variable inflammatory changes.

Diagnostic Procedures. *Biopsy of muscle. Electromyography. Blood.* LE test; rheumatoid test; sedimentation rate; blood enzymes.

Therapy. Adrenal corticoids. Treatment of associated conditions when present.

Prognosis. Very variable; a few cases of acute form have resulted in death. Usually, chronic course with or without muscle atrophy or contractures. When associated with carcinoma, excision of tumor may be followed by disappearance of myositic symptoms.

BIBLIOGRAPHY. Wagner E: Fall einer seltnen Muskelkrankheit. Arch Heilkunde 4:282–283, 1863
Adams RD, Victor M: Principles of Neurology, 3rd ed, pp 1034–1035. New York, McGraw-Hill, 1985

POLYNEUROPATHY FAMILIAL RECURRENT

Synonyms. Neuropathy hereditary; pressure palsies tomaculous neuropathy; bulbs digger palsy; see Jacob's (J.C.) (different condition).

Symptoms. Both sexes. Male more severely affected, onset at ages 15 to 20 years. After kneeling or exercising pressure in other areas of the body, attacks of pain, weakness or transient palsies of selected groups of muscle (peroneal or arms and hands) sometimes, muscle-wasting after repeated attacks. In addition to peroneal and brachial also lower cranial nerves may be affected.

Etiology. Unknown. Autosomal dominant inheritance trait.

Pathology. In the myelin sheath sausage-shaped swelling (tomaculous).

BIBLIOGRAPHY. Davies DM: Recurrent peripheral nerve palsies in a family. Lancet II: 266–268, 1954
Fewings JD, Mukherjee TM, Blumbergs PC et al: Tomaculous neuropathy: Hereditary predisposition to pressure palsies. Aust NZJ Med 15:598–603, 1985

POLYPOSIS COLI JUVENILE

Synonyms. Juvenile polyposis coli; retention polyposis; solitary polyps rectum–colon. Familial discrete polyposis, juvenile familial polyposis coli, including polyposis intestinal IV (Wolff's).

Symptoms and Signs. Slightly prevalent in young boys. Blood from anus or stool streaking; diarrhea (occasionally); constipation (rare).

Etiology. Unknown; autosomal dominant trait. Affected member of a family always shows this type of polyposis and never intestinal polyposis familial (see).

Pathology. Single or several polyps of colon. Prominent stroma; abundant vascular tissue; mononuclear infiltration; frequent eosinophils. Proliferation mucous glands and cysts with mucus.

Diagnostic Procedures. *Sigmoidoscopy. Barium enema.*

Therapy. Complete local excision; endoscopic excision.

Prognosis. Excellent; malignant potentiality of such polyps is low; however, there are several reports of older relatives over 40 years of age who had colonic cancer. Removal of polyps cures the condition.

BIBLIOGRAPHY. Woolf CM, Richards RC, Gardner EJ: Occasional discrete polyps of colon and rectum showing inherited tendency in kindred. Cancer 8:403–408, 1955
Veale AM, McColl I, Bussey HJR et al: Juvenile polyposis coli. J Med Genet 3:5–6, 1966
Rozen P, Baratz M: Familial juvenile colonic polyposis with associated colon cancer. Cancer 49:1500–1503, 1982

POLYSPLENIA

Symptoms and Signs. Prevalent in females. Signs related to (possibly) associated lung and cardiac malformations.

Etiology. Unknown. Suggested identity of this syndrome with Ivemark (see). Family occurrence reported with possible autosomal recessive inheritance.

Pathology. Accessory spleens vary from two to six or more. Associated bilateral, bilobed (left) lungs with symmetric bilateral left bronchi; bilateral morphologic left atria; bilateral superior vena cava with atrial and ventricular defects.

Diagnostic Procedures. *Blood.* Occasionally, presence of Howell–Jolly and Heinz bodies. *CT scan.*

Therapy. Correction of associated cardiac defect when indicated.

Prognosis. Variable.

BIBLIOGRAPHY. Moller JH, Nekib A, Anderson RC et al: Congenital cardiac disease associated with polysplenia. Circulation 36:789–799, 1967
Rose V, Izukawa I, Moes CAF et al: Syndromes of asplenia and polysplenia. A review of cardiac and non cardiac malformations in 60 cases with special reference to diagnosis and prognosis. Br Heart J 37:840–852, 1975
De la Monte SM, Hutchins GM: Sisters with polysplenia. Am J Med Genet 21:171–173, 1985

POMPE'S

Synonyms. Acid maltase deficiency; Alpha-1, 4-glucoside deficiency; Cori's type II glycogenosis; generalized glycogenosis; glycogenosis (type II). Four clinical varieties are recognizable according to the degree of involvement of different organs, although overlapping of symptoms and signs occur:
1. Cardiomegalic variety
2. Generalized variety
3. Muscular variety
4. Late infantile acid maltase deficiency variety.

CARDIOMEGALIC, GENERALIZED, AND MUSCULAR VARIETIES

Symptoms. Both sexes affected; clinical onset in first month of life. Vomiting; anorexia; drooling; profound weakness; failure to thrive. Severe mental retardation (may be present); repeated respiratory infections. Later, dyspnea.

Signs. Severe muscle hypotonia; macroglossia (occasional); cardiomegaly (of various degrees). Apical systolic murmur present; hepatosplenomegaly absent. Various neurologic defects (generalized variety). Later, cyanosis.

Etiology. Autosomal recessive inheritance. Absence of lysosomal alpha-1, 4-glucosidase activity.

Pathology. Generalized glycogen accumulation in heart, muscles, central and peripheral nervous systems, reticuloendothelial system, kidney, liver, adrenal glands.

Diagnostic Procedures. *Blood.* Normal; leukocytes reveal massive glycogen deposits, absence of alpha-1, 4-glucosidase activity. Blood sugar, glucose, and galactose tolerance; glucagon and epinephrine response normal. *X-ray.* Globular heart enlargement. *Electrocardiography. Electromyography. Biopsy of muscle.* Enzymes studies.

Therapy. Trial with vitamin A (to increase lysis of lysosomes).

Prognosis. Death within 1 year.

LATE INFANTILE ACID MALTASE DEFICIENCY SYNDROME

Symptoms and Signs. Clinical onset later than preceding forms. Weakness of hip muscles; Gower's signs. Contraction of Achilles tendons; muscles firm and rubbery; anal sphincter may be patulous; defective bladder contraction. Mental retardation or normal development.

Etiology. See above.

Pathology. Muscle fibers vacuolated (glycogen deposits); liver glycogen concentration normal; no gross cardiac abnormalities. Glycogen deposit in anterior horn cells of sacral cord.

Diagnostic Procedures. *Biopsy of muscle and liver.* Lack of acid maltase. *Electromyography. Blood.* Leukocytes; absence of alpha-1, 4-glucosidase activity.

Therapy. Trial with vitamin A. Epinephrine injections over long period.

Prognosis. This variant allows survival beyond infancy.

BIBLIOGRAPHY. Pompe JC: Over idiopatischehypertrophie von het hart. Ned Tidjdschr Geneeskd 76:304–305, 1932
Roth CJ, Williams HE: The muscular variant of Pompe's disease. J Pediatr 71:567–573, 1967
Swaiman KF, Kennedy WR, Sauls HS: Late infantile acid maltase deficiency. Arch Neurol 18:642–648, 1968
Howell RR, Williams JC: The glycogen storage diseases. In Stanbury JB, Wyngaarden JB, Fredrickson DS et al: The Metabolic Basis of Inherited Disease, 5th ed, p 141. New York, McGraw-Hill, 1983

POMPHOLYX

Synonyms. Cheiropompholyx; dyshidrosis.

Symptoms. Both sexes affected; onset after 10 years of age; maximal incidence between 20 and 40 years. Intense itching, usually limited to palms or soles bilaterally or unilaterally. Attacks are precipitated by such factors as warm weather, stress.

Signs. Sudden appearance of crops of vesicles, which may become confluent in bullae. After repeated attacks, dystrophic nail changes.

Etiology. Form of hyperhidrosis or dyshidrosis; emotional stress is frequently the precipitating factor. In some cases, fungus infection has been proven; in other cases, focal infection, food allergies have been suspected.

Pathology. Eczemalike changes.

Diagnostic Procedures. Evaluation of possible etiologic factors.

Therapy. Soaking in normal saline opens larger bullae; if infection, antibiotics. Mild sedatives helpful.

Prognosis. Recurrent condition, every 2 to 3 weeks for months or years, or only in warm weather. Recovery if sporadic irregular attacks.

BIBLIOGRAPHY. Simons RDGP: Eczema of the Hand, 2nd ed. Basel, Karger, 1966
Rook A, Wilkinson DS, Ebling FJG et al: Textbook of Dermatology, 4th ed, pp 394–398. Oxford, Blackwell Scientific Publications, 1986

POPLITEAL ARTERY ENTRAPMENT

Synonyms. See Peroneal compartment and anterior tibial compartment syndromes.

Symptoms. Rare; prevalent in young males; onset at an average of 24 to 26 years of age. Intermittent unilateral claudication; pain relieved by standing still or sitting; paresthesias when sitting with sharply flexed knee. Absence of signs of generalized atherosclerosis. During crisis, absence of dorsalis pedis pulse, weakness of the posterior tibial pulse. Feet skin throphic conditions good. Various types of congenital anomalies may be associated.

Etiology. Entrapment of popliteal artery in relation to medial head of gastrocnemius muscle, generally due to congenital anomaly.

Pathology. Artery loops medially to the medial head of gastrocnemius, instead of passing between lateral and medial heads. Medial head of muscle may be attached in anomalous fashion to the femur. Intermittent compression causes thrombosis and sclerosis or aneurysm of popliteal artery. Early arteriosclerotic muscle changes.

Diagnostic Procedures. *Blood.* Normal. *Electrocardiography.* Normal. *Arteriography.* Medial deviation of popliteal artery and, possibly, collateral circulation. *Oscillometry.* Normal tracing on inferior third of leg when foot is forced in plantar hyperextension.

Therapy. Surgical correction to bypass or reconstruct vessel and remove cause of compression.

Prognosis. Good with proper treatment.

BIBLIOGRAPHY. Stuart TPA: Note on a variation in the course of popliteal artery. J Anat 13:162–165, 1879
Turner GR, Gosney WG, Ellingson W et al: Popliteal artery entrapment syndrome. JAMA 208:692–693; 1969
Justis EJ Jr: Traumatic disorders. In Crenshaw AH (ed): Campbell's Operative Orthopedics, 7th ed, p 2223. St Louis, CV Mosby, 1987

POPLITEAL PTERYGIUM

Synonyms. Cleft palate-popliteal web–lip pit–genital; faciogenitopopliteal; "quadruple." See Bartsocas–Papas.

Symptoms and Signs. Present at birth. Intrafamilial variability of manifestations. Normal intelligence. Usually, bilateral pterygium or skin web that extends from heel to ischial tuberosity, limiting extension, abduction, and rotation of legs. Syndactyly of toes and fingers; bony malformations of legs. Club feet; toenail dysplasia. Orofacial cleft lip-palate; lip pits; oral webbing; fused eyelids. Genital-perineal anomalies. Cryptorchidism; cleft scrotum; inguinal hernia; absence of labia majora.

Etiology. Unknown; autosomal dominant inheritance with incomplete penetrance and variable expressivity.

Pathology. Pterygium formed by a hard nonelastic subcutaneous cord. Sciatic nerve is free within pterygium covered by a fibromuscular septum. Absence of muscle groups or abnormal insertions. See Symptoms and Signs.

Diagnostic Procedures. *X-ray. Chromosome studies.* Pattern normal.

Therapy. Surgical correction.

Prognosis. Depends on extent of lesions.

BIBLIOGRAPHY. Trélat V: Sur un vice conformation trésrare de la lévre inférieure. J Med Chir Prat 40:442–445, 1869
Gorlin RJ, Sedano HO, Cervenka J: Popliteal pterygium syndrome. Pediatrics 41:503–509, 1968
Bartsocas CS, Papas CV: Popliteal pterygium syndrome. J Med Genet 9:222–226, 1972
Pashayan HM, Lewis MB: A family with the popliteal pterygium syndrome. Cleft Palate J 17:48–51, 1980

PORPHYRIA CUTANEA TARDA

Synonyms. Acquired hepatic porphyria (misnomer); constitutional porphyria (misnomer); symptomatic porphyria (misnomer); latent porphyria; porphyria hepatica III: PCT.

Symptoms and Signs. Highest incidence in Bantu population. Both sexes affected (diagnosed more frequently in men); onset usually between 40 to 60 years of age, seldom in childhood. Insidious onset. Increased facial pigmentation; intermittent excretion of brown urine; increased skin fragility (in light-exposed areas). Spontaneous eruption of vesicular and then ulcerative lesions on face, neck, extremities, slowly healing and with residual scarring. Hypertricosis of forehead, malar areas, and extremities. Variable sensory neuropathy. Absence of motor disorders; dysreflexia; muscle wasting.

Etiology. Considered until recently an acquired condition, secondary to liver (alcoholic) injury. Today considered an autosomal dominant inheritance, with clinical expression secondary to liver injury. Reduced hepatic uroporphyrinogen decarboxylase (URO) activity a common defect in all members of affected families.

Pathology. *Liver.* Evidence of hepatic siderosis; cirrhosis; high concentration of porphyrins; increased liver iron. *Skin.* Scarring from repeated lesions.

Diagnostic Procedures. *Urine.* Color pink or brown; pink fluorescence after acidification; high excretion of uroporphyrin (mostly isomer type I). *Stool.* Variable excretion of porphyrin.

Therapy. Serial phlebotomy; desferrioxamine. Avoidance of ethanol intake.

Prognosis. Spontaneous remission possible (especially after alcohol abstinence). Prognosis good, but, following therapy, remission is temporary. Final outcome not related to porphyria but to cirrhosis and other coexisting pathology.

BIBLIOGRAPHY. Waldenström J: Studien ueber Porphiria. Acta Med Scand (Suppl) 82:1–254, 1937
Kushner JP, Barbuto AJ, Lee GR: An inherited enzymatic defect in porphyria cutanea tarda. Decreased uroporphyrinogen decarboxylase activity. J Clin Invest 56:661–667, 1976
Kappas A, Sassa S, Anderson KE: The porphyrias. In Stanbury JB, Wyngaarden JB, Fredrickson DS et al: The Metabolic Basis of Inherited Disease, 5th ed, p 1301. New York, McGraw-Hill, 1983

PORTER'S

Synonym. Idiopathic benign pericarditis.

Symptoms. Observed at all ages; prevalent in young adult males. Upper respiratory infection precedes, by 1 or 2 weeks, the acute onset of the syndrome. Acute pain in the chest, radiating widely, especially to neck and shoulders; more acute during deep respiration, cough, and sometimes swallowing. Recumbency increases the pain, sitting up decreases it. Cough; dyspnea; fever.

Signs. Pericardial rub; enlarged heart area. Frequently, pleurisy with effusion and pneumonitis are associated.

Etiology. Relationship with virus infection (Coxsackie B) proved only in a certain number of cases. Autoimmune reaction also considered a possible mechanism. In some cases, gout has been observed and considered in the etiology.

Pathology. Pericardial effusion with straw-colored or hemorrhagic fluid.

Diagnostic Procedures. *Blood.* Moderate leukocytosis; increased sedimentation rate. *Electrocardiography.* No destructive changes; sometimes simulates acute myocardial infarction. *Pericardiocentesis. X-ray of chest. Echocardiography.*

Therapy. Analgesic and rest often adequate. In severe cases, rapid response to corticosteroids. Pericardiocentesis seldom necessary.

Prognosis. Benign; cardiac tamponade, however, may occur and subside spontaneously in a few weeks. Multiple recurrences frequent, especially when corticosteroids are withheld.

BIBLIOGRAPHY. Hodges RM: Idiopathic pericarditis. Boston Med Surg J 51:140–141, 1854
Porter WB, Clark O, Porter RR: Nonspecific benign pericarditis. JAMA 144:749–753, 1950
Shabetai R: Diseases of pericardium. In Hurst JW: The Heart, 6th ed, p 1249. New York, McGraw-Hill, 1986

POSTABORTIVE METRORRHAGIA

Synonym. Functional postabortive metrorrhagia.

Symptoms. Vaginal bleeding occurring in the reproductive period of women after either a clinical or unsuspected abortion.

Signs. Signs of early pregnancy (*i.e.,* enlarged uterus, soft cervix) and blood clot in vagina.

Etiology. Due to the persistence of chorionic villi with a variable degree of viability, most often identified by histologic examination. The slowly regressing corpus luteum maintains an estrogen–progesterone imbalance leading to hyperestrinism and disturbance of menstrual rhythm.

Pathology. *Ovaries.* (Findings are not consistent.) Small with degenerative corpora lutea; normal size with cystic or degenerative corpora lutea; enlarged with cystic corpora lutea; normal or enlarged with multiple atretic follicles. *Endometrium.* Hyperplasia.

Diagnostic Procedures. Estimation of gonadotropin in urine and blood is not helpful and is negative in the conventional concentration (2000–100,000 IU/liter). It is possible that minute amounts are present, and are detectable only by special techniques.

Therapy. Curettage is curative.

Prognosis. Good after curettage.

BIBLIOGRAPHY. Aschoff L: Tratado de Anatomia Pathologica, Vol 11, p 927. Barcelona, Labor, 1934
Botella–Llusia J, Nogales–Ortiz F, Matinez H et al: Postabortive functional metrorrhagia: A clinical and histopathologic study. Am J Obstet Gynecol 100:987–996, 1968

POSTCARDIOTOMY, DIPHASIC

This syndrome, occurring after heart surgery, runs a diphasic course. A first phase a few days after surgery characterized by fever and unusual lesions of the mouth (nonulcerative, small, painful induration) disappearing in 2 weeks. A second phase occurs after 3 to 6 weeks with hepatosplenomegaly, pleural and pericardial friction rubs with a benign course but long lasting (months). This syndrome seems to represent a combination of the postperfusion syndrome (see), and the postpericardiotomy syndrome (see).

BIBLIOGRAPHY. Kahn DR, Ertel PY, Murphy WH et al: Pathogenesis of the postcardiotomy syndrome. J Thorac Cardiovasc Surg 54:682–687, 1968
Hurst JW: The Heart, 6th ed, p 1276. New York, McGraw-Hill, 1986

POSTCHOLECYSTECTOMY

Synonyms. Recurrent biliary tract; cholecystectomized painful tomorrow.

Symptoms. Recurrence of same symptoms present before operation, or postoperative occurrence of symptoms such as colicky pain, bloating, nausea, vomiting.

Signs. Pain on palpation of right upper quadrant; sometimes, jaundice.

Etiology and Pathology. Mechanisms of much different natures cause this syndrome. They may be classified in three groups. (1) Unrelated to surgery: (a) erroneous diagnosis for previous operation (symptoms of extrabiliary origin); (b) concomitant pathology (liver, pancreas, neoplasia, stenosis of Oddi's sphincter, stenosing choledo-

chitis, cholangitis). (2) Postoperative sequelae: (a) common duct injury or calculi; (b) intrahepatic calculi; (c) cystic duct or gallbladder remnant; (d) adhesion; (e) removal of functioning gallbladder. (3) Functional biliary disorders.

Diagnostic Procedures. *X-ray. Liver and pancreatic function studies.*

Therapy. According to etiology.

Prognosis. Variable according to diagnosis and further treatment.

BIBLIOGRAPHY. Meyers SG, Sandweiss DJ, Saltzstein HC: End results after gallbladder operations. Am J Dig Dis 5:667–674, 1938
Roth JLA, Berk JE: Symptoms after cholecystectomy (postcholecystectomy syndrome). In Bockus HL: Gastroenterology, 3rd ed, Vol III, p 900–913. Philadelphia, WB Saunders, 1976
Roberts-Thomson IC, Pannall PR, Toouli S: Relationship between morphine responses and sphincter of Oddi motility in undefined biliary pain after cholecystectomy. J Gastroenterol Hepatol 4:316–324, 1989

POSTCOARCTATION

Symptoms. Occur following surgery for resection of coarcted aorta segment. On second postoperative day, anorexia, increased temperature. On fourth day, abdominal pain, vomiting.

Signs. From eighth day, signs of mild peritoneal irritation. Exploration shows petechiae diffused over small bowel. Delayed hypertension (lasting 10 days).

Etiology. Removal of obstructing stenosis subjects vascular bed below coarctation to increased pulse pressure, and greater constant distention of arteries. Vasospasm and ischemia of bowel.

Pathology. Disruption and fragmentation of internal elastic lamina; intimal damage; necrotizing thrombosis; inflammatory reaction.

Therapy. Symptomatic. Prevention of syndrome by control of diastolic blood pressure (sodium nitroprusside, propanolol, reserpine) and insertion of nasogastric tube for decompression of gastrointestinal tract for 48 hours.

Prognosis. Guarded; death from necrotizing mesenteric arteritis or other unrelated postoperative causes.

BIBLIOGRAPHY. Mays ET, Sergeant CK: Postcoarctectomy syndrome. Arch Surg 91:58–66, 1965
Fox S, Pierce WS, Waldhausen JA: Pathogenesis of paradoxical hypertension after coarctation repair of the aorta during infancy. Ann Thorac Surg 29:135–141, 1980

Hurst JW: The heart, 6th ed, p 633. New York, Mc-Graw-Hill, 1986

POSTDYSENTERIC

Symptoms. Occur in patients recovered from acute dysenteric infections. Recurrence of episodes of abdominal pain and diarrhea.

Signs. Pain and tenderness predominant in lower right abdominal quadrant (in postamebic syndrome) on left side (in postbacillary syndrome).

Etiology. Loss of resistance of bowel to irritation and psychogenic influences are postulated after ruling out residual or recurrent infection.

Pathology. Atrophic changes and ulceration sometimes observed.

Diagnostic Procedures. *Stool.* Function and culture studies. *X-ray of bowel. Gastric analysis.*

Therapy. Symptomatic.

Prognosis. Symptoms may gradually disappear or persist for many years.

BIBLIOGRAPHY. Fierst SM, Werner A: Postdysenteric syndrome. Gastroenterology 27:281–291, 1954

POSTERIOR FOSSA COMPRESSION

Symptoms and Signs. Patient collapses, respiration stops, heart continues to beat vigorously, cyanosis develops, and heart eventually stops. Artificial respiration restores the heartbeat.

Etiology and Pathology. Increased tension into posterior fossa: hemorrhage from fracture of the base of skull, tumor, or abscess. Greater vulnerability of respiratory center than of cardioinhibitory center.

Therapy. Artifical respiration and prompt surgical relief of posterior fossa hypertension.

Prognosis. Lack of prompt surgical intervention is followed by death. Surgical intervention relieves the condition and offers the possibility of dealing with its determining cause.

BIBLIOGRAPHY. Rogers L: The posterior fossa compression syndrome. Br Med J 2:100–101, 1933

POSTGASTRECTOMY DUMPING SYNDROMES

Synonyms. Postcibal; postcibal hypoglycemia. Dumping.

EARLY POSTPRANDIAL DUMPING SYNDROME

Symptoms and Signs. Onset immediately after a meal or within 20 to 30 minutes. Occur in 20% to 30% of gastrectomized patients. Some patients have symptoms with every meal; some only with heavy meal or with only a single meal during the day. Excessive fullness; sometimes nausea and vomiting. Borborygmi and sudden diarrhea. Vasomotor symptoms: weakness; palpitation; pallor; sweating; sometimes, syncope.

Etiology. In gastrectomized patient, rapid filling of jejunum with undigested, hyperosmotic food solution. Other mechanism also postulated.

Diagnostic Procedures. *Blood.* Hyperglycemia coinciding with onset of symptoms; somewhat later, slight potassium and phosphorus fall in the plasma and electrocardiographic changes.

Therapy. Individualized according to severity of symptoms. Dietary planning (small feeding; low-carbohydrate, fat-rich diet). Recumbent position after eating or surgical reintervention.

Prognosis. Good in majority of cases.

LATE DUMPING SYNDROME

Symptoms. Occur in gastrectomized patients 2 to 3 hours after a meal. Symptoms of hypoglycemia (see Hypoglycemic syndromes).

Etiology. Hypoglycemia following a sharp rise of postprandial blood sugar and exaggerated pancreas response.

Therapy. Symptoms relieved by food. Dietary planning or surgical reintervention.

Prognosis. Good.

BIBLIOGRAPHY. Denecheau D: Les suites médicales éloignées de la gastroenterostomie au cours de l'ulcère de l'estomac et de ses complications. Thèses de Paris, 1907; Semaine Méd 27:316–322, 1907
Meyer JH: Chronic morbidity after ulcer surgery. In Sleisenger HM, Fordtran JS (eds): Gastrointestinal disease, 3rd ed, p 757–779. Philadelphia, WB Saunders, 1983
Caufild M, Willie R, Firor HV, Mickener W: Dumping syndrome in children. J Pediatr 110:212–215, 1987

POSTGONOCOCCAL URETHRITIS

Synonym. PGU.

Symptoms and Signs. Occur usually within 20 days of treatment with penicillin and probenecid for gonorrheal urethritis, with no possibility of heterosexual reinfection. Recurrence of urethral exudate or pyuria. Syndrome seldom occurs in patient whose gonorrhea was treated with tetracycline.

Etiology. Associated to a significant degree with mycoplasma infection of the urethra.

Pathology. Mild urethritis.

Diagnostic Procedures. *Smear and cultures of urethral exudate.*

Therapy. Tetracycline.

Prognosis. Cured by tetracycline.

BIBLIOGRAPHY. Shepard MC, Alexander CE Jr, Lunceford CD et al: Possible role of T-strain mycoplasma in nongonococcal urethritis: A sixth venereal disease? JAMA 188:729–735, 1964
Treatment of sexually transmitted diseases. (editorial) Med Let Drugs Ther 28:21, 1986

POSTHEPATITIS

Synonyms. Prolonged hepatitis; convalescent hepatitis.

Symptoms. Onset after an average of 56 days of disease, 85% of patients with viral hepatitis recover completely. The remaining 15% experience different complications. The majority of cases present persistent lassitude, fatigue, depression, sleep disturbances, anorexia, incompatibility for fatty foods, weight loss, and pain in upper right quadrant.

Signs. Subicterus; slight, tender hepatomegaly.

Etiology. Sequelae of viral hepatitis. The rare cases where subacute yellow atrophy or postnecrotic cirrhosis (see Marchand's) occur must be excluded from this diagnosis.

Pathology. In the majority of cases, completely normal liver parenchyma; in about 15% of these cases, transition to chronic hepatitis (persistent inflammatory reaction and fibrosis).

Diagnostic Procedures. *Blood.* All tests revert to normal except for a moderate persistent hyperbilirubinemia (indirect reacting fraction); slight elevation of serum cholesterol. *Stool.* Moderate steatosis. *Biopsy of liver.* See Pathology.

Therapy. Symptomatic; diet; multivitamins.

Prognosis. Majority recover completely within a few months; in about 15% (2% of total hepatitis group) transition to chronic liver diseases (chronic hepatitis, chronic persistent hepatitis, chronic active hepatitis: lupoid type, Hbs Ag-positive type, delta agent, non A, non B type, etc). Transition to chronic form higher in elderly female patients.

BIBLIOGRAPHY. Caravati CM: Posthepatitis syndrome. South Med J 37:251–257, 1944
Weissberg JI, Andres LL, Smith CI et al: Survival in chronic hepatitis B: An analysis of 379 patients. Ann Intern Med 101:613–616, 1984
Rugge M, Brollo L, Pontisso P et al: Clinical virological and histologic outcome following seroconversions from HB e Ag to anti-HBe in chronic hepatitis type B. Hepatology 6:167–172, 1986

POSTHERPETIC

Synonym. Neuralgia postherpetica.

Symptoms and Signs. Occur in patients (especially elderly ones) after herpes zoster infections. Paresthesia; itching; pain of area affected; spontaneous or following change in temperature.

Etiology. Degenerative changes and incomplete regeneration of nerves.

Therapy. Cazbamazepine (Tegretol), amitriptyline and perphenazine, useful. Analgesics (poor results). Interruption of pain fibers.

BIBLIOGRAPHY. Bannister R: Brain's Clinical Neurology, III ed, p 291. London, Oxford University Press, 1969
Adams RD, Victor M: Principles of Neurology, 3rd ed, pp 551–553. New York, McGraw-Hill, 1985

POSTHYPOXIC SYNDROMES

To severe hypoxia a combination or overlapping of the following syndromes may result:
1. Persistent coma or stupor
2. Dementia
3. Visual agnosia
4. Parkinsonism with mental deterioration
5. Choreoathetosis
6. Cerebellar ataxia
7. Epilepsy
8. Impairment of memory and of recent facts acquisition

BIBLIOGRAPHY. Adams RD, Victor M: Principles of Neurology, 3rd ed, pp 790, 868. New York, McGraw-Hill, 1985

POSTIRRADIATION VASCULAR INSUFFICIENCY

Symptoms and Signs. Occur following (remotely), radiation therapy, especially after treatment of acromegaly by radiation of pituitary. Symptoms of vascular obstruction with hemiparesis and other signs of reduced or arrested circulation in area involved.

Etiology. Radiation vascular changes. See also Radiation, acute.

Pathology. Not specific; changes of vessels involved; segmental lesions; thickening and fibrosis of vessel wall with marked endothelial proliferation.

Diagnostic Procedure. *Arteriography.*

Therapy. Anticoagulant.

Prognosis. Guarded.

BIBLIOGRAPHY. Darmondy WR, Thomas LM, Gurdjian ES: Postirradiation vascular insufficiency syndrome. Neurology 17:1190–1192, 1967

POSTOBSTRUCTIVE DIURESIS

Synonym. Water-losing nephritis.

Symptoms and Signs. Occur 24 or more hours after removal of obstruction from urinary tract. Generally mild and physiologic diuresis, resulting from the correction of the established imbalances; in several cases, however, a "pathologic" diuresis occurs and may last for weeks or longer, causing dehydration, electrolyte imbalance, and hypotension. In the initial phase, hemorrhages from the bladder walls are frequently seen.

Etiology. Defect of sodium reabsorption, causing a solute diuresis; defect in water reabsorption; cellular lack of response to vasopressin.

Diagnostic Procedures. *Blood.* Electrolytes; osmolarity; hematocrit. *Urine.* Volume; electrolytes; osmolarity. *Body weight.* Loss.

Therapy. Fluid and electrolyte balance.

Prognosis. Usually, spontaneous resolution; in some cases, it may be a life threatening event and last weeks or longer.

BIBLIOGRAPHY. Howard SS: Postobstructive diuresis: A misunderstood phenomenon. J Urol 110:537–745, 1973

POSTPARTUM BLUES

Synonyms. Postpartum dysphoria; milk fever; milk blues; postpartum psychosis; puerperium depression (50–70% of parturients); third day blues.

Symptoms. Brief crying episodes, without obvious precipitating factors, not associated with feeling of depression. Usually starting the third day postpartum and ending at the tenth day. Fatigue; increased irritability; sleep disturbances; restlessness; feeling of estrangement from the husband and undue concern for the baby. In other cases the baby is rejected as not belonging.

Etiology. Unknown; stressful psychological factors; endocrine factors. Altered target organ function (failure of alpha adrenoceptor capacity to fall after delivery). In some cases pregnancy and delivery may precipitate a pre-existing manic depressive condition or prepsychotic schizoid personality.

Therapy. Seldom requires treatment. It has been reported that administration of estrogen for suppression of lactation prevents postpartum depression. In few cases severe form may require electroconvulsive treatment.

Prognosis. Relatively benign self-limited condition: 2 of 1000 women develop psychosis after delivery. Instances of infanticide have been reported.

BIBLIOGRAPHY. Marcè LV: Traite de la follie des femmes enceintes, de nouvelles accouchèes des nourices. Paris Ballière 1858
Savage G: Observation on the insanity of pregnancy and childbirth. Guy's Hosp Rep 20:83–117, 1875
Yalom ID, Lunde DT, Moos RH et al: "Post-partum blues" syndrome; A description and related variables. Arch Gen Psychiatry 18:16–17, 1968
Adams RD, Victor M: Principles of Neurology, 3rd ed, pp 1153–1154. New York, McGraw-Hill, 1985
Swyer GIM: Postpartum mental disturbances and hormone changes. Br Med J 290:1232–1233, 1985

POSTPERFUSION

Synonym. Postcardiotomy lymphocytic splenomegaly.

Symptoms. Occur in young patients operated on for cardiac disease, using cardiopulmonary bypass technique; onset 2 to 4 weeks after surgery. Fever; absence of chest pain and of definite malaise.

Signs. Splenomegaly (70%); exudative transient pharyngitis (5%); shotty lymphadenopathy (20%); hepatomegaly (30%). Anemia and increased bilirubin in some cases. Maculopapular rash.

Etiology. Unknown; possibly, infective viral nature because of apparently seasonal distribution. Leukocyte graft-versus-host reaction (?). Probably due to the Epstein–Barr virus or to the cytomegalovirus from transfused blood.

Pathology. Scanty information; in spleen, decreased follicular pattern. Small follicular germinal centers. Congestion of the pulp. Presence of large mononuclear cells. Irregular structures within the nuclei of these cells (inclusion bodies ?). Bone marrow hyperplasia; liver passive congestion.

Diagnostic Procedures. *Blood.* Cultures (repeated) negative; lymphocytosis (60%) with atypical cells (virocytes). Serum glutamic-oxaloacetic transaminase (SGOT), serum glutamic-pyruvic transaminase, (SGPT) and lactic dehydrogenase (LDH) and mild and transient elevation. *Hepatic function tests.* Abnormal. *Heterophil antibodies.* Moderate elevation or negative.

Therapy. Corticosteroids.

Prognosis. Benign course and spontaneous resolution in 1 to 4 weeks.

BIBLIOGRAPHY. Kreel I, Zaroff LI, Canter JW et al: A syndrome following total body perfusion. Surg Gynecol Obstet 111:317–321, 1961
Reyman TA: Postperfusion syndrome. Am Heart J 72:116–123, 1966
Hurst JW: The Heart, 6th ed, p 954. New York, McGraw-Hill, 1986

POSTPERFUSION LUNG

Synonyms. Pump lung; postperfusion pulmonary vasculitis.

Symptoms. Occur in patients operated on for cardiac disease using cardiopulmonary bypass technique; onset immediately after operation (different from postperfusion syndrome, see). Fever; dyspnea.

Signs. Cyanosis; hypotension; signs of pulmonary edema.

Etiology.
1. Arterial mean pressure decreased during bypass.
2. Anoxia.
3. Reaction to denaturation or destruction of blood elements resulting from turbulence in pumping system.
4. Reaction to protein or proteinlike materials remaining in heart–lung machine from previous perfusion.

Pathology. Lung dark red, congested; zones of collapse and parenchymal hemorrhages; blood in the bronchi. In-travascular polymorphonuclear leukocytosis. In other organs, diffuse hyperemia.

Diagnostic Procedures. *X-ray of chest.* Diffuse clouding of pulmonary fields. *Blood.* Electrolytes.

Therapy. Antibiotic. Corticosteroids. Symptomatic.

Prognosis. Guarded.

BIBLIOGRAPHY. Dodrill FD: The effects of total body perfusion upon the lungs, extracorporeal circulation, p 327. Springfield, CC Thomas, 1958
Neville WE, Kontaxis A, Gavin T et al: Postperfusion vasculitis. Arch Surg 86:126–137, 1963
Hurst JW: The Heart, 6th ed, p 954. New York, McGraw-Hill, 1986

POSTPERICARDIOTOMY

Synonyms. Postcardiotomy; postcommissurotomy. See Dressler's.

Symptoms. Postcardiac operative complication appearing several weeks or months after surgical intervention. Patient usually presents slight constitutional disturbance. Pleuropericardial pain, sometimes sharp, radiated to epigastrium, shoulders, and back; aggravated by change of posture and inspiration. Fever; cough (occasional); muscle and joint pain (occasional).

Signs. Pericardial friction rub; features of pleural (unilateral or bilateral) and pericardial effusion. Signs of congestive heart failure, pulmonary infarction, or thrombosis; peripheral veins are absent.

Etiology. Unknown; possibly, a response to surgical trauma. Following incision of pericardium. Release of autogenous antigen and hypersensitivity reaction(?).

Diagnostic Procedures. *X-ray of chest. Electrocardiography. Blood.* High sedimentation rate; leukocytosis with absolute neutrophilia; occasionally, eosinophilia; occasionally, anemia.

Therapy. Responds to corticosteroids, not to salicylates.

Prognosis. Benign condition, subsiding spontaneously in a few days or weeks. Frequently recurs.

BIBLIOGRAPHY. Soloff LA, Zatuchni J, Janton OH et al: Reactivation of rheumatic fever following mitral commissurotomy. Circulation 8:481–493, 1953
Engle MA, Zabriskie JB, Senterpt LB et al: Viral illness and the postpericardiotomy syndrome. A prospective study in children. Circulation 62:1151–1158, 1980
Hurst JW: The Heart, 6th ed, p1267. New York, McGraw-Hill, 1986

POSTPHLEBITIC

Synonyms. Postphlebitic leg; postthrombotic; venous ulcer; chronic venous insufficiency; ulcus varicosum. See Lower leg stasis.

Symptoms and Signs. Sequelae appearing with 3 to 10 years of episodes of venous thrombosis; affecting mostly females in middle age. Affecting lower extremities, bilaterally in 25% of cases. Swelling, edema, pain on walking, discoloration, sometimes varicose veins, and ulceration.

Etiology. Venous hypertension due to postphlebitic incompetence of communicating veins.

Pathology. *Skin.* Epidermis: low degree of intercellular edema with few lymphocytes and granulocytes. Upper dermis: marked edema of connective tissue; swelling of collagen; fragmentation of elastic fibers; dense inflammatory infiltration (lymphocytes and plasma cells). *Blood vessels.* Thickened and dilated. The incompetent veins present uniform thinning of one half of vein wall and fibrosclerotic thickening of other half.

Diagnostic Procedures. *Serial phlebography. Trendelenburg's test. Perthes' test. Determination of venous pressure. Ultrasonography.*

Therapy. Sympathectomy (only with cyanosis, causalgia); ligatures of popliteal veins; superficial femoral veins; valved venous transplants; grafting of internal saphenous vein.

Prognosis. All surgical measures only palliative, but of considerable benefit when specifically indicated.

BIBLIOGRAPHY. Blalock A: Oxygen content of blood in patients with varicose veins. Arch Surg 19:898–905, 1929
Negus D: Calf pain in the post-thrombotic syndrome. Br Med J 2:156–158, 1968
Rook A, Wilkinson DS, Ebling FJG et al: Textbook of Dermatology, 4th ed, pp 1201–1203. Oxford, Blackwell Scientific Publications, 1986

POSTPHLEBITIC NEUROSIS

Symptoms. Misconception in patient of harboring "clots" that may become free and menace life. Refusal to leave the bed or bear weight or conduct a normal life. Alleged extreme pain and tenderness of the legs.

Etiology. Frequently, iatrogenic. Basic apprehensiveness.

Therapy. Convince patient that danger of embolism has disappeared with recovery.

Prognosis. Frequent conversion to other type of health apprehension.

BIBLIOGRAPHY. Hurst JW: The Heart, 6th ed, p 1887. New York, McGraw-Hill, 1986

POSTURAL

Symptoms. Functional type prevalent in children; structural type present at all ages. Only fatigue and backache (in functional type) or significant back pain (in structural type).

Signs. Increase of cervical lordosis; dorsal spine rounded and motion decreased. Exaggerated lordotic lumbar curve; abdominal muscles relaxed and overstretched; pelvis tilted anteriorly and hip flexors shortened. Increase of lumbosacral angle. When patient bends forward, lumbar curve is not properly obliterated.

Etiology. Functional or structural: frequently, pregnancy and obesity determining or accelerating factors.

Diagnostic Procedures. *X-ray.* Spinous processes and facets in contact with each other; secondary degenerative bone changes.

Therapy. Corrective exercises to increase strength of back and abdominal muscles. Weight loss when obesity. Supporting belt or other orthopedic devices to correct curvature of spine.

Prognosis. Persistence of syndrome leads to vertebral column sprain or, when associated with obesity, to emphysema and cardiorespiratory failure.

BIBLIOGRAPHY. Kerr WJ, Lagen JB: The postural syndrome related to obesity leading to postural emphysema and cardiorespiratory failure. Ann Intern Med 10:569–595, 1936
Kuhns JG: Posture and its relationship to orthopedic disabilities. Ann Arbor, Edward Brothers, 1942

POSTVACCINIAL SYNDROMES

Synonym. Smallpox vaccination complication.

Symptoms.
1. *Accidental infection.* The accidental implantation of vaccinia virus in the eye, mouth, or other parts of the body in the absence of eczema or other preexisting skin disorder.
2. *Generalized vaccinia.* The generalized spread of vaccinial lesions in the absence of eczema or other preexisting skin lesion.
3. *Eczema vaccinia.* The generalized spread of vaccinial lesions or local implantation of vaccinia in a person

who has eczema or a past history of eczema. This person may be the patient who was vaccinated or a contact of someone recently vaccinated.

4. *Vaccinia necrosum (progressive vaccinia)*. Spreading necrosis at the site of vaccination with or without metastatic necrotic lesions occurring elsewhere on the body.

5. *Encephalitis*. Postvaccinial central nervous system involvement including (separately or in combination) the following symptoms: meningeal signs; ataxia; muscular weakness; paralysis; lethargy; coma or convulsions.

6. *Other*. Vaccinial lesions complicating skin conditions other than eczema in addition to miscellaneous complications not listed above, such as generalized urticarial reactions, bullous erythema multiforme, and secondary bacterial infections.

BIBLIOGRAPHY. Rosen E: A postvaccinial syndrome. Am J Ophthalmol 31:1443–1453, 1948
Neff JM, Lane JM, Pert JH et al: Complications of smallpox vaccination. 1. National survey in the United States, 1963. N Engl J Med 276:125–132, 1967
Neff JM, Levine RH, Lane JM et al: Complications of smallpox vaccination in the United States, 1963. II. Results obtained by four statewide surveys. Pediatrics 39:916–923, 1967

POTATO NOSE

Synonym. Nose potato shaped.

Symptoms and Signs. Both sexes. Typical shape of nose. Lack of hypertelorism. Developmental field defect. Autosomal dominant inheritance. Same category of bifid nose (autosomal recessive trait also reported).

BIBLIOGRAPHY. Benjamins CE, Stibbe FH: Sur un cas extraordinaire de difformite congenitale de la pyramide nasale. Acta Otolaryngol 11:274–284, 1927
Toriello HV, Higgins JV, Wallen A et al: Familial occurrence of a developmental defect of the medial nasal processes. Am J Med Genet 21:131–135, 1985

POTTER'S

Synonyms. Bilateral kidney agenesis; dysplasia renofacialis; facial-renal dysplasia; oligohydramnios tetrad; renofacial dysplasia.

Symptoms and Signs. Newborn: low-set and malformed ears, long epicanthal folds, flattened nose bridge, small mandible, renal agenesis, pulmonary hypoplasia. Oligohydramnios and amnion nodosum. Associated skeletal malformations include hands and feet clubbing.

Etiology. Autosomal dominant. This syndrome does not show chromosomal abnormalities, although some syndromes, such as 18 trisomy syndrome, present very similar clinical pattern.

Pathology. Renal agenesis or malformation; typical facial alterations.

Diagnostic Procedures. *Chromosome studies. CT scan.*

Therapy. None.

Prognosis. Live-born but dying in a short time.

BIBLIOGRAPHY. Potter EL: Bilateral renal agenesis. J Pediatr 29:68–76, 1946
Passarge E, Sutherland JM: Potter's syndrome. Am J Dis Child 109:80–84, 1965
Bankier A, De Campo M, Newell R et al: A pedigree study of perinatally lethal renal disease. J Med Genet 22:104–111, 1985

POTT'S I

Synonym. Dupuytren's fracture.

Symptoms and Signs. Pain; swelling; tenderness in affected foot, which results in shortening it.

Etiology. Direct or indirect trauma.

Diagnostic Procedures. *X-ray.* Transverse fracture of medial malleolus, ankle diastasis; fibula bent inward; both distal fragments displaced laterally.

BIBLIOGRAPHY. Pott P: Some Few General Remarks of Fractures and Dislocations, pp 57–64. London, Howes, 1769
Dupuytren G: Sur la fracture de l'extremité inferieure du peroné, les luxations e les accidents qui en sont la suite. Ann Med Chir Paris 1:2–212, 1819

POTT'S II

Synonym. Gangrene senilis. Eponym used to indicate the "mortification of toes and feet" due to arterial obstruction. See Möenckeberg's.

BIBLIOGRAPHY. Pott P: Chirurgical Observation Relative to the Cataract, the Polypus of the Nose, the Cancer of the Scrotum, the Different Kinds of Ruptures, and the Mortification of the Toes and Feet. London, Howes, 1775

POTT'S III

Synonyms. David's; spine tuberculosis; tuberculous spondylitis. Pott's paraplegia.

Symptoms. Occur in both sexes; onset at all ages. Clinically subdivided in three types: (1) Pott's without paraplegia; (2) paraplegia of early onset, initially during the florid phase of spinal disease (first 2 yr); (3) paraplegia of late onset, even after many years, after the disease has become quiescent (also in absence of signs of relapse). Onset gradual. Changes in gait; pain and weakness in the back; abdominal pain, occasionally of buttocks and knee; weight loss; rigidity and upright position of spine; muscular spasm of area involved, followed by acute curvature with backward convexity; reduction of spine length; paralysis.

Etiology. *Mycobacterium tuberculosis.*

Pathology. Tubercular (caseous) lesion of vertebral bodies and intervertebral disks. Collapse producing angulation. Cold abscess formation localized or extended along anatomic path.

Diagnostic Procedures. *X-ray of spine.* See Pathology and Signs. Of thorax. Presence of specific lesions in the lungs. *Blood.* Anemia; increased sedimentation rate. *Stool.* Presence of *M. tuberculosis.*

Therapy. Specific: streptomycin, amino salicylic acid (PAS); neomycin; rifampin. Ethionamide, and surgical and orthopedic treatment.

Prognosis. According to time of onset of treatment.

BIBLIOGRAPHY. Pott P: Remarks on that Kind of Palsy of the Lower Limbs Which is Frequently Found to Accompany a Curvature of the Spine and is Supposed to be Caused by it, Together with a Method of cure. London, Johnson, 1779

David JP: Dissertation sur les Effets du Mouvement et du Repos dans les Maladies Chirurgicales. Paris 1779

Clark GM: Tuberculous arthritis. In Hollander JL, McCarty DJ: Arthritis and Allied Conditions, 8th ed, p 1248. Philadelphia, Lea & Febiger, 1975

Wood GW: Infections of spine. In Crenshaw AH (ed): Campbell's Operative Orthopedics. 7th ed, pp 3226–3229. St Louis, CV Mosby, 1987

POUTEAU'S

Eponym used to indicate a variant of the Colles' fracture (see).

BIBLIOGRAPHY. Pouteau C: Oeuvres Posthumes de M Pouteau, Vol 2, p 251. Paris, Pierres, 1783

PRADER–WILLI

Synonyms. Cryptorchidism–dwarfism–obesity–subnormal mentality; hypotonia–hypomentia–hypogonadism–obesity; HHHO; H₃O; Labhart–Willi; Prader–Labhart–Willi–Fanconi; Willi–Prader.

Symptoms. Occur most often in males, born after normal pregnancy and delivery (prolonged gestation reported by some authors). Weight at birth slightly below normal. *First Phase.* At birth hypotonia or atonia, sleepy, convulsions (very seldom) feeding difficulty (tube feeding frequently required). *Second phase.* After about 6 mo hypotonia decreases, feeding difficulty disappears to be replaced by hyperphagia and development of obesity. Slow height growth, mental retardation; walking after 2 years of age; speech development poor; emotional disturbances. Frequently observed: polydipsia, polyuria.

Signs. Blue eyes and blond hair frequently observed. First 6 months areflexia, poor or absent response to painful stimuli, Moro reflex absent. After 6 months, reflexes active. Obesity; short stature; small penis; bilateral or unilateral cryptorchidism; lack of development of secondary sexual characteristic. In female, delayed or absent development of puberal changes. Other abnormalities occasionally observed; strabismus; micrognathia; abnormal ears; hand and finger abnormalities; teeth defects.

Etiology. Unknown; hypothalamic disturbance suggested; chromosomal diseases excluded. Absence of familial incidence. Autosomal hereditary recessive nature also suggested (lack of evidence).

Pathology. *Biopsy of testicle.* Normal. *Of brain and spinal cord.* Normal. *Of muscle.* Normal.

Diagnostic Procedures. *X-ray.* Delayed maturation of bones. *Blood.* Hyperglycemia; acetonemia (usually developing after 10th yr of life). All tests usually within normal limits, including studies of endocrine functions. *Electromyography.* Normal. *Electroencephalography.* Slow waves; spiky activity; absent sleep spindles.

Therapy. Symptomatic. Diabetic manifestation responds readily to antidiabetic agents. Amphetamine controls hyperphagia. Testosterone replacement. Low calorie intake. Vagotomy might be worthy of trial for the correction of obesity.

Prognosis. No adequate information; death from vascular complications of diabetes reported. Possibly increased risk of leukemia.

BIBLIOGRAPHY. Prader A, Labhart A, Willi H: Ein Syndrom von Adipositas, Kleinwuchs, Kryptorchidismus, und Oligophrenia nach myatonieartigem Zustand im Neugeborenenalter. Schweiz Med Wochenschr 86:1260–1261, 1956

Zellweger H, Schneider HJ: Syndrome of hypotonia, hypomentia, hypogonadism, obesity (HHHO) or Prader–Willi syndrome. Am J Dis Child 115:588–598, 1968

Cohen MM Jr, Gorlin RJ: Prader–Willi syndrome. Am J Dis Child 117:213–218, 1969

Pipes PL, Halm VA: Weight control of children with Prader–Willi syndrome. J Am Diet Assoc 62:520–524, 1973

Greel DJ, Bendel CM, Wiesner GL et al: Abnormalities of the central visual pathways in Prader–Willi syndrome associated with hypopigmentation. N Engl J Med 314:1606–1609, 1986

Gavranich J, Salikowitz M: A survey of 22 individuals with Prader–Willi syndrome in New South Wales. Aust Pediatr J 25:43–46, 1989

PRASAD'S

Synonyms. Anemia–hepatosplenomegaly–dwarfism–geophagia; dwarfism–geophagia–iron deficiency; Sarrovy's; zinc deficiency.

Symptoms. Prevalent almost exclusively in males, in Iran and Turkey. Geophagia for several years; retarded growth; low-grade fever. In the United States, the geophagia is sometimes observed among black women, especially when pregnant.

Signs. Pallor; apparent age not corresponding with chronologic age; lack of development of primary and secondary sexual characteristics; hepatosplenomegaly.

Etiology. Not clearly understood. Among possible mechanisms; alimentation deficient in animal proteins; predominant wheat diet (rich in phosphates interfering with iron absorption) relative deficiency of vitamin C. Zinc deficiency possibly responsible for hypogonadism. Geophagia interfering with iron absorption. Zinc deficiency apparently not related to hypochromic anemia.

Pathology. *Biopsy of liver.* Normal or moderate fat infiltration. Of testes. Lack of development.

Diagnostic Procedures. *Blood.* Severe hypochromic anemia; liver tests normal; high alkaline phosphatase; low serum iron and zinc; rapid disappearance of zinc after its injection. *X-ray.* Bone age inferior to chronologic age. *Gastric analysis.* Gastric achylia in all patients. *Iron absorption test.* Normal.

Therapy. Oral iron and zinc administration; adequate diet.

Prognosis. With iron and diet, anemia and lack of development are corrected and hepatosplenomegaly regresses.

BIBLIOGRAPHY. Prasad AS, Halsted JA, Nadimi M: Syndrome of iron deficiency anemia, hepatosplenomegaly, hypogonadism, dwarfism, and geophagia. Am J Med 31:532–546, 1961

Wintrobe MM (ed): Clinical Hematology, 8th ed, p 622. Lea & Febiger, Philadelphia, 1981

PRECHTL–STEMMER

Synonyms. Choreiform in children; choreatiform hyperactivity, hyperkinetic.

Symptoms and Signs. Part of hyperactivity in children syndrome. Normal intelligence, little sleep, wriggling restlessness, continuous exploratory activity.

Etiology. See Cocktail party.

Therapy. Prednisone (1–2 mg/kg/day) or Haloperidol (0.02–0.1 mg/kg/day) in 2 divided doses. Do not use phenobarbital (paradoxical effect).

Prognosis. From good response to treatment to remedial education or institutionalization.

BIBLIOGRAPHY. Prechtl HFR, Stemmer CJ.: The choreatiform syndrome in children. Dev Med Child Neurol 4:119–127, 1962

Adams RD, Victor M: Principles of Neurology, 3rd ed, p 444. New York, McGraw-Hill, 1985

PREINFARCTION

Synonyms. Angina decubitus; angina intermedia; preinfarctional angina; coronary failure; acute coronary insufficiency; coronary intermediate; ischemic heart; impending myocardial infarction; prethrombotic; progressive angina. Unstable angina.

Symptoms. Occur most often in males, in executive-managerial class. Evidence of preexisting disease such as hypertension, diabetes, obesity, and past symptoms suggestive of cardiovascular disease in good percentage of cases. Presenting symptoms: chest pain, anginalike, infarctionlike, or ill-defined, usually substernal, parasternal, precordial, or anomalously located and radiating to arm, epigastrium, jaw, or back. Shortness of breath; palpitation; fatigue; paresthesia; vomiting; gastrointestinal flatulence. (1) Prolonged attack at rest (in succession or progressively increasing); (2) intensification (with change of pattern) of pain in established angina pectoris; (3) anginal pain at rest after a pain-free period (in cases of old myocardial infarction).

Signs. Usually none except for arrhythmia or gravitational edema.

Etiology. Forerunner of attack of myocardial infarction. Incomplete artherosclerotic obstruction and spasm of coronary arteries. Includes several clinical variants where the patient has been found susceptible to myocardial infarction (symptoms may even be absent). Some patients thus classified may even have had small myocardial infarctions. Angina decubitus is the variety where the pain attacks occur at rest.

Diagnostic Procedures. *Blood.* Leukocytes, sedimentation rate, SGOT normal or show moderate elevation. *X-ray.* Heart size normal. *Electrocardiography.* Myocardial ischemic pattern almost constantly present (95%), RS-T segments downward displacement; T wave abnormalities. *Coronary angiography.*

Therapy. Rest as for myocardial damage. Monitoring for arrhythmias until crisis over. Pain relievers; prevention and management of anxiety; heparin and antiarrhythmic (not routinely but as needed) plus (as indicated) other drugs used in the treatment of classic angina (see Heberden's.) By-pass surgery or angioplasty when surgery not possible and other therapies fail. Methimazole or radioactive iodine (to reduce metabolism) may be tried. Educational before and after resuming activity.

Prognosis. In 50% of cases, development of myocardial infarction. Occasionally, death. Recovery after a variable number of attacks with restoration of normal electrocardiographic pattern.

BIBLIOGRAPHY. Sampson JJ, Eliaser M: The diagnosis of impending acute coronary artery occlusion. Am Heart J 13:675–686, 1937
Feil H: Preliminary pain in coronary thrombosis. Am J Med Sci 193:42–48, 1937
Hurst JW: The Heart, 6th ed, p 962. New York, McGraw-Hill, 1986
Sherman TC, Litvack F, Grundfest W et al: Coronary angioscopy in patients with unstable angina pectoris. N Engl J Med 351:913–919, 1986
Cowley MJ, Di Sciascio G, Rehr RB, Vetrovec GW: Angiographic observations and clinical relevance of coronary thrombus in unstable angina pectoris. Am J Cardiol 63:108E–113E, 1989

PREISER'S

Synonym. Scaphoid bone necrosis. See Epiphyseal ischemic necrosis.

Symptoms. Pain and mobility reduction of the wrist.

Etiology. Trauma of the wrist causing avascular necrosis of scaphoid bone.

BIBLIOGRAPHY. Preiser G: Zur Frage der typischen traumatischen Ernaetrungsstoerungen der kurken Hand und Fuss-wurzelknochen., Fortsch Geb Roentgenol 17:360–362, 1911

PREMATURE OVARIAN FAILURE

Synonyms. Premature menopause; premature familial ovarian failure included, resistant ovary syndrome included.

Symptoms and Signs. Onset of menopause before 40 years of age.

Etiology. Various causes may determine the syndrome: (1) idiopathic; (2) antiovarian or antireceptor antibodies; (3) viral infections (mumps) (4) cytotoxic drugs; (5) radiation; (6) familial cases due to partial deletion of long arm of X chromosome (Xq 26-27).

Diagnostic Procedures. *Blood.* High gonadotropin levels. Genetic analysis and chromosome mapping (DNA hybridization techniques).

Therapy. None.

Prognosis. Limited fertility.

BIBLIOGRAPHY. Board JA, Redwine FO, Moncure CW et al: Identification of differing etiologies of clinically diagnosed premature menopause. Am J Obstet Gynecol 134:936–944, 1979
Talbet LM, Ray MH, Hammond MG et al: Endocrine and immunological studies in a patient with resistant ovary syndrome. Fertil Steril 42:741–744, 1984
Krauss CM, Nurant Turksoy R, Atkins L et al: Familial premature ovarian failure due to an interstitial deletion of the long arm of the X chromosome. N Engl J Med 317:125–131, 1987

PREMENSTRUAL

Symptoms. Exaggerated manifestation of normal premenstrual phenomena. It may be considered to occur in about 80% of women. Symptoms begin about 10 days before menstrual period and stop abruptly within 24 hours of menstruation. They begin to recur in a similar fashion on the next cycle. Symptoms of different intensity may be subdivided by systems. *Central nervous system.* Emotional instability; onset of psychotic manifestations; cyclic headache; nymphomania; visual disturbances. *Genital area and breast.* Lower abdominal heaviness; distention; low back pain or pain in the legs; anorectal symptoms of pressure and pruritus; mastalgia and swelling of breasts. *Nongenital manifestations.* Nausea; vomiting; constipation; diarrhea; asthma; rhinorrhea; epistaxis; periocular pigmentation; cyclic localized acneiform eruption; greasy or dry scalp and hair.

Etiology. Not completely assessed; predisposing constitutional factors; evidence of water–salts metabolism involvement; relative excess of estrogen or deficiency of progesterone; overcompensating secretion of aldosterone or antidiuretic hormone (or both) and other causes and mechanisms proposed.

Therapy. Sedative such as phenobarbital. Diuretic such as hydrochlorothiazide. Hormonal: medroxyprogesterone starting 5 to 10 days before cycle. Prostaglandin synthetase inhibitors. Psychotherapy.

Prognosis. Influenced favorably by treatment.

BIBLIOGRAPHY. Frank FT: Hormonal causes of premenstrual tension. Arch Neurol Psychiatr 26:1053–1057, 1931

Abplanalp JM: Psychologic components of the premenstrual syndrome: Evaluating the research and choosing the treatment. J Reprod Med 28:517–524, 1983

Budoff PW: The use of prostaglandin inhibitors for the premenstrual syndrome. J Reprod Med 28:469–478, 1983

Rossing AM: Caffeine-containing beverage and premenstrual syndrome in young women. Am J Pub Health 75:1335–1337, 1985

Pariser SF, Stern SL, Shank ML et al: Premenstrual syndrome: Concerns, controversies and treatment. Am J Obstet Gynecol 153:599–604, 1985

Spiegel A: Temporary insanity and premenstrual syndrome: Medical testimony in an 1865 murder trial. New York State J Med 88:482–492, 1988

PRETIBIAL FEVER

Synonym. Fort Bragg fever.

Symptoms. Sporadic occurrence in North Carolina and Georgia. Sudden onset. Malaise; mild general aching headache; photophobia mild, not persistent; respiratory symptoms; chills; spiking fever (two or more peaks a day) subsiding within 4 to 8 days.

Signs. On fourth day of illness, patchy erythematous rash usually limited to anterior part of both legs. Usually lasting 2 or a few more days and leaving residual pigmentation for 2 weeks. Splenomegaly; relative bradycardia.

Etiology. *Leptospira autumnalis, L. pomona* also observed in association with similar syndrome of pretibial as well as generalized rash.

Diagnostic Procedures. *Blood.* Initially leukopenia and then moderate leukocytosis, with moderate relative lymphocytosis; complement fixation for *Leptospira.* Microscopic agglutination and culture studies.

Therapy. Doxycycline 200 mg orally the first day, then 100 mg per day for 4 days. Prophylaxis by tetracyclines or penicillin given in first 4 days of disease.

Prognosis. Course of 5 to 10 days and complete recovery.

BIBLIOGRAPHY. Bowdoin CD: A new disease entity (?). J Med Assoc Ga 31:437–438, 1942

Daniels WB, Grennan HA: Pretibial fever. JAMA 122:361–365, 1943

Takafuji ET, Kirkpatrick JW, Miller RV et al: An efficacy trial of doxycycline chemoprophylaxis against leptospirosis. N Engl J Med 310:497–500, 1984

PRIEUR–TRENEL

Eponym used to designate the association of cataract and Sabouraud's syndrome (see).

BIBLIOGRAPHY. Prieur M, Trénel M: Monilethrix et cataracte précoce. Bull Soc Ophthalmol Fr 42:794–799, 1930

PRINGLE–BOURNEVILLE

Signs. Subungual and periungual warty fibromas in patient affected by Bourneville's syndrome (see).

BIBLIOGRAPHY. Pringle JJ: A case of congenital adenoma seboreum. Br J Dermatol 2:1–14, 1890

PRINZMETAL'S II

Synonym. Angina pectoris variant.

Symptoms. Precordial angina attacks with the following characteristics:
1. Onset at rest or during normal activity; not induced by strain or emotions.
2. Occur at the same time each day.
3. During each single attack, time of waxing of pain equal to time of waning (in regular angina waxing time longer than waning one).
4. Intensity and duration of attack greater than that of regular angina.
5. Nitroglycerine protects from crisis and arrests one in progress.

Signs. None.

Etiology and Pathology. Anatomic-pathologic studies have shown the single narrowing of a major coronary branch, in contrast with that found in classic angina, where several minor arteries are involved. Consequently, in this type of angina there is only one single area of ischemia, while in classical angina several small areas are involved.

Diagnostic Procedures. *Electrocardiography.* Between attacks, normal; during attack, ST elevation in determinated derivations; increase of R voltage in some derivations; ventricular arrythmias (50%) during pain acme; in rare cases where ECG is abnormal between attacks, it may paradoxically revert to normal during crisis. Effort test does not cause attack or ECG modifications; in rare cases it may induce ST depression. *X-ray of chest.* Normal. *Cineangiocardiography.* See Etiology.

Therapy. Does not differ from that of classic angina; anticoagulants useful. Surgical revascularizion particularly indicated.

Prognosis. The ischemic area of the Prinzmetal's angina frequently (33%) becomes site of myocardial infarction (and the angina pain disappears). In remaining patients, variable outcome; spontaneous resolution to progressive aggravation. Prognosis is always more severe than in the classic angina.

BIBLIOGRAPHY. Prinzmetal M, Ekmek A, Keimamer R et al: Variant form of angina pectoris. JAMA 174:1794–1800, 1960

Hurst JW: The Heart, 6th ed, pp 963–964, 1011. New York, McGraw-Hill, 1985

Polese A, De Cesare N, Bartorelli A, Fabbiocchi F, Loaldi A, Montorsi P, Guazzi MD: Different vasomotor action of nifedipine on dynamic coronary obstructions and therapeutic response in effort and prinzmetal angina. Am J Med Sci 297:73–79, 1989

PROFICHET'S

Synonyms. Calcinosis circumscripta; calcinosis cutis; hypodermolithiasis. See also Calcinosis universalis.

Symptoms. Most commonly reported in elderly females; onset insidious. Calcareous deposits, primarily affecting extremities. Usually, lesion not painful; stiffness and aching of joints; coldness of extremities.

Signs. Symmetric hard nodular or plaque formations over pressure points or joints. Skin overlying lesions is dry, red and hardened. Calcinosis of scrotum and penis reported.

Etiology. Unknown; possible association with variable conditions: collagen diseases; trauma; neoplasma. Some authors refuse to consider this form an entity and believe it is a part of the calcinosis universalis syndrome.

Pathology. Chalky material in subcutaneous fat associated with collagenous bundles.

Diagnostic Procedures. *X-ray.* To evidence nodules. *Blood.* Hypercalcemia and hyperphosphoremia. *Biopsy.* Calcium phosphate and carbonate deposits.

Therapy. None or surgical removal. Medical treatment usually useless.

Prognosis. Spontaneous recession possible. Variable degree of incapacitation.

BIBLIOGRAPHY. Profichet GC: Sur une Variété de Concretion Phosphatique Subcutanée (Pierre de la Peau). Paris, 1890

Reines S: Petrificatio cutis circumscripta. Arch Dermatol Syph (Wein) 88:267–289, 1907

Leistyna JA, Hassan AH: Interstitial calcinosis: Report of a case and a review of the literature. Am J Dis Child 107:96–101, 1964

Moss RL, Shewmake SW: Idiopathic calcinosis of the scrotum. Int J Dermatol 20:134–136, 1981

PROLIDASE DEFICIENCY

Synonyms. Lathyritic. See also lathyrism.

Symptoms and Signs. From birth. Mental retardation. Characteristic features: prominent skull sutures, ptosis eyelids, ocular proptosis, splenomegaly, chronic dermatitis, leg ulcers, recurrent respiratory infections. Joint laxity, waddling gait, protuberant abdomen, osteoporosis.

Etiology. Autosomal recessive. Deficiency of prolidase which metabolizes proline (collagen).

Diagnostic Procedures. *Urine.* peptidemia.

Therapy. None.

Prognosis. Poor *quoad vitam.*

BIBLIOGRAPHY. Goodman SI, Solomons CC, Muschenheim F et al: A syndrome resembling lathyrism associated with imidopeptiduria. Am J Med 45:152, 1968

Scriver CH, Smith RJ, Phang JM: Disorders of proline and hydroxyproline metabolism. In Stanbury JB, Wyngaarden JB, Fredrickson DS et al: The Metabolic Basis of Inherited Disease. 5th ed, p 360. New York, McGraw-Hill, 1983

PRONATOR TERES

Synonyms. Anterior interosseous; median.

Symptoms. Two clinical patterns according to level of nerve compression (see Etiology).

1. Median nerve: sensory and motor changes in area of nerve distribution.
2. Interosseous nerve: no sensory loss, weakness limited to pronator quadratus, flexor pollicis, flexor digitorum to II and III fingers.

Etiology. Trauma or fibrous band compressing median nerve before it gives off the anterior interosseous nerve or of the interosseous nerve at the elbow as it passes between the two heads of pronator teres muscle.

Therapy. Decompression surgery, sometimes required.

Prognosis. Variable.

BIBLIOGRAPHY. Dawson DM, Hallett M, Millender LH: Entrapment Neuropathies. Boston, Little, Brown & Co, 1983

PROPIONIC ACIDEMIAS

Synonyms. Glycinemia ketotic I, glycinemia ketotic II, hyperglycinemia–ketoacidosis–leukopenia I and II; PPC I and II.

Symptoms and Signs. The clinical picture is that of the ketotic hyperglycinemia syndrome (see) but the metabolic defects can be various.
1. Propionyl CoA carboxylase deficiency (beta-methylcrotonyl glycinuria II) I and II.
2. Multiple carboxylase deficiency.

PROTEUS

Synonyms. See Klippel–Trenaunay–Weber, Ollier's, and Maffucci's.

Symptoms and Signs. In male. Partial gigantism of hands and feet, nevi, hemihypertrophy, subcutaneous tumors (lipomas) macrocephaly or other skull anomalies, visceral manifestations from abdominal and pelvic lipomatosis.

Etiology. Unknown. Perhaps genetic. Autosomal dominant (?).

BIBLIOGRAPHY. Wiedeman HR, Burgio GR, Aldenhoff P et al: The proteus syndrome: Partial gigantism of the hand or feet, nevi, hemihypertrophy subcutaneous tumors, macrocephaly or other skull anomalies and possible accelerated growth and visceral affection. Eur J Pediatr 140:5–12, 1983
Costa T, Fitch N, Azouz EM: Proteus syndrome: Report of two cases with pelvic lipomatosis. Pediatrics 76:984–989, 1985

PROTHROMBIN DEFICIENCY SYNDROMES

CONGENITAL

Synonyms. Factor II deficiency, hypoprothrombinemia. Including constitutional dysthrombinemia.

Symptoms and Signs. Both sexes affected; present usually from infancy (latest onset at 13 yr). Mild hemorrhagic manifestations.

Etiology. Autosomal recessive inheritance. Two variants are recognized: (1) cross-reacting material (CRM) positive (rare) constitutional dysprothrombinemia (2) CRM-negative (more common).

Pathology. Effects and sequelae of hemorrhagic diathesis.

Diagnostic Procedures. *Form 1. Blood.* Immunoelectrophoresis normal amount of antigenically competent prothrombin, which does not yield normal amount of thrombin. Prothrombin time about 10% of normal. *Form 2. Blood.* One-stage prothrombin time normal or almost normal. Two-stage reveals true hypothrombinemia.

Therapy. No specific treatment available. Vitamin K no effect. Plasma transfusion some effect on bleeding.

Prognosis. Poor. Death from bleeding at different ages. See also Owren's and Hemophilia, classic.

ACQUIRED HYPOPROTHROMBINEMIA SYNDROMES

Symptoms and Signs. Hemorrhagic manifestation.

Etiology.
1. Vitamin K deficiency (deficiency of prothrombin; Factor VII, X, occasionally also IX).
2. Hepatocellular diseases (deficiency of prothrombin, Factor V, VII, X, occasionally IX).
3. Dicumarol medication (deficiency of prothrombin, Factor VII; slower fall also of IX and X).
4. Hemorrhagic, neonatal (see).

Diagnostic Procedures. See Etiology.

Therapy. Vitamin K; fresh plasma.

Prognosis. Depends on etiology.

BIBLIOGRAPHY. Josso F, Prou–Wartelle O, Soulier JP: Étude d'un Cas D'Hypoprothrombinemie congenitale. Nouv Rev Fr Hematol 2:647–672, 1962
McKee PA: Hemostasis and disorders of blood coagulation. In Stanbury JB, Wyngaarden JB, Fredrickson DS et al: The Metabolic Basis of Inherited Disease, 5th ed, p 1531. New York, McGraw-Hill, 1983

PRUNE BELLY

Synonyms. Abdominal muscle deficiency; Obrinsky's.

Symptoms. Almost exclusively in males, where the full syndrome is seen. Inability to move from lying to sitting position without the help of the arms. Frequent respiratory infections (unable to cough effectively). Frequently, urinary obstruction and infections.

Signs. Absence of abdominal muscles in lower and medial region of abdomen. Lower ribs flared outward; testicles retained; kidney palpable. Possibly, association of other congenital defects: lower extremities deformities; gastrointestinal anomalies; cardiac abnormalities.

Etiology. Unknown; possibly sex-linked recessive trait. Chromosomal pattern normal in subject studied. Recent studies indicate that the urogenital anomalies can be attributed to a functional urethral obstruction which in turn is the result of prostatic hypoplasia. Prostatic maldevelopment causes weakness of the prostatic wall with resultant sacculation of the prostatic urethra.

Pathology. *Abdomen.* Abdominal wall formed by skin, superficial fascia, and peritoneum, (the abdominal muscle hypoplasia is a nonspecific lesion, resulting from fetal abdominal distention secondary to early bladder distention), bilateral cryptorchidism. Absence of inguinal canal and gubernaculum. *Urinary tract.* Lower urinary obstruction (in some cases). Dysplastic kidney, sometimes cystic; dilatation and elongation of ureters; enlargement of bladder.

Diagnostic Procedures. *Cystography. Blood.* Blood urea nitrogen (BUN) determination. The syndrome can be diagnosed prenatally by means of ultrasonography.

Therapy. Abdominal belt; orchiopexy (if feasible). Urinary tract surgery to allow micturition when indicated. Fetal therapy *in utero*: drainage of the distended urinary tract.

Prognosis. About 20% stillborn; 50% die within 2 years. Record of occasional patients who reach old age (70 yr).

BIBLIOGRAPHY. Fröhlich F: Der Mangel der Muskeln, insbesondere der Seitenbauchmuskelnn. Wurzburg, Dissert, 1839.
Parker RW: Case of an infant in whom some of the abdominal muscles were absent. Trans Clin Soc (London) 28:201–203, 1895
Williams DI, Burkholder GV: The prune belly syndrome. J Urol 98:244–251, 1967
Moerman P, Fryns JP, Godderis P, Lauweryns J: Pathogenesis of the prune belly syndrome: A functional urethral obstruction caused by prostatic hypoplasia. Pediatrics 73:470–475, 1984

PRURITUS GRAVIDARUM

Synonyms. Pregnancy pruritus (including early onset pruritus pregnancy or Besnier's pruritus gestationis).

Symptoms and Signs. *Besnier's pruritus gestationis.* 1 of 300 pregnancies, onset about 25th week of pregnancy. Itching, absence of urticated lesions on the extensor aspect of limbs and shoulders; groups of crusted papules. *Pregnancy pruritus.* Onset in the third month increasing during all pregnancy. Localized in the abdominal region, may become generalized.

Etiology. Bound to cholestasis due to estrogen increases.

Diagnostic Procedures. Liver function tests.

Therapy. Choleretics. Antihistamines.

Prognosis. When severe sign of increased occurrence of cholelithiasis.

BIBLIOGRAPHY. Rook A, Wilkinson DS, Ebling FJG et al: Textbook of Dermatology, 4th ed, pp 276–277. Oxford, Blackwell Scientific Publications, 1986

PSEUDOACANTHOSIS NIGRICANS

See Acanthosis nigricans syndromes.

Symptoms and Signs. Affects both sexes equally; onset in adulthood (25–60 yr of age). Frequent association with obesity and dark complexion. Patches of pigmentation and thickening present in any body fold, inner and upper thighs.

Etiology. Unknown. Not to be confused with acanthosis nigricans. Association with obesity and moderate extension of lesion are the differential diagnostic elements.

Diagnostic Procedures. None.

Therapy. Hypocaloric diet.

Prognosis. Regression and thickening with weight loss; pigmentation reduces or may persist.

BIBLIOGRAPHY. Ollendorff–Curth H: Pseudo-acanthosis nigricans. Ann Dermatol Syph 78:417–429, 1951
Rook A, Wilkinson DS, Ebling FJG et al: Textbook of Dermatology, 4th ed, p 1462. Oxford, Blackwell Scientific Publications, 1986

PSEUDOACHONDROPLASIA

Synonym. Spondyloepiphyseal dysplasia.

Symptoms. Both sexes affected. Short stature becoming evident during adolescence. Short trunk variety. Precocious osteoarthrosis of hips, occasionally also of knees and shoulders. Absence of clinical abnormality of face and skull.

Etiology. Unknown; autosomal dominant and recessive inheritances. Still debated, abnormal synthesis or processing of cartilage protein core. Four types, two autosomal dominant (I and III) and two recessive (II and IV) types have been classified.

Pathology. Fragmentation of epiphyseal ossification centers.

Diagnostic Procedures. *X-ray of skull.* Absence of lesion. In children, fragmentation of epiphyseal ossification center. Spinal change characteristic in adult. Lumbar vertebrae formed by eburnated bone in central and posterior parts of superior and inferior plates. Osteoarthrosis. In the two dominant forms x-ray changes more severe.

Pathology. In type III cytoplasmic metachromasia of fibroblasts and specific ultramicroscopic alteration in the chondrocytes.

Therapy. None.

Prognosis. Final height 130 to 150 cm.

BIBLIOGRAPHY. Maroteaux P, Lamy M: Les formes pseudo-achondroplastiques des dysplasies spondyloépiphysaires. Presse Méd 67:383–386, 1959
McKusic VA: Heritable Disorders of Connective Tissue, 4th ed, p 798. St Louis, CV Mosby, 1972
Stanescu V, Maroteaux P, Stanescu R: The biochemical defect of pseudoachondroplasia. Eur J Pediatr 138:221–225, 1982
Young ID, Moore JR: Severe pseudoachondroplasia with parental consanguinity. J Med Genet 22:150–153, 1985

PSEUDOARTHROGRYPOSIS

Synonyms. Elbow–knee congenital rigidity; ankylosis elbow knee, Siwon's.

Symptoms and Signs. From birth. Females. Rigidity of elbows and knees.

Etiology. Autosomal dominant.

Pathology. Ankylosis and proximal fusion of tibia and fibula or humerus, radius, and ulna.

BIBLIOGRAPHY. Siwon P: Kongenital, hereditaere, doppelseitige Ankylosen der Ellenbogengelenke. Dtsch Z Chir 209:338–349, 1928
Pasina A, Wildervank LS: Hereditary occurrence of congenital rigidity of elbows and knees (congenital multiple arthrogryposis). Arch Chir Neurol 8:43–56, 1956

PSEUDOBULBAR PALSY

Symptoms. Occur in patients over 40 years of age. Dysarthria (but not dysphasia); temporary complete aphonia; dysphagia; disorder of gait; disturbed reflex; emotional reactions; spontaneous crying and laughing that cannot be controlled. Neurogenic bladder (see); intelligence affected or not.

Signs. Paresis of voluntary motion; exaggeration of automatic and reflex movements. Facial expression may be similar to that in parkinsonism; voice nasal without intonation; volume low; whispering; drooling of saliva.

Etiology. Arteriosclerosis with multiple areas of softening. Syphilis, infections, trauma, and degenerative diseases may also be responsible.

Pathology. Softening in any place where supranuclear fibers pass through: cortical; subcortical; corona radiata; internal capsula zone. Supranuclear fibers must be destroyed on both sides to produce this syndrome. Vascular lesions.

Diagnostic Procedures. None specific. *Electroencephalography. Angiography. Blood.* Cholesterol may be elevated.

Therapy. None specific; antibiotic for frequent pulmonary complications.

Prognosis. Remission of this syndrome rare, especially after emotional component becomes manifested. Rehabilitation of patient extremely difficult. Death from pulmonary complications or inanition.

BIBLIOGRAPHY. Magnus A: Fall von Aufhebung des Willenseinflusses auf einige Hirnnerven. Arch Anat Physiol Wissensch Med 258:567, 1837
Vick NA: Grinker's Neurology, 7th ed. Springfield, CC Thomas, 1976

PSEUDOCHROMHIDROSIS

See Chromhidrosis.

Symptoms and Signs. Similar to those of chromhidrosis.

Etiology. Differing from chromhidrosis in that the sweat changes color after having reached the skin, from the activity of chromogenic bacteria, especially *Corynebacterium,* usually located in hairy areas.

Therapy. Hygiene and topical antibacterial agents.

Prognosis. Condition disappears with adequate treatment.

BIBLIOGRAPHY. Hurley HJ, Shelley WB: The Human Apocrine Gland in Health and Disease. Springfield, CC Thomas, 1960

PSEUDO-CUSHING'S

Symptoms. Seen especially in young subjects. Overeating.

Signs. Truncal obesity; purple striae on abdomen and thighs.

Etiology. Unknown; possibly, psychological maladjustment or constitutional factors. Hypercortisolism secondary to alcoholism.

Pathology. Obesity.

Diagnostic Procedures. *Urine.* Increased secretion of cortisol (greater than normal, less than in Cushing's). Increased excretion of hydrocortisone metabolites. Plasma cortisol level in low-normal range. Adrenocorticotropic hormone (ACTH) test, metyrapone test, and adrenal suppression tests (Decadron) normal (see Cushing's).

Therapy. Treatment of obesity; diet; psychotherapy.

Prognosis. Weight loss, disappearance of striae, and return to normal adrenal function with treatment.

BIBLIOGRAPHY. Carpenter PC: Cushing's syndrome: Update of diagnosis and management. Mayo Clin Proc 61:49–58, 1986

PSEUDOCYESIS

Synonyms. Fantasized pregnancy; false pregnancy.

Symptoms. Occur usually in later fertile period. Amenorrhea; morning sickness; appetite variation; breast sensitivity; constipation; impression of fetal movements.

Signs. Abdominal enlargement, which disappears after anesthesia; cervis firm; uterus normal size.

Etiology. Delusion of pregnancy. Psychogenic mechanisms.

Diagnostic Procedures. *Pregnancy test.* Negative.

Therapy. Psychiatric.

Prognosis. Possible conversion to other delusional states.

BIBLIOGRAPHY. Freedman AM, Kaplan HI, Sadock BJ: Comprehensive Textbook of Psychiatry, 2nd ed, p 1656. Baltimore, Williams & Wilkins, 1975

PSEUDODIASTROPHIC DWARFISM

Symptoms and Signs. Both sexes affected; present from birth. Normal weight; reduced length; various malformations (in order of incidence): constant joint incongruity; soft tissue contractures; coxa vara; radial head subluxation; clubfoot (very common); genu valgum; flexion contractures; patellar dislocation or absence; lumbar lordosis; proximal interphalangeal joints stiffness; red swollen ears; pinnal calcifications. Common: short metatarsals; scoliosis; cubitus valgus; metacarpophalangeal and interphalangeal stiffness; pigmentation. Occasional: flat foot; genu recurvatum; clinodactyly.

Etiology. Autosomal dominant inheritance.

Diagnostic Procedures. *Blood and urine.* Usually, normal. *X-ray.* See Symptoms and Signs.

Therapy. Orthopedic correction and surgery (to feet and knees).

Prognosis. Patient remains below third percentile in height, with disproportionate features. Mental development normal.

BIBLIOGRAPHY. Bailey JA: Disproportionate Short Stature: Diagnosis and Management, p 149. Philadelphia, WB Saunders, 1973

PSEUDOGOUT

Synonyms. Chondrocalcinosis; calcium gout; crystal synovitis; synovitis crystal.

Symptoms. Occur most often in females over 40. Articular symptoms from mild arthralgias to acute arthritis mimicking gout attack (lasting from 21 hr to 50 days). Joints most frequently affected: knees, hands, and feet; 20% polyarthralgias.

Sign. Mild or acute inflammation of joints involved.

Etiology. Metabolic defect; precipitation of crystal of calcium pyrophosphate in synovial fluid cartilage and periarticular structures.

Pathology. Possibly, genetically determined or subacute inflammation due to the presence of calcium crystals.

Diagnostic Procedures. *Synovial fluid aspiration.* (Diagnostic). Intracellular and extracellular. Calcium crystal in some cases. *Blood.* Hyperuricemia and diabetes findings or alteration of glucose tolerance curve. Sedimentation rate usually elevated. Serum calcium and phosphorus normal in majority of patients. Serum alkaline phosphatase normal. *X-ray.* Articular calcification as a thin line paralleling contour of bone or granular deposit in fibro-chondral structures; degenerative changes of joints.

Therapy. Colchicine gives good to fair response; aspirin, corticosteroid good to fair. Aspiration of synovial fluid also may give relief from symptoms.

Prognosis. Relatively benign condition; articular degeneration develops, but not as severe as in rheumatoid arthritis.

BIBLIOGRAPHY. McCarty DJ, Kohn NN, Faires JS: Significance of calcium phosphate crystals in the synovial fluid arthritic patients: The "pseudogout syndrome". I. clinical aspects. Ann Intern Med 56:711–737, 1962
Moskowitz RW, Katz D: Chondrocalcinosis and chondrocalsynovitis (pseudogout syndrome). Am J Med 43:322–334, 1967
Riestra JL, Sanchez A, Rodriguez-Valverde V, Castillo E, Calderon J: Roentgenographic features of the arthropathy associated with CPPD crystal deposition disease. A comparative study with primary osteoarthritis. J Rheumatol 12:1154–1158, 1985
Doherty M, Dieppe P: Crystal deposition disease in the elderly. Clin Rheum Dis 12:97–116, 1986
McCarty DJ (ed): Cristalline Deposition Diseases. Rheum Dis Clin N America (14):2. Philadelphia, WB Saunders, 1988

PSEUDO-GRAEFE'S

Synonym. Fuchs' sign.

Symptoms and Signs. While the eye may be adducted and lid elevated, no movement up or down occurs when the vertical recti contract together.

Etiology and Pathology. Trauma or tumor at the base of skull. Regenerating fibers growing to wrong muscles, or spreading of a localized stimulation to an injured third nucleus so that when one tries to move the eye in one direction, impulses also flow into all other muscles innervated by oculomotor (III) nerve.

Diagnostic Procedures. *X-ray of skull. Spinal. Electroencephalography. Angiography. CT brain scan.*

Therapy and Procedures. According to etiology.

BIBLIOGRAPHY. Bender MB: Nerve supply to orbicularis muscle and physiology of movement of upper eyelid, with particular reference to the Pseudo-Graefe phenomenon. Arch Ophthalmol 15:21–30, 1936
Walsh FB, King AB: Ocular signs of intracranial saccular aneurysms. Arch Ophthalmol 27:1–33, 1942
Anderson JR: Ocular vertical deviations. Br J Ophthalmol (Suppl) 12:7–99, 1947

PSEUDOHERMAPHRODITISM, MALE, DEFICIENCY OF 17–20 DESMOLASE TESTIS

Synonyms. 17–20 lyase deficiency. See also pseudohermaphroditism male–gynecomastia.

Symptoms and Signs. At birth: females, normal internal and external genitalia; at puberty, lack of pubertal development and infertility. Males, pseudohermaphroditism.

Etiology. Possibly X-linked; deficiency of 17–20 desmolase of testis.

Diagnostic Procedures. Females: inability to form estrogens. Males, urine: increased pregnanetriolone; testosterone and DHEA do not increase following ACTH stimulation.

BIBLIOGRAPHY. Zachmann M, Hamilton W, Vollmin JA et al: Testicular 17–20 desmolase deficiency causing male pseudohermaphroditism. Acta Endocrinol (Suppl) 155:65–80, 1971
Forest MG, Lecosnu M, De Peretti E: Familial male pseudohermaphroditism due to 17–20 desmolase deficiency I: In vivo endocrine studies. J Clin Endocrinol Metab 50:826, 1980

PSEUDOHERMAPHRODITISM MALE–GYNECOMASTIA

Synonyms. 17-Hydroxysteroid deficiency, 17-ketosteroid reductase deficiency testis, 17-KSR deficiency, 17-β-HSD deficiency.

Symptoms and Signs. At birth. External genitalia female type with or without moderate ambiguity. Testis palpable in inguinal canal or labial folds. At puberty development of male body habitus and secondary sexual characteristics. Gynecomastia not always present.

Etiology. Autosomal recessive inheritance. 17-ketosteroid reductase deficiency limited to the testis.

Therapy. Diagnosis before puberty: removal of abnormal testis.

Prognosis. According to therapy. Female habitus is best.

BIBLIOGRAPHY. Saez JM, De Peretti E, Morera AM et al: Familial male pseudohermaphroditism with gynecomastia due to a testicular 17-ketosteroid reductase defect I: Studies in vivo. J Clin Endocrinol 32:604–610, 1971
Balducci M, Toscano V, Wright F et al: Familial male pseudohermaphroditism with gynecomastia due to 17-

beta-hydroxysteroid dehydrogenase deficiency: A report of three cases. Clin Endocrinol 23:439–444, 1985

PSEUDOHERMAPHRODITISM, MALE, INCOMPLETE HEREDITARY (TYPE I)

Synonym. Androgen resistance (type I).

Symptoms. Clinically includes a variety of subsyndromes (previously considered autonomous entities): from the extreme feminine end of the spectrum with Lub's through Gilber-Dreyfus and Reifenstein's to the other extreme of the Rosewaters,' which presents an almost complete male phenotype. Each form will present its own relative psychological problems and different needs of role adjustment.

Signs. From phenotypic female with pseudovagina (Lub's) to normal sterile male (common hypospadias). Normal body hair; scanty or absent beard.

Etiology. X-linked inheritance. See Seabright-Bantam.

Pathology. See individual syndromes. Normal gonads; incomplete spermatogenesis. Wolffian ducts vary in development; absence of ducts derivatives.

Diagnostic Procedures. *Chromatin studies.* Male sex chromatin 46XY karyotype. *Blood.* Testosterone production normal or increased. Estrogen production greater than in normal men. Gonadotropin levels elevated.

Therapy. See individual syndromes. Resistance to androgenic and anabolic effects of testosterone.

Prognosis. Good *quoad vitam.* See individual syndromes.

BIBLIOGRAPHY. Wilson JD, Griffin JE, Leshin M et al: The androgen resistence syndromes: 5-α-reductase deficiency, testicular feminization and related disorders. In Stanbury JB, Wyngaarden JB, Fredrickson DS et al: The Metabolic Basis of Inherited Disease, 5th ed, p 1001. New York, McGraw-Hill, 1983

PSEUDO-HIRSCHSPRUNG'S

Synonyms. Colonic inertia; acquired functional megacolon; idiopathic megacolon; psychogenic megacolon; sluggish colon.

Symptoms and Signs. Occur in children. Symptoms and signs of partial intestinal obstruction.

Etiology. Unknown.

Pathology. No signs of gross mechanical obstruction or disease that may cause secondary symptomatic megacolon. Histologically, intramural plexes are normal, and there is no evidence of degenerative changes.

Diagnostic Procedures. *Barium enema.* Proximal megacolon with undilated distal segment. *Biopsy of intestinal mucosa.* Normal.

Therapy. Rectosigmoidectomy. Cases treated with temporary colostomy recovered after closure of colostomy.

Prognosis. Excellent with treatment.

BIBLIOGRAPHY. Bill AH Jr, Creighton SA, Stevenson JK: The selection of infants and children for the surgical treatment of Hirschsprung's disease. Surg Gynecol Obstet 104:151–156, 1957
Ehrenpreis T: Pseudo-Hirschsprung's disease. Arch Dis Child 40:177–179, 1965
Sleisenger MH, Fortran JS (ed): Gastrointestinal Disease: Pathophysiology, Diagnosis, Management, 3rd ed. Philadelphia, WB Saunders, 1983

PSEUDO-HURLER POLYDYSTROPHY

Synonyms. ML III; mucolipidosis III.

Symptoms and Signs. Both sexes affected; onset usually at 2 to 4 years of age. Hands and shoulder stiffness, progressing to clawhand deformity (at 6–8 yr of age) and striking dwarfism. Carpal tunnel syndrome (see). Coarse facies. Fine peripheral corneal clouding (progressive). Cardiac murmurs. Mild mental retardation. Occasionally inguinal hernia; acne. Clinical picture is similar to Maroteaux–Lamy of intermediate severity.

Etiology. Autosomal recessive inheritance. Multiple enzyme defects apparently confined to connective tissue. Defect allelic to the one for Leroy's I cell disease (see). Defect of phosphorylation of hydrolases, which does not enable them to enter lysosomes and thus become active. Many mucopolysaccharides are not metabolized.

Pathology. Histologic changes similar to those of Leroy's I cell syndrome (see); inclusions not as prominent in I cells.

Diagnostic Procedures. *Fibroblast culture.* See Pathology. *Urine.* Absent or moderate mucopolysacchariduria. *Blood.* Increased lysosomal enzymes value. *X-ray.* Dysostosis multiplex; particularly striking changes in the hip.

Therapy. Orthopedic.

Prognosis. Adulthood reached with severe dysostosis.

BIBLIOGRAPHY. Maroteaux P, Lamy M: La pseudopolydystrophie de Hurler's. Presse Med 74:2889–2892, 1966

Neufeld EF, McKusick VA: Disorders of lysosomal enzyme synthesis and localization: I-cell disease and pseudo-Hurler polydystrophy. In Stanbury JB, Wyngaarden JB, Fredrickson DS et al: The Metabolic Basis of Inherited Disease, 5th ed, p 778. New York, McGraw-Hill, 1983

PSEUDOHYPOALDOSTERONISM

Synonym. Salt-wasting.

Symptoms. Onset almost immediately after birth. Vomiting; anorexia; failure to gain weight; cyanotic attacks when exposed to elevated temperature.

Signs. Poor weight gain; dehydration.

Etiology. Unknown; possibly insensitivity of the tubules to action of aldosterone. It may overlap with the Thorn's syndrome and inappropriate antidiuretic hormone syndrome.

Pathology. Unknown; in one case, renal biopsy showed 25% of small glomeruli and glomerulosclerosis of varying degrees, no major tubular changes.

Diagnostic Procedures. *Blood.* Hyponatremia; hyperkalemia. *Urine.* Normal 17-ketosteroids; high aldosterone level. Good response to adrenocorticotropic hormone (ACTH) with increased excretion of aldosterone.

Therapy. Unresponsive to desoxycorticosterone (Doca) and aldosterone; aggravated by spironolactone. Responding optimally to administration of salt.

Prognosis. Unknown; good response and weight gain with salt administration.

BIBLIOGRAPHY. Cheek DB, Perry JW: A salt wasting syndrome in infancy. Arch Dis Child 33:252–256, 1958
Royer P, Bonnette J, Mathieu H et al Pseudo-hypoaldosteronism. Ann Pediatr 10:596–605, 1963
Schrier RW: Treatment of hyponatremia. Editorial retrospective. N Engl J Med 312:1122–1123, 1985

PSEUDOLYMPHOMA

Synonym. Anticonvulsant drug sensitivity.

Symptoms. Onset 1 week to 2 years after exposure to one of these drugs. Fever, malaise, and arthralgia.

Signs. Polymorphic skin eruption; generalized lymphadenopathy; hepatosplenomegaly; joint swelling.

Etiology. Sensitivity to anticonvulsant. Diphenylhydantoin (Dilantin) and mephenytoin (Mesantoin) are most common offenders.

Pathology. Lymph node biopsy shows complete loss of normal architecture and replacement of germinal center by reticuloendothelial cells of monstrous size. Skin biopsy normal or myocosis fungoideslike pattern of infiltration with eosinophils. In liver, moderate or minimal fat metamorphosis; eosinophilic infiltration. In bone marrow, marked eosinophilic hyperplasia.

Diagnostic Procedures. *Blood.* Mild anemia, leukopenia, or leukocytosis; eosinophilia. Serum glutamic-oxaloacetic acid (SGOT), lactic dehydrogenase, alkaline phosphatase high. *X-ray of chest.* Normal. *Lupus erythematosus (LE) test.* Negative.

Therapy. Discontinuation of anticonvulsant drug.

Prognosis. Good if drug is suspended (cure in 7–14 days) and substituted. Cross-sensitization possible. If condition not identified, death may result.

BIBLIOGRAPHY. Coope R, Burrows RGR: Treatment of epilepsy with sodium diphenyl hydantoinate. Lancet 1:490–492, 1940
Schreiber MM, McGregor JG: Pseudolymphoma syndrome. A sensitivity to anticonvulsant drugs. Arch Dermatol 97:297–300, 1968

PSEUDO-MEIGS'

Term given by Meigs. Same as true Meigs' syndrome, except that in the pseudo-Meig's syndrome the tumor may be in the ovary, tubes, uterus, or round ligament. After removal of the tumor, ascites and hydrothorax do not necessarily disappear as in the case of true Meig's syndrome.

Therapy. Removal of the tumor.

Prognosis. Depends on nature of tumor, metastasis.

BIBLIOGRAPHY. Meigs JV: Pelvic tumors other than fibromas of the ovary with ascites and hydrothorax. Obstet Gynecol 3:471–486, 1954
Brenner WE, Scott RB: Meigs'-like syndrome secondary to Krukenberg's tumor. Obstet Gynecol 31:40–44, 1968

PSEUDOMEMBRANOUS ENTEROCOLITIS

Synonyms. Hemorrhagic enterocolitis; ischemic enterocolitis; necrotizing colitis; postoperative enterocolitis; staphylococcal enterocolitis; toxic pseudomembranous intestinal inflammation; uremic colitis, including Janbon's.

Symptoms and Signs. Both sexes affected. Usually a severe underlying disease of extremely variable nature.

Abrupt onset (usually after 2 days from beginning of anti-biotics up to 3 wk after their discontinuation). Nausea; vomiting; abdominal cramps and distention; watery, oc-casionally hemorrhagic, diarrhea; shock. Absence of ab-dominal tenderness and frequently also of bowel sounds. Frequently, same symptoms as in paralytic ileus.

Etiology. Antibiotics and metronidazole the most fre-quent causative agents (Janbon's syndrome) of the en-hanced development of *Clostridium difficile* (a normal resident of the intestine).

Pathology. Multiple isolated or confluent white yellow-ish plaques, slightly elevated, from 1 to 3 mm to 20 mm in diameter, covering superficial ulceration. Remaining mu-cosa edematous and hyperemic. Histologically, pseudo-membranes are composed of fibrin, mucus, desquamated cells, and leukocytes.

Diagnostic Procedures. *Sigmoidoscopy.* See Pathology. *X-ray.* Plain film reveals edema and distortion of haustra. *Blood.* Leukocytosis. *Stools.* Culture of *C. difficile* and detection of *C. difficile* cytotoxin.

Therapy. Cessation of antibiotic therapy. Fluid–elec-trolyte balance. Albumin or blood replacement or both. Vancomycin (500 mg × 4/day × 7–10 days), orally me-tronidazole (1.5–2 g/day p os), avoid antidiarrheals. Sur-gery for perforation or toxic dilatation.

Prognosis. Overall mortality 15%.

BIBLIOGRAPHY. Janbon M et al: Le syndrome choleriforme de la terramycine. Montpellier Med 41:300–311, 1952
Stergachis A, Perera DR, Schnell MM, Jick H: Antibi-otic-associated colitis. West J Med 140:217–219, 1984

PSEUDOMETATROPIC DWARFISM

Synonyms. SMED; spondylometaepiphyseal dysplasia. Spondyloepimetaphyseal dysplasia.

Symptoms and Signs. Occur in males; onset at birth. Peculiar face; short limbs; kyphoscoliosis; clubfoot. Later, inadequate length of digits. Recurrent otitis media; deaf-ness.

Etiology. Unknown; autosomal dominant or recessive inheritance.

Diagnostic Procedures. *X-ray.* Changes in spine, hands, and feet. *Blood and urine.* Normal.

Therapy. Orthopedic for kyphoscoliosis, clubfoot, or metatarsus adductus.

Prognosis. Good *quoad vitam.*

BIBLIOGRAPHY. Maloney FP: A distinctive type of spon-dylometaepiphyseal dysplasia (SMED). Birth Defects 5:360–367, 1969
Bailey JA: Disproportionate Short Stature: Diagnosis and Management, p 158. Philadelphia, WB Saunders, 1973
Sillence DO, Horton WA, Rimoin DL: Morphologic studies in the skeletal dysplasias. A Review. Am J Pathol 96:813–870, 1979
Murray LW, Rimoin DL: Type II collagen abnormalities in the spondyloepi- and spondyloepimetaphyseal dys-plasias. Am J Hum Genet 37:A13, 1985

PSEUDOPANCREATIC CHOLERA

Synonym. Chronic idiopathic secretory diarrhea.

Symptoms and Signs. In patients with or without in-testinal resections. Symptoms and signs like those of Verner–Morrison (see).

Etiology. Unknown or endocrine tumor or elevated plasma level secretagogue.

Diagnostic Procedures. Same as Verner–Morrison. Blood research for VIP negative.

Therapy. Somatostatin.

Prognosis. Good with therapy.

BIBLIOGRAPHY. Read NW, Read MG, Krejs GJ et al: A report of five patients with large volume secretory diar-rhea, but no evidence of endocrine tumor or laxative abuse. Dig Dis Sci 27:193–201, 1982
Krejs GJ, Fordtran JS: Diarrhea. In Sleisinger M, Ford-tran JS (eds): Gastrointestinal Diseases, 3rd ed, pp 257–280. Philadelphia, WB Saunders, 1983

PSEUDOPELADE

Symptoms and Signs. Sex and age incidence according to etiology. Idiopathic cases usually occur in females in third to fifth decades. Onset insidious. Formation of small, round, bald areas, smooth, soft, without signs of inflammation (moderate erythema may be present), en-larging and confluent. Vertex most frequently affected.

Etiology. Lupus erythematosus; lichen planus; sclero-derma; keratosis pilaris; idiopathic.

Pathology. Lymphocytic infiltrate around hair follicle; bulb spared; followed by atrophy of hair follicles and sebaceous glands. Sweat glands spared.

Diagnostic Procedures. *Biopsy.* (In early stage). Diag-nosis of associated disorder.

Therapy. Lesion irreversible. Treatment of underlying condition prevents spreading. Autograph from other areas of scalp.

BIBLIOGRAPHY. Degos R, Rabut R, Duperrat B et al: L'état pseudo-peladique, réflexions à propos de cent cas d'alopécies cicatricielles en aires, d'appearance primitive du type pseudopelade. Ann Dermatol Syph 81:5–26, 1954

Rook A, Wilkinson DS, Ebling FJG et al: Textbook of Dermatology, 4th ed, pp 2001–2002. Oxford, Blackwell Scientific Publications, 1986

PSEUDOPSEUDOHYPO-PARATHYROIDISM

Synonym. Albright's II.

Symptoms and Signs. All those of Martin–Albright (see) except there are normal calcium and phosphate values and lack of related symptomatology.

Etiology. Unknown; probably inherited as X-linked disorder. Coexistence of pseudohypoparathyroidism (PHP) and pseudopseudohypoparathyroidism in the same families indicates that anatomy and lack of hormonal response, although related, are not interdependent.

Diagnostic Procedures. *Blood and urine.* Normal. *X-ray.* Calcification seen in PHP not seen in this form.

BIBLIOGRAPHY. Albright F, Forbes AP, Henneman PH: Pseudopseudohypoparathyroidism. Trans Assoc Am Physicians 65:337–350, 1952

Drezler MK, Neelon FA: Pseudopseudohypoparathyroidism. In Stanbury JB, Wyngaarden JB, Fredrickson DS et al: The Metabolic Basis of Inherited Disease. 5th ed, p 1509. New York, McGraw-Hill, 1983

PSEUDO-VITAMIN D DEFICIENCY RICKETS

Synonyms. Rickets, autosomal recessive; Prader's vitamin D-dependent rickets; pseudodeficiency rickets; autosomal recessive vitamin D deficiency (ARVDD). Classified in type I and type II.

TYPE I

Symptoms and Signs. The same as in ordinary rickets due to vitamin D deficiency. Both sexes affected; onset in first 6 to 9 months of life. Growth deficiency; hypotonia; skeletal changes typical of rickets; seizures (hypocalcemia); occasionally fractures. Teeth enamel hypoplasia.

Etiology. Autosomal recessive. Genetic defect of 25-hydroxylcholecalciferol 1-α-hydroxylase that converts 25-(OH) to 1,25-(OH$_2$) D.

Diagnostic Procedures. *Blood.* Hypocalcemia, serum 1,25-(OH$_2$) D low. PTH high. Plasma phosphate normal or low.

Therapy. Vitamin D in daily doses or 1,25-(OH$_2$) D3.

Prognosis. Good with therapy.

TYPE II

Symptoms and Signs. Same as above. Frequent association with alopecia totalis.

Pathology. Probably autosomal recessive. Abnormal function of target organs: intestinal mucosa and bone.

Diagnostic Procedures. *Blood.* Hypocalcemia, hypophosphatemia, high PTH; 1,25-(OH$_2$) D level high.

Therapy. Resistance to treatment with vitamin D at high doses because of end-organ refractoriness. Patients without alopecia are more responsive to pharmacologic doses than patients with alopecia.

BIBLIOGRAPHY. Prader A, Illig R, Hirerli E: Eine besondere Form der primaeren Vitamin D resistenten Rachitis mit Hypocalcaemie und autosomal-dominanten Erbgana: die hereditaere Pseudo-Mangelrachitis. Helv Paediatr Acta 16:456–458, 1961

Rosen JF, Fluschman AR, Finberg L et al: Rickets with alopecia: An inborn error of vitamin D metabolism. J Paediatr 94:729, 1979

PSEUDO-WILLEBRAND

Synonyms. Platelet Willebrand, Willebrand–Jurgens.

Symptoms and Signs. In Puerto Ricans. Those of von Willebrands' (see).

Etiology. X-linked or autosomal dominant inheritance. Platelets remove factor VIII at abnormal rate because of augmented glycoprotein I b.

Diagnostic Procedures. *Blood.* Diminished platelets; large in size. Increased ristocetin—induced platelet aggregation, decreased plasma FV III–VWF.

Therapy. Fresh blood transfusions.

Prognosis. Good. See von Willebrand's.

BIBLIOGRAPHY. Miller JL, Castella A: Platelet type von Willebrand's disease: Characterization of a new bleeding disorder. Blood 60:790–794, 1982

Weiss HJ, Meyer D, Rabinowitz R et al: Pseudo von Willebrand's disease. An intrinsic platelet defect with aggregation by unmodified human factor VIII, von Willebrand factor and enhanced absorption of its high molecular weight multimers. N Engl J Med 306:326–333, 1982

PSOAS MYOSITIS–FIBROSIS

Symptoms. Onset insidious or sudden. Unilateral or bilateral pain in lower quadrants of abdomen, dull and aching, lasting from days to years with periodic exacerbations and remissions. Pain is enhanced by activity and is partly relieved by rest. Fibrositis of different muscles frequently associated (see Fibrositis). Anxiety manifestations.

Signs. Tenderness over psoas muscle. Contraction or stretching of muscles reproduces symptoms. When bilateral, pain stronger on one side.

Etiology. Unknown; trauma, postural defects, acute infections, pregnancy may be the exciting factor.

Pathology. See Fibrositis.

Diagnostic Procedures. Rule out abdominal, urinary tract, gynecologic, and vertebral pathology conditions. *Blood.* Leukocytosis. *X-ray.*

Therapy. See Treatment of Fibrositis. Diagnosis important to prevent useless surgery. Treatment of anxiety manifestation: psychotherapy and tranquilizers.

Prognosis. Generally good response to treatment. See Prognosis in Fibrositis.

BIBLIOGRAPHY. Greene JA: The syndrome of psoas myositis and fibrositis: Its manifestations and its significance in the differential diagnosis of lower abdominal pain. Ann Intern Med 23:30–34, 1945

PSYCHOGENIC CHEST PAIN

Synonyms. Cardiac psychosis, chest discomfort. See Anterior chest wall syndromes.

Symptoms. Gradual onset of a vague distress, usually related to a very limited area (apex of heart, nipple [finger tip sign]) or extensive area covering left anterior and lateral chest. May or may not be associated with arm symptoms. Headache, weakness, fatigability in the morning that disappear with activity or distraction are often associated. Description of type of pain extremely variable. No relation with activity, posture, or meals.

Signs. None.

Etiology. Anxiety reaction often precipitated by death or illness of relative or friend or other psychologic deep-seated derangements. Sometimes iatrogenic. Sometime chest discomfort bound to depression, self-gain motivations, or could be a real cardiac psychosis (with obsessive idea).

Therapy. Psychotherapy according to intensity and functional manifestation of the condition.

Diagnostic Procedures. Rule out cardiogenic origin. In borderline cases a coronary arteriogram may be needed.

Prognosis. Good response to psychotherapy. Frequent conversion to other psychosomatic conditions.

BIBLIOGRAPHY. Senay E, Offenkrantz WC: A case study of psychosomatic symptoms. Consultant 9:42–47, 1969
Hurst JW: The Heart, 6th ed, pp 907–908. New York, McGraw-Hill, 1986

PSYCHOGENIC POLYDIPSIA

Symptoms. Occur usually in women (80%); age at onset 8 to 60, most often between 35 and 60 years. Onset sudden or vague, usually associated with menopause, delusional illness, stress of various kinds. Neurotic trait common in childhood; frequent history of sleep walking. No stable and satisfactory sex life; stormy and dramatic medical history for psychological and organic illness. Excessive fluid intake fluctuating irregularly by the hour or day; polyuria. Periods of remission and relapses lasting months.

Signs. Few physical signs. In some, scars from multiple operations; generally, obesity; fluctuation of blood pressure.

Etiology. Psychotic compulsion associated with other psychotic manifestations, from severe to minor neurotic behavior.

Pathology. Unknown.

Diagnostic Procedures. *Blood.* Plasma osmolality significantly lower than normal. *Urine.* Ability to concentrate urine varies considerably and in most patients is impaired. Vasopressin makes the patient sick, without affecting polydipsia.

Therapy. Continuous narcosis or electroconvulsive therapy.

Prognosis. Spontaneous remissions and relapses. Transient improvement with therapy.

BIBLIOGRAPHY. Bralow ED, de Wardener HE: Compulsive water drinking. QJ Med 28:235–258, 1959
Goldberg M: Abnormalities in the renal excretion of water. Med Clin North Am 47:915–933, 1963

PSYCHOMOTOR ATTACKS

Synonym. Psychomotor convulsion; psychomotor epilepsy; precursive epilepsy, psychomotor equivalent; temporal lobe epilepsy. Complex partial seizures. See Grand mal and Petit mal.

Symptoms. Onset at any age. Change in consciousness with alteration of thoughts and feelings. Motor activity partially correlated. Aura of hallucinogenic type may precede the attack. Patient acts and talks as if partially conscious; his behavior is erratic and he may commit strange acts, sometimes violent. Occasionally, he may fall asleep after the attack and have partial amnesia of events. These patients also may have a deep alteration of their personality between attacks: paranoid; homicidal tendency; various types of psychoses.

Etiology. Idiopathic or cerebral lesion (temporal) and frontal or amygdaloid-hippocampal.

Diagnostic Procedure. *Electroencephalography.*

Therapy. Diphenylhydantoin; primidone; phenobarbital. Surgical removal of temporal lobe lesion.

Prognosis. Poor for emotional and psychic stability.

BIBLIOGRAPHY. Falconer MA, Serafetinides EA, Corsellis JAN: Etiology and pathogenesis of temporal lobe epilepsy. Arch Neurol 10:233–248, 1964

Adams RD, Victor M: Principles of Neurology, 3rd ed, p 237. New York, McGraw-Hill, 1985

PSYCHOPHONASTHENIA

Symptoms. Frequently starting in late adolescence or following some crisis in private or professional life. Occur in a person, usually cultured (singer; minister; lawyer), intelligent, but with strong, withdrawn personality, who is timid and highly sensitive. Sensitivity of the throat; choking sensation when attempting to speak, paresthesias of head and neck; dryness or excessive secretion of mouth. Cracking of the voice and, when speaking for some time, aching of vocal cords.

Signs. Occasionally, accompanying signs are tachycardia, palpitation, and sweating.

Etiology. Neurotic manifestation deriving from feeling of inadequacy. To be differentiated from true phonasthenia, where local pathology exists.

Therapy. Psychotherapy.

Prognosis. Good with treatment. Relapse or other neurotic manifestations may appear.

BIBLIOGRAPHY. Greene JS: Psychophonasthenia syndrome. Ann Otol Rhinol Laryngol 50:1177–1184, 1941

PTEROGOPALATINE FOSSA

Synonym. Sphenomaxillary fossa; see Foix–Jefferson.

Symptoms. More or less continuous, severe pain in the upper jaw (mistaken for toothache) in the region of upper back molar teeth; disturbed sensitivity on the cheek and infraorbital foramen. Distribution second branch of trigeminal (V) nerve. Later, extension of pain to lower jaw. Homolateral deafness (middle ear type). Later, palate paralysis and anesthesia and paralysis of pterygoid muscles (deviation of jaw on opening the mouth); homolateral blindness.

Signs. On posterior rhinoscopy, fullness of lateral wall of nasopharynx. Fullness of temporal fossa visible externally (late). Unilateral or bilateral enlargment of cervical and retropharyngeal glands. Later, antral lavage may show bleeding.

Etiology. More frequently, metastatic lesion in the pterygopalatine fossa; less frequently, primary lesions spreading from lateral wall of posterior part of nose or from sinus of Morgagni. In the latter case, Trotter's syndrome is included; this syndrome may precede, follow, or occur in combination.

Pathology. Neoplastic, metastatic, or primary lesion in the pterygopalatine fossa, successively invading antrum, pterygoid lamina, eustachian tube, alveolus, temporal fossa, optic (II) nerve, interior of orbit. Metastasis in lymph node, liver, and skeleton.

Diagnostic Precedures. *X-ray.* Involvement of foramen. Foramen ovale normal at first. *Biopsy.*

Therapy. Deep x-ray; radium implantation; chemotherapy.

Prognosis. Poor; treatment only palliative.

BIBLIOGRAPHY. Asherson N: Trotter's syndrome and associated lesions. J Laryngol Otol 65:349–366, 1951

Adams RD, Victor M: Principles of Neurology, 3rd ed, p 1009. New York, McGraw-Hill, 1985

PUGH

Synonyms. Pseudouveitis, glaucoma, hyphema. See UGH.

Symptoms and Signs. Pseudouveitis, glaucoma, and hyphema (UGH syndrome) plus neovascular membrane over iris and occlusion of central retinal veins.

Etiology. Unknown, unrelated to presence of intraocular lens.

BIBLIOGRAPHY. Pallin SL: Condition mimicking UGH syndrome said unrelated to presence of IOL. Ophthal Times, Aug, 1983, p 50

PULMONARY ARTERIES STENOSIS

Synonyms. Pure pulmonary arteries stenosis; supravalvular pulmonic stenosis.

Symptoms. Age at onset from infancy to adulthood. Usually, asymptomatic for a long time; sooner or later fatigue, exertional dyspnea, occasionally chest pain, or syncope on effort.

Signs. High-pitched ejection type of systolic murmur ending before second sound. Maximal on second left interspace. Administration of amyl nitrate intensifies murmur. Palpable thrill in area of maximal intensity of sound. Increased split of second sound. Occasionally, hemoptysis.

Etiology. Unknown; congenital cardiac anomaly. Familial association with autosomal dominant pattern in some cases. This syndrome may also be simulated by external compression of pulmonic artery. Occasionally, rubella infection in the mother (see Gregg's).

Pathology. Pulmonic stenosis at level of infundibulum, valve, or main pulmonary artery.

Diagnostic Procedures. *X-ray.* Early, normal size of heart; later; right ventricular enlargement. Pulmonary fields clear. *Angiocardiography.* Moderate or absent dilatation of pulmonary trunk, poststenotic dilatation of intrapulmonary vessels. *Electrocardiography. Cardiac catheterization. Pressures. Oximetry.*

Therapy. Surgical enlargement of stenotic passage. Balloon angioplasty, pericardial or synthetic patch angioplasty.

Prognosis. Surgical mortality below 10%, with mild or moderate stenosis; usually, no sign of deterioration. In severe stenosis, progressive deterioration. Median age of death from pure pulmonic stenosis 20 years. Half do not reach adult life; but survival beyond 70 years in some cases reported.

BIBLIOGRAPHY. Oppenheimer EH: Partial atresia of main branches of pulmonary artery occurring in infancy and accompanied by calcification of pulmonary artery and aorta. Bull Johns Hopkins Hosp 63:261–277, 1838
Currens JH, Kinney TD, White PD: Pulmonary stenosis with intact interventricular septum. Am Heart J 30:491–510, 1945
Friedberg CK: Diseases of the Heart, 3rd ed. Philadelphia, WB Saunders, 1966

Lock JE, Castaneda–Zuniga WR, Fuhrman BP et al: Balloon dilatation angioplasty of hypoplastic and stenotic pulmonary arteries. Circulation 67:962–967, 1983
Hurst JW: The Heart, 6th ed, pp 680–681. New York, McGraw-Hill, 1986

PULMONARY ARTERIOVENOUS FISTULA

Synonyms. Pulmonary arteriovenous aneurysm; arteriovenous varix; lung hemangioma. See Rendu–Osler–Weber.

Symptoms. Occur usually in young adults of both sexes; may be observed in infancy and childhood. Symptoms depend on size of shunt: from asymptomatic to exertional dyspnea, chest pain, dizziness, syncopal or epileptiform seizures, Morgagni–Adams–Stokes syndrome, hemoptysis.

Signs. Cyanosis; clubbing of fingers and toes. Continuous murmur may be heard over affected lung; heart enlarged (but not as much as in acquired arteriovenous fistula). Hemangiomas of skin and mucosae frequently associated.

Etiology. Unknown; inherited familial condition in cases where Rendu–Osler–Weber is present.

Pathology. Single or multiple arteriovenous fistulas in the lung, more common in right lower lobe.

Diagnostic Procedures. *Blood.* Polycythemia. *X-ray.* Pulmonary density. *Fluoroscopy.* Pulsating or nonpulsating masses. *Tomography.* Spherical lesion attached to a vessel. *Angiocardiography.*

Therapy. Resection of aneurysm; lobectomy or pneumonectomy; bilateral resection reported.

Prognosis. Cure obtained by resection of fistula(s).

BIBLIOGRAPHY. Churton T: Leeds and West-Riding Medico-Chirurgical Society: Multiple aneurysm of pulmonary artery. Br Med J 1:1223, 1897
Smith HL, Horton BT: Arteriovenous fistula of lung associated with polycythemia vera: Report of case in which diagnosis was made clinically. Am Heart J 18:589–592, 1939
Perloff JK: The Clinical Recognition of Congenital Heart Disease, p 723. 2nd ed, Philadelphia, WB Saunders, 1978
Mattila S, Meurala H, Jarvinen A et al: Pulmonary arteriovenous fistulas. Scand J Thorac Cardiovasc Surg 16:165–168, 1982
Hurst JW: The Heart 6th ed, pp 680–681. New York, McGraw-Hill, 1986

PULMONARY ARTERY COMPRESSION ASCENDING AORTA ANEURYSM

Symptoms and Signs. Occur in syphilitic patients. Aortic incompetence; right ventricular hypertrophy; single second sound.

Etiology. Syphilitic aneurysm of ascending aorta compressing pulmonary artery.

Diagnostic Procedures. *X-ray.* Enlargement of heart; marked enlargement of pulmonary artery with clear lung fields (one lung more oligemic than the other); calcification of the aneurysm. *Electrocardiography.* Right axis deviation; vertical position; biventricular hypertrophy. *Catheterization.* Right ventricle displaced to the left; failure to push the tip on compressed pulmonary artery. *Angiocardiography.* Demonstration of compression and absence of valvular stenosis. *Aortogram. Blood.* Serology positive. *Echocardiography.*

Therapy. Penicillin; surgery to correct aneurysm.

Prognosis. Progressive disease leading to death. Good results with surgery.

BIBLIOGRAPHY. Pearson JR, Nichol ES: The syndrome of compression of the pulmonary artery by a syphilitic aortic aneurysm resulting in chronic cor pulmonale, with a report of a case. Ann Intern Med 34:483–492, 1951

Kulkarni TP, Gandhi MJ, Datey KK: The syndrome of compression of the pulmonary artery by an aneurysm of the ascending aorta. Am Heart J 65:678–682, 1963

DeBakey ME, Noon GP: Aneurysm of the thoracic aorta. Mod Concepts Cardiovasc Dis 44:53–58, 1975

Bickerstaff LX, Pairoleno PC, Hollier DC et al: Thoracic aortic aneurysms: A population-based study. Surgery 92:1103–1108, 1982

Hurst JW: The Heart, 6th ed, pp 1324–1328. New York, McGraw-Hill, 1986

PULMONARY CYSTIC LYMPHANGIECTASIS

Synonyms. CPCL; pulmonary lymphangiectasia.

Symptoms. Onset at birth (some stillborn) or in first day of life. Cyanosis and respiratory distress. Conditions associated with pulmonary hypertension particularly when the pulmonary venous pressure chronically exceeds 30 mm Hg.

Signs. Numerous rales in both lungs; heart sounds normal; associated pleural effusion in some cases. Lymphedema of other organs also occasionally seen. Occasion-ally, associated with congenital cretinism or congenital heart disease (one third of cases).

Etiology. Autosomal recessive inheritance.

Pathology. Lungs larger than normal; pale firm, numerous small cysts with tense walls, transparent and glistening, containing clear colorless serous fluid. Localized lung atelectasis. Cyst wall lined with flat endothelium. No signs of inflammation in connective tissue. No connection between air passage and cysts.

Diagnostic Procedures. *X-ray of lung. Respiratory function tests.*

Therapy. Symptomatic.

Prognosis. Poor; death in early infancy.

BIBLIOGRAPHY. Virkow R: Gesammelte Abhandlungen zur Wissenschaflichen Medicin. Frankfurt, 1851

Laurence KM: Congenital pulmonary cystic lymphangiectasis. J Pathol Bacteriol 70:325–333, 1955

Felman AH, Rathigan RM, Pierson KK: Pulmonary lymphangiectasia: Observation in 17 patients and proposed classification. Am J Roentgenol 116:548–553, 1972

Scott–Emnakpor AB, Warren ST et al: Familial occurrence of congenital pulmonary lymphangiectasis: Genetic implication. Am J Dis Child 135:532–534, 1981

PULMONARY STENOSIS–PATENT FORAMEN OVALE OR OSTIUM SECUNDUM DEFECT

Synonyms. Fallot's trilogy (with reversed shunt).

Symptoms. Cyanosis especially on exertion may appear shortly after birth, but more frequently occurs later; occasionally, after puberty or in adult life; eventually becoming persistent. Squatting posture occasionally; inadequate weight gain; frequent pulmonary infections; fatigue; exertional dyspnea.

Signs. Clubbing of fingers and toes; high-pitched ejection murmur (briefer and earlier than that observed in pure pulmonic stenosis, see); second sound single. Administration of amyl nitrate decreases murmur.

Etiology. Unknown congenital heart malformation.

Pathology. Pulmonary stenosis with patent foramen ovale.

Diagnostic Procedures. *X-Ray of chest. Angiocardiography. Electrocardiography. Cardiac catheterization. Pressure. Oximetry. Echocardiography. Frank vectocardiogram.*

Therapy. Surgery.

Prognosis. Mortality from surgery 10%. Right-sided heart failure appears in third or fourth decade and is main cause of death. Occasionally subacute bacterial endocarditis (SBE) and cerebral abscesses causes of death.

BIBLIOGRAPHY. Selzer A, Carnes WH, Noble CA et al: The syndrome of pulmonary stenosis with patent foramen ovale. Am J Med 6:3–23, 1949
Friedberg CK: Diseases of the Heart, 3rd ed. Philadelphia, WB Saunders, 1966
Hurst JW: The Heart 6th ed, pp 654–658. New York, McGraw-Hill, 1986

PULMONARY SUBVALVULAR STENOSIS

Synonyms. Infundibular pulmonary stenosis; subinfundibular pulmonary stenosis.

Symptoms and Signs. Rare as isolated defect. Both sexes affected; present from birth. Same characteristics as pulmonary valve stenosis with the following differentiating signs: right ventricular impulse does not reach third left interspace; murmur and thrill maximal in fourth interspace; ejection sound absent.

Etiology. Congenital sporadic malformation. Hypertrophy of infundibular muscle may be responsible for stenosis.

Pathology. Infundibular stenosis more frequent than subinfundibular. Absence of poststenotic dilatation. Infundibulum may be dilated. Defect usually associated with ventricular septal defect, pure form seldom seen.

Diagnostic Procedures. *X-ray.* Absence of dilatation of pulmonary trunk; right aortic arch; local indentation at ostium of infundibulum. *Electrocardiography. Angiocardiography. Echocardiography. Cardiac catheterization. Right ventricular angiography.*

Therapy. Surgical valvotomy in cardiopulmonary bypass.

Prognosis. Good with surgery.

BIBLIOGRAPHY. Perloff JK: The Clinical Recognition of Congenital Heart Disease, 2nd ed, p 185. Philadelphia, WB Saunders, 1978
Hurst JW: The Heart, 6th ed, pp 658–659. New York, McGraw-Hill, 1986

PULMONARY TRUNK IDIOPATHIC DILATATION

Symptoms. Absent.

Signs. Characteristic auscultatory and phonocardiographic findings: split apical first sound; first component

of equal or greater intensity than second component; systolic click ushers in a systolic ejection murmur louder in pulmonary area. Second sound widely split. A short diastolic murmur may be present in the second intercostal space.

Etiology. Unknown; possibly a *forme fruste* of Marfan's. Criteria for diagnosis of this rare form are (1) simple dilatation of pulmonary artery or its main branches; (2) occasionally, association of hypoplasia of aorta; (3) absence of heart congenital anomalies, lung diseases, rheumatism, and syphilis.

Pathology. In some cases cystic medial necrosis of wall of pulmonary artery may be found. Medial degeneration can be severe enough to result in aneurysm, rupture, or dissection that is found in the main pulmonary arteries.

Diagnostic Procedures. *Electrocardiography.* Normal. *X-ray.* Dilatation of pulmonary artery. *Phonocardiography. Cardiac catheterization.* Normal right ventricular systolic pressure and systolic pressure difference across pulmonic valve of 15 mm Hg or less during stress (diagnostic).

Therapy. None.

Prognosis. Pulmonic valve insufficiency may develop over a period of years. Benign prognosis.

BIBLIOGRAPHY. Wessler H, Jackes L: Clinical Roentgenology of Disease of the Chest, pp 26–29. Troy (NY), Southworth, 1923
Ramsey HW, De la Torre A, Linhart JW et al: Idiopathic dilatation of the pulmonary artery. Am J Cardiol 20:324–330, 1967
McKusick VA: Heritable Disorders of Connective Tissue, 4th ed, p 61. CV Mosby, St Louis, 1972
Perloff JK: The Clinical Recognition of Congenital Heart Disease, 2nd ed, p 222. Philadelphia, WB Saunders, 1978
Hurst JW: The Heart, 6th ed, p 1322. New York, McGraw-Hill, 1986

PULMONARY VALVE ATRESIA–INTACT VENTRICULAR SEPTUM

TYPE I

Symptoms and Signs. Cyanosis from birth; distress and acute illness from first days of life. On heart auscultation, soft systolic murmur, maximal intensity mid-left sternal border, or high frequency and located in lower left sternal border. Diastolic murmur absent; quiet, single second sound. Hepatomegaly; seldom, liver pulsation.

Etiology. Unknown.

Pathology. Pulmonary valvular atresia with intact ventricular septum, small volume, thick-walled right ventricle, and hypoplastic tricuspid orifice (Type I).

Diagnostic Procedures. *X-ray.* Transverse heart configuration with moderate enlargement; concavity in main pulmonary segment; decreased vascularity. *Electrocardiography. Catheterization. Angiocardiography. Echocardiography.*

Therapy. Surgery.

Prognosis. Death from first day to 15 months; when operated, from 2 days to 5 years. High mortality at surgery.

TYPE II

Symptoms and Signs. Impossible to differentiate from Ebstein's (see) on clinical data. Only difference, more severe respiratory distress.

Etiology. Unknown.

Pathology. Pulmonary valvular atresia with intact ventricular septum, normal-sized or dilated right ventricle, and tricuspid orifice regurgitation (Type II).

Diagnostic Procedures. *X-ray. Electrocardiography. Cardiac catheterization. Angiocardiography. Echocardiography.* Sometimes allow differentiation between this syndrome and the Ebstein's syndrome.

Therapy. Differential diagnosis important because emergency pulmonary valvotomy may benefit this condition while surgery is contraindicated in Ebstein's.

Prognosis. Poor.

BIBLIOGRAPHY. Neufeld EA, Cole RB, Paul MH: Ebstein's malformation of the tricuspid valve in the neonate. Am J Cardiol 19:727–731, 1967
Cole RB, Muster AJ, Lev M et al: Pulmonary atresia with intact ventricular septum. Am J Cardiol 21:23–31, 1968
Lewis BS, Amitai N, Simcha A et al: Echocardiographic diagnosis of pulmonary atresia with intact ventricular septum. Am Heart J 97:92–95, 1983
Freedom RM, Wilson G, Trusler GA et al: Pulmonary atresia and intact ventricular septum. Scand J Thorac Cardiovasc Surg 17:26–36, 1983
Hurst JW: The Heart, 6th ed, pp 660–662. New York, McGraw-Hill, 1986

PULMONARY VALVE DYSPLASIA

Synonyms. Congenital pulmonary valve dysplasia. See Pulmonary valve stenosis.

Symptoms and Signs. Abnormal facies, hypertelorism, ptosis, low-set ears, and mental retardation. Growth re-tardation. No ejection sound or pulmonic component of second sound. Is especially common in patients with Noonan's syndrome.

Etiology. Congenital hereditary disorder.

Pathology. Pulmonary valve characterized by three distinct cusps, absence of commissural fusion, and annular hypoplasia. Cusps contain myxomatous tissue.

Diagnostic Procedures. *X-ray.* See Pulmonary valve stenosis, plus absence of poststenotic dilatation. *Electrocardiography. Echocardiogram. Cardiac catheterization. Vectocardiogram.*

Therapy. Surgical valvotomy.

Prognosis. Fair with surgery.

BIBLIOGRAPHY. Koretzky ED, Moller JH, Korus ME et al: Congenital pulmonary stenosis resulting from dysplasia of the valve. Circulation 40:43–53, 1969
Linde LM, Turner SW, Sparkes RS: Pulmonary valve dysplasia. A cardiological syndrome. Br Heart J 35:301–304, 1973
Hurst JW: The Heart, 6th ed, p 654. New York, McGraw-Hill, 1986

PULMONARY VALVE INSUFFICIENCY

Symptoms. Characteristically absent or nonspecific; mild exertional dyspnea. Hyperdynamic right ventricular impulse.

Signs. Diastolic murmur of low frequency, heard best at pulmonary area or a little lower along left sternal border, increasing in intensity during inspiration. Short systolic ejection murmur may also be present.

Etiology. Congenital valve defect, or idiopathic dilatation of pulmonary artery.

Diagnostic Procedures. *Electrocardiography.* Normal or right ventricular hypertrophy. *Phonocardiography and intracardiac phonocardiography. Cardiac catheterization.* (Diagnostic). *X-ray of chest. Echocardiography. Angiocardiography.*

Therapy. None specific; antibiotic prophylaxis during dental procedures and conditions leading to bacteremia.

Prognosis. Patients asymptomatic. They may reach adulthood free of limitation. Increased incidence of bacterial endocarditis.

BIBLIOGRAPHY. Kezdi P, Priest WS, Smith JM: Pulmonic regurgitation. Q Bull Northwest Univ Med School 29:368–373, 1955
Criscitiello MG, Harvey WP: Clinical recognition of congenital pulmonary valve insufficiency. Am J Cardiol 20:765–772, 1967

Perloff JK: The Clinical Recognition of Congenital Heart Disease, 2nd ed, p 228. Philadelphia, WB Saunders, 1978

Keith JD, Rowe RD, Vlad P: Heart Disease in Infancy and Childhood, 3rd ed, pp 841–843. New York, Macmillan, 1978

PULMONARY VALVE STENOSIS

Synonym. Valvular pulmonic stenosis.

Symptoms and Signs. Both sexes equally affected; present from birth; diagnosis usually suspected, however, during first year of life. Frequent malformation. From asymptomatic to fatigue, dyspnea with exertion (according to degree of obstruction), squatting, seldom syncope. Prominent midsystolic murmur and thrill maximal in second left interspace; pulmonic ejection sound. History of unimpaired growth; acyanosis; occasionally, high colored cheeks. Hepatomegaly.

Etiology. Congenital defect. Rarely, acquired (*e.g.*, rheumatic fever, bacterial endocarditis). Familial cases reported.

Pathology. Heart conical or dome-shaped structure with a narrow outlet. Poststenotic dilatation of pulmonary trunk and left pulmonary artery dilatation. In adults calcification. In case of dome-shaped stenosis with patent foramen ovale or atrial septal defect, the term trilogy of Fallot is applied.

Diagnostic Procedures. *Electrocardiography.* Right atrial and ventricular hypertrophy. *X-ray.* Normal or reduced pulmonary arteries. *Blood.* Hematocrit elevated; normal oxygen saturation. *Ultrasonography. Vector cardiography. Cardiac catheterization.*

Therapy. Surgical correction. Valvotomy.

Prognosis. According to degree of stenosis. Generally, survival into adulthood (average age at death 26 yr).

BIBLIOGRAPHY. Edwards JE: Pulmonary stenosis with intact ventricular septum. In Gould SE: Pathology of the Heart, 2nd ed. Springfield, CC Thomas, 1960

Perloff JK: The Clinical Recognition of Congenital Heart Disease, 2nd ed, p 185. Philadelphia, WB Saunders, 1978

Srinivasan V, Konyer A, Broda JJ, et al: Critical pulmonary stenosis in infants less than 3 months of age: A reappraisal of closed transventricular pulmonary valvotomy. J Thorac Cardiovasc Surg 83:375, 1983

Williams RG, Bierman FZ, Sanders SP: Echocardiographic Diagnosis of Cardiac Malformations, 1st ed, pp 111–112. Boston, Little Brown & Company, 1986

Hurst JW: The Heart, 6th ed, pp 654–658. New York, McGraw-Hill, 1986

PULMONARY VEIN STENOSIS

Synonyms. Congenital pulmonary vein stenosis. See Pulmonary vein stenosis–patent foramen ovale. The obstruction in the venules and small veins is designated as pulmonary veno-occlusive disease.

Symptoms and Signs. Uncomplicated vein stenosis rare. Both sexes affected; present from birth. Dyspnea; tachypnea; failure to thrive. Repeated respiratory infections. Hemoptysis.

Etiology. Congenital malformation.

Pathology. Two varieties recognized: (1) narrowing near junction with left atrium (extrapulmonic); (2) narrowing at various distances in extrapulmonary or intrapulmonary sections. Usually, several veins involved.

Diagnostic Procedures. *X-ray.* Symmetric or asymmetric pulmonary congestion; absence of left atrial enlargement. Cardiomegaly (right atrium and ventricle). *Electrocardiography.* Sinus rhythm; right atrial enlargement and right axis deviation. P waves left atrial absent; occasionally, normal. *Cardiac catheterization and echocardiography.* To exclude mitral stenosis and cor triatriatum. Stenosis of individual pulmonary veins (first variety).

Therapy. Medical management of congestive heart failure. Surgical management: discrete stenosis of pulmonary veins has seldom been relieved by operation or balloon dilatation.

Prognosis. Death range from 5 months to 10 years. Pulmonary veno-occlusion disease (second variety) average survival from onset: 20 months.

BIBLIOGRAPHY. Nakib A, Moller JH, Kanjuh VI et al: Anomalies of the pulmonary vein. Am J Cardiol 20:77–90, 1967

Driscoll DJ, Hesslein PS, Mullins CE: Congenital stenosis of individual pulmonary veins: Clinical spectrum and unsuccessful treatment by transvenous balloon dilatation. Am J Cardiol 49:1767–1773, 1982

Hurst JW: The Heart, 6th ed, pp 652–653. New York, McGraw-Hill, 1986

PULMONARY VENOUS ANOMALOUS DRAINAGE– MITRAL STENOSIS

Symptoms and Signs. Clinical impression of interatrial septal defect and tight mitral stenosis.

Etiology. Congenital defect.

Pathology. Pulmonary vein entering superior vena cava or right atrium determining a left-to-right shunt. Mitral stenosis; absence of interatrial septal defect.

Diagnostic Procedures. *Electrocardiography.* Right ventricular hypertrophy. *X-ray of chest.* Enlargement of right ventricle; hypoplastic aorta. *Cardiac catheterization.* Pulmonary wedge pressure elevated; large left-to-right shunt; high oxygen saturation in right atrium. *Echocardiogram. Cardiac catheterization.* Findings of high or low pulmonary artery wedge pressure in different parts of lungs may be additional evidence for presence of partial anomalous venous drainage.

Therapy. Surgery with correction of mitral stenosis and resection of pulmonary lobe if correction of left-to-right shunt not otherwise possible.

Prognosis. Good with surgery. Decrease subjective and objective symptoms.

BIBLIOGRAPHY. Hughes CW, Rumore PC: Anomalous pulmonary veins. Arch Pathol 37:364–366, 1944

Wassermil M, Hoffman MS: Partial anomalous pulmonary venous drainage associated with mitral stenosis with an intact atrial septum. Am J Cardiol 10:894–899, 1962

Hurst JW: The Heart, 6th ed, pp 603–605. New York, McGraw-Hill, 1986

PULMONARY VENOUS ANOMALOUS DRAINAGE TO HEPATIC VEIN

Synonym. Anomalous pulmonary venous drainage to hepatic vein.

Symptoms. Both sexes affected; present from birth. Dyspnea.

Signs. Cyanosis; edema; second pulmonic sound accentuated; absence of murmurs; pulsating hepatomegaly.

Etiology. Congenital defect.

Pathology. Pulmonary veins united entering the hepatic vein. Left atrium and ventricle very small; right atrium and ventricle enlarged. Marked pulmonary congestion.

Diagnostic Procedures. *Electrocardiography.* Right axis deviation; right ventricle hypertrophy. Peaked, high P waves. *Angiocardiography.* Shows dye below diaphragm. *Echocardiography.*

Therapy. Symptomatic. Early surgical correction.

Prognosis. Fatal; congestive failure in first month of life.

BIBLIOGRAPHY. Perloff JK: The Clinical Recognition of Congenital Heart Disease, 2nd ed, p 284. Philadelphia, WB Saunders, 1978

Hurst JW: The Heart, 6th ed, pp 603–605. New York, McGraw-Hill, 1986

PULMONARY VENOUS ANOMALOUS DRAINAGE TO RIGHT ATRIUM

Synonyms. Anomalous pulmonary venous drainage; anomalous pulmonary venous connection (Taussig–Snellen–Alberts); partial anomalous pulmonary venous connection; Taussig–Snellen–Alberts.

Symptoms. Both sexes affected; present from birth. Dyspnea; asthenia; easy fatigability; recurrent respiratory infections.

Signs. Cyanosis absent; skin semitranslucent; occasionally, deformity of left side of thorax; tachypnea; distended veins of neck; pulsating hepatomegaly; right atrium and ventricle enlarged; accentuation of second pulmonic sound; precordial systolic and midsystolic apical murmurs; arrhythmias.

Etiology. Congenital defect.

Pathology. Right pulmonary veins join the left atrium close to the rim of ostium secundum defect; or one or more pulmonary veins enter the right atrium or a systemic vein (anomalous connection). Atrial septal defect of patency of foramen ovale frequently associated. Right lung preferentially involved (10 : 1).

Diagnostic Procedures. *Electrocardiography.* Right axis deviation; right ventricle hypertrophy; P waves elevated. *Cardiac catheterization.* Oxygen saturation of right auricle greater than superior vena cava. Pulmonary artery increased pressure. *Cineangiography. Echocardiography. Cardiac catheterization.*

Therapy. Surgical correction. Early surgical correction when large pulmonary blood flow, congestive failure or pulmonary arterial hypertension is present.

Prognosis. Possibly, cardiac failure. Survival into adulthood.

BIBLIOGRAPHY. Snellen HA, Alberts FH: The clinical diagnosis of anomalous pulmonary venous drainage. Circulation 8:801–816, 1952

Taussig HB: Congenital Malformation of the Heart. Cambridge, The Commonwealth Fund, Harvard University Press, 1960

Lucas RV Jr: Anomalous venous connections, pulmonary and systemic. In Adams FH, Emmanonillides GC (eds): Mass Heart Diseases in Infants, Children and Adolescents, p 458. Baltimore, Williams & Wilkins, 1983

Hurst JW: The Heart, 6th ed, p 603–605. New York, McGraw-Hill, 1986

PULPOSUS

Synonyms. Traumatic discopathy; herniated disk; intervertebral disk protrusion; herniated nucleus pulposus.

Symptoms and Signs. Both sexes affected; onset in vigorous subjects of middle age. *Minimal form.* Asymptomatic or minor symptoms (see below) subsiding with bed rest (diagnosed by myelography). *Classical form.* History of backache. Initial episode usually follows a minor traumatic injury (following a snap); progressive increase of pain and then distal radiation. Backache that subsides, while the full sciatica syndrome (see Cotugno's) develops with all its sensorial and eventually motor features.

Etiology. Single trauma or more frequently minor trauma or strain acting on already partly degenerated annulus, which causes a prolapse of nucleus pulposus and of degenerated annulus toward the weakest point (left or right of posterior midline). According to the degree of protrusion and extrusion of the nucleus, various clinical patterns are elicited.

Pathology. Most frequent sites of herniation are L4–L5, L5–S1, less frequently L3–L4; rarely other locations.

Diagnostic Procedures. *Myelography.* To be reserved for atypical cases and when contemplating intervention. *X-ray.* In various projections and positions. *CT scan.*

Therapy. Bed rest; analgesics; anti-inflammatory agents; vitamin B_{12}. Operative treatment with or without vertebral fusion.

Prognosis. Attacks usually subside in 2 to 3 weeks with treatment or may assume subchronic or chronic evolution.

BIBLIOGRAPHY. Mixter WJ, Barr JS: Rupture of intervertebral disc with involvement of spinal canal. N Engl J Med 211:210–215, 1934
Wilson PD, Levine DB: Low back pain and sciatica. In Hollander JL, McCarty DJ: Arthritis and Allied Conditions, 8th ed. Philadelphia, Lea & Febiger, 1972
Weinstein J, Stratt KF, Lehman T et al: Lumbar disc herniation: a comparison of the results of chemonucleolysis and open discectomy after ten years. J Bone Joint Surg (Am) 68A:43–54, 1986
Nyström B: Experience of microsurgical compared with conventional techniques in lumbar disc operations. Acta neurol Scand 76:129–141, 1987

PUPILLOTONIC PSEUDOTABES

Synonyms. Argyll Robertson's with mydriasis; myotonic pupil; pupillotonia; Ross'; iridoplegia interna. If combined with altered deep tendon reflexes: Adie's; Holmes' IV; Holmes–Adie; Markus'; Reys Holmes'; Saengers'; Weill's.

Symptoms. Relatively sudden impairment of vision, with blurring, difficulty in reading, and headache. More frequent in females in the second and third decades.

Signs. Dilatation of affected pupil (80% unilateral); absent or delayed light accommodation and less severely involved convergence accommodation response. The pupil may occasionally after contracting slowly become smaller than the normal one. Diminution or absence of tendon reflexes may be present. Tonic pupil dilates with atropine. Differential diagnosis with Argyll Robertson pupil (see Argyll Robertson).

Etiology. Unknown; occasionally, in association with posttraumatic conditions or infective diseases; autosomal dominant inheritance also reported.

Pathology. Partial degeneration of postganglionic fibers to the sphincter muscles from ciliary ganglion.

Diagnostic Procedures. *Methacholine test.* Solution (2.5%) instilled into conjunctival sac gives rapid constriction of miotic pupil; pupil reacts normally to epinephrine and cocaine.

Therapy. Trial with parenteral administration of mecholyl.

Prognosis. Once developed, the syndrome remains; benign condition. The pupil tends to become smaller with increasing years.

BIBLIOGRAPHY. Mylius NI: Ueber familiacres Vorkommen der Pupillotonic. Klin Monatsbl Augenheilkd 101:598–599, 1938
See Adie's. Lowenstein O, Loewenfeld IE: Pupillotonic pseudotabes (syndrome of Markus–Weill and Reys–Holmes–Adie): A critical review of the literature. Survey Ophthalmol 10:129–185, 1965
Richwien R: Pathophysiology of tonic pupil and other stages of iridoplegia along with observation on the iridoplegia-areflexia syndrome (Weill–Reys–Holmes–Adie syndrome). Adv Ophthalmol 25:166–187, 1972
Agbeja AM, Dutton GM: Adie's syndrome as a cause of amblyopia. J Pediatr Ophthalmol Strabismus, 24:176–177, 1987

PURE RED CELL APLASIA

Synonym. Acquired erythrocytic hypoplasia.

Symptoms and Signs. Male-to-female ratio 2:1. All findings similar to pure red cell aplasia–thymoma syndrome (see), with the exception of the presence of the tumor. Onset at birth or within the first 2 years of life.

Etiology. Unknown. Possible mechanisms proposed include: a metabolic defect in the handling of tryptophan; the direct action of a virus; an immunologic response to a viral infection.

BIBLIOGRAPHY. Tsai SY, Levin WC: Chronic erythrocytic hypoplasia in adults. Am J Med 22:322–331, 1957
Wintrobe MM (ed): Clinical Hematology, 8th ed, p 837. Philadelphia, Lea & Febiger, 1981

PURE RED CELL APLASIA–THYMOMA

Synonyms. Erythrocytic hypoplasia–thymoma. Thymoma–erythrocytic hypoplasia.

Symptoms. In patients with thymoma, the aregenerative anemia association is present in 5% to 10% of cases. In adult patients with aregenerative anemia, thymoma is present in 50% of cases. Average age of onset 60 years (range 20–78 yr). Prevalent in females (4 : 1). Fatigue; weakness; shortness of breath; hemorrhagic manifestations in some cases progressive. Symptoms of myasthenia gravis may be associated.

Signs. Pallor; no lymphadenopathy or splenomegaly. Retrosternal dullness when tumor sufficiently enlarged.

Etiology. Unknown; possibly autoimmune disorder.

Pathology. Thymomas, almost always benign. Usually, spindle cell or spindle cell-lymphocytic varieties; less frequently lymphoepithelioma, lymphocytic, fibrous, and cystic.

Diagnostic Procedures. *Blood.* Hemoglobin level usually below 6 g; normocytic-normochromic type. Reticulocytes low or absent. Thrombocytopenia (10%), pancytopenia (10%); neutropenia and anemia (8%); hypogammaglobulinemia (10%); hypergammaglobulinemia (8%). *Bone marrow.* Marked hypoplasia of erythroid series; lymphocytosis.

Therapy. Chest x-rays; thymectomy; corticosteroids; testosterone.

Prognosis. Thymectomy induces remission of symptoms, permanent or temporary, in about 25% of cases. Steroids may induce remission; more effective after thymectomy. Some cases may respond to testosterone. All cases of complete cure belong to the pure red cell type.

BIBLIOGRAPHY. Matras A, Priesel A: Ueber einige Gewächse des Thymus. Beitr Pathol Anat 80:270–306, 1928
Rogers GH, Manaligod JR, Blazek WV: Thymoma associated with pancytopenia and hypogammaglobuline-

mia: Report of a case and review of the literature. Am J Med 44:154–164, 1968
Kranz SR, Kao V: Studies on red cell aplasia. II. Report of a second patient with an antibody to erythroblast nuclei and a remission after immunosuppressive therapy. Blood 34:1–13, 1969
Wintrobe MM (ed): Clinical Hematology, 8th ed, pp 725, 1396–1397. Philadelphia, Lea & Febiger, 1981

PURETIĆ'S

Synonyms. Mucopolysaccharidosis variant; hyalinosis systemic.

Symptoms. Painful contractures of joints, developing at 3 months of age. Usually death in infancy or stunted growth.

Signs. Skull and face deformed. Multiple subcutaneous nodules at joints (elbow; shoulder; knees); osteolysis of terminal phalanges.

Etiology. Unknown. Considered a variant of mucopolysaccharidosis. Possibly autosomal recessive inheritance.

BIBLIOGRAPHY. Murray J: On three peculiar cases of molluscum fibrosum in one family. Med Chir Trans London 56:235–238, 1873
Puretić S, Puretič B, Fiser–Herman M, Adamcic M: A unique form of mesenchymal dysplasia. Br J Dermatol 74:8–19, 1962
Ishikawa H, Hori Y: Systematisierte Hyalinose in Zusammenhang mit Epidermolysis bullosa polydystrophica und Hyalinosis cutis et mucosae. Arch Klin Exp Dermatol 218:30–51, 1964

PURINE NUCLEOSIDES PHOSPHORYLASE DEFICIENCY

Synonyms. PNP deficiency, NP deficiency, purine nucleoside: orthophosphate ribosyl transferase deficiency.

Symptoms and Signs. From birth defect of cellular immunity. Infections of skin, lung, ears, and urinary tract. Candida and virus infections. Anemia. Increased susceptibility to vaccinations.

Etiology. Autosomal codominant inheritance of the variants. Deficiency of PNP of various degrees leads to altered function of T cells.

Diagnostic Procedures. Tests for cellular immunity. *Blood.* Anemia, hypouricemia. *Urine.* Hypouricosuria, excessive amounts of purines. Polynucleates BC activity: low or absent.

Therapy. Attempted correction of immune deficiency with bone marrow, embryonal thymus transplants, and thymosine.

Prognosis. Fatal in some cases for infections and blood transfusions. In some patients who are surviving, vaccination may be fatal.

BIBLIOGRAPHY. Giblett ER, Ammann AJ, Wara DW et al: Nucleoside phosphorylase deficiency in a child with severely defective T cell immunity and normal B cell immunity. Lancet 1:1010–1013, 1975
Kredich NM, Hershfield MS: Immunodeficiency diseases caused by adenosine deaminase deficiency and purine nucleoside phosphorylase deficiency. In Stanbury JB, Wyngaarden JB, Fredrickson DS et al: The Metabolic Basis of Inherited Disease, 5th ed, p 1157. New York, McGraw-Hill, 1983

PURPLE PEOPLE

Synonym. Chronic chlorpromazine toxicity.

Symptoms. Both sexes affected (previously thought to occur only in women). Occur in psychiatric patients on long-term, high doses of chlorpromazine. Peculiar purplish grey pigmentation of sun-exposed skin areas, progressing to permanent blue black or purplish grey metallic color. In some patients, corneal and lens opacities may also develop.

Etiology. Deposition in the skin of a chlorpromazine metabolite that reacts with sunlight. Ultraviolet light with wavelengths above 320 nm seems to be primarily responsible for the effects.

Therapy. Special window glass to reduce ultraviolet light in institutions where this treatment is conducted.

BIBLIOGRAPHY. Greiner AC, Berry K: Skin pigmentation and corneal and lens opacities with prolonged chlorpromazine therapy. Can Med Assoc J 90:663–665, 1964
Goodman LS, Gilman A: The Pharmacological Basis of Therapeutics, 7th ed, p 408. New York, Macmillian, 1985

PURPURA, MECHANICAL

Synonym. Orthostatic purpura (included).

Symptoms and Signs. Localized cutaneous hemorrhagic manifestations: petechiae and ecchymoses. In the mechanical form, localization prevalent on head, neck, and upper extremities; in orthostatic form, on lower extremities.

Etiology. Miopragia of capillaries and small arteries.

Diagnostic Procedures. *Blood.* Frequently associated, mild thrombocytopenia.

Therapy. Vitamin C; rutin; sodium carbazochrome sulfonans.

Prognosis. Benign persistent condition.

BIBLIOGRAPHY. Wintrobe MM (ed): Clinical Hematology, 8th ed. Philadelphia, Lea & Febiger, 1981

PURPURA, PSYCHOGENIC

Synonyms. Psychosomatic; bleeding stigmata hysteric purpura.

Symptoms and Signs. Occur in subjects with strong emotional involvement or other psychotic manifestations; most often in females. Occurrence of hematomas or bleeding in connection with certain complex psychic experiences. Spontaneous reproduction of wounds and bodily suffering of Christ, of battle wounds of Mohammed, or unrelated to religious experiences; repeated spontaneous bleeding in old healed scars associated with strong emotional experiences when memory of the experience is elicited, or symbolic of repressed sexual or aggressive feelings. Menstruation equivalent in various parts of the body (axilla, nose) or bloody hand.

Etiology. Unknown; opinions divided about the pathogenesis of these manifestations, from supernatural origin, hysteric conversion phenomena and self-induced.

Pathology. Ecchymosis or blood oozing through apparently normal skin.

Diagnostic Procedures. Psychoanalysis reproduces symptomatology by reproduction of stimulating psychic conditions. Rule out self-induction by protection or observation. Rule out Werlof's (see). Coagulation study.

Therapy. Psychotherapy.

Prognosis. Recurrence of phenomena. Difficult treatment. Conversion in some cases to other hysterical manifestations.

BIBLIOGRAPHY. Hyde JH: A contribution to the study of bleeding stigmata. J Cutan Dis 15:557, 1897
Agle DP, Ratnoff OD: Purpura as a psychosomatic entity. Arch Intern Med 109:685–694, 1962
Wintrobe MM (ed): Clinical Hematology. 8th ed. Philadelphia, Lea & Febiger, 1981

PURPURA SIMPLEX

See Purpura, psychogenic.

Symptoms and Signs. Prevalent in females. Mild purpura; small ecchymoses in the legs. Exacerbation during menstrual periods.

Etiology. Unknown.

Diagnostic Procedures. Diagnosis by exclusion. *Blood.* Normal platelets; normal clotting factors; tourniquet test occasionally shows abnormality.

BIBLIOGRAPHY. Wintrobe MM (ed): Clinical Hematology. 8th ed. Philadelphia, Lea & Febiger, 1981

PURPURA SIMPLEX, HEREDITARY

Symptoms and Signs. Females almost exclusively affected. Spontaneous ecchymoses; positive tourniquet test. Rheumatic fever, rheumatoid arthritis, and ptosis frequently associated.

Etiology. Autosomal dominant trait.

Therapy. None. Deficit of only esthetic significance.

BIBLIOGRAPHY. Davis E: Hereditary familial purpura simplex. Lancet 1:145–146, 1941
Wintrobe MM (ed): Clinical Hematology, 8th ed. Philadelphia, Lea & Febiger, 1981

PURTSCHER'S

Symptoms. Duane's retinopathy; traumatic retinal angiopathy; Valsalva's retinopathy. Fat embolism. Traumatic lymphorrhagia.

Symptoms. Occur following trauma of different degrees. Transient visual impairment.

Signs. Retinal and preretinal hemorrhages, exudates, edema, venous congestion; papilledema.

Etiology. Sudden rise in blood pressure; head and chest congestion. Fat embolism to be considered.

Pathology. Possibly, partial retinal vein obstruction. See Signs.

Therapy. Antiedema treatment.

Prognosis. Usually good.

BIBLIOGRAPHY. Purtscher O: Angiopathie retinae traumatica. Lymphorrhagien des Augengrundes. Albrecht Von Graefes Arch Ophthalmol 82:341–371, 1912
Hoare GW: Traumatic retinal angiopathy resulting from chest compression by safety belt. Br J Ophthalmol 54:667–674, 1970
Geeraets WJ: Ocular Syndromes, 3rd ed. Philadelphia, Lea & Febiger, 1976

PUTSCHAR–MANION

Synonyms. Splenogonadal fusion, limb defects, micrognathia.

Symptoms. In male (only one female reported). Ectromelia, micrognathia, numerous unerupted teeth, crowding of upper incisors, V-shaped palate (no cleft).

Etiology. Autosomal dominant inheritance.

Pathology. See Signs. Fusion of spleen and gonads.

Prognosis. Death in infancy.

BIBLIOGRAPHY. Putschar WGJ, Manion WC: Splenicgonadal fusion. Am J Path 32:15–35, 1956
Pauli RM, Greenlaw A: Limb deficiency and splenogonadal fusion. Am J Med Genet 13:81–90, 1982

PUTTI–CHAVANY

Synonyms. Paralyzing sciatica; sciatica paralysant.

Symptoms and Signs. Unilateral sciatica (see Cotugno's) associated with paralysis of the foot.

Etiology. See Cotugno's.

Prognosis. Rapid resolution of painful episode followed by onset of sensory troubles.

BIBLIOGRAPHY. Putti V: Lomboartrite e Sciatica Vertebrale. Bologna, 1936.
Chavany JA: Petite histoire de la sciatique paralysant. Prog Med 86:427–435, 1958

PYLE'S

Synonyms. Bakwin–Krida; metaphyseal dysplasia; leontiasis ossea. See Craniometaphyseal dysplasia.

Symptoms. Both sexes affected; onset in early infancy. Progressing headache; vomiting; irritability. Late motor development; vacuous expression; blindness; deafness; facial muscle paralysis.

Signs. Large head; nasal bridge broad and flat; hypertelorism; open mouth.

Etiology. Unknown; autosomal recessive inheritance.

Pathology. Cranium enlarged and heavier; bone ivory-like; diploë eliminated; paranasal sinuses obliterated; suture lines indistinct; reduction of foramina. Microscopically, compact bone, dilated Haversian canals, no osteoclasts. Long bones (femur in particular) flask-shaped in metaphyseal region; decreased density.

Diagnostic Procedures. *Blood.* Normal; calcium, phosphorus, alkaline phosphatase normal. *X-ray of skull and long bones.*

Therapy. Surgical decompression of nerves at foramina (surgery at multiple stages).

Prognosis. Poor; death from bone encroachment in area of foramen magnum.

BIBLIOGRAPHY. Smith GE, Jones FW: The archeologic survey of Nubia, report for 1907–1908. Rep Remains Cairo 2:289, 1910

Pyle E: A case of unusual bone development. J Bone Joint Surg 13:874–876, 1931

Gorlin RJ, Koszalka MF, Spranger J: Pyle's disease (familial metaphyseal dysplasia). J Bone Joint Surg 52:347–354, 1970

Raad MS, Beighton P: Autosomal recessive inheritance of metaphyseal dysplasia (Pyle disease). Clin Genet 14:251–256, 1978

PYODERMA GANGRENOSUM

Synonyms. Brocq's phagedena geometricum; Meleney's undermining burrowing ulcer; phagedena geometricum; Cullen's postoperative serpiginosus ulceration; burrowing phagedenic ulcer.

Symptoms. Both sexes equally affected; onset generally in adult life, seldom in childhood. It occurs frequently in association with ulcerative colitis, rheumatoid arthritis, chronic infections, malnutrition.

Signs. Extremely variable manifestations due to the pyoderma gangrenosum and associated condition. On the lower limbs or trunk, usually at the site of insect bite, needle puncture or trauma, appearance of single or multiple tender nodules, which evolve in pustules and then, breaking down, form ulcers slowly enlarging to 10 cm or more. Ulcers assume various shapes (round; oval; serpiginous) and present a bluish reddish edge, central, and necrotic base.

Etiology. Unknown. Various aspecific germs isolated, but not considered responsible. (Defective immune response?)

Pathology. No specific changes.

Diagnostic Procedures. *Biopsy and culture.* To exclude other diagnosis. *Blood.* In several cases, hypoproteinemia

or presence of paraglobulins; assessment of nutritive status; rheumatoid factor. *X-ray of intestine.* To search for ulcerative colitis.

Therapy. In cases without demonstrable underlying diseases, trials with antibiotics, gamma globulins, corticosteroids (of relative benefit).

Prognosis. Extremely variable. Ulcers may last for weeks or years; successive crops recur at variable intervals. Usually, in previously healthy subjects, course with slower progression and faster recovery and general health not affected; with associated condition, the course follows the evolution of the basic pathology.

BIBLIOGRAPHY. Brocq JL: Nouvelle contribution à l'étude du phagédénisme géométrique. Ann Dermatol Syph 5° sr. 6:1–39, 1916

Goldgraher MB, Korsner JB: Gangrenous skin lesion associated with chronic ulcerative colitis. A case study. Gastroenterology 39:94–103, 1960

Rook A, Wilkinson DS, Ebling FJG et al: Textbook of Dermatology, 4th ed, pp 1148–1150. Oxford, Blackwell Scientific Publications, 1986

PYODERMA VEGETANS

Synonyms. Dermatitis vegetans including: genitocrural dermatitis and intertrigo. See also Hallopeau's II.

Symptoms and Signs. Both sexes affected; onset at all ages. Several clinical variants, but the general characteristics are shared by all forms. Occur in subjects with normal skin and good health, or in malnutrition and chronic alcoholism, but most frequently in individuals with preexisting eczema or infective dermatitis. Generally, in flexures and genitalia, appearance of small pustules and granulomatous reaction that form foul-smelling, moist plaques; in other variants, formation of red crusted plaques, surrounded by vesiculopustules; if mucosae (oral cavity) involved, term pyostomatitis is used.

Etiology. Unknown; nonspecific skin reaction.

Pathology. Nonspecific chronic granulomatous reaction and pseudoepitheliomatous hyperplasia. Abscess may contain many eosinophils.

Diagnostic Procedures. *Biopsy. Blood, urine, and stool.* In cases of associated or underlying pathology, evidence of ulcerative colitis, hepatopathies, malnutrition.

Therapy. That of underlying conditions. Moist compresses. Antibiotics (systemic or topical) unpredictable response.

Prognosis. Chronic condition. Possibly, spontaneous remission with residual scars. If cure of identified underlying condition achieved, fast recovery.

BIBLIOGRAPHY. Nanta A, Bazex A: Formes cliniques des pyodermites végétantes. Ann Dermatol Syph 8:609–623, 1937

Melezer N: Zur Kenntnis der chronishcen vegetierenden Pyodermien. Minerva Dermatol 34:308–313, 1959

Rook A, Wilkinson DS, Ebling FJG et al: Textbook of Dermatology, 4th ed, pp 2167–2168. Oxford, Blackwell Scientific Publications, 1986

PYRAMIDAL DECUSSATION

Synonyms. Hemiplegia cruciata; ventromedial.

Symptoms. Paralysis of one upper extremity and contralateral paralysis of lower extremity. Face is spared.

Signs. Spasticity; increase in tone of affected muscles; hyperreflexia; ankle clonus; Babinski sign; absent abdominal reflexes on side of involved leg.

Etiology. Usually, trauma and causes other than softening. Seldom, softening.

Pathology. Lesion (see Etiology) in lower part of medulla at specific point distal to decussation of arm fibers, and proximal to decussation of leg fibers.

Diagnostic Procedures. *Spinal tap. Angiography, serology.*

Therapy. Symptomatic.

Prognosis. Depends on etiology.

BIBLIOGRAPHY. Chavany JA, Taptas JN, Haggenmueller D: Les faux syndromes alternes d'origine hémisphérique; l'"hemiplegia cruciata" par lésions corticales bilatérales. Presse Med 60:1126–1128, 1952

Alpers BJ: Clinical Neurology, 6th ed. Philadelphia, FA Davis, 1971

Adams RD, Victor M: Principles of Neurology, 3rd ed, p 49. New York, McGraw-Hill, 1985

PYRIFORMIS

Symptoms. Occur in patients with history of trauma to the sacroiliac or gluteal region (sometimes forgotten because of long gap in time between trauma and onset of symptoms). Pain in zone of sacroiliac joint; greater sciatic notch and pyriformis muscle; radiating in the leg and causing difficulty in walking. Acute reexacerbation of chronic pain by stooping or lifting weight.

Signs. Palpable, sausage-shaped mass over pyriformis (during attack of pain), and tenderness, Lasègue's sign; gluteal atrophy according to duration of condition.

Etiology. Lesion of pyriformis muscle affecting sciatic nerve in cases where close relation between this muscle and nerve exist.

Pathology. Adhesion between pyriformis and sciatic nerve.

Diagnostic Procedures. *X-ray.* To rule out other pathologic conditions of lumbar, sacral, and hip articulation areas.

Therapy. Sectioning of pyriformis muscle and separation of sciatic nerve from any attachment to the muscle.

Prognosis. Excellent result with treatment indicated. Immediate and permanent relief of syndrome. Section of muscle does not interfere with any movement of hip joint and does not cause disability.

BIBLIOGRAPHY. Yoemans W: The relation of arthritis of the sacroiliac joint to sciatica. Lancet 2:1119–1122, 1928

Robinson DR: Pyriformis syndrome in relation to sciatic pain. Am J Surg 73:355–358, 1947

PYRUVATE CARBOXYLATE DEFICIENCY

Synonyms. PC deficiency. See Leigh's.

Symptoms and Signs. Rare, both sexes. Two different clinical presentations. In the first one, onset is soon after birth with chronic lacticacidemia and delayed neurologic development and seizures. Normal lactate/pyruvate ratio. The second one presents early lactico-acidosis with elevated levels of ammonia, citrulline, proline, lysine, and elevated lactate/pyruvate ratio. Progressive psychomotor retardation.

Etiology. Autosomal recessive inheritance. Deficiency of pyruvate carboxylate.

Pathology. Autopsy: reduction of white matter, hepatic fibrosis.

Diagnostic Procedures. *Blood.* Lactic acidosis, elevated pyruvate levels, intermittent hypoglycemia and ketosis.

Therapy. Reported benefits with thiamine and lipoic acid.

Prognosis. Death at early age.

BIBLIOGRAPHY. Delvin E, Neal JL, Scriver CR: Pyruvate carboxylase: Two forms of human liver. Pediatr Res 6:392 (only), 1972

Atkin B–M, Buist NRM, Utter MF et al: Pyruvate carboxylase deficiency and lactic acidosis in a retarded child without Leigh's disease. Pediatr Res 13:109–120, 1979

Robinson BH, Oci J, Sherwood WG et al: The molecular basis for two different clinical presentations of classical pyruvate carboxylase deficiency. Am J Hum Genet 36:283–294, 1984

PYRUVATE DEHYDROGENASE COMPLEX DEFICIENCY

Synonyms. PDHC deficiency, PDC deficiency.

Symptoms and Signs. Both sexes. Failure to thrive, severe psychomotor retardation, ataxia, microcephaly, optic atrophy, hypotonia.

Etiology. Autosomal recessive inheritance. Deficiency of pyruvate dehydrogenase complex in all tissue.

Pathology. At autopsy brain with reduced white and gray matter.

Diagnostic Procedures. *Blood.* Lactate acidosis. Assay for PDHC.

Therapy. Low carbohydrate diet.

Prognosis. In severe cases death in first decade. In less severe cases normal life expectancy.

BIBLIOGRAPHY. Blass JP: Pyruvate decarboxylase deficiency. In Burman D, Holton JB, Pennock CA (eds): Inherited Disorders of Carbohydrate Metabolism, p 239. Lancaster UK, MTP Press, 1980
Blass JP: Inborn errors of pyruvate metabolism. In Stanbury JB, Wyngaarden JB, Fredrickson DS et al: The Metabolic Basis of Inherited Disease, 5th ed, p 193. New York, McGraw-Hill, 1983

PYRUVATE KINASE DEFICIENCY HEMOLYTIC ANEMIA

Synonym. Dacie's anemia (type).

Symptoms. Both sexes equally affected; onset in infancy or early childhood, seldom in adulthood. Weakness; fatigue. Exacerbation of symptoms with intercurrent diseases or surgery.

Signs. All signs may appear from very mild to very severe. Jaundice; pallor; splenomegaly; hepatomegaly (rare); chronic leg ulcers (rare); prominent frontal bosses (in severe cases). Cholelithiasis at relatively early age.

Etiology. Specific erythrocyte deficiency of pyruvate kinase. Autosomal recessive inheritance with variable penetrance.

Pathology. In bone marrow, normoblastic hyperplasia, increased hemosiderin. Spleen enlarged; no specific changes; hyperplasia of reticulum; ischemia of red pulp. Absence of extramedullary hyperplasia.

Diagnostic Procedures. *Blood.* Anemia; relative macrocytosis; reticulocytosis; variable number of nucleated red cells. Leukocytes and platelets normal; moderate hyperbilirubinemia; serum haptoglobulin absent or decreased. Osmotic fragility normal. Incubated fragility test: various abnormalities. Autohemolysis test positive; not corrected by addition of glucose and adenosine. Coombs' test negative; Heinz's bodies absent. Ferrokinetic study (^{59}Fe): rapid plasma clearance. Survival time of cells shortened. *Stool.* Fecal urobilinogen increased.

Therapy. Splenectomy. Hyperbilirubinemia in newborn may require blood exchange tranfusion.

Prognosis. Extremely variable, from fulminating cases to long survival with minimal manifestations. Splenectomy partially beneficial in most cases.

BIBLIOGRAPHY. Dacie JV, Mollison PL, Richardson N et al: Atypical congenital haemolytic anaemia. QJ Med 22:79–98, 1953
Valentine WN, Tanaka KR, Miwa S: A specific erythrocyte glycolytic enzyme defect (pyruvate kinase) in three subjects with congenital non-spherocytic hemolytic anemia. Trans Assoc Am Physicians 74:100–110, 1961
Valentine WN, Tanaka KR, Paglia DE: Pyruvate kinase and other enzyme deficiency disorders of the erythrocyte. In Stanbury JB, Wyngaarden JB, Fredrickson DS: The Metabolic Basis of Inherited Disease, 5th ed, p 1606. New York, McGraw-Hill, 1983

QUARELLI'S

Eponym used to indicate Parkinson's syndrome (see) that follows chronic intoxication with carbon disulfide.

BIBLIOGRAPHY. Quarelli G: Del tremore parkinsonsimile dell'intossicazione cronica da disolfuro di carbonio. Med Lavoro 21:58–64, 1930

QUEYRAT'S

Synonyms. Queyrat's erythroplasia. See also Bowen's. Erythroplasia Queyrat's.

Symptoms. It is not observed in circumcised males. Painless thickening of external genitalia, usually on penis, less frequently on vulva, and described also in mouth and tongue.

Signs. Slightly raised, intense red, glistening plaque with sharply outlined edge; later, scaling.

Etiology. Unknown. Intraepithelial carcinoma, not associated with internal cancer (Bowen's).

Pathology. Cutaneous surface of stratum corneum stripped and covered by parakeratosis. Epidermis thick with interpapillary ridges extending into dermis which is edematous and inflamed. Acanthosis with variety of abnormal cells; increased mitosis.

Diagnostic Procedures. *Biopsy and bacteriologic exams.* In case of doubt.

Therapy. Topical application of antiirritating agents (colchicine analogues); if tendency to invasion, surgical excision. Thiocalciran cream; 5-fluorouracil cream; radium mold.

Prognosis. Lesion usually tends to remain unlimited; in some cases, diffusion and possibility of metastasis.

BIBLIOGRAPHY. Queyrat A: Erythroplasie du gland. Bull Soc Fr Dermatol Syph 22:378–382, 1911
Rook A, Wilkinson DS, Ebling FJG et al: Textbook of Dermatology, 4th ed, pp 2199–2200. Oxford, Blackwell Scientific Publications, 1986

QUINCKE'S I

Synonyms. Angioderma; Bannister's; circumscribed edema; Milton–Quincke; giant urticaria; wandering edema; angioedema–urticaria.

Symptoms. Both sexes affected. Frequently associated with urticaria. Nausea; vomiting; cephalalgia; diarrhea; severe respiratory distress according to areas involved. Polyuria, in some cases, at termination of attacks.

Signs. Rapid onset of single or multiple nonpitting, tense swellings, from dime to palm size. Any part of body may be affected; most frequently involved areas: lips; eyelids; genitalia. Tongue and larynx may be involved.

Etiology. Allergy to various agents; possibly, emotional factors are involved.

Pathology. Capillary stasis in subcutaneous tissue.

Diagnostic Procedure. *Allergy tests.*

Treatment. Antihistamines. Epinephrine and related drugs; corticosteroids. Endotracheal intubation if larynx involved. Trials of specific desensitization if allergy proven.

Prognosis. Attacks usually last 1 to 2 hours, but may persist for 2 to 3 days before spontaneous or therapeutic remission. Recurrent attacks. Life-threatening in case of laryngeal involvement. Prognosis for life usually not as serious as in angioneurotic edema, hereditary (see).

BIBLIOGRAPHY. Quincke HI: Über akutes umbeschriebenes Hautderm. Mhefte Prakt Dermatol 1:129–131, 1882
Bannister HM: Acute angioneurotic edema. J Nerv Ment Dis 21:627–631, 1894
Milton JL: On giant urticaria. Edinburgh Med J 22:513–526, 1976
Rook A, Wilkinson DS, Ebling FJG et al: Textbook of Dermatology, 4th ed, p 1099. Oxford, Blackwell Scientific Publications, 1986

QUINQUAUD'S

Synonyms. Acne decalvans; Arnozan's; Brocq's lupoid sycosis; Feldman's; folliculitis decalvans; Little's; ulerythema sycosiformis. See Taenzer's. Taenzer's; Unna's (PG) II. According to old classification: Quinquaud's: predominant involvement of scalp; Brocq's and Unna's: beard; Arnozan's: legs.

Symptoms and Signs. In scalp form, both sexes equally affected. All other forms more prevalent in men. Age of onset in males from infancy to adult life (generally); in females from third to sixth decade. Any hairy region may be involved; loss of hair in round, oval patches (scar), surrounded by perifollicular pustules. Pruritus occasionally. Slow extension over years. Association with atopic manifestations frequent.

Etiology. Unknown; seborrheic dermatitis frequently associated.

Pathology. Follicular abscesses, followed by granulomatous formation with prevalence of lymphocytes, plasma cells, and, occasionally, giant cells. Atrophic scarring with disappearance of hair follicles and sweat glands.

Diagnostic Procedures. *Culture.* Rule out ringworm infections and lupus vulgaris.

Therapy. Steroid and chlortetracycline (3%).

Prognosis. Variable; severe disfiguration may result.

BIBLIOGRAPHY. Quinquaud CS: Folliculite destructive des régions vellues. Bull Soc Med Hop 5:95–98, 1888

Taenzer P: Uber das Ulerythema ophryogenes, eine noch nicht beschriegene Hautkrankheit. Mschr Prak Derm 8:197–208, 1889

Unna PG: The Histopathology of the Diseases of the Skin, p 1086. New York, CLAY, 1896

Mertens RLJ: Ulerythema ophryogenes and atopy. Arch Dermatol 97:662–663, 1968

Rook A, Wilkinson DS, Ebling FJG et al: Textbook of Dermatology, 4th ed, pp. 2002–2003. Oxford, Blackwell Scientific Publications, 1986

QUINSY

Term derived from Greek *kynagche*, which means a bad sore throat.

Synonym. Peritonsillar abscess.

Symptoms. Malaise; chills; pain radiating from one side of throat to ear and neck; dysphagia; dysphonia; malodorous breath; trismus; drooling; stiff neck; hyperthermia.

Signs. Tonsillitis; edema and displacement prevalent in one side; tongue coated; difficulty in inspecting pharynx.

Etiology. Tonsillitis initially due to streptococcal infection, then to gram-negative microorganisms.

Pathology. Abscess into tonsil and extending into surrounding neck tissue.

Diagnostic Procedures. *Blood.* Leukocytosis. *Throat culture.* Mixed flora, usually of gram-negative type.

Therapy. Antibiotics. After fluctuation, drainage of abscess.

Prognosis. Much improved by antibiotics and surgery.

BIBLIOGRAPHY. Harley EH: Quinsy tonsilectomy as the treatment of choice for peritonsillar abscess. Ear Nose Throat J 67:84–87, 1988

RABE–SALOMON

Synonyms. Congenital afibrinogenemia; congenital fibrinogenopenia; congenital hypofibrinogenemia; Salomon's. See Dysfibrinogenemia and Hypofibrinogenemia.

Symptoms. Occur in both sexes; manifestations from birth. Bleeding from umbilical cord usually profuse. After trauma or surgery, severe bleeding. Episodes of ecchymosis, hematomas, epistaxis, hemoptysis, hematuria, hemorrhage in central nervous system, alternated with long periods of freedom from hemorrhages. Menses may be normal.

Signs. Very rarely, hemarthroses; seldom, permanent damage to tissue after hemorrhage; pseudocyst in the bone may occur.

Etiology. Failure to synthetize fibrinogen. Autosomal recessive inheritance.

Diagnostic Procedures. *Blood.* Anemia at time of hemorrhages; blood does not clot spontaneously or after addition of thrombin. Absence of fibrinogen (traces may be revealed with immunologic method). All other coagulation factors normal (slight depression of proaccelerin seldom observed). Bleeding time prolonged. Tourniquet test normal. Sedimentation rate nonexistent (after 24 hr red cells still floating). Fibrinogen antibodies (appearing after repeated transfusions).

Therapy. Bleeding treated by injection of fibrinogen. Infusion of cryoprecipitate.

Prognosis. Patients may reach adulthood; death from bleeding into vital area or severe blood loss. Possible thrombosis of pulmonary district.

BIBLIOGRAPHY. Rabe F, Salomon E: Ueber Faserstoffmangel im Blute bei einem Falle von Haemophilie. Dtsch Ark Klin Med 132:240–244, 1920
Mammen EF: Congenital abnormalities of the fibrogen molecule. Semin Tromb Hemost 1:184, 1974

RACINE'S

Synonyms. Premenstrual salivary; premenstrual sialorrhea.

Symptoms and Signs. Tumefaction of one or more salivary glands, beginning 4 to 5 days prior to menstrual cycle and disappearing at its onset.

Etiology. Unknown; part of the premenstrual syndrome (see).

Pathology. Interstitial edema and temporary dilatation of excretory canals of salivary glands.

Therapy. See Premenstrual.

BIBLIOGRAPHY. Racine W: Le syndrome salivaire prémenstruel. Schweiz Med Wochenschr 69:1204–1207, 1939

RADIATION, ACUTE

Synonyms. Radiation injuries; accidental radiation.

Symptoms and Signs. Sequential stages of the radiation syndrome as well as the characteristic forms of the syndrome (cerebral, gastrointestinal, hematopoietic) develop according to the amount of radiation received, and to a lesser extent, to individual susceptibility. "Typical" radiation-induced syndrome evolves after whole body doses of 2 or more Sv (200 rem) according to the following pattern:
1. *Prodromal stage.* Within 2 hours of exposure, anorexia, nausea, malaise, listlessness, fatigue. Progressing to prostration and culminating at about 8 hours, and then subsiding rapidly. Or second day nausea and (occasionally) vomiting, but marked improvement of general situation.
2. *Latent stage.* Third day, asymptomatic and able to return to normal activity about the 20th day. Epilation starts at second week if dose greater than 3 Sv (300 rem).
3. *Bone marrow depression stage.* Anemia; leukopenia; thrombocytopenia. Abrupt malaise; fatigue; exertional dyspnea; frank hemorrhages; purpura; stomatitis; fever. This stage culminates at the 30th day.
4. *Recovery phase.* After having survived the crisis, progressive recovery and subsidence of symptoms within another 30 days.
5. *Convalescence.* Starting approximately at the 60th day and complete by 90th day.

Etiology. Exposure to penetrating x-ray, gamma, or neutron radiation. See table for relation between dose and effect. Depending upon dose received, three main clinical forms result:
1. *Hematopoietic form* (1 Sv). Already described in stage 3; death may result within 2 months.

2. *Gastrointestinal form* (>5 Sv). Prodromal: nausea within a few minutes, vomiting, diarrhea. Latent: asymptomatic up to sixth day. Third stage: hematologic changes plus nausea, vomiting, diarrhea, paralytic ileus, circulatory collapse, death. Pathology. small intestine distended; congestion of wall; mucosa edematous, hemorrhagic; erosion of epithelial lining, and ulceration with superimposed infection. Bone marrow and lymphatic system aplasia.

3. *Cerebral form* (20 Sv). Prodromal: weakness, drowsiness within 1 hour progressing to apathy, lethargy. Within 3 hours, seizures, ataxic movements. If surviving this phase, prostration and death in 2 to 3 days. Pathology: brain edema; pyknosis of granule cell layer of cerebellum.

Diagnostic Procedures. *Blood.* Leukopenia; anemia; thrombocytopenia chromosomal aberrations (dyantrics, rings).

Therapy. *Prodromal stage.* Psychological reassurance.

Dose (Sv)	Clinical Effect
<0.5	Asymptomatic or trivial effects (moderate bone marrow depression).
0.5–1	Trivial and transitory clinical manifestations.
1.0–1.5	30% of patients: prodromal phase and bone marrow depression phase. Ambulatory; no major medical problem.
1.5–2.0	80% show typical four stages of radiation syndrome. Hospitalization required at third stage on. Generally good prognosis, recovery to normal life.
2–4	Typical acute radiation syndrome; serious manifestation requiring hospitalization and intensive care. Recovery, possibly to normal life, depending on prompt and adequate treatment.
4–6	Typical picture of acute radiation syndrome or fulminating course: up to 5 Sv, hematopoietic changes determine clinical effects and outcome (see): up to 6 Sv, gastrointestinal form of acute radiation syndrome (see).
10–20	Fulminating course, cerebral form of acute radiation syndrome.

If necessary, sedation. *Hematopoietic form.* Antibiotic as soon as signs of infection appear. (CAUTION: bone marrow depression). Transfusion of blood or separated platelets (or both) and leukocytes. Injection of compatible bone marrow (on well-defined conditions). *Gastrointestinal form.* Parenteral nutrition; fluid and electrolyte balance. Antibiotics; aseptic environment; blood transfusion. *Cerebral form.* Heavy sedation to prevent seizures.

Prognosis. See above.

BIBLIOGRAPHY. Gerstner HB: Acute radiation syndrome in man: Military and civil defense aspects. US Armed Forces Med J 9:313–354, 1958

Upton AC: Radiation injury. The University of Chicago Press, 1969

Milory NC: Management of irradiated and contaminated casualty victims. Emerg Med Clin North Am 2:667–686, 1984

American Medical Assoc: A Guide to the Hospital Management of Injuries Arising from Exposure to or Involving Ionizing Radiation. Chicago, AMA, 1985

Strambi E: Accidental radiation injuries whole-body radiation syndrome. In Manni C, Magalini SI, (eds): Emergency and Disaster Medicine, pp 355–360. Berlin, Springer-Verlag, 1985

Tubiana M, Dutreix J, Wambersie A: Radiobiologie. Hermann, Paris, 1986

RADIATION ARTHROPATHY

Symptoms and Signs. Occur after radiation exposure. Asymptomatic for years; then pain and swelling and erythema of tender areas.

Etiology. Roentgen radiation.

Pathology. Degenerative changes of cartilage. Chondrocalcinosis; ankylosis; rheumatoidlike changes; osteochondritis.

Diagnostic Procedures. *X-ray.* Narrowing of articular spaces; periarticular osteoporosis; marginal bone formation.

Therapy. None.

Prognosis. Variable evolution with final ankylosing of degeneration changes.

BIBLIOGRAPHY. Kolar J, Urabe CR, Chyba J: Arthropathies after irradiation. J Bone Joint Surg [Am] 49:1157–1166, 1967

RADIATION FIBROMATOSIS

Synonyms. Postradiation pseudosarcoma. See Pinkus (H.) I.

Symptoms and Signs. Onset usually 5 years after radiotherapy (from 16 mo to 27 yr). Firm small nodule developing at the radiation site.

Etiology. Exaggerated response to previous radiation.

Pathology. Histology varies greatly: poorly differentiated fibroblastic lesions with bizarre mitotic figures giant nuclei, to orderly interlacing bundles of spindle cells of connective tissue.

Therapy. Excision.

Prognosis. Benign; lack of recurrence after excision. No metastasis.

BIBLIOGRAPHY. Pettit VD, Chamness JT, Ackerman LV: Fibromatosis and fibrosarcoma following irradiation therapy. Cancer 7:149–158, 1954
Samitz MH: Pseudosarcoma, pseudomalignant neoplasm as a consequence of radiodermatitis. Arch Dermatol 96:283–285, 1967
Schneider AB, Shore–Freedman E, Ryo UV et al: Radiation induced tumors of the head and neck following childhood irradiation: Prospective study. Medicine 64:1–15, 1984

RADIATION PNEUMONITIS

Synonym. Irradiation pneumonia.

Symptoms. Insidious onset 1 to 6 months after completion of roentgen therapy. Dry nonproductive cough; asthenia; fever; exertional dyspnea. Inability to inhale at full lung capacity; seldom, hemoptysis.

Signs. Tachycardia; crepitation at inspiration; signs of consolidation; seldom, friction rubs.

Etiology. From doses of 20 Gy, possibility of radiation pneumonitis; dose of 50 to 60 Gy (in 5–6 wk) always causes the syndrome.

Pathology. Initially, electron microscopy shows loss of type II alveolar cells and surfactant depletion; then pulmonary hypertension develops from obliteration of vascular bed. Effects from superimposed infections and heart failure are difficult to separate from primary x-ray effects. The acute pneumonic reaction is characterized by exudation and desquamation of cells into alveolar space, vascular lesions, deposit of connective tissue and lymphocytes into septa. The late or fibrotic stage is characterized by replacement of normal tissue by fibrous tissue.

Diagnostic Procedures. *X-ray.* Consolidation of lung parenchyma, patchy or confluent; volume loss; in rare cases, hyperlucent lung (see Burke's). *Pulmonary function tests.*

Therapy. Symptomatic. Prednisolone or mustine hydrochloride.

Prognosis. Acute pneumonia may last 1 month and regress completely or evolve into pulmonary fibrosis and chronic respiratory insufficiency. Radiation therapy may be responsible for successive development of carcinomas.

BIBLIOGRAPHY. Gross NJ: Pulmonary effects of radiation therapy. Ann Intern Med 86:81–92, 1977

Staufer JL, Carbone JE: Pulmonary disease. In Krupp MA, Schroeder SA, Tierney LM Jr (eds): Current Medical Diagnosis and Treatment 1987, pp 170–171. Norwalk (Conn), Lange Medical Publications, 1987

RAEDER'S

Synonyms. Horner's incomplete; paratrigeminal paralysis; oculopupillary paratrigeminal paralysis. See Horton's and Orbital apex.

Symptoms. Reported almost exclusively in males. Unilateral, deep, severe pain concentrated around the eyes, sometimes self-limited, with complete recovery. Other times, continuous with exacerbations or relapsing after free periods. Occasionally with various combinations of parasellar nerve involvements: optic (II), oculomotor (III), trochlear (IV), abducens (VI).

Signs. Ptosis and myosis (sometimes not easily noticeable). Absence of facial sweating (differentiates this syndrome from Horner's); conjunctival injection and lacrimation (usually present).

Etiology. Neoplastic, traumatic, inflammatory, vascular, or idiopathic lesion that damages the oculosympathetic fibers distally to the bifurcation of the external carotid artery (in this way sparing the sweating fibers).

Pathology. Tumor; abscess; aneurysms. When parasellar involvement, (Raeder's paratrigeminal syndrome group I lesion in anterior part of middle cranial fossa), same causes with various localization in group II (without parasellar nerves involvement), such as abscessed tooth, internal carotid aneurysms.

Diagnostic Procedures. *X-ray of skull and neck. Arteriography.*

Prognosis. According to etiology.

BIBLIOGRAPHY. Raeder JG: Paratrigeminal paralysis of oculopupillary sympathetic. Brain 47:149–158, 1924
Law WR, Nelson ER: Internal carotid aneurysm as a cause of Raeder's paratrigeminal syndrome. Neurology 18:43–46, 1968
Adams RD, Victor M: Principles of Neurology 3rd ed, p 503. New York, McGraw-Hill, 1985

RAPE TRAUMA

Symptoms and Signs. Begin with the physical assault; however, weeks may elapse between the assault and the emergence of reaction. Phase 1. Disorganization (acute). Phase 2. Reorganization (long-term process).

Etiology. Distress of psychological trauma, compounded by added medical and legal stresses.

BIBLIOGRAPHY. Burgess A, Hofmstrom L: Rape trauma syndrome. Am J Psychiatry 131:981–986, 1974

Hicks DJ: Rape: Sexual assault. Am J Obstet Gynecol 137:931–935, 1980

RAPIDLY PROGRESSING NEPHRITIC

Synonyms. Nephritis, rapidly progressing; this condition includes three types of disease: see Idiopathic diffuse crescenting glomerulonephritis types I, II, and III.

Symptoms. Extracapillary proliferative glomerulonephritis; rapidly progressing nephritis.

Symptoms. Prevalent in males; onset in adolescence and young adulthood (in women at any age). Onset seldom acute, usually insidious. Anorexia; diarrhea; smoky urine; oliguria (more severe than in acute nephritic syndrome).

Signs. Blood hypertension (less severe than in acute nephritic).

Etiology. Usually idiopathic. In 30% of cases preceding streptococcal infection. This syndrome may be associated also with other conditions, *e.g.*, Goodpasture's; infective endocarditis; Schönlein–Henoch; vasculitis; lupus erythematosus.

Pathology. See Idiopathic diffuse crescenting glomerulonephritis.

Therapy. Anticoagulants; adrenocorticosteroids. Chronic dialysis. Kidney transplantation. Plasmapheresis may be helpful.

Prognosis. See specific diseases.

BIBLIOGRAPHY. Oredugba O, Mazumdar DC, Meyer JS et al: Pulse methylprednisolone therapy in idiopathic rapidly progressive glomerulonephritis. Ann Intern Med 92:504–506, 1980

Brenner BM, Rector FC Jr (eds): The Kidney, 3rd ed, p 940. Philadelphia, WB Saunders, 1986

RAPP–HODGKIN

Synonyms. Ectodermal hypohidrotic dysplasia. Anhidrotic ectodermal dysplasia. See also Christ–Siemens.

Symptoms and Signs. Both sexes affected; recognized in early infancy. Hyperthermia (episodes); hypohidrosis; variable growth deficiency. Low nasal bridge; narrow nose; hypoplastic maxilla; small mouth; cleft lip, palate, uvula. Thin skin; sparse fine hair; small dysplastic nails; hypodontia; conical teeth. Hypospadias. Purulent conjunctivitis and otitis media.

Etiology. Autosomal dominant inheritance. Of doubtful autonomy; appears to be a mild variant of Christ–Siemens (see).

Pathology. See Symptoms and Signs. Sweat pores present but reduced in number.

BIBLIOGRAPHY. Rapp RS, Hodgkin WE: Anhidrotic ectodermal dysplasia. Autosomal dominant inheritance with palate and lip anomalies. J Med Genet 5:269–272, 1968

Stasiowska B, Sartoris S, Goitre M et al: Rapp–Hodgkin ectodermal dysplasia syndrome. Arch Dis Child 56:793–795, 1981

RAPUNZEL

Synonyms. Bezoar; phytobezoar; trichobezoar.

Symptoms. Dragging or fullness in upper abdominal quadrant; epigastric pain (70%); nausea and vomiting (64%).

Signs. Mass palpable in epigastric region of phytobezoar (54%) and of trichobezoar (88%). Signs of peritonitis (7–10%).

Etiology. Food or ingurgitated matter that has formed a compact body, occasionally assuming the aspect of long strands of twisted hair extending from the bezoar through the intestine.

Diagnostic Procedures. *X-ray*. Direct demonstration of the presence of foreign body. *Gastroscopy*. Best diagnostic tool. *Endoscopic biopsy*. *Blood*. Hypochromia; microcytic anemia; slight white blood cell elevation.

Therapy. Surgery.

Prognosis. Good with treatment.

BIBLIOGRAPHY. Vaugh EE Jr, Sawyers JL, Scott HW Jr: The Rapunzel syndrome. An unusual complication of intestinal bezoar. Surgery 63:339–343, 1968

Diettrich NA, Gau FC: Postgastrectomy phytobezoars: Endoscopic diagnosis and treatment. Arch Surg 120:432–435, 1985

RAUCH'S

Synonyms. Adiposity–hyperthermia–oligomenorrhea–parotid swelling; AOP; AHOP.

Symptoms. Occur in women; onset at puberty. Bilateral parotid swelling and occasionally, also of submandibular glands. Within 5 years, slow progression of obesity (Fröhlic type), oligomenorrhea, melancholia, oligophrenia.

Etiology. Attributed by one author to hereditary alteration of diencephalon. Not confirmed by other reports.

BIBLIOGRAPHY. Rauch S: Die diencephale Parotitis recidivous bilateral (das AOP Syndrom). Arch Ohren-Nasen Kehlkopfh 168:377–394, 1955–56
Gorlin R, Pindborg JJ, Cohen MM Jr: Syndromes of the Head and Neck, 2nd ed. New York, McGraw-Hill, 1976

RAVENNA'S

Synonyms. Achondroplasia tarda; atypical achondroplasia; hypochondroplasia; Leri's hypochondroplasia.

Symptoms and Signs. Both sexes affected; evident at birth or within third year of age. At birth height 47.7 cm and weight 2.9 kg. Characteristic sign; a block just short of full extension of elbow. Head larger than rest of body. Shortened limbs; leg bowing less frequent than in achondroplasia. Mild motor delay; unusual mental retardation; behavioral problem common. Slow growth eventually determining a mild disproportionate dwarfism (with short limbs); final height 127 to 152.4 cm; joint relaxation; small but normal hands and feet.

Etiology. Autosomal dominant inheritance with complete penetrance. This syndrome probably is caused by an allele of achondroplasia (see).

Pathology. See Diagnostic Procedures.

Diagnostic Procedures. *X-ray.* Normal bones of skull, hands, and feet. Long bone short and larger, with exaggerated physiologic bowing. Femoral neck length shortened; greater trochanters prominent. Knee epiphyses squared aspect. Fibulas longer, causing mild varus ankle. Vertebral canal narrowed. Sacrum hypoplastic. *Blood, urine.* Normal.

Therapy. Minor orthopedic correction for feet, knees. Physical therapy. Cesarean section for pregnancy.

Prognosis. Adults report myofascial pain, bursitis, lumbosacral strain. No neurologic alteration. IQ reduced to 50 to 80 points.

BIBLIOGRAPHY. Ravenna F: Achondroplasia et chondrohypoplasie. Contribution clinique. Nouv Iconogr Salpetriere 26:157–184, 1913
Leri A, Linossier M: Hypochondroplasie hereditaire. Bull Méd Soc Med Hop (Paris) 48:1780–1787, 1924

Bailey JA: Disproportionate Short Stature: Diagnosis and Management, p 117. Philadelphia, WB Saunders, 1973
Sillence DO, Horton WA, Rinoin DL: Morphologic studies in the skeletal dysplasias. A review. Am J Pathol 96:813–870, 1979

RAYMOND–CÉSTAN

Synonyms. Céstan's; dissociation of lateral gaze; pontine.

Symptoms and Signs. Unilateral abducens paralysis; paralysis of lateral conjugate gaze; contralateral hemiplegia; anesthesia of face, extremities, and trunk.

Etiology. Hemorrhage; thrombosis tumor with nuclear lesion involving pyramidal tract. The post longitudinal bundle and the medial lemniscus may also be involved.

BIBLIOGRAPHY. Raymond F, Céstan R: Trois observations de paralysie des mouvements associés des globes oculaires. Rev Neurol (Paris) 9:70–77, 1901
Vick NA: Grinker's Neurology, 7th ed. Springfield, CC Thomas, 1976

RAYNAUD'S

Synonyms. Symmetric gangrene; symmetric asphyxia. See also Raynaud's phenomenon.

Symptoms. Prevalent in females (5 : 1); usually begins in first or second decade. Reported in five children in whom no clinical, hematologic, or immunologic evidence of a collagen disorder was found. As a rule, cold is the precipitating factor for onset of symptoms. Emotional stress also may be a precipitating factor. Episodes of color change in fingers beginning and increasing gradually; occasionally, dramatic onset of intense manifestation (dead finger phenomenon). Usually after exposure of the fingers to cold, pallor, cyanosis, and rubor appear, followed by pain and paresthesia. Initially only the tips of one or two fingers are involved. With time, the phenomenon extends to involve all fingers and rest of the hand. Bilaterality (diagnostic criterion). Absence of systemic manifestation.

Signs. Transient changes in color of fingers; cold and slight swelling during attacks. Sclerodermatous changes of the skin after repeated attacks and occasionally minor gangrenous changes.

Etiology. Unknown; functional vasospastic condition. Raynaud's syndrome (idiopathic) has to be differentiated from Raynaud's phenomenon syndrome (see) and from thromboangiitis obliterans, arteriosclerosis obliterans, Mitchell's syndrome I, and scleroderma.

Pathology. In advanced stages, thickening of intima of digital arteries. When trophic lesion, obstructed arteries and area of necrosis eventually develop.

Diagnostic Procedures. Rule out conditions associated with Raynaud's phenomenon (see).

Therapy. Protection of extremities from cold and injuries. Moving to a warmer climate is sometimes indicated. Mild Raynaud's disease, when associated with menopausal symptoms or menstrual periods, may benefit from estrogen administration. Tolazoline hydrochloride, phenoxybenzamine hydrochloride, Hydergine, local application of glyceryl trinitrate and reserpine may be used with moderate success in mild form, but usually results are disappointing. In the reported children, oral phenoxybenzamine proved useful for maintenance treatment, while during acute attacks infusions of prostacyclin, nitroprusside, and ketanserin were used.

Prognosis. Normal life span; several patients present a nonprogressive course with periodic exacerbations. Results of sympathectomy are fairly good in idiopathic Raynaud's (60%), but are disappointing in secondary Raynaud's phenomenon. (Importance of correct diagnosis before major treatment considered).

BIBLIOGRAPHY. Raynaud AGM: De L'asphyxie Local et de la Gangrène Symétrique des Extrémités, pp 6–9. Paris, Rignoux, 1862
Fries JF: Clinical significance of Raynaud's phenomenon. Med Digest June 15–20, 1967
Burns EC, Dunger DB, Dillon MJ: Raynaud's disease. Arch Dis Child 60:537, 1985

RAYNAUD'S PHENOMENON

Episode of constriction of small arteries or arterioles (or both) of extremities, with change in color of the skin, pallor, cyanosis. This phenomenon is observed in several clinical entities.
1. *Raynaud's syndrome.*
2. *Posttraumatic conditions.*
   Frostbite
   Pneumatic hammer syndrome
   After injury or surgery
   Typists' and pianists' vasospastic phenomenon
3. *Neurogenic conditions*
   Carpal tunnel syndrome
   Diseases of nervous system
   Shoulder–girdle compression syndromes
4. *Occlusive arterial diseases*
   Arteriosclerosis obliterans
   Embolism
   Thromboangiitis obliterans
   Thrombosis

5. *Intoxications*
   Ergot
   Heavy metals
6. *Miscellaneous conditions*
   Cold hemoagglutination
   Dermatomyositis
   Lupus erythematosus
   Marchiafava–Micheli syndrome
   Rheumatoid arthritis
   Scleroderma syndromes
   Waldenström's syndrome I

BIBLIOGRAPHY. Raynaud AGM: De l'asphyxie Locale et de la Gangrene Symètrique des Extrémitiés. Paris, Rignoux, 1862

RAY'S

Synonym. Amorality.

Eponym used to indicate a lack of moral sense and of relative restraints to comply with socially accepted moral rules, and the consequent antisocial activity related to the violation of established rules. An antisocial behavior is found in several psychiatric disorders, and this eponym is of only historical value.

BIBLIOGRAPHY. Ray I: A Treatise on the Medical Jurisprudence of Insanity. London, Hendersonn, 1837
Staller RJ: Does sexual perversion exist? Johns Hopkins Med J 134:43–57, 1974
Freedman AM, Kaplan HI, Sadock BJ: Comprehensive Textbook of Psychiatry, 2nd ed, p. 582, 1465. Baltimore, Williams & Wilkins, 1975

REBEITZ–KOLODNY–RICHARDSON

Synonyms. Neural achromasia–corticodentatonigral degeneration; RKR

Symptoms. Occur in late middle age. Clumsiness and slowness of movement of left limbs (presenting symptoms), then widespread. Severe impairment in control of muscular movements, postural abnormalities, involuntary muscular activity. Moderate muscular weakness. Mental faculties relatively spared. Tremor constant but not too severe. Finally, severe contractures, dysphagia, and speech impairment.

Signs. Paralysis of ocular muscles; exaggeration of myotonic reflexes and increased resistance to passive stretching of affected muscles. Babinski sign.

Etiology. Unknown; possibly, metabolic failure at cellular level. Richardson–Steele–Oslzewski syndrome (see) bears some similarity with this syndrome, but pathologically the two syndromes appear different. Some clinical aspects of this syndrome are also shared with Pick's (see), Alzheimer's (see), Huntington's (see), Parkinson's (see), and, most of all, with Jakob–Creutzfeldt (see). So many clearly different features of each of these syndromes from the present one, however, allow this to be considered as a separate entity.

Pathology. Alterations limited to brain: convolutional atrophy, especially parietal and frontal; lateral and third ventricles enlarged. No vascular alterations. Nerve cells in anterior cortex disappear. Astrocytic gliosis; slight microglial activity; signs of inflammation absent. Some of remaining nerve cells show swelling of cell body, displacement of nucleus, achromasia, hyaline cytoplasm, and vacuolization. Substantia nigra also shows loss of pigmented cells; corpus of Louys, dentate, and roof nuclei of cerebellum also loss of cells. Cerebellar cortex unaffected.

Diagnostic Procedures. *Cerebrospinal fluid.* Normal. *Electroencephalography.* Unspecific slow and sharp waves activity. *CT brain scan.* Cerebral atrophy.

Therapy. None.

Prognosis. Years of slowly progressing incapacity. Death within 6 to 8 years of onset.

BIBLIOGRAPHY. Rebeitz JJ, Kolodny H, Richardson EP: Corticodentatonigral degeneration with achromasia. Arch Neurol 18:20–33, 1968

RECLUS' II

Synonyms. Cooper's; ligneous phlegmon.

Symptoms and Signs. Abscess on the neck that causes a woody induration of subcutaneous connective tissue; pain; fever; general malaise.

Etiology. Infective.

Pathology. Suppuration with secondary fibrosis of subcutaneous tissue.

Therapy. Surgery and antibiotics.

Prognosis. According to the adequacy of treatment.

BIBLIOGRAPHY. Reclus P: Phlégmon ligneux du cou. Rev Chir (Paris) 16:522–531, 1896

RECTUS MUSCLE

Synonym. Rectus muscle hematoma.

Symptoms. Occur in late middle life; more frequent in women than in men. Sudden, severe pain on either side of midline, always below the level of umbilicus; moderate increase in temperature, prostration; vomiting; hyper-

pnea; shock. In some cases, slow development of a mass without acute symptoms.

Signs. Very tender mass at site of pain, remaining fixed; ecchymotic discoloration; tachycardia. If patient partially sits up, the mass cannot be moved laterally. No tenderness elicited in tissues surrounding the mass. Localized tonic contraction; absence of generalized rigidity.

Etiology. Sudden muscular contraction (cough; sneeze; vomiting; movement); associated frequently with infections or other conditions (pregnancy; intoxication) that result in weakening and atrophy of muscle. Degeneration of blood vessels; blood dyscrasia. In many spontaneous cases, no causes found.

Pathology. Vascular hyaline degeneration; muscle granulation and hyaline degeneration suggesting degenerative process prior to rupture. Hematoma formed by blood extravasated among degenerated fibers, or may be completely separated.

Diagnostic Procedures. See Signs. *Needle aspiration. Laboratory.* Noncontributory. *X-ray and/or xerography of abdominal wall. Surgical exploration.*

Prognosis. Good, depending on underlying or concurrent disease. Mortality 4% to 5%; in pregnancy, maternal mortality 12% and fetal mortality 25% to 50%.

BIBLIOGRAPHY. Payne RL: Spontaneous rupture of the superior and inferior epigastric arteries within the rectus abdominal sheath. Ann Surg 108:757–768, 1938
Jones TW, Merendino KA: The deep epigastric artery: Rectus muscle syndrome. Am J Surg 103:159–169, 1962

RED DIAPER

Synonym. Serratia marcescens gastrointestinal.

Symptoms. None.

Signs. Diaper turns red 24 to 36 hours after soiling.

Etiology. *Serratia marcescens* established as predominant gastrointestinal bacterial species.

Pathology. None.

Diagnostic Procedures. *Stool.* Culture.

Therapy. Sulfasalazine, gentamycin, and revision of diet.

Prognosis. *Serratia marcescens* is overgrown by usual bacterial intestinal flora as soon as change in diet is begun and sulfa treatment given.

BIBLIOGRAPHY. Waisman H, Stone WH: The presence of *Serratia marcescens* as the predominating organism in the intestinal tract of the newborn: The occurrence of the "red diaper syndrome." Pediatrics 21:8–12, 1958

REDLICH'S

Synonyms. Abortive disseminated encephalomyelitis; epidemic cerebrospinal meningitis; encephalomyelitis funicularis infectiosa; Flatau's; Munch–Patersen's. Eponym obsolete; could be considered as a variant of von Economo's encephalitis (see).

BIBLIOGRAPHY. Redlich E: Ueber abortive Formen der Encephalomyelitis disseminata. Dtsch Med Wochenschr 55:562–563, 1929

RED MAN

Synonym. Rifampin toxicity.

Symptoms and Signs. Orange and red "glowing" discoloration of the skin, facial or periorbital edema, pruritus of the head, vomiting.

Etiology. It is a toxic reaction among children inadvertently given excessive doses of rifampin for chemoprophylaxis of *Haemophilus influenzae* disease (from 20–200 times normal dose) or suicidal attempt in adults.

Diagnostic Procedures. *Serum.* Transient liver enzymes alteration.

Therapy. Symptomatic. Prevention: attention to detail in calculating the dose to be given and in the preparation and administration of the drug. Corticosteroids.

Prognosis. Rapid remission.

BIBLIOGRAPHY. Newton RW, Forrest ARW: Rifampicin overdosage. "The red man syndrome." Scot Med J 20:55–56, 1975
Bolan G, Laurie RE, Broome CV: Red man syndrome: Inadvertent administration of an excessive dose of rifampin. Pediatrics 77:633–635, 1986

REDUNDANT CAROTID ARTERY

Synonyms. Redundant carotid artery; kinking carotid artery; intermittent carotid obstruction. See Carotid system ischemia.

Symptoms. Vertigo or transient hemiparesis or episodes of blindness of one eye, when turning the head to one side. Return of vision or disappearance of paresis when turning the head to the midline.

Etiology and Pathology. Tortuosity of carotid artery. Turning of the head produces artery obstruction through kinking of the vessel. Possibly, congenital malformation of carotid artery or acquired arterial dilatation and tortuosity.

Diagnostic Procedures. *Arteriography.*

Therapy. Surgical resection of tortuous vessel with end-to-end anastomosis.

Prognosis. Treatment will usually completely relieve the symptoms.

BIBLIOGRAPHY. Riser M, Geraud J, Ducoudray J et al: Dolicho-carotide interne avec syndrome vertigineux. Rev Neurol (Paris) 85:145–147, 1951
Kellogg DR, Smith LL: Recurrent monocular blindness due to a redundant carotid artery. Arch Surg 95:908–910, 1967
Adams RD, Victor M: Principles of Neurology, 3rd ed, p 576. New York, McGraw-Hill, 1985

REED'S

Synonyms. Tietz–Reed; Reed's. See also Woolf's and Albinism oculocutaneous.

Symptoms. Both sexes affected. Profound deafness and piebaldness (large white forelock and symmetric white spots on arms, legs, and abdomen). Albinism does not affect the eyes (blue iris). Affected subjects tan normally.

Etiology. Autosomal dominant inheritance.

BIBLIOGRAPHY. Tietz WA: Syndrome of deaf-mutism associated with albinism showing autosomal dominant inheritance. Am J Med Genet 15:259–264, 1963
Reed WB, Stone VM, Boder E et al: Pigmentary disorders in association with congenital deafness. Arch Dermatol 95:176–186, 1967

REESE–BLODI

Synonym. Retinal dysplasia.
Eponym to indicate ophthalmic hypoplasia as most characteristic feature of Bartholin–Patau.

BIBLIOGRAPHY. Reese AB, Blodi FC: Retinal dysplasia. Am J Ophthalmol 33:23–32, 1950
Geeraets WJ: Ocular Syndromes, 3rd ed. Philadelphia, Lea & Febiger, 1976

REESE–ELLSWORTH

Synonym. Anterior chamber cleavage. See also Axenfeld's and Rieger's.

Symptoms. Both sexes affected; present at birth (80% bilaterally). Decreased visual acuity according to anatomic lesions of cornea. Mental retardation.

Signs. Adhesion between iris and cornea. Mesenchymal tissue in chamber angle. Shallow anterior chamber. Iris coloboma and hypoplasia; corneal opacities of variable density; sclerocornea; anterior pole cataract. Cleft palate, syndactyly, craniofacial dysostosis, myotonic dystrophy may be present.

Etiology. Abnormalities of embryologic development of anterior chamber because of failure of normal migration of mesodermal cells or failure of their differentiation. Virus (rubella) is one of the most frequent agents responsible.

Diagnostic Procedures. Increased intraocular pressure. Remains of hyaloid artery in retina.

Therapy. Surgery according to lesions.

Prognosis. Variable.

BIBLIOGRAPHY. Reese AB, Ellsworth RM: The anterior chamber cleavage syndrome. Arch Ophthalmol 75:307–318, 1966
Holmark J, Jensen OA: Anterior chamber cleavage syndrome. A typical case of Peter's anomaly with primary aphakia. Acta Ophthalmol 50:877–886, 1972

REFETOFF'S

Synonym. Thyroid hormone resistance; see Seabright–Bantam syndrome.

Symptoms and Signs. Both sexes. From infancy: recurrent goiter. No history to suggest thyrotoxicosis or hypothyroidism; other physical signs negative. Growth, development, and intelligence normal.

Etiology. Autosomal dominant inheritance. Particular resistance of peripheral tissue to the action of thyroid-stimulating hormone (TSH), pituitary also partially resistant to thyroid hormone's suppressive action.

Pathology. Thyroid: follicles of unequal size, lined by flat to cuboidal cells with round-oval nuclei; abundant colloid in areas of epithelium projecting into lumen. No lymphocytic infiltration.

Diagnostic Procedures. Markedly elevated serum total and free T_3 and T_4 levels; normal or elevated serum TSH. X-ray skeleton survey: stippled epiphyses.

Therapy. No evidence that treatment with thyroid hormone is useful. Thionamides, radioactive iodine or surgery could induce subclinical hypothyroidism.

Prognosis. Except for goiter no other manifestations affect life or functions.

BIBLIOGRAPHY. Refetoff S, DeWind LT, DeGroot LJ: Familial syndrome combining deaf-mutism, stippled epiphyses, goiter and abnormally high PBI: Possible target organ refractoriness to thyroid hormone. J Clin Endocrinol 27:279–294, 1967
Oppenheimer JH: Thyroid hormone action at nuclear level. Ann Intern Med 102:374–384, 1985

REFLEX EPILEPSIES

Symptoms. Seizures following a specific external photic stimulus (example television watching); particular sounds; music; some particular movement; somatosensory; reading. See Sensory seizures syndromes.

BIBLIOGRAPHY. Hall M: Synopsis of Cerebral and Spinal Seizures of Inorganic Origin and of Paroxysmal Form as a Class: and of Their Pathology as Involved in the Structures and Action of the Neck, 2nd ed. London, Mallett, 1851
Hishikawa Y, Yamamoto J, Furuya E et al: Photosensitive epilepsy: Relationships between the visual evoked responses and the epileptiform discharges induced by intermittent photic stimulation. Electroencephalogr Clin Neurophysiol 23:320–334, 1967

REFSUM'S

Synonyms. Ataxia hereditaria hemeralopia polyneuritiformis; hemeralopia heredoataxia polyneuritiformis; heredopathia atactica polyneuritiformis; phytanic acid storage; Refsum–Thiebaut.

Symptoms. Children develop the condition between 4 to 7 years of age, in some persons, however, as late as fifth decade. Progressive nerve deafness; concentric constriction of visual fields; night blindness; chronic polyneuropathy; involving motor and sensory nerves; cerebellar ataxia; loss of sense of smell. Dramatic exacerbation following febrile episodes, surgery, pregnancy; gradual partial recovery at the end of precipitating episodes.

Signs. Ichthyosis; atypical retinitis pigmentosa; pupillary abnormalities. Reported also, epiphyseal dysplasia, pes cavus, long metacarpal and metatarsal bones, signs of cardiomyopathy.

Etiology. Autosomal recessive inheritance. Defect of alpha-oxidation of phytanic acid of exogenous (plant) origin which accumulates principally in nervous system altering the myelin sheath.

Pathology. Nerves enlarged; accumulation of exudate between nerve bundles and beneath perineurium. Increased amount of fibrous tissue periaxon and thickening of perineural sheath (secondary changes).

Diagnostic Procedures. *Blood and tissues.* Increased content of phytanic acid. *Cerebrospinal fluid.* Increased protein without pleocytosis.

Therapy. Diet free of chlorophyll, phytol, and phytanic acid.

Prognosis. Spontaneously progressing; terminating with death after several years. Improvement reported with treatment. Early treatment may prevent or minimize symptoms.

BIBLIOGRAPHY. Refsum S: Heredo-ataxia hemeralopia polyneuritiformis-et tidligere ikke beskrevet familiaert syndrom?, en fozeløbig moddelelse. Nord Med 28:2682–2685, 1945

Steinberg D: Phytanic acid storage disease (Refsum's disease). In Stanbury JB, Wyngaarden JB, Fredrickson DS et al: The Metabolic Basis of Inherited Disease, 5th ed, p 737. New York, McGraw-Hill, 1983

REICHEL'S

Synonyms. Synovial chondromatosis; tenosynovial periarticular chondrometaplasia; Henderson–Jones; synovial osteochondromatosis.

Symptoms. More common in males; onset in youth or middle age. Asymptomatic, or pain, swelling, and motion limitation of affected joint (in order of frequency: knee; hip; elbow; shoulder). Rarely, polyarticular.

Signs. Often, presence of loose bodies in joint and increased synovial fluid.

Etiology. Unknown.

Pathology. Cartilage nodules originating from synovia and loose bodies in cavity. Histologically, metaplastic transformation of synovial tissue. Occasionally, it calcifies (osteochondromatosis).

Diagnostic Procedures. *X-ray.* Typical pattern in case of calcification; otherwise negative.

Therapy. None, or surgery.

Prognosis. Benign condition; very rarely, malignant evolution.

BIBLIOGRAPHY. Reichel P: Chondromatose der Kniegelenkkapsel. Arch Klin Chir 6:717–724, 1900

Carnesale PG: Soft tissue tumors. In Crenshaw AH (ed): Campbell's Operative Orthopedics 8th ed, p 814. St. Louis, CV Mosby, 1987

REICHERT'S

Synonyms. Geniculate ganglion neuralgia; Jacobson's nerve neuralgia; tympanic plexus neuralgia. See Hunt's I and Weisenburg's.

Symptoms. Paroxysm of stabbing pain in external auditory meatus, associated with other pains in the face and postauricular zone. It may be differentiated from Weisenburg's by the fact that it is not induced by eating, swallowing, or talking, and no increase in salivation is observed.

Etiology and Pathology. Neoplastic, inflammatory irritation of the tympanic branch of the glossopharyngeal (IX) nerve (Jacobson's nerve).

Therapy. Intracranial division of the glossopharyngeal (IX) nerve.

Prognosis. Cured by division of the glossopharyngeal (IX) nerve. After section of this nerve, unilateral loss of sensation of soft palate-pharyngeal wall from eustachian tube to epiglottis and posterior third of tongue.

BIBLIOGRAPHY. Reichert FL: Tympanic plexus neuralgia. True tic douloureux of the ear or so-called geniculate ganglion neuralgia: Cure effected by intracranial section of the glossopharyngeal nerve. JAMA 100:1744–1746, 1933

Reichert FL: Neuralgias of the glossopharyngeal nerve with particular reference to the sensory, gustatory and secretory functions of the nerve. Arch Neurol Psychiatry 32:1030–1037, 1934

Adams RD, Victor M: Principles of Neurology, 3rd ed, pp 1011–1012. New York, McGraw-Hill, 1985

REIFENSTEIN'S

Synonyms. Gynecomastia–hypospadias. Androgen insensitivity partial. See Male pseudohermaphroditism, incomplete hereditary (type I).

Symptoms and Signs. Occur in males; developing at puberal age. Gynecomastia; small penis; normal testes; high-pitched voice; sparse beard; small prostate; female pelvic development; female fat distribution. Some men in the family may be infertile but phenotypically normal.

Etiology. Unknown; sex-linked recessive inheritance. Increase of estriol level.

Pathology. Gynecomastia compatible with estrogen stimulation. Testes normal size; biopsy shows decreased Leydig's cell. Spermatozoal maturation onset with normal number of primary and secondary spermatocytes, few or no spermatids or sperm.

Diagnostic Procedures. *Blood.* Normal 17-ketosteroids; Plasma concentration of testosterone and luteinizing hormones high; low gonadotropins; receptor deficiency in cultured fibroblasts. *Sperma.* Oligo or azoo-spermia. *Chromosome studies.* Normal karyotype.

Therapy. Resistance to androgenic and anabolic effects of testosterone.

Prognosis. Good *quoad vitam;* poor *quoad functionem.*

BIBLIOGRAPHY. Reifenstein EC Jr: Hereditary familial hypogonadism. Recent Prog Horm Res 3:224, 1948

Rosewater S, Gwinup G, Hamwi GJ: Familial gynecomastia. Ann Intern Med 63:377–385, 1965

Grifin JF, Wilson JD: The syndromes of androgen resistance. N Engl J Med 302:198–209, 1980

REIMANN–ANGELIDES

Synonyms. Bone pain, periodic; periodic arthralgia.

Symptoms and Signs. Both sexes. From infancy episodes of pain localized in the shafts of long bones.

Etiology. Unknown. Autosomal dominant inheritance. Sporadic cases in the experience of the author (SIM), in which episodes disappear after adolescence.

Pathology. Unknown.

Prognosis. In congenital form persistence for life.

BIBLIOGRAPHY. Reimann HA, Angelides AP: Periodic arthralgia in 23 members of five generations of a family. JAMA 146:713–716, 1951

Thompson BH, Merritt AD: Dominantly inherited period of bone pain. Birth Defects 10:245–248, 1974

REIMANN'S

Synonyms. Hyperviscosity; purpura hyperglobulinemia; rheologic.

Symptoms. Visual troubles; epistaxis and mucosal bleeding; vertigo; weakness; fatigability; anorexia; dyspnea; syncope and convulsions.

Signs. Eyes dilated; sausage-shaped veins; retinal hemorrhage; nystagmus. Peripheral edema; decreased pulse pressure.

Etiology. Increase in blood viscosity above a certain threshold level. Increase in viscosity due to the presence of abnormal amount of macroglobulins or other dysproteinemias that affect blood viscosity.

Pathology. That of primary Waldenström's II (macroglobulinemia) syndrome (see) or secondary macroglobulinemia due to lymphomas, reticulum cell sarcoma, tumors, multiple myeloma. Diffuse mucosal bleeding; retinopathy.

Diagnostic Procedures. *Blood.* Anemia; white blood cells normal or increased lymphocytes; thrombocytes normal. Viscosity determination; protein electrophoresis. Sia test, and other indirect and direct studies for quantitative and qualitative determination of pathologic proteins. *Biopsy of bone marrow and lymph node. Electroencephalography.* Aspecific changes.

Therapy. The specific symptoms due to hyperviscosity may be well controlled by plasmapheresis. To be repeated as symptoms return or once individual threshold established every time this is approached. Treatment with support. Treatment of basic disorders: penicillamine; corticosteroids; chemotherapy for lymphomas.

Prognosis. Symptomatic relief. Natural progress of the basic condition.

BIBLIOGRAPHY. Reimann HA: Hyperproteinemia as cause of autonomous agglutination: Observations in a case of myeloma. JAMA 99:1411–1414, 1932

Fulton JE, Hurley HJ, Kennedy R: Purpura hyperglobulinemia. Arch Dermatol 97:446–449, 1968

Dine ME, Guay AT, Snyder LM: Hyperviscosity syndrome with IgA myeloma. Am J Med Sci 264:111–115, 1972

Wintrobe MM (ed): Clinical Hematology, 8th ed, pp 1732–1733. Philadelphia, Lea & Febiger, 1981

REIS–BUECKLERS

Synonyms. Corneal dystrophy (Reis–B. uecklers) including Grayson–Wilbrandt.

Symptoms. Onset variable age from 8 to 20 years. Increased severity after 40 years of age. Infrequent episodes of eye pain, reduction of vision. Frequent strabismus. In Grayson–Wilbrandt variety: variable effect on vision, normal corneal sensitivity.

Signs. Corneal changes: dusty opacity and mottled scarring with peripheral condensation ring separated from limbs by a strip of normal cornea. In Grayson–Wilbrandt variety same pattern or small, macular, gray raised opacity.

Etiology. Autosomal dominant.

Pathology. Bowman membrane erosive lesions with secondary involvement of epithelium. Ultrastructural examination shows swollen mitochondria, large vacuoles, swelling and disruption of the endoplasmic reticulum of epithelial cell, especially of the basal ones. Bowman membrane replaced by clusters of disoriented collagen fibrils and electron dense fibrils.

Therapy. Corneal transplant when needed.

Prognosis. Progressive vision reduction; in some cases vision has minimal reduction or is not affected.

BIBLIOGRAPHY. Buecklers M: Ueber eine weitere familiaere Hornhautdystrophie (Reis). Klin Monatsbl Augenheilkd 114:386–397, 1949

Grayson M, Wilbrandt H: Dystrophy of anterior limiting membrane of the cornea (Reis–Buecklers type). Am J Ophthalmol 61:345–349, 1966

Hall P: Reis–Buecklers dystrophy. Arch Ophthalmol 91:170–173, 1974

REITER'S

Synonyms. Blennorrheal idiopathic arthritis; arthritis urethritica; venereal arthritis; conjunctivourethrosynovial; Fiessinger–Leroy–Reiter; polyarthritis enterica; Ruhr's; urethro-oculo-articular; Waelsch's.

Symptoms and Signs. Prevalent in males; onset between second and fourth decades. *Urethritis.* May pass unnoticed or severe painful micturition; hematuria; purulent discharge. Usually first manifestation of the triad. In enteric form, usually mild. Balanitis circinata develops later. *Conjunctivitis.* In over 50% of cases; usually follows after 10 days from onset of urethritis. Intensity varies from simple congestion to purulent discharge. Iritis and keratitis seldom occur concomitantly. *Arthritis.* Most constant element of the triad. Symmetrical; involving mostly knees, ankle, metatarsal and midtarsal joints, seldom wrists. Swelling; skin pale and warm; arthralgia; mild fever.

Some cases present diarrhea as first symptom. Other elements of the triad follow, isolated or at the same time, after 2 or 3 weeks or much later (years), usually in a mild fashion. Skin lesions: keratoderma, limited or generalized; oral muscosal lesions may also occur as part of the syndrome, occurring concomitantly with the arthritis or later onset.

Etiology. Numerous agents are suspected of being responsible for this syndrome: pleuropneumonialike organisms (PPLO), *Chlamydia*, *Shigella flexneri* (for the enteric form). Autoimmune condition.

Pathology. Dermatologic lesions similar to pustular psoriasis, hyperparakeratosis, spongiform pustules. Synovial changes aspecific, later similar to rheumatoid arthritis lesions.

Diagnostic Procedures. *Culture and serology.* To rule out venereal diseases and possibly to identify agent (usually sterile culture). *X-ray of joints.* Early cortical erosion; new bone formation and articular destruction, followed by osteoporosis. *Blood.* Sedimentation rate increased during acute stage. HLA-B27 positive in 80% of white patients and in 30% of blacks.

Therapy. Symptomatic. Antibiotics ineffective, most effective nonsteroidal anti-inflammatory drugs; gold. Induced hyperthermia (pyrotherapy) (prolonged remission).

Prognosis. Symptoms may remit spontaneously. Conjunctivitis usually lasts 5 to 10 days, occasionally 1 month. Recurrences usually unilateral. Arthritis lasts for months. Recurrences frequent and lead to ankylosis. Complications include myocarditis, pericarditis, pleurisy,

aortic valve lesions, heart block, pulmonary infiltration, glaucoma, and thrombophlebitis.

BIBLIOGRAPHY. Brodie BC: Pathological and Surgical Observations on Diseases of Joint, 2nd ed, p 54. London, Longman, 1818

Reiter H: Ueber eine bisher unerkannte Spirochäteninfektion (Spirochaetosis arthritica). Dtsch Med Wochenschr 42:1535–1536, 1916

Fiessinger N, Leroy E: Contribution à l'étude d'une épidémie de dysenterie dans la Somme (juillet-octobre 1916). Bull Mem Soc Med Hôp Paris 40:2030–2069, 1916

Kaine JL: Reiter's syndrome and enteropathic arthritis. In Orland MJ, Saltman RJ (eds): Manual of Medical Therapeutics, 25th ed, p 382. Boston, Little, Brown & Co, 1986

REJCHMAN'S

Synonyms. Gastrosuccorrhea; hypertrophic-hypersecretory gastropathy.

Symptoms and Signs. Those of gastritis with acid regurgitation.

Etiology. Unknown.

Pathology. Florid gastric mucosa presenting mammillary or cobblestone surface between folds, associated with large parietal cell mass and otherwise normal histologic findings.

Diagnostic Procedures. *Gastric endoscopy and biopsy.*

Therapy. Antacids; cimetidine.

Prognosis. Good.

BIBLIOGRAPHY. Rejchman M: Przpadek chorobowo wzmozonego wydzielania sokn zaladkowego. Gaz Lek Warszawa 2:516–522, 1882

Stempien SJ, Daradi AE, Reingold MM et al: Hypertrophic hypersecretory gastropathy. Am J Dig Dis 9:471–493, 1964

Silvis SE, Blackwood WM, Vennes J: The selection of gastric hypersecretory patients by blind gastroscopy film review. Gastrointest Endosc 19:116–119, 1972

Weinstein VW: Gastritis. In Sleisenger MH, Fordtram JS (eds): Gastrointestinal Disease: Pathophysiology, Diagnosis, Management, 3rd ed, p 599. Philadelphia, WB Saunders, 1983

RELAPSING POLYCHONDRITIS

Synonyms. Chondromalacic arthritis; cartilagineous-arthritic deafness; systemic chondromalacia; Jaksch Wartenhorst's; Meyenburg–Altherz–Vehlinger; perichondritis; diffuse perichondritis; chronic atrophic poly-chondritis; rheumatic perichondritis; von Meyenberg's II. Granulomatous arteritis–polyarthritis.

Symptoms. Both sexes affected; onset usually in middle life (but reported in all ages). Onset acute. Recurrent episodes of malaise, fever, occasionally polyarthritic pains; occasionally, dyspnea, visual trouble, changes of pitch of voice. Hearing impairment; vertigo.

Signs. After subsidence of inflammatory phase, various cartilage changes take place at various involved sites. *Ears* (88%). Pinnas thickened, deformed; perceptive deaf-ness (48%). Labyrinthine vertigo (25%). *Nose* (82%). Cartilage atrophy; saddle deformity with dropping and softening of the tip. *Joints* (78%). In hands and feet, multiple articular dislocation. Big joints (synovial) usu-ally spared, but all cartilages may be involved (symphysis pubis; manubrium sterni; vertebrae). *Chondrocostal carti-lage* (47%). Softening with sternum retraction in deep inspiration. *Larynx and trachea* (70%). Flatness in an-teropostero direction. *Eye.* Episcleritis and conjunctivitis (47%); iritis (27%). *Heart.* Signs of aortic valve insuffi-ciency (14%).

Etiology. Unknown. Lysosomal labilizing factor of esogenous or exogenous toxic nature implied. Immuno-logic reactions considered. Familial occurrence has been reported (autosomal dominant).

Pathology. Dissolution and lysis of cartilage; loss of ba-sophilia; acidophilic coloration of the matrix. Lympho-cyte and plasma cell infiltration in perichondral tissue plus fibroblastic granulation.

Diagnostic Procedures. *Blood.* During attacks, in-creased sedimentation rate; anemia; low titer of rheuma-toid factor, aspecific protein fractions alterations. *X-ray of joints.* Moderate destruction. *Of heart.* Enlargement (if aortic insufficiency). *Of chest* (tomography). Tracheal ste-nosis.

Therapy. Corticosteroids suppress acute inflammatory reactions; if respiratory involvement, long-term treat-ment. Azathioprine; cyclophosphamide (early manage-ment).

Prognosis. Average life span from onset 7 years (range 10 mo to 10 yr). Death from airway stenosis, respiratory complications, and cardiovascular insufficiency.

BIBLIOGRAPHY. Jaksch R, Wartenhorst R: Polychondro-pathia. Wien Arch Inn Med 6:93–100, 1923
von Meyenburg H: Ueber Chondromalacia. Schweiz Med Wochenschr 66:1239–1240, 1936
Altherz F: Ueber einen Fall von systematisierter Chon-dromalacie. Virchows Arch Pathol 297:445–479, 1936
Di Liberti JH: Granulomatous vasculitis. N Engl J Med 306:1365, 1982
Rotestein D, Gibbas DL, Majunder B et al: Familial gran-ulomatous arteritis with polyarthritis of juvenile onset. N Engl J Med 306:86–90, 1982
Michet CJ Jr, McKenna CH, Luthra HS et al: Relapsing polychondritis: Survival and predictive role of early disease manifestations. Ann Int Med 104:74–78, 1986

RENAL GLYCINURIA

Synonym. Iminoglycinuria type II.
Several conditions may affect glycine transport through the kidney, traits that must be distinguished from prere-nal hyperglycinuria.
1. Renal hyperglycinuria and nephrolithiasis (DeVries)
2. Renal hyperglycinuria, autosomal dominant (Käser); type B renal diabetes and glucoglycinuria
3. Hypophosphatemic rickets and glucoglycinuria (Scriver); type A diabetes

BIBLIOGRAPHY. DeVries A, Kochwa S, Lazebuik J et al: Glycinuria: A hereditary disorder associated with nephrolithiasis. Am J Med 23:408–414,1957
Käser H, Cottier P, Antener J: Glucoglycinuria: A new familial syndrome. J Pediatr 61:386–394,1962
Scriver CR, Goldbloom RB, Ray CC: Hypophosphatemic rickets with renal hyperglycinuria, renal glucosuria and glycyloprolinuria: A syndrome with evidence for renal tubular secretion of phosphorus. Pediatrics 34:357–371, 1964
Oberiter V, Puretic Z, Fabecic–Sabadi V: Hyperglycinu-ria with nephrolithiasis. Eur J Pediatr 127:279–285, 1978

RENAL TUBULAR ACIDOSIS TYPE I

Synonyms. Persistent primary renal tubular acidosis; distal renal tubular acidosis; RIA 1; classic renal tubular acidosis; hyperchloremic renal tubular acidosis; renal tu-bular acidosis "gradient" defect; San Francisco, Okla-homa, Atlanta, Philadelphia; see Lightwood–Albright.

Symptoms. Predominant in females (70%) due to strong association with autoimmune disease. Onset from second year of life to early adulthood. Exertional dys-pnea, anorexia; lethargy; failure to thrive; bone pain and pathologic fractures, rickets; nephrocalcinosis; uretheral colics; polyuria; flaccid paralysis; mild fever.

Signs. Stunted growth. Blood hypertension; cardiac ar-rhythmias.

Etiology. Can be primary in hereditary or sporadic form and secondary to autoimmune disorders, nephrocalcino-sis, drug- or toxin-induced nephropathy, renal diseases, genetically transmitted systemic diseases and hepatic cirrhosis. Different genetic forms of hereditary RIA 1 have been described: *San Francisco syndrome*: prevalent characteristics from birth are hypercalcinuria and hypocitraturia with relevant metabolic acidosis. *Philadelphia syndrome*: may be an incomplete form of San Francisco in which nephrocalcinosis may not be present until adulthood and only then can cause metabolic acidosis. *Atlanta syndrome*: prevalent manifestation is hypercalcinuria accompained or not by nephrocalcinosis and impairment of renal function. *Oklahoma syndrome*: hypercalcinuria is primary defect, that only over time damages the tubule, impairs acidification, and causes nephrocalcinosis.

Pathology. Osteomalacia; nephrocalcinosis, renal stones, pyelonephritis.

Diagnostic Procedures. *Blood*. Acidosis, hyperchloremia, hyponatremia, hypokalemia; hypocalcemia, hypophosphatemia, elevated alkaline phosphate, decreased ammonia and titrable acid, increased excretion of potassium, calcium, and phosphorus. *X-ray*. Osteomalacia, nephrocalcinosis; kidney stones.

Therapy. Sodium and potassium bicarbonate and citrate in daily doses of 1–3 mEg/kg. Therapy must be continued for life.

Prognosis. With therapy good. Tendency to permanent condition with progression of the disease and its complications partially controlled and prevented by treatment.

BIBLIOGRAPHY. Lightwood R: Calcific infarction of the kidney in infants. Communication Proc Br Paediatr Soc Arch Dis Child 10:205–206, 1935
Albright F: Metabolic studies and therapy in a case of nephrocalcinosis with rickets and dwarfism. Bull Johns Hopkins Hosp 66:7–33, 1940
Morris RC Jr, Sebastian A: Renal tubular acidosis and Fanconi syndrome. In Stanbury JB, Wyngaarden JB, Fredrickson DS et al (eds): The Metabolic Basis of Inherited Disease, 5th ed, p 1808. McGraw-Hill, New York, 1983
Graef JW, Cone TE: Manual of Pediatric Therapeutics, 3rd ed. Boston, Little, Brown, 1985

RENAL TUBULAR ACIDOSIS TYPE II

Synonyms. Soriano's (J.R.). RIA 2; proximal tubular acidosis. Fanconi's (see). RIA 2 occurs almost always as part of Fanconi's syndrome. See Lightwood-Albright.

Symptoms and Signs. In the congenital form most (or all) cases are males. As an isolated defect: growth retardation. Also reported: mental retardation, nystagmus, cataract, corneal opacities, glaucoma, teeth defects. Tubular dysfunction similar to that of Fanconi's syndrome.

Etiology. Primary form autosomal recessive inheritance possible or sporadic. Caused also by: congenital malabsorption causing vitamin D deficiency, hypocalcemia, secondary hyperparathyroidism, hypophosphatemia. Observed also as feature of several genetically transmitted diseases: cystinosis, Lowe's; Wilson's; etc., or nongenetic condition: nephrosis, renal transplant, renal vein thrombosis; amyloidosis, etc.

Diagnostic Procedures. *Urine*. pH down to 5 during acidosis. *Blood*. Hyperchloremic acidosis; opokaliemia; red cells with increased osmotic resistance; failure of bicarbonate administration to correct acidosis; bicarbonate titration curve grossly impaired. *X Ray*. Seldom nephrocalcinosis.

Therapy. Vitamin D; correction of hyperparathyroidism; bicarbonate and potassium.

Prognosis. In congenital form: transitory condition, with growth retardation or in secondary forms persisting condition and evolving according to specific renal defects and basic condition.

BIBLIOGRAPHY. Worthey HG, Good RA: The de Toni–Fanconi syndrome with cystinosis. Am J Dis Child 95:653, 1958
Soriano JB, Boichis H, Stark H et al: Proximal renal acidosis. A defect in bicarbonate reabsorption with normal urine acidification. Ped Res 1:81–98, 1967
Lamy M, Freza J, Rey J et al: Etude metabolique du syndrome de Lowe. Rev Eur Etud Clin Biol 7:271, 1962
Morris RC Jr, Sebastian A: Renal tubular acidosis and Fanconi syndrome. In Stanbury JB, Wyngaarden JB, Fredrickson DS et al (eds): The Metabolic Basis of Inherited Disease, 5th ed, p 1808. New York, McGraw-Hill, 1983

RENAL TUBULAR ACIDOSIS TYPE IV

Synonyms. RIA 4; hyperkalemic distal renal tubular acidosis.

Symptoms and Signs. Those of hyperkalemia and underlying condition determining renal insufficiency.

Etiology. Aldosterone deficiency, diabetic nephropathy, pseudohypoaldosteronism, other causes of renal insufficiency.

Diagnostic Procedures. Renal bicarbonate reabsorption is reduced at normal plasma bicarbonate concentration. *Urine*. Low pH; low K^+.

Therapy. Mineralocorticoids, restriction of dietary potassium, resins, sodium bicarbonate, loop diuretics.

Prognosis. That of underlying condition.

BIBLIOGRAPHY. Morris RC Jr, Sebastian A: Renal tubular acidosis and Fanconi syndrome. In Stanbury JB, Wyngaarden JB, Fredrickson DS et al: The Metabolic Basis of Inherited Disease, 5th ed, p 1808. New York, McGraw-Hill, 1983

RENDU–OSLER–WEBER

Synonyms. Hemorrhagic familial angiomatosis; Babington's; Goldstein's; Osler–Rendu–Weber; hemorrhagic telangiectasia hereditaria.

Symptoms. Both sexes affected equally. Repeated epistaxis often beginning in childhood. Occult or frank gastrointestinal bleeding (melena; hematemesis) manifest in middle or later life. Hemophthisis also occurs at various ages. In older age group, weakness, pallor, and dyspnea are the presenting symptoms.

Signs. During second or third decade, circumscribed punctiform lesions in the skin and mucous membranes; bluish reddish capillary and venous telangiectasis and spider angiomas may appear. If pulmonary aneurysm syndrome, clubbing, cyanosis, polycythemia, and other typical signs.

Etiology. Unknown; autosomal dominant hereditary transmission.

Pathology. No complete agreement. Dilated capillaries and venules without muscular or elastic layer; new formation of vessels; congenital anomalies with weak capillary endothelium; lesion of mesenchymal tissue in which capillaries are imbedded.

Diagnostic Procedures. *Blood.* Coagulation studies negative, except when in association with (1) other coagulation defects as in Minot–von Willebrand syndrome or (2) hypochromic anemia. *Biopsy of lesions.*

Therapy. Treatment of bleeding and correction of anemia (iron). Caustic agents, electrocautery, x-ray treatment of lesions that may be easily reached, produce temporary relief. Recurrences frequent and occasionally more severe. Administration of ethynyl estradiol has been reported to give good results. If pulmonary aneurysm, surgery may cure the manifestations.

Prognosis. The severity of this syndrome is extremely variable; 4% mortality for severe uncontrollable bleeding has been reported. Some members of affected family found to have the condition only when carefully interrogated and examined.

BIBLIOGRAPHY. Sutton HG: Epistaxis as an indication of impaired nutrition, and of degeneration of the vascular system. Med Mirror 1:769–781, 1864
Rendu M: Epistaxis répétées chez un sujet porteur de petits angiomes cutanés et muquex. Bull Mem Soc Méd Hôp Paris 13:731–733, 1896
Osler W: On a family form of recurring epistaxis, associated with multiple telangiectases of the skin and mucous membranes. Bull Johns Hopkins Hosp 12:333–337, 1901
Weber FP: Haemorrhagic telangiectasia of the Osler-type "telangiectatic dysplasia" and isolated case, with discussion on multiple pulsating stellate telangiectases and other striking haemangiectatic conditions. Br J Dermatol 48:182–193, 1936
Chomette G, Auriol M: Classification des angiodysplasies et tumeurs vasculaires. Rev Stom et Chir Maxillo Fac 87:1–13, 1986

RENON–DELILLE

Synonym. Acromegaly–thyroid-ovarian deficiency, obsolete. See Launois'.

Symptoms and Signs. Hypotension; tachycardia; hyperhidrosis; intolerance to heat; insomnia; oliguria; acromegaly.

Etiology. Unknown. See Multiple endocrine deficiency.

BIBLIOGRAPHY. Rénon L, Delille A: Insuffisance thyro-ovarienne et hyperactivité hypophysaire (troubles acromégaliques). Amélioration par l'opothérapie Thyro-ovarienne; Augmentation de l'acromégalie par la médication hypophysaire. Bull Mem Soc Med Hôp Paris 25:973–979, 1908

RESIDUAL OVARY

Symptoms. Occur in patients who have had hysterectomy and salvage of one or both ovaries. Continuous or intermittent pelvic pain and tenderness; occasionally dyspareunia.

Signs. Persistent pelvic mass usually larger than 5 cm.

Etiology. Continued or attempted ovarian function.

Pathology. Ovary cystic, atretic, hemorrhagic follicles, corpora lutea, perioophoritis. Occasionally, endometriosis and neoplasia.

Therapy. When indicated, exogenous hormone treatment; if this treatment does not relieve symptoms, consider correction of adhesions and, as last resort, oophorectomy.

Prognosis. Neoplasia and malignant degeneration present in 8% of residual ovaries indicate the necessity of a definite diagnosis and adequate surgical procedure.

BIBLIOGRAPHY. Grogan RH: Reappraisal of residual ovaries. Am J Obstet Gynecol 97:124–129, 1967

RESPIRATORY DISTRESS SYNDROME

Synonym. Hyaline membrane disease.

Symptoms. (Over one half of infants have difficulty in initiating normal respiration.) Expiratory grunting or whining, sternal and intercostal retractions, nasal flaring, cyanosis.

Signs. Auscultation: diminished air entry.

Etiology. The disease is due to the absence, deficiency, or alteration of the pulmonary surfactant. Alteration or absence of surfactant results in decreased compliance and reduced alveolar ventilation. Right-to-left shunt, because of large lung areas not perfused.

Pathology. Gross: the lung is collapsed, firm, dark red, and liverlike. Microscopic: alveolar collapse, overdistention of the dilated alveolar ducts, pink-staining membrane on alveolar ducts. Electron microscopy: damage of alveolar epithelial cells, swelling of capillary endothelial cells.

Diagnostic Procedures. *X-Ray*. Reticulogranular, ground-glass appearance with air bronchograms. *Blood gas analysis*. Hypoxemia, often hypercarbia, metabolic acidosis.

Therapy. Neutral thermal environment, oxygen administration, assisted ventilation, continuous positive airways pressure (CPAP), no oral feeding, continuous monitor of respiration, ECG, and temperature.

Prognosis. Poor. Intensive care may completely reverse the outcome.

BIBLIOGRAPHY. Strang LB, Mac Leishm MH: Ventilatory failure and right to left shunt in newborn infants with respiratory distress. Pediatrics 98:17–27, 1961
Klaus M: Respiratory function and pulmonary disease of the newborn. In Barnett H (ed): Pediatrics, 15th ed, pp 1255–1261. New York, Appleton–Century–Crofts, 1972
Farrel P, Avery M: Hyaline membrane disease. Am Rev Resp Dis 111:657–688, 1975
Charon A, Taeusch W, Fitzgibbon C et al: Factor associated with surfactant treatment response in infants with severe respiratory distress syndrome. Pediatrics 83:348–354, 1989

RETINAL CONE DEGENERATION

Symptoms and Signs. Progressive loss of vision. Photophobia, defective color vision. Rarely loss of side vision and night blindness.

Etiology. Autosomal dominant.

Diagnostic Procedures. *Fundus*. Macular lesion with bull's eye appearance (edema). *Electroretinography*. Distinctive findings.

BIBLIOGRAPHY. Davis CT, Hollenhorst RW: Hereditary degeneration of the macula, occurring in five generations. Am J Ophthalmol 39:637–643, 1955
Krill AE, Deutman AF, Fishman M: The cone degeneration. Doc Ophthalmol 35:1–80, 1973

RETINAL NECROSIS ACUTE

Symptoms and Signs. Anterior uveitis, vitreous opacity, cementlike retinal exudates.

Etiology. Viral infection (herpes simplex virus type 1 and varicella zoster virus).

Diagnostic Procedures. Slit-lamp examination.

Pathology. Uveitis, vasculitis, vitritis, and necrosis of retina. Periarteritis, peripheral exudates, and necrosis.

Therapy. Large doses of steroid and antiherpes agents (acyclovir).

Prognosis. Retinal detachment possible.

BIBLIOGRAPHY. Culbertson W, Blumenkranz M, Haines H et al: The acute retinal necrosis syndrome. Ophthalmology 89:1317–1325, 1982
Hayreh SS: So-called "acute retinal necrosis syndrome": An acute panuveitis syndrome. Dev Ophthalmol 10:40–77, 1985
Matsno T, Makayama T, Koyama T et al: Mild type acute retinal necrosis: Syndrome involving both eyes of three-year interval. Jpn J Ophthalmol 31:455–460, 1987

RETINAL PIGMENT EPITHELIUM HYPERTROPHY

Synonyms. Congenital hypertrophy retinal pigment epithelium; CHRPE. See Gardner's syndrome.

Symptoms and Signs. Retinal lesions, "pigmented scar," unilateral, solitary of 1 or 2 disc diameters. In the center chorioretinal atrophy, and at periphery hyperpigmentation surrounded by depigmentation. Frequently found in patients affected by Gardner's syndrome and may represent a valuable clue for the presence of the latter.

Etiology. Autosomal dominant inheritance. Possibly identical genetic lesion of Gardner's.

BIBLIOGRAPHY. Blair NT, Trempe CL: Hypertrophy of the retinal pigment epithelium associated with Gardner syndrome. Am J Ophthalmol 90:661–667, 1980

Bull MJ, Ellis FD, Sato S et al: Hypertrophy of retinal pigment epithelium in Gardner syndrome. Proc Greenwood Genet Center 4:136, 1985

RETINA: POSTPOLE COLLOIDAL DEGENERATION

1. Hutchinson's. Guttate choroiditis
2. Wagner's. "Malattia levantinese"
3. Doyne's. Honeycombed degeneration (typical)
4. Holthose–Batten. Honeycombed degeneration.

RETINOSCHISIS

Synonyms. Blessing–Iwanoff; Iwanoff's; Sorby's macular dystrophy; retinal cystoid degeneration. Including ablatio falciformis congenita.

Symptoms. Sex predominance according to inheritance type. Visual handicap mild up to age 40 to 50 years. Then sudden impairment of vision.

Signs. Retinal cystic degeneration, splitting, detachment, and finally atrophy.

Etiology. Unknown. X-linked and autosomal dominant and recessive families reported.

Pathology. Cystic degeneration mainly of deep nerve layer of retina, all layers involved, cystic areas coalesce with adjacent areas splitting in two layers, detachment and atrophy with sclerosis of choroid.

Diagnostic Procedures. *Ophthalmoscopy.* On retinal periphery small translucent areas or branching channels. *Electroretinogram.* From normal to various abnormalities.

Prognosis. Variable according to evolution.

BIBLIOGRAPHY. Forsius HR, Erikson AW: Retinoschisis X-chromosomalis. In Erikson AW, Forsing HR, Nevaullinna HR et al (eds): Population Structure and Genetic Disorders, p 673. New York, Academic Press, 1900

Mann I, McRae A: Congenital vascular veils in the vitreous. Br J Ophthalmol 22:1–10, 1938

Wave H: Ablatio falciformis congenita (retinal fold). Br J Ophthalmol 22:456–470,. 1938

Hogan MJ, Zimmerman LE: Ophthalmic Pathology. Philadelphia, WB Saunders, 1962

Yassur Y, Nissenkorn I, Ben–Sira I et al: Autosomal dominant inheritance of retinoschisis. Am J Ophthalmol 94:338–343, 1982

RETIREMENT

Symptoms. Affecting people before or after retirement from jobs or careers (especially military personnel who retire at an early age). Irritability; loss of interest; lack of energy; increased alcohol intake; somatic complaints without physical basis (gastrointestinal tract, cardiovascular system).

Etiology. Psychic maladjustment to a changed status, resulting in depression–anxiety complex.

Therapy. Opportunity for activity that will provide new ambitions and goals.

BIBLIOGRAPHY. Freedman AM, Kaplan HI, Sadock BJ: Comprehensive Textbook of Psychiatry, 2nd ed. Baltimore, Williams & Wilkins, 1975.

RETT'S

Synonyms. Cerebroatrophic hyperammonemia; hyperammonemia cerebroatrophic.

Symptoms and Signs. Occurs in females. After normal initial development up to 7 to 18 months combination of psychic deterioration that in a year and a half leads to: severe dementia, autism, loss of finalized use of hands, truncal ataxia, and lack of progression of head growth (acquired microcephaly). Situation remains stable for decades except for insidious appearance of the additional symptoms: seizures, spastic paraparesis, vasomotor disturbances of legs.

Etiology. X-linked inheritance with lethality for males. No chromosomal abnormality is found. Other hypotheses have been advanced: metabolic interference.

Diagnostic Procedures. *Blood.* Mild hyperammonemia. *Pneumoencephalography. Cerebral CT brain scan.* Cerebral atrophy.

BIBLIOGRAPHY. Rett A: Ueber ein cerebral-atrophisches Syndrom bei Hyperammonaemie. Monatsschr Kinderheilkd 116:310–311, 1968

Nomura Y, Hasegawa M: Rett's syndrome. Clinical studies and pathophysiologic consideration. Brain Dev 6:475–486, 1984

Hagberg B: Rett's syndrome: Prevalence and impact on progressive severe mental retardation in girls. Acta Paediatr Scand 74:405–408, 1985

REYE'S

See Reye's (R.K.D.) II; encephalopathy-fatty hepatomegaly. Reye-Johnson.

Symptoms. Occur in children and adolescents of both sexes. Tends to occur in outbreaks following a mild infection (usually upper respiratory tract). Vomiting; convulsions; coma; fever; seldom, rash.

Signs. Hepatomegaly; hypertonia; dilated pupils; abnormal reflexes; flexed elbows, extended legs, and clenched hands.

Etiology. Unknown. Described associated with many viral infections: influenzae B (mostly) A, echo virus, reovirus, rubella, rubeola, herpes simplex, Epstein-Barr, and toxins especially salicilate.

Pathology. *Liver.* Hepatomegaly; fatty degeneration; focal necrosis; mild inflammation; inclusion bodies in some cases. *Brain.* Edema; nonspecific, noninflammatory changes. *Kidney.* Fatty changes. *Lung.* Occasionally, pneumonia.

Diagnostic Procedures. *Blood.* Transaminases increased. Hypoglycemia (in 50% of cases); hyperazotemia; cephalin flocculation and other protein lability tests positive, metabolic acidosis. *Urine.* Ketonuria; aminoaciduria. *Cerebrospinal fluid.* Hypoglycorrhachia (50%). *Electroencephalography.* Diffuse arrhythmic delta activity progressing in cases to silence (cerebral death). *Spinal fluid.* Increased pressure, acellular.

Therapy. Correction of dehydration and electrolyte and metabolic alternations; antibiotics.

Prognosis. With good treatment death 5% to 10%; once in coma, death inevitable. In some cases (minor symptomatology) spontaneous recovery with absence of sequelae.

BIBLIOGRAPHY. Brain WR, Hunter D, Turnbull HM: Acute meningo-encephalomyelitis of childhood. Lancet 1:221–227, 1929

Reye RDK, Morgan G, Baral J: Encephalopathy and fatty degeneration of the viscera: A disease entity in childhood. Lancet 2:749, 1963

Johnson GM, Scurletis TD, Carrol NB: A study of sixteen fatal cases of encephalitis-like disease in North Carolina children. NC Med J 24:464, 1963

Bradford WD, Latham WC: Acute encephalopathy and fatty hepatomegaly. Am J Dis Child 114:153–156, 1967

DeVivo DC: Reye's syndrome. Neurol Clin 3:95–115, 1985

REYE'S (R.K.D.) II

Synonyms. Hepatic encephalopathy; liver degeneration–encephalopathy.

Symptoms. Both sexes affected; onset from 6 months to 10 years. Upper respiratory infection (50%); seldom gastrointestinal involvement. Onset 3 to 21 days after recovery from infection. Progressive vomiting, frequently hemorrhagic; dyspnea; fever; hypotonia; coma; convulsions.

Signs. Some patients have characteristic posture: flexion of elbows, hands clenched, legs extended. Fluctuating liver enlargement.

Etiology. Probably due to aspirin or salicylate use during viral illness. Possibly, hepatoxic substance or virus. Several reports indicate that an association may exist between salicylate therapy and this syndrome.

Pathology. *Liver.* Massive fatty metamorphosis, without necrotic changes. *Kidney.* Fat changes. *Brain.* Edema; no inflammatory changes.

Diagnostic Procedures. *Blood.* Leukocytosis with neutrophilia; hypoglycemia; hyperammonemia; metabolic acidosis; high serum glutamic-oxaloacetic transaminase (SGOT), serum glutamic-pyruvic transaminase (SGPT), and blood urea nitrogen (BUN). *Cerebrospinal fluid.* Normal, except for marked hypoglycorrhachia.

Therapy. Intensive care based on fluid restriction, dexamethasone, neomycin, vitamin K, dextrose (25%). Integrated with endotracheal intubation, mechanical ventilation, hypothermia, and, if intracranial pressure increased, mannitol. Exchange transfusions have been used with success.

Prognosis. Greatly improved by intensive treatment; mortality about 25%. Some spontaneously recover without sequelae.

BIBLIOGRAPHY. Brain WR, Hunter D: Acute meningoencephalomyelitis of childhood: Report of six cases. Lancet 1:221–227, 1929

Reye RDK, Morgan G, Baral J: Encephalopathy and fatty degeneration of the viscera. A disease entity in childhood. Lancet 2:749–752, 1963

Starkok M, Mullick FG: Hepatic and cerebral pathology findings in children with fatal salicylate intoxication: Further evidence for causal relationship betwen salicylate and Reye's syndrome. Lancet 1:326–329, 1983

Hansen JR, McCray PB, Bale JF, Corbett AJ, Flanders DJ: Reye syndrome associated with aspirin therapy for systemic lupus erythematosus. Pediatrics 76:202–205, 1985

Banett MJ, Hurwitz ES, Schonberger LB, Rogers M: Changing epidemiology of Reye's syndrome in the United States. Pediatrics 77:598–602, 1986

RHABDOMYOLYSIS, EXERTIONAL

Synonym. March hemoglobinuria. See Anterior tibial, and peroneal compartment.

Symptoms and Signs. Onset at all ages; more frequently occurring in young men just enrolled in the military service or in athletic clubs. The attacks follow stressing calisthenics executed without previous gradual preparation. Severe myalgia of stressed muscles (tender, crampy, and swelling), lasting from a few days to 1 month, or original capacity for exercise returns in 1 to several months. The subjects notice emission of dark brown urine 24 to 38 hours after the exercise and preceded by malaise and oliguria.

Etiology. Rhabdomyolysis following strenuous exercise, particularly when to the point of exhaustion. Attack onset seems related to muscle glycogen depletion caused by alteration of muscle lipid metabolism including carnitine palmitoyl transferase deficiency. Familial cases reported (autosomal recessive?).

Pathology. Muscular inflammatory changes; coagulation necrosis of muscle fibers.

Diagnostic Procedures. *Urine.* Myoglobinuria; proteinuria. *Blood.* Creatine phosphokinase (CPK) aldolase, serum glutamic-oxaloacetic transaminase (SGOT), lactic dehydrogenase increased; blood urea nitrogen (BUN) may increase.

Therapy. Rest; prevention through gradual exercise, especially with subject in sedentary occupation. Possibility of kidney damage and anuria to be considered, and eventually treated.

Prognosis. Good; no physical impairment left after complete disappearance of symptoms.

BIBLIOGRAPHY. De Langen CD: Myoglobin and myoglobinuria. Acta Med Scand 124:213–226, 1946

Bowden DH, Fraser D, Sackson SH et al: Acute recurrent rhabdomyolysis (paroxysmal myohemoglobinuria). Medicine 35:335–393, 1956

Christensen TE, Saxtrup O, Hansen TI et al: Familial myoglobinuria: A study of muscle and kidney pathophysiology in three brothers. Dan Med Bull 30:112–115, 1983

Arcangeli A, Cavaliere F, Carducci P, Proietti R, Magalini SI: Acute rhabdomyolysis during heroin abuse. Italian J Med Vol II n 23, 1986

Ziskind A: Jet-ski rhabdomyolysis. JAMA 225:1879–80, 1986

Justis EJ Jr: Traumatic disorders. In Crenshaw AH (ed): CampBell's Operative Orthopedics. 7th ed, pp 2223–2224. St. Louis, CV Mosby, 1987

RHIZOMELIC CHONDRODYSPLASIA PUNCTATA

Synonyms. Koala bear recessive; chondrodystrophia calcificans punctata. See also Conradi–Huenermann.

Symptoms and Signs. Both sexes affected; present from birth. Rhizomelic dwarfism; joint contractures. *Head.*

Flat facies; low nasal bridge; nonconstant upward palpebral slanting; microcephaly. Cataracts (72%). *Skin.* Ichthyosiform dermatosis with alopecia (28%). Mental deficiency. Spasticity (not constant).

Etiology. Unknown; autosomal recessive inheritance.

Diagnostic Procedures. *X-ray.* Present only in early infancy: punctate epiphyseal ossification centers stippling. Later: symmetric short humeri and femora; metaphyseal splaying and cupping; vertical clefting of vertebrae on lateral projection; trapezoid dysplasia of ileum.

Therapy. None.

Prognosis. Poor; death by 2 years of age. Rarely longer survival.

BIBLIOGRAPHY. Putschar WGJ: Chondrodystrophia calcificans congenita (dysplasia epiphysialis punctata). Bull Hosp Jt Dis Orthop Inst 11:514–527, 1951

Spranger JW, Opitz JM, Bidder U: Heterogeneity of chondrodysplasia punctata. Hum Genet II:190-212, 1971

Heymans HSA, Oorthuys JWE, Nelck G et al: Rhizomelic chondrodystrophia punctata: Another peroxisomal disorder. N Engl J Med 313:187–188, 1985

RICCARDI'S (NF III)

Synonym. Neurofibromatosis mixed.

Symptoms and Signs. Those of von Recklinghausen (NF I) (freckling and cutaneous neurofibromas are pale, scarcer and relatively larger) and familial acoustic neuromas (NF II) (bilateral acoustic neuroma, meningiomas and spinal neurofibromas giving symptoms in the second or early third decade and developing rapidly); absence of optical gliomas.

Etiology. Autosomal dominant inheritance.

BIBLIOGRAPHY. Riccardi VM, Eichner JE: Neurofibromatosis: Phenotype, Natural History and Pathogenesis, Baltimore, Johns Hopkins Univ Press, 1986

RICCARDI'S (NF IV)

Synonyms. Neurofibromatosis variant forms. Neurofibromatosis atypical.

Symptoms and Signs. Heterogeneous groups of cases that do not present sufficient clinical features to be included in NF I, NF II, NF III.

Etiology. Unknown.

Prognosis. Different evolution and requiring different genetic counseling from other groups.

BIBLIOGRAPHY. Riccardi VM, Eichner JE: Neurofibromatosis: Phenotype, Natural History and Pathogenesis, Baltimore, Johns Hopkins Univ Press, 1986

RICHARD–RUNDLE

Synonyms. Ketoaciduria–mental deficiency; ataxia–deafness–retardation–ketoaciduria; Sylvester's (PE).

Symptoms and Signs. From infancy. Underdevelopment of sexual characteristics; ataxia; deafness; mental retardation; peripheral muscle wasting.

Etiology. Unknown. Autosomal recessive inheritance.

Diagnostic Procedures. *Urine.* Ketoaciduria.

Prognosis. No risk to life.

BIBLIOGRAPHY. Koennecke W: Friedreichsche Ataxia und Taubstummheit. Z Neurol Psychiat 53:161–165, 1920
Richard BW, Rundle AT: A familial hormonal disorder associated with mental deficiency, deafmutism and ataxia. J Ment Def Res 3:33–55, 1959
Sylvester PE: Spinocerebellar regeneration hormone disorder, hypogonadism, deafmutism and mental deficiency. J Ment Def Res 16:203–214, 1972

RICHARDSON–STEELE–OSLZEWSKI

Synonyms. Dementia–nuchal dystonia; supranuclear palsy; progressive supranuclear palsy.

Symptoms and Signs. Occur mostly in males; onset during sixth decade. Insidious, vague changes in personality; visual, speech alteration; unsteady gait; altered facies: deeply lined; spastic with jaw and facial jerks. Dementia with changes in personality appear early but remain usually mild. Constant pseudo-ophthalmoplegia affecting chiefly vertical gaze; pseudobulbar palsy; dysarthria; dystonic rigidity of neck and upper trunk and various inconstant cerebellar and pyramidal symptoms and signs. No forced laughter and crying. No parkinsonian tremor; tendon hyperreflexia; Babinski (inconstant).

Etiology. Unknown; possibly, degenerative conditions or virus infections. To be differentiated from paralysis agitans, cerebellar degeneration, creutzfeldt–Jakob; presenile dementia syndromes, Parkinson's. It may overlap to some extent with Lhermitte's, Cruetzfeldt–Jakob, Hirano's parkinsonism-dementia, and corticodental degenerative with neuronal achromasia. Difference in clinical manifestations or anatomic-pathologic changes, however, do not permit unifying all these syndromes under a single label at the present time.

Pathology. Neurofibrillary tangles (Hirano's globose type); granulovacuolar degeneration; occasionally torpedoes on the axons of Purkinje's cells. Loss of nerve cells in basal ganglia, brain stem, cerebellum. Fibrillary gliosis in all areas with loss of nerve cells and fibrillary tangles. Demyelinization in various tracts; saccules in substantia nigra and subthalamic nucleus; perivascular cuffing.

Diagnostic Procedures. *Cerebrospinal fluid.* Normal. *Electroencephalography. X-ray of skull.*

Therapy. L-Dopa and anticholinesterase drugs give temporary benefit.

Prognosis. Steady progressive course leading to death in 5 to 7 years.

BIBLIOGRAPHY. Chavany JA, von Bogaert L, Godlewski S: Sur un syndrome de rigidité à prédominance axiale avec perturbation des automatismes oculo-palpébraux d'origine encéphalitique. Presse Med 59:958–962, 1951
Richardson JC, Steele J, Oslezwski J: Supranuclear opthalmoplegia, pseudobulbar palsy, nuclear dystonia and dementia. Trans Am Neurol Assoc 88:25–30, 1963
Mastaglia FL, Grainger K, Kee F et al: Progressive supranuclear palsy (Steele–Richardson–Olszewsky syndrome). Clinical and electrophysiological observation in eleven cases. Proc Aust Assoc Neurol 10:35–44, 1973
Adams RD, Victor M: Principles of Neurology, 3rd ed, pp 880–881. New York, McGraw–Hill, 1985

RICHNER–HANHART

Synonym. Tyrosinemia type II.

Symptoms. Affects closely inbred families from Italy, Australia, Canada, Switzerland, and United States. From birth: lacrimation, photophobia redness; painful nonpruritic lesions of palms and soles which blister and become hyperkeratotic.

Signs. Corneal herpetiform erosions, dendritic ulcers corneal and conjunctival plaques, nystagmus, glaucoma. Mental retardation, self-mutilating behavior.

Etiology. Autosomal recessive inheritance. Deficiency of hepatic tyrosine aminotransferase (TAT).

Diagnostic Procedures. *Blood.* Tyrosinemia. *Urine.* Tyrosiluria and tyrosine metabolites over normal levels.

Therapy. Low tyrosine, low phenylalanine diet.

Prognosis. Good with early diet. If not treated, mental retardation.

BIBLIOGRAPHY. Richner H: Hornhaul affection bei Keratoma palmare et plantare hereditarium. Klin Monatsbl Augenheilkd 100:580–588, 1938

Hanhart E: Neuse Sondeformen von Keratosis palmo-plantaris, u.a.eine regelmass g-dominanten mit system-atisierten, Lipomen, ferner 2 einfach-rezessive mit Schwachsinn und Z.T. mit Hornhautveranderun-gen des Auges (Ektadermal syndrome). Dermatologica 94:286–308, 1947

Goldsmith LH: Tyrosinemia and related disorders. In Stanbury JB, Wyngaarden JB, Fredrickson DS et al: The Metabolic Basis of Inherited Disease, 5th ed, p 287. New York, McGraw–Hill, 1983

RIDDOCH'S

Synonym. Visual disorientation II. See Head–Holmes.

Symptoms and Signs. Patient not aware of defect. Visual disorientation in homonymous half field with preservation of stereoscopic vision and visual attention. Ability to fix gaze on an object and to maintain it on contralateral side, but less so on affected side. Pupillary and convergence reflexes normal. Visual acuity normal or slightly reduced.

Etiology and Pathology. Unilateral lesion of parietal lobe (neoplastic; traumatic; infective).

Diagnostic Procedures. *CT brain scan. Angiography.*

Therapy. Surgery or according to etiology.

Prognosis. Depends on etiology. After removal of cause, symptoms recede.

BIBLIOGRAPHY. Riddoch G: Dissociation of visual percep-tions due to occipital injuries, with especial reference to appreciation of movement. Brain 40:15–57, 1917

Riddoch G: Visual disorientation in homonymous half fields. Brain 58:376–382, 1935

Adams RD, Victor M: Principles of Neurology, 3rd ed, pp 191–192. New York, McGraw-Hill, 1985

RIDLEY'S

Eponym used to indicate cardiac asthma.

BIBLIOGRAPHY. Ridley H: Observationes quaedam med-ico-praticae et physiologicae; inter quas aliquanto fu-sius agitur, de asthmate et hydrophobia. Quarum etiam decem ultimis subjiciuntur administrationes totidem corporum morbis quorum tituli observationibus iis praesigunture affectorum anatomicae, cum particulari, et non ante observata, de cordis in embryone vasorum structura, et sanguinis juxta eam circuitu, disserta-tione, pp 224. Lugduni Batavorum, G Langerak et LT Lucht, 1738

Hope J: A Treatise on Diseases of the Heart and Great Vessels. London, 1833

Osler W: Lectures on Angina Pectoris and Allied States, p 81. New York, Appleton, 1897

Friedberg CK: Diseases of the Heart, 3rd ed. Philadel-phia, WB Saunders, 1966

RIEDEL'S

Synonyms. Ligneous thyroiditis; Riedel's struma; chronic fibrous thyroiditis; woody thyroiditis.

Symptoms. Female to male ratio 2:1. Onset most frequently between 30 and 60 years of age. Onset insidious; occasionally, asymptomatic. Dyspnea; dysphagia; hoarseness; aphonia. Later (and not constantly) signs of hypothyroidism (see Gull's).

Signs. Thyroid normal size or enlarged, usually symmetrically, and of hard consistency.

Etiology. Unknown.

Pathology. Thyroid tissue replaced by dense fibrotic tissue, where scattered follicular cells and acini remain; the fibrotic tissue is adherent to trachea and muscle.

Diagnostic Procedures. *Thyroid tests.* Usually normal; later T_4 concentration and ^{131}I uptake are depressed. *Blood.* Normal sedimentation rate and white blood cell count. *Biopsy.* See Pathology.

Therapy. Surgery usually only to relieve obstruction. Medical treatment if hypothyroidism.

Prognosis. Process may remain stable for years or progress slowly and produce hypothyroidism.

BIBLIOGRAPHY. Riedel BM: Die chronische zur Bildung eisenharter Tumoren fuehrende Entzuendung der Schilddruese. Verh Dtsch Ges Chir 25:101–105, 1896

Hamburger J: The various presentations of thyroiditis: Diagnostic considerations. Ann Intern Med 104:219–224, 1986

RIEGER'S

Synonyms. Axenfeld's posterior embryotoxon-juvenile glaucoma; dysgenesis mesodermalis cornae et iridis; iris dysplasia–hypodontia–myotonic dystrophy; iris dysplasia–hypertelorism–psychomotor retardation.

Symptoms. Juvenile glaucoma beginning in childhood with great oscillation in tension; frequently associated with neurologic manifestations.

Signs. Various anterior segment disturbances: dyscoria; pseudopolycoria; corectopia; iridotasis; iris dehiscences; prominence of iris sphincter; aplasia of the mesodermal leaf of the iris; ectropion uveae; corneal opacification;

anterior polar cataract; ectopia lentis. Frequently associated, microphthalmos, strabismus, ptosis palpebralis, and hemangioma conjunctivalis. Extraocular associated manifestations: absence of or irregular teeth; hypertelorism; partial absence of facial bones; myotonic dystrophy, and umbilical hernia.

Etiology. Unknown; hereditary autosomal dominant condition. Chromosomal aberrations (4, 6, 9, 13, 18, 21) have been reported in association with this syndrome.

Pathology. Elevated intraocular pressure. Embryotoxon (prominent anterior border ring of Schwalbe), associated with anterior segment disturbances (see signs).

Diagnostic Procedure. *Gonioscopy.*

Therapy. Limboscleral trephination; miotics.

Prognosis. With trephination; ocular tension usually becomes regulated and visual deterioration does not progress.

BIBLIOGRAPHY. Brailey WA: Double microphthalmos with defective development of iris, teeth and anus. Glaucoma at an early age. Trans Ophthalmol Soc UK 10:139, 1890
Axenfeld T: Embriotoxon corneal posterius. Berl Dtsch Ophthalmol Ges 42:301, 1920
Rieger H: Beiträge zur Kenntnis seltener Missbildungen der Iris: über Hypoplasie des Irisvorderblattes mit Verlagerung und Entrundung der Pupille. Albrecht Von Graefes Arch Ophthalmol 133:602–635, 1935
Friedman JM: Umbilical dysmorphology: The importance of contemplating the belly button. Clin Genet 28:343–347, 1985

RIEHL'S

Synonyms. Jute spinner melanosis; Riehl's melanosis; reticulated pigmented poikiloderma; tar melanosis; war melanosis. See Civatte's.

Symptoms. More frequent in women; onset at any age. Mild constitutional (unexplained) symptoms.

Signs. Brownish gray pigmentation of the face, more intense in forehead and temples, occasionally extension to neck and scalp, chest, seldom, hands and forearms.

Etiology. Unknown; tar derivatives, cosmetic, nutritional factors suspected.

Pathology. Degenerative changes of basal layer; perivascular dermal infiltrates; melanin free in dermis and in melanophores. Horny plugs in follicles.

Therapy. None

Prognosis. Chronic condition, slowly fading.

BIBLIOGRAPHY. Riehl G: Ueber eine eigenartige Melanose Vorläufige Mitterung. Wien Klin Wochenschr 30:780–781, 1917
Civatte A: Poikiloderma réticulée du visage et du cou. Ann Dermatol Syph 4:605–609, 1923
Nakayama H, Narada R, Toda M: Pigmented, cosmetic dermatitis. Int J Dermatol 15: 673–675, 1976

RIETTI–GREPPI–MICHELI

Synonym. Microelliptopoikilocytic anemia. See also Thalassemia syndromes. Clinical classification used prior to the discovery of the characteristic physiochemical behavior of hemoglobins. This eponym indicated the presence of hypochromic iron-resistant anemia, hemolytic jaundice, and decreased osmotic fragility.

BIBLIOGRAPHY. Rietti F: Sugli itteri emolitici primitivi. Atti Acc Sci Med Nat Ferrarae, 1925
Greppi E: Ittero emolitico familiare con aumento della resistenza dei globuli. Minerva Med (Pt 2) 8:1–11, 1928
Micheli F: Le splenomegalic emolitiche. Att 35th Congr Soc Ital Med Int, 1929

RIGA–FEDE

Synonyms. Cachectic aphthae; Cardarelli's; diphtheroid subglossitis; Fede's; subglossitis diphtheroides; sublingual fibrogranuloma.

Symptoms. Sublingual pain arising in children affected by whooping cough or diphtheria.

Signs. Small sublingual ulcerated tumor.

BIBLIOGRAPHY. Riga A: Di una Malattia Della Prima Infanzia, Probabilmente non Trattata, di Movimenti Patologici. Napoli, 1881
Fede F: Della produzione sottolinguale, malattia di Riga. I Congr Pediatr Ital Napoli, pp 251–260, 1890–1891

RIGHT RECTUS

Synonyms. Right rectus muscle; pseudoappendiceal.

Symptoms. Severe pain localized from onset to right lower quadrant. Nausea but no vomiting (absence of crampiform generalized abdominal pain).

Signs. Marked tenderness, spasticity over McBurney's point. No rebound tenderness. Persistence of tenderness when rectus muscle tenses (patient raising neck or trying to sit without the help of hands). Signs of rheumatic fever may be present.

Etiology and Pathology. Rheumatic myositis; strain of right rectus muscle.

Diagnostic Procedures. *Blood.* In rheumatic fever, elevated sedimentation rate, moderate leukocytosis, normal differential antistreptolysine titer. *Electrocardiogram.* In rheumatic fever. In strain, normal blood findings. *Echography; xerography.*

Therapy. That of rheumatic fever. Topical infection with procaine.

Prognosis. According to etiology.

BIBLIOGRAPHY. Geptill P: Differential diagnosis of abdominal manifestations of acute rheumatic fever from acute appendicitis. Ann Surg 99:650–660, 1934
Babbage ED, McLaughlin CW Jr, Fruin RL: Strain of right rectus muscle simulating acute appendicitis. War Med 5:280–282, 1944
Reitman N: Abdominal manifestations of rheumatic fever: Description of a right rectus syndrome. Ann Intern Med 22:671–687, 1945
Steinheber FV: Medical conditions mimicking the acute surgical abdomen. Med Clin North Am 57:1559–1567, 1974.
Way LW: Abdominal pain and acute abdomen. In Sleisenger MH, Fordtran JS (eds): Gastrointestinal Disease, 3rd ed, chap 20. Philadelphia, WB Saunders, 1983

RILEY–DAY

Synonyms. Familial dysautonomia; hereditary sensory autosomal neuropathy III; HSAN III.

Symptoms. Almost completely confined to Ashkenazic Jews. Condition often manifested in first days of life. Defective lacrimation; corneal hypoalgesia; relative insensitivity to pain; defective taste sensation; defective swallowing; orthostatic hypotension; paroxysmal hypertension; attacks of unexplained pyrexia; poor muscular coordination and dysarthria; emotional lability; cyclic vomiting; frequent pulmonary infections.

Signs. Frequent ulceration of cornea (50%); absence of vallate and fungiform papillae of tongue (pathognomonic); kyphoscoliosis; neuropathic joints (may also be observed). Areflexia; Romberg's sign.

Etiology. Unknown; hereditary condition (autosomal recessive inheritance).

Pathology. Hypoplasia and cytologic changes of autonomic ganglia; cytologic alterations in hypothalamus and brain stem.

Diagnostic Procedures. Characteristic response to certain drugs: absence of flushing to histamine injection and exaggerated response to methacholine and norepinephrine; potentiated miosis following instillation of methacholine into conjunctival sac. *X-ray of bones and joints. Electroencephalography. Urine.* Elevated ratio of homovanillic acid to vanillylmandelic acid.

Therapy. No satisfactory treatment available. Tarsorrhaphy. Anesthesia high risk.

Prognosis. Poor. Aspiration pneumonia, hyperpyrexia, nephrosclerosis as causes of death.

BIBLIOGRAPHY. Riley CM, Day RL, Greeley DM et al: Central autonomic dysfunction with defective lacrimation. I. Report of five cases. Pediatrics 3:468–478, 1949
Howard RO: Familial dysautonomia (Riley–Day syndrome). Am J Ophthalmol 64:392–398, 1967
Kaplan M, Schiffmann R, Shapira Y: Diagnosis of familial dysautonomia in the neonatal period. Acta Paediatr Scand 74:131–132, 1985

RILEY–SHWACHMAN

Symptoms. Described in two children. Anorexia; cachexia; asthenia.

Signs. Characteristic ambulation with stiff legs, wide base, and calcaneal limp. Deep reflexes increased; ankle clonus.

Etiology. Unknown.

Diagnostic Procedures. *X-ray.* Generalized osteoporosis and increased density at the base of the skull.

BIBLIOGRAPHY. Riley CM, Shwachman H: Unusual osseous disease with neurologic changes: Report of two cases. Am J Dis Child 66:150–154, 1943

RILEY–SMITH

Synonym. Macrocephaly–pseudopapilledema–multiple hemangiomas.

Symptoms and Signs. Noted at birth. Macrocephaly; subcutaneous hemangiomas may be present at birth or appear later in childhood. Unimpaired visual acuity; normal central visual fields; blurred disks (pseudopapilledema). Absence of bleeding tendency or manifestations. Recurrent pulmonary infections; no mental retardation.

Etiology. Unknown; possibly, heterozygous condition (single autosomal gene).

Pathology. Skin hemangiomas.

Diagnostic Procedures. *X-ray of chest.* Evidence of pulmonary fibrosis. *X-ray; CT brain scan., angiography.* Absence of hydrocephalus or vascular abnormalities.

Therapy. None.

Prognosis. Good.

BIBLIOGRAPHY. Riley HD, Smith WR: Macrocephaly, pseudopapilledema, and multiple hemangiomata. Pediatrics 26:293–300, 1960

Burke EC, Winkelmann RK, Strickland MK: Disseminated hemangiomatosis. Am J Dis Child 108:418–424,1964

RIMOIN–MCALISTER

Synonyms. Metaphyseal dysplasia (type A·V); dysostosis metaphyseal (type A·V).

Symptoms and Signs. Occur in males; present from birth. Recurrent ear infections. Conductive hearing loss; mental retardation; short limb dwarfism.

Etiology. Autosomal recessive inheritance.

Diagnostic Procedures. *X-ray.* Widening, shortening, and irregularity of metaphyses of long bones of upper and lower extremities.

BIBLIOGRAPHY. Rimoin DL, McAlister WH : Metaphyseal dysostosis, conductive hearing loss and mental retardation: A recessive inherited syndrome. Birth Defects 7:116–122, 1971

RING D$_2$ CHROMOSOME

Symptoms and Signs. Aplasia of thumbs; mental and physical retardation; trigonocephaly. Other similarities in common among patients with this syndrome are microcephaly, ptosis of eyelids, epicanthal folds, malrotation of ears, micrognathia, hypoplastic nipple, widely spaced first and second toes.

Etiology. Chromosomal deletion associated with ring D$_2$ chromosome. Clinical differences associated with variable degrees of chromosomal loss or differences in genetic background. Lack of thumbs a common feature.

Diagnostic Procedures. *Chromosome study.*

BIBLIOGRAPHY. Bain AD, Gauld IK: Multiple congenital abnormalities associated with ring chromosome. Lancet 2:304–305, 1963

Sparkes RS, Carrel RE, Wright SW: Absent thumbs with a ring D$_2$ chromosome: A new deletion syndrome. Am J Hum Genet 19:644–659, 1967

RING DERMOID

Symptoms and Signs. Usually bilateral amblyopia, astigmatism (irregular cornea), strabismus, dermoid choristoma, conjunctival plaque of keratinization and hairs growing from tumor mass.

Etiology. Unknown. Autosomal dominant.

BIBLIOGRAPHY. Henkind P: Bilateral corneal dermoids. Am J Ophthalmol 76:972–977, 1973

Mattos J: Ring dermoid syndrome. Arch Ophthalmol 98:1059–1061, 1980

RITTER'S

Synonyms. Exfoliative neonatal dermatitis; keratolysis neonatorum; Lyell's; staphylococcal-scalded skin; SSS.

Symptoms. Occur in infants around seventh day of life. Male to female ratio 4:1. Irritability; pain.

Signs. Erythema beginning in the face and spreading all over the body, followed by desquamation of epidermis in large sheets. Nikolsky's sign. Red, weeping areas result from desquamation.

Etiology. Unknown; association with staphylococcal infection (hemolytic, coagulase positive). Possibly identical with Lyell's syndrome.

Pathology. Epidermal necrosis; lack of involvement of corium.

Diagnostic Procedure. *Culture.* To identify bacteria.

Therapy. Antibiotics; cortisone. General supportive treatment.

Prognosis. Healing of the skin quite complete 10 days after onset of desquamation in more than two thirds of cases. Fatality in the remaining cases with high fever, severe toxicity, and shock.

BIBLIOGRAPHY. Ritter von Rittershain G: Die exfoliative Dermatitis jungerer Sauglinge. Ztsahr Kinderheilk 2:3–23, 1878

Lyell A: The staphylococcal-scalded skin syndrome in historical perspective: Emergence of dermopathic strains of *Staphylococcus aureus* and discovery of the epidermolytic toxin. A review of events up to 1970. J Am Acad Dermatol 9:285–294, 1983

Blanc MF, Jarnier M: Staphylococcies exfoliantes (SSSS) de l'audulte. Ann Dermatol Venerol 113:833–843, 1986

ROAF'S

Symptoms and Signs. (1) Bilateral detachment of retina occuring during first year of life; blindness. (2) Hearing loss between 6 and 12 years (marked increased of loss in high frequency and good deal of variation between one ear and the other). (3) Splaying of metaphyseal and epiphyseal regions of long bone, resulting in shortening of long bones in coxa vara deformity of femoral neck; kyphoscoliosis; flattening of vertebrae, and distortion of pelvis. Condition progressive with growth.

Etiology. Unknown.

Pathology. Unknown. Sporadic cases of spondyloepiphyseal dysplasia (see).

Diagnostic Procedures. *X-rays.* Loss of normal trabecular pattern and ground-glass appearance. *Routine biochemical findings.* Normal. *Chromosome study.* Normal.

Therapy. None.

Prognosis. Blindness; deafness; dwarfism; life expectancy unknown.

BIBLIOGRAPHY. Roaf R, Longmore JB, Forrester RM: A childhood syndrome of bone dysplasia, retinal detachment, and deafness. Dev. Med Child Neurol 9:464–473, 1967

ROBERTS'

Synonyms. Appelt–Gerken–Lenz; cleft lip-palate-tetraphocomelia; facial hemangioma–hypomelia–hypotrichosis; pseudothalidomide; SC.

Symptoms and Signs. Present from birth. At birth, length 40 cm, weight 1.5 to 2 kg; microbrachycephaly; hypertelorism; shallow orbit; prominent eyes; midfacial capillary hemangiomas; thin nares; malformed ears; cleft lip, occasionally left palate; micrognathia. Sparse, silver blond hair. Hypomelia (of all degrees from phocomelia to minor and variable alterations); cryptorchidism. In the few survivors, severe mental defect. Occasionally, hydrocephalus, cardiac and renal defects.

Etiology. Autosomal recessive inheritance.

Therapy. Not advisable in cases of severe defects in midfacial and severe limbs defects.

Prognosis. Frequently, stillbirth or early death. Survivors show severe growth defects and mental deficiency.

BIBLIOGRAPHY. Krueger R: Die Phocomelie und ihre Uebergaenga (case 87), p 92. Berlin, A Hirschwald, 1906
Roberts JB: A child with double cleft of lip and palate, protrusion of the intermaxillary portion of the upper jaw and imperfect development of bones of the four extremities. Ann Surg 70:252; 1919
Freeman MVR, Williams DW, Schimke N et al: The Roberts' syndrome. Clin Genet 5:1–16, 1974
Da Silve EO, Bezzerra LHGE: The Roberts' syndrome. Hum Genet 61:372–374, 1982

Grundy HO, Burlbaw J, Walton S, Dannar C: Roberts syndrome: Antenatal ultrasound-a case report. J Perinat Med 16:71–75, 1988

ROBINOW–SORAUF'S

Synonyms. Craniosynostosis–bifid hallux: acrocephalosyndactyly RS.

Symptoms and Signs. Facies equal to Saethre–Chotzen (see) plus bilaterally broad toes (duplication of distal phalanx).

Etiology. Autosomal dominant.

BIBLIOGRAPHY. Robinow M, Sorauf TJ: Acrocephalopolysyndactyly (type Noack) in a large kindred. Birth Defects XI (5):99–106, 1975
Young ID, Harper PS: An unusual form of acrocephalosyndactyly. J Med Genet 19:286–288, 1982

ROBINOW'S

Synonyms. Achondroplasialike dwarfism; achondroplastic dwarfism; mesomelic dwarfism; fetal face-mesomelic dwarfism.

Symptoms and Signs. Both sexes affected; present from birth. Mild shortness. *Head.* Macrocephaly; frontal bossing; hypertelorism; small upturned nose; small mouth; micrognathia; crowded teeth. *Extremities.* Brachymelia; brachydactyly. *Genitalia.* Penis or clitoris and labia majora hypoplasia. Cryptorchidism. Other associated anomalies.

Etiology. Autosomal dominant or sporadic.

Diagnostic Procedures. *Blood and urine.* Normal. *Chromosome study.* Normal. *X-ray of skeleton.* Does not confirm clinical impression of achondroplastic changes.

Pathology. See Signs; hemivertebrae.

Therapy. Question of sex rearing because penile hypoplasia.

Prognosis. Usually, normal mental performance.

BIBLIOGRAPHY. Robinow M, Silverman FN, Smith HD: A newly recognized dwarfing syndrome. Am J Dis Child 117:649–651, 1969
Saal HM, Poole HE, Lodeiro JG et al: Autosomal recessive Robinow syndrome: Evidence for genetic heterogeneity. Am J Hum Genet 37:A74, 1985

ROBINSON'S (A.R.)

Synonym. Hidrocystoma.

Symptoms. Prevalent in females; onset in middle age. Occurs in persons exposed to heat (*e.g.*, cooks). Lesion of cheeks and eyelids of cystic aspect, which progressively enlarges with repeated heat exposure.

Etiology. Unknown.

Pathology. Dilated and convoluted sweat ducts, containing amorphous debris, not connected with surface.

Therapy. Excision. Avoidance of exposure to heat.

Prognosis. Benign.

BIBLIOGRAPHY. Robinson AR: Hidrocystoma. J Cutan Dis 11:293–303, 1893
Rook A, Wilkinson DS, Ebling FJG et al: Textbook of Dermatology, 4th ed. Oxford, Blackwell Scientific Publications, 1986

ROBINSON'S (E.M.)

Synonyms. Dysmenorrhea–unilateral genital atresia.

Symptoms. Occur in patients between 12 and 27 years. Dsymenorrhea setting in shortly after menarche, increasing in severity with subsequent menstruations. Concomitant symptoms; nausea; vomiting; constipation or diarrhea; dysuria.

Signs. Unilateral pelvic tumor.

Etiology. Incomplete fusion of müllerian ducts or faulty adaptation of the müllerian ducts resulting in atresia of one side and therefore accumulation of the menstruation flow on that side with each menstruation.

Pathology. Pelvic cystic mass filled with blood occupying either the left or right lower quadrant. The mass on section represents one side of the ovary, tube, uterine cavity, and cervix.

Therapy. Early surgical removal of mass and surgical correction of the defect.

Prognosis. Good.

BIBLIOGRAPHY. Robinson EM: Supernumerary uterus in a girl eighteen years old: Removal; recovery. Ala Med J 23:152–154, 1910–11
Merckel GC, Sucoff MC, Sender B: The syndrome of dysmenorrhea and unilateral gynatresia in a double uterus: Report of a case and review of literature. Am J Obstet Gynecol 80:70–75, 1960
Way LW: Abdominal pain and acute abdomen. In Sleisenger MH, Fordtran JS (eds): Gastrointestinal Disease 3rd ed, chap 20. Philadelphia, WB Saunders, 1983

ROBINSON'S (G.C.)

Synonyms. Deafness–nail dystrophy; Robinson's ectodermal dysplasia.

Symptoms and Signs. Nonconstant presence of all features: partial anodontia; peg-shaped teeth; hypoplasia and dystrophy of nails (altered dermatoglyphics); mental retardation; seizures; moderate deafness (sensorineural type); less frequently, syndactyly, polydactyly.

Etiology. Autosomal dominant inheritance (Robinson's) and autosomal recessive (DOOR).

Diagnostic Procedures. *Sweat test.* Increase of sweat electrolytes. *Skin biopsy. Plasma and urine.* Increase of organic 2-oxoglutarate.

BIBLIOGRAPHY. Robinson GC, Miller JR, Bensimon JR, Bensimon JR: Familial ectodermal dysplasia with sensorineural deafness and other anomalies. Paediatrics 30:797–802, 1962
Feinmessers M, Zelig S: Congenital deafness associated with onycodystrophy. Arch Otolaryngol 90:474–477, 1969
Qazy QH, Nangia BS: Abnormal distal phalanges and nails, deafness, mental retardation and seizures disorder: A new familial syndrome. J Pediat 104:391–394, 1984

ROENHELD'S

Synonyms. Postprandial cardiogastric; postprandial gastrocardiac; hysteric tympanism.

Symptoms. Following a meal, atypical chest pain lasting several hours, palpitations.

Etiology. Unknown.

Diagnostic Procedures. *Electrocardiography.* Normal before meal; 30 minutes after feeding; sinus tachycardia, linear ST depression, flat T waves; 2 to 3 hours after meal, normal. In cases with heart block, bradycardia after meal.

Therapy. In many cases atropine prevents manifestations.

BIBLIOGRAPHY. Roenheld L: Der gastrocardiale Symptomenkomplex, eine besondere Form sogenannter Herzneurose. Z Phys Diat Ther 16:339–349, 1912
Gilbert NC, Fenn GK, LeRoy GV: The effect of disten-

tion of abdominal viscera. JAMA 115:1962–1967, 1940

Utsu F, Enescu V, Boszormenyi E et al: Postprandial syndrome. New Physician 15:102–103, 1966

Hersh T: Gastrointestinal causes of chest discomfort. In Hurst JW: The Heart, 6th ed, pp 911–915. New York, McGraw-Hill, 1986

ROGER'S

Synonym. Small septal ventricular heart defect. Two types of this defect are recognized:

WITH MILD PULMONIC STENOSIS

Symptoms. Asymptomatic; absence of cyanosis.

Signs. Murmur of ventricular septal defect.

Diagnostic Procedures. *Electrocardiography.* Mild right ventricular hypertrophy. *X-ray.* Normal.

Therapy. None.

Prognosis. Good.

WITH SEVERE PULMONIC STENOSIS

Symptoms and Signs. See Pulmonary subvalvular stenosis (infundibular with intact ventricular septum).

BIBLIOGRAPHY. Roger H: Reserches cliniques sur le communication congénitale des deux coeurs, par inocclusion des septum interventriculare. Bull Acad Med 8:1074–1094, 1879

Perloff JK: The Clinical Recognition of Congenital Heart Disease, 2nd ed, p 486. Philadelphia, WB Saunders, 1978

ROGERS' (L.E.)

Synonyms. Megaloblastic anemia–thiamine responsive–diabetes mellitus–sensory neural deafness; thiamine responsive anemia.

Symptoms and Signs. Both sexes. Megaloblastic anemia responding to thiamine therapy. Sensory neural deafness; situs viscerum inversus. Hepatosplenomegaly: generalized subedema, hoarseness, cardiac and neurologic disturbances. Those of diabetes.

Etiology. Autosomal recessive. Reduced α-ketoglutarate dehydrogenase activity.

Diagnostic Procedures. *Blood.* Megaloblastic anemia; hyperglycemia. *Bone marrow.* Megaloblastic erythropoiesis and many ringed sideroblasts. *Electrocardiography.* Variable patterns. *X-rays.* Situs inversus viscerum reported.

Therapy. Thiamine corrects anemia but not diabetes.

Prognosis. Fair with treatment. Relapses with discontinuation of thiamine.

BIBLIOGRAPHY. Rogers LE, Poster FW, Sidbury JB Jr: Thiamine-responsive megaloblastic anemia. J Pediat 74:494–504, 1969

Duran M, Wadman SK: Thiamine-responsive inborn errors of metabolism. J Inherit Metab Dis 8 (Suppl 1) 70–75, 1985

ROLLAND–DESBUQUOIS

Synonym. Kniestlike nonlethal.

Symptoms and Signs. Those of Kniest's (see).

Etiology. Autosomal recessive inheritance.

Prognosis. Nonlethal in neonatal period (see Kniestlike lethal).

BIBLIOGRAPHY. Rolland JC, Langier J, Grenier B et al: Nanisme chondrodystrophie et division palatine chez un nouveau-ne. Ann Pediatr 19:139–142, 1972

Stevenson RE: Micromelic chondrodysplasia: Further evidence for autosomal recessive inheritance. Proc Greenwood Genet Center 1:52–57, 1982

ROMANO–WARD

Synonyms. Long QT; LQT; QT syndrome. Ward–Romano; ventricular fibrillation prolonged QT interval. See also Jervell–Lange–Nielson.

Symptoms and Signs. Include all those present in Jervel's and Lange–Nielsen with and without deafness.

Etiology. Unknown; possibly, congenital subnormal activity of right stellate ganglion combined with reflex overactivity of left stellate ganglion. Autosomal dominant inheritance reported.

Diagnostic Procedures. See Jervell–Lange–Nielson.

Therapy. Quinidine or procainamide. Proposed therapy with beta-blocking agents. Automatic implantable defibrillator.

Prognosis. Repeated automatic attacks of dysrhythmias, syncope, and sudden death after psychologic or physical stress.

BIBLIOGRAPHY. Locati E, Moss AJ, Schwartz PJ et al: The long QT syndrome. Am J Cardiol 3:516, 1948

Romano C, Gemma G, Pongiglione R: Aritmie cardiache rare dell'età pediatrica. II. Accessi sincopali per fibrillazione ventricolare parossistica. Clin Pediatr 45:656–683, 1963

Ward OC: A new familial cardiac syndrome in children. J Irish Med Assoc 54:103–106, 1964

Bhandari AK, Scheinman M: The long QT syndrome. Mod Concepts Cardiovasc Dis 54:45–50, 1985

Wilton NCT, Hantler CB: Congenital long QT syndrome: Changes in QT interval during anesthesia with thiopental, vecuronium, fentanyl and isoflurane. Anesth Analg 66:357–360, 1987

ROMBERG–WOOD

Synonym. Primary pulmonary hypertension.

Symptoms. Female-to-male ratio 5 : 1 (in childhood equal incidence); onset usually between 12 to 40 years of age; but ranging from early infancy to eighth decade. Effort syncope; angina pectoris; dyspnea; asthenia; fatigue (in otherwise healthy young women) after exertion, cold exposure, or excitement, or spontaneously. Raynaud's phenomenon (see) occasionally associated.

Signs. In infants asthenia and cough may lead to malnutrition and failure to thrive. Occasionally, mild acrocyanosis. Pulse small; large vein (cervical) pulsation. Palpation of right ventricular systolic impulse and of main pulmonary artery: presystolic distention of right ventricle. Auscultation; loud pulmonic component of second sound with ejection sound; right-sided fourth sound. Hepatomegaly.

Etiology. Idiopathic instrinsic obstructive disease of small arteries and arterioles of pulmonary bed. Multiple causes, mostly unknown, but resulting in vicious cycle (pulmonary hypertension begets pulmonary hypertension). Both autosomal dominant and recessive inheritance reported. Associated in some cases angiitis or Marfan's.

Pathology. Histology: in small arteries and arterioles, medial hypertrophy, intima proliferation, fibrous vascular occlusion, secondary dilatation (angiomatoid lesions), necrotic and thrombotic changes.

Diagnostic Procedures. *Electrocardiography.* Initially, normal sinus rhythm; later, atrial flutter or fibrillation and various degrees of systolic overload of right atrium; up to frank right axis deviation. *X-ray.* Variable from mild to extreme enlargement of pulmonary trunk and branches; lung fields clear: *Fluoroscopy.* Pulsation of pulmonary arteries. *Catheterization.* Pulmonary arterial hypertension; without left-to-right or right-to-left shunt; normal pulmonary wedge pressure.

Therapy. No satisfactory therapy. Long-term anticoagulants. Symptomatic.

Prognosis. Variable according to course. Death in 4 to 5 years from onset of symptoms. Reported a persistent familial neonatal form with death in a few days.

BIBLIOGRAPHY. Romberg E: Ueber Sklerose der Lungernarterie. Dtsch Arch Klin Med 48:197–206, 1891–1892

Wood P: Pulmonary hypertension. Mod Concepts Cardiovasc Dis 28:513–518, 1959

Loyd JE, Primm RK, Newman JH: Familial primary pulmonary hypertension: Clinical patterns: Am Rev Respir Dis 129:194–197, 1984

Shohet I, Reichman B, Schiby G et al: Familial persistent pulmonary hypertension. Arch Dis Child 59:783–785, 1984

RONCHESE'S

Synonyms. Pili torti, twisted hair.

Symptoms and Signs. In females, from infancy. Shafts of hair, flat and twisted at regular intervals through 180 degrees, dry, coarse, lusterless, and fragile. Occasionally hypoplastic tooth enamel.

Etiology. Unknown. Autosomal recessive inheritance. This condition is observed also in Menkes' syndrome (see).

Prognosis. Usually hair becomes normal at puberty.

BIBLIOGRAPHY. Ronchese F: Twisted hairs (pili torti). Arch Dermatol Syph 26:98–109, 1932

Gedda L., Cavalieri R.: Rilievi genetici della distrofia congenita dei capelli. Proc Sec Intern Cong Hum Genet Roma Sept 6/12/61, 2:1070–1077, 1963

ROQUES'

Eponym used to indicate the combination of effects of pulmonary and cardiac sclerosis observed in old patients with cor pulmonale secondary to chronic respiratory insufficiency.

BIBLIOGRAPHY. Roques R: Les scléroses parallèles du coeur et du poumon. Sem Hop Paris 25:721–724, 1949

ROSACEA

Synonym. Acne rosacea (misleading). Couperose.

Symptoms. In adolescence, more common in males; in adulthood, male-to-female ratio 1 : 3; onset usually between 30 and 40 years of age. Variable according to different variants of the syndrome: heat and congestion in areas involved; soreness and irritability of eye (ocular rosacea). Recurrence of symptoms in the spring or following stress or fatigue.

Signs. Progressive, initially intermittent flushing, becoming a permanent erythema on the cheeks, chin, forehead; associated with papules and pustules and telangiectasis. In some cases, thickening of skin of affected areas, and association of edema of the eyelids.

Etiology. Unknown; gastrointestinal, nutritional, psychological, endocrine and infective factors, seborrheic status and vasomotor reactivity considered.

Pathology. Initially, vasodilatation; then, edema of dermal vessels, ectasia with lymphocytic infiltration followed by formation of epithelial cell foci.

Diagnostic Procedures. Psychological treatment; rest; sedation. If sunlight aggravates the symptoms, antimalarial drugs. Cycles of antibiotics: tetracyclines or chlortetracyclines. Centrifugal massage. Topical cream (sulfur ichthammol).

Therapy. Tetracycline *per os* or topical when *per os* contraindicated (pregnancy). Metronidazole *per os* or topical (1%). Corticosteroid may make rosacea worse (use of bland type for short period may be helpful).

Prognosis. Unpredictable. Recurrence of minor manifestations in spring for years (10 or more) then thickening of lesions without further remission. Many cases may subside spontaneously in a shorter period. In adolescent males the milder form lasts 4 to 5 years.

BIBLIOGRAPHY. Kissmeyer A: Sur la kératite et autres affections oculaires de la couperose. Ann Dermatol Syph 5:22–48, 1934
Pendelesco C, Valdeman J: La kératite rosacée. Arch Ophthalmol 2:1080–1087, 1938
Miescher G: Rosacea und rosacea: ähnliche Tuberkulide. Dermatologice 88:150–170, 1943
Rook A, Wilkinson DS, Ebling FJG et al: Textbook of Dermatology, 4th ed, pp 1605–1611. Oxford, Blackwell Scientific Publications, 1986

ROSENBERG–BARTHOLOMEW

Synonym. Hyperuricemia–ataxia–deafness.

Symptoms and Signs. Females: full expression: ataxia and deafness. Males: less severely affected.

Etiology. Possibly consistent with autosomal recessive or X-linked inheritance.

Diagnostic Procedures. *Blood.* Hyperuricemia. Alteration related to renal impairment. Red cell: hypoxanthineguanine phosphoribosyl transferase normal.

BIBLIOGRAPHY. Rosenberg AL, Bartholomew BA: Hyperuricemia neurologic deficits: A family study abstracted. Arthritis Rheum 17:837, 1968

Rosenberg AL, Bergstrom L, Troost BT et al: Hyperuricemia and neurologic deficits: A family Study. N Engl J Med 282:992–997, 1970

ROSENBERG–CHUTORIAN

Synonym. Optic atrophy–polyneuropathy–deafness.

Symptoms and Signs. Males. Distal muscular atrophy (type Charcot–Marie–Tooth, see), progressive optic atrophy and hearing loss.

Etiology. Unknown. Suggested X-linked semidominant inheritance.

BIBLIOGRAPHY. Rosenberg RN, Chutorian A: Familial opticoacoustic nerve degeneration and polyneuropathy. Neurology 17:827–832, 1967
Konigsmark BM, Garlin RJ: Genetic and Metabolic Deafness. Philadelphia, WB Saunders, 1976

ROSEN–CASTLEMAN–LIEBOW

Synonyms. Alveolar proteinosis; lung alveolar proteinosis; pulmonary alveolar proteinosis.

Symptoms. Onset at all ages, most often in adult males. Majority of patients chronically exposed to sawdust, fumes, or other irritating substances. Onset insidious. In half of cases, prodromal febrile illness considered pneumonia. Progressive dyspnea; productive cough; sputum thick, chunky, and yellow whitish, seldom red streaked. Fever usually absent. Fatigability, chest pain, and weight loss.

Signs. Few; pulmonary rales (rare); finger clubbing (rare); cyanosis (terminally).

Etiology. Idiopathic. Reported associated with hematologic malignancies; lymphoma; infection (bacterial, fungal, viral). Possible familial occurrence (autosomal dominant?).

Pathology. Beneath pleura, multiple yellow grayish nodules firm on palpation, size from a few millimeters to 2 cm, areas of consolidation; marked increase in weight. Microscopically, alveoli filled by PAS-positive proteinaceous material, rich in lipid; aveolar cell ghosts. Alveolar septa and interstitial tissue and capillaries normal. Interstitial fibrosis may occur in some cases.

Diagnostic Procedures. *X-ray.* Fine, diffuse, perihilar, radiating nodular or reticular pattern of increased density. Calcification does not occur; lymph nodes not enlarged. *Blood.* Moderate tendency to polycythemia. Leukocytes normal or moderate neutrophilia. *Sputum.* Culture negative. *Skin test.* Negative.

Therapy. Antibiotics for superimposed infections. No specific treatment. Corticosteroid ineffective.

Prognosis. Chronic course. Cases of spontaneous recovery in 5 months to 5 years. Clinical remission with persistence of radiographic features frequent. Progressive dyspnea, cyanosis, and death after chronic course in 25% of cases.

BIBLIOGRAPHY. Rosen SH, Castleman B, Liebow AA: Pulmonary alveolar proteinosis. N Engl J Med 258:1123–1142, 1958

Teja K, Cooper PH, Squires JE et al: Pulmonary alveolar proteinosis in four siblings. N Engl J Med 305:1390–1392, 1981

ROSENTHAL–KLOEPFER

Synonym. Acromegaloid changes–cutis verticis gyrata–corneal leukoma. See Cutis verticis gyrata and Touraine–Solente–Gole syndromes.

Symptoms and Signs. Both sexes affected; onset in early childhood. Visual troubles due to corneal leukomas; acromegaloid development; hornlike projection of lateral supraorbital ridges. From fourth decade hyperplasia and furrowing of skin of face and scalp. Normal mental development.

Etiology. Unknown; autosomal dominant inheritance.

Therapy. None.

Prognosis. Good *quoad vitam.*

BIBLIOGRAPHY. Rosenthal JW, Kloepfer HW: An acromegaloid cutis verticis gyrata, corneal leukoma syndrome. A new medical entity. Arch Ophthalmol 68:722–726, 1962

McKusick VA: Heritable Disorders of Connective Tissue, 4th ed, p 378. St Louis, CV Mosby, 1972

Rook A, Wilkinson DS, Ebling FJG et al: Textbook of Dermatology, 4th ed. Oxford, Blackwell Scientific Publications, 1986

ROSENTHAL'S (C.)

Synonyms. Sleep paralysis. Sensory paroxysm. See pavor nocturnus.

Symptoms. Occur at moment of falling asleep or awaking. Anxiety usually accompanied by hypnagogic hallucinations. Inability to talk or shout, and moaning, being half asleep and half awake with a dim awareness of environment. Attacks last 1 or 2 minutes, but subjectively seem to last a long time. May be interrupted by a sudden movement or by somebody touching the patient. Some differences from pavor nocturnus (see).

Signs. None.

Etiology. Unknown; related to narcolepsy (see Gelineau's) or of no special clinical significance.

Therapy. None specific.

Prognosis. Variable; some people may experience the attack only once or twice in life; some have repeated attacks for life.

BIBLIOGRAPHY. Mitchell SW: On some of the disorders of sleep. Virginia Med Monthly 2:769–781, (Feb) 1876

Rosenthal C: Ueber das verzoegerte psychomotorische Erwachen, seine Entspehung und seine nosologische Bedentung. Arch Psychiatr 81:159–171, 1927

Wilson SAK: The narcolepsies. Brain 51:63–109, 1928

Schneck JM, Fuseli H: Nightmare and sleep paralysis. JAMA 207:725–726, 1969

Adams RD, Victor M: Principles of Neurology, 3rd ed, p 291. New York, McGraw-Hill, 1985

ROSENTHAL'S (R.L.)

Synonyms. Factor XI deficiency; hemophilia C; plasma thromboplastin antecedent deficiency; PTA deficiency.

Symptoms. Both sexes affected. Common in European Jews and Japanese. Clinical manifestation similar to hemophilia but milder. Rarely, spontaneous bleeding, purpura, or hemarthrosis. Usually, manifestation secondary to trauma or surgery. Important feature is bleeding, occasionally occurring 2 to 3 days after surgery. Severe form exists.

Etiology. Congenital deficiency of Factor XI. Incompletely recessive autosomal inheritance; major manifestation in homozygous, minor in heterozygous individuals.

Diagnostic Procedures. *Blood.* Normal bleeding time; slightly prolonged clotting time; increased partial thromboplastin time, corrected by normal absorbed plasma or aged serum; abnormal thromboplastin generation test when all reagents are from patient; abnormal prothrombin consumption test; normal one-stage prothrombin time.

Therapy. Plasma; stored plasma effective.

Prognosis. Variable according to severity of form. Surgical or postsurgical bleeding most threatening feature.

BIBLIOGRAPHY. Rosenthal RL, Dreskin OH. Rosenthal N: New hemophilia-like disease caused by deficiency of a third plasma thromboplastin factor. Proc Soc Exp Biol Med 82:171–174, 1953

Muir WA, Ratnoff OD: The prevalence of plasma thromboplastin antecedent (PTA, factor X1 deficiency). Blood 44:569, 1974

ROSEWATER'S

Synonym. Familial gynecomastia. See Male pseudohermaphroditism, incomplete hereditary (type I); gynecomastia familial.

Symptoms and Signs. Gynecomastia; sterility. External genitalia normal.

Etiology. X-linked inheritance. Resistance to androgen action. Gwinup denies this interpretation because of the rapid masculinization apparently obtained by testosterone admistration (200 mg monthly).

Pathology. Normal internal genital system.

Diagnostic Procedures. *Blood.* Testosterone level increased; estrogens (for men) increased. Gonadotropins increased.

BIBLIOGRAPHY. Rosewater S, Gwinup G, Hamwi G: Familial gynecomastia. Ann Intern Med 63:377–385, 1965

Gwinup G: Incomplete male pseudohermaphroditism. N Engl J Med:308, 1974

Wilson SD, Griffin JE, Leshin M et al: The androgen resistance syndrome: 5-α-reductase deficiency, testicular feminization and related disorders. In Stanbury JB, Wyngaarden JB, Fredrickson DS et al: The Metabolic Basis of Inherited Disease, 5th ed, p 1001. New York, McGraw-Hill, 1983

ROSS'

Synonyms. Holmes–Adie–segmental hypohidrosis; progressive selective sudomotor denervation.

Symptoms and Signs. Time of onset of pupillotonia, hypoactive deep tendon reflexes, and hypohidrosis is variable. Localized progressive hypohidrosis to anhidrosis, following a dermatomal pattern; no vasoconstriction or alteration of blood flow.

Etiology. Unknown; the coexistence of hypohidrosis and Holmes-Adie syndrome appears not to be a chance association.

Pathology. Unknown; skin biopsy of affected areas normal.

Diagnostic Procedures. *Sweat test.* Localized hypohidrosis (quinizarin compound test, pilocarpine test). Tests indicated for pupillotonic-pseudotabes (see).

Therapy. None.

Prognosis. Usually progressive hypohidrosis.

BIBLIOGRAPHY. Ross AT: Progressive selective sudomotor denervation: A case with coexisting Adie's syndrome. Neurology 8:809–817, 1959

Lucy DD, Van Allen MW, Thompson HS: Holmes-Adie syndrome with segmental hypohidrosis. Neurology 17:763–769, 1967

ROSTAN'S

Synonyms. Cardiac asthma; paroxysmal dyspnea. Eponym used to indicate dyspneic attacks generally occurring during the night in patients with congestive heart failure.

BIBLIOGRAPHY. Rostan LL: Mémoire sur cette question, l'asthme des veillards est-il une affection nerveuse? Nouv J Med Chir Pharm 3:3–30, 1818

ROTENSTEIN'S

Synonym. Arteritis familial granulomatous polyarthritis–uveitis. See Job's.

Symptoms and Signs. Both sexes, fever, erythematous rash, hypertension, uveitis. Large vessel nodules; hand, knee, and ankles warm and red, pericardial and pleural effusion, seizures.

Etiology. Autosomal dominant.

Pathology. Systemic noncaseating granulomatous lesions. Periarticular osteoporosis.

Diagnostic Procedures. *Arteriography:* stenosis and poststenotic dilatations. *Skin liver biopsy:* see Pathology.

Therapy. Prednisone, cyclophosphamine.

Prognosis. Improvement with prolonged treatment. Fatal outcome at various ages.

BIBLIOGRAPHY. Rotenstein D, Gibbas DL, Majmudar B et al: Familial granulomatous arteritis with polyarthritis of juvenile onset. N Engl J Med 306:86–90, 1982

ROTH–BIELSCHOWSKY

Synonym. Pseudo-ophthalmoplegia.

Symptoms and Signs. Complete paralysis of all conjugate movements of eyes in one or more directions, except those under labyrinthine control. Vertical movements are relatively or preferentially affected. Stimulation of one labyrinth induces reflex deviation of eyes to side opposite that of paralysis; stimulation of other labyrinth induces deviation of eyes to side of paralysis.

Etiology and Pathology. Lesion of basal ganglia or tectum.

Therapy. According to etiology.

Prognosis. Depends on etiology.

BIBLIOGRAPHY. Roth W: Demonstration von kranken mit Ophthalmoplegie. Neurol Centralbl 20:921, 1901

Bielschowsky A: Das klinische Bild der assoziierten Blick-lähmung und seine Bedeutung für die topischen Diagnostik. MMW 50:1666–1670, 1903

Cogan DG, Adams RD: Type of paralysis of conjugate gaze (ocular motor apraxia). Arch Ophthalmol 50:434–442, 1953

Adams RD, Victor M: Principles of Neurology, 3rd ed, p 1081. New York, McGraw-Hill, 1985

ROTHMANN–MAKAI

Synonyms. Lipogranulomatosis subcutanea; Makai's syndrome.

Symptoms and Signs. Both sexes affected; prevalent in children. Appearance (usually symmetric) of nodules or plaques, slightly tender, firm, elastic consistency in subcutaneous tissue (up to 10 or 15 cm in diameter) on the trunk, occasionally on limbs and face as well. Area most affected front of thighs. No systemic symptoms.

Etiology. Unknown; possibly trauma or vascular damage.

Pathology. At onset; vasodilatation; fat cell necrosis infiltration with neutrophils. Intermediate: histiocytes with foamy cytoplasm. Terminal: fibrosis with lobular atrophy.

Diagnostic Procedures. *Biopsy.*

Therapy. None.

Prognosis. Slowly evolving condition; duration 6 months to 1 year; seldom longer (years).

BIBLIOGRAPHY. Rothmann M: Ueber Entzündung und Atrophie des subcutanen Fettgewebes Virchows Arch [Pathol Anat Physiol] 136:159–169, 1894

Makai E: Über Lipogranulomatosis subcutanea. Klin Wochenschr 7:2343–2346, 1928

Laymon CW, Peterson WC Jr: Lipogranulomatosis subcutanea (Rothmann–Makai), an appraisal. Arch Dermatol 90:288–292, 1964

Niemi KM, Forström L, Hannuksela M et al: Nodules on the legs. A clinical, histological and immunohistological study of 82 patients representing different types of nodular panniculitis. Acta Dermatol Venerol 57:145, 1977

ROTHMUND–THOMSON

Synonyms. Bloch–Stauffer; cataract-telangiectasia pigmentation; poikiloderma atrophicans-cataract juvenilis; Thomson–Rothmund. See Werner's.

Symptoms and Signs. Prevalent in females (2 : 1); appearing 3 to 6 months after birth. Cutaneous changes: telangiectasia; brownish pigmentation; atrophy of skin; lesions appearing on the face, ears, buttocks, extremities. At 4 to 6 years of age, development of bilateral cataracts (50%); occasionally later and in some cases do not develop (see Thomson's). Mental and physical development normal or deficient. In some cases, sexual retardation (1 : 4).

Etiology. Unknown; recessive hereditary familial trait.

Pathology. *Skin.* Thin and pliable; no ulceration. Distended veins form a characteristic netlike arrangement around atrophic scaling areas. Brownish pigmented spots in the vicinity of telangiectasia. No inflammatory reaction or homogenization of subcutaneous tissue. *Other organs and tissues.* Normal. In some cases, hypogenitalism (25%) and bone defect (1 : 3).

Diagnostic Procedures. *Biopsy of skin. Blood.* Low vitamin A.

Therapy. Cataract extraction.

Prognosis. Progressive in first years of life, then tends to remain static. Average life span, even to old age. Possibly, carcinomatous changes of skin.

BIBLIOGRAPHY. Rothmund A: Über Cataracten in Verbindung mit einer eigenthümlichen Hautdegeneration. Albrecht Von Graefes Arch Ophthalmol 14:159–182, 1868

Thomson MS: Poikiloderma congenitale. Br J Dermatol 48:221–234, 1936

Silver HK: Rothmund–Thomson syndrome: An oculocutaneous disorder. Am J Dis Child 111:182–190, 1966

Dechenne C, Chantraine JM, Davin JC: A Rothmund–Thomson case with hypertension. Clin Genet 24:266–272, 1983

ROTHMUND–WERNER

Cases in which features of Rothmund's and Werner's syndromes overlap.

BIBLIOGRAPHY. Thannhauser SJ: Werner's syndrome (progeria of the adult) and Rothmund's syndrome: Two types of closely related heredofamilial atrophic dermatosis with juvenile cataracts and endocrine features. Ann Intern Med 23:559–626, 1945

Merz EH, Tausk K, Dukes E: Mesoecto-dermal dysplasia and its variants. Am J Ophthalmol 55:488–504, 1963

ROTOR'S

Synonym. Idiopathic hyperbilirubinemia.

Symptoms and Signs. Both sexes affected; onset shortly after birth or in childhood. Mild fluctuating jaundice. Attacks of intermittent epigastric discomfort and occasionally abdominal pain, fever, and hepatomegaly.

Etiology. Unknown; a defect in hepatic anion uptake or storage suggested. Possibly, autosomal recessive inheritance.

Pathology. Liver: normal histology.

Diagnostic Procedures. *Blood.* No evidence of hemolysis. Serum bilirubin (conjugated) slight to moderate increase. Sulfobromophthalein in serum sample taken at 45 minutes shows a marked elevation (in Dubin–Johnson the same elevation has been seen at 90–120 min). *Urine.* Bilirubinuria. Increased total urinary coproporphyrin; absent increase of fraction III. *Cholangiography.* Normal.

Therapy. None.

Prognosis. Good.

BIBLIOGRAPHY. Rotor AB, Manahan L, Florentin A: Familial non-hemolytic jaundice with direct van den Bergh reaction. Acta Med Philippina 5:37–49, 1948
Wolkoff AW, Chowdhury JR, Arias IM: Hereditary jaundice and disorders of bilirubin metabolism. In Stanbury JB, Wyngaarden JB, Fredrickson DS et al: The Metabolic Basis of Inherited Disease, 5th ed, p 1385. New York, McGraw-Hill, 1983

ROUSSET'S

Synonym. Anodontia–monilethrix. See Sabouraud's.

Symptoms and Signs. Association of various tooth abnormalities (pointed; development limited to few permanent teeth; absence of permanent dentition) and monilethrix.

Etiology. Unknown. Monilethrix could have autosomal or recessive inheritance and is one feature of many syndromes: Menkes'; argininosuccinicaciduria; Pollit's; hairbrain; Netherton's.

BIBLIOGRAPHY. Strandberg J: A contribution to our knowledge of aplasia moniliformis. Acta Dermatol Venereol 3:650–655, 1922
Rousset J: Génodermatose difficilement classable (trichorrhexis nodosa) predominant chez les males dan quatre générations. Bull Soc Fr Dermatol Syph 59:298–300, 1952
Gorlin RJ, Pindborg JJ: Syndromes of the Head and Neck. New York, McGraw-Hill, 1964

ROUSSY–CORNIL

Synonyms. Hypertrophic neuropathy sporadic; interstitial hypertrophic neuritis; polyradiculoneuropathy.

Symptoms. Onset in second to third decade or later. Wide distribution of lancinating pains (not constant); peripheral weakness; fasciculation; disturbed vision; ataxia.

Signs. Nerves are occasionally palpable and tender when touched; peripheral atrophy; tendon reflexes diminished or abolished; myosis; sluggish pupils; scoliosis.

Etiology. Unknown; regarded as form of von Recklinghausen's neurofibromatosis, associated with cerebellar diseases. (To be differentiated from Charcot–Marie–Tooth, leprosy, polyneuritis, amyloid, and collagen diseases). Its autonomous entity doubted by some authors. It may be considered also as the adult type of Dejerine–Sottas.

Pathology. Uniform nerve trunk thickening; hypertrophy of Schwann sheaths (onionlike laminated structure). Secondary lesions: thickening of spinal roots; degeneration of posterior columns.

Diagnostic Procedures. *Laboratory.* Normal (occasionally increase in protein in cerebrospinal fluid). *Biopsy of sensory nerve.*

Therapy. None; general care and splinting of weak muscles. Corticosteroids.

Prognosis. Progressive; occasionally remissions and exacerbations.

BIBLIOGRAPHY. Roussy G, Cornil L: Névrite hypertrophique progressive non-familial de l'adulte. Ann Med 6:296–305, 1919
Dyck PJ, Lambert EH: Lower motor and primary sensory neuron diseases with peroneal muscular atrophy. Arch Neurol 18:603–618, 1968
Adams RD, Victor M: Principles of Neurology, 3rd ed, pp 979–980. New York, McGraw-Hill, 1985

ROUSSY-LÉVY

Synonyms. Hereditary ataxia-muscular atrophy; Symonds–Show.

Symptoms. Onset early in childhood. Difficulty in walking; clumsiness and tremor of hands, mental deficiency.

Signs. Muscular wasting of legs and hands. Ataxia; bilateral pes cavus; tendon areflexia; kyphoscoliosis. Sensory changes and cerebellar signs minimal or absent.

Etiology. Unknown; autosomal dominant inheritance.

Pathology. Degeneration of spinal cord radicular areas and posterior roots (see Friedreich's ataxia, Pathology).

Diagnostic Procedures. *Electromyography. Spinal tap.*

Therapy. None.

Prognosis. Slowly progressive; spontaneous remission observed. Death from intercurrent diseases.

BIBLIOGRAPHY. Roussy G, Lévy G: Sept cas d'une maladie familiale particuliére: troubles de la marche, pieds bots et aréfléxia tendineuse généralisée, avec accessoirement, légère maladresse des mains. Rev Neurol (Paris) 33:427–450, 1926

Symonds CP, Show ME: Familial claw-foot with absent tendon jerks: A forme fruste of the Charcot–Marie–Tooth disease. Brain 49:387–403, 1926

Rombold GR, Riley HA: The abortive type of Friedreich's disease. Arch Neurol Psychiatr 16:301–302, 1926

Yudell A, Dyck PJ, Lambert EA: A kinship with Roussy–Levy syndrome. Arch Neurol 13:432–440, 1965

ROWELL'S

Synonym. Multiformlike erythema-lupus erythematosus.

Symptoms and Signs. Without precipitating factors, episodic development of annular multiformlike erythema lesions on the face, mouth, neck, and chest, in patients affected by lupus erythematosus, discoid (see) or lupus erythematosus, systemic (see). Initially, lesions are papular, than ringform and, finally, bullous and necrotic.

Etiology. Unknown. See Lupus erythematosus.

Diagnostic Procedures. *Blood.* Typical serologic abnormalities. Speckled type of antinuclear factor associated with precipitine antibody to saline extract of human tissues and rheumatoid factor. Homogeneous type of antinuclear antibody may be present.

Therapy. That of lupus erythematosus.

Prognosis. Episodes last few days up to over 1 month. According to intensity, various degrees of scarring.

BIBLIOGRAPHY. Rowell NR, Beck JS, Anderson JR: Lupus erythematosus and erythema multiformlike lesions. A syndrome with characteristic immunological abnormalities. Arch Dermatol 88:176–180, 1963

Rook A, Wilkinson DS, Ebling FJG et al: Textbook of Dermatology, 4th ed, pp 1294–1295. Oxford, Blackwell Scientific Publications, 1986

ROWLAND PAYNE'S

Synonyms. Horner's ipsilateral vocal cord–phrenic nerve palsies.

Symptoms. In women with metastatic breast tumor between 6 to 42 months after first recurrence after chemo- or roentgen therapy. Scarce: pain and weakness in the shoulder, change in voice.

Signs. Horner's syndrome (see) plus ipsilateral vocal cord and phrenic nerve palsies. Nonconstant motor involvement in cervical distribution. Lymphoadenopathy of ipsilateral supraclavicular fossa.

Etiology. Metastatic lesion from breast cancer. Possibility that other malignancies (lung) can elicit same manifestations.

Pathology. Neoplastic infiltration at the level of sixth cervical vertebra.

Diagnostic Procedure. *CT brain scan.*

Treatment. That of breast cancer.

Prognosis. Preterminal syndrome. All patients died within 6 months from onset.

BIBLIOGRAPHY. Rowland Payne CME: Newly recognized syndrome in the neck: Horner's syndrome with ispilateral vocal cord and phrenic nerve palsies. J R Soc Med 74:814–818, 1981

Vaghadia H, Splitte M: Medical letter. J R Soc Med 76:7, 1983

ROWLEY–ROSENBERG

Synonyms. Renal aminoaciduria–growth retardation–cor pulmonale; Dwarfism–renal aminoaciduria–cor-pulmonale. Growth retardation–pulmonary hypertension–aminoaciduria. Busbi syndrome (family name).

Symptoms. Rate of growth begins to slow at 1 year of age, in spite of apparently normal nutritional intake; slow motor development; waddling gait; frequent respiratory infections; normal mental development.

Signs. Growth retardation; reduced muscle and adipose tissue. Signs of recurrent pulmonary infections of various degrees (*e.g.,* pneumonia; bronchitis); right ventricular hypertrophy.

Etiology. Unknown; familial recessive disorders; renal etiology for aminoaciduria; several factors in the growth disturbance. Aminoaciduria without other signs of the condition may exist in other members of the family.

Pathology. Poor muscular development; diffuse changes; fatty infiltration; loss of cross striation; foci of flocculation suggestive of nonspecific primary myopathic lesion. Subcutaneous fat practically absent. Left lung weight below average. Cardiomegaly with marked right ventricular hyperplasia (absence of congenital defects); kidney normal.

Diagnostic Procedures. *Blood.* Increase of free fatty acids; normal amino acid level; P_{CO_2} elevated, S_{O_2} decreased. *Urine.* Aminoaciduria: increased excretion of alpha-amino nitrogen (serine, threonine, histidine, lysine, tyrosine primarily). *Electrocardiography.* Right ventricular hypertrophy. *X-ray.* Minimal osteoporosis.

Therapy. None.

Prognosis. Death of patient with full syndrome before 12 years of age. Simple aminoaciduria results in a normal life.

BIBLIOGRAPHY. Rowley PT, Mueller PS, Watkin DM et al: Familial growth retardation, renal aminoaciduria, and cor pulmonale. Am J Med 31:187–204, 1961
Rosenberg LE, Mueller PS, Watkin DM: Familial growth retardation, renal aminoaciduria, and cor pulmonale. Am J Med 31:205–214, 1961
Fraser RG, Paré JAP: Diagnosis of Diseases of the Chest, 2nd ed, p 1765. Philadelphia, WB Saunders, 1977

ROYER'S

Eponym to indicate the association of diabetes mellitus and Prader–Willi syndrome (see).

BIBLIOGRAPHY. Royer P: Le diabéte sucré dans la syndrome de Willi-Prader. Journ Annu Diabetol Hôtel Dieu 4:91–99, 1963

ROYER–WILSON

Eponym used to indicate ventricular septal defect and absent pulmonary valve. See Kurtz–Sprague–White.

BIBLIOGRAPHY. Royer BF, Wilson JD: Incomplete heterotaxy with unusual heart malformations. A case report. Arch Pediatr 25:881–896, 1908

RUBINSTEIN–TAYBI

Synonyms. Broad digits; broad thumb-great toe.

Symptoms. Psychomotor retardation; history of respiratory infections. Mental deficiency (IQ 17–86).

Signs. Facial features: (variable) high arched eyebrows; down- and medially-slanting palpebral fissures (with or without epicanthic folds); ptosis; exophthalmos; strabismus; broad nose bridge; prolonged nasal septum; maxillary hypoplasia; anomalies of size, shape, and position of ears; high-arched palate. Broad thumbs and great toes; changes of dermatoglyphic pattern-low ridge count, extra triradius on tip of thumb, characteristic pattern of thenar area, ulnar loop at base of hypothenar area and in allucal area lateral displacement of f triradius with or without e triradius. Dwarfism; cryptorchidism; nevus flammeus (see). Keloid scars easily form.

Etiology. Unknown; normal karyotype. Possibly polygenic or multifactorial inheritance or autosomal recessive inheritance.

Pathology. See Signs.

Diagnostic Procedures. *Electroencephalography.* Abnormal. *X-ray.* Skeletal age retarded; large foramen magnum; low acetabular angle.

Therapy. Symptomatic.

Prognosis. Good *quoad vitam* except when associated with defect such as congenital cardiac anomalies. Ability to walk with typically abnormal gait; poor speech development.

BIBLIOGRAPHY. Rubinstein JH, and Taybi H: Broad thumbs and toes and facial abnormalities. A possible mental retardation syndrome. Am J Dis Child 105:588–608, 1963
Giroux J, Miller JR: Dermatoglyphics of the broad thumb and great toe syndrome. Am J Dis Child 113:207–209, 1967
Gillies DRN, Roussounis SH: Rubinstein–Taybi syndrome: Further evidence of a genetic aetiology. Dev Med Child Neurol 27:751–755, 1985

RUDIMENTARY TESTES

Synonyms. Microgenitosomia–normal male chromosome; Wilkins–Bergada; primary testicular hypoplasia; Leydig cell deficiency.

Symptoms and Signs. From birth, only males, small gonads either in the scrotum or inguinal channel, small penis and hypospadias. Not associated other anomalies.

Etiology. Probably familial with X-linked inheritance. The syndrome is part of congenitally hypoplastic testes that range from pure XY gonadal dysgenesis to congenital anorchia.

Pathology. Testes: small with differentiated tubules interstitial fibrosis. Internal genitalia in some cases, persistence of structures with vagina and uterus.

Diagnostic Procedures. *LHRH test.* Normal. Testosterone production: low. In postpuberal age: gonadotropins high. Karyotype: 46 XY.

Therapy. Sex assignment according to external genitalia.

Prognosis. Good *quoad vitam.* Sex assignment may be difficult. No fertility.

BIBLIOGRAPHY. Wilkins L: The Diagnosis and Treatment of Endocrine Disorders in Childhood and Adolescence, pp 276–277. Springfield Ill, Charles C Thomas Publisher, 1965

Bergada C, Cleveland WW, Jones HW et al: Variants of embryonic testicular dysgenesis: Bilateral anorchia and the syndrome of rudimentary testes. Acta Endocrinol 40:521–536, 1962

Acquafredda A, Vassal J, Job J–C: Rudimentary testes syndrome revisited. J Paediatr 80:209–214, 1987

RUD'S

Synonyms. Dwarfism–ichthyosiform erythroderma-mental deficiency. Ichthyosis–neurologic disorder–hypogonadism.

Symptoms and Signs. Both sexes affected (M/F ratio 2 : 1); onset in infancy. Erythroderma ichthyosiform; dwarfism; mental deficiency; hypogonadism; epilepsy; chronic anemia; muscular atrophy; arachnodactyly.

Etiology. Unknown; not yet completely established clinical entity. Possibly, X-linked recessive.

Pathology. In brain, immature nerve cells; beta cells show chronic chromatolysis; increased oligodendroglia in frontal cortex; binucleated cells in cortex and basal ganglia.

Diagnostic Procedures. *Blood.* Anemia, megaloblastic type. *Biopsy of skin.*

Therapy. Symptomatic.

Prognosis. Poor.

BIBLIOGRAPHY. Rud E: Et Tilfaelde af Infantilisms med Tetani, Epilepsy, Polyneuritis, Ichthiosis og Anaemia of Pernicios type. Hospitalstidende 70:525–538, 1927

York–More ME, Rundle AT: Rud's syndrome. J Ment Def Res 6:108–118, 1962

Wisniewski K, Lewis AR, Shanske AL: X-linked inheritance of the Rud syndrome. Am J Hum Genet 37:A83, 1985

RUDIGER'S

Synonym. See hand–foot–uterus.

Symptoms and Signs. A brother and a sister described. Present from birth. *Facies.* Coarse; clefting of soft palate. *Extremities.* Flexion contracture of hands; thick palmar creases; small fingers and nails, arches in all fingers. Ureteral stenosis; retarded growth. The girl had bicornuate uterus and cystic ovaries, the boy small penis and large inguinal hernia.

Etiology. Possibly, autosomal recessive inheritance.

Prognosis. Death within first year of life.

BIBLIOGRAPHY. Rudiger RA, Schimdt W, Loose DA et al: Severe developmental failure with coarse facial features, distal limb hypoplasia, thickened palmar creases, bifid uvula, and urethral stenosis: A previously undescribed familial disorder with lethal outcome: J Pediatr 79:977–981, 1971

RUFOUS ALBINISM

Symptoms and Signs. In black inhabitants of New Guinea. Mahogany skin and red hair. Irides reddish brown. Mild nystagmus and photophobia.

Etiology. Autosomal recessive inheritance.

Diagnostic Procedures. *Hairbulbs test.* Accumulation of tyrosine.

Therapy. None.

Prognosis. Stable condition.

BIBLIOGRAPHY. Pearson K, Nettleship E, Usher CH: A monograph on albinism in man: Drapers Company Research Tumors. Biometric Series 6,8,9; parts 1,2,4, London, Dulan 1911–1913

Harvey RG: The "red skins" of Lufa sub-district. Further observations on the distinctive skin pigmentation of some New Guinea indigenes. Hum Biol Oceania 1:103, 1971

RUKAVINAS'

Synonyms. Amyloid neuropathy (type II); Indiana type amyloidosis neuropathy; Maryland type amyloidosis neuropathy.

Symptoms. Both sexes affected; onset in third and fourth decades. Symptoms of peripheral neuropathy most severely affecting upper limbs. Same symptoms as in carpal tunnel syndrome. Gastrointestinal symptoms are minor (if compared with above form).

Signs. Impairment of sensation in the distribution of median nerve; little motor involvement. Sclerodermalike changes in skin of hands and arms. Vitreous opacities in eyes.

Etiology. Unknown; autosomal dominant inheritance.

Pathology. Diffuse parenchymal infiltration with amyloid substance.

Diagnostic Procedures. *Blood.* Serum electrophoresis shows unusual peak in Alpha-2-globulin area. *Congo Red test. Electrocardiography. Biopsy of rectum and nerve.*

Therapy. Symptomatic. Carpal tunnel decompression.

Prognosis. Extremely slow progression, usually leading normal life. Death 14 to 40 years after onset of symptoms.

BIBLIOGRAPHY. Falls HF, Jackson J, Carey JH, et al: Ocular manifestations of hereditary primary systemic amyloidosis. AMA Arch Ophthalmol 54:660–664, 1955

Rukavinas JB, Block WD, Jackson CE, et al: Primary systemic amyloidosis: A review and an experimental genetic and clinical study of 29 cases with particular emphasis on the familial form. Medicine 35:239–334, 1956

Benson MD, Duwler FE: Prealbumin and retinol binding protein serum concentration in the Indiana type hereditary amyloidosis. Arthritis Rheum 26:1493–1498, 1983

RUMINATION

IN INFANTS

Symptoms. Ingested food is regularly regurgitated and rechewed and partially reswallowed. Associated with failure to thrive, marasmus.

Etiology. Attributed to psychological causes. Abnormal mother–infant relationship, with immaturity of the mother and attempted autogratification of the infant (?). Considered also a conditioned response.

Therapy. In severe form, hospitalization and care of psychic aspect. In the past, conditioning therapy even by electroshock.

Prognosis. Good if habit broken, otherwise may even lead to death.

IN ADULTS

Symptoms. Onset 15 to 30 minutes after a meal, for about 1 hour, regurgitation of food, one mouthful at a time, chewing and reswallowing it, without effort, involuntarily. The practice is not associated with nausea, pyrosis, or abdominal pain. Rumination stops when food regurgitated becomes acid. In some cases, the practice may be stopped voluntarily.

Etiology. Unknown. Attributed to psychogenetic mechanism.

Diagnostic Procedures. Rule out hiatal hernia.

Therapy. None. Psychological counseling.

Prognosis. Embarassing, nondebilitating habit.

BIBLIOGRAPHY. Wivship DH, Zboralske FF, Weber WN et al: Esophagus in rumination. Am J Physiol 207:1189–1194, 1964

Hallowele JG, Gardner LI: Rumination and growth failure in male fraternal twin. Associated with disturbed family environment. Pediatrics 36:565–571, 1969

Brown WR: Rumination in the adult. A study of two cases. Gastroenterology 54:933–939, 1968

Sleisenger MH, Fordtran JS (eds): Gastrointestinal Disease, 3rd ed. Philadelphia, WB Saunders, 1983

RUMMO'S

Eponym used to indicate cardioptosis.

BIBLIOGRAPHY. Rummo G: Sulla cardioptosis, primo abbozzo anatomoclinico. Arch Med Int 1:161–183, 1898

RUNDLES–FALLS

Synonyms. Pyridoxine-responsive anemia; sideroblastic anemia, X-linked; iron loading, hereditary, anemia.

Symptoms. Occur most often in males. Females, carrier status with minor manifestations. In a minority, anemia is congenital or discovered during childhood. In the majority, discovered between 12 to 87 years. Weakness; tiredness; occasionally, leg pain and paresthesias of feet. Symptoms associated with pyridoxine deficiency, such as mental retardation, convulsions, peripheral neuropathy, glossitis, dermatitis lacking in these patients.

Signs. Pallor, hepatomegaly, and splenomegaly. Occasionally, pretibial edema and skin pigmentation.

Etiology. In some cases X-linkage inheritance. The enzyme defect may involve δ-aminolevulinic acid synthetase.

Pathology. See Diagnostic procedures.

Diagnostic Procedures. *Blood.* Anemia from mild to severe; hypochromia; microcytosis frequent; normocytosis and macrocytosis less frequently observed. Marked anisopoikilocytosis. Hemoglobin electrophoresis normal. Reticulocytes low, siderocytes frequently increased, rate of destruction of erythrocytes moderately increased. Coombs test negative. Osmotic fragility, increased resistance to hypotonic saline. White blood cell number normal or decreased, in some cases increased; platelets normal or occasionally thrombocytopenia or thrombocytosis. Serum iron increased; iron-binding capacity saturated; associated hypolipemia and hypocholesterolemia. *Bone marrow.* Marked normoblastic hyperplasia; reduction of myeloerythroid ratio. Evolution to myelofibrosis possible. Increased iron-staining granules in the erythroblasts and reticuloendothelial cells. *Tryptophan load-xanthurenic acid excretion test.* Increased excretion in many cases.

Therapy. Pyridoxine (100–200 mg/day): good response for the anemia; complete remission seldom occurs. Crude liver extract or androgen or both enhance the therapeutic effect of pyridoxine in some cases. Splenectomy.

Prognosis. Optimal or suboptimal response of the anemia and defective tryptophan metabolism. No consistent changes in associated leukocyte abnormalities. In rare cases, thrombotic episodes coincident with pyridoxine response. Relapses usually recurring with discontinuation of treatment. In some cases, spontaneous temporary remission after a period of treatment. Death occurs from overwhelming infections or hemochromatosis with liver insufficiency or both.

BIBLIOGRAPHY. Cooley TB: A severe type of hereditary anemia with elliptocytosis interesting sequence of splenectomy. Am J Med Sci 209:561–568, 1945

Rundles RW, Falls HF: Hereditary (sex linked) anemia. Am J Med Sci 211:641–658, 1946

Pasanen AVO, Eklof M, Tenhumen R: Coproporphyrinogen oxidase activity and porphyrin concentrations in peripheral red blood cells in hereditary sideroblastic anaemia. Scand J Haematol 34:235–237, 1985

RUNEBERG'S

Eponym to indicate a particular form of Addison–Biermer disease (see), where the course is characterized by spontaneous complete remissions followed by progressively more severe relapses.

BIBLIOGRAPHY. Runeberg JW: Zur Kenntnis der sogenannten progressiven perniciösen Anämie. Dtsch Arch Klin Med 28:499–520, 1880–81

RUSSELL'S

Synonym. Diencephalic infantilis.

Symptoms. Both sexes affected; onset at 3 months to 2 years. Good to increased appetite; apparent well-being; euphoria; hyperkinesia; vomiting.

Signs. Pallor of skin, not of mucosae; emaciation. Blindness or severe visual loss; homonymous hemianopia; nystagmus present in 50% of cases. The autonomic disturbance consists of excessive sweating, easy flushing of the skin, tachycardia, and vomiting. No other physical signs.

Etiology and Pathology. "Silent" neoplasm of hypothalamic region and floor of third ventricle or adjacent structures causing compression of hypothalamus. The tumor can be astrocytoma, glioma, or craniopharyngioma.

Diagnostic Procedures. *Blood.* Paradoxically, normal values; increase in eosinophils sometimes observed; hypoglycemia (occasional). *Cerebrospinal fluid.* Protein elevation (not constant). *X-ray of skull.* Erosion under anterior clinoid processes. Radiographic appearance of extremity: normal fat lines more completely obliterated than in severe emaciation or starvation. *Isotope brain scan, echoencephalography, CT brain scan.* Diagnostic.

Therapy. Cobalt irradiation; condition usually not amenable to surgery because of location.

Prognosis. Grave; 2- to 4-year remission with irradiation treatment and fatal outcome.

BIBLIOGRAPHY. Russell A: A diencephalic syndrome of emaciation in infancy and childhood. Arch Dis Child 26:274, 1951

Carradori R, Miele A, Ricci C: Su di un caso di craniofaringioma con sindrome diencefalica cachetizzante (Sindrome di Russell). Aggiornamento Pediatrico 37:117–119, 1986

RUSSELL'S III

Synonyms. Hyperammonemia (type II); OCT: ornithine carbamyl transferase deficiency.

Symptoms and Signs. Both sexes affected. Difference of severity: very severe in males, milder in females. *Male.* Normal at birth; within few hours or 1 to 2 days, lethargy, poor feeding, dyspnea, ataxia, convulsions, hyperthermia, rapid progression to coma and respiratory failure. *Female.* Onset in early infancy. Variable symptoms from dislike of protein food, to recurrent vomiting, with or without screaming, headache, confusion, ataxia, dyslalia, progressing or not progressing to coma, and seizures.

Recurrent hepatomegaly during attacks. Patients with minor symptoms are mentally normal; those with intermediate or severe symptoms have variable degrees of mental retardation. Pattern of recurrent episodes is similar to that of migraine.

Etiology. Sex-linked dominant inheritance. Ornithine carbamyl transferase (OCT) deficiency.

Pathology. Minimal and nonspecific changes.

Diagnostic Procedures. *Blood.* Postprandial blood hyperammonemia: elevation directly correlated to degree of enzyme deficiency and clinical manifestations (from simple increase in postprandial period to constant extreme elevation). Serum glutamic-oxaloacetic transaminase (SGOT) and serum glutamic-pyruvic transaminase (SGPT) increased, plasma amino acids normal; pyrimidine metabolites increased (also increased urinary excretion). *Enzyme studies.* Deficiency of OCT in liver biopsy.

Therapy. Reduction of protein from diet.

Prognosis. *Males.* Death in neonatal period. *Females.* Death at later age or survival, generally, with mental and physical retardation.

BIBLIOGRAPHY. Russell A, Levin B, Oberhalzer VG et al: Hyperammoniemia: A new instance of an inborn enzymatic defect of the biosynthesis of urea. Lancet 2:699–700, 1962

Walser M: Urea cycle disorders and other hereditary hyperammoniemic syndromes. In Stanbury JB, Wyngaarden JB, Fredrickson DS et al: The Metabolic Basis of Inherited Disease, 5th ed, p 408. New York, McGraw-Hill, 1983

RUSSELL–SILVER

Synonyms. Asymmetry-dwarfism; Silver's.

Symptoms and Signs. No sex preponderance. Small size for gestational age. Significant congenital asymmetry (78%) from marked hemihypertrophy to limited asymmetry involving skull, spine, extremity. Shortness of stature (93%); pattern of growth parallel to normal but below the third percentile. Usually, small at birth; variation in sexual development (34%): precocious sexual development; dissociation between physical evidence of maturation and epiphyseal development. Other occasional manifestations: *cafe au lait* areas of skin; short and incurved fifth fingers; downturning of mouth; triangular shape of face; syndactyly of toes; mental retardation; renal anomaly; hypospadias.

Etiology. Unknown; may arise from different causes; sporadic, autosomal dominant in one family. Six cases of this syndrome with growth hormone deficiency have been reported, three of which had additional pituitary abnormalities.

Diagnostic Procedures. *Blood.* Elevated gonadotropins, evidence of estrogenic stimulation in desquamated cells; tendency toward fasting hypoglycemia (from 10 mo to 3 yr); investigation for pituitary abnormalities. *X-ray.* In some cases, dissociation between epiphyseal age and physical evidence of sexual development.

Therapy. Symptomatic; high replacement doses of growth hormone may be required to overcome deficiency.

Prognosis. Tendency toward improvement in growth and appearance in childhood and adolescence; 10% association with Wilms' tumor (see Wilms' tumor–hemihypertrophy).

BIBLIOGRAPHY. Silver HK, Kiyasu W, George J et al: Syndrome of congenital hemihypertrophy, shortness of stature, and elevated urinary gonadotropins. Pediatrics 12:368–376, 1953

Russell A: A syndrome of "intrauterine" dwarfism recognizable at birth with craniofacial dysostosis disproportionately short arms and other anomalies (5 examples). Proc R Soc Med 47:1040–1044, 1954

Cassidy SB, Blonder O, Courtney VW et al: Russell–Silver syndrome and hypopituitarism. Am J Dis Child 140:155–159, 1986

RUST'S

Synonyms. Malum suboccipitale; suboccipital vertebral.

Symptoms and Signs. Pain in suboccipital area, which the patient tries to reduce by keeping the head in flexed position. Trigeminal neuralgia; hypoglossal and vagus paralysis; tongue atrophy; cardiac arrhythmias. Localized swelling or suboccipital region.

Etiology. Variable: traumatic, rheumatic, neoplastic, infective (*e.g.,* tuberculosis, syphilis).

Therapy. According to etiology.

BIBLIOGRAPHY. Rust JN: Aufsaetze und Abhändlungen aus dem Gebiete der Medizin. Chirurgie und Staatsarzneikunde, Vol 1, p 196. Berlin, Enslin, 1834

RUTHERFURD'S

Synonyms. Oculodental. Corneal dystrophy–gum hypertrophy; gingival hypertrophy–corneal dystrophy. See also Gorlin–Chaudhry–Moss, Peter's, Rieger's, and Meyer–Schwickerath–Weger.

Symptoms. Both sexes affected; present from birth. Iris anomalies; oligodontia; microdontia; hypoplastic enamel; gum hypertrophy; mental retardation.

Etiology. Autosomal dominant inheritance.

BIBLIOGRAPHY. Rutherfurd ME: Three generations of inherited dental defects. Br Med J 2:9–11, 1931.

Houston IB, Shotts N: Rutherfurd's syndrome. A familial oculo-dental disorder. A clinical and electrophysiologic study. Acta Paediatr Scand 55:233–238, 1966.

RUVALCABA'S

Synonym. Brachymetapody–hypogenitalism–retardation.

Symptoms and Signs. Occur in males; present from birth. Microcephaly; hypoplastic genitalia; mental (not invariably) and physical retardation; variable skeletal anomalies. Antimongoloid slant; narrow small nose; micrognathia with crowded teeth. Pectus carinatum; kyphoscoliosis; elbow limited motion; short metacarpals and metatarsals; inguinal hernia.

Etiology. Unknown. Type of inheritance not yet assessed.

BIBLIOGRAPHY. Ruvalcaba RH, Reichert A, Smith DW: A new familial syndrome with osseous dysplasia and mental deficiency. J Pediatr 79:450–455, 1971.

Hunter A: Ruvalcaba syndrome. Am J Med Genet 21:785–786, 1985.

RUVALKABA–MYHRE–SMITH

Synonyms. RMSS; see Sotos'.

Symptoms and Signs. Both sexes. From birth. Severe mental deficiency; macrosomy; macroencephaly; symptoms related to ileal and colon polyposis. At adolescence: tanned flat spots on shaft and glans penis. Reported also myopathy.

Etiology. Unknown. Autosomal dominant inheritance proposed.

Pathology. In cases with myopathy: lipid storage predominantly in type 1 fibers. Type 2 smaller than normal.

Diagnostic Procedures. *Electromyography. X-Ray of intestine. Muscle biopsy.* Lipid storage myopathy.

Therapy. Partial colectomy (in one case).

Prognosis. Fair. Normal adult stature.

BIBLIOGRAPHY. Ruvalkaba V, Myhre S, Smith DW: Sotos syndrome with intestinal polyposis and pigmentary changes of the genitalia. Clin Genet 18:413–416, 1980.

Di Liberti JH, D'Agostino AN, Ruvalkaba RHA et al: A new lipid storage myopathy observed in individual with the Ruvalkaba–Myhre–Smith syndrome. Am J Genet 18:163–167, 1984.

SABIN–FELDMAN

Synonyms. Cerebral damage–chorioretinopathy; pseudotoxoplasmosis. Microcephaly–chorioretinopathy.

Symptoms and Signs. Onset in early infancy. Variable neurologic symptoms, related to extensive destruction of cerebral tissue. Hydrocephalus; chorioretinopathy and degenerative changes of small retinal vessels.

Etiology. Unknown. The clinical pattern is identical to that caused by toxoplasmosis, but this agent was not identified in these patients. Familial cases reported (autosomal recessive?).

Diagnostic Procedures. *Blood.* No toxoplasma antibodies. *X-ray of brain.* Scattered calcifications.

Therapy. Symptomatic.

Prognosis. Fatal.

BIBLIOGRAPHY. Sabin AB, Feldman HA: Chorioretinopathy associated with other evidence of cerebral damage in childhood. A syndrome of unknown etiology separable from congenital toxoplasmosis. J Pediatr St Louis 35:296–309, 1949

Parke JT, Riccardi VM, Lewis RH et al: A syndrome of microcephaly and retinal pigmentary abnormalities without mental retardation in a family with coincidental autosomal dominant hyperreflexia. Am J Med Genet 17:585–594, 1984

SABOURAUD'S

Synonyms. Beaded hair; monilethrix. See Pollitt's.

Symptoms. Both sexes affected; onset usually in first 2 months, but later onset up to adult life also reported. No clinical features except higher incidence of cataracts and related visual impairment.

Signs. Hair normal at birth, progressively thinning up to second month, when there is complete loss. In the entire scalp or selected zones (*e.g.,* nape, occipital), from small follicular, horny papules, development of brittle, beaded hairs easily breakable before they reach 1 to 2 cm in length. Other hairy regions may also be affected, with resulting areas of alopecia.

Etiology. Unknown; autosomal dominant inheritance. Families with recessive inheritance also described. A metabolic disorder (enzyme defect) suggested.

Pathology. *Hair.* Beading, elliptical nodes 1 mm apart, separated by constricted zone lacking medulla. *Follicles.* Horny plugging; otherwise normal.

Diagnostic Procedures. *Urine.* Arginoaminic aciduria not consistently found.

Therapy. None.

Prognosis. Variable. Increasing severity through childhood; improvement in summer; persistence or regression in adult life.

BIBLIOGRAPHY. Sabouraud R: Sur les cheveux moniliformes. (Trichorhexies et monilethrix). Ann Dermatol Syph 3:781–793, 1892

Shaap T, Even–Paz Z, Hodes ME et al: The genetic analysis of monilethrix in a large inbred kindred. Am J Med Genet 11:469–474, 1982

SACCHAROPINURIA

Synonyms. Saccharopine dehydrogenase deficiency; Carson's AASS deficiency. See Hyperlysinemia.

Symptoms and Signs. Mental retardation in some cases; short stature, no seizures, spastic diplegia.

Etiology. Autosomal recessive inheritance supposed. Disease due to mutation of a single locus that codes for aminoadipic semialdehyde synthetase (AASS) causing altered lysine degradation.

Pathology. Not reported.

Diagnostic Procedures. *Urine.* Excretion of large quantity of lysine, citrulline, histidine, and saccharopine. *Blood.* Serum saccharopine and homocitrulline, present in small quantity. Lysine 4 to 5 times higher than normal, and similar increase for the citrulline. *Cerebrospinal fluid.* High concentration of saccharopine. *Electroencephalography* abnormalities.

Therapy. None.

Prognosis. Good *quoad vitam.* Neurologic abnormalities.

BIBLIOGRAPHY. Carson NAJ, Scally BB, Neill DW et al: Saccharopinuria: A new inborn error of lysine metabolism. Nature 218:679, 1968

Sim Ell O, Johansson T, Aula P: Enzyme defect in saccharopinuria. J Pediatr 82:54–57, 1973

Ghadini H: The hyperlysinemias. In Stanbury JB, Wyngaarden JB, Fredrickson DS et al: The Metabolic Basis of Inherited Disease, 5th ed, p 439. New York, McGraw-Hill, 1983

SACK–BARABAS

Synonyms. Ehler–Danlos IV type; polyaneurysmatic.

Symptoms and Signs. Early appearance: aneurysm in skin, bowel, uterus, and major blood vessels. Bruises, recurrent abdominal pain and eventual intestinal perforation, uterine rupture in pregnancy.

Etiology. Autosomal recessive or dominant. Altered synthesis of type III collagen.

Diagnostic Procedures. Microscopy alteration of elastic lamina of vessels, absence of myofilaments in smooth muscle cells. Derma: scarce elastin. *Urine.* Increased excretion of hydroxyproline. *Blood.* Sometimes anti smooth muscle antibodies.

Therapy. Surgery.

Prognosis. Poor due to complications.

BIBLIOGRAPHY. Sack G: Status Dysvascularis, ein Fall von besonderer Zerreisslichkeit der Blutgefässe. Dtsch Arch Klin Med 178:663–669, 1936
Barabas AP: Vascular complications in the Ehler–Danlos syndrome. J Cardiovasc Surg 13:160–167, 1972
Stella A, Gessaroli M, Cifiello BI et al: Sack–Barabas (Ehler–Danlos IV type) (Clinical and histopathologic ultrastructural correlations). Vasc Surg 20:67–73, 1986

SAETHRE–CHOTZEN

Synonyms. Acrocephalosyndactyly (type III); Chotzen's; ACS III; SCS, acrocephaly–skull asymmetry–mild syndactyly.

Symptoms. Both sexes affected; present from birth. Mild to moderate mental retardation; convulsions; multiple respiratory infections.

Signs. Short stature (primary or secondary?). *Head.* Flat occiput; prognathism; hypertelorism; deviated nasal septum; ear deformity; strabismus. Defective teeth (primary or secondary?). *Limbs.* Partial syndactyly of second and third or fourth and fifth fingers and toes; radioulnar synostoses; simian palmar creases. Cryptorchidism. Heart murmur (cardiac anomaly?). *Forme fruste* possible in relatives.

Etiology. Unknown; autosomal dominant transmission, with variable expression suggested.

Pathology. See Signs. Also, renal anomalies.

Diagnostic Procedures. *Blood.* Normal; absence of amino acid abnormalities. *X-ray of skeleton. Chromosome studies.* Apparently normal.

Therapy. None.

Prognosis. Permanent condition. Facial appearance tends to improve during childhood.

BIBLIOGRAPHY. Saethre H: Ein Beitrag zum Turmschädelproblem. Dtsch Z Nervenheilk 117–119; 533–555, 1931
Chotzen F: Eine eigenartige familiäre Entwicklungsstörung (Akrocephalosyndaktlylie, Dystostosis craniofacialis und Hyperteloismus). Monatsschr Kinderheilkd 55:97–122, 1932
Bianchi E, Arico M, Potesta F et al: A family with Saethre–Chotzen syndrome. Am J Med Genet 22:649–658, 1985

ST. HELENIAN CELLULITIS

Synonym. Helenia's.

Symptoms. Cases observed on St. Helena's Island. Female-to-male ratio 3 : 1. Intense burning pain in legs, accompanied by headache and rigor and sometimes by pulmonary edema.

Signs. After 24 hours, unilateral leg lesion, accompanied by redness from calf to ankle; development of small blisters, which may coalesce in large blisters or burst.

Etiology. Unknown; probably, infective.

Diagnostic Procedures. *Blood.* Neutrophilic leukocytes increased.

Therapy. None.

Prognosis. The lesions dry, scab, and resolve in 6 weeks. Brown discoloration may remain. The episodes may recur.

BIBLIOGRAPHY. Shine IB: St. Helenia's cellulitis. Br J Dermatol 76:357–361, 1964
Rook A, Wilkinson DS, Ebling FJG et al: Textbook of Dermatology, 4th ed, p 751. Oxford, Blackwell Scientific Publications, 1986

ST. LOUIS

Term refers to "first" epidemic observed in St. Louis in July 1933; actually observed previously in Paris in 1932.

Synonyms. St. Louis encephalitis.

Symptoms. Onset in late summer and early fall; occur in infancy and later. From asymptomatic to severe. Prodromal: lassitude; malaise; cephalalgia; sore throat. Or acute onset. Severe cephalalgia; hyperthermia; stiff neck; mental confusion, delirium; transitory blurring of vision.

Signs. Increase in deep reflexes; absence of abdominal reflexes; Kernig's sign. Cranial nerves may be involved; ocular signs rare.

Etiology. Arbovirus transmitted by *Culex* mosquito vector.

Pathology. Cerebral edema; diffuse hemorrhages in all central nervous system areas. Focal lymphocyte infiltration of meninges; neuronal degeneration; glial proliferation.

Diagnostic Procedures. *Blood.* Leukocytosis; presence of neutralizing antibodies. *Cerebrospinal fluid.* Leukocytes, proteins, and pressure increased.

Therapy. Symptomatic. Sedation.

Prognosis. Mortality 20%; prolonged period of convalescence and possible sequelae.

BIBLIOGRAPHY. Vick NA: Grinker's Neurology, 7th ed. Springfield, CC Thomas, 1976
Kennard C, Swash M: Acute viral encephalitis: Its diagnosis and outcome. Brain 104:129–148, 1981

SAINT SYNDROMES

1. *St. Agatha's.* Mastopathic inflammatory
2. *St. Aignan's* or *Agnan's.* Favus ringworm; tinea
3. *St. Arman's.* Pellagra
4. *St. Anthony.* Eponym applied to several different conditions:
   A. *St. Anthony's dance.* Chorea (see) also called *St. Vitus' dance.*
   B. *St. Anthony's fire.* Ergotism (epidemic gangrene and psychotic alterations).
   C. *St. Anthony's fire.* Erysipelas
   D. *St. Anthony's fire.* Herpes zoster
5. *St. Apollonia.* Toothache
6. *St. Avertin's.* Epilepsy (see)
7. *St. Avidus'.* Deafness
8. *St. Blasius'.* Quinsy (see) (or Blaize's)
'9. *St. Dymphna's.* Mental derangements
10. *St. Erasmus'.* Colic pain
11. *St. Fiacre's* or *Flacre's.* Hemorrhoids
12. *St. Francis'.* Erysipelas
13. *St. Gervasius'.* Juvenile or adult rheumatic pains
14. *St. Gete's.* Carcinoma
15. *St. Giles'.* Leprosy
16. *St. Gothard's.* Ancylostomiasis
17. *St. Guy's dance.* Chorea
18. *St. Hubert's.* Rabies
19. *St. Ignatius'.* Pellagra
20. *St. Louis'.* Encephalitis (see)
21. *St. Kilda's.* Colds, infection
22. *St. Main.* Scabies
23. *St. Martin's.* Alcoholism
24. *St. Mathurin's.* Idiocy
25. *St. Modestus'.* Chorea (see)
26. *St. Roch's* or *Roche's.* Plague
27. *St. Sebastian's.* Plague
28. *St. Valentine's.* Epilepsy (see)
29. *St. Vitus' dance.* Chorea
30. *St. Zachary's.* Mutism

SAINT'S TRIAD

Synonyms. Hiatus hernia–gall stones–diverticulosis.

Symptoms. Occur in both sexes, prevalent in females; onset in middle to late life. 1. Those of Bochdalek's diaphragmatic hernia: vague, intermittent abdominal pain; bloating; regurgitation or chest pain or both; dyspnea and cardiovascular symptoms or those of acute intestinal obstruction. 2. Those of cholelithiasis: right upper abdominal pain with typical back irradiation; vomiting; nausea; fatty food intolerance. 3. Those of diverticulosis: abdominal pain in various areas; constipation or diarrhea.

Etiology. Unknown.

BIBLIOGRAPHY. Hueller CJB: Hiatus hernia diverticulosis coli and gallstones. Saint's triad. South Afr Med J 22:376, 1948
Palmer ED: Saint's triad (hiatus hernia, gallstones, and diverticulosis coli): The problem of properly directing surgical therapy. Am J Dig Dis 22:314–315, 1955
Small LD: Cholelithiasis. In Bockus HL: Gastroenterology, 3rd ed. Vol 3, p 774. New York, WB Saunders, 1976

SAKATI–NYHAN–TISDALE

Synonyms. Acrocephalopolysyndactyly III, ACPS, ACPS-leg hypoplasia.

Symptoms and Signs. One case reported in a boy of 8 years. Multiple abnormalities noted at birth: craniosynostosis with acrocephaly; brachydactyly; polydactylysyndactyly of toes; bowed femora; hypoplastic tibias; posterior displacement of fibulas on the femora; congenital heart disease; inguinal hernia; areas of alopecia and cutaneous atrophy of scalp; lineal submental scars resembling clefts. In the first year, difficult breathing, with frequent respiratory infections, attacks of cyanosis. Development slow, eventually with help, patient partially overcame difficulty of ambulation, learned to walk with special crutches at 5 years of age. Intelligence normal despite signs of increased intracranial pressure.

Etiology. Unknown; possibly, single gene mutation. Not to be excluded the action of teratogen. It shares elements with Apert's, (see) Laurence–Moon–Bartet–Biedl (see) and other acrocephalosyndactyly syndromes (see).

Pathology. See Symptoms and Signs.

Diagnostic Procedures. *X-rays.* Described bone anomalies; signs of increased intracranial pressure. Epiphyseal center frequently missing. Generalized osteoporosis. *Electrocardiography.* Left axis deviation; incomplete right bundle branch block. *Urine.* Amino acid normal. *Cytology.* Normal. *Dermatoglyphic pattern.* Altered.

Treatment. None. Physical therapy.

Prognosis. Fair *quoad vitam.*

BIBLIOGRAPHY. Sakati N, Nyhan WL, Tisdale WK: A new case with acrocephalopolysyndactyly, cardiac disease, and distinctive defects of the ear skin and lower limbs. J Pediatr 79:104–109, 1971

SALZMANN'S

Synonym. Nodular cornea dystrophy.

Symptoms and Signs. Both sexes affected; onset at any age in persons with corneal disease. Vision impairment; ocular pain.

Etiology. Complication of phlyctenular keratitis or trachoma.

Pathology. Nodular dystrophy of cornea with progressive vascularization and degeneration of epithelium and Bowman's membrane.

Therapy. Lamellar keratoplasty.

Prognosis. Slow progression.

BIBLIOGRAPHY. Salzmann M: Ueber eine eigentümliche Form von Hornhautentzündung. Mitt Verein Aertze Steiermark 53:194–198, 1916

SANCHEZ–CORONA'S

Synonyms. Spinocerebellar ataxia–dysmorphism. See Friedreich's ataxia.

Symptoms and Signs. Both sexes (one family reported). Hair: abundant, rough; mild palpebral ptosis; thick lips with down-curved angles. Dysarthria, ataxia, psychomotor development delayed; scoliosis; foot deformity.

Etiology. Autosomal recessive inheritance probable.

BIBLIOGRAPHY. Sanchez–Corona J, Garcia–Cruz D, Gonzales–Angulo A et al: A distinct dysmorphic syndrome with spinocerebellar ataxia and probable autosomal recessive inheritance. Hum Genet 69:243–245, 1985

SANDERS'

Synonyms. Epidemic keratoconjunctivitis; macular keratitis; shipyard keratoconjunctivitis.

Symptoms. Both sexes affected; onset at all ages; high incidence in factories, shipyards, and eye clinics. Malaise; cephalalgia; pain in the affected eyes; photophobia; lacrimation; no increase in temperature.

Signs. Unilateral preauricular adenopathy.

Etiology. Virus infections, possibly by adenovirus 8–11.

Pathology. Edema and hyperemia of conjunctiva; hypertrophy of affected lymph nodes.

Diagnostic Procedures. *Smear of tears.* Mononuclear cells.

Therapy. Antibiotics.

Prognosis. Spontaneous remission. Possible complications: keratosis and persistent visual impairment.

BIBLIOGRAPHY. Sanders M: Epidemic keratoconjunctivitis ("shipyard conjunctivitis"). I. Isolation of a virus. Arch Ophthalmol 28:581–586, 1942

SANDHOFF'S

Synonyms. Gangliosidosis (type 2); GM-2; Jatzkewitz–Pilz.

Symptoms. Onset at 6 months of age. Motor weakness; startle reaction to sound; early blindness; progressive mental and motor deterioration. Frequent respiratory infections.

Signs. Macrocephaly; doll-like facies; cherry red spots in macula.

Etiology. Autosomal recessive inheritance. Enzyme defect (deficiency of hexosaminidase A and B).

Pathology. Brain cortex, cerebellar, spinal, and autonomic neuronal lipoidosis; cytoplasm of neurons ballooned and enlarged with nucleus displacement. Accumulation of osmiophylic cytoplasmic bodies. Secondary demyelinization. Gliosis. Presence of vacuolated histiocytes in viscera, with possible preeminence of Henle's renal loop localization.

Diagnostic Procedures. *Body tissues and fluids.* Activity of hexosaminidase A and B deficiency. *Blood.* Hexosaminidase assay of serum (lymphocytes vacuolization scarce). *Bone marrow.* Rarely, foamy histiocytes. *Biopsy.* Not necessary.

Therapy. No specific therapy. Enzyme replacement therapy hazardous.

Prognosis. Death by 3 years of age from respiratory infections.

BIBLIOGRAPHY. Sandhoff K, Harzer K: Total hexosaminidase deficiency in Tay–Sachs disease (variant O). In Hero HG, Van Hoff F (eds): Lysosomes and Storage Diseases, p 345. New York, Academic 1973
O'Brien JS: The gangliosidoses. In Stanbury JB, Wyngaarden JB, Fredrickson DS et al: The Metabolic Basis of Inherited Disease, 5th ed, p 945. New York, McGraw-Hill, 1983

SANDIFER'S

Synonym. Hiatus hernia–torticollis.

Symptoms. Prevalent in males; onset in infancy. Epigastric pain; vomiting. In infancy; asthenia.

Signs. Pallor. Head rotation with neck stretching, which is enhanced during eating or reading. Strabismus. Malnutrition.

Etiology. Unknown. All manifestations seem correlated to the presence of the hiatus hernia.

Diagnostic Procedures. *Blood.* Iron deficiency anemia. *X-ray of stomach.* Hiatus hernia.

Therapy. Surgical correction of hernia.

Prognosis. Anemia, torticollis, strabismus, malnutrition disappear with treatment of hernia.

BIBLIOGRAPHY. Sutcliffe J: Torsion spasms and abnormal posture in children with hiatus hernia: Sandifer's syndrome. Prog Pediatr Radiol 2:190–197, 1969
O'Donnell JJ, Howard RO: Torticollis associated with hiatus hernia (Sandifer's syndrome). Am J Ophthalmol 71:1134–1137, 1971

SANFILIPPO'S

Synonyms. Heparinuria; mucopolysaccharidosis III, MPS III; polydystrophic oligophrenia; Sanfilippo–Good types A, B, C, D.

Symptoms. Both sexes affected. Severe mental retardation, becoming fully evident at school age. Minor somatic changes in facial features and joints. Good body strength.

Signs. Dwarfism and stiff joints (less severe than in other mucopolysaccharidoses); moderate hepatospleno-

megaly. Absence of corneal opacification. Generalized hirsutism.

Etiology. Autosomal recessive inheritance. Four forms of enzymatic defect in degradation of heparan sulfate have been distinguished.
Type A: heparan N-sulfatase
Type B: α-N-acetylglucosaminidase
Type C: specific N-acetyl transferase
Type D: α-N-acetylglucosamine-6-sulfatase
These different enzymopathies share the same clinical picture.

Pathology. Presence of metachromatic inclusion positive for mucopolysaccharide and acid phosphatase in cells of all types. Heparan sulfate found in brain.

Diagnostic Procedures. *Urine.* Excretion of heparan sulfate only; in some cases, absence of this finding. *Enzymes assay.* In fibroblasts and other cells or serum. *X-rays.* Mild dysostosis multiplex.

Therapy. None. Institutionalization required in most cases.

Prognosis. Death in second decade in majority of cases.

BIBLIOGRAPHY. Sanfilippo SJ, Podosin R, Langer LO Jr et al: Mental retardation associated with acid mucopolysacchariduria (heparin sulfate type). J Pediatr 63:837–838, 1963
McKusick VA, Neufeld EF: The mucopolysaccharide storage diseases. In: Stanbury JB, Wyngaarden JB, Fredrickson DS et al: The Metabolic Basis of Inherited Disease. 5th ed, p 751. New York, McGraw-Hill, 1983

SANTAVUORI'S

Synonyms. Finnish type ceroid lipofuscinosis. Neuronal ceroid–lipofuscinosis, infantilis, Finnish; INCL. See Batten's.

Symptoms and Signs. Both sexes affected; onset at 8 to 18 months. Mental development arrest; hypotonia; ataxia; seizures; early visual impairment. Fundus oculi hypopigmentation, atrophy; discoloration of macula.

Etiology. Autosomal recessive inheritance (see Batten's).

Pathology. See Batten's. Severe brain atrophy.

Prognosis. Within 3 years, total incapacitation.

BIBLIOGRAPHY. Santavuori P, Haltia M, Rapola J et al: Infantile type of so-called neuronal ceroid-lipofuscinosis. A clinical study of 15 patients. J Neurol Sci 18:257–267, 1973

Santavuori P: Infantile type of neuronal ceroid–lipofuscinosis (INCL). In Eriksson AW, Forsing HR, Nevaulinna HR et al: Population Structure and Genetic Disorders, pp 626–632. New York, Academic Press, 1980

SARCOID MYOPATHY

See Besnier–Boeck–Schaumann.

Symptoms. Onset most often in middle and old age. Muscular pain; weakness of legs or, less frequently, of arms.

Signs. Muscle wasting or firm enlargement of muscles with nodules; contractures.

Etiology. Unknown; see Besnier–Boeck–Schaumann.

Pathology. On muscle biopsy, appearance of changes described in sarcoidosis: interstitial infiltration with giant cells; epithelioid cells and lymphocytes; palisadelike and reticular collagen fiber network, replacing tissue; muscle fiber degeneration with floccular necrosis.

Diagnostic Procedures. *Blood.* Intermittent monocytosis and eosinophilia; leukopenia and increased calcium; hyperproteinemia; increased alkaline phosphatases. Kveim test (60% positive).

Therapy. Corticosteroids.

Prognosis. Good response to treatment.

BIBLIOGRAPHY. Licharew A: Demonstration. Dermatol Centralbl 11:253–254, 1908
Talbot PS: Sarcoid myopathy. Br Med J 4:465–466, 1967
Adams RD, Victor M: Principles of Neurology. 3rd ed, p 1033. New York, McGraw-Hill, 1985

SATURDAY NIGHT PALSIES

Synonym. Alcoholic neuropathy.

Symptoms. Occur in heavy drinkers. Discovered when awaking after alcohol intoxication and having fallen asleep or "passed out" in various positions with arm abducted, resting over edge of a chair or with head over arm. Most frequently, paralysis of muscle innervated by radial nerve (extension of elbow, wrist, fingers); also peripheral nerve of lower extremities affected; especially peroneal nerve.

Etiology. Compression neuritis. Frequently, pre-existing alcoholic neuritis.

Therapy. Abstention from alcohol. Thiamine; vitamin B_{12}; pyridoxine; diet rich in carbohydrates and protein. Physical therapy.

BIBLIOGRAPHY. Mayer RF: Recent studies in man and animal of peripheral nerve and muscle dysfunction associated with chronic alcoholism. Ann NY Acad Sci 215:370–372, 1973
Adams RD, Victor M: Principles of Neurology, 3rd ed, p 984. New York, McGraw-Hill, 1985

SAUNDERS–SUTTON

Synonym. Delirium tremens.

Symptoms. Occur in chronic alcoholic patients; onset associated with alcohol withdrawal or intercurrent trauma or infection. Irritability; food aversion; insomnia; constant confabulation; hallucinations of terrifying objects or animals; generalized tremor and seizures (occasional).

Signs. Perspiration; coated tongue; tachycardia.

Etiology. In chronic alcoholic condition, dehydration associated with any condition is usually the precipitating cause.

Pathology. Brain edema. Swelling and granular degeneration of ganglion cells. Perivascular hemorrhages.

Diagnostic Procedures. *Body fluid.* Presence of alcohol. *Blood.* Leukocytosis. *Urine.* Albuminuria.

Therapy. Prevent self-injury (physical restraints). Drugs for sedation: diazepam; Chlordiazepoxide. High-caloric intake; thiamine and multivitamins containing folic acid. Maintenance of fluid and electrolyte balance (hypomagnesemia and hypoglycemia are frequent).

Prognosis. Easy collapse and death from exhaustion; heart failure; pneumonia. After period of rest, treatment, and long period of sleep, gradual improvement.

BIBLIOGRAPHY. Sutton T: Tracts on Delirium Tremens, on Peritonitis and on Some Other Internal Inflammatory Affections on the Gout. London, Underwood, 1813
Seixas FA, Williams K, Eggleston S (eds): Medical consequences of alcoholism. Ann NY Acad Sci 252:1–399, 1975
Fox PT: Neurologic emergencies in internal medicine. In Orland MJ, Saltman RJ (eds): Manual of Medical Therapeutics, 25th ed, p 394. Boston, Little, Brown Co, 1986

SAVAGE

Synonyms. Pure gonadal dysgenesis (XX); pure ovary failure (XX); including Swyer's syndrome.

Symptom. Amenorrhea.

Signs. Good breast development; normal axillary and pubic hair.

Etiology. Ovarian tissue resistant to follicle-stimulating hormone (FSH). Stimulation (see Seabright–Bantam) or failure of normal ovarian development due to environmental factors or imperceptible deletion of part of long arm of one X chromosome. (46 XX sex chromatin positive or 46 XY sex chromatin negative, Swyer's syndrome.)

Pathology. Ovary resembling "fat" streak; presence of numerous primordial follicles; none showing development beyond antrum stage; stromal cell hyperplastic in some areas and luteinized in others.

Diagnostic Procedures. *Urine.* Total gonadotropins elevated both FSH and luteinizing hormone (LH), estrogen 5 to 10 ug/24 h, pregnanediol 1 mg/24 h. *Chromosome study.* Normal pattern. (46 XX sex chromatin positive or 46 XY sex chromatin negative, Swyer's syndrome).

Therapy. Steroid withdrawal induces bleeding. Trial with clomiphene citrate 100 mg daily, which does not change FSH or LH values. Human chorionic gonadotropin, 10,000 IU after previous treatment has been completed, however, results in an increased evidence of estrogenic activity. In case of Swyer's syndrome streak gonads have to be removed because of potential neoplastic development.

BIBLIOGRAPHY. Solivar AR: The syndrome of pure gonadal dysgenesis. Am J Med 38:615–619, 1965
Jones GS, Ruehsen–DeMoraes M: Communication to AMA, San Francisco Meeting, 1968
Ross GT: Diagnosis and treatment of primary amenorrhea, secondary amenorrhea and dysfunctional uterine bleeding. In De Groot LJ, Cahill FG Jr, Odell WD et al (eds): Endocrinology, p 1428. New York, Grune & Stratton, 1979

SCAPULOCOSTAL

Synonym. Postural drag paradox.

Symptoms. Occur in middle-aged individuals; insidious onset. Deep shoulder pain with different patterns of irradiation: neck, occiput, chest, or combinations.

Signs. Trigger point at or under medial angle of scapula at posterior thoracic wall.

Etiology and Pathology. Traumatic or nontraumatic factors (arthritis; bursitis; myositis).

Diagnostic Procedures. *X-ray of shoulder, cervical spine. Electrocardiogram.* To rule out cardiopathy.

Therapy. Physical therapy: massage, exercises. Injection of procaine or hydrocortisone at the trigger point. Firm digital pressure of trigger point often followed by mitigation of acute symptoms.

Prognosis. Spontaneous remission 70%.

BIBLIOGRAPHY. Michele AA: Scapulocostal syndrome: Its mechanism and diagnosis. NY J Med 55:2485–2493, 1955
Hurst JW, King SB, Frisinger GE et al: Atherosclerotic coronary heart disease. In Hurst JW (ed): The Heart, 6th ed, p 918. New York, McGraw-Hill, 1985

SCASSELLATI–SFORZOLINNI

Synonym. Vertical bilateral retraction.
See Duane's and A and V syndromes.

Symptoms and Signs. Unilateral or bilateral partial or almost complete loss of upward gaze; some limitation of downward gaze; retraction upon depression and pseudoptosis. A exotropia or V exotropia can be found. Associated congenital anomalies include unilateral partial ptosis, facial asymmetry, and anomalies of the optic (II) nerve heads.

Etiology. Unknown; congenital inherited condition.

Pathology. Unknown.

Diagnostic Procedures. *Electromyography.*

BIBLIOGRAPHY. Scassellati–Sforzolini G: Una sindrome molto rara: Difetto congenito monolaterale della elevazione con retrazione del globo. Riv Otoneurooft 33:431–439, 1958
Khodadoutst AA, von Noorden GK: Bilateral vertical retraction syndrome: A family study. Arch Ophthalmol 78:606–612, 1967

SCHAEFER–SOERENSEN

Synonyms. Bagolini's, plagiocephaly–superior oblique deficiency; ocular torticollis.

Symptoms and Signs. Prevalent in females. Combination of plagiocephaly (unilateral coronal sutures stenosis) strabismus (particularly dissociation of conjugate movements), torticollis.

Etiology. Various intrauterine influences on developing cranial sutures. Possible pathogenetic mechanism proposed for strabismus: palsy or motor imbalance due to shortened length of superior oblique muscle and variation of its mechanical effect on rotation of eyeball because of enlarged angle.

Diagnostic Procedures. *X-ray of skull; Bielchowsky head-tilt test.*

BIBLIOGRAPHY. Archer DB, Gordon DS, Maguire CJF et al: Ophthalmic aspects of craniosynostosis. Trans Ophthalmol Soc UK 94:172–196, 1974

Schaefer WD, Sorensen N: Motilitatsstorungen bei Koronarnaht-Synostosen. Meeting of Berufsverband Augenarzte. Wiesbaden, Germany, 1979

Bagolini B, Campos EC: Plagiocephaly causing superior oblique deficiency and ocular torticollis: A new clinical entity. Arch Ophthalmol 100:1093–1096, 1982

SCHÄFER'S

Synonym. Keratosis palmoplantaris variant.

Symptoms and Signs. Disseminated follicular keratosis of skin; leukokeratosis of oral mucosa; small foci of alopecia; dysonychia; congenital cataracts; microcephaly; mental retardation; hypogenitalism and dwarfism.

Etiology. Unknown; autosomal dominant inheritance.

BIBLIOGRAPHY. Schäfer E: Zur Lehre von den congenitalen Dyskeratosen. Arch Dermatol Syph 148:425–432, 1925

Silver HK: Rothmund-Thompson syndrome: An oculocutaneous disorder. Am J Dis Child 111:182–190, 1966

SCHAMBERG'S

Synonyms. Purpuric pigmentary dermatosis; pigmentary progressive dermatosis.

Symptoms and Signs. Occur more often in males; onset at any age. Irregular plaques, orange brownish with "cayenne pepper" spots, within and at edges of lesions, erupting most frequently on the legs, occasionally other parts of the body. Occasionally, slight pruritus. No systemic symptoms.

Etiology. Unknown; stasis may play a role. Autosomal dominant trait.

Pathology. Slight changes in epidermis; hemosiderin deposits.

Therapy. None.

Prognosis. Chronic recurrences; years' duration.

BIBLIOGRAPHY. Schamberg JF: A peculiar progressive pigmentary disease of the skin. Br J Dermatol 13:1–5, 1901

Rook A, Wilkinson DS, Ebling FJG et al: Textbook of Dermatology, 4th ed, pp 1116–1117. Oxford, Blackwell Scientific Publications, 1986

SCHANZ'S II

Synonym. Spinal insufficiency.

Symptoms. Moving from erect to a prone position causes a feeling of fatigue and lumbar pain.

Etiology. Lumbar spine pathology of different etiologies: rheumatic, inflammatory, neoplastic, muscle weakness congenital, or acquired.

BIBLIOGRAPHY. Schanz A: Eine typische Erkrankung der Wirbelsaeule (insufficientia vertebrale). Klin Wochenschr 44:989–992, 1907

SCHATZKI'S

Synonyms. Esophagogastric ring; lower esophageal ring.

Symptoms. Both sexes affected; onset after 50 years of age. Asymptomatic or episodes of substernal pain, dysphagia on swallowing solid food, and pyrosis.

Signs. Diameter of lower esophageal ring normal or reduced.

Etiology. Unknown. Motor disorder of lower esophageal ring or anatomic malformation, associated frequently with diaphragmatic hernia.

Pathology. Mucosal strands of connective muscular tissue 4 or 5 cm above diaphragm at the gastroesophageal area.

Diagnostic Procedures. *Fluoroscopy.* With barium swallow. *Esophageal manometry.*

Therapy. Repair of an associated hernia insufficient to control dysphagia. Bougienage or excision of the ring followed by treatment of esophagitis.

BIBLIOGRAPHY. Schatzki R, Gary JE: Dysphagia due to a diaphragmlike localized narrowing in lower esophagus ("lower esophageal ring"). Am J Roentgenol 70:911–922, 1953

Blanchon P, Dupuis J, Babok D: L'anneau de Schatzki. Atlas Radiol Clin 47:1–4, 1968

Pope CE II: Physiology. In Sleisenger MH, Fordtran JS: Gastrointestinal Disease, p 504. Philadelphia, WB Saunders, 1978

Wilkins EW Jr: The lower esophageal ring: How unique? (editorial). Ann Thorac Surg 37:101–102, 1984

SCHEIE'S

Synonyms. Alpha-L-iduronidase deficiency; Hurler's late; mucopolysaccharidosis V (formerly); MPSV (formerly); MPS IS; mucopolysaccharidosis. IS: Spat–Hurler.

Symptoms. Both sexes affected. Visual impairment; normal intelligence; cases with psychosis reported.

Signs. Stiff joints; claw hand; carpal tunnel syndrome; facies characteristically "broad mouthed." Clouding of cornea, uniform in early stage, later becoming densest peripherally. Retinitis pigmentosa. Stature normal or low-normal range; excessive body hair; aortic valve regurgitation.

Etiology. Autosomal recessive inheritance; Alpha-L-iduronidase deficiency.

Pathology. Same alterations as in Hurler's (see). Cortical neuron normal (different from Hurler's).

Diagnostic Procedures. Same as in Hurler's. Differential diagnosis on clinical basis only.

Therapy. Surgery for correction of carpal tunnel, glaucoma; aortic valve prothesis.

Prognosis. Good *quoad vitam;* normal intelligence and stature.

BIBLIOGRAPHY. Scheie HG, Hambrick GW Jr, Barness LA: A newly recognized forme fruste of Hurler's disease (gargoylism). Am J Ophthalmol 53:753–769, 1962
McKusick VA, Neufeld EF: The mucopolysaccharide storage diseases. In: Stanbury JB, Wyngaarden JB, Fredrickson DS et al: The Metabolic Basis of Inherited Disease. 5th ed, p 751. New York, McGraw-Hill, 1983
Madhava Rao B, Gupta SK, Abraham KA et al: Rare multivalvular involvement in a family of Scheie syndrome. Indian J Pediatr 55:317–322, 1988

SCHEUERMANN'S

Synonyms. Kyphosis dorsalis juvenilis; epiphyseal osteochondritis; vertebral osteochondrosis; osteochondrosis spinal.

Symptoms. Both sexes affected; early manifestation from 12 years of age. Backache.

Signs. Kyphosis originating in late childhood in which there is a rigid arcuate backward curvature. In many cases, however, absence of kyphosis and presence of flat thoracic area (with loss of lordosis in lumbar tract) and the localized scoliosis (thoracic or lumbar) are the only clinical signs.

Etiology. Unknown. Growth disorder: transition from cartilage to bone irregular and patchy. Families with autosomal dominant inheritance.

Pathology. Osteochondrosis of affected vertebral bodies.

Diagnostic Procedures. *X-ray of spine.* Increased anteroposterior diameter of vertebral bodies (wedge shaped); disk spaces reduced; kyphosis; Schmorl's nodes.

Therapy. Orthopedic and medical.

Prognosis. Early manifestations mild, but have serious effects on future capacity for sports and physical activities.

BIBLIOGRAPHY. Scheuermann H: Kyphosis dorsalis juvenilis. Über geshkrift Laeger 82:385–393, 1920
Stoddard A, Osborn JF: Scheuermann's disease or spinal osteochondrosis. J Bone Joint Surg 61:56–58, 1979
Bjersand AJ: Juvenile kyphosis in identical twins. Am J Roentgenol 134:598–599, 1980

SCHILDER–FOIX

Synonym. Centrilobar symmetric sclerosis. See Schilder's.

Eponym used to indicate variable neurologic manifestations related to sclerosis of white matter; nonprogressive lesions possibly due to anoxic encephalopathy.

BIBLIOGRAPHY. Schilder P: Zur Frage der Enzephalitis periaxialis diffusa (sogenannte diffuse Sklerose). Z Ges Neurol 15:359, 1913
Foix C, Marie J: La sclérose cérébrale centrolobulaire à tendence symetrique; ses rapports avec l'encephalite periaxiale diffuse. Encephale 22:81, 1927

SCHILDER'S

Synonyms. Myelinoclastic diffuse sclerosis, Heubner-Schilder, Sudanophilic leukodystrophy, encephalitis periaxialis diffusa (incorrect term).

Symptoms. Very rare. Affects both children and adults. Onset in prepuberty. Headache, cerebral blindness, central deafness, mental changes, dullness, apathy progressing to stupor. Bilateral or monolateral spastic weakness progressing to paralysis. Multiple neurologic symptoms (motor and sensorial according to areas involved).

Signs. Eyes: nystagmus; extranuclear palsy (occasional); hemianopia; papilledema (15–20%). Seldom, bronzing of skin or jaundice.

Etiology. Unknown; possibly variety of etiologic agents; toxic; infectious; abiotrophic neural defects. The disease is considered a variant of multiple sclerosis.

Pathology. Affects centrum semiovale: perivascular lymphocytes infiltration, vacuolated cells containing oil red O-positive material, osmophilic bodies.

Diagnostic Procedures. *Spinal tap.* Increased pressure, slight pleocytosis, high immunoglobin G content with oligoclonal bands. *Blood and urine.* Rule out adrenoleukodystrophy by analysis of long-chain fatty acids of plasma cholesterol esters. *CT scan.* Hypodense lesions with contrast enhancement.

Therapy. Corticosteroids.

Prognosis. Early manifestations mild, but have serious effects on future capacity for sports and physical activities.

BIBLIOGRAPHY. Schilder P: Zu Kenntnis der sogenannten diffusen Sklerose. Ueber Encephalitis periaxialis diffusa. Z Ges Neurol Psychiatr, (Berlin) Leipzig 10:1–60, 1912

Poser CM, Goutieres F, Carpentier M, Aicardi J: Schilder's myelinoclastic diffuse sclerosis. Pediatrics 77:107–112, 1986

SCHIRMER'S

Eponym used to indicate the association of early glaucoma (hydrophthalmia) and Sturge–Weber (see).

BIBLIOGRAPHY. Schirmer R: Ein Fall von Teleangiektasie. Arch Ophthalmol 7:119–121, 1860

SCHMID'S (B.J.)

Synonym. Spondylometaphyseal dysplasia (type C-III).

Symptoms and Signs. Both sexes affected; onset of clinical manifestations in early infancy. Abnormalities of sternum and ribs; altered gait. Later becoming more evident; short neck; prognathism; kyphoscoliosis; genu valgum.

Etiology. Unknown; karyotypic alterations of chromosomes questionable.

Pathology. Normal structure of bone; proliferation of connective and osteoid tissue with increased osteoblasts in medullary space.

Diagnostic Procedures. *Blood and urine.* Normal. *X-rays of spine, hips, and metaphyses of long bones.* Dorsolumbar kyphosis; acetabular "blowout"; delayed ossification metaphyseal defects of ossification; major vertical streaks in upper extremities.

Therapy. Corrective osteotomy. Trials with vitamin D.

Prognosis. Poor *quoad functionem.*

BIBLIOGRAPHY. Schmid BJ, Becak W, Becak ML et al: Metaphyseal dysostosis. Review of literature, study of a case with cytogenetic analysis. J Pediatr 63:106–112, 1963

Kozlowski K, Beemer FA, Bens G et al: Spondylometaphyseal dysplasia: Report of 7 cases and essay of classification. In Papadatos CI, Bartsocas CS (eds): Skeletal Dysplasias, pp 89–101. New York, Alan R. Liss, 1982

SCHMID'S (F.)

Synonyms. Chondrodystrophia adolescentium sui tarda; dysostosis enchondralis metaphysaria; Schmid's metaphyseal chondrodysplasia; metaphyseal dysostosis (type BI).

Symptoms and Signs. Both sexes affected; onset in early childhood. Clinically, no characteristic features: retarded growth with bow legs and short diaphyses. Leg pains in childhood. No face and skull involvement. Trunk may be normal or short. Metaphysis less affected than in Jansen's. Hands and feet not involved or minimally involved. Women affected have children with little difficulty.

Etiology. Unknown; autosomal dominant inheritance.

Pathology. Cartilage hypoplasia. *Biopsy.* Rough-surfaced endoplasmic reticulum cisternae of chondrocytes from accumulation of a protein (?). Osteoid: normal.

Diagnostic Procedures. *X-ray.* Changes described. Vertebrae may show same features as in Jansen's syndrome. Epiphyses close prematurely.

Therapy. High doses of vitamin D have been tried, with doubtful success. Orthopedic measures limited to major deformities.

Prognosis. In adult, metaphyseal lesions appear healed. Sequelae of coxa vara and shortening of bones. Osteoarthritic manifestations minimal or absent.

BIBLIOGRAPHY. Schmid F: Beitrag zur Dysostosis enchondralis metaphysaria. Monatsschr Kinderheilkd 97:393–397, 1949

Bailey JA: Disproportionate Short Stature: Diagnosis and Management, p 283. Philadelphia, WB Saunders, 1973

SCHMIDT'S (A.)

Synonym. Vagoaccessory.

Symptoms. Stiff neck; inability to turn the head; speech disorders, swallowing disorders.

Signs. Unilateral and ipsilateral paralysis of soft palate, vocal cords, sternocleidomastoid and trapezius muscles (partial or total).

Etiology and Pathology. Most frequently, vascular lesion affecting cranial nerves within medulla oblongata or at their point of exit from skull. Neoplasm and infections less frequently.

Diagnostic Procedures. *X-ray. Angiography. Spinal tap. Serology.* For syphilis.

Therapy. According to etiology.

Prognosis. Guarded; according to etiology.

BIBLIOGRAPHY. Schmidt A: Doppelseitige Accessorms-lähmung bei Syringomyelie. Dtsch Med Wochenschr 18:606–608, 1892

Adams RD, Victor M: Principles of Neurology, 3rd ed, pp 1016–1017. New York, McGraw-Hill, 1985

SCHMIDT'S (M.B.)

Synonyms. Thyroid-adrenocortical-pancreatic insufficiency; polyglandular autoimmune II.

Symptoms and Signs. Onset at all ages; predominantly in females. Manifestations of hypothyroidism may precede or follow the manifestations of Addison's syndrome. Diabetic conditions very often coexist; their onset may precede or follow hypothyroidism and hypoadrenalism. Possible anemia (pernicious).

Etiology. Unknown; an autoimmune mechanism postulated with common antibodies against thyroid and adrenal and possibly pancreas. Possibly autosomal dominant inheritance.

Pathology. *Adrenal.* Changes consistent with slowly progressive necrosis of cortex, with lymphocytic plasma cells and macrophage infiltration. *Thyroid.* Extensive lymphocytic infiltration; fewer plasma cells than in adrenals; mild fibrosis; no frank necrosis of epithelium. Generalized changes: those observed in Addison's and hypothyroidism.

Diagnostic Procedures. See Addison's and hypothyroidism, diabetes. *Antibody studies.* Against thyroid and adrenals.

Therapy. That of Addison's disease and hypothyroidism.

Prognosis. Variable according to degree of involvement and treatment.

BIBLIOGRAPHY. Schmidt MB: Eine biglanduläre Erkrankung (Nebennieren und Schilddrüsse) bei Morbus Addisonii. Verh Dtsch Pathol Ges 21:212–221, 1926

Carpenter CC, Solomon N, Silverberg SG et al: Schmidt's syndrome (thyroid and adrenal insufficiency): A review of the literature and a report of fifteen new cases including ten instances of co-existent diabetes mellitus. Medicine 43:153–180, 1964

Butler MG, Hodes ME, Conneally PM et al: Linkage analysis in a large kindred with autosomal dominant transmission of polyglandular autoimmune disease type II (Schmidt's syndrome). Am J Med Genet 18:61–65, 1984

SCHMITT–WIESER

Synonym. Clay shoveler's.

Symptoms and Signs. Occur following overstraining in shoveling or performing similar activity. Lesion of spinous process of first thoracic vertebra and displacement of apophysis.

Prognosis. Spontaneous repair within a few months.

BIBLIOGRAPHY. Schmitt HG, Wieser P: Die Schipperkrankenkheit bei Jugendlichen. Arch Klin Chir (Berl) 268:333–340, 1961

SCHNEIDER'S

Synonym. Central cervical spinal cord injury.

Symptoms. Weakness prevalent in upper extremities up to paresis, and paralysis; sensory loss of variable degree; radicular pain.

Signs. Paralysis of fingers and arms, and paresis of upper part of legs; feet spared.

Etiology. Arthritis; trauma causing compression of cervical cord between osteophytes and ligamentum flavum; associated with vascular insufficiency because of compression of vertebral artery on hyperextension of cervical spine.

Diagnostic Procedures. *X-ray of spine.* Fractures or osteoarthritic changes. *Cerebrospinal fluid.* Abnormal proteins.

Therapy. Orthopedic measures for spine stabilization. Corticosteroids to reduce edema.

Prognosis. Variable.

BIBLIOGRAPHY. Schneider HC: Trauma to the spine and spinal cord. In Kahn EA, Basset RC, Scheined RC et al: Correlative Neurosurgery. Springfield, CC Thomas, 1955

Adams RD, Victor M: Principles of Neurology. 3rd ed, pp 667–671. New York, McGraw-Hill, 1985

SCHNYDER'S

Synonyms. Crystalline corneal dystrophy; corneal-crystalline dystrophy; crystalline dystrophy.

Symptoms. Both sexes affected; onset early in life. Moderate decrease of visual acuity.

Signs. Arcus juvenilis appearing early in life as oval or annular cloudy opacification of central part of cornea with clear periphery. Progressive extension of opacity toward periphery, but never reaching the limbus.

Etiology. Unknown; autosomal dominant inheritance.

Pathology. Normal epithelium; small needlelike crystal (unknown composition) in opaque area located in anterior portion of stroma posterior to Bowman's membrane.

Diagnostic Procedures. *Slit-lamp examination. Biopsy of cornea.*

BIBLIOGRAPHY. Van Went JM, Wibaut F: Hereditary anomaly in cornea. Ned Tijdschr Geneeskd 1:2996–2997, 1924

Schnyder W: Mitteilung ueber einen neuen Typus von familiaerer Hornhauterkrankung. Schweiz Med Wochenschr 10:559, 1929

Schnyder W: Scheibenförmige Kristalleinlagerungen in der Hornhautmitte las Erbleiden (degeneratio cristallinea corneal hereditaria). Klin Monatsbl Augenheilkd 103:494–502, 1939

Bron AJ, Williams HP, Carruthers ME: Hereditary crystalline stromal dystrophy of Schnyder. I. Clinical features of family with hyperlypoproteinemia. Br J Ophthalmol 56:383–399, 1972

SCHÖNENBERG'S

Synonym. Cardiopathy–dwarfism.

Symptoms and Signs. Present from birth. Symptoms and signs of various types of congenital cardiac defects. Blepharophimosis; epicanthal folds; pseudoptosis of eyelids. Proportionate dwarfism.

Etiology. Unknown; consanguinity of parents and familial occurrence reported.

BIBLIOGRAPHY. Schönenberg H: Über ein neues Kombinationsbild multipler Abartungen. (Minderwuchs, Vitium cordis, beiderseitige congenitale Ptose). Ann Pediatr 182:229–240, 1954

François J: L'heredité en ophthalmologie. Bull Soc Belge Ophthal 94:300, 1958

Buffoni L, Chiossi FM: Presentatione di un caso di' una rara sindrome malformativa-la sindrome di Schönenberg. Minerva Pediatr 23:1549–1554, 1971

SCHÖNLEIN–HENOCH

Synonyms. Anaphylactoid purpura; hemorrhagic capillary toxicosis; Henoch–Schönlein; peliosis rheumatica.

Symptoms and Signs. Most often seen in childhood and young adulthood, seldom later in life; prevalent in males. Onset variable: headache; anorexia; fever (moderate and irregular); abdominal pains or pain on the joint (cutaneous manifestation) may each be first complaint. Abdominal pain (35–60% of patients) have colicky character and come frequently at night; occasionally, vomiting, diarrhea, and melena or severe constipation accompany the colic. No abdominal rigidity. Rheumatoid pains affecting all joints, most frequently legs; periarticular effusion frequent. Cutaneous mainfestations may present different types of lesions: purpura; urticaria wheals; angioneurotic edema; diffuse erythema; necrotic ulcer, most frequently affecting legs, seldom oral mucosa. Nervous system and special sense organs may be affected: paresis; convulsions; optic atrophy; ophthalmitis. Hematuria, progressive renal failure.

Etiology. Allergic reaction to bacteria, food, drugs. A case is reported in which the syndrome, in a 9-year-old girl, was associated with selective IgA deficiency.

Pathology. In skin, perivascular inflammation, necrotizing arteriolitis (in severe cases), plasma and cells pericapillary extravasation. Gastrointestinal mucosae may show some of the lesions described. Kidney biopsy: light microscopy mesangial proliferative glomerulonephritis. Electron microscopy: electron dense deposits. Immunofluorescence: granular deposits of IgA IgG and IgM. Skin biopsy immunofluorescence: deposits of IgA C3 and C5.

Diagnostic Procedures. *Blood.* Normal platelet number or only very moderate decrease. *X-rays of gastrointestinal tract.* May initially reveal "spiking" of bowel outline and later "thumb-print" or rigid effacement of mucosa; these changes disappear with recovery.

Therapy. Symptomatic; bed rest; removal of cause if identified. Corticosteroids and adrenocorticotrophic hormone (ACTH) less effective than expected.

Prognosis. Generally good. Edema of glottis the main life-threatening feature. Intestinal intussusception not a rare complication.

BIBLIOGRAPHY. Schönlein JL: Allgemeine und specielle Pathologie und Therapie. Nach dessen Vorlesungen niedergeschrieben und hrsg. von einigen seiner Zuhörer. 3 aufl, Herisou, Lit-Comp 1837

Henoch E: Über eine eigenthumliche Form von Purpura. Klin Wochenschr 11:641–643, 1874

Martini A, Ravelli A, Notarangelo RD et al: Henoch–Schönlein syndrome and selective IgA deficiency. Arch Dis Child 60:160, 1985

SCHÖNLEIN'S

This eponym is sometimes used in place of the term Schönlein–Henoch syndrome (see) when the rheumatoid pain and cutaneous lesions are predominant.

SCHOEPF'S

Synonym. Hypotrichosis-oligodontia-palmoplantar keratosis. Could be assimilated in the Papillon–Lefevre syndrome (see).

Symptoms and Signs. Hypospadias; oligodontia. At puberty, palmoplantar hyperkeratosis. At 25 years of age, hair loss; at 50 years of age, rosacea; at 60, cysts of both eyelids.

Etiology. Possibly, autosomal recessive inheritance.

BIBLIOGRAPHY. Schoepf E, Schulz HJ, Passage E: Syndrome of cystic eyelids, palmoplantar keratosis; hypospadias and hypotrichosis as a possible autosomal recessive trait. Birth Defects 7:219–221, 1971

SCHROEDER'S (C.H.)

Synonyms. Congenital hereditary luxation; humeroradial synostosis. See Larsen's and Pfeiffer's.

Symptoms and Signs. Bizarre pinnas; bilateral radial luxation; radiohumeral ankylosis; bilateral hip, shoulder, and knee dislocation: camptodactyly.

Etiology. Unknown. Autosomal recessive inheritance.

BIBLIOGRAPHY. Schroeder CH: Familiaere kongenitale Luxationem. Z Orthop Chir 57:500–596, 1932
Kentel J, Kindermann J, Mockel H: Eine wahrscheinlich autosomal recessiv vererbte Skeletmissbildung mit Humeroradialsynostose. Humangenetik 9:43–53, 1970

SCHROEDER'S I (H.A.)

Synonym. Acute "lowsalt". See Hyponatremic syndromes.

Symptoms and Signs. Occur in patients treated intensively for congestive heart failure. Rapid physical and mental deterioration. Further unresponsiveness to diuretics; thirst; anorexia; nausea; prostration; calf cramps; tendency to syncope in the erect position; narrowing of pulse pressure (rise of diastolic level); oliguria and finally renal failure.

Etiology. Acute dehydration as hyponatremia or as hypochloremia developing after iatrogenic profuse diuresis. Not to be confused with chronic dilution hyponatremia (see).

Diagnostic Procedures. *Blood.* Predominant decrease of chloride or depression of sodium as well as chloride; azotemia increased.

Therapy. In the acute form with dehydration, oral administration of water and salt. Parenteral administration only in emergency or with inability to take fluid by mouth.

Prognosis. Guarded.

BIBLIOGRAPHY. Schroeder HA: Renal failure associated with low extracellular sodium chloride: The low salt syndrome. JAMA 141:117–124, 1949
Vogl A: The low-salt syndromes in congestive heart failure. Am J Cardiol 3:192–198, 1959
Schrier RW: Treatment of hyponatremia. Editorial retrospective. N Engl J Med 312:1121–1123, 1985

SCHROEDER'S II (H.A.)

Synonyms. Endocrine hypertensive. Including maternal obesity syndrome.

Symptoms. Prevalent in females; seldom in males; relatively sudden onset of obesity, occurring at menarche, menopause, after multiple pregnancies or gynecologic operations. Headache; menstrual irregularity; aversion to salty food and high fluid intake. Tendency to easy bruising and ecchymosis.

Signs. Obesity of central type with pale striae on thighs; mild hirsutism. Blood hypertension occurring after the weight gain; fundus oculi changes. In no instance should the above signs and symptoms be confused with those of Cushing's syndrome.

Etiology. The pathogenesis and etiology of this syndrome are obscure. A hereditary factor may predispose to this variety of hypertension. See Cohen's syndrome.

Pathology. Left ventricular hypertrophy; slight to moderate arteriolar nephrosclerosis; polyps or myomas of uterus; adenomas or focal hyperplasia of the adrenal cortex.

Diagnostic Procedures. *Blood.* Mild polycythemia; abnormal carbohydrate metabolism; several abnormally low concentrations of sodium and chlorides. Differential diagnosis: (1) The maternal obesity syndrome, characterized by the rapid gain in weight observed in women during pregnancy or after childbirth. (2) Large baby diabetic syndrome. (3) Cushing's syndrome.

Therapy. The hypertension responds favorably to severe restriction of dietary salt, and lesions in the ocular fundi may regress.

Prognosis. Good.

BIBLIOGRAPHY. Schroeder HA, Davies DF, Clark HE: A syndrome of hypertension, obesity. Menstrual irregularities and evidence of adrenal cortical hyperfunction. J Lab Clin Med 34:1746, 1949

Schroeder HA, Davies DF: Studies on "essential" hypertension. V. An endocrine hypertensive syndrome. Ann Intern Med 40:516–539, 1954

SCHROETTER'S

Synonyms. Diaphragmatic chorea; laryngeal chorea.

Symptoms. Nonpainful tics that cause utterance of a peculiar cry.

BIBLIOGRAPHY. von Schroetter L: Uber "Chorea laryngis." Allg Wien Med Ztg 24:67–68, 1879

SCHULTZ'S (W.)

Synonyms. Acute agranulocytosis; agranulocytic angina; primary granulocytopenia; pernicious leukopenia; malignant neutropenia; pernicious granulocytopenia.

Symptoms. More frequent in adults and in females (3 : 1); onset in middle age. Acute onset. Prostration; chills; fever. Ulceration of mucous membranes, principally of mouth and throat.

Etiology. Hematopoietic disorders: aleukemic leukemia; chemical agents as hematopoietic depressants; ionizing radiation; idiopathic.

Pathology. Gangrenous ulceration of mucosae.

Diagnostic Procedures. *Blood.* Extreme leukopenia (1000); almost complete absence of neutrophil leukocytes. The few present show toxic granulation and nuclear and cytoplasmatic changes. Usually no anemia and thrombocytopenia. *Bone marrow.* May be hypoplastic, normal, or hyperplastic. When hypoplastic, only immature myeloid elements present.

Therapy. Find, if possible, the offending agent and avoid exposure of the patients to it; smears and cultures to identify the organism causing infection, and then administration of the most suitable antibiotics, general care of the patient, with particular emphasis on oral hygiene; neutrophil transfusion. Adrenocorticosteroids and ACTH are not indicated.

Prognosis. Continuously improving with the constant development of potent antibiotics, and with the progress in general intensive care.

BIBLIOGRAPHY. Brown PK, Ophuls WA: A fatal case of acute primary infectious pharyngitis. Am Med 3:649–651, 1902
Tuerk W: Septische Erkrankungen bei verkuemmerung des Granulocytensystems. Wien Klin Wochenschr 20:157, 1904

Schultz W: Über eigenartige Halserkrankungen. Dtsch Med Wochenschr 48:1495–1496, 1922
Wintrobe MM (ed): Clinical Hematology, 8th ed, p 1304, Philadelphia, Lea & Febiger, 1981

SCHUTZ–HAYMAKER

Synonym. Olivopontocerebellar atrophy IV.

Symptoms and Signs. Both sexes. Adult onset. High variability of symptomatology: spinocerebellar ataxia to spastic paraplegia, involvement of cranial nerves (IX, X, XII).

Etiology. Autosomal dominant inheritance. Deficiency of glutamic dehydrogenase in some patients.

Pathology. High variability of data. Changes in inferior olivary nucleus and cerebellum with different degree of pontine involvement, loss of anterior motor cells of spinal cord in the spinocerebellar tracts and posterior funiculus.

BIBLIOGRAPHY. Schutz JW: Hereditary ataxia: Clinical study through six generations. Arch Neurol Psychiatr 63:535–568, 1950
Schutz JW, Haymaker W: Hereditary ataxia: Pathologic study of 5 cases of common ancestry. J Neuropath Clin Neurol 1:183–213, 1951
Plaitakis A, Nicklas WJ, Dresnick RJ: Glutamate dehydrogenase deficiency in the patients with spinocerebellar syndrome. Ann Neurol 7:297–303, 1980

SCHWARTZ–BARTTER

Synonyms. ADH; inappropriate antidiuretic hormone; Bartter–Schwartz; cerebral hyponatremia; cerebral salt-wasting.

Symptoms. Headache; confusion; disorientation; hostility and other mental aberrations without motor or sensory defects.

Signs. Normal reflexes; no dehydration; no edema; no signs of renal, hepatic, or cardiac disease.

Etiology. Syndrome associated with carcinoma of lung or following head trauma, brain tumor, cerebral vascular disease, encephalitis, tuberculosis, meningitis. This syndrome is the result of electrolyte imbalance, namely hyponatremia due to inappropriate secretion by neoplastic tissues of antidiuretic hormone (ADH) or other chemical substances which have ADH-like effect on renal collecting tubule.

Diagnostic Procedures. *Blood.* Hyponatremia, moderate or severe. Normal blood urea nitrogen (BUN). *Urine.* Hypertonic; increased sodium and chloride excretion.

Poor response of hyponatremia to hypertonic saline infusion. *X-ray. CT scan.* Demonstration of malignancy, infection, trauma. *Spinal tap. Electroencephalography.* Different types of abnormality.

Therapy. Restriction of fluid intake. In severe hyponatremia: furosemide diuresis plus electrolyte replacement; demeclocycline to correct antidiuresis.

Prognosis. Depends on association with malignant or benign etiology. Water restriction sufficient in inducing remission of symptoms. Recurrence with increase of fluid intake.

BIBLIOGRAPHY. Leaf A, Bartter FC, Santos RF et al: Evidence in man that urinary electrolyte loss induced by pitressin is function of water retention. J Clin Invest 32:868–878, 1953

Schwartz WB, Bennett W, Curelop S et al: A syndrome of renal sodium loss and hyponatremia probably resulting from inappropriate secretion of antidiuretic hormone. Am J Med 23:259–542, 1957

Lipscomb HS, Retiene WK, Matsen F et al: The syndrome of inappropriate secretion of antidiuretic hormone. Cancer Res 28:378–383, 1968

Ayus JC, Olivero JJ, Frommer JP: Rapid correction of severe hyponatremia with intravenous hypertonic saline solution. Am J Med 72:43–48, 1982

SCHWARTZ–JAMPEL–ABERFELD

Synonyms. Blepharophimosis–myopathy–dwarfism; osteochondromuscular dystrophy. SIA; myotonic myopathy–dwarfism–chondrodystrophy–oculofacial abnormalities; Aberfeld's; chondrodystrophic myotonic.

Symptoms. Onset within first month of life. Myotonia; contractures.

Signs. Short stature; hypoplastic facial bones; micrognathia. Eyes upward slanting; blepharophimosis; exotropia; myopia; microcornea; low-set auricles; hypertrichosis; arachnodactyly; hypoplastic larynx; abnormal epiglottis; short neck; pectus carinatum; kyphoscoliosis; abnormal acetabulum.

Etiology. Postulated membrane defect with inability to maintain proper gradient of Na and K. Autosomal recessive inheritance, possibility of heterozygote manifestation in some cases (?).

Pathology. Muscle biopsy shows diffuse atrophy with replacement of muscle fibers by adipose and connective tissue. Skeletal lesions similar to that of Morquio's (see).

Diagnostic Procedures. *Blood.* Serum enzymes. *Urine.* Amino acids. *Chromosome studies.* Pattern normal. *X-ray.* Osteoporosis. *Electromyography.*

Therapy. Procainamide helps muscular function.

BIBLIOGRAPHY. Pinto LM, de Spuza JS: Un caso de "doenca muscular" de difficil classificacao. Rev Port Pediatr Pueric 6:1, 1961

Schwartz O, Jampel RS: Congenital blepharophimosis associated with a unique generalized myopathy. Arch Ophthalmol 68:52–57, 1962

Aberfeld DS, Hinterbuchner LP, Schneider M: Myotonia, dwarfism, diffuse bone disease and unusual ocular and facial abnormalities (a new syndrome). Brain 88:313–322, 1965

Edwards WC, Root AW: Chondrodystrophia myotonica (Schwartz–Jampel syndrome): Report of a new case and follow-up of patients initially reported in 1969. Am J Med Genet 13:51–56, 1982

SCHWARZ–LELEK

Synonym. Frontal bossing-Genu varum. See Pyle's.

Symptoms and Signs. Two cases reported. Onset from birth. Frontal bossing; genu varum.

Etiology. Unknown. Sporadic.

Diagnostic Procedures. *X-ray of head.* Hyperostosis and sclerosis, more marked in frontal, occipital, maxillary, and mandibular areas. Paranasal sinuses obliterated. *Of clavicles, ribs, humeri, hands.* Hyperostosis (see Pyle's). *Of femur.* Bowing; radiolucency of metaphyseal area. *Blood.* Alkaline phosphatases elevated.

BIBLIOGRAPHY. Schwarz E: Craniometaphyseal dysplasia. Am J Roentgenol 94:461–466, 1960

Lelek I: Camurati–Engelmannische Erkrangungen. Fortschr Roentgenst 94:702–712, 1961

Gorlin RJ, Spranger JW, Koszalka MF: Genetic craniotubular bone dysplasia and hyperostose: A critical analysis. Birth Defects V (4):79–95, 1969

SCHWENINGER–BUZZI

Synonym. Anetoderma. See Jadassohn–Pellizzari syndrome.

Symptoms and Signs. Occur almost exclusively in females; onset usually in third to fifth decades. Symmetric crops of round or oval skin-colored papules, eventually becoming bluish, soft protuberances (1–2 cm in diameter). Back of shoulders and extensor surfaces of arms preferred locations.

Etiology. Unknown. See Jadassohn–Pellizzari.

Pathology. No inflammatory changes; fragmentation and disappearance of elastic fibers; collagen fibers narrowed.

Diagnostic Procedures. *Biopsy.*

Therapy. None.

Prognosis. Involution of lesion with formation of depressed scars.

BIBLIOGRAPHY. Schweninger E, Buzzi S: Multiple benigne geschwulstartige Bildundgen der Haut. Internat. Atlas seltener Hautkrankht. Heft V. Hamburg und Leipzig, Voss, 1891

Korting GW, Cabré J, Holzmann H: Zur Kenntnis der Kollagenveränderungen bei der Anetodermie von Typus Schweninger-Buzzi. Arch Klin Exp Dermatol 218:274–297, 1964

SCIMITAR

Synonyms. Hypogenetic lung; turkish sabre; scimitar vein.

Symptoms. Prevalent in females; 25% of cases are diagnosed in early infancy; they suffer from recurrent respiratory infections. Can be completely asymptomatic or paucisymptomatic. Fatigue; dyspnea; history of pneumonia; cough, chest pain; wheezing. Seldom, growth failure.

Signs. Right displacement of heart; infrequently, decreased size and motion of right chest; rales; loud cardiac murmurs over the sternum or on either side of it; occasionally physical examination normal.

Etiology. Congenital malformation (see Pathology). Some familial cases reported.

Pathology. Anomalous venous drainage through abnormal pulmonary vein of the right lung that joins the inferior vena cava. Right pulmonary artery frequently hypoplastic. Lung lobation or bronchial distribution frequently abnormal. Diverticula and cysts of bronchi. Small right lung; heart displacement to the right. Diaphragmatic defects and congenital heart defect may also be associated.

Diagnostic Procedures. *X-ray.* Displacement of heart to the right; abnormal venous trunk "scimitar sign" lying parallel to right heart border distally, broader and curving medially and anteriorly. *Fluoroscopy.* Absence of pulsation. Opacity of right lung. *Tomography. Bronchoscopy. Bronchography. Angiocardiography. Catheterization. Pulmonary function tests. Echocardiography.*

Therapy. Physiologically corrective operations: connection of anomalous vein to right atrium, plus creation of atrial septal defect, or direct transplantation to left atrium, or, if a branch leading to left atrium is present, simple ligation between the branch and the inferior vena cava. Pneumonectomy or lobectomy in some cases with severe pulmonary disease.

Prognosis. Condition is frequently without serious symptoms and with good prognosis. Association with pulmonary and cardiac malformations makes the prognosis guarded.

BIBLIOGRAPHY. Cooper G: Case of malformation of the thoracic viscera: Consisting of imperfect development of right lung and transposition of the heart. Lond Med Gaz 18:600–602, 1836

Chassinat R: Observations d'anomalies anatomiques remarquables de l'appareil circulatoire, avec hépatocéle congéniale, symptom particulier. Arch Gen, Med 11:80–91. 1836

Mardini MK, Sakati NA, Lewall DB, Christie R, Nyhan L: Scimitar syndrome. Clin Pediatr, 21:350–354, 1982

Oakley D, Naik D, Verel D, Rajan S: Scimitar vein syndrome: Report of nine new cases. Am Heart J 107:596–598, 1984

Hurst JW: The Heart, 6th ed, pp 604–605. New York, McGraw-Hill, 1986

SCLERODERMA

Synonyms. Acrosclerosis; hidebound skin; progressive systemic sclerosis; PSS.

Symptoms and Signs. Predominantly in females (4 : 1); onset usually in fourth decade in females; later in males. Raynaud's phenomenon (see) usually presenting symptoms; less frequently, hand swelling or joint swelling; ulceration of fingers or legs. Weight loss; dyspnea; gastroesophageal reflux; diarrhea or constipation; abdominal pain. *Skin changes.* Face and hands usually involved; lesion spreading to forearm, chest. Typical faces: smooth, shiny forehead; skin thickened; lines cancelled; nose becoming small; radial furrows around the mouth; mouth opening reduced; hardening of skin prevents depression of eyelids. Telangiectases. *Hand.* Swelling initially; bulbous appearance, then atrophy; painful ulcer; gangrene; retraction holding the hand in semiflexion. *Feet.* Similar but usually less severe changes. Calcinosis localized or generalized. *Gastrointestinal.* Esophageal reflux; dysphagia; colicky abdominal pains; malabsorption (see). *Respiratory.* Dyspnea; dry or productive cough; cyanosis; recurrent pneumothorax. *Cardiac.* Arrhythmia; cardiomegaly. *Muscular.* Weakness. *Joint.* Arthralgia; rheumatoid arthritis typical changes.

Etiology. Unknown; collagen disorder, autoimmunity. Rare instances of familial occurrence reported.

Pathology. Sclerotic changes in skin, lungs, heart, submucosa, muscularis of gastrointestinal tract, and skeletal muscles. Vascular intimal proliferation; occlusive thrombosis; hyalinization; perivascular infiltration with lymphocytes.

Diagnostic Procedures. *Biopsy of skin and muscle. Blood.* Increased sedimentation rate (50%), and globulin level (50%), false-positive serology (5%); cold agglutinins (25%); rheumatoid factor test positive (30%); antinuclear antibodies (78%). *Urine.* Proteinuria (moderate); may develop Epstein's syndrome (see). *X-ray of bones and joints.* Lesion equal to rheumatoid arthritis. *Of gastrointestinal tract.* Esophageal dilatation; abnormal peristalsis strictures; stomach seldom affected; duodenum may have ulceration; jejunum and ileum seldom involved; colon frequently involved; widemouthed diverticula; appearance of ulcerative colitis. *Of chest.* Diffuse reticular infiltration, usually in lower two-thirds; cystic changes; pleurisy; pneumonia (frequent). *Electrocardiography.* Usually abnormal. *Kidney and pulmonary function tests.*

Therapy. Corticosteriods (as symptomatic); low molecular weight dextran intravenously. (No consistent benefit.) Prostaglandin E_1, prostacyclin, reserpine, guanethidine ketanserin, nifedipine, prazosin to decrease Raynaud's phenomenon intensity and frequency. D penicillamine: to decrease skin thickness and rate of further visceral involvement. Azathioprine: useful in 30% of cases: Symptomatic treatment: minoxidil, captopril, hemodialysis. Hyperbaric O_2.

Prognosis. Variable, from death in 1 to 2 years, to many years after onset. Men have poorer prognosis than women. Carcinoma of lungs develops frequently in cases with pulmonary involvement; malignant hypertension, carcinoma, or perforation of gastrointestinal tract.

BIBLIOGRAPHY. Curzio C: Discussioni anatomo-pratiche di un raro e stravagante morbo cutaneo in una giovane donna felicemente curato in questo gŕande ospedale degli Incurabili. Napoli G di Simone, 1753
Gintrac E: Note sur la sclerodermie. Rev Med Chir (Paris) 2:263–267, 1847
Rook A, Wilkinson DS, Ebling FJG et al: Textbook of Dermatology, 4th ed, pp 1347–1366 Oxford, Blackwell Scientific Publications, 1986

SCLEROSTEOSIS

Synonyms. Cortical hyperostosis–syndactyly; see van Buchem's.

Symptoms and Signs. See van Buchem's plus greater severity of manifestations and presence of syndactyly.

Etiology. Autosomal recessive inheritance. It may represent a modification of the same genes responsible for the van Buchem's syndrome.

BIBLIOGRAPHY. Hirsh IS: Generalized osteitis fibrosa. Radiology 13:44–84, 1929

Beighton P, Barnard A, Hamersma H et al: The syndromic status of sclerosteosis and van Buchem disease. Clin Genet 25:175–181, 1984

SCLEROTYLOSIS

Synonyms. Scleroatrophic–keratotic dermatosis limbs. Mennecier's.

Symptoms and Signs. Present at birth. Both sexes. Atrophic fibrinosis of skin of limbs, nail hypoplasia, tylosis palms and soles. Frequently associated cancer of skin and bowel.

Etiology. Autosomal dominant trait.

BIBLIOGRAPHY. Mennecier M: Individualisation d'une nouvelle entite: la genodermatose sclero-atrophiante et keratodermique des extremities frequemment degenerative. Etude clinique et genetique (possibilite de linkage avec le system MNSS). M.D. Thesis Univ de Lille, 1967
Fisher S: La genodermatose scleroatrophiante et keratodermique des extremites (au sujet de trois nouveaux cas familieux). Ann Dermatol Venerol 105:1079–1082, 1978

SCOTOMA, HOMONYMOUS HEMIANOPTIC

Symptoms. Sudden onset of difficulty in reading and fixing objects located close to the central field of the affected eye. No reduced visual acuity; homonymous scotoma that excludes the macula; maintenance of peripheral field in such a manner that unaffected part of the field lies between periphery and scotoma.

Signs. Normal ophthalmologic findings.

Etiology. Unknown; possibly, a vascular accident, embolus, toxic condition, infection(?).

Pathology. Unknown; lesion of lateral geniculate bodies or above that point.

Therapy. None.

Prognosis. Good for visual acuity; the patient accommodates to the presence of blindspot in his field of vision.

BIBLIOGRAPHY. Wilbrand H: Ueber die makulärhemianopische Lesestörung und die von Monakowsche Projektion der Makula auf die Sehsphäre. Klin Monatsbl Augenheilkd 45:1–39, 1907
Allen T, Carman H: Homonymous hemianoptic paracentral scotoma. Arch Ophthalmol 20:846–849, 1938
Adams RD, Victor M: Principles of Neurology, 3rd ed, pp 191–192. New York, McGraw-Hill, 1985

SCOTT'S

Synonym. Craniodigital–mental retardation.

Symptoms and Signs. Present from birth. Brachycephaly; pointed nose; micrognathia; long lashes; prominent and arched eyebrows; hirsutism; cutaneous syndactyly of second, third, and fourth fingers. Mental and somatic retardation.

Etiology. X-linked recessive inheritance (?).

BIBLIOGRAPHY. Scott CR, Bryant JL, Graham CB: A new craniodigital syndrome with mental retardation. J Pediatr 78:658–663, 1971

SCRIVER'S

Synonyms. HBD; hypophosphatemic nonrachitic bone disease.

Symptoms and Signs. Both sexes. From birth osteomalacia with minimal rickets, growth retardation less severe than simple vitamin D-resistant rickets.

Etiology. Autosomal dominant disorder of phosphate transport in the kidney.

Diagnostic Procedures. *Blood.* Hypophosphatemia. Normal phosphaturic response to PHT (different from simple vitamin D-resistant rickets) (see). Reduced TMP/GFR.

Therapy. Treatment by 1,25-(OH)2 D3 at low doses alone without phosphate.

Prognosis. Good. Rapid correction of rickets by therapy.

BIBLIOGRAPHY. Scriver CR, MacDonald W, Reade T et al: Hypophosphatemic nonrachitic bone disease: An entity distinct from X-linked hypophosphatemia in renal defect, bone involvement and inheritance. Am J Med Genet 1:101–117, 1977
Scriver CR, Reade T, Halal F et al: Autosomal hypophosphatemic bone disease responds to 1,25-(OH)2 D3. Arch Dis Child 56:203–207, 1981

SEA-BLUE HISTIOCYTE

Synonyms. Sawitsky's; Silverstein; bleu histiocyte.

Symptoms. Both sexes affected; onset from infancy to old age, usually in subjects under 40. Asymptomatic or increased bleeding tendency.

Signs. Marked splenomegaly; mild purpura; occasionally, liver cirrhosis.

Etiology. Autosomal recessive inheritance (?). Secondary form associated with several conditions: idiopathic thrombocytopenic purpura; thalassemia; chronic myeloid leukemia; Vaquez's disease; Besnier–Boeck–Schaumann; Wolman's; various lipidoses.

Pathology. In bone marrow, diffuse infiltration by a distinct histiocyte ($20-60\mu$ in diameter), single eccentric nucleolus; cytoplasm granules staining (Giemsa or Wright's) sea-blue. Granules are stainable with Sudan black B; para-aminosalicylic acid (PAS) and acid-fast staining. Spleen similarly infiltrated. Other organs occasionally infiltrated.

Diagnostic Procedures. *Bone marrow.* See Pathology. *X-rays.* Lung infiltration in 30% of patients.

Therapy. None. Corticosteriods tried.

Prognosis. Usually benign and uncomplicated course; possibility, however, of extension of infiltration and involvement of various organs and fatality. The younger the age of onset, the poorer the prognosis.

BIBLIOGRAPHY. Silverstein MN, Young DG, ReMine WH et al: Splenomegaly with rare morphologically distinct histiocyte. A syndrome. Arch Intern Med 114:251–257, 1964
Lee RE: Histiocytic disease of bone marrow. Hematol Oncol Clin North Am 2:657–667, 1988

SEABRIGHT–BANTAM SYNDROMES

Used restrictively as eponym for pseudohypothyroidism, or, more correctly to indicate a failure of a tissue to respond to a specific endocrine stimulation. In the Seabright–Bantam rooster, the tail feathers have the appearance of female plumage, and represent a failure of an organ to respond to a specific stimulation, in this case androgenic hormone. This lack of response of a target organ to hormonic stimulation is observed in many syndromes. (i.e.)

1. In pseudohypothyroidism, the failure of response of the biochemical changes to the administration of parathyroid hormone.
2. ADH-resistant diabetes insipidus (see)
3. De Morsier's II
4. Dwarfism (Seabright–Bantam type) (see)
5. Savage (see)
6. Goldberg–Maxwell (see)
7. Pseudohypohermaphroditism, male, incomplete hereditary (see)
8. Thyroidal insensitivity to TSH
9. Rosewater's (see)

10. Nowakowski–Lenz (see)
11. Reifenstein's (see)
12. Laron's

BIBLIOGRAPHY. Albright F, Burnett, CH, Smith PH et al: Pseudo-hypoparathyroidism—Example of "Seabright-Bantam syndrome"; report of 3 cases. Endocrinology 30:922–932, 1942

SEAT BELTS

Not a clinical entity. Under this heading are included all injuries resulting directly from wearing the belt during a car accident. Many types of abdominal injury have been reported, as well as injury in the chest caused by shoulder belts.

BIBLIOGRAPHY. LeMire JR, Earley DE, Hawley C: Intra-abdominal injuries caused by automobile seat belts. JAMA 201:735–737, 1957

Garrett JW, Braunstein PW: The seat belt syndrome. J Trauma 2:220–238, 1962

Doersch KB, Dozier WE: The seat belt syndrome, the seat belt sign, intestinal and mesenteric injuries. Am J Surg 116:831–833, 1968

SECKEL'S

Synonyms. Bird-headed dwarfism; nanocephaly; microcephalic primordial dwarfism. Virchow–Seckel.

Symptoms. Both sexes affected; present at birth. Low birth weight; failure to grow; mental retardation; sweet disposition. Recently a case has been described in which all the features of the syndrome were present, but not the dwarfism. This could be an incomplete form of the syndrome or a variant.

Signs. Dwarfism; small head; prominent beaked nose, strabismus; sparse hair; different congenital malformations: dislocation of hip; clubfoot; absent thumb; cloaca-like malformation of genitourinary tract and rectum.

Etiology. Unknown; autosomal recessive inheritance.

Pathology. See Signs. Small brain with primitive convolutional pattern; ectopic and small kidney; deformed liver.

Diagnostic Procedures. *Chromosome studies. Virus studies.* Cytomegalic. *X-ray. Biochemical studies.* Blood and urinary excretions.

Therapy. Symptomatic.

Prognosis. Good *quoad vitam;* patient may survive to advanced age, but with moderate to severe mental retardation.

BIBLIOGRAPHY. Mann TP, Russel A: Study of microcephalic midget of extreme type. Proc R Soc Med 52:1024–1029, 1959

Seckel HPG: Bird-headed Dwarfs: Studies in Developmental Anthropology Including Human Proportions. Springfield, CC Thomas, 1960

Majewski F, Goecke T: Studies of microcephalic primordial dwarfism I: Approach to a delineation of the Seckel Syndrome. Am J Med Genet 12:7–21, 1982

Thompson E, Dembry M: Seckel syndrome: An over-diagnosed syndrome. J Med Genet 22:192–201, 1985

Rico S, Skinner C, Salamea F, Cañizares JC, Casanova Bellido M: Sindrome de Seckel: a proposito de una observacio. Acta Pediatr Esp 44:214–217, 1986

SECRETAN'S

Symptoms and Signs. Posttraumatic, marked restriction of digital flexion (except the thumb), or edema of dorsal metacarpal region and base of fingers. If trauma on the foot, posttraumatic edema of the dorsum of foot.

Etiology. Overload and dilatation of lymphatics caused by constricting band, tourniquet on wrist, base of finger, above the knee.

Pathology. Edema of dorsum of hand or foot.

Therapy. Psychiatric advice, if no response to conservative measures, closed lymphangioplasty.

Prognosis. Treatment prevents permanent deformity and achieves excellent cosmetic and functional results. Possible conversion to other neurotic manifestation.

BIBLIOGRAPHY. Secretan H: Oedeme dur et hyperplasie traumatique du metacarpe dorsal. Rev Med Suisse Rom 21:409–416, 1901

Grobmyer AJ III, Bruner JM, Dragstedt LR II: Closed lymphangioplasty in Secretan's disease. Arch Surg 97:81–83, 1968

Rook A, Wilkinson DS, Ebling FJG et al: Textbook of Dermatology, 4th ed, pp 1199–1236. Oxford, Blackwell Scientific Publications, 1986

SEELIMUELLER'S

Synonym. Syphilitic neuralgia.
It is a sign rather than a syndrome: pain elicited by pressure on cranial areas associated with diffused neuralgic pains.

Etiology. Syphilis.

BIBLIOGRAPHY. Seelimueller OLG: Ueber syphilitische Neuralgien. Dtsch Med Wochenschr 9:624–625, 1883

SEEMANOVA'S

Synonyms. See Paine syndrome.

Symptoms and Signs. Similar to those of Paine's (see) except for: absence of abdominal reflexes; normality of level of amino acid in cerebrospinal fluid, absence of hypoplasia of cerebellum, pons, and inferior olive.

Etiology. X-linked inheritance. Debated if same condition as that described by Paine.

BIBLIOGRAPHY. Seemanova E, Lesny I, Hyanek J et al: X-chromosomal recessive microcephaly with epilepsy spastic tetraplegia and absent abdominal reflex. New variety of "Paine syndrome?" Humangenetik 20:113–117, 1973

Opitz JM, Sutherland GR: International workshop on the fragile X and X-linked mental retardation. Am J Med Genet 17:5–94, 1984

SEIDLMAYER'S

Synonyms. Postinfection purpura; purpura postinfectiva.

Symptoms and Signs. Occur especially in children after episodes of infections, which may have been mild or ignored. Appearance of a purpuric eruption characterized by coinlike elevations.

Etiology. Direct vascular damage or allergic mechanism.

BIBLIOGRAPHY. Seidlmayer H: Die fruehinfantile, postinfektiose Kokarden-Purpura. Z Kinderheilkd 61:217–255, 1939

SEITELBERGER'S

Synonym. Infantile neuroaxonal dystrophy. See Pelizaeus–Merzbacher.

Symptoms and Signs. Both sexes affected; normal at birth; normal development up to second year of life. Then difficulty in standing and walking; progressive deterioration of neurologic function; speech; incontinence during sleep; nystagmus; strabismus; blindness; seizures; tendon hyporeflexia or areflexia; or initially pathologic reflexes, flexion, and deformities.

Etiology. Unknown; still undetermined metabolic disorder. Familial tendency suspected (autosomal dominant inheritance), but not proved. Relationship with Hallenvorden–Spatz (adult) is postulated.

Pathology. Widespread lesions in central nervous system with the appearance of eosinophilic round or oval structures (Schollen or spheroids) mostly in the grey matter; swelling of axons and dendrites; degeneration of nerve cells; accumulation of fat granules in parts of basal ganglia; cerebellar atrophy with sclerosis; degeneration of optic pathway; degeneration of tracts of spinal cord.

Diagnostic Procedures. *Urine.* Creatine increased; creatinine decreased. Possible diabetes insipidus. *Blood.* Thyroid-stimulating hormone decreased. *CT brain scan.* Acoustical and visual evocated potentials. *Electroencephalographic brain mapping. Electromyography. Electrocardiography. Spinal tap. Biopsy of muscle.*

Prognosis. Poor; death from complications within months or a few years of onset.

BIBLIOGRAPHY. Seitelberger F: Eine unbekannte Form von infantiler lipoidspeicher Krankheit des Geshirns. In Proc 1st Inter Cong Neuropath (Rome Sept 8–13, 1952) Vol. 3, p 323. Turin, Rosenberg-Sellier, 1952

Nagashima K, Suzuki I, Ichikawa E et al: Infantile neuroaxonal dystrophy: Perinatal onset with symptoms of diencephalic syndrome. Neurology 35:735–738, 1985

SELIGMAN'S

Synonyms. Alpha-heavy chain; alpha HCD.

Symptoms and Signs. Both sexes affected; onset in childhood and adolescence. Severe malnutrition; diarrhea; failure to thrive or weight loss; asthenia; respiratory complications; bleeding. Digital clubbing. Affects individuals in poor hygienic environment.

Etiology. Unknown. Probably a true intestinal sarcoma with Sternberglike cells. Infective disease hypothesized.

Pathology. Infiltration of lamina propria of intestine, visceral lymph nodes, respiratory tract by plasma cells, lymphocytes, reticular cells; occasionally, bone marrow also infiltrated. Peripheral lymph nodes are not involved.

Diagnostic Procedures. *Blood.* Hypocalcemia; rise in alkaline phosphatase. Electrophoresis: increased alpha-2 beta fractions. Immunoelectrophoresis reaction with anti-alpha sera. Anemia. *Bone marrow.* Usually normal. *Biopsy of small bowel.* Typical infiltration. *Lymphography, barium enema.* Hypertrophic folds and pseudopolyposis of duodenal and jejunal mucosa.

Therapy. Radiotherapy. Corticosteroids; cyclophosphamide; antibiotics. For patients with immunoblastic infiltration of the intestine combination chemotherapy: nitrogen mustard, vincristine, prednisone and procarbazide (MOPP), or cyclophosphamide, adriamicin, vincristine and prednisone (CHOP).

Prognosis. Poor.

BIBLIOGRAPHY. Seligman M, Davon F, Hurer D: Alpha chain disease: A new immunoglobulin abnormality. Science 162:1396–1397, 1968

Broudet JC: Les maladies des chaines lourdes. In Encycl Med Chir, Paris Sang, 13013 F10, 1980

SELYE'S

Synonyms. Adaptation; GAS; general adaptation stress.

Eponym in use to indicate the sum of all reactions that follow a prolonged stress (independent from its nature). The typical pathologic findings are represented by adrenal cortical hyperplasia, thymic and lymphatic involution, gastrointestinal erosion or ulcers.

BIBLIOGRAPHY. Selye H: The Physiology and Pathology of Exposure to Stress; a Treatise Based on the Concepts of the General-Adaptation Syndrome and the Disease of Adaptation. Montreal, 1950

Selye H: The Stress of Life. New York, McGraw-Hill, 1956

SEMINAL VULVITIS

Symptoms and Signs. Vulvar edema, itching and erythema after intercourse, occasionally followed by generalized urticaria.

Etiology. In atopic subjects with allergy to human seminal plasma or other antigens transmitted that way. A case of interest, attacks after the partner had eaten walnuts.

BIBLIOGRAPHY. Mathias CG, Frick OL, Caldwell TM, et al: Immediate hypersensitivity to seminal fluid and atopic dermatitis. Arch Dermatol 116:209–212, 1980

SENEAR–USHER

Synonyms. Ormsby's; pemphigus erythematosus.

Symptoms and Signs. Bullae appearing in normal skin of trunk and limbs, which, after breaking, result in crusted lesions similar to seborrheic dermatitis. Lesion on the face; erythematous scaling and crusts; butterfly distribution on malar areas; transient mucosal involvement possible.

Etiology. Unknown; possibly autoimmune, viral infection, but not proved. In most cases it is suggested the combination of lupus erythematosus (LE) and pemphigus; in some cases observed combination with Erb–Goldflam.

Pathology. Acantholysis; dark-staining cells (acantholytic), but smaller than cells of pemphigus vulgaris (pyknotic acantholytic cells).

Diagnostic Procedures. *Biopsy of skin. LE test.*

Therapy. Corticosteroids. Immunosuppressive agents (azathioprine, cyclophosphamide, methotrexate). Gold sodium thiomalate.

Prognosis. Better than in pemphigus vulgaris. Localized lesions may continue for years before becoming generalized, bullous reactions recurrent at different times. Patient reported by Senear and Usher was alive and well at the age of 78.

BIBLIOGRAPHY. Senear F, Usher B: An unusual type of pemphigus; combining features of lupus erythematosus. Arch Dermatol Syph 13:761–781, 1926

Rook A, Wilkinson DS, Ebling FJG et al: Textbook of Dermatology, 4th ed, pp 1636–1637. Oxford, Blackwell Scientific Publications, 1986

SENILE DEMENTIA

Synonyms. Diffuse brain atrophy; senile psychosis; see Alzheimer; Pick's (A.); brain–bone–fat.

Symptoms. Occur in both sexes; onset over 60 years of age. Insidious onset. Deficit of immediate memory, and interest focused on the past. Power of concentration decreased; change in behavior and paranoid tendency; depression. Lack of interest and disregard for personal appearance; occasionally, hallucination, delirium. (see Brain syndrome, chronic). Focal symptoms may be present.

Signs. Decreased reflexes; sluggish pupil, loss of vibratory sensibility.

Etiology. Unknown; to be considered genetically different from arteriosclerotic dementia. Autosomal dominant gene with low penetrance. Today considered same as Alzheimer's presenile dementia (see); although in some families this diagnosis has been ruled out by cerebral biopsy.

Pathology. Shrinking of brain; thickening of meninges. Alteration of cortex; dilatation of ventricles. Shrinking of basal ganglia; alteration of nerve cells.

Diagnostic Procedures. *Electroencephalography. CT scan. Magnetic resonance. Arteriography. Leukocyte culture and chromosomal count.* Loss of chromosomal material. Increased loss of chromosomes, mainly X chromosomes in female patients. *Cerebrospinal fluid.* Normal.

Therapy. None.

Prognosis. Poor; death after chronic progression of mental and focal symptomatology.

BIBLIOGRAPHY. Larsson T, Sjögren T, Jacobson G: "Senile dementia," a clinical, sociomedical and genetic study. Acta Psychiatr Scand [Suppl 167] 39:1–259, 1963

Nielsen J: Chromosomes in senile dementia. Br J Psychiatr 114:303–309, 1968

Morris JC, Cole M, Bauker BQ et al: Hereditary dysphasic dementia and the Pick–Alzheimer spectrum. Ann Neurol 16:455–466, 1984

Mesulman MM: Dementia: its definition, differential diagnosis and subtypes. JAMA 253:2559–2561, 1985

SENIOR–LOKEN

Synonyms. Letterer–Senior–Loken; nephropathy–tapetal-retinal degeneration; oculorenalretinal degeneration; tubulointerstitial nephropathy–retinal degeneration.

Symptoms. Both sexes affected; onset in early childhood. Thirst; polyuria; mental retardation. Visual loss progressing to complete blindness.

Signs. In eyes, tapetoretinal degeneration. Arterial hypertension (late development).

Etiology. Unknown; familial condition, possibly induced by pleotropic gene with variable expression.

Pathology. *Kidneys.* Tubulointerstitial nephropathy. *Eyes.* Tapetoretinal degeneration similar to Leber's type (see).

Diagnostic Procedures. *Urine.* Minimal hematuria and albuminuria. *Blood.* Anemia, blood urea nitrogen (BUN), and creatinine increased.

Therapy. Symptomatic. Diet, dialysis.

Prognosis. Poor; death before adulthood.

BIBLIOGRAPHY. Senior B, Friedmann AI, Brando JL: Juvenile familial nephropathy with tapetoretinal degeneration. A new oculorenal dystrophy. Am J Ophthalmol 52:625–633, 1961

Schuman JS, Lieberman KV, Friedman AH et al: Senior-Loken syndrome (familial renal retinal dystrophy) and Coat's disease. Am J Ophthalmol 100:822–827, 1985

SENSENBRENNER'S

Symptoms and Signs. Both sexes affected. Dolichocephaly; frontal bossing; hypertelorism; antimongoloid slant; epicanthal fold; full cheeks; elevated lower lip. Short hair; teeth small and spaced; multiple frenula. Short thorax; short limbs; abnormal distal phalanges; fifth finger clinodactyly.

Etiology. Autosomal recessive inheritance (?).

Diagnostic Procedures. *X-ray of long bones.* Flattening epiphyses. *Of hands.* Bones short.

BIBLIOGRAPHY. Sensenbrenner JA, Dorst JP, Owens RP: New syndrome of skeletal, dental and hair anomalies. Birth Defects 11:372–379, 1975

Gorlin JK, Pindborg JJ, Cohen MM Jr: Syndromes of the Head and Neck, 2nd ed. New York, McGraw-Hill, 1976

SENSORY SEIZURES SYNDROMES

Synonym. Seizures sensory.
Several types of this form of epilepsy are known:
1. Auditory
2. Vertiginous
3. Visual
4. Olfactory (uncinate seizures)
5. Gustatory
6. Cutaneous

Symptoms. According to the form the patient experiences, hallucination of different senses, usually of unpleasant nature. Movement of mouth and lips occurs sometimes, followed by major seizure. Memory may be disturbed.

Etiology. Lesions of different cerebral centers or idiopathic. In uncinate seizures, lesions are usually found.

Diagnostic Procedures. *Electroencephalography. X-ray of skull. Angiography. CT scan. Magnetic resonance. Auditory, sensorial, visual evoked potential.*

Therapy. See Grand mal.

BIBLIOGRAPHY. Vick NA: Grinker's Neurology, 7th ed. Springfield, CC Thomas, 1976

Adams RD, Victor M: Principles of Neurology, 3rd ed, pp 239–240. New York, McGraw-Hill, 1985

SENTER'S

Synonyms. Keratosis–ichthyosis–deafness; ichthyosiform erythroderma–sensorineural deafness.

Symptoms and Signs. Those of Ichthyosiform erythroderma (see), plus sensorineural deafness; vascularized corneas; cryptorchidism, variable flexion contractures. In some cases in middle age: hepatomegaly, hepatic cirrhosis, glycogen storage.

Etiology. Unknown. Possibly autosomal recessive inheritance.

Prognosis. May not reach middle age.

BIBLIOGRAPHY. Desmond F, Bar J, Chevillard Y: Erythrodermic ichthyosiforme congenitale seche, surdi-mutite, hepatomegalie de transmission recessive autosomique. Bull Soc Fran Derm Syph 78:585, 1971

Senter TP, Jones KL, Sakati N et al: Atypical ichthyosiform erythroderma and congenital sensorineural deafness. A distinct syndrome. J Pediatr 92:68–72, 1978

SEPTO-OPTIC DYSPLASIA

Synonyms. De Morsier's II; dwarfism–septo-optic dysplasia. See also Lorain–Levi and Gilford–Burnier.

Symptoms. Visual impairment. Partial to complete amblyopia. Symptoms related to partial or complete panhypopituitarism. Usually, normal intelligence.

Signs. Growth deficiency and other signs related to pituitary deficiencies. Pendular nystagmus.

Etiology. Unknown; usually sporadic.

Pathology. Association of optic (II) nerve and pellucid septum hypoplasia.

Diagnostic Procedures. *Funduscopic evaluation.* Hypoplasia of optic disk. *Pituitary function test.* Hormone studies.

Therapy. Pituitary single hormone deficiency replacement.

Prognosis. Fair with therapy. In severe cases, poor.

BIBLIOGRAPHY. De Morsier G: Etudes sur les dysraphies crânioencéphaliques; agénésie du septum lucidum avec malformation du tractus optique. La dysplasie septo-optique. Schweiz Arch Neurol Psychiatr 77:267–292, 1956
Blethen SL, Weldon VV: Hypopituitarism and septo-optic dysplasia in first cousins. Am J Med Genet 21:123–129, 1985
Hanna CE, Mandel H, La Franchi SH: Puberty in the syndrome of septo-optic dysplasia. AJDC 143:186–189, 1989

SERUM SICKNESS

Synonym. Inoculation reaction.

Symptoms. Onset 7 to 15 hours (or up to 2 wk) after exposure (injection) to a foreign antigen (heterologous protein) for prophylaxis of infections (*e.g.,* rabies, diphtheria, *Clostridium,* snake venom) or administration of certain drugs (*e.g.,* penicillin; sulfa compounds). Fever; myalgia; arthralgia. Rare complication: laryngeal edema.

Signs. Arthritis; urticaria; lymphadenopathy; splenomegaly.

Etiology. Antigen excess causing the formation of soluble antigen–antibody complexes which, diffusing into tissues and activating the complement, cause the inflammatory response.

Diagnostic Procedures. *Blood.* Increased sedimentation rate; leukocytosis; occasionally, eosinophilia. Hemoagglutinating antibodies level rises and complement level decreases. *Urine.* Hematuria; proteinuria; *Synovial fluid.* Leukocytosis (20,000), mostly polynucleated.

Therapy. Epinephrine; antihistamines; salicylates; in severe form, corticosteroids.

Prognosis. Good; self-limited condition; no residua.

BIBLIOGRAPHY. Patterson R, Anderson J: Allergic reactions to drugs and biologic agents. JAMA 248:2637–2645, 1982
Antiallergic, antiviral, and immunologic agents. In AMA Drug Evaluations, 5th ed, chap 9. AMA, 1983

SETLEIS'

Synonyms. Forceps marks–unusual face; temporal forceps marks–unusual face; facial ectodermal dysplasia.

Symptoms and Signs. Present from birth. Bitemporal aplasia of skin (forceps marklike scarring); vertical groove below lip; polystichia of upper eyelids; lower eyelid astichia and absence of meibomian glands; widow's peak; wrinkling of skin around eyes; rubbery consistency of nose and chin; flattening of thenar and hypothenar areas.

Etiology. Possibly, autosomal recessive.

BIBLIOGRAPHY. Setleis H, Kramer B, Valcarcel M et al: Congenital ectodermal dysplasia of the face. Pediatrics 32:540–548, 1963
Rudolph RI, Schwartz W, Leyden JJ: Bitemporal aplasia cutis congenita. Arch Dermatol 110:615–618, 1974

SEVER'S

Synonyms. Calcaneous apophysitis; osteochondrosis os calcis.

Symptoms and Signs. Occur in children. Pain and tenderness over posterior part of heel.

Etiology. See Epiphyseal ischemic necrosis.

BIBLIOGRAPHY. Gordon BL: Current Medical Information and Terminology, 4th ed. Chicago, American Medical Association, 1971

SEXUAL IMPOTENCE-LOW BACK INJURY

Symptoms. Occur in male patients with back injuries. Development of impotence (complete or partial). This group of patients, when compared with potent counterpart, presents double amount of subjective physical complaints, requests for hospitalization, surgical procedures.

Etiology. Unknown; psychological factors partially involved. History reveals that patient was an only child or youngest child in a family of many siblings, came from unstable home, or suffered parental loss or separation.

BIBLIOGRAPHY. LaBan MM, Burk RD, Johnson EW: Sexual impotence in men having low-back syndrome. Arch Phys Med 47:715–723, 1966

SEZARY–BOUVRAIN

Synonyms. Erythrodermia with Sezary cells.

Symptoms and Signs. In adult sudden appearance of recurring eczematous, erythematous lesions similar to lesions observed in the Alibert–Bazin syndrome (see). Lesion may be dry and scaly, but frequently it is associated with edema localized or diffuse to the entire surrounding area. Occasionally: pigmentation (10–20%), palmoplantar keratoderma, alopecia, nail disorders, adenomegaly (66% of cases), hepatomegaly (rare), splenomegaly (exceptional).

Etiology. Unknown. The syndrome may be located between the Alibert–Bazin and the lymphoid leukemia (T-lymphocytes type).

Pathology. *Skin biopsy.* Band of infiltration by macrophages, lymphocytes, and typical Sezary cells (two types have been identified—the large and the small). The first 12 to 20 μ in diameter with basophilic cytoplasm, irregular, frequently multilobulated nucleus without nucleoli. The second 8 to 10 μ in diameter with less irregular nucleus.

Diagnostic Procedures. *Blood.* Moderate leukocytosis from 10% to 99% of lymphocytes are Sezary cells. *Bone marrow.* For long time respected by neoplastic cells. Moderate presence of Sezary cells (number not related to circulating cells).

Prognosis. Subacute or chronic evolution, with good general conditions. Between 2 to 10 years from onset, death from complications (infections, heart, kidney failure, conversion into malignant lymphoma). The small type variety has a more favorable outcome.

BIBLIOGRAPHY. Sezary A, Bouvrain Y: Erythrodermie avec presence de cellules monstrueuses dans le derme et le sang circulant. Bull Soc Fr Dermatol Syphylogr 45:254–260, 1938
Guilhon JJ, Meynadier J, Clot J: Le syndrome de Sezary. Conceptions actuelles. Nouv Presse Med 7:29–34, 1979
Flaudrin G, Daniel MJ: Sezary syndrome cytochemistry and ultrastructure. In Polliack A (ed): Human Leukemia, p 327–330. Boston, Grune & Stratton, 1984

SHAVER'S

Synonyms. Bauxite pneumoconiosis; Shaver–Ridell; nonnodular silicosis.

Symptoms. Onset gradual. Nonproductive cough; expectoration, dyspnea; anorexia; asthenia; retrosternal pain.

Signs. Cyanosis; pulmonary rales.

Etiology. Inhalation of aluminium oxide, silicone dioxide fumes produced by melting of bauxite.

Pathology. In lungs, nonnodular fibrosis; emphysematous bullous areas. Intraalveolar fibrosis; bronchiolectasis; typical particles (double refracting).

Diagnostic Procedures. *X-ray.* Reticulation of lungs; fine spotting. Lymph node enlargement. In advanced cases cystic shadows. *Pulmonary function tests.* Decrease in diffusing capacity.

Therapy. None.

Prognosis. Progression with rapid aggravation of symptoms.

BIBLIOGRAPHY. Shaver CG, Ridell AR: Lung changes associated with manufacture of alumina abrasives. J Indust Hyg 29:145–157, 1947
Fraser RG, Paré JAP: Diagnosis of Diseases of the Chest, p 1528. Philadelphia, WB Saunders, 1977

SHEEHAN'S

Synonyms. Postpartum; panhypopituitarism; postpartum hypopituitarism; Reye–Sheehan; Simmonds–Sheehan. See Simmonds and Pituitary apoplexy.

Symptoms. Onset postpartum. Acute initial shock; failure of lactation; asthenia; hypoglycemic crisis; amenorrhea or menstrual irregularity.

Signs. Pallor out of proportion to anemia; loss of pubic and axillary hair; dryness of skin; atrophy of vaginal mucosa; return phase of tendon reflexes slow.

Etiology. Spasm of infundibular arteries, which are drained by hypophyseal portal vessels. If spasm persists for several hours, most of tissue in the anterior lobe necrotizes; when blood starts to flow, stasis or thrombosis occurs in the stalk and adenohypophysis.

Pathology. Pituitary thrombosis, necrosis, and scar formation; secondary atrophy of thyroid, adrenal cortex, and ovaries.

Diagnostic Procedures. *Basal metabolic rate.* Low. *Blood.* High cholesterol; low protein-bound iodide. *Urine.*

Low excretion of corticosteroids, estrogen, and pituitary gonadotropins.

Therapy. Replacement therapy.

Prognosis. Remarkably improved by replacement therapy.

BIBLIOGRAPHY. Simmonds M: Ueber Hypophysis-schwund mit tödlichem Ausgang. Dtsch Med Wochenschr 40:322–323, 1914

Sheehan HL: Post-partum necrosis of the anterior pituitary. J Pathol Bacteriol 45:189–214, 1937

Grimes HG, Brooks MH: Pregnancy in Sheehan's syndrome. Report of a case and review. Obstet Gynecol Surv 35:481–488, 1980

Hickstein D, Chaundler WF, Marshall JC: The spectrum of pituitary adenoma hemorrhage. West J Med 144:433–436, 1986

Lakhdar AA, McLaren EH, Davda NS, McKay EJ, Rubin PC: Pituitary failure from Sheehan's syndrome in the puerperium. Two case reports. Br J Obstet Gynaecol 94:998–999, 1987

SHELL NAIL

Signs. Atrophy of nail bed; atrophic bony changes. Mirror image of clubbing, where there is proliferation of soft tissue and periostitis, with new bone formation and bulging of nail.

Etiology. Unknown. This type of lesion has been found associated with bronchiectasis.

BIBLIOGRAPHY. Cornelius CE III, Shelley WB: Shell nail syndrome associated with bronchiectasis. Arch Dermatol 96:694–695, 1967

SHEPHERD'S

Synonym. Astragaloid (talar) fracture.

Eponym used to indicate a fracture of the astragalus with separation of the external margin.

BIBLIOGRAPHY. Shepherd FJ: A hitherto undescribed fracture of the astragalus. J Anat Physiol (Lond) 17:79–81, 1882

SHIN SPLINT

Synonyms. Charley horse; quadriceps femoris contusion.

Symptoms. Occur in athletes (with absence of direct injuries). Pain and discomfort in the leg gradually increasing from repetitive running on a hard surface or forcible, excessive use of foot flexors. Usual sites of pain in lower half of postmedial border of tibia, tibial compartment, interosseous membranes. At first, pain is relieved by rest, then becomes continuous and incapacitating to the point of forcing discontinuation of sport.

Signs. Tenderness over area involved; moderate swelling. Anterior tibial pulse good.

Etiology and Pathology. Sterile mechanical inflammation of muscle–tendon determined by overexertion of leg muscles. Minimal tears of periosteum, interosseous membrane, muscle, or muscle–tendon junction. To be differentiated from fractures and ischemic disorders, fascial hernias.

Diagnostic Procedures. *X-ray. Electromyography.* Normal.

Therapy. Rest. Athletes try to prevent it by ingesting NaCl. Quinine sulfate (300 mg *tid*) or diphenhydramine hydrochloride (50 mg) may prevent it in subjects prone to cramps.

Prognosis. From 10 to 24 days' duration.

BIBLIOGRAPHY. Rachun A, Allman FL, Blazina ME et al: Standard Nonmenclature of Athletic Injuries. Chicago, American Medical Association, 1966

Slocum DB: The shin splint syndrome: Medical aspects and differential diagnosis. Am J Surg 114:875–881, 1967

Adams RD, Victor M: Principles of Neurology, 3rd ed, pp 1090–1091. New York, McGraw-Hill, 1985

SHONE'S

Synonyms. Parachute mitral valve. Heart malformation complex including the following:
1. Parachute mitral valve (chorda tendineae of both leaflets inserted into single left ventricular papillary muscle obstructing valve flow)
2. Supravalvular stenosing ring
3. Subvalvular aortic stenosis
4. Coarctation of aorta. In individual patients, each of the malformations mentioned may be missing from the complex.

Symptoms and Signs. Those of mitral valve stenosis (see) or regurgitation if chordae are elongated and not fused.

BIBLIOGRAPHY. Shone JD, Sellers RD, Anderson RC et al: The development complex of "parachute mitral valve" supraventricular ring of left atrium, subaortic stenosis and coarctation of aorta. Am J Cardiol 11:714–725, 1963

Perloff JK: The Clinical Recognition of Congenital Heart Disease, 2nd ed, p 156. Philadelphia, WB Saunders, 1978

SHORT BOWEL

Synonym. Small intestinal insufficiency.

Symptoms and Signs. Occur in patients in whom a long portion of the intestine has been removed. A spectrum of deficiency patterns. Overall result of malabsorption consisting of weight loss, muscle wasting weakness, lassitude, diarrhea, pallor.

Etiology. Lack of adequate absorbing surface causes selective deficiencies resulting from removal of specialized areas of the intestine. This syndrome appears and persists when more than half of small bowel is removed. Removal of two thirds usually is compatible with life, but severe deficiencies occur and survival is not certain. Permanence of 3 to 4 feet is the minimal length for reasonable health.

Diagnostic Procedures. *Blood.* Anemia; glucose tolerance test; low protein; low cholesterol; electrolytes studies. *Stool.* Steatorrhea and undigested product.

Therapy. Supportive: diet high in calories and supplying all essential elements; low in residue. Integrated with or substituted by parenteral administration. Anemia treated with vitamin B_{12}, folic acid, and iron according to type. Drugs to prolong transit time (codeine paregoric). Surgical: reversing of a segment of small intestine to slow transit; vagotomy.

Prognosis. When this syndrome is present after surgery, it has to be kept in mind that spontaneous recovery usually occurs because of improvement of absorption and eventual increase of transit time through remaining tract. As pointed out before, pathologic manifestations are directly related to extent of intestine removed, from minor transient symptoms to a severe progressive pathology and death.

BIBLIOGRAPHY. Colcock BP, Braasch JW: Surgery of Small Intestine in the Adult. Philadelphia, WB Saunders, 1968
Jeejeebhoy KN: Therapy of the short gut syndrome. Lancet 1:1427–1430, 1983
Lin CH, Rossi TM, Heitlinger LA et al: Nutritional assessment of children with short bowel syndrome receiving home parenteral nutrition. Am J Dis Child 141:1093–1098, 1987

SHORT'S

Synonyms. Laslett–Short; tachycardia–bradycardia.

Symptoms. Affects females in higher (but not significant) percentage; onset usually after sixth decade (average 68 yr). Syncope (55%); palpitations (12%); vertigo (6%); ingravescent angina (12%); other symptoms due to ingravescent congestive cardiac insufficiency (15%).

Signs. Not diagnostic. Out of crisis, heart frequency at 60 beats; asystole after tachycardia episodes; also, episodes of isolated bradycardia and tachycardia.

Etiology. Sick sinus node abnormally susceptible to suppressive influence of ectopic atrial activity. Coronaropathy; hypertension; cardiopathies (*e.g.*, rheumatic, congenital, idiopathic).

Diagnostic Procedures. *Electrocardiography.* Prolonged registration to document episodes (usually 6–12 hr adequate). Reported to be of diagnostic value, but discussed: massage of carotid sinus or injection of atropine during ECG to evidentiate sinus malfunction; atrial stimulation with evaluation of recovery time.

Therapy. Poorly responding to pharmacologic treatments: digitalis plus propanolol; quinidine plus propanolol; diuretics; antihypertensive agents. Permanent artificial pacemaker usually required.

Prognosis. Chronic, progressive; uncomfortable condition. With pacemaker, good results.

BIBLIOGRAPHY. Laslett EE: Syncopal attacks associated with prolonged arrest of whole heart. Q J Med 2:347, 1909
Short DS: The syndrome of alternating bradycardia and tachycardia. Br Heart J 16:208–214, 1954
Hurst JW: The Heart, 6th ed, p 489. New York, McGraw-Hill, 1986

SHOULDER MUSCULOTENDINOUS CUFF

Symptoms. History of trauma to the shoulder; sensation of "snap"; sudden pain, frequently followed by a pain-free period and then recurrence. Disability; inability to raise arm or initiate abduction. Chronic symptoms; soreness of shoulder; impaired mobility; night discomfort.

Signs. Local discoloration; tenderness over shoulder; crepitation.

Etiology. Trauma of periarticular soft tissue of the shoulder; "aging" tissues.

Pathology. Rupture of supraspinatus and other shoulder tendons; degenerative, inflammatory changes.

Diagnostic Procedures. *X-ray.* Negative.

Therapy. Conservative measures when possible, and surgical measures when indicated by evidence of tear or rupture of tendons.

Prognosis. Depends on etiology and degree of lesions.

BIBLIOGRAPHY. Hollander JL, McCarty DJ: Arthritis and Allied Conditions, 8th ed. Philadelphia, Lea & Febiger, 1972

SHPRINTZEN'S

Synonyms. Velo-cardio-facial; VCF.

Symptoms. From birth. Both sexes. Hypotonia in infancy. Conductive hearing loss, learning disability, intellectual impairment (50%).

Signs. Shorter stature; microsomy (30–40% of patients) microcephaly; long facies; retracted mandible; cleft of secondary palate; prominent nose; narrow palpebral fissures; abundant hair; minor auricular deformities; slender and hypotonic limbs; ventricular septal defect (70%); right aortic arch (45%); tetralogy of Fallot (see) (15%); aberrant left subclavian artery (15%).

Etiology. Probably autosomal dominant (X-linked dominancy not excluded).

Therapy. Correction of cleft and cardiosurgery.

Prognosis. Reduced learning ability and intellectual skills. Depends on cardiac anomalies.

BIBLIOGRAPHY. Shprintzen RJ, Goldberg RB, Lewin ML et al: A new syndrome involving cleft palate, cardiac anomalies, typical facies, and learning disabilities: Velo-cardio-facial syndrome. Cleft Palate J 15:56–59, 1978
Shprintzen RJ, Goldberg RB, Young D et al: The velo-cardio-facial syndrome: A clinical and genetic analysis. Pediatrics 67:167–172, 1981
Wraith JE, Super M, Watson GH et al: Velo-cardio-facial syndrome presenting as holoprosencephaly. Clin Gen 27:408–410, 1985

SHULMAN'S

Synonyms. Posttransfusion purpura; purpura posttransfusion.

Symptoms and Signs. Rare reaction reported only in middle-aged females after repeated blood transfusions. Onset about 1 week after blood transfusion. Severe purpura.

Etiology. Possibly, formation of a cross-reacting antibody that destroys patient's platelets.

Diagnostic Procedures. *Blood.* Severe thrombocytopenia; presence of platelet isoantibody in plasma. Platelet agglutination test; inhibition of clot retraction; complement fixation test.

Therapy. Adrenocorticotropic hormone (ACTH); prednisone; exchange transfusion in extremely severe cases.

Prognosis. Thombocytopenia persists for 24 hours to 44 days, except if exchange transfusion is done. Antibody titer also falls in weeks. After recovering, injection of platelets has no untoward effect and antibodies are not recalled.

BIBLIOGRAPHY. Van Loghem JJ, Dorfmeijer H, Van der Hart M: Serological and genetical studies on platelet antigen (Zw.) Vox Sang 4:161–169, 1959
Shulman NR, Aster RH, Leitner A et al: Immunoreactions involving platelets. V. Posttransfusion purpura due to a complement fixing antibody against a genetically controlled platelet antigen. A proposed mechanism for thrombocytopenia and its relevance in "autoimmunity." J Clin Invest 40:1597–1620, 1961
Morrison FS, Mollison PL: Posttransfusion purpura. N Engl J Med 275:243–248, 1966
Weisberg LJ, Linker CA: Prednisone therapy and posttransfusion purpura. Ann Intern Med 100:76–77, 1985

SHWACHMAN'S

Synonyms. Burke's (V); metaphyseal dysostosis (type B IV); neutropenia–pancreatic insufficiency; Shwachman–Bodian; pancreatic insufficiency–bone marrow dysfunction; lipomatosis of pancreas, congenital.

Symptoms and Signs. Onset at 2 to 10 months of age. In childhood, may be asymptomatic, or one or both features of the syndrome: (1) malabsorption, steatorrhea; (2) recurrent infections. Bleeding tendency. Absence of chronic respiratory diseases.

Etiology. Unknown; a familial incidence observed, but not an adequate number of cases to establish mode of inheritance; autosomal recessive inheritance presumed.

Pathology. Small intestine biopsy shows mild inflammatory changes. *Pancreas.* Hypoplasia of exocrine tissue with normal islets. *Bone marrow.* Myeloid series hypoplasia; occasionally, megakaryocyte deficiency. Bone marrow findings may drastically change according to cyclic phase of proliferation and depression of myeloid series. *Bone.* Metaphyseal chondrodysplasia; focal lack of mineralization in epiphyses.

Diagnostic Procedures. *CT scan. Blood.* Neutropenia; hypochromic anemia in some cases; thrombocytopenia (occasionally). *Stool.* Steatorrhea; decrease of serum pancreatic enzymes (lipase, amylase, trypsine). Fat balance study. *X-ray.* In some cases, metaphyseal dysostosis. *Sweat studies.*

Therapy. Pancreatic enzymes; antibiotic for infections.

Prognosis. Steatorrhea decreases as patient grows older; however, pancreatic exocrine secretion remains low. Tendency to hematologic malignancies.

BIBLIOGRAPHY. Shwachman H, Diamond LK, Oski FA et al: Pancreatic insufficiency and bone marrow dysfunction. A new clinical entity. J Pediatr 63:835–843, 1963

Shwachman H, Diamond LK, Oski FA et al: The syndrome of pancreatic insufficiency and bone marrow dysfunction. J Pediatr 65:645–663, 1964

Burke V, Colebatch JH, Anderson CM et al: Association of pancreatic insufficiency and chronic neutropenia in childhood. Arch Dis Child 42:147–157, 1967

Genieser NB, Halac ER, Greco MA et al: Shwachman–Bodian syndrome. J Comput Assist Tomogr 6:1191–1192, 1982

Dossetor JFN, Spratt HC, Rolles CJ, et al: Immunoreactive trypsin in Shwachman's syndrome. Arch Dis Child 64:395–406, 1989

D'Angio CT, Lloid JK: Nephrocalcinosis in Shwachman's syndrome. Arch Dis Child 64:614–615, 1989

SHY–DRAGER

Synonyms. Orthostatic hypotension–neurologic; orthostatic hypotension variant; Shy–McGee–Drager; multiple system atrophy, MSA.

Symptoms. Occur in adults; onset gradual. Orthostatic hypotension; impotence; general or localized anhidrosis; loss of sphincter control; visual troubles; rigidity; tremor; adiadochokinesis; fasciculations; muscle wasting leading to severe invalidism. Occasionally, dysphagia. Central nervous system manifestations may be identical to those of Parkinson's (see).

Signs. Iris atrophy; external ophthalmoparesis; hyperactive muscle stretch reflexes; pathologic reflexes.

Etiology. Unknown; progressive degenerative process of nervous system. Inflammatory nature cannot be completely excluded. A slowly evolving familial form of this condition has been reported. The autonomic defect appears to be located centrally or partially in the afferent pathways controlling reflex adjustment to postural changes.

Pathology. Nonspecific; bilaterally symmetric neuronal loss and demyelinization of basal ganglia, cerebellar system, corticospinal motor system and autonomic nervous system.

Diagnostic Procedures. *Blood.* Electrolyte alterations. In recumbent position normal plasma level of norepinephrine; failure of the level to be modified by change in position or exercise. Low level of dopamine betahydroxylase. Significant vasoconstrictor response to intraarterial tyramine, and normal response to norepinephrine. *Urine.* Increased excretion of deaminated metabolites of norepinephrine. Injection of acetyl methylcholine; absence of any change. *Electromyography. Electroencephalography.*

Therapy. Administration of 9-fluorohydrocortisone and salt may correct the orthostatic hypotension, but the neurologic symptoms continue to progress. Mechanical measures; volume expanders; pharmacologic agents (sympathomimetics, vasoconstrictors, β-receptor blockers, α₂-receptor agonists, prostaglandin synthesis inhibitors, antiserotoninergics, MAO inhibitors, vasopressin). Atrial tachypacing (100 rate).

Prognosis. Progressive, general debilitation leading to fatal complications.

BIBLIOGRAPHY. Shy GM, Drager GA: A neurological syndrome associated with orthostatic hypotension. Arch Neurol 2:511–527, 1960

Goaverts J, Verfaillie C, Fagard R et al: Effect of prenalteral on orthostatic hypotension in the Shy–Drager syndrome. Br Med J 288:817–818, 1984

Hurst JW: The Heart, 6th ed, pp 511–513. New York, McGraw-Hill, 1986

Lee S, Chen CN: Clinical diversity of the Shy-Drager syndrome: A case in Hong Kong. Journal of the Royal Society of Medicine, 82:225–226, 1989.

SHY–GONATAS

Synonyms. Oculopharyngeal-muscular dystrophy. See also Hunter's and Refsum's.

Symptoms. Onset in middle age, high variability among families where any one of the symptoms may be dominating. Pharyngeal symptoms. Weight loss up to starvation. Weakness of proximal section of extremities; ataxia (cerebellar); double vision and decreased acuity; especially in night vision; dementia.

Signs. Gargoylism; reflexes absent; cardiac arrhythmias; proptosis; hypertelorism; keratopathy.

Etiology. Unknown; metabolic defect in myelinization. Autosomal dominant trait. Membrane abnormalities suggested. According to Gonatas, pathologic findings distinguish the form from gargoylism.

Pathology. Accumulation of lipids and mitochondrial inclusion bodies in muscles. Extensive demyelinization and pathologic cytosomes (zebra bodies) in Schwann's cells and axons. In liver cells, inclusion bodies. In cornea, ulcers. Retinal pigmentary degeneration.

Diagnostic Procedures. *Electromyography.* Suggests myopathy. *Blood.* Normal enzymes.

Therapy. None specific; if pharyngeal symptoms prevent feeding: artificial alimentation; if cardiologic: pacing may be required.

Prognosis. Progressing condition to starvation and motor incapacitation.

BIBLIOGRAPHY. Shy GM, Silberberg DH, Appel SM et al: A generalized disorder of the nervous system, skeletal muscle and heart resembling Refsum's disease and Hurler's syndrome. I. Clinical, pathologic, and biochemical characteristics. Am J Med 42:163–169, 1967

Gonatas NK: A generalized disorder of the nervous system, skeletal muscle and heart resembling Refsum's disease and Hurler's syndrome. II. Ultrastructure. Am J Med 42:169–178, 1967

Appel SH, Roses AD: The muscular dystrophy. In Stanbury JB, Wyngaarden JB, Fredrickson DS et al: The Metabolic Basis of Inherited Disease, 5th ed, p 1483. New York, McGraw-Hill, 1983

SHY–MAGEE

Synonyms. Central core; muscle core; nonprogressive congenital myopathy. See Floppy infant syndromes.

Symptoms. Both sexes affected; onset in first year of life or later; cases reported of onset in adult life. Proximal muscular weakness; delayed physical development in walking, climbing (some patients take 5 years to start to walk). Normal mental development. Association with malignant hyperthermia syndrome reported in some families.

Signs. Symmetric hypotonia of proximal muscles, greater in lower extremities than upper. No fasciculation or myotonia. Minor wasting; tendon flexes normal or diminished.

Etiology. Unknown; autosomal, dominant inheritance, with variable penetrance or expression.

Pathology. *Muscle.* Densely packed core of altered striated myofibrils on the center of muscle fiber. Partial disorganization of normal striation and irregular Z disk in the core. Occasionally, floccular changes in isolated muscle fibers.

Diagnostic Procedures. *Biopsy of muscle.* See Pathology. *Biochemical studies of muscle metabolism. Blood.* Creatine index increased. Serum glutamic-oxalacetic transaminase (SGOT) normal. *Electromyography.* Decreased duration of action potential.

Therapy. Symptomatic.

Prognosis. Defect remains without progression.

BIBLIOGRAPHY. Shy GM, Magee KR: A new congenital non-progressing myopathy. Brain 79:610–621, 1956

Stanbury JB, Wyngaarden JB, Fredrickson DS: The Metabolic Basis of Inherited Disease, 2nd ed. New York, McGraw-Hill, 1966

Gamstrop I: Non-dystrophic myogenic myopathies with onset in infancy or childhood: A review of some characteristic syndromes. Acta Pediatr Scand 71:881–886, 1982

SIALIDOSIS

Synonyms. Cherry red spot–myoclonus. Mucolipidosis I, ML I; neuraminidase deficiency. Distinguished type I and II. See Goldberg's.

Symptoms and Signs. Type I: more frequent in Italians. From second decade. Myoclonus, decreased vision, night blindness, painful neuropathy (see Fabry's), nystagmus ataxia, grand mal. Cherry red spot in macula. Type II: dysmorphic type, divided into juvenile and infantile forms. *Juvenile form:* in Japanese from second decade: coarse facies, dysostosis multiplex, myoclonus, same ocular symptoms of type I. Angiokeratoma and glucosidosis. Vacuolated lymphocytes. *Infantile form:* normal at birth then development of mucopolysaccharidosis phenotype. Abnormal renal function. Congenital form with hydrops fetalis and ascites reported in family groups.

Etiology. Autosomal recessive inheritance. Defect of α-neuraminidase.

Pathology. *Biopsies.* Vacuolated cells.

Diagnostic Procedures. *Urine.* High sialic acid containing oligosaccharides. *Blood.* Vacuolated lymphocytes (except in type I).

Therapy. None.

Prognosis. Death in second decade for infantile form. Later (4th to 5th) for other forms.

BIBLIOGRAPHY. Lowden JA, O'Brien JS: Sialidosis: A review of human neuraminidase deficiency. Am J Hum Genet 31:1–18, 1979

Matsuo T, Igawa I, Okada S et al: Sialidosis type II in Japan: Clinical study in two siblings: Cases and review of literature. J Neurol Sci 58:45–55, 1983

SICCA

Synonym. Sjögren's group E, A, B. See Alacrima. Association of keratoconjunctivitis sicca and xerostomia without an associated collagen disease (see Sjögren's).

BIBLIOGRAPHY. Deutsch HJ: Sjögren's syndrome and pseudolymphoma. Ann Otol 76:1074–1084, 1967

SICK SINUS

See Short's.

Symptoms. Symptoms of periodic mild cerebral artery insufficiency. Slight changes in personality; irritability; fleeting memory losses; sleep alterations. Fatigue; weakness; mild digestive troubles; modest periodic oliguria. In more severe form, speech slurring, paresis, judgment alterations.

Signs. Persistent, severe, sudden sinus bradycardia; cessation of sinus rhythm for short intervals with other rhythms supervening; long periods of sinus arrest resulting in cardiac arrest; bouts of ventricular rhythm following chronic atrial fibrillation with slow ventricular rate. Failure to resume sinus rhythm after cardioversion.

Etiology. Considered an inadequate descriptive term since it includes any form of sinus nodal depression; it is applied as synonym of Short's; it implies disease of the atrioventricular (AV) junction. the pathogenetic mechanism is represented by transient pressure injury of the sinus, from catheter or destruction of nodal tissue by ischemic, sclerotic, or inflammatory process. Symptoms are due to hypoperfusion of brain, kidney, and heart.

Pathology. Lesion of sinoatrial node. Other features of preexisting cardiac pathology.

Diagnostic Procedures. *Electrocardiography.*

Therapy. Electrical pacing. Isoproterenol not practical. Atropine may not be effective.

Prognosis. With electrical pacing, fair.

BIBLIOGRAPHY. Ferrer MI: The sick sinus syndrome in atrial disease. JAMA 206:645–646, 1968
Hurst JW: The Heart 6th ed, p 489. New York, McGraw-Hill, 1986

SICKLE CHEST

Symptoms and Signs. Complication of sickle cell disease (see Herrick). Chest pain, fever, leukocytosis.

Etiology. Intravascular sickling in lung that causes alveolar necrosis. Infection is usually secondary.

Diagnostic Procedures. *Blood.* Sickle cell anemia. *Angiography.* Occlusion of distal pulmonary vessels. *Pulmonary artery pressure measurement.* Increased.

Therapy. Exchange transfusion: artificial ventilation with positive pressure or prepulmonary oxygenation with extracorporeal membrane.

Prognosis. High mortality in spite of good intensive treatment.

BIBLIOGRAPHY. Davies SC, Luce PJ, Riordan PJ et al: Acute chest syndrome in sickle cell disease. Lancet i:36–38, 1984
Gillett DS, Gunning KEJ, Sawicka EH et al: Life-threatening sickle chest syndrome treated with extracorporeal membrane oxygenation. Br J Med 294:81–82, 1987

SIEGAL–CATTAN–MAMOU

Synonyms. Armenian; benign paroxysmal peritonitis; familial Mediterranean fever; Mediterranean fever; FMF; periodic amyloid; periodic peritonitis; recurrent polyserositis; Reimann's.

Symptoms. Peculiar ethnic distribution in people of Mediterranean ancestry; more frequent in males. Onset most frequently in late adolescence, also in early age, seldom after 40 years of age. Complete syndrome of subsyndromes may represent the clinical manifestation of this disease. Paroxysmal attacks, most frequently accompanied by fever, are the common feature for this condition. Frequency of attack variable from once a year to once a week. Cycles of repeated attacks with periods of complete remission. In women, attack may be largely limited to the menstrual periods. *Abdomen.* Pain most frequently in right lower quadrant, lower left quadrant, upper left quadrant, with stooped posture. *Thorax.* Stabbing unilateral pain; chest or shoulder dyspnea. *Joints.* Arthralgias (2–3 days' duration); occasionally monoarthralgia of big articulations. *Skin.* Urticaria (rare).

Signs. *Abdomen.* Tenderness, spasm, and guarding; distention; occasionally, moderate splenomegaly. *Chest.* No function sound; tenderness of chest wall; decreased sound transmission of minor degree. *Joints.* Local erythema; swelling.

Etiology. Unknown; congenital familial autosomal recessive trait; possibly, an inherited error in metabolism of one or more steriod hormones.

Pathology. Transient peritonitis with simple hyperemia of peritoneum or extended to abdominal organs; scattered deposit of fibrinous material. Small amount of free fluid. In microscopic study of exudate, fibrin mesh with neutrophils. Typical lack of peritoneal adhesions in spite of recurrent attacks. Liver and spleen may show adhesions. In kidney, progressive lesion consistent with amyloidosis or in some cases, with chronic glomerulonephritis.

Diagnostic Procedures. Symptoms may be elicited by 10 mg metacaminol. *Blood.* During attack leukocytosis (15,000, seldom higher); neutrophilia; moderate anemia. Sedimentation rate increased. Glycoprotein increased; α-2 globulin increased. Fibrinogen increased. Evanescent minimal signs of hepatic involvement may be recorded; bilirubin; flocculation test. *Peritoneal and pleural fluid.* Serofibrinous, predominantly polymorphonuclear or mixed response. *Joint fluid.* Polymorphic cytology. *X-ray.* During attack, presence of fluid in abdomen or chest or both. Gastrointestinal tract may show transient abnormalities of mucosa of small bowel.

Therapy. Attack dramatically responds to adrenal steroid. Low-fat diets seem to benefit a great number of patients. Rest, treatment of tension also effective in large number of cases. Colchicine (preventive).

Prognosis. Essentially benign condition, despite the recurrence of attacks. Amyloidosis and renal failure complications.

BIBLIOGRAPHY. Siegal S: Benign paroxysmal peritonitis. Ann Intern Med 23:1–21, 1945

Mamou H, Cattan R: La maladie périodique (sur 14 cas personnels dort 8 compliqués de néphropathies). Sem Hop Paris 28:1062–1070, 1952

Janeway TC, Mosenthal HO: An unusual paroxysmal syndrome probably allied to recurrent vomiting with a study of the nitrogen metabolism. Trans Assoc Am Phys 23:504–518, 1968

Barakat MH, El–Chawad AO, Gumaa KA et al: Metaraminol provocative test: A specific diagnostic test for familial Mediterranean fever. Lancet 656–657, 1984

Knecht A, Debeer FC, Pras M: Serum amyloid: A protein in familial Mediterranean fever. Ann Intern Med 102:71–72, 1984

Pras M, Bronshfigel N, Zemer D, Gafni J: Variable incidence of amyloidosis in familial Mediterranean fever among different ethnic groups. Johns Hopkins Med J 150:22–26, 1982

SIEGRIST'S

Synonyms. Pigmented choroidal vessels; Siegrist-Hutchinson.

Symptoms and Signs. Prevalent in females; onset in advanced age. Decreasing vision; exophthalmos; granular pigmented areas in the choroid that follows the path of the larger choroidal vessels. Blood hypertension.

Etiology. Unknown.

Pathology. Changes of choroid and other manifestations related to arteriosclerotic changes.

Diagnostic Procedures. *Urine.* Albuminuria.

Therapy. None.

Prognosis. The occurrence of these choroidal changes indicate an unfavorable prognosis.

BIBLIOGRAPHY. Siegrist A: Zur Kenntnis der Arteriosclerose der Augengefässe. IX Cong. internat D'Opht d'Utrecht pp 131–139, 1900.

Geeraets WJ: Ocular Syndromes, 3rd ed Philadelphia, Lea & Febiger, 1976

SIEMEN'S

Synonyms. Congenital ectodermal defect; keratosis follicularis spinulosa decalvans; ichthyosis follicularis.

Symptoms and Signs. Present from birth. Complete picture only in males; in heterozygous females, partial expression. Variable occurrence of associated symptoms and signs. Complete pattern includes follicular hyperkeratosis, especially in the extensor surfaces of extremities; generalized alopecia on head (particularly under occipital protuberances), face, axillae, pubic area, and lanugo; sparse eyelashes and eyebrows (particularly on the later portion); photophobia; lacrimation; corneal abnormalities (punctate lesions). Associated findings: blepharitis; ectropion; telangiectasis in the cheeks; hypoplasia of mandible.

Etiology. Unknown; X-linked transmission. Autosomal dominant trait also reported.

Pathology. See Symptoms and Signs.

Diagnostic Procedures. *Slit-lamp examination.* Corneal lesions. *Urine.* Amino acid excretion pattern.

Therapy. Symptomatic.

Prognosis. *Quoad vitam* good.

BIBLIOGRAPHY. Lameris: Ichthyosis follicularis. Ned Tijdschr Geneeskd 41:1524, 1905

Siemens HW: Ueber einen in der menschlichen Pathologie noch nicht beobachteten. Vererbungsmodus: Dominant-geschlechtsgebundene Vererbung. Arch Rass U Ges Biol 17:47–61, 1925

Siemens HW: Keraton; follicularis spinulosa decalvans. Arch Dermatol Syph 151:384–386, 1926

Adler RC, Nyhan WL: An oculocerebral syndrome with aminoaciduria and keratosis follicularis. J Pediatr 75:436–442, 1969

Knops HJ: Siemens's syndrome I (keratosis follicularis spinulosa decalvans). Br J Dermatol 100:611, 1979

SILFVERSKIÖLD'S

Synonyms. Grudzinski's; Morquio's variant; extremity osteochondrodystrophy. Possibly a variant of Morquio's syndrome. Term obsolete in modern nomenclature.

BIBLIOGRAPHY. Silfverskiöld N: A forme fruste of chondrodystrophia, with changes simulating several of the known local malacias. Acta Radiol 4:44–57, 1925

Helweg–Larsen HF, Morch ET: Hereditary of osteochondrodystrophy: Silfverskiöld and Morquio syndromes. Nord Med 30:377–882, 1946

SILLENCE'S

Synonym. Brachydactyly symphalangism.

Symptoms and Signs. Brachydactyly, distal symphalangism (chess pawn), scoliosis, pes equinus, normal stature.

Etiology. Autosomal dominant inheritance.

BIBLIOGRAPHY. Sillence DO: Brachydactyly, distal symphalangism, scoliosis, tall stature, and club feet: A new syndrome. J Med Genet 15:208–211, 1978

SILVESTRINI–CORDA

Synonym. Endocrine deficiency–hepatic cirrhosis.

Symptoms. Occur in patients with liver cirrhosis. Anorexia; asthenia; loss of libido; impotence; menstrual disorders (menorrhagia; amenorrhea; postmenopausal bleeding.)

Signs. Gynecomastia (Silvestrini); testicular atrophy (Corda). Loss of axillary hair; vascular arterial "spider" plus all signs of liver cirrhosis (*e.g.,* liver enlarged at onset; reduced and nodular, later ascites).

Etiology. Secondary endocrinologic changes due to failure of liver to metabolize different hormones.

Pathology. That of liver cirrhosis; gynecomastia; atrophy of testicular germinal epithelium; prostatic nodular hyperplasia. Decrease of lipoid content of adrenals.

Diagnostic Procedures. *Blood.* Typical changes of liver cirrhosis. *Urine.* Increased excretion of estrogen and decrease of 17-ketosteroids and androgen.

Therapy and Prognosis. That of liver cirrhosis.

BIBLIOGRAPHY. Corda L, Sulla CD: Reviviscenza della mammella maschile nella cirrosi epatica. Minerva Med 5:1067–1069, 1925
Silvestrini R: La reviviscenza mammaria nell'uomo affetto da cirrosi del Laennec. Riforma Med 42:701–704, 1926
Lloyd CW, Williams RH: Endocrine changes associated with Laennec's cirrhosis of the liver. Am J Med 4:315–330, 1948
Callen JP: Cutaneous Aspects of Internal Disease, p 530. Chicago, Year Book Medical Publishers, 1981

SILVESTRONI–BIANCO

Synonyms. Microdrepanocytosis; sickle cell–thalassemia.

Symptoms. Variable pattern including features of Herrick's and thalassemia syndromes. From mild anemia to severe anemia; abdominal crisis; splenomegaly.

Etiology. Combination of two pathologic genes usually inherited one from each parent, seldom both from same parent.

Diagnostic Procedures. *Blood.* Findings of sickling and thalassemia. Hemoglobin electrophoresis usually shows 60% to 80% of hemoglobin S, 20% of hemoglobin F, and balance hemoglobin A; hemoglobin A_2 usually increased.

Prognosis. Variable according to biochemical defect. Death in infancy or childhood, or survival into adulthood.

BIBLIOGRAPHY. Silvestroni E, Bianco I: Ricerche cliniche, genetiche et dermatologiche sui malati di anemia microcitica constituzionale e di morbo di Cooley. Haematologica 3:135–190, 1948
Silvestroni E, Bianco I: Genetic aspects of sickle cell anemia and microdrepanocytic disease. Blood 7:429–435, 1952
Serjeant GR, Sommerveux AM, Stevenson M et al: Comparison of sickle cell β°-thalassemia with homozygous sickle cell disease. Br J Haematol 41:83–93, 1979

SIMELL–TAKKI

Synonyms. Gyrate atrophy of choroid and retina; retinitis pigmentosa atypical, Jacobsohn's, hyperornithinemia Finnish type.

Symptoms and Signs. Both sexes, prevalent in Finnish people. From childhood progressive loss of vision, blindness reached in fourth decade. Posterior subcapsular cataracts. Sometimes associated anomalies of body hair.

Etiology. Autosomal recessive. Defect in ornithine-δ-aminotransferase which causes accumulation of ornithine which inhibits creatine synthesis.

Diagnostic Procedures. In childhood: demarcated circular areas of chorioretinal degeneration which enlarge and coalesce in adult life. *Electroretinography.* Reduced conduction with progression of disease. *Muscle biopsy.* Abnormalities of muscle fibers (type II). *Body fluids.* Elevation of ornithine level.

Therapy. Exogenous creatine and pyridoxine give some results.

Prognosis. Progressive condition.

BIBLIOGRAPHY. Jacobsohn E: Ein Fall von Retinitis pigmentosa atypica. Klin Monatsbl Augenheilkd 26:206, 1888
Simell O, Takki K: Raised plasma ornithine and gyrate atrophy of the choroid and retina. Lancet 1:1031, 1973
Kennaway NG, Weleber RG, Buist NRM: Gyrate atrophy of the choroid and retina, with hyperornithinemia: Biochemical and histological studies and response to vitamin B_6. Am J Hum Genet 32:529–541, 1980

SIMMONDS'

Synonyms. Glinski–Simmonds; hypopituitarism; panhypopituitarism; postpuberal panhypopituitarism. See Sheehan's.

Symptoms. Prevalent in females; onset in postpuberal period. Asthenia; prolonged inanition to emaciation. Loss of libido and potency.

Signs. Weight loss; atrophy of all body tissues; loss of body hair; atrophic skin gives the appearance of premature aging. Atrophy of genital organs. Sensitivity to cold; bradycardia. Low blood pressure may reach shock level with patient in upright position. Psychic changes.

Etiology. Lesion and hypofunction or atrophy (or both) of anterior pituitary gland (idiopathic; tumor; infections; x-rays; surgery).

Pathology. *Pituitary.* See Etiology. *Thyroid adrenal, gonads.* Secondary atrophy.

Diagnostic Procedures. *Blood.* Thyroid-stimulating hormone (TSH) and adrenocorticotropic hormone (ACTH) level. Anemia of various degrees according to degree of hypofunction. Basic metabolic rate low. *Urine.* Low 17-ketosteroids, 11-oxysteroids, and gonadotropins.

Therapy. ACTH, gonadotropins, thyroid, and other deficient hormones.

Prognosis. With treatment, dramatic improvement.

BIBLIOGRAPHY. Simmonds M: Ueber Hypophysisschwund mit tödlichem Ausgang. Dtsch Med Wochenschr 40:322–323, 1914
Hickstein DD, Chaundler WF, Marshall JC: The spectrum of pituitary adenoma. West J Med 144:433–436, 1986

SIMPLE VITAMIN D-RESISTANT RICKETS

Synonyms. Familial hypophosphatemic rickets; X-linked hypophosphatemia; rickets–x-linked hypophosphatemia.

Symptoms. Occur in males; in females, only hypophosphatemia or less severe clinical manifestations. Normal at birth. Onset when beginning to walk. Waddling gait.

Signs. Mild growth deficiency; bowing of legs; coxa vara.

Etiology. X-linked inheritance. Defect of proximal tubular phosphate transport coupled with rate of 1,25-(OH)2 D3 synthesis.

Pathology. See Rickets.

Diagnostic Procedures. *Blood.* Hypophosphatemia; hyperphosphatasemia alkaline; calcium and urea normal. *Urine.* Hyperphosphaturia; amino acid excretion normal. Occasionally, renal glycosuria. *X-ray.* Typical changes of rickets.

Therapy. Phosphate supplement (1–4 g); vitamin D (25,000–75,000 IU).

Prognosis. Partially responsive to combined phosphate-vitamin D treatment. Deformities may progress into adult life. Final adult height 130 to 160 cm.

BIBLIOGRAPHY. Winters RW, Graham JB, Williams TF et al: A genetic study of familial hypophosphatemia and vitamin D-resistant rickets. Trans Assoc Am Physicians 70:234–242, 1957
Rasmussen H, Anast C: Familial hypophosphatemic rickets and vitamin D-dependent rickets. In Stanbury JB, Wyngaarden JB, Fredrickson DS et al: The Metabolic Basis of Inherited Disease, 5th ed, p 1743. New York, McGraw-Hill, 1983

SIMPSON'S

Synonym. Hysterical abdominal bloating.

Symptoms. Occur in women or occasionally men (see Couvade). Abdominal swelling; pseudocyesis.

Signs. Depression of diaphragm and lordosis of spine.

Etiology. Unknown; delusion of pregnancy a symptom of many psychotic states.

Diagnostic Procedures. Under anesthesia abdominal swelling disappears, and returns as soon as patient awakes.

BIBLIOGRAPHY. Simpson J: Clinical Lectures on Diseases of Women, p 363. Edinburgh, Black, 1872
Enock MD, Trethouan WH, Barker JC: Some uncommon psychotic syndromes. Baltimore, Williams & Wilkins, 1967

SIMPSON'S (S.L.)

Synonym. Adipose gynandrism. Adipose gynism (equivalent syndrome in female). See Pseudo-Cushing's.

Symptoms and Signs. Onset in preadolescence. Tendency toward obesity and delayed sexual maturation. Some morphologic features suggesting female habitus (due to fat distribution and delayed sexual development). Patient somewhat taller than average.

Etiology. Unknown; genetic factor: endocrine changes possibly secondary to obesity. One of the many shades of the hypogenitalism group of syndromes.

Diagnostic Procedures. See Pseudo-Cushing's.

Therapy. Diet.

Prognosis. Good. Eventually, normal development and fertility.

BIBLIOGRAPHY. Simpson SL: Clinical and pathological aspects of adrenal glands. Proc R Soc Med 27:383–387, 1934
Simpson SL: Adrenal hyperfunction and function. Bull NY Acad Med 27:723–742, 1951
Paschkis KE, Rakoff AE, Cantarow A et al: Clinical Endocrinology. New York, Harper & Row, 1967

SINGLE ATRIUM

Synomyms. Common atrium; cor triloculare biventriculare.

Symptoms. Both sexes affected; present from early age. Effort dyspnea; frequent respiratory infections; cardiac failure (in severe form).

Signs. Mild cyanosis; constant or transitory crying on exercise. In mild form, red cheeks and digital redness. In severe form, physical underdevelopment. Frequently associated with Ellis–van Creveld (see) and asplenia (see Ivemark's) and polysplenia (see). On auscultation, pulse and precordial movements are those characterizing the large atrial septal defect.

Etiology. Congenital malformation.

Pathology. Complete absence of atrial septum; right and left sides of the common cavity have the respective characteristics of the right and left atrium.

Diagnostic Procedures. *Electrocardiography.* Tendency for leftward deviation of P wave axis; QRS similar to those observed in endocardial cushion defect. Volume overload of right ventricle. *X-ray.* Size of right atrium unimpressive.

Therapy. Surgical correction.

Prognosis. Extremely variable according to type and intensity of left-to-right shunts or right-to-left shunts and pulmonary vascular resistance.

BIBLIOGRAPHY. Cunningham GJ: Trilocular heart with bilateral aneurysmal dilatation of pulmonary arteries. J Pathol Bacteriol 60:379–386, 1948
Hurst JW: The Heart, 6th ed, p 612. New York, McGraw-Hill, 1986

SINGLETON–MERTEN

Synonym. Aortic arch calcification-osteoporosis–tooth buds hypoplasia.

Symptoms and Signs. Occur in both sexes. Failure of some teeth eruption; reduction in number; widening of hand bones; cardiomegaly; muscular weakness and poor physical development. Occasionally psoriatic skin manifestation.

Etiology. Unknown. Possibly autosomal dominant inheritance.

Diagnostic Procedures. *X-ray.* Cardiomegaly; calcification of aortic arch; osteoporosis of cranial vault and long bones.

Prognosis. In two cases, death from ventricular fibrillation.

BIBLIOGRAPHY. Singleton EB, Merten DF: An unusual syndrome of widened medullary cavities of the metacarpals and phalanges, aortic calcification and abnormal dentition. Pediatr Radiol 2:2–4, 1973
Gay B Jr, Kuhn JP: A syndrome of widened medullary cavities of bone, aortic calcification, abnormal dentition and muscular weakness (The Singleton–Merten syndrome). Radiology 118:389–395, 1976

SINGLE VENTRICLE

Synonyms. Cor triloculare biatriatum. Common ventricle; univentricular heart. See Holmes'.

Symptoms. Male predominance 2 to 4:1; present from birth. Frailty; orthopnea.

Signs. Moderate or absent cyanosis; edema; left sternal edge; holosystolic murmur of low pitch; blurred middiastolic or late diastolic murmur; accentuated second pulmonic sound. Cardiomegaly.

Etiology. Congenital malformation.

Pathology. Single ventricle with anatomic features of left ventricle; associated with two atria; two separated atrioventricular A-V valves enter the single ventricle, occasionally, joined to form a single valve. Possibly, stenosis or narrowing of pulmonary trunk.

Diagnostic Procedures. *Blood.* Polycythemia. *X-ray.* Cardiomegaly with globular shape. *Angiocardiography. Electrocardiography. Echocardiography. Cardiac catheterization.*

Therapy. Medical management for congestive heart failure and anoxic periods; bacterial endocarditis prevention. Palliative surgery frequently needed.

Prognosis. Sixty percent of patients require hospital admission within first month of life.

BIBLIOGRAPHY. Perloff JK: The Clinical Recognition of Congenital Heart Disease, 2nd ed, p 641. Philadelphia, WB Saunders, 1978

Hurst JW: The Heart 6th ed, pp 703–706. New York, McGraw-Hill, 1986

SIPPLE'S

Synonyms. Familial chromaffinomatosis; multiple endocrine neoplasia II; MEN II; MEN IIa; multiple neuroma; pheochromocytoma–thyroid medullary carcinoma; PCT.

Symptoms and Signs. The association of medullary thyroid carcinoma (frequently bilateral) and pheochromocytoma (frequently bilateral) constitutes a definite syndrome, which is further characterized by occasional coexistence of parathyroid tumors, neurofibromas, diabetes mellitus, and diarrhea. Both sexes affected. The symptoms and signs depend on the various phases of development of the tumors, and the eventual predominance of one of them or of the associated lesions in different periods.

Etiology. Both familial (with a dominant autosomal inheritance) and sporadic types have been described. Chromosome 20 alteration not consistently observed by various authors.

Pathology. Medullary carcinoma of thyroid: group of cells varying in size and shape from small and round, to large ovoid or spindle cells, sometimes palisaded, indistinct cellular outline, scanty cytoplasm. In all cases amyloid is found in various amounts up to the point of dominating the pattern, or to exclude cellular elements. Metastasis to cervical nodes in two thirds of the cases and distant sites in one third. Pheochromocytoma frequently bilateral, seldom malignant.

Diagnostic Procedures. *Radioactive iodine uptake.* Studies for pheochromocytoma (see).

Therapy. Surgery. Chemotherapy.

Prognosis. Patient with medullary carcinoma of thyroid or pheochromocytoma should be followed for development of other lesions or manifestations of the syndrome.

BIBLIOGRAPHY. Eisenberg AA, Wallerstein H: Pheochromocytoma of the suprarenal medulla (paraganglioma): Clinicopathological study. Arch Pathol 14:818–836, 1932
Beer EC, King FM, Prinzmetal M: Pheochromocytoma with demonstration of pressor (adrenalin) substances in the blood preoperatively during hypertensive crises. Ann Surg 106:85–91, 1937
Sipple JH: The association of pheochromocytoma with carcinoma of the thyroid gland. Am J Med 31:163–166, 1961
Zatterale A, Stabile M, Nunziata V et al: Multiple endocrine type 2 (Sipple's syndrome): Clinical and cytogenetic analysis of a kindred. J Med Genet 21:108–111, 1984

SJAASTAD–DALE

Synonym. Hemicrania chronic, paroxysmal.

Symptoms and Signs. Those of cluster headache (see). Unilateral pains of temporo-orbital are paroxysmal of short duration (20–30 min). Differently from cluster headache, episodes occur many times each day, for years.

Etiology. Unknown. See Migraine classic.

Therapy. Different from cluster headache, attacks are stopped dramatically by indomethacin.

BIBLIOGRAPHY. Sjaastad O, Dale I: A new clinical headache entity: Chronic paroxysmal hemicrania. Acta Neurol Scand 54:140–156, 1976
Nappi G, Savoldi F: Headache: diagnostic system and taxonomic criteria. J Libbey Eurotext, London-Paris 1985

SJÖGREN–LARSSON

Synonyms. Spastic diplegia–ichthyosis–oligophrenia; ichthyosiform erythroderma. See Ichthyosis syndromes and Rud's.

Symptoms. No sex predilection. Consanguinity between parents; high incidence in siblings. Neurologic disorders seldom diagnosed at birth, usually within first year. Stiff awkward movement of legs, then in the arms (spastic diplegia). Severe mental deficiency (idiocy or imbecility). No patients reported with low or normal intelligence.

Signs. Usually evident at birth; scalp hair normal or thin; moderate hyperkeratosis face and scalp; slightly scaling ichthyosis of trunk, back, neck, and extremities (more marked in flexural areas). Erythema of various degrees; moderate hyperkeratosis of palms and soles, but no keratoderma. Dysplasia of tooth enamel may be present. Macular lesions and recurrent corneal ulceration may be observed. Deep hyperreflexia for the legs; ankle clonus; Babinski sign; minor or no hyperreflexia for the arms.

Etiology. Unknown; autosomal recessive inheritance.

Pathology. On skin biopsy, hyperkeratosis and acanthosis; stratum granulosum diminished or absent. No reported autopsy studies.

Diagnostic Procedures. *Biopsy of skin* (see Pathology). *CT scan.* Hydrocephalus; sclerotic cortical atrophy; no intracerebral calcifications. *Electroencephalography.* Slow paroxysmal activity.

Therapy. Symptomatic, corneal graft to save sight when there are corneal ulcerations.

Prognosis. Spastic diplegia usually remains stationary after 5 years of life.

BIBLIOGRAPHY. Pardo–Castello V, Faz H: Ichthyosis–Little's disease. Arch Dermatol 26:915, 1932

Sjögren T, Larsson T: Oligophrenia in combination with congenital ichthyosis and spastic disorders: A clinical and genetic study. Acta Psychiatr Neurol Scand 32 [Suppl 113]: 1–112, 1957

Jagell S, Linden S: Ichthyosis in the Sjögren–Larsson syndrome. Clin Genet 21:243–252, 1982

SJÖGREN'S I

Synonyms. Dacryosialoadenopathia atrophicans; Gougerot–Sjögren; Gougerot–Houwer–Sjögren; keratoconjunctivitis sicca–xerostomia; secreto-inhibitor-xerodermatostenosis.

Symptoms and Signs. Prevalent in females (80–90%); onset in middle age (36% before menopause; 64% at or after menopause). In male patients, average age at onset 47 years. Insidious onset. Diminution or cessation of lacrimation (keratoconjunctivitis sicca) (A); of salivary gland secretion (xerostomia) (B); pharyngitis; laryngitis; rhinitis sicca; swelling of parotid gland (50% initial symptoms). Polyarthritis (C). Combinations of AB, AC, BC diagnostic. Other possible components of syndrome: excessive dental cavities; tracheobronchitis; vaginitis; achlorhydria; Raynaud's phenomenon; purpura; arteritis; focal myositis; neuropathy; alopecia; splenomegaly; hepatomegaly.

Etiology. Unknown. Possible factors; endocrine; infectious; allergic; autoimmune; congenital or familial (autosomal or recessive); associated with collagen disorders.

Pathology. In parotid gland, lymphocytic infiltration with recognizable architecture of gland, not folliculoid pattern, proliferation of myoepithelial cells, atrophy of some acini (pattern similar to Mikulicz's pattern, see). Alacrimal keratoconjunctivitis with lymphocytic infiltration. In submandibular, tracheal, esophageal, vaginal, subepithelial mucous glands, similar pattern with parotid gland. In kidney (occasional), chronic interstitial nephritis. Focal myositis (occasional); focal peripheral arteritis (occasional).

Diagnostic Procedures. *Schirmer's test.* Measure of extent to which a thin paper strip inserted into conjunctival sac is moistened. *Sialography. Blood.* Leukopenia; eosinophilia; thrombocytopenia; hyperglobulinemia; cephalin flocculation; thymol turbidity; rheumatoid factor; tissue antibodies; increased sedimentation rate.

Therapy. Corticosteroids; adrenocorticotropic hormone (ACTH); occlusion of the puncta by electrocautery may alleviate keratoconjunctivitis. Topical fibronectin.

Prognosis. Chronic disease, only partially responsive to treatment. Usually, mild form for years, then some patients may develop lymphoma or reticular cell sarcoma or simple generalized adenopathy (pseudolymphoma). Other cases complicated by various collagen diseases.

BIBLIOGRAPHY. von Graefes AF: Demonstration in der Berliner Medizinischen Gesellschaft. Klin Wochenschr 5:127, 1868

Sjögren H: Zur Kenntnis der Keratoconjunctivitis sicca (Keratitis filiformis bei Hypofunktion der Tramendrüsen). Acta Ophth [Suppl II] 1–151, 1933

Sjögren H: A new conception of kerato-conjunctivitis sicca. Hamilton JB (trans), Sidney, Australasian Medical, 1943

Reveille JD, Wilson RW, Provost TT et al: Primary Sjögren's syndrome and other autoimmune diseases in families: Prevalence and autoimmunogenetic studies in six kindreds. Ann Intern Med 101:748–756, 1984

Bone RC, Fox RI, Howell FV, Fantozzi R: Sjogren's syndrome: A persistent clinical problem. Laryngoscope 95:295–299, 1985

Kono I, Matsumoto Y, Konok et al: Beneficial effect of topical fibronectin in patients with keratoconjunctivitis sicca of Sjögren's syndrome. J Rheumatol 12:487–489, 1985

SLEEP APNEA

Symptoms and Signs. All ages. Three varieties of syndromes identified.

1. *Predominant obstructive type.* Frequently overweight, short and fat neck. Average age 46 years; daytime fatigue.
2. *Predominantly central sleep apnea.* Usually normal or under weight; average age 63 years; no daytime fatigue. Apneic events lead to cardiac arrhythmias and to arousal.
3. *Mixed type.* Features of type 1 and 2. Frequently hypertension. Type 1 subjects awake: normal pulmonary function; subject sleeping: apneic events, frequently accompanied by cardiac arrhythmias and hemodynamic changes.

Etiology. Multifactorial.

Diagnostic Procedures. Type I sleep-induced airway obstruction or upper airway apnea. Type II decreased diaphragmatic activity during sleep. During sleep various techniques noninvasive or invasive (in severe forms) to document number and predominant type of apneic events. *Electrocardiography 24-hour monitoring.* Progressive sinus bradycardia during episodes, followed by abrupt reversal and sinus acceleration at termination; may occur also atrioventricular blocks, prolonged sinus pause, ventricular tachycardia, atrial fibrillation. Systemic and pulmonary arterial pressure: rise during episodes.

Therapy. Atropine sulfate and oxygen blunt the marked sinus variations. Propanolol no obvious effect.

Prognosis. Life-threatening arrhythmias and sudden death during sleep possible. It seems however that the prevalence of serious arrhythmias and conduction defects during sleep in patients with this syndrome is lower than reported.

BIBLIOGRAPHY. Bond WC, Ebey J Jr, Welf S: Rhythm heart rate variability (sinus arrhythmias) related to stages of sleep. Cond Reflex 8:98–107, 1973

Tilkian AG, Guillemninault C, Schroeder KL et al: Sleep induced apnea syndrome: Prevalence of cardiac arrhythmias and their reversal after tracheostomy. Am J Med 63:348–358 1977

Miller WP: Cardiac arrhythmias and conduction disturbances in the sleep apnea syndrome. Prevalence and significance. Am J Med 73:317–321, 1982

SLIM DISEASE

Symptoms and Signs. Fever, itching maculopapular, general malaise, prolonged diarrhea, occasional respiratory symptoms. Maculopapular rash, oral candidiasis; extreme wasting and weight loss. Lymphadenopathy and Kaposi's sarcoma are not as common in slim disease as found among Western homosexual patients with AIDS. Kaposi's sarcoma is commoner among slim disease patients than among western hemophiliacs infected with AIDS virus.

Etiology. HTLV-III infection, transmitted by heterosexual contact, homosexual contact, insect vectors such as mosquitos, bed bugs or lice, and injections.

Diagnostic Procedures. HTLV-III serum ELISA assay.

Therapy. Antibiotics. Symptomatic treatment.

Prognosis. Not known (a very new disease).

BIBLIOGRAPHY. Serwadda D, Mugerwa R, Sewan–Kambo N et al: Slim disease: A new disease in Uganda and its association with HTLV-III infection. Lancet 2:849–852, 1985

SLIT VENTRICLE

Symptoms and Signs. *Acute form.* Symptoms of increased intracranial pressure; symptoms of cerebral edema; decrease of the consciousness level. *Subacute form.* Increased tendency to convulsions; headache; ataxia; balance disturbances; changed sleeping patterns and drowsiness; nausea. *Chronic form.* Recurrent and postural symptoms, as in the subacute form.

Etiology. Overdrainage of cerebrospinal fluid (CSF) in patients with hydrocephalus who had a ventriculoatrial or ventriculoperitoneal shunt.

Pathology. *Acute form.* Subdural effusion and epidural hemorrhage. *Subacute and chronic forms.* Collapsed ventricles, ventricular catheter closed by the ventricular wall, no CSF drained through the shunt. The chronically collapsed ventricle loses its flexibility and does not reinflate easily.

Diagnostic Procedures. *CT scan.* Acute and subacute form: collapsed ventricles, periventricular lucency, subarachnoid accumulation of CSF; chronic form: recurrent, total, or partial collapse of ventricles. *Electroencephalography.* Increased abnormality.

Therapy. Replacement of the valve with a high resistance one; use of an antisiphon device; full neurosurgical evaluation.

BIBLIOGRAPHY. Hide–Brown MD, Rekate HL, Nulsen FE: Re-expansion of previously collapsed ventricles: The slit ventricle syndrome. J Neurosurg. 56:536–539, 1981

Serlo W, Heikkinem E, Saukkonen AL, Wendt L: Classification and management of the slit ventricle syndrome. Child's Nerv Syst 1:194–199, 1985

Epstein F, Lapras C, Wisoff JH: Slit ventricle syndrome: etiology and treatment. Pediatr Neurosci 14:5–10, 1988

SLUDER'S

Synonyms. Lower facial neuralgia; sphenopalatine neuralgia; sphenopalatine ganglion neuralgia.

Symptoms. Episodic recurrences of vague head pains, in nose and orbit and other parts. Also, shoulder and neck pains, never extending over the ear. Associated congestion of nose and eye; lacrimation. Attacks last minutes, hours, or days.

Etiology. Sphenopalatine ganglion irritation. Little reason to believe that such condition exists (Grinker) as an autonomous entity; variant of cluster headache.

Therapy. Injection of the ganglion with alcohol or application of cocaine over the ganglion reported effective by some Authors. Others were not successful with this treatment.

BIBLIOGRAPHY. Sluder G: The role of sphenopalatine (Meckel's) ganglion in nasal headaches. NY Med J 87:989–990, 1908

Vick NA: Grinker's Neurology, 7th ed. Springfield, CC Thomas, 1976

SLY'S

Synonyms. Mucopolysaccharidosis VII; MPS VII; beta-glucuronidase deficiency.

Symptoms. Both sexes affected; onset in early infancy or later. Repeated respiratory infections. Visual impairment; mental and physical retardation (not constant).

Signs. From delayed growth to normal stature. Facies coarse. Gross corneal clouding (not constant); other occasional findings are hepatosplenomegaly, umbilical or inguinal hernias, anterior chest deformities, vertebral column deformities, extremity deformities (*e.g.,* club foot, genu valgum, metatarsus adductus).

Etiology. Autosomal recessive inheritance. Several alleles postulated as responsible for different phenotypes. Deficiency of beta-glucuronidase responsible for block of degradation of heparan sulfate.

Diagnostic Procedures. *Test for beta-glucuronidase.* In fibroblast leukocytes and serum. *Blood.* Inclusion bodies in leukocytes.

Therapy. None.

Prognosis. Variable; periods of survival not yet assessed.

BIBLIOGRAPHY. Sly WS, Quinton BA, McAlister WN et al: Beta-glucuronidase deficiency. Report of clinical, radiological and biochemical features of a new mucopolysaccharidosis. J Pediatr 82:249–257, 1973
McKusick VA, Neufeld EF: The mucopolysaccharide storage diseases. In Stanbury JB, Wyngaarden JB, Fredrickson DS et al: The Metabolic Basis of Inherited Disease, 5th ed, p 751. New York, McGraw-Hill, 1983

SMALL CUFF

Synonym. Nonhypertension.

Symptoms and Signs. When a small cuff is used to determine arterial pressure, gross error may result in the auscultatory systolic and diastolic values. Erroneous diagnosis may result with unnecessary anxiety and possibly therapeutic mismanagement. To determine the blood pressure in infants and children where this situation may more easily arise, the use of cuffs of different sizes is suggested. In newborn; 2.5 cm cuff; in infants (2 wk to 1 yr), 5.0 cm cuff; in children, (1–13 yr), 9.0 cm cuff. The same concept applies to extremely obese patients where a larger cuff has to be used instead of the regular one.

BIBLIOGRAPHY. Robinow M, Hamilton WF, Woodbury RA et al: Accuracy of clinical determination of blood pressure in children with values under normal and abnormal conditions. Am J Dis Child 58:102–118, 1939

Hansen RL, Stickler GB: The "nonhypertension" or "small-cuff" syndrome. Clin Pediatr 5:579–580, 1966
O'Rourke RA: Physical examination of the arteries and veins (including blood pressure determination). In Hurst JW: The Heart, 6th ed, p 139. New York, McGraw-Hill, 1986

SMALL'S

Synonyms. Coat's disease–deafness–muscular dystrophy mental retardation.

Symptoms and Signs. Both sexes. From birth. Visual impairment, neural deafness, immobile facies, muscular weakness, accentuated spinal curvature, mental retardation.

Etiology. Unknown. Autosomal recessive trait.

Diagnostic Procedures. *Fundus oculi.* Tortuosity of retinal vessels, exudative retinitis.

Prognosis. Muscle disease progresses from childhood.

BIBLIOGRAPHY. Small RG: Coat's disease and muscular dystrophy. Trans Am Acad Ophthalmol Otolaryngol 72:225–231, 1968

SMITH–LEMLI–OPITZ

Synonyms. Cerebrohepatorenal. SLO, RSH.

Symptoms. Onset in fetal life. (Feeble fetal activity; at birth short stature.) Prevalent in males. Growth retardation; failure to thrive; mental retardation; vomiting in infancy.

Signs. Several combinations of the following features: short stature; moderate muscle hypertonicity or, more rarely, hypotonicity; microcephaly. Epicanthal folds; ptosis of eyelids; strabismus; broad nose; upturned nares; micrognathia; arched palate; posterior palatal cleft. Ear auricles low set, abnormal shape; small external canal. Hypospadias; cryptorchidism. Hands with horizontal upper palmar creases; dermal pattern 10/10 whorls; distal palmer axial triradius; short third fingers; short thumb and toes; cutaneous syndactyly of second and third toes; metatarsus adductus.

Etiology. Unknown; autosomal recessive inheritance.

Pathology. See Signs. Small brain, kidneys; duplication of pelvis; cortical renal cysts; congenital pyloric stenosis in some cases. Hepatomegaly; intrahepatic biliary dysgenesis. Congenital heart diseases may be associated.

Diagnostic Procedures. *Electroencephalography. X-ray. Chromosome studies.*

Therapy. Symptomatic.

Prognosis. Death from complications at early age. Survival to adulthood reported.

BIBLIOGRAPHY. Smith DW, Lemli L, Opitz JM: Newly recognized syndrome of multiple congenital anomalies. J Pediatr 64:210–217, 1964
Passarge E, McAdams AJ: Cerebrohepato-renal syndrome: A newly recognized hereditary disorder of multiple congenital defects, including sudanophilic leukodystrophy, cirrhosis of the liver and polycystic kidneys. J Pediatr 71:691–702, 1967
Fine RN, Gwin JL, Young EF: Smith–Lemli–Opitz syndrome, radiologic and postmortem findings. Am J Dis Child 115:483–488, 1968
Smith DH: Recognizable Patterns of Human Malformation. Philadelphia, WB Saunders, 1976
Greene C, Pitts W, Rosenfeld R et al: Smith–Lemli–Opitz syndrome in two 46 XY infants with female external genitalia. Clin Genet 25:366–372, 1984

SMITH'S (J.F.)

Synonyms. Smith's keratoacanthoma; Ferguson-Smith; epithelioma, self-healing, squamous; multiple keratoacanthomas; multiple molluscum sebaceum; multiple molluscum pseudocarcinomatosum.

Symptoms. Male-to-female ratio 3 : 1; onset in middle life. Asymptomatic or according to location (anus, scrotum, etc). On the face, less frequently on hands, back of wrists, and forearm, seldom on thighs and chest, rarely on anogenital areas: firm, round, reddish papules that rapidly enlarge and in 1 month reach to 1 to 2 cm in diameter; the center contains a horny plug, covered more or less by a crust. The lesion evolves or spontaneously resolves in 3 months.

Etiology. Unknown. Autosomal dominant inheritance. Relationship with keratoacanthoma (single) still uncertain.

Pathology. Intradermal tumors of symmetric, globular shape; the epidermis over lesions is thinned. Early lesion formed by multiplying squamous cells; central cells keratinize. Initially similar to a squamous cell carcinoma. In mature form, decrease of peripheral mitosis, enlarging of the core, invasion by inflammatory cells and opening like a flower leaving, finally, a scar.

Diagnostic Procedures. *Biopsy.*

Therapy. Curettage or excision. Radiotherapy. Trial with 13-cis-retinoic acid (teratogenic in pregnant women).

Prognosis. Benign. Spontaneous resolution or therapeutic resolution.

BIBLIOGRAPHY. Fergusson–Smith J: A case of multiple primary squamous celled carcinomata of the skin in a young man, with spontaneous healing. Br J Dermatol 46:267–272, 1934
Hayday RP, Reed ML, Dzubow LM et al: Treatment of keratoacanthomas with oral 13-cis-retinoic acid. N Engl J Med 303:560–562, 1980

SMITH'S (R.W.)

Synonym. Reversed Colles' fracture.

Symptoms. Pain in the wrist following fall on dorsum of flexed hand.

Signs. Tenderness. Spade handle deformity.

Pathology. Nonarticular fracture of distal radius with dorsal angulation and volar displacement.

Therapy. Open reduction seldom indicated except in young adult.

BIBLIOGRAPHY. Smith RW: Fractures of the Bones of the Fore-arm in the Vicinity of the Wrist Joint in His: A Treatise on Fracture in the Vicinity of Joint and on Certain Forms of Accidental and Congenital Dislocations, pp 129–175. Dublin, Hodges Smith, 1847
Sisk FD: Fractures in shoulder girdle and upper extremities. In Crenshaw AH (ed): Campbell's Operative Orthopedics, 7th ed, p 1828. St. Louis, CV Mosby, 1987

SMITH–THEILER–SCHACHENMANN

Synonyms. Cerebrocostomandibular; rib gap defects–micrognathia.

Symptoms. Both sexes affected; evident from birth. Mental handicap; severe unusual cough.

Signs. Palatal defect; micrognathia; severe costovertebral defect (rib segmentation—fusion of ribs to vertebrae). In one case, elbow hypoplasia, defect of sacrum and coccyx. In another, webbing of the neck and area of skin redundance.

Etiology. Unknown. Autosomal dominant or recessive inheritance.

Pathology. See Signs. Malformed tracheal cartilages.

Diagnostic Procedures. *X-ray of chest.* Deficiency of posterior portion of affected ribs (diagnostic).

Therapy. Symptomatic.

Prognosis. In most cases, early fatality.

BIBLIOGRAPHY. Smith DW, Theiler K, Schachenmann G: Rib-gap defect with micrognathia, malformed tracheal

cartilages, and redundant skin: A new pattern of defective development. J Pediatr 69:799–803, 1966
Langer LO, Herrmann J: The cerebrocostomandibular syndrome. Birth Defects 10:167–170, 1974
Schroer RJ, Meyer LC: Cerebro-costo-mandibular syndrome. Proc Greenwood Genet Center 4:55–59, 1985

SMOKER'S RESPIRATORY

Synonym. Tabagism.

Symptoms. Occur in smokers of all ages. Chronic condition with exacerbation after increase in smoking. Chronic pharyngitis; hoarseness; cough and expectoration; wheezing relieved by expectoration. Occasionally, dyspnea, chest constriction, and pain may be observed.

Signs. Those of chronic pharyngitis and bronchitis.

Etiology. Tobacco smoke.

Pathology. Chronic bronchitis and inflammatory changes and edema of pharynx and larynx.

Diagnostic Procedures. *X-ray of chest.*

Therapy. Eliminate cause (stop smoking). Antibiotics in acute stage.

Prognosis. Excellent if smoking is stopped.

BIBLIOGRAPHY. Fogg AH: Queries and minor notes: Allergy to tobacco smoke. JAMA 144:810–811, 1950
Waldbott GL: Smoker's respiratory syndrome: A clinical entity. JAMA 151:1398–1400, 1953
Hunninghake GW, Crystal RG: Cigarette smoking and lung destruction. Am J Respir Dis 128:833–838, 1983

SNEDDON–WILKINSON

Synonyms. Duhring–Sneddon–Wilkinson; subcorneal pustular dermatosis.

Symptoms and Signs. Predominantly in women (4 : 1); onset after 40 years of age. Seldom in children. Eruption of pustules in the groin, axillae, submammary areas, flexor surfaces of limbs, occasionally palms and soles. Face and mucosae spared. Erythema around pustules at onset. Pustules are usually oval, flaccid, turbid. They dry in a few days, leaving superficial crusts. Their grouping produces a serpiginous outline.

Etiology. Unknown; possibly a variant of Stevens–Johnson. Reported in association with IgA and IgG gammopathy pyoderma gangrenosum and ulcerative colitis.

Pathology. Subcorneal pustule, covered by thin keratin layer; base formed by granular tissue or prickle cells layer. In the fluid, many neutrophils and red cells, scanty eosinophils. Mild acanthosis; questionable acantholysis; no bacteria.

Diagnostic Procedures. *Biopsy.*

Therapy. Dapsone 100 mg a day. If gammopathy found vitamin A acid, and corticosteroid topically.

Prognosis. Benign condition of several years duration. Possible myeloma appearance in older patients.

BIBLIOGRAPHY. Sneddon IB, Wilkinson DS: Subcorneal postular dermatosis. Br J Dermatol 68:385–394, 1956
Sneddon IB, Wilkinson DS: Dermatose pustuleuse sous-cornée. Bull Soc Fr Dermatol Syph 64:226–233, 1957
Rook A, Wilkinson DS, Ebling FJG et al: Textbook of Dermatology, 4th ed, pp 1659–1661. Oxford, Blackwell Scientific Publications, 1986

SOLAR ELASTOSIS SYNDROMES

Synonyms. Actinodermatosis; chronic lucite.

Symptoms. Both sexes; occurring usually at late age (fourth decade) in people subjected to prolonged exposure to the sun.

Signs. May be different and combinations have been designed by various eponyms:
1. *Acrokeratoelastosis.* Small, warty papules, yellowish or pinkish, in narrow bands; occasionally, telangiectasic at the border or palmodorsal skin of hand, from tip of thumb to radial side of index finger.
2. *Debreuilh's.* Yellow plaques, more or less marginated on face or neck.
3. *Favre-Racouchot.* See.
4. *Jadassohn's cutis rhomboidalis nuchal.* Skin of back of neck thickened by yellowish infiltration subdivided by furrows in a networklike pattern; occasionally lesion extends to the sides and upper chest.
5. *Milian's citron skin.* Yellowish thickening and wrinkling of the skin.
6. *Path's.* Multiple keratotic lesions of the skin with pattern similar to squamous carcinomas; spontaneously disappear.

Etiology. Sun exposure; trauma; possibly, genetic factors also involved.

Pathology. Elastotic degeneration of collagen.

Therapy. Sunscreens for susceptible persons.

BIBLIOGRAPHY. Debreuilh MW: De la melanose circonscrite precancereuse. Ann Dermatol Syph (Paris) 3:129–151, 205–230, 1912
Milian G, Manson M: Erytheme polymorphe photobiotrophique avec localization préternale. Bull Soc Fr Dermatol 39:651–652, 1932

Path DD: Tumorlike keratosis: Report of a case. Arch Dermatol 39:228–238, 1936

Rook A, Wilkinson DS, Ebling FJG et al: Textbook of Dermatology, 4th ed, pp 1847–1848. Oxford, Blackwell Scientific Publications, 1986

SOLITARY HUNTER

Synonyms. Lonely hunter; pain-prone; psychogenic pain. See Women who fall syndrome.

Symptoms. Average age at onset 28 years. Intractable pain, not organic, with evidence of psychogenic nature; solitary hunting; conflict over the expression of aggression and depression; tendency to drive fast cars; accident proneness; unrealistic ambitions and problem with work.

Etiology. Patients with this syndrome do not belong to any definite psychiatric category. Character disorders with problems of impulse, control, and conversion symptoms. Hunting and solitude may be considered defense against murderous impulses. Pain as atonement for guilt feeling. Different clinical syndromes (masochism, pain proneness, phantom limb pain, primary atypical facial neuralgia, and some painful posttraumatic states) belong (with others) to this entity, (psychogenic pain).

Therapy. Difficult; positive approach and showing that pains are real; cautious referral to psychiatrist. Hospitalization may be necessary.

Prognosis. Progressively unable to perform work, and progressive depression.

BIBLIOGRAPHY. Engel GL: "Psychogenic" pain and the pain-prone patient. Am J Med 26:899–918, 1959

Tinling DC, Klein RF: Psychogenic pain and aggression: The syndrome of solitary hunter. Psychosom Med 28:738–748, 1966

Freedman AM, Kaplan HI, Sadock BJ: Comprehensive Textbook of Psychiatry, 2nd ed, p 1704. Baltimore, Williams & Wilkins, 1975

SOLUTE LOADING–HYPERTONICITY

Synonym. Water loss-solute excess.

Symptoms and Signs. The same as in pure water depletion syndrome with two exceptions: (1) Patient gains, instead of loses, weight. (2) Patient is polyuric with low specific gravity urine instead of oliguric.

Etiology and Pathology. Nasogastric feeding with inadequate water. Bleeding ulcer patient treated with milk and alkali, without adequate water. Infants fed with too-concentrated milk. Diabetic with polyuria or when over-treated with unnecessary electrolyte replacement and insulin.

Diagnostic Procedures. *Urine.* Polyuria with low specific gravity.

Therapy. The same as in pure water depletion syndrome (see) plus the correction of iatrogenic causes.

Prognosis. If condition not recognized and treated early, death occurs.

BIBLIOGRAPHY. Goldberger E: A Primer of Water, Electrolyte, and Acid-base Syndromes, 3rd ed. Philadelphia, Lea & Febiger, 1965

Jamison RL, Kritz W: Urinary Concentrating Mechanisms. Oxford Univ Press, 1972

SOMATOSTATINOMA

Symptoms and Signs. Rare. Malabsorption and steatorrhea. Weight loss.

Etiology. Tumor producing somatostatin (tetradecapeptide) substance with neurocrine or paracrine activity: suppression of secretion of growth hormone, of thyrotropin, and inhibition of numerous intestinal endocrine and exocrine functions (all intestinal hormones release). It is produced by the D cells of pancreas and gut and found in ganglia and nerve cells of intestine. May be also associated with other endocrine tumor of gastroenteropancreatic axis.

Pathology. The presence of elevated somatostatin in insulinoma and gastrinoma may be evidenced by immunohistochemical staining. Frequently metastatic at time of discovery.

Diagnostic Procedures. *Blood.* Diabetes mellitus (nonketotic). Somatostatic levels increased (RIA methodology). *X-ray.* Cholelithiasis and gallbladder reduced contractility. *Gastric juice.* Hypochlorhydria, decreased gastrin release. *Stool.* Steatorrhea, evidence of exocrine pancreatic secretion.

Therapy. Surgery with tumor debulking, followed by chemotherapy.

BIBLIOGRAPHY. Larson LI, Holst JJ, Kuhl C et al: Pancreatic somatostatinoma: Clinical features and physiological implications. Lancet 1:666–668, 1977

Ganda OP, Weir GC, Soeldner JS et al: Somatostatinoma. A somatostatin-containing tumor of the endocrine pancreas. N Engl J Med 296:963–967, 1977

Pipellers D, Couturier E, Gepts W: Five cases of somatostatinoma: Clinical heterogeneity and diagnostic usefulness of basal and tolbutamide induced hypersomatostatinemia. J Clin Endocrinol 56:1236–1242, 1983

SORIANO'S (M.)

Synonym. Periostitis deformans. See Leri–Joanny.

Symptoms and Signs. Both sexes affected. Recurrent pains in areas of bone where the formation of pseudotumoral masses occurs. The attack may recur several times. During more severe episodes anorexia and general debilitation may be associated.

Etiology. Unknown.

Pathology. Hyperplastic osteogenic osteoperiostitis.

Diagnostic Procedures. *X-ray of bones.*

Therapy. Analgesics.

Prognosis. In 2 to 12 months, regression of the masses. Each individual attack is less severe than the previous one.

BIBLIOGRAPHY. Soriano M: Periostitis deformans. Ann Rheum Dis 11:154–161, 1952

SORSBY'S I

Synonyms. Macular hereditary coloboma. Coloboma of macula–brachydactyly B. See also Laurence–Moon and Biemond's.

Symptoms. Both sexes affected; onset from birth. Reduced visual acuity.

Signs. *Hands and feet.* Dystrophy; rudimentary or absent nails of index fingers; bifurcation of distal phalanges of thumbs; absence of big toes; hallux valgus. *Face.* Cleft palate. *Eye.* Hyperopia; nystagmus; bilateral macular colobomas with variable pigmentation and sharp borderline.

Etiology. Autosomal dominant inheritance.

Pathology. See Signs. Kidney aplasia. Chondrocytes surrounded by densely packed staining material.

Therapy. Symptomatic.

Prognosis. Poor.

BIBLIOGRAPHY. Sorsby A: Congenital coloboma of the macula; together with an account of the familial occurrence of bilateral macular coloboma in association with apical dystrophy of hands and feet. Br Ophthalmol 19:65–90, 1935
Smith RD, Fineman RM, Sillence et al: Congenital macular colobomas and short-limb skeletal dysplasia. Am J Med Genet 5:365–371, 1980

SORSBY'S II

Synonym. Fundus dystrophy–pseudoinflammatory.

Symptoms and Signs. Both sexes affected. Onset in third and fourth decades of life, occasionally in fifth decade. Visual trouble with clouding of central vision, first in one eye and then in the other one. Fundus shows hemorrhages and exudates on central areas, with scar and pigmentary deposits; eventually, evolution into choroid atrophy with disappearance of vessels.

Etiology. Unknown; autosomal dominant inheritance.

BIBLIOGRAPHY. Sorsby A et al: A fundus dystrophy with unusual features (late onset and dominant inheritance of a central retinal lesion showing oedema, haemorrhage and exudates developing into generalized choroidal atrophy with massive pigment proliferation). Br J Ophthalmol 33:67–100, 1949
Kalmus H, Seedburgh D: Probable common origin of a hereditary fundus dystrophy (Sorsby's familial) pseudoinflammatory macular dystrophy in an English and Australian family. J Med Genet 13:271–276, 1976

SOTOS'

Synonym. Cerebral gigantism in childhood.

Symptoms and Signs. Both sexes. Birth weight and length greater than normal; accelerated growth during the first 4 to 5 years of life; then growth seems to approach normal, remaining, however, two standard deviations above means for chronologic age. Macrocrania, dolichocephaly; prognathism; hypertelorism; antimongoloid obliquity of palpebral fissures; characterizing facies; high-arched palate; mental retardation; clumsiness or ataxia. Occasionally, obesity, convulsions, abnormal dermatoglyphic pattern.

Etiology. Unknown; possibly, pathogenic mechanism operating in uterus or impaired function of hypothalamic-pituitary axis. Failure of growth hormone to rise following hypoglycemia. Possibly, variant of Lawrence–Seip and Russell's syndromes. The three forms are parts of the same spectrum. Most cases sporadic; autosomal dominant inheritance reported.

Pathology. See Signs.

Diagnostic Procedures. *CT brain scan.* Dilated ventricular system (mainly lateral and third). *Chromosome studies.* Normal. *Oral glucose tolerance test.* Abnormal in some cases; fasting plasma growth hormone levels normal. Increase of 17-ketosteroids; normal OHCS. *Electroencephalography.* Abnormal.

Therapy. Symptomatic.

Prognosis. Generally, good health after childhood. Problem of social adjustment due to aggressiveness.

BIBLIOGRAPHY. Sotos JF, Dodge PR, Muirhead D et al: Cerebral gigantism in childhood, a syndrome of excessively rapid growth with acromegalic features and a nonprogressive neurologic disorder. New Engl J Med 271:109–116, 1964

Stephenson JN, Mellinger RC, Manson G: Cerebral gigantism. Pediatrics 41:130–138, 1968

Bale AE, Drum MA, Parry DM et al: Familial Sotos syndrome (cerebral gigantism): Craniocephalic and psychological characteristics. Am J Med Genet 20:613–624, 1985

Beermer F, Veenema H, De Pater JM: Cerebral gigantism (Sotos syndrome) in two patients with Fra (X) chromosomes. Am J Med Genet 23:221–226, 1986

Verloes A, Sacré J–P, Guebelle F: Sotos syndrome and fragile X chromosomes. Lancet II: 329, 1987

SPAET–DAMESHEK

Synonym. Chronic hypoplastic neutropenia.

Symptoms. Onset between 14 and 67 years of age. Repeated severe, prolonged infections of the skin, mouth, throat, ears, paranasal sinuses, and lungs.

Signs. No characteristics except for scar of previous infections; splenomegaly of moderate degree.

Etiology. Unknown; bone marrow selective (neutrophil) hypoplasia.

Diagnostic Procedures. *Blood.* Severe neutropenia; almost constant monocytosis. Only occasionally, moderate anemia, and thrombocytopenia. *Bone marrow.* Marked selective granulocytic hypoplasia. Other series normal.

Therapy. Antibiotics. This neutropenia is not affected by splenectomy, corticosteroids, adrenocorticotropic hormone (ACTH), and immunosuppressive agents.

Prognosis. Good; extremely chronic condition, very lengthy course.

BIBLIOGRAPHY. Hattersley PG: Chronic neutropenia. Report of case not cured by splenectomy. Blood 2:227–234, 1947

Spaet TH, Dameshek W: Chronic hypoplastic neutropenia. Am J Med 13:35–45, 1952

Wintrobe MM (ed): Clinical Hematology, 8th ed, p 1330. Philadelphia, Lea & Febiger, 1981

SPAHR'S

Synonyms. Metaphyseal dysplasia (type A·1); metaphyseal dysostosis (type A·1).

Symptoms and Signs. Marked bowing of legs.

Etiology. Possibly autosomal recessive inheritance.

Therapy. If needed, osteotomy.

BIBLIOGRAPHY. Spahr A, Spahr–Hartmann I: Dysostose metaphisaire familiale étude de 4 cas dans une fratrie. Helv Paediatr Acta 16:836–849, 1961

Bailey JA: Disproportionate Short Stature: Diagnosis and Management, p 273. Philadelphia, WB Saunders, 1973

SPANLANG–TAPPEINER

Synonyms. Alopecia–hyperhidrosis–corneal dystrophy; keratosis palmoplantaris–corneal dystrophy.

Symptoms and Signs. Both sexes affected; onset between 5 and 20 years. Alopecia partial, total, or localized; nail dystrophy; hyperkeratosis of palms and soles. Teeth normal, visual impairment because of tongue-shaped corneal opacities.

Etiology. Unknown; autosomal dominant inheritance.

BIBLIOGRAPHY. Unna PG: Über das Keratoma Palmare et Plantare Heretitatium. Vjschr Dermatol 15:231, 1883

Spanlang H: Beiträge zur Klinik und Pathologie seltener Hornhauterkrankungen (Dystrophia adiposa corneal, Dystker atosis corneae congenital). Z Augenheilk 62:21–41, 1927

Stevanovic DV: Alopecia congenita: The incomplete dominant form of inheritance with varying expressivity. Acta Genet 9:127–132, 1959

Rook A, Wilkinson DS, Ebling FJG et al: Textbook of Dermatology, 4th ed. Oxford, Blackwell Scientific Publications, 1986

SPASMODIC LAUGHTER

Synonyms. Forced laughter; Homeric laughter; sham mirth.

Symptoms. Uncontrollable laughter without the emotion of pleasure (mirthless): spontaneous or following different slight stimulations that normally arouse no emotional response, such as pointing the finger or a normal sound.

Etiology. It must be considered a symptom more than a syndrome. It is observed in the following conditions: multiple sclerosis; pseudobulbar palsy; epilepsy; intracranial hemorrhages; after premotor lobotomy. May be caused by release of paleothalamus from phylogenetically younger thalamic structures, suprasegmental, frontal cerebral cortex. Observed also in Kuru (see).

Pathology. Severe diffuse organic brain lesions. See Etiology.

Prognosis. Poor; bad omen symptoms.

BIBLIOGRAPHY. Homer: Iliad and Odyssey: "an unextinguished laugher shakes the skies."
Martin JP: Fits of laughter (sham mirth) in organic cerebral disease. Brain 73:453–464, 1950
Vick NA: Grinker's Neurology, 7th ed. Springfield, CC Thomas, 1976

SPASMODIC TORTICOLLIS

Synonym. Wry neck.

Symptoms. Both sexes affected. The head is suddenly intermittently pulled and turned to one side. Slight movement at first gradually increasing in intensity. Emotions, stress, make them more severe. During sleep, movements cease. With time muscle may become permanently contracted and the head deviated to one side. With special maneuver the patient may decrease or stop movements. See also Torticollis.

Signs. Contraction and hypertrophy of muscles involved (especially sternocleidomastoid, posterior, and lateral muscles of neck, upper part of trapezii).

Etiology. Unknown; as localized dystonia part of the dystonic lenticular syndrome; as sequela of chronic encephalitis.

Therapy. Psychotherapy does not help. Supporting padded collar of some help. Section of intraspinal portion of spinal accessory nerves and upper three or four anterior roots of spinal cord gives good results.

Prognosis. Usually progressing; 10% show involvement of other muscles of body; may become static or spontaneously regress.

BIBLIOGRAPHY. Poppen JL, Martinez–Niochet A: Spasmodic torticollis. Clin North Am 31:883–890, 1951
Adams RD, Victor M: Principles of Neurology, 3rd ed, pp 85–86, 882–883. New York, McGraw-Hill, 1985

SPASMUS NUTANS

Symptoms. Both sexes affected; onset between 6 and 18 months. Aggravated by cold weather. Rhythmic movements of the head in the upright position associated with rapid, horizontal bilateral nystagmus. Attempt at gaze fixation intensifies manifestations. During sleep, it disappears.

Etiology. Unknown.

Prognosis. Spontaneous disappearance by the age of 3 or 4 years; in this period remission and relapses possible. No residue.

BIBLIOGRAPHY. Vick NA: Grinker's Neurology, 7th ed. Springfield, CC Thomas, 1976

SPIEGHEL'S

Synonyms. Spiegelian hernia, hernia Spieghel's.

Symptoms and Signs. Pain of hernia site, usually above level of the inferior epigastric vessels level on the linea semilunaris. Pain is enhanced by increase in intraabdominal pressure. The mass is made more evident with patient standing and straining, and may disappear with gurgling sound on pressure, thus allowing the palpation of the orifice. Occasionally the mass is not evident.

Etiology. Acquired condition.

Diagnostic Procedures. *Ultrasound* and *CT scan*.

Therapy. Aponeurotic repair of the orifice.

Prognosis. High incidence of incarceration. Good with repair.

BIBLIOGRAPHY. Spieghel A: Opera quae extore omnia, p 103. Amsterdam, John Bloew, 1645
Spangen L: Spieghelian hernia. Surg Clin North Am 64:351–366, 1984

SPIEGLER–FENDT

Synonyms. Bäfverstedt's, Kaposi–Spiegler; lymphadenosis benigna cutis; miliary lymphocytoma.

Symptoms and Signs. Prevalent in females (3 : 1); onset any age (more frequently second and third decades). *Variety 1.* Circumscribed lymphocytoma cutis. No systemic symptoms, except secondary to lesion displacing genitourinary structures. One or several purple yellowish, rubbery, elevated nodules, usually appearing on the face (60%), earlobes, and tip of nose. Nipple, scrotum, vagina less frequently affected. Regional lymph nodes seldom enlarged; no splenomegaly. *Variety 2.* Miliary eruption of several bluish nodules on face, trunk, and limbs. Itching especially in summer months. No lymph node or spleen enlargement.

Etiology. Benign hyperplasia of reticuloendothelial tissue of the skin. Trauma, insect bite, photosensitivity among precipitating causes.

Pathology. Lymphocyte infiltration of dermis separated from epidermis by normal connective tissue. Occasionally assuming a follicular pattern. Eosinophil accumulation at the periphery (occasional).

Diagnostic Procedures. *Biopsy. Blood.* Normal.

Therapy. Radiotherapy (effects not substantiated). Topical steroids for miliary lesions.

Prognosis. Good response to treatment. Circumscribed form may disappear spontaneously. Generalized form may persist for life or regress and relapse, without affecting general health or life expectancy.

BIBLIOGRAPHY. Spiegler E: Ueber die sogenannte Sarkomatosis cutis. Arch Dermatol Syph 27:163–174, 1894
Fendt H: Beiträge zur Kenntnis der sogenannten sarcoiden Geswülsteder Haut. Arch Dermatol Syph 53:213–242, 1900
Höfer W: Lymphadenosis benigna cutis. Arch Klin Exp Dermatol 203:23–40, 1956
Rook A, Wilkinson DS, Ebling FJG et al: Textbook of Dermatology, 4th ed, pp 1713–1716. Oxford, Blackwell Scientific Publications, 1986

SPILLER'S

Synonyms. Charcot–Joffroy; epidural ascending paralysis; hypertrophic spinal meningitis. Obsolete. See also Erb–Charcot.

Symptoms and Signs. Severe pain in the neck, back of the head, upper shoulder, chest, and arms; enhanced by movement of the neck. Atrophy and fasciculation of muscles of those regions develop in weeks or months. Hyporeflexia or areflexia of tendons of arms and hands first; later weakness and spasticity of legs and sensory loss below level of lesions. Vasomotor and atrophic changes, and sphincter insufficiency may develop.

Etiology. Nonspecific etiology; syphilis in some cases.

Pathology. Granulomatous infiltration of dura mater usually of the cervical region, sometimes of thoracic region. Roots of cervical cord constricted and inflamed.

Diagnostic Procedures. *Lumbar puncture.* Complete, partial or no block of spinal subarachnoid space. *Myelography, electromyography.*

Therapy. Extirpation of dura mater from posterior portion of affected part.

Prognosis. Dramatic improvement if treatment is not delayed.

BIBLIOGRAPHY. Charcot JM, Joffroy A: Deux cas d'atrophie musculaire progressive avec lésions de la substance grise et des faisceaux antérolatéraux de la moelle épinière. Arch Physiol 2:354–367, 1869
Spiller WG: Epidural ascending spinal paralysis. Rev Neurol Psychiatry 9:494–498, 1911
Vick NA: Grinker's Neurology, 7th ed. Springfield, CC Thomas, 1976

SPINAL CHRONIC ARACHNOIDITIS

Synonyms. Hypertrophic cervical pachymeningitis; arachnoiditis spinal; meningitis circumscripta spinalis.

Symptoms and Signs. Insidious onset. Pain, weakness, sensorimotor loss (paralysis, paresthesias) involving lower extremities asymmetrically, then ascending. Prominent fasciculation.

Etiology. It follows one of the chronic infective processes; or occasionally, after intrathecal injection. A family with autosomal inheritance of this syndrome reported (analogy with Peyronie's and Dupuytren's proposed).

Pathology. Fibrous tissue proliferation in delimited areas or diffused with chronic type of inflammatory reactions. Interference with cerebrospinal fluid flow.

Diagnostic Procedures. *Blood.* Leukocytosis. *Cerebrospinal fluid.* Partial or complete spinal block; xanthochromia or Froin's syndrome (see); increased proteins. *Myelography.* May reveal single or multiple locations of process.

Therapy. No effective medical or surgical treatment. Corticosteriods not beneficial.

Prognosis. Progressing condition.

BIBLIOGRAPHY. Winkelman NW, Eckel JL: Focal lesions of the spinal cord due to vascular disease. JAMA 99:1919–1926, 1932
Duke RJ, Hashimoto SA: Familial spinal arachnoiditis: A new entity. Arch Neurol 30:300–303, 1974
Adams RD, Victor M: Principles of Neurology, 3rd ed, pp 683–684. New York, McGraw-Hill, 1985

SPINAL CORD INJURY-PROGRESSIVE CONFUSIONAL

Symptoms. Occur in patients with fracture of cervical vertebrae and in nontraumatic injury of spinal cord. Mental symptoms: loss of memory; hallucination; delirium.

Signs. Those of spinal cord lesion. In some patients, circulation appears to fail before respiration (opposite to posterior fossa compression, see); slight cyanosis.

Etiology. Unknown; previously considered as result of cerebral contusion. Interruption of vasomotor pathways and sensory tracts in nontraumatic cases.

Pathology. Traumatic or pathologic fractures of vertebrae, hematomyelia, or sarcoma and other pathology of spinal cord. Atelectasis of lungs.

Diagnostic Procedures. X-ray. Spinal tap.

Therapy. Symptomatic. Corticosteroids, naloxone. If compression, surgery.

Prognosis. All patients who developed this syndrome died shortly after.

BIBLIOGRAPHY. Putnam T: The progressive confusional syndrome following injuries to cervical portion of the spinal cord. Science 86:542–543, 1937

SPINAL SHOCK

Synonyms. Riddock's, including "autonomic dysreflexia."

Symptoms and Signs. All ages. After spinal cord injury. Clinically divided in two stages:
Areflexia. The symptomatology present in this stage is of variable degree from fully manifested or minimal. All neural elements below the lesion fail. Tetraplegia (if lesion at C4–C5 segments); paraplegia (if lesion at thoracic level); accompanied by bladder (overflow incontinence) and bowel paralytic ileus, atonic paralysis, gastric atony; sensory loss, muscular flaccidity; loss of reflexes, loss of autonomic activity (sweating, vasomotor, tone, etc). Skin pale and dry, decubital ulcerations; depression of genital reflexes.
Hyperreflexic activity. After a few weeks reflexes return and become gradually stronger and finally exaggerated up to flexor spasms "mass reflex" elicited by stimulation, variety of paresthesias or dull pain. Above lesion successively may develop the "autonomic dysreflexia" syndrome: episodic response to specific stimuli (*i.e.,* distended bladder) or exaggerated sweating, flushing, headache, blood hypertension, bradycardia.

Etiology. Spinal trauma.

Pathology. Functional (edema) or anatomic interruption of corticospinal tracts.

Therapy. Usually symptomatic and conservative. Avoid movement especially flexion and traction (surgical fixation may be adopted in a second stage) or early decompression may be adopted. Spinal cord cooling. In acute phase: corticosteroids, naloxone; endogenous opiate antagonists, bladder catheterization, enemas. In chronic phase: physiotherapy according to evaluation.

Prognosis. Complete areflexia duration varies from hours to permanent. In the majority minimal activity returns within 1 to 6 weeks. Paresis and hyperreflexic activity duration extremely variable according to intensity of trauma and treatment.

BIBLIOGRAPHY. Riddock G: The reflex functions of the completely divided spinal cord in men, compared with less severe lesions. Brain 40:264, 1917
Guttman L: Spinal Cord Injuries: Comprehensive Management and Research. Oxford, Blackwell Scientific Publications, 1976
Albin MS, Babinski MF: Acute cervical spinal cord injuries. In Repin M, Tinker J (eds): Care of the Critically Ill Patient, p 653. New York, Springer-Verlag, 1983

SPIRA'S

Synonym. Fluorine toxicity.

Symptoms and Signs. Onset in late childhood to early adulthood. Mottling or brown discoloration of teeth. Nausea; anorexia; vomiting; constipation. In older patients, possibly, stiffness, rheumatalgia. Osteosclerotic changes in the skeleton and rarely central nervous system involvement.

Etiology. Fluoride chronic intoxication from water, food, dust (in cryolite mines), or dusts and vapors (industry and agriculture).

Pathology. Hypoplasia of dental enamel and defective bone calcification.

Therapy. None specific. Cessation of exposure or consumption.

Prognosis. Rheumatalgia and stiffness may regress. Teeth lesions remain.

BIBLIOGRAPHY. Spira D: Br Med Rev 5:61, 1928
Dean HT: Chronic endemic fluorosis. JAMA 107:1269–1273, 1936
Hodge HC, Smith FA: Biological effects of inorganic fluorides. In Simons SH (ed): Fluorine Chemistry, Vol 4. New York, Academic Press, 1965
Hodge HC, Smith FA: Occupational fluoride exposure. J Occup Med 19:12–39, 1977

SPLIT NOTOCHORD

Synonyms. See Meckel–Gruber. Includes the malformation previously reported as posterior enteric sinus, posterior enteric cyst, posterior spina bifida, diastematomyelia or diplomyelia, anterior spina bifida, prevertebral enteric cyst, rachischisis. Caudal dysplasia, see Mermaid.

Symptoms. Variable according to nature and extent of malformation.

Signs. Posterior enteric cysts or sinuses; small protrusion of distal end of the intestine dorsal to the split vertebrae. Split spine without herniation of alimentary canal observed.

Etiology. Unknown. Autosomal dominant inheritance reported.

Pathology. See Synonyms and Signs.

Diagnostic Procedures. X-ray.

Therapy. Surgery when feasible.

Prognosis. Several of the manifestations of this syndrome compatible with life, but syndrome often fatal.

BIBLIOGRAPHY. Meckel JR: Beschreibung zweier durch sehrähnliche Bildungsabweichung entstellter Geschwister. Dtsch Arch Phys 7:99–172, 1822

Gruber GB: Zur Frage der neurenterischen Offnung bei Früchten mit vollkommener Wirbelspaltung. Z Anat Entwicklungsgesch 80:433–453, 1926

Denes J, Gonti J, Leb J: Dorsal herniation of gut: A rare manifestation of the split notochord syndrome. J Pediatr Surg 2:359–363, 1967

Welch JP, Alterman K: The syndrome of caudal dysplasia: A review, including etiologic considerations and evidence of heterogeneity. Pediatr Pathol 2:313–327, 1984

SPOTTED LEG

Symptoms and Signs. Occur in diabetic patients; onset at a mean age of 50 to 60 years. Most patients showing evidence of neuropathy or retinopathy or both. A few or many bilateral, asymmetric, round or oval, circumscribed, shallow lesions covered by atrophic, shiny, pigmented skin. Lesions not painful, not ulcerated. Distributed over anterior, lateral, and medial aspects of legs below the knees. Patient aware of lesions; no recollection of trauma; usually ignores them and does not call the physician's attention to them. Associated neuropathy of hypoesthesia type and diminished or absent reflexes.

Etiology. Manifestation of vascular disease in diabetes; possibly, trauma a factor in the development of lesions.

Pathology. Atrophy of epidermis; slight fibrosis; separation of collagen fibers of dermis; pigmentation due to hemosiderin and increased evidence of melanin (because of atrophy). Abnormal capillaries with thick walls and obliteration of lumen.

Therapy. Diabetes treatment. Surgery with distal revascularization gives good results.

Prognosis. That of diabetes and its complications.

BIBLIOGRAPHY. Melin H: An atrophic circumscribed skin lesion in the lower extremities of diabetics. Acta Med Scand 176 [Suppl 423]. 1–75, 1964

Murphy RA: Skin lesions in diabetic patients: the "spotted leg" syndrome. Lahey Clin Found Bull 14:10–14, 1965

SPRANGER'S

Synonyms. Geleophysic dwarfism; mucopolysaccharidoses variant.

Symptoms. Present from birth. Unusual, pleasant, and happy face; dwarfism. Dysostosis: multiflexlike alteration primarily involving the hands and feet. Frequently evidence of cardiac valvulopathies.

Etiology. Unknown; autosomal recessive inheritance. Possibly, a variant of mucopolysaccharidosis.

Pathology. Heart valves. Striking abnormalities. Focal accumulation of mucopolysaccharides in the liver and cardiovascular system.

Therapy. Symptomatic. Heart valve prothesis.

Prognosis. Poor. Death in infancy.

BIBLIOGRAPHY. Vanace PW, Friedman S, Wagner BM: Mitral stenosis in an atypical case of gargoylism: A case report with pathologic and histochemical studies of the cardiac tissues. Circulation 21:80–98, 1960

Spranger JW, Filbert EF, Tuffli GA et al: Geleophysic dwarfism: A "focal" mucopolysaccharidosis? Lancet 2:97–98, 1960

Koiffman CP, Wajntal A, Uzsich MJM et al: Familial recurrence of geleophysic dysplasia. Am J Med Genet 19:483–486, 1984

SPRENGEL'S

Synonyms. High scapula congenita; shoulder elevation.

Symptoms and Signs. One scapula (seldom both) short in vertical axis and wider in transverse and closer to the midline than the other one. Retracted during movement, except when fixed to thoracic spine or ribs. Because of this malformation, the shoulder on affected side is elevated and advanced. Scoliosis is frequently present, and torticollis may occasionally be associated. Abduction of shoulder beyond 90 degrees is impossible.

Etiology. Unknown. Autosomal dominant inheritance.

Pathology. Bands of connective tissue or bony bridge between scapula and ribs or spine. Trapezius or serratus magnus muscle may be replaced by connective tissue.

Diagnostic Procedures. *X-ray.*

Therapy. None, or attempted orthopedic correction.

Prognosis. Nonprogressive condition.

BIBLIOGRAPHY. Sprengel: Die angeborene Verschiebung des Schulterblattes nach oben. Arch Klin Chir Berl 42:545–549, 1891
Hodgson SV, Chin DC: Dominant transmission of Sprengel's shoulder and cleft palate. J Med Genet 18:263–265, 1981

SPRUE, TROPICAL

Synonyms. Aphthae tropical; Ceylon sore mouth; Cochin China diarrhea; tropical diarrhea; Hill diarrhea.

Symptoms. More common in certain tropical and subtropical regions, affecting particularly recently immigrated Caucasians. Onset usually insidious. Explosive diarrhea with foul smelling, bulky, pale, greasy, frothy stools during day and night. Weight loss; nausea; vomiting; anorexia; paresthesia; pain in the mouth and anal region; disinterest in self and surroundings.

Signs. Pallor; cheilosis; stomatitis; aphthae; glossitis with smooth, beefy red tongue; teeth partially or totally absent; bleeding manifestations; moderate to severe wasting; premature aging; hair dry. Heart frequently small; hypotension; abdomen protuberant (especially on standing). Liver smooth, soft, easily palpable, but not enlarged. Neurologic examination in some cases: Lichtheim's syndrome (see).

Etiology. Unknown. Possibly, specific infectious agent not yet clearly identified. It could be the alpha-Prototheca partoricensis in zygote form.

Pathology. External and internal wasting with disappearance of fat deposits, viscera reduced in size and weight. Intestinal villi shortened and thick; tendency to fuse together; blunted edematous free margins. Infiltration of mucosa with inflammatory cells, especially eosinophils.

Diagnostic Procedures. *Blood.* Macrocytic anemia; leukopenia; moderate or severe thrombocytopenia; occasionally, hypoprothrombinemia; hypocholesterolemia; hypoproteinemia; hyperbilirubinemia. Serum iron normal; liver function usually normal. *Bone marrow.* Megaloblastosis; giant metamyelocytes. *Gastric fluid.* Anacidity. Cytologic changes similar to those of pernicious anemia. *Stool.* See Symptoms. Increase in fatty acids. Vitamin A tolerance curve, flat curve, D-xylose test generally depressed. *X-ray.* Sprue pattern. *Biopsy of small intestine.* See Pathology.

Therapy. Folic acid (15 mg/day); vitamin supplement; antibiotics. Diet complete and compatible with diet to which the patient was previously accustomed. Vitamin B_{12} (parenteral). Treatment of symptomatic complications or other coexisting conditions (*e.g.,* parasistosis).

Prognosis. Excellent recovery following treatment; maintenance treatment necessary. Most sprue patients remain lean. Without treatment, poor prognosis.

BIBLIOGRAPHY. Ketelaer V: Commentarius medicus, de aphthis nostratibus, seu Belgarum sprouw. Ludg Bat, 1672
Hillary W, Severini A: Observations on the Changes of the Air, and the Concomitant Epidemical Diseases in the Island of Barbados, 2nd ed, p 103. London, Hawkes, Clarke, and Collins, 1766
Klipstein FA: Tropical sprue in travelers and expatriates living abroad. Gastroenterology 80:590–600, 1981
Tier JS: Celiac sprue. In Sleisenger MH, Fortrau JS (eds): Gastrointestinal Disease. Pathophysiology, Diagnosis, Management, 3rd ed, pp 1050–1067. Philadelphia, WB Saunders, 1983

SRB'S

Synonym. Costosternal malformation.

Symptoms and Signs. Present from birth. Neuralgic pains of scapulohumeral girdle. Aplasia and synostosis of first two ribs; horniform protrusion of manubrium; secondary atrophy of muscles supplied by first two thoracic nerves; local venous congestion.

Etiology. Unknown.

Diagnostic Procedures. *X-ray.* See Symptoms and Signs.

Therapy. Surgical decompression of nerves and blood vessels.

BIBLIOGRAPHY. Srb J: Ueber Missbildung en der ersten Rippe. Med Jahrb Wien 5:75, 1862–65
Wenz W, Geipert G: Röntgenologie und Klinik der erbschen rippen-sternum anomalie. Radiologie 7:53–58, 1967

STANESCU'S

Synonyms. Osteochondrosis–osteopetrosis. Craniofacial dystosis–Diaphyseal hyperplasia. See also Maroteaux–Lamy II.

Symptoms. Present from birth; both sexes affected. Slow growth. Normal intelligence and normal fertility.

Signs. Small stature (short limbs especially, upper arms and hands). Brachycephaly; depression at frontoparietal sutures; exophthalmos; narrow maxilla; small mandible; crowded teeth. Possible: exostoses; fractures.

Etiology. Autosomal dominant inheritance.

Pathology. Osteopetrosis.

Diagnostic Procedures. *X-ray.* Bone tends to become denser with age and to show thick cortex. Diaphyseal hyperplasia. Thin skull. Occasionally, sacralization S1.

Therapy. None.

Prognosis. Good *quoad vitam.*

BIBLIOGRAPHY. Stanescu V, Maximilian C, Poenaru S et al: Syndrome héréditaire dominant, réussissant une dyostose cranio-faciale de type particulier, une insuffisance de croissance d'aspect chondrodystrophique et un épaississement massif de la corticale des os longs. Rev Fr Endocrinol Clin 4:219–231, 1963
Dipierri JE, Guzman JD: A second family with autosomal dominant osteosclerosis typical Stanescu. Am J Med Genet 18:13–18, 1984

STAPHYLOCOCCAL SCALDED SKIN

Synonyms. SSSS; Lyell's; Debré-Lamy-Lyell; dermatitis medicomentosa; acute toxic epidermolysis; epidermolysis necroticans combustiformis; bullous erythroderma epidermolysis; Fuchs-Lyell (drug reaction variety); Fuchs-Salzmann-Terrier; toxic epidermal necrolysis; scalded skin. All the synonyms have been used to indicate a generalized erythema-inflammation-necrosis of epidermis following a bullous phase. Today two different syndromes have been classified: the Ritter's (see) that represents the proper Staphylococcal scalded syndrome and the Toxic epidermal necrolysis.

BIBLIOGRAPHY. Fuchs E: Ueber Knoechenfoermige Hornhautruebung. debrecht Von Graefes. Arch Ophthalmol 53:423–435, 1902
Fuchs E: Ueber Knochenförnige Horhauttrübungen. Arch Ophthalmol 89:337–349, 1915
Debré R, Lamy M, Lamotte M: Un cas d'erythrodermie avec epidermolyse chez un enfant de 12 ans. Bull Soc Pediatr 37:231–238, 1939
Lyell A: Toxic epidermal necrolysis: eruption resembling scalding of the skin. Br J Dermatol 68:355–361, 1956
Niederle J: Akute toxische Epidermolyse (Lyell-Syndrom). Dtsch Med Wochenschr 93:1005–1013, 1968
Rook A, Wilkinson DS, Ebling FJG, et al: Textbook of Dermatology. 4th ed, pp 1656–1657. Oxford, Blackwell Scientific Publications, 1986

STARGARDT'S

Synonyms. Macular degeneration juvenile. Stargardt's type; fundus flavimaculatus-atrophic macular dystrophy.

Symptoms. Onset between 6 and 20 years of age. Gradual bilateral decrease of vision (previously reported as normal).

Signs. Initially, no ophthalmologic changes. Later, disappearance of foveal reflex (first signs) and then changes in the pigmented epithelium (greyish yellow spots); fovea granulated, covered by a snail slimelike material; perifoveal flecks beneath vessels; later, horizontal oval area of atrophy of pigment "beaten bronze atrophy," surrounded by flecks, which progressively enlarges with its halo of flecks without, however, reaching the periphery. Disk and vessels are spared.

Etiology. Primary defect is in the pigment epithelium or in neuroepithelium. Autosomal recessive inheritance; possibly, dominant in some families. It has been suggested that Stargardt's syndrome be used only to refer to the atrophic form with flecks and not to include in it all forms of juvenile macular dystrophies.

Pathology. Disappearance of visual elements in the macular and perimacular areas. The substance accumulated seems to be of mucopolysaccharide nature.

Diagnostic Procedures. *Fluorescein angiography and photography. Retinal function studies.*

Therapy. None.

Prognosis. Slowly evolving condition.

BIBLIOGRAPHY. Stargardt K: Ueber familiäre, progressive Degeneration in der Maculagegende des Auges. Albrecht von Graefes Arch Klin Ophthalmolol 71:540–550, 1909
Pearce WG: Hereditary macular dystrophy: A clinical and genetic study of two specific forms. Canad J Ophthalmol 10:319–325, 1975
Cibis GW: Dominantly inherited macular dystrophy with flecks (Stargardt) Arch Ophthalmol 98:1785–1789, 1980
Smith BF, Smith JB, Low J: Stargardt's disease: The evolution of a diagnosis. J Pediatr Ophthalmol Strabismus 24:259–262, 1987

STATUS DYSRAPHICUS

Association of Morvan's with external congenital malformations such as cervical rib syndrome, Klippel–Feil, and Arnold–Chiari.

STATUS EPILEPTICUS

Symptom. Successive seizures without regaining consciousness between attacks.

Signs. Exhaustion; stupor; coma; tachycardia; dyspnea. If patient recovers, hemiplegia may follow.

Etiology. Complication of epilepsy, *grand mal* or *petit-mal,* usually following withdrawal of medication or change in therapy.

Therapy. Support vital functions. Phenytoin, intravenous infusion without exceeding 50 mg/minute (loading dose 15–18 mg/Kg). Diazepam, 5–10 mg intravenously for a rapid stop of the seizures while waiting for the phenytoin to have effect. In very severe cases: sodium thiopental 0.5–1 mg/Kg.

Prognosis. Severe; death if situation is not brought under control.

BIBLIOGRAPHY. Adams RD, Victor M: Principles of Neurology, 3rd ed, p 252. New York, McGraw-Hill, 1985
Orland MJ, Saltman RJ (eds): Manual of Medical Therapeutics. 25th ed, Boston, Little, Brown, 1986

STEAKHOUSE

Synonyms. Lower esophageal ring; café coronary.

Symptoms. Intermittent, complete esophageal obstruction often during rapid eating, commonly at steak dinner. The symptoms may arise also when a person aspirates food, sometimes by eating peanut butter, bubble gum, honey. The victim clutches the chest, becomes cyanotic and may die.

Signs. Endoscopy frequently does not show any esophageal stricture.

Etiology. Passive fibrous stricture at the esophagogastric junction uniformly with hiatus herniation.

Pathology. Shell consisting of connective tissue without inflammation and overgrowth of muscularis mucosae, esophageal mucosa on upper, and gastric mucosa on the lower surface.

Diagnostic Procedures. *X-ray of esophagus.* Smooth, sharp, concentric narrowing of the distal part of esophagus, not easily seen at routine fluoroscopy. Seen when esophagus is fully distended by thick barium.

Therapy. Change of eating habit. A blow over the back to produce expulsion of bolus of food, manual removal of obstructing bolus (in case of meat) or the "bear clutch" maneuver over the abdomen with repeated quick thrusts

until food is expelled. Bougienage and pneumatic dilatation or endoscopic punch biopsy; direct surgical approach for severe cases and repair of hiatus hernia.

Prognosis. Good; dilatation usually adequate; surgery in more severe cases prevents recurrences.

BIBLIOGRAPHY. Ingelfinger FJ, Kramer P: Dysphagia produced by contractile ring in lower esophagus. Gastroenterology 23:419–430, 1953
Schatzki R, Gary JE: Dysphagia due to diaphragm-like localized narrowing in the lower esophagus ("Lower esophageal ring"). Am J Roentgenol 70:911–922, 1953
Atlas DH: Cafe coronary from peanut butter. N Engl J Med 296:399, 1977

STEATOCYSTOMA MULTIPLEX

Synonyms. Multiple atheromas; sebaceous cystis multiple.

Symptoms. Both sexes equally affected; onset in adolescence or adult life. Asymptomatic.

Signs. Smooth, yellowish swellings on the skin. Diameter 1 or 2 mm to 2 cm, distributed on proximal parts of limbs and presternal region. Absence of punctum on lesions; some inflammation and suppuration.

Etiology. Autosomal dominant inheritance.

Pathology. Dermoid cysts formed by keratinizing epithelium with oily content, some containing hair.

Therapy. Excision when feasible, mostly for cosmetic reasons.

Prognosis. Benign; permanent conditions. One case of malignant transformation reported.

BIBLIOGRAPHY. Mount LB: Steatocystoma multiplex. Arch Dermatol Syph 36:31–39, 1937
Hodes ME, Norins AL: Pachonychia congenita and steatocytoma multiplex. Clin Genet 11:359–364, 1977

STEATORRHEA–IgA DEFICIENCY

Symptoms. Cases reported in adults. Steatorrhea; general fatigue; bone pain.

Signs. Moderate abdominal distention; pitting edema of ankle.

Etiology. Unknown.

Pathology. Diffuse nodules in the intestinal mucosa consisting of enlarged lymphoid follicles within lamina propria. Intense mitotic activity; large germinal center. Plasma cells almost absent.

Diagnostic Procedures. *Blood.* Anemia; hypogammaglobulinemia (absence of IgA; moderate depression of IgG). *X-ray.* Lymphoid hyperplasia diffuse in all intestinal tract, evident as multiple mucosal nodules. *D-xylose absorption test.*

Therapy. Some cases will improve on gluten-free diet and vitamin supplementation.

Prognosis. Long-range prognosis not established.

BIBLIOGRAPHY. Hermans PE, Huizenga KA, Hoffman HN et al: Dysgammaglobulinemia associated with nodular lymphoid hyperplasia of the small intestine. Am J Med 40:78–89, 1966
Sell S: Immunological deficiency diseases. Arch Pathol 86:95–107, 1968
Rosen FS: Genetic defects in gamma-globulin synthesis. In Stanbury JB, Wyngaarden JB, Fredrickson DS et al: The Metabolic Basis of Inherited Disease, 5th ed, p 1928. New York, McGraw-Hill, 1983

STEIDELE'S

Synonyms. Aortic arch atresia; aortic arch interruption; Steidele's complex.

Symptoms. According to different combinations of associated defects.
1. *Aortic arch atresia, patent ductus arteriosus, and ventricular septal defect.* Prevalent in males. May appear normal at birth; then cardiac failure and death within first month of life, seldom later. Clinical recognition difficult. Cyanosis mild or inconspicuous.
2. *Aortic arch atresia without supracardiac or intracardiac shunts.* Seldom, congestive heart failure in infancy. In postadolescence or early adulthood, dyspnea, cephalalgia, epistaxis, leg fatigue, and soreness on walking.

Signs. Usually no difference between upper and lower arterial pulses in type 1. Marked difference in type 2.

Etiology. Congenital malformation.

Pathology. Complete anatomic interruption of aortic arch. A patent ductus arteriosus virtually always present. A ventricular septal defect is frequently present. Other malformations may coexist.

Diagnostic Procedures. *Electrocardiography.* Right ventricular hypertrophy with high peaked P waves. In older patients without shunts, also left ventricular hyperplasia. *Two dimensional echocardiography. Cardiac catheterization. X-ray.* Cardiomegaly; pulmonary venous congestion; in type without shunt, rib notching possible.

Therapy. Prevention of bacterial endocarditis. Medical management. Palliative surgery attempted in type 1. In type 2 surgical correction when indicated.

Prognosis. In type 1 death within first month; a few may reach early adulthood. In type 2 survival into third decade.

BIBLIOGRAPHY. Steidele RJ: Sammlg. Verschiedener in der chirurg. prakt. Lehrshule Germachten Beobb 2:114, 1777–78.
Hurst JW: The Heart, 6th ed, pp 634–635. New York, McGraw-Hill, 1985

STEINBACK–BROWN

Synonyms. Acrodysplasia IV; epiphyseal dysplasia; diastrophic dwarfism variant (?); epiphyseal dysostosis.

Symptoms and Signs. Normal height; acromelic shortening.

Etiology. Unknown.

Diagnostic Procedures. *X-ray.* Axial skeletal changes. Malsegmentation of hands and feet.

BIBLIOGRAPHY. Steinback HI, Brown RA: Epiphyseal dysostosis. Am J Roentgenol 105:860–869, 1969
Bailey JA: Disproportionate Short Stature: Diagnosis and Management, p 197. Philadelphia, WB Saunders, 1973

STEINBROCKER'S

Synonyms. Coronary scapular; shoulder–hand; sympathetic reflex dystrophy. See Sudeck's.

Symptoms and Signs. Affects both sexes, slight predominance of females; onset after 50 years of age (90%). Gradual stiffness, discomfort, weakness in shoulder and hand. Sudden severe pain and stiffness, swelling, hyperesthesia of hand. Three stages. (1) Lasting 3 to 6 months; complete hand and shoulder involvement. (2) Lasting 3 to 6 months; partial or total resolution of swelling and vasospasm or vasodilatation. Early trophic changes and contractures, and muscle atrophy. (3) Varying duration (in some cases years); atrophic and dystrophic changes; contractures of fingers; "frozen" shoulder; residual pain infrequent.

Etiology. Reflex dystrophy secondary to internal lesions; postmyocardial infarction (20%); cervical disk or intraforaminal spurs (20%); posttraumatic (10%); posthemiplegic (6%); miscellaneous causes (Herpes zoster, vasculitis, tumor, arthritis) (10%), or idiopathic (25%).

Pathology. *Shoulder tissue.* Inflammatory aspecific changes similar to those seen in capsulitis, periarthritis.

Skin of finger. Edema; fat depletion, small hemorrhages (see Sudeck's).

Diagnostic Procedures. To rule out rheumatoid arthritis (*X-ray, RA test, sedimentation rate*). *Electrocardiography. X-ray of chest, cervical spine, and shoulder.*

Therapy. Treatment of underlying condition: analgesic; physical therapy; exercise; corticosteroids; stellate ganglionic blocks; sympathectomy.

Prognosis. Variable and unpredictable; lack of correlation with extent and nature of etiology. Residual contractures observed frequently.

BIBLIOGRAPHY. Steinbrocker O: Painful homolateral disability of the shoulder and hand, with swelling and atrophy of the hand. Ann Rheum Dis 6:80–84, 1947
Hurst JW: The Heart, 6th ed, p 987. New York, McGraw-Hill, 1986

STEINDLER'S

Eponym used for sacralgia. See Fibrositis.

BIBLIOGRAPHY. Steindler AV, Luck JV: Differential diagnosis of pain low in the back. Allocation of the source of pain by procaine hydrochloride method. JAMA 110:106–113, 1938

STEINERT'S

Synonyms. Batten-Gibb; Curshmann-Batten-Steinert; myotonic dystrophy; myotonia atrophica.

Symptoms. Appear slightly more frequently in male between 20 and 30 years of age. Weakness; myotonia (inability to relax the grasp properly due to abnormal, delayed relaxation of skeletal muscles); motions slow and inefficient. Loss of libido; impotence, oligomenorrhea to amenorrhea. Frequent pulmonary infection. Development of myotonic dystrophy personality: whining dependency. Feeblemindedness and onset in childhood tends to occur in second generation.

Signs. Atrophy of muscles (facial, sternocleidomastoideus, quadriceps femoris, distal forearm and hand). Frontal alopecia; myotic pupils that react sluggishly to light and accommodation; ptosis; cataracts. Percussion of a muscle stimulates contraction of many fibers determining a prolonged localized contraction of the muscle. Tendon reflexes diminished or absent; cardiac conduction defects with arrhythmias.

Etiology. Unknown; dominant inheritance.

Pathology. Atrophy of muscle fibers, replaced by fat and connective tissue interposed with normal and hypertrophic fibers. No pathology in brain. Atrophy of testis (80%) or ovary.

Diagnostic Procedures. *Blood, urine, cerebrospinal fluid.* Normal. *Electromyography.* Characteristic pattern. *Electrocardiography.* Reveals abnormality. *Pulmonary function studies. Endocrine studies. X-ray of skull.* Radiologic abnormalities (60%).

Therapy. Symptomatic. Quinine relieves the myotonic symptoms; specific endocrine deficiency corrected by administration of hormones. Cataracts corrected surgically.

Prognosis. Slowly progressive; patient may reach old age.

BIBLIOGRAPHY. Steinert H: Myopathologische Beitrage: Ueber das klinische und anatomische Bild des Muskelschwunds der Myotoniker. DPtsch Z Nervenheilk 37:58–104, 1909
Batten FE, Gibbs HP: Myotonia atrophica. Brain 32:187–205, 1909
Curshmann H: Ueber familiaere atrophische Myotonia. Dtsch Z Nervenheilk 45:161–202, 1912
Moorman JR, Coleman RE, Packer DL, et al: Cardiac involvement in myotonic muscular dystrophy. Medicine 64:371–387, 1985

STEINER–VOERNER

Synonyms. Angiomatosis miliaris; miliary angiomatosis.

Symptoms. Prevalent in females; onset at all ages, especially in adolescence. In patients with vasomotor and thermal lability. Frequently concurrent with eruptions (see Signs); cephalalgia; vertigo; nausea; vomiting; diarrhea; tachycardia; anhidrosis; polyuria; various visual impairments; fever.

Signs. Appearance of small diffuse angiomas on cutaneous and mucosal areas.

Etiology. It represents one of the forms of *miliaria* according to recent classification: *crystallina* (sudamina); *rubra* (prickly heat); *profunda* (mamillaria) due to epidermal injury in susceptible individuals, where due to sweat the skin flora produces a toxin that damages luminal sweat cells and causes obstruction of the sweat glands by a PAS-positive material.

Therapy. Sedatives. Antiserotonin compounds.

BIBLIOGRAPHY. Steiner L, Voerner H. Angiomatosis miliaris. Eine idiopathische Gefaesserkrankung. Dtsch Arch Klin Med 96:105–116, 1909
Rook A, Wilkinson DS, Ebling FJG et al: Textbook of Dermatology, 4th ed, pp 234–235, 1891–1893. Oxford, Blackwell Scientific Publications, 1986

STEIN–LEVENTHAL

Synonyms. Polycystic bilateral ovarian. See ovarian hyperthecosis.

Symptoms. Onset after puberty or in late teenage years. Menstruation normal at onset and for some time; then progressive oligomenorrhea and finally amenorrhea. Sometimes, primary amenorrhea and menorrhagic episodes. Sterility. Minor voice change.

Signs. Obesity, hypertrichosis, and sometimes virilism; ovaries are usually enlarged and often described as "oyster-like." In familial form, males abnormally hairy.

Etiology. Still not quite settled, but numerous researchers think it might be an abnormality in the steroidogenesis of ovarian hormone: a block in the conversion of androstenedione to estrogen, due to enzymatic deficiencies concerned with aromatization of androstenedione into estrogens. If primary abnormality resides in hypothalamus or pituitary still not clear. Autosomal dominant inheritance reported in some families.

Pathology. Numerous cystic follicles underneath a thickened ovarian capsule; usually enlarged ovaries; hyperplastic fibrosis of cortical stroma; hypertrophy and hyperplasia of endometrium. Hyperplasia of theca cells in atretic follicles, sparse primordial and developing follicles stromal hyperplasia.

Diagnostic Procedures. *Blood, urine.* Slight elevation of 17-ketosteroids in urine; slight elevation of plasma androstenedione or testosterone level, slight elevation of luteinizing hormone levels. Estradiol and follicle-stimulating hormone low. *X-ray. Gynecography. Culdoscopy. Exploratory laparotomy.*

Therapy. Induction of ovulation is the key to success. Trial with cortisone for a minimum of 6 months; induction of ovulation with clomiphene. Wedge resection of both ovaries; should be last method. Bromocriptine for the treatment of hirsutism.

Prognosis. Eighty percent cured with wedge resection in well-selected patients; recurrences are common.

BIBLIOGRAPHY. Stein IF, Leventhal ML: Amenorrhea associated with bilateral polycystic ovaries. Am J Obstet Gynecol 29:181–191, 1935

Stein IF: The Stein–Leventhal syndrome. A curable form of sterility. N Engl J Med 259:420–423, 1958

Yen SSC: The polycystic ovary syndrome: Review. Clin Endocrinol 12:177–208, 1980

Zumoff B, Freeman R, Coupey S et al: A chronobiologic abnormality in luteinizing hormone secretion in teenage girls with polycystic ovary syndrome. N Engl J Med 309:1206–1209, 1983

Murdoch AP, McClean KG, Watson MJ et al: Treatment of hirsutism in polycystic ovary syndrome with bromocriptine. Br J Obstet Gynaecol 94:358–365, 1987

Schwartz M, Gindoff PR, Jewelewicz R: Polycystic ovary syndrome: An enigma awaiting solution. Bull NY Acad Med 63:134–155, 1987

STEVENS–JOHNSON

Synonyms. Baader's; erythema multiforme exudativum; Fissinger–Rendu; Klauder's; respiratory mucosa; mucocutaneocular; Neumann's II. See erythema multiforme. Lyell's.

Symptoms. Affects all ages, greatest incidence in first and third decades; moderate prevalence in men. Occur (1) in individuals in good general health, without exogenous factors evident (17%); (2) in individuals presenting vague symptomatology of headache, upper respiratory or urinary tract infections (prodromata?) and where some drugs (see Etiology) have been given (50%); (3) in individuals to whom drugs were given for symptoms not suggesting prodromata of Stevens–Johnson syndrome. Malaise; mild pruritus; burning sensation; arthralgia; myalgia; fever.

Signs. Vesiculobullous lesions of skin and two or more mucous membrane sites (oral cavity; genitourinary tract; conjunctiva). Nikolsky's signs negative.

Etiology. Unknown; only some cases of unequivocal correlation with drug administration. Viral infections, allergic mechanism suspected. Drugs most frequently involved: sulfonamides; penicillin; phenolsulfophthalein; sedatives; also many other unrelated drugs.

Pathology. Hyperkeratosis; acanthosis; vesicles with eosinophils, fibrin precipitate, lymphocytes and neutrophils. Lymphocyte perivascular infiltrate in dermis.

Diagnostic Procedures. *Cytology and culture of bullae aspirate. X-ray of chest.* Frequently, finding of pneumonitis. *Blood.* Sedimentation rate, white blood cells increased.

Therapy. Bed rest; liquid diet; gargles; calamine lotion; bacitracin ointment for skin; corticosteroid eye drops.

Prognosis. Approximately 10-day course with severe manifestations; 15 to 30 days for healing lesions. Usual recovery; possible recurrence. In some cases, persistent corneal lesions; loss of vision. Fatal in some cases.

BIBLIOGRAPHY. Stevens AM, Johnson FC: A new eruptive fever associated with stomatitis and ophthalmia: Report of two cases in children. Am J Dis Child 24:526–533, 1922

Bianchine JR, Macaraeg PVJ, Lasagna L et al: Drugs as etiologic factors in the Stevens-Johnson syndrome. Am J Med 44:390–405, 1968

Rook A, Wilkinson DS, Ebling FJG et al: Textbook of Dermatology, 4th ed, pp 1085–1090. Oxford, Blackwell Scientific Publications, 1986

Savill JS, Barrie S, Ghosh S et al: Fatal Stevens-Johnson syndrome following urography with iopamidol in systemic lupus erythematosus. Postgraduate Medical J 64:392–394, 1988

STEWART–BERGSTROM

Synonyms. Arthrogryposiclike   hands–sensorineural deafness.

Symptoms. Both sexes; onset early after birth. Hand abnormalities (arthrogryposiclike), and minor abnormalities of feet. Sensorineural deafness with external ear canal, tympanic membranes normal.

Etiology. Autosomal dominant inheritance with complete penetrance and variable expressivity.

Diagnostic Procedures. *Blood.* Normal. *X-ray.* Hand abnormalities and occasional minor alterations of acetabulum. *Palmar dermatoglyphics.* Similar to those observed in arthrogryposis. *Audiography.*

Therapy. Orthopedic correction.

Prognosis. Nonprogressive condition.

BIBLIOGRAPHY. Stewart JM, Bergstrom L: Familial hand abnormality and sensorineural deafness. A new syndrome. J Pediatr 78:102–110, 1971

Akbarnia BA, Bowen JR, Doegherty J: Familial arthrogryptotic hand abnormality and sensorineural deafness. Am J Dis Child 113:403–405, 1979

STEWART–HOLMES

See Jackson's cerebellar fits.

Symptoms. Attacks last 2 to 3 minutes. Jerking movements of one arm (unilateral); irregular in sequence and distribution; occasionally affecting the contralateral arm to a slighter degree; frequently associated with vertigo. Other signs of cerebellar lesion may be observed.

Etiology and Pathology. Lesion in cerebellum; traumatic; vascular; neoplastic.

Diagnostic Procedures. *Electroencephalography. Angiography. CT brain scan.*

Therapy. Surgery if indicated.

Prognosis. According to nature of lesion.

BIBLIOGRAPHY. Stewart TG, Holmes G: Symptomatology of cerebellar tumours: A study of forty cases. Brain 27:522–591, 1904

Dow RS, Moruzzi G: The Physiology and Pathology of the Cerebellum. Minneapolis, University of Minnesota Press, 1958

STEWART–TREVES

Synonyms. Extremity lymphangiosarcoma; postmastectomy lymphangiosarcoma.

Symptoms and Signs. Occur in patients with chronic lymphedematous extremity; majority of cases in women with breast cancer after mastectomy. Reported in cases (male and female) of groin dissection and radiation for cancer, and in cases of congenital lymphedema without evidence of previous malignancy. Appearance on edematous extremity of a mass, usually dark, slightly tender, enlarging.

Etiology. Alteration in lymphatic circulation, due to surgery or irradiation or idiopathic, causing neoplastic changes of vascular cells.

Pathology. Lymphangiosarcoma. In postmastectomy cases, the sarcomatous nature of tumor has been challenged by some authors, and considered instead as retrograde metastasis from carcinoma.

Diagnostic Procedures. *Biopsy.*

Therapy. Amputation. External radiotherapy. Intraarterial ^{90}y in ceramic microspheres.

Prognosis. Generally poor; frequent widespread metastasis.

BIBLIOGRAPHY. Stewart FW, Treves N: Lymphangiosarcoma in postmastectomy lymphedema. Report of 6 cases of elephantiasis chirurgica. Cancer 1:64–81, 1948

Gray GF, Gonzalez–Licea A, Hartmann WH et al: Angiosarcoma in lymphedema, an unusual case of Stewart–Treves syndrome. Bull Johns Hopkins Hosp 119:117–128, 1966

Rook A, Wilkinson DS, Ebling FJG et al: Textbook of Dermatology, 4th ed, p 2470. Oxford, Blackwell Scientific Publications, 1986

STIFF BABY

Synonyms. Hyperreflexia, startle disease. The syndrome is different from the stiff-man syndrome.

Symptoms and Signs. Stiffness immediately after birth; delayed locomotor development; diaphragmatic, umbilical and inguinal hernias; exaggerated startle response to sudden noises or movement, that may persist into adulthood; choking, vomiting, and difficulty in swallowing possible. The motor development of these infants is delayed but intelligence is normal.

Etiology. The syndrome is transmitted in a genetic dominant fashion with variable penetrance.

Pathology. Histologic examination of muscle has not been reported.

Diagnostic Procedures. *Electromyography.* Demonstrates continous muscle activity with only rare periods of quiescence. Action potentials and nerve conduction studies are normal.

Therapy. Oral diazepam. The syndrome is associated with resistance to succinylcholine.

Prognosis. Good, the symptoms ameliorate with time.

BIBLIOGRAPHY. Klein R, Haddow JE, De Luca C: Familial congenital disorder resembling stiff-man syndrome. Am J Dis Child 124:730–731, 1972
Lingam S, Wilson J, Hart E: Hereditary stiff-baby syndrome. Am J Dis Child 135:909–911, 1981
Cook W, Kaplan R: Neuromuscular blockade in a patient with stiff-baby syndrome. Anesthesiology 65:525–528, 1986

STIFF HEART

Synonyms. Restrictive cardiac; restrictive hemodynamic. See Pick's (F.).

Symptoms. Exertional dyspnea; finally orthopnea; occasionally, pain in the chest.

Signs. Elevation of systemic venous pressure; pulsus paradoxus; Kussmaul's sign may be present; heart sound faint or normal; additional diastolic sounds (strong evidence for the condition); hepatomegaly; ascites and edemas.

Etiology and Pathology. Chronic constrictive pericarditis (tuberculosis; trauma; radiation; rheumatoid arthritis; mycosis; idiopathic). Primary and secondary myocardiopathies (myocardial fibrosis; subendocardial fibroelastosis). Loeffler's subendocardial fibroelastosis; amyloidosis hemochromatosis.

Diagnostic Procedures. *Electrocardiography.* Normal or some abnormalities. *X-ray.* Helpful in differential diagnosis. *Cardiac catheterization.* Diagnostic. *Other tests.* As needed, according to etiology and symptoms.

Therapy. Not specific; according to etiology and symptoms. Digitalization of little benefit.

Prognosis. Chronic evolution; results according to etiology.

BIBLIOGRAPHY. Shabetai R, Fowler NO, Fenton JC: Restrictive cardiac disease, pericarditis and the myocardiopathies. Am Heart J 69:271–280, 1965
Kilpatrick TR, Horack HM, Moore CB: "Stiff heart" syndrome. An uncommon cause of heart failure. Med Clin North Am 51:959–966, 1967
Hurst JW: The Heart, 6th ed, pp 1263–1266. New York, McGraw-Hill, 1986

STIFF SKIN

Synonym. Mucopolysaccharidosis variant.

Symptoms. Rare. Both sexes affected; congenital or noticed in early childhood. Limited mobility of various joints.

Signs. Localized areas of stony-hard skin involving primarily buttocks and upper thighs. Lordotic stance.

Etiology. Unknown; probably, autosomal dominant inheritance. Could belong, as a variant, in mucopolysaccharidosis group.

Pathology. Epidermis unremarkable; in the upper dermis interstitial ground substance granular and eosinophilic; abnormal amount of hyaluronidase-digestible acid mucopolysaccharide; appendages are normal.

Diagnostic Procedures. *Biopsy of skin.* See Pathology. *Blood.* Normal. *Urine.* Normal; no increased excretion of mucopolysaccharides. *X-ray of skeleton.* Normal.

Therapy. None.

Prognosis. Stable condition.

BIBLIOGRAPHY. Pichler E: Hereditaere Kontrakturen mit sclerodermieartigen Hantveraenderungen. Z Kinderheilkd 104:349–361, 1968
Esterly NB, McKusick NA: Stiff skin syndrome. Pediatr 47:360–369, 1971
Stevenson RE, Lucas TL Jr, Martin JB Jr: Symmetrical lipomatosis associated with stiff-skin and systemic manifestations in four generations. Proc Grenwood Genet Center 3:56–64, 1984

STILLER'S

Synonyms. Asthenia universalis congenita; morbus asthenicus.

Symptoms. Asthenia; gastric atonia; pallor. Tall and skinny individual; scarce subcutaneous tissue; splanchnoptosis.

Etiology. Unknown.

Prognosis. In the past, this habitus was associated with a high incidence of tubercular diseases.

BIBLIOGRAPHY. Stiller B: Die asthenische Konstitutionskrankheit (Asthenia universalis congenita. Morbus asthenicus). Stuttgart, Enke, 1907

STILL'S

Synonyms. Juvenile rheumatoid arthritis; Chauffard–Ramon; Chauffard–Still; Dreier's; acute polyarthritis. Eponym also used for subacute and chronic juvenile rheumatoid arthritis.

Symptoms and Signs. More frequent in females; onset before puberty (never before 6 mo of age). High fever; skin rash (erythema multiformlike); pneumonitis; pericarditis; iridocyclitis; failure to thrive; lymphadenopathy; splenomegaly. Eventually monoarticular or polyarticular arthritis becomes evident.

Etiology. Unknown; possibility of genetic origin not assessed. Relation with collagen and autoimmune diseases.

Pathology. Nonspecific synovitis in joint with granulation tissue, erosion of cartilage, fibrosis, bony ankylosis. Nonspecific lymph node hyperplasia. Myocarditis.

Diagnostic Procedures. *Blood.* Leukocytosis (50%); moderate anemia; high sedimentation rate. Lupus erythematosus test negative. Test for rheumatoid arthritis positive (20%). *X-ray of joints.* Demineralization; erosions; reduction of joint space.

Therapy. Corticosteroids. Phenylbutazone; aspirin; chloroquine; intramuscularly.

Prognosis. Persistent activity for 2 or 3 years. Pain disappearing 10 years after onset. Ankylosis and failure to grow.

BIBLIOGRAPHY. Cornil V: Mémoire sur les coïncidences pathologiques du rhumatisme articulaire chroniques. C R Soc Biol 1 (2):3–25, 1864–65
Still GF: On a form of chronic joint disease in children. Proc R Med Chir Soc (Lond) 9:10–15, 1896
Fink CW: Treatment of juvenile arthritis. Bull Rheumat Dis 32:21–24, 1982
Larson EB: Adult Still's disease: Evolution of a clinical syndrome and diagnosis. Treatment and follow-up of 17 patients. Medicine 63:82–93, 1984

STIMMLER'S

Synonyms. Alaninuria–microcephaly–dwarfism–diabetes mellitus.

Symptoms and Signs. At birth. Female. Microcephaly, small teeth, low weight. Then physical (dwarfism) and mental retardation.

Etiology. Autosomal recessive inheritance.

Diagnostic Procedures. *Blood.* Alanine, pyruvate, lactate increased. *Urine.* Alanine excretion increased.

BIBLIOGRAPHY. Stimmler L, Jensen N, Toseland P: Alaninuria associated with microcephaly, dwarfism, enamel hypoplasia, and diabetes mellitus in two sisters. Arch Dis Child 45:682–685, 1970

STOKVIS–TALMA

Synonyms. Autotoxic cyanosis; enterogenous cyanosis; idiopathic methemoglobinemia; van den Bergh's. Eponym obsolete; no longer considered an entity. The symptoms are today attributed to ingestion of a product that produces methemoglobinemia. The possibility, however, persists that bacterial overgrowth in the intestine may damage the red cells' metabolism and make them more sensitive to the action of ingested products, with oxidant properties (e.g., analgesics, antipyretics).

BIBLIOGRAPHY. Stokvis BJ: Kihdrage tot de casuistick der autotoxiche enterogene Cyanosen, (Methaemoglobinaemia ?) et Enteritis parassitaria. Med Tschr Geneesk 36:678–693, 1902
Talma S: Intraglobulare Methaemoglobinaemia beim Menschen. Berl Klin Wochenschr 39:865–867, 1902
Wintrobe MM (ed): Clinical Hematology, 7th ed, p 1010. Philadelphia, Lea & Febiger, 1976

STOMATOCYTOSIS

Synonym. Hydrocytosis.

Symptoms and Signs. A peculiar morphologic feature of red cells which are uniconcave, with slitlike area of central pallor. These erythrocytes show shorter survival and increased osmotic fragility resulting in hemolytic anemia.

Etiology. Stomatocytes are found in more than one type of congenital hemolytic anemia both on autosomal and recessive inheritance. Defect is caused by a potassium–sodium disorder, higher Na and lower K content in red cells. A cold-sensitive variety has also been described.

Therapy. Splenectomy may be beneficial in severe forms.

BIBLIOGRAPHY. Lock SP, Smith R, Hardisty RM: Stomatocytosis: A hereditary red cell anomaly associated with haemolytic anaemia. Br J Haemat 7:303–314, 1961

Oski FA, Naiman JL, Blum SF et al: Congenital hemolytic anemia with high-sodium low-potassium red cells. N Engl J Med 280:909–916, 1969
Townes PL, Miller G: Further studies on cold-sensitive variant of stomatocytosis. Am J Genet 32:57A, 1980

STONE HEART

Synonym. Ischemic contracture of heart.

Symptoms. Occur in both sexes; onset at any age in people with acquired severe heart disease (class III or IV) after cardiac surgery. Sudden development of myocardial failure due to a small spastic heart, stopped in systole, where not even vigorous manual massage succeeds in producing an adequate stroke volume. The contracted state is irreversible.

Etiology. Unknown. State of rigor of the ischemic myocardium failing to relax, attributed to loss of myocardial energy stores, leading to depletion of adenosine triphosphate (ATP) in the region occupied by the myofilaments.

Pathology. Heart hypertrophy of concentric type; presence of fibrosis; small left ventricular chamber.

Therapy. Attempt to prevent by ensuring continued oxygen supply to myocardium during surgery, perfusion with low-calcium solutions, maintaining a relative condition of acidosis, and administration of ATP and potassium. The best management in preventing stone heart is the reduction of aortic clamping time; a corrected myocardial protection with cardioplegic solution during clamping time and finally, after declamping, adequate coronaric reperfusion.

Prognosis. Once developed, the condition presently appears irreversible.

BIBLIOGRAPHY. Cooley DA, Reul GJ, Wukasch DC: Ischemic contraction of the heart: "Stone heart". Am J Cardiovasc 29:575–577, 1972
Katz AM, Tada M: The "stone heart": A challenge to the biochemist. Am J Cardiol 29:578–580, 1972

STORMORKEN'S

Synonyms. Thrombocytopathy–asplenia–miosis.

Symptoms. From early infancy. Asthenia, cephalea, dyslexia, easy bleeding.

Signs. Ichthyosis, miosis.

Etiology. Unknown. Familial occurrence (autosomal dominant?).

Diagnostic Procedures. *CT scan.* Absence of spleen. *Blood.* Red cells with Howell–Jolly bodies. Platelets in normal number.

BIBLIOGRAPHY. Stormorken H, Sjaastad O, Langslet A et al: A new syndrome: Thrombocytopathy, muscle fatigue, asplenia, miosis, migraine, dyslexia, and ichthyosis. Clin Genet 28:367–374, 1985

STRACHAN'S

Synonyms. Ariboflavinosis; amblyopia–painful neuropathy–orogenital dermatitis. Howes–Pallister–Landor; Strachan–Scott.

Symptoms. Amblyopia; paresthesias of feet, hands, trunk, and occasionally face. Dizziness; deafness; hoarseness; spasticity; ataxia.

Signs. Reflex loss; genital dermatitis; corneal degeneration; glossitis; stomatitis. Features of chronic malnutrition.

Etiology. Chronic malnutrition.

Pathology. Bilateral symmetric loss of myelinated fibers in central part of optic nerves. Loss of ganglion cells in the macula (in severe form).

Diagnostic Procedures. *Blood.* Hypoproteinemia; hypochromic, microcytic, or macrocytic anemia; reduced level of B_2 and B_{12} (occasional); low transketolase activity. *Urine.* Abnormal excretion of methylmalonic acid.

Therapy. Oral or parenteral B vitamin group; improved nutrition.

Prognosis. Degree of recovery according to degree of amblyopia and time of onset of treatment.

BIBLIOGRAPHY. Strachan H: On a form of multiple neuritis prevalent in the West Indies. Practitioner (Lond) 59:477–484, 1897
Adams RD, Victor M: Principles of Neurology, 3rd ed, p 733. New York, McGraw-Hill, 1985

STRAIGHT BACK

Synonym. Back straight.

Symptoms. Delusion of heart disease (because of faulty diagnosis) affecting activities and employment of the patient. In some cases, dyspnea.

Signs. Loss of kyphotic curve of upper dorsal spine (flattened palm of examiner's hand on the area does not have normal deviation of fingers). Heart auscultation: harsh, late systolic murmur, ejection type from grade IV to grade I at the base. Increased pulmonic closure sounds.

Etiology and Pathology. Congenital abnormality of upper dorsal spine that decreases anteroposterior diameter of chest and causes spurious heart enlargement and mechanical murmurs. In some cases, pulmonary obstruction with elevation of pulmonary arterial pressure.

Diagnostic Procedures. *Echocardiography. X-ray of chest, frontal and lateral view.* Anterior concavity of vertebral column in upper dorsal region absent, with compression of heart against the sternum and kinking of great vessels. *Fluoroscopy, electrocardiography.* Normal.

Therapy. None. If dyspnea and signs of pulmonary hypertension, surgery to correct chest cage deformity.

Prognosis. Benign condition; correct diagnosis avoids iatrogenic heart disease.

BIBLIOGRAPHY. Ravlings MS: The "straight back" syndrome: A new cause of pseudoheart disease. Am J Cardiol 5:333–338, 1960

Leinbach RC, Harthorne JW, Dinsmore RE: Straight back syndrome with pulmonary venous obstruction. Am Cardiol 21:588–592, 1968

Hurst JW: The Heart, 6th ed, p 134. New York, McGraw-Hill, 1986

STRANSKY–REGALA

Synonym. Chronic congenital hemolytic anemia. Eponym obsolete; used to indicate a variety (?) of congenital chronic hemolytic anemias occurring in the Philippines; splenectomy controlled the hemolytic component but not the anemia.

BIBLIOGRAPHY. Stransky E, Regala A: New type of familial congenital chronic hemolytic anemia. Am J Dis Child 71:492–505, 1946

STRAUSS–CHURG–ZAK

Synonyms. Churg–Strauss; allergic granulomatosis–angiitis.

Symptoms and Signs. Prevalent in women. Asthmatic attacks; recurrent eruptions on trunk and limbs of erythema multiformlike; hemorrhagic and nodular lesions in the skin.

Etiology. Unknown; related to vasculitis syndrome and collagen diseases. Differing from periarteritis nodosa (See Kussmaul–Maier) because of lung involvement and peculiar granulomatous skin lesions.

Pathology. Endothelial necrosis; edema; fibrinoid necrosis of collagen; granulomas with prevalence of eosinophils, histiocytes, giant cells.

Diagnostic Procedures. *Blood.* Anemia; eosinophilia; high sedimentation rate. *Biopsy of skin.*

Therapy. Corticosteroids.

Prognosis. Very poor; high mortality.

BIBLIOGRAPHY. Strauss L, Churg J, Zak FG: Cutaneous lesions of allergic granulomatosis: Histopathologic study. J Invest Dermatol 17:349–359, 1951

Lenham JG, Elkan KB, Pusey CD et al: Systemic vasculitis with asthma and eosinophilia: A clinical approach to Churg–Strauss syndrome. Medicine 63:65–81, 1984

Leavitt RV, Fauci AF: Pulmonary vasculitis. Am Rev Respir Dis 134:149–166, 1986

Rook A, Wilkinson DS, Ebling FJG et al: Textbook of Dermatology, 4th ed, p 1186. Oxford, Blackwell Scientific Publications, 1986

STRAW PETER

Synonyms. Cerebral dysfunction infantilis; hyperkinetic; hypokinetic; minimal brain dysfunction; slovenly Peter; Struwwelpeter. See Prechtel–Stemmer and cocktail party.

Symptoms. Estimated to affect between 5% and 20% of general school population. In preschool age, manifested as clumsiness (general coordination deficits); abnormal activity level (hyperkinetic; restless; fidgety; disorganized thought processes; or hypokinetic); impulsivity; emotional lability. At school, excessive distractibility, specific learning disability (reading, spelling, arithmetic, abstract concepts), perceptual motor deficits (poor drawing, printing).

Signs. Transient strabismus, poor coordination of fingers, impaired auditory or visual (or both) perceptual systems; motor awkwardness.

Etiology. Variable: Prechtel–Stemmer syndrome (see). From psychosociologic environmental factors to minimal brain dysfunction; genetic predisposition.

Pathology. Unknown.

Diagnostic Procedures. Multidisciplinary approach. *Electroencephalography.* Borderline or minimal abnormalities observed. *Otologic, ophthalmologic, psychological, psychiatric,* and *educational evaluations.*

Therapy. Home management: routinized and scheduled program, decrease in environmental stimulation. School management: close cooperation between doctors and teachers; special tutorial education, if needed. Medication to reduce hyperactivity and increase attention: Captodiamine hydrochloride, thioridazine hydrochloride, and amphetamines.

Prognosis. Usually symptoms subside by puberty. Mild degree of mental retardation; epilepsy, other disabilities may become evident.

BIBLIOGRAPHY. Clements SD, Peter JE: Minimal brain dysfunctions in school-age child. Arch Gen Psychiatr 6:185–197, 1962

Peiper A: Cerebral Function in Infancy and Childhood. New York Consultant Bureau, 1963

Pincus JH, Glaser GH: The syndrome of "minimal brain damage" in childhood. N Engl J Med 275:27–35, 1966

Hoffmann H: "Struwwelpeter" (quoted by ed). JAMA 202:28–29, 1967

de la Cruz FF, Fox BH, Roberts RH (eds): Minimal brain dysfunction. Ann NY Acad Sci 205:1–396, 1973

Barlow C: Mental Retardation and Related Disorders. Philadelphia, Davis, 1977

STRESS FRACTURE OF FIBULA

Synonym. Fibular fatigue-fracture. See Shin splint.

Symptoms. Common in athletes and in children. Abrupt onset; severe pain above and behind lateral side of ankle. Insidious onset (more frequent); gradually increasing pain during or following activity. Frequently limp. Running or climbing stairs causes severe pain.

Signs. Tenderness above lateral ankle and occasionally swellings that become bone-hard with time.

Etiology. Fracture of fibula usually at tibiofibular joint due to excessive stress during sports activity.

Pathology. Fracture of fibula; formation of callus (see also Stress fracture of tibia).

Diagnostic Procedures. *X-ray.* Fracture seldom seen at onset except with special studies (macrograph). Typical appearance may not be seen before 4 weeks.

Therapy. Rest from sport; adhesive elastic strapping.

Prognosis. With treatment, usually cure in about 6 weeks; then gradual return to sport activity. Without treatment, the entire sport season may be lost.

BIBLIOGRAPHY. Burrows HJ: Fatigue fractures of fibula. J Bone Joint Surg [Br] 30:266–279, 1948

Devas MB, Sweetnam R: Stress fractures of the fibula: A review of 50 cases in athletes. J Bone Joint Surg [Br] 38:818–829, 1956

Slocum DB: The shin splint syndrome: Medical aspects and differential diagnosis. Am J Surg 114:875–881, 1967

STRESS FRACTURE OF TIBIA

Synonym. Periostitis tibiae ab excercitio.

Symptoms. Occur in athletes (runners); insidious onset of dull pain in the shin at the end of a run. It increases over the days or months until it prevents continuation of sport activities. At beginning pain is relieved by rest; later pain remains after activity. Abrupt onset also observed, although less frequently.

Signs. Tenderness and swelling over tibia (lower third). Absence of inflammatory reaction. Good tibial pulse.

Etiology. Repeated stress fractures of cortex at first, then spreading to the bone. To be differentiated from shin splint syndrome and other overuse syndromes.

Pathology. At onset localized osteoclastic reabsorption, then linear fracture, then periosteal and endosteal callus.

Diagnostic Procedures. *X-ray.* Changes appear usually late, 3 to 4 weeks after onset.

Therapy. Rest from sport; adhesive strapping.

Prognosis. After 3 to 4 months, complete recovery.

BIBLIOGRAPHY. Aleman O: Tumors of foot from long marches. Tidskr Militar Hälsovard 54:191–208, 1929

Devas MB: Stress fractures of the tibia in athletes or "shin soreness." J Bone Joint Surg [Br] 40:227–239, 1958

Slocum DB: The shin splint syndrome: medical aspects and differential diagnosis. Am J Surg 114:875–881, 1967

STRING

Symptoms and Signs. Appears as a complication of cerclage suture used to oppose choroid and retina and retinal detachment. Onset between 4th and 19th postoperative day. Intense pain in the eye; edema of eyelids; proptosis of the globe; chemosis of conjunctiva; uveitis; ocular hypertension. Cornea remains clear; anterior chamber is very deep; iris is fixed and assumes green color.

Etiology and Pathology. Complication of cerclage operation. Suture causing vascular obstruction; configuration of eye predisposing factor.

Therapy. Responds slowly to steroids. Application of diathermy in conjunction with cerclage suture may prevent the occurrence of the syndrome.

Prognosis. Persists for weeks, ultimately resolves; secondary changes persist and result in complete detachment of retina.

BIBLIOGRAPHY. Mason N: The "string syndrome": Seen as a complication of Arruga's cerclage suture. Br J Ophthalmol 48:70–74, 1964

Pauh H: Differential Diagnosis of Eye Disease. Philadelphia, WB Saunders, 1978

STROKE SYNDROMES

Three types or stages clinically distinguished.
1. Transient ischemic attacks
2. Stroke in evolution
3. Completed stroke

STROKE IN EVOLUTIONS

Synonym. Progressive stroke.

Symptoms. Sudden onset of relentless progression of symptoms. Sensorial alterations from stupor to coma.

Signs. Breathing irregular (Cheyne–Stokes or other anomalies). Focal signs of lesions; flaccidity; hemiplegia. This stage is the cerebral shock.

COMPLETE STROKE

Symptoms. Partial or total recovery of consciousness; lessening of paralysis; flaccidity converted to spasticity.

Etiology. Cerebrovascular accident: hemorrhagic or thrombotic.

Pathology. Focal injury of brain and peripheral or general edema.

Diagnostic Procedures. *Cerebrospinal fluid.* Increased pressure. Red cells in some cases. *Electroencephalography.* Focal signs. *Angiography. CT scan.* Evidence of area of lesion.

Therapy. General supportive measures. Antiedema treatment. Consideration and evaluation of neurosurgical intervention. Antibiotics.

Prognosis. Variable from deepening of coma and death, to recovery and partial to almost complete remission of symptoms.

BIBLIOGRAPHY. Vick NA: Grinker's Neurology, 7th ed. Springfield, CC Thomas, 1976

STRONG'S

Synonyms. Right-sided aortic arch–mental deficiency–facial dysmorphism. Aortic arch anomaly–peculiar facies–mental retardation. See Rubinstein–Taybi, Russell-Silver, and Floppy infant.

Symptoms and Signs. Evident from birth; both sexes affected. Low birth weight; mental retardation; micro-cephaly; hypotonia; hyperactive patellar reflexes. *Facies.* Asymmetric, triangular. Nose, prominent; septal deviation. Antimongoloid slant. Large ears; rotated posteriorly. Broad forehead. Small, downturned mouth. Teeth abnormalities. *Hands.* Syndactyly. *Heart.* Significant murmur.

Etiology. Unknown; genetic mutation, followed by dominant inheritance without apparent sex-linkage.

Pathology. See Signs. Fourth and sixth aortic arch abnormalities.

Diagnostic Procedures. *X-ray of chest,* with barium swallow. Right-sided aortic arch and esophageal indentation. Bone age normal. Asymmetry of facial bones; deviation of nasal septum; slight hypertelorism. *Electrocardiography.* Normal. *Psychometric evaluation.* Mental retardation or subnormality. *Karyotype study.* Normal. *Urine.* Amino acid chromatogram normal.

Therapy. Symptomatic.

Prognosis. *Quoad vitam,* good. A few patients may grow normally, complete schooling, and hold skilled jobs; however, majority fail to be promoted a grade at least once.

BIBLIOGRAPHY. Strong WB: Familial syndrome of right-sided aortic arch mental deficiency and facial dysmorphism. J Pediatr 73:882–888, 1968

STRUDWICK'S*

Synonyms. Murdock-Walker; dappled metaphysis; KO2 Lowsky-Zychowicz; metaphyseal dysostosis (type B-II); Sutcliffe's; spondylometaphyseal dysplasia (type C-V); spondylometaphyseal dysostosis (type C-IV).

Symptoms and Signs. Both sexes affected; present from birth. Short trunk and extremities. Normal weight. Nose broad and flat. Eye problems. Sternum prominent. Breathing short and impaired (rib retraction), hyperpneic. Moderate hepatosplenomegaly; protuberant abdomen. Delayed growth and motor milestones. Joint laxity; elbows do not extend fully; coxa vara; knock-knee; scoliosis and lordosis. Other possible malformations: cleft palate; hemangiomas; hernias; foot malformations.

Etiology. Autosomal recessive trait.

Diagnostic Procedures. *Blood, urine.* Normal. *X-rays.* Metaphyseal irregularities; "paint brush" and radiologic hyperlucency. "Dappling" alternated zones of osteosclerosis and osteopenia maximal in the ulna and fibula.

---

* Name of prototype patient.

Therapy. Control of respiratory infections. Surgical correction of cleft palate, hernias, and significant sternum deformities, and nonsurgical orthopedic measures to correct various defects.

Prognosis. Fair *quoad vitam;* increased mortality in early age. Poor for function; frequently, episodic polyarthritis in later life. Severe scoliosis and cord compression in early adulthood.

BIBLIOGRAPHY. Kozolowsky K, Zichowicz C: Metaphyseal dystosis of mixed type in a female child. Am J Roentgen 88:443–449, 1962
Sutcliffe J: Metaphyseal dystosis. Am Radiol 9:219–223, 1966
Murdock JL, Walker BA: A new form of spondylometaphyseal dysplasia. Birth Defects 5:368–370, 1969
Kousseff BG, Nichols P: Autosomal recessive spondylometaepiphyseal dysplasia type Strudwick. Am J Med Genet 17:547–550, 1984

STRÜMPELL–LEICHTENSTERN

Synonyms. Acute hemorrhagic encephalitis. Weston Hurst acute hemorrhagic leukoencephalitis. Includes hemorrhagic necrotizing encephalomyelitis.

Symptoms. Both sexes affected; onset at all ages, prevalent in children. Onset rapid or apoplectiform (necrotizing). Prodromata of cephalalgia and fever. Convulsions; mental dullness; delirium; coma.

Signs. Focal manifestations; tachypnea; neck rigidity; myoclonus; aphasia; optic atrophy; ataxia.

Etiology. Multiple: viral; postvaccinal; drug-induced; hypersensitive mechanisms.

Pathology. In brain, scattered hemorrhagic foci usually in white matter (intranuclear inclusion bodies in some cases). In necrotizing variety, liquefaction of white matter.

Diagnostic Procedures. *Blood.* Usually, leukocytosis and high sedimentation rate. *Cerebrospinal fluid.* Normal or lymphocytic pleocytosis and a few scattered red cells. *Angiography.* May suggest presence of occupying lesion. *Electroencephalography.*

Therapy. Symptomatic. Trial with antibiotics; corticosteroids.

Prognosis. Usually fatal; the few recoveries will show severe residuals. In necrotizing form, death may supervene in 24 hours.

BIBLIOGRAPHY. von Strümpell A: Ueber primaere acute Encephalitis. Dtsch Arch Klin Med 47:53–74, 1890
Leichtenstern O: Ueber primaere acute haemorrhägische Encephalitis. Dtsch Med Wochenschr 18:39–40, 1892
Hurst EW: Acute haemorrhagic leukoencephalitis: Previously undefined entity. Med J Australia 2:1–6, 1941
Adams RD, Victor M: Principles of Neurology, 3rd ed, pp 715–716. New York, McGraw-Hill, 1985

STRUEMPELL–LORRAIN

Synonyms. Spastic infantile paralysis; spastic familial paraplegia. See Kugelberg–Welander and Behr's I.

Symptoms. Prevalent in males; onset in early life. Lower extremities hypertonicity and weakness, followed by involvement of upper limbs, dysarthria, and dysphagia.

Signs. Clumsy ambulation; pes cavus (frequent); exaggerated deep reflexes; Babinski's sign; decreased or abolished abdominal reflexes; sphincters slightly affected (later).

Etiology. Autosomal (usually) recessive inheritance or sex linked. Could be considered a variant of Friedreich's ataxia (see) and some heredoataxias with cerebellar atrophy.

Pathology. Degeneration of corticospinal and spinocerebellar tracts of cord, greatest in lumbar and thoracic segments. Possibly, agyria.

Diagnostic Procedures. *Cerebrospinal fluid.* Normal. *Electromyography. Blood.* Creatine phosphokinase (CPK) normal or slightly elevated.

Therapy. None. Orthopedic measures.

Prognosis. Slowly progressive in years; finally, confines patient to bed. Death from intervening conditions.

BIBLIOGRAPHY. Struempell A: Beitraege zur Pathologie des Rueckenmarks. Arch Psychiatr 10:676–717, 1880
Lorrain M: Contribution a l'étude de la paraplégie spasmodique familiale (thesis). Paris, 1898
Merritt HH: A Textbook of Neurology, 6th ed, p 561. Philadelphia, Lea & Febiger, 1979
Adams RD, Victor M: Principles of Neurology, 3rd ed, p 886. New York, McGraw-Hill, 1985

STRUMA OVARY

Synonym. Ovary–thyroid tumor.

Symptoms. Onset usually between 30 and 50 years of age. Sensation of abdominal pressure and fullness. In 10% of patients, variable combinations of symptoms of hyperthyroidism (see Flajani's).

Signs. Movable mass in adnexal area; occasionally, bilateral masses.

Etiology. Unknown.

Pathology. Benign teratoma, nodular surface, small cystic spaces. Typical thyroid follicle.

Diagnostic Procedures. *X-ray. Abdominal scan.* See Flajani's.

Therapy. Surgery.

Prognosis. Hyperthyroidism signs disappear after surgery.

BIBLIOGRAPHY. Kempers RD, Dockerty MB, Hoffman DL et al: Struma ovarii ascites, hyperthyroid and asymptomatic syndromes. Ann Intern Med 72:883–893, 1970
Kaplan M, Kamli R, Lubin E et al: Ectopic thyroid gland. J Pediatr 92:205–209, 1978

STRYKER–HALBEISEN

Synonym. Erythroderma–macrocytic anemia. Obsolete.

Symptoms. Weakness; fatigue; intense pruritus.

Signs. Late feature: patchy, scaly, vesicular erythroderma on face, neck, and upper chest.

Etiology. There are no absolute cutaneous markers of pernicious anemia except a frequent association with vitiligo (10 times more frequent occurrence than in normal population).

Diagnostic Procedures. *Blood.* Macrocytic anemia.

Therapy. Pyridoxine and other B complex vitamins; crude liver extract.

Prognosis. Skin lesions and blood changes corrected by treatment.

BIBLIOGRAPHY. Stryker GV, Halbeisen WA: Determination of macrocytic anemia as an aid in diagnosis of certain deficiency dermatoses. Arch Dermatol Syph 51:116–123, 1945
Rook A, Wilkinson DS, Ebling FJG et al: Textbook of Dermatology, 4th ed, p 2365. Oxford, Blackwell Scientific Publications, 1986

STUART–PROWER FACTOR DEFICIENCY

Synonym. Factor X deficiency. See Prothrombin deficiency syndromes.

Symptoms and Signs. Same manifestations as factor VII deficiency (see). Childhood bleeding from mild to severe resembling hemophilia. Thromboembolism.

Etiology. Autosomal recessive. An abnormal factor X (Factor X Friuli) also reported.

Diagnostic Procedures. *Blood.* Prolonged prothrombin time and partial thromboplastin time. Different from factor VII deficiency because thromboplastin generation and viper venom (Stypven) time abnormal. Immunodiffusion techniques and antibody neutralization show two variants of this defect: (cross-reacting material) CRM positive and CRM negative.

Therapy. Blood, plasma, plasma concentrate. Trial with progestational agents.

Prognosis. Good; but death from hemorrhage may occur.

BIBLIOGRAPHY. Telfle TP: A new coagulation defect. Br J Haematol 2:308–316, 1956
Denson KWE, Lurie A, De Cataldo F et al: The factor X defect: Recognition of abnormal forms of factor X. Br J Haematol 18:317, 1970

STUB THUMB

Synonyms. Brachydactyly type D, Potter thumbs, murder thumb. Brachymegalodactylism.

Symptoms and Signs. Both sexes. Unilateral 25% or bilateral 75%. Both sexes. Short and large terminal phalanx of digits.

Etiology. Autosomal dominant with variable penetrance.

BIBLIOGRAPHY. Breitenbecher JK: Hereditary shortness of thumbs. J Hered 14:15–21, 1923
Gray E, Hurt BK: Inheritance of brachydactyly type D. J Hered 75:297–299, 1984

STUEHMER'S

Synonyms. Balanitis xerotica obliterans; penis kraurosis.

Symptoms. Usually young adult men. Pain during erection. Pruritus.

Signs. May present different aspects: ivory white patches on the penis; hemorrhagic periurethral bullae; parchmentlike membrane covering glans; with progression, shrinkage and atrophy of penis, with meatal narrowing and fissuring of prepuce. Regional lymphadenopathy.

Etiology. May be an advanced stage of several conditions; for example lichen sclerosus, chronic balanitis.

Pathology. Atrophic epidermis; collagen homogenization; infiltration under collagen by lymphocytes and histiocytes.

Therapy. Corticosteroid ointments; intralesional corticosteroid injections; circumcision; dorsal slit; urethral dilatation.

Prognosis. Evolving form toward atrophy of penis. Occasionally, malignant transformation.

BIBLIOGRAPHY. Stuehmer A: Pigmentnaevi und ihre Behandlung. Medizinische 735–739, May 30, 1953
Rook A, Wilkinson DS, Ebling FJG et al: Textbook of Dermatology, 4th ed, pp 2190–2192. Oxford, Blackwell Scientific Publications, 1986

STURGE–WEBER

Synonyms. Encephalofacial angiomatosis; encephalotrigeminal angiomatosis; Dimitri's hemoangiomatosis; Jahnke's (variant without glaucoma); Kulisher's; Krabbe's II: Lawford's (variant with glaucoma, without increased ocular pressure) meningocutaneous; neurooculocutaneous; Parkes Weber's; phacomatosis; vascular encephalotrigeminal; Weber–Dimitri. See Klippel–Trenaunay–Weber.

Symptoms. Usually promising start, even intellectual precocity, before onset of mental retardation and epileptic seizures. Convulsions are of focal type and on the contralateral side of facial nevus. Seldom hemorrhage from angiomas.

Signs. Unilateral facial nevus (port wine) along area of distribution of trigeminal (V) nerve. Atrophy or spasticity on contralateral side of nevus. Increase or decrease of intraocular tension. Glaucoma, enophthalmos, exophthalmos, optic atrophy, and vascular malformation frequently observed. Limb hypertrophy. Obesity (not constant).

Etiology. Congenital; dysplasia of embryonic vascular system occurring during sixth week of embryonic life, affecting vessels between those surrounding the brain wall and those of membranous skull and integument.

Pathology. Hemangioma of face and brain. Mesodermal defect of capillary or cavernous blood vessels; arteriovenous aneurysm.

Diagnostic Procedures. *X-ray.* Radiologic evidence of intracerebral calcifications same side as nevus (becoming detectable at age 2). *Electroencephalography.* Gross dysrhythmia.

Therapy. Cerebral lobectomy has to be considered in infancy before epilepsy occurs. In cases with hemiparesis, promising results with hemispherectomy. Symptomatic treatment of epilepsy when surgery not feasible. Alternative forms of treatment include injection of sclerosing solution, radiation therapy or radium implant, carbon di-

oxide snow, electrodissection, or insertion of steel wire electrodes.

Prognosis. Mental retardation and hemiparesis eventually develop if surgery does not prevent them.

BIBLIOGRAPHY. Sturge WA: A case of partial epilepsy, apparently due to a lesion of one of the vaso-motor centers of the brain. Trans Clin Soc Lond 12:162–167, 1879; Br Med J 1:704, 1879
Weber FP: Right-sides, hemi-hypotrophy resulting from right-sided congenital spastic hemiplegia with a morbid condition of the left side of the brain revealed by radiogram. J Neurol Psychopathol Lond 37:301–311, 1922
Dimitri V: Tumor cerebral congénito (angioma cavernosum). Rev Assoc Med Argent 36:63, 1923
Susac JO, Smith JL, Scelfo RJ: The "Tomato-catsup" fundus in Sturge–Weber syndrome. Arch Ophthalmol 92:69–70, 1974
Chomette G, Auriol M: Classification des angiodysphasies et tumeurs vasculaires. Rev Stomatol Chir Maxillofac 87:1–15, 1986

SUBDURAL HEMATOMA SYNDROMES

ACUTE

Synonym. Hemorrhagic internal pachymeningitis.

Symptoms. Onset immediately after trauma. Unconsciousness; coma.

Signs. Dilated pupil on one side; loss of corneal reflexes; fundic venous congestion; progressive weakness of contralateral arm and leg.

Etiology. Trauma.

Pathology. Laceration of veins crossing to superior longitudinal sinus.

Diagnostic Procedures. *Angiography. CT scan.*

Therapy. Immediate operation.

Prognosis. Poor; high mortality.

SUBACUTE

Symptoms. Appear 1 week or longer after trauma. Headache; irritability; neck stiffness; hemiplegia and aphasia.

Signs. Hemiplegia; Babinski's sign; changes in pulse and respiration; strabismus.

Pathology. Laceration of brain or veins crossing superior longitudinal sinus (or both). Hematoma with membranous capsule containing hemorrhagic fluid and clots.

Diagnostic Procedures. *X-ray. Angiography. CT scan.*

Therapy. Surgical evacuation.

Prognosis. Mortality 25%.

CHRONIC

Symptoms. Occur in infants and in adults, especially in alcoholics. Onset weeks or months after severe or mild trauma of the head. Gradual progression. Severe unremitting headache. Some patients present convulsions as first symptoms. Irritability; inattention; lethargy; finally stupor. Hemiplegia (usually contralateral, occasionally ipsilateral). Hemianopsia (seldom). Sensory changes not frequent.

Signs. Frequently absent; papilledema (in only 20% of cases). Dilated fixed pupil; external ophthalmoplegia.

Etiology. Trauma.

Pathology. Not true hematomas but hemorrhagic cysts. Small bleeding cysts in which disintegration increases the osmotic pressure and attracts fluid so that the volume of the cyst progressively enlarges. Content of cyst chocolate-colored fluid.

Diagnostic Procedures. *Spinal tap.* Frequently, normal pressure and chemistry. Fluid clear or slightly xanthochromic; normal cell count; protein slightly increased. *X-ray.* Often negative (shift of Pineal body). *Echoencephalography. Angiography. Ventriculography. Electroencephalography. CT scan.*

Therapy. Removal of fluid through trephine opening or, if needed, removal of capsule and clotted content.

Prognosis. According to time of removal. In some cases, spontaneous regression. If symptomatic, surgery indicated.

IN INFANTS

Symptoms. Onset during first 6 months of life. Vomiting; failure to eat; irritability; convulsions; stupor.

Signs. Low-grade fever; bulging of fontanelles and head enlargement; distention of scalp veins; retinal hemorrhages; seldom papilledema.

Etiology. Trauma or clotting defect.

Pathology. Accumulation of blood and fluid.

Diagnostic Procedures. Puncture of subdural space through lateral angle of anterior fontanelle or coronal suture.

Therapy. According to need: (1) daily tapping and drainage of 10 ml of fluid; (2) bilateral holes and evacuation of hematoma; (3) craniotomy with excision of membrane and evacuation of clot.

Prognosis. Fair; good response to treatment.

BIBLIOGRAPHY. Adams RD, Victor M: Principles of Neurology, 3rd ed, pp 641–662. New York, McGraw-Hill, 1985

SUBDURAL HYGROMA

Symptoms and Signs. Similar to those of subdural hematoma. In order of frequency: headache, nervousness and irritability; stupor; loss of memory and confusion; hemiparesis or hemiplegia; dizziness.

Etiology. Cranial trauma (tearing of arachnoid). Subdural effusion secondary to infections. Rupture of arachnoid at basal cistern in communicating hydrocephalus.

Pathology. Collection of clear or yellowish fluid in subdural space, with high concentration of protein.

Diagnostic Procedures. See Subdural hematoma syndromes.

Therapy. See Subdural hematoma syndromes.

Prognosis. See Subdural hematoma syndromes.

BIBLIOGRAPHY. Naffziger HC: Subdural fluid accumulation following head injury. JAMA 82:1751–1752, 1924
Wycis HT: Subdural hygroma: Report of seven cases. J Neurosurg 2:340–357, 1945
Adams RD, Victor M: Principles of Neurology, 3rd ed, pp 645, 904. New York, McGraw-Hill, 1985

SUBMERSION

Symptoms. Occur in individuals who have been near drowning. Tachypnea; mild fever; restlessness; vertigo; confusion and occasionally nausea; vomiting; shock.

Signs. Cyanosis, signs of pulmonary congestion and edema, and abdominal distention.

Etiology. Unknown; possibly related to asphyxia and effect of stress.

Pathology. No evidence of aspiration of water into the lung. Lung congestion and edema.

Diagnostic Procedures. *Blood.* White blood cells increased.

Therapy. Rest; symptomatic.

Prognosis. Good; transitory condition.

BIBLIOGRAPHY. Saline M, Baum GL: The submersion syndrome. Ann Intern Med 41:1134–1138, 1954
Conn AW, Modell JH: Current neurological considerations in near-drowning. Can Anaesth Soc J 27:197–198, 1980

Tabeling BB, Modell JH: Drowning and near-drowning. In Tinker J, Rapin M (eds): Care of the Critically Ill Patients, p 697. Berlin, Springer–Verlag, 1983

SUCROSE-DEXTRINOSE DEFICIENCY

Synonyms. Sucrose-isomaltose malabsorption, disaccharide intolerance I, Sucrose-isomaltose deficiency.

Symptoms and Signs. Early childhood. Symptoms of alactasia (see) evoked by table sugar or sweetened foods. Association of renal calculi (oxalate) possible.

Etiology. Autosomal recessive.

Diagnostic Procedures. *Small intestine biopsy.* Low activity of sucrose and isomaltose. *Oral sucrose tolerance test.* Oral administration of a test dose (1–2 mg/kg) of lactose, glucose, or galactose and of maltose produces a normal rise of blood sugar concentration. Ingestion of sucrose is followed by explosive diarrhea. *Stool.* pH is low.

Therapy. Suspension of sucrose from diet. Enzyme of fungal origin may be tried. Sucrose-free diet is provided by milk, meat, fish, fowl, eggs, animal fat, glucose, vegetables, and cheese.

Prognosis. Good with therapy.

BIBLIOGRAPHY. Moore D, Lichtman S, Durie P et al: Primary sucrose-isomaltase deficiency: Importance of clinical judgment. Lancet II:164–165, 1985

SUDDEN DEATH ADULT

Synonyms. See Mort d'amour; voodoo death.

Symptoms and Signs. In subjects of all ages in apparent good health. Clinically unexplainable sudden death.

Etiology. Pathologic findings retrospectively will indicate the previously unidentified causes as: congenital cardiac malformations, infective-immune, thrombolytic, atherosclerotic, or other degenerative processes.

Therapy. Early: attempt to resuscitate.

BIBLIOGRAPHY. Lancisi GM: De subitaines mortibus. Buegni Roma 1707 Translation: White PD, Boursey AV, St John's Univ Press, New York, 1971
Hurst JW: The Heart, 6th ed, pp 529–537. New York, McGraw-Hill, 1986

SUDDEN INFANT DEATH

Synonyms. Crib death; cot death.

Symptoms. Distinctive age distribution. Almost never occurs before 2 weeks or after 8 months of age. Higher incidence among nonwhite and poor families and in lower-weight-range babies. Seasonal: highest incidence late autumn, winter, and spring. It occurs almost exclusively during sleep. Babies who are completely healthy and normal occasionally, except for history of minor respiratory symptoms for 1 to 2 weeks, are discovered dead in the morning, lying in a characteristic abdominal position, with face to side.

Etiology. Unknown; parathyroid insufficiency theory rejected; thymolymphaticus habitus theory rejected; suffocation excluded. Death may result from the combination of many interrelated factors in which possibly virus infections, low birth weight, and laryngospasm seem to play a role. To be differentiated from other forms of unexpected death, where etiologic findings may be identified.

Pathology. Petechial hemorrhages (93%) appearing only in the thoracic contents. Pulmonary edema; heart dilated, containing fluid blood. Urinary bladder empty; redness of pharynx and minor inflammatory changes of airway.

Diagnostic Procedures. *Autopsy.* Cannot explain death or presence of described findings.

Prognosis. Sudden death syndrome represents 10% of deaths occurring in first year of life. Prophylaxis unknown.

BIBLIOGRAPHY. Beckwith JB, Bergman AB: The sudden death syndrome of infancy. Hosp Pract 2:44–52, 1967
Proceedings of the first Australian Rotary Health Research Fund Conference on "cot death." Aust Paediatr J 22:Suppl 1, 1986
Nelson EAS, Taylor BJ, Weatherall IL: Sleeping position and infant bedding may predispose to hyperthermia and the sudden infant death syndrome. Lancet 1:199–200, 1989

SUDECK'S

Synonyms. Posttraumatic atrophy; posttraumatic bone atrophy; posttraumatic sympathetic dystrophy; Kienboeck's; posttraumatic osteoporosis; peripheral trophoneurosis; posttraumatic osteoporosis; reflex dystrophy; Sudeck–Leriche. See Mitchell's I and Causalgia.

Symptoms and Signs. Prevalent in old people and in women. Those of Steinbrocker's (see). Typical bone changes, however, are not always associated with trauma.

Etiology. Unknown (see Steinbrocker's syndrome).

Pathology. Patchy osteoporosis, especially around joints.

Diagnostic Procedures. *X-ray.* Typical pattern of localized osteoporosis.

Therapy. See Steinbrocker's.

Prognosis. Osteoporosis sometimes remains after the patient has recovered from other symptoms of Steinbrocker's syndrome.

BIBLIOGRAPHY. Sudeck P: Ueber die acute enzündliche Knockenatrophie. Arch Klin Chir 62:147–156, 1900
Sudeck P: Ueber die acute enzündliche Knochenatrophie. Verh Dtsch Ges Chir 29:673–682, 1900
Hurst JW: The Heart, 6th ed, p 987. New York, McGraw-Hill, 1986

SUGARMAN'S

Synonym. Brachydactyly–major proximal phalanges shortening.

Symptoms and Signs. Short fingers with no motility at proximal interphalangeal joints. Hallux more proximal and dorsal than usual.

Etiology. Possibly autosomal recessive inheritance or dominant with reduced penetrance.

Diagnostic Procedures. *Rx hand.* Double first metacarpal bilaterally.

Therapy. Amputation of big toe.

BIBLIOGRAPHY. Sugarman GI, Hager D, Kulik WJ: A new syndrome of brachydactyly of hands and feet with duplication of the first toes. Birth Defects 5:1–8, 1974
Fujimoto A, Smolensky LS, Wilson MG: Brachydactyly with major involvement of proximal phalanges. Clin Genet 21:107–111, 1982

SULZBERGER–GARBE

Synonyms. Exudative discoid lichenoid dermatosis; lichenoid chronic dermatosis; polymorphic prurigo. Savill's.

Symptoms. Prevalent in men (especially Jews); abrupt onset in fourth to sixth decade. Cyclothymic or neurotic personalities. Severe pruritus, nocturnal and paroxysmal,

localized on genitals, under breast, around the mouth or extremities, often following a local infection.

Signs. Ephemeral exudative lesions; follicular papules and urticarialike lesions. Lichenification, crusting and serous discharge may develop.

Etiology. Unknown; emotional disturbances and secondary reaction to rubbing and scratching the lesion. Infectious eczematoid dermatitis has been described under this term.

Pathology. Similar to seborrheic dermatitis with greater crusting and lichenification. Cocci in corneal layer of epidermis not constantly found.

Diagnostic Procedures. *Biopsy of skin. Psychiatric evaluation. Blood.* Eosinophilia.

Therapy. If infection, treat topically; psychiatric treatment; antipruritics; anesthetics and combinations. Systemic steroids (temporary effect).

Prognosis. Control of superimposed infection and psychotherapy may give good results. Usually, chronic and difficult to control. Relapses frequent; spontaneous remissions occasional, usually after months or years.

BIBLIOGRAPHY. Savill T: On an epidemic skin disease. Br Med J 2:1197–1202, 1891
Sulzberger MB, Garbe W: Nine cases of a distinctive exudative discoid and lichenoid chronic dermatosis. Arch Dermatol Syph 36:247–278, 1937
Rook A, Wilkinson DS, Ebling FJG et al: Textbook of Dermatology, 4th ed, pp 387–388. Oxford, Blackwell Scientific Publications, 1986

SUMMERSKILL–WALSHE

Synonyms. Recurrent benign intrahepatic cholestasis; Tygstrup's. Intrahepatic cholestasis benign.

Symptoms. Prevalent in males. First episode usually before 20 years of age; number of attacks very variable. Duration 2 weeks to 18 months. Fatigue; nervous tension; anorexia; occasionally, nausea and vomiting; weight loss; pain in upper right abdominal quadrant (50%); bleeding tendency.

Signs. Jaundice; occasionally, abdominal tenderness; liver enlargement; easy bruising; pruritus.

Etiology. Benign intrahepatic disorder; cholestasis resulting from defect of excretion of conjugated bilirubin from liver cells and canaliculi. Possibility of recessive genetic condition with poor penetrance. Features to distinguish it from cholestasis, intrahepatic hereditary recurrences are not clear, except for milder course and later age of onset.

Pathology. Liver biopsy during jaundice: bile stasis in the canaliculi; round cell infiltration in portal tracts. No changes indicating extrahepatic obstruction; no irreversible change of hepatic architecture. In asymptomatic periods: no changes. Electromicroscopic studies during attack: numerous vescicles containing low-medium density material present in many cells. Following recovery they disappear.

Diagnostic Procedures. *Blood.* Increase of conjugated bilirubin; high alkaline phosphatase; normal protein and electrophoretic pattern; colloidal lability tests normal; prothrombin time prolonged in some cases. Abnormal findings reverting to normal during remission. *Urine.* Urobilin present. *Stool.* Steatorrhea. *X-ray of gallbladder.* Good visualization.

Therapy. None specific. Correction of malabsorption (vitamins). Steroids and phenobarbital may reduce bilirubin level without affecting course of disease; cholestyramine relieves some symptoms (pruritus).

Prognosis. Good, with recurrence of condition.

BIBLIOGRAPHY. Summerskill WHJ, Walshe JM: Benign recurrent intrahepatic "obstructive" jaundice. Lancet 2:686–690, 1959
Wolkoff AW, Chowdhury JR, Arias IM: Hereditary jaundice and disorders of bilirubin metabolism. In Stanbury JB, Wyngaarden JB, Fredrickson DS et al: The Metabolic Basis of Inherited Disease, 5th ed, p 1385. New York, McGraw-Hill, 1983

SUMMITT'S

Synonyms. Summitt's acrocephalosyndactyly; craniosynostosis–syndactyly–obesity.

Symptoms and Signs. Present from birth. *Head.* Acrocephaly; occipital irregularity; epicanthal folds; strabismus; narrow palate; delayed teeth eruption. *Extremities.* Syndactyly from mild to severe; genu valgum and coxa valga (occasional). *Trunk.* Obesity; moderate gynecomastia. Normal mental development.

Etiology. Autosomal recessive (?) inheritance.

BIBLIOGRAPHY. Summit RL: Recessive acrocephalosyndactyly with normal intelligence. Birth Defects 5:35–38, 1969
Sells CJ, Hanson JW, Hall JG: The Summitt syndrome: Observation of a third case. Am J Med Genet 3:27–33, 1979

SUPERIOR LONGITUDINAL SINUS THROMBOSIS

Symptoms. More frequent in children. Headache; nausea; vomiting; general prostration; aplasia, urinary incontinence (in bilateral cases); convulsions. Occasionally, symptoms of spastic paraplegia.

Signs. Scalp edema; distention of veins near fontanelles. Homonymous hemianopsia or quadrantanopia, paralysis of conjugate gaze.

Etiology. Infective or aseptic thrombosis of superior longitudinal sinus (less frequent than in lateral sinus, see); extension of infection or reaction from paranasal sinuses; skull infection; brain abscess or because of extension from other cerebral venous sinuses.

Pathology. See Etiology. Frequent intracranial hemorrhagic complications.

Diagnostic Procedures. Difficult diagnosis. *X-ray.* Direct injection of radiopaque dye into longitudinal sinus.

Therapy. Antibiotics. Surgery.

Prognosis. Frequently fatal or severe residual neurologic manifestations; in some cases, complete recovery.

BIBLIOGRAPHY. Vick NA: Grinker's Neurology, 7th ed. Springfield, CC Thomas, 1976
Adams RD, Victor M: Principles of Neurology, 3rd ed, pp 521–522. New York, McGraw-Hill, 1985

SUPINE HYPOTENSIVE

Synonym. Inferior vena cava.

Symptoms. Occur in last month of pregnancy in 3% to 11%. Sudden fall of systolic blood pressure; circulatory collapse; retching and nausea when assuming supine position.

Signs. Tachycardia; fall of arterial pressure over 30 mm Hg. A few patients presenting this syndrome have premature separation of placenta because of sudden increase in venous pressure when lying down causing compression of vena cava.

Etiology and Pathology. Compression of inferior vena cava by flaccid full-term pregnant uterus, thus reducing venous return to heart and decreasing cardiac output.

Therapy. Lying down on left lateral position. If drop of pressure occurs on delivery table, tilting the right pelvis to the left.

Prognosis. Good; spontaneously corrected after termination of pregnancy.

BIBLIOGRAPHY. Runge H: Venous pressure during pregnancy, delivery, and puerperium. Arch Gynäkol 122:142–157, 1924
Robbins RA, Estrara T, Russell C: Supine hypotensive syndrome and abruptio placenta. Am J Obstet Gynecol 80:1207–1208, 1960
Hurst JW (ed): The Heart, Arteries and Veins, 4th ed, p 1726. New York, McGraw-Hill, 1978
Hurst JW: The Heart, 6th ed, p 1379. New York, McGraw-Hill, 1986

SURVIVOR

Synonyms. Concentration camp II; postconcentration camp.

Symptoms. Occur in victims who survived concentration camp or physical and mental distress due to persecution (hiding and striving for survival). Chronic state of tension; vigilance; irritability; depression; unrest and fear; sleep disturbances; nightmares. Headache; fatigue; excessive sweating. Avoidance of company and, in severe cases, complete withdrawal. Feeling of guilt (especially if only survivor of family) because of survival. Memory defects; parapraxia.

Etiology. Persistence of after-effect of psychological trauma.

Therapy. Psychotherapy. Group therapy in some cases indicated.

Prognosis. Difficult therapy.

BIBLIOGRAPHY. Niederland WG: Psychiatric disorders among persecution victims. A contribution to the understanding of concentration camp pathology and its after-effects. J Nerv Ment Dis 139:458–474, 1964

SUSPENDED HEART

Synonym. Vasoregulatory asthenia.

Symptoms. Onset at all ages; no sex preference. Chest pain or palpitation or both.

Signs. Usually, asthenic habitus; no evidence of cardiovascular disease.

Etiology. Alteration of position of heart so that it appears elongated and vertical or disturbance of the autonomic nervous system with hyperdynamic circulation.

Diagnostic Procedures. *Electrocardiography.* Depression of the ST segment in leads III and IIIR (during deep inspiration); lesser depression in II and CR7; not changed by change to upright position. *X-ray.* Anterior view: apparently normally located heart. During deep inspiration left cardiophrenic junction moves toward the middle. Right oblique view: during inspiration, heart and diaphragm separated widely. Left oblique view: during inspiration, gap between heart and diaphragm.

Therapy. None.

Prognosis. Excellent. This syndrome represents only an innocuous electrocardiographic variation. Its importance is due to the fact that an ST depression (in absence of digitalization) usually indicates the presence of a myocardial infarction.

BIBLIOGRAPHY. Evans W, Lloyd-Thomas HG: The syndrome of the suspended heart. Br Heart J 19:153–158, 1957
Hurst JW: The Heart, 6th ed, p 910. New York, McGraw-Hill, 1986

SUTTON'S I

Synonyms. Halo leukoderma; leukoderma acquisitum centrifugum; halo nevus.

Symptoms. Both sexes affected; onset in young adulthood, (range 4 to 45 yr). Asymptomatic.

Signs. Halo of hypomelanosis (0.5–1.0 cm) developing around a cutaneous nevus (benign or malignant). The phenomenon is observed usually with lesion on the trunk; less frequently on the head; seldom on the extremities. The central nevus tends to disappear slowly. In 30% of patients development of vitiligo.

Etiology. Unknown. Part of process of involution of melanotic nevi; genetic defect in melanogensis. Familial occurence (autosomal recessive reported).

Pathology. The histology of central lesions shows the substitution of the melanocytes by lymphocytes and reticular cells.

Diagnostic Procedures. *Biopsy of central lesion.*

Therapy. None, except if malignancy confirmed.

Prognosis. Good in most instances.

BIBLIOGRAPHY. Sutton R: An unusual variety of vitiligo (leucoderma acquisitum centrifugum). J Cutan Dis 34:797–800, 1916
Rook A, Wilkinson DS, Ebling FJG et al: Textbook of Dermatology, 4th ed, p 1595. Oxford, Blackwell Scientific Publications, 1986

SUTTON'S II

Synonym. Periadenitis–mucosa–necrotica–recurrent II. See Zahorsky's.

Symptoms and Signs. Onset in childhood or adolescence. Painful nodular lesions in the mucosa of mouth, frequently affecting the tongue also. Occasionally, vagina may be involved. After 3 or 4 days, detachment of necrotic plug and ulceration.

Etiology. Unknown; variant of aphthosis.

Pathology. See Zahorsky's.

Therapy. See Zahorsky's.

Prognosis. Chronic recurrent lesions.

BIBLIOGRAPHY. Sutton RL Jr: Recurrent scarring painful aphthae. Amelioration with sulfathiazole in two cases. JAMA 117:175–176, 1941
Rook A, Wilkinson DS, Ebling FJG et al: Textbook of Dermatology, 4th ed, pp 2099–2100. Oxford, Blackwell Scientific Publications, 1986

SWAN'S I

Synonyms. Blindspot; squint; monofixation.

Symptoms and Signs. Periodic diplopia; concomitant compensating esotropia of 12 to 18 degrees. No other clinical findings.

Etiology. Physiological mechanism to project the image of nondeviating eye onto blindspot of the deviating one, thus allowing its plotting as a central scotoma for the latter. There is criticism against considering such mechanism as a syndrome.

Therapy. Optical correction suggested.

Prognosis. Of no significant clinical importance.

BIBLIOGRAPHY. Swan KC: The blind spot syndrome. Arch Ophthalmol 40:371–388, 1940
Verhaeff FC: The so-called blindspot syndrome. Am J Ophthalmol 40:802–808, 1955
Bolet RV: Development of monofixation syndrome in congenital atropia. J Pediatr Ophthalmol Strabismus 18:49–51, 1981

SWAN'S II

Synonym. Congenital epiblepharon-inferior oblique insufficiency.

Symptoms and Signs. Observed in infants. (1) Epiblepharon, bilateral or unilateral; little irritation of cornea or occasionally keratitis. (2) Little or no eye deviation except in the field of action of the affected inferior oblique muscle (involved only unilaterally). Lack of contraction of the antagonists.

Etiology. Unknown; rare combination: 4 : 5000 cases examined at the University of Oregon Medical School.

Therapy. Control the inversion of the lash line, possibly by nonsurgical means. Antibiotic for irritation.

Prognosis. Patient learns to avoid rotation of his eyes to superior gaze (left or right according to eye involved); he is rarely aware of diplopia and carries his head in a normal position.

BIBLIOGRAPHY. Swan K: The syndrome of congenital epiblepharon and inferior oblique insufficiency. Am J Ophthalmol 39:130–136, 1955
Duke–Elder S: System of Ophthalmology, vol 3, p 2. St Louis, CV Mosby, 1963

SWANSON'S

Synonyms. Anhidrosis-pain insensitivity; hereditary sensory-autonomic neuropathy IV, HSAN IV; familial dysautonomia II; pain insensitivity anhidrosis.

Symptoms and Signs. Present from birth. Analgesia (loss of superficial and deep sensitivity); hyporeflexia; mild mental retardation; pupillary abnormalities from partial to complete Horner's syndrome (see); vasomotor instability; anhidrosis; aplasia of dental enamel; blond hair; blue eyes; both sexes.

Etiology. Suggested abnormality in differentiation of neural crest. See also Christ-Siemens-Touraine. Autosomal recessive inheritance.

Pathology. Normal sweat glands; meningeal thickening and cystic changes.

Diagnostic Procedures. *Urine.* Abnormal vanillylmandelic and homovanyllic acid assays.

Therapy. Symptomatic.

Prognosis. Poor.

BIBLIOGRAPHY. Swanson AG: Congenital insensitivity to pain with anhidrosis: a unique syndrome in two male siblings. Arch Neurol 8:299–306, 1963
Brown JW, Podosin R: A syndrome of the neural crest. Arch Neurol 15:294–301, 1966
Axelrod FB, Pearson J, Tapperby J, et al: Congenital sensory neuropathy with skeletal dysplasia. J Pediatr 102:727–730, 1983

SWANSON'S

Synonyms. Neuropathy sensory–anhidrosis; dysautonomia familial II; pain insensitivity–anhidrosis; sensory-autonomic neuropathy IV; SAN–IV; see Biemond's.

Symptoms. Both sexes. From infancy. Unexplained episodes of fever; self-mutilating behavior, congenital insensibility to pain. Low IQ (70).

Signs. Thermal and traumatic injuries when child begins to crawl.

Etiology. Unknown. Developmental defect; autosomal recessive trait.

Pathology. No uniform findings. Absence of small myelinated and unmyelinated fibers. Sweat glands present in the skin but not innervated.

Diagnostic Procedures. Lack of sweating also after intense stimulation physical or pharmacologic. Spontaneous lacrimation, but lack of response to Mecholyl or neostigmine.

Therapy. Careful handling of child. Padding of area susceptible to trauma.

Prognosis. Poor. Infection, traumatic lesion, self-mutilation.

BIBLIOGRAPHY. Swanson AG: Congenital insensitivity to pain with anhidrosis. A unique syndrome in two male siblings. Arch Neurol 8:299–306, 1963
Matsuo M, Kurakawa T, Goya N et al: Congenital insensitivity to pain with anhidrosis in a 2-month-old boy. Neurology 31:1190–1192, 1981

SWEAT RETENTION

Synonyms. Anhidrosis; hypohidrosis; thermogenic anhidrosis.

Symptoms. Occur when patient exposed to high temperature and high humidity. Malaise; weakness; flushing; pruritus; headache; nausea.

Signs. Tachycardia; tachypnea; fever.

Etiology. All causes that prevent sweating (inability to produce or to deliver to skin surface). Congenitally absent or deficient sweat glands; dermatitis; ectodermal dysplasia scars; neurogenic factors; miliaria; endocrine and metabolic conditions. Usually inherited as X-linked trait (see Christ–Siemens–Tourine); autosomal recessive inheritance reported as well.

Diagnostic Procedures. *Colorimetric test.* Absence of sweating.

Therapy. Removal to cooler, dryer place with breeze. Treatment, when feasible, of determining causes.

Prognosis. Severe hyperthermia may develop, sometimes with fatal consequences.

BIBLIOGRAPHY. Wolkin J, Goodman JI, Kelley WE: Failure of sweat mechanism in desert. JAMA 124:478–482, 1944
Mahloudji M, Livingston KE: Familial and congenital simple anhidrosis. Am J Dis Child 113:477–479, 1967
Crump IA, Danks DM: Hypohidrotic ectodermal dysplasia: A study of sweatpore in the X-linked forms and in a family with probable autosomal recessive inheritance. J Pediatr 78:466–473, 1971

SWEDISH TYPE PORPHYRIA

Synonyms. Intermittent acute porphyria; IAP; porphyria hepatica I; porphyria intermittens acuta; pyrroloporphyria; Waldenström's I.

Symptoms. Both sexes affected; female-to-male ratio 3:2; usual onset in young adulthood. *Abdominal symptoms.* Intermittent, recurrent attack of pain (colicky type); localized or generalized constipation. Vomiting occasionally severe. Attacks may last days or months. During attack, slight fever may be present. Weight loss, emaciation, electrolyte imbalance with dehydration may result. *Neurologic symptomatology.* Highly variable; polyneuritis including cranial nerves; autonomic system abnormalities; cerebral function derangement with motor, sensorial, and psychotic manifestations. Absence of photosensitivity and of increased mechanical fragility of skin.

Signs. Abdomen usually soft; no rebound tenderness; stomach distended. Neurologic findings highly variable. Blood hypertension (not constant). During attack, sinus tachycardia.

Etiology. Autosomal dominant inheritance. Deficiency of porphobilinogen (PBG) deaminase with which concomitant factors (steroid hormones, drugs, nutrition) determine clinical syndrome. Women probably have more frequent episodes because of menstrual cycles.

Pathology. High concentration of PBG in liver.

Diagnostic Procedures. *Blood.* During attack, leukocytosis may be present. Electrolyte imbalance (when severe vomiting); hyponatremia. *Urine.* Excretion of high amount of PBG and d-aminolevulinic acid (ALA) (rough correlation of their amounts with attacks); in intermittent periods values may approach normality). *X-ray of gastrointestinal tract.* Areas of distention proximal to areas of spasm.

Therapy. Avoid dangerous drugs (especially barbiturates). Symptomatic: narcotic analgesics for pain relief.

High carbohydrate intake ameliorates symptoms; hematin IV.

Prognosis. Attacks may last for various lengths of time; occasionally fatal. Usually followed by periods of latency lasting weeks or years. Death rate highest in third decade. Some of these patients undergo repeated abdominal operations before the diagnosis is made.

BIBLIOGRAPHY. Günther H: Die Haematoporphyrie. Dtsch Arch Klin Med 105:89–146, 1911
Waldenström J: Studien über Porphyrie. Acta Med Scand [Suppl] 82:1–254, 1937
Kappas A, Sassa S, Anderson KE: The porphyrias. In Stanbury JB, Wyngaarden JB, Fredrickson DS et al: The Metabolic Basis of Inherited Disease, 5th ed, p 1301. New York, McGraw-Hill, 1983

SWEET'S

Synonym. Acute febrile neutrophilic dermatosis.

Symptoms and Signs. Occur in women; onset in middle age. Infection precedes onset. High persistent fever; eruption of painful plaques on skin of limbs, face, and neck. Later, pustules.

Etiology. Unknown; possibly, hypersensitivity to infective agent.

Pathology. *Skin.* Focal infiltration of neutrophils and lymphocytes; moderate leukocytolysis. Moderate vascular endothelial swelling and vasodilatation.

Diagnostic Procedures. *Blood.* Culture; moderate leukocytosis.

Therapy. Antibiotics ineffective. Steroids effective as long as administered.

Prognosis. Condition lasts 2 weeks or more. Repeated relapses (usually preceded by infections).

BIBLIOGRAPHY. Sweet RD: An acute febrile neutrophilic dermatosis. Br J Dermatol 76:349–356, 1964
Spector JI, Zimbler H, Levine R et al: Sweet's syndrome, association with acute leukemia. JAMA 244:1131–1132, 1980
Rook A, Wilkinson DS, Ebling FJG et al: Textbook of Dermatology, 4th ed, p 1151. Oxford, Blackwell Scientific Publications, 1986

SWYER–JAMES

Synonyms. Unilateral pulmonary emphysema; unilateral hyperlucent lung; pulmonary artery functional hypoplasia; MacLeod's.

Symptoms. Onset in childhood and adolescence. Recurrent pulmonary infections.

Signs. Unilateral diminished pulmonary expansion, faint breath sounds, and fine rales.

Etiology. Acquired condition, secondary to necrotizing bronchitis, probably viral in origin, with onset in early infancy, damaging peripheral bronchial passages with consequent emphysema and bronchiolectasis and functional insufficiency of pulmonary artery and its branches. Agenesis and congenital hypoplasia of pulmonary artery are usually accompanied by major symptomatology due to cardiovascular and pulmonary anomaly, which allows the differentiation of the two conditions.

Pathology. Obliteration of peripheral capillaries of affected lung. Bronchiolectasis; some alveolar emphysematous zones are collapsed. Chronic inflammatory changes.

Diagnostic Procedures. *X-ray of chest.* Must be done in inspiration and forced expiration. Hyperlucency of affected lung or lobe; decreased peripheral vascular marking with small hilar shadow. *CT scan.* Reinforces the findings of radiography. *Fluoroscopy.* Heart and mediastinum shift toward affected lung in inspiration and away in expiration. *Bronchoscopy.* No obstruction of major bronchi. *Bronchography.* Decreased or absent filling at periphery. Unusual bronchial pattern; small bronchioles terminating in clubs or pools. *Angiography.* In the affected side, decreased filling of pulmonary artery. Isotopic V/Q study shows hypoperfusion.

Therapy. Antibiotic for acute or chronic pulmonary infections. When syndrome does not react to treatment and interferes with work and well-being of patient because of persistence of definite syndrome, surgery is indicated.

Prognosis. Variable according to intensity of symptoms and response to treatment.

BIBLIOGRAPHY. Swyer PR, James GCW: Case of unilateral pulmonary emphysema. Thorax 8:133–136, 1953
Guillem Lanuza F, Roig Riu M, Villaroja Luna J, Vila Martinez R: Sindrome de Swyer–James. Revision y presentacion de un caso. Acta Pediatr Esp 44:454–462, 1986
Avital A, Shulman DL, Baryishay E et al: Differential lung function in an infant with the Swyer-James syndrome. Thorax 44:298–302, 1989

SYDENHAM'S

Synonyms. Acute chorea; minor chorea; rheumatic chorea; Saint Vitus' dance.

Symptoms. Occur in children from 5 to 13; more frequently in females. Involuntary, purposeless, irregular, short-lasting movements (choreiform) initially in one limb. Anxiety; irritability; weakness; face movements that simulate smirking expressions. Voice changes may also be observed; dysarthria may be severe. Movements cease during sleep. Emotional instability.

Signs. Hypotonic musculature; flaccidity; passive motion that allows unusual and otherwise uncomfortable positions. Tendon reflexes variable; no sensory changes; psychological changes; possibly fever.

Etiology. Unknown; association with rheumatic fever, tonsillitis, less frequently typhus, malaria, or other infections, or completely independent. Phenothiazine drugs, haloperidol may cause chorea.

Pathology. Diffuse cerebral edema; congestion of corpus striatum. Three orders of changes: inflammatory, degenerative, and vascular. But no precise localization of lesions.

Diagnostic Procedures. *Cerebrospinal fluid.* Mildly increased pressure; mild pleocytosis; increased glucose. *Blood.* Sedimentation rate; antistreptolysin titer; C-reactive protein.

Therapy. Rest; quiet; protection from harmful movements. Phenobarbital; paraldehyde; phenothiazine; haloperidol. Salicylates or other specific therapy if rheumatic fever present.

Prognosis. Variable; mild form recovers in weeks; exacerbation may prolong form for years. Death may result from exhaustion or associated cardiac complication. Relapses after months or years in 33% of cases.

BIBLIOGRAPHY. Sydenham T: Schedula monitoria de novae febris ingressu Londini, Kettilby, 1636
Begbie J: Remarks on rheumatism and chorea; their relation and treatment. Month J Med Sci 7:740–754, 1847
Adams RD, Victor M: Principles of Neurology, 3rd ed, p 61. New York, McGraw-Hill, 1985

SYLVESTER'S (P.E.)

Synonym. Friedreich's ataxia–optic atrophy–sensorineural deafness.

Symptoms and Signs. Both sexes, from childhood. Neural deafness, optic atrophy, ataxia; muscle wasting of shoulder girdle and arms; mental dullness.

Etiology. Unknown. Autosomal dominant inheritance.

Pathology. Degeneration of optic nerves, posterior columns, spinocerebellar and corticospinal tracts.

Prognosis. Variable progressivity.

BIBLIOGRAPHY. Sylvester PE: Some unusual findings in a family with Friedreich's ataxia. Arch Dis Child 33:217–221, 1958

SYMMETRIC ADENOLIPOMATOSIS

Synonyms. Launois-Bensaude; Buschke's II; Madelung's II; Brodie's; cephalothoracic lipodystrophy; lipomatosis multiple symmetric, LMS, MSL.

Symptoms. Onset between 35 to 40 years of age; prevalent in males. At first the patient notices that he cannot button the collar of his shirt and discovers large diffuse tumefaction in the posterior part of the neck; then the appearance of symmetric masses in the submandibular region and successively other lipomas on the chest and rest of body, with the exclusion of limbs. Asthenia and apathy are usually present. Compression of peripheral nerve results in pain (seldom paresis); dyspnea and cough may also develop. High frequency of neuropathies. Alteration of vibratory sensation.

Signs. Round lipomas, doughy consistency, egg or melon size, diffuse margins, free from superficial and deep planes. Cyanosis, exophthalmos may develop. Trophic ulcers, Charcot's arthropathy.

Etiology. Unknown; ectodermal anomaly. Autosomal dominant inheritance observed.

Pathology. Normal fat tissue (fat cells smaller than normal) expanding without cyst formation.

Diagnostic Procedures. *Biopsy. Blood.* Liver function tests slightly abnormal; lipidogram slightly abnormal; increase of HDL, decrease of LDH. *Basal metabolism.* Occasionally increases. *Urine.* 17-ketosteroid excretion occasionally decreased.

Therapy. Plastic surgery to remove some of the most disfiguring lipomas.

Prognosis. Absence of spontaneous degeneration of the lipomatous masses. After plastic surgery no hematoma, necrosis, infection, or superficial sclerosis develops.

BIBLIOGRAPHY. Brodie BC: Clinical Lectures on Surgery. Delivered at St. George Hospital, pp 201–202. Philadelphia, Lea & Blanchard 1846
Madelung OW: Ueber den Fetthals (diffuses Lipom des Halses). Arch Klin Chir Berlin 37:106–130, 1888
Launois-Bensaude PE: L'adenolipomatose symetrique. Bull Soc Med Hôp. Paris 15:298–318, 1898
Enzi G, Angelini C, Negrin P et al: Sensory, motor, and autonomic neuropathy in patients with multiple symmetric lipomatosis. Medicine 64:388–393, 1985

SYNBLEPHARON

Symptoms and Signs. Partial or complete adherence of the eyelid to the eyeball. Inability to close eyelids effectively. Diplopia.

Etiology. Defect due to inflammation, injury, or burns. Congenital type, usually of recessive inheritance, possibly dominant. Frequently associated with ankyblepharon, microphthalmos, ankyloblepharon filiforme adnatum or with cleft palate. This manifestation is present in various congenital syndromes.

Pathology. Affects lower lid more frequently. Bands of fibrous tissue between globe and lid.

Therapy. Prevention by daily probing. Mucous membrane grafts.

Prognosis. Frequent recurrence. Disfigurement, lagophthalmus.

SYNCOPAL MIGRAINE

Symptoms and Signs. More frequent in adolescent females, frequently associated with menstrual cycle. Premonitory aura of migraine is followed by consciousness loss. Slow onset. At awaking severe headache (occipital area).

Etiology. Unknown. Postulated brain stem ischemia or prolonged localized basilar artery spasm. Hyperresponsiveness of dopamine receptors is an alternative explanation.

Therapy. See Migraine.

Prognosis. That of migraine.

BIBLIOGRAPHY. Bickerstaff ER: Impairment of consciousness in migraine. Lancet 2:1057–1070, 1961

Sicuteri F, Boccuzzi M, Fanciullacci M et al: A new nonvascular interpretation of syncopal migraine. Adv Neurol 33:199–210, 1982

SYPHILID, TUBEROSERPIGINOUS

Synonym. Lewis'.

Symptoms and Signs. Both sexes affected; skin lesions similar to those of lupus vulgaris affecting eyelids, nose, and ears and, possibly, also extremities and trunk. Lower eyelids more frequently affected. Conjunctival lesions; corneal ulcers.

Etiology. Syphilis.

Therapy. Specific.

Prognosis. Lesions could be arrested by treatment.

BIBLIOGRAPHY. Schreck E: Veraenderungen des Sehorgans bei Haut-und-Geschlechtskrankheiten. In: Gottron HA, Schoenfeld V (eds). Dermatologie und Venerologie (IV) Stuttgart, Thieme 1960

Korting GW: The Skin and Eye, p 26. Philadelphia, WB Saunders, 1973

T

TACHYPNEA TRANSIENT NEWBORN

Synonym. Respiratory distress type II.

Symptoms and Signs. Usually full-term infants. Elevated respiratory rate on first day of life; some retraction and grunting; slight cyanosis; no rales or rhonchi. Respiratory rate remains elevated for 2 to 5 days.

Etiology. Unknown; it may represent a delay in resorption of fluid from lungs.

Pathology. Postulated reduction of compliance of the lung from delay of resorption of alveolar fluid and distention of periarterial space.

Diagnostic Procedures. *Electrocardiography.* Normal. *X-ray of chest.* Suggestive of vascular engorgement or passive vascular congestion (poorly defined margins). Lack of reticulogranular pattern. Slight cardiomegaly (mean ratio 0.60). *Blood.* pH and Pco_2; standard bicarbonate within normal limits.

Therapy. Symptomatic; oxygen.

Prognosis. Recovery with disappearance of radiologic findings between first and fifth days.

BIBLIOGRAPHY. Avery ME, Gatewood OB, Brumley G: Transient tachypnea of newborn. Possible delayed resorption of fluid at birth. Am J Dis Child 111:380–385, 1966
Rawlings JS, Smith FR: Transient tachypnea of the newborn: An analysis of neonatal and obstetric risk factors. Am J Dis Child 138:869–871, 1984
Shohat M, Levy G, Levy I et al: Transient tachypnoea of the newborn and asthma. Arch Dis Child 64:277–279, 1989

TAENZER'S

Synonyms. Ulerythema sycosiforme; Unna's (PG) II. See Brocq's (lupoid sycosis), Quinquaud's, and Folliculitis decalvans. Considered today a variant of folliculitis decalvans in its various stages of evolution. Prevalent in males; onset in adult life, less frequently in adolescence and childhood.

BIBLIOGRAPHY. Taenzer PR: Über das Ulerythema ophryogenes. Eine noch nicht bescriebene Hautkrankheit. Wochenschr Prakt Dermatol 8:197–208, 1889
Unna PG: The Histopathology of the Diseases of the Skin, p 1086. New York, Clay, 1896

TAFFY CANDY

Synonyms. Mitral regurgitation–chordal elongation; primary chordal dysplasia; secondary chordal dysplasia. See also Papillary muscle.

Symptoms and Signs. Gradual or sudden, severe mitral regurgitation symptomatology.

Etiology. Inappropriate elongation of anterior leaflet chordae. In course of rheumatic fever, myocardial infarction; without underlying abnormalities.

Pathology. Chordae of anterior leaflet elongated and thinned out, especially in the middle; all the features of mitral regurgitation.

Diagnostic Procedures. *Electrocardiography. Angiocardiography. X-ray of chest. Echocardiography. Cardiac catheterization.*

Therapy. Medical or surgical.

Prognosis. Fair with treatment; may evolve into chordal rupture.

BIBLIOGRAPHY. Cobbs BW Jr: In Hurst JW, Logue RB (eds): The Heart, 1st ed, p 88. New York, McGraw-Hill, 1966
Hurst JW: The Heart, 6th ed, p 767. New York, McGraw-Hill, 1986

TAKAHARA'S

Synonyms. Acatalasia; acatalasemia.

Symptoms. Common in Japanese and Koreans; reported in Caucasians as well. Asymptomatic (50%). Chronic, severe infection of mouth; gangrenous lesions, including alveolar destruction.

Etiology. Deficiency of enzyme catalase in tissues and cells, including blood, erythrocytes. Genetic recessive inheritance.

Pathology. Gangrenous lesion of mouth due to lack of resistance to normal flora.

Diagnostic Procedures. Addition of hydrogen peroxide to whole acatalasic blood produces methemoglobin, black-brown color (normal blood remains pink).

Therapy. Antibiotics; local surgical excision, tooth extraction. Whole blood transfusion to raise catalase level in period of need. Crystalline catalase suspension for topical treatment.

Prognosis. Lesions respond in part to antibiotic treatment and measures to prevent infections. After healing, lesions may produce scarring that may impair mouth opening.

BIBLIOGRAPHY. Takahara S: Progressive oral gangrene probably due to lack of catalase in the blood. Lancet 2:1101–1104, 1952
Matsunaga T, Seger R, Hoger P et al: Congenital acatalasemia: A study of neutrophil functions after provocation with hydrogen peroxide. Pediatr Res 19:1187–1190, 1985

TAKAYASU'S

Synonyms. Aortic arch arteritis; brachiocephalic arteritis; reversed coarctation; Martorell's II; Martorell–Fabre; pulseless; Raeder–Arbitz; young female aortic arch arteritis.

Symptoms. Prevalent in young women; symptoms may be intermittent. Usually, unilateral transient amblyopia or persistant blindness. Aphasia; transient hemiparesis; headache; vertigo; syncope, convulsions. Weakness and pain in the muscles of mastication; occasionally, weakness, numbness, or pain exertion of upper limb.

Signs. Atrophy and pigmentation on skin of face; ulceration of nose and palate. Cataracts. In fundus: anastomosis about the disk; atrophy of iris, optic nerve, atrophy or pigmentation of retina. Weakness of pulse in the arm; decrease of blood pressure on the arm; tendency to hypertension of the legs. Bruit on upper chest and neck. Marked pulmonary hypertension can occur, in the absence of symptoms referrable to systemic vasculitis.

Etiology. Unknown; idiopathic arteritis; possibly autoimmune condition.

Pathology. Arteritis confined to first few centimeters of innominate, common carotid, and subclavian arteries, adjacent thoracic aorta. The pulmonary vessels can be the principal vessels involved. Microscopically, all layers of arteries are involved; round cell (and occasionally giant cell) infiltration. Elastica disrupted; medial atrophy and fibrosis.

Diagnostic Procedures. *Blood.* Normal red cell and white cell number; sedimentation rate increased; hypergammaglobulinemia. *X-ray.* Notching of upper ribs; occasionally, calcification of ascending arch and descending aorta. *Aortography.*

Therapy. Chronic anticoagulation and corticosteroid (result not unequivocal). Surgery with excision and graft replacement of part of artery involved; bypass for multiple occlusions.

Prognosis. Poor; survival varies from 1 to 15 years from onset of symptoms.

BIBLIOGRAPHY. Takayasu M: A case with peculiar changes of the central retinal vessels. Acta Soc Ophthalmol (Jpn) 12:554, 1908
Domingo RT, Maramba TP, Torres LF et al: Acquired aorto-arteritis. A worldwide vascular entity. Arch Surg 95:780–790, 1967
Haas A, Stiehm R: Takayasu's arteritis presenting as pulmonary hypertension. Am J Dis Child 140:372–374, 1986.

TALMA'S

Synonyms. Acquired myotonia. Myotonia, percussion.

Symptoms and Signs. Onset in adult life. Prolonged contraction of some muscles after electric or mechanical stimulation, with delayed relaxation. Strong voluntary contraction also followed by delayed relaxation.

Etiology. Unknown. It follows or is associated with acute infections, intoxications, and traumas.

Therapy. Symptomatic. Quinine; procaine.

Prognosis. Variable. Usually, regression of the myotonic phenomenon.

BIBLIOGRAHY. Talma S: Over myotonia acquisita. Med Tschr Geneesk 28:321–328, 1892
Adams RD, Victor M: Principles of Neurology, 3rd ed, p 1025. New York, McGraw-Hill, 1985

TANGIER

Named after the Chesapeake Bay Island where first cases were identified.

Synonyms. Alpha-lipoprotein deficiency; analphalipoproteinemia; familial HDL deficiency; high-density lipoprotein deficiency.

Symptoms. Both sexes affected; age of detection from childhood to fourth or fifth decade. Usually asymptomatic. In some cases, intermittent diarrhea; recurrent mild sensory symptoms, at distal part of extremities (pain and temperature); bilateral motor weakness, usually proximal, occasionally also distal.

Signs. Enlargement of tonsils with typical orange color. If tonsils removed, remaining follicles show the same color. Occasionally, splenomegaly and moderate lymphadenopathy, and, still less frequently, moderate hepatomegaly, corneal infiltration (in adult). Premature coronary heart condition in some patients. Abnormal rectal mucosa.

Etiology. Unknown; characterized by almost complete absence of plasma high-density lipoproteins and cholesterol esters storage in many tissues. Lipoprotein instability causes cholesterol deposit in reticuloendothelial macrophages. Autosomal recessive with different penetrability.

Pathology. Storage of large amount of cholesterol esters in reticuloendothelial tissues. Tonsil, pharyngeal, and rectal mucosae show typical orange color. Spleen, liver, and lymph nodes may be enlarged with the presence of foam cells. Muscle biopsy shows neurogenic myopathy changes.

Diagnostic Procedures. *Blood.* Plasma cholesterol below 120 mg/100 ml; phospholipids reduced; triglycerides normal or elevated. Lipoproteins study shows practically an absence of high-density lipoprotein. Hyperuricemia (only in adults). *Biopsy of lymph node and bone marrow.* Presence of foam cells. *Electromyography.*

Therapy. No treatment presently indicated.

Prognosis. Benign course; to date has not affected longevity. Possibility of increased incidence of vascular pathology considered.

BIBLIOGRAPHY. Fredrickson DS, Altrocchi PH, Avioli LV et al: Tangier disease. Ann Intern Med 55:1016–1031, 1961
Herbert PW, Assman G, Gotto AM, Fredrickson DS: Familial lipoprotein deficiency: Abetalipoproteinemia, hypobetalipoproteinemia and Tangier disease. In Stanbury JB, Wyngaarden JB, Fredrickson DS et al: The Metabolic Basis of Inherited Disease, 5th ed, p 589. New York, McGraw-Hill, 1983

TAPETALLIKE REFLEX

Synonym. See Flecked retina.

Symptoms and Signs. In females (heterozygous) no visual defect. Ring scotoma; retina and choroid: bright yellow greenish spots in posterior polar region. Retinitis pigmentosa may be associated.

Etiology. Unknown; sex-linked heterozygous transmission.

Pathology. Degenerative changes in Bruch's membrane (?).

Therapy. None.

Prognosis. Benign lesion.

BIBLIOGRAPHY. Niccol W: A family with bilateral developmental defects of the macula. Trans Ophthalmol Soc UK 58:763, 1938
Ciccarelli EC: A new syndrome of tapetal-like fundic reflexes with ring scotomata; report of two cases. Arch Ophthalmol 67:316–320, 1962
Nussbaum RL, Lewis RA, Lesko JG et al: Mapping X-linked ophthalmic diseases II: Linkage relationship of X-linked retinitis pigmentosa to X chromosomal short arm markers. Hum Genet 70:45–50, 1985

TAPIA'S

Synonym. Nucleus ambiguus-hypoglossal; vagohypoglossal.

Symptoms. Dysarthria and dysphagia.

Signs. Ipsilateral paralysis of tongue, soft palate, vocal cord; hemiatrophy of tongue.

Etiology. Trauma; aneurysm of carotid artery, malignancy determining paralysis of the hypoglossal (XII) nerve and partial paralysis of the vagus (X) nerve. Occasional involvement of the XI.

Pathology. Extracranial lesion of hypoglossal (XII) and vagus (X) (partial) nerves. Fracture of skull; luxation of atlas; aneurysm or malignancy.

Diagnostic Procedures. *X-ray of skull. Angiography.*

Therapy. Symptomatic.

Prognosis. Depends on etiology.

BIBLIOGRAPHY. Tapia AG: Un nouveau syndrome; quelques cas d'hémiplégie du larynx et de la langue avec ou sans paralysie du sternocléido-mastoïdien et du trapèze. Arch Int Laryngol 22:780–785, 1906
Andrioli G, Rigobello L, Mingrino S.: Tapia's syndrome caused by a neurofibroma of the hypoglossal and vagus nerves. J Neurosurg 52:730–732, 1980

TARSAL TUNNEL

Synonym. Jogger's foot.

Symptoms. Intermittent burning pain, paresthesias, cyanosis, coldness, and numbness of foot following prolonged standing or walking; sometimes progressing in intensity during the day; occasionally, pain at night. Usually more pronounced in toes and sole. Removal of shoe, massage and sometimes walking relieve pain. Radiation of pain to calf occasionally experienced.

Signs. Presence of area of hypoesthesia and diminished two-point discrimination. Tinel's sign or formication sign (percussion over or just below the point of original nerve section gives rise to tingling sensation in the periphery) positive. Atrophy of abductor hallucis (in advanced state) or occasionally hypertrophy of abductor hallucis. In some patients, fat ankle and foot.

Etiology and Pathology. Posttraumatic fibrosis; presence of accessory of hypertrophic abductor hallucis muscle; tenosynovitis or spontaneous entrapment resulting in chronic compression from fascial bands of posterior tibial nerve beneath flexor retinaculum and deep fascia along medial border of foot.

Diagnostic Procedures. *Electromyography. Nerve conduction studies. Local injection with cortisone, tourniquet test.* To produce temporary passive congestion and an ischemic element.

Therapy. Local steroid injection; weight reduction; surgical decompression of nerve.

Prognosis. Good with treatment.

BIBLIOGRAPHY. Pollock LJ, Davis L: Peripheral Nerve Injuries, pp 32; 484–493. New York, Hoeber, 1933
Keck C: The tarsal tunnel syndrome. J Bone Joint Surg [Am] 44:180–182, 1962
Edwards WG, Lincoln CR, Bassett FH III et al: The tarsal tunnel syndrome, diagnosis and treatment. JAMA 207:716–720, 1969
Richardson EG: The foot in adolescents and adults. In Crenshaw AH (ed): Campbell's Operative Orthopedics, 7th ed, pp 952–954. St. Louis, CV Mosby, 1987

TARUI'S

Synonyms. Glycogen storage defect (type VII); glycogenosis (type VII); muscle phosphofructokinase deficiency.

Symptoms and Signs. Both sexes affected. Identical to McArdle's syndrome (see). Occasionally, myoglobinuria.

Etiology. Autosomal recessive inheritance.

Diagnostic Procedures. *Blood.* Reticulocytosis; reduced red cell life span; reduction of red cell phosphofructokinase activity. Ischemic exercise does not cause rise in venous lactate. *Biopsy of muscle.* Increase of glucose 6-phosphate and fructose 6-phosphate and decrease of fructose, 1, 6-diphosphate. Phosphofructokinase activity equal to 1% to 3% of normal. Glycogen storage.

Therapy. None.

Prognosis. Good.

BIBLIOGRAPHY. Tarui S, Okuno G, Ikura Y et al: Phosphofructokinase deficiency in skeletal muscle. A new type of glycogenosis. Biochem Biophys Res Com 19:517–523, 1965

Howell RR, Williams JC: The glycogen storage diseases. In Stanbury JB, Wyngaarden JB, Fredrickson DS et al (eds): The Metabolic Basis of Inherited Disease, 5th ed, p 741. New York, McGraw-Hill, 1983

TAUSSIG–BING

Synonyms. Double outlet right ventricle III; pulmonic stenosis absence–right ventricle origin of both great arteries-supracrystal septal defect.

Symptoms and Signs. Onset at birth. Cyanosis; dyspnea on exertion; underdevelopment; cardiomegaly; systolic murmur in left third intercostal space; loud second pulmonic sound.

Etiology. Congenital vascular malformation.

Pathology. Ventricular septal defect anterosuperior to the crista supraventricularis, close to the pulmonary valve, without pulmonary stenosis. Aorta completely transposed arising from right ventricle, levoposition of large pulmonary artery that overrides left ventricle without arising completely from it. High ventricular septal defect; right ventricular hypertrophy.

Diagnostic Procedures. *Electrocardiography. X-ray of chest. Angiocardiography. Cardiac catheterization. Echocardiography. Blood.* Moderate polycythemia.

Therapy. Medical treatment and surgical correction.

Prognosis. Permanent and progressive cyanosis. Clubbing of fingers becomes evident after survival for a few years. Patient may live to second to fourth decade.

BIBLIOGRAPHY. Taussig HB, Bing RJ: Complete transposition of aorta and levoposition of pulmonary artery. Am Heart J 37:551–559, 1949
What is the Taussig-Bing Malformation? (editorial). Circulation 38:445–449, 1968
Hurst JW: The Heart, 6th ed, pp 696–699. New York, McGraw-Hill, 1986

TAYBI'S

Synonyms. Otopalatodigital; OPD.

Symptoms. Both sexes affected; females show variable degrees of expression. Moderate deafness (conductive); mild mental deficiency; limited elbow extension.

Signs. Small stature; frontal and occipital prominence; hypertelorism; small nose and mouth; partial anodontia; cleft soft palate; short trunk. Short broad phalanges of thumbs and toes; short nails.

Etiology. Unknown; X-linked semidominant inheritance.

Diagnostic Procedures. *X-ray.* Thick cranial bones; absence of frontal and sphenoidal sinuses; failure of neural arch fusion. Accessory ossification center at base of second metatarsal; short metacarpals third, fourth, fifth.

BIBLIOGRAPHY. Taybi H: Generalized skeletal dysplasia with multiple anomalies. Am J Roentgenol Rad Ther Nucl Med 88:450–457, 1962

Gall JC Jr, Stern AM, Poznanski AK et al: Oto-palato-digital syndrome: Comparison of clinical and radiographic manifestations in males and females. Am J Hum Genet 24:24–36, 1972

Gorlin RJ, Poznanski AK, Heudon I: The oto-palato-digital (O.P.D.) syndrome in females. Oral Surg 35:218–224, 1973

TAYLOR'S

Synonyms. Congestion fibrosis; congestive dysmenorrhea; pelvic congestion; pelvic sympathetic.

Symptoms. Affects women of childbearing age. Onset of symptoms especially in premenstrual period. Menometrorrhagia; ill-defined pelvic pain; emotional lability.

Signs. Cervix: soft, bluish; excess of cervical mucus. Uterus; symmetric enlargement; pain on uterus examination. Congested painful breasts; frequently varicosities of legs.

Etiology. Diagnosis of exclusion once chronic inflammatory disease ruled out. Possibly a "stress disease," psychogenic in origin, manifested in women who (1) had insecure family life in childhood, (2) are unable to function adequately as women, (3) reveal signs of immaturity and dependency. May be a result of pregnancy and its excessive hormonal effects on the vessels of reproductive organs.

Pathology. Circulatory engorgement of pelvic viscera; slight boggy hypertrophy of uterus; telangiectasia and lymphectasia involving also the cervix. Varicosity of veins of broad ligaments; ovaries enlarged, soft, edematous.

Therapy. Reassurance and symptomatic treatment. Understanding that it may be treated by psychotherapy. Hysterectomy if severe pain and incapacitation.

Prognosis. Responding to treatment.

BIBLIOGRAPHY. Taylor HC Jr: Vascular congestion and hyperemia. Their effect on structure and function in the female reproductive system. Am J Obstet 57:211–230; 637–653; 654–668, 1949

Stearus HC, Sneeden VD: Observations on the clinical and pathologic aspects of the pelvic conditions syndrome. Am J Obstet Gynec 94:718–732, 1966

TAY'S

Synonyms. Ichthyosis–trichothyodystrophy; Trichothyodystrophy–congenital ichthyosis.

Symptoms. Both sexes. From birth. Nonbullous ichthyosiform erythroderma, growth and mental retardation, progerioid lack of subcutaneous fat; short brittle hair; dysplastic nails; photosensitivity; congenital cataracts; spasticity; ataxia; decreased fertility.

Etiology. Unknown. Autosomal recessive inheritance.

Pathology. Ichthyosis (see), typical sulfur deficiency in the hair.

Therapy. Symptomatic.

Prognosis. Poor.

BIBLIOGRAPHY. Tay CH: Ichthyosisform erythroderma, hair shaft abnormalities and mental and growth retardation: A new recessive disorder. Arch Dermatol 104:4–13, 1971

Happle R, Grobe H et al: The Tay syndrome (congenital ichthyosis with trichothyodystrophy). Eur J Pediatr 141:147–152, 1984

TAY–SACHS

Synonyms. Amaurotic familial infantile idiocy; cerebromacular degeneration; ganglioside infantile lipoidosis GM-2 gangliosidoses (type S).

Symptoms. Affects Jewish population 100 times more frequently than other ethnic groups. The sexes are equally affected. Onset between birth and 10 months (average 6 mo) in apparently normal infants. Insidious progression of feeding difficulties, weakness, growth retardation, restlessness, to motor deterioration. Abnormal movements; convulsions; hyperacusis; visual difficulty.

Signs. Doll-like facies. Fine hair. Macrocephaly (after 16 mo of life). Extremities spastic hyperreflexic initially, then flaccid and paralyzed. Blindness. Fundus shows typical cherry-red spot in the macula.

Etiology. Autosomal recessive inheritance. Severe deficiency of hexosaminidase A.

Pathology. *Brain.* Atrophic with ventricular dilatation (initially); marked atrophy and smaller ventricles (later). Consistency firm or leathery. Ballooning of ganglion cells. Astrocyte and microglia hypertrophic (foamy or fat granule cells) Myelin degeneration. *Visceral organs.* No evidence of pathologic changes, except for (occasionally) lipid inclusion.

Diagnostic Procedures. *Blood.* Serum and leukocytes assay of hexosaminidase (absence of hexosaminidase A). *Fibroblast culture.* Assay of hexosaminidase. *X-ray.* No significant changes. *Urine.* Absence of mucopolysaccharide.

Therapy. No specific therapy. Symptomatic and general intensive case.

Prognosis. Invariably fatal by the age of 3 or 4 years.

BIBLIOGRAPHY. Tay W: Symmetrical changes in the region of the yellow spot in each eye of an infant. Trans Ophthalmol Soc UK 1:55–57, 1881

Sachs B: On arrested cerebral development, with special reference to its cortical pathology. J Nerv Ment Dis 14:541–553, 1887

O'Brien JS: The gangliosidoses. In Stanbury JB, Wyngaarden JB, Fredrickson DS et al: The Metabolic Basis of Inherited Disease, 5th ed, p 945. New York, McGraw-Hill, 1983

TELFER'S

Synonym. Piebald–neurologic defect.

Symptoms and Signs. Both sexes. Piebald trait. Leukoderma of dorsal and ventral areas. Cerebellar ataxia; mental and physical development impaired; deafness.

Etiology. Autosomal dominant inheritance.

BIBLIOGRAPHY. Telfer MA, Sugar M, Jaeger EA et al: Dominant piebald trait (white forelock and leukoderma) with neurological impairment. Am J Hum Genet 23:383–389, 1971

Konigsmark BW: Hereditary diseases of the nervous system with hearing loss. In Vinken PJ, Bruyn GW (eds): Handbook of Clinical Neurology, Vol 22, pp 499–526. Amsterdam, (N Holland), 1975

TEMTAMY'S

Synonyms. Brachydactyly type A4; brachymesophalangy II and V.

Symptoms and Signs. Brachymesophalangy of second and fifth digits. Absence of middle phalanges of lateral four toes. Mild radial clinodactyly of fifth and fourth fingers.

Etiology. Autosomal dominant inheritance.

BIBLIOGRAPHY. Jeanselme B, Joannon NI: Brachydactylie symmetrique familiale. Rev Anthrop 33:1–23, 1923

Temtamy SA, McKusick VA: The Genetics of Hand Malformation. New York, Alan R. Liss, 1978

TENNIS ELBOW

Synonyms. Golfer elbow; tennis elbow; epicondylitis; radiohumeral bursitis.

Symptoms. Pain in the elbow, at first, intermittent, then persistent. Radiating to forearm, occasionally to the hand. Stabs of pain cause weakness of hand and object dropping. Limited functions.

Signs. Tenderness on pressure over radiohumeral area of elbow; pain with resisted extension; no pain with flexion.

Pathology. Inflammatory signs in aponeurosis, bursa, periosteum. Fibrosis; tear of common extensor tendon in median epicondyle area.

Etiology. Strain of arm extensors, frequently associated with tennis (backhand).

Therapy. Massage; physical therapy; antiinflammatory agents, or in severe cases, injection of hydrocortisone into tendon distal to epicondyle. Or surgery: section of orbicular ligament of radius and division of common extensor.

Prognosis. Tennis elbow with medical treatment, recovery in 12 months; golfer elbow faster recovery.

BIBLIOGRAPHY. Wright PE: Shoulder and elbow injuries. In Crenshaw AH (ed): Campbell's Operative Orthopedics, 7th ed, p 2515. St. Louis, CV Mosby, 1987

TENNIS LEG

Synonym. Calf muscle rupture.

Symptoms. During strong exercise (tennis) audible snap in the leg, sudden intense pain in the calf that may extend to popliteal space, enhanced by passive dorsiflexion of ankle.

Signs. Marked tenderness on the calf; local discoloration.

Etiology. Sudden muscular contraction with rupture of one of calf muscles during violent exercise.

Therapy. Strapping to immobilize ankle in plantar flexion; after weeks, massage and gradual exercises.

Prognosis. Several weeks before all symptoms subside.

BIBLIOGRAPHY. Pinals RS: Traumatic arthritis and allied conditions. In Hollander JL, McCarty DJ: Arthritis and Allied Conditions, 8th ed, p 1407. Philadelphia, Lea & Febiger, 1978

TERRIEN'S

Synonyms. Marginal degeneration of Terrien; gutter dystrophy; peripheral furrow keratitis; senile marginal atrophy.

Symptoms and Signs. Onset at all ages (the youngest case described was age 9), two-thirds were more than 40 years old. Acute onset of severe ocular pain, usually associated with conjunctival hyperemia, lacrimation, and photophobia. The attacks last 2 days to a week; the durations are consistent for each individual patient. The attack usually recurs, and can affect one eye or both.

Etiology. Unknown. The condition is believed to be degenerative in origin, with secondary inflammatory symptoms.

Pathology. Peripheral, fine, yellow punctate stromal opacities frequently associated with mild superficial corneal vascularization. Progressive thinning leads to peripheral gutter formation.

Diagnostic Procedure. *Slit-lamp examination.*

Therapy. None. Topical corticosteroids have not relieved the symptoms or halted the attacks.

Prognosis. Recurrent episodes can interfere with the patients' normal life. Vision can gradually deteriorate because of increasing corneal astigmatism.

BIBLIOGRAPHY. Duke–Elder S: Textbook of Ophthalmology, Vol 8, p 909. London, Kingston, 1965
Austin P, Brown SI: Inflammatory Terrien's marginal corneal disease. Am J Ophthalmol 92:189–192, 1981

TERRIEN–VIEL

Synonyms. Unilateral recurrent glaucoma; glaucomatocyclitic critis; Posner–Schlossman.

Symptoms. Both sexes affected; occur in subjects presenting allergic diathesis. Periodic slight blurring of vision, and colored halos, without visual field losses. Occasionally, eye pain during episodes.

Signs. Possibly, heterochromia. Features of (usually) unilateral benign glaucoma: high intraocular pressure; enlarged pupil, anisocoria; trace of aqueous flare; chamber angle open; possible presence of keratitic precipitates.

Etiology. Unknown. Allergy, hypothalamic disturbances with neurosympathetic functional impairment considered.

Diagnostic Procedures. *Ophthalmoscopy. Tonometry. Gonioscopy. Allergy test.*

Therapy. Diuretics; topical treatment with antiinflammatory agents and antibiotics.

Prognosis. Crises last from few hours to few weeks.

BIBLIOGRAPHY. Terrien F, Viel P: De certaines glaucomes soi-disant primitifs. Bull Soc Fr Ophthalmol 42:349–368, 1929
Posner A, Schlossman A: Syndrome of unilateral recurrent attacks of glaucoma with cyclic symptoms. Arch Ophthalmol 39:517–535, 1948

TERRY'S

Synonyms. Prematurity retinopathy; retrolental fibroplasia.

Symptoms. Occur in premature underweight infants who are exposed to atmosphere with increased oxygen content. Visual disturbances, up to blindness.

Signs. Pupillary light reflexes absent. Ophthalmoscopic examination shows bilateral opaque retrolental membrane. Vessels are dilated, tortuous, later obliterated. Ciliary body drawn anteriorly; ciliary process around dilated pupil; shallow anterior chamber.

Etiology. Immaturity and periods of retinal hyperoxia are considered to be major factors in the development of the syndrome. The syndrome can develop (in rare instances) in the premature or the full-term healthy infant who has received little or no oxygen therapy.

Pathology. Hemorrhages; retinal edema; proliferation of vascular retinal tissue and successive organization and substitution with fibrous tissue and contraction. Retinal detachment.

Therapy. Prevention by control of amount of oxygen given (the least concentration and for short periods). The biologic antioxidant tocopherol (vitamin E) is being studied as a means of protecting infants who are at risk for the syndrome (premature); preliminary studies suggest that use of tocopherol can be successful.

Prognosis. Blindness may result from this lesion. Before etiology was discovered 5 out of 25 premature infants developed this condition. Unfortunately this complication has not yet completely disappeared.

BIBLIOGRAPHY. Terry TL: Extreme prematurity and fibroblastic overgrowth of persistent vascular sheath behind each crystalline lens; preliminary report. Am J Ophthalmol 25:203–204, 1942
Johnson L: Retrolental fibroplasia: A new look at an unsolved problem. Hosp Pract 16:109–121, 1981
Merritt JC, Sprague DH, Merritt WE et al: Retrolental fibroplasia: A multifactional disease. Anesth Analg 60:109–111, 1981

Nelson WE: Textbook of Pediatrics, 12th ed. Philadelphia, WB Saunders, 1983.

Bachynski BN, Kincaid MC, Nussbaum J, Green WR: A hemorrhagic form of zone I retinopathy of prematurity. J Pediatr Ophtalmol Strabismus 26:56–60, 1989

TERSON'S

Synonym. Subarachnoid hemorrhage–ocular hemorrhage.

Symptoms. Onset at all ages; both sexes affected. Sudden loss of consciousness; reduced vision.

Signs. Weakness of extraocular muscles and, occasionally, uncoordinated gaze; anisocoria; intraocular hemorrhages; papilledema.

Etiology. Syndrome may be spontaneous, follow trauma or rupture of brain aneurysm. Subarachnoid hemorrhages are associated in 5% of cases with intraocular hemorrhages, in 6% of cases with papilledema.

Pathology. Subarachnoid hemorrhage; preretinal, peripapillary hemorrhages; papilledema; secondary hemorrhage in the optic nerve.

Diagnostic Procedures. *Cerebrospinal fluid.* Presence of red cells. *CT scan. Angiography.*

Therapy. Control of cerebral edema: osmotic diuretics, corticosteroids. Surgery for clipping of brain aneurysm; intensive care.

Prognosis. The association subarachnoid-intraocular hemorrhages: unfavorable prognosis. Death rate double that in single subarachnoid hemorrhage.

BIBLIOGRAPHY. Paton L: Ocular symptoms in subarachnoid hemorrhage. Trans Ophthalmol Soc UK 44:110–126, 1924

Tureen LL: Lesions of the fundus associated with brain hemorrhage. Arch Neurol Psychiatr 42:664–678, 1939

Castren GA: Pathogenesis and treatment of Terson's syndrome. Acta Ophthalmol 41:430–434, 1963

Fahmy JA: Vitreous hemorrhage in subarachnoid hemorrhage. Terson's syndrome. Report of a case with macular degeneration as a complication. Acta Ophthalmol 50:137–143, 1972

TESTOTOXICOSIS, FAMILIAL

Synonyms. Precocious puberty–male limited; gonadotropin–independent sexual precocity.

Symptoms and Signs. Male. Sexual development at 1 year of age, accelerated growth and development of secondary sexual characteristics. Final: short stature (150–160 cm), normal size penis, small soft testis, normal reproduction.

Etiology. Unknown. Autosomal dominant inheritance (sisters normal), X-linked mutation cannot be excluded.

Pathology. Testis biopsy: Leydig cells: nuclear and cytoplasmic characteristics of fully differentiated normal cells. Adrenals normal.

Diagnostic Procedures. *Blood.* Testosterone level high; gonadotropins low. Absence of suppressive effects of potent gonadotropin-releasing hormone analogs. *X-ray of skeleton.* Bone age superior.

Prognosis. Good. Short stature; normal reproduction.

BIBLIOGRAPHY. Schedewie HK, Reiter EO, Beitins IZ, et al: Testicular Leydig cell hyperplasia as cause of familial sexual precocity. J Clin Endocrinol Metabol 52:271–278, 1981

Gondos B, Egli CA, Rosenthal SM et al: Testicular changes in gonadotropin-independent familial male sexual precocity: Familial testotoxicosis. Arch Pathol Lab Med 109:990–995, 1985

THALASSEMIA SYNDROMES

Various classifications of these syndromes exist.

CLINICAL CLASSIFICATIONS
1. THALASSEMIA MINIMA

Synonym. Microcythemia minima.

Symptoms. Asymptomatic with barely detectable erythrocyte anomaly. See Silvestroni–Bianco.

2. β-THALASSEMIA MINOR

Synonym. Heterozygous β-thalassemia. See Rietti–Greppi–Micheli, also Jaksch–Hayem–Luzet.

Symptoms. Wide spectrum of symptoms and signs, all related to chronic moderate anemia; hemolysis and splenomegaly. Chronic ulcers in the legs may be observed.

Etiology. Heterozygous beta chain defects.

Pathology. Increased red cell production, medullary and occasionally extramedullary; secondary bone changes. Generalized hemochromatosis; splenomegaly.

Diagnostic Procedures. *Blood.* Hypochromic microcytic, moderate anemia; anisopoikilocytosis; schistocytosis; target cells; reticulocytosis; moderate hyperbilirubinemia; increased low osmotic resistance. *Bone marrow.* Erythroid hyperplasia. *X-ray of skeleton.* Osteoporosis. *Hemoglobin electrophoresis.* Increased A_2 fraction, occasionally increased hemoglobin F.

Therapy. Symptomatic.

Prognosis. Variable from normal life span to symptoms associated with chronic anemia.

3. THALASSEMIA INTERMEDIA

Symptoms. Intermediate between thalassemia minor and Cooley's syndrome.

4. COOLEY'S SYNDROME

Synonyms. Beta-thalassemia (type I); erythroblastic anemia; thalassemia major; Mediterranean; homozygous β-thalassemia.

Symptoms and Signs. Both sexes affected, clinical onset insidious at 3 to 6 months of age. Severe weakness; pallor; mongoloid facies; large head; oxycephaly; enlargement of abdomen; splenomegaly; hepatomegaly; stunted growth; jaundice; recurrent febrile episodes; cardiac dilatation; hemorrhagic manifestation.

Etiology. Homozygous beta chain defects. True homozygosity for one or another thalassemia gene or double heterozygosity for any two different β-thalassemia genes.

Pathology. Marked medullary and extramedullary erythropoiesis; hepatosplenomegaly; hematochromatosis. Bone changes secondary to the erythropoietic proliferation.

Diagnostic Procedures. *Blood.* Severe anemia. Marked anisopoikilocytosis, poor in pigment; target cells; marked distortion and deformation of cells; nucleated red cells with various degrees of immaturity. Marked reticulocytosis; osmotic fragility usually markedly decreased. Usually, leukocytosis with some immature forms; hyperbilirubinemia; serum iron high; iron-binding capacity markedly decreased or absent. *Urine.* Increased urobilinogen and urobilin; increased aminoaciduria. *Stool.* High coproporphyrin. *X-ray of skeleton.* Marked thickening of diploë of skull with perpendicular striations between thinned tables. Long bones, decreased density of medulla and thinning of cortex, mosaic pattern.

Therapy. Symptomatic; blood transfusion. Splenectomy moderately beneficial in some cases. Corticosteroids in some cases. Desferrioxamine plus vitamin C.

Prognosis. Very severe; ultimately fatal in few months to years.

Biochemical classification. Various classifications of these syndromes exist. We report the last classification. For individual syndromes see clinical and hematologic classification under specific titles.

5. ALPHA-THALASSEMIA SYNDROMES

1. Heterozygous α-thalassemia 2 or "silent carrier" state (no symptoms)
2. Heterozygous α-thalassemia 1 or α-thalassemia trait (no symptoms)
3. HbH disease: double heterozygosity for α-thalassemia 1 + α-thalassemia 2 (see)
4. Hydrops fetalis with Hb Bart's: homozygous α-thalassemia 1
5. Hb constant spring syndromes (see)
6. $\alpha + \beta$ thalassemia

6. BETA-THALASSEMIA SYNDROMES

1. Heterozygous β-thalassemia, β-thalassemia trait, or β-thalassemia minor (see).
   a. With elevated HbA_2 + elevated HbF
   b. With normal HbA_2 + elevated HbF: delta-thalassemia (δ-thalassemia) or F-thalassemia
      1. $G\gamma^A\gamma(\delta\beta)°$ thalassemia
      2. $G\gamma(^A\gamma\delta\beta)°$ thalassemia
   c. With normal HbA_2 and HbF
      1. "Silent carrier" including Hb Knossos
      2. Concomitant $\delta + \beta$ thalassemia, in cis or trans
      3. $\gamma\delta\beta$-thalassemia
      4. Other: atypical $\delta\beta$-thalassemia; concomitant iron deficiency
   d. Hb Lepore trait
2. Homozygous β-thalassemia, Cooley's anemia or β-thalassemia major (see Cooley's)
   a. True homozygosity for one or another β-thalassemia gene
   b. Double heterozygosity for any two different β-thalassemia genes
3. β-thalassemia intermedia (see)

7. RARE FORMS OF THALASSEMIA

1. γ-thalassemia
2. δ-thalassemia
3. $\gamma\delta\beta$-thalassemia

8. INTERACTING THALASSEMIA

1. α-thalassemia + α-chain variant
   a. HbQ/α-thalassemia (like HbH disease)
   b. HbG/α-thalassemia (mild anemia)
2. α-thalassemia + β-chain variant
   a. Sickle/β-thalassemia (see sickle)
   b. HbC/β-thalassemia (mild anemia)
   c. HbE/β-thalassemia (like homozygous thalassemia)

9. HEREDITARY PERSISTENCE OF FETAL HEMOGLOBIN

1. Pancellular (no symptoms)
   a. $G\gamma^A\gamma(\delta\beta)°$ HPFH
   b. Hb Kenya (G γ HPFH)
   c. Black G $\gamma\beta$-HPFH with high HbF
   d. Greek A γ-HPFH
   e. Chinese A γ-HPFH
2. Heterocellular (no symptoms)
   a. Swiss type G $\gamma_A\gamma$ HPFH
   b. British type Aγ-HPFH
   c. Other: Seattle type G$\gamma^A\gamma$-HPFH; Atlanta type-Black G$\gamma\beta$ +HPFH with low HbF; Saudi high HbF determinant

BIBLIOGRAPHY. Cooley TB, Lee P: Series of cases of splenomegaly in children with anemia and peculiar bone change. Trans Am Pediatr Soc 37:29, 1925

Marks PA: Thalassemia syndromes. Biochemical, genetic and clinical aspects. New Engl J Med 275:1363–1369, 1966

Wintrobe MM (ed): Clinical Hematology, 7th ed. Philadelphia, Lea & Febiger, 1974

Bunn HF, Forget BG: Hemoglobin: Molecular Genetic and Clinical Aspects, pp 333–335. Philadelphia, WB Saunders, 1986

THANATOPHORIC DWARFISM

Symptoms and Signs. Male-to-female ratio 2 : 1; onset in fetal life. Feeble fetal activity and polyhydramnios. At birth, reduced length (40 cm average), shortened limbs. Head enlarged; small face; enlarged fontanelles; high forehead; frontal bossing; bulging eyes; saddle nose. Abdomen protuberant. Thorax narrow; short ribs. Absence of primitive reflexes. Marked hypotonia. Respiratory distress and cardiac failure.

Etiology. Unknown; sporadic. Genetics still confused. Various possibilities of inheritance. Possibly various conditions reported under this heading. One variety associated with cloverleaf skull (possibly autosomal dominant) and one called Glasgow variant (possibly autosomal recessive) have been reported.

Pathology. Nodular masses epiphyseal cartilage; slanting of bony trabeculae of growth plates; fibrous band interposed between epiphyses and metaphyses. In brain, microgyria, absent corpus callosum, temporal lobe, and cerebellum disorganized. Extramedullary hematopoiesis.

Diagnostic Procedures. *X-ray of spine.* Short flattened vertebrae ("H configuration"); wide intervertebral disk of pelvis; squarish; reduced height; small sciatic notch; medial spurs. *Of limbs.* Marked bowing of femora.

Prognosis. Death usually within first 3 days of life.

BIBLIOGRAPHY. Maroteaux P, Laury M, Robert JM: Le nanisme thanatophore. Presse Med 75:2519–2522, 1967

Bailey JA: Disproportionate Short Stature: Diagnosis and Management, p 169. Philadelphia, WB Saunders, 1973

Isaacson G, Blakemore KJ, Chervenak FA: Thanatophoric dysplasia with cloverleaf skull. Am J Dis Child 137:896–898, 1983

Connor JM, Connor RAC, Sweet EM et al: Lethal neonatal chondrodysplasia in the West of Scotland 1970–1983 with description of a thanatophoric dysplasialike, autosomal recessive disorder, Glasgow variant. Am J Med Genet 22:243–253, 1985

Elejalde BR, de Elejalde MM: Thanatophoric dysplasia:

Fetal manifestations and prenatal diagnosis. Am J Med Genet 22:669–693, 1985.

THIBIERGE–WEISSENBACH

This eponym is used to describe different diseases included in a spectrum that goes from progressive systemic sclerosis with calcinosis to the CRST syndrome (see).

BIBLIOGRAPHY. Thibierge G, Weissenbach RJ: Concrétions calcaires sou-cutanées et sclérodermie. Ann Dermatol Syph 2:129–155, 1911

Dellipiani AW, George M: Syndrome of sclerodactyly, calcinosis. Raynaud's phenomenon, and telangiectasia. Br Med J 4:334–345, 1967

THIEFFRY AND SORRELL–DEJERINE

Synonyms. Hereditary osteolysis; hyperhydroxyprolinemia–osteolysis; Thieffry–Kohler. Osteolysis hereditary–carpal bones–nephropathy.

Symptoms and Signs. Both sexes affected. Marfanoid appearance; frontal bossing; micrognathia; scoliosis; pes cavus; overlapping toes; plantar cysts. During childhood, onset of a progressive painless osteolysis beginning in the carpal and tarsal bones and spreading distally and proximally to other bones. Occasionally, osteolysis may be asymmetric. Hypertension and signs of renal failure.

Etiology. Sporadic and autosomal dominant cases reported.

Diagnostic Procedures. *Blood.* Elevated hydroxyproline and alkaline phosphatase levels. *Urine.* Hydroxyproline.

BIBLIOGRAPHY. Thieffry S, Sorrell–Dejerine J: Forme spéciale d'ostéolysis essentielle héréditaire et familiale a stabilization spontanée, survenant dans l'énfance. Presse Méd 66:1858–1861, 1958

Kohler E, Babbitt D, Huizenga B et al: Hereditary osteolysis. Radiology 108:99–105, 1973

Fryns JP: Osteolyse essentielle a debut carpien et tarsien. J Genet Hum 30(Suppl 5):423–428, 1982

THIEMANN'S

Synonyms. Phalangeal avascular necrosis; digital osteoarthropathy; metaphyseal dysplasia–epiphyseal tarda; MEDT IIIa; Thiemann–Fleischer. See also Multiple epiphyseal dysplasia syndromes.

Symptoms. Both sexes affected; onset in infancy and up to 18 years of age. In finger joints, pain with limitation of movements.

Signs. Fusiform enlargement of proximal interphalangeal joints, especially of medial finger, less frequently of other digits. Later, possible digital shortening.

Etiology. Unknown. In some cases autosomal dominant inheritance proved; in others, the recessive type suspected.

Pathology. Avascular osteolysis in epiphyseal-diaphyseal zone of digits.

Diagnostic Procedures. *X-ray of hands and feet.* Destruction of cartilages; lacunae of bone reabsorption; hazy outline; shortening of phalangeal epiphyses.

Therapy. None. Symptomatic.

Prognosis. Severe deformities. Spontaneous arrest after closure of epiphyses. Eventual regeneration of cartilage.

BIBLIOGRAPHY. Thiemann H: Juvenile Epiphysenstoerungen, idiopathische Erkrankung der Epiphysenknoepel der Fingerphalangen. Fortschr Roengtenol 14:79–87, 1909–10
Gewanter H, Baum J: Thiemann's disease. J Rheum 12:150–153, 1985

THIES–SCHWARZ

Synonym. Eruptive milia.

Symptoms. Onset in adult life. Development of nodules without apparent reason.

Signs. Milialike nodules on face and upper trunk, 1 to 5 mm, symmetric; some show a central black comedo.

Etiology. Unknown. Sporadic; (original T–S) also reported possible autosomal dominant inheritance.

Pathology. Deformed follicles joined by epitheliomal strands with dermis and epidermis. Occasionally, horn cysts. The affected follicles are enclosed in a sheath of connective tissue.

Diagnostic Procedure. *Biopsy of skin.*

Therapy. Comedo may be removed but will re-form. Dermabrasion.

Prognosis. Some cases develop a trichoepitheliomalike tumor.

BIBLIOGRAPHY. Thies W, Schwarz E: Multiple eruptive milia. An organoid follicle hamartoma. Arch Klin Exp Dermatol 214:21–34, 1961
Rook A, Wilkinson DS, Ebling FJG et al: Textbook of Dermatology, 4th ed, p 2401. Oxford, Blackwell Scientific Publications, 1986

THOMAS'

Symptoms and Signs. Occur in subjects who underwent partial thyroidectomy. Association of clinical manifestations of hypothyroidism and Marie–Bamberg.

BIBLIOGRAPHY. Thomas HMJ: Acropachy. Secondary superiosteal new bone formation. Arch Intern Med 51:571–588, 1933

THOMPSON'S (A.H.)

Synonyms. Congenital optic atrophy. Eponym used to indicate a congenital type (autosomal dominant inheritance) of atrophy of optic nerve characterized by nystagmus and blindness.

BIBLIOGRAPHY. Thompson AH, Cashell GTW: A pedigree congenital optic atrophy entrancing sixteen affected cases in six generations. Proc R Soc Med 28:1415–1426, 1935

THOMSEN'S

Synonyms. Myotonia congenital dominant; myotonia dystrophica.

Symptoms. Prevalent in males; onset at birth or shortly after, or at puberty with sudden onset. After a period of rest, difficulty in relaxing muscles. Frequently limited to extremities only. Difficulty in initiating walking, then normal ambulation. Difficulty in releasing grip. Masticatory, laryngeal, and ocular muscles may also be affected. Emotions and cold enhance symptoms. Warmth decreases them. Five varieties have been described: first, the Thomsen's classic; the others with partial symptomatology to end in the fifth with isolated myotonia on percussion of the tongue.

Signs. Firm and solid muscle.

Etiology. Autosomal dominant inheritance. Possibly excessive production of acetylcholine at neuromuscular junction.

Pathology. In muscles, increase of myofibril number and sarcoplasm. Sarcolemmal nuclei and also the connective interstitial tissue increased. Later stages, atrophic changes appear.

Diagnostic Procedures. *Biopsy of muscle. Electromyography.*

Therapy. Symptomatic; quinine; procainamide. Cortisone and chlorothiazide (to cause K^+ depletion).

Prognosis. Cataracts, muscular wasting may develop, and other features of myotonic dystrophy, now considered identical disease.

BIBLIOGRAPHY. Thomsen J: Tonische Krämpfe in willkürlich beweglichen Muskeln in Folge von ererbter psychischer Disposition (Ataxia muscularis ?). Arch Psychiatr Nervenkr 76:706–718, 1875–76
Becker RE: Myotonia congenita and syndromes associated with myotonia. VIII, Top Hum Genet, Stuttgart, George Thieme, 1977

THOMSEN'S (O.)

Synonyms. Polydactyly (preaxial IV). Polysyndactyly; preaxial polysyndactyly; syndactyly. See Greig's syndrome.

Symptoms and Signs. Preaxial polydactyly of hands or feet more severe of variable grade.

Etiology. Autosomal dominant with variable expression.

Diagnostic Procedures. *X-ray of hand.* Dysplastic distal phalanges with a central hole (specific finding of this form).

BIBLIOGRAPHY. Thomsen O: Einige Eigentumlichkeiten der Erblichen Poly und Syndaktylie bei menschen. Acta Med Scand 65:609, 1927
Baraitner M, Winter RM, Brett EM: Greig cephalopolysyndactyly: Report of 13 individuals in three families. Clin Genet 24:257–265, 1983
Reynolds JF, Sommer A, Kelly TE: Preaxial polydactyly type 4: Variability in a large kindred. Clin Genet 25:267–272, 1984

THOMSON'S (M.S.)

Synonym. Atrophic heredofamilial dermatosis.

Symptoms and Signs. Skin changes identical to those observed in Rothmund's (see). Cataracts were not reported in any of the cases described by Thomson.

Etiology. Unknown; autosomal recessive trait. Likely represents a *forme fruste* of Rothmund's.

BIBLIOGRAPHY. Thomson MS: A hitherto undescribed familial disease. Br J Dermatol 35:455–462, 1923
Silver HK: Rothmund–Thomson syndrome. An oculocutaneous disorder. Am J Dis Child 111:182–190, 1966

THORACIC OUTLET

Synonyms. Shoulder girdle compression; neurovascular shoulder compression. This eponym includes various syndromes previously described as separate entities which all share the same physiopathology and characteristics:

1. Naffziger or Adson's; cervical rib-without cervical rib; Coote–Hanauld; Haven's; Nonne's II; scalenus anticus.
2. Cervical rib or first thoracic rib, Rust's.
3. Falconer–Weddell. Costoclavicular; military posture.
4. Wright's; hyperabduction; subcoracoid-pectoralis minor.
5. Law's ligaments simulating cervical ribs.

Symptoms. Usually in adult life after trauma to the shoulder (cervical rib), stretching of arm (cervical rib, Wright's–Falconer's–Weddell's), pregnancy, military service (Falconer–Weddell described cases in soldiers carrying military packs) or not in relation to particular posture (Naffziger's). More frequent in females (cervical rib), usually unilateral. Exercise increases pain, rest reduces it. Pain from neck to hand, usually on the ulnar side, or pain over deltoid extending to the arm, greatest at the elbow. Paresthesia, weakness of affected arm, occasionally hyperesthesia in painful areas, vasomotor alterations.

Signs. Edema, venous congestion of arm, pulse decreased particularly in fourth-fifth finger (Falconer–Weddell), Adson's maneuver induces symptoms. Reflexes reduced or absent on affected arm. Tender point at scalenus anticus (Naffziger), supraclavicular bruit if axillary artery aneurysm, bony mass palpable in supraclavicular fossa (cervical rib).

Etiology. Compression of neurovascular bundle at thoracic outlet (first rib, clavicle, scalenus muscle) due to various causes: cervical rib, muscular malformation (scalenus anticus, Naffziger's), ligaments simulating scalenus anticus (Law's) forced hyperabduction with weight load (Falconer–Weddell, Wright's). Some cases with familial incidence reported.

Pathology. Atrophy of muscles, neuritis, possible occurrence of aneurysm of axillary artery, or thrombosis of vein.

Diagnostic Procedures. *Adson's test.* (Costoclavicular and hyperabduction maneuvers) positive. *X-ray.* Shows supernumerary rib. *Electromyography. Arteriography.*

Therapy. In case of hyperabduction simple correction of posture is sufficient. In other cases surgery with resection of first thoracic rib, which is usually done by subaxillary approach (Roos technique).

Prognosis. Good with therapy.

BIBLIOGRAPHY. Hunauld FJ: Communication to the Royal Academy of Sciences in 1740. Amsterdam, 1744
Willshire: Supernumerary first rib. Lancet 2:633, 1860
Naffziger HC: The scalenus syndrome. Surg Gynecol Obstet 64:119–120, 1937

Murphy T: Brachial neuritis caused by pressure of first rib. Aust Med J 15:582–585, 1910

Law AA: Adventitious ligaments simulating cervical ribs. Ann Surg 72:497, 1920

Adson AW, Caffey IR: Cervical rib. A new method of approach for relief of symptoms by division of the scalenus anticus. Ann Surg 85:839–857, 1927

Haven H: Neurocirculatory scalenus anticus syndrome in the presence of developmental defect of the first rib. Yale J Biol Med 11:443–458, 1938–1939

Falconer MA, Weddell G: Costoclavicular compression of subclavian artery and vein: Relation to scalenus anticus syndrome. Lancet 2:539–543, 1943

Wright IS: The neurovascular syndrome produced by hyperabduction of the arms. Am Heart J 29:1–19, 1945

Roos DB: Transaxillary approach for first rib resection to relieve thoracic outlet syndrome. Ann Surg 163:354, 1966

THORN'S

Synonyms. Pseudo-Addison; renal tubular salt-wasting; salt-losing nephritis.

Symptoms. Prevalent in males; onset at all ages; most often in young adulthood. Polyuria and nocturia present in 50% of cases before diagnosis. Thirty percent of patients had history of gastritis and prolonged intake of large amount of alkali. Salt-craving only in a few cases. During acute episodes: nausea; vomiting; anorexia; weakness; muscle cramps; fainting; mental confusion.

Signs. Increased skin pigmentation (bronzing); dehydration; blood pressure usually normal.

Etiology. Not a separate disease entity but a syndrome observed in chronic renal diseases. When salt intake falls below level of urinary salt loss.

Pathology. *Kidney.* Chronic pyelonephritis. *Adrenal.* Enlargement. *Parathyroid.* Hyperplasia. Calcification of vessels and nephrolithiasis occasionally.

Diagnostic Procedures. *Urine.* Specific gravity fixed; albuminuria and altered tests of renal function. High urinary aldosterone; 17-ketosteroids normal or elevated. Lack of response to administration of desoxycorticosterone acetate (DOCA). *Blood.* Moderate to severe azotemia; acidosis; low serum sodium; serum potassium frequently elevated; occasionally, depressed.

Therapy. A mixture of NaCl and NaHCO3 in equal parts, 1–2 g 2–3 times daily with meals. Monitoring of serum sodium levels: with the progression of the disease, sodium restriction may become necessary.

Prognosis. Varies according to degree of renal impairment. With treatment, prompt relief of symptoms and survival of 20 more years in relative comfort. If no treatment, death may ensue following attack. With progression of renal pathology, loss of salt decreases and patient develops edema, hypotension, cardiac failure.

BIBLIOGRAPHY. Thorn GW, Koepf GF, Clinton M Jr: Renal failure simulating adrenocortical insufficiency. N Engl J Med 231:76–85, 1944

Hughes JM: Salt-losing nephritis: A case report and a review. Arch Intern Med 114:190–195, 1964

Berl T, Anderson RJ, McDonald KM: Clinical disorders of water metabolism. Kidney Int 10:117–132, 1976

3/B TRANSLOCATION

Synonym. Chromosome 3/B translocation

Signs. Affected offspring comprise 41% of the progeny of female carriers. In contrast, only 12% of the progeny of male carriers were affected, and these included miscarriages only and no congenitally malformed children. The newborn will present with the following congenital anomalies: low birth weight; micrognathia; small ears; cleft lip and palate; coloboma; cloudy cornea; proptosis; strabismus; cardiac defects: ventricular septal defect, atrial septal defect, absent ductus arteriosus, pulmonary arterial diverticulum, right aortic arch, absent pulmonic valve.

Etiology. Chromosomal anomaly. It is associated with a translocation between a chromosome No. 3 and member of the B group (no. 4–5). The anomaly is transmitted by the female carrier but not, for some unknown reason, by the male carrier. This differential transmission is similar to that associated with that for Down's syndrome with a familial 13–15/21 (D/G) translocation.

Pathology. See Signs.

Therapy. Symptomatic.

Prognosis. Guarded.

BIBLIOGRAPHY. Walzer S, Favara B, Ming PM et al: A new translocation syndrome (3/B). N Engl J Med 275:290–298, 1966

THROMBOCYTOPENIA, HYPERSPLENIC PRIMARY

Synonym. Primary hypersplenism.

Symptoms and Signs. Both sexes affected; onset at all ages. Variable degree of hemorrhagic manifestations; splenomegaly.

Etiology. Unknown; selective dysfunction of spleen with trapping and destruction of platelets. Often associated with other feature of hypersplenism, anemia, neutropenia (see Doan–Wright).

Therapy. Splenectomy.

Prognosis. Return to normal platelet value after splenectomy.

BIBLIOGRAPHY. Cooney DP, Smith BA: The pathophysiology of hypersplenic thrombocytopenia. Arch Intern Med 121:332–337, 1968
Bowdler AJ: Splenomegaly and hypersplenism. Clin Haematol 12:467–488, 1983

THURMAN–HILLIER

Synonyms. LV-RA communication; left ventricular to right atrial communication; right atrial from left ventricular communication.

Symptoms and Signs. Both sexes equally affected; present at birth. Holosystolic murmur located over sternum or right sternal edge; apical or tricuspid midsystolic murmur occasionally present. On palpation, right ventricular impulse extremely prominent.

Etiology. Congenital cardiac defect.

Pathology. Communication between left ventricle and right atrium in the region of membranous septum inferior to the crista supraventricularis, in some cases below level of tricuspid annulus (Thurman) and in others above the insertion of septal leaflets of tricuspid valve.

Diagnostic Procedures. *Electrocardiography.* Peaked P waves in right atrial enlargement. Possibly, atrial arrhythmias. Similar pattern with normal septal defect. *X-ray.* Prominent pulmonary trunk; small aorta; large left ventricle; right ventricle and atrium extremely enlarged (ball-like shape in frontal position). *Echocardiography.*

Therapy. Medical management for intercurrent respiratory infections; prevention of bacterial endocarditis and failure. Surgery if indicated.

Prognosis. Fair.

BIBLIOGRAPHY. Thurman J: Aneurysms of the heart; with cases. Med Chir Trans Lond 21:187–265, 1838
Hillier T: Congenital malformation of the heart. Perforation of the septum ventriculorum, establishing a communication between the left ventricle and the right auricle. Trans Pathol Soc Lond 10:110, 1858–1859
Hurst JW: The Heart, 6th ed, pp 613–614. New York, McGraw-Hill, 1986

THYGESON'S

Synonyms. Keratitis superficialis punctata; punctata superficial keratitis.

Symptoms and Signs. Small punctiform lesions spread on superficial layers of cornea.

Etiology. Unknown; viral origin suspected.

Therapy. Symptomatic.

Prognosis. Recurrence every 3 to 4 years.

BIBLIOGRAPHY. Thygeson P: Superficial punctate keratitis. JAMA 144:1544–1549, 1950

THYROID HORMONE RESISTANCE

Synonyms. Familial thyroid hormone resistance; see Seabright-Bantam.

Symptoms and Signs. Both sexes. From infancy: recurrent goiter. No history to suggest thyrotoxicosis or hypothyroidism; other physical signs negative. Growth, development, and intelligence normal.

Etiology. Autosomal dominant inheritance. Particular resistance of peripheral tissue to the action of thyroid-stimulating hormone (TSH), pituitary also partially resistant to thyroid hormones' suppressive action.

Pathology. *Thyroid.* Follicles of unequal size, lined by flat to cuboidal cells with round-oval nuclei; abundant colloid in areas of epithelium projecting into lumen. No lymphocytic infiltration.

Diagnostic Procedures. Markedly elevated serum total and free T_3 and T_4 levels; normal or elevated serum TSH.

Therapy. No evidence that treatment with thyroid hormone is useful. Thionamides, radioactive iodine, or surgery could induce subclinical hypothyroidism.

Prognosis. Except for goiter no other manifestations affect life or functions.

BIBLIOGRAPHY. Refetoff S, De Groot LJ, Barsano CP: Defective thyroid hormone feedback regulation in the syndrome of peripheral resistance to thyroid hormone. J Clin Endocrinol Metab 51:41–45, 1980
Brooks H, Barbato L et al: Familial thyroid hormone resistance. Am J Med 71:414–421, 1981

TIÈCHE–JADASSOHN

Synonyms. Blue nevus; chromatophoroma; Jadassohn-Tièche; melanofibroma.

Symptoms. Both sexes affected; (female-to-male, 2.5:1). Onset in infancy or adolescence.

Signs. On the face, forearms, hands, or thighs (less frequently on other areas) appearance of a solitary nevus, dark blue, round or oval, with sharp border, smooth and slightly raised.

Etiology. Unknown.

Pathology. Mixture of melanocytes, fibrous and collagen fibers and dendritic, bipolar, and fusiform cells.

Therapy. Excision and plastic surgery (for cosmetic reasons).

Prognosis. Benign.

BIBLIOGRAPHY. Tièche M: Uber Melanome ("chromatophorome") der Haut. "Blaue Naevi." Virchows Arch 186:212–228, 1906
Jadassohn J: Dermatologie, p 429. Wien, 1938
Rook A, Wilkinson DS, Ebling FJG et al: Textbook of Dermatology, 4th ed, pp 2443–2444. Oxford, Blackwell Scientific Publications, 1986

TIETZE'S

Synonyms. Costal chondritis; chondropathia tuberosa; chondrocostal junction.

Symptoms. Pain in one or more costal cartilages, enhanced by motion, coughing, sneezing; radiation to neck shoulder, and arm.

Signs. Swelling of upper costal cartilage; tenderness and slight hyperemia of skin overlying fusiform swelling. Second rib most frequently affected.

Etiology. Unknown.

Pathology. Nonsuppurative inflammation of rib cartilage; perichondritis.

Diagnostic Procedures. *Electrocardiography.* To rule out cardiac conditions. *X-ray of chest.*

Therapy. Steroid infiltration when pain is severe.

Prognosis. Benign condition, lasting weeks or months; relapses possible.

BIBLIOGRAPHY. Tietze A: Ueber eine eigenartige Häufung von Fällen mit Dystrophie der Rippenknorpel. Berl Klin Wochenschr 58:829–831, 1921
Kayser HL: Tietze's syndrome. A review of literature. Am J Med 21:982–989, 1956
Hurst JW: The Heart, 6th ed, p 918. New York, McGraw-Hill, 1986

TIXIER'S

Synonyms. Childhood hemolytic anemia; Hutinel–Tixier. Obsolete term. Acute fulminating hemolytic crisis in debilitated newborns.

BIBLIOGRAPHY. Hutinel VH: La pseudo-chlorose des nourrissons. Med Mod Paris 19:193, 1908
Tixier L: Les anémies infantiles. Pediatrie Prat (Lille) 10:526–535, 1912; 11:512–517, 1913
Tixier L: Les anémies. Paris, Flammarion, 1923

TODD'S POSTEPILEPTIC PARALYSIS

A sequela of Jacksonian attacks, manifested by temporary weakness or paralysis of arm or leg, lasting a few hours or days.

BIBLIOGRAPHY. Todd RB: Clinical Lectures on Paralysis, 2nd ed. London, Churchill, 1856
Adams RD, Victor M: Principles of Neurology, 3rd ed, pp 246, 514, 929. New York, McGraw-Hill, 1985

TODESERWARTUNG

Synonym. Death expectancy. See Survivor syndrome.

Symptoms. Occur in residents of old-age homes. Hypochondriasis; hysteria; dependency and impulsivity; varieties of somatic complaints purely functional or elaboration of existing deficit. Attitude of not getting involved with other residents; lack of communication between residents; loss of self-esteem; assumption of role of passive child and exploitation of the advantages deriving from it.

Etiology. Attitude assumed to repress thoughts of death and withdrawal from reality.

Therapy. Find ways to substitute meaningful social interaction and feeling of self-esteem and utility.

BIBLIOGRAPHY. Berman MI: The Todeserwartung syndrome. Geriatrics 21:187–192, 1966

TOGLIA'S

Synonym. Toglia's dysostosis.

Symptoms and Signs. *Skull.* Open suture. *Facies.* "Oldish"; deep set eyes; flat nose; prognathism. *Limbs.* Spadelike hands and short fingers.

Etiology. Unknown. Familial occurrence. Single report. Unclassifiable.

BIBLIOGRAPHY. Toglia JU: Hereditary dysostosis. Tex J Med 62:23–41, 1966
Aita JA: Congenital Facial Anomalies with Neurological Defects. Springfield, CC Thomas, 1969

TOLOSA–HUNT

Synonyms. Ophthalmoplegia dolorosa; painful ophthalmoplegia.

Symptoms. Both sexes affected; onset most frequent in fifth decade. Unilateral, steadily progressive retro-orbital pain. May also be of recurrent type (remission for months or years) of scintillating scotoma. Blurred vision up to complete blindness.

Signs. Paresis of oculomotor (III), trochlear (IV), abducens (VI) and first branch of trigeminal (V) nerves (may follow or be concomitant with manifestation of pain). Decrease of corneal sensitivity; decreased pupillary reaction or fixity. Absence of systemic signs.

Etiology. Various causes that result in inflammatory lesions of cavernous sinus.

Pathology. According to etiology. Inflammatory changes of cavernous sinus; no other structure involved.

Therapy. According to etiology. Corticosteroids for granulomatous lesions.

Prognosis. May last days or weeks. Spontaneous or therapeutic remission (residual neurologic defects possible). Recurrence in months or years.

BIBLIOGRAPHY. Tolosa E: Periarteritic lesions of carotid siphon with clinical features of carotid infraclinoidal aneurysm. J Neurol Neurosurg Psychiatry 17:300–302, 1954
Hunt WE, Meacher JN, Le Fever HE et al: Painful ophthalmoplegia: Its relation to indolent inflammation of the cavernous sinus. Neurology 11:56–62, 1961
Spector R, Fiandaca M: The 'sinister' Tolosa–Hunt syndrome. Neurology 36:198–203, 1986

TORIELLO'S

Synonym. Brachial arch–X-linked.

Symptoms and Signs. Male; microcephaly, downslanting palpebral fissures, high palate, low-set ears, bilateral deafness, moderately webbed neck, short stature, mental retardation. Occasional cryptorchidism and subvalvular pulmonic stenosis.

Etiology. Autosomal X-linked inheritance.

Pathology. See Signs. Defects of brachial arch.

BIBLIOGRAPHY. Toriello HV, Higgins JV, Abrahamson J et al: X-linked syndrome of brachial arch and other defects. Am J Med Genet 21:137–142, 1985

TORN ANTERIOR CRUCIATE LIGAMENT

Synonyms. Anterior cruciate ligament tear; knee anterior cruciate ligament tear.

Symptoms and Signs. Usually occur during athletic competition, following a deceleration twisting of the knee: "pop" from deep within the joint, preventing further activity and followed within hour by tense effusion.

Etiology. Trauma causing an isolated tear of the anterior cruciate ligament.

Diagnostic Procedures. *Surgical exposure.* Through enlarged anterior medial incision.

Therapy. Surgical repair.

Prognosis. If undiagnosed beyond 10 days lesion is rarely amenable to repair.

BIBLIOGRAPHY. Feagin JA: Jr: The syndrome of torn anterior cruciate ligament. Orthop Clin North Am 10:81–90, 1979

TORNWALDT'S

Synonyms. Chronic nasopharyngitis; pharyngeal bursitis; Tornwaldt's syndromes.

Symptoms. Occipital headache; sensation of mucus accumulation back of the nose; expectoration.

Signs. Nasopharynx covered by mucopurulent material.

Etiology. Chronic inflammation of infected pharyngeal bursa or median recess extending to fauces and pharynx.

Pathology. Nasopharyngeal mucosa congested, with signs of chronic inflammation. Abscess of pharyngeal tonsils.

Diagnostic Procedures. *Culture and antibiotic sensitivity of agents involved.*

Therapy. Antibiotics; surgery occasionally indicated.

Prognosis. Prompt recovery with adequate treatment.

BIBLIOGRAPHY. Tornwaldt GL: Ueber die Bedeutung der Bursa pharyngea für die Erkennung und Behandlung gewisser Nasenrachenraum Krankheiten. Wiesbaden, Bergmann, 1885
Hollender AR, Szanto PB: Tornwaldt's syndrome. Ann Otol Rhinol Laryngol 54:575–581, 1945
James AE, MacMillan AS, MacMillan AS Jr et al: Tornwaldt's cyst. Br J Radiol 41:902–904, 1968

TORTICOLLIS

Synonyms. Caput obstinatum; crooked neck; stiff neck; twisted neck. See also Spasmodic torticollis.

CONGENITAL

Symptoms and Signs. Onset in first months of life. Inclination of head and rotation of occiput. Palpation of exostosis on clavicle at point of insertion of sternocleidomastoid muscle; eyebrow of affected side slopes downward; face broadened and vertically shortened; cranial vault deformed.

Etiology. Many causes are responsible for this condition: (1) intrauterine theory; (2) birth trauma theory; (3) infections theory; (4) neurogenic theory; (5) ischemic theory; (6) combinations of the above. Autosomal dominant inheritance reported.

Pathology. In early phase: vacuolization and degeneration of muscle fibers of lower half of sternocleidomastoid muscle. Later: connective tissue replacement with normal muscle fiber left.

Therapy. Tenotomy.

Prognosis. Good response to early treatment.

ACQUIRED

Symptoms and Signs. Painful contraction of sternocleidomastoid muscle, with inclination and deviation of head.

Etiology. Infection, neoplastic, traumatic, psychogenic, paralytic factors.

Pathology, Therapy, and Prognosis. According to etiology.

BIBLIOGRAPHY. Taylor F: Induration of sternomastoid muscle. Trans Pathol Soc Lond 26:224–227, 1875

Lidge RT, Bechtol RC, Lambert CN: Congenital muscular torticollis; etiology and pathology. J Bone Joint Surg 39:1165–1182, 1957

Gilbert GJ: Familial spasmodic torticollis. Neurology 27:11–13, 1977

Adams RD, Victor M: Principles of Neurology, 3rd ed, pp 882–883, 1066. New York, McGraw-Hill, 1985

TOURAINE'S I

Eponym used to indicate the association of retinal angioid streaks and cardiovascular lesions. Today recognized as manifestation (or subsyndrome) of Groenblod–Strandberg–Touraine (see).

BIBLIOGRAPHY. Touraine MA: L'élastorrhexie systématisée. Bull Soc Fr Dermatol 47:255–273, 1940

TOURAINE'S III

Synonym. Purpura telangiectasica arciformis.

Symptoms and Signs. Variant of Majocchi's (see). Fewer, larger arciform lesions.

BIBLIOGRAPHY. Touraine A: Le purpura annulaire télangiectasique de Majocchi et ses parentes (less capillarites ectasiantés). Presse Med 57:934–936, 1949

TOURAINE–SOLENTE–GOLÉ

Synonyms. Acropachyderma; Audry's II; Brugsch's (same condition plus acromicria); Friedreich–Erb–Arnold; megalia cutis et osseum; primary hypertrophic osteoarthropathy; osteodermopathic; pachydermoperiostitis; Roy's; Roy–Jutras; Hehlinger's. See Cutis verticis gyrata syndrome.

Symptoms and Signs. Prevalent (almost exclusively) in males; onset after puberty, up to third decade. Skin of forehead, face, scalp, hands, and feet becomes thick and furrowed. Hyperhidrosis of hands and feet; increased sebaceous secretion. Hands and feet become enormous; nails are watch-crystallike. Arms and legs appear cylindrical. Effusions of ankles, knees, and occasionally other joints. General health, mental status not affected.

Etiology. Unknown; primary form autosomal dominant (?) inheritance with variable expressivity; sex influenced. Hypertrophic osteoarthropathy (secondary form) is a form closely related or identical (see Marie–Bamberg).

Pathology. *Bones.* Peripheral periostitis with diffuse irregular periosteal ossification (usually leg bones); in severe forms all bones may be involved (except cranium). *Skin.* Hypertrophy of connective tissue and epidermis.

Diagnostic Procedures. *X-ray of skeleton and chest. Biopsy of skin. Blood.* Low sodium. *Urine.* Normal sodium excretion.

Therapy. None.

Prognosis. Progressing for 5 to 10 years, and then remaining stabilized for rest of life. Reduced activity capacity. Life expectancy normal.

BIBLIOGRAPHY. Friedreich M: Hyperostose des gesammten Skeletoes. Virchows Arch [Pathol Anat] 43:83–87, 1868

Audry C: Pachydermia occipitale vorticalée (cutis verticis gyrata). Ann Dermatol Syph 10:257–258, 1909

Labbe M, Renault P: Hypertrophic osteodermopathy. Bull Mem Soc Med Hop Paris 1:1065–1067, 1926

Touraine A, Solente G, Golé L: Un syndrome ostéodermopathique: La pachyderme plicaturée avec pachypériostose des extrémités. Presse Med 42:1820–1824, 1935

Brugsch HG: Acropachyderma with pachyperiostitis. Report of case. Arch Intern Med 68:687–700, 1941

Hadayati H, Barmade R, Skosey JL: Acrolysis in pachydermoperiostosis (primary or idiopathic hypertrophic osteoarthropathy). Arch Intern Med 140:1087–1088, 1980

Rook A, Wilkinson DS, Ebling FJG et al: Textbook of Dermatology, 4th ed, pp 157–159. Oxford, Blackwell Scientific Publications, 1986

TOURNIQUET PARALYSIS

Synonym. Pressure paralysis.

Symptoms. Paralysis with hypotonia or atonia but no atrophy distal to application of tourniquet. No paresthesia after tourniquet is removed; real hyperalgesia.

Signs. Sensory examination shows loss of touch, light pressure sensations, vibration, and position sense while cold and warmth sensations, pain and pilomotor reflexes are preserved. Color and temperature of skin normal.

Etiology. Compression of nerves.

Pathology. Absence of neuroma at the point of injury.

Diagnostic Procedures. *Electric stimulation of nerves.* Block of conduction: in motor nerve lack of stimulation above and good response below the injury. Sensory fibers tingling sensation when stimulation above the lesion and no tingling when stimulation below lesion.

Therapy. None.

Prognosis. Good; return to function in short time. When paralysis complete, impairment of motor and sensory function can last 3 months or longer.

BIBLIOGRAPHY. Duchenne de Boulogne GBA: De l'électrisation localisée et son Application à la Pathologic et à la Thérapeutique, 2nd ed. Paris, Bailière, 1861

Moldaver J: Tourniquet paralysis syndrome. Arch Surg 58:136–144, 1954

TOWNES–BROCKS'

Synonyms. Anus imperforate–hand, foot, ear anomalies; deafness sensorineural–imperforate anus–hypoplastic thumbs. See Vater.

Symptoms and Signs. Both sexes. From birth. Anus imperforate; anomalies of hands (triphalangeal thumb and others) and feet (absent bones, supernumerary thumbs, fusion of metatarsal bones). Sensorineural deafness (mild), satyr ears. Possibly associated hypoplastic kidney, radial dysplasia.

Etiology. Autosomal dominant inheritance.

Pathology, Diagnostic Procedures, Therapy, and Prognosis. See Anus, imperforate; orthopedic and ORL consultation.

BIBLIOGRAPHY. Townes PL, Brocks E: Hereditary syndrome of imperforate anus with hand, foot and ear anomalies. J Pediatr 81:321–326, 1972

Aylsworth AS: The Townes–Brock syndrome: A member of the anus–hand–ear family of syndromes. Am J Hum Genet 37:A43, 1985

TOXIC MEGACOLON

Synonym. Megacolon toxic.

Symptoms and Signs. Systemic toxicity, fever, tachycardia, abdominal distention.

Etiology. Complication of idiopathic, ulcerative colitis, Crohn's disease; observed also in intestinal infections (amebiasis, typhoid, cholera, etc). Other contributing causes cathartics, opiates, anticholinergics.

Pathology. Mucosal denudation and inflammatory changes of submucosal strata.

Diagnostic Procedures. *Blood.* Leukocytosis. Frequently hypokalemia. *X-rays.* Dilatation of colon.

Therapy. Colon decompression (intestinal tube). Fluid and electrolytes balance. Cortical steroid (attention to K^+ depletion). Broad-spectrum antibiotics. Intensive therapy and eventually surgery (subtotal colectomy).

Prognosis. Severe.

BIBLIOGRAPHY. Grant CSA, Dozois RR: Toxic megacolon: Ultimate fate of patients after successful medical managements. Am J Surg 147:106–110, 1984

TRANSFERASE DEFICIENCY GALACTOSEMIA

Synonyms. Galactosemia I; Mason–Turner; von Reuss'.

Symptoms. Both sexes affected; onset after few days or weeks of milk ingestion. Vomiting; diarrhea; dehydration; hypoglycemic crisis; failure to grow. In fulminating cases; death. In intermediate cases, hypotonia, lethargia, severe mental and neurologic manifestations. In mild cases, only milk intolerance.

Signs. Jaundice; ascites (found in infants who died); hepatomegaly between 4 and 8 weeks of life, formation of cataracts.

Etiology. Inability to metabolize galactose because of deficiency of galactose 1-phosphate uridyl transferase. Autosomal recessive inheritance. Various allelic types have been detected that cause intermediate syndromes. *Negro, Duarte, Münster, Indiana, Rennes, Los Angeles, Chicago, variants.*

Pathology. In liver, typical acinar formation, cirrhosis, galactose infiltration.

Diagnostic Procedures. *Blood.* Elevated galactose; decreased glucose (especially evident during crisis); abnormal galactose tolerance. Red cell screening test for determination of deficiency of galactose 1-phosphate uridyl transferase. Hemoglobinemia; immature red blood cells. *Bone marrow.* Erythroblastosislike pattern (occasionally). *Urine.* Galactose; albumin; aminoaciduria (several amino acids).

Therapy. Galactose-free diet. Liver transplantation.

Prognosis. Continuation of administration of galactose-containing food leads to death. If galactose-free diet is started promptly, all symptoms and signs disappear. Cirrhosis and cataract also may regress. If mental retardation already established, no improvement. Preventable only by very early withdrawal of galactose from diet.

BIBLIOGRAPHY. von Reuss A: Zuckerausscheidung im Säuglingsalter. Wien Med Wochenschr 58:799–803, 1908

Mason HH, Turner ME: Chronic galactemia. Report on a case with studies on carbohydrates. Am J Dis Child 50:359–374, 1935

Segal S: Disorders of galactose metabolism. In Stanbury JB, Wyngaarden JB, Fredrickson DS et al: The Metabolic Basis of Inherited Disease, 5th ed, p 167. New York, McGraw-Hill, 1983

TRANSIENT CUSHING'S

Symptoms and Signs. Occur mostly in young patients, but reported also in older patients. Frank symptoms and signs of Cushing's syndrome (see) followed by intense weight gain, loss and disappearance of other features of the syndrome spontaneously or as a result of dietary or dehydration therapy.

Etiology and Pathology. Possibly, hypothalamic functional alteration; idiopathic or secondary to adjacent or indirect mechanical alteration (increased intracranial pressure; meningioma). See also periodic hypothalamic discharge syndrome and inappropriate antidiuretic hormone secretion syndrome.

Diagnostic Procedures. See Cushing's, Periodic hypothalamic discharge, and Conn's.

Therapy. Diet; diuretics.

Prognosis. Guarded.

BIBLIOGRAPHY. Zondek H: Die Krankeiten der endokrinen Drusen, p 371. Berlin, Springer, 1923

Zondek H, Leszynsky HE: Transient Cushing syndrome with report of a case. Br Med J 1:197–200, 1956

Wolff SM, Adler RC, Buskirk ER et al: A syndrome of periodic hypothalamic discharge. Am J Med 36:956–967, 1964

TRANSIENT THYROTOXICOSIS

Synonym. Levi's. See Flajani's.

Symptoms and Signs. Those of typical thyrotoxicosis (see Flajani's) without significant ocular signs; spontaneously regress within weeks or months (occasionally passing through a phase of hypothyroidism and of single or repeated relapses).

Etiology. Unknown. Could be considered a form of painless thyroiditis (?).

Pathology. *Biopsy.* Fibrosis and lymphocyte infiltration, not typical for Hashimoto's (see) or De Quervain's (see).

Diagnostic Procedures. *Antithyroglobulin and antimicrosomal antibodies.* Normal.

BIBLIOGRAPHY. Taft AD (ed): Hyperthyroidism (Symposium). Clin Endocrinol Metab 14(2), (All issue), 1985

TRANSPLANT LUNG

Symptoms and Signs. Occur in patients after homotransplantation; onset follows a rejection crisis or decrease in dose of corticosteroids. Fever; at onset absence of malaise or fatigue. Symptoms and signs of diffuse bilateral pulmonary infiltrates, mostly at bases and hilus.

Etiology. Unknown; immune mechanism (virus, fungi, infection ?).

Pathology. Thickened alveolar membranes; features of infection (fungal, bacterial). Frequently observed, presence of cytomegalic inclusions.

Diagnostic Procedures. *X-ray.* Diffuse bilateral pulmonary infiltrates. *Pulmonary function tests.* Abnormalities consistent with alveolar-capillary block, demonstrable before clinical and x-ray findings. *Blood and sputum to demonstrate virus or fungus.*

Therapy. (1) Increase dose of corticosteroid or other immunosuppressing agents; (2) reduce hypoxia; (3) specific antibiotic treatment.

Prognosis. With prompt and adequate treatment, possibility of recovery high.

BIBLIOGRAPHY. Rifkind D, Starzl TE, Marchioro TL et al: Transplantation pneumonia. JAMA 189:808–812, 1964

Slapak M, Lee HM, Hume DM: Transplant lung: A new syndrome. Br Med J 1:80–84, 1968

TRANSSEXUALISM

Synonyms. Paranoia metamorphosis sexualis; psychopathia transsexualis; psychosexual inversion; "Scythes maladie des."

Symptoms. Prevalent in males (3–7 times). Intense desire for sexual transformation with procedures to accomplish a complete identification of the male with the female sex or vice versa, by surgical and hormonal means. Cooperation of the physician is sought to reach such transformation: castration, penectomy, and plastic construction of an artificial vagina or mastectomy and hysterectomy, and hormone administration.

Etiology. No organic or genetic etiology (as general rule); some patients show some sexual underdevelopment. Psychological and sociological factors in early parent–child relationship play an important role in etiology, plus some unknown biologic factor (possibly). It may, in some cases, be considered a paranoid state.

Diagnostic Procedures. *Chromosome and hormone studies. Psychological evaluation.*

Therapy. Psychotherapy. In some cases, decision to operate and treat this patient to accomplish his aim is prompted by uncontrollable suicide or self-mutilation tendency.

Prognosis. Variable; some individuals, once measures are taken, become deluded that metamorphosis has been accomplished, and that they really belong to different sex. Integrate if new role is not challenged. Many keep insisting on new operations to further transformation, such as ovary or uterus transplantation to become pregnant.

BIBLIOGRAPHY. Friedreich J: Versuch Einer Lieterargeschichte der Pathologic und Therapie der psychischen Krankheiten. Wurzburg, 1830

Pauly IB: Male psychosexual inversion: Transsexualism. A review of 100 cases. Arch Gen Psychiatry 13:172–181, 1965

Freedman AM, Kaplan HI, Sadock BJ: Comprehensive Textbook of Psychiatry, 2nd ed, p 1603. Baltimore, Williams & Wilkins, 1975

The physician's guide to sexual counseling (special issue). Med Aspects Hum Sex 20:(All/issue), 1986

TRAUMATIC MYOSITIS OSSIFICANS

Synonyms. Calcified hematoma; myositis ossificans traumatica; myositis ossificans circumscripta; ossifying hematoma.

Symptoms. Both sexes affected; onset at all ages. More frequent in young active persons with athletic habits or occupations requiring exertion and physical contact that may injure muscles. A particular type (myositis ossificans circumscripta) is determined by repeated minor traumas. From asymptomatic to painful mass and motion limitation becoming evident 1 to 4 weeks after traumatic event. Minor traumas type is responsible for minor motor limitation and discomfort.

Signs. Palpable mass at site of injury. Most frequent sites are quadriceps femoris, brachialis anticus.

Etiology. Unknown; trauma of periosteum and displacement of osteoblasts into muscle: activation of osteoblasts, present metaplastic change.

Pathology. Hematoma followed by aseptic inflammation, proliferation of connective tissue, and formation of cartilage and bone island containing residual muscle fibers.

Therapy. Rest. Symptomatic. Surgery. Diphosphonate 5 mg/kg/day orally for no more than 6 months to prevent and reduce swellings. Prednisone can also be tried.

Prognosis. Spontaneous regression possible

BIBLIOGRAPHY. Fay OJ: Traumatic periosteal bone and callus formation: The so-called traumatic ossifying myositis. Surg Gynecol Obstet 19:174–190, 1914

Adams RD, Kakulas BA: Disease of the muscle: Pathological Foundation of Clinical Myology, Vol IV. Philadelphia, Harper & Row, 1985

TREACHER–COLLINS'

Synonyms. Collins'. Mandibulofacial; Treacher–Collins–Franceschetti. See Franceschetti's, Pierre Robin's, and Nager–Reynier.

Symptoms and Signs. Prevalent in Caucasians, but occur in all major ethnic groups. Notching of lower eyelids with antimongoloid obliquity of palpebral fissures; flattening of malar bones. When associated with mandible defects, external ears defect, and deafness, it is more exactly called Franceschetti's syndrome (see); when associated with micrognathia, glossoptosis, and cleft palate, Pierre Robin's syndrome.

Etiology. See First arch syndrome(s). Autosomal dominant inheritance proposed.

Pathology. Absence or hypoplasia of zygomatic arch.

Diagnostic Procedures. *Chromosomal studies.* Normal pattern. *X-ray.*

Therapy. Symptomatic.

Prognosis. In syndrome with only the classic signs, good.

BIBLIOGRAPHY. Berry GA: Note on congenital defect (coloboma) of lower lid. Lond Ophthalmol Hosp Rep 12:255–277, 1889

Collins E: Case with symmetrical congenital notches in outer part of each lower lid, and defective development of malar bones. Trans Ophthalmol Soc UK 20:190–192, 1900

Halal F, Herrmann J, Pallister PD et al: Differential diagnosis of Nager acrofacial dysostosis syndrome: Report of 4 patients with Nager syndrome and discussion of other related syndromes. Am J Med Genet 14:209–224, 1983

TREFT

Synonym. Optical atrophy–deafness.

Symptoms and Signs. Visual loss by age 11, deafness by age 14. Myopathic changes, difficulty of balance. Ptosis of lids, ophthalmoplegia.

Etiology. Unknown. Autosomal dominant.

BIBLIOGRAPHY. Treft RL: Unique hereditary syndrome found, involves vision and hearing loss. Ophthalmol Times, July 12–13, 1983

TREVOR'S

Synonyms. Dysplasia epiphyseal hemimelia.

Symptoms and Signs. Male/female 3:1 ratio. Asymmetric excessive growth of one or several epiphyses of carpal and tarsal bones and less frequently of other bones, occasionally associated chondromas and osteochondromas.

Etiology. Unknown. Sporadic cases or familial occurrence.

BIBLIOGRAPHY. Trevor D: Tarsoepiphysealis aclasis: A congenital error of epiphyseal development. J Bone Joint Surg 32B:204–213, 1950

Wiedemann HR, Mann M, von Kreudenstein PS: Dysplasia epiphysealis hemimelia. Trevor disease: Severe manifestation in a child. Eur J Pediatr 136:311–316, 1982

TRICEPS SURAE

Symptoms and Signs. This disorder may be simple or may represent a combination of several functional and anatomic disturbances of ambulation. Spasticity or actual shortening of gastrocnemius and soleus.

Etiology. Involvement of gastrocnemius and soleus, which form the triceps surae, in cerebral palsy patient with spasticity or with marked tension; associated with athetosis. It may also occur as compensatory in response to disturbance of other antigravity muscles, or be evidence of overflow mechanism initiated in other part of the body or extremities.

Therapy. Surgical correction: to decrease spasticity; eliminate clonus; restore functional or anatomic length; restore knee extension; correct pes planus or equinus; decrease overflow to or from the muscles by neurectomies; tendon lengthening, or transplant.

Prognosis. Surgery in well-evaluated patient may offer great advantages over conservative therapy.

BIBLIOGRAPHY. Baker LD: Triceps surae syndrome in cerebral palsy. Operation to aid its relief. Arch Surg 68:216–221, 1954

TRICHODENTO-OSSEOUS

Synonyms. Amelogenesis imperfecta; osteosclerosis; taurodontism–curly hair–osteosclerosis; TDO.

Synonyms. Both sexes affected; present from birth. Asymptomatic.

Signs. *Hair.* Kinky, strikingly curly. *Nails.* Brittle; desquamating. *Head.* Frontal bossing, dolichocephaly; square jaw; small, spaced teeth, with deficient enamel and periapical abscesses. Teeth are lost in second or third decade.

Etiology. Autosomal dominant inheritance.

Diagnostic Procedures. *X-ray of skeleton.* Moderate increase of bone density; increased pulp chamber of teeth. Occasionally, partial craniosynostosis. *Blood.* Serum acid phosphatase increased.

Therapy. Care of teeth.

Prognosis. Good except for eventual teeth loss.

BIBLIOGRAPHY. Robinson GC, Miller JR, Worth HM: Hereditary enamel hypoplasia. Its association with characteristic hair structure. Pediatrics 37:489–502, 1966

Lichtenstein J, Warson R, Jorgenson R et al: The tricho-dento-osseous (T.D.O.) syndrome. Am J Hum Genet 24:569–582, 1972

Shapiro SD, Quattromani FL, Jorgenson RJ et al: Tricho-dento-osseous syndrome: Heterogeneity or clinical variability. Am J Med Genet 16:225–236, 1983

TRICHORHINOPHALANGEAL

Synonym. Giedion's. See also Langer–Giedion.

Symptoms and Signs. Both sexes affected; present from birth. Repeated respiratory infections. *Head.* Sparse hair (especially in frontotemporal zone), fine and brittle; eyebrows broad and medially narrowing; cilia scant; ears large; nose bulbous and flabby; philtrum prominent; upper lip thin; mild micrognathia; occasionally, oral malformations. *Skeleton.* Variable growth retardation; in middle childhood, fingers deform (swelling at proximal interphalangeal joints, clinobradydactyly). Thumbs and great toes short. Nails thin.

Etiology. Unknown; both autosomal dominant and recessive inheritance reported; chromosome rearrangement also described.

Diagnostic Procedures. *Blood.* Hypoglycemia. *X-ray.* Typical cone-shaped epiphyses of fingers and toes. Scoliosis and lordosis in some cases. Bone age usually retarded.

Therapy. None.

Prognosis. Hand deformation tends to arrest itself at puberty. Mental retardation, occasionally cerebrovascular accident.

BIBLIOGRAPHY. Klingmüller G: Ueber eigentümliche Konstitutionsanomalien der 2 Schwestern und ihre Beziehungen zu neneun entwicklungspathologischen Befunden. Hautarzt 7:105–113, 1956

Giedion A: Das Tricho-rhino-phalangeal syndrome. Helv Paediatr Acta 2:475–482, 1966

Sanchez JM, Labarta JD, De Negrotti TC et al: Complex translocation in a boy with trichorhinophalangeal syndrome. J Med Genet 22:314–318, 1985

TRICUSPID ATRESIA

Symptoms. Both sexes affected; male predominance. Extremely variable according to associated defects or lack of them. Retarded growth and development; from birth progressive cyanosis, after crying or feeding, hypoxic spells, dyspnea, lethargy, consciousness loss.

Signs. Underdevelopment; edema; clubbing. Pulse normal. On palpation, left ventricular impulse without right ventricular impulse. First and second heart sounds usually single. Absence of pulmonic ejection sound. Murmur absent or variable according to coexisting malformations. Prominent third sound (increased pulmonary blood flow and left failure).

Etiology. Congenital malformation.

Pathology. Atresic tricuspid valve; hypoplasia of right ventricle; interatrial communication; large left ventricle. Variable presence or absence of pulmonary blood flow; and origin and spatial relation of great arteries.

Diagnostic Procedures. *Electrocardiography.* Sinus rhythm; P waves abnormal; PR interval normal or short, seldom prolonged; QRS axis left deviation. *X-ray.* Reduction of pulmonary vessels; aorta enlarged. Heart size normal (initially); absence of right ventricle; hypertrophy of left ventricle; apex elevated above diaphragm; various differences according to associated malformations. *Echocardiogram.* Hypoplastic right side of heart, no record of tricuspid valve. *Cardiac catheterization.*

Therapy. Surgery for palliation; repeated if symptoms return (see Prognosis).

Prognosis. Longevity according to adequacy of interatrial communication and pulmonary arteries flow. From death in first few months (60–75%) to (seldom) longer survival. Return of symptoms 5 to 10 years after intervention indicates need for second operation.

BIBLIOGRAPHY. Holmes WF: Case of malformation of the heart. Trans Med Chir Soc Edinb 1:252–259, 1824

Perloff JK: The Clinical Recognition of Congenital Heart Disease, 2nd ed, p 619. Philadelphia, WB Saunders, 1978

Hurst JW: The Heart, 6th ed, pp 675–676. New York, McGraw-Hill, 1986

TRICUSPID REGURGITATION-PROTEIN-LOSING ENTEROPATHY

See Gordon's.

Symptoms and Signs. Occur in patients with tricuspid regurgitation secondary to rheumatic heart. Development of protein-losing enteropathy; edema.

Etiology. Suggested that elevated systemic venous pressure leads to congestion of bowel lymphatics and loss of lymph in gastrointestinal tract.

Diagnostic Procedures. *Blood.* Hypoproteinemia; lymphocytopenia. *Skin.* Anergy; inability to reject skin graft and other immunologic deficiencies. *X-Ray of chest. Car-*

diac catheterization. Echocardiography. Electrocardiography.

Therapy. Correction of venous hypertension.

Prognosis. Poor.

BIBLIOGRAPHY. Strober W, Cohen LS, Waldmann TA et al: Tricuspid regurgitation. A newly recognized cause of protein-losing enteropathy, lymphocytopenia and immunologic deficiency. Am J Med 44:842–850, 1968

TRIGGER FINGER AND THUMBS

Symptoms. In children younger than 2 years or adults usually after age 45. Local tenderness (not prominent complaint) on the thumbs or one or more fingers (middle and ring more frequently).

Signs. Nodule or fusiform swelling on the flexor tendon that moves with tendon, causing a relative stenosis of the sheath (triggering) and snapping.

Etiology. Congenital, collagen diseases, rheumatoid arthritis.

Therapy. Congenital form usually resolves within first 2 years. In adult, sectioning of the proximal annulus.

BIBLIOGRAPHY. Fahey JJ, Bellinger JA: Trigger in adult and children. J Bone Joint Surg 36A:1200–1212, 1954

TRIGGER POINT

Used to designate any of the syndromes where a local area of tenderness exists, and the stimulation of such areas elicits the pain or symptoms of a referred area thus simulating many different conditions.

Injection of procaine into trigger area leads to relief of pain in most instances.

TRIHYDROXYCOPROSTANIC ACID

Synonym. Cholestasis intrahepatic–trihydroxycoprostanic acid.

Symptoms and Signs. Neonatal jaundice.

Etiology. Autosomal recessive. Impaired transformation of trihydroxycoprostanic acid to cholic acid.

Diagnostic Procedures. *Bile.* Absence of primary bile acid, cholic acid and presence of trihydroxycoprostanic acid.

BIBLIOGRAPHY. Eyssen H, Parmentier G, Campermolle F et al: Trihydroxycoprostanic acid in the duodenal fluid

of two children with intrahepatic bile duct anomalies. Biochim Biophys Acta 273:212–221, 1972

TRIOSEPHOSPHATE ISOMERASE DEFICIENCY

Synonyms. Enzymopathic hemolytic anemia (TPI); TPI deficiency.

Symptoms and Signs. Both sexes affected; onset in infancy. Chronic hemolysis or hemolytic crisis. In homozygous, atypical progressive neurologic syndrome after first year of life; splenomegaly; recurrent infections; sudden death.

Etiology. Deficiency of triosephosphate isomerase in red cells and leukocytes.

Pathology. Not specific.

Diagnostic Procedures. *Blood.* Red cell and leukocyte deficiency of TPI. Slight macrocytosis; some red cells with fingerlike projection. Autohemolysis almost completely corrected by glucose or ATP.

Therapy. Symptomatic.

Prognosis. Poor; unexplained death.

BIBLIOGRAPHY. Schneider AS, Valentine WN, Hattori M et al: Hereditary hemolytic anemia with triosephosphate isomerase deficiency. N Engl J Med 272:229–235, 1965
Clay SA, Shore NA, Landing BH: Triosephosphate isomerase deficiency: A case report with neuropathological findings. Am J Dis Child 136:800–802, 1982
Rosa R, Prehu MO, Calvin MC et al: Hereditary triosephosphate isomerase deficiency. Seven new homozygous cases. Hum Genet 71:235–240, 1985

TRIPLE X

Synonyms. Jacob's (P.A.); superfemale; XXX.

Symptoms and Signs. Incidence 1 : 800 live female births. Often asymptomatic and not associated with characteristic phenotype. Occasionally, mental retardation; sometimes, menstrual irregularities, early menopause; microcephaly; hypertelorism; strabismus; abnormal dentition.

Etiology. Presence of an extra X chromosome, due to nondisjunction. Frequently associated with autosomal trisomies. Single trisomy X may not be considered a characteristic syndrome.

Pathology. Presence of double chromatin bodies.

Prognosis. Majority of individuals exist unrecognized. Many have proved fertile, and all conceived children are normal, phenotypically and cytogenetically.

BIBLIOGRAPHY. Jacobs PA, Baikie AG, Court–Brown WM et al: Evidence for the existence of the human "superfemale." Lancet 2:423–425, 1959

Kohn G, Winter JSD, Mellman WJ: Trisomy X in three children. J Pediatr 72:248–252, 1968

Gorlin RJ, Pindborg JJ, Cohen MM: Syndromes of the Head and Neck, 2nd ed. New York, McGraw–Hill, 1976

TRIPLOIDY

Symptoms and Signs. Variable associations of severe malformations. More frequent: large placenta; prenatal growth deficits; large posterior fontanelle; eye (microophthalmia; iris coloboma) and ear malformations; syndactyly; equinovarus; heart defects; genital, brain, and kidney malformations. Less frequent: anomalous skull; cleft lip; micrognathia; hypertelorism; meningomyelocele.

Etiology. Extra set of chromosomes due to diandry or digyny.

Diagnostic Procedures. *Chromosome studies* XXY (two thirds of cases); XXX (one third). Diploid/triploid mosaic.

Prognosis. Stillbirth or early neonatal death. Mosaics may survive with variable degree of mental impairment.

BIBLIOGRAPHY. Bernard R, Stahl A, Goignet J et al: Triploide chromosomique chez un nouveau-né polymalformé. Ann Genet (Paris) 10:70–74, 1967

Beatty RA: The origin of human triploidy: An integration of qualitative and quantitative evidence. Ann Hum Genet 41:229–314, 1978

Harris MJ, Poland BJ, Dill FJ: Triploidy in 40 human spontaneous abortuses: Assessment of phenotype in embryos. Obstet Gynecol 57:600–606, 1981

TRISOMY 4p

(Trisomy for the short arm of chromosome 4.)

Synonym. Wilson (M.G.).

Symptoms and Signs. Prenatal onset growth deficiency. Hypertonia during infancy followed by hypotonia. Seizures. Abnormal EEG. Microcephaly, prominent forehead, bulbous nose with depressed or flat nasal bridge; macroglossia, irregular teeth, small pointed mandible; frequently enlarged ears with abnormal helix and anthelix; short neck. Clinodactyly of fifth fingers, campodactyly, hypoplastic finger and toe nails. Micropenis, hypospadias, cryptorchidism. Kyphoscoliosis.

Etiology. Trisomy for part of most of the short arm of chromosome 4.

Pathology. Various malformation findings as outlined above.

Diagnostic Procedures. *Chromosome study.*

Therapy. Symptomatic.

Prognosis. One-third of reported cases died during early infancy. Severe mental deficiency is present in 100% of those who survive (without visceral anomalies, such as cardiac or renal defects occasionally present). Life span does not seem to be impaired. Feeding problems are frequent in the neonatal period, and respiratory difficulties are a common complication.

BIBLIOGRAPHY. Wilson MG, Towner JW, Coffin GS, Forsman I: Inherited pericentric inversion of chromosome no. 4. Am J Hum Genet 22:679–683, 1970

Smith DW: Recognizable Patterns of Human Malformation. Philadelphia, WB Saunders, 1982

Dallapiccola B, Mastroiacovo PP, Montali E et al: Trisomy 4p: Five new observations and overview. Clin Genet 12:344–356, 1977

TRISOMY 8

Synonym. C-group trisomy.

Symptoms. Both sexes affected; present from birth. Variable degrees of mental deficiency; poor coordination.

Signs. Forehead prominent; hypertelorism; eyes deeply set; strabismus; nasal root broad; nares enlarged; lips full; micrognathia; ears cupped. Camptodactyly of fingers and toes. Other occasional defects of bones and urogenital system.

Etiology. Trisomy 8 full or in majority mosaics C/normal.

Diagnostic Procedures. *Chromosome studies. Blood.* Occasionally anemia or leukopenia or both.

Therapy. None.

Prognosis. Variable according to ratio of trisomal-to-normal cells. Survival is less restricted than in most other chromosome aberrations: less than one tenth of all patients died during the first 2 years of life, and most of these were victims of cardiac failure, hydrocephalus internus or infections. Some cases with normal karyotype from cultured leukocytes but trisomy 8 in skin fibroblasts can have an IQ estimated in the 70s and can lead a nearly normal life.

BIBLIOGRAPHY. Stalber GR, Buhler EM, Weber JR: Possible trisomy in chromosome group 6-12. Lancet 1:1379–1381, 1963

Caspersson T, Lindsten J, Zeck L et al: Four patients with trisomy 8 identified by the fluorescence and giemsa bonding techniques. J Med Genet 9:1–7, 1972

Pfeiffer RA: Trisomy 8. In Yunis GJ (ed): New Chromosomal Syndromes. New York, Academic Press, 1977

Anneren G, Frodis E, Jorulf H: Trisomy 8 syndrome. The rib anomaly and some new features in two cases. Helv Paediatr Acta 36:465–472, 1981

TRISOMY 9/MOSAIC

Synonym. Haslam's.

Symptoms and Signs. Prenatal onset growth deficiency; severe mental deficiency; craniofacial anomalies: sloping forehead with narrow bifrontal diameter; upslanting, short palpebral fissures, deeply-set eyes; prominent nasal bridge with short root, small fleshy tip, and slitlike nostrils; micrognathia, low-set, posteriorly rotated and misshapen ears. Skeletal anomalies: joint anomalies including abnormal position or function of hips, knees, feet, elbows, and digits; kyphoscoliosis; narrow chest. Other abnormalities: heart defects in about two-thirds of cases, micropenis, cryptorchidism, renal malformations, cystic dilatation of fourth ventricle with lack of midline fusion of cerebellum.

Etiology. Trisomy for chromosome 9.

Diagnostic Procedures. *Chromosome study.*

Pathology. The anomalies listed above.

Therapy. Symptomatic.

Prognosis. Poor.

BIBLIOGRAPHY. Haslam R, Broske SP, Moore CM et al: Trisomy 9 mosaicism, with multiple congenital anomalies. J Med Genet 10:180–184, 1973

Smith DW: Recognizable Pattern of Human Malformation. Philadelphia, WB Saunders, 1982

Sanchez JM, Fijtman N, Migliorini AM: Report of a new case and clinical delineation of mosaic trisomy 9 syndrome. J Med Genet 19:384–386, 1982

TRISOMY 9p

Synonym. Rethore's.

Symptoms and Signs. Growth deficiency, primarily of postnatal onset. Delayed puberty such that some patients continue to grow up to the middle of their third decade; severe mental deficiency; microcephaly, hypertelorism; downslanting palpebral fissures, deep-set eyes, prominent nose, downturned corners of the mouth, cup-shaped ears; short fingers and toes with dystrophic nails; kyphoscoliosis, usually developing during the second decade; congenital heart defects in 5% to 10% of cases and cleft lip or palate in 5%.

Etiology. Trisomy for the entire short arm of chromosome 9. If only the distal half of 9p is duplicated, the clinical picture is less severe.

Pathology. Malformation findings as outlined above.

Diagnostic Procedures. *Chromosome study.*

Therapy. Symptomatic.

Prognosis. Of reported patients 5% to 10% have died in early childhood. The others survived but with mental deficiency and variable degree of handicaps.

BIBLIOGRAPHY. Rethore MO, Larget–Piet L, Abony D et al: Sur quatre cas de trisomie pour le bras court du chromosome 9. Individualisation d'une nouvelle entité morbide. Ann Genet (Paris) 13:217–232, 1970

Smith DW: Recognizable Patterns of Human Malformation. Philadelphia, WB Saunders, 1982

Shih L, Diamond N, Searle B et al: Pure 9p trisomy resulting from maternal mosaicism. Am J Hum Genet 31:110A, 1979

Eydoux P, Jumien C, Despoisse S et al: Gene dosage effect for GALT in 9p trisomy and in 9p tetrasomy with an improved technique for GALT determination. Hum Genet 57:142–144, 1981

Ginsberg J, Soukup S, Bendon RW: Further observations of ocular pathology in Trisomy 9. J Pediatr Ophthalmol Strabismus 26:146–149, 1989

TRISOMY 10p

Symptoms and Signs. Pre- and postnatal growth retardation; dolichocephaly, defective ossification of the calvarian bones, with wide sutures and fontanelles, craniofacial disproportion, narrow face with high forehead, flat nasal bridge, long philtrum, retroposition of the mandible, low-set, posteriorly rotated prominent and dysplastic ears, low hair line; dislocated lips, clubfeet; fine, dry hair, atrophic skin; male genital hypoplasia. Other malformations frequently associated are: cleft lip and palate, heart defects, hypoplasia of the diaphragm, bile duct atresia, cystic kidneys.

Etiology. Trisomy for the short arm of chromosome 10.

Prognosis. Almost half of the patients described died perinatally or during the early postnatal course of asphyxia, prolonged jaundice, feeding difficulties, seizures.

The survivors showed muscular hypotonia and underdevelopment, hyporeflexia, diminished activity, and motor and mental deficiency.

BIBLIOGRAPHY. Yunis E, Silva R, Giraldo A: Trisomy 10p. Ann Genet (Paris) 19:57–60, 1976

Stall C, Willard D: La trisomie 10p. A propos d'une observation d'une translocation maternelle. Pediatrie 35:251–255, 1980

TRISOMY PARTIAL 10q

Synonym. Yunis–Sanchez.

Symptoms and Signs. Prenatal onset growth deficiency; mean birth weight 2.7 kg; microcephaly; flat face with high forehead and high arched eyebrows; ptosis; short palpebral fissures; microphthalmia; broad and depressed nasal bridge, bow-shaped mouth with prominent upper lip; cleft palate; malformed; posteriorly rotated ears; campodactyly, proximally placed thumbs, syndactyly between second and third toes, foot position anomalies; heart and renal malformations; kyphoscoliosis; pectus excavatum; cryptorchidism. Occasional abnormalities: brain malformations, ocular anomalies, malrotation of the gut, hypospadias, vertebral malformations.

Etiology. Trisomy 10q24 qter, the distal segment of the long arm of chromosome 10.

Pathology. Various malformations as outlined above.

Diagnostic Procedures. *Chromosome study.*

Therapy. Symptomatic.

Prognosis. Poor. One half of the reported patients died of heart defects; surviving children showed marked mental deficiency.

BIBLIOGRAPHY. Yunis J, Sanchez O: A new syndrome resulting from partial trisomy for the distal third of the long arm of chromosome 10. J Pediatr 84:567–570, 1974

Klep-de Pater JM, Bijlsma JB, de France HF et al: Partial trisomy 10q. A recognizable syndrome. Hum Genet 46:29–40, 1979

Smith DW: Recognizable Patterns of Human Malformation. Philadelphia, WB Saunders, Philadelphia, 1982

TRISOMY 12p

Synonym. Duplication of the short arm of chromosome 12.

Symptoms and Signs. Midface hypoplasia, shallow orbits, epicanthal folds, flat, wide bridge and upturned tip of the nose and small ears; turribrachycephaly with high forehead, irregular and bushy eyebrows, a long, poorly modeled philtrum, everted lower lip, large tongue, full cheeks; short, broad hands and fingers, and clinodactyly of little fingers; congenital heart defects; microphthalmia, aniridia; cleft palate; and atresia; mental retardation.

Etiology. Duplication of the short arm of chromosome 12.

BIBLIOGRAPHY. Alfi OS, Lange M: Trisomy 12p, a clinically recognizable syndrome. Birth Defects XIII (3b):231–232, 1977

Qazi QH, Kanachanapoomi R, Cooper R et al: Duplication (12p) and hypoplastic left heart. Am J Med Genet 9:195–199, 1981

TRISOMY 20

Symptoms and Signs. In most cases, normal growth; mild to moderate mental deficiency, hypotonia, poor coordination, ataxia, tremor. Craniofacial anomalies: brachycephaly, upslanting palpebral fissures, blepharophimosis, hypotelorism or hypertelorism; flat nasal bridge with anteverted nares, large and poorly formed ears. Limb anomalies: cubitus valgus, small and tapering fingers, foot position defects. Other: vertebral defects, kyphoscoliosis, umbilical or inguinal hernias, genital hypoplasia with cryptorchidism. Occasional abnormalities: cardiac defects, renal malformations, atretic ear canals, iridal colobomata, myopia, strabismus, cataract, hydrocephalus.

Etiology. Trisomy 20.

Therapy. Symptomatic.

Prognosis. Depends on the presence of major anomalies (cardiac). In some cases, patients with mild mental deficiency and no major malformations were not detected before the birth of a second affected sibling.

BIBLIOGRAPHY. Pan SF, Fatora SR, Haas JE et al: Trisomy of chromosome 20. Clin Genet 9:449–453, 1975

Nevin NC, Nevin J, Thompson W: Trisomy 20 mosaicism in amniotic fluid cell culture. Clin Genet 15:440–443, 1979

TROCHANTERIC

Symptoms and Signs. Deep aching pain in the region of great trochanter, usually radiated to the thigh. Occasionally, radiation to the hip, and dorsolateral aspect of foot. In other instances, radiation to lower part of back, lower portion of abdomen, and medial portion of buttock.

Etiology. Trauma.

Diagnostic Procedures. *X-ray. Blood.* To assess lesions and evaluate any coexisting disease.

Treatment. Ultrasound therapy may aggravate the syndrome; infiltrations (procaine–hydrocortisone) usually relieve the symptoms.

Prognosis. According to etiology.

BIBLIOGRAPHY. Hays MB: Trochanteric syndrome. J Bone Joint Surg 45:657, 1963

TROELL–JUNET

Synonym. Acromegaly–goiter–skull hyperostosis–diabetes.

Symptoms and Signs. Reported only in females. Those of acromegaly, toxic goiter (usually nodular type), and Morgagni's (see); diabetes mellitus also frequently associated.

Etiology. See multiple endocrine adenomatosis.

Pathology. Pituitary adenoma (eosinophilic, and in one case chromophobic). Nodular type of goiter. Acromegalic and Morgagni's syndrome changes.

Diagnostic Procedures. *X-rays. Hormonal studies.* See Acromegaly.

Therapy. Removal of pituitary adenoma and symptomatic.

Prognosis. Poor.

BIBLIOGRAPHY. Troell A: "Syndroma morgagni" hos patienter med samtidig akromegali och tyreotoxikos. Seven Lak Tidn 35:763–771, 1938
Junet RM: Histopathologic du squelette acromegalique et ses modifications sous l'influence de l'hyperthroidisme Geneva, Thése No. 1681, 1938
Moore S: Troell–Junet syndrome. Acta Radiol 39:485–493, 1953

TROISIER–HANOT–CHAUFFARD

Synonyms. Bronze diabetes; diabetes–hemochromatosis; Hanot–Chauffard; primary hemochromatosis; iron storage; Leschke's; Recklinghausen–Applebaum. Hemochromatosis idiopathic.

Symptoms. Greatest frequency in men (80%) between 40 and 60 years of age. Lassitude; weakness; weight loss; upper right abdominal quadrant sharp pain; dyspnea; loss of libido. Occasionally, specific progressive polyarthropathy.

Signs. Skin pigmentation of two types: (1) Addisonlike or (2) grayish hue on (genitals, face, arms, skinfolds, seldom mucosae 15%); edema; ascites. Later, jaundice, loss of body hair, gynecomastia, hepatomegaly, splenomegaly, testicular atrophy; eventually, signs of heart failure.

Etiology. *Idiopathic.* Autosomal recessive inheritance. Linkage disequilibrium with HAL-A$_3$. Complete expression only in males; females and sibs have only altered metabolism of iron. Various cell sites of anomalies of iron absorption: gut, plasma transferrin, liver, and reticuloendothelial system. Symptoms appear when iron overload reaches 20 to 40 gamma and hemosiderin deposits lead to organ impairment. *Secondary forms due to erythropoietic.* Chronic defect of hemoglobin synthesis, ineffective erythropoiesis, hemolytic processes. *Iron loading.* Medication; diet (Bantu siderosis); transfusions.

Pathology. *Skin.* Thin; melanin pigment in basal layer. *Liver.* Nodular cirrhosis; hemosiderin deposits. *Pancreas.* Nodular fibrosis. *Testes.* Atrophic. *Heart.* Deposit of hemosiderin.

Diagnostic Procedures. *Blood.* At onset high hemoglobin concentration; later macrocytic anemia, increased serum iron and serum-bound iron. Hyperglycemia; hyperbilirubinemia; liver function test altered. *Biopsy of liver.*

Therapy. Diabetes treatment (insulin resistant in most cases). Phlebotomies. Chelate; desferrioxamine intramuscularly.

Prognosis. With adequate treatment; reversal of symptoms according to the amount of damage.

BIBLIOGRAPHY. Troisier CE: Diabète sucré. Bull Soc Anat Paris 16:231, 1871
Hanot VC, Chauffard AM: Cirrhose hypertrophique pigmentaire dans le diabète sucrè. Rev Med 3:385–403, 1882
Bothwell TH, Charlton RW, Motulsky AG: Idiopathic hemochromatosis. In Stanbury JB, Wyngaarden JB, Fredrickson DS et al: The Metabolic Basis of Inherited Disease, 5th ed, p. 1269. New York, McGraw-Hill, 1983

TROPICAL EOSINOPHILIA

Synonyms. Tropical eosinophilic lung; Frimodt–Moller's; Weingarten's. See Eosinophilic lung, secondary.

Symptoms. Occur in Near and Far East, primarily in Indians. May appear in persons of other races coming back from the Orient. Chronic productive cough, malaise, and wheezing, with spontaneous remissions and relapses.

Signs. In chest, bilateral rales localized to middle and basilar areas.

Etiology. An atypical host response to various filariae including *Wuchereria bancrofti* and *Brugia malayi*.

Pathology. Eosinophilic bronchopneumonia; histiocytic infiltration often associated with fibrosis; mixed cell exudate with eosinophils, lymphocytes; marked fibrosis.

Diagnostic Procedures. *Blood.* Eosinophilia. High titers of filarial antibodies: IgE levels more than 1000 U ml. *Sputum.* Eosinophils. *X-ray of lung.* Symmetric middle and basilar zone infiltrations.

Therapy. Diethylcarbamazine, preceded by antihistamines; corticosteroids.

Prognosis. Chronic course; rapid improvement with treatment; some patients develop chronic pulmonary insufficiency and failure from development of pulmonary fibrosis. Not as benign as previously considered.

BIBLIOGRAPHY. Frimodt–Moller C, Barton RM: Pseudotuberculous condition associated with eosinophilia. Indian Med Gaz 75:607–613, 1940
Weingarten RJ: Tropical eosinophilia. Lancet 1:103–105, 1943
Udwadia FE: Tropical eosinophilia. A correlation of clinical, histopathologic and lung function studies. Dis Chest 52:531–538, 1967
Ottesen EA: Tropical eosinophilia. In Cecil Textbook of Medicine, p 1776. Philadelphia, WB Saunders, 1982

TROPICAL SPLENOMEGALY

Synonyms. African macroglobulinemia; Bengal splenomegaly; cryptogenic splenomegaly; idiopathic splenomegaly. Big spleen.

Symptoms. Found in tropical and subtropical regions with endemic malaria. Predominant in females. Asthenia; fatigue.

Signs. Marked splenomegaly.

Etiology. Unknown; malaria considered a direct or indirect agent, but no conclusion reached. Abnormal immune response.

Pathology. In spleen different findings in different regions. In New Guinea, more sinus dilatation and less lymphatic proliferation than in cases in Africa. Reticuloendothelial biopsy shows lack of malarial pigment.

Diagnostic Procedures. *Blood.* Anemia a constant feature; search for malaria parasites negative, or few parasites. In Nigeria, peripheral blood and bone marrow lymphocytosis. In Uganda and New Guinea, absence of lymphocytosis. Increased concentration of IgM immunoglobulin in serum.

Therapy. Proguanil (also if malarial parasites are absent), life-long treatment. Splenectomy not indicated because of risk of bacterial infections and fatal attacks of malaria, although in selected cases has been beneficial.

Prognosis. With proguanil, slow and progressive decrease in size of spleen and improvement of general health (over months). With cessation of treatment, full relapse in 3 months.

BIBLIOGRAPHY. Conferences and Meeting: Tropical splenomegaly syndrome. Br Med J 4:614, 1967
Wintrobe MM (ed): Clinical Hematology, 8th ed, pp 1432–1433. Philadelphia, Lea & Febiger, 1981.

TROTTER'S

Synonyms. Morgagni's sinus; peritubal.

Symptoms. Predominant in males; onset from adolescence to old age. Deafness (first or early symptom), middle ear type; severe neurologic pain in the ear, side of head, lower jaw, side of tongue (third branch of trigeminal nerve); anesthesia of lower jaw (later symptoms) in the region of the mental foramen; defective mobility of soft palate, trismus (later stage).

Signs. (1) Fullness without ulceration in the lateral wall of nasopharynx (firm thickening) that eventually extends to adjacent muscles. (2) Asymmetry of soft palate (observed when it is relaxed). (3) Eustachian catheterization may produce bleeding, temporary relief of deafness. (4) Unilateral or bilateral cervical and retropharyngeal glands (frequently, first sign).

Etiology. Lateral nasopharyngeal lesion of neoplastic nature. Also occurring as development of the Jacod's syndrome (for extension of an intracranial lesion) or of the pterigopalatine fossa syndrome. The Trotter's syndrome may precede or follow the pterigopalatine syndrome, or occur in combination.

Pathology. Neoplastic lesion not invading the mucous membrane, spreading into sinus of Morgagni, and involving adjacent muscles. Cervical lymph nodes, liver, and skeleton metastasis.

Diagnostic Procedures. *X-ray of skull.* Involvement of foramen ovale. *Biopsy.*

Therapy. Deep x-ray therapy; surgery to reach lesion for radium implantation.

Prognosis. Very poor; treatment only palliative.

BIBLIOGRAPHY. Trotter W: On certain clinically obscure malignant tumours of the nasopharyngeal wall. Br Med J 2:1057–1059, 1911
Asherson N: Trotter's syndrome and associated lesions. J Laryngol Otol 65:349–366, 1951
Bingas B: Tumors of the base of skull. In Vinken PJ, Bruyn GW (eds): Handbook of Clinical Neurology,

vol 17, chap 4, pp 136–233. Amsterdam (North Holland), 1974

TROUSSEAU'S

Synonyms. Carcinogenic thrombophlebitis; thrombophlebitis migrans; recurrent thrombophlebitis.

Symptoms. Repeated episodes of pain extending over a period of months or years. Extremities most frequently affected areas.

Signs. Red, tender, raised, short cordlike nodules under the skin, usually disappearing with little or no residual damage before next lesions appear.

Etiology. Unknown; frequent association with carcinoma (especially of the pancreas, lung, breast, colon, stomach). Possibly, release of thromboplastinlike substance from neoplasia.

Pathology. Segmental thrombosis of veins; infiltration of media and of adventitia; clot firmly attached.

Diagnostic Procedures. Search for hidden malignancy.

Therapy. No specific treatment necessary.

Prognosis. The thrombi disappear spontaneously. Low incidence of pulmonary thrombosis. In idiopathic form, disappearance of condition without treatment. If sign of malignancy, according to nature and degree of development of this lesion.

BIBLIOGRAPHY. Trousseau A: Lectures delivered in 1862.
Thompson AV: Thrombosis of visceral veins in visceral cancer. Clin J 67:137–140, 1938
Sibrack LA, Gouterman IH: Cutaneous manifestations of pancreatic disease. Cutis 21:763–768, 1978
Rio B: Manifestations Lématologiques des tumeurs malignes non hematopoiétiques. Encyl Med Chir. Paris France Sang 13036 F 207, 1986
Malamani GD, Agata G, Grandi A et al: Trombocitosi secondarie e reattive. Significato clinico-epidemiologico a proposito di 385 casi di osservazione personale. Rec Prog Med 79:15–18, 1988

TRYPSINOGEN DEFICIENCY

Symptoms and Signs. Present from birth. Severe growth failure; edema; pallor; hypochromotrichia.

Etiology. Unknown; specific deficiency of trypsinogen. Autosomal recessive inheritance.

Diagnostic Procedures. *Blood.* Anemia; moderate reticulocytosis; severe neutropenia; severe hypoproteinemia; all protein fractions low. *Sweat chloride test.* Negative. *Urine.* Normal. *Duodenal aspirate.* Complete lack of trypsinogen.

Therapy. Protein hydrolysate.

Prognosis. Optimal response to treatment. Growth progresses regularly and all clinical and hematologic features disappear.

BIBLIOGRAPHY. Townes PL: Trypsinogen deficiency disease. J Pediatr 66:275–285, 1965
Townes PL, Bryson MF, Miller G: Further observations on trypsinogen deficiency disease: Report of a second case. J Pediatr 71:220–224, 1967
Anderson CM, Burke V (eds): Pediatric Gastroenterology. Oxford, Blackwell Scientific Publications, 1975

TUCKER'S

Synonyms. Pagetlike amyotrophic sclerosis; Pagetoid neuroskeletal.

Symptoms and Signs. Both sexes equal distribution. Onset insidious after 30 years of age. Weakness and then atrophy of muscles of legs and proximal part of arms. Progression to total motor incapacitation: tetraparesis and dementia. Respiratory insufficiency.

Etiology. Unknown. Possibly autosomal dominant inheritance.

Pathology. *Bone.* Thickening and spotty sclerosis.

Diagnostic Procedures. *Blood:* Increased alkaline phosphatases. *X-ray.* Skeleton (see Pathology). *Nerve conduction studies.* Normal. *Electromyogram.* Muscle denervation. *Muscle biopsy.* Atrophy from muscle denervation.

Therapy. None. Prognosis: death at about age 60.

BIBLIOGRAPHY. Tucker WS Jr, Hubbard WH, Stricker JD et al: A new familial disorder of combined lower motor neuron degeneration and skeletal disorganization. Trans Assoc Am Physicians 95:126–134, 1982

TUFFLI–LAXOVA

Synonym. Ectodermal dysplasia adrenal cyst.

Symptoms and Signs. One case (male) reported: aplasia cutis verticis, hypohidrosis, nipple hypoplasia; onychodysplasia, delayed teeth eruption. Large adrenal cyst. Mother presented analogous features.

Etiology. Autosomal dominant inheritance.

BIBLIOGRAPHY. Tuffli GA, Laxova R: New autosomal dominant form of ectodermal dysplasia. Am J Med Genet 14:381–384, 1983

TÜRK'S

See Duane's.

Symptoms and Signs. Limitation of abduction of affected eye beyond midline; retraction of bulb on abduction.

Etiology. Birth injury (?). Considered incomplete Duane's syndrome.

Pathology. Fibrous degeneration of external rectus muscle.

Therapy. Surgery to correct strabismus.

BIBLIOGRAPHY. Türk S: Ueber Retractionsbewegungen der Augen. Dtsch Med Wochenschr 22:199–201, 1896

TUOMAALA–HAAPANEN

Synonym. Brachymetapody – anodontia – hypotrichosis–albinoidism.

Symptoms and Signs. Finnish family. Both sexes. *Facies.* Oxycephaly; alopecia; antimongoloid lid fissures; hypoplastic tarsus; nystagmus; strabismus; cataract; fovea hypoplasia; myopia; wide nose bridge; micrognatia; anodontia. *Limbs.* Short digits. *Skin.* Depigmentation.

Etiology. Unknown; familial occurrence reported.

BIBLIOGRAPHY. Tuomaala P, Haapanen E: Three siblings with similar anomalies of the eyes, bones and skin. Acta Opthalmol 46:365–371, 1968

TURCOT'S

Synonyms. Colon polyposis–brain tumor; glioma polyposis; Turcot–Després–St. Pierre. See Gardner's.

Symptoms and Signs. Those of colon polyposis (see intestinal polyposis, familial) and central nervous system tumor. *Skin. Cafe au lait* spots.

Etiology. Autosomal recessive condition; only two cases (in brother and sister born from consanguineous marriage) reported.

Pathology. Polypoid adenomatosis of colon; medulloblastoma of spinal cord in one case; glioblastoma of frontal lobe in the other one. Various types of brain tumors reported.

Diagnostic Procedures. *X-rays. Intestine. Endoscopic examination. Cerebral CT scan.*

Prognosis. Poor.

BIBLIOGRAPHY. Turcot J, Després MP, St. Pierre F: Malignant tumors of central nervous system associated with familial polyposis of colon: Report of two cases. Dis Colon Rectum 2:465–468, 1959
McKusick VA: Genetic factors in intestinal polyposis. JAMA 182:271–277, 1962
Chowdhary VM, Boehme DH, AL–Jishi M: Turcot syndrome (glyoma–polyposis): Case report. J Neurosurg 63:804–807, 1985

TURNBRIDGE–PALEY

Synonym. Optic atrophy–deafness–diabetes.

Symptoms and Signs. Onset in childhood. Primary optic atrophy and perceptive hearing loss in patients with juvenile diabetes mellitus.

Etiology. Unknown. Familiar. Frequent association with Friedreich, Refsum, Laurence–Moon–Biedel syndromes, dementia and epilepsy.

Pathology. Optic atrophy, retinal pigmentation.

Therapy. None.

Prognosis. Poor.

BIBLIOGRAPHY. Turnbridge RE, Paley RG: Primary optic atrophy in diabetes mellitus. Diabetes 5:295–296, 1956
Ikkos DG: Association of juvenile diabetes mellitus, primary optic atrophy, and perceptive hearing loss in 3 sibs, with additional diabetes insipidus in one case. Acta Endocrinol 65:95–102, 1970

TURNER–KIESER

Synonyms. Arthro-osteo-onychodysplasia–iliac horns; Chatelain's; Fong's; HOOD (hereditary osteo-onychodysplasia); nail patella; congenital iliac horns; Oesterreicher–Turner; osteo-onychodysostosis; Touraine's II.

Symptoms. Usually not discovered until second or third decade; males and females equally affected. Usually asymptomatic or (in a few cases) weakness, difficulty in climbing stairs, dislocation of patella.

Signs. *Nails.* Large spectrum of symmetric abnormalities from anonychia to minimal longitudinal ridging, hypoplasia, thinness affecting all of patients. *Elbow.* Inability to extend fully, pronate, or supinate. Flexion usually normal; prominence of medial epicondyle (90%). *Knees.* Patellae usually smaller than normal or absent. Frequent dislocation; prominence of medial femoral condyles and decrease in the size of lateral femoral condyles (90%). *Pelvis.* Palpable iliac horns arising from central area of external iliac fossa, bilateral, symmetric (70%). *Eyes.* Anomalies of iris pigmentation (darker around inner margin; lighter at the periphery, 45%). Other abnormalities occasionally observed: anomalies of scapula; lumbar lordosis; clinodactyly; early arthritic joint changes.

Etiology. Unknown; genetic defect, autosomal dominant (single gene ?), variable expression with possible linkage with loci for determination of ABO blood group.

Pathology. Information fragmentary. In knee, absence of anterior cruciate ligament, osteoarthritic changes. In kidney, glomerulonephritis in different phases.

Diagnostic Procedures. *Urine.* Proteinuria (in about 40%); increased mucoproteins. *X-ray of elbow.* Prominence of medial epicondyle of humerus; dysplasia with or without luxation. *Of knee.* Hypoplasia of lateral femoral condyle and hypoplasia or absence of patella. *Of pelvis.* Iliac horns (pathognomonic).

Therapy. Symptomatic.

Prognosis. Very good.

BIBLIOGRAPHY. Little EM: Congenital absence or delayed development of patella. Lancet 2:781–784, 1897

Turner JW: Hereditary arthrodysplasia associated with hereditary dystrophy of nails. JAMA 100:882–884, 1933

Kieser W: Die Sog. Flughaut beim ihre Beziehung Zum Status dysraphicus und ihre Erbichkleit. Z Menschl Vererb 2:594–619, 1939

Palacios E: Hereditary osteo-onychodysplasia; the nail patella syndrome. Am J Roentgenol 101:842–850, 1967

McKusick VA: Heritable Disorders of Connective Tissue, 4th ed, p 835. St Louis, CV Mosby, 1972

Sabnis SG, Autonovych TT, Argy WP et al: Nail patella syndrome. Clin Nephrol 14:148–153, 1980

TURNER'S

Synonyms. Bonnevie–Ullrich; ovarian dwarfism; genital dwarfism; gonadal dysgenesis (XO); monosomy X; Morgagni–Turner–Albright; pterygolymphangiectasia; Schereshevkii–Turner; Turner–Ullrich; XO.

Symptoms. Female phenotype; onset in childhood. Retardation of linear growth; primary amenorrhea; lack of development of secondary sex characteristic.

Signs. Short stature (105–130 cm). Lack of axillary hair and very scanty or absent pubic hair. Breasts underdeveloped. Congenital abnormalities of various nature associated: webbed neck; cubitus valgus; ptosis; strabismus; nystagmus; cardiac abnormalities: coarctation of aorta (70%), or other cardiovascular lesions almost constantly affecting left heart. Lymphedema of extremities (30–40%). Occasionally, anomalies of bone development such as protuberance of sternum, high palate, underdeveloped mandible.

Etiology. Genetic abnormality due to sex chromatin abnormalities. Karyotype generally XO (80%): lack of one of the sex chromosomes. In 20%, sex chromatin positive for various chromosomal abnormalities: XX (one chromosome abnormal); mosaicism XO (XX and even XO [XX]-XXX).

Pathology. Absent, or rudimentary, gonads. Usually, absence of proliferation of epithelial layer. In some cases, germinal element of cortical (ovary) or medullary (testicular) origin may be found. The gonadal dysgenesis syndrome and its variants represent a continuum that ranges from typical pattern (see above) to normal male or female.

Diagnostic Procedures. *Sex chromatin study. Chromosome determination. Culposcopy.*

Therapy. Estrogen replacement either by continuous method or cyclic fashion. Therapy should be started as early as age 14 or 15 and should be continued as long as menstrual period is needed.

Prognosis. Use of estrogen prevents premature aging and decreases incidence of cardiovascular and coronary heart diseases.

BIBLIOGRAPHY. Morgagni GB: Epistola Anatomica Medica, XLVII: Article 20, 1768

Ullrich O: Über typische Kombinationsbilder multiple Abartungen. Z Kinderheilkd 49:271–276, 1930

Turner HH: A syndrome of infantilism, congenital webbed neck and cubitus valgus. Endocrinology 23:566–574, 1938

Carothers AD, Frackiewicz A, De Mey R et al: A collaborative study of the aetiology of Turner syndrome. Ann Hum Genet 43:355–368, 1980

Chen H, Faigenbaum D, Weiss H: Psychosocial aspects with the Ullrich–Turner syndrome. Am J Med Genet 8:191–203, 1981

Lin AE, Lippe BM, Geffner ME et al: Aortic dilation, dissection and rupture in patients with Turner syndrome. J Pediatr 109:820–826, 1986

Massarano AA, Brook CGD, Hindmarsh PC et al: Growth hormone secretion in Turner's syndrome and influence of oxandrolone and ethinyl oestradiol. Arch Dis Child 64:587–592, 1989

TURPIN'S

Synonym. Bronchiectasis-megaesophagus-osteopathy.

Symptoms and Signs. Present from neonatal period. Repeated respiratory infections with chronic respiratory insufficiency, cough, and purulent sputum. Coughing on swallowing liquids.

Etiology. Congenital malformation.

Pathology. Association of bronchiectasis, megaesophagus, and osteopathy (vertebral and costal malformations). Frequently, tracheobronchial fistula.

Diagnostic Procedures. *X-ray of lung, gastrointestinal tract, and skeleton.* See Pathology.

Therapy. Surgery when indicated and feasible. Antibiotics.

Prognosis. Poor.

BIBLIOGRAPHY. Turpin R et al: Image claire, cervicale, traduction radiographique d'un mégaoesophagus groupment dysmorphique particulier. J Fr Med Chir Thor 3:436–439, 1949

TWIN-TO-TWIN TRANSFUSION

Synonyms. Neonatal arteriovenous transfusion; intrauterine parabiotic.

Symptoms and Signs. One of the twins (recipient) is bigger, polycythemic, hypervolemic. He shows increased cardiac size with myocardial hyperplasia and arterial hypertension, both systemic and pulmonary. The other twin (donor) is pale, with hypovolemia, undersized visceral organs. Disparity of body growth between the two twins. The recipient twin is usually associated with polyhydramnios. Two cases of the syndrome have been described in which the donor twin exhibited blueberry muffinlike macules and papules associated with cutaneous erythropoiesis (that is considered to be due to persistence or reactivation of fetal dermal erythropoiesis secondary to prolonged, severe intrauterine anemia).

Etiology. Unknown, results from transfusion of blood from one fetus to the other; occurs only in monozygous twins. The transfusion occurs via anastomotic channels between the two circulations. These channels are artery-to-artery, artery-to-vein, vein-to-vein.

Pathology. See Symptoms and Signs.

Diagnostic Procedures. *Examination of placenta on delivery.* Suspicion if (1) hydramnios with twin pregnancy is noticed and (2) disparity of growth between two twins is observed. *Placentography.* With radioactive isotopes. *Skin biopsy.* Of blueberry muffin lesion.

Therapy. Blood transfusion to donor (undersized) twin. Removal of blood from recipient twin.

Prognosis. Increased perinatal mortality. Good response if adequate treatment.

BIBLIOGRAPHY. Schotz F: Die Gefassverbindunger der Placenta kreislaufe eineuger Zwillinge, ihre Entwick-

elung und ihre Flogen. Arc Gur Gynaekol 30:335–381, 1887
Simopoulas AP: Arteriovenous transfusion syndrome in newborn twins. GP 33:141, 1966
Schwartz JL, Maniscalco WM, Lane AT, Currao WJ: Twin transfusion syndrome causing cutaneous erythropoiesis. Pediatrics 74:527–529, 1984

TYLOSIS–ESOPHAGUS CARCINOMA

Synonym. Keratosis palmo-plantaris-esophagus carcinoma.

Symptoms and Signs. Both sexes affected; onset between third and sixth decades. Keratosis of palms and soles; development of symptoms and signs of carcinoma of the esophagus.

Etiology. Unknown; autosomal dominant inheritance.

Pathology. Hyperkeratosis of palms and soles. Squamous cell carcinoma of esophagus (usually lower third).

Diagnostic Procedures. *Esophagoscopy. X-ray. Biopsy.*

Therapy. Surgery if feasible.

Prognosis. Poor.

BIBLIOGRAPHY. Howel–Evans W, McConnell RB, Clarke CA et al: Carcinoma of the esophagus with keratosis palmaris et plantaris (tylosis). A study of two families. Q J Med 27:413–429, 1958
Shine I, Allison PR: Carcinoma of the esophagus with tylosis (keratosis palmaris et plantaris). Lancet 1:951–953, 1966
Yesudian P, Premalatha S, Thambiah AS: Genetic tylosis with malignancy: A study of a South Indian pedigree. Br J Dermatol 102:597–600, 1980

TYLOSIS–OPTIC ATROPHY

Symptoms. Prevalent in females. Thickening of skin of palms and soles (tylosis), occasionally of the ears as well. Development of optical atrophy late in life.

Etiology. Unknown; possibly, sex-linked dominant inheritance.

BIBLIOGRAPHY. Dimsdale H: Hereditary optic atrophy in family with keratodermia palmaris et plantaris (tylosis). Proc R Soc Med 42:796, 1949

TYROSINEMIA, NEONATAL

Symptoms and Signs. Occur usually in premature infants. Apparently asymptomatic and harmless.

Etiology. Temporarily delayed development of enzymes necessary to metabolize tyrosine. The importance of this syndrome is in relation to differential diagnosis with the hereditary tyrosinemia-tyrosiluria syndrome.

Pathology. None.

Diagnostic Procedures. *Plasma and urine.* High tyrosine level.

Therapy. Vitamin C.

Prognosis. Excellent; metabolic defect disappears with treatment or spontaneously.

BIBLIOGRAPHY. Avery ME, Clow CL, Menkes JH et al: Transient tyrosinemia of the newborn: Dietary and clinical aspects. Pediatrics 39:378–384, 1967

Goldsmith LA: Tyrosinemia and related disorders. In Stanbury JB, Wyngaarden JB, Fredrickson DS et al: The Metabolic Basis of Inherited Disease, 5th ed. p 287, New York, McGraw-Hill, 1983

TYROSINEMIA–TYROSILURIA, HEREDITARY SYNDROMES

TYROSINEMIA TYPE I OR TYROSINOSIS

Synonyms. Tyrosiluria, hypemethioninemia, inborn hepatorenal dysfunction.

Symptoms. Prevalence in French Canadian population of Québec. Both sexes affected; normal at birth; onset 2 to 8 weeks of age. Fever; lethargy; irritability; drowsiness; anorexia; vomiting; diarrhea; hematuria; epistaxia; melena; hematemesis.

Signs. Peculiar (cabbage) urine odor; jaundice; ecchymosis; abdominal distention; hepatosplenomegaly; edema.

Etiology. Deficiency of fumaril acetoacetate (FAA) hydrolase.

Pathology. Generalized edema and hemorrhages. *Liver.* Degenerative changes; vacuolization. *Kidney.* Interstitial edema; marked renal tubular dilatation. *Pancreas.* Islet cell hyperplasia.

Diagnostic Procedures. *Blood.* Anemia; high reticulocytes; leukocytosis; thrombocytopenia; prothrombin de-

ficiency; partial thromboplastin generation prolonged. Bilirubin high; alkaline phosphatase high; esterified cholesterol low; sulfobromophthalein abnormal; total protein low; glucose low. Tyrosine increased; other amino acids in normal range. *Urine.* High excretion of tyrosine and methionine.

Therapy. Diet with low tyrosine and phenylalanine. High doses of vitamin C.

Prognosis. Poor; death in months. If patients survive, they develop Baber's syndrome.

BABER'S SYNDROME

Symptoms and Signs. Occur in patients initially presenting the chronic form or survivors of the acute form. Same as above, but with reduced intensity. Failure to thrive and dwarfism develop. Rickets.

Etiology. As above.

Pathology. *Liver.* Firmer than normal; nodular cirrhosis; various degree of fibrosis; inflammatory (lymphmono) infiltration; bile stasis. *Kidney.* Edema; marked tubular dilatation; foci of calcium deposits. *Pancreas.* Hyperplasia of Langerhans islets (50%).

Diagnostic Procedures. As above. Most cases develop Fanconi's syndrome (see), hypophosphatemic rickets, and disturbance of water and electrolyte metabolism.

Therapy. As above. Rickets resistant to vitamin D.

Prognosis. Unknown if patients may survive into adulthood.

TYROSINEMIA TYPE II

See Richner–Hannart.

BIBLIOGRAPHY. Medes G: A new error of tyrosine metabolism: Tyrosinosis. Biochem J 26:917–940, 1932

Baber MD: A case of congenital cirrhosis of the liver with renal tubular defects akin to those in the Fanconi syndrome. Arch Dis Child 31:335–339, 1956

Conference on Hereditary Tyrosinemia, Hosp for Sick Children, Toronto, Ontario. Can Med Assoc J 97:1045–1101, 1967

Goldsmith LA: Tyrosinemia and related disorders. In Stanbury JB, Wyngaarden JB, Fredrickson DS: The Metabolic Basis of Inherited Disease. 5th ed, p 287. New York, McGraw-Hill, 1983

U

UGH

Synonym. Uveitis-glaucoma-hyphema.

Symptoms and Signs. Uveitis; glaucoma; hyphema.

Etiology. Defective anterior chamber lens, or caused by toxics incorporated into plastic of the lens, or warped intraocular lens.

BIBLIOGRAPHY. Pallin SL: Condition mimicking UGH syndrome said unrelated to presence of IOL. Ophthal Times, Aug 1983, p 50

UHL'S

Synonym. Parchment heart.

Symptoms. Age of clinical presentation from 1 to 57 years. Dyspnea; fatigue; chest pain and syncope on exertion.

Signs. Cyanosis; widely split and soft second heart sound; nonspecific systolic murmur.

Etiology. Congenital malformation.

Pathology. Normal tricuspid valve; atrophy of right ventricular wall; chamber dilatation. Fibrosis of right ventricular wall with irregular islands of myocardial tissue. Right ventricular thrombi found at death.

Diagnostic Procedures. Prominent α wave in jugular venous pulse. *X-ray of chest.* Cardiomegaly. *Angiography.* Excludes Ebstein's anomaly and shows large noncontractile right ventricle. *Electrocardiography. Echocardiography. Cardiac catheterization.*

Therapy. Medical management. Surgery not generally recommended; only palliative, attempts to be evaluated.

Prognosis. Only one 14-year-old alive reported.

BIBLIOGRAPHY. Uhl HMS: A previously undescribed congenital malformation of the heart: almost total absence of the myocardium of right ventricle. Bull Johns Hopkins Hosp 91:197–205, 1952
Hurst JW: The Heart, 6th ed, p 680. New York, McGraw-Hill, 1986

ULCERATIVE COLITIS, IDIOPATHIC

Synonyms. Colitis gravis; thromboulcerative colitis.

Symptoms. Both sexes affected with equal incidence; onset at all ages, more frequently between 20 and 40 years of age. Occasionally, insidious onset with simple appearance of bloody mucus on outside of stool. Usually, abrupt onset with diarrhea (day and night), soft, mushy, or loose with mixed blood. Tenesmus; abdominal pain of various degrees relieved by defecation. Gastric symptoms and anorexia may occur. Anxiety manifestation usually precipitating and accompanying attacks. Weight loss frequent; fever occasional. Frequently, rheumatoid arthritis manifestations; less frequently, erythema multiforme, pyoderma gangrenosum. In children, infantilism may be found. Three clinical patterns may be recognized: (1) *Relapsing, remitting type.* (a) Mild; without fever; self-limited; each attack lasting 1 to 3 months; (b) severe; fever; blood loss; toxemia. (2) *Chronic, continuous type.* Duration; 6 months or longer mild or severe. (3) *Acute, fulminating type* (rare, 5%); fever; hemorrhages; perforation or obstruction.

Signs. During attacks, pallor, weakness, weight loss, tenderness over colon. Rectal examination painful; nutritional deficiency.

Etiology. Unknown; autoimmunity suspected. Psychosomatic pathogenesis possible.

Pathology. *Colon.* Gross: ulceration of colon with island of normal mucosa (pseudopolyps); microscopic: microabscesses in crypts of mucosal glands; aspecific inflammatory reaction around ulcers; metadysplastic mucosal regeneration and fibrotic changes.

Diagnostic Procedures. *Sigmoidoscopy.* Reveals typical lesions. *Blood.* Microcytic anemia; hypoproteinemia; electrolytes alteration. *X-ray.* Colon shortened; hose appearance; loss of haustral marking.

Therapy. According to clinical type: diet; salicylazosulfapyridine; antibiotics; corticosteroids; sedatives; azathioprine; nitrogen mustard. Surgical resection of affected part. In fulminating type: blood replacement, electrolyte balance, parental alimentation.

Prognosis. Spontaneous remission and relapses characterize course of the condition. In chronic continuous type, development of carcinoma after 5 years frequent. Death from complications, circulatory collapse, hemorrhage, hypokalemia, liver cirrhosis, perforation, marasmus.

BIBLIOGRAPHY. Wilks W, Moxon W: Lectures on Pathological Anatomy. London, Churchill, 1875
Sales DJ, Kirsner JB: The prognosis of inflammatory

bowel disease (review). Arch Int Med 143:294–299, 1983

Sandberg-Gertzen H, Jänerot G, Kraaz W: Azodisal sodium in the treatment of ulcerative colitis: a study of tolerance and relapse-prevention properties. Gastroenterology 90:1024–1030, 1986

ULICK'S

Synonyms. Aldosterone deficiency 2; 18-dehydrogenase of 18-hydroxycorticosterone deficiency; corticosterone methyl oxidase type II deficiency; CMO II.

Symptoms and Signs. High incidence in Iranian Jews. From birth. Hypotension that leads to death or just short stature and postural hypotension.

Etiology. Autosomal recessive inheritance. Deficiency of 18-dehydrogenase or 18-hydroxycorticosterone with impaired production of aldosterone. Sex hormones and glucocorticoids are unaffected.

Diagnostic Procedures. *Blood.* Variable levels of aldosterone; plasma renin activity; elevated hyponatremia. *Urine.* Ratio of 18-hydroxycorticosterone metabolites to aldosterone greater than 100 (n.v. less than 3.0).

Therapy. Substitutive.

Prognosis. From death in infancy to normal life span.

BIBLIOGRAPHY. Royer P, Lestradet H, de Menibus CH et al: Hyperaldosteronisme familial chronique à debut neo-natal. Ann Paediat 8:133–138, 1961
Ulick S, Gautier E, Vetter KK et al: An aldosterone biosynthetic defect in a salt-losing disorder. J Clin Endocrinol Metab 24:669–672, 1964
Lee PDK, Patterson BD, Hintz RL et al: Biochemical diagnosis and management of corticosterone methyl oxydase type II deficiency. J Clin Endocr Metab 61:225–229, 1986

ULLRICH-BONNEVIE

Obsolete.

Synonyms. Bonnevie-Ullrich; pterygolymphangiectasia. See Turner's; Noonan's.

Symptoms. Present from birth. Pterygium colli; lymphedema of the hands and feet; various congenital disorders of bones, muscle, and viscera; dwarfism.

Etiology. To be identified with Turner's (see) and/or Noonan's (see).

BIBLIOGRAPHY. Ullrich O: Ueber typiche kombinationsbilder Multipler Abartungen. Z Kinderheilkd 49:271–276, 1930

Bonnevie K: Embryological analysis of gene manifestation in Little and Bagg's abnormal mouse tribe. J Exp Zool 67:443–520, 1934

ULLRICH-FEICHTEIGER

Obsolete.

Synonyms. Anophthalmia-cleft lip-palate-polydactyly; Bortholin's; dyscraniopylophalangy. See also Fraser's.

Symptoms and Signs. Anophthalmia or microphthalmia; cleft lip or palate (or both); polydactyly.

Etiology. Unknown. Sporadic occurrence. (Some cases reported are likely D1 trisomy.)

BIBLIOGRAPHY. Ullrich O: Der Status Bonnevie-Ullrich in Rahmenanderer "Dyscranio-Dysphalangien." Ergebn Inn Med Kinderheilkd NF2:412–420, 1951
Warburg M: Anophthalmos complicated by mental retardation and cleft palate. Acta Ophthalmol 38:394–404, 1960
Gorlin RJ, Pindborg JJ, Cohen MM Jr: Syndromes of the Head and Neck, 2nd ed. New York, McGraw-Hill, 1976

ULNA-FIBULA HYPOPLASIA

Synonyms. Brachymelia; Clyde's mesomelic dwarfism. See Langer's and Nievergelt's.

Symptoms and Signs. At birth, short forearms and ulnar deviation of hands. Height remaining below zero percentile.

Etiology. Suggestive of autosomal dominant inheritance.

Pathology. Short ulna and fibula; dislocated radial heads.

Diagnostic Procedures. See Pathology. Skeletal architecture of hands and humeri relatively normal.

Therapy. Night splints for correction of hand deviation.

BIBLIOGRAPHY. Pfeiffer RA: Beitrag zur erblichen Verkuerzung von Ulna und Fibula. In Weidemann HR (ed): Dysostosen, Stuttgart, G Fisher Verlag, 1966
Bailey JA: Disproportionate Short Stature; Diagnosis and Management, p 259. Philadelphia, WB Saunders, 1973

ULNAR-NERVE COMPRESSION (WRIST AND HAND) SYNDROMES

Synonyms. Ulnar tunnel; Guyon's canal; ulnar-carpal canal. See also Entrapment and Gessler's. Frequently affects gold polishers, oyster openers, cutlery workers, motorcyclists, bowlers (bowler's thumb). According to the site of compression, three different syndromes result.

ULNAR NERVE COMPRESSION (TYPE I)

Symptoms and Signs. Gradual onset. Motor weakness of all hand muscles innervated by ulnar nerve, with sensory deficit of palmar surfaces of hypothenar eminence and index and little fingers, on dorsum of medial side of the hand.

Etiology. Pressure on the ulnar nerve just proximal to or within the ulnar tunnel.

Pathology. Any of the following lesions may cause the compression and relative syndromes: ganglion (28.7%); occupational neuritis (23.5%); laceration (10.3%); arteritis, thromboangiitis (8.1%); fracture of metacarpal (2.9%); other bone fractures; aberrant muscles, bursitis.

Diagnostic Procedures. *X-ray of hand and wrist, cervical spine, shoulder and elbow* if indicated. *Electromyography and nerve conduction studies. Blood.* For evidence of generalized disorders: diabetes mellitus rheumatoid arthritis; scleroderma.

Therapy. Conservative therapy: immobilization; cortisone injection; change of occupation. If unsuccessful, surgical decompression and exploration of nerve and its branches.

Prognosis. Good with adequate treatment.

ULNAR NERVE COMPRESSION (TYPE II)

Symptoms and Signs. Motor weakness of muscles innervated by deep branch of ulnar nerve; normal sensation in the hand.

Etiology. Pressure on the deep branch of ulnar nerve at the exit from the ulnar tunnel or at the hook of hamate at origin of abductor and flexor digiti minimi brevis manus and in opponens digiti minimi muscles.

Pathology. See type I.

Diagnostic Procedures. See type I.

Therapy. See type I.

Prognosis. See type I.

ULNAR NERVE COMPRESSION (TYPE III)

Symptoms and Signs. Sensory deficits in the volar surface of hypothenar eminence and in the ring and little

fingers; absence of muscle weakness or atrophy. On dorsum, normal sensation.

Etiology. Pressure on the superficial branch of the ulnar nerve in the ulnar tunnel or at hook of hamate or in palmaris brevis. Arteritis of ulnar artery and direct trauma along the ulnar border of the hand are among the causes of compression of this particular type of the syndrome.

Pathology. See type I.

Diagnostic Procedures. See type I.

Therapy. See type I. If arteritis is responsible for the syndrome, resection of affected segment of the artery.

Prognosis. See type I.

BIBLIOGRAPHY. Guyon F: Note sur une disposition anatomique propre à la face antérieure de la région du poignet et non encore décrite par le docteur. Boll Soc Anat Paris 6:184–186, 1861

Hunt JR: Thenar and hypothenar types of neural atrophy of the hand. Am J Med Sci 141:224–241, 1911

Shea JD, McClain EJ: Ulnar nerve compression syndromes at and below the wrist. J Bone Joint Surg 51:1095–1103, 1969

Milford L: Carpal tunnel and ulnar tunnel syndrome. In Crenshaw AH (ed), Campbell's Operative Orthopedics, 7th ed, p 461 St. Louis, CV Mosby, 1987

UMBER'S

Synonyms. Nonketotic hyperosmolar coma; hyperglycemic dehydration; Sament-Schwartz.

Symptoms and Signs. Most frequent in middle-aged patients with no previous history of diabetes; in most cases iatrogenic precipitating causes (e.g., drugs, fluid restrictions) applied to the treatment of variable associated illness. Dehydration; weakness (leading symptoms); polyuria and polydipsia (may persist for weeks before becoming appreciated and correctly interpreted). Consciousness alterations from drowsiness to frank coma; focal neurologic findings (transitory). Shock, infections frequently associated.

Etiology. Persistent osmotic diuresis leading to dehydration; sodium and potassium deficits and severe hyperglycemia in absence of marked hyperketonemia.

Pathology. In brain, findings still debated: edema; localized brain infections; subdural hemorrhages. Increased frequency of pancreatitis, pulmonary embolus, and thromboembolic phenomena.

Diagnostic Procedures. *Blood.* Hyperosmolarity; hyperglycemia; absence of marked elevation of ketone bodies; high blood urea nitrogen; creatinine ratio exceeds 30.

Therapy. Rapid partial correction of dehydration and shock prevention or treatment; Potassium balance. Specific treatment for basic illness. Insulin in graduated doses (20–25 IU) intramuscularly or intravenously in albumin to produce a more sustained, gradual fall of plasma glucose over a period of hours.

Prognosis. Very variable according to reported series. Mortality approximately 40–50%.

BIBLIOGRAPHY. Umber F: Stoffwechsel krankheiten. II. Diabetes mellitus. Med Wochenschr (Munich) 71:1324–1326, 1924
Sament S, Schwartz MB: Severe diabetic stupor without ketosis. S Afr Med J 31:893–894, 1957
Crapo LM, Reaven G: Hyperosmolar non-ketotic diabetic coma. Med Grand Rounds 2:344–356, 1983
Khardori R: Soler NG: Hyperosmolar hyperglycemic non-ketotic syndrome. Am J Med 77:899–904, 1984

UNDERWOOD'S

Synonyms. Sclerema adiposum; sclerema neonatorum.

Symptoms. Both sexes affected; onset during first week of life (in premature or debilitated children) or later associated with severe disorders. Prodromata represented by respiratory or gastrointestinal manifestations.

Signs. Small, weak infant. Cyanosis; progressive hardening of skin of buttocks, thighs, and calves, then of rest of body, with the exception of genitalia, palms, and soles. Skin assumes a mottled white color. Body temperature progressively decreases.

Etiology. Unknown. Exposure to cold is frequently the precipitating factor of shock, circulatory failure, and temperature fall.

Pathology. Hardening of subcutaneous fat; scanty histologic changes. Swollen trabeculae.

Diagnostic Procedures. Identification of basic pathology.

Therapy. Incubator. Antibiotics (for treatment of underlying condition). Corticosteroids (of doubtful utility).

Prognosis. Extremely severe. The 80% mortality may be reduced to 50% with adequate treatment. The outcome, however, is bound to the basic pathology.

BIBLIOGRAPHY. Underwood M: A Treatise on the Diseases of Children. London, Matthews, 1784
Rook A, Wilkinson DS, Ebling FJG et al: Textbook of Dermatology, 4th ed, p 256–257. Oxford, Blackwell Scientific Publications, 1986

UNNA'S (P.G.)

Synonyms. Seborrheic dermatitis; seborrheic eczema.

Symptoms. Pruritus most frequently affecting scalp, external ear, and retroauricular area, or less frequently, generalized with localizations between scapulae and over sternal region and groin.

Signs. Scales of scalp (dandruff) and seborrheic dermatitis of areas indicated; exfoliative dermatitis with or without secondary eczematization may superimpose.

Etiology. Unknown.

Pathology. Hyperkeratosis; parakeratosis; intracellular and extracellular edema; slight or moderate acanthosis. Frequently, perifolliculitis, cutis infiltrates with polymorphs, lymphocytes (occasionally, plasma cells); presence of clumps of cocci in epidermis and stratum corneum. Elastic and connective tissues not affected.

Diagnostic Procedures. *Biopsy of skin* (area not scrubbed too vigorously, so that scales are not removed). *Blood.* Normal.

Therapy. Regular washing and frequent use of a detergent shampoo. Corticosteroids alone or with antibiotics. Ketonazole (temporary action). Salicylic acid to reduce scaling.

Prognosis. No effective treatment except in those cases where the condition is manifestation of a reversible systemic process.

BIBLIOGRAPHY. Unna PG: Das sebborhoische Ekzem Mschr Pract Derm 6:829–846, 1887
Rook A, Wilkinson DS, Ebling FJG et al: Textbook of Dermatology, 4th ed, pp 375–381. Oxford, Blackwell Scientific Publications, 1986

UNVERRICHT'S

Synonyms. Lundborg-Unverricht; familial myoclonia; myoclonus epilepsy.

Symptoms and Signs. Irregular, fast contraction of groups of muscles. Seizures starting at puberty and associated with myoclonus, precipitated by slight stimulus. Loss of mental power; amaurosis. Terminal stage: parkinsonism and muscle innervated by bulbar centers affected.

Etiology. Unknown; hereditary condition autosomal recessive (see Lafora). Possibility of X-linked inheritance.

Pathology. Numerous intracellular bodies found in extrapyramidal center. Degenerative changes in Purkinje cells and neurons in the medial part of thalamus.

Diagnostic Procedures. *Electroencephalography.* Wave and spike formation 3/sec in all cortical leads, associated with jerks. *Blood.* Decrease of mucoprotein content reported in a patient and siblings.

Therapy. Diphenylhydantoin; phenobarbital; L-5 hydroxytryptophan; clonazepam.

Prognosis. Incapacitation by the age of 20 years in severe cases. Death in young adulthood.

BIBLIOGRAPHY. Unverricht H: Die Myoclonie. Berlin, Franz Dewticke, 1891

Merritt HH: A Textbook of Neurology, 6th ed, p 473. Philadelphia, Lea & Febiger, 1979

Wienker TF, Von Reutern GM, Ropers HH: Progressive myoclonus epilepsy: a variant with probable X-linked inheritance. Hum Genet 49:83–89, 1979

URBACH-WIETHE

Synonyms. Hyalinosis cutis et mucosae; lipoid proteinosis; proteinosis-lipoidosis. Rössle-Urbach-Wiethe.

Symptoms. Both sexes affected; onset in infancy. Inability to cry. Itching of the eyes. Hoarseness.

Signs. Generalized papules; plaques and ulcers of skin and mucosae. Predilection for lips, mouth, pharynx, vocal cords, eyelids, neck, hands, fingers, knees, elbows, and scrotum. Apparently no visceral symptoms or signs. Possibly, macrocheilia, macroglossia.

Etiology. Lysosomal storage disease. Autosomal recessive inheritance. Association with diabetes mellitus.

Pathology. Early lesions: hyaline thickening of capillary walls. Intermediate lesions: eosinophilic hyalinosis bands around capillaries in dermis and hyaline wrapping around sweat glands. Late lesions: substitution of dermal collagen and elastic tissue by hyaline material, with atrophy of glands. Lipid deposits in hyalinized areas. Epithelium overlying lesions usually becomes hyperplastic and hyperkeratotic.

Diagnostic Procedures. *Blood.* Phospholipids increased. *Urine.* Increased excretion of amino acids (tyrosine). *X-ray.* Possibly, calcification of sella turcica. *Biopsy of skin.* See Pathology.

Therapy. Insulin indicated also in absence of hyperglycemia. Surgical removal of growths on vocal cord.

Prognosis. Relatively benign, progressive course.

BIBLIOGRAPHY. Urbach E, Wiethe C: Lipoidosis cutis et mucosae. Virchows Arch [Pathol Anat] 273:285–319, 1929

Haneke E, Hornstein OP, Meisel-Stosiek M et al: Hyalinosis cutis et mucosae in siblings. Hum Genet 68:342–345, 1984

UREA ENZYMOPATHIES

Synonym. Hyperammonemia
1. N-acetylglutamate synthetase deficiency (AGA deficiency). One case described. Mental retardation; ataxia.
2. Carbamoyl phosphate synthetase deficiency (CPS deficiency).
3. Ornithine carbamoyl transferase deficiency (OCT deficiency) see Russell's III.
4. Citrullinemia (ASAS deficiency) (see).
5. Argininosuccinate lyase deficiency (argininosuccinic aciduria) (ASAL deficiency) (see).
6. Arginase deficiency (see).
7. Hyperornithinemia syndromes (see Simell-Takki); hyperornithinemia-hyperammonemia-homocitrullinuria.
8. Lysinuric protein intolerance (hyperdibasic aciduria). Perheentupa-Visakorpi (see).
9. Hyperlysinemia periodic (see); persistent hyperlysinemia that is not associated with hyperammonemia.
10. Rett's (see).

Hyperammonemia may be present also in other disorders of amino acid metabolism.

UREMIC CARDIAC

Synonym. Cardiouremica.

Symptoms and Signs. Occur in patients with chronic uremia, treated with a selected low-protein diet. Pronounced cardiomegaly; gallop rhythm; severe hypotension; pericarditis with or without pericardial effusion; arrhythmias; marked sensitivity to cardiac glycosides.

Etiology. Unknown; considered a progression of the uremia or secondary to dietetic factors, prolonged anemia, or prolonged hypertension.

Diagnostic Procedures. *Blood and urine.* All features of chronic uremia. Low hematocrit (which remains low after recovery from syndrome). *X-ray of chest.* Cardiomegaly. *Electrocardiography. Venous pressure.*

Therapy. Hemodialysis or kidney homotransplantation.

Prognosis. Recovery. Abnormal findings disappear or markedly improve as soon as treatment with hemodialysis or peritoneal dialysis is started.

BIBLIOGRAPHY. Bailey GL, Hampers CL, Merrill JP: Annual Meeting of American Society Artificial Internal Organs. JAMA 200:8–30, 1967

Hurst JW: The Heart, 6th ed, pp 1462–1483. New York, McGraw-Hill, 1986

UREMIC-NEUROMYOPATHIC

Synonyms. Uremic myopathy; uremic polyneuropathy; tetanic uremic neuromyopathy. Still not well defined or universally accepted symptom complexes that develop in patients with chronic uremia. Four different syndromes may be recognized.

UREMIC POLYNEUROPATHY

Symptoms. Occur in young males with chronic uremia. Initially, painful burning sensation of feet; followed by progression to lower extremities, paresthesias, painful cramps, and weakness. Same symptoms but much milder in upper extremities. Distal segment more affected than proximal. Trunk and face spared.

Signs. Feet sensitive to light touch and pressure. Atrophy of leg muscles. Sensory loss of feet and legs, less pronounced on arms and hands. Tendon reflexes abolished.

Etiology. Unknown; possibly, metabolic defect resulting in polyneural alteration (specific nature not determined).

Pathology. Disappearance of a proportion of large medullated fibers, maximal degree on feet. Less pronounced lesions on proximal part of nerves. Anterior horn cells of spinal cord; chromatolysis limited to lumbosacral and cervical enlargements. No evidence of regeneration. Atrophic muscles (denervation atrophic type).

Diagnostic Procedures. *Blood.* All findings of chronic uremia. *Electromyography. Biopsy of muscle and peripheral nerve.*

Therapy. Dialysis; renal transplantation.

Prognosis. Progressive form; treatment results in slow improvement of nerve function.

UREMIC MYOPATHY

Symptoms. Occur in older subjects than previous syndrome; not prevalent in males. Asthenia and weakness of muscles of both pelvic and scapular region. Alteration of subjective sensitivity.

Signs. Atrophy of scapular and pelvic girdle muscles. Tendon reflex normal; idiomuscular reflexes abolished.

Etiology. Unknown; muscular atrophy secondary to metabolic defect (specific nature not determined).

Pathology. Muscular tissue fiber atrophy; degenerative changes, occasional disintegration, and necrosis of muscle fibers; moderate hyperplasia of sarcolemma. Lack of inflammatory changes. Fibroadipose involution.

Diagnostic Procedures. *Blood.* All features of chronic uremia. *Biopsy of muscle.* See Pathology. *Electromyography.*

Therapy. Symptoms do not respond to dialysis.

Prognosis. Poor.

UREMIC NEUROMYOPATHY

Combination of symptoms, signs, and pathologic findings of the two previously described syndromes.

TETANIC NEUROMYOPATHY

Symptoms and Signs. Severe, painful, and unrelenting tonic contraction of muscles. Myoclonus and convulsions may also be present.

Signs. Rigid extension of the legs; plantar flexion, internal rotation of the feet. Abdomen rigid and painful. Injection of calcium and magnesium does not affect symptomatology (in one patient myospasm so intense as to tear abdominal rectus muscle: blue discoloration simulating Cullen's signs).

Etiology. Unknown; neuromyopathy due to chronic renal failure.

Pathology. Chronic uremia.

Diagnostic Procedures. *Blood.* High blood urea nitrogen; calcium, magnesium normal. *Urine.* Findings of chronic renal failure.

Prognosis. Syndrome preceding death by hours or months.

BIBLIOGRAPHY. Merklen P, Gounelle H: Uremie musculaire. Medicine 12:225–229, 1931

Tenckhoff HA, Boen FST, Jebsen RH et al: Polyneuropathy in chronic renal insufficiency. JAMA 192:1121–1124, 1965

Serratrice G, Toga M, Roux H et al: Neuropathies, myopathies et neuromyopathies chez des urémiques chroniques. Presse Med 75:1835–1838, 1967

Biasioli S, D'Andree G, Feriani S et al: Uremic encephalopathy: an updating. Clin Nephrol 25:57–63, 1986

UROGENITAL TRACT AND EAR MALFORMATIONS

Synonym. Renal–genital–middle ear (Winter's).
1. Urogenital tract and external ear (Potter's syndrome (see)).
2. Urogenital tract and middle ear (Winter's). Combination of renal hypoplasia, internal genital, and middle ear malformations, possibly caused by autosomal recessive gene inheritance.

BIBLIOGRAPHY. Longenecker CG, Ryan RF, Vincent RW: Malformations of the ear as a clue to urogenital anomalies: report of six additional cases. Plast Reconstr Surg 35:303–309, 1965

Winter JSD, Millman WJ: A familial syndrome of renal, genital, and middle ear anomalies. J Pediatr 72:88–93, 1968

Turner GA: Second family with renal, vaginal, and middle ear anomalies. J Pediatr 76:641, 1970

Warkany J: Congenital Malformations, p 1037. Chicago, Year Book Medical Publishers, 1971

USHER'S

Synonyms. Hereditary deafness-retinitis pigmentosa; Von Graefe; Graefe-Sjögren; retinitis pigmentosa-deafness. See Graef-Sjögren.

Symptoms. Time of onset unknown. Family history of poor night vision, blue-green color blindness, or total blindness. During childhood, progressive hearing loss (evident at age 4 to 6) and secondary lack of speech development. Usually, a few years later (average age 9) progressive poor night vision, degeneration of peripheral visual fields, tunnel vision, blindness.

Signs. Physical examination normal (see Diagnostic Procedures).

Etiology. Unknown; anatomic and metabolic conditions causing deafness and retinitis are unknown. Autosomal recessive inheritance and X-linked.

Four types have been subclassified (Davenport):

Type I. Profound congenital deafness; onset of retinitis by age 10.
Type II. Moderate to severe progressive congenital deafness; onset of retinitis in the teens.
Type III. Retinitis at puberty with progressive hearing loss.
Type IV. A possible X-linked form.
Another classification (Fishman) has two types: the first with earlier and more severe: night blindness, vision loss, hearing loss; unintelligible speech, vestibular reflexes, and ataxia. The second with less severe and delayed manifestations.

Pathology. In eyes, rod degeneration preceding the typical pigment deposits on the retina. No adequate microscopic studies of cochlear lesions.

Diagnostic Procedures. *Audiography.* Pure tone threshold losses of variable severity. Intracochlear defect. *Electroretinography.* Early signs of retinal degeneration detected by abnormal dark- adapted electroretinogram.

Therapy. Early diagnosis of hearing loss allows prevention of lack of speech development and improves secondary retarded speech.

Prognosis. Hearing loss is usually not rapidly progressing. Eye lesions may progress to total blindness.

BIBLIOGRAPHY. Von Graefe AF: Demonstration in der Berliner Medizinischen Gesellschaft. Berlin Klin Wochenschr 5:127, 1868
Usher CH: On the inheritance of retinitis pigmentosa with notes of cases. Roy Lond Ophthalmol Hosp Rep 19:130–236, 1914
Davenport SLH, Omenn GS: The heterogeneity of Usher syndrome. Fifth International Conference on Birth Defects, Montreal, Aug 1977
Fishman GA, Kumar A, Joseph ME et al.: Usher's syndrome: ophthalmic and neuro-otologic findings suggesting genetic heterogeneity. Arch Ophthal 101:1367–1374, 1983
Fulton AB, Hansen RM: Foveal cone pigments and sensitivity in young patients with Usher's syndrome. Am J Ophthalmol 103:150–160, 1987

UYEMURA'S

Synonyms. Fundus albipunctatus-hemeralopia-xerosis; night blindness I; nyctalopia-xerosis-fundus albipunctatus.

Symptoms. More often in males; onset in childhood or young adulthood. Night blindness; (transitory); conjunctival xerosis.

Signs. Fundus oculi grayish white appearance and densely covered by yellowish white spots.

Etiology. Deficiency of vitamin A. To be differentiated from retinitis punctata albescens, fundus albipunctatus, and Oguchi's. Unclear whether etiology is genetic.

Therapy. Vitamin A.

Prognosis. Quick recovery with treatment.

BIBLIOGRAPHY. Uyemura M: Ueber eine merkwürdige Augenhintergrundveräderung bei zwei Fällen von idiopathischer Hemeralopie Klin Monatsbl Augenheilkd 81:471–473, 1928
Fuchs A: White spots of the fundus combined with night blindness and xerosis (Uyemura's syndrome). Am J Ophthalmol 48:101–103, 1959
Krill AE, Martin D: Photopic-abnormalities in congenital stationary nightblindness. Invest Ophthalmol 10:625–636, 1971
Krill AE: Hereditary retinal and choroidal diseases. Hagerstown, Md, Harper & Row, 1977

VAANDRAGER–PENA

Synonyms. Spondylometaphyseal dysplasia type C-IV; spondylometaphyseal dysostosis type C-IV. Metaphyseal chondrodysplasia.

Symptoms and Signs. Present from birth. Metaphyseal dysostosis primarily involving vertebrae and pelvis (coxa vara) and resulting in dwarfism.

Etiology. Probably, autosomal recessive inheritance.

BIBLIOGRAPHY. Vaandrager GJ: Metafysaire dystosis? Nederl T Geneesk 104:547–552, 1960

Pena J: Dysostosis metafisaria. Una revision, con aportacion de una observation familiar. Una forma nueva de la enfermaded? Radiologia (Madrid) 47:3–22, 1965

Kozlowski K, Sikorska B: Dysplasia metaphysaria Typ Vaandrager–Pena. Z Kinderheilkd 108:165–170, 1970

VAGAL BODY TUMOR

Symptoms. Relatively equal sex distribution; average age at onset 37 years. Frequently asymptomatic. Duration of symptoms and signs before diagnosis variable, up to 3 years. Sudden hoarseness; dull pain on side of the neck; syncope; difficulty in swallowing; disturbed balance.

Signs. Mass in high anterolateral side of neck (more frequently the right side). Peritonsillar structures displaced medially (50%); hemiatrophy of tongue (rare); Horner's syndrome (rare).

Etiology. Unknown; tumor of vagal body.

Pathology. Nodular, ovoid, encapsulated mass, 2 to 6 cm in diameter, below base of skull, near foramen jugulare, contiguous with vagus (X) nerve. Infiltration of jugular foramen occasionally observed. Microscopically, chemodectoma cluster of "balls" of polyhedral cells, thin vascular fibrus septa. Metastasis rare.

Therapy. Surgical excision; X-ray treatment.

Prognosis. May be cured by surgical excision. This tumor seems to have more of a tendency to metastasize than glomus jugular tumor and carotid body tumor.

BIBLIOGRAPHY. White EG: Die Structur des Glomus caroticum, seine Pathologie und Physiologie und seine Beziehung zum Nerven-system. Beitr Pathol Anat 96:177–227, 1935

Oberman HA, Holtz F, Sheffer LA et al: Chemodectomas (nonchromaffin paragangliomas) of the head and neck: a clinicopathologic study. Cancer 21:838–851, 1968

VAHLQUIST-GASSER

Synonyms. Gasser's I; benign infantile granulocytopenia; chronic infantile granulocytopenia; chronic granulocytopenia of childhood.

Symptoms. Negative family history. Onset at infancy or early childhood. Trivial infections; paronychia; gingivitis; ulcerations; furunculosis; respiratory tract infection. Child appears healthy in intervals between infections.

Signs. None or moderate lymphadenopathy in connection with infections. Moderate splenomegaly in some cases.

Etiology. Unknown; disturbance of leukocytogenesis; no familial tendency.

Pathology. Cytologic examination of pus reveals the presence of neutrophils.

Diagnostic Procedures. *Blood.* Moderate leukopenia; absolute and relative neutropenia; no anemia or thrombocytopenia. Leukocyte response to epinephrine variable, occasionally normal. Protein electrophoretic pattern: no consistent changes. *Bone marrow.* Cellularity normal or slightly increased. Variable lymphocytosis. Erythroid series normal; myeloid-erythroid ratio normal. Myeloid series normal, except for almost total absence of mature neutrophils. Megakaryocytic series normal. Histoid series normal. Response to local stimulus (window technique) absence of neutrophils.

Therapy. Antibiotics; no response to steroids or splenectomy.

Prognosis. Good; infections controlled by antibiotics. Spontaneous recovery frequent at 1 to 3 years of age.

BIBLIOGRAPHY. Hotz A: Zur Differentialdiagnose-Agranulocytose-Leukamie. Z Kinderheilkd 65:529–540, 1949

Vahlquist B, Anjou N: Granulocytopénie chronique bénigne. Acta Haematol (Basel) 8:199–208, 1952

Gasser C, Vrtilek MR: Essentielle chronische Granulocytopenie in Kindersalter. Schweiz Med Wochenschr 52:1122–1123, 1952

Zuelzer WW, Bajoghli M: Chronic granulocytopenia in childhood. Blood 23:359–374, 1964

Wintrobe MM (ed): Clinical Hematology, 8th ed, p 1327. Philadelphia, Lea & Febiger, 1981

Wintrobe MM (ed): Clinical Hematology, 8th ed, p 550. Philadelphia, Lea & Febiger, 1981

VAIL'S

Synonym. Vidian neuralgia. See Horton's II.

Symptoms. Prevalent in adult females. Usually unilateral, often nocturnal, severe pain in nose, face, eyes, ears, head, neck, and shoulders. Nasal sinusitis symptoms frequent.

Etiology and Pathology. Irritation or inflammation of vidian nerve, secondary to infection of sphenoidal sinus. Relationship of this syndrome with Sluder's not clear.

Diagnostic Procedures. Cocainization of sphenopalatine ganglion.

Therapy. Therapy of sinus disease; procaine alcohol injection of sphenopalatine ganglion.

Prognosis. Good result with injection.

BIBLIOGRAPHY. Vail HH: Vidian neuralgia, with special reference to eye and orbital pain in suppuration of petrous apex. Ann Otol Rhinol Laryngol 41:837–856, 1932

Vick NA: Grinker's Neurology, 7th ed. Springfield, Ill, CC Thomas, 1976

Adams RD, Victor M: Principles of Neurology, 3rd ed, p 139. New York, McGraw-Hill, 1985

VALSUANI'S

Synonyms. Pernicious anemia gravidica; gravidic pernicious anemia; pregnancy pernicious anemia; Wills–Metha.

Symptoms and Signs. Those of Addison–Biermer (see) appearing during pregnancy and receding after its termination.

Etiology. Deficiency of folic acid.

Pathology. See Addison-Biermer.

Therapy. Folic acid plus iron. Diagnosis and proper treatment of infections.

Prognosis. Prompt remission with treatment.

BIBLIOGRAPHY. Valsuani E: Cachessia puerperale raccolta nella clinica ginecologica dell'ospedale Maggiore di Milano, Bernardoni, 1870

Wills L, Metha MM: Studies in "pernicious anemia" of pregnancy. I. Preliminary report. Indian J Med Res 17:777–792, 1930

VAN ALLEN'S

Synonyms. Amyloid neuropathy IV; Iowa type amyloidosis neuropathy.

Symptoms and Signs. Occur in patients of English-Scottish-Irish descent. Both sexes involved; age at onset 26 to 44 years (average 35). Neuropathy dominates at onset, involving all four extremities. Severe peptic ulcer disease; frequently, hearing loss and blurred vision (cataracts but no vitreous opacities). Commonly, impotence and sphincter disturbances. Seldom, foot ulcers or cardiomegaly. Later evidence of nephropathy.

Etiology. Autosomal dominant inheritance suggested.

Pathology. Widespread amyloidosis.

Diagnostic Procedures. *Blood.* Normal; later, evidence of nephropathy.

Therapy. None.

Prognosis. Average survival 12 years. Usual cause of death: amyloid nephropathy.

BIBLIOGRAPHY. Van Allen MW, Frolich JA, Davis JR: Inherited predisposition to generalized amyloidosis. Neurology 19:10–25, 1969

Glenner GG, Ignaczak TF, Page DL: The inherited systemic amyloidosis and localized amyloid deposits. In Stanbury JB, Wyngaarden JB, Fredrickson DS: The Metabolic Basis of Inherited Disease, 4th ed, p 1326. New York, McGraw-Hill, 1978

VAN BOGAERT-HOZAY

Synonyms. Hozay's; acro-osteolysis–facial dysplasia.

Symptoms and Signs. Both sexes affected; onset at 3 years of age. *Facies.* Asymmetric; nose flat and wide with broad bridge; pronounced zygomatic arcs; hypertelorism; hypoplasia of cilia and eyebrows; eyelid ptosis; alternating squint; astigmatism and myopia; arched palate. *Extremities.* Short; sudden arrest of growth; acrocyanosis; short, thick phalangeal joints. From normal to mild mental retardation.

Etiology. Unknown. Possible autosomal recessive inheritance.

BIBLIOGRAPHY. Van Bogaert L: Essai de classement et d'interprétation de quelques acro-ostéolyses mutilantes et non mutilantes actuelment connues. Acta Neurol Psych Belg 53:90–115, 1953

Hozay J: Sur une dystrophie familiale particulière. Inibition précoce de la croissance et osteolyse non mutilante acrales avec dysmorphie faciale. Rev Neurol (Paris) 89:245–258, 1953

Durner W: Das van Bogaert-Hozay syndrom. Eine Falldemonstration. Klin Monatsbl Augenheilkd 162:658–660, 1973

VAN BOGAERT–SCHERER–EPSTEIN

Synonyms. Cerebrotendinous cholesterolosis; spinal cholesterolosis; Thiébaut's; CTX

Symptoms and Signs. Both sexes affected; onset at different ages. Onset in childhood with dementia; evolving in adolescence with progressive ataxia, spasticity, and cataracts, and finally in adulthood with tendinous xanthoma, severe spastic ataxic syndrome, bulbar paralysis, and distal muscle wasting. Hepatosplenomegaly. Palmar and plantar xanthomas.

Etiology. Autosomal recessive inheritance. Defect in bile acid synthesis with incapacity to form cholic and chenodeoxycholic acids. Enterohepatic recirculation is thus defective, the liver synthetizes increased quantities of cholesterol and cholestanol, which are deposited in tissues.

Pathology. *Tendon.* Granulomatous lesions with deposits of cholesterol. *Brain.* Atrophy with granulomatous lesions in the white matter; demyelinization; cystic spaces with foamy cells, crystals of cholesterol. Cerebellum and brain stem similar lesions. *Eyes.* Cataract. Xanthomas also in lungs.

Diagnostic Procedures. *Blood.* Cholesterol triglyceride and phospholipid normal in most cases, elevated in others, especially at later stages. Cholestanol levels range from 1.3 to 15 mg/dl (3 to 20 times higher than normal value in plasma). Measurement of cholestanol levels in xantomatous tissue.

Therapy. Good results with chenodeoxycholic acid. Cholestyramine absolutely not indicated.

Prognosis. See Symptoms and Signs. Patient may reach 5th or 6th decade. Arrest of disease with therapy.

BIBLIOGRAPHY. Van Bogaert L, Scherer HJ, Epstein E: Une forme cerébralé de cholestérinose généralisée. Paris, Masson, 1937

Thiébaut F: Paraplégies spasmodiques et xanthomes tendineux associés. Des rapports de ce syndrome avec le cholestérinose cérébrospinal. Rev Neurol (Paris) 74:313–315, 1942

Salen G, Shefer S, Berginer VM: Familial diseases with storage of sterol other than cholesterol: cerebrotendinous xanthomatosis and sitosterolemia with xanthoma-

tosis. In Stanbury JB, Wyngaarden JB, Fredrickson DS, et al: The Metabolic Basis of Inherited Disease, 5th ed, p 713. New York, McGraw-Hill, 1983

VAN BUCHEM'S

Synonyms. Buchem's; endosteohyperostosis; hyperostosis corticalis generalisata; leontiasis ossea generalisata; hyperphosphatasemia tarda.

Symptoms. More frequent in males; onset in puberty; onset of clinical manifestation between 20 and 50 years of age. Usually asymptomatic for long period except in cases where mental retardation is associated. In due course patients may present paralysis of facial nerve, optic atrophy, and perceptive deafness.

Signs. Prognathism absent; wide chin; occasionally, mild exophthalmos.

Etiology. Unknown; autosomal recessive inheritance.

Pathology. *Cranium, jaw, clavicles, and ribs.* Thickened compact aspect and absence of diplöe. *Long bones.* Thickening of cortical zone and periosteal irregularities.

Diagnostic Procedures. *Blood.* Normal or minor anemia. *Urine.* Normal. *Ophthalmoscopy.* Papillary edema. *X-ray.* See Pathology.

Therapy. None. When signs of compression become manifest, decompression of nerves.

Prognosis. Does not limit physical activity. Its progression involves facial (VII) nerve paralysis, optic (II) and acoustic (VIII) nerve damage.

BIBLIOGRAPHY. Van Buchem FSP, Hadders HN, Ubbens R: Uncommon familial systemic disease of skeleton: hyperostosis cortical generalisata familiaris. Acta Radiol 44:109–120, 1955

Turner HV, Kelly DH Jr: Osteodysplasia with mental deficiency. J Iowa Med Soc 58:260–268, 1968

Beighton P, Barnard A, Hamersham H et al: The syndromic status of sclerostenosis and Van Buchem disease. Clin Genet 25:175–181, 1984

VAN DER BOSH

Symptoms and Signs. From birth. Mental deficiency; choroideremia; acrokeratosis verruciformis; anhidrosis; skeletal deformities.

Etiology. Possibly X-linked recessive inheritance.

BIBLIOGRAPHY. Van der Bosh J: A new syndrome in three generations of a Dutch family. Ophthalmologica 137:422–423, 1959

VANISHING LUNG SYNDROMES

See also Swyer-James, Wilson-Mikity, and Burke's. Eponym used to indicate a radiologic sign common to many diseases: decrease of roentgenographic density. This may be due to the following physiopathologic conditions:

1. Increased air. Unchanged blood and tissue (local, due to bronchial obstruction or general asthma, bronchiolitis).
2. Increased air. Decreased blood and tissue (due to diffuse obstructive emphysema, or bullae and cysts).
3. Normal amount of air. Decreased blood and tissue (local: lobar emphysema, embolism without infarction; general: decreased blood flow).
4. Reduction of all three components.
5. Pulmonary artery agenesis.

BIBLIOGRAPHY. Burke RN: Vanishing lung: A case report of bullous emphysema. Radiology 28:367–371, 1937

Fraser RG, Paré JAP: Diagnosis of Diseases of the Chest, 2nd ed, p 536. Philadelphia, WB Saunders, 1977

VANISHING TESTES

Synonyms. Anorchism; castrate; functional castrate; testicular agenesis; embryonic testicular regression.

Symptoms. In childhood, normal development including external genitalia; no development of secondary sex characteristics at puberal age and acquisition of typical eunuchoid phenotype.

Etiology. Unknown. Destruction of testis between 7th and 14th week of intrauterine life (infection ?, torsion ?, vascular accident ?); X-linked inheritance in some cases.

Pathology. Residual derivatives of Wolffian ducts; prepuberal testes hyalinization.

Diagnostic Procedures. *Blood.* Highest gonadotropin level of all testicular disorders and extremely low testosterone. Administration of human chorionic gonadotropin (HCG) fails to enhance testosterone production.

Therapy. Long-acting testosterone for life.

Prognosis. Correction of all functional and metabolic deficits by adequate treatment.

BIBLIOGRAPHY. Koopman J: Congenital anorchia: case. Geneesk Gids 8:309–330, 1930

Josso N, Briard ML: Embryonic testicular regression syndrome. J Pediatr 97:200–204, 1980

Abeyaratue MR, Aherne WA, Scott JES: The vanishing testis. Lancet II:822–826, 1969

VAN LOHUIZEN'S

Synonyms. Cutis marmorata telangiectatica; congenital generalized phlebectasia. See Cutis marmorata.

Symptoms and Signs. Present from birth. Localized or generalized network of dilated veins in the skin, associated with spider nevi and small ulcers.

Etiology. Unknown. Usually sporadic. Autosomal recessive occurrence also reported.

Prognosis. Spontaneous improvement. Seldom, lesions may persist and develop varicose veins and hypertrophy of extremities involved.

BIBLIOGRAPHY. Van Lohuizen CHJ: Ueber eine seltene angeborene Hautanomalie (cutis Marmorata Telangiectatica Congenita). Acta Derm Venereol 3:202–211, 1922

Kurczynski TW: Hereditary cutis marmorate telangiectasica congenita. Pediatrics 70:52–53, 1982

VAN NECK'S

Synonyms. Ischiopubic osteochondropathy; Odelberg's; osteitis pubis.

Symptoms. Onset few weeks after prostate or bladder intervention, herniorrhaphy in children, or childbirth. Pain in pubic symphysis area, radiating down the inner side of thighs. Cough and strains may enhance the pain. Analgesis gait; low fever.

Signs. Point tenderness. Spasm of abdominal and hip muscles.

Etiology. Osteomyelitis of pubic bones secondary to adjacent areas trauma. Various factors implied in the pathogenesis (neurovascular; endocrine; infective).

Pathology. Erosion of bone, with sclerosing and periosteal reaction.

Diagnostic Procedures. *X-ray.* Normal initially; signs of osteolysis perisymphyseal within 2 to 4 weeks.

Therapy. Antiinflammatory drugs; immobilization; surgery.

Prognosis. Possible spontaneous remission; however symptoms may last many months.

BIBLIOGRAPHY. Odelberg A: Some cases of destruction of the ischium of doubtful etiology. Arch Chir Scand 56:273–284, 1923

Van Neck M: Ostéocondritis du pubis. Arch Fr Belg Chir 27:238–240, 1924

Richardson EG: Miscellaneous nontraumatic disorders. In Crenshaw AH (ed): Campbell's Operative Orthopedics. 7th ed, pp 1060–1062. St Louis, CV Mosby, 1987

VAQUEZ-OSLER

Synonyms. Erythremia; erythrocytosis megalosplenica; myelopathic polycythemia; Osler's II; cryptogenic polycythemia; polycythemia rubra; polycythemia vera; splenomegalic polycythemia.

Symptoms. Slightly more prevalent in males; onset middle or late life, reported occasionally in childhood (see Erythrocytosis in childhood). Insidious onset. Headache; dizziness; transitory syncope; visual disturbances; ringing in the ears; fatigue; exertional dyspnea; intense itching after bath; sensitivity to cold; epistaxis and gum bleeding; pain in the limbs; paresthesia. Sense of weight or swelling in the abdomen and occasional pain in left quadrant.

Signs. Color of face "rubor"; change in color also on distal extremities of limbs, with cyanotic hue. Ecchymoses of various sizes; purpura (8%). Eyes congested; conjunctiva and mucosae deep red; in eye grounds; engorgement of vessels. Clubbing of fingers and toes (rare). Hepatomegaly (40% to 50%), see Mosse's and Budd-Chiari. Splenomegaly (90%), hard and smooth.

Etiology. Unknown; belongs to the group of myeloproliferative syndromes (see).

Pathology. Plethoric engorgement of all organs; enlarged thrombosed veins; diffuse hemorrhages in skin, membranes, serosa, meninges, and various organs. *Spleen.* Enlarged; infarct; thrombosis; cysts; atrophic follicles; hypertrophic pulp; foci of extramedullary hematopoiesis. *Liver.* Enlarged and hyperemic; occasionally, extramedullar hematopoiesis. *Stomach and duodenum.* Frequently, ulcers are found.

Diagnostic Procedures. *Blood.* Red cells 7 to 10 million; hemoglobin increased to 18 to 24 g/100 ml; leukocytes over 10,000 with shift to the left. Leukocyte alkaline phosphatase values above normal; platelets increased as high as 3 to 6 million; blood viscosity markedly increased; sedimentation rate greatly delayed. Total blood volume typically increased. Uric acid normal or elevated. *Bone marrow.* Hypercellular; hyperplasia of all series. *Urine.* Normal or seldom proteinuria.

Therapy. Phlebotomies; radioactive phosphorus (^{32}P); busulfan; antihistamines (for pruritus).

Prognosis. The disease has a progressive, rather prolonged course. Hemorrhages, cardiovascular insufficiency among leading cases of death. Transformation (or evolution) into myeloid leukemia or erythroleukemia rather frequent.

BIBLIOGRAPHY. Vaquez H: Sur une forme spéciale de cyanose s'accompagnant d'hyperglobulie excessive et persistente. C R Bull Med Paris 44:384–388, 1892
Osler W: Chronic cyanosis with polycythemia and enlarged spleen: a new clinical entity. Am J Med Sci 126:187–201, 1903
Wintrobe MM (ed): Clinical Hematology, 8th ed, p 1596. Philadelphia, Lea & Febiger, 1981

VARIOT-PIRONNEAU

Obsolete.

Symptoms and Signs. Similar to Hutchinson-Gilford syndrome (see).

Etiology. Adrenal or pluriglandular deficiency. Familiar occurrence. See multiendocrine deficiency syndromes.

BIBLIOGRAPHY. Variot & Pironneau: Nanisme avec dystrophie osseuse et cutanée speciales: Soupçon d'agénésie des capsules surrénales. Bull Soc Pédiatr Paris 12:307–314, 1910
Valenzano L, Valenzano G: Osservazioni su due casi di: "Sindrome di Rummo e Ferrarini." Boll Ist Dermatol S Gallicano 6:55–72, 1970

VASA PREVIA

Synonym. Placenta vasa previa.

Symptoms. Occur during the 3rd trimester of pregnancy. Usually rupture of the amniotic sac and slight to moderate vaginal bleeding.

Signs. Irregularities in the fetal heart tones; bradycardia during uterine contractions; vaginal bleeding.

Etiology. Velamentous insertion of the umbilical vessels torn with rupture of the amniotic sac, or rupture because of pressure of the presenting part.

Pathology. Placenta pale; velamentous insertion of the umbilical vessels; rupture in one or more of the umbilical vessels.

Diagnostic Procedures. *Vaginal blood.* Tested for fetal hemoglobin, which is alkaline resistant (adult hemoglobin is not).

Therapy. Once diagnosed, rapid delivery, either vaginally or abdominally.

Prognosis. Maternal: excellent. Fetal: poor, associated with increased mortality.

BIBLIOGRAPHY. Torrey WE Jr: Vasa previa. Am J Obstet Gynecol 63:146–152, 1952

Naftolin F, Mishell DR Jr: "Vasa previa," report of 3 cases. Obstet Gynecol 26:561–565, 1965

Dougall A, Baird CH: Vasa praevia-report of three cases and review of literature. Br J Obstet Gynaecol 94:712–715, 1987

VASOVAGAL

Synonyms. Gowers'; Nothnagel's II; vasodepressor syncope. See orthostatic syncope; Da Costa's and Weisenburg's.

Symptoms. Most common form of syncope. Onset at any age. Precipitating factors: emotion; fatigue; minor trauma with pain; lack of food or sleep; indigestion; close environment; the sight of blood; or no factor. Patient before syncope is standing, occasionally sitting, never lying down. Warning symptoms: sudden weakness; sweating; dizziness; epigastric discomfort; paresthesia; palpitation; sialorrhea. Syncope may be prevented by lying down when warning symptoms appear. Syncope: loss of consciousness for a few seconds or minutes; occasionally, tonic and clonic movements. After regaining consciousness usually no residue; occasionally nervousness, dizziness, headache. Some patients may experience all symptoms and signs without, however, reaching the complete loss of consciousness.

Signs. Pallor; cold skin; sweating; moderate cyanosis; weak pulse. Bradycardia (sometimes preceded by tachycardia); hypotension.

Etiology. Sudden reflex; loss of peripheral resistance creating a temporary cerebral anoxia.

Pathology. None.

Diagnostic Procedures. Rule out epilepsy, heart conditions.

Therapy. None. Sympathomimetic drugs only in severe cases.

Prognosis. Good; attack appears at irregular intervals or according to precipitating factors. During attack patient may injure himself.

BIBLIOGRAPHY. Foster M: Textbook of Physiology, pp 297; 345. London, Macmillan, 1888

Weissler AM, Warren JV: Syncope pathophysiology and differential diagnosis. In Hurst JW: The Heart, 6th ed, p 516. New York, McGraw-Hill, 1986

VATER

Synonyms. Vertebral defects–anal atresia–TE fistula-radial-renal dysplasia; VATERS (V for both vertebral and ventricular defects and S for single umbilical artery).

Symptoms. Both sexes affected; present from birth. Failure to thrive; slow development, normal intelligence.

Signs. Association of three or more of the following defects:

Vertebral anomalies (70%)

Ventricular septal defects (53%)

Anal atresia (80%)

Tracheoesophageal (T-E) fistula (esophageal atresia) (70%)

Radial dysplasia (69%)

Renal anomalies (53%)

Single umbilical artery (39%)

Other abnormalities: inguinal hernias; small intestinal malformations; choanal atresia; cleft lip and/or palate.

Etiology. Unknown. Sporadic occurrence.

Therapy. Symptomatic, medical, and surgical.

Prognosis. Variable. If surviving, normal brain function.

BIBLIOGRAPHY. Say B, Gerald PS: A new polydactyly, imperforate anus, vertebral anomalies syndrome. Lancet II:688, 1968

Quan L, Smith DW: The VATER association Vertebral defects, anal atresia, T-E fistula, with esophageal atresia, Radial and Renal dysplasia: A spectrum of associated defects. J Pediatr 82:104–107, 1973

Weaver DD, Mapstone CL, Yu Pao-lo: The VATER association: analysis of 46 patients. Am J Dis Child 140:225–229, 1986

VENA CAVA, INFERIOR, OBSTRUCTION

Symptoms. According to site and rapidity of obstruction. Vomiting; diarrhea.

Signs. Edema in legs; enlargement of superficial veins of legs, abdomen, chest; occasionally, ascites.

Etiology and Pathology. *Congenital;* aneurysm; thrombosis; intra-abdominal malignancy; infection; trauma; cirrhosis. Retroperitoneal fibrosis; primary or metastatic (renal cell carcinoma) tumors.

Diagnostic Procedures. *Urine. Albuminuria. Blood.* Hyperbilirubinuria, and other liver function tests altered; increased blood urea nitrogen.

Therapy. Surgery difficult. According to etiology. Symptomatic.

Prognosis. Depends on etiology and site of obstruction. Rapid obstruction above renal artery usually fatal.

BIBLIOGRAPHY. Pleasants J: Obstruction of the inferior vena cava with a report of eighteen cases. Johns Hopkins Hosp 16:363–558, 1911

Hurst JW: The Heart, 6th ed, p 1379. New York, Mc-Graw-Hill, 1986

VENA CAVA, SUPERIOR, OBSTRUCTION

Synonym. Superior mediastinal.

Symptoms. Predominant in males; observed at all ages, maximum frequency between 40 and 50 years of age. Neck and face: venous distention and edema. Dyspnea; orthopnea; dysphagia; hoarseness; epistaxis; headache; vertigo; tinnitus; somnolence; syncope.

Signs. Edema and cyanosis of face, neck, shoulder, and arms; suffused conjunctivae. Varicose veins over shoulder, upper thorax. No edema of lower parts of the body or marked preference of edema for upper part so that a clear line of demarcation may be noticed (short cape edema). Edema and cyanosis of mucous membrane of mouth, pharynx, larynx, hydrothorax; occasionally hydropericardium.

Etiology and Pathology. Any cause compressing or infiltrating superior vena cava and obstructing its circulation. Mediastinal neoplasms and aneurysm of aorta, carcinoma of lung or adjacent structures, thyroid adenoma, and idiopathic causes. Ormond's syndrome (see).

Diagnostic Procedures. *X-ray of chest. CT scan. Angiography. Electrocardiography.*

Therapy. Surgery with decompression whenever feasible. Roentgen therapy.

Prognosis. Depends on etiology and degree of damage.

BIBLIOGRAPHY. Corvisart: Essai sur les Maladies et les Lesions Organiques du Coeur, p 350. Paris, 1806

McArt BA, Ramsey FB, Tosik WA et al: Surgical reversal of superior vena cava syndrome; report of a case caused by intrathoracic goiter and associated with roentgenographic hilar vascular shadow simulating neoplasm of chest. Arch Surg 69:4–11, 1954

Vanker VP, Maddison FE: Superior vena cava syndrome secondary to aortic disease; report of two cases and review of the literature. Dis Chest 51:656–662, 1967

Lokich JJ, Goodman R: Superior vena cava syndrome: Clinical management. JAMA 231:58–61, 1975

Parish JM, Marschke RF Jr, Dines DE et al: Etiologic considerations in superior vena cava syndrome. Mayo Clin Proc 56:407–413, 1981

VENTRICULAR SEPTAL ANEURYSM

Symptoms and Signs. Both sexes affected; usually asymptomatic; however, defect may cause complication: conduction disturbances; systemic embolism; aortic or tricuspid regurgitation; obstruction or right ventricular outflow; perforation causing a shunt; subacute bacterial endocarditis.

Etiology. Congenital malformation.

Pathology. Membranous septum continuous with aorta lies above muscular septum; the formed aneurysm protrudes into right ventricle or atrium or both.

Diagnostic Procedures. *Electrocardiography. Cardiac catheterization; X-ray.* Variable findings.

Therapy. If needed, surgical correction.

Prognosis. Extremely variable. Occasionally, autopsy finding in old persons.

BIBLIOGRAPHY. Baron MG, Wolf BS, Grisham A et al: Aneurysm of membraneous septum. Am J Roentgen 91:1303, 1964

Hoeffel JC, Henry M, Flizet M et al: Radiologic patterns of aneurysm of the membranous septum. Am Heart J 91:450–456, 1976

Perloff JK: The Clinical Recognition of Congenital Heart Disease, 2nd ed, p 397. Philadelphia, WB Saunders, 1978

VERALLO-HASERICK

Synonym. Lymphomatoid pityriasis lichenoides.

Symptoms and Signs. Those of Mucha-Habermann (see) with papules, and purpura, plaques, and edema.

Etiology. Unknown.

Pathology. Histology of skin shows colonization with atypical lymphocytes (high nucleus: cytoplasm ratio) and abnormal mitosis.

Therapy. Topical steroids; photochemotherapy (PUVA).

Prognosis. Chronic course; small number of patients proceed to full Alibert-Bazin (see).

BIBLIOGRAPHY. Verallo VM, Haserick JR: Mucha-Habermann's disease simulating lymphoma cutis: report of two cases. Arch Derm 94:295–299, 1966

Rook A, Wilkinson DS, Ebling FJG et al: Textbook of Dermatology, 4th ed, p 1750. Oxford, Blackwell Scientific Publications, 1986

VERBOV'S

Synonym. Anonychia-flexural pigmentation.

Symptoms and Signs. Both sexes. *Extremities.* Nails of fingers and toes absent; palmar and plantar skin dry, thin, and peeling. *Hair.* Coarse and sparse. *Teeth.* Early caries. *Axillae, groins.* Mottled hyperhypopigmentation.

Etiology. Autosomal dominant inheritance.

BIBLIOGRAPHY. Verbov J: Anonychia with bizarre flexural pigmentation: an autosomal dominant dermatosis. Br J Derm 92:469–474, 1975

VERBRYCKE'S

Synonym. Cholecystohepatic flexure adhesion.

Symptoms. In upright position, dull pain in epigastrium or upper right quadrant; nausea.

Signs. Tenderness and some protective splinting of muscles on right upper quadrant (nonconstant).

Etiology and Pathology. Adherence between gallbladder and hepatic flexure of colon.

Diagnostic Procedures. *Cholecystography.* Normal function of gallbladder. *Simultaneous examinations of colon (barium) and gallbladder (dye).* Reveal the lesion.

Therapy. Cholecystectomy.

Prognosis. Excellent with surgery.

BIBLIOGRAPHY. Verbrycke JR Jr: Adhesions of cholecystohepatic flexure, new syndrome with specific test. JAMA 114:314–316, 1940
Matolo NM (ed): Symposium on biliary disease. Surg Clin N Am 61:765 (whole issue), 1981

VERMIS AGENESIS

Synonyms. Dandy-Walker (see); Eisenring-Robb-Andermann; Rossi's (V).

Symptoms and Signs. The simple agenesis of vermis is not responsible for the clinical manifestations. Patients with vermis agenesis may have intelligence, development, and life span within normal limits. The clinical manifestations are due to the associated defects. Psychomotor retardation, hypotonia, incoordination, headache, convulsions, and other signs related to obstruction of ventricular system (when present) such as hydrocephalus, midline central nervous system malformations; cranioschisis, myelomeningocele. A better defined syndrome

associated with agenesis of vermis has been reported (see Joubert's.

Etiology. Unknown. Both agenesis of vermis and associated malformations may be due in some cases to primitive maldevelopment (familial and sporadic), in others to internal hydrocephalus that has led to the abnormalities during fetal life. Autosomal recessive inheritance to be considered.

Pathology. Two types of defects: complete or partial agenesis. Other midline malformations often encountered, but not necessarily associated (see Symptoms and Signs).

Diagnostic Procedures. *X-ray. CT brain scan.*

Therapy. Symptomatic or neurosurgical.

Prognosis. Extremely variable according to degree of associated lesions: from death few days after birth to normal life span. The agenesis of vermis per se is not responsible for neurologic or psychic development disorders.

BIBLIOGRAPHY. Rossi V: Un caso di mancanza del lobo mediano del cervelletto con presenza della fossetta occipitale media. Sperimentale 45:518–528, 1891
Joubert M, Eisenring JJ, Robb JP et al: Familial agenesis of the cerebellar vermis. Neurology 19:813–825, 1969

VERNER-MORRISON

Synonyms. Water diarrhea-hypokalemia-pancreatic adenoma, WDHA; vipoma; pancreatic cholera.

Symptoms. May occur as part of MEN I or may coexist with bronchogenic carcinoma. Onset from 2nd to 6th decades, predominant in 5th decade. Diarrhea of variable severity and duration, usually progressive. In acute stages, watery diarrhea, abdominal pain, nausea, and vomiting. In quiescent state, mushy stools and weight loss. Generalized weakness progressing to paralysis and then to stupor. Duration of symptoms from months to years. Spontaneous remission during pregnancy.

Signs. Weight loss; hypotonia; sigmoidoscopy negative.

Etiology. Islet cell adenoma. In a few cases more than one endocrine adenoma observed (thyroid; parathyroid). Production of a vasoactive intestinal peptide (VIP) that stimulates intestinal fluid and electrolyte secretion, decreases acid secretion, relaxes smooth muscle, and keeps stool moist.

Pathology. Islet cell adenoma. In some cases metastasis to the liver. Secondary effects of chronic severe diarrhea (e.g., weight loss). VIP secretion tumors usually originate in the pancreas (84%) but may also originate in other organs (16%) especially along the sympathetic chain.

Diagnostic Procedures. *Blood.* Hyperchloremia (metabolic acidosis); hyperglycemia; hypercalcemia, plasma VIP levels. *Stool.* Cultures negative. Alkaline, isotonic more than 500 ml/day. *X-ray.* Absence of peptic ulceration and gastric hypersecretion. *CT scans and ultrasound.* Most useful identifying techniques.

Therapy. Surgical removal of pancreatic islet cell tumor. Oral glucose-electrolyte solutions. Pharmacologic agents to control diarrhea: prednisone. Trials with alpha adrenergic agonists; norepinephrine; indomethacin; lithium carbonate; somatostatin; phenothiazine; propanolol.

Prognosis. Cessation of all symptoms with removal of tumor. Occasional recurrence when metastases are present. If no surgery or if tumor unexcisable, death from dehydration and shock.

BIBLIOGRAPHY. Moldawer MP, Nardi GL, Raker JW: Concomitance of multiple adenomas of the parathyroids and pancreatic islets with tumor of the pituitary: a syndrome with familial incidence. Am J Med Sci 228:190–206, 1954

Verner JV, Morrison AB: Islet cell tumor and a syndrome of refractory watery diarrhea and hypokalemia. Am J Med 25:374–380, 1958

O'Dorisio TM, Mekhjian HS: Vipoma syndrome. In Cohen S, Soloway RD (eds): Hormone-Producing Tumors of the Gastrointestinal Tract, 5th ed, pp 101–116. Edinburgh, Churchill-Livingstone, 1984

Krejs GJ: Vipoma syndrome. Am J Med (suppl 5B):37–47, 1987

VERNET'S

Synonyms. Foramen lacerum posterior; jugular foramen.

Symptoms. Hoarseness; taste alterations; dysphagia for solid food; nasal regurgitation of fluids.

Signs. Paralysis of palate, pharynx, and larynx. Posterior wall of pharynx deviates to unaffected side when tongue is protruded. Tachycardia; paralysis and atrophy of sternocleidomastoid and upper portion of trapezius muscles.

Etiology and Pathology. Trauma; aneurysm; neoplasia involving glossopharyngeal (IX), vagus (X), spinal accessory (XI) nerves in the region of the jugular foramen.

Diagnostic Procedures. *X-rays of skull and esophagus. Angiography. Brain isotope scan. CT scan.*

Therapy. Surgery when indicated to remove pressure.

Prognosis. Depends on etiology.

BIBLIOGRAPHY. Vernet M: Les paralysies laryngées associés (thesis), p 233. Lyon, 1916

Vernet M: The classification of syndromes of associated laryngeal paralysis. Med Rev NY: 449–458, 1918

Adams RD, Victor M: Principles of Neurology. 3rd ed, p 504. New York, McGraw-Hill, 1985

VESICA PUDICA

Synonym. Shy bladder.

Symptoms and Signs. Inability to initiate urinary flow, (or a long delay) when other person is watching or waiting in line in public toilets; or when the micturition has to be performed in unusual places (train, airplane, or in the open country).

Etiology. Psychoneurologic reflex. Of interest only because it may help some people once they hear about its existence in other people.

VESICOURETERAL REFLUX

Synonyms. Innes Williams; megaureter-megacystis; primary ureteral reflux.

Symptoms. Repeated urinary tract infections in children, temporarily cured by antibiotics.

Signs. Dilated, refluxing ureters and a large, thin-walled bladder.

Etiology. Primary ureteral reflux. The ureteral reflux may be due to lack of development of trigonal muscles, or other mechanisms. The so-called megacystis with thin-walled bladder is secondary and due to the distensibility of the bladder walls of children. Multifactorial or mendelian (autosomal dominant) trait reported.

Diagnostic Procedures. *Urine.* Culture. *Excretory urography.* Normal or scarred dilated calices and irregular ureters. *Cystourethrography.* Large, thin-walled bladder extending outside bony pelvis; ureters and pelvis ballooned out; normal voiding of urethra and emptying of bladder.

Therapy. Assessment of degree of reflux. *Grade 1* (lower ureteral filling) and *Grade 2* (ureteral and pelvicaliceal without pelvic dilatation). Antibiotics (1 year trial); if failure, surgery. *Grade 3* (grade 2 plus pelvic dilatation). Antibacterial agents or surgery debated. *Grade 4.* Direct surgery followed by antibiotics. Tunnel reimplantation of ureters, anchoring the bladder wall near the neck, without revising the bladder neck (Politano-Leadbetter technique).

Prognosis. Good with adequate and timely treatment.

BIBLIOGRAPHY. Kretschmer HL, Greer JR: Insufficiency at the ureterovesical junction. Surg Gynecol Obstet 21:228–231, 1915

Politano VH, Leadbetter WF: An operative technique for correction of the vesicoureteral reflux. J Urol 79:932, 1958

Paquin AJ Jr, Marshal VF, McGovern JH: The megacystis syndrome. J Urol 83:634–646, 1960

Harrow BR: The myth of the megacystis syndrome. J Urol 98:205, 1967

Chapman CJ, Bailey RR, Janus ED et al: Vesicoureteral reflux: segregation analysis. Am J Med Genet 20:577–584, 1985

VESTIBULAR PARALYSIS, BILATERAL

Symptoms and Signs. Patients stagger and walk zigzag, more so after dark; cannot swim and become disoriented in the water; have no sense of depth with the eyes closed but no difficulty with eyes open. Loss of hearing is often associated.

Etiology and Pathology. Infective process bilaterally affecting the vestibular system in any site between the semicircular canals and the vestibular nuclei in the brain. Usually, vasculitic type of lesions (e.g., scrub typhus, scarlet fever, syphilis). Neoplasms.

Diagnostic Procedures. *Rotation and caloric stimulation.* Does not elicit vertigo, unsteadiness, nausea; nystagmus because of inability to maintain ocular fixation. *Galvanic stimulation.* Elicits nystagmus and unsteadiness in semicircular canal lesions but not in central lesions (ganglion, nerves, nuclei). Hearing lost in central lesions, not in semicircular canal lesions. Search for specific agent of infection. *Culture, complement fixation, antibodies.*

Therapy. Specific for infection or neoplasm.

Prognosis. Lesions may be persistent.

BIBLIOGRAPHY. James W: The sense of dizziness in deaf-mutes. Am J Otol 4:239–254, 1882

Chusid J, DeGutierrez-Mahoney CG: Syndrome of bilateral vestibular paralysis. J Nerv Ment Dis 103:172–180, 1946

Plum F: Ataxia and related gait disorders. In Cecil Textbook of Medicine p 1966. Philadelphia, WB Saunders, 1982

VESTMARK-VESTMARK

Synonyms. Sex-linked thrombocytopenia; Wiskott-Aldrich variant. Canales-Mauer. See also Bernard-Soulier.

Symptoms and Signs. Appear only in males; a female reported (lyonization); onset in childhood. Purpura; epistaxis; easy bruising; pallor; absence of eczema.

Etiology. Sex-linked inheritance. Raised question of its distinctness from Wiskott-Aldrich.

Diagnostic Procedures. *Blood.* Hypochromic anemia; thrombocytopenia; leukoctyes normal or decreased Evidence of immunologic defect. *Bone marrow.* Normal or moderate erythroid hyperplasia.

Therapy. Moderate response to corticosteroids. Occasional benefit from splenectomy.

Prognosis. Greatest severity in childhood, then chronic course.

BIBLIOGRAPHY. Vestmark B, Vestmark S: Familial sex-linked thrombocytopenia. Arch Pediatr 53:369–370, 1964

Ata M, Fisher OD, Holman CA: Inherited thrombocytopenia. Lancet 1:119–123, 1965

Canales L, Mauer AM: Sex-linked hereditary thrombocytopenia as a variant of Wiskott-Aldrich syndrome. N Engl J Med 277:899–901, 1967

Cohn J, Hange M, Andersen V, et al: Sex-linked hereditary thrombocytopenia with immunologic defect. Hum Hered 25:309–317, 1975

VIBRATORY ANGIOEDEMA

Synonym. Angioedema vibratory.

Symptoms and Signs. Stimulation of frictional or vibratory type triggers severe local reaction followed by generalized erythema and cephalea.

Etiology. Autosomal dominant inheritance.

Diagnostic Procedures. *Venous blood.* From area submitted to stimulation, increase of amine levels.

BIBLIOGRAPHY. Patterson R, Mellies CJ, Blankenship ML et al: Vibratory angioedema: a hereditary type of physical hypersensitivity. J Allergy Clin Immun 50:174–182, 1972

VIDAL'S

Synonyms. Pityriasis circinata; pityriasis rotunda; acquired pseudoichthyosis. Toyama's, Brocq's I.

Symptoms. Common in Far East populations, less in South Africans, Bantus, Egyptians, and West Indians; onset between 7 and 76 years of age. Pregnancy or infection may precipitate onset.

Signs. Appearance of solitary or multiple round patches of dry scaling, without inflammatory changes, on the buttocks, thighs, abdomen, back, arms.

Etiology. Unknown; genetic factors postulated.

Pathology. Mild hyperkeratitic changes in areas affected.

Treatment. None. Keratin stripping: temporary effect.

Prognosis. Life-long lesions.

BIBLIOGRAPHY. Vidal E: Du lichen (Lichen, prurigo, strophulus) Ann Dermatol Syph (Paris) 7:133–154, 1866

Toyama I: Isshu no Kasshoku enkei rakushosei hifubyo ni tsnite. Jpn Derm 6:91–105, 1906

Aguilera Maruri C, Aguilera Diaz L: Le pityriasis circiné et marginé de Vidal, Maladie autonome. Ann Dermatol Syph 95:49–57, 1968

Arndt KA, Pane BS, Stern RS et al: Treatment of pityriasis rosea with UV radiation. Arch Dermatol 9:381–382, 1983

VIGNES'

Synonyms. Blepharophimosis-ptosis-epicanthus inversus-lacrimal stenosis, BPES: Komoto's triad; Kohn-Romano; conjunctival eyelid tedra (CET).

Symptoms. Male predominance, onset from birth. Visual impairment; occasional amblyopia. Normal mental development. Female infertility.

Signs. Telecanthus; microphthalmus; ptosis; epicanthus inversus; blepharophimosis; elongated lid margin. Divergent strabismus; nystagmus; esotropia. Ductus lacrimalis anomalies. Fundus oculi normal. Low-set ears; deformed pinnae. High-arched palate.

Etiology. Unknown, autosomal dominant inheritance. Possibly two types: (1) with infertility of affected females, (2) transmission from both males and females.

Therapy. Plastic surgery; canthoplasty for aesthetic and ocular functional reasons.

BIBLIOGRAPHY. Vignes L: Epicanthus héréditaire. Rev Gen Ophthalmol, 8:438, 1889

Komoto J: Ptosis operation. Klin Monatsbl Augenheilkd 66:952, 1921

Kohn R, Romano PE: Blepharoptosis, blepharophimosis, epicanthus inversus, and telecanthus: a syndrome with no name. Am J Ophthalmol 72:625–632, 1971

Zlotogora J, Sagi M, Cohen T: The blepharophimosis, ptosis and epicanthus inversus syndrome: delineation of two types. Am J Med Genet 35:1020–1027, 1983

VILANOVA-AGUADÉ

Synonyms. Nodular migratory panniculitis; sclerodermiform panniculitis; erythema nodosum migrans. See Bazin's and Whitfield's syndromes.

Symptoms. Seldom in males; previous history of acute tonsillitis frequent. Trauma often preceding first lesion. Nodule or plaque (singly or in crops) on one leg (usually ankle region) expanding or joining to form a large erythematous plaque of hard successive eruptions. Consistent for weeks or months; always limited to legs.

Etiology. Unknown; variant of erythema nodosum (see).

Pathology. *Early.* Epithelial proliferation occluding capillaries and small vessels. Infiltration with lymphocytes, monohistiocytes and fibroblasts. *Later.* Only giant cells. Skin and subcutaneous *restitutio ad integrum* as lesion regresses.

Therapy. Treatment of focal infections if identified.

Prognosis. Spontaneous remission after variable time. Recurrences also after long periods.

BIBLIOGRAPHY. Vilanova X, Piñol Aguadé JP: Hypodermite nodulaire subaiguë migratrice. Ann Derm Syph 83:369–404, 1956

Vilanova X, Piñol Aguadé JP: Subacute nodular migratory panniculitis. Br J Derm 71:45–50, 1959

Rook A, Wilkinson DS, Ebling FJG, et al: Textbook of Dermatology, 4th ed, pp 1164–1165. Oxford, Blackwell Scientific Publications, 1986

VILLARET—DESOILLES

Synonyms. Maxillofacial dysostosis; dysostosis maxillofacial dysplasia; Peters-Hoevels.

Symptoms and Signs. Bilateral hypoplasia of malar bones; antimongoloid obliquity of lids without colobomas; open bite; excessive development of lower jaw.

Etiology. Unknown. Autosomal dominant inheritance.

BIBLIOGRAPHY. Villaret R, Desoilles H: L'hypoplasie primitive familiale du maxillare supérieur. Ann Med 32:378–381, 1932

Peters A, Hoevels O: Die dysostosis maxillofacialis, eine erbliche, typische Fehlbildung des I. Visceral Bogens. Z Meuschl Vererb Kostitutionslehre 35:434–444, 1960

Melnick M, Eastman JR: Autosomal dominant maxillofacial dysostosis. Birth Defects Orig Art Series XIII (3B):39–44, 1977

VILLARET'S

Synonyms. Parotid posterior space; retroparotid space. See Collet-Sicard.

Symptoms and Signs. Ipsilateral paralysis of soft palate, pharynx, and vocal cords, associated with Horner's syndrome.

Etiology and Pathology. Trauma, infections, neoplasm involving last four cranial nerves (9th through 12th) and cervical sympathetic chain.

Diagnostic Procedures. *X-ray of skull. Angiography CT brain scan. Culture.* If infection.

Therapy. Surgical, according to etiology, to relieve nerve involved.

Prognosis. Depends on etiology.

BIBLIOGRAPHY. Villaret M: Le syndrome nerveux de l'espace rétro-parotidien postérieur. Rev Neurol (Paris) 23:188–190, 1916
Adams RD, Victor M: Principles of Neurology, 3rd ed, p 504. New York, McGraw-Hill, 1985

VISCEROSPINAL SYNDROMES

This term designates confusing intra-abdominal symptoms that are manifestations of a radiculitis or myositis (see Trigger point). Symptoms of appendicitis, gallbladder disease, ureteral colic, and cardiovascular diseases may be found. Treatment of nerve irritation, once the trigger point is identified, leads to the disappearance of all symptoms.

BIBLIOGRAPHY. Ussher NT: Spinal curvatures-visceral disturbances in relation thereto. Calif West Med 38:423–428, 1933
Ussher NT: The viscerospinal syndrome: a new concept of visceromotor and sensory changes in relation to deranged spinal structures. Ann Intern Med 13:2057–2090, 1940
Strong EK, Davila JC: The cluneal nerve syndrome: a distinct type of low back pain. Indust Med S 26:417–429, 1957

VISSER'S

This syndrome is actually part of the adrenogenital syndromes (see), but alterations of sexual characteristics are not present.

Synonyms. Aldosterone deficiency I; 18-hydroxylase deficiency; salt-wasting; hypoaldosteronism, primary; corticosterone methyloxidase, type I deficiency; CMOI deficiency.

Symptoms and Signs. Rare. From birth. Dehydration; intermittent fever.

Etiology. Autosomal recessive inheritance. Deficiency of 18-hydroxylase; which converts corticosterone to aldosterone, hence no aldosterone production.

Diagnostic Procedures. *Blood.* Hyponatremia; hyperkalemia.

Pathology. *At autopsy.* Adrenals grossly normal. *Histology.* Glomerulosa with tubular empty areas.

Therapy. Desoxycorticosterone acetate.

Prognosis. Good results with therapy.

BIBLIOGRAPHY. Visser HKA, Cost WS: A new hereditary defect in the biosynthesis of aldosterone: urinary C21—corticosteroid pattern in three related patients with salt losing syndrome suggesting an 18-oxidation defect. Acta Endocrinol 47:589–612, 1964
Jean R, Legrand JC, Meylan F et al: Hypoaldosteronism primaire par anomalie probable de la 18-hydroxylation. Arch Franc Pediatr 26:769, 1969
Drp SLS, Frohn-Mulder IME, Visser HKA et al: The effect of ACTH stimulation on plasma steroids in two patients with congenital hypoaldosteronism and their relatives. Acta Endocrinol 99:245–250, 1982

VITROCORNEAL TOUCH

Synonyms. Cataract extraction; postcataract extraction.

Symptoms. Onset usually 2 to 3 weeks after cataract extraction.

Signs. Central cornea shows area of diminished transparency and edema; iris bombé; bullous keratopathy.

Etiology. Vitreous, bulging through pupillary space touching and adhering to corneal endothelium, promotes aqueous collection into vitreous body.

Therapy. According to some authors, destruction of anterior vitreous hyloid surface allows liquid vitreous to touch cornea. Others recommend posterior sclerectomy aspiration of liquid vitreous and air injection into anterior chamber, respecting anterior hyloid membrane.

Prognosis. Fair with treatment.

BIBLIOGRAPHY. Leahey BD: Bullous keratitis vitreous from contact. Arch Ophthalmol 46:22–28, 1951
Gostin SB: Vitrocorneal touch syndrome. South Med J 65:741–766, 1972
Geeraets WJ: Ocular Syndromes, 3rd ed. Philadelphia, Lea & Febiger, 1976

VOERNER'S I

Synonyms. Haloderma; knuckle pads—keratosis palmoplantaris.

Symptoms and Signs. The association of knuckle pads and keratosis palmoplantaris.

Etiology. Familial occurrence (autosomal dominant) reported. Possibly, a feature of more than one syndrome in the complex group of keratoderma syndromes.

BIBLIOGRAPHY. Voerner H: Zur kenntnis des Keratomas hereditarium palmare et plantare. Arch Dermatol Syph 56:3–31, 1901
Schwann J: Keratosis palmaris et plantaris cum surditate congenita et leukonychia totaly unguium. Dermatologica 126:335–353, 1963

VOERNER'S II

Synonyms. Nevus anemicus; nevus avasculosus.

Symptoms. Both sexes affected; onset at birth or in early childhood. Asymptomatic.

Signs. On face, chest, or back of neck, irregularly shaped area of pale skin, occasionally multiple areas. Diascopic pressure cancels difference with surrounding skin, cold-heat application does not produce erythema, in contrast with surrounding skin.

Etiology. Unknown. Developmental (functional) anomaly. Consistent with autosomal dominant inheritance. Impaired blood supply.

Pathology. Normal histology.

Diagnostic Procedures. *Iontophoresis.* With acetylcholine. No dilatation, epinephrine does not increase pallor of the affected area.

Therapy. None. Cosmetic cream.

Prognosis. Lesion persisting for life.

BIBLIOGRAPHY. Piorkowski FO: Nevus Anemicus (Voerner). Arch Derm Syph 54:374–377, 1944
Butterworth T, Walter JD: Observation on pharmacologic responses of Voerner's nevus anemicus. Arch Derm Syph 66:333–339, 1952
Cardoso H, Vignale R, Abren de Sastre H: Familial naevus anemicus. Am J Hum Genet 27:24A, 1975

VOGT-KOYANAGI-HARADA

Synonyms. Alopecia-poliosis-uveitis-vitiligo-deafness; cutaneous-uveo-oto; VKH. See Harada's.

Symptoms and Signs. Onset between 20 and 50 years; no sex or race preference. *Prodromal phase (meningeal).* Nausea; emesis; fever; headache; drowsiness; vertigo. Various other neurologic signs may appear during this phase, or later; Kernig's, Brudzinski's signs; acute brain syndrome; paresis of cranial nerves (usually unilateral); hemiparesis; aphasia. *Ophthalmic phase.* One or two weeks later, eye irritation, photophobia, and rapid vision loss. Signs of granular inflammation of iris, ciliary body, and retina. According to degree of inflammation, edema, secondary glaucoma, and partial or total detachment of retina may develop. *Convalescent phase.* During the course of several weeks, intermittent symptoms and progression after the subsidence of acute stage, the following additional manifestations appear: poliosis; leukoderma; alopecia; skin pigmentation, sensitive, easily sunburned, paresthetic; canities; dysacusia; tinnitus. Acute neurologic signs and ocular symptoms and signs remit while neurologic and ophthalmic damage may persist unchanged or improve (see Prognosis).

Etiology. Unknown; viral inflammation theory. Allergic sensitivity of pigmented structures.

Pathology. *Central nervous system.* During acute stage diffuse adhesive inflammatory arachnoiditis in the brain and spinal cord. *Eyes.* Typical acute bilateral uveitis; retinal detachment. After convalescent stage, from complete remission and reattachment of retina, to permanent detachment, cataracts, scarring, and retraction of entire globe. *Skin.* Irregular spot of depigmentation (neurotrophic type); hair depigmentation frequently following distribution of cutaneous nerves.

Diagnostic Procedures. Acute phase. *Cerebrospinal fluid.* Pleocytosis and increase of protein and pressure. *Electroencephalography.* Changes. *Blood.* Normal; serology negative. *Urine.* Normal. *X-rays.* Negative. *Skin tests.* For tuberculosis, coccidioidomycosis, and blastomycosis: negative.

Therapy. Large doses of steroids.

Prognosis. Through the different phases, the natural course of the disease is of about 1 year with possible relapse during this period and no further progression or relapses later. From complete remission to serious sequelae: blindness; total or partial deafness; personality changes and psychosis; persistent aphasia. Neurologic deficit and endocrine complications from involvement of pituitary gland. Steroids may shorten the course and prevent most of the complications.

BIBLIOGRAPHY. Vogt A: Fruhzeitiges ergrauen der Zilien und bemerkungen über den sogenannten plotzlichen Eintritt dieser Veranderung. Klin Augenheilkd 44:228–242, 1906
Harada E: Beitrage zur klinischen Kernitis von nichteitri-

ger Choroiditis. Nippon Ganka Gakkai Zasshi 30:356–361, 1926

Koyanagi Y: Dysakusis, Alopecia und Poliosis bei schwerer Uveitis nichttraumitischen Ursprunges. Klin Monatsbl Augenheilkd 82:194–211, 1929

Rook A, Wilkinson DS, Ebling FJG, et al: Textbook of Dermatology. 4th ed, pp 1590–1591. Oxford, Blackwell Scientific Publications, 1986

VOGT'S (A.) I

Synonym. Frosted cataract. Aculeiform cataract including coralliform cataract (Nettleship's)

Symptoms. Variable degree of visual impairment.

Signs. Frostlike, whitish threads in superficial layers of embryonic nucleus.

Etiology. Unknown; autosomal dominant inheritance; recessive also suspected.

Therapy. Corneal transplantation.

BIBLIOGRAPHY. Nettleship E: Seven new pedigrees of hereditary cataract. Trans Ophthal Soc UK 29:188–211, 1909

Vogt A: Weitere Ergebmisse der Spaltlampen mikroscopie des vorden Bulbusatschnittes (Cornea, Vorderkrammer, Iris, vorder Glaskorper, Conjunctive, Lidrendev). Albrecht Von Graefes Arch Ophthalmol 106:63–103, 1921

Gifford SR, Puntenney I: Coralliform cataract and a new form of congenital cataract with crystals in the lens. Arch Ophthalmol 17:885–892, 1937

Jordan M: Stammbaumuntersuchungen bei Cataracta stellata coralliformis. Klin Monatsbl Augenheilkd 126:467–469, 1955

VOGT'S (A.) II

Synonym. Cornea guttata.

Symptoms and Signs. Both sexes affected with equal incidence; onset after 40 years of age (70%). Variable visual impairment. Cornea with numerous central fine, wartlike excrescences on Descemet's membrane, which spread progressively toward periphery.

Etiology. Autosomal dominant inheritance (?).

Pathology. Endothelium of cornea hexagonal aspect disturbed; cells irregular in shape and size; golden brown pigmentation; pigment deposition on corneal posterior surface.

BIBLIOGRAPHY. Vogt A: Weitere Ergebmisse der Spaltlampen mikroscopie des vorden Bulbusabschnittes. III.

Augeborene und Fruherworbene linsenveranderung. Albrecht von Graefes Arch Ophthalmol 107:196–240, 1922

Goldberg MF: Genetic and Metabolic Eye Disease, p 302. Boston, Little Brown, 1974

VOGT'S (A.) III

Synonyms. Cornea farinata; floury cornea.

Symptoms and Signs. Both sexes affected; onset in old age. Variable visual impairment. In the cornea, fine, floury, dusty layer in a restricted area of posterior stroma, anterior to Descemet's membrane.

Etiology. Unknown. Type of heredity not established.

BIBLIOGRAPHY. Vogt A: Neure Ergebnisse der Spaltlampen mikroscopie. Schweiz Med Wochenschr 53:989–995, 1923

Goldberg MF: Genetic and Metabolic Eye Disease, p 302. Boston, Little Brown, 1974

VOGT'S (A.) IV

Synonyms. Crocodile shagreen; mosaic corneal degeneration.

Symptoms and Signs. Both sexes affected; onset in old age. Variable visual impairment. Cornea showing flat, gray, polygonal opacities at Bowman's membrane level (axial mosaic).

Etiology. Autosomal dominant inheritance; acquired form.

BIBLIOGRAPHY. Vogt A: Lehrbuch und Atlas der Spaltlampen Mikroscopie des Lebenden Augens. Berlin, Springer, 1930

Goldberg MF: Genetic and Metabolic Eye Disease, p 290. Boston, Little Brown, 1974

VOGT–VOGT

Synonym. Status dysmyelinatus.

Symptoms and Signs. Onset in first year of life. Athetoid movements replaced successively by rigidity.

Etiology. Unknown.

Pathology. Shrinkage of caudate nucleus, globus pallidus, subthalamic nucleus. Myelin sheaths in affected areas are absent.

Therapy. Symptomatic.

Prognosis. Death in second decade.

BIBLIOGRAPHY. Vogt C, Vogt O: Zum Lehre der Erkrankungen des striäten systems. J Psychol Neurol 18:627–846, 1920

Adams RD, Victor M: Principles of Neurology, 3rd ed, p 745. New York, McGraw-Hill, 1985

VOHWINKEL'S

Synonyms. Mutilating keratoderma; keratoderma mutilating hereditarium; deafness-keratopachydermia-ainhum.

Symptoms. Both sexes affected. Hyperhidrosis; keratosis pilaris; hourglass nail; development of tylosis and fissure with ainhumlike constriction (see Ainhum) with spontaneous amputation of fingers. Deafness. Symptoms and signs of hypogonadism. Years after onset of tylosis, development of symptoms and signs of syringomyelia.

Etiology. Unknown; autosomal dominant inheritance.

BIBLIOGRAPHY. Vohwinkel KH: Keratoma hereditarium mutilans. Arch Derm Syph 158:354–364, 1929

Tatz K: Pityriasis rubra pilaris with ainhum and syringomyelia. Br J Derm 58:123–126, 1946

Aku F, Mietens C: Keratopachydermie mit Schnuerfurchen in Fingern und Zehen und Innenohzschwerhoerikeit. Paediatr Prox 23:303–310, 1980

VOLKMANN'S I

Eponym used to indicate tibiotarsal dislocation causing a congenital deformity of the foot.

BIBLIOGRAPHY. Volkmann R: Ein Fall von hereditaerer kongenitaler Luxation beider Sprunggelekne. Dtsch Z Chir 2:538–542, 1873

VOLKMANN'S II

Synonyms. Ischemic contracture; myositis fibrosa; posttraumatic muscle contraction.

Symptoms. Burning pain, weakness or paralysis or paresthesia in hand and forearm.

Signs. Hand cyanosis; swelling; coldness. Fingers in fixed contracted flexion. Radial pulse absent or weak. Atrophic changes of skin of forearm and hand.

Etiology. Spastic or organic occlusion of artery or vein of arm. Fracture; extrinsic compression (splint-tourniquet).

Pathology. Muscle fibers degenerated and necrotic; fibrotic changes. Ischemic degeneration of nerve fibers.

Diagnostic Procedures. X-rays. Arteriography.

Therapy. Removal of obstruction. Splitting the deep fascia in front of the elbow within 36 hours after injury.

Prognosis. Good if immediately treated. If unrecognized, it results in chronic, permanent deformity with atrophy of forearm and hand, abduction of thumb and flexion of fingers.

BIBLIOGRAPHY. Volkmann R: Die ischaemischen Muskellahmungen und Kontracturen. Zentralbl Chir 8:801–803, 1881

Milford, L: Volkmann's contracture and compartment syndrome. In Crenshaw AH (ed), Campbell's Operative Orthopedics, 7th ed, pp 409–418. St Louis, CV Mosby, 1987

VOLTOLINI'S

Synonym. Acute labyrinthitis. See Pedersen's and Menière's.

Symptoms. Occur in young children; onset after infectious diseases. Intense otalgia; bilateral deafness; delirium; loss of consciousness; meningeal irritation signs.

Etiology. Infection.

Diagnostic Procedures. Lack of labyrinth excitability.

Therapy. Antibiotics.

Prognosis. Severe. Progressive, leading to permanent deafness.

BIBLIOGRAPHY. Voltolini FER: Die acute Entzuendung des hauetigen Labyrinthes, gewoehlich irrthuemlich fuer Meningitis gehalten. Mschr Ohrenh 1:9–14, 1867

Adams RD, Victor M: Principles of Neurology. 3rd ed, p 229. New York, McGraw-Hill, 1985

VON BEKHTEREV-STRÜMPELL

Synonyms. Ankylosing spondylitis; Bekhterev's; juvenile spondylitis; Marie-Strümpell; rheumatoid spondylitis; rhizomelic spondylitis; spondylitis ossificans ligamentosa II; spondylosis deformans.

Symptoms. Prevalent in males, onset insidious in 2nd or 3rd decade. Lumbar pain with radiation, limited flexibility of spine; pain in the chest (pleuritic type); generalized arthralgia. Back stiff after a period of inactivity.

Signs. Loss of normal lumbar lordosis; reduced mobility of spine. Other articulations eventually become involved. Kyphosis, scoliosis, forward displaced head and total rigidity of spine eventually develop.

Etiology. Unknown; autosomal hereditary transmission reported in some cases.

Pathology. Minimal chronic inflammatory changes, fibrosis, and eventually calcification of capsules and intervertebral ligaments. Ankylosis and periarticular osteoporosis.

Diagnostic Procedures. *X-ray.* Bamboo spine; extensive spondylosis. *Blood.* Rheumatoid arthritis (R.A.) test.

Therapy. Corticosteroids, analgesic, roentgen therapy. Physical therapy.

Prognosis. Chronic course evolving to complete spinal rigidity in 10 to 15 years (bamboo spine) with temporary remission and exacerbation. Rapid progressive course in some cases. Pulmonary diseases frequently develop.

BIBLIOGRAPHY. Connor B, Marie P: Les rheumatismes deformants. Trib Med 27:27–30, 1895 Phil Trans 19:21, 1695

Bekhterev VM: Oderevenelast' pozvonochikas iskrivleniemego, kak osobia forma zabolevaniia. Vrach St Petersburg 13:899–903, 1892

Strümpell A: Bemerkung über die chronische Ankylosirende Entzündung der Wirbelsäule un der Hüftgelenke. Dtsch Z Nervkr 11:338–342, 1897

Moller P, Berg K: Ankylosing spondylitis is part of multifactorial syndrome: hereditary multifocal relapsing inflammation (HEMRI). Clin Genet 26:187–194, 1984

VON BERGMANN'S

Synonyms. Bergmann's diaphragmatic hernia; gastrocardiac; hiatus hernia; paraescphageal hernia; sliding diaphragmatic hernia.

Symptoms. Sliding hernia prevalent in males; onset in old age. Paraesophageal hernia in females; onset in middle age. Symptoms of variable nature and intensity. Epigastric or midthoracic pain; radiation to left costal margin or shoulder and arm. Frequently manifested when lying down or after meals. Symptoms may mimic coronary, colic, duodenal pains.

Signs. On chest auscultation, gurgling sounds.

Etiology. Autosomal recessive or X-linked inheritance. Sudden weight loss; increase of intra-abdominal pressure; chronic inflammation of esophagus; emphysema.

Pathology. Paraesophageal hernia with or without herniation of cardias into thoracic cavity.

Diagnostic Procedures. *X-ray of digestive tract. Blood.* Usually, hypochromic anemia.

Therapy. Surgery.

Prognosis. Good with surgical correction.

BIBLIOGRAPHY. von Bergmann G: Das "Epiphrenale syndrom" seine Beziehung zue Angina pectoris und zum Kardiospasmus. Dtsch Med Wochenschr 58:605–609, 1932

Cunha F: Recurrent "hiatus hernia" syndrome of von Bergmann. Am J Dig Dis Nutrition 1:170–172, 1934

Norio R, Kaariainen H, Rapola J et al: Familial congenital diaphragmatic defects: aspects and etiology, prenatal diagnosis and treatment. Am J Med Genet 17:471–483, 1984

VON ECONOMO'S

Synonyms. Economo's; Economo-Cruchet; encephalitis lethargica; sleeping sickness (African).

Symptoms. Occur in epidemic form; both sexes affected; onset at all ages. Febrile onset. Headache; dizziness; fatigue; irritability; choreiform movements. Later, parkinsonism (see). Oculogyric crisis; disorder of behavior.

Signs. Variable in different patients and course of the disease according to neurologic lesions and degree of recovery. Motor, sensorial lesions, and alterations.

Etiology. Trypanosomiasis (in African sleeping sickness).

Pathology. *Brain.* hyperemia; petechiae in basal ganglia of midbrain; pons; destruction of nerve fibers; lymphocytic infiltration.

Diagnostic Procedures. *Cerebrospinal fluid.* Increase in pressure, proteins, and cells. Viral cultures.

Therapy. Symptomatic. L-Dopa and other antiparkinsonian agents.

Prognosis. Variable course and sequelae.

BIBLIOGRAPHY. von Economo C: Encephalitis lethargica. Wien Klin Wochenschr 30:581–585, 1917

Adams RD, Victor M: Principles of Neurology, 3rd ed, p 560. New York, McGraw-Hill, 1985

VON EULENBERG'S

Synonyms. Eulenberg's; normokalemic periodic paralysis (type B); paramyotonia; see Gamstrop's.

Symptoms. Both sexes equally affected; onset in 1st decade. Between attacks asymptomatic. Precipitating factors: sleeping; rest after exertion; alcohol; cold and dampness; mental stress. Attack: flaccid paralysis of all muscles except facial expression, mastication, deglutition, speech, and respiration. In some cases, jaw muscle may be affected. Limited muscle groups may be affected.

Signs. Hyporeflexia of affected muscles.

Etiology. Unknown; simple autosomal dominant inheritance. Paramyotonia (or cold-sensitive myotonia), according to majority of myologists, represents an end of a spectrum extending to periodic paralysis (see Gamstrop's), since many cases show both conditions. In addition it does not appear justifiable to separate normokalemic from hyperkalemic paralysis since, in these two syndromes, serum potassium levels do not (always) correlate with muscle weakness.

Pathology. Subsarcolemmal vacuolization observed. No degenerative changes.

Diagnostic Procedures. Administration of potassium chloride precipitates attack. *Blood.* Serum potassium normal during and between attacks. Occasionally hypocalcemia during attacks. *Electromyography.*

Therapy. If mild, no treatment required. In severe attacks calcium gluconate may restore power; if unsuccessful, glucose plus insulin and chlorothiazide must be tried. Continuous use of diuretics (chlorothiazide) prevents attacks; if myotonic symptoms prevail: procainamide or phenytoin are beneficial.

Prognosis. Chronic recurrent condition. Some patients develop polymyopathy with persistent weakness.

BIBLIOGRAPHY. Von Eulenberg A: Ueber eine familiare, durch 6 Generationen Verfolgbare. Form Kongenitaler Paramyotonic. Neurol Zentralbl 5:265–272, 1886
Poskauzer DC, Kerr DNS: A third type of periodic paralysis with normokalemia and favorable response to sodium chloride. Am J Med 31:328–342, 1961
Adams RD, Victor M: Principles of Neurology, 3rd ed, p 1087. New York, McGraw-Hill, 1985

VON GIERKE'S

Synonyms. Cori's type I glycogenosis; glucose 6-phosphate deficiency; glycogen storage (type I); glycogenosis (type I); Gierke's; hepatorenal glycogenosis; hepatonephromegalia glycogenica; von Creveld-von Gierke.

Symptoms. Both sexes affected; clinical onset during first year of life. Convulsion (hypoglycemic); failure to thrive. Bleeding tendency. Epistaxis; oozing after surgery. Occasionally, steatorrhea.

Signs. Retarded growth without disproportion, lumbar lordosis; adiposity; skin yellowish xanthomas over joints and buttocks. Large abdomen; marked hepatomegaly; no spleen enlargement. Kidney enlarged. Bilateral, symmetric, yellow paramacular lesions of eye fundus. Gout-related signs.

Etiology. Deficiency of glucose 6-phosphatase. Autosomal recessive inheritance.

Pathology. Accumulation of glycogen in various tissues. Liver becomes markedly enlarged and kidneys are particularly involved.

Diagnostic Procedures. *Blood.* Mild anemia; marked hypoglycemia; marked hyperglyceridemia; hypercholesterolemia; increase of fatty acids; acetonemia; hyperuricemia; low serum phosphate; normal alkaline phosphatases. *Urine.* Acetonuria; glucosuria; occasionally, aminoaciduria. *Biopsy of liver.*

Therapy. Correction of hypoglycemia (multiple feedings day and night). Prevention of acidosis and infections. L-Thyroxine-glucagon. Good results with portal diversions, portocaval shunting, and liver transplantation.

Prognosis. Poor. If treated and death is prevented for 4 years, disease becomes less severe.

BIBLIOGRAPHY. von Gierke E: Hepato-Nephromegalia glykogenica (Glykogenspeicherkrankheit der Leber und Nieren). Beitr Pathol Anat 82:497–513, 1929
Howell RR, Williams JC: The glycogen storage diseases. In Stanbury JB, Wyngaarden JB, Fredrickson DS, et al: The Metabolic Basis of Inherited Disease. 5th ed, p 141. New York, McGraw-Hill, 1983

VON HERRENSCHWAND'S

Synonyms. Herrenschwand's; Passow's; sympathetic heterochromia. See also Fuch's III.

Symptoms and Signs. Hemifacial decreased sweating; enophthalmos; ptosis; heterochromia (unilateral iris): myosis.

Etiology. Represents the combination of heterochromia and Horner's. May be caused by sympathetic palsy (traumatic, surgical, or due to secondary infections), or transmitted as irregular autosomal dominant trait. Associated also with other syndromes: Waarderburg's; Marfan's, etc.

Pathology. See Horner's.

Diagnostic Procedures. Differential diagnosis with Fuch's III: typical architecture and trabeculae of deeper iris layers remain well outlined.

Therapy. Once the cause is found the same as in Horner's.

Prognosis. According to etiology.

BIBLIOGRAPHY. von Herrenschwand F: Ueber verschiedene Arten von Heterochromia iridis. Klin Monatsbl Augenheilkd 60:467–494, 1918
Gladstone RM: Development of significance of heterochromia of the iris. Arch Neurol 21:184–192, 1969

VON HIPPEL–LINDAU

Synonyms. Angiomatosis retinae; cerebello retina angiomatosis; hemoangioblastomatosis cerebello retinae; Hippel's; Hippel–Czermak; Lindau–von Hippel; retinocerebello angiomatosis.

Symptoms. Onset in young adulthood. Headache; dizziness; unilateral ataxia; mental changes; blindness.

Signs. In eyes, tortuous aneurysms of retinal vessels, exudates on fundus, subretinal yellowish spot.

Etiology. Unknown; autosomal dominant inheritance.

Pathology. *Brain.* Cystic, hemorrhagic lesion in lateral lobes of cerebellum with mural nodules; vascular epithelialized channels; foamy fat cells. *Retina.* Subretinal hemorrhages; aneurysm with dilatation and tortuosity of vessels; destruction of nerve elements. Frequently associated, simple renal cyst or renal carcinoma, pancreatic cysts, and solid or cystic tumors of epididymis; pheochromocytoma.

Diagnostic Procedures. *Spinal tap.* Increased in pressure. *Angiography. Brain isotope scan. CT scan. Blood.* Polycythemia. *Ophthalmoscopy.* Papilledema.

Therapy. Photocoagulation; cryotherapy of retinal lesions. Neurosurgery; aspiration of cyst and removal of nodules.

Prognosis. Blindness; permanent brain damage.

BIBLIOGRAPHY. von Hippel E: Vorstellung eines Patienten mit einem sehr ungewöhnlichen Aderhautleiden. Bericht 24 Versammlung Ophthalmol Ges. 269, 1895
Lindau A: Studien über Kleinhincysten. Acta Pathol Microbiol Scand [suppl] 1–128, 1926
Chomette G, Auriol M: Classification des angiodysplasias et tumeurs vasculaires. Rev Stom Clin Maxillo Fac 87:1–5, 1986

VON MIKULICZ'S

Synonyms. Dacryosialoadenopathy; Mikulicz–Sjögren; Mikulicz–Radecki; Mikulicz's.

Symptoms. Dryness of mouth and absent or decreased lacrimation; vision blurring.

Signs. Symmetric, painless, hard tumefactions of lacrimal and salivary glands, gradually progressing.

Etiology. Lymphoid leukemia; lymphomas; sarcoidosis; tuberculosis; syphilis; idiopathic; associated with thiouracil treatment; familial possible.

Pathology. Atrophy of acinar parenchyma and replacement with lymphoid cells.

Diagnostic Procedures. *Blood.* For diagnosis of leukemia. *Bone marrow. X-ray of chest. Sputum.* Smear and culture. *Mantoux skin test. Kveim's test. Serology. Sialography.*

Therapy. According to etiology: roentgen; chemotherapy; corticoids; antibiotics.

Prognosis. That of primary condition. Remissions and relapses or cure of the syndrome may be observed according to the response to the specific treatment.

BIBLIOGRAPHY. von Mikulicz J: Ueber eine eigenartige symmetrische Erkrankung der Tränen und Mundspeicheldrüsen. Beitr Chir Fortschr Gewidmet, Stuttgart, Theodor Billroth, pp 610–630, 1892
von Mikulicz J: Concerning a peculiar symmetrical disease of the lacrimal and salivary glands. Med Classics 2:165–186, 1937
Rubin P, Besse BE Jr: The sialographic differentiation of Mikulicz's disease and Mikulicz's syndrome. Radiology 68:477–487, 1957

VON RECKLINGHAUSEN'S I

Synonyms. Neurofibromatosis, NF1; Recklinghausen's phakomatosis; Recklinghausen's I;

Symptoms. Onset in childhood; becomes more active at puberty, during pregnancy, and at menopause. Asymptomatic or pain when tumor produces pressure on adjacent structures. Occasionally, mental retardation, cretinism, and growth abnormalities; delay in sexual development; spontaneous fractures; hemifacial hypertrophy.

Signs. *Café au lait* skin pigmentation. Multiple tumors of different consistencies along the course of cutaneous nerves; kyphoscoliosis; acromegaly. Occasionally (not rarely), proptosis, ptosis, ocular muscle palsy, unilateral hydrophthalmos, optic atrophy.

Etiology. Unknown; congenital autosomal dominant inheritance. In some families or in isolated cases, male linkage and recessive inheritance.

Prognosis. Benign tumor (fibroma mollusca) arising from covering cells of peripheral nervous system; tumor of meninges, optic (II) nerve, and central nervous system frequent. Osteodysgenesis; subperiosteal tumors. Possible association with gliomatous tumors of brain or spinal cord.

Diagnostic Procedures. *Biopsy. Electroencephalography. Brain scan. X-ray of skeleton.*

Therapy. Removal of tumors that produce symptoms.

Prognosis. Tumor benign and usually does not regrow after removal. Prognosis depends on ocular and central nervous system involvement. Malignant change (5–10%) mostly in males.

BIBLIOGRAPHY. von Recklinghausen FD: Ueber die multiplen Fibrome der Haut und ihre Beziehung zu den multiplen Neuromen. Festschr. Feier Funfundzwanzigjahrigen Best Pathol Inst Berlin. Berlin, A. Hirschwald, 1882

Riccardi VM, Eichner JE: Neurofibromatosis: Phenotype, Natural History and Pathogenesis. Baltimore, Johns Hopkins, University Press, 1986

Crozier WC: Upper airway obstruction in neurofibromatosis. Anaesthesia 42:1209–1211, 1987

VON ROKITANSKY–CUSHING

Synonyms. Cushing's ulcer; neurogenic gastrointestinal bleeding; Rokitansky-Cushing.

Eponym used to indicate the gastrointestinal hemorrhagic complication arising after head injury or neurosurgery. See Curling's ulcer.

BIBLIOGRAPHY. Von Rokitansky CV: Handbuch der pathologischen Anatomie kien Braumueller-Seidel, Vol 8, 1842

Cushing H: Peptic ulcers and the interbrain. Surg Gynecol Obstet 55:1–34, 1932

VON ROKITANSKY'S

Synonyms. Corrected great arteries transposition; Rokitansky's II.

Symptoms. Male predominance. Pure defect (rare). Asymptomatic.

Signs. Second sound accentuated at left of sternum.

Etiology. Congenital heart defect.

Pathology. Mirror images of atrioventricular valves (resembling normal contralateral valves); aorta arises from a morphologic right ventricle and pulmonary trunk arises from a morphologic left ventricle. Common associated condition (80%): ventricular septal defect.

Diagnostic Procedures. *Electrocardiography.* Left ventricular hypertrophy; prolonged P-R interval; in lead I, high P waves; II or III heart block. *Angiocardiography.* Pulmonary main artery medial to aorta; right ventricle smooth outline. *Cardiac catheterization. Echocardiography.*

Therapy. Surgical approach and correction of associated defects are dictated by anatomic reversal of ventricles and conduction system.

Prognosis. Normal survival (in pure form); some patients may, however, develop "spontaneous" heart failure.

BIBLIOGRAPHY. Von Rokitansky KF: Die Defecte der Scheidewande des Hertzens. Vienna, W Braumiller, 1875

Perloff JK: The Clinical Recognition of Congenital Heart Disease, 2nd ed, p 57. Philadelphia, WB Saunders, 1978

Hurst JW: The Heart, 6th ed, pp 700–703. New York, McGraw-Hill, 1986

VON SALLMAN–PATON–WITKOP

Synonyms. Intraepithelial benign hereditary dyskeratosis, HBID; Sallman's. Witkop–von Sallman.

Symptoms. Both sexes affected; onset in infancy or childhood, progressing to adolescence. Photophobia; lacrimation, especially in the summer months.

Signs. Eye, oral, and labial mucosae smooth; opalescent plaques; thicker lesions folded (see Cannon's). Eyes small; pingueculae or foamy gelatinous plaques over conjunctiva.

Etiology. Unknown; autosomal dominant inheritance.

Pathology. Acanthosis; vacuolated cells; eosinophilic cells; parakeratosis and hyperkeratosis.

Diagnostic Procedures. *Biopsy. Conjunctival cell smears.* Presence of waxy eosinophilic cells and "cell within cell" pattern.

Therapy. None.

Prognosis. Lesions progress to adolescence, then remain stable. Benign condition.

BIBLIOGRAPHY. Witkop CJ Jr, Shankle CH, Graham JB et al: Hereditary benign intraepithelial dyskeratosis. Arch Pathol 70:696–711, 1960

Von Sallman L, Paton D: Hereditary benign intraepithelial dyskeratosis. Arch Ophthalmol 63:421–429, 1960

Yanoff M: Hereditary benign intra-epithelial dyskeratosis. Arch Ophthalmol 79:291–293, 1968

McLean IW et al. Hereditary benign intraepithelial dyskeratosis. Ophthal 88:164–168, 1981

VON WILLEBRAND

Synonyms. Angiohemophilia; vascular hemophilia; Minot–von Willebrand; pseudohemophilia; constitutional thrombopathy.

Symptoms. Frequency per million, 5–10. Both sexes affected, more frequent in women. Onset usually in early childhood. Manifestation of the bleeding among affected individuals extremely variable in intensity. Bleeding tendency; easy bruising; epistaxis; bleeding from gums and female genitalia; occasionally, also from urinary and gastrointestinal tracts. Hemathrosis rare. Inconstant, prolonged bleeding from trauma or surgery.

Etiology. Autosomal dominant transmission with variable penetrance and expressivity; 70 to 90% autosomal dominant, the rest autosomal recessive. Certain families have both kinds of transmission, indicating a double heterozygosity. Reduction of von Willebrand factor (vWF) or anomalies; reduction of factor VIII. According to the deficit, various forms have been described:
Type I. Concomitant reduction of all activities of factor VIII and vWF. Autosomal dominant or double heterozygotes.
Type II. Discordant reduction of elements of factor VIII and vWF. Factor VIII C or factor VIII R : Ag are normal or high while vWF is low. Autosomal dominant or recessive inheritance.

Diagnostic Procedures. In full expression, morphologic and functional alteration of platelets and deficiency of factor VIII; however, any combination of these abnormalities may be observed. Usually the following pattern is observed: tourniquet test usually normal; bleeding time may be prolonged; partial thromboplastin time (PPT), and clotting time pathologic; prothrombin consumption impaired; thromboplastin generation test (TGT) plasma defect; thrombin and prothrombin time normal; vWF decreased (75% of cases) or normal (25%); ristocetine platelet aggregation decreased.

Therapy. Whole blood, plasma, or plasma fraction containing factor VIII. New synthesis of factor VIII seems to follow transfusion. Fresh frozen plasma, cryoprecipitate; DDAVP (only in mild cases). In women sex hormones to ameliorate menometrorrhagias.

Prognosis. Severity of bleeding tendency decreases with age and during pregnancy.

BIBLIOGRAPHY. Von Willebrand EA, Jürgen R: Ueber eine neue vererbbares Bluterkrenkheit; Die konstitutionelle Thrombopathie. Dtsch Arch Klin Med 175:453–483, 1933
Minot GR: Familial hemorrhagic condition associated with prolongation of bleeding time. Am J Med Sci 175:301–306, 1928
Von Willebrand EA: Hereditary pseudohemofilia; description; previously observed cases. Finska LakSallsk Handl 68:87–112, 1926
Zimmermann TS, Ruggieri ZM: Von Willebrand's disease. Clin Haemat 12:175–200, 1983

Weiss JH, Pietu G, Rabinowitz R et al: Heterogenous abnormalities in the multimeric structure, antigenic properties, and plasma-platelet content of factor VIII von Willebrand factor in subtypes of classic (type I) and variant (type II A) von Willebrand disease. J Lab Clin Med 101:411–425, 1983

VOODOO DEATH

Synonyms. Curse death; wish dying.

Symptoms. Occur in African and West Indian societies, particularly in Haiti. Short, ritual-induced hysterical states; convulsions; twilight states; excitement. Voodoo death in people who, believing they are under magic spells, die.

Etiology. Unknown. Explanation for voodoo death: state of hopeless resignation that through sympathetic or parasympathetic imbalance reduces resistance to shock (?). Possibility of poisoning, organic illness, or refusal of food or water must be considered.

BIBLIOGRAPHY. Richter CP: On the phenomenon of sudden death in animals and men. Psychosomat Med 19:191–198, 1967
Freedman AM, Kaplan HI: Comprehensive Textbook of Psychiatry, 2nd ed, p 1732. Baltimore, Williams & Wilkins, 1975

VOORHOEVE'S

Synonym. Osteopathia striata.

Symptoms and Signs. Asymptomatic. Radiologic syndrome.

Etiology. Unknown. Condition differs from osteoporosis, Engelmann's, Ribbing's, and other bone affections since only cancellous bone is involved. Occurs as a feature in Goltz's, in Pierre Robin's (see), and in two specific syndromes; osteopathia striata-cranial stenosis (see) and osteopathia striata-pigmentary dermopathy (see).

Diagnostic Procedures. X-ray. Multiple condensations of cancellous bone tissue, beginning at the epiphyseal line and extending into diaphysis. Any of long bones may be involved; in the ilium "sunburst" aspect around acetabulum.

BIBLIOGRAPHY. Voorhoeve N: L'image radiologique non encore décrite d'un anomalie du squelette. Les rapports avec la dyschondroplasie et l'osteopathia condensans disseminata. Acta Radiol (Stockh) 3:407–427, 1924

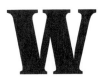

W

Synonym. Pallister's W.

Symptoms. Mental retardation; seizures.

Signs. *Facies.* Frontal bossing; hypertelorism; antimongoloid palpebral fissures; broad, flat nose bridge; notch of upper lip and submucous cleft of hard palate; absence of upper incisors. *Limbs.* Subluxation of elbow; camptodactyly; pes cavus.

Etiology. Unknown; X-linked trait.

BIBLIOGRAPHY. Pallister PD, Hermann J, Springer JW et al: The W syndrome. Birth Defects Orig Art Ser X (7):51–60, 1974

WAARDENBURG'S

Synonyms. Embryonic fixation; interoculoiridodermatoauditory dysplasia; Klein-Waardenburg; Mende's; ptosis-epicanthus; Van der Hoeve–Halberstam–Gualdi. Including Fisch-Renwick. See Albinism syndromes and Meesmann's (possibly the same).

Symptoms. No sex preference; reported in all ethnic groups. Complete form rare; various combinations of various characteristics (*forme fruste* or incomplete found in different members of affected families). Evident at birth. Deafness (in 20% of cases).

Signs. The syndrome has been divided into type WS1 with dystopia canthorum and type WS2 without dystopia and with higher frequency of deafness; there is also a WS III (see Klein-Waardenburg), and a pseudo Waardenburg's with unilateral congenital ptosis and without dystopia canthorum. *Other signs.* High nose bridge (78%); hypertrichosis of the eyebrows tending to join at midline (45%); hypopigmentation and hypoplasia of iris stroma in one or both eyes (25%); median white forelock of varying size, from a few hairs to obvious large forelock (17%) (this sign may be evident at birth and disappear during first year of life, or begin after puberty). Some patients may also present white patches of the skin or areas of increased pigmentation.

Etiology. Unknown; congenital familial ectodermal dysplasia; autosomal dominant transmission.

Pathology. Not many reports; examination of auditory pathway in one case with deafness revealed absence of Corti's organ and atrophy of spiral ganglion and nerve.

Diagnostic Procedures. *Chromosome studies.* Normal. No biochemical (blood, urine) abnormalities.

Therapy. Eye surgery for cosmetic reason and epiphora.

Prognosis. Good *quoad vitam.*

BIBLIOGRAPHY. Van der Breggen FA: Een familiare oogafwijking en een aangeboren symmetrische misvorming van handen en voeten. Ned Tijdschr Geneeskd 59:1874–1876, 1915
Van der Hoeve J: Abnorme Länge der Tränenrohrchen mit Ankyloblepharon. Klin Monatsbl Augenheilkd 56:232; 238, 1916
Klein D: Albinisme partial (leucism) avec surdimutité, blépharophimosis ey dysplasie myo-ostéo-articulaire. Helv Paediatr Acta 5:38–58, 1950
Waardenburg PJ: A new syndrome combining developmental anomalies of the eyelids, eyebrows and nose root with pigmentary defects of the iris and head and with congenital deafness. Am J Hum Genet 3:195–253, 1951
Goodman RN, Lewithal I, Solomon A et al: Upper limb involvement in the Klein-Waardenburg syndrome. Am J Med Genet 11:425–433, 1982
Nork TM, Shihab ZM, Young RSL, and Price J: Pigment distribution in Waardenburg's syndrome: a new hypothesis. Graefe's Arch Clin Exp Ophthalmol 224:487–492, 1986

WAARDENBURG-JONKERS

Synonyms. Corneal dystrophy; Waardenburg-Jonkers.

Symptoms. Both sexes affected; present from 1st year of life. Eye irritation episodes; progressive vision reduction, and reduction of corneal sensibility.

Signs. Cornea stroma shows multiple opacities similar to snowflakes or hailstones that increase with age in number to involve the epithelium.

Etiology. Autosomal dominant inheritance.

Therapy. Corneal transplantation.

Prognosis. Progressive vision loss.

BIBLIOGRAPHY. Waardenburg PJ, Jonkers GA: A specific type of dominant progressive dystrophy of the cornea developing after birth. Acta Ophthalmol (Copenh). 39:919–923, 1961

WADIA'S

Synonym. Cerebellar degeneration-slow eye movement. See Jervis's.

Symptoms and Signs. Described in India and the United States. Manifestations of spinocerebellar degeneration plus abnormal eye movements: absent scanning, and slow tracking. Progressive mental deterioration.

Etiology. Unknown. Cerebellar degeneration and possibly also paramedian pontine reticular formation.

BIBLIOGRAPHY. Wadia NH, Swami RK: A new form of heredo-familial spinocerebellar degeneration with slow eye movements. (nine families). Brain 94:359–374, 1971
Starkman S, Kaul S, Fried J, et al: Unusual abnormal eye movements in a family with hereditary spino-cerebellar degeneration. Neurology 22:402, 1972

WAGENER-KEITH

Obsolete eponym used to indicate the symptom complex: headache; monoplegia or hemiplegia; seizures; variable degree of visual impairment; asthenia; dyspnea and peripheral edemas associated with blood hypertension.

BIBLIOGRAPHY. Wagener HP, Keith NM: Cases of marked hypertension, adequate renal function and neuroretinitis. Arch Intern Med 34:374–387, 1924

WAGNER'S

Synonyms. Cervenka's; clefting; hyaloid-retina degeneration-palatoschisis; David-Stickler's; Stickler's. See Favre and Marshall's.

Symptoms. Both sexes affected; onset variable according to presence or development of findings. Loss of visual acuity. In 2nd decade, myopia, scotomas.

Signs. *Facies.* Anomalies; hypoplastic maxilla; saddle nose; palatoschisis. Epicanthus. *Eyes.* Nystagmus; abnormal anterior chamber angle; iris atrophy; vitreous degeneration with streaks in posterior hyaloid membrane; cataract; keratopathy. *Extremities.* Joint hyperextensibility (finger, elbow, knee); tapering fingers; genu valga; hip deformities; talipes equinovarus.

Etiology. Irregular dominant inheritance with variable expression.

Diagnostic Procedures. *X-ray of skeleton.* See Signs. *Ophthalmoscopy.* Various types of retinal degeneration (after 19 years of age); choroidal sclerosis, pseudoedema, and pale optic disk.

Therapy. Symptomatic.

Prognosis. Poor. Frequently, death before full syndrome becomes manifest.

BIBLIOGRAPHY. Wagner H: Ein bisher unberkauntes Erbleiden des Auges (Degeneratio hyaloideo-retinalis hereditaria), beobachtet in Kanton Zuerich. Klin Monatsbl Augenheilkd 100:840–857, 1938
Daniel R, Kanski JJ, Claaspool MG: Hyalo-retinopathy in the clefting syndrome. Br J Ophthalmol 58:96–102, 1974
Libergarb RM, Hirose T, Holmes LB: The Wagner-Stickler syndrome: a study of 22 families. J Pediatr 99:394–399, 1981

WAGNER-UNVERRICHT

Synonyms. Dermatomyositis; dermatomucomyositis; neuromyositis; polymyositis gregarina.

Symptoms. Prevalent in females (2 : 1); onset in infancy rare, in childhood usually before 10 years; in adult, predominant in 4th to 6th decades. Variable symptoms according to prevalent skin or muscular involvement. Malaise; fever; weakness. Erythematous rash; edema of eyelids and periorbital. Erythema usually involves face, forearms, upper back. Hands present scaly reddish plaques, especially periungually and over back of joints. Visible capillary loops under nail. When acute phase fades, telangiectatic erythema and pigmentation or depigmentation remains. Other types of skin lesions occasionally seen: bullous urticaria, erythema nodosum, or multiforme type, hypertrichosis. Muscle weakness, especially shoulder and pelvic girdles; difficulty in swallowing; respiratory difficulty; tachycardia (in 30% of cases).

Etiology. Unknown; possibly, autoimmune mechanism; association with neoplastic disease (15–20% of adult cases).

Pathology. In skin lesion, lymphocytic infiltration, perivascular or in clusters (histiocytes, plasma cells, and eosinophils may be present). Later, homogenization and sclerosis of collagen leading to atrophic changes. Calcification occasionally seen. Muscle involvement frequently localized (seen on biopsy of affected muscles): paleness; flabbiness; fibrosis; calcification according to stage. Vacuolar degeneration of fibers; lymphocytic infiltration. In blood vessels, eosinophilic thickening and thrombosis.

Diagnostic Procedures. *Biopsy of skin and muscle. Blood.* Serum glutamic-oxaloacetic transaminase (SGOT) elevated; sedimentation rate slightly elevated; lupus erythematosus (L.E.) test negative. *X-ray.* Skin and muscle calcification; search for malignancy. *Electrocardiography. Electromyography.*

Therapy. If malignancy, surgery or chemotherapy. Rest in acute phase. Corticosteroids (high doses, then maintenance). Physical therapy to prevent contracture.

Prognosis. In fulminating cases (20%), death during first year. In children 5 to 16 years survival (75%). Removal of cancer may cure dermatomyositis. In chronic forms, survival variable from 2 to several years. Death from respiratory infections, malnutrition, cardiac failure.

BIBLIOGRAPHY. Wagner E: Fall Einer Seltener Muskelkrank-Heit. Arch Theilk 4:282–283, 1863
Unverricht H: Ueber eine eigentnemliche Form von akuten Muskelentzuendung mit einem der Trichinose aehnelden. Krankheitsbilde Munch Med Wochenschr 4:488–492, 1887
Rook A, Wilkinson DS, Ebling FJG et al: Textbook of Dermatology, 4th ed, pp 1376–1388. Oxford, Blackwell Scientific Publications, 1986

WALDENSTRÖM'S II

Synonym. Primary macroglobulinemia.

Symptoms. More common in males; onset in 6th and 7th decades. Lassitude; weakness; weight loss; frequent infections; visual troubles (often first chief complaint); hemorrhagic manifestation (see Raynaud's syndrome).

Signs. Pallor; microlymphadenopathy; hepatosplenomegaly (variable), fundus oculi, hemorrhagic lesions.

Etiology. Unknown. Primary plasma cell dyscrasia. Genetic predisposition and role of various inflammatory and nonreticular neoplasms discussed. To be differentiated from a stable gamma globulin production abnormality; gammopathy, benign monoclonal. A genetic basis (autosomal dominant) reported in some families.

Pathology. Hemorrhagic lesions. In bone marrow, presence of small atypical lymphomonocytoid cells, increase of mast cells.

Diagnostic Procedures. *Blood.* Anemia; leukopenia; thrombocytopenia. Rouleau formation; Sia test and formol-gel test positive. High sedimentation rate; in some varieties (macrocryogel globulins) low sedimentation rate. Increased serum viscosity and presence of cold agglutinin. Electrophoresis demonstration of homogeneous typical protein fraction in globulin zone (more frequently in gamma zone). Ultracentrifugation of protein, demonstration of macroglobulin: IgM sedimentation 19S and other fractions more rapidly sediment. *Bone marrow.* In-

filtration by abnormal lymphoid cells; demonstration by immunofluorescence of monoclonal IgM on their cytoplasm and surface. *Urine.* Bence-Jones protein in some cases.

Therapy. Chlorambucil; cyclophosphamide, penicillamine; plasmapheresis; corticosteroids. In secondary form, specific treatment.

Prognosis. Poor; progressive condition with death in months or years.

BIBLIOGRAPHY. Waldenström J: Incipient myelomatosis or "essential" hyperglobulinemia with fibrinogenopenia—a new syndrome? Acta Med Scand 117:216–247, 1944
O'Reilly RA, MacKenzie MR: Primary macrocryoglobulinemia. Remission with adrenal corticosteroid therapy. Arch Intern Med 120:234–238, 1967
Wintrobe MM (ed): Clinical hematology, 8th ed. pp 1419–1420. Philadelphia, Lea & Febiger, 1981
San Roman C, Ferro T, Guzman N et al: Clonal abnormalities in patients with Waldenström's macroglobulinemia with special reference to a Burkitt-type (8; 14). Cancer Genet Cytogenet 18:155–158, 1985

WALDENSTRÖM'S III

Synonyms. Acute thyrotoxic encephalopathy; thyroid storm.

Symptoms. Occur in patients affected by Flajani's syndrome (see); onset usually in advanced age. The crisis is precipitated by various medical, surgical, or metabolic factors. Severe vomiting; diarrhea; rapid weight loss; fever that is slightly elevated at onset and that rapidly rises to extreme values; severe dyspnea. This variety of thyrotoxic storm is characterized by a neurologic component represented by dysphagia, dysphonia, labioglossopharyngeal paralysis, oculomotor paralysis; choreiform movements, and transitory palsies.

Signs. Those of Flajani's (see).

Etiology. Excessive production of thyroid hormones and particular sensitivity of central nervous system and peripheral nervous system.

Diagnostic Procedures. See Flajani's syndrome.

Therapy. *It is a major medical emergency* and needs intensive treatment and continuous monitoring of vital functions. Methymazole (15 mg every 6 hours) orally or parenterally. Propylthiuracil (150 to 250 mg every 6 hours) 1 hour after the administration of one of the above mentioned drugs. Sedation; oxygen; digitalization; rehydration; cooling by physical means (mattress); antibiotics; if hypoadrenalism suspected, hydrocortisone (100–200 mg) or equivalent must be given before initiating the specific (above mentioned) treatment. Other useful drugs are reserpine or guanethidine (every 8 hours), propanolol (every 6 hours).

Prognosis. Severe; may be improved by the above mentioned treatment, which brings the crisis under control.

BIBLIOGRAPHY. Waldenström J: Acute thyrotoxic encephalo or myopathy, its cause and treatment. Acta Med Scand 121:251–294, 1945
Mackin JF, Canary JJ, Pittman CS: Thyroid storm and its management. N Engl J Med 29:1396–1398, 1974
Mazzaferri EL: The thyroid. In Mazzaferri EL (ed.) Textbook of Endocrinology, 3rd ed, pp 207–209. New York, Medical Examination Publishing, 1985
Toft AD (ed). Hyperthyroidism (Symposium). Clin Endocrinol Metab (whole issue), 1985

WALDENSTRÖM-UVEOPAROTITIS

Synonym. Waldenström's uveoparotitis. See also Heerfordt's.

Symptoms and Signs. Variety of Heerfordt's (see), with addition of hallucinatory manifestations, lethargy, peripheral polyneuritis, areflexia of patella and Achilles' tendon. Babinski's sign.

Etiology. See Heerfordt's.

BIBLIOGRAPHY. Waldenström J: Some observations on uveoparotitis and allied conditions with special references to the symptoms from the nervous system. Acta Med Scand 91:53–68, 1937

WALKER–CLODIUS

Synonyms. EEC; ectrodactyly–ectodermal dysplasia–clefting; lobster claw deformity–nasolacrimal obstruction; Walker-Clodius; Rosselli's.

Symptoms. Both sexes affected; onset from birth. Photophobia.

Signs. *Facies.* Hypertelorism; constant epiphora; mucopurulent conjunctival discharge; cleft palate and lips. Partial anodontia, microdontia. *Extremities.* Deformities of hands: syndactyly; absence of 2nd metacarpal of index and middle finger; and rudimentary 3rd metacarpal of same digits; and feet: absence of 1st and 5th metacarpal and occasionally of the toe; mild nail dysplasia. Hair sparse, thin, light colored. Occasionally: deafness; ear malformation; renal anomalies.

Etiology. Autosomal dominant inheritance.

Therapy. Surgery.

Prognosis. Good *quoad vitam*.

BIBLIOGRAPHY. Rosselli D, Giulienetti R: Ectodermal dysplasia. Br J Plas Surg 14:190–204, 1961.
Walker JC, Clodius L: The syndrome of cleft lip, cleft palate and lobster claw deformities of hand and feet. Plast Reconstr Surg 32:627–636, 1963
Preus M, Fraser FC: The lobster claw defect with ectodermal defects, cleft lip-palate, tear duct anomaly and renal anomalies. Clin Genet 4:369–377, 1973
Kuster W, Majewski F, Meinecke P: EEC syndrome without ectrodactyly? Report of 8 cases. Clin Genet 28:130–135, 1985

WALLENBERG'S

Synonyms. Posteroinferior cerebellar artery; cerebellar peduncle; dorsolateral medullary; lateral bulbar; lateral medullary; Vieseaux-Wallenberg.

Symptoms. Occur usually in patients over 40 years of age. Sudden or gradual onset. Vertigo; vomiting; hiccup; dysphagia; diplopia, ipsilateral course; ataxia; pain or analgesia; loss of temperature sensitivity ipsilateral side of the face; contralateral hypoesthesia for pain and temperature of extremities and trunk. Seldom, contralateral hemiparesis.

Signs. Ipsilateral enophthalmos; ptosis; coarse nystagmus; loss of corneal reflex; miosis; lack of coordination; ipsilateral hypotonia; ipsilateral paralysis soft palate, pharynx, vocal cord.

Etiology. Thrombosis of posterior inferior cerebellar or vertebral artery or both. Arteriosclerotic vascular disease, syphilis, and other types of occlusive disease.

Pathology. Infarction of lateral medulla, inferior part of cerebellum, spinal tract, nucleus ambiguous, restiform body, vestibular nucleus.

Diagnostic Procedures. *Spinal tap. Electroencephalography. Angiography. CT Scan.*

Therapy. Anticoagulant.

Prognosis. Symptoms may disappear abruptly; complete recovery usually in months. Facial neuralgia, crossed neuralgia of extremities and trunk persist for a longer time.

BIBLIOGRAPHY. Wallenberg A: Acute bulbäraffection (Embolie der Art. Cerebellar post, inf. sinstr. ?). Arch Psychiatry 27:504–540, 1895
Hoernsten G: Wallenberg's syndrome. I. General symptomatology with reference to visual disturbance and imbalance. Acta Neurol Scand 50:834–846, 1974
Adams RD, Victor M: Principles of Neurology, 3rd ed, p 587. New York, McGraw-Hill, 1985

WALTER-BOHMANN'S

Eponym reported to indicate symptoms complex occurring after cholecystectomy or cholecystoduodenostomy: pallor; cold sweat; hypothermia; tachycardia and polypnea (see Postcholecystectomy).

BIBLIOGRAPHY. Akel S: Kolesistektomiden soura goeruelen bir Walter-Bohmann syndrom V. Tuerk tip Cem Mec 21:255–256, 1956
Way LW, Sleisenger MH: Postoperative syndrome. In Sleisenger MH, Fordtran JS: Gastrointestinal Disease, p 1336. Philadelphia, WB Saunders, 1978

WALTON'S

Synonyms. Benign congenital hypotonia; congenital benign muscular hypoplasia; muscular benign hypoplasia. See Floppy infant syndromes.

Symptoms. Onset in neonatal period. Extreme muscular weakness. Same symptoms as in Werdnig-Hoffmann (see), but late in developing, however, patients obtain a good range of spontaneous movements. Arms affected to a lesser degree than legs.

Signs. Reflexes may be depressed or normal; no fasciculations. Muscles extremely flabby.

Etiology. Unknown; delay of development of neuromuscular apparatus.

Pathology. *Biopsy of muscle.* Smallness of all muscle fibers; increase of connective tissue or fat, or degenerative changes.

Diagnostic Procedures. Difficult to differentiate at early stage from Werdnig-Hoffmann, except with muscle biopsy.

Therapy. Symptomatic.

Prognosis. Good; seldom persists beyond first decade. Progressive improvement. Some contortionists may have had this syndrome in infancy.

BIBLIOGRAPHY. Sobel J: Essential or primary hypotonia in young children. Med J Rec 124:225–230, 1926
Walton J: Amyotonie congenita. Lancet I:1023–1028, 1956
Zellweger H, Afifi A, McCormick WF et al: Benign congenital muscular dystrophy: a special form of congenital hypotonia. Clin Pediatr 6:544–553, 1967
Adams RD, Victor M: Principles of Neurology, 3rd ed, p 1072. New York, McGraw-Hill, 1985

WANDERING PACEMAKER

Synonyms. Atrioventricular nodal rhythm; shifting pacemaker.

Symptoms. Frequently asymptomatic. Occasionally, palpitation, choking from sensation of fullness in neck.

Signs. Bradycardia. Undue variations of 1st heart sound; irregularity may induce suspicion of presence of atrial fibrillation.

Etiology. Suppression of successive pacemakers and successive takeover by following centers. Usually, shifting back and forth between sinus and A-V nodes. In normal heart, caused by fluctuating vagal tone.

Diagnostic Procedures. *Electrocardiography.* Changes in size, shape of P waves; P-Q intervals shortened to less than 0.10 sec; rate alterations.

Therapy. None. Decrease of vagal tone.

Prognosis. Transitory phenomenon of no clinical importance.

BIBLIOGRAPHY. Hurst JW: The Heart, 6th ed, pp 468–469. New York, McGraw-Hill, 1986

WARDROP'S

Synonym. Onychia maligna.

Symptoms and Signs. Fetid ulceration of fingertips with eventual loss of nails.

Etiology. Primary or secondary infective process of nail beds.

BIBLIOGRAPHY. Wardrop H: An account of some diseases of the toes and fingers, with observation on their treatment. Med Chir Trans 5:129–143, 1814
Barak R, Dawber RPR (eds): Diseases of the Nail and Their Management. Oxford, Blackwell Scientific Publications, 1984

WATERHOUSE-FRIEDERICHSEN

Synonyms. Adrenal apoplexy; adrenal hemorrhage; Marchand-Waterhouse-Friederichsen; meningococcal adrenal; purpura meningococcemia. See Addisonian syndromes.

Symptoms. Occur usually in infants or children, occasionally in adults. Increased irritability; headache; nausea; vomiting; abdominal pain; diarrhea. Fever initially moderate, then high.

Signs. Pallor; clammy skin; cyanosis; petechial rash; neck stiffness; convulsion; dyspnea; tachycardia; hypotension; coma; dehydration; oliguria.

Etiology. In large majority of cases, meningococcemia. Seen also with other infections (diphtheria; pneumococcus; staphylococcus; smallpox).

Pathology. That of acute infection; necrosis and hemorrhage of adrenal cortex; large skin hemorrhage.

Diagnostic Procedures. *Blood.* Culture; serology; low sodium and chlorides; high potassium.

Therapy. Treatment of sepsis; control of collapse; adrenal hormone therapy.

Prognosis. Death in 24 to 48 hours if treatment not given rapidly. Permanent adrenal insufficiency not recorded in patients who survive.

BIBLIOGRAPHY. Marchand F: Ueber eine eigentümliche Erkrankung des Sympathicus, der Nebennieren der peripherischen Nerven (ohne Bronzehaut). Virchows Arch [Pathol] 81:477–502, 1880

Waterhouse R: A case of suprarenal apoplexy. Lancet I:577–578, 1911

Friederichsen C: Nebeunieren-apoplexie bei Kleinen Kinderh. Jahrb Kinderheilkd 87:109–125, 1918

Burke CW: Adrenocortical insufficiency. Clin Endocrinol Med 14:947–976, 1985

WATER INTOXICATION

Synonyms. Dilution; overhydration. See Hyponatremia and Schwartz-Bartter syndromes.

Symptoms. *Chronic type.* Slow accumulation of water; weakness; sleepiness; apathy; anorexia; nausea; vomiting; sialorrhea; lacrimation; watery diarrhea; perspiration not excessive; progression to behavioral changes, seizures, and coma. *Acute type.* Decreased attention; strange behavior; confusion; aphasia; incoordination; apathy alternated with violent behavior; marked muscle weakness.

Signs. Skin warm, moist; pitting edema. Muscle twitching; tendon hyporeflexia; Babinski's sign (later). Hemiplegia may develop. Signs of pulmonary edema, especially if heart condition preexists.

Etiology. Administration of water in excess of kidney excretion capacity. Psychogenic water drinker. Usually iatrogenic excessive water administration, especially in patients with excessive antidiuretic hormone (ADH) secretion, in postoperative stage with low renal blood flow, or with Addisonian syndromes (see), acute renal insufficiency, congestive heart failure. May occur from large enema in hyponatremic patients, and in infants with megacolon.

Diagnostic Procedures. *Blood.* Hemoglobin, hematocrit decreased; macrocytosis with decrease of mean hemoglobin concentration. Sodium low; potassium low, normal or high in severe form. Blood urea nitrogen normal, or low (except if previously increased). Bicarbonates low. *Urine.* Volume variable; specific gravity low; sodium and chloride low or normal.

Therapy. *Acute treatment.* Initiate and maintain rapid diuresis with IV furosemide; replace the sodium and potassium lost in urine (3% saline seldom required). *Chronic treatment.* Restrict water; discontinue hypotonic solutions; administer demeclocycline, furosemide.

Prognosis. Guarded. Varies in accordance with the etiology and the general fitness of the patient.

BIBLIOGRAPHY. Goldberger E: A Primer of Water, Electrolyte, and Acid-base Syndromes, 3rd ed. Philadelphia, Lea & Febiger, 1965

Brenner BM, Rector FC: The Kidney, 3rd ed, p 444. Philadelphia, WB Saunders, 1986

Berl T: Psychosis and water balance. N Engl J Med 318(7):441–442, 1988

WATSON-MILLER

Synonyms. Hepatofacial-neurocardiac-vertebral; hepatic ductal hypoplasia-multiple malformations. Alagille's; arterio-hepatic dysplasia, AHD; cholestasis-pulmonary artery stenosis.

Symptoms. Onset during first 3 months of life. Pruritus.

Signs. Prominent forehead; mongoloid slant; mild hypertelorism; straight or bulbous nose; hepatomegaly (from 3rd month); occasionally diffuse xanthomas (palms; extensor areas; creases). Harsh mesosystolic murmur. Growth and mental retardation. In males, hypogonadism.

Etiology. Unknown. Autosomal dominant inheritance.

Pathology. Liver cholestasis and inflammation; pulmonary valve and peripheral pulmonary artery stenosis.

Diagnostic Procedures. *Blood.* From 3rd month, moderate hyperbilirubinemia. From 2nd year, hypercholesterolemia and hypertriglyceridemia; depressed or absent alpha-lipoproteins and increased beta-lipoproteins. *Urine.* Dark. *Stool.* Clay colored. *Cardiac function test.* Normal. *X-rays.* Vertebral defects (spina bifida) frequent.

Therapy. Cardiosurgery may be considered according to conditions. Medical treatment of cholestasis.

Prognosis. Patients reach adult age.

BIBLIOGRAPHY. Watson GH, Miller V: Arteriohepatic dysplasia, familial pulmonary artery stenosis with neonatal liver disease. Arch Dis Child 48:459–466, 1973

Alagille D et al: Hepatic ductular hypoplasia associated with characteristic facies, vertebral malformation, retarded physical, mental and sexual development and cardiac murmur. J Pediatr 86:63–71, 1975

Alagille D, Odievre M, Gautier M et al: Hepatic ductural hypoplasia associated with characteristic facies, vertebral malformation, retarded physical, mental, and sexual development and cardiac murmur. Digest Dis Sci 26:485–497, 1981

Shulman SA, Hyams JS, Gunta R et al: Arteriohepatic dysplasia (Alagille syndrome). Am J Med Genet 19:325–332, 1984

WATSON'S

Synonyms. *Café-au-lait* spots-mental retardation-pulmonic stenosis; Pulmonic stenosis-*café au lait* spots. See Leopard.

Symptoms and Signs. Association of *café-au-lait* spots with pulmonic stenosis and mental retardation. Both sexes.

Etiology. It may represent an incomplete form of leopard syndrome. (see)

BIBLIOGRAPHY. Watson GH: Pulmonary stenosis, *café au lait* spots and dull intelligence. Arch Dis Child 42:303–307, 1967

Partington MW, Burggraf GW Jr., Fay JE et al: Pulmonary stenosis, *café au lait* spots and dull intelligence: the Watson syndrome revisited. Proc Greenwood Genet Center 4:105, 1985

WEATHERALL'S

Synonyms. Hemoglobin H disease-mental retardation; HbH with multiple congenital anomalies.

Symptoms and Signs. Rare. In North European families. From birth, mental retardation (IQ 50–70) or multiple congenital anomalies.

Etiology. Heterogenous molecular basis. Inheritance of HbH disease (see). Spontaneous mutation of loci on chromosome 16 which are near alpha globin gene cluster and codeleted may lead to mental retardation with alpha thalassemia.

Diagnostic Procedures. *Hemoglobin electrophoresis.*

Therapy. None.

Prognosis. Poor.

BIBLIOGRAPHY. Weatherall DJ, Higgs DR, Bunch C et al: Hemoglobin H disease and mental retardation: a new syndrome or a remarkable coincidence? N Engl J Med 305:607, 1981

Bowcock AM, Van Ionder S, Jenkins T: The hemoglobin H disease mental retardation syndrome: molecular studies on the South African case. Br J Haematol 56:69, 1984

WEAVER'S

Symptoms and Signs. Large birth size and accelerated growth; mild hypertonia; hoarse cry. Loose skin; thin hair. *Head.* Wide frontal area; flat occiput; hypertelorism; large ears; long philtrum; micrognathia; hoarse voice. *Extremities.* Elbow and knee reduced extension; broad distal femur and ulna; broad thumbs; camptodactyly; thin nails. Umbilical hernia.

Etiology. Sporadic. A mesenchymal defect resulting in early mineralization of the ossification centers has been suggested. Males are affected three times as frequently as females? Females may have a milder form of the syndrome.

Diagnostic Procedures. *X-rays.* Accelerated bone maturation, and splaying of distal part of long bones (femur; ulna).

Prognosis. Accelerated physical growth continuing in infancy; however, overgrowth seems to be a variable in both onset and duration.

BIBLIOGRAPHY. Weaver DD, Graham CB, Thomas IT et al: A new overgrowth syndrome with accelerated skeletal maturation, unusual facies, and camptodactyly. J Pediatr 84:547–552, 1974

Ardinger HH, Hanson JW, Harrod MJ et al: Further delineation of Weaver syndome. J Pediatr 108:228–235, 1986

WEBER-CHRISTIAN

Synonyms. Nodular nonsuppurative panniculitis; Pfeifer-Weber-Christian; spondylopanniculitis.

Symptoms. Occur in every age group; no sex dominance. Prodromal symptoms; malaise; low fever; oropharyngeal infections; mild arthralgia or arthritis.

Signs. Subcutaneous nodules of various diameters (from 1 to 12 cm) in all parts of body, more frequently on the thighs. Hands, face, and feet usually spared. Usually tender; seldom painful. Redness of overlying skin; after acute phase, pigmentation and then atrophy of skin. Nodules (seldom) rupture with extrusion of yellow fatty fluid. Splenomegaly; anterior uveitis, and acute exudative central choroiditis in some cases. Relapses frequent.

Etiology. The syndrome is probably the result of an inborn error in the regulation of the inflammatory response leading to uncontrolled fever, leukocytosis, and local inflammatory reactions directed mainly, but not exclusively, against fat.

Pathology. Early lesion: fat-laden macrophages. Larger lesion: small central area of fat necrosis with halo of lymphocytes, polymorphonuclear and macrophages. Old lesions: decrease of necrotic material and fibrotic changes. Blood vessels in the nodules usually normal; occasionally moderate vasculitic changes or thrombosis or both. Liver usually shows fatty changes and necrosis. Macrophages may be found in many organs (lymph nodes; spleen; pancreas; lung).

Diagnostic Procedures. *Blood.* During acute phase, moderate to marked leukopenia with moderate relative lymphocytosis and moderate anemia. Leukocytosis in involution phase. *Biopsy of subcutaneous node. X-ray.* Occasionally, calcification of nodules has been reported.

Therapy. Symptomatic. Corticosteroids: methylprednisolone dosages of up to 2 mg/kg 4 times a day during acute episodes of fever, pain, and pulmonary symptoms; during remissions, 0.25–0.5 mg/kg/day. Attempts to further reduce the dosage or to use alternate-day therapy have often resulted in recurrence of panniculitis.

Prognosis. Febrile period (acute) of different lengths (weeks); then spontaneous regression. Frequent relapses in months or years. Myocardosis, coronary occlusion, granulomatous pneumonitis, ileus, liver cirrhosis, myelofibrotic pancytopenia, glaucoma, and retroperitoneal fibrosis may develop as complications of this syndrome.

BIBLIOGRAPHY. Pfeifer V: Ueber einen Fall von herdweiser Atrophie des subkutanen Fettgewebes. Dtsch Arch Klin Med 50:438–449, 1892
Weber FP: A case of relapsing nonsuppurative nodular panniculitis showing phagocytosis of subcutaneous fat cells by macrophages. Br J Derm 37:301–311, 1925
Christian HA: Relapsing, febrile, nodular nonsuppurative panniculitis. Arch Intern Med 42:338–351, 1928
Sorensen R, Abramowsky C, Stern RC: Ten-year course of early-onset Weber-Christian syndrome with recurrent pneumonia: a suggestion for pathogenesis. Pediatrics 78:115–120, 1986

WEBER-COCKAYNE

Synonyms. Acanthosis bullosa; epidermolysis bullosa localized; hand-feet epidermolysis bullosa; Cockayne-Touraine. See also Fox's, Goldscheider's, and Herlitz's syndromes.

Symptoms and Signs. Both sexes affected; onset in infancy, especially in warm season. After minor trauma formation of bullae on palms and soles. Sharp pain when bullae rupture. Hyperhidrosis.

Etiology. Autosomal dominant inheritance.

Pathology. Subepidermal bullae with clear fluid; scarce or absent signs of inflammation. Elastic tissue broken or frayed.

Diagnostic Procedures. *Biopsy of skin.* See Pathology.

Therapy. Protection from trauma, especially during warm season.

Prognosis. Chronic condition.

BIBLIOGRAPHY. Elliot GT: Two cases of epidermolysis bullosa. J Cutan Genitourin Dis 13:10–18, 1895
Weber FP: Recurrent bullous eruption of the feet in a child. Proc Roy Soc Med 19:72, 1926
Cockayne EA: Recurrent bullous eruption of the feet. Br J Derm 50:358–362, 1938
Montgomery H: Dermatopathology. New York, Harper & Row 1967
Haldane JBS, Poole RA: A new pedigree of recurrent bullous eruption on the feet: four generations of foot blister. J Hered 33:17–18, 1985

WEBER-GUBLER

Synonyms. Alternating oculomotor; cerebellar peduncle; superior alternating hemiplegia; Leyden's oculomotor alternating paralysis; ventral medial midbrain; Weber's (H).

Symptoms and Signs. Ipsilateral oculomotor (III) nerve paresis; contralateral spastic paresis of lower face, tongue, and extremities. External strabismus; fixed dilated pupil; ptosis.

Etiology. Vascular occlusion of paramedian area of midbrain; parasellar aneurysm tumor.

Pathology. Hemorrhage; thrombosis of ventral part of midbrain with involvement of nucleus or oculomotor (III) nerve.

Diagnostic Procedures. *Spinal tap. Angiography. CT brain scan.*

Therapy. According to etiology.

Prognosis. Variable, usually poor.

BIBLIOGRAPHY. Weber H: A contribution to the pathology of the crura cerebri. Med Chir Tr (Lond) 46:121–139, 1863

Adams RD, Victor M: Principles of Neurology, 3rd ed, pp 582–583. New York, McGraw-Hill, 1985

WEBINO

Synonym. Wall-eyed bilateral internuclear ophthalmoplegia.

Symptoms and Signs. Distinctive disordered ocular motility of bilaterally impaired adduction and dissociated nystagmus of the abducting eye on horizontal gaze in either direction.

Etiology. The condition has been observed in demyelinating diseases, arteriosclerotic cerebrovascular disease, trauma, Arnold-Chiari malformation, syphilis, periarteritis nodosa, glioma, and cryptococcal meningitis, and lymphoma after intrathecal chemotherapy and cranial irradiation.

Diagnostic Procedures, Therapy, Prognosis. Those of the underlying disorder.

BIBLIOGRAPHY. Daroff RB, Hoyt WF: Supranuclear disorders of ocular control systems in man. In Bach YR, Rita P, Collins CC (eds): The Control of Eye Movements, p 223. New York, Academic Press, 1971
Lepore FE, Nissenblatt MJ: Bilateral internuclear ophthalmoplegia after intrathecal chemotherapy and cranial irradiation. Am J Ophthalmol 92:851–853, 1981

WEFRING-LAMVIK

Synonym. Alpers-hepatic cirrhosis.

Symptoms and Signs. Both sexes. In early life, seizures, spasticity, myoclonus, and dementia; later, jaundice, ascites.

Etiology. Recessive inheritance.

Pathology. Diffuse anoxic encephalopathy. Liver cirrhosis.

Therapy. Symptomatic.

Prognosis. Death in early infancy.

BIBLIOGRAPHY. Wefring KW, Lamvik JD: Familial progressive polydystrophy with cirrhosis of liver. Acta Paediatr Scand 56:295–300, 1967

WEGENER'S

Synonyms. Arteritis-pulmonary-nephropathy; granulomas-arteritis-glomerulonephritis; granulomatosis pathergic; Klinger's; necrotizing respiratory granulomatosis.

Symptoms. Occur in individuals of both sexes; onset at all ages. Persistent rhinitis; malaise; fever; cough; severe weight loss; hemoptysis.

Signs. Ulceration of midline structure of face. Pulmonary infiltration signs. Hypertension, purpura, and telangiectasia (late stage).

Etiology. Unknown; possibly, an autoimmune disease. It is considered the generalized form of the lethal midline granuloma (see).

Pathology. In skin; necrotic granulomatous lesions, necrotizing vasculitis (artery and veins). Hyaline and fibrinoid thrombi in all organs, but always predominantly involving upper respiratory tract, lungs, and kidneys.

Diagnostic Procedures. *Biopsy. X-ray of chest. Urine.* Albuminuria; casts; hematuria. *Blood.* Anemia, high blood urea nitrogen and creatinemia; transient eosinophilia; hyperglobulinemia. *Sputum cytology.*

Therapy. Relative effectiveness of steroids, nitrogen mustard, azathioprine, chlorambucil, cyclophosphamide. Antibiotics for secondary infections.

Prognosis. Progressive. Death in a month, occasionally in 2 to 3 years. Uremia and arteritis cause death. Spontaneous remissions of 2 or 3 months that temporarily interrupt progressive fatal course are occasionally observed.

BIBLIOGRAPHY. Klinger H: Grenzformen der Periarteritis nodosa. Frank Zt Pathol 42:455–480, 1931
Wegener F: Ueber generalisierte septische gefosser Krankungen. Verhandl Dtsch Pathol Ges 29:202–210, 1936
Douglas AG, Anderson TJ, MacDonald M et al: Midline and Wegener's granulomatosis. Ann New York Acad Sci 278:618–635, 1976
Lê Thi Huong Du, Wechsler B, Cabane J et al: Granulomatose de Wegener. Aspects cliniques, problèmes nosologiques. Revue de la Littérature à propos de 30 observations. Ann Med Intern 139:169–182, 1988

WĘGIERKO'S

Synonym. Third diabetic coma. See Umber's.

Symptoms. Eponym used to indicate a cluster of neurologic symptoms: vomiting; anorexia; insomnia; restlessness; hallucination; depression; coma, which occur in diabetic patients without hyperketonemia or hyperglycemia. A hypothalamic lesion suspected by the author, but no autopsy findings are reported. The author reported also a mortality of 100% in his cases.

BIBLIOGRAPHY. Węgierko H: Typowy Zespòl objawów klinicznych u chorych na cukrzyce, zakońcozony s'miercią w śpiaczce bez zakwaszenia Ketonowegą ("trzecia śpiączka"). Pol Typ Lek 11:2020–2033, 1956

WEILL-MARCHESANI

Synonyms. Brachymorphia-spherophakia; Marchesani's; Marfan's inverted; mesodermal hypoplastic dystrophy.

Symptoms. Onset of ocular symptoms in 1st decade, myopia with or without glaucoma; blindness in one-third of cases. Inability to flex the fingers completely, or to make a fist. Possibly, defective hearing.

Signs. In eyes; spherophakia, microphakia, subluxated lenses (50%). Short stature (average 148 cm), short extremities, and brachydactyly. In some cases, cardiac murmur. Teeth malformed; maxillary hypoplasia.

Etiology. Unknown; considered a result of a basic embryologic mesodermal defect. Marchesani considers this syndrome to be the opposite of Marfan's and represents the hyperplastic (brachydactyly) variant of the latter. Inherited condition of homozygous recessive genotype; dominant inheritance also suggested. Full form or partial form may be manifested.

Diagnostic Procedures. X-ray of hand. Symmetric shortening and widening of metacarpals and phalanges and retardation of carpal ossification. Feet and toes may share in the process of delayed ossification. Ophthalmoscopy. See Signs; retinal pigment degeneration; optic atrophy.

Therapy. Ophthalmologic procedures to correct myopia and pressure. Medical and surgical (removal of lens).

Prognosis. The patients are short. Eye pathology sometimes corrected, sometimes proceeding to blindness.

BIBLIOGRAPHY. Weill G: Ectopie des cristallins et malformations génèrales. Ann Ocul (Paris) 169:21–44, 1932
Marchesani O: Brachydaktylie und angeborene Kugellinse als Systemar-Krankung. Klin Monatsbl Augenheilkd 103:392–406, 1939
Ferrier S, Nussle D, Friedlei B et al: Le syndrome de Marchesani (sphenophakicbrachymorphic). Helv Paediatr Acta 35:185–198, 1980

WEIL'S II

Synonyms. Fielder's II; spirochetal jaundice; Landouzy-Mathieu-Weil; Landouzy's II icterohemorrhagic leptospirosis; Mathieu's; spirochetosis; Vasilev's.

Symptoms and Signs. Prevalent in male, teen-age, and young to middle-age adults. Onset during hot months, in people directly or indirectly exposed to excretions of any of a wide variety of domestic and wild animals. Biphasic illness; acute infection manifestation at onset: headache; fever; muscle aching. Distinct features appear on 3rd to 6th day and slowly progress: jaundice; generalized hemorrhages (epistaxis; hemoptysis, GI gastrointestinal bleeding); and a combination of hepatic and renal manifestations (with one of the two predominating). Hepatic tenderness and enlargement; renal involvement (see Diagnostic Procedures).

Etiology. Usually due to Leptospira icterohaemorrhagiae, occasionally other leptospirae. Direct toxic damage due to leptospiral antigens.

Pathology. Hemorrhages and bile staining of skeletal muscles, kidney, liver, adrenals, stomach, spleen, lung, and brain. Focal microscopic, vacuolization of sarcoplasm with neutrophilic infiltrations. In kidney, hemoglobin, myoglobin casts, interstitial neutrophilic infiltration of cortex and medulla; glomeruli usually spared. Other tissue changes not diagnostic.

Diagnostic Procedures. Blood. From leukopenia to marked leukocytosis (neutrophilia 70%); anemia; demonstration of hemolysis. Seldom, thrombocytopenia. Hyperbilirubinemia; azotemia. Cultural and serologic studies for identification of Leptospira. Dark-field examination. Urine. Proteinuria; red cell casts; urobilinuria.

Therapy. Penicillin; streptomycin; tetracyclines (given within first 4 days). Doxycycline (as prophylactic agent 200 mg per os once a week). Fluid and electrolytes balance.

Prognosis. Average mortality 10%. Severity of form correlates with duration of disease: in anicteric patients, no deaths reported; with jaundice, 15% to 40% mortality.

BIBLIOGRAPHY. Landouzy LTJ: Typhus hépatique. Gaz Hôp Paris 56:913–914, 1883
Weil A: Ueber eine eigenthümliche, mit Milztumor, Icterus und Nephritis einhergehende, acute Infektionskrankheit. Dtsch Arch Klin Med 39:209–232, 1886
McClain JB, Ballou WR, Harrison SM et al: Doxycycline therapy for leptospirosis. Ann Int Med 100:696–698, 1984

WEINBERG-HIMELFARB

Synonyms. Endocardial dysplasia; endocardial fibroelastosis, EFE; subendocardial sclerosis; primary endocardial fibroelastosis.

Symptoms. Both sexes equally affected; onset in infancy or early childhood, seldom at older age. Dyspnea; cough;

irritability; anorexia; vomiting; weakness; chest pain; failure to thrive.

Signs. Diaphoresis; tachypnea; tachycardia; pulmonary rales; hepatomegaly; acyanosis; absence of cardiac murmurs.

Etiology. Two forms described. *Primary* or idiopathic with no other heart disease; *secondary* with left-sided congenital heart condition (aorta coarctation, stenosis, mitral stenosis, or atresia). Has been discussed as separate entity.

Pathology. Diffuse opaque thickening of endocardium. Proliferation of collagenous and elastic tissue. Left ventricle exclusively or predominantly involved. Two types described: dilated heart type; nondilated type (rare). In first type, possibly, association with mitral insufficiency with chordae tendinae short and thick; seldom, aortic valve insufficiency.

Diagnostic Procedures. *Electrocardiography.* Sinus rhythm; left ventricular hypertrophy. *X-ray.* Cardiomegaly (dilated type); hilar and intrapulmonary vessels show venous congestion. *Angiography. Fluoroscopy.* Pulsation on cardiac margin; weak wavy contraction. *Echocardiography.* Markedly dilated left ventricle, a thin free wall and greatly decreased contractility. *Biopsy.*

Therapy. Symptomatic. L-Carnitine, steroids, digitalis, diuretics. Antibiotics for pulmonary complications. Heart transplantation.

Prognosis. Death usually before completion of 2nd year of life. Survival after 5 years of age unusual. Particularly poor if condition becomes manifest in 1st month of life.

BIBLIOGRAPHY. Weinberg T, Himelfarb AJ: Endocardial fibroelastosis (so-called fetal endocarditis). Bull Johns Hopkins Hosp 72:299–306, 1943
Perloff JK: The Clinical Recognition of Congenital Heart Disease, 2nd ed, p 174. Philadelphia, WB Saunders, 1978
Wenger NK, Goodwin JF, Roberts WC: Cardiomyopathy and myocardial involvement In Hurst JW: The Heart., 6th ed, pp 1215–1216. New York, McGraw-Hill, 1986

WEINBERG'S

Synonyms. Dysplasia tarda of lower limb; MEDT (type IIa); lower limbs dysplasia.

Symptoms and Signs. Present from birth. Epiphyseal dysplasia of lower limbs. Occasionally, minor abnormality of vertebrae.

Etiology. Autosomal dominant inheritance.

BIBLIOGRAPHY. Weinberg H, Frankerl M, Mekin J et al: Familial epiphyseal dysplasia of lower limbs. J Bone Joint Surg [Br] 42:313–332, 1960.

WEISENBURG'S

Synonym. Glossopharyngeal neuralgia. See Reichert's.

Symptoms. Unilateral lancinating, paroxysmal pain usually starting in the tonsillar region, lateral pharynx, or base of tongue, radiating deeply into the ear. Irritated by eating, talking, or movement of pharynx or tongue with occasionally increased salivation. Rarely recurrent episodes of syncope. Sinus bradycardia, hypotension.

Signs. Induction of the symptoms by stimulating one of the trigger points.

Etiology and Pathology. Irritation of entire glossopharyngeal (IX) nerve. Neoplasia; inflammation.

Therapy. Intracranial section of glossopharyngeal (IX) nerve. Carbamazepine. To control syncopal episodes: atropine or, if uncontrollable, a pacemaker.

Prognosis. Cured by treatment. Sectioning of the glossopharyngeal (IX) nerve results in unilateral anesthesia of soft palate and pharyngeal wall, and anesthesia and loss of taste of posterior third of the tongue.

BIBLIOGRAPHY. Weisenburg TH: Cerebellopontine tumor diagnosed for six years as a tic douloureux. The symptoms of irritation of ninth and twelfth cranial nerves. JAMA 54:1600–1604, 1910
Dykman TR, Montgomery IB, Gastenberger PD et al: Glossopharyngeal neuralgia with syncope secondary to tumor. Am J Med 71:165–170, 1981
St John JN: Glossopharyngeal neuralgia associated with syncope and seizures. Neurosurgery 10:380–383, 1982

WEISMANN-NETTER'S

Synonyms. Tibioperoneal diaphyseal pachyperiostosis; Weismann-Netter-Stuhl; toxopachyostéose diaphysaire tibio-péronière.

Symptoms and Signs. Equal distribution both sexes. Dwarfism; mental retardation; bowing of legs, minor alterations of the arms.

Etiology. Familial incidence (autosomal dominant) reported.

Diagnostic Procedures. *X-ray.* Selective thickening of affected bones. Diaphyseal bowing may be present in other long bones; squaring of iliac bones. Dural calcification.

BIBLIOGRAPHY. Weismann-Netter R, Stuhl I: D'une osteopathie congénitale éventuellement familiale surtout définie par l'incurvation antéro-postérieure et l'épaississement des deux os de la jambe (toxopachyostéose diaphysaire tibiopéronière). Presse Med 62:1618–1622, 1954

Amendola MA, Brower, AC, Tisnado J: Weismann-Netter-Stuhl syndrome: toxopachypériostéose diaphysaire tibio-péronière. Am J Roentgen 135:1211–1215, 1980

WEISS'

Synonym. Storage pool deficiency.

Symptoms and Signs. Mild or moderate hemorrhagic tendency.

Etiology. Autosomal dominant inheritance. Hereditary condition frequently associated with other platelet anomalies: Hermanski-Pudlak (see); Chediak-Higashi (see); Wiskott-Aldrich (see).

Diagnostic Procedures. *Blood.* Decrease of adenosine diphosphate in the dense granules of platelets. It may either affect the delta or the alpha granules or the two types.

Prognosis. Fair.

BIBLIOGRAPHY. Weiss HJ, Chervenick PA, Zalusky R et al: A familial defect in platelet function associated with impaired release of adenosine diphosphate. New Engl J Med 281:1264–1270, 1969

Weiss HJ, Lages BA: Platelet malondialdehyde production and aggregation responses induced by arachidonate, prostaglandin-G2, collagen and epinephrine in 12 patients with storage pool deficiency. Blood 58:27–33, 1981

WEISS-BAKER

Synonym. See Carotid sinus.

Symptoms. With patient in any position, loss of consciousness.

Signs. No change in pulse rate or arterial pressure. Attacks may be preceded or accompanied by focal neurological signs.

Etiology. See Carotid sinus.

Diagnostic Procedures. See Carotid sinus.

Therapy. See Carotid sinus.

Prognosis. See Carotid sinus.

BIBLIOGRAPHY. Weiss S, Baker JP: The carotid sinus re-

flex in health and disease: its role in the causation of fainting and convulsions. Medicine 12:297–354, 1933

Hurst JW: The Heart, 6th ed, p 515. New York, McGraw-Hill, 1986

WEISSENBACHER-ZWEYMULLER

Synonym. W-Z. See Wagner's.

Symptoms and Signs. At birth. Micrognathia; rhizomelic chondrodysplasia (dumbbell-shaped femora and humeri).

Etiology. Autosomal dominant inheritance. Considered neonatal expression of Wagner's syndrome (see).

Prognosis. Regression of bone changes and successive normal growth.

BIBLIOGRAPHY. Weissenbacher G, Zweymuller E: Gleichzeitiges Vorkommen eines Syndromes von Pierre Robin und einer fetalen Chondrodysplasie. Monatsschr Kinderh 112:315–317, 1964

Kelly TE, Wells HH, Tuck KB: The Weissenbacher-Zweymuller syndrome: possible neonatal expression of the Stickler's syndrome. Am J Med Genet 11:113–119, 1982

WELLS'

Synonyms. Eosinophilia-granulomatous dermatitis; granulomatous dermatitis.

Symptoms and Signs. Both sexes affected. Variable age (29–70). *First stage.* Localized redness and edema of skin that in 2 or 3 days spreads, with central involution and, possibly, blistering. *Second stage.* Formation of dermal mass, overlying skin slate colored, with violet edge. *Third stage.* Evolution toward a pale solid, morphealike mass and, finally, regression.

Etiology. Unknown. Related to allergic vasculitis, Schulman's, and other hypereosinophilic syndromes.

Pathology. Three stages: *First.* Dermal edema; intradermal leukocytes (eosinophils prevalent) masses. *Second.* Granulomatous dermatitis; eosinophil infiltrates around fibrinoid flame masses, surrounded by a palisade of histiocytes and giant cells. *Third.* Histiocyte necrobiosis and persistence of flame figures. No evidence of vasculitis at any stage, but evidence of eosinophilic infiltration in fascia and muscles as well.

Diagnostic Procedures. *Blood and bone marrow.* Increase in eosinophils. *Biopsy of skin.* See Pathology.

Therapy. Steroids.

Prognosis. Duration 1 year with variability of severity.

BIBLIOGRAPHY. Wells GC: Recurring granulomatous dermatitis with eosinophilia. Trans St Johns Hosp Dermatol Soc 37:46–56, 1971

Spigel GT, Ninikelmann RK: Wells' syndrome: recurrent granulomatous dermatitis, with eosinophilia. Arch Derm 119:611–613, 1979

WERDNIG-HOFFMANN

Synonyms. Hoffmann's (J.) I; spinal muscular atrophy infantile, SMAI; muscular atrophy, infantile; PHYI. See Kugelberg-Welander. See Floppy infant syndromes.

Symptoms. Present at birth or onset in newborn in half of cases. In other half, onset within 1st year of life. Symmetric paralysis of trunk and limbs, so that head cannot be turned, and infant cannot turn over. Loss of sucking ability.

Signs. Tendon reflexes depressed or absent; muscular wasting; fasciculation of tongue and other muscles. Respiratory embarrassment.

Etiology. Unknown; autosomal recessive inheritance; possibly, dominant with incomplete expression.

Pathology. In central nervous system, paucity of cells on anterior horn, no glial or inflammatory reaction, demyelinized anterior root and peripheral nerves. Muscle thin with atrophic fibers.

Diagnostic Procedures. *Biopsy of muscle. Electromyography.*

Therapy. Symptomatic.

Prognosis. Death between 3rd month and end of 4th year.

BIBLIOGRAPHY. Werdnig G: Zwei frühinfantile hereditäre Fälle von progressive Muskelatrophie unter dem Bilde der Dystrophie aber auf neurotischer Grundlage. Arch Psychiatr Nervenkr 22:437–480, 1891

Hoffmann J: Ueber chronische spinale Muskelatrophie im Kindersalter, auf familiarer Basis. Dtsch Z Nervenkr 3:427–470, 1893

Brandt S: Hereditary factors in infantile progressive muscular atrophy: study of one hundred and twelve cases in seventy families. Am J Dis Child 78:226–236, 1949

Hausmanowa-Petrusewics I, Zaremba J, et al: Chronic proximal spinal muscular atrophy of childhood and adolescence: problems of classification and genetic counselling. J Med Genet 22:350–353, 1985

WERLHOF'S

Synonyms. Idiopathic thrombocytopenic purpura; ITP; purpura hemorrhagica.

ACUTE IDIOPATHIC THROMBOCYTOPENIA

Symptoms. Both sexes equally affected; prevalent in children (85% under 8 years of age). Usually, infection 1 or 2 weeks prior to onset. Sudden skin and mucosa purpura.

Signs. Purpura; ecchymosis; no palpable spleen.

Etiology. Idiopathic; following infection (in children) or drug administration or exposure to chemicals (in adult).

Pathology. Generalized hemorrhagic manifestation.

Diagnostic Procedures. *Blood.* Anemia (occasionally secondary to blood loss), normal leukocytes; thrombocytopenia; shortened platelet survival time; demonstration of antiplatelet factors. *Bone marrow.* Normal number of megakaryocytes.

Therapy. Transfusion if needed; corticosteroid or adrenocorticotropic hormone (ACTH); intravenous IgG.

Prognosis. Self-limited course of 1 week or a few months in 90% of cases; 10% of cases become chronic.

CHRONIC IDIOPATHIC THROMBOCYTOPENIC PURPURA

Symptoms. Prevalent in females (3 : 1); onset usually in adult life, except the cases with acute onset (see above). The onset is usually insidious. Increased bruisability; prolonged menses; mild bleeding manifestations.

Signs. Spleen normal or slightly enlarged.

Etiology. Unknown; possibly, autoimmune disorder.

Diagnostic Procedures. *Blood.* Moderate anemia may be present, leukocytes normal. Moderate thrombocytopenia (40,000 to 80,000); platelet survival shortened. Demonstration of serum antiplatelet factors.

Therapy. Corticosteroids; ACTH; splenectomy; intravenous IgG.

Prognosis. Chronic condition. Complete cure probably never occurs spontaneously. Clinical remission and relapses (occasionally, at time of menses or with infection, vaccination, or other stressing situations), with or without variation of platelet number; however, platelet numbers never reach normal values, and they always show a shortened life span. Cure by splenectomy in almost 70% of cases. Mortality from this condition 6.8% in one large series.

RECURRENT IDIOPATHIC THROMBOCYTOPENIC PURPURA

Symptoms. As above, recurrent episodes with complete clinical and hematologic remissions (return to normal of platelet number and to normal life span).

BIBLIOGRAPHY. Werlhof PG: Disquisitio Medica et Philologica ed Variolis et Anthracibus. Brunswick, 1735

Frank E: Die essentielle Thrombopenie. Berl Klin Wochenschr 52:454–458, 1915

Imbert CL, Shaison G: Interet des immunoglobines dans le traitment du purpura thrombopenique idiopathique. Encycl Med Chir Sang 13019 A 10:7, 1987

WERMER'S

Synonyms. Endocrine adenoma-peptic ulcer complex; MEA; MEN I; multiple endocrine adenomatosis I; multiple endocrine neoplasias I; pluriglandular adenomatosis I.

Symptoms and Signs. Both sexes affected with same frequency; onset at all ages, after 1st decade. Protean symptomatology according to glands involved and function of adenomas. Hyperfunction of any single gland for some time, usually at onset. Peptic ulcer symptoms most common initial feature. Hypoglycemic crisis; headache; visual field defects; amenorrhea; diarrhea; weight loss. Acromegaly; Cushing's syndrome; hyperthyroidism features.

Etiology. Genetic basis. Transmitted by single dominant autosomal gene; high degree of penetrance (according to Wermer).

Pathology. Adenomas or hyperplasia of multiple glands: parathyroid (88%); pancreas (81%); pituitary (65%); adrenals (19%). Lesions of nonendocrine organs found in the same patients are also manifestations of the syndrome (e.g., gastrointestinal tract pathology).

Diagnostic Procedures. *Blood and urine. X-ray of skull and gastrointestinal tract.* According to clinical manifestation.

Therapy. Surgery when feasible and medical treatment of specific hormonal and secondary metabolic alterations.

Prognosis. Cause of death frequently related to syndrome manifestations such as hypoglycemic coma or to complications of surgery.

BIBLIOGRAPHY. Erdheim J: Zur normalen und pathologischen Histologie der Glandula thyroidea, parathyroidea und Hypophysis. Beitz Pathol Anat Allg Pathol 33:158–236, 1903

Wermer P: Genetic aspects of adenomatosis of endocrine glands. Am J Med 16:363–371, 1954

Schimke RN: Genetic aspects of multiple endocrine neoplasia. Am Rev Intern Med 35:25–31, 1984

WERNER'S (C.W.O.)

Synonym. Adult progeria.

Symptoms. Fully developed during 2nd and 3rd decades of life, tendency to occur in brother and sister. Normal birth; early physical and mental development. In adolescence, growth failure, hypogonadism, lack of sexual desire, and appearance of typical signs.

Signs. Short stature; sexual underdevelopment; canities (hair becoming gray); premature baldness; development of atrophic dermatitis (see Pathology) of lower legs, feet, upper arms, hands, and partially on the face. Nose beaked; eyes prominent; extremities slender (atrophy of subcutaneous fat and muscles); development of bilateral cataracts and finally signs of arteriosclerosis, completing the picture of presenility. This syndrome may also occur in *forme fruste* with only some of the signs present.

Etiology. Unknown; inherited condition, autosomal type.

Pathology. Skin: circumscribed areas of hyperkeratosis and atrophy; skin becoming tightly pulled over bony prominence; hair follicle and sweat glands scarce and not well developed; no proliferative or necrotizing arteritis; elastic fiber of corium loose but unaltered. Generalized arteriosclerotic changes; hypertrophic arthritis; osteoporosis; tissue calcification.

Diagnostic Procedures. *Biopsy of skin. X-ray. Hormone excretion studies. Blood.* Sugar (frequently diabetes mellitus develops). Increased number of both anti-double-stranded and anti-single-stranded DNA antibodies in the IgG class.

Therapy. Surgery for cataract; skin grafting for ulcer; none specific.

Prognosis. Average life span of 47 years.

BIBLIOGRAPHY. Werner CWO: Ueber Katarakt in Verbindung mit Sclerodermie Inaug Disser Kiel, 1904

Thannhauser SJ: Werner's syndrome (progeria of adult) and Rothmund's syndrome; two types of closely related heredofamilial atrophic dermatoses with juvenile cataracts and endocrine features: Critical study with five new cases. Ann Intern Med 23:559–626, 1945

Goto M, Tanimoto K, Aotsuka S et al: Age-related changes in auto- and natural antibody in the Werner syndrome. Am J Med 72:607–614, 1982

Gebhart E, Schinzel M, Ruprecht KW: Cytogenetic studies using clastogens in two patients with Werner syndrome and control individuals. Hum Genet 70:324–327, 1985

Bauer EA, Uitto J, Tan EM et al: Werner's syndrome: evidence for preferential regional expression of a generalized mesenchymal cell defect. Arch Derm 124:90–101, 1988

WERNER'S (P.)

Synonym. Werner's mesomelic dwarfism. See ulna-fibula hypoplasia and Nievergelt's.

Symptoms and Signs. Both sexes affected; present from birth. Polydactyly (hands and feet); absent thumbs; short legs (absence of tibia); reduced knee movements.

Etiology. Autosomal dominant inheritance with variable expressivity.

Diagnostic Procedures. *X-ray.* Absence or short tibias; altered growth of arm bones. Spine and head normal.

Therapy. Surgical: amputation of extra finger. Pollicization. Feet bracing; prosthesis.

Prognosis. According to degree of lesions. Corrective measures may improve mobility and height of patient.

BIBLIOGRAPHY. Werner P: Ueber einen seltenen Fall von Zwergwuchs. Arch Gynaekol 104:278–300, 1919
Bailey JA: Disproportionate Short Stature: Diagnosis and Management, p 269. Philadelphia, WB Saunders, 1973

WERNICKE-KORSAKOFF

Synonyms. Association of Wernicke's (see) and Korsakoff's (see) syndromes frequently observed in alcoholic, nutritionally deficient patients. Cerebral beriberi; encephalopathy hemorrhagica superioris; Gayet-Wernicke; hemorrhagica superior polyencephalitis; Wernicke I: transketolase defect; alcohol-induced encephalopathy; anamnestic confabulatory; Meynert's; Korsakoff's.

Symptoms. More frequent in Europeans. Anorexia; insomnia; anxiety; confusion; drowsiness; vomiting; progressive dementia.

Signs. Nystagmus; partial to complete ophthalmoplegia (most commonly, external recti); paralysis of conjugate gaze; ptosis; impairment of pupil reactions; ataxia; prostration; coma. Peripheral neuritis frequently associated. Severe form (Gayet's).

Etiology. Inborn error of metabolism of transketolase that makes cells more susceptible to thiamine deficiencies. This defect is presumably autosomal recessive. In alcoholics and chronic hemodialysis patients.

Pathology. *Brain.* Generalized production of new blood vessels (granulation tissuelike); proliferation of vascular endothelium; thickening of blood walls; dilatation of vessels; small hemorrhages; fibroblasts into scars; destruction of nervous tissue and invasion by neuroglia. Hemorrhage and scar widespread in corpora mammilari.

Diagnostic Procedures. *Blood.* Hypochromic anemia (usually); elevated pyruvic acid. *Isoenzyme studies. Spinal tap. Electroencephalography.*

Therapy. Thiamine. Propranolol has been tried with some success.

Prognosis. Early treatment with thiamine reverses condition rapidly and completely. If untreated, coma and death.

BIBLIOGRAPHY. Gayet M: Affection encéphalique (Encéphalique diffuse probable). Localisée aux étages supérieurs des pédoncules (cerébraux et aux couches optiques, ainsi qu'au plancher du quatrième ventricule et aux parosis latérales du troisème. Observation recueille. Arch Physiol Norm Pathol Paris 2:341–351, 1875
Wernicke C: Lehrbuch der Gehirnkrankeiten fur Aerzte und Studirende. Kassel, T Fisher, 1881
Korsakoff SS: Ob alkogol' nour paraliche. Vest Psikhiat (Moskva) 4:1887
Victor M: Alcohol and nutritional diseases of the nervous system. JAMA 167:65–71, 1958
Lopez RI, Collins GH: Wernicke's encephalopathy. Arch Neurol 18:248–259, 1968
Dreyfus PM: Thoughts on the physiopathology of Wernicke disease. Am New York Acad Sci 215:367–369, 1973
Nixon PF, Kaczmarek MJ, Tate J et al: An erythrocyte transketolase isoenzyme pattern associated with Wernicke Korsakoff syndrome. Eur J Clin Invest 14:278–281, 1984
Yudofsky SC, Stevens L, Silver J et al: Propranolol in the treatment of rage and violent behavior associated with Korsakoff's psychosis. Am J Psychiatry 141:114–115, 1984
Adams RD, Victor M: Principles of Neurology, 3rd ed, pp 761–768. New York, McGraw-Hill, 1985

WERNICKE'S APHASIA

Synonyms. Receptive aphasia; sensory aphasia; Bastian's; Pick-Wernicke; temporoparietal.

Symptoms and Signs. Lack of comprehension of spoken language, alexia, and agraphia. Voluble speech; paraphasia.

Etiology and Pathology. Lesion on posterior temporoparietal lobe of dominant hemisphere. Vascular, infective, traumatic, neoplastic etiology.

Diagnostic Procedures. *X-ray. Angiography. Brain isotope scan.*

Therapy. According to etiology.

Prognosis. Depends on etiology. When vascular lesion, progressive improvement is frequently noticed.

BIBLIOGRAPHY. Wernicke K: Der Aphasische Symptomekomplex. Breslau, M Chohn und Weigert, 1874
Adams RD, Victor M: Principles of Neurology, 3rd ed, p 357–358. New York, McGraw-Hill, 1985

WERNICKE'S (C.) II

Synonym. Neurosis cramps.

Symptoms. In state of fear or anxiety painful, muscular cramps in various parts of the body.

Etiology. Psychogenic mechanism the precipitating factor.

BIBLIOGRAPHY. Wernicke C: Ein Fall von Crampus-Neurose. Klin Wochenschr 41:1121–1124, 1904

WEST INDIES ATAXIC –SPASTIC

Synonyms. Jamaican paraplegic ataxic-spastic. See Leber's II. See Grierson-Gopalan.

ATAXIC GROUP

Described originally in the West Indies; observed also in besieged population during wars in Europe, the Middle and Far East, and Africa. Presently considered part of an enlarged Grierson-Gopalan syndrome (see).

Symptoms. Either sex; insidious onset. Bilateral symptoms; deafness; decrease in vision; central or paracentral scotoma (never complete blindness). Other symptoms precede leg symptoms by years. Weakness; unsteadiness of gait; numbness and burning of lower legs and feet.

Signs. Ataxia, mild spasticity, Babinski's sign; symmetric, confined to or exclusive of lower extremities. Wasting of leg muscles and foot drop (in long-lasting cases). Fundus oculi: various degrees of bilateral optic atrophy, marked temporal pallor.

Etiology. Unknown; no vitamin deficiency or consistent spirochetal infections demonstrated.

Pathology. Unknown.

Diagnostic Procedures. *Cerebrospinal fluid.* Normal. *Gastric analysis.* Achlorhydria or hypochlorhydria. *Blood.* Occasionally hypochromic anemia. *X-ray.* Normal. *Serology.* For syphilis; positive only in some cases.

Prognosis. Relatively benign condition. All symptoms and signs progress steadily for months, then become stationary.

SPASTIC GROUP

Symptoms. Occur in early middle age, in both sexes. Sudden onset. First symptoms unilateral. Mild nerve deafness (infrequent); weakness; pain and numbness of legs; lumbar backache; occasionally, severe paraplegia developing in a few days. Later, bladder dysfunction.

Signs. Leg spasticity; Babinski's sign, loss of abdominal reflexes (not constant); mild spasticity of upper limbs.

Jaw jerk reflex exaggerated. Eyes; pupils may be slightly irregular and reaction is sluggish to light and accommodation.

Etiology. Unknown; possible role of syphilis and yaws considered, but features of this syndrome are atypical. Toxins, vitamin deficiencies also may play a role.

Pathology. Inflammatory changes of variable degree; destruction of myelin; particularly in pyramidal, spinocerebellar; dorsomedial tracts and thickening of blood vessels.

Diagnostic Procedures. *Cerebrospinal fluid.* Moderate increase (in 40%) in lymphocytes or proteins, or both; abnormal colloidal gold reactions. *Blood.* Hypergammaglobulinemia. *Gastric analysis.* Hypochlorhydria or achlorhydria. *X-ray.* Negative. *Serology.* For syphilis. Positive only in some cases. Negative in spinal fluid.

Therapy. Symptomatic; physical therapy.

Prognosis. Progression of symptoms for weeks or months, occasionally for years. Variable degree of impairment. Bladder dysfunction in most cases. (Described also, a group with both ataxic and spastic features.)

BIBLIOGRAPHY. Montgomery RD, Cruickshank EK, Robertson WB et al: Clinical and pathological observations on Jamaican neuropathy; a report on 206 cases. Brain 87:425–462, 1964
Adams JH, Blackwood W, Wilson J: Further clinical and pathological observations on Leber's optic atrophy. Brain 89:15–26, 1966
Adams RD, Victor M: Principles of Neurology, 3rd ed, p 773. New York, McGraw-Hill, 1985

WESTPHAL-LEYDEN

Synonyms. Acute ataxia; chorea-akinetic-rigidity variety; Westphal's ataxia; Leyden's ataxia; Goekay-Tuekel. See Choreiform.

Symptoms and Signs. Both sexes affected; onset in childhood. Vomiting; vertigo; proximal muscle rigidity; convulsive seizures; mental abnormalities. Choreic movements (rare).

Etiology. Unknown. Nosologic confused condition. Possibly autosomal dominant inheritance.

Diagnostic Procedures. *Electroencephalography. Angiography. CT brain scan.*

Therapy. Haloperidol; chlorpromazine.

Prognosis. Death within 10 years. Final stage indistinguishable from Huntington's chorea (see).

BIBLIOGRAPHY. Westphal C: Eigenthümliche mit Einschlafen verbundene Anfälle. Arch Psychiatr 7:631–635, 1877

Leyden E: Ueber akute Ataxia. Z Klin Med 18:576–587, 1890

Diseases of the Nervous System in Infancy, Childhood and Adolescence, 6th ed. Springfield Ill, CC Thomas 1973

WESTPHAL-PILTZ

Synonyms. Neurotonic pupillary reaction; Piltz-Westphal.

Symptoms and Signs. Pupillary contraction occurring after vigorous closing of eyes. Delayed reaction to light, followed by slow dilatation of pupil.

Etiology. Unknown. See Pupillotonic syndrome.

BIBLIOGRAPHY. Westphal A: Ueber ein bischer nicht beschriebene Pupillenphänomen. Neurol Centralbl (Leipz) 18:161–164, 1899

Piltz J: Das vagotonische Pupillenphänomen, von Somogyi. (Wiener Klin Wschr 1913 NR 33). Neurol Centralbl (Leipz) 33:1124, 1914

WEST'S

Synonyms. Generalized flexion epilepsy; infantile spasm; jackknife convulsion; massive myoclonia; salaam spasms.

Symptoms. Onset during first year of life. Convulsion in infancy, characterized by fast recurrence, nodding of the head, with or without bending of entire body. Occasionally, opisthotonos with or without rapid movements of arms (less frequently legs) reminiscent of Moro's reflex. Mental retardation; visual problems.

Etiology. Many causes suggested. Brain damage from trauma, anoxia, or degenerative, metabolic factors and infective agents. Possibly X-linked inheritance.

Pathology. According to etiology.

Diagnostic Procedures. *Electroencephalography.* Hypsarrhythmia. *Blood and cerebrospinal fluid.* Cultures. *Metabolic studies.*

Therapy. Anticonvulsive therapy: diphenylhydantoin; phenobarbital; trimethadione. Cortical steroids. ACTH initiated early.

Prognosis. Poor for mental development.

BIBLIOGRAPHY. West WJ: On a peculiar form of infantile convulsions. Lancet I:724–725, 1840–41.

Feldman RA, Schwartz JF: Possible association between cytomegalovirus infection and infantile spasms. Lancet I:180–181, 1968

Pavone L, Mollica F, Incorpora C et al: Infantile spasms

syndrome in monozygotic twins. Arch Dis Child 55:870–872, 1980

WEYERS' II

Synonyms. Acrodysostosis; Weyers'; acrodysplasia Weyers'; dysostosis acrofacialis; Miller's; Neger-De Reyner; Treacher Collins. See Meyer-Schwicherath, Weyers', Curry-Hall.

Symptoms and Signs. Both sexes affected; present from birth. Postaxial hands and feet hexadactyly and fusion of 5th and 6th metatarsals and metacarpals. Cleft of mandibular symphysis; anomalies of lower incisors and oral vestibule.

Etiology. Autosomal dominant inheritance.

BIBLIOGRAPHY. Weyers H: Ueber eine Korrehierte Missbildung der Kiefer und Extremitaetenakren. (Dysostosis acro-facialis) Fortsch Roentgen 77:562–567, 1952

Roubicek M, Spranger J: Weyers' acrodental dysostosis in a family. Clin Genet 26:587–590, 1984

WEYERS' IV

Synonyms. Iridodental dysplasia; dentoiridial dysplasia.

Symptoms and Signs. Present from birth. Dysplasia and small perforation of iris; pupillary synechiae; microphthalmia; corneal opacity. Later microdontia, oligodontia, and hypoplasia of dental enamel. Later, dwarfism and myotonic dystrophy become evident.

Etiology. Unknown; Autosomal dominant inheritance.

Diagnostic Procedures. *X-ray of skeleton. Electromyography.*

BIBLIOGRAPHY. Weyers H: Dysgenesis iridodentalis. En neues Syndrom mit abweichdendem chromosomalen Geschlecht bei weiblichen Merkmaltraegern. Meeting of Deutsche Gessellschaft fuer Kinderheilkunde, Kassel, 1960

Gorlin RJ, Pindborg JJ, Cohen MM Jr: Syndromes of the Head and Neck, 2nd ed, p 735. New York, McGraw-Hill, 1976

WHIPPLE'S

Synonyms. Lipophagic intestinal granulomatosis; intestinal lipodystrophy. See Malabsorption syndromes.

Symptoms. Predominant in males, onset usually between 4th and 7th decades. Migratory arthralgia; diffuse abdominal discomfort; intermittent diarrhea with frothy, bulky, foul-smelling stool. Cough; dyspnea; weakness; weight loss; intermittent fever.

Signs. Grayish pigmentation of skin; occasionally, purpura; edema; emaciation. Abdomen: generalized tenderness; doughy consistency. Lymphadenopathy; ascites; polyserositis.

Etiology. Unknown. Host susceptibility factors and not yet identified or confirmed organism.

Pathology. Thickening of intestinal wall; white patches; bluish discoloration of serosa. Enlarged mesenteric lymph nodes. Mucosa: velvety; clubbed villi. Presence of macrophage containing periodic acid-Schiff (PAS)-positive material in jejunal lamina propria and in various organs: heart; adrenals; lymph nodes, subcutaneous fat. With high magnification many bacilli may be seen.

Diagnostic Procedures. *Stool.* Rich in fat and fatty acid. *Blood.* Hypochromic anemia; increased sedimentation rate; hypoproteinemia; hypocholesterolemia; glucose tolerance test normal or flat. *Gastric analysis.* Decreased free acid. *Biopsy of lymph node and jejunae mucosa* (see Pathology). *X-ray.* Deficiency in small intestine.

Therapy. Antibiotics (continued indefinitely, intermittently). Corticosteroids give temporary remission.

Prognosis. Dramatic response to treatment with disappearance of symptoms and signs. Weight gain; increased well-being.

BIBLIOGRAPHY. Whipple, GH: A hitherto undescribed disease characterized anatomically by deposits of fat and fatty acids in the intestinal and mesenteric lymphatic tissues. Bull Johns Hopkins Hosp 18:382–391, 1907

Kinath RD, Merrell DE, Vlietstra R et al: Antibiotic treatment and relapse in Whipple's disease: long term follow up of 88 patients. Gastroenterology 88:1867–1873, 1985

Fleming JL, Wiesner RH, Shorter RG: Whipple's disease: Clinical, biochemical and histopathologic features and assessment of treatment in 29 patients. Mayo Clin Proc 63:539–551, 1988

WHITE LIVER

Synonyms. Fatty metamorphosis viscerae; steatosis of liver; visceral steatosis.

Symptoms and Signs. Both sexes. Onset congenital. Progressive muscle hypotonia; lethargy; coma; hemorrhagic condition; jaundice.

Etiology. Possibly lack of one of the mechanisms of excretion of triglycerides formed in hepatocytes. Autosomal recessive inheritance.

Pathology. Heart, liver, kidney fatty infiltration (fatty acids 15 times normal amount) and increase of triglycerides.

Diagnostic Procedures. *Blood.* Milky serum with chylomicrons and high pre-beta and high quantity of high-density lipoproteins; hypoglycemia; hypocalcemia.

Therapy. None specific.

Prognosis. Death in first days after birth or within a few weeks.

BIBLIOGRAPHY. Peremans J, Degraef PJ, Strubbe G et al: Familial metabolic disorder with fatty metamorphosis of the viscera. J Pediatr 69:1108–1112, 1966

Chesney RW, Sveum RJ, Lacey M et al: A three months old infant with seizures, hypoglycemia, and apnea. Am J Med Genet 16:373–388, 1983

WHITFIELD'S

Synonym. Erythema induratum Whitfield's. See Bazin's, Vilanova-Aguadé.

Symptoms. Predominant in women; onset in middle age. Aching of legs after prolonged standing; generalized malaise; minor systemic complaints.

Signs. Edema of ankles; crops of painful tender nodules erupting after exposure to cold, minor traumas, general infections. No erythrocyanosis; no ulceration.

Etiology. Unknown; venous stasis may play a role. Allergic mechanism possible. See Bazin's and Villanova-Aguadé.

Pathology. Vasculitis of different degrees. Pattern clouded by venous involvement with edema and fibrosis and thrombosis of small vessels.

Therapy. Elevation of legs; rest; elastic stockings. Elimination infective foci.

Prognosis. Chronic recurrences with precipitating factors.

BIBLIOGRAPHY. Whitfield A: On the nature of the disease known as erythema induratum scrofulosorum. Am J Med Sci 122:828–834, 1901

Rook A, Wilkinson DS, Ebling FJG et al: Textbook of Dermatology. 4th ed, p 1168. Oxford, Blackwell Scientific Publications, 1986

WHITMORE'S

Synonyms. Melioidosis (means "similar to distemper in asses"); pneumoenteritis; pseudocholera; Stanton's.

Symptoms. Endemic in Southeast Asia; rare in Western Europe. Men more frequently affected than women, onset 2 or more days after exposure. From asymptomatic to acute, subacute, and chronic. Chills; cough; bloody sputum; abdominal pain; diarrhea; prostration.

Signs. *Acute* (most frequent). Signs of pneumonia; empyema; lung abscess; splenomegaly; jaundice; hyperthermia. *Subacute.* Lymphadenitis; signs of osteomyelitis; numerous abscesses (pulmonary, cutaneous, liver, spleen); occasionally, pyelonephritis. *Latent.* For years recrudescent; may become activated after long periods of latency by intercurrent trauma, burns, surgery.

Etiology. *Pseudomonas pseudomallei* (Whitmore's bacillus).

Pathology. Lesions prevalent in the lung; extensive abscesses: outer border hemorrhagic; medial zone neutrophilic leukocytes; inner core formed by necrotic debris with multinucleated histiocytes (giant cells), marked karyorrhexis. Similar abscesses (but less frequently) in any other viscera or organs (e.g., subcutaneous, brain, eye, heart, liver, spleen, lymph node).

Diagnostic Procedures. *Pus culture.* Presence of specific agents. *Isotope scan of affected organ. Blood.* Bacteriemia; leukocytosis (up to 20,000); complement fixation; hemoagglutination.

Therapy. Choice of antibiotics for acute form based on sensitivity studies; tetracycline, chloramphenicol, kanamycin, sulfadiazine for at least 30 days. TMS-SMX (trimethoprim/sulfamethoxalole 1/5). Surgical drainage.

Prognosis. Variable. Without treatment, mortality from apparent infection 95%; with treatment, in septicemic form mortality 50%.

BIBLIOGRAPHY. Whitmore A: An account of glanderlike disease occurring in Rangoon. J Hygiene 13:1–34, 1913
The choice of antimicrobial drugs. Med Lett Drugs Ther 26:19, 1984

WIDAL-RAVAUT

Synonyms. Abrami's; Hayem-Widal; hemolytic anemia. These syndromes are now recognizable as Coombs' test-positive immunohemolytic anemia.

Eponym now obsolete. As a group, all syndromes present variable degrees of hemolytic anemia, different times of onset but usually evident in infancy and childhood, absence of spherocytosis or increased osmotic fragility, as a rule not benefiting, or only mildly benefiting, from splenectomy. Dacie described two types. *Dacie's type I hemolytic syndrome.* Oval macrocytosis; normal autohemolysis, with addition of glucose decreased autohemolysis to a lesser extent than in normal cells. *Dacie's type II hemolytic syndrome.* Round macrocytosis, autohemolysis and potassium loss greater than normal, and unaffected by addition of glucose.

BIBLIOGRAPHY. Hayem G: Sur une variéte particulière d'ictère chronique. Ictère infectieux chronique splénomégalique. Press Méd 6:121, 1898
Widal F, Ravaut P: Ictère chronique acholurique congénital chez un homme de vingt-neuf ans. Bull Mem Soc Med Hôp Paris 19:984–991, 1902
Dacie JV, Mollison PL, Richardson N et al: Atypical congenital haemolytic anaemia. Q J Med 22:79–98, 1953
Engelfriet CP, Van Tveer MB, Maas Nel et al: Autoimmune haemolytic anaemias. In Clinical Immunology and Allergy, Vol 1, p 251. London, Philadelphia, Baillière Tindall, 1987

WIEDEMANN'S

Synonyms. Thalidomide phocomelia; Lenz's.

Symptoms and Signs. Occur in newborns of mothers who took thalidomide during gestation period (most critical period between 37th and 50th day after last menstrual period). No sex preference. Varying degrees of limb deformities from amelia to minor thumb anomalies. Deformities prevalent in upper extremities; involvement bilateral but generally asymmetric. Other associated anomalies include cranial malformation, hydrocephalus, meningomyelocele, macrophthalmia or anophthalmia, saddle nose, cleft palate, webbed neck, capillary hemangioma of the face, cardiovascular anomalies, and malformation of gastrointestinal and genitourinary tracts. Usually normal intelligence.

Etiology. Ingestion of thalidomide during gestational period.

Pathology. See Signs.

Diagnostic Procedures. *X-ray. Chromosome studies.* Pattern normal.

Therapy. Orthopedic and surgical procedures.

Prognosis. Depends on degree and type of the lesions.

BIBLIOGRAPHY. Weidenbach A: Total Phocomelie. Zentralbl Gynaekol 81:2048–2052, 1956
Wiedemann HR: Hinweis auf eine derzeitige Häufung hypo—und aplastischer Fehlbildungen der Gliedmassen Med Welt 2:1863–1866, 1961
Mellin GW, Katzenstein M: The saga of thalidomide (concluded), neuropathy to embryopathy, with case reports of congenital anomalies. New Engl J Med 267:1238–1244, 1962
Smithells RW: The thalidomide syndrome. Comprehensive care. Clin Pediatr 5:255–258, 1966

Dukes MN: Meyler's Side Effects of Drugs, 10th ed, p 89, Amsterdam, Excerpta Medica, 1984

WILDERVANCK'S

Synonyms. Acoustic cervico-oculo; cervico-oculo-acoustic. See also Klippel-Feil.

Symptoms. Prevalent in females; present from birth. Deafness or deaf-mutism. Epileptic attacks. Mental retardation.

Signs. Torticollis and short, webbed neck. Orbit: bulbar retraction. Nystagmus; paresis of abducens (VI) nerve. Heterochromia iridis. Cleft palate. Dextrocardia.

Etiology. Unknown. Hereditary polygenic with limitation to females.

BIBLIOGRAPHY. Wildervanck LS: Klippel-Feil syndrome associated with abducens paralysis, bulbar retraction and deaf-mutism. Ned Tijdschr Geneeskd 96:2751–3122, 1952
Wildervanck LS: Een Cervico-oculo-acoustic Nerve Syndroom Ned Tijdschr Geneeskd 104:2600–2605, 1960
Cremers CWRJ, Hoogland GA, Kuypers W: Hearing loss in the cervico-oculo-acoustic (Wildervanck) syndrome. Arch Otolaryngol 110:54–57, 1984

WILLAN-PLUMBE

Synonyms. Alphos; lepra alphos; lepra Willan; psora; psoriasis.

Symptoms. Both sexes equally affected; onset at any age. Very rare before age of 3 years; peak at puberty and following childbirth. Typical lesions appear occasionally after infective diseases or trauma, or in any part of the skin (face usually spared). Skin lesions: uniform, thick, typically intense red, scaling. Lesions may present different morphology: guttate; nummular; rupioid; exfoliative; pustular. Some features are present according to site of involvement. Nail involvement: pitting; discoloration; subungual keratosis; onycholysis. Nail involvement frequently associated with arthritis. Two clinical syndromes recognized. (1) *Stable erythrodermic psoriasis.* Exfoliative phase appearing suddenly or as an evolution of chronic form; involving all skin; sparing only limited areas. Itching mild or absent. Local treatment well tolerated. (2) *Unstable erythrodermic psoriasis.* Sudden or following infection, treatment, or complicating arthropathic form. Entire skin surface involved; fever; severe malaise; severe itching. Intolerance to treatment.

Etiology. Unknown. Autosomal dominant trait.

Pathology. Upper dermis: micropustules; acanthosis; absent or reduced granular layer; hyperparakeratosis; polymorph invasion; parakeratotic scaling.

Diagnostic Procedures. *Biopsy. Blood.* Hypocalcemia or hyperuremia (or both) in some cases.

Therapy. Methotrexate; triacetyl azauridine; corticosteroids (danger of rebound). Local treatment: ultraviolet light; tar baths; coal-tar ointment; dithranol paste; salicylic acid ointment; local corticosteroids. (In acute form: bland application; in chronic form: stronger application.)

Prognosis. Unpredictable; spontaneous or therapeutic remission. Frequent relapses. Stable form has best prognosis. Unstable form may be fatal or convert to stable form.

BIBLIOGRAPHY. Willan R: Description and Treatment of Cutaneous Diseases, pp 132–188. London, 1796–1808
Plumbe S: A Practical Treatise of the Skin. London, Underwood, 1824
Propping P, Hohenschutz C, Voigtlander V: Increased birth weight in psoriasis—another expression of a "thrifty genotype"?. Hum Genet 71:92, 1985

WILLIAMS-BEUREN

Synonyms. Supravalvular aortic stenosis, SAS; Beuren's; elfin face; hypercalcemia-supravalvular aortic stenosis; hypercalcemic face. See Hypercalcemia, infantile.

Symptoms. Affects both sexes; onset at birth or early infancy. Feeding problem, anorexia; vomiting; slow weight gain; retarded physical and mental development. Various degrees of hypotonia; easy fatigability; occasionally, chest pain and syncope. Reduction of exercise tolerance.

Signs. Height and weight below 3rd percentile. Facial abnormalities: elfin face (broad forehead, heavy cheeks, pointed chin). Bilateral corneal opacities. Tooth enamel hypoplasia; malocclusion; cavities. Unequal blood pressure between two arms. In heart; harsh ejection systolic murmur, with thrill maximum at 2nd intercostal space. Absent aortic systolic click; occasionally, aortic diastolic murmur.

Etiology. Unknown; primary disturbance begins *in utero.* Familial tendency (no genetic basis is apparent). Possibly, abnormality of vitamin D metabolism.

Pathology. See Signs; supravalvular aortic stenosis associated with some degree of generalized hypoplasia of entire aorta or normal aorta caliber. Coexistence of multiple peripheral pulmonary stenosis. Hypoplasia of several organs. In kidney, calcium deposition, arterial hyperplasia.

Diagnostic Procedures. *Blood.* Hypercalcemia (frequently present in this condition) or normal calcium and phosphorus. Hypercholesterolemia (occasional). Hypercalcemia and hypercholesterolemia usually disappear during 2nd or 3rd decade of life. *X-ray.* Metaphyseal osteosclerosis and craniostenosis. *Angiocardiography. Cardiac catheterization. Electrocardiography. Urine.* Endogenous creatine clearance decreased. *Chromosome study.* Normal pattern. *Echocardiography.*

Therapy. Vascular surgery; low calcium and vitamin D diet.

Prognosis. Depends on degree of malformations and surgical correction.

BIBLIOGRAPHY. Langdon-Down JLH: Observations on an Ethnic Classification of Idiots. Clinical Lectures and Report. London, 1866

Fanconi G, Girardet, P, Sclesinger B, et al: Chroniche Hypercalcaemia, Kombiniert mit Osteosklerose, Hyperazotaemia, Minderwunhs und Kongenitalen Missbildungen. Helv Paediatr Acta 7:314–341, 1952

Williams JCP, Barratt-Bayes BG, Lowe JB: Supravalvular aortic stenosis. Circulation 24:1311–1318, 1961

Beuren AJ, Apitz J, Harmianz B: Supravalvular aortic stenosis in association with mental retardation and certain facial appearance. Circulation 26:1235–1240, 1962

Pagon RA, Bennet FC, Laveek B et al: Williams syndrome: features in late childhood. J Pediatr 80:85–91, 1987

WILLIAMS-CAMPBELL

Synonyms. Bronchial cartilage absence-bronchiectasis; bronchomalacia.

Symptoms and Signs. Onset in early childhood. Pneumonia as complication of exanthematous disease of infancy, followed by pulmonary infections with cough and purulent sputum.

Etiology. Absence of bronchial annular cartilage causing development of bronchiectasis. Familial occurrence reported (autosomal recessive type).

Diagnostic Procedures. *X-ray. Pulmonary function studies.*

Therapy. Antibiotics. Fluidification of secretions.

Prognosis. Poor

BIBLIOGRAPHY. Williams H, Campbell P: Generalized bronchiectasis associated with deficiency of cartilage in the bronchial tree. Arch Dis Child 35:182–191, 1960

Mitchell RE, Bury RG: Congenital bronchiectasis due to deficiency of bronchial cartilage (Williams-Campbell syndrome): a case report. J Pediatr 87:230–234, 1975

Davis PB, Hubbard VS, McCoy et al: Familial bronchiectasis. J Pediatr 102:177–185, 1983

WILLIGE-HUNT

Synonyms. Hunt's corpus striatum juvenile parkinsonism; Hunt's (JR) II; pallidopyramidal paralysis agitans; See Parkinson's and Hunt's (J.R.) II; striatonigral degeneration.

Symptoms and Signs. Both sexes affected; onset between 10 and 30 years of age or earlier. Tremor; bradykinesia; dysarthria; rigidity; fixed facies. Symptoms less intense than in Parkinson's. Tendency to faint. Mental function intact; no reflex changes. Orthostatic hypotension (frequent association with Shy-Drager syndrome, see).

Etiology. Autosomal dominant and recessive inheritance. Sporadic or multifactorial inheritance.

Pathology. Decrease of large cells and increase of glial cells in the globus pallidus; same findings, but less evident, in other basal ganglia.

Diagnostic Procedures. See Parkinson's.

Therapy. Except in few early cases levodopa has no effect or makes the patient worse (lack of dopamine receptors?).

Prognosis. Slower progression of symptoms than in Parkinson's. Long survival; possibly normal life expectancy.

BIBLIOGRAPHY. Willige H: Ueber Paralysis agitans im Hugendlichen Alter Z Ges Neurol Psychiatr 4:520, 1911

Hunt JR: Progressive atrophy of the globus pallidus (primary of the pallidal system). A system disease of the paralysis agitans type, characterized by atrophy of the motor cells of the corpus striatum. A contribution to the functions of the corpus striatum. Brain 40:58–148, 587, 1917

Adams RD, Victor M: Principles of Neurology, 3rd ed, p 880. New York. McGraw-Hill, 1985

WILMS'

Synonyms. Embryonal kidney adenomyosarcoma; Birch-Hirschfeld's; embryonal kidney carcinosarcoma; embryonal mixed tumor; embryonal kidney; nephroblastoma.

Symptoms. Both sexes affected; onset before 5 years of age in 75% of cases, reported also in adults. Initially, asymptomatic; later, moderate local pain, nausea, vomiting, apathy, fever.

Signs. Pallor; weight loss; abdominal distention; blood hypertension (75–95%); palpable mass in kidney lodge; peripheral edema; ascites; varicocele.

Etiology. Unknown. Neoplasia of kidney. Autosomal recessive inheritance suggested.

Pathology. Neoplastic kidney invasion of great variety of cells like abortive renal element of mesodermal and epithelial type; occasionally bilateral.

Diagnostic Procedures. *Urine.* Albuminuria; increased lactic dehydrogenase (LDH). *Biopsy of kidneys.* See Pathology. *Renal function tests.* Altered. *X-ray.* Mass related to kidney; variously deformed kidney structures.

Therapy. Surgical excision. Chemotherapy. Roentgen therapy.

Prognosis. Very poor. Rapid diffusion of neoplasia; diffuse metastasis to all organs. In firm nonmetastatic tumor treated within first year, the prognosis is better, with possibility of cure in 60% of cases, and in children younger than 1 year of age close to 90%.

BIBLIOGRAPHY. Birsh-Hirschfeld FV: Sarkomatoese Druesengeschwueste der Niere im Kindersalter (Embryonales Adenosarcom). Deitr Pathol Anat 24:343–362, 1898
Wilms M: Die Mischgeschwueste. I. Die Mischgeschwuelste der Niere. Leipzig, 1899
D'Angio GJ, Beckwith JB, Breslow NE, et al: Wilms' tumor: An update. Cancer 45 (7 suppl):1791–1798, 1980

WILSON-MIKITY

Synonyms. Cystic pulmonary emphysema; interstitial prematurity fibrosis; lung cystic emphysema; neonatal cystic pulmonary emphysema. Bubbly lung, chronic neonatal pulmonary disease, pulmonary dysmaturity, bronchopulmonary dysplasia.

Symptoms. Seen most commonly in premature infants usually of less than 32 weeks' gestation and birth weight below 1500 g, onset occurring between birth and end of 1st month of life (average at 8th day). The syndrome is characterized by insidious onset of dyspnea, tachypnea, retractions, and cyanosis.

Signs. Cyanosis; auscultation of lung clear or rales, rhonchi, or wheezing; tachypnea; rib recession.

Etiology. Unknown; no infective causes could be found.

Pathology. Lung histology: inequality of terminal airspace size; variation of alveolar walls (increase of reticulum and elastic fibers and increased cellularity). Occasionally, unusual prominent bands of muscle in the wall of terminal bronchioles. Absence of clear-cut increase of pulmonary fibrosis.

Diagnostic Procedures. *X-ray of chest.* This is essentially a radiologic diagnosis. Three stages of the condition may be recognized: (1) *Acute.* Bilateral diffuse reticulonodular pattern with small, round, radiolucent foci; generalized hyperaeration. (2) *Intermediate* (in weeks or months). Coarse streaking from hilus into upper lobe; focal lucent areas disappear; generalized hyperaeration persists. (3) *Clearing.* Complete disappearance of findings between 4th and 11th months of age. *Pulmonary function tests.* Dynamic lung: "compliance" significantly reduced; static lung: "Compliance" within normal limit. *Sputum.* Culture. *Biopsy of lung* (only with severe symptoms).

Therapy. Treatment consists of supportive measures: oxygen for cyanosis, digitalization and diuretics for cardiac failure, acid-base correction, and assisted ventilation when indicated. Prophylaxis with vitamin E does not decrease the incidence or severity of bronchopulmonary dysplasia.

Prognosis. A few patients may die during acute stage; majority slowly recover completely. Radiologic findings disappear as well within 4 to 11 months.

BIBLIOGRAPHY. Wilson MC, Mikity VG: A new form of respiratory disease in premature infants. Am J Dis Child 99:489–499, 1960
Nelson Textbook of Pediatrics, 12th ed. Philadelphia, WB Saunders, 1983

WILSON'S (S.A.K.)

Synonyms. Kinnier Wilson's; lenticular progressive degeneration; pseudosclerosis; Westphal-Strümpell. Hepatolenticular degeneration.

Symptoms. Slightly more prevalent in males; onset in childhood to early adulthood. Occasionally acute onset with fulminant hepatic failure (jaundice, vomiting), hemolytic crisis, arthritis, renal colics with emission of stones, renal tubular acidosis. Females more often present with hepatic failure, males more often with neurological symptoms. In group of Eastern Europe extraction, later onset. Tremor beginning on extremity and successively extending to head and body. Weakness; drooling; dysarthria; mental changes. Later stage: anarthria, dysphagia.

Signs. *Eyes.* Pigmentation of periphery of cornea (Kayser-Fleischer ring). *Skin.* Discoloration; occasionally, jaundice; spider angiomas. Hepatosplenomegaly. Bone or joint changes and muscular wasting. From mild to severe incoordination; choreic movements; dystonic spasm convulsions; plastic rigidity of extremities.

Etiology. Autosomal recessive inheritance. Specific defect is not known but the two chief disturbances are (1) reduction of rate of incorporation of copper in ceruloplasmin and (2) reduced biliary excretion of copper. The accumulated metal deposits in hepatocytes and successively in central nervous system.

Pathology. *Brain.* Basal ganglia brown pigmentation and cavitation. Increased number of glial cells throughout brain. *Liver.* Coarse nodular cirrhosis, postnecrotic type with active regeneration. Esophageal varices; ascites. Copper content increased in brain, liver (> 100 mg/g of tissue), kidney, and cornea.

Diagnostic Procedures. *Blood.* Hemolytic anemia; hypocupremia; hypoceruloplasminemia (less than 20 mg/dl of serum. *Liver function test.* Cirrhosis pattern. *Urine.* Hypercupriuria (variable); hyperaminoaciduria; hematuria. *Biopsy of liver. X-ray.* Osteoporosis.

Therapy. Dietary restriction of copper. Dimercaprol intramuscularly and (better) penicillamine (orally 1 g/day over 10 years of age and adult; 0.5 to 0.75 under this age). Continue treatment in spite of lack of apparent clinical improvement; triethylene tetramine dihydrochloride is another nontoxic, good, potential drug. Zinc sulfate can be a low toxic and well tolerated alternative for D-penicillamine. Liver transplant successfully attempted.

Prognosis. Progressive; fatal. Benefit of treatment directly correlated to time treatment was initiated. Good results with transplantation and penicillamine reported.

BIBLIOGRAPHY. Westphal C: Ueber eine dem Bilde der cerebrospinalen graven Degeneration ähnliche Erkrankung des centralen Nervensystems ohne anatomischen Befund, nebst einigen Bemerkungen öcüber paradoxe Contraction. Arch Psychiatr Berl 14:87–134, 1883

Wilson SAK: Progressive lenticular degeneration: a familial nervous disease associated with cirrhosis of the liver. Brain 34:295–509, 1911–12

Danks DM: Hereditary disorders of copper metabolism in Wilson's disease and Menkes' disease. In Stanbury JB, Wyngaarden JB, Fredrickson DS, et al: The Metabolic Basis of Inherited Disease, 5th ed, p 1251. New York, McGraw-Hill, 1983

Van Caillie-Bertrand M, Degenhart HJ et al: Wilson's disease: assessment of D-penicillamine treatment. Arch Dis Child 60:652, 1985

Van Caillie-Bertrand M, Degenhart HJ, Visser HKA et al: Oral zinc sulphate for Wilson's disease. Arch Dis Child 60:656, 1985

WINCKEL'S

Synonyms. Charrin-Winckel; cyanosis afebrilis icterica perniciosa cum hemoglobinuria; neonatal hemoglobinuria.

Symptoms and Signs. Occur in newborns. Recurrent crises of jaundice, cyanosis, hemorrhagic manifestation, and hemoglobinuria.

Etiology. Unknown. It appears to be an obsolete entity.

BIBLIOGRAPHY. Charrin S: Maladie bronzée hematique des enfants nouveau-nés (tubulhematie renale de M. Parrot) (thesis). Paris, 1873

Winckel F: Ueber eine bisher miet bescheriebene endemisch aufgetretene Erkrankung Neugeborener. Dtsch Med Wochenschr 5:303–307, 415–418; 431–436; 447–450, 1879

Rook A, Wilkinson DS, Ebling FJG et al: Textbook of Dermatology. 4th ed, pp 2134–2135. Oxford, Blackwell Scientific Publications, 1986

WINDSHIELD WIPER

Symptoms and Signs. May follow cataract extraction with a posterior chamber J Loop intraocular lens. The intraocular lens is too short and moves like a windshield wiper.

Etiology and Pathology. Ruptured zonules; lateral tilt and decentration of intraocular lens.

BIBLIOGRAPHY. Simcoe CW: Simcoe posterior chamber lens: therapy, techniques and results. Am Intraocular Implant Soc J 7:154–157, 1981

WINKLER'S

Synonym. Chondrodermatitis helicis.

Symptoms. Ten times more frequent in men; onset after 40 years of age. Severe pain in the ear initiated by pressure, interfering with sleep (in women less intense). In men (90%) the helix in the right ear more frequently involved.

Signs. Single and occasionally multiple globular nodules of 1 cm or larger and raised 0.5 cm hyperemia of surrounding skin. Skin usually scaly or crusty. In women both ears equally affected and localization is usually in the antihelix and tragus.

Etiology. Predisposing factors: anatomical development defects of vascular supply; age. Causative factors: trauma; cold.

Pathology. Acantholysis and hyperkeratosis of epidermis with parakeratosis in center of nodule. Edema; homogenization; fibrinoid necrosis; vascular granulation of dermis. Perichondral tissue: fibrinoid degeneration and, according to involvement, various degrees of degeneration and reactive changes.

Therapy. Surgical excision.

Prognosis. Recurrences possible.

BIBLIOGRAPHY. Winkler M: Knoetchenfoermige Erkrankung am Helix. (Chondrodermatitis nodularis chronica helicis). Arch Derm Syph 121:278–285, 1915–16.
Rook A, Wilkinson DS, Ebling FJG et al: Textbook of Dermatology. 4th ed, pp 2134–2135. Oxford, Blackwell Scientific Publications, 1986.

WISKOTT-ALDRICH

Synonyms. Aldrich's; Aldrich-Huntley; Aldrich-Dees; eczema–infections–thrombocytopenia triad.

Symptoms. Occur in infancy and childhood, only in males. Eczema; easy bruisability; hemorrhage; recurrent infections, especially otitis media; bloody diarrhea.

Signs. Petechiae and hematomas; eczema; otitis media; periosteal hemorrhages.

Etiology. Unknown; sex-linked recessive condition. Primary inability to process certain polysaccharide antigens as required for normal induction of an immunoresponse (Cooper et al.).

Pathology. Manifestation of a broad spectrum of infective diseases: viral; bacterial; fungal; pneumocystis carinii. Hemorrhagic manifestation affecting all organs. If surviving, widespread malignancies of lymphoreticular type develop at later age.

Diagnostic Procedures. *Blood.* Anemia; thrombocytopenia; lymphopenia; hypogammaglobulinemia (IgM and isoagglutinins levels low; IgA and IgE elevated); impaired delayed hypersensitivity. *Bone marrow.* Normal megakaryocytes; decreased platelet production; microplatelets; thrombi in lymph node vessels.

Therapy. Bone marrow transplantation has been performed with success. The transplantation was preceded by high-dose immunosuppression with cyclophosphamide.

Prognosis. A patient treated with bone marrow transplantation is still alive and in good health after 15 years.

BIBLIOGRAPHY. Wiskott A: Familiarer Angeborener Morbus Werlhoffi. Monatsschr Kinderheilkd 68:212–216, 1937
Aldrich RA, Steinberg AG, Campbell DC: Pedigree dem-

onstrating a sex-linked recessive condition characterized by draining ears, eczematoid dermatitis and bloody diarrhea. Pediatrics 13:133–139, 1954
Stiehm ER, Fulgiti VA (eds.): Immunologic Disorders in Infants and Children. Philadelphia, WB Saunders, 1973
Meuwissen H, Bortin M, Bach F, et al: Long term survival after bone marrow transplantation: a 15-year follow-up report of a patient with Wiskott-Aldrich syndrome. J Pediatr 105:365–369, 1984

WISSLER-FANCONI

Synonyms. Subsepsis hyperergia; subsepsis allergica; Wissler's.

Symptoms. Most frequent in children and young adults. Intermittent fever; recurring exanthemas of various types; transient rheumatoid arthralgia and occasionally pleuritic pain.

Signs. Slight transient jaundice; nonpalpable or slightly enlarged spleen; no lymph node enlargement; occasionally, pleuritic and pneumonic signs.

Etiology. Unknown; supposed allergic reaction to moderate bacteremia. Possibly, allied to rheumatic fever and rheumatoid arthritis. Diagnosis reached by exclusion of other known fever-producing diseases.

Pathology. Not reported.

Diagnostic Procedures. *Blood.* High sedimentation rate; anemia; leukocytosis (neutrophilia; normal number of eosinophils); blood and throat cultures negative; antistreptolysin titer frequently elevated; lupus erythematosus (L. E.) test negative. Transient signs of myocardial involvement (electrocardiographic) or liver or kidney involvement.

Therapy. Lack of response to antibiotics (except for an initial temporary moderate decrease of temperature). Steroids in moderate or high dose not always effective; antihistamines helpful to alleviate symptoms.

Prognosis. Spontaneous recovery and recurrences. Possibility that this syndrome represents a prodromal stage of rheumatoid arthritis that will eventually develop its full-blown pattern. See Cheshire cat syndrome.

BIBLIOGRAPHY. Wissler H: Ueber eine Besondere Form sepsisahnlicher Krankheiten (subsepsis hyperergica). Monatsschr Kinderheilkd 94:1–15, 1943
Fanconi G: Über einen Fall von Subsepsis allergica Wissler. Helv Paediatr Acta 1:532–537, 1946
Bottiger LE, Landegren J: Wissler's syndrome. Acta Med Scand 174:415–420, 1963
Bywaters FGL: Still's disease in the adult. Ann Rheum Dis 30:121–133, 1971

WITCH'S MILK

Symptoms and Signs. Galactorrhea in the newborn, both sexes.

Etiology. Unknown. Former theories about an association between this disorder and hypothyroidism with other endocrinopathies are not accepted today.

Pathology. Breast nodules significantly larger than those of children without galactorrhea.

Therapy. None. Pressing the infant's breast can be dangerous (inflammation and breast abscesses).

Prognosis. Good. Galactorrhea may persist for 2 months.

BIBLIOGRAPHY. Forbes TR: Witch's milk and witches' marks. Yale J Biol Med 22:219–225, 1950
Madlon-kay DJ: Witch's milk. Galactorrhea in the newborn. Am J Dis Child 140:252–253, 1986

WITHDRAWAL EMERGENT

Synonym. Neuroleptic dyskinetic.

Symptoms and Signs. In children and adolescents after discontinuation or reduction of neuroleptics. Choreoathetoid and myoclonic movements of the trunk, extremities, and orofacial region.

Etiology. Neuroleptic removal. Dopamine receptor hypersensitivity.

Therapy. Discontinuation of medication.

Prognosis. Good after weeks; spontaneous regression of signs.

BIBLIOGRAPHY. Gualtieri CT, Quade D, Hicks RE et al: Tardive dyskinesia and other clinical consequences of neuroleptic treatment in children and adolescents. Am J Psychiatry 141a:20–23, 1984

WITKOP'S I

Synonyms. Amelogenesis imperfecta; hypoplastic type; Steinberg's; microdontia.

Symptoms and Signs. Clusters of enamel defects: smooth, rough, pitted; failure to erupt of many teeth.

Etiology. Six forms recognized: 4 autosomal dominant, 2 X-linked.

BIBLIOGRAPHY. Witkop CJ Jr, Sauk JJ Jr: Heritable defects of enamel Cp 7. In Stewart RE, Prescott GH, Oral facial genetics. St. Louis, CV Mosby, 1976

WITKOP'S II

Synonyms. Amelo-onychohypohidrotic; nails-teeth; hypodontic-nail dysgenesis.

Symptoms and Signs. Hypocalcified enamel hypoplasia; onycholysis; subungual hyperkeratosis; hypohidrosis.

Etiology. Autosomal inheritance.

BIBLIOGRAPHY. Witkop CJ Jr, Brearly LJ, Gentry WC Jr: Hypoplastic enamel, onycholysis and hypohidrosis inherited as an autosomal dominant trait: a review of ectodermal dysplasia syndromes. Oral Surg, 39:71–86, 1975

WITTMAAK-EKBOM

Synonyms. Anxietas tibialis; asthenia crurum paresthetica; Ekbom's; leg jitter; restless legs; acromelalgia-painful legs-moving toes.

Symptoms. Recurrent, unpleasant, peculiar creeping or crawling sensation in the legs, occasionally in the thighs or feet, felt deep inside the muscle or bones, which prevents the patient from keeping the involved extremities still. Bilateral and symmetric involvement or preponderant on one side; seldom affecting the arms and hands in "tono minor." Seldom true pain. Worst in the evening and at night or when the patient rests for some time. Sometimes lasting only a short period, sometimes hours. Sensation is relieved by movement, but reappears a short time after patient returns to bed. Important cause of severe insomnia.

Signs. None or cold feet and lower legs.

Etiology. Unknown; psychic factor of some importance (symptoms appearing especially during boring programs, movies, television, theater). Iron-deficiency anemia a possible etiologic factor. Hereditary (dominant transmission) implicated. In pregnancy present in 10% of cases; disappears after delivery.

Diagnostic Procedures. *Blood.* Moderate anemia; serum iron low in some cases.

Therapy. If anemia and iron deficiency, correction of condition will relieve symptoms. Most patients will not need treatment; reassurance of the benign nature of the syndrome may suffice. For those who require drug therapy, a trial with one of the following drugs can be suggested: levodopa, benserazide, carbidopa, clonazepam, carbamazepine, and for resistant cases chlorpromazine.

Prognosis. In some cases, spontaneous remission. Some cured by treatment of anemia. In pregnancy, symptoms disappear after delivery. Patient with aching pain is resistant to all kinds of treatment.

BIBLIOGRAPHY. Willis T: The London Practice of Physick, p 404. London, Bassett Crooke, 1685

Wittmaak T: Pathologie und Therapie der Sensibilitat-Neurosen, p 459. Leipzig, Schafer, 1861

Ekbom KA: Asthenia crurum paraesthetica ("irritable legs"): A new syndrome consisting of weakness, sensation of cold and nocturnal paresthesia in legs, responding to certain extent to treatment with priscol and doryl. Note on paresthesis in general. Acta Med Scand 118:197–209, 1944

Bogen D, Peyronnard JM: Myoclonus in familial restless legs syndrome. Arch Neurol 33:368–370, 1976

Gibb WRG, Lees AJ: The restless legs syndrome. Postgrad Med J 62:329–333, 1986

Clough C: Restless legs syndrome. Br Med J 294:262–263, 1987

WOLCOTT-RALLISON

Synonyms. Epiphyseal dysplasia-early diabetes mellitus. Diabetes mellitus-epiphyseal dysplasia.

Symptoms. Both sexes. Symptoms become evident during first weeks of life.

Signs. Normal facies. Tooth discoloration; skin abnormalities; hepatosplenomegaly; multiple bone fractures, dwarfism.

Etiology. Autosomal recessive inheritance; abnormality in collagen synthesis.

Pathology. *Bone.* Demineralization. *Liver and spleen.* Fat infiltration.

Diagnostic Procedures. *X-Rays.* Spondyloepiphyseal dysplasia. *Blood.* Insulin dependent diabetes.

Therapy. Slow-acting insulin. Symptomatic.

Prognosis. That of juvenile diabetes. Dwarfism.

BIBLIOGRAPHY. Wolcott CD, Rallison ML: Infancy onset diabetes mellitus and multiple epiphyseal dysplasia. J Pediatr 80:292–297, 1972

Stoss H, Pesch HJ, Poptiz B et al: Wolcott-Rallison syndrome: diabetes mellitus—spondyloepiphyseal dysplasia. Eur J Pediatr 138:120–129, 1982

WOLFF-PARKINSON-WHITE

Synonyms. WPW; anomalous atrioventricular excitation; false bundle-branch block; preexcitation.

Symptoms and Signs. Most patients asymptomatic. Onset at young age. Episodes of paroxysmal tachycardia in 10% of cases.

Etiology. Congenital variation in the heart conduction system; bypassing of the delay at A-V node and early excitation of a portion of ventricles.

Pathology. None.

Diagnostic Procedures. *Electrocardiography.* WPW pattern: short P-R interval with prolonged QRS complex. *Vectorcardiography. Echocardiography.*

Therapy. Response to drugs usually unpredictable. Most paroxysms resolve spontaneously. Digitalis, while contraindicated by many authors, found useful. Digitalis plus quinidine best results; propranolol (considered by others as drug of choice). Counter-shock if paroxysm is persistent; procainamide or lidocaine considered useful. As last resort, surgical division of accessory path.

Prognosis. Usually benign condition, but severe condition in some cases. Patients who develop tachyarrhythmia present atrial flutter (4%), atrial fibrillation (16%); atrial tachycardia (70%), and unidentified supraventricular tachycardia (10%).

BIBLIOGRAPHY. Wolff L, Parkinson J, White PD: Bundle branch block with short P-R interval in healthy young people prone to paroxysmal tachycardia. Am Heart J 5:685–704, 1930

Lamb LE: Wolff-Parkinson-White syndrome. Postgrad Med 43:173–176, 1968

Weissler AM, Warren JV: Syncope: Pathophysiology and differential diagnosis. In Hurst JW: The Heart, 6th ed, p 523. New York, McGraw-Hill, 1986

WOLFRAM'S

Synonyms. Marquardt-Loriaux; diabetes insipidus-diabetes mellitus-optic atrophy-deafness, DIDMOAD; Turnbridge-Paley.

Symptoms and Signs. Both sexes affected; present from childhood. Bilateral optic atrophy; extensive visual loss, with small paracentral islands of remaining function; diabetes mellitus; diabetes insipidus, later, development of neurosensory deafness; in some cases, neurogenic bladder and autonomic dysfunction; blood hypertension.

Etiology. Hereditary condition. Retrograde or anterograde trans-synaptic degeneration (?). Autosomal recessive inheritance suggested. Possible linkage with brachydactyly type E (see).

Diagnostic Procedures. *Blood.* Hyperglycemia. *Urine.* Hyperalaninuria. *Electroretinography.* Primary lesion of central optic pathway, with relative sparing of the external retinal layers located more in the cone than in the rod system. *Electroencephalography.* Abnormal pattern (?).

Prognosis. Poor *quoad functionem* and *quoad vitam.*

BIBLIOGRAPHY. Wolfram DJ, Wagener HP: Diabetes mellitus and simple optic atrophy among siblings: Report of four cases. Mayo Clinic Proc 13:715–718, 1938

Niemeyer G, Marquardt JL: Retinal function in a unique syndrome of optic atrophy, juvenile diabetes mellitus, diabetes insipidus, neurosensory hearing loss autonomic dysfunction and hyperalaninenuria. Invest Ophthalmol 11:617–624, 1972

Friedman E, Blau A, Fargel Z: A variant of the DIDMOAD syndrome (diabetes insipidus, diabetes mellitus, optic atrophy and deafness). Clin Genet 29:79–82, 1986

WOLF'S

Synonyms. Partial deletion chromosome 4; partial monosomy 4; 46; 4B; XX; Wolf-Hirschhorn.

Symptoms. Present from birth. Slow growth; repeated respiratory infections; seizures (minor or grand mal—characteristic); severe mental deficiency; hypotonia.

Signs. *Head.* Microcephaly; hypertelorism; lids antimongoloid slant; broad nasal root; beaked nose; strabismus; iris coloboma; speckled irides; cleft lip or palate (characteristic); fishlike mouth; micrognathia; ear malformations. Absence of cat cry (characteristic). *Extremities.* Simian creases; altered dermal ridges. Talipes equinovarus. *Genitals.* Hypospadias; cryptorchidism. Cardiac malformations.

Etiology. Partial deletion of chromosome 4 of B group.

Diagnostic Procedures. *Chromosome studies.* See Etiology.

Therapy. Symptomatic.

Prognosis. Short life expectancy (one-third die before 3 years of age). Survivors show slow growth and repeated infections.

BIBLIOGRAPHY. Sidbury JB, Schmickel RD, Gray M: Findings in a patient with apparent deletion of short arms on one of the B group chromosomes. J Pediatr 65:1098, 1964

Wolf U, Porsch R, Baitsch H et al: Deletion on short arms of a B-chromosome without "cri du chat" syndrome. Lancet I:769, 1965

Van Kempen C, Jongbloet PH: Partial deletion of the short arm of a chromosome no. 4. Wolf's syndrome. Maandschr Kindergeneesk 35:252–269, 1967

Centerwall WR, Thompson WP, Allen IE et al: Translocation 4p-Syndrome; a general review Am J Dis Child 129:366–370, 1975

Iino Y, Toriyama M, Sarai Y et al: A histological study of the temporal bones and the nose in Wolf-Hirschhorn Syndrome. Arch Otolaryngol Head Neck Surg 113:1325–1329, 1987

WOLMAN'S

Synonyms. Adrenal calcification—familial xanthomatosis; acid lipase deficiency (fatal form); xanthomatoses-

calcified adrenals. See also Cholesteryl ester hydrolase deficiency.

Symptoms. Both sexes affected; onset in first weeks of life. Forceful vomiting; abdominal distention; watery diarrhea; failure to thrive. Occasionally low fever. Initially mentally bright and alert; by 9th or 10th week reduction of activity.

Signs. Hepatomegaly; from 6th week progressive pallor. Optic fundus normal; occasionally, tendon hyperreflexia, clonus, positive Babinski's.

Etiology. Autosomal recessive inheritance. Deficient activity of acid cholesteryl ester hydrolase (or acid lipase) causing accumulation of cholesteryl esters and triglycerides in tissues.

Pathology. *Adrenal glands.* Normal configuration; enlarged, bright yellow, firm, containing calcified tissue. Zona glomerulosa and fasciculata well preserved; cells swollen; vacuolated. Zona inner fasciculata and reticularis replaced by large cells with vacuolated foamy cytoplasm, with necrosis, lipid infiltration, and calcifications. *Medulla.* Narrow but normal. *Liver.* Hepatomegaly; yellow; architecture variably distorted; cells large and vacuolated. *Spleen, lymph nodes, thymus.* Large foamy cells. *Other organs and tissues.* Variable degree of cell vacuolization.

Diagnostic Procedures. *Blood.* Total lipids, cholesterol, and triglycerides normal or low. Anemia. Lymphocyte vacuolization. *Tissue extracts.* Qualitative and quantitative cholesterol and triglyceride alterations. *Fibroblast culture.* Severe deficiency of acid ester hydrolase activity. *X-ray.* Adrenal calcification.

Therapy. None.

Prognosis. Death in first few months of life.

BIBLIOGRAPHY. Alexander WS: Nieman-Pick disease. Report of a case showing calcification in the adrenal glands. NZ Med J 45:43–45, 1946

Abramov A, Schorr S, Wolman M: Generalized xanthomatosis with calcified adrenals. Am J Dis Child 91:282–286, 1956

Assman G, Fredrickson DS: Acid lipase deficiency Wolman's disease and cholesteryl ester storage disease. In Stanbury JB, Wyngaarden JB, Fredrickson DS et al: The Metabolic Basis of Inherited Disease, 5th ed, p 803. New York, McGraw-Hill, 1983

WOMEN WHO FALL

Symptoms. Occur only in females; usually begins in late childhood and persists in adulthood. Stumbling and falling without any apparent reason.

Signs. None.

Etiology. Psychiatric disturbance. Precipitating factors are emergence into consciousness of aggressive or erotic impulses. To be differentiated from myoclonic syndrome and epileptic syndromes.

Pathology. None.

Diagnostic Procedures. *Psychoanalysis. Electroencephalography.*

Therapy. Psychiatric treatment.

Prognosis. When properly recognized and treated, good result. Correction of the basic personality derangement more difficult.

BIBLIOGRAPHY. Leuba J: Women who fall. Int J Psychoanalysis 31:6–7, 1950

WOOLF'S

Synonym. Deafness-piebaldism. See Albinism, oculocutaneous.

Symptoms and Signs. Reported in two males of the Hopi Indian tribe (southwestern part of United States). Present from birth. Subtotal nerve deafness; piebaldism; patch of hair whiter than in Indians with generalized albinism, and rest of hair normal color. Irides do not have the characteristic transparency observed in albinism; nystagmus absent; fundus oculi normal except for the presence of pigmented clumping on the retina; mild astigmatism; normal intelligence.

Etiology. Unknown type of inheritance. Autosomal recessive (?) or X-linked (?).

BIBLIOGRAPHY. Woolf CM, Dolowitz DA, Aldous HE: Congenital deafness associated with piebaldism. Arch Otolaryngol 82:244–250, 1965

WOOLLY HAIR

Symptoms and Signs. Hair, short, curled, woolly in Caucasian subjects.

Etiology. Dominant and recessive forms.

BIBLIOGRAPHY. Mohr OL: Woolly hair, a dominant mutant character in man. J Hered 23:467–473, 1985
Mortimer PS: Unruly hair. Br J Derm 113:467–473, 1985

WORINGER-KOLOPP

Synonyms. Epidermotropic lymphoblastoma; pagetoid reticulosis. See also Alibert-Bazin.

Symptoms and Signs. Rare. Asymptomatic. Affects young adults. Isolated plaque on distal part of legs, slowly expanding.

Etiology. Unknown. Particular form of T-cell lymphoma (may be a variant of Alibert-Bazin).

Pathology. Acanthotic epidermis colonized by two populations of cells; small lymphocytes with surface membrane markers of suppressor cells or T helper subsets (T4 + T8 +); second type larger and paler cells (related to histocytes, Langerhans cells or Merkel cells ?). These cells show strong staining for lysozyme.

Diagnostic Procedures. *Biopsy of skin.*

Therapy. Surgical excision and low-dose radiotherapy.

Prognosis. Very slow local extension.

BIBLIOGRAPHY. Woringer F, Kolopp P: Lesion erythemato-squameuse polycyclique de l'avantbras evoluant depuis 6 ans chez un garconnet de 13 ans histologiquement infiltrant intraepidermique d'apparence tumorale. Ann Derm Syph 10:945, 1939
Denean JG, Wood GS, Becksverd J et al: Woringer-Kolopp disease (pagetoid verticulosis): four cases with histopathologic, ultrastructural and immunohistologic observations. Arch Derm 120:1045, 1984

WRINKLY SKIN

See also Ehler-Danlos.

Symptoms. Onset from birth. Muscle hypotonia. Severe myalgia and decreasing visual acuity. Delayed growth.

Signs. Normal face. Body skin, including palms and soles, is markedly wrinkled and shows a decreased elasticity. Venous pattern over chest. Dwarfism; kyphosis; scapular winging.

Etiology. Autosomal recessive inheritance.

Pathology. Absence of abnormality of elastic fibers and collagen of skin.

Therapy. None.

Prognosis. Dwarfism. Mental retardation.

BIBLIOGRAPHY. McKusick VA: Heritable Disorders of Connective Tissue, 4th ed. St Louis, CV Mosby, 1972
Gazit E, Goodman RM, Bat-Miriam Katznelson M et al: The wrinkly skin syndrome: a new heritable disorder of connective tissue. Clin Genet 4:186–192, 1973
Adams RD, Victor M: Principles of Neurology, 3rd ed, p 1847. New York, McGraw-Hill, 1985

WUNDERLICH'S

Synonyms. Perirenal hematoma; perirenal apoplexy.

Symptoms and Signs. Both sexes affected; onset at all ages. Usually secondary to direct trauma, causing contusion or compression of kidney, acting on the lumbar region or on the hypochondrium. Hematuria. Abdominal mass. Contraction makes the physical demonstration of the perirenal hematoma difficult, but in severe cases, inspection and palpation confirm the presence of the mass, which usually progressively enlarges to reach even the iliac fossa. In the following days wide lumbar zone discoloration; occasionally, the hematoma may emerge in the inguinoscrotal region. Shock is frequent.

Etiology. Trauma direct or (seldom) indirect or other lesions causing a perirenal hematoma.

Pathology. Simple ecchymosis: subcapsular hemorrhage, with parenchymal ecchymosis and capsula intact. Interstitial fracture: capsula intact and parenchymal lesions.

Diagnostic Procedures. *Blood.* Central venous pressure decreased. Anemia. *Blood pressure.* Hypotension. *Urine.* Hematuria. *CT scan.*

Therapy. Treatment and stabilization of patient; if persistent, hematuria and shock progressing in spite of treatment, surgical intervention.

Prognosis. Variable according to degree, speed of progression, and treatment.

BIBLIOGRAPHY. Wunderlich CA: Grundriss der speziellen Pathologie und Therapie. Stuttgart, Ebner Seubert, 1858

WYBURN-MASON'S

Synonym. Cerebroretinal arteriovenous aneurysm. See Bonnet-Dechance-Blanc, Klippel-Trenaunay-Weber, Sturge-Weber, and von Hippel-Lindau.

Symptoms. More frequently in males; present from birth. Onset of symptons in 3rd decade, gradual or sudden. Loss of vision in one eye; severe headache; vomiting; sudden proptosis. When hemorrhage of midbrain, neck rigidity, meningitis symptoms, loss of consciousness, tinnitus, deafness, aphasia, cerebellar signs may be present. In some patients, mental retardation, psychotic symptoms.

Signs. Multiple cutaneous facial nevi, vascular, occasionally pigmented, usually ipsilateral to affected eye and in area of distribution of trigeminal (V) nerve. Eye: papilledema; nystagmus; ptosis; fundus shows arteriovenous aneurysm between veins and arteries. Signs of increased intracranial pressure or brain hemorrhage according to location. Other congenital anomalies may be associated.

Etiology. Unknown; autosomal dominant inheritance.

Pathology. Arteriovenous aneurysm of one or both sides of midbrain. Arteriovenous aneurysm or other types of congenital anomalies of retina. Vascular (pigmented or not) facial nevi.

Diagnostic Procedures. *X-ray of skull. Angiography. CT brain scan.*

Therapy. Symptomatic; surgery occasionally indicated.

Prognosis. When hemorrhages occur in mid-brain, poor.

BIBLIOGRAPHY. Wyburn-Mason R: Arteriovenous aneurysm of midbrain and retina, facial naevi and mental changes. Brain 66:163–203, 1943
Burke EC, Winkelmann RK, Strickland MK: Disseminated hemangiomatosis: the newborn with central nervous system involvement. Am J Dis Child 108:418–424, 1964
Chouette G, Auriol M: Classification de angiodysplasies et tumeurs vasculaires. Rev Stom Clin Maxillo Fac 87:1–5, 1986

XANTHINURIA

Two types.

CLASSICAL XANTHINURIA

Synonym. Isolated deficiency of xanthine oxydase.

Symptoms and Signs. Rare. Prevalent in males. Usually from 2nd decade, excretion of renal calculi, myopathy, arthropathy. Some cases can be completely asymptomatic.

Etiology. Autosomal recessive inheritance. Deficiency of xanthine oxydase.

Diagnostic Procedures. *Blood.* Hypouricemia. *Urine.* Hypouricosuria; increased excretion of oxypurines (xanthine, hypoxanthine).

Pathology. *Calculi.* Xanthine.

Therapy. Alkali; light liquid intake.

Prognosis. From asymptomatic to renal failure due to stone formation.

XANTHINURIA ASSOCIATED WITH DEFICIENCY OF SULFITE OXYDASE

Synonym. Molybdenum metabolism defect.

Symptoms and Signs. Few cases described. Those of the classical form plus neurologic signs.

Etiology. Acquired (prolonged parenteral therapy with consequent molybdenum deficiency). Molybdenum is a cofactor for both xanthine oxydase and sulfite oxydase.

Therapy. Administration of molybdenum.

Prognosis. In congenital case poor.

BIBLIOGRAPHY. Dent CE, Philpot GR: Xanthinuria, an inborn error (or deviation) of metabolism. Lancet I:182, 1954

Holmes EW, Wyngaarden JB: Hereditary xanthinuria. In Stanbury JB, Wyngaarden JB, Fredrickson DS et al: The Metabolic Basis of Inherited Disease, 5th ed, p 1192. New York, McGraw-Hill, 1983

XANTHURENIC ACIDURIA

Synonym. Kynureninase deficiency. See Hunt's (A.D.), Rundles-Falls, and Hartnup's.

Symptoms and Signs. Both sexes affected; present from infancy. Mental retardation; variable symptoms; mild stomatitis or cheilosis; high occurrence of urticaria, anemia, bronchial asthma, and diabetes in the families of affected probands.

Etiology. Autosomal recessive inheritance. Defect of kynureninase (a vitamin B_6 dependent enzyme) in tryptophan metabolism.

Diagnostic Procedures. *Urine.* Excessive excretion of xanthurenic acid, kynurenic acid, 3-hydroxy-kynurenine and kynurenine following tryptophan loading. Urinary abnormalities temporarily abolished by large dose of pyridoxine.

Therapy. Pyridoxine. Responsive and unresponsive forms are unknown.

Prognosis. Mental retardation; may reach adulthood.

BIBLIOGRAPHY. Knapp A: Ueber eine neue hereditäre, von Vitamin-B_6 abhängige Störung im Tryptophan-Stoffwechsel. Clin Chim Acta 5:6–13, 1960.

Tada K, Yokoyama Y, Nakagawa H et al: Vitamin B_6 dependent xanthurenic aciduria. Tohoku J Exp Med 93:115–124, 1967

XEROCYTOSIS

Synonym. Desiccosis. See Black Heel and Purpura traumatica.

Symptoms and Signs. Both sexes. After activities, based on impact of hands and feet on unyielding surface (marching, jogging, karate, freestyle swimming): fatigue, pallor, jaundice, darkened urine.

Etiology. Membrane protein of red cell abnormality with increased permeability to cations and higher loss of K than Na. Autosomal dominant trait proposed.

Diagnostic Procedures. *Blood.* Increased mechanical fragility of red cells. Free hemoglobin in plasma; hyperbilirubinuria. *Urine.* Hematuria after exercise.

BIBLIOGRAPHY. Glader BE, Fortier N, Albala MM et al: Congenital hemolytic anemia associated with dehydrated erythrocytes and increased potassium loss. New Engl J Med 191:491–496, 1974

Platt OS, Lux SE, Nathan DG. Exercise-induced hemolysis in xerocytosis: erythrocyte dehydration and shear sensitivity. J Clin Invest 68:631–638, 1981

XIPHOID PROCESS

Synonyms. Hypersensitive xiphoid; xiphoidadenia; xiphoidalgia.

Symptoms. Deep, slightly nauseating, dull pain in differing intensity from mild to agonizing in anterior chest; occasionally radiating to epigastrium, back, shoulders, arm, or precordium. Occurs also during night and interferes with sleep. Onset not instantaneous, lasting from minutes to days; recurrences for weeks or months, rarely for years. Precipitating causes: bending; stooping; lifting; head turning; eating large meal; walking.

Signs. Palpation of xiphoid process reproduces typical pain and associated manifestations (*sine qua non* sign for the diagnosis).

Etiology. Unknown; xiphoidalgia may be present without association with other diseases or in concomitance with coronary artery, gallbladder, gastrointestinal diseases.

Pathology. Unknown. In cases in which the process was removed, perichondritis and periostitis have been described.

Diagnostic Procedures. All studies to rule out concomitant conditions. *Electrocardiography. X-ray of gastrointestinal tract, cholecystography.* According to other symptoms and signs of these diseases.

Therapy. Procaine infiltration of xiphoid area; ethyl chloride spray. If underlying disease, specific treatment. Psychological reassurance on benign nature of the process. Surgery in refractory cases.

Prognosis. Responds optimally to treatment (especially procaine infiltration). Untreated, lasts for months. Recurrences are common.

BIBLIOGRAPHY. Junghanns H: Der Schwertfortsatzschemerz (Xyphoideodinie). Zentralbl Chir 67:628–629, 1940
Lipkin M, Fulton LA, Wolfson EA: The syndrome of the hypersensitive xiphoid. N Engl J Med 253:591–597, 1955

XXXXY

Symptoms and Signs. Males affected; present from birth. Variable pattern of features. Most common elements in over 50% of cases: at birth, low weight and stature; muscle hypotonia; joint laxity; mental retardation (average IQ 34). *Head.* Hypertelorism; upward slanted eyelids; inner epicanthic folds; strabismus; depressed nasal bridge; wide nose tip; prognathism; ear deformations; short neck. *Extremities.* Limited elbow pronation; clinodactyly; coxa vara and genu varum; pes planus. Abnormal dermal ridge count. *Genitalia.* Cryptorchidism, small testis. Possibly numerous other abnormalities.

Etiology. XXXXY aneuploidy.

Diagnostic Procedures. *Chromosome studies.* Three X-chromatin masses in all nuclei of buccal smear of subject with 49 chromosomes. *X-ray.* Retarded bone maturation; sclerotic cranial sutures; thick sternum; radioulnar synostosis; and other signs indicated above.

Therapy. Testosterone.

Prognosis. Dwarfism. Sterility. Lack of development of secondary sexual characteristics.

BIBLIOGRAPHY. Fraccaro M, Kaijser K, Lindsten J: A child with 49 chromosomes. Lancet II:724–726, 1960
Penrose LS: Finger-print pattern and sex chromosomes. Lancet I:298–300, 1967
Christensen MF, Therkelsen AJ: A case of the XXXXY chromosome anomaly with maternal X chromosomes and diabetic glucose tolerance. Acta Paediatr Scand 59:706–710, 1970

XYY

Synonym. YY.

Symptoms. Onset in early childhood. Behavioral problems (tantrum; aggressivity); psychic dullness; weakness and poor coordination; later, psychosexual derangements.

Signs. At birth, occasionally increased length; in childhood, accelerated growth (at 5 to 6 years). Chest and shoulder, poor development. In adolescence, nodulocystic acne. Facial asymmetry; long ears; large teeth; long fingers.

Etiology. Chromosomal abnormality: XYY.

Diagnostic Procedures. *X-ray of skeleton.* Increased length; relatively reduced breadth; occasionally, synostosis. *Electroencephalography.* Occasionally, altered. *Electrocardiography.* Occasionally, prolonged P-R.

Therapy. Institutionalization for delinquency frequently required.

BIBLIOGRAPHY. Sanderberg AA, Koepf GF, Ishihara T et al: XYY Human male. Lancet II:488–489, 1961
Harrison MJG, Tennent TG: Neurological anomalies in XYY males. Br J Psychiatry 120:447–448, 1972
Baghdassarian A, Bayard F, Digamber S et al: Testicular function in XYY men. Johns Hopkins Med J 136:15–29, 1979

YELLOW NAIL

Synonyms. Bronchiectasis-lymphedema-yellow nails; Samman's.

Symptoms and Signs. Onset at all ages, usually becoming apparent late in life. Slow-growing nails of fingers and toes, usually remaining smooth. Cross-ridging and hump may be present, becoming progressively curved from side to side, with insufficient cuticles. Color change to pale yellow or slightly green with darker border; proximal part remains of normal color. Onycholysis of one or more fingernails may occur. Edema of the ankle usually becoming evident (occasionally years) after nail changes have been noticed. Facial edema or Nonne–Milroy–Meige syndrome in both legs may be observed. Thoracic signs related to presence of bronchiectasis and recurrent pleural effusion at later stage.

Etiology. Unknown.

Pathology. Hypoplasia or atresia of lymphatics.

Diagnostic Procedures. *Lymphangiography.* Shows lymphatic abnormalities.

Therapy. Symptomatic. Recurrent infections from bronchiectasis and pleural effusion may indicate surgical treatment.

Prognosis. Fair.

BIBLIOGRAPHY. Heller J: In Jadassohn: Handbuch der Haut-und Geschlechtskrankheiten XIII. Berlin, Springer, 1927
Samman PD, White WF: The "yellow nail" syndrome. Br J Derm 76:153–157, 1964
Zerfas AJ, Wallace HJ: Yellow nail syndrome with bilateral bronciectasis. Proc Roy Soc Med 59:448, 1966

YESUDIAN'S

Synonym. Ichthyosis–split hair–aminoaciduria. See Netherton's.

Symptoms and Signs. Both sexes. From birth. Ichthyosis (lamellar) and split hairs. Mental retardation.

Etiology. Unknown. Autosomal recessive inheritance.

Diagnostic Procedures. *Blood* and *Urine.* Increase of arginine, alanine, lysine, serine, absence of proline and hydroxyproline.

BIBLIOGRAPHY. Yesudian P, Srinivas K: Ichthyosis with unusual hair shaft abnormalities in siblings. Br J Derm 96:199–203, 1977

YOUNG-PAXSON

Synonyms. Obstetric-gynecological crush: Paxson's.

Symptoms and Signs. Occur following obstetric conditions: retroplacental hemorrhage; trauma of labor; rupture of uterus; observed also in twisted ovarian cyst with bloody extravasation. Tissue injury; shock, at times absent or minimal; urinary suppression progressing to anuria; hypertension; symptoms and signs of uremia.

Etiology. Extensive trauma and prolonged tissue ischemia (same as in Bywater's).

Pathology. In kidney, pigmentary casts occluding tubules with degeneration of tubular epithelium.

Diagnostic Procedures. *Blood.* Hyperkalemia; hyperazotemia (peak at 5th to 9th day following injury). *Urine.* Hematuria; pigmentary and granular casts. *Electrocardiography.* Signs of hyperkalemia.

Therapy. Fluid balance and liquid diet with minimum protein and potassium, calcium intravenously, cation exchange enemas (to remove potassium). If transfusion indicated, removal of plasma to avoid administration of potassium; if acidosis, small amount of sodium bicarbonate. Hemodialysis with artificial kidney often indicated. When diuresis starts, liberal amount of fluid and careful control of electrolyte balance.

Prognosis. Guarded; less severe than in the past because of medical management and prevention of complications: infection, lung edema, cardiac insufficiency.

BIBLIOGRAPHY. Young J: Renal failure after utero-placental damage. Br Med J 2:715–718, 1942
Paxson NF, Golub LJ, Hunter RM: The crush syndrome in obstetrics and gynecology. JAMA 131:500–504, 1946

YUNIS–VARON

Synonym. Cleidocranial dysplasia–micrognathia–absent thumbs and distal aphalangia.

Symptoms and Signs. From birth. *Head.* macrocrania (diastasis of sutures); micrognathia; retracted and poorly delineated lips. *Limbs.* absent thumbs and distal phalanges of fingers; hypoplasia of proximal phalanx of big toe. Absent clavicles; pelvic dysplasia; bilateral hip dislocation.

Etiology. Unknown. Autosomal recessive inheritance.

BIBLIOGRAPHY. Yunis E, Varon H: Cleidocranial dysostosis, severe micrognathism; bilateral absence of thumbs and first metatarsal bone and distal aphalangia: a new genetic syndrome. Ann J Child 134:649–653, 1980

Z

ZAHN'S

Synonyms. Zahn's infarct; pseudoinfarct of liver. See also Liver peliosis.

Eponym used to indicate a pseudoinfarct resulting from the occlusion of small branches of portal vein formed by dilatation of sinusoids and atrophy of neighboring lobules and hepatocytes, without necrotic component. They are seen after splenectomy. Usually asymptomatic.

BIBLIOGRAPHY. Zahn FW: Ueber die Folgen des Verschusses der Lungenar terien und Fortaderäste durch Embolie. Verh Ges Dtsch Natur Aerzt 2 (2 part):9–11, 1898

ZAHORSKY'S II

Synonyms. Angina herpetica, aphthosis; canker sores; herpes angina; Mikulicz's aphthae.

Symptoms. Both sexes equally affected before puberty; after, more prevalent in females. Onset from late childhood to 3rd decade, increased incidence, then decreased. Small red macules in oral mucosa, seldom genital location, which rapidly break, leaving shallow painful ulcers.

Etiology. Unknown; Coxsackie A virus.

Pathology. Early lymphocytic infiltration around lobules and ducts of salivary glands; no primary vascular changes.

Therapy. Topical tetracycline suspension and steroid applied every 2 to 3 hours; levamisole; metronidazole; chlorhexidine gel; topical tetracycline.

Prognosis. Extremely variable; lesions last 7 to 10 days; no scar. Recurrence more or less periodic.

BIBLIOGRAPHY. Zahorsky J: Herpangina. Arch Pediatr NY 41:181–184, 1924
Graykowski EA, Barile MF, Lee WB, et al: Recurrent aphthous stomatitis. Clinical, therapeutic, histopathologic, and hypersensitivity aspects. JAMA 196:637–644, 1966
Rook A, Wilkinson DS, Ebling FJG et al: Textbook of Dermatology. 4th ed, pp 2098–2099. Oxford, Blackwell Scientific Publications, 1986

ZANGE–KINDLER

Synonym. Cisternal block. Eponym used to indicate a block of spinal fluid circulation at the level of the cisterna magna, caused by any space-occupying lesion of posterior cranial fossa with the classic symptoms of increased intracranial tension: nausea; vomiting; cephalalgia; choked disks; stupor and mental clouding.

BIBLIOGRAPHY. Zange J: Ueber Subarchnoidealblock, insbesondere den der Cisterna cerebellomedullaris ("Zisternenblock"). (Entstehungsbedingungen des letzteren, klinische Feststel lung und liquor-diagnostische Bedeutung, namentlich bei entzuendlichen Erkrankungen im Schaedel). Munch Med Wochenschr 73:1150–1152, 1926
Kindler W: Vorteile und Gefahren des diagnostischen Zinternenstiches. Wien Klin Wochenschr 41:632–634, 1928
Vick NA: Grinker's Neurology, 7th ed. Springfield, Ill, CC Thomas, 1976

ZANOLI-VECCHI

Synonyms. Convulsive post-spinal-operative; postoperative spinal hemorrhage. See Spinal cord injury-progressive confusional. Spinal shock.

Symptoms and Signs. Occur after surgical intervention on the spine. Convulsion; loss of consciousness; apnea.

Etiology. Spinal hemorrhage and siphoning of blood into cerebral ventricles.

Therapy. Diazepam for the control of convulsions; intensive care; tracheal intubation and respiratory assistance. Treatment of circulatory shock with fluids, atropine, and dopamine.

BIBLIOGRAPHY. Zanoli R, Vecchi B: Sindrome convulsiva postoperatoria da emorachide. Gaz Sanit 27:421–423, 1956

ZAPPERT'S

Synonyms. Acute cerebellar ataxia in children; cerebellar ataxia in children; hypertonic-dyskinetic infantile cerebral ataxia.

Symptoms and Signs. Onset at age 1 to 12 years. Symptoms developing in healthy children or following infections (e.g., measles, chickenpox, scarlet fever) Ataxia of station and gait; intentional tremor; slurred speech; vomiting, convulsion; unconsciousness; delirium; nystagmus.

Etiology. Unknown. Hypoxia and hypoglycemia (?). Hyperthermia most frequent cause; hypothermia usually better tolerated.

Pathology. Unknown. Loss of some of Purkinje cells, swelling pyknosis, if survive longer complete degeneration of Purkinje cells and gliosis and degeneration of the dental nuclei.

Diagnostic Procedures. *Cerebrospinal fluid.* Normal or pleocytosis and increased protein. *CT brain scan.* Diffuse atrophy of various degrees. *Electroencephalography.* Normal or diffuse activity.

Therapy. Symptomatic.

Prognosis. Variable, from death to recovery usually in 3 to 6 weeks, rarely exceeding 3 months. In some cases, residual mental deficiency.

BIBLIOGRAPHY. Zappert J: Ueber den acuten zerebralen Tremor im frühen Kindesalter. Monatsschur Kinderh 8:133–149, 1909

Goldwyn A, Waldman AM: Acute cerebellar ataxia in children: a report of three cases. J Pediatr 42:75–79, 1953

Dow RS, Moruzzi G: The Physiology and Pathology of the Cerebellum. Minneapolis, University of Minnesota Press, 1958

Adams RD, Victor M: Principles of Neurology, 3rd ed, p 803. New York, McGraw-Hill, 1985

ZEEK'S

Synonym. Hypersensitivity angiitis. See Kussmaul–Maier.

Symptoms and Signs. Male-to-female ratio 1.3:1. Respiratory disease in previous year (56%); drug reaction in previous year (38%); middle ear infection (31%) hypertension (25%). Except for the variation in frequency above mentioned, all symptoms and signs overlap with Kussmaul–Maier syndrome (see).

Etiology. Hypersensitivity arteritis. See Kussmaul–Maier. The Zeek's varity of polyarteritis has been differentiated on the basis of anatomopathologic findings (see) and the frequent pulmonary involvement.

Pathology. The main features differentiating Zeek's from Kussmaul–Maier syndrome are the lack of involvement of large muscular arteries and no predilection for

sites of bifurcation. Presence of vasculitis of pulmonary arteries; frequent splenic hilar vasculitis and splenic follicular arteriolitis; interstitial inflammation; focal necrosis; extravascular granulomas.

Diagnostic Procedures. Same as Kussmaul–Maier. *Blood.* More prominent eosinophilia.

Therapy. See Kussmaul–Maier.

Prognosis. Slightly better than in Kussmaul–Maier.

BIBLIOGRAPHY. Zeek PM, Smith CC, Weeter JC: Studies on periarteritis nodosa; differentiation between vascular lesions of periarteritis nodosa and of hypersensitivity. Am J Pathol 24:889–917, 1948

Moskowitz RW, Baggenstoss AH, Slocumb CH: Histopathologic classification of periarteritis nodosa: a study of 56 cases confirmed at necropsy. Proc Staff Meet Mayo Clinic 38:345–357, 1963

Winkelmann RK, Ditto WB: Cutaneous and visceral syndromes of necrotizing or "allergic" angiitis: a study of 38 cases. Medicine 43:59–89, 1964

ZELLWEGER'S

Synonyms. Cerebrohepatorenal; hepatocerebrorenal; renohepatocerebral; CHR. See Adrenoleukodystrophy, autosomal neonatal.

Symptoms. Onset in fetal life; prevalent in females. Feeble fetal activity. After birth (breech presentation prevalent), marked generalized hypotonia (poor or absent Moro's reflex). Respiratory problems. Failure to thrive; vomiting; mental retardation; variable seizures.

Signs. Several combinations of the following features: low birth weight; jaundice; short stature; moderate muscle hypotonicity or (rarely) hypertonicity. Abnormal craniofacial development: microcephaly; high forehead; hypertelorism; shallow supraorbital ridges: bilateral cataracts; broad nose; upturned nares; micrognathia; arched palate; posterior palatal cleft; abnormal ears; hypospadias; cryptorchidism. Hands with horizontal upper palmar creases; short fingers and toes; camptodactyly; syndactyly. Limited extension of knee; equinovarism. Hepatomegaly. Occasionally, heart signs consistent with septal defect or patent ductus arteriosus.

Etiology. Unknown; autosomal recessive inheritance.

Pathology. *Brain.* Small; macrogyria and polymicrogyria; sudanophilic leukodystrophy. Neuropathologic studies have revealed disturbed neuronal migration resulting in a malformed cerebral cortical plate. *Liver.* Variable unspecific findings; in some cases, cirrhosis; intrahepatic biliary dysgenesis. *Kidneys.* Cortical cysts. Extramedullary hematopoiesis. Tissue iron increased. Congenital heart disease may be associated.

Diagnostic Procedures. *Blood.* Hyperbilirubinemia; hypoprothrombinemia; hypoproteinemia; elevated serum iron and iron-binding capacity. Hyperpipecolic acid. Screening for the presence of coprostanic acids and the C29 dicarboxylic bile acid in serum or urine is a reliable method for detection of syndrome and confirmation of diagnosis. *Electromyography.* Normal. *Chromosome studies.* Normal. *Nerve conduction.* Velocity normal. *X-ray.* See Signs; pattern of chrondrodystrophia calcificans characterized by multiple punctate calcifications in the epiphyses. *Isotope scan (of kidney) and pyelography.*

Therapy. Symptomatic.

Prognosis. Death within few weeks or months of life, often due to hemorrhages.

BIBLIOGRAPHY. Bowen P, Lee CSN, Zellweger H et al: A familial syndrome of multiple congenital defects. Bull Johns Hopkins Hosp 114:402–414, 1964
Kelley RI: The cerebro-hepatorenal syndrome of Zellweger, morphologic and metabolic aspects. Am J Med Genet 16:503–517, 1983
Barth PG, Schutgens RBH, Bakken JAJM et al: A milder variant of Zellweger syndrome. Eur J Pediatr 144:338–342, 1985
Eyssen H, Eggermont E, Van Eldere J et al: Bile acid abnormalities and the diagnosis of cerebro-hepato-renal syndrome (Zellweger syndrome). Acta Paediatr Scand 74:539–544, 1985
Suzuki Y, Shimozawa N, Orii T et al: Zellweger-like syndrome with detectable hepatic peroxisomes: a variant form of peroximal disorder. J Pediatr 113:841–845, 1988

ZIEGLER'S

Synonyms. Cachectic endocarditis; nonbacterial thrombotic endocarditis; indeterminate endocarditis; marantic endocarditis.

Symptoms. Both sexes affected; age range 18 to 90 years. Usually occur in patients with prolonged disease or cachexia, but observed also in early stage of many other diseases. Symptoms due to peripheral arterial embolization. Fever may be present.

Signs. Usually systolic murmur (33%).

Etiology. Unknown. Associated with malignancy or other acute or chronic disease, even psychosis. Attempted correlation also with disseminated intravascular coagulation.

Pathology. Five types of lesions described: small single node along edge of closure of valve; large nonverrucous node on valve; small multiverrucous friable lesions on valve edge; (embolizing); fibrous tab, result of collagen degeneration on valve edge (nidus for thrombus).

BIBLIOGRAPHY. Lebman E: Characterization of various forms of endocarditis. JAMA 80:813, 1923
Gross L, Friedberg C: Nonbacterial thrombotic endocarditis. AMA Arch Intern Med 58:620–640, 1936
Hurst JW: The Heart, 6th ed, p 1137. New York, McGraw-Hill, 1986

ZIEHEN–OPPENHEIM

Synonyms. Dystonia lenticularis; dystonia musculorum deformans; torsion dystonia; torsion spasm. See Paraspasm, bilateral and Spasmodic torticollis, which may be considered localized forms of this syndrome.

Symptoms. Onset between 5 and 15 years of age, frequently in Semitic peoples. Usually unilateral; gradual onset; foot becomes flexed, inverted, or adducted; abnormal movements spread to entire leg and then spread to other one, and finally to whole musculature, particularly of trunk and neck. During sleep the patient relaxes; while awake, continuously turns and twists.

Signs. Reflexes difficult to elicit or exaggerated. Babinski's sign absent.

Etiology. Unknown or symptomatic of infections or vascular, toxic, neoplastic lesions of extrapyramidal system. The autosomal dominant variety (not ethnic background) onset at later age and slower and more benign course. Hereditary autosomal recessive and autosomal dominant (this variety correlated with elevation of serum dopamine-beta-hydroxylase).

Pathology. Degenerative changes of putamen, caudate nuclei, and other extrapyramidal centers. In symptomatic lesion, according to etiology.

Diagnostic Procedures. Establishment of idiopathic or secondary type. *Cerebrospinal fluid. Blood. X-ray of skull. Arteriography.*

Therapy. Disappointing. Early in the course beneficial: L-dopa and belladonna groups of drugs; bromocriptine. Diazepam; chlorpromazine; haloperidol; carbomazepine. Various neurosurgical procedures: root sections; spinal cord operations; thalamus lesions. Attempts to utilize biofeedback mechanisms.

Prognosis. Progressing to confinement in bed.

BIBLIOGRAPHY. Ziehen GT: Demonstrationen im Psychiatrischen Verein zu Berlin. Zentralbl Nervenkr 30:109–112, 1911
Oppenheim H: Ueber eine eigenartige Krampfkran: Kheit des Kindlichen und jugendliche Alters. (Dysbasia lordotica progressiva, Dystonia musculorum deformans). Zentralbl Nervenkr 30:1090–1109, 1911
Thomalla C: Ein Fall von Torsionsspasmus mit Sektionsbefund und seine Beziehungen zur Athétose doppel

Wilsoncheni Krankheit und Pseudosklerose. Z Ges Neurol Psychiatr 41:311–343, 1918

Denny-Brown D: The Basal Ganglia. London, Oxford University Press, 1962

Adams RD, Victor M: Principles of Neurology, 3rd ed, pp 881–882. New York, McGraw-Hill, 1985

ZIEVE'S

Synonyms. Alcoholic hyperlipemia; hemolytic anemia-hyperlipemic alcoholic; hepatopancreatic alcoholic; transitory alcoholic hyperlipemia.

Symptoms. More prevalent in middle-aged male patients. History of recent alcohol intake; onset insidious; weakness; fatigability; anorexia; nausea; vomiting and pain (dull cramps) in upper part of abdomen; varying in intensity, changing location. More frequent on right side than left. The acute pain lasts from minutes to hours and never subsides completely.

Signs. Moderate hepatomegaly; occasionally, mild splenomegaly. Weight loss; jaundice.

Etiology. Alcoholic intake with specific liver and pancreas damage. It has not been shown that all the features of the syndrome are causally interrelated.

Pathology. *Liver.* Minimal to moderate cirrhotic findings, and fatty infiltration. *Pancreas.* Cellular and obstructive type of pancreatitis.

Diagnostic Procedures. *Blood.* Anemia hemolytic type (shorter survival time; increased reticulocytes; increased bilirubin). Hyperlipemia: milky, cloudy plasma; hypercholesterolemia; hyperphospholipemia; increase of neutral fat and fatty acids; hyperuricemia; amylase normal; white blood cells usually increased. Platelets usually increased. *Bone marrow.* Marked normoblastic hyperplasia; presence of large phagocytic histiocytes with lipid granules. *Biopsy of liver.*

Therapy. Abstinence from alcohol; adequate diet.

Prognosis. Spontaneous remission of hemolytic anemia, hyperlipemia, jaundice, and pains with abstinence from alcohol occurs within 4 to 6 weeks.

BIBLIOGRAPHY. Zieve L: Jaundice, hyperlipemia and hemolytic anemia: a heretofore unrecognized syndrome associated with alcoholic fatty liver and cirrhosis. Ann Intern Med 48:471–496, 1958

Balcerzak SP, Westerman MP, Heinle EW: Mechanism of anemia in Zieve's syndrome. Am J Med Sci 255:277–287, 1968

Dickson AP, O'Neil J, Imrie CW: Hyperlipemia, alcohol abuse and acute pancreatitis. Br J Surg 71:685–688, 1984

ZINSSER–COLE–ENGMAN

Synonyms. Cole's; Cole–Rauschkalb–Toomey; Engman's; dyskeratosis congenita. See Fanconi's anemia.

Symptoms. Almost exclusively in males; onset between 5 and 13 years. Dysonychia with shedding, complete destruction; repeated suppurative paronychia. Later development of reticulate grayish pigmentation, mostly on neck and thighs but also involving entire trunk. Atrophy and telangiectases. Face red, atrophic; maculated skin. Macules on back of hands and feet. Palmar and sole keratosis; hyperhidrosis; bullae. Mucosal lesions: oral; small erosions evolving to leukoplakia; on conjunctiva similar lesions; excessive lacrimation. Defect of teeth. Hypotrichia-cicatricial alopecia. Physical and mental development may be retarded. In the majority of cases testicular atrophy.

Etiology. Unknown; sex-linked recessive inheritance.

Pathology. Skin changes not specific; parakeratosis; hyperkeratosis; acanthosis. Gastrointestinal tract mucosa may show same lesions as the oral.

Diagnostic Procedures. *Blood.* (In some cases) anemia or pancytopenia; Fanconi's type (see Fanconi's).

Therapy. Symptomatic.

Prognosis. Malignant transformation in areas of leukoplakia, occasionally also from atrophic zone. Death from carcinoma between 30 to 50 years of age. In *forme fruste* (only dysonychia and pigmentation), normal life expectancy.

BIBLIOGRAPHY. Zinsser F: Atrophia cutis reticularis cum pigmentatione, dystrophia unguium et leukoplakia oris (poikilodermia atrophicans vascularis Jacobi). Ikonogr Derm (Kyoto), 219–223, 1906

Engman MF: A unique case of reticular pigmentation of the skin with atrophy. Arch Derm Syph Suppl 13:685, 1926

Cole HN, Rauschkolb JE, Toomey J: Dyskeratosis congenita with pigmentation, dystrophia unguis and leukokeratosis oris. Arch Derm Syph 21:71–95, 1930

Garb J: Dyskeratosis congenita with hypoplastic anemia: a stem cell defect. Am J Hemat 20:85–87, 1985

ZIPOKOWSKI-MARGOLIS

Synonyms. Albinism-deaf-mutism (sex-linked); Albinism–deafness, sex-linked; Woolf's (see); Reed's.

Symptoms and Signs. Only males. Those of oculocutaneous albinism; piebaldism is possible. Sensorineural deafness from birth.

Etiology. Sex-linked inheritance.

BIBLIOGRAPHY. Zipokowski LA, Krakowski A, Adam A et al: Partial albinism and deaf mutism due to a recessive sex-linked gene. Arch Derm 86:530–539, 1962

Margolis E: A new hereditary syndrome: sex-linked deaf-mutism associated with total albinism. Acta Genet (Basel) 12:12–19, 1962

Woolf CM, Dolowitz DA, Aldous HE: Congenital deafness associated with piebaldism. Arch Otolaryngol 82:244–250, 1965

Reed WB, Stone VM, Boder E et al: Pigmentary disorders in association with congenital deafness. Arch Derm 95:176–186, 1967

ZOLLINGER–ELLISON

Synonyms. Z–E; multiple partial adenomatosis; multiple partial endocrine adenomatosis; pancreatic ulcerogenic tumor; polyglandular adenomatosis; Strøm-Zollinger–Ellison. See Wermer's.

Symptoms. Males affected slightly more frequently than females; peak of onset 3rd to 5th decades (10% in first 2 decades of life). Peptic ulcer pain (in 90% of cases), severe, refractory to usual medical or surgical measures (short of total gastrectomy); hematemesis or melena (45%); vomiting (25%); diarrhea (36%); abdominal pain (50%). Pancreatic tumor seldom produces local symptoms.

Signs. Dehydration (60%).

Etiology. Islet cell adenoma of pancreas secreting a gastrinlike material. Usually malignant, metastasizing tumor; in 10% of cases syndrome determined by simple diffuse islet cell hyperplasia; autosomal dominant inheritance.

Pathology. Malignant or benign tumor of islet cell of pancreas (difficult to differentiate microscopically) but distinguished by the presence of invasion and metastasis, or simple diffuse hyperplasia of islet cells. In many patients primary tumor located in stomach or duodenum, classified as non-beta cell tumor. Stomach: hypersecretion; multiple stomach and duodenal or proximal jejunal ulcers.

Diagnostic Procedures. *Gastric aspiration.* Massive hypersecretion of acid gastric juice. *Stool.* Diarrhea with steatorrhea frequently observed. Relieved by gastric aspiration. *X-ray.* Multiple ulcers or abnormally located ulcers; marked hypertrophy of gastric folds; duodenal ileus; small bowel pattern; rapid barium transit through small bowel. *CT brain scan* (20% of cases), *angiography* (20% of cases). To detect gastrinoma. Percutaneous transhepatic portal-venous sampling with gastrin measured in blood samples (not useful).

Therapy. *Medical.* H2-receptor blockers, cimetidine or ranitidine, acid inhibition of parietal cells (measures highly effective 90% of cases). Surgery not routinely recommended (as in the recent past), but (except in case with precise localization) limited to surgical exploration. Total gastrectomy recommended for patients who do not respond to medical treatment.

Prognosis. According to size, localization, and metastasis of tumor, association with other tumors (MEN–I, see). Removal of tumors: cure of hypersecretion and ulcers.

BIBLIOGRAPHY. Strøm R: A case of peptic ulcer and insuloma. Acta Chir Scand 104:252–260, 1952–1953

Zollinger RM, Ellison EH: Primary peptic ulcerations of the jejunum associated with islet cell tumors of the pancreas. Ann Surg 142:709–728, 1955

Ellison EH, Wilson SD: The Zollinger–Ellison syndrome updated. Surg Clin N Am 47:1115–1124, 1967

Mee AS, Ismail S, Boruman PC et al: Changing concepts in the presentation diagnosis and management of the Zollinger–Ellison syndrome. GI Med 206:256–267, 1983

Zollinger RM, Ellison EL, O'Dorisio TM et al: Thirty years experience with gastrinoma. World J Surg 8:552–560, 1984

Delcore R Jr, Cheung LY, Friesen SR: Outcome of lymphnode involvement in patients with the Zollinger–Ellison syndrome. Ann Surg 208:291–298, 1988

ZONDEK–BROMBERG–ROZIN

Synonym. Anterior pituitary hyperhormonotrophic.

Symptoms. Occur in female patients 20 to 30 years old; not seen in nulliparae. Prolonged, abundant uterine bleeding; anemia; galactorrhea; thyroidotoxic manifestation (tachycardia; perspiration; diarrhea); nervous symptoms; weight loss; secondary sterility.

Signs. Pallor; emaciation; enlargement of thyroid with signs of thyrotoxicosis (exophthalmos). *Breast.* Areolar hyperpigmentation with flaccid breast. *Uterus.* Enlargement; palpable cystic ovaries.

Etiology and Pathology. Overproduction of estrogenic, thyrotropic, lactotrophic hormones due to hyperplasia of the hypophysis or to hypothalamic pathology (?).

Diagnostic Procedures. *Blood.* Anemia; hypoglycemia with occasionally flat curve in glucose tolerance test. *Urine.* Increased urinary estrogens and no increase in gonadotropin (FSH); hyperestrogenic. *Vaginal smear.* *Hysterosalpingography.* Normal. *Milk.* Does not coagulate on boiling. *Basal metabolic rate.* Increased. *X-ray of skull.* Normal with no alteration of sella.

Therapy. X-ray or ablation of hypophysis seems to be indicated for the treatment of this rare syndrome.

BIBLIOGRAPHY. Zondek B, Bromberg YM, Rozin S: Anterior pituitary hyperhormonotrophic syndrome (excessive uterine bleeding, galactorrhea, hyperthyroidism). J Obstet Gynaecol B Emp 58:525–537, 1951
Dowling JT, Richards JB, Freinkel N et al: Nonpuerperal galactorrhea. Arch Intern Med 107:885–893, 1961
Christy MP, Warren MP: Disease syndromes of the hypothalamus and anterior pituitary. In De Groot LJ, Cahill FG Jr, Odell WD et al (eds.): Endocrinology, p 237. New York, Grune & Stratton, 1979

ZOON'S

Synonyms. Plasma cell balanitis; pseudo-erythroplasmic balanitis.

Symptoms and Signs. Occur in middle-aged and old men. Indolent plaques on glans and prepuce with shiny, moist skin, stippling of skin, "cayenne pepper" on the surface.

Etiology. Unknown; possibly, aspecific chronic balanitis.

Pathology. Plasma cell infiltration and deposit of hemosiderin.

Therapy. Topical cortisone ointment; gentamycin ointment. Circumcision permanent cure.

Prognosis. Chronic benign condition that temporarily disappears with application of steroids.

BIBLIOGRAPHY. Zoon JJ: Balantis circumscripta chronica met plasmacellen-infiltrant. Ned Tijdsch Geneesk 94:1529–1530, 1950
Rook A, Wilkinson DS, Ebling FJG et al: Textbook of Dermatology, 4th ed, pp 2189–2190. Oxford, Blackwell Scientific Publications, 1986

ZUELZER–OGDEN

Obsolete. The term refers to megaloblastic anemia with a superimposed infection and deficiency of vitamin C, observed in children.

BIBLIOGRAPHY. Zuelzer WW, Ogden FN: Megaloblastic anemia in infancy. Am J Dis Child 71:211–243, 1946

Index

The word *syndrome* is implied after most entries. Words in parentheses indicate main dictionary entries.

ISBN 0-397-50882-4

9 780397 508822

90000